Handbook of
BIOCHEMISTRY and MOLECULAR BIOLOGY

Fifth Edition

Handbook of
BIOCHEMISTRY and
MOLECULAR BIOLOGY

Fifth Edition

Handbook of
BIOCHEMISTRY and MOLECULAR BIOLOGY

Fifth Edition

Edited by
Roger L. Lundblad
Fiona M. Macdonald

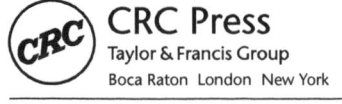
CRC Press
Taylor & Francis Group
Boca Raton London New York

CRC Press is an imprint of the
Taylor & Francis Group, an **informa** business

CRC Press
Taylor & Francis Group
6000 Broken Sound Parkway NW, Suite 300
Boca Raton, FL 33487-2742

First issued in paperback 2020

ISBN-13: 978-1-138-03309-2 (hbk)
ISBN-13: 978-0-367-78113-2 (pbk)

Library of Congress Cataloging-in-Publication Data

Names: Lundblad, Roger L., editor. | Macdonald, M. (Fiona), 1960- editor.
Title: Handbook of biochemistry and molecular biology / editors, Roger L. Lundblad,
Fiona M. Macdonald.
Description: Fifth edition. | Boca Raton : Taylor & Francis, 2018. | Includes
bibliographical references and index.
Identifiers: LCCN 2017055451 | ISBN 9781138033092 (hardback : alk. paper)
Subjects: | MESH: Biochemical Phenomena | Tables
Classification: LCC QH345 | NLM QU 16 | DDC 572--dc23
LC record available at https://lccn.loc.gov/2017055451

Visit the Taylor & Francis Web site at
http://www.taylorandfrancis.com

and the CRC Press Web site at
http://www.crcpress.com

This work is dedicated to the many scientists of the "The Greatest Generation" who contributed to the base of our knowledge of biochemistry and molecular biology.

Roger L. Lundblad, Ph.D.

Dedicated to James Ivan Yanchak, my husband

Fiona M. Macdonald, Ph.D., F.R.S.C.

This work is dedicated to the many scientists of DNA... The Genetic Generation, who contributed to the base of our knowledge of biochemistry and molecular biology.

Robert J. Brooker, PhD

Dedicated to Gene... and Sarah. As my best and...

TABLE OF CONTENTS

Table of Contents

PREFACE

This is the fifth edition of the *Handbook of Biochemistry and Molecular Biology*. The first edition was published as a single volume in 1968 under the guidance of Herbert Sober. The second edition appeared in 1970 and the third, with Gerald Fasman as editor, appeared in eight volumes published in 1975–6. This increase in size reflected the rapid advances in knowledge in the then relatively new field of molecular biology. The 4th edition of the *Handbook of Biochemistry and Molecular Biology* was published in 2010 with the goal of retaining material from the previous editions as well as incorporating some new material.

It is intended that current *Handbook of Biochemistry and Molecular Biology* be a companion volume to the *CRC Handbook of Chemistry and Physics*—a single volume ready-reference work that will find a home on the bookshelves of biochemists and molecular biologists everywhere. We have retained material from the fourth edition as well as including a large amount of material from the third edition. It is recognized that some of this material is dated but it was our intent to convert this material to electronic copy with the goal of revising such for the 6th edition. We do not expect to go back again to previous volumes for additional material. It is intended that the *Handbook of Biochemistry and Molecular Biology* serve as repository of data on the properties of biochemicals and it is not intended to serve as textbook. As such, some exciting areas of molecular biology are not included. There is comfort in that such work is extensively covered in other reviews. The advent of electronic media allows for more frequent updating and it is hoped that any infelicities in our selection may be readily rectified. Additionally, suggestions on new topics for this Handbook and notification of errors are always appreciated. Address all comments to Editor, *Handbook of Biochemistry and Molecular Biology*, Taylor & Francis Group, 6000 Broken Sound Parkway NW, Suite 300, Boca Raton, FL 33487.

Roger L. Lundblad
University of North Carolina

Fiona M. Macdonald
University of London

ACKNOWLEDGMENTS

This work would not have been possible without the outstanding support of the various research librarians at the University of North Carolina at Chapel Hill. The work of Max Bowman and her colleagues in Interlibrary Loan was critical. Danielle Zarfati of CRC Press pulled all the "stuff" together for production and without the skill and arduous work of Glenon Butler, also of CRC Press, production would not have happened. Professor Bryce Plapp of the University of Iowa provided insight and support. We also acknowledge the useful comments of Professor Ed Dennis of the University of California at San Diego as well as Professor Michael Boutros of the German Cancer Research Center and Heidelberg University. However, the editors take all responsibility for the selection of content.

EDITORS

Roger L. Lundblad is a native of San Francisco, California. He received his undergraduate education at Pacific Lutheran University and his PhD in biochemistry from the University of Washington. After postdoctoral work in the laboratories of Stanford Moore and William Stein at the Rockefeller University, he joined the faculty of the University of North Carolina at Chapel Hill. He joined the Hyland Division of Baxter Healthcare in 1990. Currently Dr. Lundblad is an independent consultant and writer in biotechnology in Chapel Hill, North Carolina. He is an adjunct professor of pathology at the University of North Carolina at Chapel Hill. He is the author of more than 150 journal publications and a number of reference texts and an editor of several books. He is the past editor-in-chief of several biotechnology journals.

Fiona M. Macdonald received her BSc in chemistry from Durham University, UK. She obtained her PhD in inorganic biochemistry from Birkbeck College, University of London, studying under Peter Sadler. Having spent most of her career in scientific publishing, she is now at Taylor & Francis Group and is involved in developing chemical information products.

Section I
Amino Acids, Peptides, and Proteins

PROPERTIES OF AMINO ACIDS

This table gives selected properties of some important amino acids and closely related compounds. The first part of the table lists the 20 "standard" amino acids that are the basic constituents of proteins. The second part includes other amino acids and related compounds of biochemical importance. Within each part of the table the compounds are listed by name in alphabetical order. Structures are given in the following table.

Symbol: Three-letter symbol for the standard amino acids

M_r: Molecular weight

t_m: Melting point

pK_a, pK_b, pK_c, pK_d: Negative of the logarithm of the acid dissociation constants for the COOH and NH_2 groups (and, in some cases, other groups) in the molecule (at 25°C)

pI: pH at the isoelectric point

S: Solubility in water in units of grams of compound per kilogram of water; a temperature of 25°C is understood unless otherwise stated in a superscript. When quantitative data are not available, the notations sl.s. (for slightly soluble), s. (for soluble), and v.s. (for very soluble) are used.

V_2^0: Partial molar volume in aqueous solution at infinite dilution (at 25°C)

Data on the enthalpy of formation of many of these compounds are included in the table "Heat of Combustion, Enthalpy and Free Energy of Formation of Amino Acids and Related Compounds" on p. 69 of this Handbook. Absorption spectra and optical rotation data can be found in Reference 3. Partial molar volume is taken from Reference 5; other thermodynamic properties, including solubility as a function of temperature, are given in References 3 and 5. Most of the pK values come from References 1, 6, and 7.

References

1. Dawson, R. M. C., Elliott, D. C., Elliott, W. H., and Jones, K. M., *Data for Biochemical Research*, Third Edition, Clarendon Press, Oxford, 1986.
2. O'Neil, Maryadele J., Ed., *The Merck Index, Fourteenth Edition*, Merck & Co., Rahway, NJ, 2006.
3. Sober, H. A., Ed., *CRC Handbook of Biochemistry. Selected Data for Molecular Biology*, CRC Press, Boca Raton, FL, 1968.
4. Voet, D., and Voet, J. G., *Biochemistry, Second Edition*, John Wiley & Sons, New York, 1995.
5. Hinz, H. J., Ed., *Thermodynamic Data for Biochemistry and Biotechnology*, Springer–Verlag, Heidelberg, 1986.
6. Fasman, G. D., Ed. *Practical Handbook of Biochemistry and Molecular Biology*, CRC Press, Boca Raton, FL, 1989.
7. Smith, R. M., and Martell, A. E., *NIST Standard Reference Database 46: Critically Selected Stability Constants of Metal Complexes Database*, Version 3.0, National Institute of Standards and Technology, Gaithersburg, MD, 1997.
8. Ramasami, P., *J. Chem. Eng. Data*, 47, 1164, 2002.

Symbol	Name	Mol. Form	M_r	t_m/°C	pK_a	pK_b	pK_c	pK_d	pI	S/g kg⁻¹	V_2^0/cm³ mol⁻¹
Ala	L-Alanine	$C_3H_7NO_2$	89.09	297	2.33	9.71			6.00	166.9	60.54
Arg	L-Arginine	$C_6H_{14}N_4O_2$	174.20	244	2.03	9.00	12.10		10.76	182.6	127.42
Asn	L-Asparagine	$C_4H_8N_2O_3$	132.12	235	2.16	8.73			5.41	25.1	78.0
Asp	L-Aspartic acid	$C_4H_7NO_4$	133.10	270	1.95	9.66	3.71		2.77	5.04	74.8
Cys	L-Cysteine	$C_3H_7NO_2S$	121.16	240	1.91	10.28	8.14		5.07	v.s.	73.45
Gln	L-Glutamine	$C_5H_{10}N_2O_3$	146.14	185	2.18	9.00			5.65	42.5	
Glu	L-Glutamic acid	$C_5H_9NO_4$	147.13	160	2.16	9.58	4.15		3.22	8.6	89.85
Gly	Glycine	$C_2H_5NO_2$	75.07	290	2.34	9.58			5.97	250.2	43.26
His	L-Histidine	$C_6H_9N_3O_2$	155.15	287	1.70	9.09	6.04		7.59	43.5	98.3
Ile	L-Isoleucine	$C_6H_{13}NO_2$	131.17	284	2.26	9.60			6.02	34.2	105.80
Leu	L-Leucine	$C_6H_{13}NO_2$	131.17	293	2.32	9.58			5.98	22.0	107.77
Lys	L-Lysine	$C_6H_{14}N_2O_2$	146.19	224	2.15	9.16	10.67		9.74	5.8	108.5
Met	L-Methionine	$C_5H_{11}NO_2S$	149.21	281	2.16	9.08			5.74	56	105.57
Phe	L-Phenylalanine	$C_9H_{11}NO_2$	165.19	283	2.18	9.09			5.48	27.9	121.5
Pro	L-Proline	$C_5H_9NO_2$	115.13	221	1.95	10.47			6.30	1622	82.76
Ser	L-Serine	$C_3H_7NO_3$	105.09	228	2.13	9.05			5.68	250	60.62
Thr	L-Threonine	$C_4H_9NO_3$	119.12	256	2.20	8.96			5.60	98.1	76.90
Trp	L-Tryptophan	$C_{11}H_{12}N_2O_2$	204.23	289	2.38	9.34			5.89	13.2	143.8
Tyr	L-Tyrosine	$C_9H_{11}NO_3$	181.19	343	2.24	9.04	10.10		5.66	0.46	
Val	L-Valine	$C_5H_{11}NO_2$	117.15	315	2.27	9.52			5.96	88	90.75
	N-Acetylglutamic acid	$C_7H_{11}NO_5$	189.17	199						s.	
	N⁶-Acetyl-L-lysine	$C_8H_{16}N_2O_3$	188.22	265	2.12	9.51					
	β-Alanine	$C_3H_7NO_2$	89.09	200	3.51	10.08				723.6	58.28
	2-Aminoadipic acid	$C_6H_{11}NO_4$	161.16	207	2.14	4.21	9.77		3.18	2.2⁴⁰	

PROPERTIES OF AMINO ACIDS (Continued)

Name	Mol. Form	M_r	$t_m/°C$	pK_a	pK_b	pK_c	pK_d	pI	$S/\text{g kg}^{-1}$	$V_2^0/\text{cm}^3 \text{mol}^{-1}$
DL-2-Aminobutanoic acid	$C_4H_9NO_2$	103.12	304	2.30	9.63			6.06	210	75.6
DL-3-Aminobutanoic acid	$C_4H_9NO_2$	103.12	194.3	3.43	10.05			7.30	1250	76.3
4-Aminobutanoic acid	$C_4H_9NO_2$	103.12	203	4.02	10.35				971	73.2
10-Aminodecanoic acid	$C_{10}H_{21}NO_2$	187.28	188.5							167.3
7-Aminoheptanoic acid	$C_7H_{15}NO_2$	145.20	195						v.s.	120.0
6-Aminohexanoic acid	$C_6H_{13}NO_2$	131.17	205					7.29	863	104.2
L-3-Amino-2-methylpropanoic acid	$C_4H_9NO_2$	103.12	185						s.	
2-Amino-2-methylpropanoic acid	$C_4H_9NO_2$	103.12	335	2.36	10.21			5.72	137	77.55
9-Aminononanoic acid	$C_9H_{19}NO_2$	173.26	191							151.3
8-Aminooctanoic acid	$C_8H_{17}NO_2$	159.23	192							136.1
5-Amino-4-oxopentanoic acid	$C_5H_9NO_3$	131.13	118	4.05	8.90					
5-Aminopentanoic acid	$C_5H_{11}NO_2$	117.15	157 dec						s.	87.6
o-Anthranilic acid	$C_7H_7NO_2$	137.14	146	2.05	4.95				3.5[14]	
Azaserine	$C_5H_7N_3O_4$	173.13	150		8.55				v.s.	
Canavanine	$C_5H_{12}N_4O_3$	176.17	172	2.50	6.60	9.25		7.93	v.s.	
L-γ-Carboxyglutamic acid	$C_6H_9NO_6$	191.14	167	1.70	9.90	4.75	3.20			
Carnosine	$C_9H_{14}N_4O_3$	226.23	260	2.51	9.35	6.76			322	
Citrulline	$C_6H_{13}N_3O_3$	175.19	222	2.32	9.30			5.92	s.	
Creatine	$C_4H_9N_3O_2$	131.13	303	2.63	14.30				16	
L-Cysteic acid	$C_3H_7NO_5S$	169.16	260	1.89	8.70	1.30			v.s.	
L-Cystine	$C_6H_{12}N_2O_4S_2$	240.30	260	1.50	8.80	2.05	8.03		0.11	
2,4-Diaminobutanoic acid	$C_4H_{10}N_2O_2$	118.13	118.1	1.85	8.24	10.44		9.27	s.	
3,5-Dibromo-L-tyrosine	$C_9H_9Br_2NO_3$	338.98	245						2.72	
3,5-Dichloro-L-tyrosine	$C_9H_9Cl_2NO_3$	250.08	247						1.97	
3,5-Diiodo-L-tyrosine	$C_9H_9I_2NO_3$	432.98	213	2.12	9.10	6.16			0.62	
Dopamine	$C_8H_{11}NO_2$	153.18			10.36	8.88			s.	
L-Ethionine	$C_6H_{13}NO_2S$	163.24	273	2.18	9.05	13.10				
N-Glycylglycine	$C_4H_8N_2O_3$	132.12	263	3.13	8.10				225	
Guanidinoacetic acid	$C_3H_7N_3O_2$	117.11	282	2.82					5	
Histamine	$C_5H_9N_3$	111.15	83		9.83	6.11			v.s.	
L-Homocysteine	$C_4H_9NO_2S$	135.19	232	2.15	8.57	10.38		5.55	s.	
Homocystine	$C_8H_{16}N_2O_4S_2$	268.35	264	1.59	9.44	2.54	8.52		0.2	
L-Homoserine	$C_4H_9NO_3$	119.12	203	2.27	9.28			6.17	1100	
3-Hydroxy-DL-glutamic acid	$C_5H_9NO_5$	163.13	209					3.28		
5-Hydroxylysine	$C_6H_{14}N_2O_3$	162.19		2.13	8.85	9.83		9.15		
trans-4-Hydroxy-L-proline	$C_5H_9NO_3$	131.13	274	1.82	9.47			5.74	361	84.49
L-3-Iodotyrosine	$C_9H_{10}INO_3$	307.08	205	2.20	9.10	8.70			sl.s.	
L-Kynurenine	$C_{10}H_{12}N_2O_3$	208.21	194						sl.s.	
L-Lanthionine	$C_6H_{12}N_2O_4S$	208.24	294						1.5	
Levodopa	$C_9H_{11}NO_4$	197.19	277	2.32	8.72	9.96	11.79		5[20]	
L-1-Methylhistidine	$C_7H_{11}N_3O_2$	169.18	249	1.69	8.85	6.48			200	
L-Norleucine	$C_6H_{13}NO_2$	131.17	301	2.31	9.68			6.09	15	107.7
L-Norvaline	$C_5H_{11}NO_2$	117.15	307	2.31	9.65				107	91.8
L-Ornithine	$C_5H_{12}N_2O_2$	132.16	140	1.94	8.78	10.52		9.73	v.s.	
O-Phosphoserine	$C_3H_8NO_6P$	185.07	166	2.14	9.80	5.70				
L-Pyroglutamic acid	$C_5H_7NO_3$	129.12	162	3.32						
Sarcosine	$C_3H_7NO_2$	89.09	212	2.18	9.97				428	
Taurine	$C_2H_7NO_3S$	125.15	328	-0.3	9.06				105	
L-Thyroxine	$C_{15}H_{11}I_4NO_4$	776.87	235	2.20	10.01	6.45			sl.s.	

STRUCTURES OF COMMON AMINO ACIDS

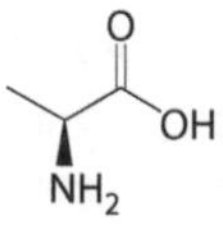

L-Alanine (Ala)

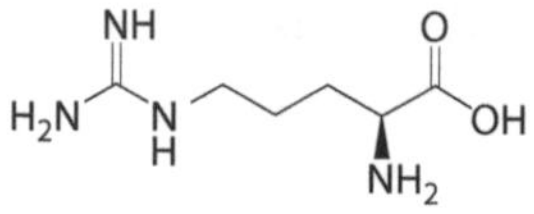

L-Arginine (Arg)

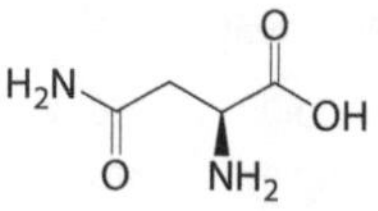

L-Asparagine (Asn)

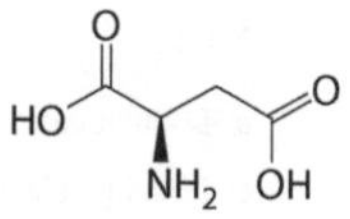

L-Aspartic acid (Asp)

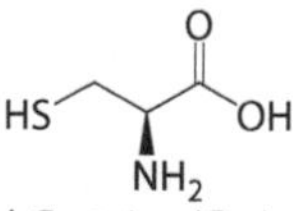

l-Cysteine (Cys)

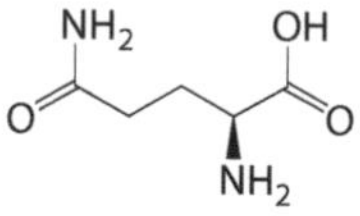

l-Glutamine (Gln)

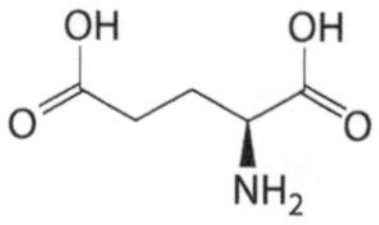

L-Glutamic acid (Glu)

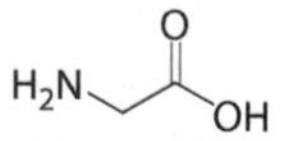

Glycine (Gly)

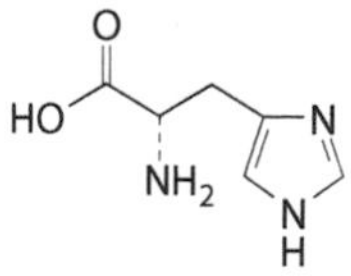

L-Histidine (His)

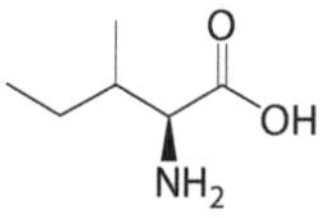

L-Isoleucine (Ile)

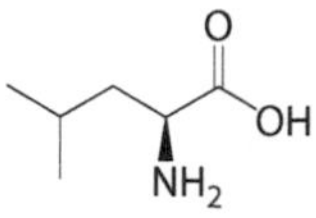

L-Leucine (Leu)

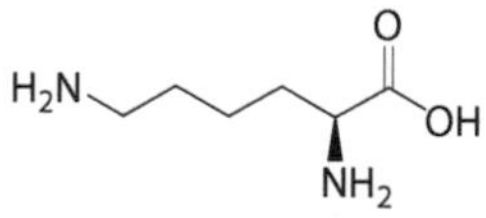

L-Lysine (Lys)

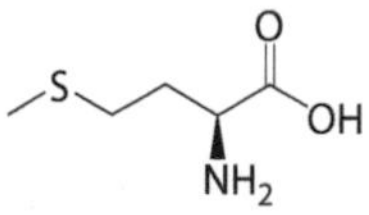

L-Methionine (Met)

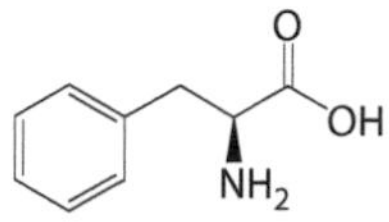

L-Phenylalanine (Phe)

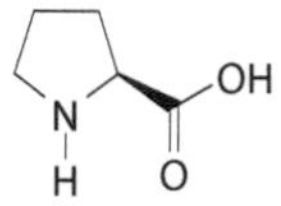

L-Proline (Pro)

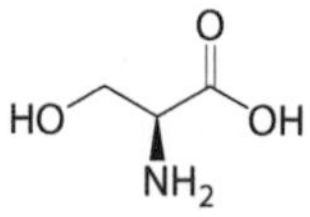

L-Serine (Ser)

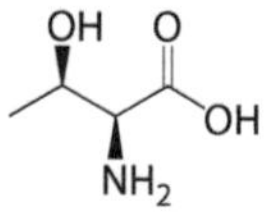

L-Threonine (Thr)

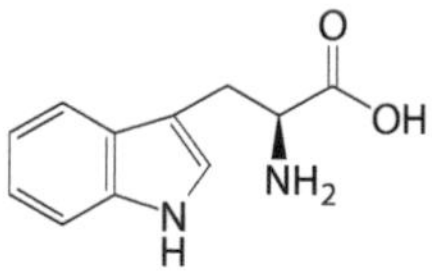

L-Tryptophan (Trp)

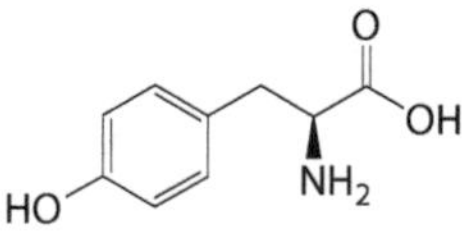

L-Tyrosine (Tyr)

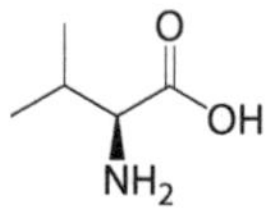

L-Valine (Val)

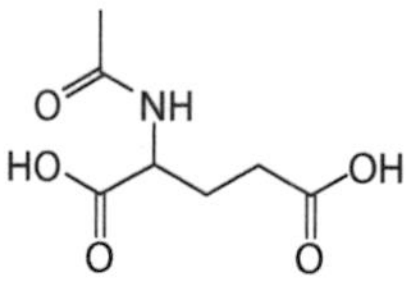

N-Acetylglutamic acid

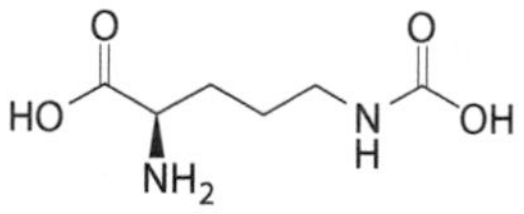

N6-Acetyl-L-lysine

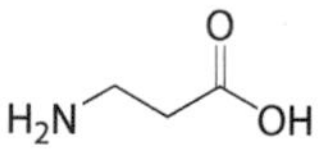

β-Alanine

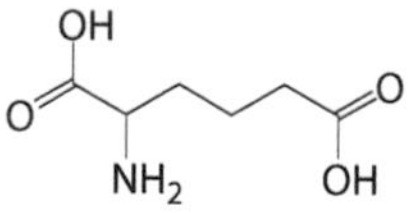

2-Aminoadipic acid

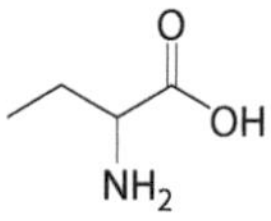

DL-2-Aminobutanoic acid

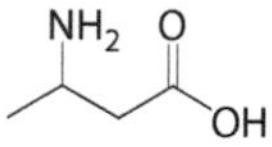

DL-3-Aminobutanoic acid

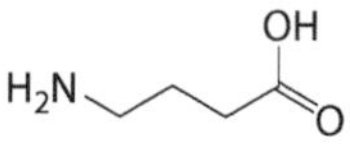

4-Aminobutanoic acid

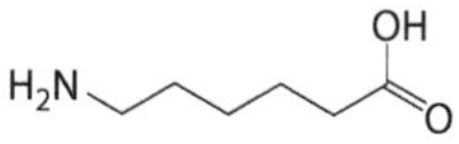

6-Aminohexanoic acid

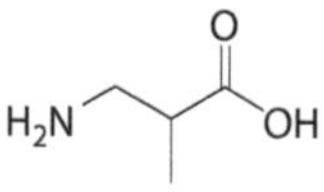

L-3-Amino-2-methylpropa-noic acid

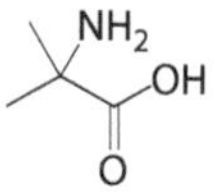

2-Amino-2-methylpropanoic acid

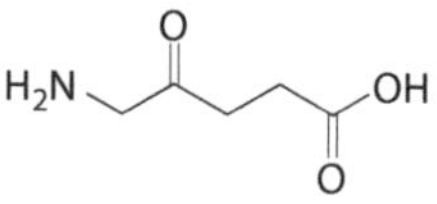

5-Amino-4-oxopentanoic acid

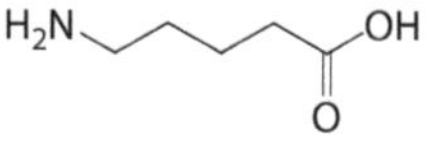

5-Aminopentanoic acid

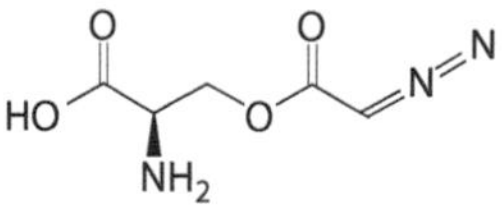

Azaserine

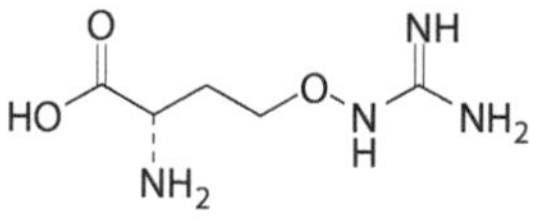

Canavanine

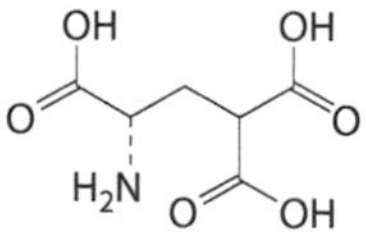

L-γ-Carboxyglutamic acid

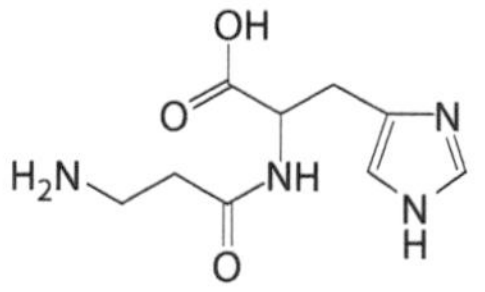

Carnosine

STRUCTURES OF COMMON AMINO ACIDS (Continued)

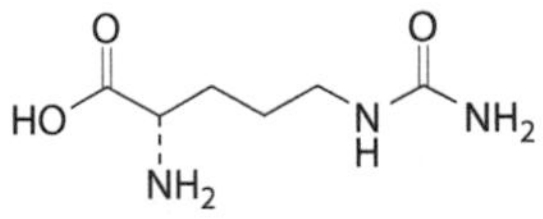

Citrulline

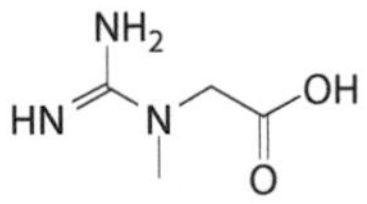

Creatine

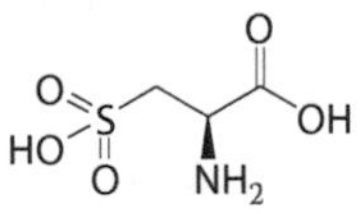

L-Cysteic acid

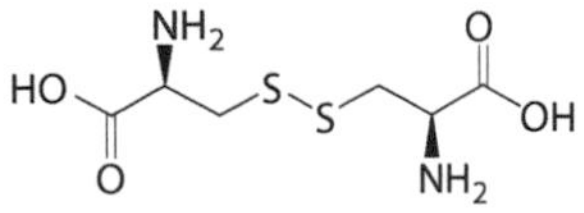

L-Cystine

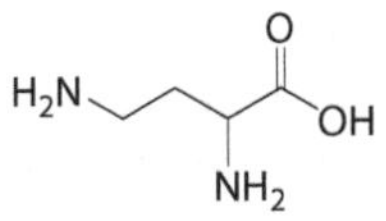

2,4-Diaminobutanoic acid

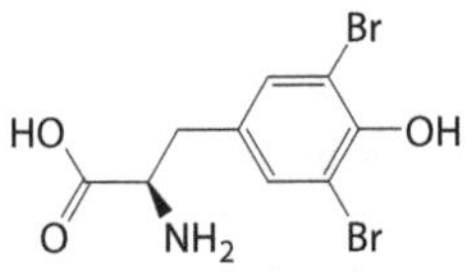

3,5-Dibromo-L-tyrosine

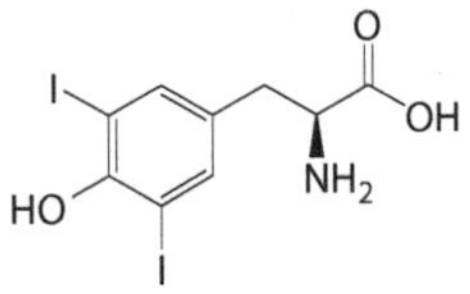

3,5-Diiodo-L-tyrosine

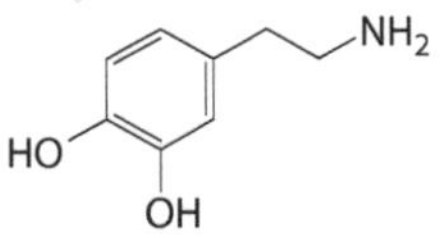

Dopamine

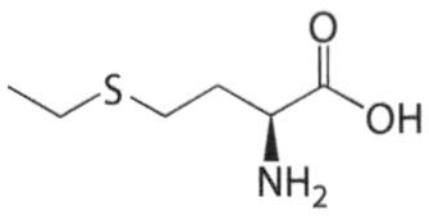

L-Ethionine

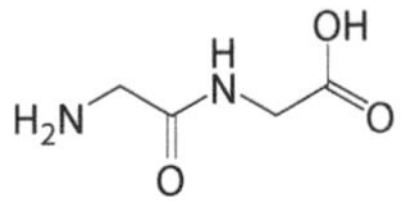

N-Glycylglycine

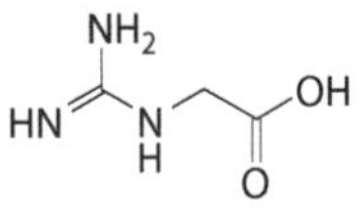

Guanidinoacetic acid

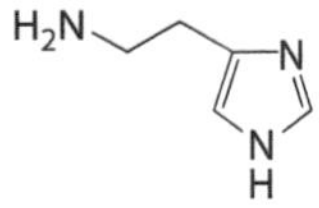

Histamine

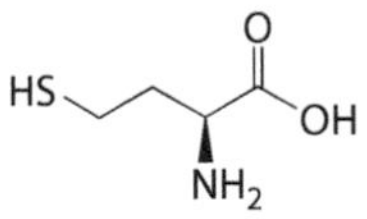

L-Homocysteine

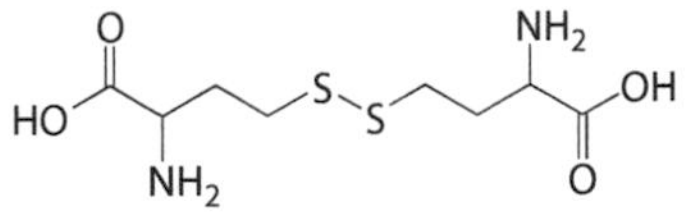

Homocystine

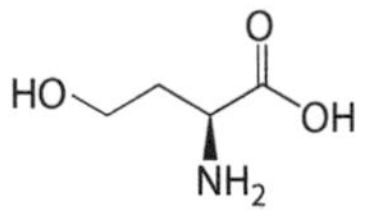

L-Homoserine

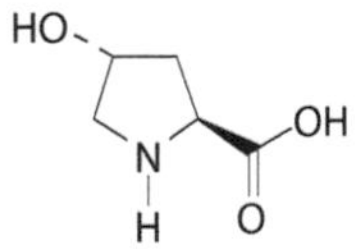

trans-4-Hydroxy-L-proline

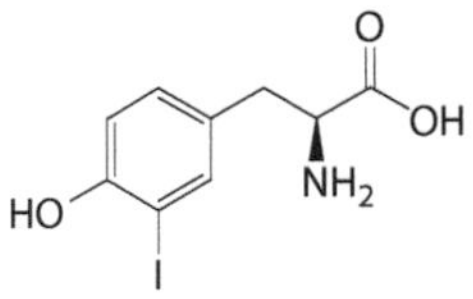

L-3-Iodotyrosine

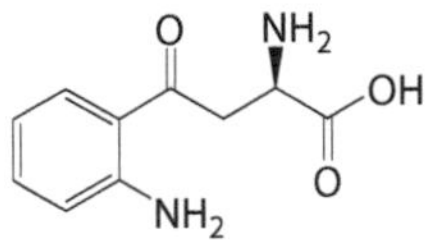

L-Kynurenine

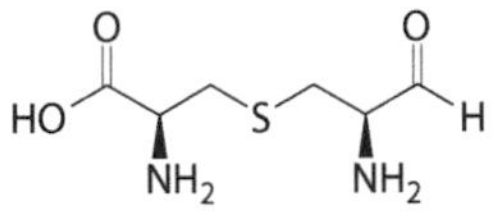

L-Lanthionine

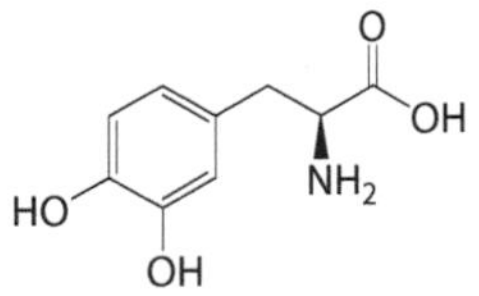

Levodopa

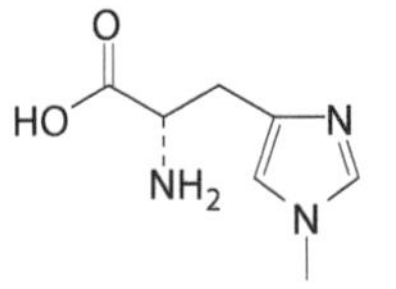

L-1-Methylhistidine

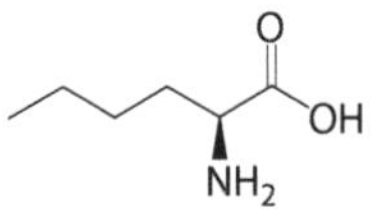

L-Norleucine

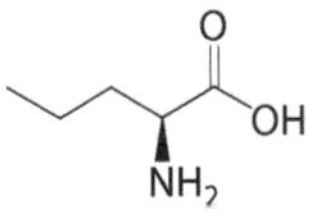

L-Norvaline

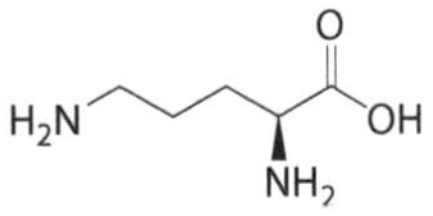

L-Ornithine

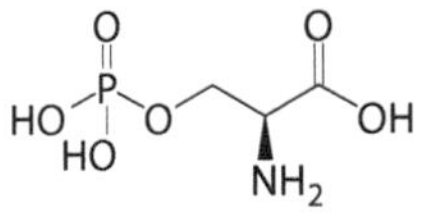

O-Phosphoserine

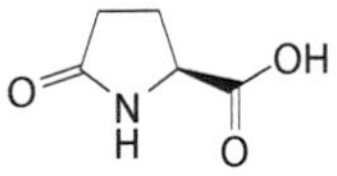

L-Pyroglutamic acid

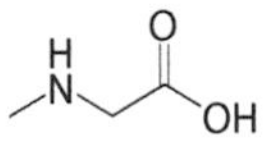

Sarcosine

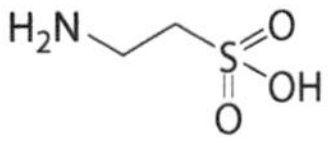

Taurine

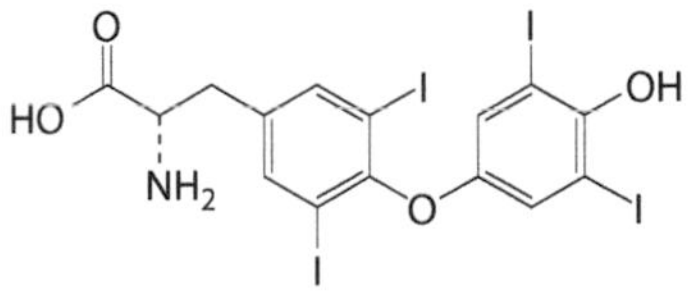

L-Thyroxine

DATA ON THE NATURALLY OCCURRING AMINO ACIDS

Elizabeth Dodd Mooz

The amino acids included in these tables are those for which reliable evidence exists for their occurrence in nature. These tables are intended as a guide to the primary literature in which the isolation and characterization of the amino acids are reported. Originally, it was planned to include more factual data on the chemical and physical properties of these compounds; however, the many different conditions employed by various authors in measuring these properties (i.e., chromatography and spectral data) made them difficult to arrange into useful tables. The rotation values are as given in the references cited; unfortunately, in some cases there is no information given on temperature, solvent, or concentration.

The investigator employing the data in these tables is urged to refer to the original articles in order to evaluate for himself the reliability of the information reported. These references are intended to be informative to the reader rather than to give credit to individual scientists who published the original reports. Thus not all published material is cited.

The compounds listed in Sections A to N are known to be of the l configuration. Section O contains some of the d amino acids which occur naturally. This last section is not intended to be complete since most properties of the d amino acids correspond to those of their l enantiomorphs. Therefore, emphasis was placed on including those d amino acids whose l isomers have not been found in nature. The reader will find additional information on the d amino acids in the review by Corrigan[263] and in the book by Meister.[1]

Compilation of data for these tables was completed in December 1974. Appreciation is expressed to Doctors L. Fowden, John F. Thompson, Peter Müller, and M. Bodanszky who were helpful in supplying recent references and to Dr. David Pruess who made review material available to me prior to its publication. A special word of thanks to Dr. Alton Meister who made available reprints of journal articles which I was not able to obtain.

DATA ON THE NATURALLY OCCURRING AMINO ACIDS (Continued)

A. L-MONOAMINO, MONOCARBOXYLIC ACIDS

No.	Amino Acid (Synonym)	Source	Formula (Mol Wt)	Melting Point °C[a]	$[\alpha]_D$[b]	pKa	References Isolation and Purification	Chromatography	Chemistry	Spectral Data
1	Alanine (α-aminopropionic acid)	Silk fibroin	$C_3H_7NO_2$ (89.09)	297°	+1.8^25 (c 2, H2O) (1) +14.6^25 (c 2, 5 N HCl) (1)	2.34 9.69	2	3	4	4
2	β-Alanine (β-aminopropionic acid)	Iris tingitana	$C_3H_7NO_2$ (89.09)	196° (dec)	—	3.55 10.24	5	5	5	—
3	α-Aminobutyric acid	Yeast protein	$C_4H_9NO_2$ (103.12)	292° (dec)	+20.5^25 (c 1–2, 5 N HCl) (290) +9.3^25 (c 1–2, H2O) (290) +42^25 (c 1–2, gl acetic) (290)	2.29 9.83	6	7	6	—
4	γ-Aminobutyric acid (piperidinic acid)	Bacteria	$C_4H_9NO_2$ (103.12)	203° (dec)	—	4.03 10.56 (290)	8–10	9, 10	11	—
5	1-Aminocyclopropane-1-carboxylic acid	Pears and apples	$C_4H_7NO_2$ (101.11)	—	—	—	11	11	12	12
6	2-Amino-3-formyl-3-pentenoic acid	Bankera fulgineoalba (a mushroom)	$C_6H_9NO_3$ (143.15)	—	—	—	13	13	13	13
7	α-Aminoheptanoic acid	Claviceps purpures	$C_7H_{15}NO_2$ (145.21)	—	—	—	14	14	—	—
7a	2-Amino-4,5-hexadienoic acid	Amanita solitaria	$C_6H_9NO_2$ (127.16)	200° (dec) (14a)	—	—	14a	—	—	14a
8	2-Amino-4-hexenoic acid	Ilamycin	$C_6H_{11}NO_2$ (129.17)	—	—	—	15	15	—	—
8a	2-Amino-4-hydroxyhept-4-ynoic acid	Euphoria longan	$C_7H_{11}NO_3$ (157.19)	—	−27^20 (c 2, H2O) −8^20 (c 1, 5 N HCl) (15a)	—	15a	15a	—	15a
8b	2-Amino-6-hydroxy-4-methyl-4-hexenoic acid	Aesculus California seeds	$C_7H_{13}NO_3$ (159.21)	—	−31^20 (c 2.2, H2O) +2^20 (c 1.1, 5 N HCl) (23b)	—	23b	23b	—	15b
8c	2-Amino-4-hydroxy-5-methylhexenoic acid	Euphoria longan	$C_7H_{11}NO_3$ (157.19)	—	−27^20 (c 2, H2O) −13^20 (c 1, 5 N HCl) (15a)	—	15a	—	15a	15a
8d	2-Amino-3-hydroxy-methyl-3-pentenoic acid	Bankera fulgineoalba	$C_6H_{11}NO_3$ (145.18)	150–161° (dec) (13)	+182^25 (c 0.8, H2O) +201^25 (c 0.8, 0.3 N HCl) (13)	—	13	13	13	13
9	α-Aminoisobutyric acid	Iris tingitana, muscle protein	$C_4H_9NO_2$ (103.12)	200° (dec)	—	2.36 10.21 (290)	16	16	—	—
10	β-Aminoisobutyric acid	Iris tingitana	$C_4H_9NO_2$ (103.12)	179° (17)	−21^26 (c 0.43, H2O) (17)	—	17	17	17	17
10a	2-Amino-4-methoxy-trans-3-butenoic acid	Pseudomonas aeruginosa	$C_6H_9NO_3$ (131.15)	—	—	—	17a	17b	—	17a, 17b
11	γ-Amino-α-methylenebutyric acid	Arachis hypogaea (groundnut plants)	$C_4H_9NO_2$ (115.13)	152° (18)	—	—	18	18	18	—
12	2-Amino-4-methylhexanoic acid (homoisoleucine)	Aesculus californica seeds	$C_7H_{15}NO_2$ (145.21)	—	−2^20 (c 1, H2O) (19) +24^20 (c 0.87, 5 N HCl) (19)	—	19	19	19	19
13	2-Amino-4-methyl-4-hexenoic acid	Aesculus californica seeds	$C_7H_{13}NO_2$ (143.19)	—	−61^20 (c 2.4, H2O) (19) −36 (c 1.2, 6 N HCl) (19)	—	19	19	19	19
13a	2-Amino-4-methyl-5-hexenoic acid	Streptomyces species	$C_7H_{13}NO_2$ (143.21)	260° (dec) (19a)	−9.6° (c 1.78, H2O) +5.7° (c 0.7, 1 N HCl) (99a)	—	19a	19a	—	19a

DATA ON THE NATURALLY OCCURRING AMINO ACIDS (Continued)

No.	Amino Acid (Synonym)	Source	Formula (Mol Wt)	Melting Point °C[a]	$[\alpha]_D^b$	pK_a	References — Isolation and Purification	Chromatography	Chemistry	Spectral Data
14	2-Amino-5-methyl-4-hexenoic acid	Leucocortinarius bulbiger	$C_7H_{13}NO_2$ (143.19)	260–270° (dec) (22a)	-45.9^{23} (c 0.47, H_2O) -7^{23} (c 0.4, 1 N HCl) (22a)	–	22, 22a	22a	–	22a
14a	2-Amino-4-methyl-5-hexenoic acid	Euphoria longan	$C_7H_{11}NO_2$ (141.19)	–	-33^{20} (c 2, H_2O) -27^{20} (c 1, 5 N HCl) (15a)	–	15a	–	15a	15a
15	α-Aminooctanoic acid	Aspergillus atypigue	$C_8H_{17}NO_2$ (159.23)	–	–	–	23	23	23	23
15a	2-Amino-4-pentynoic acid	Streptomyces sp. #6-4	$C_5H_7NO_2$ (113.13)	241–242° (dec) (23a)	-31.1^{25} (c 1, H_2O) -5.5^{25} (c 1, 5 N HCl) (23a)	–	23	23a	23a	23a
15a′	cis-α-(Carboxycyclopropyl)glycine	Aesculus parviflora	$C_6H_9NO_4$ (159.16)	–	$+25^{20}$ (c 1, H_2O) +58 (c 0.5, 5 N HCl) (23a′)	–	23a′	23a′	–	23a′
15b	trans-α-(Carboxycyclopropyl)glycine	Blighia sapida	$C_6H_9NO_4$ (159.16)	–	$+107^{20}$ (c 2, H_2O) $+146^{20}$ (c 1, 5 N HCl) (23a′)	–	23a′	23a′	–	23a′
15b′	trans-α-(2-Carboxymethylcyclopropyl)glycine	Blighia unijugata	$C_7H_{11}NO_4$ (173.19)	–	$+12^{20}$ (c 1, H_2O) $+45^{20}$ (c 0.5, 5 N HCl) (99a)	–	99a	99a	–	99a
15c	γ-Glutamyl-2-amino-4-methylhex-4-enoic acid	Aesculus californica seeds	$C_{12}H_{20}N_2O_5$ (272.34)	–	$+17^{20}$ (c 3, H_2O) (23b)	–	23b	23b	–	–
	B. L-MONOAMINO, DICARBOXYLIC ACIDS									
16	Glycine (α-aminoacetic acid)	Gelatin hydrolyzate	$C_2H_6NO_2$ (75.07)	290° (dec) (1)	–	2.35 9.78 (290)	24	3	25	25
17	Hypoglycin A [α-amino-β-(2-methylene cyclopropyl)propionic acid]	Blighia sapida	$C_7H_{11}NO_2$ (141.18)	280–284° (26)	$+9.2$ (c 1, H_2O) (26)	–	26	26	27	27
18	Isoleucine (α-amino-β-methylvaleric acid)	Sugar beet molasses	$C_6H_{13}NO_2$ (131.17)	284° (1)	$+39.5^{25}$ (c 1, 5 N HCl) (290)$+12.4^{25}$ (c 1, H_2O) (290)	2.36 9.68	3	9	29	1
19	Leucine (α-aminoisocaproic acid)	Muscle fiber, wool	$C_3H_{13}NO_2$ (131.17)	337° (1)	-11^{25} (c 2, H_2O)$+16^{25}$ c 2, 5 N HCl) (1)	2.36 960 (1)	30	3	31	31
19a	N-Methyl-γ-methyl-alloisoleucine	Etamycin	$C_8H_{17}NO_2$ (159.26)	–	–	–	31a	31a	–	–
19b	β-Methyl-β-(methylenecyclopropyl)alanine	Aesculus californica seeds	$C_8H_{13}NO_2$ (155.22)	–	1.5^{20} (c 2, H_2O)$+45^{20}$ (c 1, 5 N HCl) (23b)	-960 (1)	23b	23b	–	15b
20	α-(Methylenecyclopropyl)glycine	Litchi chinensis	$C_6H_9NO_2$ (127.15)	–	$+43^{22.5}$ (c 0.5, 5 N HCl) (32)	–	32	32	32	32
21	β-(Methylenecyclopropyl)-β-methylalanine	Aesculus californica	$C_8H_{13}NO_2$ (155.19)	–	$+1.5^{20}$ (c 2, H_2O)$+45^{20}$ (c 1, 5 N HCl)	–	19	19	19	19, 21
21a	β-Methylenenorleucine	Amanita vaginata	$C_7H_{13}NO_2$ (143.21)	171° (35a)	$+158^{20}$ (c 0.51, 1 N HCl)$+149^{20}$ (c 0.56, H_2O) (35a)	–	–	35a	35a	–
22	Valine (α-aminoisovaleric acid)	Casein	$C_5H_{11}NO_2$ (117.15)	292–295° (1)	$+28.3^{25}$ (c 1, 2, 5 N HCl)$+5.63^{25}$ (c 1–2, H_2O) (290)	2.32 9.62 (1)	35	3	35, 36	36
23	α-Aminoadipic acid	Pisum sativum	$C_6H_{11}NO_4$ (161.18)	195° (37)	$+3.2^{25}$ (c 2, H_2O (290)$+23^{22}$ (c 2, 6 N HCl) (37)	2.14 4.21 9.77 (290)	37	37	37	–
24	3-Aminoglutaric acid	Chondria armata	$C_5H_9NO_4$ (162.13)	280–282° (38)	$\pm0^c$ (c 2, 5 N HCl) (38)	–	38	38	38	38
25	α-Aminopimelic acid	Asplenium septentrionale	$C_7H_{13}NO_4$ (175.19)	204° (39)	–	–	39	39	39	–
26	Asparagine (α-aminosuccinamic acid)	Asparagus	$C_4H_8N_2O_3$ (132.12)	236° (1)	$+5.06^{25}$ (c 2, H_2O) (290)$+33.2$ (3 N HCl) (1)	2.02 8.80 (1)	40	3	41	42

DATA ON THE NATURALLY OCCURRING AMINO ACIDS (Continued)

No.	Amino Acid (Synonym)	Source	Formula (Mol Wt)	Melting Point °C[a]	$[\alpha]_D$[b]	pK_a	References — Isolation and Purification	References — Chromatography	References — Chemistry	References — Spectral Data
27	Aspartic acid (α-aminosuccinic acid)	Conglutin, legumin	$C_4H_7NO_4$ (133.10)	270° (1)	$+5.05^{25}$ (c 2, H_2O)$+25.4^{25}$ (c 2, 5 N HCl) (1)	1.88, 3.65, 3.60 (1)	43	3	41	41
28	Ethylasparagine	*Ecballium elaterium*, *Bryonia dioica*	$C_6H_{12}N_2O_3$ (160.19)	—	—	—	45	45	45	45
29	γ-Ethylideneglutamic acid	*Mimosa*	$C_7H_{11}NO_4$ (173.18)	—	$+21^{20}$ (c 2.8, H_2O) (47)$+38.3^{20}$ (c 1.4, 6 N HCl) (47)	—	46	46	—	46
30	N-Fumarylalanine	*Penicillium recticulosum*	$C_7H_9NO_5$ (187.16)	229° (48)	—	—	48	—	48	—
31	Glutamic acid (α-aminoglutaric acid)	Gluten-fibrin hydrolyzates	$C_5H_9NO_4$ (147.13)	249° (1)	$+12^{25}$ (c 2, H_2O)$+31.8^{28}$ (c 2, 5 N HCl) (1)	2.19, 4.25, 3.67 (1)	49	3	50	50
32	Glutamine (α-aminoglutaramic acid)	Beet juice	$C_5H_{10}N_2O_3$ (146.15)	185° (1)	$+6.3^{25}$ (c 2, H_2O)$+31.8^{25}$ (c 2, 1 N HCl) (1)	2.17, 3.13 (1)	51	3	50	50
33	N-Isopropylglutamine	*Lunaria annua*	$C_8H_{16}N_2O_3$ (188.23)	—	$+7.1^{22}$ (c 1.7, H_2O) (53)	—	53	53	53	—
34	N-Methylasparagine	—	$C_5H_{10}N_2O_3$ (146.15)	241–244° (54)	-4.2 (c 5.5, H_2O) (54)	—	—	54	—	—
35	β-Methylaspartic acid	*Clostridium tetanomorphum*	$C_5H_9NO_4$ (147.13)	—	-10 (c 0.4, H_2O)$+12.4$ (c 3, 1 N HCl)$+13.3$ (c 3, 5 N HCl) (55)	3.5, 3.9 (290)	55	55	55	—
36	γ-Methylglutamic acid	*Phyllitis scolopendrium*	$C_6H_{11}NO_4$ (141.17)	—	—	—	56	56	—	—
37	γ-Methyleneglutamic acid	*Arachis hypogaea*	$C_6H_9NO_4$ (159.15)	196° (57)	—	—	57	57	57	—
38	γ-Methyleneglutamine	*Arachis hypogaea*	$C_6H_{10}N_2O_3$ (158.17)	173–182° (57)	—	—	57	57	57	—
39	Theanine (α-amino-γ-N-ethylglutaramic acid)	*Xerocomus hadius*	$C_7H_{14}N_2O_3$ (174)	—	—	—	59	59	59	59
39a	β-N-Acetyl-α, β- diaminopropionic acid (β-acetamido-L-alanine)	*Acacia armata* seeds	$C_5H_{10}N_2O_3$ (146.17)	—	-87^{20} (c 8, H_2O)-35^{20} (c 4, 6 N HCl) (59a)	—	59a	59a	59a	59a

C.L-DIAMINO, MONOCARBOXYLIC ACIDS

No.	Amino Acid (Synonym)	Source	Formula (Mol Wt)	Melting Point °C[a]	$[\alpha]_D$[b]	pK_a	References — Isolation and Purification	References — Chromatography	References — Chemistry	References — Spectral Data
40	N-Acetylornithine	*Asplenium* species	$C_7H_{14}N_2O_3$ (174.11)	200° (dec) (60)	—	—	60	60	60	—
41	α-Amino-γ-N-acetylaminobutyric acid	Latex of *Euphorbia pulcherrima*	$C_6H_{12}N_2O_3$ (160.18)	220–222° (dec) (61)	—	≈.45 (33)	61	61	—	—
42	N-ε-(2-Amino-2-carboxyethyl)lysine	Alkali-treated protein	$C_9H_{19}N_3O_4$ (233.28)	—	—	≈2, 6.5, ≈8, ≈9.9 (62)	62	62	62	—
43	N-δ-(2-Amino-2-carboxyethyl)ornithine	Alkali-treated wool	$C_8H_{17}N_3O_4$ (273.72)	—	—	—	63	63	63	63
44	2-Amino-3-dimethylaminopropionic acid	*Streptomyces neocaliberis*	$C_5H_{12}N_2O_2$ (117.15)	—	-17.8^{25} (c 1, H_2O)$+18.1$ (c 1, HCl pH 3) (64)	—	64	64	64	64
45	α-Amino-β-methylaminopropionic acid	*Cycas circinalis*	$C_4H_{11}N_2O_2$ (105.15)	165–167° (65)	—	—	65	65	65	65
45a	α-Amino-β-oxalylaminopropionic acid	*Crotalaria*	$C_5H_8N_2O_5$ (176.15)	—	—	—	—	65a	—	—
46	Canaline	*Canavalia ensiformis*	$C_4H_{10}N_2O_3$ (134.14)	—	—	≤40, ≤70, ≤20 (20)	66	—	67	—
46a	threo-α,β-Diaminobutyric acid	Amphomycin hydrolyzate	$C_4H_{10}N_2O_2$ (118.16)	213–214° (dec) (67a)	$+27.1^{25}$ (c 2, 5 N HCl) (67a)	—	67b	67b	67a	67b

DATA ON THE NATURALLY OCCURRING AMINO ACIDS (Continued)

No.	Amino Acid (Synonym)	Source	Formula (Mol Wt)	Melting Point °C[a]	$[\alpha]_D$[b]	pK$_a$	Isolation and Purification	Chromatography	Chemistry	Spectral Data
							References			
47	α,γ-Diaminobutyric acid (γ-aminobutyrine)	Glumamycin	$C_4H_{10}N_2O_2$ (134.14)	–	+7.2^{25} (c 2, H$_2$O)	1.85 / 10.50 (20)	68	68	68	–
48	3,5-Diaminohexanoic acid	Clostridium stricklandii	$C_6H_{14}N_2O_2$ (146.19)	204–208° (69)	+14.6^{18} (c 3.67, H$_2$O)^g (290)	–	69	69	69	69
48a	2,6-Diamino-7-hydroxyazelaic acid	Bacillus brevis (edeine A and B)	$C_9H_{18}N_2O_{15}$ (234.29)	–	+14.6^{10} (c 3.67, H$_2$O)^g (290)	–	69a	69a	69a	–
49	α,β-Diaminopropionic acid (β-aminoalanine)	Mimosa	$C_3H_8N_2O_2$ (104.11)	–	–	1.23 / 6.73 / 9.56 (20)	70	70	70	–
49a	N^ε,N^ε-Dimethyllysine	Human urine	$C_8H_{18}N_2O_3$ (174.28)	214–216° (dec) (70a)	–	–	70a	70a	–	70a
49b	N^δ-Iminoethylornithine	Streptomyces broth	$C_7H_{15}N_3O_2$ (173.25)	226–229° (70b)	+20.6^{25} (c 1, 5 N HCl) (70b)	1.97 / 8.86 / 11.83 (70b)	70b	70b	–	70b
50	Lathyrus factor (β-N-(γ-glutamyl) aminopropionitrile)	Lathyrus pusillus	$C_8H_{13}N_3O_3$ (199.22)	193–194° (72)	+28^{18} (c 1, 6 N HCl) (72)	2.2 / 9.14	71	72	72	72
51	Lysine (α,ε-diaminocaproic acid)	Casein	$C_6H_{14}N_2O_2$ (146.19)	224–225° (dec) (73)	+14.6^{20} (H$_2$O) (73)	2.16 / 9.18 / 10.79 (290)	74	3	75	–
52	β-Lysine (isolysine; β,ε-diaminocaproic acid)	Viomycin	$C_6H_{14}N_2O_2$ (146.19)	240–241° (76)	–	–	76	76	76	76
53	Lysopine N^2-(D-1-carboxyethyl)-lysine	Calf thymus histone	$C_9H_{18}N_2O_4$ (204.25)	157–160° (77)	+18 (c 1.4, H$_2$O) (77)	–	78	78	77	77
54	ε-N-Methyllysine	Calf thymus histone	$C_7H_{16}N_2O_2$ (160.23)	–	–	–	79	79	–	79
55	Ornithine (α,δ-diaminovaleric acid)	Asplenium nidus	$C_5H_{12}N_2O_2$ (132.16)	–	+12.1 (c 2, H$_2$O)	1.71 / 8.69	60	60	81	81
55a	4-Oxalysine	Streptomyces	$C_5H_{12}N_2O_3$ (148.19)	–	+28.4 (c 2, 5 N HCl) (1)	10.76 (290)	81a	81a	–	81a
56	β-N-Oxalyl-α,β-diaminopropionic acid	Lathyrus sativus	$C_5H_8N_2O_3$ (176.13)	206° (dec) (82)	–36.9^7 (c 0.66, 4 N HCl) (82)	1.95 / 2.95 / 9.25 (82)	82	82	82	82
56a	β-Putreanine [N-(4-aminobutyl)-3-aminopropionic acid]	Bovine brain	$C_7H_{16}N_2O_2$ (160.25)	250–251° (dec) (82a)	–	3.2 / 9.4 / 11.2 (82a)	82a	82a	–	82a
	D. L-DIAMINO, DICARBOXYLIC ACIDS									
57	Acetylenic dicarboxylic acid diamide	Streptomyces chibaensis	$C_4H_4N_2O_2$ (112.09)	216–218° (dec)	–	–	83	83	83	83
58	α,ε-Diaminopimelic acid	Pine pollen	$C_7H_{14}N_2O_4$ (190.20)	–	+8.1^{25} (c 5, H$_2$O) / +45^{26} (c 1, 1 N HCl) / +45.1^{24} (c 2.6, 5 N HCl) (290)	1.8 / 2.2 / 9.9 / 8.8 (290)	84	84	85	–

DATA ON THE NATURALLY OCCURRING AMINO ACIDS (Continued)

No.	Amino Acid (Synonym)	Source	Formula (Mol Wt)	Melting Point °C[a]	$[\alpha]_D$[b]	pKa	References Isolation and Purification	Chromatography	Chemistry	Spectral Data
59	2,3-Diaminosuccinic acid	Streptomyces rimosus	C4H8N2O4 (148.10)	240–290° (dec)	—	—	86	86	86	86
			E. L-KETO, HYDROXY, AND HYDROXY SUBSTITUTED AMINO ACIDS							
60	O-Acetylhomoserine	Pisum	C6H11NO4 (161.17)	—	—	—	87	87	87	—
60a	Threo-α-amino-β,γ-dihydroxybutyric acid	Streptomyces	C4H9NO4 (135.14)	210°(dec)	−13.3²⁵ (c 1, H2O) −1.1²⁵ (c 1, 2.2 N HCl) (87a)	—	87a	—	—	—
61	2-Amino-4,5-dihydroxypentanoic acid	Lunaria annua	C5H11NO4 (149.15)	—	—	—	88	88	88	—
61a	2-Amino-3-formyl-3-pentenoic acid	Bankera fuligineoalba	C6H9NO3 (143.16)	—	—	—	88a	88a	88a	88a
62	α-Amino-γ-hydroxyadipic acid	Vibrio comma	C6H11NO5 (177.17)	—	—	—	89	—	—	—
63	2-Amino-6-hydroxyaminohexanoic acid	Mycobacterium phlei	C6H14N2O3 (162.19)	—	+6.3²⁰(c 5, H2O)+23.9¹⁰ (c 5.1, 1 N HCl) (90)	—	90	90	90	—
64	α-Amino-γ-hydroxybutyric acid	Escherichia coli mutants	C4H9NO3 (119.12)	199° (91)	—	—	91	91	91	—
65	γ-Amino-β-hydroxybutyric acid	Escherichia coli mutants	C4H9NO3 (119.12)	—	—	—	—	92	—	—
66	2-Amino-6-hydroxy-4-methyl-4-hexenoic acid	Aesculus californica	C7H13NO3 (159.19)	—	−30²⁰(c 2.2, H2O) +2²⁰ (c 1.1, 5 N HCl) (19)	—	19	19	19	19, 21
67	2-Amino-3-hydroxymethyl-3-pentenoic acid	Bankera fuligineoalba	C6H11NO3 (145.17)	160–161° (13)	+182²⁵ (c 0.8, H2O) +201²⁵ (c 0.8, 0.3N HCl) (13)	—	13	13	13	13
68	α-Amino-γ-hydroxypimelic acid	Asplenium seplentrionale	C7H13NO5 (191.19)	—	—	—	96	96	—	—
69	α-Amino-δ-hydroxyvaleric acid	Canavalia ensiformis	C5H11NO3 (133.15)	216° (dec) (97)	+6²⁵ (c 2.65, H2O) +2.4²⁵₃₆₅ (c 2.65, H2O) (97)	—	97	97	97	97
70	α-Amino-β-ketobutyric acid	Mikramycin A	C4H7NO3 (117.11)	—	—	—	98	—	—	—
71	α-Amino-β-methyl-γ, δ-dihydroxyisocaproic acid	Phalloidin	C7H15NO4 (177.21)	208–210° (99)	—	—	99	99	99	99
71a	2-Amino-5-methyl-6-hydroxyhex-4-enoic acid	Blighia unijugata	C7H13NO3 (159.21)	—	—	—	99a	99a	—	99a
72	O-Butylhomoserine	Soil bacterium	C8H17NO3 (175.23)	267° (100)	—	—	100	100	100	100
72a	Dihydrorhizobitoxine [O-(2-amino-3-hydroxypropyl)homoserine]	Rhizobium japonicum	C7H16N2O4 (192.25)	—	—	7.2 8.6 (100b)	100a	—	—	100
73	β,γ-Dihydroxyglutamic acid	Rheum rhaponticum	C5H9NO6 (179.13)	—	—	—	101	101	101	—
74	β,γ-Dihydroxyisoleucine	Thiostrepton	C6H15NO4 (165.20)	—	—	—	102	—	—	—
75	γ,δ-Dihydroxyleucine	Phalloin	C6H13NO4 (163.18)	—	—	—	103	—	103	103
75a	δ,ε-Dihydroxynorleucine	Bovine tendon	C6H13NO4 (163.20)	—	—	—	103a	—	103a	—
76	O-Ethylhomoserine	Soil bacterium	C6H13NO3 (147.18)	262° (100)	−14³⁰ (c 2.5, H2O) (100)	—	100	100	100	100
76a	β-Guanido-γ-hydroxyvaline	Viomycin	C6H14N4O3 (190.24)	182°(dec) (104a)	−8.8²⁵ (c1–2, H2O)	—	—	—	—	104a
77	Homoserine (α-amino-γ-hydroxybutyric acid)	Pisum sativum	C4H9NO3 (119.12)	—	+18.3²⁶ (c 2, 2 N HCl) (290)	2.71 9.62 (290)	105	105	—	—

DATA ON THE NATURALLY OCCURRING AMINO ACIDS (Continued)

No.	Amino Acid (Synonym)	Source	Formula (Mol Wt)	Melting Point °C[a]	$[\alpha]_D$[b]	pK_a	Isolation and Purification	Chromatography	Chemistry	Spectral Data
78	α-Hydroxyalanine	Peptides of ergot	$C_3H_7NO_3$ (105.10)	–	–	–	106	–	–	–
79	α-Hydroxy-γ-aminobutyric acid	E. coli mutants	$C_4H_9NO_3$ (119.12)	–	–	–	91	91	–	–
80	β-Hydroxy-γ-aminobutyric acid	Mammalian brain	$C_4H_9NO_3$ (119.12)	–	–	–	–	108	–	–
81	α-Hydroxy-ε-aminocaproic acid	Neurospora crassa	$C_6H_{13}NO_3$ (147.18)	–	–	–	109	109	–	–
82	β-Hydroxyasparagine	Human urine	$C_4H_8O_4N_2$ (148.12)	238–240° (dec) (110)	–	2.09 8.29 (20)	110	110	110	110
83	β-Hydroxyaspartic acid	Azotobacter	$C_4H_7NO_5$ (149.10)	–	+41.4 (c 2.42, H_2O) +53.0 (c 2.46, 1 N HCl) (290)[d]	1.91 3.51 9.11 (20)	111	111	–	–
83a	N'-(2-Hydroxyethyl)alanine	Rumen protozoa	$C_5H_{11}NO_3$ (133.17)	–	–	–	111a	–	–	111a
84	N'-(2-Hydroxyethyl)asparagine	Bryonia dioica	$C_6H_{12}N_2O_4$ (176.20)	199–200° (112)	-2.9^{20} (c 5, H_2O) (112)	–	112	112	112	112
85	N'-(2-Hydroxyethyl)glutamine	Lunaria annua	$C_7H_{14}N_2O_4$ (190.23)	–	$+5.8^{19}$ (c 1.8, H_2O) (88)	–	88	88	88	–
86	β-Hydroxyglutamic acid	Mycobacterium tuberculosis	$C_5H_9NO_5$ (163.13)	187° (dec) (290)	+8.69 (H_2O)+30.8^{20} (c 2, 20% HCl) (290)[d]	–	114	114	–	–
87	γ-Hydroxyglutamic acid	Linaria vulgaris	$C_5H_9NO_5$ (163.13)	–	–	–	115	115	115	–
88	γ-Hydroxyglutamine	Phlox decussata	$C_5H_{10}N_2O_4$ (162.15)	163–164° (dec) (116)	–	–	116	116	116	–
89	ε-Hydroxylaminonorleucine (α-amino-ε-hydroxyaminohexanoic acid)	Mycobacterium phlei	$C_5H_{12}N_2O_3$ (148.17)	223–225° (dec) (117)	$+6.3^{20}$ (c 5, H_2O)+23.9^{18} (c 5.1, N HCl) (117)	–	117	117	117	–
89a	4-Hydroxyisoleucine	Trigonella foenumgraecum	$C_6H_{13}NO_3$ (147.20)	–	$+31^{20}$ (c 1, H_2O) (117a)	–	117a	117a	–	117a
90	δ-Hydroxy-γ-ketonorvaline	Streptomyces akiyoshiensis novo	$C_5H_9NO_4$ (147.13)	–	-8.2^{17} (c 3.4, H_2O) (118)	2.0 9.1	118	118	118	118
91	δ-Hydroxyleucenine (δ-ketoleucine)	Phalloidin	$C_6H_{11}NO_3$ (145.17)	–	–	–	119	119	119	119
92	β-Hydroxyleucine	Antibiotic from Paecilomyces strain	$C_6H_{13}NO_3$ (147.17)	–	–	–	16	16	16	–
93	δ-Hydroxyleucine	Paecilomyces	$C_6H_{13}NO_3$ (147.17)	–	–	–	121	121	121	121
94	threo-β-Hydroxyleucine	Deutzia gracilis	$C_6H_{13}NO_3$ (147.17)	–	–	–	122	122	122	122
95	α-Hydroxylysine (α,ε-diamino-α-hydroxycaproic acid)	Silvia officinalis	$C_6H_{15}N_2O_3$ (162.19)	–	–	2.13 8.62 9.67 (20)	123	123	–	–
96	δ-Hydroxylysine (α,ε-diamino-δ-hydroxycaproic acid)	Fish gelatin	$C_6H_{15}N_2O_3$ (162.19)	–	–	–	124	111	–	–
96a	β-Hydroxynorvaline	Streptomyces species	$C_5H_{11}NO_3$ (133.17)	244° (dec) (124a)	–	–	124a	124a	–	124a
97	γ-Hydroxynorvaline	Lathyrus odoratus	$C_5H_{11}NO_3$ (133.15)	–	$+22^{20}$ (c 5, H_2O)+32 (c 2.5, gl. acetic) (126)	–	126	126	126	–
98	γ-Hydroxyornithine	Vicia sativa	$C_5H_{12}N_2O_3$ (148.16)	–	–	–	127	127	–	–
99	α-Hydroxyvaline	Ergot	$C_5H_{11}NO_3$ (133.15)	–	–	2.55 9.77 (20)	106	–	–	–

DATA ON THE NATURALLY OCCURRING AMINO ACIDS (Continued)

No.	Amino Acid (Synonym)	Source	Formula (Mol Wt)	Melting Point °C[a]	$[\alpha]_D$[b]	pK_a	References: Isolation and Purification	Chromatography	Chemistry	Spectral Data
100	γ-Hydroxyvaline	Kalanchoe daigremontiana	$C_5H_{11}NO_3$ (133.15)	228° (dec) (129)	+1020 (H_2O) (129)	–	129	129	–	–
100a	Hypusine	Bovine brain	$C_{10}H_{23}N_3O_3$ (233.27)	234–238° (dec) (129a)	–	–	129a	–	129a	129a
100b	Isoserine	Bacillus brevis (edeine A and B)	$C_3H_7NO_3$ (105.11)	–	–	–	129b	129b	129b	–
101	4-Ketonorleucine (2-amino-4-ketohexanoic acid)	Citrobacter freundii	$C_6H_{11}NO_3$ (145.17)	142–143° (130)	–	–	131	131	130	130
102	γ-Methyl-γ-hydroxyglutamic acid	Phyllitis scolopendrium	$C_6H_{11}NO_5$ (157.17)	–	–	–	56	56	–	–
103	Pantonine (α-amino-β,β-dimethyl-γ-hydroxybutyric acid)	Escherichia coli	$C_6H_{13}NO_3$ (147.18)	–	–	–	132	132	132	–
103a	threo-β-Phenylserine	Canthium eurysides	$C_9H_{11}NO_3$ (181.21)	–	–	–	–	–	–	252a
103b	Pinnatanine [N^5-(2-hydroxymethylbutadienyl)-allo-γ-hydroxyglutamine]	Staphylea pinnata	$C_{10}H_{16}N_2O_5$ (244.28)	165° (dec) (132a)	+3.2^{27} (c 0.5, H_2O) (132a)	9.1 (132a)	132a	132a	–	132a
104	O-Propylhomoserine	Soil bacterium	$C_7H_{15}NO_3$ (161.21)	285° (100)	–11^{30} (c 2, H_2O) (100)	–	100	100	100	100
104a	Rhizobitoxine [2-amino-4-(2-amino-3-hydroxypropoxy)but-3-enoic acid]	Rhizobium japonicum	$C_7H_{15}N_2O_4$ (191.24)	–	–	–	132b	–	–	132c
105	Serine (α-amino-β-hydroxypropionic acid)	Silk fibroin	$C_3H_7NO_3$ (105.09)	228° (dec) (1)	–7.5^{25} (c2, H_2O)+15.1^{25} (c2. 5 N HCl) (290)	2.19 9.21 (290)	134	3	134	134
106	O-Succinylhomoserine	Escherichia coli	$C_8H_{13}NO_6$ (219.20)	130–181° (135)	–	4.4 9.5 (135)	135	135	135	–
107	Tabtoxinine (α,ε-diamino-β-hydroxypimelic acid)	Pseudomonas tabaci	$C_7H_{14}N_2O_5$ (186.20)	–	–	–	136	137	137	–
108	Threonine (α-amino-β-hydroxybutyric acid)	Fibrin hydrolyzate	$C_4H_9NO_3$ (119.12)	253° (1)	–28^{25} (c 1–2, H_2O) –15^{25} (c 1–2, 5 N HCl) (290)	2.09 9.10 (290)	138	3	138, 139	139
	F. L-AROMATIC AMINO ACIDS									
109	α-Amino-β-phenylbutyric acid	Streptomyces bottropensis	$C_{10}H_{13}NO_2$ (187)	176–177° (140)	–	–	140	140	140	140
109a	β-Amino-β-phenylpropionic acid	Roccella canariensis hydrolyzate	$C_9H_{11}NO_2$ (165.21)	–	–	–	–	–	–	140a
110	3-Carboxy-4-hydroxyphenylalanine (m-carboxytyrosine)	Reseda odorata	$C_{10}H_{11}NO_5$ (165.15)	–	–7.7^{25} (c 0.9, 1 N NaOH)–29.9^{24} (c 0.6, 0.2 M PO_4, pH 7) (297)	2 3.4 9.3 12–13 (297)	141	141	141	141
111	m-Carboxyphenylalanine	Iris bulbs	$C_{10}H_{11}NO_4$ (191.26)	–	–	1.5 3.9 (142)	142	142	142	142
111a	2,3-Dihydroxy-N-benzoylserine	Escherichia coli	$C_{10}H_{11}NO_6$ (241.22)	193–194° (142a)	–	–	142a	142a	–	142a
112	2,4-Dihydroxy-6-methylphenylalanine	Agrostemma githago	$C_{10}H_{13}NO_4$ (211.23)	252° (144)	+19.7^{18} (1 N HCl) (144)	–	144	144	144	144

DATA ON THE NATURALLY OCCURRING AMINO ACIDS (Continued)

No.	Amino Acid (Synonym)	Source	Formula (Mol Wt)	Melting Point °C[a]	$[\alpha]_D$[b]	pK_a	Isolation and Purification	Chromatography	Chemistry	Spectral Data
113	3,4-Dihydroxyphenylalanine (DOPA)	Vicia faba	$C_9H_{11}NO_4$ (209.21)	–	-14.3 (1 N HCl) (146)	2.32e 8.68e 9.88e	145	–	146	–
114	3,5-Dihydroxyphenylglycine	Euphorbia helioscopia	$C_8H_9NO_4$ (183.16)	230–232° (147)	–	–	147	147	147	147
114a	γ-Glutaminyl-4-hydroxybenzene	Agaricus bisporus	$C_{11}H_{14}N_2O_4$ (238.27)	225–226° (147a)	+42.5^25 (c 0.67, 0.1 N NaOH) (147a)	–	147a	–	–	147a
114b	3-Hydroxymethylphenylalanine	Caesalpinia tinctoria	$C_{10}H_{13}NO_3$ (195.24)	–	-36^20 (c 1, H₂O)—4^20 (c 0.67, 1 N NaOH) (147b)	–	147b	147b	–	147b
114c	4-Hydroxy-3-hydroxymethylphenylalanine	Caesalpinia tinctoria	$C_{10}H_{13}NO_4$ (211.24)	–	–	–	147b	147b	–	147b
115	3-Hydroxykynurenine	Human urine	$C_{10}H_{12}N_2O_4$ (224.21)	–	–	–	148	148	–	–
115a	p-Hydroxymethylphenylalanine	Escherichia coli	$C_{10}H_{13}NO_3$ (195.24)	231–233° (dec) (148a)	-32.5^20 (148a)	–	–	148b	148b	148a
116	m-Hydroxyphenylglycine	Euphorbia helioscopia	$C_8H_9NO_3$ (177.16)	212–214° (147)	–	–	147	147	147	147
117	Kynurenine (β-anthraniloyl-α-aminopropionic acid)	Rabbit urine	$C_{10}H_{12}N_2O_3$ (208.21)	191° (dec) (290)	-30.5^25 (c 1, H₂O) (290)	–	148	–	148	148
118	O-Methyltyrosine (β-(p-methoxyphenyl)alanine)	Puromycin	$C_{10}H_{13}NO_3$ (195.22)	191° (150)	-5—9_546 (HCl) (150)—3.2_546 (1 N NaOH) (150)	–	149	–	150	–
119	Phenylalanine	Lupinus luteus	$C_9H_{11}NO_2$ (165.19)	284° (1)	-34.5^25 (c 1–2, H₂O) (290)	2.16 9.18 (290)	151	3	152	152
120	Tyrosine (α-amino-β-hydroxyphenylpropionic acid)	Casein, alkaline hydrolyzate	$C_9H_{11}NO_3$ (181.19)	344° (1)	-10^25 (c 2, 5 N HCl)(1) -4.5^25 (c 1–2, 5 N HCl) (290)	2.20 9.11 (1) 10.13 (290)	153	3	154	154
120a	β-Tyrosine	Bacillus brevis (edeine A and B)	$C_9H_{11}NO_3$ (181.21)	–	–	–	129b	129b	129b	–
121	m-Tyrosine	Euphorbia myrsinites L	$C_9H_{11}NO_3$ (181.19)	272–274° (155)	-14.5^22 (70% EtOH) +8.9 (70% EtOH, 2 N HCl) (155)	–	155	155	155	155

G. L-UREIDO AND GUANIDO AMINO ACIDS

No.	Amino Acid (Synonym)	Source	Formula (Mol Wt)	Melting Point °C[a]	$[\alpha]_D$[b]	pK_a	Isolation and Purification	Chromatography	Chemistry	Spectral Data
121a	N-Acetylarginine	Cattle brain	$C_7H_{16}N_4O_3$ (204.27)	270° (155a)	–	–	155a	155a	155a	155a
122	Albizziine (2-amino-3-ureidopropionic acid)	Mimosaceae	$C_4H_9N_3O_3$ (119.12)	–	-66^26 (c 2, H₂O) (157)	–	156	157	157	157
123	Arginine (amino-δ-guanidinovaleric acid)	Lupinus luteus	$C_6H_{14}N_4O_2$	238° (1)	+12.5^25 (c 2, H₂O) +27.6^25 (c 2, 5 N HCl) (1)	1.82 8.99 12.48 (290)	158	3	159	159
124	Canavanine (α-amino-(O-guanidyl)-γ-hydroxybutyric acid)	Canavalia ensiformis	$C_5H_{12}N_4O_3$ (176.19)	172° (160)	+18.6^18.5 (c 7.8, H₂O) (160)	2.50 6.60 9.25 (33)	161	160	160	162
125	Canavanosuccinic acid	Canavalia ensiformis	$C_9H_{16}N_4O_7$ (292.27)	–	+4^25 (c 2, H₂O)	–	163	163	–	–
126	Citrulline	Watermelon	$C_6H_{13}N_3O_3$	202° (164)	+24.2^25 (c 2, N HCl) +10.8 (c 1.1, 0.1 N NaOH) (290)	2.43 9.41 (290)	164	165	164	–

DATA ON THE NATURALLY OCCURRING AMINO ACIDS (Continued)

No.	Amino Acid (Synonym)	Source	Formula (Mol Wt)	Melting Point °C[a]	$[\alpha]_D$[b]	pK_a	References Isolation and Purification	Chromatography	Chemistry	Spectral Data
127	Desaminocanavanine	Canavanine	$C_5H_9N_3O_3$	256–257° (166)	+26.61²¹ (H₂O) (166)	–	166	166	166	–
127a	N^G, N^G-Dimethylarginine	Bovine brain	$C_8H_{18}N_4O_2$ (202.30)	198–201° (70a)	–	–	166a	166a	–	166a
127b	N^G, N'^G-Dimethylarginine	Bovine brain	$C_8H_{18}N_4O_2$ (202.30)	237–239° (dec) (70a)	–	–	166a	166a	70a	166a
128	Gigartinine (α-amino-δ-(guanylureido)valeric acid)	Gymnogongrus flabelliformis	$C_7H_{15}N_5O_3$ (217.25)	–	–	–	167	167	167	167
129	Homoarginine	Lathyrus species	$C_7H_{16}N_4O_2$ (188.25)	–	+42.4⁻ (c 0.452, 1.02 N HCl)[y] (168)	–	168	168	168	168
130	Homocitrulline	Human urine	$C_7H_{14}N_3O_3$ (189.22)	–	–	–	169	169	–	–
131	γ-Hydroxyarginine	Vicia sativa	$C_6H_{14}N_4O_3$ (190.20)	–	–	–	170	170	170	170
131a	N^5-Hydroxyarginine	Bacillus species	$C_6H_{14}N_4O_3$ (190.24)	206–212° (dec) (170a)	+21²⁵ (c 1, 5 N HCl) (170a)	–	170a	170a	170a	170a
132	γ-Hydroxyhomoarginine (α-amino-ε-guanidino-γ-hydroxyhexanoic acid)	Lathyrus tingitanus	$C_7H_{16}N_4O_3$ (204.23)	–	–	–	171	171	171	171
133	Indospicine (α-amino-ε-amidinocaproic acid)	Indigofera spicata	$C_7H_{15}N_3O_2$ (173.23)	131–134° (173)	+18²² (c 1.1, 5 N HCl) (173)	–	173	173	173	–
133a	ω-N-Methylarginine (guanidinomethylarginine)	Bovine brain	$C_7H_{16}N_4O_2$ (188.27)	–	–	–	166a	166a	–	166a
H. L-AMINO ACIDS CONTAINING OTHER NITROGENOUS GROUPS										
134	Alanosine [2-amino-3-(N-nitrosohydroxyamino)propionic acid]	Streptomyces alanosinicus	$C_3H_7N_3O_4$ (149.11)	–	+8 (1 N HCl)-46 (0.1 N NaOH) (174)	(174)	174	–	174	174
135	Azaserine (O-diazoacetylserine)	Streptomyces	$C_5H_7N_3O_4$ (173.14)	146–162° (175)	-0.5²⁷·⁵ (c 8.46, H₂O) (175)	8.55 (34)	175	175	175	175
136	β-Cyanoalanine	Vicia sativa	$C_4H_6N_2O_2$ (114.11)	214.5° (176)	-2.9²⁶ (c 1.4, 1 N acetic acid) (177)	1.7 / 7.4 (177)	176	176	177	177
136a	γ-Cyano-α-aminobutyric acid	Chromo-bacterium violaceum	$C_5H_8N_2O_2$ (128.15)	221–223° (177a)	+32.1²¹ (c 0.38, 1 N HOAc) (177a)	–	177a	177a	177a	177a
137	ε-Diazo-δ-ketonorleucine	Streptomyces	$C_6H_9N_3O_3$ (171.17)	145–155° (178)	21²⁶ (c 5.4, H₂O) (178)	–	178	178	178	178
138	Hadacidin (N-formyl-N-hydroxyaminoacetic acid)	Penicillium frequentans	$C_3H_5NO_4$ (119.08)	205–210° (179)	–	–	179	–	179	179
I. L-HETEROCYCLIC AMINO ACIDS										
138a	2-Alanyl-3-isoxazolin-5-one	Pea seedlings	$C_6H_8N_2O_4$ (172.16)	203–205° (dec) (180b)	–	–	180b	180b	180b	180b
139	Allohydroxyproline	Santalum album	$C_5H_9NO_3$ (131.13)	248° (180)	-57²⁵ (c 0.65, H₂O) (180)	–	180	180	180	–
140	Allokainic acid (3-carboxymethyl-4-isopropenyl proline)	Digenea simplex	$C_{10}H_{15}NO_4$ (213.24)	–	+8²⁶ (H₂O) (184, 185)	–	184, 185	–	184, 185	184, 185
140a	1-Amino-2-nitrocyclopentanecarboxylic acid	Aspergillus wentii	$C_6H_{10}N_2O_4$ (174.18)	150° (dec) (185a)	–	–	185a	185a	185a	185a
141	4-Aminopipecolic acid	Strophanthus scandens	$C_6H_{11}N_2O_2$ (143.18)	–	–	–	186	186	–	–
141a	cis-3-Aminoproline	Morchella esculenta	$C_5H_{10}N_2O_2$ (130.17)	215° (dec) (186a)	+5.8²⁰ (c 2, H₂O) / +23.0²⁰ (c 2, 5 N HCl) (186a)	–	186a	186a	186a	186a
141b	Anticapsin	Streptomyces griseoplanus	$C_9H_{13}NO_4$ (199.23)	240° (dec) (186b)	+125²⁵ (c 1, H₂O) (186b)	4.3 / 10.1 (186b)	186b	186b	186b	186b

DATA ON THE NATURALLY OCCURRING AMINO ACIDS (Continued)

No.	Amino Acid (Synonym)	Source	Formula (Mol Wt)	Melting Point °C[a]	$[\alpha]_D$[b]	pK_a	Isolation and Purification	Chromatography	Chemistry	Spectral Data
142	Ascorbigen	Cabbage	$C_{15}H_{15}NO_6$ (305.30)	–	–	–	187	188	189	–
143	Azetidine-2-carboxylic acid	Convallaria majalis	$C_4H_7NO_2$ (101.11)	–	–	–	190	190	190	190
143a	Azirinomycin (3-methyl-2-hydroazirine carboxylic acid)	Streptomyces aureus	$C_4H_5NO_2$ (99.10)	–	–	–	189a	189a	–	189a
144	Baikiain (1,2,3,6-tetra-hydropyridine-α-carboxylic acid)	Baikiaea plurijuga	$C_6H_9NO_2$, (127.15)	273–274° (183)	–	–	181	182	183	183
144a	N-Carbamoyl-2-(p-hydroxyphenyl)glycine	Vicia faba	$C_9H_{10}N_2O_4$ (210.21)	194–195° (dec) (190a)	–	–	190a	–	–	190a
144b	3-Carboxy-6,7-dihydroxy-1,2,3,4-tetrahydroisoquinoline	Mucuna mutisiana	$C_{10}H_{11}NO_4$ (209.22)	286–288° (190b)	-114.9^{25} (c 1.65, 20% HCl) (190b)	–	190b	–	190b	190b
144c	Claviciptic acid	Claviceps (ergot fungus)	$C_{16}H_{18}N_2O_2$ (270.36)	262° (dec) (190c)	–	–	190c	–	–	190c
145	Cucurbitine (3-amino-3-carboxypyrrolidine)	Cucurbita moschata	$C_5H_{10}N_2O_2$ (116.14)	–	-19.76^{27} (c 9.3, H_2O) (191)	–	191	191	191	191
145a	N-Dihydrojasmonylisoleucine	Gibberella fujikuroi	$C_{18}H_{31}N_3O_4$ (325.50)	140–141° (191a)	–	–	–	191a	191a	191a
145b	2,5-Dihydrophenylalanine (1,4-cyclohexadiene-1-alanine)	Streptomycete X-13, 185	$C_9H_{13}NO_2$ (167.23)	206–208° (191b)	-33.7^{25} (c 1, 5 N HCl) (191b)	–	191b	–	–	191b
145c	2-N,6-N-Di-(2,3-dihydroxybenzoyl)lysine	Azobacter vinelandii	$C_{20}H_{22}N_2O_8$ (418.44)	–	–	4.8, 9 (191c)	191c	191c	–	191c
145d	cis-3,4-trans-3,4-Dihydroxyproline	Diatom cell walls	$C_5H_9NO_4$ (147.15)	262° (dec) (191d)	-61.2^{20} (c 0.5, H_2O) (191d)	–	191d	191d	–	191e
145e	β-(2,6-Dihydroxypyrimidin-1-yl)alanine	Pea seedlings	$C_7H_9N_3O_4$ (199.19)	230° (dec) (191f)	–	–	191f	–	191f	191f
145f	4,6-Dihydroxyquinoline-2-carboxylic acid	Tobacco leaves	$C_{10}H_7NO_4$ (205.18)	287° (dec) (191g)	–	–	191g	191g	191g	191g
146	Dihydrozanthurenic acid (8-hydroxy-1,2,3,4-tetrahydro-4-ketoquinaldic acid)	Lepidoptera	$C_{10}H_9NO_4$ (207.19)	185–190° (192)	-45^{20} (c 0.9, MeOH)$+18^{20}$ (c 0.9, MeOH-HCl) (192)	–	192	192	192	192
147	Domoic acid (2-carboxy-3-carboxymethyl-4-1-methyl-2-carboxy-1,3-hexadienylpyrrolidine)	Chondria armata	$C_{15}H_{21}NO_6$ (311.35)	217° (193)	-109.6^{12} (c 1.314, H_2O) (193)	2.20, 3.72, 4.93, 9.82 (193)	193	193	193	193
148	Echinine (2-tert-pentenyl-5,7-diisopentenyltryptophan)	Aspergillus glaucus	$C_{26}H_{36}N_2O_2$ (408.50)	169–172° (194)	–	–	194	–	194	194
148a	Enduracidine [α-amino-β-(2-iminoimidazolidinyl)propionic acid]	Enduracidin hydrolyzate	$C_6H_{12}N_4O_2$ (172.22)	–	$+63.3^{22}$ (1 M HCl)$+57.6^{22}$ (1 M NaOH) (194a)	2.5, 8.3, 12 (94a)	–	194a	–	194a
148a'	Furanomycin (α-amino(2,5-dihydro-5-methyl)furan-2-acetic acid]	Streptomyces L-803	$C_7H_{11}NO_3$ (157.19)	220–223° (dec) (194a')	$+136.1^{27}$ (c 1, H_2O) (194a')	2.4, 9.1 (194a')	194a'	194a'	194a'	194a'
148a"	Furosine [ε-N-(2-furoylmethyl)lysine]	Heated milk	$C_{12}H_{18}N_2O_4$ (254.32)	–	–	–	194a"	194b	–	194a"
148b	γ-Glutaminyl-3,4-benzoquinone	Agaricus bisporus	$C_{11}H_{12}N_2O_5$ (252.25)	–	–	–	194b	194b	–	194b
149	Guvacine	Areca cathecu	$C_6H_9NO_2$ (127.15)	–	–	–	195, 196	–	–	–
150	Histidine	Protamine from sturgeon sperm	$C_6H_9N_3O_2$ (155.16)	277° (1)	-38.5^{25} (H_2O)$+11.8$ (5 N HCl)(1)	1.82, 6.00, 9.17 (1)	197	3	198	198

DATA ON THE NATURALLY OCCURRING AMINO ACIDS (Continued)

No.	Amino Acid (Synonym)	Source	Formula (Mol Wt)	Melting Point °C[a]	$[\alpha]_D$[b]	pK_a	Isolation and Purification	Chromatography	Chemistry	Spectral Data
150a	β-Hydroxyhistidine	Bleomycin A₂ (antibiotic)	$C_6H_9N_3O_3$ (171.18)	205° (dec) (198a)	$+40^{28}$ (c 1, H₂O) (198a)	<2.0 / 198a / 5.5 / 8.8 (198a)	198a	–	198a	–
151	4-Hydroxy-4-methylproline	Apples	$C_6H_{11}NO_2$ (145.16)	–	–	–	199	199	–	200
152	Hydroxyminaline	Penicillium aspergillus	$C_5H_5NO_3$ (127.10)	–	–	–	201	–	201	201
153	4-Hydroxypipecolic acid	Acacia pentadenia	$C_6H_{11}NO_3$ (145.16)	250–270° (202)	-12.5^{21} (H₂O)$+0.34^{21}$ (1 N HCl) / -18.5^{21} (1 N NaOH) (202)	–	202	202	202	203
154	5-Hydroxypipecolic acid	Rhapis excelsa	$C_6H_{11}NO_3$ (145.16)	–	–	–	203	203	–	203
154a	5-Hydroxypiperidazine-3-carboxylic acid	Monamycin hydrolyzate	$C_5H_{10}N_2O_3$ (146.17)	201–202° (DNP cerv.) (204a)	$+21.4^{24}$ (c 0.39, H₂O) (204b)	–	204a	204a	204a	204, 204a
155	3-Hydroxyproline (3-hydroxypyrrolidine-2-carboxylic acid)	Telomycin	$C_5H_9NO_3$ (131.13)	225–235° (206)	-17.4^{20} (c 1, H₂O)$+13.3^{20}$ (c 0.5, 1 N HCl) (206a)	–	206	206	206	206a
156	4-Hydroxyproline (4-hydroxypyrrolidine-2-carboxylic acid)	Gelatin hydrolyzate	$C_5H_9NO_3$ (131.13)	273–274° (290)	-76.0^{25} (c 2, H₂O) / -50.5^{25} (c 2, 5 N HCl)(290)	1.82 / 9.66 (290)	207	3	208	208
157	2-Hydroxytryptophan	Phalloidin	$C_{11}H_{12}N_2O_3$ (220.22)	257° (210)	$+40.8$ (c 4.2, 1 N NaOH) (210)	–	209	–	210	–
158	5-Hydroxytryptophan	Chromobacterium violaceum	$C_{11}H_{12}N_2O_3$ (220.22)	273° (dec) (290)	-32.5^{22} (c 1, H₂O)	–	211	211	–	–
159	Ibotenic acid (α-amino-3-keto-4-isoxazoline-5-acetic acid)	Amanita strobiliformis	$C_5H_6N_2O_4$ (114.10)	177–178° (212)	$\pm0°$ (212)	5.1 / 8.2 (212)	212	–	212	212
160	4-Imidazoleacetic acid	Polyporus sulfureus	$C_5H_7N_2O_2$ (125.11)	–	–	2.96 / 7.35 (20)	213	–	–	–
161	N-(Indole-3-acetyl)aspartic acid	Magnolia	$C_{14}H_{14}N_2O_5$ (290.29)	–	–	–	214	214	–	–
162	Indole-3-acetyl-ε-lysine	Pseudomonas savastanoi	$C_{16}H_{21}N_3O_3$ (303.36)	259–261° (215)	$+22^{23}$ (2 N HCl) (215)	–	215	215	215	215
162a	N-Jasmonoylisoleucine	Gibberella fujikuroi	$C_{18}H_{29}NO_4$ (323.48)	147–149° (191a)	–	–	–	191a	191a	191a
163	Kainic acid (3-carboxymethyl-4-isopropenyl proline)	Digenea simplex	$C_{10}H_{15}NO_4$ (213.25)	251° (216)	-15^{17} (H₂O) (185, 216)	–	216	216	–	–
164	4-Keto-5-methylproline	Actinomycin	$C_6H_9NO_3$ (143.18)	215° (217)	–	–	217	217	217	217
165	4-Ketopipecolic acid	Staphylomycin	$C_6H_9NO_3$ (143.15)	–	–	–	218	–	–	–
166	4-Ketoproline	Actinomycin	$C_5H_9N_4O_2$ (181.00)	–	–	–	219	–	219	–
167	Lathytine (tingitanine)	Lathyrus tingitanus	$C_7H_{10}N_4O_2$ (182.00)	215° (220)	-55.9^{21} (H₂O) (220)	2.4 / 4.1 / 9.0 (220)	220	220	–	220
167a	exo-3,4-Methanoproline	Aesculus parviflora	$C_6H_9NO_2$ (127.16)	–	-132^{20} (c 2, H₂O) / -104^{20} (c 1, 5 N HCl) (23a)	–	23a	23a	–	23a
168	4-Methyleneproline	Eriobotrya japonice	$C_6H_9NO_2$ (127.15)	225° (221)	$\pm0^c$	–	221	221	222	–

DATA ON THE NATURALLY OCCURRING AMINO ACIDS (Continued)

No.	Amino Acid (Synonym)	Source	Formula (Mol Wt)	Melting Point °C[a]	$[\alpha]_D^b$	pK_a	References: Isolation and Purification	Chromatography	Chemistry	Spectral Data
168a	1-Methyl-6-hydroxy-1,2,3,4-tetrahydroisoquinoline-3-carboxylic acid	Euphorbia myrsinites	$C_{11}H_{13}NO_3$ (207.25)	–	–	–	222a	222a	–	222a
169	4-Methylproline	Apples	$C_6H_{11}NO_2$ (129.16)	232–234° (224)	-52 (c 0.3, H_2O) (224)	–	223	223	224	224
170	N-Methylproline (hygric acid)	Apples	$C_6H_{11}NO_2$	–	–	–	223	223	223	–
170a	N-Methylstreptolidine	Streptothricin	$C_7H_{14}N_4O_3$ (202.25)	–	–	–	224a	224a	–	–
171	β-Methyltryptophan	Telomycin	$C_{12}H_{14}N_2O_2$ (218.25)	–	–	–	226	–	226	226
172	Mimosine	Mimosa pudica	$C_8H_{10}N_2O_4$ (198.18)	228–229°; 227	-21^{22} (H_2O); $+10^{22}$ (1% HCl)(227)	–	227a	–	227	227
173	Minaline (pyrrole-2-carboxylic acid)	Diastase	$C_5H_5NO_2$ (111.10)	180° (228)	–	–	228	–	228	228
174	Muscazone	Amanita muscaria	$C_5H_6N_2O_5$ (174.12)	190° (229)	–	–	229	–	230	231
174a	Nicotianamine [1-(3'-{γ-amino-α-γ-dicarboxypropylamino)propylazetidine-2-carboxylic acid]	Tobacco leaves	$C_{12}H_{21}N_3O_6$ (303.36)	240° (dec) (231a)	-60.5^{23} (c 2.7, H_2O) (231a)	–	231a	–	231a	231a
175	β-3-Oxindolylalanine	Phalloidin	$C_{11}H_{12}N_2O_3$ (220.24)	249–253° (209)	$+39.2^{20}$ (1 N NaOH) (209)	–	209	–	209	–
176	Pipecolic acid	Apples	$C_6H_{11}NO_2$ (129.17)	260° (dec) (290)	-25.4^{18} (c 5, H_2O) -13.3^{25} (c2, 5 N HCl) (290)	–	233	233	m	–
176a	Piperidazine-3-carboxylic acid	Monamycin hydrolyzate	$C_5H_{10}N_2O_2$ (130.17)	153–155° (DNP derv.) (204b)	$+307^{25}$ (c 0.18, CH_3OH) (204b)	–	–	–	–	204a
177	Proline (pyrrolidine-2-carboxylic acid)	Casein hydrolyzate	$C_5H_9NO_2$ (115.13)	222° (1)	-86.2^{25} (c 1–2, H_2O) -60.4 (c 1–2, 5 N HCl) (1)	1.95 10.64 (290)	234	3	235	235
178	β-Pyrazol-1-ylalanine	Citrullus vulgaris	$C_6H_9N_3O_2$ (155.17)	236–238° (236)	-7.3^{20} (c 3.4, H_2O) (236)	2.2 (236)	236	236	236	236
178a	Pyridosine [ε-(1,4-dihydro-6-methyl-3-hydroxy-4-oxo-1-pyridyl)lysine]	Heated milk	$C_{12}H_{19}N_3O_4$ (269.34)	–	–	–	236a	–	–	236a
178b	Pyrrolidonecarboxylic acid (5-oxoproline)	Human plasma	$C_5H_7NO_3$ (129.13)	–	–	–	236b	236b	–	–
179	Roseanine	Roseothricin	$C_6H_{12}N_4O_3$ (188.21)	–	$+56.8^{22}$ (c 2.35, H_2O) (238)	–	237	238	238	238
179a	Stendomycidine	Stendomycin (from Streptomyces)	$C_8H_{16}N_4O_2$ (200.28)	–	–	–	238a	238a	238a	238a, 238b
180	Stizolobic acid [β-(3-carboxypyran-5-yl)alanine]	Stizolobium hassjoo	$C_9H_9NO_6$ (227.18)	231–233° (239)	–	–	239	239	239	239
181	Stizolobinic acid [β-(6-carboxy-α-pyran-3-yl)alanine]	Stizolobium hassjoo	$C_9H_9NO_6$ (207.18)	–	–	–	239	239	240	240
181a	Streptolidine	Streptothricin	$C_6H_{12}N_4O_3$ (188.22)	215° (dec) (224a)	$+55.3^{25}$ (c 1.01, H_2O) (224a)	–	224a	224a	224a	224a
182	Tricholomic acid (α-amino-3-keto-5-isoxazolidineacetic acid)	Tricholoma muscarium	$C_5H_8N_2O_4$ (160.13)	207° (242)	m	6.0 8.6 (242)	242	m	242	242
183	Tryptophan (α-amino-β-3-indolepropionic acid)	Casein	$C_{11}H_{12}N_2O_2$ (204.24)	282° (1)	-33.7^{25} (c 1–2, H_2O) $+2.8^{25}$ (c 1–2, 1 N HCl) (1)	2.43 9.44 (290)	243	3	244	244
183a	Tuberactidine (2-imino-4-hydroxyhexahydro-6-pyrimidinylglycine)	Streptomyces griseoverticillatus	$C_6H_{12}N_4O_3$ (188.22)	182° (dec) (244a)	-25.8^{15} (c 0.5, H_2O) (244a)	–	244a	–	–	244a

DATA ON THE NATURALLY OCCURRING AMINO ACIDS (Continued)

No.	Amino Acid (Synonym)	Source	Formula (Mol Wt)	Melting Point °C[a]	$[\alpha]_D$[b]	pK_a	Isolation and Purification	Chromatography	Chemistry	Spectral Data
184	Viomycidine (guanidine-1-pyrroline-5-carboxylic acid)	Viomycin	$C_6H_{10}N_4O_2$ (170.19)	181–182° (dec) (246a)	$-151^{32.2}$ (c 1.25, H_2O) $-38^{22.2}$ (c 0.8, HCl) (246a)	1.3 5.5 12.6 (246)	76, 246a	246, 246a	246, 246a	246a
185	Willardine [3-(1-uracyl)alanine]	Mimosa	$C_7H_9N_3O_4$ (199.18)	–	-12.1^{22} (c 1.2, 1 N HCl) (248)	–	247	247	247, 248	248
				J. L-N-SUBSTITUTED AMINO ACIDS						
186	Abrine (N-methyltryptophan)	Abrus precatorius	$C_{12}H_{14}N_2O_3$ (218.41)	297° (dec) (249)	–	–	250	–	249	–
186a	N-Acetylalanine	Human brain	$C_5H_9NO_3$ (131.15)	–	–	–	250a	250a	250a	–
186a'	N-Acetylglutamic acid	Mammalian liver	$C_7H_{11}NO_5$ (189.19)	–	–	–	250a'	250a'	–	–
186b	N-Acetylaspartic acid	Extract of cat brain	$C_6H_9NO_5$ (175.16)	123–125° (250b)	-11.8^{27} (2% methyl cellosolve) (250b)	–	250b	250b	–	250b
187	2,3-Dihydro-3,3-dimethyl-1H-pyrrolo[1,2-a]-indole-9-alanine	Etamycin	$C_{16}H_{20}N_2O_2$ (272.34)	170–175° (dec) (251)	–	–	251	251	251	251
188	β,N-Dimethylleucine	Etamycin	$C_8H_{17}NO_2$ (159.23)	315–316° (dec) (252)	+33.15 (c 2, H_2O) $+39.2^{29}$ (c 2.2, 5 N HCl)(252)	–	252	252	252	–
188a	N,N-Dimethylphenylalanine	Canthium eurysides	$C_{11}H_{15}NO_2$ (193.27)	–	–	–	–	–	–	252a
189	γ-Formyl-N-methylnorvaline	Ilamycin	$C_7H_{13}NO_3$ (159.19)	–	–	1.8 10.2 (253)	253	–	253	253
190	Fusarinine [δ-N-(cis-5-hydroxy-3-methylpent-2-enoyl)-δ-N-hydroxyornithine]	Fusarium	$C_{11}H_{20}N_2O_4$ (244.30)	–	–	–	254	254	254	254
191	Homarine (N-methylpicolinic acid)	Arenicola marina	$C_7H_7NO_2$ (137.15)	–	–	–	255	255	–	–
192	4-Hydroxy-N-methylproline	Afrormosia elata heartwood	$C_6H_{11}NO_3$ (145.16)	238–240° (dec) (256)	−86.6 (c 1.5, H_2O) (256)	–	256	–	256	256
193	Merodesmosine	Elastin	$C_{18}H_{34}N_4O_6$ (420)	–	–	–	257	257	257	257
194	N-Methylalanine	Dichapetalum cymosum (Gifblaar)	$C_4H_9NO_2$ (103.12)	–	–	–	258	258	258	258
195	1-Methylhistidine	Cat urine	$C_7H_{11}N_3O_2$ (169.18)	245–247° (259)	-25.8^{18} (c 3.9, H_2O) (290)	1.69 6.48 (imidazole) 8.85 (290)	259	259	–	–
196	3-Methylhistidine	Human urine	$C_7H_{11}N_3O_2$ (169.18)	–	-26.5^{26} (c 2.1, H_2O) (290) $+13.5^{27}$ (c 1.9, 1 N HCl)(260)	–	260	260	260	260
197	N-Methylisoleucine	Enniatin A	$C_7H_{15}NO_2$ (145.21)	–	$+28.6^{22}$ (c 1.034, H_2O) $+44.8^{22}$ (c 1.162, 5 N HCl) (261)	–	261	261	261	–
198	N-Methylleucine	Enniatin A	$C_7H_{15}NO_2$ (145.21)	–	$+21.4^{15}$ (c 0.77, H_2O) $+31.3^{15}$ (c 0.86, 5 N HCl)(262)	–	262	262	262	–
199	N-Methyl-β-methylleucine	Etamycin	$C_8H_{17}NO_2$ (159.23)	–	$+26^{30}$ (c 1.8, H_2O) $+33.2^{30}$ (c 1.9, 5 N HCl)(252)	–	252	252	252	–
200	N-Methyl-O-methylserine	Mycobacterium butyricum	$C_5H_{11}NO_3$ (133.14)	203–205° (dec) (264)	–	–	264	264	264	264
201	N-Methylphenylglycine (α-phenylsarcosine)	Etamycin	$C_9H_{12}NO_2$ (166.21)	–	$+118^{31}$ (c 4.8, 1 N, HCl) (252)	–	252	252	252	–

DATA ON THE NATURALLY OCCURRING AMINO ACIDS (Continued)

No.	Amino Acid (Synonym)	Source	Formula (Mol Wt)	Melting Point °C[a]	$[\alpha]_D^b$	pK_a	References Isolation and Purification	References Chromatography	References Chemistry	References Spectral Data
201a	N-Methylthreonine	Stendomycin hydrolyzate	$C_5H_{11}NO_3$ (133.17)	–	-17^{25} (c 2, 5 N HCl) (264a)	–	–	–	–	264a
202	N-Methyltyrosine (Surinamine)	Andira	$C_{10}H_{13}NO_3$ (195.22)	280–300° (267)	–18.6 (267)	–	266	–	267	–
203	N-Methylvaline	Actinomycin	$C_6H_{13}NO_2$ (131.18)	–	+17.5 (H_2O) +30.9 (5N HCl) (269)	–	268	268	269	–
204	Saccharopine (N^6-(2-glutaryl)lysine)	Saccharomyces	$C_{11}H_{20}N_2O_6$ (276.30)	–	$+33.6^{23}$ (c 1, 0.5 N HCl) (271)	2.6 4.1 9.2 10.3 (270)	270	270	271	271
205	Sarcosine (N-methylglycine)	Cladonia silvatica	$C_3H_7NO_2$ (89.10)	210° (dec) (290)	–	2.21 10.20 (270)	272	272	–	–

K. L-SULFUR AND SELENIUM CONTAINING AMINO ACIDS

No.	Amino Acid (Synonym)	Source	Formula (Mol Wt)	Melting Point °C[a]	$[\alpha]_D^b$	pK_a	Isolation and Purification	Chromatography	Chemistry	Spectral Data
206	N-Acetyldjenkolic acid	Acacia farnesiana	$C_9H_{16}N_2O_5S$ (264.32)	170° (273)	-49.0^{25} (c 2, 1% HCl) -60.2^{25} (c 1, 1 N HCl)(273)	–	273	273	273	273
207	Alliin	Allium sativum	$C_6H_{11}NO_3S$ (177.24)	163–165° (274)	$+62.8^{21}$ (H_2O) (274)	–	274	–	356	–
208	S-Allylcysteine	Allium sativum	$C_6H_{11}NO_2S$ (161.24)	218° (275)	-8.7^{20} (275)	–	275	275	275	–
209	S-Allylmercaptocysteine	Allium sativum	$C_6H_{11}NO_2S_2$ (193.31)	188° (276)	$-95.3\pm10^{23.5}$ (c 0.19, 6 N HCl) (276)	–	276	276	276	276
210	α-Amino-β-(2-amino-2-carboxyethylmercaptobutyric acid)	Subtilin	$C_7H_{14}N_2O_4S$ (222.28)	–	-34.7^{24} (c 5.4, 1 N HCl) (277)	–	277	277	277	277
211	Cystathionine S-(2-amino-2-carboxyethylhomocysteine)	Human brain	$C_7H_{14}N_2O_4S$ (222.28)	301° (279)312° (290)	$+(26.4^{25}$ (c 0.8, 1 N HCl) (279)	–	279	279	279	279
212	3-Amino-(3-carboxypropyldimethylsulfonium)	Cabbage	$C_6H_{14}NO_2S$ (164.26)	–	–	–	280	280	280	–
212a	α-Amino-γ-[2-(4-carboxy)thiazolylbutyric acid	Xeromus subtomentosus (mushroom)	$C_8H_{10}N_2O_4S$ (230.26)	237–238° (280a)	–	3.7 (280a)	280a	280a	280a	280a
213	Carbamyltaurine	Cat urine	$C_3H_8N_2O_3S$ (152.17)	–	–	–	281	–	–	–
214	2-[S-(β-Carboxy-β-aminoethyltryptophan)]	Amanita phalloides	$C_{14}H_{17}N_3O_4S$ (323.40)	–	–	–	–	119	–	–
215	S-(β-Carboxyethyl)cysteine	Albizia julibrissin	$C_6H_{11}NO_4S$ (193.17)	218° (282)	-9.33^{20} (c 3, 1 N HCl) (283)	–	283	283	282	283
216	N-(1-Carboxyethyl)taurine	Red algae	$C_5H_{11}NO_5S$ (197.22)	258° (283)	-1.15^{13} (c 5, 1 N NaOH) (284)	–	284	284	284	284a
216a	S-(Carboxymethyl)homocysteine	Human urine	$C_6H_{11}NO_4S$ (193.24)	223–225° (dec) (284a)	–	–	284a	–	–	284a
217	S-(2-Carboxyisopropyl)cysteine	Acacia	$C_7H_{13}NO_4S$ (207.26)	202° (284)	$+6.6^{22}$ (c 2, H_2O) $+31^{25}$ (c 1.94, 1 N NaOH) (285)	–	285	285	285	285
218	S-(2-Carboxypropyl)cysteine	Onions	$C_7H_{13}NO_4S$ (207.26)	191–194° (285)(286)	-50.1^{21} (H_2O) (286)	–	286, 287	286, 287	286, 287	286, 287
219	Chondrine (1,4-thiazane-5-carboxylic acid 1-oxide)	Chondria crassicaulis	$C_5H_9NO_3S$ (163.20)	255–257° (287)	$+20.9^{16}$ (c 2, H_2O) (288) $+30.2^{16}$ (c 2, 6 n HCl) (288)	–	288	288	288	–
220	Cycloallin (3-methyl-1,4-thiazane-5-carboxylic acid oxide)	Onions	$C_6H_{11}NO_3S$ (177.24)	–	-17.4^{20} (H_2O) (289)	–	289	289	289	–
221	Cysteic acid (β-sulfo-α-aminopropionic acid)	Sheep's fleece	$C_3H_7NO_5S$ (169.17)	289° (dec) (290)	+8.66 (c 7.4, H_2O) (290)	1.3 (SO_3H) 1.9 8.7 (290)	291	292	–	–

DATA ON THE NATURALLY OCCURRING AMINO ACIDS (Continued)

No.	Amino Acid (Synonym)	Source	Formula (Mol Wt)	Melting Point °C[a]	$[\alpha]_D$[b]	pK_a	Isolation and Purification	Chromatography	Chemistry	Spectral Data
								References		
222	Cysteine (α-amino-β-mercaptoprcpionic acid)	Cystine	$C_3H_7NO_2S$ (121.15)	178° (1)	-16.5^{25} (c 2, H_2O) $+6.5^{25}$ (c 2, 5 M)	1.92 8.35 10.46 (SH)	293	3	294	294
223	Cysteinesulfinic acid (β-sulfinyl-α-aminopropionic acid)	Rat brain	$C_3H_7NO_4S$ (153.17)	—	+11 (H_2O) +24 (c 1, 1 N HCl)	ca 2.1 (290)	295	295	—	—
224	Cystine [β,β'-dithiodi(α-aminopropionic acid)]	Urinary calculi	$C_6H_{12}N_2O_4S_2$ (240.29)	261° (1)	-232^{25} (c 1, 5 N HCl) (1)	<1 2.1 8.02 8.71 (290)	296	3	294	294
225	Cystine disulfoxide	Rat tissue	$C_6H_{12}N_2O_6S_2$ (272.33)	—	—	—	—	298	298	298
226	S-(1,2-Dicarboxyethyl)cysteine	Bovine lens	$C_7H_{11}NO_6S$ (237.25)	—	—	—	299	299	299	—
227	Dichrostachinic acid [S-(β-hydroxy-β-carboxyethanesulfonyl methyl)cysteine]	Mimosa	$C_7H_{13}NO_7S$ (255.27)	201° (300)	$+9.2^{24}$ (c 2.2, 1 N HCl) (300)	—	300	300	300	300
228	Dihydroalliin (S-propylcysteine sulfoxide)	Allium cepa	$C_6H_{13}NO_3S$ (179.26)	—	—	—	301	301	301	—
229	Djenkolic acid	Djenkol beans	$C_7H_{14}N_2O_4S_2$ (254.32)	300–350° (303)	$-65^{20.5}$ (c 1, 1 N HCl) (303)	—	302	—	303	—
230	Ethionine	Escherichia coli	$C_6H_{13}NO_2S$ (163.23)	—	—	—	304	304	—	—
231	Felinine	Cat urine	$C_8H_{17}NO_3S$ (207.30)	177° (305)	$+23^{20}$ (c 2.2, H_2O) (305)	—	305	305	305	—
232	N-Formyl methionine	Escherichia coli	$C_6H_{11}NO_3S$ (177.22)	—	—	—	306	306	—	—
233	Glucobrassicin [S-β-1-(glucopyranosyl)-3-indolylacetothiohydroximye-O-sulfate]	Brassica species	$C_{16}H_{20}N_2O_9S_2$ (447.47)	—	-13.3^{23} (c 3, H_2O) (189)	—	189	189	189	189
234	Guanidotaurine	Arenicola marina	$C_3H_9N_3O_3S$ (167.20)	228–230° (308)	—	—	308	308	308	—
235	Homocysteine	Neurospora	$C_4H_9NO_2S$ (135.18)	—	—	2.22 8.87 10.86 (290)	278	310	—	—
236	Homocystine	Human urine	$C_8H_{16}N_2O_4S_2$ (268.36)	282–3° (dec) (290)	-16^{21} (c 0.06, H_2O) $+78^{25}$ (c 1–2, 5N HCl) (290)	1.59 2.54 8.52 9.44 (290)	311	311	—	—
237	Homocysteinecysteine disulfide	Human urine	$C_7H_{14}N_2O_4S_2$ (254.35)	—	-52.2^{25} (1 N HCl) (312)	—	312	—	312	312
238	Homolanthionine	Escherichia coli	$C_8H_{16}N_2O_4S$ (236.29)	—	$+37.3^{24}$ (C 1, 1 N HCl) (363)	—	313	313	313	—
239	Homomethionine (5-methylthionorvaline)	Cabbage	$C_6H_{13}NO_2S$ (163.25)	223–225° (314)	$+(21^{25.5}$ (c 0.3, 6 N HCl)(314)	—	314	314	314	314
239a	β-6-(4-Hydroxybenzothiazolyl)alanine	Chicken feather pigment	$C_{10}H_9N_2O_3S$ (237.27)	—	—	—	314a	314a	—	314a
239a'	S-(2-Hydroxy-2-carboxyethyl)homocysteine	Human urine	$C_7H_{13}NO_5S$ (223.27)	—	—	—	284a	—	—	—
239a''	S-(2-Hydroxy-2-carboxyethylthio)-homocysteine	Human urine	$C_7H_{13}NO_5S_2$ (223.27)	—	—	—	377	377	377	—
239b	S-(3-Hydroxy-3-carboxy-n-propylthio)cysteine	Human urine	$C_7H_{13}NO_5S_2$ (255.33)	176–177° (dec) (377)	-96.3^{26} (c 2.3, 1 N HCl) (377)	—	377	377	377	377
239c	S-(3-Hydroxy-3-carboxy-n-propyl)cysteine	Human urine	$C_7H_{13}NO_5S$ (223.27)	—	—	—	284a	—	—	—
239c'	S-(3-Hydroxy-3-carboxy-n-propylthio)homocysteine	Human urine	$C_8H_{15}NO_5S_2$ (269.36)	187–188° (dec) (377)	$+8.1^{25}$ (c 15.2, 1 N HCl) (377)	—	377	377	377	377

DATA ON THE NATURALLY OCCURRING AMINO ACIDS (Continued)

No.	Amino Acid (Synonym)	Source	Formula (Mol Wt)	Melting Point °C[a]	$[\alpha]_D$[b]	pK_a	Isolation and Purification	Chromatography	Chemistry	Spectral Data
								References		
239d	α-Hydroxycysteinecysteine disulfide	Human urine	$C_6H_{12}N_2O_5S_2$ (256.32)	181° (dec) (378)	-263^{23} (c 2.2, H_2O) (378)	–	–	378	378	–
240	Hypotaurine (2-aminoethanesulfinic acid)	Rat brain	$C_2H_7NO_2S$ (109.14)	–	–	–	295	295	–	–
241	Isovalthine (isopropylcarboxymethylcysteine)	Human urine	$C_8H_{15}NO_4S$ (221.28)	–	–	–	316	317	317	317
242	Lanthionine [β,β'-thiodi(α-aminopropionic acid)]	Wool	$C_6H_{12}N_2O_4S$ (208.23)	270–304° (318)	–	–	318	–	319	–
242a	β-Mercaptolactatecysteine disulfide	Human urine	$C_6H_{11}NO_5S_2$ (241.30)	–	–	–	–	319a	319a	–
243	S-Methylcysteine	Phaseolus vulgaris	$C_4H_9NO_2S$ (135.19)	220° (320)	-26^{25} (c 2.5) (320)	8.75 (20)	320	320	320	320
243a	S-Methylcysteine sulfoxide	Cabbage	$C_4H_9NO_3S$ (151.20)	173° (320a)	–	–	–	–	–	–
244	Methionine (α-amino-γ-methylthiobutyric acid)	Casein hydrolyzate	$C_5H_{11}NO_2S$ (149.21)	283° (1)	-10^{25} (H_2O) $+23.2^{25}$ (5 N HCl)(1)	2.28 9.21 (1)	321	3	322	322
245	3,3'-(2-Methylethylene-1, 2-dithio)dialanine	Allium shoenoprasum	$C_9H_{17}N_2O_4S_2$ (282.40)	–	–	–	323	323	323	323
246	β-Methyllanthionine	Yeast	$C_7H_{14}N_2O_4S$ (222.28)	–	–	–	277	–	277	–
247	S-Methylmethionine (α-aminodimethyl-γ-butyrothetin)	Asparagus	$C_6H_{13}NO_2S$ (164.24)	–	–	–	325	325	280	325
248	β-Methylselenoalanine (β-methylselenocysteine)	Stanleya pinnata	$C_4H_9NO_2Se$ (182.08)	–	–	–	327	327	–	–
249	Neoglucobrassicin	Brassica napus	$C_{17}H_{21}N_2O_{10}S_2$ (476.48)	175° (328)	–	–	328	328	328	328
250	S-(Prop-1-enyl)cysteine	Allium sativum	$C_6H_{11}NO_2S_2$ (161.24)	–	–	–	329	329	–	–
251	S-(Prop-1-enyl)cysteine sulfoxide	Onions	$C_6H_{11}NO_3S$ (177.22)	146–148° (330)	–	–	330	330	330	330
252	S-r-Propylcysteine	Allium sativum	$C_6H_{13}NO_2S$ (163.26)	–	–	–	331	331	–	–
253	S-r-Propylcysteine sulfoxide	Onions	$C_6H_{13}NO_3S$ (179.26)	–	–	–	301	301	–	–
254	Selenocystathionine	Stanleya pinnata	$C_7H_{14}N_2O_4Se$ (269.07)	–	–	–	327	327	327	–
255	Selenocystine	Astragalus pectinatus	$C_6H_{12}N_2O_4Se_2$ (334.11)	263–265° (334)	–	–	334	–	334	–
255a	Selenomethionine	Escherichia coli (hydrolyzate)	$C_5H_{11}NO_2Se$ (196.13)	–	–	–	334a	334a	–	–
256	Selenomethylselenocysteine	Astragalus bisulcatus	$C_3H_6NO_2Se$ (167.03)	–	–	–	335	335	335	–
257	Taurine (2-aminoethanesulfonic acid)	Plant and animal tissue	$C_2H_7NO_3S$ (125.15)	320° (dec) (290)	–	–0.3 9.06 (290)	–	292	–	–
258	β-(2-Thiazole)-β-alanine	Bottromycin	$C_6H_8N_2O_2S$ (172.22)	197.5–201.5° (337)	–	–	337	337	337	337
259	Thiolhistidine	Erythrocytes and microorganisms	$C_6H_9N_2O_2S$ (173.23)	–	-10^{25} (c 2, 1 N HCl) (339)	1.84 8.47 11.4 (290)	338	–	339	–
260	Thiostreptine	Thiostrepton	$C_9H_{14}N_2O_4S$ (246.32)	–	-4^{25} (c 1, 1 N acetic acid)(102)	–	102	102	102	102
261	Tyrosine-O-sulfate	Human urine	$C_9H_{11}NO_6S$ (261.26)	–	–	–	341	342	–	–
		I. L-HALOGEN-CONTAINING AMINO ACIDS								
262	2-Amino-4,4-dichlorobutyric acid	Streptomyces armentosus	$C_4H_7Cl_2NO_2$ (172.02)	–	$+6.7^{25}$ (c 0.74, H_2O) $+26.2^{25}$ (c 0.74, 1 N HCl)(64)	–	64	64	64	64

DATA ON THE NATURALLY OCCURRING AMINO ACIDS (Continued)

No.	Amino Acid (Synonym)	Source	Formula (Mol Wt)	Melting Point °C[a]	[α]_D[b]	pK_a	Isolation and Purification	Chromatography	Chemistry	Spectral Data
								References		
262a	5-Chloropiperidazine-3-carboxylic acid	Monamycin hydrolyzate	$C_5H_9ClN_2O_2$ (164.61)	83–85° (DNP deriv) (204a)	$+157^{33}$ (c 0.18, CHCl$_3$) (204b)	—	204b	204b	—	204a, 204b
263	3,5-Dibromotyrosine	Gorgona species	$C_9H_9NO_3Br_2$ (339.01)	245° (344)	—	2.17 6.45 (OH) 7.60	344	—	344	—
263a	2,4-Diiodohistidine	Human urine	$C_6H_7I_2N_3O_2$ (406.96)	—	—	—	344a	344a	—	—
264	3,3'-Diiodothyronine	Bovine thyroid gland	$C_{15}H_{13}I_2NO_4$ (525.11)	233–234° (dec) (345)	—	—	345	345	345	—
265	3,5-Diiodotyrosine (iodogorgoic acid)	Coral protein	$C_9H_9I_2NO_3$ (433.01)	194° (dec) (290)	+2.9 (1.1 N HCl)(1)	2.12 6.48 (OH) 7.82 (290)	346	347	348	—
266	3-Monobromotyrosine	Sea fans and sponges	$C_9H_{10}NO_3Br$ (260.10)		—	—	349	349	—	—
266a	3-Monobromo-5-monochlorotyrosine	Buccinum undatum	$C_9H_9ClNO_3Br$ (294.55)		—	—	349a	349a	—	349a
266b	5-Monochlorotyrosine	Buccinum undatum	$C_9H_{10}ClNO_3$ (215.65)		—	—	349b	349b	—	349b
267	2-Monoiodohistidine	Rat thyroid gland	$C_6H_8IN_3O_2$ (281.02)		—	—	350	350	—	—
268	Monoiodotyrosine	Nereocystis luetkeana (an alga)	$C_9H_{10}NO_3$ (307.11)		—	—	351	351	—	—
269	Thyroxine	Thyroid gland	$C_{15}H_{11}I_4NO_4$ (776.88)	236° (dec) (290) 95% EtOH) (290)	+15 (c 5, 1 N HCl, (OH) 10.1 (290)	2.2 6.45	352	353	348	348
270	3,5,3'-Triiodothyronine	Phaseolus vulgaris	$C_{15}H_{12}I_3NO_4$ (650.98)	233–234° (dec) (290)	$+23.6^{24}$ (c 5, 1 N HCl-EtOH) (290)	2.2 8.40 (OH) 10.1 (290)	355	347	—	—
	M. L-PHOSPHORUS-CONTAINING AMINO ACIDS									
271	α-Amino-β-phosphonopropionic acid	Tetrahymena pyriformis, Zoanthus sociatus	$C_2H_8NO_5P$ (157.07)	228° (dec) (357)	—	2.2 4.5 8.8 11.0 (357)	358	358	357	—
272	Ciliatine (2-aminoethylphosphonic acid)	Sea anemone	$C_2H_8NO_3P$ (125.07)	280–281° (dec) (359)	—	6.4 (359)	359	359	359	359
273	2-Dimethylaminoethylphosphonic acid	Sea anemone	$C_4H_{12}NO_3P$ (153.13)	249.5° (360)	—	—	360	360	360	360
273a	1-Hydroxy-2-aminoethylphosphonic acid	Acanthamoeba castellanii (plasma membrane)	$C_2H_8NO_4P$ (141.08)	—	—	—	360a	360a	—	360a
274	Lombricine (2-amino-2-carboxyethyl-2-guanidineethyl hydrogen phosphate)	Earthworm	$C_6H_{15}N_4O_6P$ (270.21)	223–224° (361)	$+14.5^{23.5}$ (c 0.93, H$_2$O) (362)	8.9 (20)	361	361	362	362
275	2-Methylaminoethylphosphonic acid	Sea anemone	$C_3H_{10}NO_3P$ (139.10)	291° (360)	—	—	360	360	360	360
276	O-Phosphohomoserine	Lactobacillus	$C_4H_{10}NO_6P$ (199.11)	178° (dec) (364)	$+6.25^{22.5}$(c 2.4, H$_2$O) (364)	—	364	364	364	—
277	O-Phosphoserine	Casein	$C_3H_8NO_6·P$ (185.08)	—	+7.2 (H$_2$O) (366)	—	365	366	366	—
278	2-Trimethylaminoethylbetaine phosphonic acid	Sea anemone	$C_5H_{14}NO_3P$ (167.16)	250–252° (360)	—	—	360	360	360	360

DATA ON THE NATURALLY OCCURRING AMINO ACIDS (Continued)

No.	Amino Acid (Synonym)	Source	Formula (Mol Wt)	Melting Point °C[a]	$[\alpha]_D$[b]	pK_a	Isolation and Purification	Chromatography	Chemistry	Spectral Data
				N. L-BETAINES						
279	N-(3-Amino-3-carboxypropyl)-β-carboxypyridinium betaine	Tobacco leaves	$C_{10}H_{14}N_2O_5$ (242.24)	241–243° (dec) (368)	$+24^{24}$ (c 2, H_2O)(368)	–	368	368	368	368
280	Betonicine (4-hydroxyproline betaine)	Stachys (Betonica) officinalis	$C_7H_{13}NO_3$ (159.19)	243–244° (dec) (369)	-36.6^{15}(369)	–	369	–	369	–
281	γ-Butyrobetaine (γ-aminobutyric acid betaine)	Rat brain	$C_7H_{15}NO_2$ (144.20)	180–184° (370)	–	–	370	370	–	–
282	Carnitine (γ-amino-β-hydroxybutyric acid betaine)	Vertebrate muscle	$C_7H_{15}NO_3$ (161.21)	195–197° (371)	$+23.5^{22}$ (c 5, H_2O) (374)	–	372	373	367, 371	–
283	Desmosine	Bovine elastin	$C_{24}H_{39}N_5 O_8$(879.43)	–	–	1.70 2.40 8.80 9.85 (375)	375	–	257, 375	375
284	Ergothionine (betaine of thiol histidine)	Ergot	$C_9H_{15}N_3 O_2$(229.29)	290° (340)	$+115^{27.5}$ (c 1, H_2O) (290)	–	336	340	340	340
285	Hercynin (histidine betaine)	Mushrooms	$C_9H_{15}N_3 O_2$ (203.22)	–	–	–	332	–	333	–
286	Homobetaine (β-alanine betaine)		$C_6H_{13}NO_2$ (131.18)	–	–	–	324	–		–
287	Homostachydrine (pipecolic acid betaine)	Alfalfa	$C_8H_{14}NO_2$ (156.21)	–	–	–	315	309		–
288	3-Hydroxystachydrine (3-hydroxyproline betaine)	Courbonia virgata	$C_7H_{13}NO_3$ (159.20)	210–212° (307)	$+10^{30}$ (c 2.9, H_2O) (307)	–	307	–	307	–
289	Hypaphorin (tryptophan betaine)	Erythrina subumbrans	$C_{14}H_{18}N_2 O_2$ (246.29)	–	–	–	58	–	282	–
290	Isodesmosine	Bovine elastin	$C_{24}H_{39}N_5 O_8$ (879.43)	–	–	–	375	–	257	–
291	Luminine (α-amino-ε-trimethylamino adipic acid)	Laminaria angustata	$C_9H_{20}N_2 O_4$ (220.29)	–	–	–	245	–	245	245
292	Lycin (glycine betaine)	Lycium barbarum	$C_5H_{11}NO_2$ (118.16)	–	–	–	234	–		–
293	Miokinine (ornithine betaine)	Human skeletal muscle	$C_{11}H_{25}N_2 O_2$ (217.33)	–	–	–	232	–		–
294	Nicotianine (N-3-amino-3-carboxypropyl-β-carboxypyridinium betaine)	Tobacco leaves	$C_{10}H_{14}N_4 O_5$	241–243° (dec) (156)	$+28.4^{24}$ (c 5, H_2O) (156)	–	156	156	156	156
295	Stachydrine (proline betaine)	Stachys tuberifera	$C_7H_{13}NO_2$ (157.22)	–	-20.7^{26g} (H_2O) (125)	–	128	–	128	–
296	Trigonelline (coffearin)	Foenum graceum	$C_7H_7NO_2$ (137.15)	–	–	–	120	107		–
296a	ε-N-Trimethyl-δ-hydroxylysine betaine	Diatom cell walls	$C_9H_{20}N_2 O_3$ (204.31)	243° (dec) (381)	$+15.0^{24}$ (c 0.84, H_2O) $+23.1^{24}$ (c 0.84, 2 N HCl) (381)	–	381	381		–
297	ε-N-Trimethyllysine betaine	Histone of murine ascites cells	$C_9H_{20}N_2 O_2$ (188.28)	225–226° (dec) (70a)	$+10.8^{18}$ (c 5, H_2O) (379)	–	44, 379	44, 380	380	379
				O. D-AMINO ACIDS						
297a	D-Alloenduracididine[α-amino-β-(2-iminoimidazolidinyl)propionic acid]	Enduracidin hydrolyzate	$C_6H_{12}N_4 O_2$ (172.22)	–	$+8.7^{23}$ (1 M HCl) $+13.3^{23}$ (1 M NaOH) (194)	2.5 8.3 12 (194a)	–	194a	194a	194a
297b	D-Alloisoleucine	Stendomycin hydrolyzate	$C_6H_{13}NO_2$ (131.20)	–	–	–	–	264a		–
298	D-Allothreonine	Actinomycetales species	$C_4H_9NO_3$ (119.12)	–	–	2.11 9.10 (290)	52	52		–

DATA ON THE NATURALLY OCCURRING AMINO ACIDS (Continued)

No.	Amino Acid (Synonym)	Source	Formula (Mol Wt)	Melting Point °C[a]	$[\alpha]_D$[b]	pK$_a$	References Isolation and Purification	References Chromatography	References Chemistry	References Spectral Data
299	1-Amino-D-proline	Flax seed	C$_5$H$_{10}$N$_2$O$_2$ (130.15)	155° (dec) (80)	+113^{25} (c 2, 0.5 N HCl)(80)	–	80	80	80	80
299a	O-Carbamyl D-serine	Streptomyces strain	C$_4$H$_8$N$_2$O$_4$ (148.14)	238° (dec) (384)	–19.6 (c 2, 1 N HCl) +2 (c 2, H$_2$O) (384)	–	384	384	384	–
300	D-(3-Carboxy-4-hydroxyphenyl) glycine	Reseda luteola	C$_9$H$_9$NO$_5$ (211.18)	<250° (dec) (93)	–121^{22} (c 0.75, 1 N HCl) (93)	–	93	93	93	93
301	D-Cycloserine (oxamycin, D-4-amino-3-isoxazolinone)	Streptomyces orchidaceus	C$_3$H$_5$N$_2$O$_2$ (101.09)	156° (dec) (94)	–89^{25} (c 0.6, H$_2$O)(94)	(94)	94	–	94	94
302	m-Carboxyphenylglycine	Iris bulbs	C$_9$H$_9$NO$_4$ (195.18)	215° (143)	+112^{25} (c 5, 2 N HCl)(326)	4.4 7.3 (326)	143	143	143	143
302a	N-α-Malonyl-D-alanine	Pea seedlings	C$_6$H$_9$NO$_5$ (175.16)	138–140° (dec) (382)	+33^{28} (c 0.38, H$_2$O) (382)	–	382	382	382	382
303	N-α-Malonyl-D-methionine	Tobacco	C$_8$H$_{13}$NO$_5$S (235.30)	–	–	–	95	95	95	–
304	N-α-Malonyl-D-tryptophan	Spinach	C$_{14}$H$_{13}$N$_2$O$_5$ (289.27)	–	–	–	104	–	104	–
304a	N-Methyl-D-leucine	Griselimycin hydrolyzate	C$_7$H$_{15}$NO$_2$ (145.23)	–	–19.6^{20} (c 0.9, H$_2$O) (376)	–	–	–	–	376
305	D-α-Methylserine	Streptomyces	C$_4$H$_9$NO$_3$ (119.12)	–	–	2.3 9.4 (113)	113	–	113	113
306	D-Octopine [N-α-(1-Carboxyethylarginine]	Octopus muscle	C$_9$H$_{18}$N$_4$O$_4$ (246.28)	–	+20.6^{24} (c 1, H$_2$O) 20^{25} (c 2, 5 N HCl) (290)	1.36 2.40 8.76 11.3 (290)	133	–	205	–
307	D-Penicillamine	Penicillin	C$_5$H$_{11}$NO$_2$S (149.22)	–	(225)	1.8 7.9 10.5	225	–	225	–
308	Turcine (d-allohydroxyproline betaine)	Stachys (Betonica) officinalis	C$_7$H$_{13}$NO$_3$ (159.19)	249° (241)	+36.26^{15} (241)	–	241	–	241	–

a Melting point or decomposition point in degrees, C.
b c, grams/100 mL of solution at 20 to 25°C unless specified; wavelength as subscript in millimicrons; temperature as superscript. References are 1, 3, and 290 unless indicated.
c The isolated amino acid appears to be a racemic DL mixture.
d The naturally occurring isomer is the erythro-l-form 290.
e Thermodynamic values.
f As hydrochloride of amino acid.
g For cycloalliin sulfoxide.

References

1. Meister, *Biochemistry of the Amino Acids*, 2nd ed., Academic Press, New York, 1965, 28.
2. Schutzenberger and Bourgeois, *C.R. Hebd. Seances Acad. Sci. (Paris)*, 81, 1191 (1875).
3. Greenstein and Winitz, *Chemistry of the Amino Acids*, Vol.2, John Wiley & Sons, New York, 1961, 1382.
4. Greenstein and Winitz, *Chemistry of the Amino Acids*, Vol.2, John Wiley & Sons, New York, 1961, 1819.
5. Morris and Thompson, *Nature*, 190, 718 (1961).
6. Abderhalden and Bahn, *Hoppe Seyler's Z. Physiol. Chem.*, 245, 246 (1937).
7. Virtanen and Miettinen, *Biochim. Biophys. Acta*, 12, 181 (1953).
8. Ackerman, *Hoppe Seyler's Z. Physiol. Chem.*, 69, 273 (1910).
9. Work, *Bull. Soc. Chim. Biol*, 31, 138 (1949).
10. Steward, *Science*, 110, 439 (1949).
11. Gabriel, *Chem. Ber.*, 23, 1767 (1890).
12. Vahatalo and Virtanen, *Acta Chem. Sc.*, 11, 741 (1957).
13. Doyle and Levenberg, *Biochemistry*, 7, 2457 (1968).
14. Steiner and Hartmann, *Biochem. Z*, 340, 436 (1964).
14a. Chilton, Tsou, Kirk, and Benedict, *Tetrahedron Lett.*, 6283 (1968).
15. Takita, *J. Antibiot. (Tokyo)*, 17, 264 (1964).
15a. Sung, Fowden, Millington, and Sheppard, *Phytochemistry*, 8, 1227 (1969).
15b. Millington and Sheppard, *Phytochemistry*, 7, 1027 (1968).
16. Kenner and Sheppard, *Nature*, 181, 48 (1958).
17. Asen, *J. Biol. Chem.*, 234, 343 (1959).
17a. Scannell, Pruess, Demny, Sello, Williams, and Stempel, *J. Antibiot. (Tokyo)*, 25, 122 (1972).
17b. Sahm, Knobloch, and Wagner, *J. Antibiot. (Tokyo)*, 26, 389 (1973).
18. Fowden and Done, *Biochem. J.*, 55, 548 (1953).
19. Fowden and Smith, *Phytochemistry*, 7, 809 (1968).
19a. Kelly, Martin, and Hanka, *Can. J. Chem.*, 47, 2504 (1969).
20. Perrin, *Dissociation Constants of Organic Bases in Aqueous Solution*. Butterworths, London, 1965.
21. Millington and Sheppard, *Phytochemistry*, 7, 1027 (1968).
22. Dardenne, Casimar, and Jadot, *Phytochemistry*, 7, 1401 (1968).
22a. Dardenne, Casimar, and Jadot, *Phytochemistry*, 7, 1401 (1968).
23. Staron, Allard, and Xuong, *C.R. Hebd. Seances Acad. Sci. (Paris)*, 260, 3502 (1965).
23a. Scannell, Pruess, Demny, Weiss, Williams, and Stempel, *J. Antibiot. (Tokyo)*, 24, 239 (1971).
23a'. Fowden, Smith, Millington, and Sheppard, *Phytochemistry*, 8, 437 (1969).
23b. Fowden and Smith, *Phytochemistry*, 7, 809 (1968).
24. Braconnot, *Ann. Chim. Phys.*, 13, 113 (1820).
25. Shorey, *J. Am. Chem. Soc.*, 19, 881 (1897).
26. Hassall and Keyle, *Biochem. J.*, 60, 334 (1955).
27. Carbon, *J. Am. Chem. Soc.*, 80, 1002 (1958).
28. Ehrlich, *Chem. Ber.*, 37, 1809 (1904).
29. Greenstein and Winitz, *Chemistry of the Amino Acids*, Vol.3, John Wiley & Sons, New York, 1961, 2043.
30. Proust, *Ann. Chim. Phys.*, 10, 29 (1819).
31. Greenstein and Winitz, *Chemistry of the Amino Acids*, Vol.3, John Wiley & Sons, New York, 1961, 2075.
31a. Walker, Bodanszky, and Perlman, *J. Antibiot. (Tokyo)*, 23, 255 (1970).
32. Gray and Fowden, *Biochem. J.*, 82, 385 (1961).
33. Kortrum, Vogel, and Andrussow, *Dissociation Constants of Organic Acids in Aqueous Solutions*, Butterworths, London, 1961.
34. Yukowa, *Handbook of Organic Structural Analysis*. Benjamin, New York, 1965, 584.
35. Fischer, *Hoppe Seyler's Z. Physiol. Chem.*, 33, 151 (1901).
35a. Vervier and Casimir, *Phytochemistry*, 9, 2059 (1970).
35b. Levenberg, *J. Biol. Chem.*, 243, 6009 (1968).
36. Greenstein and Winitz, *Chemistry of the Amino Acids*, Vol.3, John Wiley & Sons, New York, 1961, 2368.
37. Hatanaka and Virtanen, *Acta Chem. Scand.*, 16, 514 (1962).
38. Takemoto and Sai, *J. Pharm. Soc. Jap.*, 85, 33 (1965).
39. Virtanen and Berg, *Acta Chem. Scand.*, 8, 1085 (1954).
40. Vauqelin and Robiquet, *Ann. Chim.*, 57, 88 (1806).
41. Greenstein and Winitz, *Chemistry of the Amino Acids*, Vol.3, John Wiley & Sons, New York, 1961, 1856.
42. Davies and Evans, *J. Chem. Soc.*, p.480 (1953).
43. Ritthausen, *J. Prakt. Chem.*, 103, 233 (1868).
44. Hempel, Lange, and Berkofer, *Naturwissenschaften*, 55, 37 (1968).
45. Gray and Fowden, *Nature*, 189, 401 (1961).
46. Gmelin and Larsen, *Biochim. Biophys. Acta*, 136, 572 (1967).
46a. Nulu and Bell, *Phytochemistry*, 11, 2573 (1972).
47. Fowden, *Biochem. J.*, 98, 57 (1966).
48. Birkinshaw, Raistick, and Smith, *Biochem. J.*, 36, 829 (1942).
49. Ritthausen, *J. Prakt. Chem.*, 99, 454 (1866).
50. Greenstein and Winitz, *Chemistry of the Amino Acids*, Vol.3, John Wiley & Sons, New York, 1961, 1929.
51. Schulze and Bosshard, *Landwirtsch. Vers. Stn.*, 29, 295 (1883).
52. Ikawa, Snell, and Lederer, *Nature*, 188, 558 (1961).
53. Larsen, *Acta Chem. Scand*, 19, 1071 (1965).
54. Fowden and Gray, *Amino Acid Pools*, Holden, Ed., Elsevier, Amsterdam, 1962, 46.
55. Barker, Smyth, Wawszkiewicz, Lee, and Wilson, *Arch. Biochem. Biophys.*, 78, 468 (1958).
56. Virtanen and Berg, *Acta Chem. Scand.*, 9, 553 (1955).
56a. Przybylska and Strong, *Phytochemistry*, 7, 471 (1968).
57. Done and Fowden, *Biochem. J.*, 51, 451 (1952).
58. Greshoff, *Chem. Ber.*, 23, 3537 (1890).
59. Casimir, Jadot, and Renard, *Biochim. Biophys. Acta*, 39, 462 (1960).
59a. Seneviratne and Fowden, *Phytochemistry*, 7, 1030 (1968).
60. Virtanena and Linko, *Acta Chem. Scand.*, 531 (1955).
61. Liss, *Phytochemistry*, 1, 87 (1962).
62. Bohak, *J. Biol. Chem.*, 239, 2878 (1964).
63. Ziegler, Melchert, and Lurken, *Nature*, 214, 404 (1967).
64. Argoudelis, Herr, Mason, Pyke, and Zieserl, *Biochemistry*, 6, 165 (1967).
65. Vega and Bell, *Phytochemistry*, 6, 759 (1967).
65a. Bell, *Nature*, 218, 197 (1968).
66. Damodaran and Narayanan, *Biochem. J.*, 34, 1449 (1940).
67. Kitagawa and Monobe, *J. Biochem. (Tokyo)*, 18, 333 (1933).
67a. Bodanszky and Bodanszky, *J. Antibiot. (Tokyo)*, 23, 149 (1970).
67b. Bodanszky, Chaturvedi, Scozzie, Griffith, and Bodanszky, *Antimicrob. Agents Chemother.*, p.135 (1969).
68. Fujino, Inoue, Ueyanagi, and Miyake, *Bull. Chem. Soc. Jap.*, 34, 740 (1961).
69. Tsai and Stadtman, *Arch. Biochem. Biophys.*, 125, 210 (1968).
69a. Hettinger and Craig, *Biochemistry*, 9, 1224 (1970).
70. Gmelin, Strauss, and Hasenmaiet, *Hoppe Seyler's Z. Physiol. Chem.*, 314, 28 (1959).
70a. Kakimoto and Akazawa, *J. Biol. Chem.*, 245, 5751 (1970).
70b. Scannell, Ax, Pruess, Williams, Demm, and Stempel, *J. Antibiot. (Tokyo)*, 25, 179 (1972).
71. Dupuy and Lee, *J. Am. Pharm. Assoc. (Sci. Ed.)*, 43, 61 (1954).
72. Schilling and Strong, *J. Am. Chem. Soc.*, 77, 2843 (1955).
73. Vickery and Leavenworth, *J. Biol. Chem.*, 76, 437 (1928).
74. Drechsel, *Z. Prakt. Chem.*, 39, 425 (1889).
75. Greenstein and Winitz, *Chemistry of the Amino Acids*, Vol.3, John Wiley & Sons, New York, 1961, 2477.
76. Haskell, Fusari, Frohardt, and Bartz, *J. Am. Chem. Soc.*, 74, 599 (1952).
77. Biemann, Lioret, Asselineau, Lederer, and Polonsky, *Bull. Soc. Chim. Biol.*, 42, 979; *Biochim. Biophys. Acta*, 40, 369 (1960).
78. Lioret, *C.R. Hebd Seances Acad Sci. (Paris)*, 244, 2171 (1957).
79. Murray, *Biochemistry*, 3, 10 (1964).
80. Klosterman, Lamoureux, and Parsons, *Biochemistry*, 6, 170 (1967).
81. Greenstein and Winitz, *Chemistry of the Amino Acids*, Vol 3, John Wiley & Sons, New York, 1961, 2477.
81a. Stapley, Miller, Mata, and Hendlin, *Antimicrob. Agents Chemother.*, p.401 (1967).
82. Rao, Adiga, and Sarma, *Biochemistry*, 3, 432 (1964).
82a. Shiba, Kubota, and Kaneto, *Tetrahedron*, 26, 4307 (1970).
83. Suzuki, Nakamura, Okuma, and Tomiyama, *J. Antibiot. (Tokyo)*, 11A(81), 84 (1958).
84. Cummings and Hudgins, *Am. J. Med. Sci.*, 236, 311 (1958).

85. Sorensen and Andersen, *Hoppe Seyler's Z. Physiol. Chem.*, 56, 250 (1908).
86. Hochstein, *J. Org. Chem.*, 24, 679 (1959).
87. Grobbelaar and Steward, *Nature*, 182, 1358 (1958).
87a. Westley, Pruess, Volpe, Demny, and Stempel, *J. Antibiot. (Tokyo)*, 24, 330 (1971).
88. Larsen, *Acta Chem. Scand.*, 21, 1592 (1967).
88a. Doyle and Levenberg, *Biochemistry*, 7, 2457 (1968).
89. Blass and Macheboeuf, *Helv. Chim. Acta*, 29, 1315 (1946).
90. Snow, *J. Chem. Soc.*, 2588, 4080 (1954).
91. Virtanen and Hietala, *Acta Chem. Scand.*, 9, 549 (1955).
92. Umbreit and Heneage, *J. Biol. Chem.*, 201, 15 (1953).
93. Kjaer and Larsen, *Acta Chem. Scand.*, 17, 2397 (1963).
94. Hidy, Hodge, Yound, Harned, Brewer, Phillips, Runge, Staveley, Pohland, Boaz, and Sullivan, *J. Am. Chem. Soc.*, 77, 2345 (1955).
95. Keglevic, Ladesic, and Pokorney, *Arch. Biochem. Biophys.*, 124, 443 (1968).
96. Virtanen, Uksila, and Matikkala, *Acte Chem. Scand.*, 1091 (1954).
97. Thompson, Morris, and Hunt, *J. Biol. Chem.*, 239, 1122 (1964).
98. Okabe, *J. Antibiot. Ser. A*, 13, 412 (1961).
99. Wieland and Haufer, *Justus Liebigs Ann. Chem.*, 619, 35 (1968).
99a. Fowden, MacGibbon, Mellon, and Sheppard, *Phytochemistry*, 11, 1105 (1972).
99a'. Rudzats, Gellert, and Halpern, *Biochem. Biophys. Res. Commun.*, 47, 290 (1972).
100. Murooka and Harada, *Agric. Biol. Chem.*, 31, 1035 (1967).
100a. Giovanelli, Owens, and Mudd, *Biochim. Biophys. Acta*, 227, 671 (1971).
100b. Owens, Thompson, and Fennessey, *Chem. Commun.*, p. 715 (1972).
101. Virtanen and Ettala, *Acta Chem. Scand.*, 11, 182 (1957).
102. Bodanszky, Alicino, Birkhimer, and Williams, *J. Am. Chem. Soc.*, 84, 2004 (1962).
103. Wieland and Schopf, *Justus Liebigs Ann. Chem.*, 626, 174 (1959).
103a. Mechanic and Tanzer, *Biochem. Biophys. Res. Commun.*, 41, 1597 (1970).
104. Good and Andreae, *Plant Physiol.*, 32, 561 (1957).
104a. Takita and Maeda, *J. Antibiot. (Tokyo)*, 22, 39 (1969).
105. Saarivirta and Virtanen, *Acta Chem. Scand.*, 19, 1008 (1965).
106. Craig, *J. Biol. Chem.*, 125, 289 (1938).
107. Joshi and Handler, *J. Biol. Chem.*, 235, 2981 (1961).
108. Setsuseo, *J. Osaka Univ.*, 833 (1957).
109. Schweet, Holden, and Lowy, *J. Biol Chem.*, 211, 517 (1954).
110. Tominaga, Hiwaki, Maekawa, and Yoshida, *J. Biochem. (Tokyo)*, 53, 227 (1963).
111. Wilding and Stahlmann, *Phytochemistry*, 1, 241 (1962).
111a. Kemp and Dawson, *Biochim. Biophys. Acta*, 176, 678 (1969).
112. Fowden, *Biochem. J.*, 81, 155 (1961).
113. Flynn, Hinman, Caron, and Woolf, *J. Am. Chem. Soc.*, 75, 5867 (1953).
114. Nagao, *Bull. Fac. Fish Hokkaido Univ.*, 2, 128 (1951).
115. Hatanaka, *Acta Chem. Scand.*, 16, 513 (1962).
116. Brandner and Virtanen, *Acta Chem. Scand.*, 17, 2563 (1963).
117. Snow, *J. Chem. Soc.*, 2589 (1954).
117a. Fowden, Pratt, and Smith, *Phytochemistry*, 12, 1707 (1973).
118. Miyake, *Chem. Pharm. Bull. (Tokyo)*, 1071 (1960).
119. Wieland and Schön, *Justus Liebigs Ann. Chem.*, 593, 157 (1955).
120. Jahns, *Chem. Ber.*, 18, 2518 (1885); 20, 2840 (1887).
121. Jadot and Casimir, *Biochim. Biophys. Acta*, 48, 400 (1961).
122. Jadot, Casimir, and Alderweireldt, *Biochim. Biophys. Acta*, 78, 500 (1963).
123. Brieskorn and Glasz, *Naturwissenschaften*, 51, 216 (1964).
124. Schryver, *Proc. R. Soc.*, B98, 58 (1925).
124a. Godtfredsen, Vangedal, and Thomas, *Tetrahedron*, 26, 4931 (1970).
125. Steenbock, *J. Biol. Chem.*, 35, 1 (1918).
126. Fowden, *Nature*, 209, 807 (1966).
127. Bell and Tirimanna, *Biochem. J.*, 91, 356 (1964).
128. Planta and Schulze, *Chem. Ber.*, 26, 939 (1893).
129. Pollard, Sondheimer, and Steward, *Nature*, 182, 1356 (1958).
129a. Shiba, Mizote, Kaneko, Nakajima, and Kakimoto, *Biochim. Biophys. Acta*, 244, 523 (1971).
129b. Hettinger and Craig, *Biochemistry*, 9, 1224 (1970).

130. Barry and Roark, *J. Biol. Chem.*, 239, 1541 (1964).
131. Barry, Chen, and Roark, *J. Gen. Microbiol.*, 33, 95 (1963).
132. Ackermann and Kirby, *J. Biol. Chem.*, 175, 483 (1948).
132a. Grove, Daxenbichler, Weisleder, and van Etlen, *Tetrahedron Lett.*, 4477 (1971).
132b. Owens, Guggenheim, and Hilton, *Biochim. Biophys. Acta*, 158, 219 (1968).
132c. Owens, Thompson, Pitcher, and Williams, *Chem. Commun.*, p. 714 (1972).
133. Morizawa, *Acta Sch. Med. Univer. Kioto*, 9, 285 (1927).
134. Cramer, *J. Prakt. Chem.*, 96, 76 (1865).
135. Flavin, Delavier-Klutchko, and Slaughter, *Science*, 143, 50 (1964).
136. Wooley, *J. Biol. Chem.*, 197, 409 (1952).
137. Wooley, *J. Biol. Chem.*, 198, 807 (1953).
138. Rose, McCoy, Meyer, and Carter, *J. Biol. Chem.*, 112, 283 (1935).
139. Greenstein and Winitz, *Chemistry of the Amino Acids*, Vol. 3, John Wiley & Sons, New York, 1961, 2238.
140. Wisvisz, Van der Hoever, and Nijenhuis, *J. Am. Chem. Soc.*, 79, 4522 (1957).
140a. Bohmen, *Tetrahedron Lett.*, p. 3065 (1970).
141. Olesen-Larsen, *Biochim. Biophys. Acta*, 93, 200 (1964).
142. Thompson, Morris, Asen, and Irreverre, *J. Biol. Chem.*, 236, 1183 (1961).
142a. O'Brien, Cox, and Gibson, *Biochim. Biophys. Acta*, 177, 321 (1969).
143. Morris, Thompson, Asen, and Irreverre, *J. Am. Chem. Soc.*, 81, 6069 (1959).
144. Schneider, *Biochem. Z.*, 330, 428 (1958).
145. Guggenheim, *Z. Physiol. Chem.*, 88, 276 (1913).
146. Greenstein and Winitz, *Chemistry of the Amino Acids*, Vol. 3, John Wiley & Sons, New York, 1961, 2713.
147. Muller and Schulte, *Z. Naturforsch.*, 23b, 659 (1958).
147a. Weaver, Rajagopalan, Handler, Rosenthal, and Jeffs, *J. Biol Chem.*, 246, 2010 (1971).
147b. Watson and Fowden, *Phytochemistry*, 12, 617 (1973).
148a. Smith and Sloane, *Biochim. Biophys. Acta*, 148, 414 (1967).
148b. Sloane and Smith, *Biochim. Biophys. Acta*, 158, 394 (1968).
148. Makino, Satoh, Fujik, and Kawaguchi, *Nature*, 170, 977 (1952).
149. Waller, Fryth, Hutchings, and Williams, *J. Am. Chem. Soc.*, 75, 2025 (1953).
150. Behr and Clark, *J. Am. Chem. Soc.*, 54, 1630 (1932).
151. Schultze and Barbieri, *Chem. Ber.*, 14, 1785 (1881).
152. Greenstein and Winitz, *Chemistry of the Amino Acids*, Vol. 3, John Wiley & Sons, New York, 1961, 2156.
153. Liebig, *Justus Liebigs Ann. Chem.*, 57, 127 (1846).
154. Greenstein and Winitz, *Chemistry of the Amino Acids*, Vol. 3, John Wiley & Sons, New York, 1961, 2348.
155. Mothes, Schütte, Müller, Ardenne, and Tümmler, *Z. Naturforsch.*, 196, 1161 (1964).
155a. Ohkusu and Mori, *J. Neurochem.*, 16, 1485 (1969).
156. Noguchi, Sakuma, and Tamaki, *Phytochemistry*, 7, 1861 (1968).
157. Kjaer and Larsen, *Acta Chem. Scand.*, 13, 1565 (1959).
158. Schulze and Steiger, *Chem. Ber.*, 19, 1177 (1886); *Z. Physiol. Chem.*, 11, 43 (1886).
159. Greenstein and Winitz, *Chemistry of the Amino Acids*, Vol. 3, John Wiley & Sons, New York, 1961, 1841.
160. Fearon and Bell, *Biochem. J.*, 59, 221 (1955).
161. Kitagawa and Tomiyama, *J. Biochem. (Tokyo)*, 11, 265 (1929).
162. Bell, *Biochem. J.*, 75, 618 (1960).
163. Walker, *J. Biol. Chem.*, 204, 139 (1954).
164. Wada, *Biochem. Z.*, 224, 420 (1930).
165. Rogers, *Biochim. Biophys. Acta*, 29, 33 (1958).
166. Kitagawa and Tsukamoto, *J. Biochem. (Tokyo)*, 26, 373 (1937).
166a. Nakajima, Matsuoka, and Kakimoto, *Biochim. Biophys. Acta*, 230, 212 (1971).
167. Ito and Hashimoto, *Nature*, 211, 417 (1966).
168. Rao, Ramachandran, and Adiga, *Biochemistry*, 2, 298 (1962).
169. Gerritsen, Vaughn, and Waisman, *Arch. Biochem. Biophys.*, 100, 298 (1963).
170. Bell and Tirimanna, *Nature*, 197, 901 (1963).
170a. Maehr, Blount, Pruess, Yarmchuk, and Kellett, *J. Antibiot. (Tokyo)*, 26, 284 (1973).

171. Bell, *Biochem. J.*, 21, 358 (1964).
173. Hegarty and Pound, *Nature*, 217, 354 (1968).
174. Tamoni and Gallo, *Farmaco Ed. Sci.*, 21, 269 (1966).
175. Fusari, Bartz, and Elder, *Nature*, 173, 72; *J. Am. Chem. Soc.*, 76, 2878 (1954).
176. Ressler, *J. Biol. Chem.*, 237, 733 (1962).
177. Ressler and Ratzkin, *J. Org. Chem.*, 26, 3356 (1961).
177a. Brysk and Ressler, *J. Biol. Chem.*, 245, 1156 (1970).
178. Dion, Fusari, Jakubowski, Zora, and Bartz, *J. Am Chem. Soc.*, 78, 3075 (1956).
179. Kaczka, Gitterman, Dulaney, and Folkers, *Biochemistry*, 1, 340 (1962).
180. Radhakrishnan and Giri, *Biochem. J.*, 58, 57 (1954).
180a. Lambein and Van Parijs, *Biochem. Biophys. Res. Commun.*, 32, 474 (1968).
180b. Lambein, Schamp, Vandendriessche, and Van Parijs, *Biochem. Biophys. Res. Commun.*, 37, 375 (1969).
181. King, *J. Chem. Soc.*, p. 3590 (1950).
182. Grobbelaar, *Nature*, 175, 703 (1955).
183. Dobson and Raphael, *J. Chem. Soc.*, p. 3642 (1958).
184. Tanaka, Miyamoto, Honjo, Morimoto, Sugawa, Uchibayshi, Sanno, and Tatsuoka, *Proc. Jap. Acad.*, 33, 47 (1957).
185. Tanaka, Miyamoto, Honjo, Morimoto, Sugawa, Uchibayshi, Sanno, and Tatsuoka, *Chem. Abstr.*, 51, 1788 (1957).
185a. Burrows and Turner, *J. Chem. Soc.*, 255 (1966).
186. Schenk and Schütte, *Naturwissenschaften*, 48, 223 (1961).
186a. Hatanaka, *Phytochemistry*, 8, 1305 (1969).
186b. Shah, Neuss, Gorman, and Boeck, *J. Antibiot. (Tokyo)*, 23, 613 (1970).
187. Prochazka, *Czech. Chem. Commun.*, 22, 333–654 (1957).
188. Pironen and Virtanen, *Acta Chem. Scand.*, 16, 1286 (1962).
189. Gmelin and Virtanen, *Ann. Acad. Sci. Fenn. (Med.)*, 107, 3 (1961).
189a. Miller, Tristram, and Wolf, *J. Antibiot. (Tokyo)*, 24, 48 (1971).
190. Fowden, *Nature*, 176, 347 (1955).
190a. Eagles, Laird, Matai, Self, and Synge, *Biochem. J.*, 121, 425 (1971).
190b. Bell, Nulu, and Cone, *Phytochemistry*, 10, 2191 (1971).
190c. Robbers and Floss, *Tetrahedron Lett.*, p. 1857 (1969).
191. Fang, Li, Nin, and Tseng, *Sci. Sinica*, 10, 845 (1961).
191a. Cross and Webster, *J. Chem. Soc. (Org.)*, 1839 (1970).
191b. Scannell, Pruess, Demny, Williams, and Stempel, *J. Antibiot. (Tokyo)*, 23, 618 (1970).
191c. Corbin and Bulen, *Biochemistry*, 8, 757 (1969).
191d. Nakajima and Volcani, *Science*, 164, 1400 (1969).
191e. Karle, Daly, and Witkop, *Science*, 164, 1401 (1969).
191f. Brown and Mangat, *Biochim. Biophys. Acta*, 177, 427 (1969).
191g. Macnicol, *Biochem. J.*, 107, 473 (1968).
192. Brown, *J. Am. Chem. Soc*, 87, 4202 (1965).
193. Daigo, *J. Pharm. Soc. Jap.*, 79, 353 (1959).
194. Casnati, Quilico, and Ricca, *Gazz. Chim. Ital.*, 93, 349 (1963).
194a. Horii and Kameda, *J. Antibiot. (Tokyo)*, 21, 665 (1968).
194a'. Katagiri, Tori, Kimura, Yoshida, Nagasaki, and Minato, *J. Med. Chem.*, 10, 1149 (1967).
194a". Finot, Bricout, Viani, and Mauron, *Experimentia*, 24, 1097 (1968).
194b. Weaver, Rajagopalan, and Handler, *J. Biol. Chem.*, 246, 2015 (1971).
195. Jahns, *Chem. Ber.*, 24, 2615 (1891).
196. Freidenberg, *Chem. Ber.*, 51, 976 (1918).
197. Kossel, *Hoppe Seyler's Z. Physiol. Chem.*, 22, 176 (1896).
198. Greenstein and Winitz, *Chemistry of the Amino Acids*, Vol. 3, John Wiley & Sons, New York, 1961, 1971.
198a. Takita, Yoshioka, Muraoka, Maeda, and Umezawa, *J. Antibiot. (Tokyo)*, 24, 795 (1971).
199. Hulme, *Nature*, 174, 1055 (1954).
200. Biemann and Deffner, *Nature*, 191, 380 (1961).
201. Minagawa, *Proc. Imp. Acad. (Tokyo)*, 21, 33, 37 (1945).
202. Virtanen and Gmeim, *Acta Chem. Scand.*, 13, 1244 (1959).
203. Schoolery and Virtanen, *Acta Chem. Scand.*, 16, 2457 (1962).
204. Hassall, Morton, Ogihara, and Thomas, *Chem. Commun.*, p. 1079 (1969).
204a. Bevan, Davies, Hassall, Morton, and Phillips, *J. Chem. Soc. (Org.)*, p. 514 (1971).
205. Irvine and Wilson, *J. Biol. Chem.*, 127, 555 (1939).

206. Sheehan and Whitney, *J. Am. Chem. Soc.*, 84, 3980 (1962).
206a. Sung and Fowden, *Phytochemistry*, 7, 2061 (1968).
207. Fischer, *Chem. Ber.*, 35, 2660 (1902).
208. Greenstein and Winitz, *Chemistry of the Amino Acids*, Vol. 3, John Wiley & Sons, New York, 1961, 2018.
209. Wieland and Witkop, *Justus Liebigs Ann. Chem.*, 543, 171 (1940).
210. Kotake, Sakan, and Miwa, *Chem. Ber.*, 85, 690 (1952).
211. Mitoma, Weissbach, and Udenfriend, *Nature*, 175, 994 (1955).
212. Takemoto, Nakajima, and Yokobe, *J. Pharm. Soc. Jap.*, 84, 1232 (1964).
213. List, *Planta Med.*, 6, 424 (1958).
214. von Klämbt, *Naturwissenschaften*, 47, 398 (1960).
215. Hutzinger and Kosuge, *Biochemistry*, 7, 601 (1968).
216. Murakami, Takemoto, and Shimzu, *J. Pharm. Soc. Jap.*, 73, 1026 (1953).
217. Beockman and Staehler, *Naturwissenschaften*, 52, 391 (1965).
218. Vanderhaeghe and Parmetier, *17th Congr. Pure Appl. Chem.*, Butterworths, London, 1959, 56.
219. Brockmann, *Ann. N. Y. Acad. Sci.*, 89, 323 (1960).
220. Bell, *Biochim. Biophys. Acta*, 47, 602 (1961).
221. Gray and Fowden, *Nature*, 193, 1285 (1962).
222. Bethell, Kenner, and Shepperd, *Nature*, 194, 864 (1962).
222a. Müller and Schütte, *Z. Naturforsch.*, 236, 491 (1968).
223. Hulme and Arthington, *Nature*, 173, 588 (1954).
224. Burroughs, Dalby, Kenner, and Sheppard, *Nature*, 189, 394 (1961).
224a. Borders, Sax, Lancaster, Hausmann, Mitscher, Wetzel, and Patterson, *Tetrahedron*, 26, 3123 (1970).
225. Chain, *Ann. Rev. Biochem.*, 17, 657 (1948).
226. Sheehan, Drummond, Gardner, Maeda, Mania, Nakamura, Sen, and Stock, *J. Am. Chem. Soc.*, 85, 2867 (1963).
227. Adams and Johnson, *J. Am. Chem. Soc.*, 71, 705 (1949).
227a. Murakoshi, Kuramoto, Ohmiya, and Haginiwa, *Chem. Pharm. Bull. (Japan)*, 20, 855 (1972).
228. Minagawa, *Proc. Jap. Acad.*, 22, 130 (1946).
229. Eugster, Muller, and Good, *Tetrahedron Lett.*, 23, 1813 (1965).
230. Reiner and Eugster, *Helv. Chim. Acta*, 50, 128 (1967).
231. Fritz, Gagnent, Zbinden, Geigy, and Eugster, *Tetrahedron Lett.*, 25, 2075 (1965).
231a. Noma, Noguchi, and Tamaki, *Tetrahedron Lett.*, p. 2017 (1971).
232. Engeland and Biehler, *Hoppe Seyler's Z. Physiol. Chem.*, 123, 290 (1922).
233. Hulme and Arthington, *Nature*, 170, 659 (1952).
234. Husemann and Marme, *Justus Liebigs Ann. Chem.*, Suppl. 2, 382 (1863).
235. Greenstein and Winitz, *Chemistry of the Amino Acids*, Vol. 3, John Wiley & Sons, New York, 1961, 2316.
236. Noe and Fowden, *Biochem. J.*, 77, 543 (1960).
236a. Finot, Viani, Bricout, and Mauron, *Experimentia*, 25, 134 (1969).
236b. Wolfersberger and Tabachnik, *Experimenta*, 29, 346 (1973).
237. Nakanishi, Ito, and Hirata, *J. Am. Chem. Soc.*, 76, 2845 (1954).
238. Carter, Sweeley, Daniels, McNary, Schaffner, West, Tamelen, Dyer, and Whaley, *J. Am. Chem Soc.*, 83, 4296 (1961).
238a. Bodanszky, Marconi, and Bodanszky, *J. Antiobiot., (Tokyo)*, 22, 40 (1969).
238b. Marconi and Bodanszky, *J. Antibiot. (Tokyo)*, 23, 120 (1970).
239. Hattori and Komamine, *Nature*, 183, 1116 (1959).
240. Senoh, Imamato, Maeno, Tokyama, Sakan, Komamine, and Hattori, *Tetrahedron Lett.*, 46, 3431 (1964).
241. Schulze and Trier, *Hoppe Seyler's Z. Physiol. Chem.*, 76, 258; 79, 235 (1912).
242. Takemoto and Nakajima, *J. Pharm. Soc. Jap.*, 84, 1230 (1964).
243. Hopkins and Cole, *J. Physiol. (Lond.)*, 27, 418 (1901).
244. Greenstein and Winitz, *Chemistry of the Amino Acids*, Vol. 3, John Wiley & Sons, New York, 1961, 2316.
244a. Nakamiya, Shiba, Kaneko, Sakakibara, Take, and Abe, *Tetrahedron Lett.*, p. 3497 (1970).
245. Takemoto, Diago, and Takagi, *J. Pharm. Soc. Jap.*, 84, 1176 (1964).
246. Dyer, Hayes, Miller, and Nassar, *J. Am. Chem. Soc.*, 86, 5363 (1964).
246a. Büchi and Raleigh, *J. Org. Chem.*, 36, 873 (1971).
247. Gmelin, *Hoppe Seyler's Z. Physiol. Chem.*, 316, 164 (1959).
248. Kjaer, Knudsen, and Larsen, *Acta Chem. Scand.*, 15, 1193 (1961).

249. Gordon and Jackson, *J. Biol. Chem.*, 110, 151 (1935).
250. Ghatak and Kaul, *Chem. Zentralbl.*, 3730 (1932).
250a. Auditore and Wade, *J. Neurochem.*, 18, 2389 (1971).
250a'. Hall, Metzenberg, and Cohen, *J. Biol. Chem.*, 230, 1013 (1958).
250b. Tallan, Moore, and Stein, *J. Biol. Chem.*, 219, 257 (1956).
251. Takita, Naganawa, Maeda, and Umezawa, *J. Antibiot. (Tokyo)*, 17, 90 (9164).
252. Sheehan, Zachau, and Lawson, *J. Am. Chem. Soc.*, 80, 3349 (1958).
252a. Bouloin, Ottinger, Pais, and Chiurdoglu, *Bull. Soc. Chim. Belges*, 78, 583 (1969).
253. Takita, *J. Antibiot. (Tokyo)*, 16, 175 (1963).
254. Emery, *Biochemistry*, 4, 1410 (1965).
255. Ackerman, *Hoppe Seyler's Z. Physiol. Chem.*, 302, 80 (1955).
256. Morgan, *Chem. Ind. (Lond.)*, p. 542 (1964).
257. Starcher, Partridge, and Elsden, *Biochemistry*, 6, 2425 (1967).
258. Eloff and Grobbelaar, *J. S. Afr. Chem. Inst.*, 20, 190 (1967).
259. Searle and Westall, *Biochem. J.*, 48, 1 (P) (1951).
260. Tallan, Stein, and Moore, *J. Biol. Chem.*, 206, 825 (1954).
261. Plattner and Nager, *Helv. Chim. Acta*, 31, 665 (1948).
262. Plattner and Nager, *Helv. Chim. Acta*, 31, 2192 (1948).
263. Corrigan, *Science*, 164, 142 (1969).
264. Vilkas, Rojas, and Lederer, *C. R. Hebd. Seances Acad. Sci. (Paris)*, 261, 4258 (1965).
264a. Bodanszky, Muramatsu, Bodanszky, Lukin, and Doubler, *J. Antibiot. (Tokyo)*, 21, 77 (1968).
265. Thompson, Morris, and Smith, *Ann. Rev. Biochem.*, 38, 137 (1969).
266. Hiller-Bombien, *Arch. Pharm.*, 230, 513 (1892).
267. Winterstein, *Hoppe Seyler's Z. Physiol. Chem.*, 105, 20 (1919).
268. Brockmann and Grobhofer, *Naturwissenschaften*, 36, 376 (1949).
269. Plattner and Nager, *Helv. Chim. Acta*, 31, 2203 (1948).
270. Darling and Larsen, *Acta Chem. Scand.*, 15, 743 (1961).
271. Kjaer and Larsen, *Acta Chem. Scand.*, 15, 750 (1961).
272. Linko, Alfthan, Miettinen, and Virtanen, *Acta Chem. Scand.*, 7, 1310 (1953).
273. Gmelin, Kjaer, and Larsen, *Phytochemistry*, 1, 233 (1962).
274. Stoll and Seebeck, *Helv. Chim. Acta*, 31, 189 (1948).
275. Suzuki, *Chem. Pharm. Bull. (Tokyo)*, 9, 251 (1961).
276. Sugii, *Chem. Pharm. Bull. (Tokyo)*, 12, 1114 (1964).
277. Alderton, *J. Am. Chem. Soc.*, 75, 2391 (1953).
278. Horowitz, *J. Biol. Chem.*, 171, 255 (1947).
279. Tallan, Moore, and Stein, *J. Biol. Chem.*, 230, 707 (1958).
280. McRorie, Sutherland, Lewis, Barton, Glazener, and Shive, *J. Am. Chem. Soc.*, 76, 115 (1954).
280a. Jadot, Casimir, and Warin, *Bull. Soc. Chim. Belges*, 78, 299 (1969).
281. Salkowski, *Chem. Ber.*, 6, 744 (1873).
282. Romburgh and Barger, *J. Chem. Soc. (Lond.)*, 99, 2068 (1911).
283. Gmelin, Strauss, and Hasenmaler, *Z. Naturforsch.*, 13b, 252 (1958).
284. Kuriyama, *Nature*, 192, 969 (1961).
284a. Kodama, Yao, Kobayashi, Hirayama, Fujii, Mizuhara, Haraguchi, and Hirosawa, *Physiol. Chem. Phys.*, 1, 72 (1969).
285. Gmelin and Hietala, *Hoppe Seyler's Z. Physiol. Chem.*, 322, 278 (1960).
286. Virtanen and Matikkala, *Hoppe Seyler's Z. Physiol. Chem.*, 322, 8 (1960).
287. Mizuhara and Ohmori, *Arch. Biochem. Biophys.*, 92, 53 (1961).
288. Kuriyama, Takagi, and Murata, *Bull. Fac. Fish Hokkaido Univ.*, 11, 58 (1960).
289. Virtanen and Matikkala, *Acta Chem. Scand.*, 13, 623 (1959).
290. Dawson, Elliott, Elliott, and Jones, *Data for Biochemical Research*, Oxford University Press, Oxford, 1969, 2.
291. Martin and Synge, *Adv. Protein Chem.*, 2, 7 (1945).
292. Dent, *Biochem. J.*, 43, 169 (1948).
293. Baumann, *Hoppe Seyler's Z. Physiol. Chem.*, 8, 299 (1884).
294. Greenstein and Winitz, *Chemistry of the Amino Acids*, Vol. 3, John Wiley & Sons, New York, 1961, 1879.
295. Bergeret and Chatagner, *Biochim. Biophys. Acta*, 14, 297 (1954).
296. Wollaston, *Ann. Chim. Phys.*, 76, 21 (1810).
297. Larsen and Kjaer, *Acta Chem. Scand.*, 16, 142 (1962).
298. Sweetman, *Nature*, 183, 744 (1959).
299. Calam and Waley, *Biochem. J.*, 86, 226 (1963).
300. Gmelin, *Hoppe Seyler's Z. Physiol. Chem.*, 327, 186 (1962).
301. Virtanen and Matikkala, *Acta Chem. Scand.*, 13, 1898 (1959).
302. van Veen and Hijman, *Rec. Trav. Chem. Pays-Bas*, 54, 493 (1935).
303. Armstrong and du Vigneaud, *J. Biol. Chem.*, 168, 373 (1947).
304. Fisher and Mallette, *J. Gen. Physiol.*, 45, 1 (1961).
305. Westall, *Biochem. J.*, 55, 244 (1953).
306. Adams and Capecchi, *Proc. Natl. Acad. Sci. USA*, 55, 147 (1966).
307. Cornforth and Henry, *J. Chem. Soc.*, 597 (1952).
308. Thoai and Robin, *Biochim. Biophys. Acta*, 13, 533 (1954).
309. Robertson and Marion, *Can. J. Chem.*, 37, 1043 (1959).
310. Stock, Friedel, and Hambsch, *Hoppe Seyler's Z. Physiol. Chem.*, 305, 166 (1956).
311. Gerritson, Vaughn, and Waisman, *Biochem. Biophys. Res. Commun.*, 9, 493 (1962).
312. Frimpter, *J. Biol. Chem.*, 236, PC51 (1961).
313. Huang, *Biochemistry*, 2, 296 (1963).
314. Sugii, Suketa, and Suzuchi, *Chem. Pharm. Bull. (Tokyo)*, 12, 1115 (1964).
314a. Minale, Fattorusso, Cimino, DeStefano, and Nicolaus, *Gazzetta*, 97, 1636 (1967).
315. Wiehler and Marion, *Can. J. Chem.*, 36, 339 (1958).
316. Ohmori and Mizuhara, *Arch. Biochem. Biophys.*, 96, 179 (1962).
317. Ohmori, *Arch. Biochem. Biophys.*, 104, 509 (1964).
318. Horn, Jones, and Ringel, *J. Biol. Chem.*, 138, 141 (1941).
319. du Vigneaud and Brown, *J. Biol. Chem.*, 138, 151 (1941).
319a. Ampola, Bixby, Crawhall, Efron, Parker, Sneddon, and Young, *Biochem. J.*, 107, 16P (1968).
320. Thompson, *Nature*, 178, 593 (1956).
320a. Fujiwara, Itokawa, Uchino, and Inoue, *Experimenta*, 28, 254 (1972).
321. Mueller, *Proc. Soc. Exp. Biol. Med.*, 19, 161 (1922).
322. Greenstein and Winitz, *Chemistry of the Amino Acids*, Vol. 3, John Wiley & Sons, New York, 1961, 2125.
323. Matikkala and Virtanen, *Acta Chem. Scand.*, 17, 1799 (1963).
324. Guggenheim, Die Biogenen. Amine, S. Karger, Basel, (1951)
325. Challenger and Hayward, *Biochem. J.*, 58, 10 (1954).
326. Friis and Kjaer, *Acta Chem. Scand.*, 17, 2391 (1963).
327. Shrift and Virupaksha, *Biochim. Biophys. Acta*, 100, 65 (1965).
328. Gmelin and Virtanen, *Suomen Kemistilehti*, B35, 34 (1962); *Acta Chem. Scand.*, 16, 1378 (1962).
329. Matikkala and Virtanen, *Acta Chem. Scand.*, 16, 2461 (1962).
330. Spare and Virtanen, *Acta Chem. Scand.*, 17, 641 (1963).
331. Virtanen, Hatanaka, and Berlin, *Suomen Kemistilehti*, B35, 52 (1962).
332. Kutscher, *Zentralbl. Physiol.*, 24, 775 (1910).
333. Barger and Ewins, *Biochem.*, 7, 204 (1913).
334. Horn and Jones, *J. Biol. Chem.*, 139, 649 (1941).
334a. Tuve and Williams, *J. Biol. Chem.*, 236, 597 (1961).
335. Trelease, DiSomma, and Jacobs, *Science*, 132, 618 (1960).
336. Tanret, *C. R. Hebd. Seances Acad. Sci.(Paris)*, 149, 222 (1909).
337. Waisvisz, van der Hoeven, and Rijenhuis, *J. Am. Chem. Soc.*, 79, 4524 (1957).
338. Behre and Benedict, *J. Biol. Chem.*, 82, 11 (1929).
339. Greenstein and Winitz, *Chemistry of the Amino Acids*, Vol. 3, John Wiley & Sons, New York, 1961, 2671.
340. Heath, *Nature*, 166, 106 (1950).
341. Tallan, Bella, Stein, and Moore, *J. Biol. Chem.*, 217, 703 (1955).
342. Bettelheim, *J. Am. Chem. Soc.*, 76, 2838 (1954).
343. Partridge, Elsden, and Thomas, *Nature*, 197, 1297 (1963).
344. Morner, *Hoppe Seyler's Z. Physiol. Chem.*, 88, 138 (1913).
344a. Savoie, Massin, and Savoie, *J. Clin. Invest.*, 52, 116 (1973).
345. Gross and Pitt-Rivers, *Biochem. J.*, 53, 645 (1950).
346. Drechsel, *Z. Biol.*, 33, 96 (1896).
347. Greenstein and Winitz, *Chemistry of the Amino Acids*, Vol. 3, John Wiley & Sons, New York, 1961, 1426.
348. Greenstein and Winitz, *Chemistry of the Amino Acids*, Vol. 3, John Wiley & Sons, New York, 1961, 2259.
349. Low, *J. Mar. Res.*, 10, 239 (1951).
349a. Hunt and Breuer, *Biochim. Biophys. Acta*, 252, 401 (1971).
349b. Hunt, *FEBS Lett.*, 24, 109 (1972).
350. Roche, Lissitzky, and Michel, *C. R. Hebd. Seances Acad. Sci. (Paris)*, 232, 2047 (1951).
351. Roche and Yagi, *C. R. Soc. Biol.*, 146, 642 (1952).

352. Kendall, *J. Biol. Chem.*, 39, 125 (1919).
353. Coulson, *J. Sci. Food Agric. Abstr.*, 6, 674 (1955).
354. Butenandt, Weidel, Weicher, and Von Derjugen, *Hoppe Seyler's Z. Physiol. Chem.*, 279, 27 (1937).
355. Fowden, *Physiol. Plant*, 12, 657 (1959).
356. Stoll and Seebeck, *Helv. Chim. Acta*, 34, 481 (1951).
357. Chambers and Isbell, *J. Org. Chem.*, 29, 832 (1964).
358. Kittredge and Hughes, *Biochemistry*, 3, 991 (1964).
359. Kittredge, Roberts, and Simonsen, *Biochemistry*, 1, 624 (1962).
360. Kittredge, Isbell, and Hughes, *Biochemistry*, 6, 289 (1967).
360a. Korn, Dearborn, Fales, and Sokoloski, *J. Biol. Chem.*, 248, 2257 (1973).
361. Thoai and Robin, *Biochim. Biophys. Acta*, 14, 76 (1954).
362. Beatty, Magrath, and Ennor, *J. Am. Chem. Soc.*, 82, 4983 (1960); *J. Biol. Chem.*, 236, 1028 (1961).
363. Weiss and Stekol, *J. Am. Chem. Soc.*, 73, 2497 (1951).
364. Agren, *Acta Chem. Scand.*, 16, 1607 (1962).
365. Lipmann, *Biochem. Z.*, 262, 3 (1933).
366. Greenstein and Winitz, *Chemistry of the Amino Acids*, Vol. 3, John Wiley & Sons, New York, 1961, 2208.
367. Tomita and Sendju, *Hoppe Seyler's Z. Physiol. Chem.*, 169, 263 (1927).
368. Noguchi, Sakuma, and Tamaki, *Arch. Biochem. Biophys.*, 125, 1017 (1968).
369. Kung and Trier, *Hoppe Seyler's Z. Physiol. Chem.*, 85, 209 (1913).
370. Hosein and Proulx, *Nature*, 187, 321 (1960).
371. Carter and Bhattacharyya, *J. Am. Chem. Soc.*, 75, 2503 (1953).
372. Gulewitsch and Krimberg, *Hoppe Seyler's Z. Physiol. Chem.*, 45, 326 (1905).
373. Friedman, McFarlane, Bhattacharyya, and Fraenkel, *Arch. Biochem. Biophys.*, 59, 484 (1955).
374. Carter, Bhattacharyya, Weidman, and Fraenkel, *Arch. Biochem. Biophys.*, 38, 405 (1952).
375. Thomas, Elsden, and Partridge, *Nature*, 200, 651 (1963).
376. Terlain and Thomas, *Bull. Soc. Chim. Fr.*, p. 2349 (1971).
377. Kodama, Ohmori, Suzuki, Mizuhara, Oura, Isshiki, and Uemura, *Physiol. Chem. Phys.*, 3, 81 (1971).
378. Wälti and Hope, *J. Chem. Soc. (Org.)*, p. 2326 (1971).
379. Larsen, *Acta Chem. Scand.*, 22, 1369 (1968).
380. Delange, Glazer, and Smith, *J. Biol. Chem.*, 244, 1385 (1969).
381. Nakajima and Volcani, *Biochem. Biophys. Res. Commun.*, 39, 28 (1970).
382. Ogawa, Fukuda, and Sasaoka, *Biochim. Biophys. Acta*, 297, 60 (1973).
383. Zygmunt and Martin, *J. Med. Chem.*, 12, 953 (1969).
384. Hagemann, Pénasse, and Teillon, *Biochim. Biophys. Acta*, 17, 240 (1955).

COEFFICIENTS OF SOLUBILITY EQUATIONS OF CERTAIN AMINO ACIDS IN WATER[a]

Amino Acid	a_1	$b_1 \times 10^2$	$c_1 \times 10^5$	a_2	a_3	$b_3 \times 10^2$	$c_3 \times 10^5$	a_4	$b_4 \times 10^2$	$c_4 \times 10^5$
L-Alanine	2.1048	0.4669	—	0.1551	-2.5792	1.075	—	-6.5150	1.037	—
D,L-Alanine	2.0830	0.5608	—	0.1333	-3.2199	1.291	—	-7.1317	1.245	—
L-Asparagine H$_2$O	0.9289	2.311	-4.981	-1.2475	-25.9584	1.059	-11.47	-30.2463	11.79	-11.84
L-Aspartic acid	0.3194	1.519	—	-1.8047	-13.7113	3.499	—	-17.7370	3.502	—
D,L-Aspartic acid	0.4181	2.016	-4.999	-1.7060	-25.1918	10.93	-11.51	-29.2797	10.98	-11.61
L-Cystine	-1.299	1.357	—	-3.680	-18.643	3.125	—	-21.023	3.125	—
D,L-Cystine[c]	-1.7959	0.8013	27.89	-4.1766	19.4912	-23.66	47.61	15.4747	-23.66	47.61
D,L-Cystine[c]	-2.1087	3.367	-22.56	-4.4894	-36.9568	14.48	-16.80	-40.9733	14.48	-16.80
Meso-cystine[c]	-1.7190	0.4514	27.39	-4.0997	34.7268	-33.38	63.01	30.7013	-33.38	63.01
Meso-cystine[c]	-2.6034	5.890	-49.41	-4.9841	-133.4125	75.4125	-113.8	-137.429	-75.73	-113.8
L-Dibromotyrosine (hydrated)	0.0839	1.627	—	-2.445	-15.881	3.753	—	-19.894	3.752	—
L-Dibromotyrosine (anhydrous)	0.188	0.9884	—	-2.343	-11.610	2.276	—	-15.537	2.247	—
L-Dichlorotyrosine	0.0065	1.038	4.648	-2.392	-4.058	-3.450	1.069	-8.426	-3.215	1.030
L-Diiodotyrosine	-0.690	1.92	—	-3.326	-19.745	4.42	—	-23.761	4.43	—
D,L-Diiodotyrosine	-0.827	1.43	—	-3.464	-16.989	3.30	—	-21.006	3.30	—
D-Glutamic acid	0.5331	1.613	—	-1.6345	-13.9054	3.714	—	-17.9095	3.709	—
D,L-Glutamic acid	0.9317	1.523	—	-1.2359	-12.4244	3.507	—	-16.4071	3.495	—
Glycine	2.1516	1.087	-4.114	0.2762	-13.2619	7.676	-9.473	-17.8976	8.171	-10.50
L-Hydroxyproline	2.4603	0.3891	—	0.3428	-1.6575	0.8959	—	-5.5906	0.8514	—
L-Isoleucine	1.5787	0.07662	2.594	-0.5389	2.7190	-3.081	5.972	-1.3913	-3.020	5.866
D,L-Isoleucine	1.2616	0.2512	3.794	-0.8560	2.9651	-4.193	8.736	-1.1373	-4.134	8.632
L-Leucine[d]	1.3561	0.02233	3.727	-0.7615	4.5073	-4.683	8.582	-0.7252	-3.814	7.198
D,l-Leucine	0.9013	0.2635	4.591	-1.2163	3.4260	-5.167	10.57	-0.6258	-5.143	10.53
D,l-Methionine	1.2597	1.108	-1.221	-0.9140	-11.1682	4.086	-2.811	-15.2099	4.111	-2.871
D,l-Norleucine	0.9258	0.4524	3.402	-1.1918	0.2523	-3.236	7.833	-4.2067	-2.941	7.340
L-Phenylalanine	1.2974	0.6982	—	-0.9204	-6.510	1.608	—	-10.5103	1.601	—
D,L-Phenylalanine	0.9986	0.5252	3.140	-1.2192	-0.7184	-2.739	7.229	-5.0876	-2.495	6.808
L-Proline	3.1050	0.4206	—	1.0441	-0.2407	0.9686	—	-3.8586	0.7586	—
D,l-Serine	1.3432	1.520	-3.548	-0.6782	-17.2153	7.963	-8.169	-21.4529	8.134	-8.504
Taurine	1.5945	1.916	-8.500	-0.5029	-27.8015	15.10	-19.57	-32.1283	15.35	-20.07
L-Tryptophan	0.9156	0.4834	2.988	-1.3942	-11.3824	4.872	6.881	-15.3928	4.869	-6.879
L-Tyrosine	-0.708	1.46	—	-2.966	-10.799	3.36	—	-20.062	3.37	—
D,l-Tyrosine	-0.833	1.51	—	-3.091	-16.562	3.46	—	-20.577	3.46	—
L-Valine[b]	1.9211	8.1515	8.589	-0.1456	0.6274	-8.927	1.978	-3.4570	-8.528	1.9058
L-Valine[b]	1.6675	97.75	80.22	-0.4011	-20.8468	123.4	18.47	-24.2293	119.4	17.85
L-Valine[b]	1.8847	11.42	4.799	-0.1839	-0.3175	-3.406	1.105	-3.6570	-8.125	1.910
L-Valine[b]	1.9227	—	—	-0.1459	-0.3359	—	—	-4.3653	—	—
L-Valine[b]	1.8836	—	—	-0.1850	-0.4260	—	—	-4.4542	—	—
D,l-Valine	1.7749	0.2389	2.607	-0.2966	-2.2921	-2.729	6.003	-1.7417	-2.705	5.928

[a] Solubility equations:
Log S = $a_1 + b_1 t + c_1 t^2$ (grams per 1,000 gms water)
Log m = $a_2 + b_1 t + c_1 t^2$ (moles per 1,000 gms water)
ln m = $a_3 + b_3 T + c_3 T^2$
ln N_2 = $a_4 + b_4 T + c_4 T^2$

[b] The five sets of values which are given under L-valine refer to the various crystal forms.

[c] The first set of values refer to 273.1 K to 303.1 K and the second set to 298.1 K to 323.5 K absolute.

[d] Values are not strictly accurate due to contamination of the leucine with a small amount of methionine.

Reprinted with slight modification from *The Chemistry of the Amino Acids and Proteins*, C. L. A. Schmidt, Ed. Charles C Thomas, Publisher, Springfield, Ill., 1944, 845. Courtesy of the publisher.

HEAT CAPACITIES, ABSOLUTE ENTROPIES, AND ENTROPIES OF FORMATION OF AMINO ACIDS AND RELATED COMPOUNDS

John O. Hutchens

Heat capacity (C_p°), absolute entropy (S°), and the entropy change for formation from the elements (ΔSf°) are given for a temperature of 298.15 K. The units are cal deg^{-1} mole^{-1} for all entries except for proteins where they are cal deg^{-1} g^{-1}. 1 cal = 4.1840 absolute joules and 0°C—273.15 K. International Atomic Weights of 1959 are employed. In calculating ΔSf° the entropies of the elements used are (in cal deg^{-1} mole^{-1}) C (graphite), 1.3609; H$_2$ (gas), 31.211; O$_2$ (gas), 49.003; N$_2$ (gas), 45.767; Cl$_2$ (gas), 53.31; and S (rhombic), 7.62.[1] S° for D$_2$ (gas) is 34.620 cal deg^{-1} mole^{-1}.[2]

The references cited give heat capacities at other temperatures, and, in most cases, the additional thermodynamic functions $(H^\circ - H_0^\circ)$, $(H^\circ - H_0^\circ)/T$ and $-(F^\circ - H_0^\circ)/T$. None of the stated values is more accurate than ± 0.2%. Values obtained by extrapolating below 90 K are uncertain by ± 1–2 cal deg^{-1} mole^{-1}. Entries are listed in alphabetical order under (1) amino acids, (2) peptides, (3) proteins, and (4) miscellaneous related substances.

Compound	C_p°	S°	$-\Delta Sf^\circ$	Reference	Remarks
				AMINO ACIDS	
L-Alanine	29.22	30.88	154.33	3, 4	
D-Arginine	55.8[a]	59.9	307.3[a]	5	Extrapolated below 90 K
L-Arginine · HCl	26.37	68.43	341.01	6	
L-Asparagine	38.3[a]	41.7	207.9[a]	7	
L-Asparagine · H$_2$O	49.69	50.10	255.17	8	
L-Aspartic Acid	37.09	40.66	194.91	8	
DL-Citrulline	55.2[a]	60.8	292.4[a]	9	Extrapolated below 90 K
L-Cysteine	38.8[a]	40.6	152.2[a]	10	Extrapolated below 90 K
L-Cystine	62.60	67.06	287.38	11	
L-Glutamic Acid	41.84	44.98	223.16	8	
D-Glutamic Acid · HCl	50.0[a]	59.3	251.1[a]	12	Extrapolated below 90 K
L-Glutamine	44.02	46.62	235.51	8	
Glycine	23.71	24.74	127.90	3, 4	
L-Histidine · HCl	59.64	65.99	242.54	6	
L-Hydroxyproline	36.79	41.19	202.45	13	Transitions at 21.9 and 31.5 K
L-Hydroxyproline (deuterated)	39.40	43.04	205.72	14	Transitions at 25.9 and 28.9 K.
					From 99.6% D$_2$O. Carboxyl, hydroxyl, andimido hydrogens presumably replaced
L-Isoleucine	45.00	49.71	233.21	4	—
L-Leucine	48.03	50.62	232.30	4	—
L-Lysine · HCl	57.10	63.21	300.46	6	—
L-Methionine	69.32	55.32	202.65	11	Transition at 305.5 K
DL-Ornithine	45.6[a]	46.2	242.6[a]	9	Extrapolated below 90 K
L-Phenylalanine	48.52	51.06	204.74	15	—
L-Proline	36.13	39.21	179.93	15	—
L-Serine	32.40	35.65	174.06	16	—
L-Threonine	35.2	36.5	205.8	13	Several samples tested. Difficult to dry. Anomalous behavior 250—300 K
L-Tryptophan	56.92	60.00	237.01	15	—
L-Tyrosine	51.73	51.15	229.15	15	—
L-Valine	40.35	42.75	207.60	4	—
				PEPTIDES	
DL-Alanylglycine	43.6[a]	51.0	231.1[a]	18	Extrapolated below 90 K. MW not stated in references. C_p° given per g in references
Glycylglycine	39.19	43.09	206.47	13	—
DL-Leucylglycine	61.3[a]	67.2	312.6[a]	17	Extrapolated below 90 K. MW not stated in reference. C_p° given per g in reference
				PROTEINS	
Bovine Serum Albumin	—	—	—	18	—
Native Hydrated	0.3161	0.3249	—	—	2.14% H$_2$O. No heat of fusion noted
Native Anhydrous	0.3049	0.3175	—	—	—
Denatured Anhydrous	0.3096	0.3205	—	—	—

Compound	C_p°	S°	$-\Delta Sf^\circ$	Reference	Remarks
Bovine Zinc Insulin	—	—	—	13	
Native Hydrated	0.3155	0.3252	—	—	4.0% H_2O. No heat of fusion noted
Native Anhydrous	0.2996	0.3144	—	—	—
Collagen	—	—	—	14	Bovine serosal collagen
Native Hydrated	0.3834	0.3589	—	—	13.53% H_2O. No heat of fusion noted
Native Anhydrous	0.2921	0.3081	—	—	
α-Chymotrypsinogen	—	—	—	18	Bovine source
Native Hydrated	0.3834	0.3635	—	—	10.7% H_2O. No heat of fusion noted
Native Anhydrous	0.3090	0.3227	—	—	—
		MISCELLANEOUS RELATED SUBSTANCES			
Creatine	41.1[a]	45.3	218.2[a]	19	—
Creatinine	33.2[a]	40.0	167.8[a]	19	—
Urea	22.26	25.00	109.06	20	—

[a] Calculated by compiler, not in reference cited.

References

1. National Bureau of Standards Circular 500 (1961), Selected Values of Chemical Thermodynamic Properties, U.S. Gov. Print. Off., Washington, D.C.
2. National Bureau of Standards Report No. 8504 (1964), Preliminary Report on the Thermodynamic Properties of Selected Light-Element and Some Related Compounds, U.S. Gov. Print. Off., Washington, D.C.
3. Hutchens, Cole, and Stout, *J. Am. Chem. Soc.*, 82, 4813 (1960).
4. Hutchens, Cole, and Stout, *J. Phys. Chem.*, 67, 1128 (1963).
5. Huffman and Ellis, *J. Am. Chem. Soc.*, 59, 2150 (1937).
6. Cole, Hutchens, and Stout, *J. Phys. Chem.*, 67, 2245 (1963).
7. Huffman and Borsook, *J. Am. Chem. Soc.*, 54, 4297 (1932).
8. Hutchens, Cole, Robie, and Stout, *J. Biol. Chem.*, 238, 2407 (1963).
9. Huffman and Fox, *J. Am. Chem. Soc.*, 63, 3464 (1940).
10. Huffman and Ellis, *J. Am. Chem. Soc.*, 57, 46 (1935).
11. Hutchens, Cole, and Stout, *J. Biol. Chem.*, 239, 591 (1964).
12. Huffman, Ellis, and Borsook, *J. Am. Chem. Soc.*, 62, 297 (1940).
13. Hutchens, J. O., Cole, A. G., and Stout, J. W., unpublished data.
14. Hutchens, J. O., Kim, S., and Stout, J. W., unpublished data.
15. Cole, Hutchens, and Stout, *J. Phys. Chem.*, 67, 1852 (1963).
16. Hutchens, Cole, and Stout, *J. Phys. Chem.*, 239, 4194 (1964).
17. Huffman, *J. Am. Chem. Soc.*, 63, 688 (1941).
18. Hutchens, J. O., unpublished data.
19. Huffman and Borsook, *J. Am. Chem. Soc.*, 54, 4297 (1932).
20. Ruerhwein and Huffman, *J. Am. Chem. Soc.*, 68, 1759 (1946).

This table originally appeared in Sober, Ed., *Handbook of Biochemistry and Selected Data for Molecular Biology*, 2nd ed., Chemical Rubber Co., Cleveland, 1970.

HEAT OF COMBUSTION, ENTHALPY, AND FREE ENERGY OF FORMATION OF AMINO ACIDS AND RELATED COMPOUNDS

John O. Hutchens

Heat of combustion (ΔH_c°) is given as the enthalpy change for the reaction of burning the compound at constant pressure to produce CO_2 (gas), H_2O (liquid), N_2 (gas), and S (rhombic). The enthalpy of formation (ΔHf°) is given for formation of the compound from C (graphite), H_2 (gas), O_2 (gas), N_2 (gas), and S (rhombic). In calculating ΔHf°, the enthalpies of formation of CO_2 (gas, $p = 0$) = 94.0518 Kcal mole^{-1} and of H_2O (liquid) = 68.3174 Kcal mole^{-1} were employed.[1] Most of the heats of combustion were originally reported as the enthalpy change for the combustion reaction with all gases at $p = 1$ atmosphere. No correction has been made for further expansion of the gases. However, all heats of combustion have been corrected so that International Atomic Weights of 1959 apply. The listings are for a temperature of 298.15°K. 0°C = 273.15°K and 1 cal = 4.1840 absolute joules. The units for all entries are kcal mole^{-1}.

In calculating ΔGf° the free energy change for formation of the compound from C (graphite), H_2 (gas, f = 1); O_2 (gas, f = 1), N_2 (gas, f = 1), and S (rhombic) the entropies of formation (ΔSf°) of amino acids and peptides listed in table on page 65 were employed. $\Delta Gf^\circ = \Delta Hf^\circ - T\Delta Sf^\circ$. Where available ΔSf° for the L-isomer of an amino acid was used in calculating ΔGf° for D- and DL-form on the assumption that this entropy value was more reliable. Available entropy data on D- and DL-forms depend on extrapolation of heat capacity data below 90°K while those for the L-amino acids in most cases do not.

The table is intended to be comprehensive rather than selective. All heats of combustion which have come to the compiler's attention have been included regardless of degree of reliability. Where more than one heat of combustion has been reported for a compound, ΔHf° and ΔGf° have been calculated only from the apparently more reliable data. Where no reasonable choice could be made between apparently equally reliable recent heats of combustion (since 1930) ΔHf° and ΔGf° have been calculated from both.

Compounds are listed alphabetically under (1) Amino Acids, (2) Peptides, and (3) Miscellaneous related compounds.

Compound	$-\Delta H_c^\circ$	Reference	$-\Delta Hf^\circ$	$-\Delta Gf^\circ$	Remarks
		AMINO ACIDS			
D-Alanine	387.1	2	134.2	88.2	—
	387.1	3			—
L-Alanine	386.8[a]	4, 5	134.5	88.4	—
DL-Alanine	386.6	6	134.7	88.7	—
	387.6	3			—
	387.8	7			—
	389.5	8			—
D-Arginine	893.5	6	149.0	57.4	—
L-Asparagine	460.8	2	188.7	126.7	—
	463.5	9			—
L-Asparagine · H_2O	458.1	2	259.7	183.6	—
	459.8	10			—
L-Aspartic Acid	382.6	2	232.6	174.5	—
	382.2	10			
	385.0	11			
	385.0	12			
	385.7	8			
L-Cysteine	394.6	13	126.7	81.3	—
L-Cystine	724.6	13, 14	249.6	163.9	—
D-Glutamic Acid	537.5	2	240.2	173.7	—
L-Glutamic Acid	536.4[a]	15, 16	241.3	174.8	—
	536.9	12	—	—	—
	542.6	8	—	—	—
L-Glutamine	614.3[a]	15, 16	197.5	127.3	—
Glycine	230.5[a]	4, 5	128.4	90.3	—
	232.6	6	126.3	88.2	—
	233.4	3	—	—	—
	234.5	9	—	—	—
L-Isoleucine	855.8[a]	4, 5	152.5	83.0	—
D-Leucine	856.0	6	152.4	83.1	—
L-Leucine	856.0	6	152.4	83.1	—
	853.7[a]	15	154.6	85.4	—
DL-Leucine	855.2	6	153.2	83.9	—
	856.0	9	—	—	—
L-Methionine	664.8[a]	4, 14	181.2	120.9	—

L-Phenylalanine	1110.6	4	111.6	50.6	—
DL-Phenylalanine	1111.9	8	110.9	49.9	—
	1112.3	17	—	—	—
L-Serine	347.7	18	173.6	121.6	Calculated from structural factor -OH for -H on L-Alanine
Isoserine	343.8	3	177.5	125.5	Secondary alcohol. $-\Delta H_c^o$ lower than Serine expected
L-Threonine	490.7[a]	4	192.9	131.5	—
L-Tryptophan	1,345.2[a]	4	99.2	28.5	—
L-Tyrosine	1061.7	12	160.5	92.2	Agree with structural change-OH for -H on L-Phenylalanine
	1058.3	6	—	—	—
	1070.8	10	—	—	—
L-Valine	698.3[a]	15, 5	147.7	85.8	—
DL-Valine	701.1	3	144.9	83.0	—
PEPTIDES					
DL-Alanylglycine	625.9	19	186.0	117.1	—
DL-Alanyl-DL-Phenylalanine	1505.4	20	169.8	77.4[b]	—
DL-Alanyl-DL-Phenylalanyl-glycine	1742.7	21	223.0	107.2[b]	—
Glycycl-DL-Alanyl-DL-phenylalanine	1744.2	20	221.5	105.7	—
Glycylglycine	471.4	19	178.1	116.6	—
	470.8	8	—	—	—
di-Glycylglycine	710.0	3	230.1	145.1[b]	—
tri-Glycylglycine	946.9	3	283.7	175.3[b]	—
Glycyl-DL-Phenylalanine	1349.2	20	163.6	79.1[b]	—
Glycyl-DL-Tryptophan	1586.2	21	148.8	54.7[b]	—
Glycyl-DL-Valine	937.0	20	199.6	115.3[b]	—
DL-Leucylglycine	1093.4	19	205.6	112.4	—
	1095.8	3	—	—	—
DL-Leucylglycylglycine	1333.7	8	258.8	139.7[b]	—
DL-Serylserine	692.7	20	281.5	192.4[b]	—
DL-Valyl-DL-Phenylalanine	1816.8	21	183.1	74.9[b]	—
MISCELLANEOUS					
Creatine	555.1	2	128.4	63.3	—
Creatinine	558.1	2	57.0	7.0	—
Urea	151.0	22	79.6	47.1	—

[a] Authors give only ΔE for bomb process. ΔH_c^o calculated by compiler.

[b] Calculated assuming $\Delta_{298.15} = 10.3$ cal deg^{-1} mole^{-1} for the reaction: Amino Acid (solid) + Amino Acid (solid) → Dipeptide (solid) + H_2O (liquid).

References

1. National Bureau of Standards Circular 500 (1961), *Selected Values of Chemical Thermodynamic Properties*, U.S. Gov. Print. Off., Washington, D.C.
2. Huffman, Ellis, and Fox, *J. Am. Chem. Soc.*, 58, 1728 (1936)
3. Wrede, *Z. Phys. Chem.*, 75, 81 (1910)
4. Tsuzuki, Harper, and Hunt, *J. Phys. Chem.*, 62, 1594 (1958).
5. Hutchens, Cole, and Stout, *J. Phys. Chem.*, 67, 1128 (1963).
6. Huffman, Fox, and Ellis, *J. Am. Chem. Soc.*, 59, 2144 (1937).
7. Landrieu, *Compt. Rend.*, 142, 580 (1906).
8. Fischer and Wrede, *Sitz. Kgl. Preuss. Akad. Wiss.*, p 687 (1904).
9. Stohmann and Langbein, *J. Prakt. Chem.*, 44, 336 (1891).
10. Emery and Benedict, *Am. J. Physiol.*, 28, 301 (1911).
11. Stohmann, *Z. Phys. Chem.*, 10, 410 (1892).
12. Oka, *Nippon Seirigaku Zasshi*, 9, 365 (1944).
13. Huffman and Ellis, *J. Am. Chem. Soc.*, 57, 41 (1935).
14. Hutchens, Cole, and Stout, *J. Biol. Chem.*, 239, 591 (1964).
15. Tsuzuki and Hunt, *J. Phys. Chem.*, 61, 1668 (1957).
16. Hutchens, Cole, Robie, and Stout, *J. Biol. Chem.*, 238, 2407 (1963).
17. Breitenbach, Derkosch, and Wessely, *Nature*, 169, 922 (1952).
18. Hutchens, Cole, and Stout, *J. Phys. Chem.*, 67, 1852 (1963).
19. Huffman, *J. Phys. Chem.*, 46, 885 (1952).
20. Ponomarev, Alekseeva, and Akimova, *Russ. J. Phys. Chem.* (Engl. Transl.), 36, 457 (1963).
21. Alekseeva and Ponomarev, *Russ. J. Phys. Chem.* (Engl. Transl.), 38, 731 (1964).
22. Huffman, *J. Am. Chem. Soc.*, 62, 1009 (1940).

This table originally appeared in Sober, Ed., *Handbook of Biochemistry and Selected Data for Molecular Biology*, 2nd ed., Chemical Rubber Co., Cleveland, 1970.

SOLUBILITIES OF AMINO ACIDS IN WATER AT VARIOUS TEMPERATURES

John O. Hutchens

The table gives the solubilities of the amino acids in grams per kilogram of water at various temperatures. None of the experimental observations were made at temperatures above 70°C. In most cases the experimental values were obtained both from a colder originally unsaturated solution and a warmer originally saturated solution. Even where four significant figures are given, many of the values probably are not reliable to better than 1 to 2% as judged by agreement between investigators. Lack of a value at a given temperature indicates that, in the opinion of the compiler, extrapolation of the curve from lower temperatures could not be justified.

SOLUBILITIES OF AMINO ACIDS IN WATER AT VARIOUS TEMPERATURES 0°–100° C (g/kg)

Substance	0°	10°	20°	30°	40°	50°	60°	70°	80°	90°	100°	References
L-Alanine	127.3	141.7	157.8	175.7	195.7	217.9	242.6	270.2	300.8	335.0	373.0	1, 2
DL-Alanine	121.1	137.8	156.7	178.3	202.9	230.9	262.7	299.0	340.1	387.0	440.4	1–3
L-Arginine · HCL	400.0	553.0	718.0	931.0	1240.0	—	—	—	—	—	—	2
L-Asparagine · H₂O	8.49	14.29	23.5	37.79	59.37	91.18	136.8	200.6	287.7	403.0	551.7	4
L-Aspartic Acid	1.72	2.82	4.18	5.94	8.38	11.99	17.01	24.14	34.25	48.59	68.93	1, 3
DL-Aspartic Acid	2.62	4.12	6.33	9.50	14.0	20.0	28.0	38.4	51.4	67.3	85.9	1, 3
L-Cystine	0.0502	0.0686	0.0938	0.1281	0.1751	0.2394	0.3272	0.4472	0.612	0.836	1.142	4
L-Diiodotyrosine	0.204	0.318	0.494	0.769	1.197	1.862	2.897	4.508	7.015	10.91	16.98	1
L-Glutamic Acid	3.29	4.98	7.20	10.19	14.70	—	—	—	—	—	—	2
DL-Glutamic Acid	8.55	12.13	17.22	24.47	34.75	49.34	70.06	99.50	141.3	200.8	284.9	1, 3
Glycine	141.8	180.4	225.2	275.9	331.6	391.0	452.6	513.9	572.7	626.2	671.7	1, 3
L-Hydroxyproline	288.6	315.6	345.2	377.6	413.0	451.7	494.1	540.4	591.0	646.5	706.9	5
L-Isoleucine	—[a]	32.0	33.6	35.4	37.5	—	—	—	—	—	—	2
DL-Isoleucine	18.26	19.52	21.23	23.50	26.47	30.3	35.39	42.01	50.75	62.37	78.02	1, 3
L-Leucine	22.70	23.01	23.74	24.90	26.58	28.87	31.89	35.84	40.98	47.65	56.38	1
DL-Leucine	7.97	8.56	9.39	10.51	12.03	14.06	16.78	20.46	25.46	32.38	42.06	1, 3
L-Lysine · HCL	462.0	556.0	666.0	799.0	965.0	—	—	—	—	—	—	2
L-Methionine	36.8	43.7	51.4	60.4	70.9	—	—	—	—	—	—	2
DL-Methionine	18.19	23.41	29.95	38.12	48.23	60.70	75.95	94.52	116.9	143.9	176.0	4
DL-Norleucine	8.43	9.43	10.71	12.36	14.49	17.27	20.88	25.7	32.02	40.60	52.29	1, 3
L-Phenylalanine	19.83	23.29	27.35	32.13	37.73	44.31	52.04	61.11	71.78	84.29	99.00	4
DL-Phenylalanine	9.97	11.33	13.07	15.29	18.15	21.87	26.71	33.12	41.66	53.16	68.8	1, 3
L-Proline	1274.0	1403.0	1545.0	1703.0	1876.0	2066.0	2277.0	2508.0	2764.0	3045.0	3355.0	5
L-Serine	133.0	247.0	362.0	476.0	592.0	—	—	—	—	—	—	2
DL-Serine	22.04	31.03	42.95	58.52	78.42	103.4	134.1	171.1	214.8	265.4	322.4	4
Taurine	39.31	59.92	87.84	123.8	167.8	218.8	274.2	330.5	383.1	427.0	457.6	4
L-Tryptophan	8.23	9.27	10.57	12.23	14.35	17.06	20.57	25.14	31.16	39.14	49.87	4
L-Tyrosine	0.196	0.274	0.384	0.537	0.752	1.052	1.473	2.1	2.884	4.036	5.7	1, 3
DL-Tyrosine	0.147	0.208	0.294	0.417	0.743	0.836	1.2	1.7	2.4	3.4	4.8	6
L-Valine	—[b]	53.7	56.5	59.7	63.6	—	—	—	—	—	—	2, 7
DL-Valine	59.6	63.3	68.1	74.2	81.7	91.1	102.8	117.4	135.8	158.9	188.1	1, 3

[a] Experimental value of 33 g/kg H₂O at 1°C.[2]
[b] Experimental value of 53.4 g/kg H₂O at 1°C.[2]

References

1. Dalton and Schmidt, *J. Biol. Chem.*, 103, 549 (1933).
2. *Hade*, Thesis, University of Chicago, December 1962.
3. Dunn, Ross, and Read, *J. Biol. Chem.*, 103, 579 (1933).
4. Dalton and Schmidt, *J. Biol. Chem.*, 109, 241 (1935).
5. Tomiyama and Schmidt, *J. Gen. Physiol.*, 19, 379 (1935).
6. Winnick and Schmidt, *J. Gen. Physiol.*, 18, 889 (1935).
7. Dalton and Schmidt, *J. Gen. Physiol.*, 19, 767 (1936).

This table originally appeared in Sober, Ed., *Handbook of Biochemistry and Selected Data for Molecular Biology*, 2nd ed., Chemical Rubber Co., Cleveland, 1970.

HEATS OF SOLUTION OF AMINO ACIDS IN AQUEOUS SOLUTION AT 25° C

John O. Hutchens

Enthalpy changes are given for: (1) Solution of the solid crystalline amino acid into the infinitely dilute solution $(\bar{H}_2^\circ - \bar{H}_2)$ (2) solution of the solid crystalline substance into saturated solution $(\bar{H}_2^\circ(\text{sat}) - \bar{H}_2^\circ)$ and (3) dilution of the saturated solution to infinite dilution $(\bar{H}_2^\circ - \bar{H}_2(\text{sat}))$. All entries are Kcal mole^{-1} and are for 25° C. Columns headed "cal" indicate direct calorimetric measurement. Columns headed "soly" indicate that the value was calculated from solubility and activity data. Generally speaking the two methods agree within the limits of error of either method.

The data suffer from multiple defects. The purity of many of the amino acids used in older work[1] is subject to question. Calculations from solubility data are handicapped by poor knowledge of activity coefficients, particularly for sparingly soluble amino acids. Some amino acids form hydrates, and it is not always clear that the solubility data are for the crystalline anhydrous form or that equilibrium has been reached as regards either crystalline form or solubility.

Compound	$(\bar{H}_2^\circ - \bar{H}_2)$		$(\bar{H}_2^\circ(\text{sat}) - \bar{H}_2^\circ)$		$(\bar{H}_2^\circ - \bar{H}_2(\text{sat}))$	Reference	Remarks
	cal	soly	cal	soly			
D-Alanine	—	1.83	—	1.83	0	1	Agrees with (2). Assumed $\partial \ln \gamma_m / \partial \ln m = 0$
L-Alanine	—	1.83	—	2.0	−0.2	2	Assumes $\partial \ln \gamma_N / \partial \ln N = 0.09$
DL-Alanine	2.0	2.2	2.2	2.2	−0.2	1	—
D-Arginine	1.5	—	1.1	—	0.4	1	—
L-Arginine·HCl	—	7.9	—	7.0	0.9	2	Assumes $\partial \ln \gamma_N / \partial \ln N = -0.245$
L-Asparagine	5.8	—	5.8	–	0	1	—
L-Asparagine·H$_2$O	8.0	8.4	8.0	—	0	1	—
	—	—	—	7.7	—	2, 3	—
L-Aspartic Acid	6.0	6.2	5.8	5.6	0.2?	1	Questionable assumption that $\partial \ln \gamma_N / \partial \ln m = 0.549$
	—	6.3	—	6.3	0	2, 3	Assumes $\partial \ln \gamma_N / \partial \ln N = 0$
DL-Aspartic Acid	7.1	7.2	6.9	6.5	0.2?	1	Questionable assumption that $\partial \ln \gamma_m / \partial \ln m = 0.549$
L-Cystine	—	5.5	—	—	—	1	Too sparsely soluble for reliable activity measurements
L-Diiodotyrosine	—	7.8	—	7.8	0	1	—
D-Glutamic Acid	—	6.5	6.3	6.0	—	1	Questionable assumption that $\partial \ln \gamma_m / \partial \ln m = 0.539$
DL-Glutamic Acid	6.5	6.2	6.3	5.7	0.2?	1	Questionable assumption that $\partial \ln \gamma_m / \partial \ln m = 0.539$
Glycine	3.8	3.4	3.4	3.4	0.4	1	$\partial \ln \gamma_m / \partial \ln m = 0.06$
L-Histidine	3.3	—	3.2	—	0.1	1	$\bar{H}_2^\circ - \bar{H}_2(\text{sat})$ from dilution of 0.5 M solution
L-Histidine·HCl	—	10.2	—	—	—	2	Activity data needed $\gamma_\pm \neq 1$
L-Hydroxyproline	1.4	1.4	1.4	—	<0.1	1	$\bar{H}_2^\circ - \bar{H}_2(\text{sat})$ from dilution of 2 M solution
D-Isoleucine	—	0.8	—	—	—	1	—
L-Isoleucine	—	0.9	—	0.9	<0.l	2	—
DL-Isoleucine	—	1.8	—	1.8	—	1	—
L-Leucine	—	0.8	—	0.8	—	1	Sample contained methionine
	—	1.0	—	1.0	<0.1	2, 3	—
DL-Leucine	—	2.0	—	2.1	−0.1	1	Questionable assumption that $\partial \ln \gamma_m / \partial \ln m = 0.38$
D-Lysine	−4.0	—	−3.5	–	−0.5	1	$\bar{H}_2^\circ - \bar{H}_2(\text{sat})$ (sat) from dilution of 1 M solution
L-Lysine·HCl	—	5.0	—	7.0	−2.0	2	Assumes $\partial \ln \gamma_N \partial \ln N = 0.44$
L-Methionine	—	2.8	—	2.8	<0.1	2	—
DL-Norleucine	—	2.5	—	2.5	—	1	—
L-Phenylalanine	—	2.8	—	–	—	1	—
	—	2.7	—	2.7	—	2, 3	Forms hydrate
DL-Phenylalanine	—	2.8	—	2.8	—	1	—
L-Proline	−0.8	1.3	>0.3	—	−1.0	1	$\bar{H}_2^\circ - \bar{H}_2(\text{sat})$ from dilution of 8 M solution
L-Serine·H$_2$O	—	4.6	—	3.7	0.9	2	—
L-Serine	2.8	—	—	—	—	4	$\bar{H}_2^\circ - \bar{H}_2(\text{sat})$ includes heat of hydration
DL-Serine	5.2	5.4	—	5.0	0.1	1	Must form hydrate in solution
L-Tryptophan	—	1.4	—	—	—	1	—
	—	—	—	2.5	—	3	Possibly forms hydrate
L-Tyrosine	—	6.0	—	6.0	—	1	—
D-Valine	—	0.5	—	—	—	1	—
L-Valine	—	0.9	—	1.0	−0.1	2, 3	—
DL-Valine	1.4	1.5	1.7	1.6	−0.3	1	Assumes $\partial \ln \gamma_m / \partial \ln m = -0.549$

References

1. Huffman and Borsook, in *Chemistry of the Amino Acids and Proteins*, Schmidt, Ed., C C Thomas, Springfield, Ill., 1938. A compilation, original references are cited.
2. *Hade*, Thesis, University of Chicago, December 1962.
3. Hade, E. P. K., *personal communication.*
4. Hutchens, J. O. and Hade, E. P. K., unpublished data.

This table originally appeared in Sober, Ed., *Handbook of Biochemistry and Selected Data for Molecular Biology*, 2nd ed., Chemical Rubber Co., Cleveland, 1970.

FREE ENERGIES OF SOLUTION AND STANDARD FREE ENERGY OF FORMATION OF AMINO ACIDS IN AQUEOUS SOLUTION AT 25° C

The table lists the molality (m, moles per kg of H_2O) of the saturated solution at 25°C (298.15 K); the appropriate molal activity coefficient (γ_m or $\gamma_m^{\pm}$); the free energy change for transporting one mole of the solute from the saturated solution to a hypothetical aqueous solution at an activity of 1 molal (ΔG soln); and the free energy change for formation of the substance in hypothetical 1 molal solution from the elements ($\Delta Gf°$). The units of ΔG soln and $\Delta Gf°$ are kcal mole^{-1}.

Substance	Saturated Solution mmole/kg	Reference	γ_m	Reference	ΔG soln kcal mole^{-1}	$-\Delta Gf°$ kcal mole^{-1}	Remarks
L-Alanine	1.862	1	1.045	2	−0.368	88.8	—
L-Arginine · HCl	4.061	1	0.587[a]	3	−1.03	—	Assumes 1:1 electrolyte ΔG solution = 2RT ln $(m_{\pm}\gamma_m^{\pm})$
L-Asparagine · H_2O	0.190	1	1.0	4	0.983	182.6	—
L-Aspartic Acid	0.0375	1	1.0	4	2.06	172.4	—
L-Cystine	4.57×10^{-4}	5	1.0	—	4.53	159.4	Activity coefficient assumed
L-Glutamic Acid	0.0586	1	1.0	4	1.77	173.0	—
L-Glutamine	0.291	6	1.0	4	0.731	126.6	—
Glycine	3.33	5	0.729	7	−0.525	90.8 / 88.7	Heats of combustion disagree
L-Hydroxyproline	2.75	5	1.05	8	−0.629	—	—
L-Isoleucine	0.263	1	1.0	4	0.791	82.2	—
L-Leucine	0.165	1	1.0	4	1.07	82.0 / 84.3	Heats of combustion disagree
L-Methionine	0.377	1	0.875	4	0.656	120.2	—
L-Phenylalanine	0.167	1	1.0	4	1.06	49.5	—
L-Proline	14.1	5	3.13	8	−2.24	—	Activity coefficient from extrapolation above m = 7.3
L-Serine	4.02	1	0.602	3	−0.524	122.1	—
L-Tryptophan	0.0666	1	1.0	4	1.60	26.9	—
L-Tyrosine	2.51×10^3	5	1.0	—	3.55	88.6	Activity coefficient assumed
L-Valine	0.496	1	0.923	4	0.461	85.3	—

[a] Activity coefficient is $\gamma_m^{\pm}$.

References

1. Hade, Thesis, University of Chicago, December 1962.
2. Smith and Smith, *J. Biol. Chem.*, 121, 607 (1937).
3. Hutchens, Figlio, and Granite, *J. Biol. Chem.*, 238, 1419 (1963).
4. Hutchens, J. O. and Nancy Norton, unpublished data.
5. Borsook and Huffman, in *The Chemistry of the Amino Acids and Proteins*, Schmidt, Ed., C C Thomas, Springfield, Ill., 1938.
6. Weast, Ed., *Handbook of Chemistry and Physics*, Chemical Rubber Co., Cleveland, Ohio, 1956.
7. Smith and Smith, *J. Biol. Chem.*, 117, 209 (1937).
8. Smith and Smith, *J. Biol. Chem.*, 132, 57 (1940).

This table originally appeared in Sober, Ed., *Handbook of Biochemistry and Selected Data for Molecular Biology*, 2nd ed., Chemical Rubber Co., Cleveland, 1970.

FAR ULTRAVIOLET ABSORPTION SPECTRA OF AMINO ACIDS

The absorption of a chromophoric amino acid in this spectral region is due to the combined absorptions of the side chain chromophore and of the carboxylate group. Because the carboxylate group is consumed in polymerizing amino acids to polypeptides, an amino acid residue absorbs less intensely than a free amino acid. The magnitude of this difference can be estimated from the spectra of the nonchromophoric amino acids – leucine, proline, alanine, serine, and threonine – whose total absorption is due only to the carboxylate group. The variations between the absorptions of these amino acids reflect the variability of carboxylate absorption in slightly different environments.

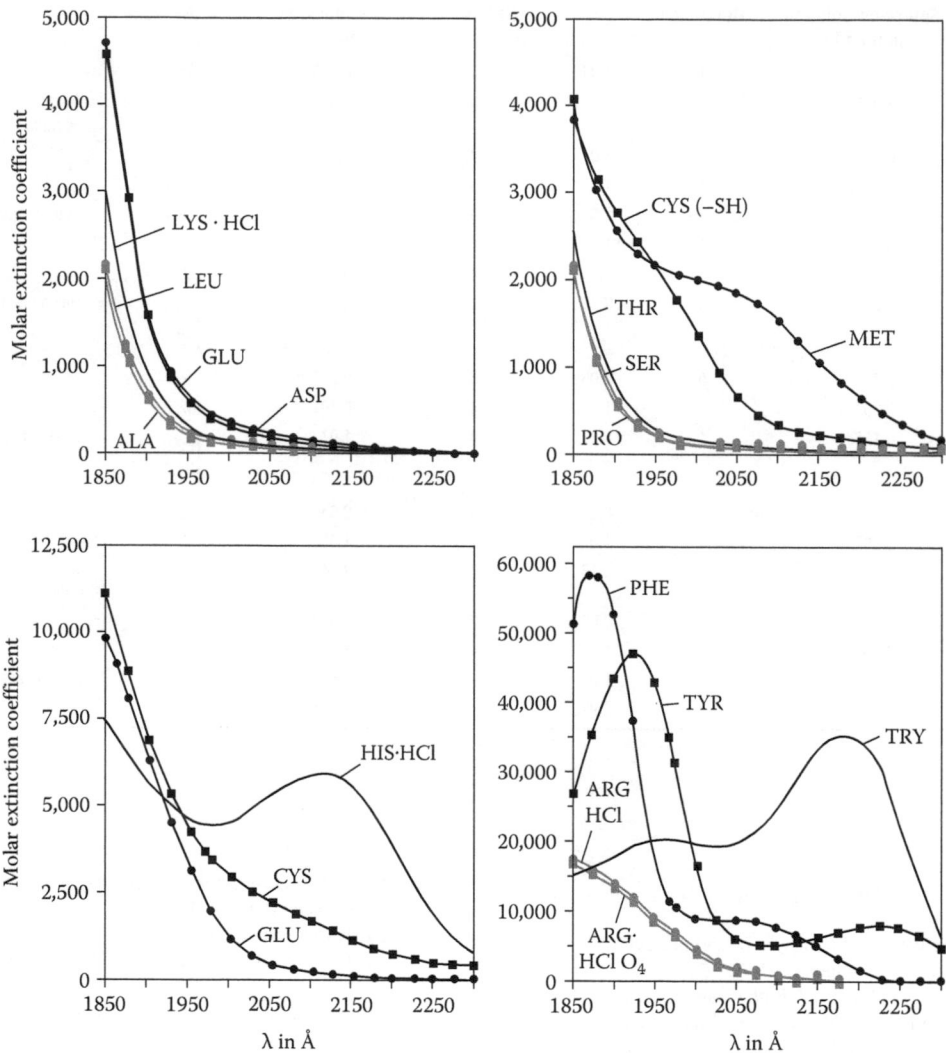

Far ultraviolet spectra of amino acids. All amino acids were in aqueous solution at pH 5, except cystine (pH 3). The dibasic amino acids were measured as hydrochlorides and the absorbance corrected by subtracting the absorbance contribution of chloride ion. Taken from Wetlaufer, *Adv. Protein Chem.*, 17, 320 (1962). With the permission of Academic Press and R. Sussman-McDiarmid and W. Gratzer.

FAR ULTRAVIOLET ABSORPTION SPECTRA OF AMINO ACIDS (Continued)

Amino Acid	$\lambda_{190.0}$	$\lambda_{197.0}$	$\lambda_{205.0}$	Maxima λ	Maxima ε	Minima λ	Minima ε	Shoulder λ	Shoulder ε
				Feature[a]					
				IN NEUTRAL WATER					
Tryptophan	17.60	20.50	19.60	196.7	20.60	203.3	19.40	–	–
	–	–	–	218.6	46.70	–	–	–	–
Tyrosine	42.80	35.50	5.60	192.5	47.50	208.0	4.88	–	–
	–	–	–	223.2	8.26	–	–	–	–
Phenylalanine	54.50	12.30	9.36	187.7	59.60	202.5	8.96	–	–
	–	–	–	206.0	9.34	–	–	–	–
Histidine[b]	5.57	4.35	5.17	211.3	5.86	198.4	4.22	–	–
Cysteine[c]	2.82	1.94	0.730	–	–	–	–	195.2	2.18
1/2 Cystine	3.25	1.76	1.05	–	–	–	–	207.0	0.96
Methionine	2.69	2.11	1.86	–	–	–	–	204.7	1.89
Arginine[c]	13.1	6.61	1.36	–	–	–	–	–	–
Acids[d]	1.61	0.460	0.230	–	–	–	–	–	–
Amides[d]	6.38	2.06	0.400	–	–	–	–	–	–
Lysine[b]	0.890	0.200	0.110	–	–	–	–	–	–
Leueine[d]	0.670	0.190	0.100	–	–	–	–	–	–
Alanine[d]	0.570	0.150	0.070	–	–	–	–	–	–
Proline[d]	0.540	0.150	0.070	–	–	–	–	–	–
Serine[d]	0.610	0.160	0.080	–	–	–	–	–	–
Threonine[d]	0.750	0.180	0.100	–	–	–	–	–	–
				IN 0.1 M SODIUM DODECYL SULFATE[d]					
Tryptophan	16.70	19.70	19.00	197.3	19.80	204.1	18.90	–	–
	–	–	–	220.0	46.60	–	–	–	–
Tyrosine	39.10	36.60	5.87	193.2	45.10	208.5	4.88	–	–
	–	–	–	223.7	7.86	–	–	–	–
Phenylalanine	54.10	11.30	8.45	188.3	57.0	201.5	7.79	–	–
	–	–	–	207.2	8.66	–	–	–	–
Histidine[b]	5.88	4.48	5.03	212.0	5.88	199.0	4.25	–	–
Cysteine[c]	2.66	1.79	0.650	–	–	–	–	194.5	2.15
1/2 Cystine	2.62	1.61	0.92	–	–	–	–	–	–
Methionine	2.67	2.10	1.84	–	–	–	–	204.1	1.89
Arginine[c]	12.50	5.70	0.94	–	–	–	–	–	–

Compiled by Ruth McDiarmid.

[a] Molar extinctions, $\varepsilon \times 10^{-3}$. Wavelength, λ, in millimicrons.

[b] The absorptions of lysine and histidine were determined for the hydrochlorides and corrected for the absorption of the chloride ion. $\varepsilon_{Cl^-} = 0.740$ ($\lambda = 190.0$), 0.050 ($\lambda = 197.0$) and $0 (\lambda = 205.0)$.

[c] The absorptions of cysteine and arginine were determined for the HClO$_4$ salt.

[d] The spectra of the carboxylic acids, the amides, the aliphatic, and the hydroxy amino acids and lysine are unchanged from those obtained in neutral water.

This figure and table originally appeared in Sober, Ed., *Handbook of Biochemistry and Selected Data for Molecular Biology*, 2nd ed., Chemical Rubber Co., Cleveland, 1970.

UV ABSORPTION CHARACTERISTICS OF *N*-ACETYL METHYL ESTERS OF THE AROMATIC AMINO ACIDS, CYSTINE, AND OF *N*-ACETYLCYSTEINE

	Water[a]		Ethanol[a]	
	λ	ε	λ	ε
Phenylalanine				
Inflection	(208)	10.20	(208)	10.40
Inflection	(217)	5.00	(217)	5.30
Minimum	240	0.080	244	0.088
Maximum	241.2	0.086	242.0	0.093
Maximum	246.5	0.115	247.3	0.114
Maximum	251.5	0.157	252.3	0.158
Maximum	**257.4**	**0.197**	**258.3**	**0.195**
Inflection	(260.7)	–	(261.2)	–
Maximum	263.4	0.151	264.2	0.155
Maximum	267.1	0.091	267.8	0.096
Tyrosine				
Maximum	193	51.70	–	–
Minimum	212	7.00	212	6.20
Maximum	224	8.80	227	10.20
Minimum	247	0.176	246	0.174
Maximum	**274.6**	**1.420**	**278.4**	**1.790**
Inflection	281.9	–	285.7	–
Tryptophan				
Minimum	205	21.40	206	21.30
Maximum	219	35.00	221	37.20
Minimum	245	1.900	245	1.560
Maximum	**279.8**	**5.600**	**282.0**	**6.170**
Maximum	288.5	4.750	290.6	5.330
Cystine				
Inflection	(250)	0.360	(253)	0.372
Inflection	260	0.280	260	0.320
Inflection	280	0.110	280	0.135
Inflection	300	0.025	300	0.035
Inflection	320	0.006	320	0.007
***N*-Acetylcysteine**				
	250	0.015	250	0.020
	280	0.005	280	0.005
	320	(nil)	320	(nil)

Compiled by W. B. Gtatzer.

[a] λ, wavelength in millimicrons; $\varepsilon \times 10^{-3}$, molar extinctions. Inflection denotes unresolved inflection.

From J. E. Bailey, Ph.D. Thesis, London University (1966).

NUMERICAL VALUES OF THE ABSORBANCES OF THE AROMATIC AMINO ACIDS IN ACID, NEUTRAL, AND ALKALINE SOLUTIONS

Molecular Absorbances of Tyrosine

nm[c]	Neutral[a]	Alkaline[b]	nm[c]	Neutral[a]	Alkaline[b]
230	4980	7752±108	276	1367±0	1206±4
232	3449	8667±38	278	1260±2	1344±5
234	1833±14	9634±19	280	1197±0	1507±5
236	1014±43	10440±20	282	1112±2	1675±5
238	571±36	11000±10	284	845±8	1850±6
240	349±34	11300±20	286	506±7	2024±4
240.5 ↑	–	11340±30	288	248±8	2179±5
242	252+20	11230±40	290	113±0	2300±7
244	209±18	10760±50	292	50±1	2367±5
245.3 ↓	202±20	–	293.2 ↑	–	2381±6
246	205±17	9918±78	294	23±1	2377±8
248	218±15	8734±72	296	13±0	2317±10
250	246±14	7382±56	298	8±1	2195±16
252	287±13	5844±77	300	6±0	2006±23
254	341±14	4471±55	302	5±1	1747±29
256	401±12	3360±46	304	3±0	1445±27
258	485±10	2476±20	306	2±1	1107±35
260	582±9	1883±17	308	1±0	800±27
262	693±13	1467±7	310	1±0	547±21
264	821±13	1204±14	312	–	346±15
266	960±14	1054±16	314	–	206±12
268	1083±13	985±13	316	–	118±9
269.3 ↓	–	974±8	318	–	67±5
270	1197±9	979±9	320	–	32±3
272	1310±9	1019±8	322	–	15±3
274	1394±6	1094±8	324	–	6±2
274.8 ↑	1405±7	–	326	–	1±1

Compiled by Elmer Mihalyi.

[a] 0.1 *M* phosphate buffer, pH 7.1.
[b] 0.1 *N* KOH.
[c] Maxima, minima, and inflection points are indicated by ↑, ↓, and ~.

Reprinted with permission from *J. Chem. Eng. Data*, 13, 179 (1968). Copyright 1968 American Chemical Society.

Molecular Absorbances of Tryptophan

nm[c]	Neutral[a]	Alkaline[b]	nm[c]	Neutral[a]	Alkaline[b]
230	6818	13200	279.0 ↑	5579±14	–
232	4037±60	7470	280	5559±12	5377±43
234	2772±71	4354±81	280.4 ↑	–	5385±34
236	2184±64	2951±50	282	5323±10	5302±34
238	1904±55	2282±29	284	4762±11	4962±42
240	1764±52	1959±30	285.8 ↓	4471±6	–
242.0 ↓	1737±49	1813±25	286	4482±11	4596±22
244	1772±48	1773±29	286.8 ↓	–	4565±27
244.4 ↓	–	1763±29	287.8 ↑	4650±12	–
246	1869±40	1792±27	288	4646±16	4634±19
248	2018±35	1877±23	288.3 ↑	–	4639±28
250	2217±32	2013±25	290	3935±5	4393±32
252	2462±19	2187±37	292	2732±5	3551±46
254	2760±27	2410±38	294	1824±5	2666±27
256	3087±20	2664±25	296	1211±10	1990±24
258	3422±18	2953±39	298	797±4	1472±19
260	3787±17	3261±34	300	510±1	1064±19
262	4142±14	3586±46	302	314±3	755±16
264	4472±10	3895±32	304	184±2	517±10
266	4777±14	4212±48	306	112±4	333±6
268	5020±15	4481±46	308	55±9	217±4
270	5220±8	4742±37	310	27±11	129±5
272	5331±5	4933±45	312	11±8	84±8
272.1 ↑	5344±5	–	314	3±2	53±7
273.6 ↓	5329±10	–	316	–	31±7
274	5341±8	5025±34	318	–	17±4
274.5 ~	–	5062±38	320	–	8±2
276	5431±8	5108±39	322	–	3±4
278	5554±12	5275±46			

Compiled by Elmer Mihalyi.

[a] 0.1 M phosphate buffer, pH 7.1.

[b] 0.1 N KOH.

[c] Maxima, minima, and inflection points are indicated by ↑, ↓, and ~.

Reprinted with permission from *J. Chem. Eng. Data*, 13, 179 (1968). Copyright 1968 American Chemical Society.

Molecular Absorbances of Phenylalanine

nm[c]	Neutral[a]	nm[c]	Alkaline[b]	nm[c]	Neutral[a]	nm[c]	Alkaline[b]
230	32.8±1.5	230	161.9±1.9	257.6 ↑	195.1±1.5	257	188.4±2.8
232	32.1±1.6	232	99.2±1.9	258	193.4±1.3	258	209.1±0.3
234	35.6±2.1	234	70.7±2.4	259	171.9±1.0	258.2 ↑	209.6±0.2
236	42.8±2.1	236	63.3±2.7	260	147.0±0.6	260	184.2±1.0
238	48.5±2.3	238	62.3±2.6	261.9 ↓	127.7±1.5	260.7 ~	178.6±0.3
240	59.4±2.0	240	68.9±3.2	262	128.1±1.4	262	157.8±0.9
242 ~	72.2±2.3	242	83.0±2.8	263.7 ↑	151.5±0.6	262.7 ↓	105.5±1.3
		243 ~	85.4±2.9	264	148.7±0.4	263.9 ↑	161.2±1.0
244	80.1±2.1	244	89.0±3.0	265	119.8±1.3	264	160.0±2.1
246	102.0±0.6	246	108.9±2.8	266	91.8±1.4	266	114.3±1.6
247.4 ↑	110.7±2.2	247	120.9±1.5	266.8 ~	85.6±1.5	266.5 ↓	109.7±1.8
248	109.8±1.9	248.0 ↑	126.1±1.4			267.7 ↑	117.7±1.8
248.3 ↓	109.5±2.0	248.7 ↓	125.1±1.7	268	74.7±1.0	268	115.0±1.0
250	123.5±2.6	250	132.7±1.8	270	30.0±1.8	270	50.2±2.0
251	143.0±2.8	251	149.3±1.9	272	14.3±1.0	272	18.7±1.1
252	153.9±1.0	252	167.0±1.1	274	5.4±0.3	274	7.4±0.3
252.2 ↑	154.1±1.0	252.9 ↑	171.5±1.3	276	2.2±0.4	276	2.6±0.4
254	139.6±1.0	254	166.3±0.8	278	1.1±0.5	278	0.7±0.3
254.5 ↓	138.5±1.4	254.9 ↓	162.8±1.7	280	0.7±0.3	280	0.4±0.2
256	156.5±2.2	256	168.4±1.9				

Compiled by Elmer Mihalyi.

[a] 0.1 *M* phosphate buffer, pH 7.1.

[b] 0.1 *N* KOH.

[c] Maxima, minima, and inflection points are indicated by ↑, ↓, and ~.

Alkaline[b] vs. Neutral[a] Difference Spectra of Tyrosine, Tryptophan, and Phenylalanine

nm	Tyrosine	Tryptophan	Phenylalanine	nm	Tyrosine	Tryptophan	Phenylalanine
230	3041	4135	123.9	280	315±1	−191±18	−
232	5440	3213	66	282	558±1	−24±4	−
234	7608	1621	35.4	284	994±10	194±3	−
236	9415	732±35	20.7	286	1513±11	110±10	−
238	10490	345±23	13.9	288	1936±1	11±3	−
240	11060	149±21	9.9	290	2196±14	467±8	−
242	11090	45±15	11.1	292	2331±15	802±3	−
244	10660	−40±15	8.8	294	2357±7	830±8	−
246	9844	−104±11	9.0	296	2307±6	755±10	−
248	8567	−172±10	16.4	298	2194±7	652±13	−
250	7205	−233±9	8.3	300	2002±3	527±5	−
252	5671	−298±16	15.3	302	1754±2	413±11	−
254	4344	−371±10	25.8	304	1437±2	300±14	−
256	3127	−435±14	11.3	306	1097±9	205±8	−
258	2142	−490±19	19.1	308	792±14	137±5	−
260	1368±37	−535±13	37.8	310	526±13	88±3	−
262	820±36	−564±8	26.9	312	334±9	55±8	−
264	420±25	−580±10	16.1	314	221±19	22±14	−
266	125±20	−573±12	22.4	316	101±7	16±10	−
268	−78±18	−539±14	42.8	318	62±2	5±2	−
270	−225	−486±12	17.4	320	28±4	0	−
272	−296	−394±12	4.0	322	12±5	−	−
274	−299	−308±7	1.7	324	3±4	−	−
276	−158	−312±16	0.3	326	1±1	−	−
278	89±5	−278±13	0	328	0	−	−

Compiled by Elmer Mihalyi.

[a] 0.1 *M* phosphate buffer, pH 7.1.
[b] 0.1 *N* KOH.

Reprinted with permission from *J. Chem. Eng. Data*, 13, 179 (1968). Copyright 1968 American Chemical Society.

Acid[b] vs. Neutral[a] Difference Spectra of Tyrosine, Tryptophan, and Phenylalanine

nm	Tyrosine	Tryptophan	Phenylalanine	nm	Tyrosine	Tryptophan	Phenylalanine
230	—	—	46.7	276	−40	128±16	0
232	576	421±49	34.1	278	−45	110±10	—
234	441	610±37	23.3	280	−34	71±11	—
236	346	590±31	16.0	282	−46	−23±7	—
238	218	512±29	10.8	284	−73	−92±9	—
240	108	432±23	6.9	286	−71	−3±9	—
242	40	358±19	3.9	288	−49	−26±4	—
244	4	305±20	3.3	290	−31	−250±5	—
246	−13	263±21	1.2	292	−20	−317±9	—
248	−18	240±16	−0.3	294	−16	−276±9	—
250	−20	223±14	2.5	296	−14	−227±5	—
252	−16	216±17	−1.8	298	−12	−177±7	—
254	−12	219±15	−1.9	300	−10	−131±9	—
256	−7	222±11	4.0	302	−9	−88±6	—
258	−5	223±14	−3.3	304	−7	−59±8	—
260	−3	225±14	−4.3	306	−6	−40±10	—
262	0	232±13	2.5	308	−4	−24±10	—
264	0	232±18	−3.1	310	−3	−13±10	—
266	−4	224±15	−3.4	312	−2	−7±7	—
268	−8	214±7	−4.4	314	−1	−4±4	—
270	−11	190±9	−2.0	316	−1	0	—
272	−13	159±12	−0.7	318	−0	—	—
274	−20	127±15	−0.3				

Compiled by Elmer Mihalyi.

[a] 0.1 *M* phosphate buffer, pH 7.1.
[b] 0.1 *N* HCl.

From *J. Chem. Eng. Data*, 13, 179 (1968). With permission of the author and copyright owner.

HYDROPHOBICITIES OF AMINO ACIDS AND PROTEINS

C. C. Bigelow and M. Channon

TABLE 1: Hydrophobicities of Amino Acids

The hydrophobicity of an amino acid side chain is derived from the measurement of the solubility of the amino acid in water and an organic solvent.[1,2] The data are converted into the molar free energy of transfer for the amino acid from an aqueous solution to a solution in the organic solvent at the same mole fraction at the limit of infinite dilution:

$$\Delta F_t = RT \ \ln \frac{N_w \gamma_w}{N_{org} \gamma_{org}}$$

The hydrophobicity of the side chain, HΦ, is then determined by subtracting ΔF_t for glycine. The thermodynamic interpretation of the hydrophobicity has been discussed by Noaki and Tanford.[2]

Amino Acid	HΦ (cal/mol)	Amino Acid	HΦ (cal/mol)
Trp	3,400	Cys/2	1,000
Ile	2,950	Arg	750
Pro	2,600	His	500
Phe	2,500	Ala	500
Tyr	2,300	Thr	400
Leu	1,800	Gly	0
Val	1,500	Asp	0[a]
Lys	1,500	Glu	0[a]
Met	1,300	Ser	−300

Compiled by C. C. Bigelow and M. Channon.

[a] Assumed values.

References

1. Tanford, *J. Am. Chem. Soc.*, 84, 4240 (1962).
2. Nozaki and Tanford, *J. Biol. Chem.*, 246, 2211 (1971).

TABLE 2: Average Hydrophobicities of Selected Proteins

The values in the table have been calculated for proteins from amino acid compositions in the literature. Proteins have been included only if the content of all the amino acids is known. The selection has been guided by a desire to include proteins of different properties (globular and fibrous, aggregating and monomeric) as well as members of some families of related proteins.

$$H\Phi_{ave} = \frac{\sum_i n_i H\Phi_i}{\sum_i n_i}$$

where

n_i = the number of residues of the ith amino acid;
$H\Phi_i$ = its hydrophobicity from Table 1.[475, 476]

	Protein	Average Hydrophobicity	Reference
1	Acetoacetic acid decarboxylase (*Clostridium acetobutylicum*)	1,140	1
2	Acetylcholine receptor (*Electrophorus electricus*)	1,060	2
3	Acetylcholinesterase (*Electrophorus electricus*)	990	3
4	*N*-Acetyl-β-D-glucosaminidase-A (beef spleen)	930	5
6	*N*-Acetyl-β-D-glucosaminidase-B (beef spleen)	930	5
7	*N*-Acetyl-β-D-glucosaminidase-A (porcine kidney)	1,040	6
8	*N*-Acetyl-β-D-glucosaminidase-B (porcine kidney)	1,030	6
9	*N*-Acetyl-β-D-glucosaminidase (human plasma)	960	7
10	Acetylornithine γ-transaminase (*Escherichia coli*)	930	8
11	O-Acetylserine sulfhydrylase A (*Salmonella typhimurium*)	1,020	9
12	α$_1$-Acid glycoprotein (human plasma)	1,040	10
13	Actin (*Acanthamoeba castellani*)	1,030	11
14	Actin (beef carotid)	1,000	12
15	Actin (beef heart muscle)	980	13

TABLE 2: Average Hydrophobicities of Selected Proteins (Continued)

	Protein	Average Hydrophobicity	Reference
16	Actin (beef skeletal muscle)	980	13
17	Actin (brown trout)	1,000	14
18	Actin (chicken)	1,010	13
19	Actin (fish)	980	13
20	Actin (frog)	980	13
21	Actin (human platelet)	950	15
22	Actin (human uterus)	980	16
23	Actin (lamb)	980	13
24	Actin (mollusc)	910	13
25	Actin (pig)	990	13
26	Actin (rabbit muscle)	1,010	17
27	Actin (rabbit muscle)	1,000	18
28	Actin (sheep uterus)	990	16
29	Acylcarrier protein (*Escherichia coli*)	830	19
30	Acylphosphatase (bovine brain)	980	20
31	Acylphosphatase (horse muscle)	900	21
32	Adenosine and adenosine monophosphate deaminase (*Aspergillus oryzae*)	890	22
33	Adenosine deaminase (calf intestinal muscle)	1,010	23
34	Adenosine deaminase (calf spleen)	990	24
35	Adenosine monophosphate deaminase (rabbit muscle)	1,060	22
36	Adenosine monophosphate nucleosidase (*Azotobacter vinelandii*)	770	25
37	Adenosine triphosphatase, (Na$^+$ + K$^+$), large chain (canine renal medulla)	1,040	26
38	Adenosine triphosphatase, (Na$^+$ + K$^+$), small chain (canine renal medulla)	1,130	26
39	Adenosine triphosphate-creatine transphosphorylase (rabbit)	980	27
40	Adenylate cyclase (*Brevibacterium liquefaciens*)	880	28
41	Adenylosuccinate – AMP-lyase (*Neurospora* sp.)	940	29
42	Adrenodoxin (bovine)	850	30
43	Adrenodoxin reductase (bovine adrenal gland)	940	31
44	Aequorin (*Aequorea*)	990	32
45	Agglutinin (wheat germ)	680	33
46	Alanine amino transferase (rat liver)	990	34
47	Albumin (bovine plasma)	1,000	35
48	Albumin (dog plasma)	990	36
49	Albumin (human serum)	960	37
50	Albumin (rat serum)	980	38
51	Alcohol dehydrogenase (horse liver)	1,030	39
52	Aldehyde dehydrogenase, protein A (Baker's yeast)	1,020	40
53	Aldolase B (rabbit liver)	940	41
54	Aldolase C (rabbit brain)	980	41
55	Aldolase, fructose-1,6 -diphosphate (*Boa constrictor constrictors*)	970	42
56	Aldolase, fructose-1,6-diphosphate (*Discostichus mawsonii*)	980	43
57	Aldolase, fructose-1,6-dophosphate (*Gallus domesticus*, brain)	920	44
58	Aldolase, fructose-1,6-diphosphate (*Gallus domesticus*, breast muscle)	960	45
59	Aldolase, fructose-1,6-diphosphate (*Gallus domestricus*, liver)	970	46
60	Aldolase, fructose diphosphate (*Micrococcus aerogenes*)	940	47
61	Aldolase, fructose-1,6-diphosphate (ox)	970	48
62	Aldolase, fructose-1,6-diphosphate (porcine)	960	48
63	Aldolase, fructose-1,6-diphosphate (rabbit liver)	960	49
64	Aldolase, fructose-1,6-diphosphate (rabbit, muscle)	960	48
65	Aldolase, fructose-1,6-diphosphate (sturgeon)	990	48
66	Aldolase, fructose-1,6-diphosphate (*Trematomus borchgrevinki*)	980	43
67	Aldolase, fructose-1,6-diphosphate (yeast)	990	50
68	Aldolase, 2-keto-3-deoxy-6-phosphogluconate (*Pseudomonas putida*)	1,090	51
69	Alkaline phosphatase (*Bacillus licheniformis* MC 14)	940	52
70	Alkaline phosphatase (*Escherichia coli*)	810	53
71	Alkaline proteinase-B (*Streptomyces rectus proteolyticus*)	820	54
72	ω-Amidase (rat liver)	980	55
73	Amino acid decarboxylase, aromatic (porcine kidney)	1,050	56
74	D-Amino acid oxidase (porcine kidney)	1,050	57
75	Aminopeptidase (*Aeromonas proteolytica*)	860	58
76	Aminotripeptidase, TP-2 (porcine kidney)	1,090	59
77	Amylase (*Bacillus macerans*)	910	60
78	Amylase (rat pancreas)	970	61
79	Amylase PI (rabbit pancreas)	940	62
80	Amylase PII (rabbit pancreas)	950	62
81	Amylase PIII (rabbit pancreas)	930	62

TABLE 2: Average Hydrophobicities of Selected Proteins (Continued)

	Protein	Average Hydrophobicity	Reference
82	Amylase (rabbit parotid)	940	62
83	α-Amylase (*Aspergillus aryzae*)	990	63
84	α-Amylase (*Bacillus stearothermophilus*)	970	64
85	α-Amylase (*Bacillus subtilis*)	970	65
86	α-Amylase (porcine pancreas)	1,040	66
87	α-Amylase (human saliva)	940	67
88	α-Amylase-I (porcine pancreas)	960	68
89	α-Amylase-II (porcine pancreas)	970	68
90	Anthranylate synthetase, component I (*Pseudomonas putida*)	1,020	69
91	Anthranylate synthetase, component II (*Pseudomonas putida*)	950	69
92	Apo-high density lipoprotein (bovine plasma)	960	70
93	Apolipoprotein – alanine-I (human plasma)	830	71
94	Apolipoprotein – alanine-II (human plasma)	830	71
95	Apolipoprotein – glutamine-I (human plasma)	870	72
96	Apolipoprotein – glutamine-I (porcine plasma)	890	72
97	Apolipoprotein – glutamine-II (human plasma)	970	73
98	Apolipoprotein-valine (human plasma)	920	74
99	Apovitellinin-I (*Dromaeus novaehollandiae*)	1,210	75
100	α-L-Arabinofuranosidase (*Aspergillus niger* K1)	900	76
101	L-Arabinose-binding protein (*Escherichia coli* B/r)	1,020	77
102	L-Arabinose isomerase (*Escherichia coli*)	990	78
103	Arginine decarboxylase (*Escherichia coli*)	980	79
104	Arginine kinase (*Callinectus sapidus*)	940	80
105	Arginine kinase (*Homarus americanus*)	980	81
106	Arginine kinase, negative (*Limulus polyphemus*)	950	80
107	Arginine kinase, neutral (*Limulus polyphemus*)	970	80
108	Arginine kinase (*Pagurus bernhardus*)	970	80
109	Asparaginase (*Escherichia coli* B)	870	82
110	Asparaginase (guinea pig)	970	83
111	L-Asparaginase (*Proteus vulgaris*)	950	84
112	Aspartate aminotransferase (ox heart)	980	85
113	Aspartate aminotransferase (rat brain, cytoplasm)	1,050	86
114	Aspartate aminotransferase (rat brain, mitochondria, fraction II)	990	86
115	Aspartate aminotransferase (rat brain, mitochondria, fraction III)	990	86
116	Aspartate-β-decarboxylase (*Alcaligenes faecalis*)	1,010	87
117	Aspartate-β-decarboxylase (*Pseudomonas dacunhae*)	1,020	88
118	Aspartate transcarbamylase, catalytic chain (*Escherichia coli*)	990	89
119	Aspartate transcarbamylase, regulatory chain (*Escherichia coli*)	980	89
120	Aspartokinase, lysine sensitive (*Escherichia coli* K-12, HfrH)	940	90
121	Aspergilliopeptidase B (*Aspergillus oryzae*)	810	91
122	Avidin (chicken egg)	930	92
123	Azurin (*Pseudomonas fluorescens*)	880	93
124	Azurin (*Pseudomonas polymyxa*)	970	94
125	Biotin carboyxyl carrier protein (*Escherichia coli*)	1,300	95
126	Blastokinin (rabbit)	1,030	96
127	Bradykininogen (bovine)	980	97
128	α-Bungarotoxin (*Bungarus multicintus*)	1,040	98
129	C_1-inactivator (human plasma)	1,020	99
130	Calcitonin (bovine)	1,080	100
131	Calcitonin (human)	1,100	101
132	Calcitonin (porcine)	1,100	102
133	Calcitonin (salmon)	860	103
134	Calcium-binding protein (bovine adrenal medulla)	780	104
135	Calcium-binding protein (chick duodenal mucosa)	930	105
136	Calcium-binding protein-B (parvalbumin) (*Cyprinus carpio* muscle)	890	106
137	Calcium-binding protein (porcine brain)	740	107
138	Carbamyl phosphate synthetase (*Escherichia coli* B)	960	108
139	Carbonic anhydrase (bovine)	1,000	109
140	Carbonic anhydrase (*Gallus domesticus*)	1,000	110
141	Carbonic anhydrase (parsley)	1,100	111
142	Carbonic anhydrase (sheep)	990	112
143	Carbonic anhydrase B (bovine)	950	113
144	Carbonic anhydrase B (equine)	940	114
145	Carbonic anhydrase B (*Macaca mulata*)	960	115
146	Carbonic anhydrase B (porcine)	1,000	116
147	Carbonic anhydrase C (equine)	960	114

TABLE 2: Average Hydrophobicities of Selected Proteins (Continued)

	Protein	Average Hydrophobicity	Reference
148	Carbonic anhydrase C (porcine)	1,010	117
149	β-Carboxy-cis,cis-muconate lactonizing enzyme (*Pseudomonas putida*)	940	118
150	γ-Carboxymuconolactone decarboxylase (*Pseudomonas putida*)	1,170	119
151	Carboxypeptidase A (bovine pancreas)	1,010	120
152	Carboxypeptidase A (*Penaeus setiferus*)	910	121
153	Carboxypeptidase B (*Penaeus setiferus*)	940	121
154	Carboxypeptidase B (*Protopterus aethiopicus*)	1,010	122
155	Procarboxypeptidase B (*Protopterus aethiopicus*)	990	122
156	Carboxypeptidase B (dogfish pancreas)	1,070	123
157	Carboxypeptidase Y (yeast)	1,050	124
158	Carboxytransphosphorylase (propionic acid bacteria)	950	125
159	Catalase (bovine liver)	1,110	126
160	Colchicine-binding protein (sea urchin)	930	127
161	Colchicine-binding protein (porcine brain)	930	128
162	Chorionic gonadotropin-α (human)	960	126
163	Chorionic gonadotropin-β (human)	1,120	130
164	Chorismate mutase-prephenate dehydratase (*Escherichia coli* K-12)	990	131
165	Chymoelastase, lysine free (*Streptomyces griseus* K-1)	720	132
166	Chymoelastase, guanidine stable (*Streptomyces griseus* K-1)	760	132
167	Chymotrypsin anionic (fin whale)	1,060	133
168	Chymotrypsin II (human)	940	134
169	Chymotrypsinogen A (dogfish)	1,010	135
170	Chymotrypsinogen B (bovine pancreas)	950	136
171	Chymotrypsinogen B (porcine pancreas)	1,010	137
172	Chymotrypsinogen C (porcine pancreas)	970	137
173	Cocoonase (*Antheraea pernyi*)	840	138
174	Cocoonase (*Antheraea polyphemus*)	860	138
175	Prococoonase (*Antheraea polyphemus*)	840	138
176	Colicin I$_a$-CA53 (*Escherichia coli*)	880	139
177	Colicin I$_b$-P9 (*Escherichia coli*)	940	139
178	Collagen (chicken tendon)	880	140
179	Collagen, α-fraction (calf skin)	880	141
180	Collagen, spongin B (sponge)	760	142
181	Collagen (sturgeon swim bladder)	770	143
182	Collagenase (*Uca pugilator*)	920	144
183	Conalbumin (chicken)	980	145
184	Corrinoid protein (*Clostridium thermoaceticum*)	890	146
185	Creatine kinase (*Cyprinus carpio* L.)	960	147
186	Creatine kinase (human)	970	148
187	Crotonase (*Clostridium acetobutylicum*)	970	149
188	Crotoxin (*Crotalus terrificus terrificus*)	970	150
189	Cystathionase (rat liver)	980	151
190	Cytochrome b$_s$ (bovine liver)	1,000	152
191	Cytochrome b$_s$ (equine liver)	970	152
192	Cytochrome b$_s$ (porcine liver)	900	152
193	Cytochrome c (horse heart)	1,050	153
194	Cytochrome c (chicken)	1,050	154
195	Cytochrome c (cow, pig, sheep)	1,020	154
196	Cytochrome c (dog)	1,070	154
197	Cytochrome c (kangaroo)	1,130	154
198	Cytochrome c (king penguin)	1,060	154
199	Cytochrome c (*Macaca mulata*)	1,060	154
200	Cytochrome c (moth)	1,060	154
201	Cytochrome c (pigeon)	1,070	154
202	Cytochrome c (rabbit)	1,070	154
203	Cytochrome c (rattlesnake)	1,050	154
204	Cytochrome c (*Saccharomyces*)	1,040	154
205	Cytochrome c (tuna)	1,050	154
206	Cytochrome c (turkey)	1,050	154
207	Cytochrome CA (*Humicola lanuginosa*)	910	155
208	Cytochrome C$_3$ (*Desulfovibrio desulfuricans*)	920	156
209	Cytochrome C$_3$ (*Desulfovibrio gigas*)	870	157
210	Cytochrome C$_3$ (*Desulfovibrio salexigens*)	840	157
211	Cytochrome C$_3$ (*Desulfovibrio vulgaris*)	840	158
212	Cytochrome 553 (*Monochysis lutheri*)	730	159
213	Daunorubicin reductase (rat liver)	1,100	160

TABLE 2: Average Hydrophobicities of Selected Proteins (Continued)

	Protein	Average Hydrophobicity	Reference
214	3-Deoxy-ᴅ-arabinoheptulosonate 7-phosphate synthetase-chorismate mutase (*Bacillus subtillis*)	1,000	161
215	Deoxycytidylate deaminase (T₂ r⁺ bacteriophage)	970	162
216	Deoxyribonuclease (bovine pancreas)	930	163
217	Deoxyribonuclease A (bovine pancreas)	970	164
218	Deoxyribonuclease B (bovine pancreas)	980	164
219	Deoxyribonuclease C (bovine pancreas)	980	164
220	Deoxyribonuclease II (porcine spleen)	1,050	165
221	Deoxyribonucleic acid ligase (*Escherichia coli*)	970	166
222	Deoxyribonucleotidase inhibitor II (calf spleen)	1,010	167
223	α-Dialkylamino transamidase (*Pseudomonas cepacia*)	930	168
224	Dihydrofolate reductase (T₄ bacteriophage)	1,030	169
225	Dihydrofolate reductase (*Escherichia coli* MB 1428)	1,030	170
226	Dihydrofolate reductase (*Lactobacillus casei*)	1,010	171
227	Dihydrofolate reductase (*Streptococcus faecium*)	1,060	172
228	3,4-Dihydroxyphenylacetate-2,3-oxygenase (*Pseudomonas ovalis*)	980	173
229	Dopamine-β-hydroxylase (bovine adrenal)	950	174
230	Elastin (bone aorta)	940	175
231	Elastin (bovine ear cartilage)	990	175
232	Elastin (bovine ligamentum nuchae)	980	175
233	Encephalitogenic A-1 protein (bovine brain)	850	176
234	Encephalitogenic A-1 protein (human brain)	820	176
235	Endopolygalacturonase (*Verticillium albo-atrum*)	850	177
236	Enolase (monkey muscle)	970	178
237	Enolase (*Onkorhynchus keta*)	980	179
238	Enolase (*Onkorhynchus kisutch*)		
239	Enolase (rabbit muscle)	990	180
240	Enolase (*Thermus* X-1)	900	181
241	Enolase (*Thermus aquaticus* YT-1)	770	182
242	Enolase (yeast)	890	183
243	Enterotoxin C (*Staphylococcus* 137)	990	184
244	Enterotoxin E (*Staphylococcus aureus* FRI-326)	940	185
245	Enterotoxin A (*Staphylococcus aureus* 13N-2909)	980	186
246	Erythrocuprein (human)	740	187
247	Esterase (pig liver)	1,100	188
248	Estradiol dehydrogenase (human placenta)	940	189
249	Factor III lac (*Staphylococcus aureus*)	850	190
250	Factor VIII (bovine plasma)	1,030	191
251	Factor VIII (human plasma)	990	192
252	Ferredoxin (*Chlorobium thiosulfatophilum*)	910	193
253	Ferredoxin (*Clostridium pasteurianium*)	920	194
254	Ferredoxin (*Chromatium*)	870	195
255	Ferredoxin (*Cyperus rotundus*)	900	196
256	Ferredoxin (*Desulfoyibrio gigas*)	930	196
257	Ferredoxin (*Spinacea*)	850	197
258	Ferredoxin (*Scenedesmus*)	800	198
259	Ferredoxin I (*Azotobacter vinelandii*)	1,050	199
260	Ferredoxin I (*Bacillus polymxa*)	920	200
261	Ferredoxin II (*Bacillus polymxa*)	920	200
262	Ferritin (horse spleen)	900	201
263	Ferritin (tadpole red blood cell)	850	202
264	Fibrinogen B (lobster)	990	203
265	Fibroin (*Bombyx mori*)	330	204
266	Fibroin (*Tussah*)	430	204
267	Ficin II (*Ficus glabrata*)	930	205
268	Ficin III (*Ficus glabrata*)	960	205
269	Flagellin (*Proteus vulgaris*)	730	206
270	Flagellin (*Salmonella* SJ 25)	680	207
271	Flagellin (*Salmonella typhimurium*)	700	208
272	Flavodoxin (*Clostridium* MP)	1,010	209
273	Flavodoxin (*Clostridium pasteurianium*)	820	210
274	Flavodoxin (*Desulfovibrio gigas*)	890	211
275	Flavodoxin (*Desulfovibrio vulgaris*)	870	212
276	Flavodoxin (*Peptostreptococcus elsdenii*)	870	213
277	Follicle stimulating hormone (ovine)	900	214
278	*N*-formimino-ʟ-glutamate iminohydrolase (*Pseudomonas* ATCC 11299b)	930	215
279	Fructose-1,6-diphosphatase (porcine kidney)	1,010	216

TABLE 2: Average Hydrophobicities of Selected Proteins (Continued)

	Protein	Average Hydrophobicity	Reference
280	β-Galactosidase (*Escherichia coli*)	970	217
281	Gastricin (human)	920	218
282	Gastricin (porcine)	1,100	219
283	Gliadin SP 2-2 (Cappelle 1966 flour)	1,300	220
284	Gliadin SP 2-1 (wheat, Wichita 1963)	1,250	220
285	Gliadin SP 2-2 (wheat, Wichita 1963)	1,180	220
286	Gliadin SP 2-3 (wheat, Wichita 1963)	1,180	220
287	Globulin, 0.6 S γ_2 (human plasma)	1,090	221
288	Glucagon (bovine)	810	222
289	Glutamate decarboxylase (*Escherichia coli*)	1,080	223
290	Glutamate dehydrogenase (bovine liver)	1,000	224
291	Glutamate dehydrogenase (*Neurospora crassa*)	880	225
292	Glutaminase-asparaginase (*Achromobacteraceae*)	960	226
293	Glutamine synthetase (rate liver)	1,010	227
294	γ-Glutamyl cyclotransferase (porcine liver)	960	228
295	Glyceraldehyde-3-phosphate dehydrogenase (*Bacillus stearothermophilus*)	940	229
296	Glyceraldehyde-3-phosphate dehydrogenase (bovine liver)	980	230
297	Glycerol-3-phosphate dehydrogenase (rabbit muscle)	1,040	231
298	Glycocyamine kinase (*Nepthys coeca*)	990	232
299	Glycogen phosphorylase (Baker's yeast)	1,050	233
300	Glycogen phosphorylase (*Carcharhinus falciformis*)	1,080	234
301	Glycogen phosphorylase (human)	1,060	235
302	Glycogen phosphorylase (rabbit liver)	1,060	236
303	Glycogen phosphorylase (rat)	1,070	237
304	Glycogen synthetase (porcine kidney)	870	238
305	γ-Glycoprotein (human plasma)	1,070	239
306	Growth hormone (human)	950	240
307	Haptoglobin, α_2-chain (human plasma)	960	241
308	Haptoglobin, α_{1S}-chain (human plasma)	990	241
309	Haptoglobin, β-chain (human plasma)	1,020	242
310	Hemagglutinin (*Lens esculenta Muench*)	1,000	243
311	Hemagglutinin I (*Pisum sativum L. var. pyram*)	990	244
312	Hemagglutinin II (*Pisum sativum L. var. pyram*)	930	244
313	Hemagglutinin (*Robina pseudoaccacia*)	990	245
314	Hemagglutinin II (snail)	1,070	246
315	Hemagglutinin (soy)	990	247
316	Hemagglutinin (*Ulex europeus*)	950	248
317	Hemerythrin (*Golfingia gouldii*)	1,170	249
318	Hemocyanin (*Cancer magister*)	1,000	250
319	Hemocyanin (*Crustaceae C. sapidus*)	980	251
320	Hemocyanin (*Crustaceae E. spinifrons*)	980	251
321	Hemocyanin (*Crustaceae H. vulgaris*)	980	251
322	Hemocyanin (*Crustaceae P. vulgaris*)	980	251
323	Hemocyanin (*Mollusca E. moschata*)	1,050	251
324	Hemocyanin (*Mollusca M. brandaris*)	1,000	251
325	Hemocyanin (*Mollusca M. tranculus*)	1,010	251
326	Hemocyanin (*Mollusca O. macropus*)	1,050	251
327	Hemocyanin (*Mollusca O. vulgaris*)	1,080	251
328	Hemocyanin (*Xiphosura L. polyphemus*)	980	251
329	Hemoglobin (*Ascaris* body wall)	980	252
330	Hemoglobin (*Entosphenus japonicus*)	1,010	253
331	Hemoglobin (*Glycera dibranchiata*)	870	254
332	Hemoglobin, α-chain (*Catostomus clarkii*)	1,100	255
333	Hemoglobin, α-chain (human)	960	256
334	Hemoglobin, γ-chain (bovine)	960	256
335	Hemoglobin, γ-chain (human)	960	256
336	Hemoglobin, F-1 (*Eptatretus burgeri*)	1,170	258
337	Hemoglobin, F-2 (*Eptatretus burgeri*)	1,160	258
338	Hemoglobin, F-3 (*Eptatretus burgeri*)	1,140	258
339	Hemoglobin, F-4 (*Eptatretus burgeri*)	1,040	258
340	Hemopexin (human)	1,020	259
341	Hemopexin (rabbit)	1,010	259
342	High potential iron sulfur protein (*Chromatium vinosum* D)	880	260
343	High potential iron sulfur protein (*Thiocapsa pfennigii*)	930	261
344	Histidine: ammonia lyase (*Pseudomonas* ATCC 11299b)	890	262
345	Histidine-binding protein (*Salmonella typhimurium*)	970	263

TABLE 2: Average Hydrophobicities of Selected Proteins (Continued)

	Protein	Average Hydrophobicity	Reference
346	Histidine decarboxylase (*Lactobacillus* 30a)	980	264
347	L-Histidinol phosphate aminotransferase (*Salmonella typhimurium*)	970	265
348	Histidyl-tRNA synthetase (*Salmonella typhimurium*)	940	266
349	Histone III (Calf thymus)	990	267
350	Histone III (*Letiobus bubalus*)	980	268
351	Histone III (pea)	980	269
352	Histone III (rainbow trout)	950	270
353	Hyaluronidase (bovine testicular)	1,030	271
354	Hydrogenase (*Clostridium pasteurianium* W5)	1,160	272
355	3-Hydroxyacyl coenzyme A dehydrogenase (porcine heart muscle)	960	273
356	β-Hydroxybutyrate dehydrogenase (bovine heart mitochondria)	930	274
357	α¹-Hydroxysteroid dehydrogenase (*Pseudomonas testosteroni*)	900	275
358	17-β-Hydroxysteroid dehydrogenase (human placenta)	910	276
359	Immunoglobulin, Eu heavy chain (human plasma)	980	277
360	Immunoglobulin, Eu light chain (human plasma)	860	277
361	Immunoglobulin, New λ-chain (human plasma)	870	278
365	Inorganic pyrophosphatase (yeast)	1,130	279
363	Insulin (bovine)	1,020	280
364	Insulin (cod)	1,110	281
365	Inverfase (*Saccharomyces* FH4C)	990	282
366	Isoamylase I (porcine pancreas)	960	283
367	Isoamylase II (porcine pancrease)	970	283
368	Isocitrate dehydrogenase (*Azotobacter vinelandii* ATCC 9104)	980	284
369	Isocitrate dehydrogenase (porcine liver)	990	285
370	Isomerase I (rabbit)	1,080	286
371	Isomerase II (rabbit)	1,100	286
372	Keratinase (*Trichophyton mentagrophytes*)	880	287
373	Δ⁵-3-Ketosteroid isomerase (*Pseudomonas testosteronii*)	910	288
374	α-Lactalbumin (bovine milk)	1,050	289
375	Lactoferrin (bovine)	920	290
376	β-Lactoglobulin (caprid)	1,040	291
377	β-Lactoglobulin A (bovine)	1,070	291
378	β-Lactoglobulin A (ovine)	1,050	291
379	β-Lactoglobulin A (bovine)	1,060	291
380	β-Lactoglobulin A (ovine)	1,050	291
381	β-Lactoglobulin C (bovine)	1,070	292
382	Lactoperoxidase (bovine milk)	1,080	292
383	Lectin, α-D-galactosyl-binding (*Bandeiraea simplicifola*)	980	293
384	Leghemoglobin I (soyaben root nodule)	1,010	294
385	Leghemoglobin II (soyaben root nodule)	1,010	294
386	Leucine aminopeptidase (bovine lens)	1,010	295
387	Lipase (rat pancreas)	980	61
388	β-Lipolytic hormone (porcine pituitary)	950	296
389	γ-Lipolytic hormone (sheep)	780	297
390	α-Lipovitellin (chicken egg yolk)	980	298
391	Luciferase (*Renilla reniformis*)	940	299
392	Luciferase-α (MAV)	880	300
393	Luciferase-β (MAV)	960	300
394	Luciferase-α (*Photobacterium fischeri*)	960	300
395	Luciferase-β (*Photobacterium fischeri*)	990	300
396	Luteinizing hormone-α chain (equine)	1,070	301
397	Luteinizing hormone-β chain (equine)	1,120	301
398	Lysine decarboxylase (*Escherichia coli*)	1,080	302
399	L-Lysine monooxygenase (*Pseudomonas fluorescens*)	1,040	303
400	Lysostaphin (*Staphylococcus aureus*)	950	304
401	Lysozyme (*Chalaropsis*)	960	305
402	Lysozyme, chick type (black swan)	970	306
403	Lysozyme, goose type (black swan)	930	306
404	Lysozyme (chicken)	890	307
405	Lysozyme (papaya)	1,080	308
406	Lysozyme (turkey)	910	309
407	Lysyl: tRNA ligase (*Escherichia coli*)	990	310
408	Lysyl: tRNA ligase (yeast)	1,040	310
409	α-Lytic protease (*Sorangium* sp.)	780	311
410	β-Lytic protease (*Sorangium* sp.)	820	311

TABLE 2: Average Hydrophobicities of Selected Proteins (Continued)

	Protein	Average Hydrophobicity	Reference
411	Melate dehydrogenase (*Bacillus subtillis*)	970	312
412	Malate-lactate transhydrogenase (*Micrococcus lactilyticus*)	960	313
413	Malate-vitamin K reductase (*Mycobacterium phleii*)	890	314
414	L-Malic enzyme (*Escherichia coli*)	1,020	315
415	β-Melanocyte stimulating hormone (bovine)	1,180	316
416	Melilotate hydroxylase (*Pseudomonas* sp.)	970	317
417	Methionyl-tRNA synthetase (*Escherichia coli*)	1,040	318
418	β-Methyl aspartase (*Clostridium tetanomorphum*)	980	319
419	β-Methylcrotonylcoenzyme A carboxylase (*Achromobacter*)	890	320
420	Methylmalonatesemialdehydedehydrogenase (*Pseudomonas aeruginosa*)	1,030	321
421	Molydbenum-iron protein (soyaben root nodule bacteroid)	1,010	322
422	Monellin (*Dioscoreophyllum cumminsii*)	1,140	323
423	Motilin (porcine intestinal mucosa)	1,020	324
424	cis,cis-Muconate lactonizing enzyme (*Pseudomonas putida*)	990	325
425	Muconolactone isomerase (*Pseudomonas putida*)	1,070	325
426	Mutarotase (bovine kidney cortex)	850	326
427	Myoglobin (human)	1,000	327
428	Myoglobin (whale)	1,040	328
429	Myoglobin (*Zalophus californianus*)	1,030	329
430	Myohemery thrin (*Dendrostamum pyroides*)	1,090	330
431	Myosin (bovine heart)	880	331
432	Myosin (cod)	860	332
433	myosin (rabbit)	890	333
434	myosin (tuna)	880	333
435	Neocarzinostatin (*Streptomyces carzinostaticus* F-41)	750	334
436	Neurophysin I (bovine pituitary)	850	335
437	Neurophysin II (bovine pituitary)	830	335
438	Neurophysin III (bovine pituitary)	820	336
439	Neurotoxin I (*Androctonus australis*)	1,070	337
440	Neurotoxin II (*Androctonus australis*)	990	337
441	Neurotoxin III (*Androctonus australis*)	1,120	337
442	Neurotoxin I (*Leiurus quinquestriatus quinquestriatus*)	1,040	337
443	Neurotoxin II (*Leiurus quinquestriatus quinquestriatus*)	970	337
444	Neurotoxin III (*Leiurus quinquestriatus quinquestriatus*)	1,030	337
445	Neurotoxin IV (*Leiurus quinquestriatus quinquestriatus*)	1,050	337
446	Neurotoxin V (*Leiurus quinquestriatus quinquestriatus*)	1,020	337
447	Nuclease (Micrococcus sodonecis ATCC 11880)	880	338
448	Nuclease (*Staphylococcus*)	980	339
449	Nucleoside diphosphokinase (Brewer's yeast)	1,030	340
450	Nucleoside phosphotransferase-A-chain (carrot)	920	341
451	Nucleoside phosphotransferase-B-chain (carrot)	860	341
452	5′-Nucleotidase (*Escherichia coli*)	930	342
453	Ornithine transcarbamylase (bovine liver)	1,040	343
454	Ornithine transcarbamylase (*Streptococcus faecalis*)	990	343
455	Ovalbumin (chicken egg)	980	145
456	Ovomacroglobulin (chiken egg)	1,040	344
457	Ovomucin (chicken egg)	990	345
458	Ovomucoid (chicken egg)	830	145
459	Ovotransferrin (chicken egg)	960	346
460	2-Oxoglutarate dehydrogenase (porcine heart)	1,010	347
461	Oxytocin (mammalian)	1,290	348
462	Papain (papaya)	1,030	349
463	Parathyroid hormone (bovlne)	900	350
464	Parvalbumin (rabbit skeletal muscle)	920	351
465	Penicillocarboxypeptidase-S (*Penicillium janthinellum*)	980	352
466	Pepsin (bovine)	940	353
467	Pepsin (human)	930	218
468	Pepsin I (*Rhizopus chinensis*)	910	354
469	Pepsin II (*Rhizopus chinensis*)	910	354
470	Pepsin A (bovine)	960	355
471	Pepsinogen A (*Mustelus canis*)	920	356
472	Pepsinogen A (porcine)	970	357
473	Pepsinogen C (porcine)	1,020	358
474	Phenylalanine ammonia lyase (*Solanum tuberosum*)	1,030	359
475	Phenylalanine ammonia lyase (*Zea mays* L.)	940	359
476	Phenylalanine hydroxylase (rat liver)	930	360

TABLE 2: Average Hydrophobicities of Selected Proteins (Continued)

	Protein	Average Hydrophobicity	Reference
477	Phosphatidyl serine decarboxylase (*Escherichia coli*)	1,050	361
478	Phosphoenol pyruvate carboxykinase (yeast)	1,030	362
479	Phosphofructokinase (chicken liver)	940	363
480	Phosphoglucomutase (rabbit muscle)	1,020	364
481	Phosphoglucose isomerase (human)	1,020	365
482	Phosphoglucose isomerase (rabbit muscle)	1,010	366
483	Phosphoglycerate kinase (human erythrocyte)	980	367
484	Phospholipase A (*Bitis gabonica* venom)	910	368
485	Phospholipase A$_1$ (*Crotalus adamanteus*)	1,030	369
486	Phospholipase A$_2$ (*Crotalus atrox*)	920	370
487	Phospholipase A (*Laticuda semifasciata*)	950	371
488	Phosphorylase (frog skeletal muscle)	1,070	372
489	Phycocyanin (*P. calothricoides*)	910	93
490	Phycocyanin (*S. lividicus*)	1,040	93
491	Phycoerythrin (*P. tenera*)	830	373
492	Phytochrome (oat)	1,010	374
493	Plastocyanin (parsley)	880	375
494	Prealbumin (human serum)	990	376
495	Prealbumin, Pt 1-1 (monkey)	990	377
496	Prealbumin, Pt 2-2 (monkey)	1,010	377
497	Procarboxypeptidase A (bovine)	1,010	378
498	Procarboxypeptidase A (*Squalus acanthias*)	1,010	379
499	Progesterone-binding protein (guinea pig plasma)	1,040	380
500	Prohistidine decarboxylase (*Lactobacillus* 30a)	990	381
501	Prolactin (ovine pituitary)	950	382
502	Protease (*Bacillus thermoprotolyticus*)	940	383
503	Protease (*Mucor miehei* CBS 370.65)	940	384
504	Protease (*Staphylococcus aureus* V8)	900	385
505	Protease – A$_1$ (*Streptomyces griseus*)	700	386
506	Protease-acid (*Rhizopus chinensis*)	950	387
507	Protein kinase modulator (lobster tail muscle)	720	388
508	Prothrombin (bovine)	960	389
509	Protyrosinase (Rana pipiens pipiens	1,100	390
510	Putidaredoxin (*Pseudomonas putida*)	910	391
511	Putrescine oxidase (*Micrococcus rubens*)	860	392
512	Pyruvate kinase (bovine skeletal muscle)	1,010	393
513	Quinonoid dihydropterin reductase (sheep liver)	890	394
514	Retinol-binding protein (human)	960	395
515	Retinol-binding protein (monkey)	960	396
516	Rhodopsin (bovine)	1,120	397
517	Riboflavin-binding protein (chicken)	910	398
518	Ribonuclease (*Aspergillus fumigatus*)	830	399
519	Ribonuclease (*Bacillus subtilis*)	1,000	400
520	Ribonuclease (bovine pancreas)	780	401
521	Rubonuclease (ovine pancreas)	750	402
522	Ribonuclease Ch. (*Chalaropsis sp.*)	940	403
523	Ribonuclease N (*Neurospora crassa*)	890	404
524	Ribonuclease R$_1$ (*Rhizopus oligosporus*)	970	405
525	Ribonuclease R$_2$ (*Rhizopus oligosporus*)	960	405
526	Ribonuclease T$_1$ (*Aspergillus oryzae*)	740	406
527	Ribonuclease U$_1$ (*Ustilago sphaerogena*)	760	407
528	Ribonucleotide reductase (*Lactobacillus leichmanii*)	960	408
529	Ribulose diphosphate carboxylase (*Hydrogenomonas eutropha*)	980	409
530	Ribulose diphosphate carboxylase (*Hydrogenomonas facilis*)	980	409
531	Ribulose diphosphate carboxylase (*Rhodospirillum rubrum*)	940	410
532	Rubredoxin (*Clostridium pasteurianum*)	990	411
533	Rubredoxin (*Micrococcus aerogenes*)	1,120	412
534	Rubredoxin (*Pseudomonas oleovorans*)	960	413
535	D-Serine dehydratase (*Escherichia coli*)	920	414
536	Streptokinase (human plasma)	980	415
537	Subtilisin BPN (*Bacillus subtilis*)	810	416
538	Succinyl coenzyme A synthetase (*Escherichia coli*)	970	417
539	Sucrose synthetase (*Phaseolus aureus*)	1,040	418
540	Superoxide dismutase (*Neurospora crassa*)	760	419
541	Thermolysin (*Bacillus thermoproteolyticus*)	890	420
542	Thioredoxin (T-4 bacteriophage)	1,150	421

TABLE 2: Average Hydrophobicities of Selected Proteins (Continued)

	Protein	Average Hydrophobicity	Reference
543	Thioredoxin II (yeast)	960	422
544	Thrombin (bovine)	1,040	423
545	Thymidylate synthetase (T-2 bacteriophage)	1,140	424
546	Thyroglobulin (calf)	950	425
547	Thyroglobulin (human)	950	425
548	Thyroglobulin (porcine)	950	425
549	Thyroglobulin (rabbit)	920	425
550	Thyroglobulin (sheep)	950	425
551	Thyroid stimulating hormone – α-chain (human)	1,010	426
552	Thyroid stimulating hormone – β-chain (human)	1,170	426
553	Toxin FVII (*Dendroaspis angusticeps*)	890	427
554	Toxin α (*Dendroaspis polylepsis*)	940	428
555	Toxin γ (*Dendroaspis polylepsis*)	1,000	428
556	Toxin 4 (*Enhydrina schistosa*)	760	429
557	Toxin 5 (*Enhydrina schistosa*)	710	429
558	Toxin (*Laticauda colubrina*)	790	430
559	Toxin (*Laticauda laticauda*)	790	430
560	Toxin a (*Laticauda semifasciata*)	880	431
561	Toxin b (*Laticauda semifasciata*)	930	431
562	Toxin (*Naja haje haje*)	830	432
563	Toxin b (*Naja melanoleuca*)	1,090	433
564	Toxin d (*Naja melanoleuca*)	830	433
565	Toxin (*Naja naja atra*)	680	434
566	Toxin (*Naja nigricollis*)	930	435
567	α-Toxin A (*Staphylococcus aureus* Woods 46)	890	436
568	α-Toxin B (*Staphylococcus aureus* Woods 46)	890	436
569	Transaminase B (*Salmonella typhimurium*)	980	437
570	Transcortin (guinea pig)	960	438
571	Transcortin (human)	970	438
572	Transcortin (rabbit)	960	440
573	Transcortin (rat)	1,030	440
574	Transferrin (bovine)	930	441
575	Transferrin (equine)	970	441
576	Transferrin (human)	930	442
577	Transferrin (porcine serum)	970	441
578	Transferrin (rabbit serum)	970	441
579	Triose phosphate dehydrogenase (*Bombus nevadensis*)	1,040	443
580	Triose phosphate dehydrogenase (honey bee)	1,020	443
581	Triose phosphate dehydrogenase (lobster)	980	443
582	Triose phosphate dehydrogenase (porcine)	990	443
583	Triose phosphate isomerase-I (human erythrocyte)	920	444
584	Triose phosphate isomerase-III (human erythrocyte)	940	444
585	Triose phosphate isomerase (rabbit muscle)	930	445
586	Triose phosphate isomerase (yeast)	970	446
587	Troponin-C (rabbit muscle)	780	447
588	Troponin-T (rabbit muscle)	1,040	447
589	Trypsin (*Evasterias trochelli*)	1,000	448
590	Trypsin (lungfish)	920	449
591	Trypsin (human)	870	450
592	Trypsin, anionic (human)	930	451
593	Trypsin (porcine)	970	452
594	Trypsin (sheep)	850	453
595	Trypsin (shrimp)	840	454
596	Trypsin (*Streptomyces griseus*)	820	455
597	Trypsin inhibitor (*Ascaris lumbricoides suis*)	970	456
598	Trypsin inhibitor (bovine pancreas)	1,150	457
599	Trypsin inhibitor (porcine pancreas)	900	458
600	Trypsin inhibitor (bovine pancreas)	1,070	459
601	Trypsin inhibitor I (*Phaseolus vulgaris*)	800	460
602	Trypsin inhibitor II (*Phaseolus vulgaris*)	780	460
603	Trypsinogen (bovine)	910	461
604	Trypsinogen (dogfish)	950	462
605	Trypsinogen (lungfish)	930	449
606	Trypsinogen, anionic (porcine)	980	463
607	Trypsinogen (sheep)	900	464
608	Tryptophan synthetase A (*Escherichia coli*)	1,060	465

TABLE 2: Average Hydrophobicities of Selected Proteins (Continued)

	Protein	Average Hydrophobicity	Reference
609	Tryptophan synthetase – α-chain (*Aerobacter aerogenes*)	1,060	466
610	Tryptophan synthetase – α-chain (*Bacillus subtilis*)	1,020	467
611	Tryptophan synthetase – α-chain (*Salmonella typhimurium*)	980	466
612	Tryptophan synthetase – β-chain (*Bacillus subtilis*)	940	468
613	Tryptophanase (*Bacillus alvei*)	980	469
614	Tryptophanase (*Escherichia coli* B/1t7-A)	1,030	470
615	Tyrosyl-tRNA synthetase (*Bacillus stearo thermophilus*)	1,060	471
616	Urease (jackbean meal)	990	472
617	Urokinase S-1 (human urine)	1,030	473
618	Urokinase S-2 (human urine)	990	473
619	Valine:tRNA ligase (yeast)	1,080	310
620	Vasopressin, lysine (mammalian)	1,210	474

Complied by C. C. Bigelow and M. Channon.

References

1. Lederer, Courts, Laursen, and Westheimer, *Biochemistry*, 5, 823 (1966).
2. Klett, Fulpius, Cooper, Smith, Reich, and Possani, *J. Biol. Chem.*, 248, 6841 (1973).
3. Rosenberry, Chang, and Chen, *J. Biol. Chem.*, 247, 1555 (1972).
4. Mega, Ikenaka, and Matsushima, *J. Biochem.* (Tokyo), 68, 109 (1970).
5. Verpoorte, *J. Biol. Chem.*, 247, 4787 (1972).
6. Wetmore and Verpoorte, *Can. J. Biochem.*, 50, 563 (1972).
7. Verpoorte, *Biochemistry*, 13, 793 (1974).
8. Forsyth, Theil, and Jones, *J. Biol. Chem.*, 245, 5354 (1970).
9. Becker, Kredich, and Tomkins, *J. Biol. Chem.*, 244, 2418 (1969).
10. Ikenaka, Ishiguro, Emura, Kaufman, Isemura, Bauer, and Schmid, *Biochemistry*, 11, 3817 (1972).
11. Weihing and Korn, *Biochemistry*, 10, 590 (1971).
12. Gosselin-Rey, Gerady, Gaspar-Godfroid, and Carsten, *Biochim. Biophys. Acta*, 175, 165 (1969).
13. Carsten and Katz, *Biochim. Biophys. Acta*, 90, 534 (1964).
14. Bridgen, *Biochem. J.*, 123, 591 (1971).
15. Booyse, Hoveke, and Rafelson, Jr., *J. Biol. Chem.*, 248, 4083 (1973).
16. Carsten, *Biochemistry*, 4, 1049 (1965).
17. Adelstein and Kuehl, *Biochemistry*, 9, 1355 (1970).
18. Elzinga, *Biochemistry*, 9 1365 (1970).
19. Vanaman, Wakil, and Hill, *J. Biol. Chem.*, 243, 6420 (1968).
20. Diederich and Grisolia, *J. Biol. Chem.*, 244, 2412 (1969).
21. Ramponi, Guerritore, Treves, Nassi, and Baccari, *Arch. Biochem. Biophys.*, 130, 362 (1969).
22. Wolfenden, Tomozawa, and Bamman, *Biochemistry*, 7, 3965 (1968).
23. Phelan, McEvoy, Rooney, and Brady, *Biochim. Biophys. Acta*, 200, 370 (1970).
24. Pfrogner, *Arch. Biochem. Biophys.*, 119, 147 (1967).
25. Schramm and Hochstein, *Biochemistry*, 11, 2777 (1972).
26. Kyte, *J. Biol. Chem.*, 247, 7642 (1972).
27. Noltmann, Mahowald, and Kuby, *J. Biol. Chem.*, 237, 1146 (1962).
28. Takai, Kurashina, Suzuki-Hori, Okamoto, and Hayashi, *J. Biol. Chem.*, 249, 1965 (1974).
29. Woodward and Braymer, *J. Biol. Chem.*, 241, 580 (1966).
30. Tanaka, Haniu, and Yasunobu, *J. Biol. Chem.*, 248, 1141 (1973).
31. Chu and Kimura, *J. Biol. Chem.*, 248, 2089 (1973).
32. Shimomura and Johnson, *Biochemistry*, 8, 3991 (1969).
33. Nagata and Burger, *J. Biol. Chem.*, 249, 3116 (1974).
34. Matsuzawa and Segal, *J. Biol. Chem.*, 243, 5929 (1968).
35. Pederson and Foster, *Biochemistry*, 8, 2357 (1969).
36. Allerton, Elwyn, Edsall, and Spahr, *J. Biol. Chem.*, 237, 85 (1962).
37. McMenamy, Dintzis, and Watson, *J. Biol. Chem.*, 246, 4744 (1971).
38. Peters, Jr., *J. Biol. Chem.*, 237, 2182 (1962).
39. Jornvall, *Eur. J. Biochem.*, 16, 25 (1970).
40. Steinman and Jakoby, *J. Biol. Chem.*, 243, 730 (1968).
41. Penhoet, Kochman, and Rutter, *Biochemistry*, 8, 4396 (1969).
42. Schwartz and Horecker, *Arch. Biochem. Biophys.*, 115, 407 (1966).
43. Komatsu and Feeney, *Biochim. Biophys. Acta*, 206, 305 (1970).
44. Marquardt, *Can. J. Biochem.*, 48, 322 (1970).
45. Marquardt, *Can. J. Biochem.*, 47, 527 (1969).
46. Marquardt, *Can. J. Biochem.*, 49, 658 (1971).
47. Lebherg, Bradshaw, and Rutter, *J. Biol. Chem.*, 248, 1660 (1973).
48. Anderson, Gibbons, and Perham, *Eur. J. Biochem.*, 11, 503 (1969).
49. Rutter, Woodfin, and Blostein, *Acta Chem. Scand.*, 17, S226 (1963).
50. Harris, Kobes, Teller, and Rutter, *Biochemistry*, 8, 2442 (1969).
51. Robertson, Hammerstedt, and Wood, *J. Biol. Chem.*, 246, 2075 (1971).
52. Hulett-Cowling and Campbell, *Biochemistry*, 10, 1364 (1971).
53. Christen, Vallee, and Simpson, *Biochemistry*, 10, 1377 (1971).
54. Mizusawa and Yoshida, *J. Biol. Chem.*, 247, 6978 (1972).
55. Hersh, *Biochemistry*, 10, 2884 (1971).
56. Christenson, Dairman, and Udenfriend, *Arch. Biochem. Biophys.*, 141, 356 (1970).
57. Tu and McCormick, *J. Biol. Chem.*, 248, 6339 (1973).
58. Prescott, Wilkes, Wagner, and Wilson, *J. Biol. Chem.*, 246, 1756 (1971).
59. Chenoweth, Brown, Valenzuela, and Smith, *J. Biol. Chem.*, 248, 1684 (1972).
60. DePinto and Campbell, *Biochemistry*, 7, 114 (1968).
61. Vandermeers and Christophe, *Biochim. Biophys. Acta*, 154, 110 (1968).
62. Malacinski and Rutter, *Biochemistry*, 8, 4382 (1969).
63. Stein, Junge, and Fischer, *J. Biol. Chem.*, 235, 371 (1960).
64. Pfueller and Elliott, *J. Biol. Chem.*, 244, 48 (1967).
65. Junge, Stein, Neurath, and Fischer, *J. Biol. Chem.*, 234, 556 (1959).
66. Caldwell, Dickey, Hanrahan, Kung, Kung, and Misko, *J. Am. Chem. Soc.*, 76, 143 (1954).
67. Muus, *J. Am. Chem. Soc.*, 76, 5163 (1954).
68. Cozzone, Paséro, Beaupoil, and Marchis-Mouren, *Biochim. Biophys. Acta*, 207, 490 (1970).
69. Queener, Queener, Meeks, and Gunsalus, *J. Biol. Chem.*, 248, 151 (1973).
70. Jonas, *J. Biol. Chem.*, 247, 7767 (1972).
71. Morrisett, David, Pownall, and Gotto, Jr., *Biochemistry*, 12, 1290 (1973).
72. Jackson, Baker, Taunton, Smith, Garner, and Gotto, Jr., *J. Biol. Chem.*, 248, 2639 (1973).
73. Lux, John, and Brewer, Jr., *J. Biol. Chem.*, 247, 7510 (1972).
74. Brown, Levy, and Fredrickson, *J. Biol. Chem.*, 245, 6588 (1970).
75. Burley, *Biochemistry*, 12, 1464 (1973).
76. Kaji and Tagawa, *Biochim. Biophys. Acta*, 207, 456 (1970).
77. Parsons and Hogg, *J. Biol. Chem.*, 249, 3602 (1974).
78. Patrick and Lee, *J. Biol. Chem.*, 244, 4277 (1969).
79. Boeker, Fischer, and Snell, *J. Biol. Chem.*, 244, 5239 (1969).
80. Blethen and Kaplan, *Biochemistry*, 7, 2123 (1968).
81. Blethen and Kaplan, *Biochemistry*, 6, 1413 (1967).
82. Ho, Milikin, Bobbitt, Grinnon, Burch, Frank, Boeck, and Squires, *J. Biol. Chem.*, 245, 3708 (1970).
83. Yellin and Wriston, Jr., *Biochemistry*, 5, 1605 (1966).

84. Tosa, Sano, Yamamoto, Nakamura, and Chibata, *Biochemistry*, 12, 1075 (1973).
85. Marino, Scardi, and Zito, *Biochem. J.*, 99, 595 (1966).
86. Magee and Phillips, *Biochemistry*, 10, 3397 (1971).
87. Tate and Meister, *Biochemistry*, 7, 3240 (1968).
88. Tate and Meister, *Biochemistry*, 9, 2626 (1970).
89. Weber, *J. Biol. Chem.*, 243, 543 (1968).
90. Lafuma, Gros, and Patte, *Eur. J. Biochem.*, 15, 111 (1970).
91. Subramanian and Kalnitsky, *Biochemistry*, 3, 1868 (1964).
92. Green and Toms, *Biochem. J.*, 118, 67 (1970).
93. Berns, Scott, and O'Reilly, *Science*, 145, 1054 (1964).
94. Ambler and Brown, *J. Mol. Biol.*, 9, 825 (1964).
95. Fall and Vagelos, *J. Biol. Chem.*, 247 8005 (1972).
96. Krishnan and Daniel Jr., *Biochim. Biophys. Acta*, 168, 579 (1966).
97. Nagawa, Mizushima, Sato, Iwanaga, and Suziki, *J. Biochem.* (Tokyo), 60, 643 (1966).
98. Clark, Macmurchie, Elliott, Wolcott, Landed, and Raftery, *Biochemistry*, 11, 1663 (1972).
99. Haupt, Heimburger, Kranz, and Schwick, *Eur. J. Biochem.*, 17, 254 (1970).
100. Brewer, Jr., Schlueter, and Aldred, *J. Biol. Chem.*, 245, 4232 (1970).
101. Neher, Riniker, Maier, Byfield, Gudmundsson, and MacIntyre, *Nature* (Lond.), 220, 984 (1968).
102. Brewer, Jr., Keutman, Potts, Jr., Reisfeld, Schlueter, and Munson, *J. Biol. Chem.*, 243, 5739 (1968).
103. O'Dor, Parkes, and Copp, *Can. J. Biochem.*, 47, 823 (1969).
104. Brooks and Siegel, *J. Biol. Chem.*, 248, 4189 (1973).
105. Bredderman and Wasserman, *Biochemistry*, 13, 1687 (1974).
106. Coffee and Bradshaw, *J. Biol. Chem.*, 248, 3305 (1973).
107. Wolff and Siegel, *J. Biol. Chem.*, 247, 4180 (1972).
108. Foley, Poon, and Anderson, *Biochemistry*, 10, 4562 (1971).
109. Nyman and Lindskog, *Biochim. Biophys. Acta*, 85, 141 (1964).
110. Bernstein and Schraer, *J. Biol. Chem.*, 247, 1306 (1972).
111. Tobin, *J. Biol. Chem.*, 245, 2656 (1970).
112. Tanis and Tashian, *Biochemistry*, 10, 4852 (1971).
113. Wong and Tanford, *J. Biol. Chem.*, 248, 8518 (1973).
114. Furth, *J. Biol. Chem.*, 243, 4832 (1968).
115. Duff and Coleman, *Biochemistry*, 5, 2009 (1966).
116. Ashworth, Spencer, and Brewer, *Arch. Biochem. Biophys.*, 142, 122 (1971).
117. Tanis, Tashian, and Yu, *J. Biol. Chem.*, 245, 6003 (1970).
118. Patel, Meagher, and Ornston, *Biochemistry*, 12, 3531 (1973).
119. Parke, Meagher, and Ornston, *Biochemistry*, 12, 3537 (1973).
120. Smith and Stockell, *J. Biol. Chem.*, 207, 501 (1954).
121. Gates and Travis, *Biochemistry*, 12, 1867 (1973).
122. Reeck and Neurath, *Biochemistry*, 11, 3947 (1972).
123. Prahl and Neurath, *Biochemistry*, 5, 4137 (1966).
124. Haberland, Willard, and Wood, *Biochemistry*, 11, 712 (1972).
125. Hayashi, Moore, and Stein, *J. Biol. Chem.*, 248, 2296 (1973).
126. Schnuchel, *Z. Physiol. Chem.*, 303, 91 (1956).
127. Shelanski and Taylor, *J. Cell Biol.*, 38, 304 (1968).
128. Weisenbug, Borisy, and Taylor, *Biochemistry*, 7, 4466 (1968).
129. Bellisario, Carlsen, and Bahl, *J. Biol. Chem.*, 248, 6796 (1973).
130. Carlsen, Bahl, and Swaminathan, *J. Biol. Chem.*, 248, 6810 (1973).
131. Davidson, Blackburn, and Dopheide, *J. Biol. Chem.*, 247, 4441 (1972).
132. Siegel and Award, Jr., *J. Biol. Chem.*, 248, 3233 (1973).
133. Koide and Matsuoka, *J. Biochem.* (Tokyo), 68, 1 (1970).
134. Coan, Roberts, and Travis, *Biochemistry*, 10, 2711 (1971).
135. Prahl and Neurath, *Biochemistry*, 5, 2131 (1966).
136. Smillie, Enenkel, and Kay, *J. Biol. Chem.*, 241, 2097 (1966).
137. Gratecos, Guy, Rovery, and Desnuelle, *Biochim. Biophys. Acta*, 175, 82 (1969).
138. Kramer, Felsted, and Law, *J. Biol. Chem.*, 248, 3021 (1973).
139. Konisky, *J. Biol. Chem.*, 247, 3750 (1972).
140. Leach, *Biochem. J.*, 67, 83 (1957).
141. Piez, Weiss, and Lewis, *J. Biol. Chem.*, 235, 1987 (1960).
142. Piez and Gross, *Biochim. Biophys. Acta*, 34, 24 (1959).
143. Eastore, *Biochem. J.*, 65, 363 (1957).
144. Eisen, Henderson, Jeffrey, and Bradshaw, *Biochemistry*, 12, 1814 (1973).
145. Lewis, Snell, Hirschman, and Fraenkel-Conrat, *J. Biol. Chem.*, 186, 23 (1950).
146. Ljungdahl, LeGall, and Lee, *Biochemistry*, 12, 1802 (1973).
147. Gosselin-Rey and Gerday, *Biochim. Biophys. Acta*, 221, 241 (1970).
148. Kumdavalli, Moreland, and Watts, *Biochem. J.*, 117, 513 (1970).
149. Waterson, Castellino, Hass, and Hill, *J. Biol. Chem.*, 247, 5266 (1972).
150. Fischer and Dorfel, *Z. Physiol. Chem.*, 297, 278 (1954).
151. Loiselet and Chatagner, *Biochim. Biophys. Acta*, 130, 180 (1966).
152. Ozols, *Biochemistry*, 13, 426 (1974).
153. Stellwagen and Rysary, *J. Biol. Chem.*, 247, 8074 (1972).
154. Margoliash and Schejter, *Adv. Protein Chem.*, 21, 113 (1966).
155. Morgan, Hensley, Jr., and Riehm, *J. Biol. Chem.*, 247, 6555 (1972).
156. Drucker, Trousil, Campbell, Barlow, and Margoliash, *Biochemistry*, 9, 1515 (1970).
157. Drucker, Trousil, and Campbell, *Biochemistry*, 9, 3395 (1970).
158. Trousil, and Campbell, *J. Biol. Chem.*, 249, 386 (1974).
159. Laycock and Cragie, *Can. J. Biochem.*, 49, 641 (1971).
160. Felsted, Gee, and Bachur, *J. Biol. Chem.*, 249, 3672 (1974).
161. Huang, Nakatsukasa, and Nester, *J. Biol. Chem.*, 249, 4467 (1974).
162. Maley, Guarino, and Maley, *J. Biol. Chem.*, 247, 931 (1972).
163. Gehrmann, and Okada, *Biochim. Biophys. Acta*, 23, 621 (1957).
164. Salnikow, Moore, and Stein, *J. Biol. Chem.*, 245, 5685 (1970).
165. Oshima and Price, *J. Biol. Chem.*, 248, 7522 (1973).
166. Modrich, Anraku, and Lehaman, *J. Biol. Chem.*, 248, 7495 (1973).
167. Lindberg, *Biochemistry*, 6, 323 (1967).
168. Lamartiniere, Itoh, and Dempsey, *Biochemistry*, 10, 4783 (1971).
169. Erickson and Mathews, *Biochemistry*, 12, 372 (1973).
170. Poe, Greenfield, Hirshfield, Williams, and Hoogsteen, *Biochemistry*, 11, 1023 (1972).
171. Gundersen, Dunlap, Harding, Freisheim, Otting, and Huennekens, *Biochemistry*, 11, 1018 (1972).
172. D'Souza, Warwick, and Freisheim, *Biochemistry*, 11, 1528 (1972).
173. Senoh, Kita, and Kamimoto, in *Biological and Chemical Aspects of Oxygenases*, Bloch and Hayaishi, Eds. Maruzen, Tokyo, 1966, 378.
174. Craine, Daniels, and Kaufman, *J. Biol. Chem.*, 248, 7838 (1973).
175. Gotte, Stern, Elsden, and Partridge, *Biochem. J.*, 87, 344 (1963).
176. Oshiro and Eylar, *Arch. Biochem. Biophys.*, 138, 606 (1970).
177. Wang and Keen, *Arch. Biochem. Biophys.*, 141, 749 (1970).
178. Winstead, *Biochemistry*, 11, 1046 (1972).
179. Ruth, Soja, and Wold, *Arch. Biochem. Biophys.*, 140, 1 (1970).
180. Holt and Wold, *J. Biol. Chem.*, 236, 3227 (1961).
181. Barnes and Stellwagen, *Biochemistry*, 12, 1559 (1973).
182. Stellwagen, Cronlund, and Barnes, *Biochemistry*, 12, 1552 (1973).
183. Malmström, Kimmel, and Smith, *J. Biol. Chem.*, 234, 1108 (1959).
184. Huang, Shih, Borja, Avena, and Bergdoll, *Biochemistry*, 6, 1480 (1967).
185. Borja, Fanning, Huang, and Bergdoll, *J. Biol. Chem.*, 247, 2456 (1972).
186. Schantz, Roessler, Woodburn, Lynch, Jacoby, Silverman, Gorman, and Spero, *Biochemistry*, 11, 360 (1972).
187. Kimmel, Markowitz, and Brown, *J. Biol. Chem.*, 234, 46 (1959).
188. Barker and Jencks, *Biochemistry*, 8, 3879 (1969).
189. Burns, Engle, and Bethune, *Biochemistry*, 11, 2699 (1972).
190. Hays, Simoni, and Roseman, *J. Biol. Chem.*, 248, 941 (1973).
191. Schmer, Kirby, Teller, and Davie, *J. Biol. Chem.*, 247, 2512 (1972).
192. Legaz, Schmer, Counts, and Davie, *J. Biol. Chem.*, 248, 3946 (1973).
193. Buchanan, Matsubara, and Evans, *Biochim. Biophys. Acta*, 189, 46 (1969).
194. Tanaka, Nakashima, Benson, Mower, and Yasunobu, *Biochemistry*, 5, 1666 (1966).
195. Sasaki and Matsubara, *Biochem. Biophys. Res. Commun.*, 28, 467 (1967).
196. Lee, Travis, and Black, *Arch. Biochem. Biophys.*, 141, 676 (1970).
197. Matsubara, Sasaki, and Chain, *Proc. Natl. Acad. Sci. USA*, 57, 439 (1967).
198. Matsubara, *J. Biol. Chem.*, 243, 370 (1968).
199. Yoch and Arnon, *J. Biol. Chem.*, 247, 4514 (1972).
200. Stombaugh, Burris, and Orme-Johnson, *J. Biol. Chem.*, 248, 7951 (1973).
201. Harrison, Hofmann, and Mainwaring, *J. Mol. Biol.*, 4, 251 (1962).

202. Theil, *J. Biol. Chem.*, 248, 622 (1973).
203. Fuller and Doolittle, *Biochemistry*, 10, 1305 (1971).
204. Lucas, Shaw, and Smith, *J. Mol. Biol.*, 2, 339 (1960).
205. Kortt, Hamilton, Webb, and Zener, *Biochemistry*, 13, 2023 (1974).
206. Kobayashi, Rinker, and Koffler, *Arch, Biochem. Biophys.*, 84, 342 (1959).
207. Hotani, Ooi, Kagawa, Asakura, and Yamaguchi, *Biochim. Biophys. Acta*, 214, 206 (1970).
208. Joys and Rankis, *J. Biol. Chem.*, 247, 5180 (1972).
209. Tanaka, Haniu, and Yasunobu, *J. Biol. Chem.*, 249, 4393 (1974).
210. Knight, Jr. and Hardy, *J. Biol. Chem.*, 242, 1370 (1967).
211. Dubourdieu and LeGall, *Biochem. Biophys. Res. Commun.*, 38, 965 (1970).
212. Tanaka, Haniu, Matsueda, Yasunobu, Mayhew, and Massey, *Biochemistry*, 10, 3041 (1971).
213. Mayhew and Massey, *J. Biol. Chem.*, 244, 794 (1969).
214. Cahill, Shetlar, Payne, Endecott, and Li, *Biochim. Biophys. Acta*, 154, 40 (1968).
215. Wickner and Tabor, *J. Biol. Chem.*, 247, 1605 (1972).
216. Mendicino, Kratowich, and Oliver, *J. Biol. Chem.*, 247, 6643 (1972).
217. Fowler and Zabin, *J. Biol. Chem.*, 245, 5032 (1970).
218. Mills and Tang, *J. Biol. Chem.*, 242, 3093 (1967).
219. Tauber and Madison, *J. Biol. Chem.*, 240, 645 (1965).
220. Booth and Ewart, *Biochim. Biophys. Acta*, 181, 226 (1969).
221. Nimberg and Schmid, *J. Biol. Chem.*, 247, 5056 (1972).
222. Behrens and Bromer, *Vitam. Horm.* (New York), 16, 263 (1958).
223. Strausbauch and Fischer, *Biochemistry*, 9, 226 (1970).
224. Moon and Smith, *J. Biol. Chem.*, 248, 3082 (1973).
225. Jacobson, Strickland, and Barratt, *Biochim. Biophys. Acta*, 188, 283 (1969).
226. Roberts, Holcenberg, and Dolowy, *J. Biol. Chem.*, 247, 84 (1972).
227. Tate, Leu, and Meister, *J. Biol. Chem.*, 247, 5312 (1972).
228. Adamson, Sewczuk, and Connell, *Can. J. Biochem.*, 49, 218 (1971).
229. Singleton, Kimmel, and Amelunxen, *J. Biol. Chem.*, 224, 1623 (1969).
230. Heinz and Kulbe, *Z. Physiol. Chem.*, 351, 249 (1970).
231. Fondy, Ross, and Sollohub, *J. Biol. Chem.*, 244, 1631 (1969).
232. Pradel, Kassab, Conlay, and Thoai, *Biochim. Biophys. Acta*, 154, 305 (1968).
233. Fosset, Muir, Nielsen, and Fischer, *Biochemistry*, 10, 4105 (1971).
234. Assaf and Yunis, *Biochemistry*, 12, 1423 (1973).
235. Appelman, Yunis, Krebs, and Fischer, *J. Biol. Chem.*, 238, 1358 (1963).
236. Wolf, Fischer, and Krebs, *Biochemistry*, 9, 1923 (1970).
237. Sevilla and Fischer, *Biochemistry*, 8, 2161 (1969).
238. Issa and Mendicino, *J. Biol. Chem.*, 248, 685 (1973).
239. Boenisch and Alper, *Biochim. Biophys. Acta*, 214, 135 (1970).
240. Dixon and Li, *J. Gen. Physiol.*, suppl. 45, 176 (1962).
241. Black and Dixon, *Nature* (Lond.), 218, 736 (1968).
242. Barnett, Lee, and Bowman, *Biochemistry*, 11, 1189 (1972).
243. Ticha, Entlicher, Kostir, and Kocourek, *Biochim. Biophys. Acta*, 221, 282 (1970).
244. Entlicher, Kostir, and Kocourek, *Biochim. Biophys. Acta*, 221, 272 (1970).
245. Bourillon and Fort, *Biochim. Biophys. Acta*, 154, 28 (1968).
246. Hammarström and Kabat, *Biochemistry*, 8, 2696 (1969).
247. Wada, Pallansch, and Liener, *J. Biol. Chem.*, 233, 395 (1958).
248. Matsumoto and Osawa, *Biochim. Biophys. Acta*, 194, 180 (1969).
249. Groskopf, Holleman, Margoliash, and Klotz, *Biochemistry*, 5, 3779 (1966).
250. Carpenter and van Holde, *Biochemistry*, 12, 2231 (1973).
251. Ghiretti-Magaldi, Nuzzolo, and Ghiretti, *Biochemistry*, 5, 1943 (1966).
252. Okazaki, Wittenberg, Briehl, and Wittenberg, *Biochim. Biophys. Acta*, 140, 258 (1967).
253. Dohi, Sugita, and Yoneyama, *J. Biol. Chem.*, 248, 2354 (1973).
254. Imamura, Baldwin, and Riggs, *J. Biol. Chem.*, 247, 2785 (1972).
255. Powers and Edmundson, *J. Biol. Chem.*, 247, 6694 (1972).
256. Schroeder, Shelton, Shelton, Cormick, and Jones, *Biochemistry*, 2, 992 (1963).

257. Babin, Schroeder, Shelton, Shelton, and Robberson, *Biochemistry*, 5, 1297 (1966).
258. Bannai, Sugita, and Yoneyama, *J. Biol. Chem.*, 247, 505 (1972).
259. Hrkal and Muller-Eberhard, *Biochemistry*, 10, 1746 (1971).
260. Dus, Tedro, and Bartsch, *J. Biol. Chem.*, 248, 7318 (1973).
261. Tedro, Meyer, and Kamen, *J. Biol. Chem.*, 249, 1182 (1974).
262. Klee and Gladner, *J. Biol. Chem.*, 247, 8051 (1972).
263. Lever, *J. Biol. Chem.*, 247, 4317 (1972).
264. Chang and Snell, *Biochemistry*, 7, 2012 (1968).
265. Henderson and Snell, *J. Biol. Chem.*, 248, 1906 (1973).
266. DeLorenzo, Di Natale, and Schechter, *J. Biol. Chem.*, 249, 908 (1974).
267. Delange, Hooper, and Smith, *J. Biol. Chem.*, 248, 3261 (1973).
268. Hooper, Smith, Sommer, and Chalkley, *J. Biol. Chem.*, 248, 3275 (1973).
269. Patthy, Smith, and Johnson, *J. Biol. Chem.*, 248, 6834 (1973).
270. Bailey and Dixon, *J. Biol. Chem.*, 248, 5463 (1973).
271. Brunish and Hogberg, *C.R. Trav. Lab. Carlsberg*, 32, 35 (1960).
272. Nakos and Mortenson, *Biochemistry*, 10, 2442 (1971).
273. Noyes and Bradshaw, *J. Biol. Chem.*, 248, 3052 (1973).
274. Menzel and Hammes, *J. Biol. Chem.*, 248, 4885 (1973).
275. Squire, Delin, and Porath, *Biochim. Biophys. Acta*, 89, 409 (1964).
276. Jarabak and Street, *Biochemistry*, 10, 3831 (1971).
277. Edelman, *Biochemistry*, 9, 3197 (1970).
278. Chen and Poljak, *Biochemistry*, 13, 1295 (1974).
279. Heinrikson, Sterner, Noyes, Cooperman, and Bruchman, *J. Biol. Chem.*, 248, 4235 (1973).
280. Corfield and Robson, *Biochem. J.*, 84, 146 (1962).
281. Grant and Reid, *Biochem. J.*, 106, 531 (1968).
282. Neumann and Lampen, *Biochemistry*, 6, 468 (1967).
283. Cozzone, Paséro, and Marchis-Mouren, *Biochim. Biophys. Acta*, 200, 590 (1970).
284. Chung and Franzen, *Biochemistry*, 8, 3175 (1969).
285. Illingworth and Tipton, *Biochem. J.*, 118, 253 (1970).
286. Yoshida and Carter, *Biochim. Biophys. Acta*, 194, 151 (1969).
287. Yu, Harmon, Wachter, and Blank, *Arch. Biochem. Biophys.*, 135, 363 (1969).
288. Kawahara, Wang, and Talalay, *J. Biol. Chem.*, 237, 1500 (1962).
289. Gordon and Ziegler, *Arch. Biochem. Biophys.*, 57, 80 (1955).
290. Castellino, Fish, and Mann, *J. Biol. Chem.*, 245, 4269 (1970).
291. Bell, McKenzie, and Shaw, *Biochim. Biophys. Acta*, 154, 284 (1968).
292. Rombauts, Schroeder, and Morrison, *Biochemistry*, 6, 2965 (1967).
293. Hayes and Goldstein, *J. Biol. Chem.*, 249, 1094 (1974).
294. Elfolk, *Acta Chem. Scand.*, 15, 545 (1961).
295. Carpenter and Vahl, *J. Biol. Chem.*, 248, 294 (1972).
296. Gilardeau and Chretien, *Can. J. Biochem.*, 48, 1017 (1970).
297. Gráf, Cseh, and Medzihradszky-Schweigher, *Biochim. Biophys. Acta*, 175, 444 (1969).
298. Bernardi and Cook, *Biochim. Biophys. Acta*, 44, 96 (1960).
299. Karkhanis and Cormier, *Biochemistry*, 10, 317 (1971).
300. Hastings, Weber, Friedland, Eberbard, Mitchell, and Gunsalus, *Biochemistry*, 8, 4681 (1969).
301. Landefeld and McShan, *Biochemistry*, 13, 1389 (1974).
302. Sabo and Fischer, *Biochemistry*, 13, 670 (1974).
303. Flashner and Massey, *J. Biol. Chem.*, 248, 2579 (1974).
304. Trayer and Buckley, *J. Biol. Chem.*, 245, 4842 (1970).
305. Shih and Hash, *J. Biol. Chem.*, 246, 996 (1971).
306. Arnheim, Hindenburg, Begg, and Morgan, *J. Biol. Chem.*, 248, 8036 (1973).
307. Canfield and Anfinsen, *J. Biol. Chem.*, 238, 2684 (1963).
308. Smith, Kimmel, Brown, and Thompson, *J. Biol. Chem.*, 215, 67 (1955).
309. Larue and Speck, Jr., *J. Biol. Chem.*, 245, 1985 (1970).
310. Rymo, Lundvik, and Lagerkvist, *J. Biol. Chem.*, 247, 3888 (1972).
311. Jurášek and Whitaker, *Can. J. Biochem.*, 45, 917 (1967).
312. Yoshida, *J. Biol. Chem.*, 240, 1113 (1965).
313. Allen and Patil, *J. Biol. Chem.*, 247, 909 (1972).
314. Imai and Brodie, *J. Biol. Chem.*, 248, 7487 (1973).
315. Spina, Jr., Bright, and Rosenbloom, *Biochemistry*, 9, 3794 (1970).
316. Li, *Adv. Protein Chem.*, 12, 270 (1957).
317. Strickland and Massey, *J. Biol. Chem.*, 248, 2944 (1973).

318. Lawrence, *Eur. J. Biochem.*, 15, 436 (1970).
319. Hsiang, Myrtle, and Bright, *J. Biol. Chem.*, 242, 3079 (1967).
320. Apitz-Castro, Rehn, and Lynen, *Eur. J. Biochem.*, 16, 71 (1970).
321. Bannerjee, Sanders, and Sokatch, *J. Biol. Chem.*, 245, 1828 (1970).
322. Israel, Howard, Evans, and Russel, *J. Biol. Chem.*, 249, 500 (1974).
323. Morris, Mortenson, Deibler, and Cagan, *J. Biol. Chem.*, 248, 534 (1973).
324. Brown, Cook, and Dryburgh, *Can. J. Biochem.*, 51, 533 (1973).
325. Meagher and Ornston, *Biochemistry*, 12, 3523 (1973).
326. Fishman, Pentchev, and Bailey, *Biochemistry*, 12, 2490 (1973).
327. Perkoff, Hill, Brown, and Tyler, *J. Biol. Chem.*, 237, 2820 (1962).
328. Edmundson, *Nature*, (Lond.), 205, 883 (1965).
329. Vigna, Gurd, and Gurd, *J. Biol. Chem.*, 249, 4144 (1974).
330. Klippenstein, Riper, and Oosterom, *J. Biol. Chem.*, 247, 5956 (1972).
331. Tada, Bailin, Bárány, and Bárány, *Biochemistry*, 8, 4842 (1969).
332. Connell and Howgate, *Biochem. J.*, 71, 83 (1959).
333. Chung, Richards, and Olcott, *Biochemistry*, 6, 3154 (1967).
334. Samy, Atreyi, Maeda, and Meienhofer, *Biochemistry*, 13, 1007 (1974).
335. Hollenberg and Hope, *Biochem. J.*, 106, 557 (1968).
336. Furth and Hope, *Biochem. J.*, 116, 545 (1970).
337. Miranda, Kupeyan, Rochat, Rochat, and Lissitzky, *Eur. J. Biochem.*, 16, 514 (1970).
338. Berry, Johnson, and Campbell, *Biochim. Biophys. Acta*, 220, 269 (1970).
339. Omenn, Ontjes, and Anfinsen, *Biochemistry*, 9, 304 (1970).
340. Palmieri, Yue, Jacobs, Maland, Yu, and Kuby, *J. Biol. Chem.*, 248, 4486 (1973).
341. Rodgers and Chargaff, *J. Biol. Chem.*, 247, 5448 (1972).
342. Neu, *J. Biol. Chem.*, 242, 3896 (1967).
343. Marshall and Cohen, *J. Biol. Chem.*, 247, 1641 (1972).
344. Donovan, Mapes, Davis, and Hamburg, *Biochemistry*, 8, 4190 (1969).
345. Donovan, Davis, and White, *Biochim. Biophys. Acta*, 207, 190 (1970).
346. Phillips and Azari, *Biochemistry*, 10, 1160 (1971).
347. Koike, Hamada, Tanaka, Otsuka, Ogasahara, and Koike, *J. Biol. Chem.*, 249, 3836 (1974).
348. DuVigneaud, Ressler, Swan, Roberts, and Katsoyannis, *J. Am. Chem. Soc.*, 76, 3115 (1954).
349. Smith, Stockell, and Kimmel, *J. Biol. Chem.*, 207, 551 (1954).
350. Rasmussen and Craig, *J. Biol. Chem.*, 236, 759 (1961).
351. Lehky, Blum, Stein and Fischer, *J. Biol. Chem.*, 249, 4332 (1974).
352. Jones and Hofmann, *Can. J. Biochem.*, 50, 1297 (1972).
353. Lang and Kassell, *Biochemistry*, 10, 2296 (1971).
354. Graham, Sodek, and Hofmann, *Can. J. Biochem.*, 51, 789 (1973).
355. Chow and Kassell, *J. Biol. Chem.*, 243, 1718 (1968).
356. Merrett, Bar-Eli, and Van Vunakis, *Biochemistry*, 8, 3696 (1969).
357. Rajagopalan, Moore, and Stein, *J. Biol. Chem.*, 241, 4940 (1966).
358. Ryle and Hamilton, *Biochem. J.*, 101, 176 (1966).
359. Havir and Hanson, *Biochemistry*, 12, 1583 (1973).
360. Fisher, Kirkwood, and Kaufman, *J. Biol. Chem.*, 247, 5161 (1972).
361. Dowhan, Wickner, and Kennedy, *J. Biol. Chem.*, 249, 3079 (1974).
362. Cannata, *J. Biol. Chem.*, 245, 792 (1970).
363. Kono, Uyeda, and Oliver, *J. Biol. Chem.*, 248, 8592 (1973).
364. Harshman and Six, *Biochemistry*, 8, 3423 (1969).
365. Tilley and Gracy, *J. Biol. Chem.*, 249, 4571 (1974).
366. Pon, Schnackerz, Blackburn, Chatterjee, and Noltmann, *Biochemistry*, 9, 1506 (1970).
367. Yoshida and Watanabe, *J. Biol. Chem.*, 247, 440 (1972).
368. Botes and Viljoen, *J. Biol. Chem.*, 249, 3827 (1974).
369. Wells and Hanahan, *Biochemistry*, 8, 414 (1969).
370. Hachimori, Wells, and Hanahan, *Biochemistry*, 10, 4084 (1971).
371. Tu, Passey, and Toom, *Arch. Biochem. Biophys.*, 140, 96 (1970).
372. Metzger, Glaser, and Helmreich, *Biochemistry*, 7, 2021 (1968).
373. Kimmel and Smith, *Bull. Soc. Chem. Biol.*, 40, 2049 (1958).
374. Mumford and Jenner, *Biochemistry*, 5, 3657 (1966).
375. Graziani, Agrò, Rotilio, Barra, and Mondovi, *Biochemistry*, 13, 804 (1974).
376. Peterson, *J. Biol. Chem.*, 246, 34 (1971).
377. von Jaarsveld, Branch, Robbins, Morgan, Kanda, and Canfield, *J. Biol. Chem.*, 248, 7898 (1973).
378. Freisheim, Walsh, and Neurath, *Biochemistry*, 6, 3010 (1967).
379. Lacko and Neurath, *Biochemistry*, 9, 4680 (1970).
380. Milgrom, Allouch, Atger, and Baulieu, *J. Biol. Chem.*, 248, 1106 (1973).
381. Recsei and snell, *Biochemistry*, 12, 365 (1973).
382. Ma, Brovetto-Cruz, and Li, *Biochemistry*, 9, 2302 (1970).
383. Ohta, *J. Biol. Chem.*, 242, 509 (1967).
384. Rickert and Elliot, *Can. J. Biochem.*, 51, 1638 (1973).
385. Drapeau, Boily, and Houmard, *J. Biol. Chem.*, 247, 6720 (1972).
386. Johnson and Smillie, *Can. J. Biochem.*, 50, 589 (1972).
387. Tsuru, Hattori, Tsuji, and Fukumoto, *J. Biochem.* (Tokyo), 67, 415 (1970).
388. Donnelly, Jr., Kuo, Reyes, Liu, and Greengard, *J. Biol. Chem.*, 248, 190 1973).
389. Heldebrant, Butkowski, Bajaj, and Mann, *J. Biol. Chem.*, 248, 7149 (1973).
390. Barisas and McGuire, *J. Biol. Chem.*, 249, 3151 (1974).
391. Tanaka, Haniu, Yasunobu, Dus, and Gunsalus, *J. Biol. Chem.*, 249, 3689 (1974).
392. DeSa, *J. Biol. Chem.*, 247, 5527 (1972).
393. Cardenas, Dyson, and Strandholm, *J. Biol. Chem.*, 248, 6931 (1973).
394. Cheema, Soldin, Knapp, Hofmann, and Scrimgeour, *Can. J. Biochem.*, 51, 1229 (1973).
395. Rask, Vahlquist, and Peterson, *J. Biol. Chem.*, 246, 6638 (1971).
396. Vahlquist and Peterson, *Biochemistry*, 11, 4526 (1972).
397. Shields, Dinovo, Henriksen, Kimbel, Jr., and Millar, *Biochim. Biophys. Acta*, 147, 238 (1967).
398. Farrell, Jr., Mallette, Buss, and Clagett, *Biochim. Biophys. Acta*, 194, 433 (1969).
399. Glitz, Angel, and Eichler, *Biochemistry*, 11, 1746 (1972).
400. Lees and Hartley, Jr., *Biochemistry*, 5, 3951 (1966).
401. Yankeelov, Jr., *Biochemistry*, 9, 2433 (1970).
402. Becker, Halbrook, and Hirs, *J. Biol. Chem.*, 248, 7826 (1973).
403. Fletcher, Jr. and Hash, *Biochemistry*, 11, 4281 (1972).
404. Uchida and Egami, in *The Enzymes*, 3rd ed., Boyer, Ed., Academic Press, New York, 1971, 205.
405. Woodroof and Glitz, *Biochemistry*, 10, 1532 (1971).
406. Takahashi, *J. Biol. Chem.*, 240, PC 4117 (1965).
407. Kenney and Dekker, *Biochemistry*, 10, 4962 (1971).
408. Panagou, Orr, Dunstone, and Blakley, *Biochemistry*, 11, 2378 (1972).
409. Kuehn and McFadden, *Biochemistry*, 8, 2403 (1969).
410. Tabita and McFadden, *J. Biol. Chem.*, 249, 3459 (1974).
411. Lovenburg and Williams, *Biochemistry*, 8, 141 (1969).
412. Bachmayer, Benson, Yasunobu, Garrard, and Whiteley, *Biochemistry*, 7, 986 (1968).
413. Lode and Coon, *J. Biol. Chem.*, 246, 791 (1971).
414. Dowhan, Jr. and Snell, *J. Biol. Chem.*, 245, 4618 (1970).
415. Brockway and Castellino, *Biochemistry*, 13, 2063 (1974).
416. Matsubara, Kaspar, Brown, and Smith, *J. Biol. Chem.*, 240, 1125 (1965).
417. Leitzmann, Wu, and Boyer, *Biochemistry*, 8, 2338 (1970).
418. Delmer, *J. Biol. Chem.*, 247, 3822 (1972).
419. Misra and Fridovich, *J. Biol. Chem.*, 247, 3410 (1972).
420. Titani, Hermodson, Ericsson, Walsh, and Neurath, *Biochemistry*, 11, 2427 (1972).
421. Sjöberg, *J. Biol. Chem.*, 247, 8058 (1972).
422. Gonzalez, Baldesten, and Reichard, *J. Biol. Chem.*, 245, 2363 (1970).
423. Batt, Mihula, Mann, Guarracino, Altiere, Graham, Quigley, Wolf, and Zafonte, *J. Biol. Chem.*, 245, 4857 (1970).
424. Galivan, Maley, and Maley, *Biochemistry*, 13, 2282 (1974).
425. Spiro, *J. Biol. Chem.*, 245, 5820 (1970).
426. Cornell and Pierce, *J. Biol. Chem.*, 248, 4327 (1973).
427. Viljoen and Botes, *J. Biol. Chem.*, 248, 4915 (1973).
428. Strydom, *J. Biol. Chem.*, 247, 4029 (1972).
429. Karlsson, Eaker, Fryklund, and Kadin, *Biochemistry*, 11, 4628 (1972).
430. Sato, Abe, and Tamiya, *Biochem. J.*, 115, 85 (1969).
431. Tu, Hong, and Solie, *Biochemistry*, 10, 1295 (1971).
432. Botes and Strydom, *J. Biol. Chem.*, 244, 4147 (1969).
433. Botes, *J. Biol. Chem.*, 247, 2866 (1972).
434. Chang and Hayashi, *Biochem. Biophys. Res. Commun.*, 37, 841 (1969).

435. Karlsson, Eaker, and Porath, *Biochim. Biophys. Acta*, 127, 505 (1966).
436. Six and Harshman, *Biochemistry*, 12, 2672 (1973).
437. Lipscomb, Horton, and Armstrong, *Biochemistry*, 13, 2070 (1974).
438. Schneider and Slaunwhite, Jr., *Biochemistry*, 10, 2086 (1971).
439. Chader and Westphal, *J. Biol. Chem.*, 243, 928 (1968).
440. Chader and Westphal, *Biochemistry*, 7, 4272 (1968).
441. Hudson, Ohno, Brockway, and Castellino, *Biochemistry*, 12, 1047 (1973).
442. Mann, Fish, Cox, and Tanford, *Biochemistry*, 9, 1348 (1970).
443. Carlson and Brosemer, *Biochemistry*, 10, 2113 (1971).
444. Sawyer, Tilley, and Gracy, *J. Biol. Chem.*, 247, 6499 (1972).
445. Norton, Pfuderer, Stringer, and Hartman, *Biochemistry*, 9, 4952 (1970).
446. Krietsch, Pentchev, Klingenburg, Hofstatter, and Bucher, *Eur. J. Biochem.*, 14, 289 (1970).
447. Greaser and Gergely, *J. Biol. Chem.*, 248, 2125 (1973).
448. Winter and Neurath, *Biochemistry*, 9, 4673 (1970).
449. Reeck and Neurath, *Biochemistry*, 11, 503 (1972).
450. Travis and Roberts, *Biochemistry*, 8, 2884 (1969).
451. Mallery and Travis, *Biochemistry*, 12, 2847 (1973).
452. Travis and Liener, *J. Biol. Chem.*, 240, 1967 (1965).
453. Travis, *Biochem. Biophys. Res. Commun.*, 30, 730 (1968).
454. Gates and Travis, *Biochemistry*, 8, 4483 (1969).
455. Jurášek and Smillie, *Can. J. Biochem.*, 51, 1077 (1973).
456. Kucich and Peanasky, *Biochim. Biophys. Acta*, 200, 47 (1970).
457. Sherman and Kassell, *Biochemistry*, 7, 3634 (1968).
458. Tschesche and Wachter, *Eur. J. Biochem.*, 16, 187 (1970).
459. Kassell, Radicevic, Berlow, Peanasky, and Laskowski, Sr., *J. Biol. Chem.*, 238, 3274 (1966).
460. Wilson and Laskowski, Sr., *J. Biol. Chem.*, 248, 756 (1973).
461. Walsh and Neurath, *Proc. Natl. Acad. Sci. USA*, 52, 884 (1964).
462. Bradshaw, Neurath, Tye, Walsh, and Winter, *Nature* (Lond.), 226, 237 (1970).
463. Voytek and Gjessing, *J. Biol. Chem.*, 246, 508 (1971).
464. Schyns, Bricteaux-Grégoire, and Florkin, *Biochim. Biophys. Acta*, 175, 97 (1969).
465. Henning, Helinski, Chao, and Yanofsky, *J. Biol. Chem.*, 237, 1523 (1962).
466. Li and Yanofsky, *J. Biol. Chem.*, 248, 1830 (1973).
467. Hoch, *J. Biol. Chem.*, 248, 2999 (1973).
468. Hoch, *J. Biol. Chem.*, 248 2992 (1973).
469. Hoch and DeMoss, *J. Biol. Chem.*, 247, 1750 (1972).
470. Kamamiyama, Wada, Matsubara, and Snell, *J. Biol. Chem.*, 247, 1571 (1972).
471. Koch, *Biochemistry*, 13, 2307 (1974).
472. Milton and Taylor, *Biochem. J.*, 113, 678 (1969).
473. White, Barlow, and Mozen, *Biochemistry*, 5, 2160 (1966).
474. DuVigneaud, Bartlett, and Johl, *J. Am. Chem. Soc.*, 79, 5572 (1957).
475. Tanford, *J. Am. Chem., Soc.*, 84, 4240 (1962).
476. Bigelow, *J. Theor. Biol.*, 16, 187 (1967).

PARTIAL VOLUMES OF AMINO ACIDS[a]

Roger L. Lundblad

						$cm^3\ m^{-1}$				
	[1][b]	[2][b]	[3][b,c]	[3][b,d]	[4][b]	[5][e]	[6][b]	[7][e]	[8][e]
Ala	60.45	60.4	63.9	60.5	60.43	60.43	60.43	60.42	60.6
Arg	123.7		123.6	127.3		127.34		123.86	
Asn	77.18		76.8	77.3				95.63	78
Asp	71.79		69	73.8		73.83		74.8	58.9
(Cys)2	148								
Cys	73.62		74.3	73.4		73.44			
Gln	94.36		93.5	93.6				93.61	
Glu	89.36		82.9	85.9		85.88		89.85	
Gly	43.25	43.12	48.8	43.2	43.14	43.19	43.14	43.19	43.5
His	99.14	98.81	94.9	98.9		98.79		98.3	99.3
Ile	105.45		105.5	105.7				195.8	
Leu	107.57		104.6	107.8	107.72		107.72	107.83	
Lys	108.71		115.5	108.5	125.9		125.9	124.76	108.5
Met	105.3		106.9	104.8		105.35		105.57	
Phe	121.92		111.8	121.5		121.48		122.2	121.3
Pro	82.65		84.7	82.5		82.83		82.63	81
Ser	60.62	60.32	66.5	60.6				60.62	60.8
Thr	76.84	76.84	81.9	76.9				76.83	
Trp	144		123.9	143.4		143.91		143.8	144.1
Tyr	123		113.1	124.3				124.4	
Val	90.79		90.6	90.8	90.39	90.78		90.65	
Hypro									84.4
NorLeu								107.93	
NorVal								91.7	

[a] Values obtained at 298.15 K (25°C).
[b] Partial molar volume.
[c] Calculated using the Kirkwood–Buff equation and a three-dimensional reference interaction site model (3D-RISM) integral equation theory for molecular liquids.
[d] Experimental value.
[e] Partial molal volume.

References

1. Jolicoeur, C., Riedl, B., Desrochers, D., *et al.*, Solvation of amino acid residues in water and urea-water mixtures: Volumes and heat capacities of 20 amino acid in water and 8 M urea at 25°C, *J. Solut. Chem.* 15, 109–128, 1986
2. Shen, J.-L., Li, Z.-F., Wang, B.-H., and Zhang, Y.-M., Partial molar volumes of some amino acids and a peptide in water, DMSO, NaCl, and DMSO/NaCl aqueous solutions, *J. Chem. Thermodynam.* 32, 805–819, 2000
3. Harano, Y., Imai, T., Kovalenko, A., Kimoshito, M., and Hirata, F., Theoretical study for partial molar volume of amino acids and polypeptides by three-dimensional reference interaction model, *J. Chem. Phys.* 114, 9506–9511, 2001
4. Singh, S.K., and Kishore, N., Volumetric properties of amino acids and hen-egg white lysozyme in aqueous Triton X-100 at 298.15 K, *J. Solut. Chem.* 33, 1411–1427, 2004.
5. Milero, F.J., and Huang, F., The partial molal volumes and compressibilities of nonelectrolytes and amino acids in 0.725 M NaCl, *Aquat. Geochem.* 22, 1–16, 2016.
6. Singh, S.K., Kundu, A., and Kishore, N., Interaction of some amino acids and glycine peptides with aqueous sodium dodecyl sulfate and cetylmethylammonium bromide at T = 298.15 K: A volumetric approach, *J. Chem. Thermodynam.* 36, 7–16, 2004.
7. Mishra, A.K., and Abluwalla, J.C., Apparent molal volumes of amino acids, N-acetylamino acids, and peptides in aqueous solution, *J. Phys. Chem.* 88, 86–92, 1984.
8. Cohn, E.J., McMeekin, T.L., Edsall, J.T., and Blanchard, M.H., Studies in the physical chemistry of amino acids, peptides and related substances. I. The apparent molal volume and electrostriction of the solvent, *J. Am. Chem. Soc.* 56, 784–794, 1934.

Partial volumes of amino acids and amino acid residues

	[1][a] x 10⁻³ nm³	[2][b,c] cm³ mol⁻¹	[3][b] cm³ mol⁻¹	[4][e,f]	[5][e]	[6][g]	[7][h] Vm/MW	[8]
Ala	87.2	17.75	17.20	13.0–15.34	12.7	0.17	0.74	
Arg	181.3		80.48	13.0–26.05		0.676	0.70	
Asn	117.4	35.43	33.93			0.344	0.62	
Asp	114.6		28.54	13.0–21.09		0.304	0.60	
Cys	106.7		105[d]	13.0–21.10			0.61	
Cys/2			30.37			0.299		
Gln	142.4		51.11			0.50	0.67	
Glu	141.4		46.11	13.0–23.24		0.467	0.66	
Gly				8.68–13.1	13.5	0.0	0.64	
His	152.4	58.0	55.89	10.8–29.40	10.8	0.555	0.67	
Ile	168.9	65.32	62.20			0.636		
Leu	168.9	65.43	64.32	13.0–23.39		0.636		
Lys	174.3		65.45		18.3	0.647	0.82	
Met	163.1	63.18	62.01	13.0–22.33		0.613	0.75	
Phe	187.9		78.67	13.3–27.44	13.7	0.774	0.77	
Pro	122.4		39.40	9.54–14.27	13.8	0.373	0.76	
Ser	91.0		17.37	12.9–17.2	12.9	0.172	0.63	
Thr	117.4		33.61			0.334	0.70	
Trp	228.5		100.71	15.1–29.15	15.1	1.0	0.74	
Tyr	192.1		80			0.796	0.71	
Val	141.4		47.54	13.1–22.33		0.476		

[a] These values are a consensus of amino acid residue volumes from six sets of data (see Ref.[1]).
[b] Partial molar amino acid residue volume.
[c] Obtained from the analysis of the tripeptide, gly-X-gly [8].
[d] Calculated data (see also Reference [1]).
[e] Value for electrorestriction. Electrorestriction, in this context, is the observed decrease in volume due to interaction of the dipolar amino acid with solvent [9, 10].
[f] Three methods were used to calculate the value for electroconstriction and the range of values is shown.
[g] *Residue volume*: It is assumed that this is amino acid residue–specific volume normal to 0–1.0 with Trp = 1.0.
[h] Specific volume of the residue obtained by dividing molal volume by molecular weight.

References

1. Perkins, S.J., Protein volumes and hydration effects. The calculation of partial specific volumes, neutron scattering matchpoints and 280-nm absorption coefficients for proteins and glycoproteins from amino acid sequences, *Eur. J. Biochem.* 157, 169–180, 1986.
2. Hedwig, G.R., Partial molar heat capacities volumes and compressibilities of aqueous solutions of some peptides that model the side chains of proteins, *Pure Appl. Chem.* 66, 387–397, 1994.
3. Jolicoeur, C., RIedl, B., Desrochers, D., *et al.*, Solvation of amino acid residues in water and urea-water mixtures: Volumes and heat capacities of amino acids in water and in 8 M urea at 25°C, *J. Solut. Chem.* 15, 109–128, 1986.
4. Millero, E.J., Lo Surdo, A., and Shin, C., The apparent molal volumes and adiabatic compressibilities of aqueous amino acids at 25°C, *J. Phys. Chem.* 82, 784–792, 1976.
5. Cohn, E.J., McMeekin, T.L., Edsall, J.T., and Blanchard, M.H., Studies in the physical chemistry of amino acids, peptides and related substances. I. The apparent molal volume and the electrostriction of the solvent, *J. Am. Chem. Soc.* 56, 784–794, 1934.
6. Goodarza, H., Katanforoush, A., Torabi, N., and Najafabadi, H.S., Solvent accessibility, residue charge and residue volume, the three ingredients of a robust amino acid substitution matrix, *J. Theoret. Biol.* 245, 715–725, 2007.
7. Cohn, E.J., and Edsall, J.T., *Density and apparent specific volume of proteins*, in *Proteins, Amino Acids and Peptides as Ion and Dipolar Ions*, eds. E.J. Cohn and J.T. Edsall, Chapter 16, pp. 370–381, Reinhold Publishing, New York, 1943.
8. Hedwig, G.R., Partial molar volumes of amino acid side chains of proteins in aqueous solution: Some comments on their estimates using partial molar volumes of amino acids and small peptides, *Biopolymers* 32, 537–540, 1992.
9. Greenstein, J.P., Wyman, J., Jr., and Cohn, E.J., Studies of multivalent amino acids and peptides. III. The dielectric constants and electrorestriction of the solvent in solutions of tetrapoles, *J. Am. Chem. Soc.* 57, 637–642, 1935.
10. Linderstrøm-Lang, K., and Jacobsen, C.F., The contraction accompanying break-down of proteins, *Enzymologia* 10, 97–126, 1941.

Effect of solvent on partial molar volume [1] (values in cm³ m⁻¹).

Amino acid	Water [2]	0.10 *M* DMSO [2]	2.0 *M* NaCl [2]	0.75 *M* NaCl [3]	8.0 *M* urea [4]
Gly	43.12	43.12	46.02	42.68	47.33
Als	60.4	60.3	62.9	60.4	64.2
Ser	60.32	60.68	63.73		64.97
Thr	76.84	76.81	79.64		81.1
I-His	98.81	98.68	101.84		103.52

DMSO, dimethyl sulfoxide; NaCl, sodium chloride.

References

1. Shen, J.-L., LI, Z.-F., Wang, B.-H., and Zhang, Y.-M., Partial molar volumes of some amino acids and a peptide in water, DMSO, NaCl, and DMSO/NaCl aqueous solutions, *J. Chem. Thermodynam.* 32, 805–819, 2000.

2. Millero, F.J., and Huang, F., The partial molar volumes and compressibilites on nonelectrolytes and amino acids in 0.725 M NaCl, *Aquat. Geochem.* 22, 1–16, 2016.

3. Jolilcoeur, C., Riedl, B., Desrochers, D., *et al.*, Solvation of amino acid residues in water and urea–water mixtures: Volumes and heat capacities of 20 amino acids in water and 8 M urea at 25°C, *J. Solut. Chem.* 15, 109–128, 1986.

DEAMIDATION OF ASPARAGINE

Roger L. Lundblad

Deamidation of asparagine in peptides and proteins.

The deamidation of asparagine with the associated formation of isoaspartic acid [1,2] and peptide bond cleavage [3] is one of the most common causes of heterogeneity in biopharmaceutical protein products. The process of deamidation of asparagine involves the formation of a cyclic succinimide which decomposes to form aspartic acid or isoaspartic acid. Deamidation results in heterogeneity of the protein which, in turn, results in a loss of potency [4,5]. Factors that affect deamidation of asparagine residues include the amino acid sequence around the asparagine residue, pH, buffer composition, and temperature. In general, asparagine in proteins is less susceptible to deamidation than peptides [6]. Glutamine is also susceptible to deamidation [7].

References

1. Song, Y., Schowen, R.L., Borchardt, R.T., and Topp, E.M., Effect of 'pH' on the rate of asparagine deamidation in polymeric formulations: 'pH'-rate profile, *J. Pharm. Sci.* 90, 141–156, 2001.
2. Reubsaet, J.L., Beijnen, J.H., Bult, A., *et al.*, Analytical techniques used to study the degradation of proteins and peptides: Chemical instability, *J. Pharm. Biomed. Anal.* 17, 955–978, 1998.
3. Catak, S., Monard, G., Aviyente, V., and Ruiz-López, M.F., Computation study on nonenzymatic peptide bond cleavage at asparagine and aspartic acid, *J. Phys. Chem.* 112, 8752–8761, 2008.
4. Zhang, L., Martinez, T., Woodruff, B., *et al.*, Hydrophobic interaction chromatography of soluble interleukin I receptor type II to reveal chemical degradations resulting in loss potency, *Anal. Chem.* 80, 7022–7078, 2008.

5. Nellis, D.F., Michiel, D.F., and Jiang, M.S., Characterization of recombinant human IL-15 deamidation and its practical elimination through substitution of asparagine 77, *Pharm. Res.* 29, 722–738, 2012.

6. Xie, M., and Schowen, R.L., Secondary structure and protein deamidation, *J. Pharm. Sci.* 88, 8–13, 1999.

7. Bischoff, R., and Kole, H.V., Deamidation of asparagine and glutamine residues in proteins and peptides: Structural determinants and analytical methodology, *J. Chromatog. B Biomed. Appl.* 662, 261–278, 1994.

Deamidation of asparagine and glutamine in peptides and proteins

Peptide/protein sequence	Reaction conditions	Rate	Reference
QNSLLWR (18–24 from recombinant human lymphotoxin)[a]	50 mM phosphate, pH 11.0 at 40°C	0.58×10^{-6} s^{-1}	[1]
QNSLLWR (18–24 from recombinant human lymphotoxin)[a]	50 mM phosphate, pH 11.0 with 4 M GuCl[b] at 40°C	17.7×10^{-6} s^{-1}	[1]
GFSLSNNSLL (contained in 30–67 from recombinant human lymphotoxin	50 mM phosphate, pH 11.0 at 40°C	0.1×10^{-6} s^{-1}	[1]
QNSLLWR (18–24 from recombinant human lymphotoxin)[a]	50 mM phosphate, pH 11.0 with 4 M GuCl[b] at 40°C	0.87×10^{-6} s^{-1}	[1]
Ac-KQNSL-NH$_2$	50 mM phosphate, pH 11.0 at 40°C	8×10^{-6} s^{-1}	[1]
Ac-KQNSL-NH$_2$	50 mM phosphate, pH 11.0 with 4 M GuCl[b] at 40°C	6.6×10^{-6} s^{-1}	[1]
Ac-LSNNGL-NH$_2$	50 mM phosphate, pH 11.0 at 40°C	8.1×10^{-6} s^{-1}	[1]
Ac-LSNNGL-NH$_2$	50 mM phosphate, pH 11.0 with 4 M GuCl[b] at 40°C	9.7×10^{-6} s^{-1}	[1]
rhVEGF	100 mM phosphate, pH 5.0 at 37°C	5×10^{-4} h^{-1}	[2]
rhVEGF	100 mM phosphate, pH 8.0 at 37°C	4.18×10^{-3} h^{-1}	[2]
GQNHH	100 mM phosphate, pH 5.0 at 37°C	6.08×10^{-3} h^{-1}	[2]
GQNHH	100 mM phosphate, pH 8.0 at 37°C	4.86×10^{-3} h^{-1}	[2]
GQNGG	100 mM sodium phosphate, pH 5.0 at 37°C	3.6×10^{-4} h^{-1}	[3]
GQNGG	100 mM sodium phosphate, pH 6.0 at 37°C	25.5×10^{-4} h^{-1}	[3]
GQNGG	100 mM sodium phosphate, pH 7.0 at 37°C	185.5×10^{-4} s^{-1}	[3]
GQNGG	100 mM sodium phosphate, pH 8.0 at 37°C	517.6×10^{-4} s^{-1}	[3]
GQNGG	100 mM sodium phosphate, pH 9.0 at 37°C	1211.5×10^{-4} s^{-1}	[3]
GQNGG	100 mM sodium phosphate, pH 10.0 at 37°C	2685×10^{-4} s^{-1}	[3]
GQNGH	100 mM sodium phosphate, pH 5.0 at 37°C	3.6×10^{-4} h^{-1}	[3]
GQNGH	100 mM sodium phosphate, pH 6.0 at 37°C	17.7×10^{-4} h^{-1}	[3]
GQNGH	100 mM sodium phosphate, pH 7.0 at 37°C	124.1×10^{-4} h^{-1}	[3]
GQNVH	100 mM sodium phosphate, pH 6.0 at 37°C	1.6×10^{-4} h^{-1}	[3]
GQNVH	100 mM sodium phosphate, pH 7.0 at 37°C	14.6×10^{-4} h^{-1}	[3]
GQNVH	100 mM sodium phosphate, pH 8.0 at 37°C	45.6×10^{-4} h	[3]
GQNHA	100 mM sodium phosphate, pH 6.0 at 37°C	19.6×10^{-4} h^{-1}	[3]
GQNHA	100 mM sodium phosphate, pH 7.0 at 37°C	116.9×10^{-4} h^{-1}	[3]
GQNHA	100 mM sodium phosphate, pH 8.0 at 37°C	122.1×10^{-4} h^{-1}	[3]
VSNGV	20 mM phosphate, pH 7.3 at 60°C	0.12 h$^{-1,c}$	[4]
VSNGV	20 mM TAPS, pH 8.0 at 60°C	4.1×10^{-2} h$^{-1,c}$	[4]
VSNGV	20 mM phosphate, pH 8.0 at 60°C	0.17 h$^{-1,c}$	[4]
VSNGV	50 mM phosphate, pH 8.0 at 60°C	0.26 h$^{-1,c}$	[4]
VSNGV	100 mM phosphate, pH 8.0 at 60°C	0.35 h$^{-1,c}$	[4]
VSNGV	20 mM CAPS, pH 10.0 at 60°C	0.11 h$^{-1,c}$	[4]
VSNGV	20 mM CAPS + 20 mM glycine, pH 10.0 at 60°C	0.46 h$^{-1,c}$	[4]
VSNGV	20 mM CAPS + 50 mM NH$_4$OH, pH 10.0	0.63 h$^{-1,c}$	[4]
VSNGV	20 mM CAPS + 250 mM triethylamine, pH 10.0	0.12 h$^{-1,c}$	[4]
VSNHV	20 mM phosphate, pH 7.3 at 60°C	2.7×10^{-2} h$^{-1,c}$	[4]
VSNSV	20 mM phosphate, pH 7.3 at 60°C	1.5×10^{-2} h$^{-1,c}$	[4]
VSNRV	20 mM phosphate, pH 7.3 at 60°C	9.1×10^{-3} h$^{-1,c}$	[4]

Deamidation of asparagine and glutamine in peptides and proteins (Continued)

Peptide/protein sequence	Reaction conditions	Rate	Reference
VSNLV	20 mM phosphate, pH 7.3 at 60°C	2.9×10^{-3} h$^{-1,c}$	[4]
VSNLV	20 mM CAPS, pH 10.0 at 60°C	2.1×10^{-2} h$^{-1,c}$	[4]
VSNAV	20 mM phosphate, pH 7.3 at 60°C	1.1×10^{-2} h$^{-1,c}$	[4]
VSNTV	20 mM phosphate, pH 7.3 at 60°C	2.9×10^{-3} h$^{-1,c}$	[4]
VSNVV	20 mM phosphate, pH 7.3 at 60°C	1.7×10^{-3} h$^{-1,c}$	[4]
VANTV	20 mM phosphate, pH 7.3 at 60°C	5.8×10^{-3} h$^{-1,c}$	[4]
VYPNGA	100 mM sodium phosphate, pH 7.4 at 37°C	2.1×10^{-2} h$^{-1,d}$	[5]
VYPNGA	100 mM sodium phosphate, pH 7.4 at 100°C	46.2 h$^{-1,d}$	[5]
VYPNLA	100 mM sodium phosphate, pH 7.4 at 37°C	9.9×10^{-3} h^{-1}	[5]
VYPNLA	100 mM sodium phosphate, pH 7.4 at 100°C	0.14 h^{-1}	[5]
VYPNPA	100 mM sodium phosphate, pH 7.4 at 37°C	6.5×10^{-3} h^{-1}	[5]
VYPNPA	100 mM sodium phosphate, pH 7.4 at 100°C	9.2×10^{-2} h^{-1}	[5]
N$_{54}$ in monoclonal antibody	100 mM Tris, pH 8.5 at 40°C	2.6×10^{-6} s$^{-1,e}$	[6]
GANAG	Phosphate, pH 7.4 ($I = 0.2$)^f at 37°C	8.4×10^{-8} s^{-1}	[7]
GRNAG	Phosphate, pH 7.4 ($I = 0.2$)^f at 37°C	4.43×10^{-7} s^{-1}	[7]
GDNAG	Phosphate, pH 7.4 ($I = 0.2$)^f at 37°C	1.83×10^{-7} s^{-1}	[7]
GCNAG	Phosphate, pH 7.4 ($I = 0.2$)^f at 37°C	1.17×10^{-7} s^{-1}	[7]
GENAG	Phosphate, pH 7.4 ($I = 0.2$)^f at 37°C	1.64×10^{-7} s^{-1}	[7]
GGNAG	Phosphate, pH 7.4 ($I = 0.2$)^f at 37°C	9.2×10^{-8} s^{-1}	[7]
GHNAG	Phosphate, pH 7.4 ($I = 0.2$)^f at 37°C	1.77×10^{-7} s^{-1}	[7]
GINAG	Phosphate, pH 7.4 ($I = 0.2$)^f at 37°C	1.6×10^{-8} s^{-1}	[7]
GLNAG	Phosphate, pH 7.4 ($I = 0.2$)^f at 37°C	3.7×10^{-8} s^{-1}	[7]
GKNAG	Phosphate, pH 7.4 ($I = 0.2$)^f at 37°C	1.32×10^{-7} s^{-1}	[7]
GMNAG	Phosphate, pH 7.4 ($I = 0.2$)^f at 37°C	1.04×10^{-7} s^{-1}	[7]
GFNAG	Phosphate, pH 7.4 ($I = 0.2$)^f at 37°C	1.69×10^{-7} s^{-1}	[7]
GPNAG	Phosphate, pH 7.4 ($I = 0.2$)^f at 37°C	8.0×10^{-8} s^{-1}	[7]
GSNAG	Phosphate, pH 7.4 ($I = 0.2$)^f at 37°C	1.53×10^{-7} s^{-1}	[7]
GTNAG	Phosphate, pH 7.4 ($I = 0.2$)^f at 37°C	1.18×10^{-1} s^{-1}	[7]
GWNAG	Phosphate, pH 7.4 ($I = 0.2$)^f at 37°C	9.2×10^{-8} s^{-1}	[7]
GYNAG	Phosphate, pH 7.4 ($I = 0.2$)^f at 37°C	9.4×10^{-1} s^{-1}	[7]
GVNAG	Phosphate, pH 7.4 ($I = 0.2$)^f at 37°C	7.2×10^{-8} s^{-1}	[7]
GAQAG	Phosphate, pH 7.4 ($I = 0.2$)^f at 37°C	1.5×10^{-8} s^{-1}	[7]
GAQRG	Phosphate, pH 7.4 ($I = 0.2$)^f at 37°C	4.2×10^{-8} s^{-1}	[7]
GAQIG	Phosphate, pH 7.4 ($I = 0.2$)^f at 37°C	7.2×10^{-9} s^{-1}	[7]
GAQKG	Phosphate, pH 7.4 ($I = 0.2$)^f at 37°C	5.1×10^{-8} s^{-1}	[7]
GRQAG	Phosphate, pH 7.4 ($I = 0.2$)^f at 37°C	2.1×10^{-8} s^{-1}	[7]
GRQRG	Phosphate, pH 7.4 ($I = 0.2$)^f at 37°C	2.8×10^{-8} s^{-1}	[7]
GDQAG	Phosphate, pH 7.4 ($I = 0.2$)^f at 37°C	3.8×10^{-8} s^{-1}	[7]
GEQAG	Phosphate, pH 7.4 ($I = 0.2$)^f at 37°C	3.5×10^{-8} s^{-1}	[7]
GGQAG	Phosphate, pH 7.4 ($I = 0.2$)^f at 37°C	1.9×10^{-8} s^{-1}	[7]
GHQAG	Phosphate, pH 7.4 ($I = 0.2$)^f at 37°C	8.3×10^{-8} s^{-1}	[7]
GIQAG	Phosphate, pH 7.4 ($I = 0.2$)^f at 37°C	7.3×10^{-9} s^{-1}	[7]
GLQAG	Phosphate, pH 7.4 ($I = 0.2$)^f at 37°C	1.2×10^{-8} s^{-1}	[7]
GKQAG	Phosphate, pH 7.4 ($I = 0.2$)^f at 37°C	2.8×10^{-8} s^{-1}	[7]
GMQAG	Phosphate, pH 7.4 ($I = 0.2$)^f at 37°C	7.8×10^{-8} s^{-1}	[7]
GFQAG	Phosphate, pH 7.4 ($I = 0.2$)^f at 37°C	7.6×10^{-9} s^{-1}	[7]
GPQAG	Phosphate, pH 7.4 ($I = 0.2$)^f at 37°C	7.2×10^{-9} s^{-1}	[7]
GSQAG	Phosphate, pH 7.4 ($I = 0.2$)^f at 37°C	9.0×10^{-9} s^{-1}	[7]

Deamidation of asparagine and glutamine in peptides and proteins (Continued)

Peptide/protein sequence	Reaction conditions	Rate	Reference
GTQAG	Phosphate, pH 7.4 ($I = 0.2$)[f] at 37°C	2.3×10^{-9} s^{-1}	[7]
GWQAG	Phosphate, pH 7.4 ($I = 0.2$)[f] at 37°C	1.1×10^{-8} s^{-1}	[7]
GYQAG	Phosphate, pH 7.4 ($I = 0.2$)[f] at 37°C	1.2×10^{-8} s^{-1}	[7]
GYQLG	Phosphate, pH 7.4 ($I = 0.2$)[f] at 37°C	9.0×10^{-8} s^{-1}	[7]
GVQAG	Phosphate, pH 7.4 ($I = 0.2$)[f] at 37°C	2.4×10^{-9} s^{-1}	[7]

Room temperature assumed to be 23°C.

rhVEGF, recombinant human vascular endothelial growth factor, CAPS; TAPS.

[a] Recombinant human lymphotoxin was incubated under the indicated solvent conditions for 43 days at which time the protein was denatured in 8.0 M urea and subjected to tryptic hydrolysis. Peptides containing asparagine were isolated and the extent of deamination determined and used for the first-order rate constants.

[b] Incubation was performed in the presence of 4.0 M guanidine hydrochloride.

[c] Calculated for $t_{1/2}$ data, $t_{1/2}$ = 0.693/K.

[d] Extrapolated from the data obtained at 70°C.

[e] N_{58} undergoes deamidation at a much slower rate (13% after 2 weeks compared to 76% for N_{54}; N_{56} is resistant to deamidation).

[f] *Buffer.* A combination of potassium dihydrogen phosphate (potassium monobasic phosphate) and sodium monohydrogen phosphate (sodium dibasic phosphate).

References

1. Xie, M., Shabrokh, X., Kadkhodayan, M., *et al.*, Asparagine deamidation in recombinant human lymphotoxin: Hindrance by three-dimensional structures, *J. Pharm. Sci.* 92, 869–880, 2003.
2. Goolcharran, C., Jones, A.J.S., Borchardt, R.T., Cleland, J.L., and Keck, R., Comparison of the rates of deamidation, diketopiperazine formation, and oxidation in recombinant human vascular endothelial growth factor and model peptides, *Pharm. Sci.* 2(E5), 2000.
3. Goolcharran, C., Stauffer, L.L., Cleland, J.L., and Bordchardt, R.T., The effects of a histidine residue on the C-terminal side of as asparaginyl residue on the rate of deamidation using model pentapeptides, *J. Pharm. Sci.* 89, 818–825, 2000.
4. Tyler-Cross, R., and Schirch, V., Effects of amino acid sequence, buffers, and ionic strength on the rate and mechanism of deamidation of asparagine residues in small peptides, *J. Biol. Chem.* 266, 22549–22556, 1991.
5. Geiger, T., and Clarke, S., Deamidation, isomerization, and racemization at asparaginyl and aspartyl residues in peptides, *J. Biol. Chem.* 262, 785–794, 1987.
6. Phillips, J.J., Buchanan, A., Andrews, J., *et al.*, Rate of asparagine deamidation in a monoclonal antibody correlating with hydrogen exchange rate at adjacent downstream residues, *Anal. Chem.* 89, 2361–2368, 2017.
7. Robinson, A.B., Scotchler, J.W., and McKerrow, J.H., Rates of nonenzymatic deamidation of glutaminyl and asparaginyl residues in pentapeptides, *J. Am. Chem. Soc.* 95, 8156–8159, 1973.

General Reference for Deamidation:

Lindner, H., and Helliger, W., Age-dependent deamidation of asparagine residues in proteins. *Exp. Gerontol.* 36(9), 1551–1563, 2001. Review. PubMed PMID: 11525877.

MICHAEL REACTIONS OF PROTEINS

Roger L. Lundblad

Michael Addition Reaction

Michael addition reaction was originally defined as the base-catalyzed addition of an active methylene compound (e.g., malonic ester) to an activated unsaturated compound such as an α,β-unsaturated ketone. There is a broad definition for the Michael reaction today as the conjugate addition of a nucleophile as across double bonds conjugated with an electron-withdrawing group [1]. Michael additions are of great importance in biochemistry and molecular biology for the chemical modification of proteins and for the manufacture of antibody–drug conjugates as well as three-dimensional matrices such as hydrogels. N-ethylmaleimide is the most extensively used reagent for the Michael addition modification of thiol groups where it serves as a Michael acceptor with the thiolate serving as the Michael donor.

Reference

1. Sharp, D.W.A., *Penguin Dictionary of Chemistry*, 2nd edn., Penguin Books, London, UK, 1990.

Rate constants for the reaction of N-ethylmaleimide with model thiol compounds and proteins.

Protein or model compound/reaction conditions	Rate (M^{-1} s^{-1})	Reference	Protein or model compound/reaction conditions	Rate (M^{-1} s^{-1})	Reference
L-Cysteine hydrochloride, pH 3.0/25°C	0.196[a]	[1]	Yeast alcohol dehydrogenase/50 mM sodium pyrophosphate, pH 6.5/20°C	0.07[d]	[4]
Cysteine, pH 3.0/25°C	0.346[a]	[2]	Myosin S_1 cysteine residue/50 mM Tris–0.5 M KCl, pH 6.0/0°C	10.2[d] 30.3[f]	[6]
Cysteine, pH 4.95/25°C	14.1[a]	[2]			
Glutathione, pH 4.95/25°C	10.6[a]	[2]	Myosin S_2 cysteine residue/50 mM Tris–0.5 M KCl, pH 7.9/0°C	1.2	[6]
Cysteine, pH 6.98/25°C	1460[b,c]	[2]	Papain/0.1 M phosphate, pH 6.0/25°C	0.661[d]	[8]
Cysteine, pH 4.75/25°C	8.1[a]	[3]	Papain/0.13 M potassium phosphate, pH 6.8/25°C	2.77[d]	[9]
Cysteine, pH 4.75/25°C/1% SDS	6.7[a]	[3]	Jack bean urease/20 mM phosphate, pH 7.4/25°C	0.92[d]	[10]
Cysteine/25 mM sodium acetate, pH 5.0,[c] 25°C	20.2[b]	[4]	Jack bean urease/20 mM phosphate, pH 8.3/25°C	3.17[d]	[10]
Glutathione/25 mM sodium acetate, pH 5.0,[c] 25°C	25.8[b]	[4]	Apo-CadC/5 mM MES–0.40 M NaCl, pH 7.0/25°C	32.2[g]	[11]
N-Acetyl-L-cysteine, pH 6.0/25°C	26.7[a]	[5]	(PbII)CadC/5 mM MES–0.40 M NaCl, pH 7.0/25°C	0.031[g]	[11]
N-Acetylcysteine/20 mM phosphate–0.1 mM EDTA, pH 6.0/0°C	5.8[a]	[6]	(CdII)CadC/5 mM MES–0.40 M NaCl, pH 7.0/25°C	0.20[g]	[11]
Cysteine, pH 5.0/25°C	15.5[a]	[7]	Chalcone isomerase, 100 mM PIPES (I = 0.15 with KCl), pH 6.8/25°C	0.14[d]	[12]
Cysteine, pH 7.0/25°C	1530[a]	[7]			
N-Acetylcysteine, pH 5.0/25°C	2.4[a]	[7]	Chalcone isomerase, 50 mM TAPS (I = 0.10 with KCl), pH 8.5/25°C	0.95[d]	[12]
N-Acetylcysteine, pH 7.0/25°C	230	[7]			
N-Acetylcysteine amide, pH 5.0/25°C	13.4[a]	[7]	Rabbit muscle L-α-glycerophosphate dehydrogenase/50 mM Tris, pH 7.0/10°C	0.043	[13]
N-Acetylcysteine amide, pH 7.0/25°C	1330	[7]			
Glutathione, pH 5.0/25°C	11.9[a]	[7]	L-Serine-activating enzyme from *Escherichia coli*/100 mM phosphate, pH 6.6/0°C	77	[14]
Glutathione, pH 7.0/25°C	1150	[7]			
4-Mercaptomethylimidazole, pH 5.0/25°C	94.5[a]	[7]	Opiate membrane receptor/50 mM Tris, pH 7.4,[h] 37°C	0.18	[15]
4-Mercaptomethylimidazole, pH 7.0/25°C	9450	[7]	Plasma membrane H⁺-ATPase (*Neurospora crassa*)/50 mM Tris, pH 8.7 with 5% dimethyl sulfoxide,[i] 0°C	205[h,j] 0.078[k]	[16]
4-(2-mercaptoethyl)imidazole, pH 5.0/25°C	11.0[a]	[7]			
4-(2-mercaptoethyl)imidazole, pH 7.0/25°C	1100	[7]	Bacterial luciferase (luminous strain MAV)/20 mM phosphate, pH 7.0/25°C	2.78[d]	[17]
N-Acetyl-Cys-His-Asp, pH 5.0/25°C	10.4[a]	[7]			
N-Acetyl-Cys-His-Asp, pH 7.0/25°C	1000	[7]	Choline acetyltransferase/50 mM potassium phosphate–100 mM KCl–0.1 mM EDTA, pH 7.4/37°C	32.5[d]	[18]
β-Lactoglobulin, pH 6.0/25°C/1% SDS	1.4[d,e]	[3]			
β-Lactoglobulin, pH 7.0/25°C/1% SDS	11.2[d,e]	[3]	Lactose permease from *Escherichia coli*/100 mM sodium phosphate, pH 7.0/23°C[l]	17.3[d]	[19]
Yeast alcohol dehydrogenase/50 mM sodium pyrophosphate, pH 7.0/20°C	0.22[d]	[4]	RNA polymerase of vesicular stomatitis virus/50 mM Tris–100 mM NaCl–5 mM $MgCl_2$, pH 8.0/0°C	8.8[d]	[20]
			Metallothionein/10 mM MOPS,[m] pH 7.4/25°C	1.09[n]	[21]

EDTA; MAV; MOPS; SDS.

[a] Reaction rates determined by changes in the spectra of NEM [22–24]. It should be noted that this method measures the disappearance of reactant rather than the formation of product. Thus, it is possible, but not likely, that reaction with amino groups might be a complication [25]. It would be useful to validate the spectrophotometric method by measurement of product(s). It is also necessary to correct for hydrolysis of the N-ethylmaleimide [12, 25]. Oxidation of the Michael donor should also be considered (at pH 9.0/25°C: 2-mercaptoethanol, 0.054 M^{-1} s^{-1}; cysteine, 0.113 M^{-1} s^{-1}) [26].

[b] Estimated value.

[c] Reaction at pH 7.0 was too fast to measure.

[d] Reaction rate determined by loss of enzyme activity.

[e] Native β-lactoglobulin is a dimer where each monomer has two disulfide bonds and a single sulfhydryl group; the sulfhydryl group is not available for modification without denaturation of the protein [27].

[f] pH-independent second-order rate constant [28].

[g] For reaction at Cys7 (determined by mass spectrometry)

[i] Fast site.

[h] The reaction of NEM with the "fast site" had to be studied in an indirect manner (by protection against modification with N-pyrenemaleimide.

[i] Slow site.

[k] The sulfhydryl reagents were introduced into the reaction mixture with dimethylsulfoxide and stated that the dimethylsulfoxide concentration was maintained at 5% (assume V/V). It is stated that the presence of 5% dimethylsulfoxide reduced the rate of NEM inhibition by 50%.

[l] Room temperature assumed as 23°C.

[m] N-ethylmaleimide is subjected to base hydrolysis to form N-ethylmaleamic acid. The rate of hydrolysis of the N-ethylmaleimide to form N-ethylsuccinamic acid is dependent on the buffer; the rate is highest in tris and bicarbonate buffers and much slower in phosphate and MOPS buffers.

[n] The alkylation is reversed by the presence of 2-mercaptoethanol. This is a reflection of the competition of zinc ions and N-ethylmaleimide for the thiolate anion.

References

1. Lee, C.C., and Samuels, E.R., The kinetics of reaction between l-cysteine hydrochloride and some maleimides, *Canad. J. Chem.* 42, 168–170, 1964.
2. Gorin, G., Martic, P.A., and Doughty, G., Kinetics of the reaction of *N*-ethylmaleimide with cysteine and some congeners, *Arch. Biochem. Biophys.* 115, 593–597, 1966.
3. Franklin, J.G., and Leslie, J., The kinetics of the reaction of *N*-ethylmaleimide with denatured β-lactoglobulin and ovalbumin, *Biochim. Biophys. Acta* 160, 333–339, 1968.
4. Heitz, J.R., Anderson, C.D., and Anderson, B.M., Inactivation of yeast alcohol dehydrogenase by *N*-alkylmaleimides, *Arch. Biochem. Biophys.* 127, 627–636, 1968.
5. Glick, B.R., and Brubacher, L.J., The reaction between *N*-ethylmalemide and ribosomes, *J. Mol. Biol.* 93, 319–321, 1975.
6. Takamori, K., Kato, K.A., and Sekine, T., Thiols of myosin IV. "Abnormal" reactivity of S1 thiol, *J. Biochem.* 80, 101–110, 1976.
7. Schneider, F., and Wenck, H., Kinetik der Reaktion von Imidazol-SH-Verbindungen mit *N*-Äthyl-malinimid, *Hoppe-Seyler's Zeit. Physiol. Chem.* 350, 1521–1530, 1969.
8. Brubacher, L.J., and Glick, B.R., Inhibition of papain by *N*-ethylmaleimide, *Biochemistry.* 13, 915–920, 1974.
9. Anderson, B.M., and Vasini, E.C., Nonpolar effects in reaction of sulfhydryl groups of papain, *Biochemistry.* 9, 3348–3352, 1970.
10. Kot, M., and Bicz, A., Inactivation of jack bean urease by *N*-ethylmaleimide: pH dependence, reversibility and thiols influence, *J. Enzyme Inhib. Med. Chem.* 23, 514–520, 2008.
11. Apuy, J.L., Busenlehner, L.S., Russell, D.H., and Giedroc, D.P., Ratiometric pulsed alkylation mass spectrometry as a probe of thiolate reactivity in different metalloderivatives of *Staphylococcus aureus* p1258 CadC, *Biochemistry.* 43, 3824–3834, 2004.
12. Bednar, R.A., Reactivity and pH dependence of thiol conjugation to *N*-ethylmaleimide: Detection of a conformational change in chalcone isomerase, *Biochemistry.* 29, 3684–3690, 1990.
13. Anderson, B.M., Kim, S.J., and Wang, C.-N., Inactivation of rabbit muscle l-α-glycerophosphate dehydrogenase by *N*-alkylmaleimides, *Arch. Biochem. Biophys.* 138, 66–72, 1970.
14. Bryce, G.F., Enzymes involved in the biosynthesis of cyclic tris-(*N*-2,3-dihydroxybenzoyl-L-seryl) in *Escherichia coli*: Kinetic properties of the l-serine-activating enzyme, *J. Bacteriol.* 116, 790–796, 1973.
15. Shahrestanifar, M.S., and Howells, R.D., Sensitivity of opioid receptor binding to N-substituted malemides and methanethiosulfonate derivatives, *Neurochem. Res.* 21, 1295–1299, 1996.
16. Davenport, J.W., and Slayman, C.W., The plasma membrane H+-ATPase of *Neurospora crassa*: Properties of two reactive sulfhydryl groups, *J. Biol. Chem.* 263, 16007–16013, 1988.
17. Nicoli, M.Z., and Hastings, J.W., Bacterial luciferase: The hydrophobic environment of the reactive sulfhydryl, *J. Biol. Chem.* 249, 2393–2396, 1974.
18. Roskoski, R., Choline acetyltransferase inhibition by thiol reagents, *J. Biol. Chem.* 249, 2156–2159, 1974.
19. Page, M.G.P., and West, I.C., Characterisation in vivo of the reactive thiol groups of the lactose permease from *Escherichia coli* and a mutant: Exposure, reactivity and the effects of substrate binding, *Biochim. Biophys. Acta.* 858, 67–82, 1986.
20. Massey, D.M., and Lenard, J., Inactivation of the RNA polymerase of vesicular stomatitis virus by *N*-ethylmaleimide and protection by nucleoside triphosphates, *J. Biol. Chem.* 262, 8734–8737, 1987.
21. Shaw, C.F., III, He, L., Muñoz, A., *et al.*, Kinetics of reversible *N*-ethylmaleimide alkylation of metallothionein and the subsequent metal release, *J. Biol. Inorg. Chem.* 2, 65–73, 1997.
22. Friedmann, E., Spectrophotometric investigation of the interaction of glutathione with maleimide and *N*-ethylmaleimide, *Biochim. Biophys. Acta.* 9, 65–75, 1952.
23. Gregory, J.D., The stability of *N*-ethylmaleimide and its reaction with sulfhydryl groups, *J. Am. Chem. Soc.* 77, 3922–3923, 1955.
24. Roberts, E., and Rouser, G., Spectrophotometric assay for reaction of *N*-ethylmaleimide with sulfhydryl groups, *Anal. Chem.* 30, 1291–1292, 1958.
25. Sharpless, N.E., and Flavin, M., The reactions of amines and amino acids with maleimides: Structure of the reaction products deduced from infrared and nuclear magnetic resonance spectroscopy, *Biochemistry.* 5, 2963–2971, 1966.
26. Schelté, P., Boeckler, C., Frisch, B., and Schuber, F., Differential reactivity of maleimide of bromoacetyl functions with thiols: Application to the preparation of liposomal diepitope constructs, *Bioconjug. Chem.* 11, 118–123, 2000.
27. Croguennec, T., Bouhallab, S., Mollé, D., *et al.*, Stable monomeric intermediate with exposed Cys-119 is formed during heat denaturation of β-lactoglobulin, *Biochem. Biophys. Res. Commun.* 301, 465–471, 2003.
28. Lindley, H., A study of the kinetics of the reaction between thiol compounds and chloroacetamide, *Biochem. J.* 74, 577–584, 1960.

Rate constants for reaction of alkyl maleimides cysteinyl residues in proteins.[a]

Reagent	YADH[b]	DAAO[c]	GPD[d]	LDH[e]	BL (MAV)[f]	MBSD[g]
N-Ethylmaleimide	0.22	0.45	0.04	6.9	27.8[h]	3.63/0.41[i]
N-Butylmaleimide	0.56	1.21	0.19	14.1	155	4.33/0.51
N-Pentylmaleimide	0.84	1.83	0.62	18.3	—	—
N-Hexylmaleimide	1.13	2.85	2.37	23.3	816	—
N-Heptylmaleimide	1.88	4.70	8.67	36.4	845	—
N-Octylmaleimide	2.16	6.72	28.8	—	—	—
N-Nonylmaleimide	—	—	91.7	—	—	—
N-Benzylmaleimide	1.34	—	—	—	—	—
N-Phenylmaleimide	—	5.33	—	—	—	—
N-Benzylmaleimide	—	—	—	—	—	15.0[j]

BL, bacterial luciferase; DAAO, D-amino acid oxidase; GPD, rabbit muscle L-α-glycerophosphate dehydrogenase; YADH, yeast alcohol dehydrogenase; EtOH.

[a] Data as rate ($M^{-1}s^{-1}$).

[b] YADH/0.1 M sodium pyrophosphate, pH 7.0 with 2% EtOH/20°C [1]. This study also showed that there is no difference in the rate of reaction of *N*-ethylmaleimide and *N*-heptymaleimide with glutathione (27.75 M^{-1} s^{-1} at pH 5.0).

[c] DAAO/50 mM sodium pyrophosphate, pH 7.0, 25°C [2].

[d] GPD /50 mM Tris-HCl, pH 7.0 with 2% EtOH/10°C [3].

[e] *Haemophilus influenza* D-lactate dehydrogenase/50 mM HEPES, pH 7.0 with 2.5% EtOH, 25°C [4].

[f] Bacterial luciferase (strain MAV)/20 mM phosphate, pH 7.0, 25°C [5].

[g] Membrane-bound succinic dehydrogenase/50 mM sodium phosphate, pH 7.6, 37°C [6].

[h] The active site sulfhydryl group in bacterial luciferase is known to be highly reactive [7, 8].

[i] Two classes of sulfhydryl groups are suggested to be involved in the activity of succinate dehydrogenase. The second-order rate constants for the two classes of sulfhydryl groups are shown here. Data are expressed as mM^{-1} min^{-1}.

[j] The increased rate of reaction with the reagents in these experiments correlated with the octanol: water partition coefficient.

References

1. Heitz, J.R., Anderson, C.D., and Anderson, B.M., Inactivation of yeast alcohol dehydrogenase by N-alkylmaleimides, *Arch. Biochem. Biophys.* 127, 627–636, 1968.
2. Fonda, M.L., and Anderson, B.M., d-Amino acid oxidase IV inactivation by maleimides, *J. Biol. Chem.* 244, 666–674, 1969.
3. Anderson, B.M., Kim, S.J., and Wang, C.-N., Inactivation of rabbit muscle L-glycerophosphate dehydrogenase by N-alkylmaleimides, *Arch. Biochem. Biophys.* 138, 66–72, 1970.
4. Denicola-Seoane, A., and Anderson, B.M., Nonpolar interactions in the maleimide inactivation of *Haemophilus influenza* d-lactate dehydrogenase, *Biochim. Biophys. Acta.* 1040, 84–88, 1990.
5. Nicoli, M.Z., and Hastings, J.W., Bacterial luciferase: The hydrophobic environment of the reactive sulfhydryl, *J. Biol. Chem.* 249, 2393–2396, 1974.
6. Lê-Quôc, K., Lê-Quôc, D., and Gaudemer, Y., Evidence for the existence of two classes of sulfhydryl groups essential for membrane-bound succinate dehydrogenase activity, *Biochemistry* 20, 1705–1710, 1981.
7. Merritt, M.V., and Baldwin, T.O., Modification of the reactive sulfhydryl of bacterial luciferase with spin-labeled maleimides, *Arch. Biochem. Biophys.* 202, 499–506, 1980
8. Baldwin, T.O., Christopher, J.A., Raushel, F.M., *et al.*, Structure of bacterial luciferase, *Curr. Opin. Struct. Biol.* 5, 798–809, 1995.

Reaction of some α,β-unsaturated carbonyl compounds (Michael acceptors) with model nucleophiles.

Michael acceptor	Michael donor/reaction conditions	Reaction rate ($M^{-1}\,s^{-1}$)	Reference
Acrylamide	GAPDH/5 mM Tris-acetate, 13.6 mM sodium arsenate, pH 7.4/30°C	0.053[a]	[1]
Acrylamide	GAPDH/5 mM Tris-acetate, 13.6 mM sodium arsenate, pH 8.5/30°C	0.267[a]	[1]
Methyl vinyl ketone	GAPDH/5 mM Tris-acetate, 13.6 mM sodium arsenate, pH 7.4/30°C	128[a]	[1]
Acrolein	GAPDH/5 mM Tris-acetate, 13.6 mM sodium arsenate, pH 7.4/30°C	297[a]	[1]
4-HNE	Ac-lysine amide/50 mM sodium phosphate, pH 7.4/23°C	1.33×10^{-3}	[2]
4-ONE	Ac-lysine amide/50 mM sodium phosphate, pH 7.4/23°C	7.46×10^{-3}	[2]
4-HNE	Ac-histamine/50 mM sodium phosphate, pH 7.4/23°C	2.14×10^{-3}	[2]
4-ONE	Ac-histamine/50 mM sodium phosphate, pH 7.4/23°C	2.21×10^{-2}	[2]
4-HNE	Ac-cystamine/50 mM sodium phosphate, pH 7.4/23°C	1.21	[2]
4-ONE	Ac-cystamine/50 mM sodium phosphate, pH 7.4/23°C	186	[2]
4-HNE	Glutathione/50 mM sodium phosphate, pH 7.4/23°C	1.33	[2]
4-ONE	Glutathione/50 mM sodium phosphate, pH 7.4/23°C	145	[2]
N-Ethylmaleimide	Cysteine/pH 7.0/25°C	1530	[3]
N-Ethylmaleimide	Cysteine/pH 6.0/25°C	153	[3]
N-Ethylmaleimide	Papain/pH 6.0/25°C	0.661	[4]

GAPDH, glyceraldehyde-3-phosphate dehydrogenase; 4-HNE, 4-hydroxy-2-nonenal; 4-ONE, 4-oxo-2-nonenal.
[a] The rate of inactivation of GAPDH is measured and assumed to reflect reaction at Cys152. The pKa of this residue is reported to be 6.03.

References

1. Martyniuk, C.J., Fang, B., Koomen, J.M., *et al.*, Molecular mechanism of glyceraldehyde-3-phosphate dehydrogenase inactivation by α,β-unsaturated carbonyl derivatives, *Chem. Res. Toxicol.* 24, 2302–2311, 2011.
2. Doorn, J.A., and Petersen, D.R., Covalent modification of amino acid nucleophiles by the lipid peroxidation products 4-hydroxy-2-nonenal and 4-oxo-2-nonenal, *Chem. Res. Toxicol.* 15, 1445–1450, 2002.
3. Gorin, G., Martic, P.A., and Doughty, G., Kinetics of the reaction of N-ethylmaleimide with cysteine and some congeners, *Arch. Biochem. Biophys.* 115, 593–597, 1966.
4. Brubacher, L.J., and Glick, B.R., Inhibition of papain by N-ethylmaleimide, *Biochemistry.* 13, 915–920, 1974.

The reaction of *N*-ethylmaleimide with amines and model sulfhydryl compounds.

Michael donor/reaction conditions	Rate (M^{-1} s^{-1})	Reference
Benzylamine, pH 8.5/25°C	0.025	[1]
Glycylglycine, pH 8.5/25°C	0.022	[1]
Piperidine, pH 8.5/25°C	0.10	[1]
L-Proline, pH 8.5/25°C	0.059	[1]
Glycine, pH 7.0/25°C	0.000062	[2]
L-Cysteine, pH 3.0/25°C	0.346	[3]
L-Cysteine, pH 4.95/25°C	14.1[a]	[3]

[a] A value of 1530 M^{-1} s^{-1} was estimated for the reaction of *N*-ethylmaleimide and L-cysteine at pH 7.0/25°C.

References

1. Sharpless, N.E., and Flavin, M., The reactions of amines and amino acids with maleimides. Structure of the reaction products deduced from infrared and nuclear magnetic resonance spectroscopy, *Biochemistry.* 5, 2963–2971, 1966.
2. Leslie, J., Kinetics of the reaction of glycine with *N*-ethylmaleimide, *Canad. J. Chem.* 48, 507–508, 1970.
3. Gorin, G., Martic, P.A., and Doughty, G., Kinetics of the reaction of N-ethylmaleimide with cysteine and some congeners, *Arch. Biochem. Biophys.* 115, 593–597, 1966.

Michael additions with fumarate

Fumarate is an intermediate of the Krebs cycle in intermediary metabolism. It has been shown that fumarate can serve as a Michael acceptor reacting with cysteine [1] and thiol groups in proteins [2]. Reaction with glutathione has also been observed [3] forming a product suggested to enhance the formation of reactive oxygen species(ROS). The formation of *S*-(2-succinyl)cysteine in glyceraldehyde-3-phosphate has been suggested to be a biomarker of mitochondrial stress [4]. Dimethyl fumarate is an active pharmaceutical ingredient of Fumaderm®—which is used to treat psoriasis; the formation of a dimethyl fumarate adduct with glutathione [5,6]. Dimethyl fumarate is rapidly hydrolyzed to monomethylfumarate which also reacts with glutathione [5]. Dimethyl fumarate has also been shown to react with amines [7]. An enzyme which catalyzes the formation of conjugates between glutathione and Michael acceptors such as diethyl fumarate was described in 1968 [8]. Other compounds of biological interest have been demonstrated to form conjugates with thiols via Michael reactions. 4-Methyleneglutamic acid [9] was observed to react with thiols [10].

References

1. Alderson, N.L., Wang, Y., Blatnik, M., *et al.*, S-(2-succinyl)cysteine: A novel chemical modification of tissue proteins by a Krebs cycle intermediate, *Arch. Biochem. Biophys.* 450, 1–8, 2006.
2. Blatnik, M., Thorpe, S.R., and Baynes, J.W., Succination of proteins by fumarate. Mechanism of inactivation of glyceraldehyde-3-phosphate dehydrogenase in diabetes, *Ann. N. Y. Acad. Sci.* 1126, 272–275, 2008.
3. Sullivan, L.B., Martinez-Garcia, E., Nguyen, H., *et al.*, The proto-oncometabolite fumarate binds glutathione to amply ROS-dependent signaling, *Mol. Cell.* 51. 236–246, 2013.
4. Blatnik, M., Frizzell, N., Thorpoe, S.R., and Baynes, J.W., Inactivation of glyceraldehyde-3-phosphate dehydrogenase by fumarate in diabetes. Formation of *S*-(2-succinyl)cysteine, a novel chemical modification of protein and possible biomarker of mitochondrial stress, *Diabetes.* 57, 41–49, 2008.
5. Schmidt, T.J., Muarrem, A., and Mrowietz, U., Reactivity of dimethyl fumarate and methyl hydrogen fumarate towards glutathione and *N*-acetyl-l-cysteine: Preparation of *S*-substituted thiosuccinic acid esters, *Bioorg. Med. Chem.* 15, 333–342, 2007.
6. Dibbert, S., Clement, B., Skak-Nielsen, T., Mrowietz, U., and Rostami-Yazdi, M., Detection of fumarate-glutathione adducts in the portal vein blood of rats: Evidence for rapid dimethylfumarate metabolism, *Arch. Dermatol.* 305, 447–451, 2013.
7. Gurjar, A., Sinha, P., and Bansal, R.K., Tandem Michael addition of amines to maleic anhydride and 1,3-prototropic shift: Experimental and theoretical results, *Tetrahedron.* 70, 5052–5056, 2014.
8. Boyland, E., and Chaseaud, L.F., Enzymes catalyzing conjugations of glutathione with αβ-unsaturated carbonyl compounds, *Biochem. J.* 109, 651–661, 1968.
9. Marcus, A., Feeley, J., and Shannon, L.M., Preparation and properties of γ-methyleneglutamic acid, *Arch. Biochem. Biophys.* 100, 80–85, 1963.
10. Powell, G.K., Winter, H.C., and Dekker, E.E., Michael addition of thiols with 4-methyleneglutamic acid: Preparation of adducts, their properties and presence in peanuts, *Biochem. Biophys. Res. Commun.* 105, 1361–1367, 1982.

Retro-Michael Additions

Retro-Michael additions of interest for antibody conjugate formation. (a) The reversible reaction of a monocyclic cyanoenones with dithiothreitol [1]. (b) The reversible reaction of a cyanoacrylamide derivative with 2-mercaptoethanol [2]. (c) The reversible reaction of benzalcyanoacetamides with a thiol [3].

The reaction of maleimide with cysteine and stability of the adduct. (a) The reaction of an *N*-alkylmaleimide with a cysteine residue in a protein and the subsequent transfer of the alkyl moiety to the sulfhydryl group in albumin or glutathione as has been observed in blood with antibody drug conjugates based on maleimide chemistry [4,5]. (b) The hydrolysis of the succinide ring in base to form an *N*-alkylsuccinimic acid [6]. (c) Acid hydrolysis under conditions used for amino acid analysis yields *S*-1,2-carboxyethylcysteine from the *N*-ethylsuccinimide derivative [7].

References

1. Zheng, S., Laxmi, Y.R.S., David, E., *et al.*, Synthesis, chemical reactivity as Michael acceptors, and biological potency of monocyclic cyanoenones, novel and highly potent anti-inflammatory and cytoprotective agents, *J. Med. Chem.* 55, 4837–4846, 2012.
2. Serafimova, I.M., Pufall, M.A., Krishnan, S., *et al.*, Reversible targeting of noncatalytic cysteines with chemically tuned electrophiles, *Nat. Chem. Biol.* 8, 471–476, 2012.
3. Zhong, Y., Xu, Y., and Anslyn, E.V., Studies of reversible conjugate additions, *Eur. J. Org. Chem.* 2013, 5021–5027, 2013.
4. Shen, B.Q., Xu, K., Liu, L., *et al.*, Conjugation site modulates the *in vivo* stability and therapeutic activity of antibody-drug conjugates, *Nat. Biotechnol.* 30, 184–189, 2012.
5. Wei, C., Zhang, G., Clark, T., *et al.*, Where did the linker-payload go? A quantitative investigation on the destination of the released linker-payload from an antibody-drug conjugate with a maleimide linker in plasma, *Anal. Chem.* 86, 4979–4986, 2016.
6. Gehring, H., and Christen, P., A diagonal procedure for isolating sulfhydryl peptides alkylated with *N*-ethylmalemide, *Anal. Biochem.* 107, 358–361, 1980.
7. Abe, Y., Ueda, T., and Imoto, T., Reduction in disulfide bonds in proteins by 2-aminothiophenol under weakly acidic conditions, *J. Biochem.* 115, 52–57, 1994.

MOLECULAR WEIGHTS OF PROTEINS AND SOME OTHER MATERIALS INCLUDING SEDIMENTATION, DIFFUSION, AND FRICTIONAL COEFFICIENTS AND PARTIAL SPECIFIC VOLUMES

Malcolm H. Smith

These tables follow earlier compilations, notably by Svedberg and Pedersen [235] and Edsall [55], and are similarly concerned primarily with information relating to ultracentrifuge studies, particularly by the sedimentation velocity technique. Such studies require direct measurement of the sedimentation coefficient, S; diffusion coefficient, D; and partial specific volume, V. From these three values, it is possible to calculate the molecular weight, M, and the frictional coefficient, f/f_0. The latter is a ratio expressing the resistance met with by the sedimenting molecule, relative to that of a smooth spherical particle of the same weight and density. It is generally assumed as a first approximation that increasing values indicate increasing axial ratios, that is, that there is departure from the spherical shape ($f/f_0 = 1$) towards something more elongated ($f/f_0 > 1$). However, the degree of hydration can also influence the frictional coefficient markedly.

The compilation is divided into index, data tables and references. The index gives an alphabetical list of entries by name of the enzyme, accompanied by an indication of the source, for example, "Cathepsin, cod spleen." Each entry in the index has one or more "entry numbers" that locate the information relating to the entry. This information is presented in the main section, consisting of a series of consecutively numbered entries divided into six parts. Tables I–VI entries are generally listed by order of sedimentation coefficient (low values first), each table starting a new sequence. Tables I and II comprise full data on globular and fibrous proteins, respectively; Tables III and IV comprise partial data on globular and fibrous proteins, respectively. The partial data may be a single S value or an S value plus either a D value or a V value. Any of the entries may also include an estimate of the molecular weight. All the entries in Tables I–IV comprise values at 20°C.

Table V is complete and distinct in itself. It comprises S values only for a large number of vertebrate serum proteins. The values were obtained from the sedimentation patterns of serum itself, during centrifugation at ambient room temperature, "very close to 20° and within the range 20–22°C" [530; Seal, personal communication].

Table VI consists of miscellaneous data—(a) entries for globular and fibrous proteins, (b) entries for viruses, (c) entries for particles and organelles, (d) entries for nucleic acids, (e) entries for carbohydrates, and (f) other entries. Some of these miscellaneous values are for temperatures other than 20°C. Such values are placed at the end of the appropriate section.

Each entry in the tables has one or more reference numbers (different from the Table numbers) which give the source of information according to the list of references which completes the compilation.

All the values quoted in the tables have been collected by personal examination of the literature, with the sole exception of a few entries in the data presented by Svedberg and Pedersen [235] and Edsall [55]. Some effort has been taken to try and ensure that calculated values of M and f/f_0 are genuinely based on measurements made by one laboratory, or on the same starting material,

rather than by combining measurements made at different times or places, or by including an assumed value. It seems that this is the only course which can enable one to evaluate such data statistically in the absence of independent knowledge of, say, the molecular weight. The entries in Tables I and II, and a few in Table VI, have met this rather stringent criterion. Tables III, IV and V, and most of Table VI, consist of entries that were inadequate in this respect.

All the molecular weights and frictional coefficients given in Tables I, II, and VI have been checked or calculated for this compilation. (Grateful acknowledgement is made to Dr. L.M. Brown for preparing a computer program and assisting with these calculations and to Dr. G.M. Birtwistle for preparing a similar program for another computer.) They are quoted to four significant figures for statistical purposes, and not because they are necessarily regarded as being of that accuracy. In contrast, all other molecular weights are as given by the authors. They are based on calculations involving the assumption of one or more values (often V), or on other methods of determining molecular weight, including sedimentation equilibrium. They are included here in order to enhance the usefulness of the tables, and their accuracy should be confirmed by reference to the original source.

The protein entries have been classed as "globular" or "fibrous," taking globular to mean approximately egg-shaped, with maximal frictional coefficient of 1.5, and fibrous to mean cigar-shaped or threadlike, with frictional coefficient above 1.5. Data presented in Tables I and II broadly support this concept, but it must be noted that there is some overlap. It is not yet clear whether the primary data are at fault or whether the general concept is too simple. It is not always clear whether a given protein is to be regarded as globular or fibrous, and any errors and anomalies in this respect are a reflection of the compiler's uncertainties in the matter.

An analysis of part of the data has shown [220] that the distribution of V is Gaussian for globular and fibrous proteins, with a mean value of about 0.74 (0.736, SD 0.020 for globular proteins). This property depends mainly on the amino acid composition, and the occurrence of a mean value is explained by the finding that there is a basic pattern of amino acid composition among proteins in general [221]. The distribution of frictional coefficient values is also Gaussian for globular proteins, with a mean value of about 1.25, suggesting an axial ratio of about 2. For fibrous proteins, there is a range of values from 1.2 to 4.7 with no clear mean. (The value of 1.5 taken as an arbitrary value to distinguish between globular and fibrous proteins suggests an axial ratio of about 6.)

Index to Protein Tables I–VI

The following index comprises an alphabetical list of entries for Tables I–VI. Entry numbers from Tables I and II, and some from Table VI, are listed in bold face. These are the entries for which full data are available.

Entry	Entry Number
A protein, *E. coli*	251
Acid proteinase, *Aspergillus*	297
Acetyl cholinesterase, *Electrophorus*	336, 803
Acetyl-CoA synthetase, bovine heart	393
F_1-Actin	878
F_2-Actin	879
G-Actin, cod	826
G-Actin, rabbit skeletal muscle	**124**
Acyl phosphatase, bovine brain	155
Acylase I, hog kidney	481
Adenine deaminase, calf intestinal mucosa	213
S-Adenine deaminase	677
Adrenocorticotropin (ACTH), pig	145, 202, 211, 214
Sheep	146, 147, 201, 207
Aequorin, *Aquorea*	209
Alanine dehydrogenase, *B. subtilis*	631
Albumin, carp serum	447
Cow	356, 358, 372, 375, 377, 394, 401, 428 429, 1059, 1088
Dog	**51**, 357
Horse	**45**, 398, 410, 1054, 1057, 1058, 1091
Human	**46**, **48**, 359, 1087
Rat	**40**, 346
Albumin esterase, mouse	392
Alcohol dehydrogenase, horse liver	**53, 56**
Yeast	584
Aldolase	615
Aldolase, bovine liver	**1099**
Rabbit liver	593
Rabbit muscle	**76**
Aldose dehydrogenase, pseudomonad	542
Alkaline phosphatase, calf	509
E. coli	512
Amandin	678, 1066
Amino acid oxidase, *Crotalus*	521
D-Amino acid oxidase, pig kidney	41, 86, 89, 583
L-Amino acid oxidase, Moccasin snake	534
Rat kidney	450, 647
δ-Aminolevulinate dehydratase, mouse	672
Amylase, malt	43
α-Amylase, *B. subtilis*	44, 68
α-Amylase, *B. stearothermophilus*	110
Pig pancreas	42
Pseudomonas	425
β-Amylase, sweet potato	633
Anthranilate synthetase, *E. coli*	648
Anticatalase	536
D-Arabinose dehydrogenase, pseudomonad	485
Arachin, *Arachis hypogaea* (ground nut)	**95**, 441, 510, 636, 641
Arginine phosphotransferase, crustacean	236
Ascorbate oxidase, *Cucurbita pepo*	490, 493, 494, 513, 531
Aspartate transaminase, ox heart	462, 466
Yeast	489
Autoprothrombin *c*, bovine	**15**
Autoprothrombin II, bovine	**39**
Azurin, *Bordetella*	165
Bacillus phlei protein	**4**
Bacteriophage—see Viruses	
Bence Jones protein, human urine	**34**, 319
Blue protein, *Pseudomonas*	195
Blue latex protein, *Rhus vernicifera*	199
C-Reactive protein	577
Canavalin, Jack bean	**67**
Carbamate kinase	**324**
Carbamyl phosphate synthetase, frog liver	656
Carbohydrates	1153-1170
Carbonic anhydrase, mammalian RBC	1098
Carbonic anhydrase, human	273

Entry	Entry Number
Carbonic anhydrase, ox blood	259
Carbonic anhydrase B	278
Carbonic anhydrase X_1, human RBC	**27**
Y, human RBC	**29**
α-Carboxylase, wheat germ	749
Carboxylesterase, pig kidney	613
Carboxypeptidase	279, 1044
Carboxypeptidase B, pig	**26**
Casein, mouse milk	874
α-Casein, cow milk	**126**
β-Casein, cow milk	**113**
Catalase, bovine liver	**91**, 654
Horse liver	**90**
Human blood	655
Micrococcus	650
Pig blood	653
Cathepsin, cod spleen	296
Cathepsin C	605
Ceruloplasmin, human	**79**, **134**, **138**, 492, 529, 550, 558
Pig	**80**, 582
Choline acetyltransferase, human placenta	423
Rabbit brain	458
Chlorocruorin, *Sabella*	770
Chloroperoxidase, *Caldariomyces fumago*	332
Chloroplast protein, spinach leaf	842
Chymopapain	254
Chymotrypsin, bovine pancreas	238, 257, 290, 1050
Chymotrypsin α, bovine pancreas	**16**, 33
Chymotrypsin β, bovine pancreas	243
Chymotrypsin inhibitor, potato	307
	18, 253, 282
Chymotrypsinogen α, bovine pancreas	**19**, 231
Chymotrypsinogen β, bovine pancreas	232
Citrate cleaving enzyme, rat liver	698
Citrate-oxalacetate lyase, *Aerobacter*	710
Clostridium toxin	862, 1101, 1105
Clupein sulfate	1108
Cobalamin protein A, hog gastric mucosa	430
Cobalamin protein B, hog gastric mucosa	403
Cocosin	669
Collagen, cod	824, 827, 831
Collagen A, earthworm	832
Collagen B, earthworm	835
Collagenase	474
Conalbumin, hen egg white	**55, 57**
Conarachin	628
Concanavalin A, Jack bean	**64, 322**
Concanavalin B, Jack bean	**32**
Creatine kinase, chicken	453, 460
Rabbit	442, 445
Crotonase	594
Crotoxin, *Crobalus benificus* (rattlesnake)	**23**
Cryptocytochrome *c*, *Pseudomonas*	245
α-Crystallin, bovine lens	863, 864, 865, 869, 870
β-Crystallin, bovine lens	857
Cytochrome, *Chlorobium*	323
Rhodopseudomonas	738
Cytochrome *a*, mammalian heart	**102**
Cytochrome b_1, *E. coli*	734
Cytochrome b_2, yeast	217, 638
Cytochrome b_3, calf liver	**112**
Cytochrome *c*, bovine heart	**2, 5, 6**, 234, 321
Chromatium	**65**
Horse heart	206, 1038
Human	177
Pig heart	221
Rust fungus	158
Vertebrate	193, 1041, 1081

Entry	Entry Number
Cytochrome c_1, bovine heart	**92**
Rhodopseudomonas	227
Cytochrome *f*	535
Cytochrome *h*	176
Cytochrome oxidase, *P. aeruginosa*	**63**
DDT dehydrochlorinase	311
DNA, T_7 bacteriophage	1152
Dehydropeptidase, bovine kidney	444
Denitrifying enzyme, bacterial (*Pseudomonas*?)	519
Dextran saccharase, *Leuconostoc*	630
Diaphorase, pig heart	470
Dihydrolipoic dehydrogenase, *E. coli*	523
Spinacea oleracea	497
Diphtheria toxin	**47**
Diphtheria antitoxin	477, 1094
Edestin	681, 1065
Enolase	**60**
Enolase, rabbit	**1096**
Elastin (urea degraded), bovine ligamentum nuchae	**108**
Erythrocuprein, human	**21**, 275
Excelsin	694, 1060
FMN, dimer	**1171**
Fatty acid synthetase system, pigeon liver	**1138**
Ferredoxin, *Clostridium*	182
Ferritin, guinea pig	719
Ferritin, horse spleen	97
Fetuin, bovine	**117, 123**
Fetuin, cow fetus	**119, 125**
Fibrinogen, bovine	852
Cod	851
Cow	1106
Horse	**139**
Human	**140**, 855, 1104
Ficin	248
Follicle-stimulating hormone, sheep	**50**, 270
Fluorokinase	645
Fumarase, hog heart	625
Galactose dehydrogenase, pseudomonad	433
β-Galactosidase, *E. coli*	**96**, 709
Ganglioside micelles, ox brain	**1137**
Globulin, *Acacia* seed	154, 159, 256, 566, 581, 590, 591, 596, 599, 601, 663, 700, 722, @@
Arachis	19@@, 621, 686
Astragalus seed	620, 690
Avena	241, 603
Cytisus	185, 600, 602, 697, 702
Dolichos	561, 664
Ervum	554, 691
Festuca	224, 617
Genista	
Glycine	598, 688
Hordeum vulgare	229, 508, 616, 670
Lathyrus	574, 576, 578, 585, 673, 683, 684, 685
Lotus	619, 689
Lupinus	562, 592, 611, 612, 618, 627, 661, 662, 675, 676, 687
Medicago	527, 660
Panicum	623
Phaseolus	360, 443, 522, 555, 567, 646, 651, 674
Phleum	609
Pisum	604, 680
Secale	240, 607
Trifolium	556, 586, 587, 657, 682, 724
Triticum vulgare	230, 608
Vicia	545, 551, 667, 668
Zea	242, 622
Globulin, bovine	723
Horse	**142**, 546, 1063, 1090
Human	**131, 141, 143**, 250, 266, 549, 861
Pig	721

Entry	Entry Number
α-Globulin, human	295, 448
α₂-Globulin	635
α-Globulin, barley	237
β-Globulin, human	479, 538, 733, 820
γ-Globulin, cow	502, 539, 570, 1061, 1082, 1085
Horse	**82**, 518, 533, 537, 1089
Human	**72, 136, 137**, 553, 559, 644
Pig	557
Rabbit	501, 526, 543
Barley	629
Gliadin	208, 1053, 1084
Glucose oxidase, *P. amagasakiense*	**84**, 614
Glucose oxidase microside protein, *Penicillium*	595
Glucose-6-phosphate dehydrogenase, human RBC	547
Glutamate dehydrogenase, bovine liver	**103**
Chicken liver	695, 703
Glutamate-aspartate transaminase	475
Glyceraldehyde phosphomutase, yeast	528
D-Glyceraldehyde-3-phosphate	649
dehydrogenase, crawfish	624
Mammalian	88
Rabbit muscle	71, 78, 81
Glycerokinase, *Candida*	
Glycoprotein, bovine plasma	320
Egg white	814
Rat	216a
α-Glycoprotein, fetal calf serum	331, 736, 868
Human	817
α₁-Glycoprotein	23a, 828
M₂-Glycoprotein, bovine	829
Gonadotrophin, human	127
Pregnant mare	301
Growth hormone, pituitary	188, 314, 1049
Pig pituitary	274
Haptoglobin type 1-1, human	833, 1102
Haptoglobin I-(methemoglobin)²	856
Haptoglobin II	128
Haptoglobin II-(methemoglobin)	846
Hemagglutinin, castor bean	515
Human cold	720
Soya bean	507, 516
Iso-hemagglutinin	732
Hemocyanin, *Achatina*	706, 784, 800
Agriolimax	796
Arion	780, 783, 793
Astacus	743
Buccinum	801, 805
Busycon	799, 804
Calocaris	753
Cancer	713, 745
Carcinus	714, 744
Chirodothea	707, 741
Eledone	756, 758, 1075
Eupagurus	717, 737
Euscorpius	752
Helix	107, 787, 792, 797, 798, 1077
Homarus	740, 1070
Hyas	742
Limax	790
Limnea	778, 791
Limulus	500, 708, 754, 765
Littorina	794, 806
Loligo	652, 727, 766, 775
Maia	748
Nephrops	747, 1069
Neptunea	802
Octopus	759, 1074
Ommatostrephes sloani pacificus	100

Entry	Entry Number
Pagurus	704
Pandalus	718
Palaemon	705
Palinurus	712, 1067
Paludina	**106**, 785, 789, 795
Rossia	764, 1076
Sepia	762
Sepiola	763
Squilla	746
Tonicella	781
Hemocyanin component, *Helix*	**101**, **105**
Paludina	**144**
Hemoglobin, *Aethelges*	729
Anadara (= Area)	302, 416
Anguilla	335
Anguis	436
Ape	326
Arenicola	769
Ascaris	666
Bufo	438, 439, 569, 588, 679
Cat	348
Chameleon	417
Chironomus	198
Chrysemys	405, 541
Coluber	418
Corvus	389
Cow	361, 420
Cyprinus	390
Daphnia	711
Dog	343, 349
Dogfish	345
Duck	379, 388
Eisenia	782
Esox	351
Eumenia	776
Frog	373, 404, 426
Gasterophilus	235
Gasterosteus	407
Glycera	306
Haemopsis	767
Hedgehog	406
Hen	350, 378
Hirudo	771
Horse	330, 385, 395, 421, 1055
Human	340, 353, 374, 397, 400, 409, 411, 412, 413, 414, 468, 531, 1051
Lacerta	419, 548
Lampetra	183, 187, 192, 1039
Lucioperca	408
Lumbricus	779, 1073
Lumbrineiris	777
Legume	**11**, **12**
Marphysa sanguinea	773, 788, 807
Mouse	344
Myxine	220
Neiris	774
Notomastus	205
Opsanus	368
Ox	339, 1093
Paramecium	162
Parus	364
Pectinaria	761
Picus	363
Pig	342
Pigeon	382, 387
Planorbis	751, 755, 1072
Pleuronectes	367
Polymnia	768
Prionotus	391

Entry	Entry Number
Protopterus	366
Rabbit	354, 386
Raja	365
Salamandra	437, 540
Salmo	334
Sheep	341
Syrnium	362
Tautoga	352
Thyone	244
Tubifex	757
Turtle	355
δ-Hemolysin, staphylococcal	505
Hemopexin	440
Heparin fraction	**116**
Histone I, calf thymus	**114**
Histone II, calf thymus	808
β-Histone	811, 859
γ-Histone	822
Homogentisate oxygenase, *Pseudomonas fluorescens*	665
Hordein	200
p-Hydroxybenzoate hydroxylase, *Pseudomonas putida*	459
Hydroxyproline epimerase, *Pseudomonas*	171
20-β-Hydroxy steroid dehydrogenase, *Streptomyces*	524
L-Iditol dehydrogenase	589
Insulin	**8**, 153, 166, 168, 178, 186, 284, 298, 303, 310, 316, 329, 1095
Interferon	432
Interstitial cell-stimulating hormone (ICSH), human pituitary	255
Iridine, *Salmo*	**109**
Iron-binding protein, cow milk	456
Isocitrate lyase, *Pseudomonas*	640
Isocitric enzyme	435
Kallikrein inactivator, bovine parotid	156
Keratinase, *Streptomyces*	223
α-Ketoglutarate dehydrogenase system, *E. coli*	**1141**
Laccase	473, 511, 520
Laccase A, *Polyporus*	434
Laccase B, *Polyporus*	427
Lactalbumin, cow	191, 1040
Human	173
Lactate dehydrogenase, chicken	**73, 75**
Bovine	**70, 74, 77**
Ox heart	478, 544
Pig heart	**69**
Lactogenic hormone	247
Lactogenic hormone, sheep	**14**, 215
Lactoglobulin	283, 1048
β-Lactoglobulin	261, 268, 277, 289
β-Lactoglobulin, goat	263
β₂-Lactoglobulin, human	267
Lactoperoxidase	**58**
Lactotransferrin	402, 424
Legumin, *Pisum sativum* (pea)	**94**
Lewis blood group substance	**132**
Lipase, milk	1
Lipoamide dehydrogenase, pig liver	503
Lipoeuglobulin III, human	853
Lipoprotein, human serum (high density)	838, 841
α-Lipoprotein, human serum	337, 840, 843
β-Lipoprotein, human	**133**
β-Lipovitellin	837
Lipovitellin	858
Lipoxidase, soya bean	**61**
β-Livetin	272, 821
α-Livetin	383
Luciferase, *Cypridina*	**299, 415**
Luteinizing hormone, pig	
Lysolecithin sol, egg	1136
Lysosome, rat liver	1148a

Entry	Entry Number
Lysozyme, chicken egg white	**7**, 180, 189, 210, 1045
Lysozyme, *Papaya*	239
α-Macroglobulin, rat serum	725
α₂-Macroglobulin, human	866
Malate-lactate transhydrogenase, *Micrococcus lactilyticus*	422
Malate dehydrogenase, *B. subtilis*	506
Bovine	369, 457
Horse	381
Ox	396, 1097
Pig heart	312, 376
Megacin	380
Merino wool protein, SCM KB1	170
SCM KB2	163
Metallothionein, horse kidney	**3**
Metapyrocatechase, *Pseudomonas*	484
Methylmalonyl racemase, *Propionibacterium*	269
Milk protein, mouse	160
Mitochondrion, rat liver	1148b
Monoamine oxidase, ox plasma	634
Plasma	639
Mucin, pig submaxillary gland	836
Mucoid, bovine cervix	873, 867
Mucoprotein, cartilage	849
Cow milk	839
Human plasma	**121**, 860
Sheep submaxillary gland	854
Urinary	739, 750, 830, 871, 875, 877
Myeloperoxidase, infected dog uterus	**85**
Myogen A, rabbit skeletal muscle	**83**
Myoglobin, *Aplysia*	203
Horse	**13**, 197
Guinea pig	204
Mammalian	**10**
Seal	190
Tortoise	179
Tunny	169
Myokinase	174
Myosin	848, 850, 1100
Myosin, bovine	844
Cod	**135**, 847
Dog heart	845
γ-Myosin	818
Myxomyosin	876
NAD glycohydrolase	327
Nerve protein, lobster	693
Neuraminase, *Vibrio cholerae*	476
Nuclear protein, chicken RBC	148
Rat carcinoma	157
Nucleic acid—see DNA, RNA	
Old yellow enzyme, brewer's yeast	**62**, 491
Ornithine transcarbamylase	568
Ovalbumin	309, 315, 1047, 1092
Oxytocic hormone	246
Papain	225
Paramyosin, *Venus mercenaria*	1110
Penicillinase, *Bacillus*	286, 1046
Pepsin	265, 271, 294, 1042, 1043, 1086
Pepsinogen	291
Peptidase A, *Penicillium*	281
Peptomyosin B	812
Peroxidase, wheat	249, 293
Peroxidase II, horse radish	**31**, **36**
Phage—see Viruses	
Phenol oxidase, *Calliphora* larva	716
Phosphoenolpyruvate carboxykinase, pig liver	463
Phosphoglycerate mutase, chicken muscle	325
Rabbit muscle	399
Yeast	514

Entry	Entry Number
Sulfate-binding protein, *Salmonella*	287
T component, horse	532
TB bacillus protein	**28**
Taka-amylase A	**49**, 328
Thetin-homocysteinase	610
Thiogalactoside transacetylase, *E. coli*	452
Thrombin, bovine	**35**, 149
Thyroglobulin, pig	728, 730, 1071, 1083
Transamidinase, hog kidney	482
Transferrin, human	446, 449, 454, 471, 480, 483, 486, 504, 1103
Monkey	461
Pig	495, 496
Rat	455
Transglutaminase, pig liver	1098a
Tropocollagen, calf skin	823
Tropomyosin, blowfly	815, 819
Pinna nobilis	**120**
Rabbit	816, 1109
Triose phosphate dehydrogenase, bovine	571
Chicken	564
E. coli	562
Halibut	580
Human	579
Lobster	573
Pheasant	563
Rabbit	560
Sturgeon	572
Turkey	565
Yeast	575
Trypsin	172, 233
Trypsinogen, bovine pancreas	**17**
Trypsin inhibitor, bovine pancreas	151
soya bean	181, 218, 219, 222, 1079
α-Trypsin inhibitor, human serum	**30**, 300
Tryptophan synthetase B, *E. coli*	451
Tryptophanase, *E. coli*	637, 642
Turnip Yellow Mosaic Virus protein	**104**
Tween hydrolysing enzyme	530
Tyrosine transaminase, rat kidney	499
Tyrosine, *Psalliota* (mushroom)	517
Tyrosinase L, *Neurospora crassa*	370
Tyrosinase S, *Neurospora crassa*	371
Urease, Jack bean	**99**
Venom substrate, bovine plasma	**38**
Vicilin, *Pisum sativum* (pea)	**87**
Viper venom coagulant	**54**
Viruses	1111–1134
Wheat germ hemoprotein 550	**24**
Yeast protein	**66**
Zein	810, 1107

Protein Tables I–VI: Conditions and Units

All values given in the following protein tables (Tables I–VI) were determined in aqueous medium. They are corrected to standard conditions (20°C, water), except for Table V and a few values in Table VI. Values extrapolated to zero concentration are quoted where possible. Names of proteins follow those given by the original authors, except where a preferred alternative has become obvious.

Sedimentation coefficients are given in Svedbergs, $S = \sec \times 10^{-13}$.

Diffusion coefficients are given in Ficks, $F = cm^2\ sec^{-1} \times 10^{-7}$.

Partial specific volumes, $V = g/ml^3$.

TABLE I: Full data—globular proteins

No.	Protein	$S_{20.w} \times 10^{13}$	$D_{20.w} \times 10^{7}$	V_{20}	Molecular Weight	f/f_0	Reference Number
1	Lipase, milk	1.14	14.48	0.7137	6,669	1.190	277
2	Cytochrome c, bovine heart	1.71	11.40	0.728	13,370	1.191	56
3	Metallothionein, horse kidney	1.75	12.42	0.648	9,720	1.264	115
4	*Bacillus phlei* protein	1.80	10.20	0.748	16,970	1.218	235, 286
5	Ferro-cytochrome c, bovine heart	1.87	12.90	0.707	12,000	1.102	171
6	Ferri-cytochrome c, bovine heart	1.91	13.20	0.707	11,980	1.077	171
7	Lysozyme, chicken egg white	1.91	11.20	0.703	13,930	1.210	227
8	Insulin	1.95	7.30	0.735	24,430	1.516	55, 287
9	Ribonuclease, bovine pancreas	2.00	13.10	0.707	12,640	1.066	55, 288
10	CO-myoglobin I, mammalian	2.01	10.30	0.743	18,400	1.177	56
11	Hemoglobin I, legume	2.01	11.18	0.740	16,760	1.120	59
12	Hemoglobin II, legume	2.04	12.35	0.740	15,400	1.043	59
13	Myoglobin, horse heart	2.04	11.30	0.741	16,890	1.105	235, 289, 290
14	Lactogenic hormone (prolactin), sheep	2.19	8.44	0.739	24,100	1.315	138
15	Autoprothrombin c, bovine	2.27	8.4	0.695	21,500	1.401	278
16	Chymotrypsin α (monomer), bovine pancreas	2.40	10.20	0.736	21,600	1.130	55, 291
17	Trypsinogen, bovine pancreas	2.48	9.70	0.737	23,560	1.154	55, 292
18	Chymotrypsinogen, bovine pancreas	2.54	9.50	0.721	23,240	1.193	55, 293
19	Chymotrypsinogen α, bovine pancreas	2.58	9.48	0.721	23,650	1.188	263
20	RHP, *Rhodospirillum rubrum*	2.70	8.65	0.731	28,130	1.223	9
21	Erythrocuprin, human	2.77	7.05	0.715	33,430	1.427	232
22	Rhodanese, bovine liver	3.00	7.50	0.742	37,570	1.275	229
23	Crotoxin, *Crotalus terrificus* (rattlesnake)	3.14	8.60	0.704	29,920	1.221	235, 294
23a	α-Glycoprotein, pleural fluid	3.15	6.75	0.75	45,230	1.327	22
24	Wheat germ hemoprotein 550	3.16	6.87[a]	0.720	39,830	1.379	279
25	RHP, *Chromatium*	3.20	7.50	0.706	35,200	1.325	9
26	Carboxypeptidase B, pig	3.23	8.16	0.720	34,280	1.220	69
27	Carbonic anhydrase X_1, human RBC	3.23	10.66	0.739	28,140	0.989	194
28	T.B. bacillus protein	3.30	8.20	0.700	32,540	1.247	235, 286
29	Carbonic anhydrase Y, human RBC	3.30	10.04	0.740	30,640	1.020	194
30	α-Trypsin inhibitor, human serum	3.41	5.2	0.646	44,980	1.813	28
31	Peroxidase II, horse radish	3.48	7.05	0.699	39,780	1.357	35
32	Concanavalin B, Jack bean	3.50	7.40	0.730	42,470	1.247	235, 295
33	Chymotrypsin α (dimer), bovine pancreas	3.50	7.40	0.731	42,620	1.245	55, 291 296
34	Bence Jones protein, human urine	3.50	9.65	0.715	30,860	1.071	50
35	Thrombin, bovine	3.76	8.76	0.69	33,590	1.161	92
36	Peroxidase II, horse radish	3.85	6.84	0.690	44,050	1.358	247
37	Proteinase, *Pseudomonas*	3.99	7.4	0.730	48,410	1.194	102
38	Venom substrate, bovine plasma	4.23	4.57	0.738	85,630	1.593	65
39	Autoprothrombin II, bovine	4.33	7.45	0.708	48,280	1.199	92
40	Albumin, rat serum	4.41	6.0	0.720	63,650	1.350	280
41	D-Amino acid oxidase apo-enzyme, pig kidney	4.50	4.50	0.789	114,700	1.435	271
42	α-Amylase, pig pancreas	4.50	8.05	0.700	45,200	1.139	41
43	Amylase, malt	4.52	6.53	0.690	54,180	1.328	42
44	α-Amylase (Zn free), *B. subtilis*	4.56	7.98	0.717	48,960	1.109	67
45	Albumin, horse serum	4.58	6.42	0.748	68,600	1.215	55, 297
46	Albumin, human serum	4.60	6.10	0.733	68,460	1.288	55, 177
47	*Diphtheria* toxin	4.60	6.00	0.736	70,390	1.296	55, 299
48	Albumin, human serum	4.67	5.93	0.736	72,300	1.300	55, 300
49	Taka-amylase A	4.67	7.37	0.700	51,240	1.193	103
50	Follicle-stimulating hormone, sheep	4.7	6.0	0.718	67,360	1.326	55, 301
51	Albumin, canine serum	4.84	6.19	0.729	69,950	1.263	253
52	Prothrombin, bovine	4.85	6.24	0.700	62,850	1.316	188
53	Alcohol dehydrogenase, horse liver	4.88	6.50	0.751	73,050	1.174	245
54	Viper venom coagulant	5.05	4.20	0.720	104,100	1.637	265
55	Conalbumin, chicken egg white	5.05	5.30	0.732	86,180	1.374	75
56	Alcohol dehydrogenase, horse liver	5.11	5.96	0.750	83,090	1.227	58
57	Fe-conalbumin, chicken egg white	5.26	5.72	0.732	83,180	1.288	75
58	Lactoperoxidase	5.37	5.95	0.764	92,620	1.178	247
59	Red protein, cow milk	5.55	5.75	0.725	85,100	1.276	86
60	Enolase	5.59	8.08	0.735	63,280	0.998	55
61	Lipoxidase, soya bean	5.62	5.59	0.750	97,440	1.240	246
62	Old yellow enzyme, brewer's yeast	5.76	6.30	0.731	82,390	1.174	235, 302
63	Cytochrome oxidase, *P. aeruginosa*	5.80	5.80	0.730	89,790	1.240	99
64	Concanavalin A, Jack bean	6.00	5.60	0.730	96,200	1.255	235, 295

TABLE I: Full data—globular proteins (Continued)

No.	Protein	$S_{20.w} \times 10^{13}$	$D_{20.w} \times 10^7$	V_{20}	Molecular Weight	f/f_0	Reference Number
65	Cytochrome c, Chromatium	6.00	5.30	0.718	97,350	1.328	9
66	Yeast protein	6.20	5.89	0.744	99,640	1.172	141
67	Canavalin, Jack bean	6.40	5.10	0.730	112,700	1.307	235, 295
68	α-Amylase, B. subtilis	6.47	5.72	0.717	96,920	1.233	67
69	Lactate dehydrogenase, pig heart	6.93	5.95	0.741	109,000	1.127	105
70	Lactic dehydrogenase H, beef heart	7.0	5.10	0.750	133,000	1.226	281
71	D-Glyceraldehyde-3-phosphate dehydrogenase, rabbit muscle	7.01	5.46	0.741	120,100	1.189	243
72	γ-Globulin, human	7.12	4.00	0.718	153,100	1.513	185
73	Lactic dehydrogenase H, chicken	7.31	4.53[b]	0.740	150,400	1.330	282
74	Lactic dehydrogenase M, beef heart	7.32	4.47[b]	0.740	152,600	1.342	282
75	Lactic dehydrogenase M, chicken	7.33	4.90	0.740	139,400	1.261	282
76	Aldolase, rabbit skeletal muscle	7.35	4.63	0.742	149,100	1.304	243
77	Lactic dehydrogenase H, beef heart	7.45	5.47[b]	0.747	130,400	1.152	282
78	D-Glyceraldehyde-3-phosphate dehydrogenase, rabbit muscle	7.50	10.00	0.731	67,590	0.790	60
79	Ceruloplasmin, human	7.50	4.70	0.730	143,300	1.309	185
80	Ceruloplasmin, pig	7.50	4.70	0.730	143,300	1.309	185
81	D-Glyceraldehyde-3-phosphate dehydrogenase (+ KCN), rabbit muscle	7.71	4.97	0.725	136,800	1.260	71
82	γ-Globulin, horse	7.75	4.80	0.739	149,900	1.257	180
83	Myogen A, rabbit skeletal muscle	7.86	4.78	0.735	150,400	1.264	81
84	Glucose oxidase, P. amagasakiense	7.93	5.02	0.750	153,100	1.188	130
85	Myeloperoxidase, infected dog uterus	7.94	4.81	0.731	148,800	1.263	57
86	D-Amino acid oxidase holo-enzyme, pig kidney	8.00	6.00	0.718	114,700	1.111	271
87	Vicilin, Pisum sativum (pea)	8.10	4.26	0.752	185,800	1.312	43
88	D-Glyceraldehyde-3-phosphate dehydrogenase, mammalian	10.00	6.80	0.737	135,500	0.919	60
89	D-Amino acid oxidase, Michaelis complex, pig kidney	11.00	6.80	0.655	113,800	1.013	270
		11.00	7.90	0.705	114,500		
90	Catalase, horse liver	11.20	4.30	0.715	221,600	1.246	3
91	Catalase, bovine liver	11.30	4.10	0.730	247,500	1.251	100, 235, 303
92	Cytochrome c_1, bovine heart	12.05	3.31	0.762	370,500	1.335	283
93	Soya bean protein	12.20	2.91	0.719	361,800	1.561	267
94	Legumin, Pisum sativum (pea)	12.64	3.49	0.735	331,300	1.330	43
95	Arachin, Arachis hypogaea (ground nut)	14.6	3.2	0.72	395,100	1.377	108
96	β-Galactosidase, E. coli ML309	15.93	3.12	0.76	515,300	1.270	284
97	Apoferritin, horse spleen	17.60	3.61	0.747	466,900	1.141	196
98	Protochlorophyll-protein complex, bean leaf	18.00	2.63	0.730	614,500	1.440	18
99	Urease, Jack bean	18.60	3.46	0.730	482,700	1.186	235, 304
100	Hemocyanin, Ommatostrephes sloani pacificus (Squid)	19.50	2.80	0.724	611,800	1.358	176
101	Hemocyanin component, Helix pomatia	19.70	1.77	0.738	1,030,000	1.795	27
102	Cytochrome a, mammalian heart	21.9	3.58	0.72	529,800	1.117	241
103	Glutamate dehydrogenase, bovine liver	26.60	2.54	0.750	1,015,000	1.250	55, 305
104	Turnip yellow mosaic virus protein	48.80	1.51	0.740	3,013,000	1.470	147
105	Hemocyanin component, Helix pomatia	65.70	1.41	0.738	4,310,000	1.398	27
106	Hemocyanin, Paludina vivipara	102.5	1.09	0.738	8,699,000	1.431	27
107	Hemocyanin, Helix pomatia	103.0	1.07	0.738	8,905,000	1.446	27

Compiled by Malcolm H. Smith.
[a] Calculated from quoted value of $S/D = 0.46 \times 10^6$.
[b] Calculated from sedimentation equilibrium data.

TABLE II: Full data—fibrous proteins

No.	Protein	$S_{20.w} \times 10^{13}$	$D_{20.w} \times 10^7$	V_{20}	Molecular Weight	f/f_0	Reference Number
108	Elastin (urea-graded), bovine ligamentum nuchae	0.71	11.33	0.778	6,830	1.466	24
109	Iridine, *Salmo*	0.74	13.0	0.66	4,064	1.605	285
110	α-Amylase, *B. stearothermophilus*	0.762	3.85	0.69	15,450	3.421	146
111	Spore peptide, *B. megaterium*	1.28	5.88	0.655	15,320	2.286	191
112	Cytochrome b_3, calf liver	1.37	8.13	0.723	14,750	1.620	233
113	β-Casein, cow milk	1.57	6.05	0.739	24,100	1.835	236
114	Histone I, calf thymus	2.03	5.13	0.74	36,890	1.877	251
115	Sialoprotein (phosphate extracted), bovine cortical bone	2.10	5.20	0.68	30,630	2.026	266
116	Heparin fraction	2.13	7.45	0.44	12,420	2.209	132
117	Fetuin, bovine	2.86	5.2	0.712	46,310	1.738	188
118	Phosvitin	2.92	4.6	0.545	33,910	2.384	113, 159
119	Fetuin, cow fetus	3.09	5.0	0.692	48,680	1.795	186
120	Tropomyosin, *Pinna nobilis*	3.1	2.21	0.736	128,800	2.877	119
121	Mucoprotein, human plasma	3.11	5.27	0.675	44,070	1.775	222
122	α₁-Seromucoid, human plasma	3.2	6.0	0.688	41,480	1.581	210
123	Fetuin, calf	3.28	5.5	0.714	50,570	1.595	186
124	G-ADP actin, rabbit skeletal muscle	3.38	5.28	0.732	57,900	1.575	156
125	Fetuin, cow fetus	3.47	5.73	0.696	48,330	1.567	230
126	α-Casein, cow milk	3.99	2.90	0.726	121,700	2.244	236
127	Gonadotrophin, human urinary	4.3	4.4	0.76	98,630	1.563	143
128	Haptoglobin II	4.3	4.7	0.720	79,230	1.602	87
129	Plasminogen, human plasma	4.30	4.31	0.71	83,440	1.725	46
130	α₃-Protein, canine	4.84	4.07	0.727	105,600	1.676	253
131	Globulin, metal-binding, human plasma	4.9	5.0	0.716	83,680	1.482	210
132	Lewis blood group substance	5.44	1.37	0.643	270,100	3.793	122
133	β-Lipoprotein, human	5.9	1.7	0.97	2,663,000	1.243	55, 306
134	Apo-ceruloplasmin, human	6.15	2.96	0.728	185,200	1.910	117
135	Myosin, cod	6.43	1.10	0.730	524,800	3.628	38
136	Pseudo γ-globulin, human plasma	6.9	4.0	0.720	149,400	1.524	210
137	Eu-γ-globulin, human plasma	6.9	4.0	0.720	149,400	1.524	210
138	Ceruloplasmin, human	7.08	3.76	0.713	159,100	1.593	117
139	Fibrinogen, horse	7.2	1.2	0.710	501,800	3.408	210
140	Fibrinogen, human	7.63	1.98	0.725	339,700	2.336	32
141	Euglobulin, human pathological	19.3	1.5	0.733	1,168,100	2.035	185
142	Globulin, horse antipneumococcus	19.3	1.80	0.715	912,400	1.857	235, 307
143	α₂-Macroglobulin, human plasma	19.5	2.3	0.735	775,500	1.520	210
144	Hemocyanin component, *Paludina vivipara*	21.8	1.79	0.738	1,127,000	1.722	27

Compiled by Malcolm H. Smith.

Table III: Incomplete data—globular proteins

No.	Protein	$S_{20.w} \times 10^{13}$	$D_{20.w} \times 10^7$	V_{20}	Molecular Weight	Reference Number
145	Adrenocorticotropin A, pig pituitary	0.54	11.3	–	4,390	137
146	Adrenocorticotropin, sheep pituitary	0.73	12.2	–	5,363	137
147	Adrenocorticotropin, sheep pituitary	0.736	13.19	–	4,790	231
148	Nuclear protein, chicken RBC	0.8	–	–	–	440
149	Thrombin, bovine	0.9	9.0	–	9,250	441
150	Proteinase, *Tetrahymena*	0.95	–	–	10,400	51
151	Trypsin inhibitor, bovine pancreas	1.0	–	–	6,513	442
152	Secretin phosphate, hog intestine	1.03	–	–	–	91, 235
153	Insulin	1.2	16	–	–	55, 308, 421
154	Globulin, *Acacia* seed	1.25	–	–	–	43
155	Acyl phosphatase, bovine brain	1.25	9.15	–	13,200	190
156	Kallikrein inactivator, bovine parotid	1.32	11.0	–	11,600	128
157	Nuclear protein, RP2-L, rat carcinoma	1.32	2.68	–	33,000	443
158	Cytochrome *c*, rust fungus	1.4	7.7	–	18,000	167
159	Globulin, *Acacia* seed	1.46	–	–	–	43
160	Milk protein, mouse	1.5	16.4	–	9,000	199
161	Ribonuclease, *B. subtilis*	1.5	–	0.703	10,500	444
162	Hemoglobin, *Paramecium*	1.50	9.8	–	13,400	225
163	Merino wool protein, SCMKB2	1.55	–	–	22,000	445
164	Proteinase, *B. subtilis*	1.58	–	–	27,000	446
165	Azurin, *Bordetella*	1.59	10.6	–	14,600	447
166	Insulin	1.6	15	–	12,000	55, 309
167	Ribonuclease T$_1$	1.62	12.0	–	11,000	252
168	Insulin	1.65	–	–	–	55, 310
169	Myoglobin, tunny	1.65	–	–	–	192
170	Merino wool protein, SCMKB1	1.65	–	–	28,000	445
171	Hydroxyproline epimerase, *Pseudomonas*	1.65	–	–	10,500	448
172	Trypsin	1.69	10.95	–	15,100	55, 297
173	Lactalbumin, human	1.7	–	0.72	23,000	144
174	Myokinase	1.7	–	–	21,600	30
175	Plastocyanin, spinach	1.72	6.6	–	21,000	118
176	Cytochrome *h*	1.73	8.4	–	–	121
177	Cytochrome *c*, human	1.73	–	0.72	12,502	449
178	Insulin	1.75	–	–	–	55, 308, 421
179	Myoglobin, tortoise	1.75	–	–	–	101
180	Lysozyme, chicken egg white	1.8	–	–	–	55, 312
181	Trypsin inhibitor, soya bean	1.80	–	0.736	14,300	450
182	Ferredoxin, *Clostridium*	1.80	–	–	–	237
183	Hemoglobin, *Lampetra*	1.80	–	–	17,200	5
184	Ribonuclease, bovine pancreas	1.82	–	–	–	451
185	Globulin, *Cytisus* seed	1.84	–	–	–	43
186	Insulin	1.85	–	–	–	55, 313
187	Hemoglobulin, *Lampetra*	1.87	–	–	17,100	235, 314
188	Growth hormone, pituitary	1.88	7.20	–	25,400	137
189	Lysozyme, chicken egg white	1.9	11.2	–	–	55, 315
190	Myoglobin, seal	1.9	–	–	–	201
191	Lactalbumin, cow	1.9	–	–	17,400	55
192	Hemoglobin, *Lampetra*	1.9	–	–	18,200	136
193	Cytochrome *c*, Vertebrate	1.9	–	–	–	235
194	Ribonuclease, pancreatic	1.9	–	0.691	13,500	444
195	Blue protein, *Pseudomonas*	1.90	11.1	–	16,300	234
196	Globulin, *Arachis* seed	1.93	–	–	–	43
197	Myoglobin, horse	1.97	–	–	–	200
198	Hemoglobin, *Chironomous*	2.0	–	–	31,500	235, 317
199	Blue latex protein, *Rhus vernicifera*	2.0	6.0	–	25,000	175
200	Hordein	2.0	6.5	–	–	235, 318
201	Adrenocorticotropin, sheep	2.00	9.0	–	20,000	55, 319
202	Adrenocorticotropin, pig	2.04	–	–	–	55, 320
203	Myoglobin, *Aplysia*	2.06	–	–	–	200
204	Myoglobin, guinea pig	2.07	11.3	–	17,100	94
205	Hemoglobin, *Notomastus*	2.1	–	–	36,400	235, 317
206	Cytochrome *c*, horse heart	2.1	13.0	–	13,400	55, 321
207	Adrenocorticotropin, sheep	2.1	10.5	–	–	55, 323
208	Gliadin	2.10	–	–	28,000	235, 322
209	Aequorin, *Aquorea*	2.1	–	–	–	452

TABLE III: Incomplete data—globular proteins (Continued)

No.	Protein	$S_{20,w} \times 10^{13}$	$D_{20,w} \times 10^{7}$	V_{20}	Molecular Weight	Reference Number
210	Lysozyme, chicken egg white	2.11	–	0.722	17,200	55, 324
211	Adrenocorticotropin, pig	2.11	–	–	–	55, 320
212	Ribonuclease, bovine pancreas	2.15	10.2	–	17,000	55, 325
213	Adenine deaminase, calf intestinal mucosa	2.15	–	–	–	25
214	Adrenocorticotropin, pig	2.16	10.8		–	223
215	Prolactin, sheep	2.17	8.62		23,400	453
216	Pomelin	2.2	–	–	–	235, 326
216a	Glycoprotein, rat	2.2	–	–	–	68
217	Cytochrome b_2, yeast	2.2	10.8	–	18,000	274
218	Trypsin inhibitor, soya bean	2.29	–	0.735	21,600	450
219	Trypsin inhibitor, soya bean	2.3	9.03	–	24,000	15
220	Hemoglobin, *Myxine*	2.3	–	–	23,100	235, 317
221	Cytochrome *c*, pig heart	2.3	12.3	–	15,500	55, 321
222	Trypsin inhibitor, soya bean	2.30	–	0.745	22,700	450
223	Keratinase, *Streptomyces*	2.4	–	–	–	454
224	Globulin, *Festuca* seed	2.4	–	–	–	43
225	Papain	2.42	10.3	–	20,700	226
226	Proteinase, *Tetrahymena*	2.45	–	–	17,500	51
227	Cytochrome c_1, *Rhodopsendomonas*	2.47	–	–	25,000	178
228	Somatotropin, human	2.47	8.88	–	27,100	137
229	Globulin, *Hordeum vulgare* seed	2.5	–	–	–	43
230	Globulin, *Triticum vulgare* seed	2.5	–	–	–	43
231	Chymotrypsinogen α, bovine pancreas	2.5	10.2	–	22,000	55, 327
232	Chymotrypsinogen β, bovine pancreas	2.5	10.4	–	21,600	55, 327
233	Trypsin	2.5	–	–	–	55, 329
234	Cytochrome *c*, bovine heart	2.5	13.3	–	15,600	55, 321
235	Hemoglobin, *Gasterophilus*	2.5	–	–	–	2
236	Arginine phosphotransferase, crustacean	2.5	5.6	–	43,000	61
237	α-Globulin, barley	2.5	7.4	–	29,000	43
238	Chymotrypsin, bovine pancreas	2.53	–	–	–	55, 330
239	Lysozyme, *Papaya*	2.57	9.35	–	24,300	224
240	Globulin, *Secale* seed	2.6	–	–	–	43
241	Globulin, *Avena* seed	2.6	–	–	–	43
242	Globulin, *Zea* seed	2.6	–	–	–	43
243	Chymotrypsin β, bovine pancreas	2.6	9.9	–	23,600	55, 327
244	Hemoglobin, *Thyone*	2.6	–	–	23,600	235, 317
245	Cryptocytochrome *c*, *Pseudomonas*	2.60	9.1	–	26,400	234
246	Oxytocic hormone	2.61	8.5	–	30,000	55, 331
247	Prolactin	2.65	7.5	–	32,000	55, 332
248	Ficin	2.66	–	–	–	37
249	Peroxidase, wheat	2.68	7.98	–	32,000	215
250	γ_1-Globulin, human plasma	2.7	–	–	–	240
251	"A" Protein, *E. coli*	2.7	–	–	29,500	95
252	Scarlet fever toxin	2.7	9.5	–	27,000	55, 333
253	Chymotrypsinogen, bovine pancreas	2.7	–	0.73	30,000	55, 330
254	Chymopapain	2.71	–	0.721	27,000	53
255	Interstitial-cell-stimulating hormone (ICSH), human pituitary	2.71	–	–	26,000	455
256	Globulin, *Acacia* seed	2.72	–	–	–	43
257	Chymotrypsin, bovine pancreas	2.74	4.14	–	64,500	55, 297
258	Somatotrophin, sheep	2.76	5.25	–	47,800	137
259	Carbonic anhydrase, ox blood	2.8	9.0	–	30,000	55, 328
260	Protease, *Streptococcus*	2.8	–	–	20,000	170
261	β-Lactoglobulin	2.83	7.34	–	–	55, 355, 430
262	Somatotrophin, whale	2.84	6.56	–	39,900	137
263	β-Lactoglobulin, goat	2.85	7.48	–	37,100	8
264	ε-Protoxin, *Clostridium*	2.85	11.5	–	23,200	456
265	Pepsin	2.88	–	–	32,700	457
266	γ-Globulin, human	2.9	–	–	25,000	359
267	β_2-Lactoglobulin, human	2.9	–	–	–	208
268	β-Lactoglobulin	2.91	–	–	–	55, 334
269	Methylmalonyl racemase, *Propionibacterium*	2.95	–	–	–	459
270	Follicle-stimulating hormone, bovine pituitary	3.0	–	–	31,000	531
271	Pepsin	3.0	–	–	–	55, 335
272	β-Livetin	3.00	–	–	45,000	150

TABLE III: Incomplete data—globular proteins (Continued)

No.	Protein	$S_{20,w} \times 10^{13}$	$D_{20,w} \times 10^7$	V_{20}	Molecular Weight	Reference Number
273	Carbonic anhydrase, human	3.01	–	–	34,000	172
274	Growth hormone, pig pituitary	3.02	6.54	–	41,600	183
275	Erythrocuprein, human RBC	3.02	9.3	–	28,000	124
276	Phospholipase A-II, *Crotalus adamanteus*	3.03	–	–	30–35,000	488
277	β-Lactoglobulin	3.05	–	–	–	55, 336
278	Carbonic anhydrase B	3.06	–	0.742	31,000	140
279	Carboxypeptidase	3.07	–	–	–	55, 337
280	Phospholipase A-I, *Crotalus adamanteus*	3.08	–	–	30–35,000	488
281	Peptidase A, *Pencillium*	3.1	8.40	–	32,000	492
282	Chymotrypsinogen, bovine pancreas	3.1	7.9	–	38,000	55, 338
283	Lactoglobulin	3.12	–	0.751	–	235, 339
284	Insulin	3.12	8.2	–	–	39
285	Protein X, human blood	3.15	–	0.747	25,000	49
286	Penicillase, *Bacillus*	3.17	5.2	–	56,000	187
287	Sulfate-binding protein, *Salmonella typhimurium*	3.18	7.4	–	34,000	532
288	Somatotrophin, beef	3.19	7.23	–	45,000	137
289	β-Lactoglobulin	3.2	–	–	–	55, 340
290	Chymotrypsin, bovine pancreas	3.2	–	–	–	55, 341
291	Pepsinogen	3.24	–	–	40,400	457
292	Pyridine nucleosidase, bull semen	3.25	–	–	–	1
293	Peroxidase, wheat germ	3.29	7.10	–	45,000	215
294	Pepsin	3.3	–	–	35,500	55, 342
295	α-Globulin, human	3.3	–	–	–	188, 343
296	Cathepsin, cod spleen	3.31	5.65	–	58,300	458
297	Acid proteinase, *Aspergillus*	3.33	–	–	34,900	413
298	Insulin	3.34	–	–	–	55, 344
299	Luciferase, *Cypridina*	3.4	7.4	–	45,000	66
300	Trypsin inhibitor, human	3.41	5.2	0.646	–	188
301	Gonadotrophin, pregnant mare	3.45	–	–	–	135
302	Hemoglobin, *Anadara* (= *Arca*)	3.46	–	–	33,500	235, 317
303	Insulin	3.47	–	–	–	55, 345
304	Proteolytic inhibitor, blood	3.48	4.35	–	72,000	82
305	Phosphoglycerokinase, chicken muscle	3.5	–	–	–	
306	Hemoglobin, *Glycera*	3.5	–	–	–	235, 317
307	Chymotrypsin inhibitor, potato	3.50	8.25	–	34,000	461
308	Proteinase, *Tetrahymena*	3.54	–	–	29,300	51
309	Ovalbumin	3.55	–	0.749	–	235
310	Insulin	3.55	7.53	–	46,000	55, 346
311	DDT dehydrochlorinase	3.6	–	–	36,000	142
312	Malic dehydrogenase, pig heart	3.6	8.47	–	40,000	268
313	Protease, *Bacillus thermoproteolyticus*	3.6	–	–	37,500	533
314	Growth hormone, pituitary	3.60	7.36	–	49,200	55, 347
315	Ovalbumin	3.66	–	–	43,500	55, 348
316	Insulin	3.68	7.45	–	47,800	55, 311
317	Phosphoglucomutase	3.69	4.83	–	74,000	243
318	Protease, bacterial	3.7	–	–	–	158
319	Bence Jones protein	3.7	–	0.769	35,000	235, 349
320	Glycoprotein, bovine plasma	3.8	–	–	39,000	14
321	Cytochrome *c*, beef heart	3.9	–	–	52,000	20
322	Concanavalin A, Jack bean	3.9	5.43	–	68,000	298
323	Cytochrome, *Chlorobium*	3.90	–	–	–	78
324	Carbamate kinase	3.92	–	–	–	85
325	Phosphoglycerate mutase, chicken muscle	3.92	6.1	–	65,690	462
326	Hemoglobin, ape	4.0	–	–	–	235, 317
327	NAD glycohydrolase	4.0	–	–	60,000	463
328	Taka-amylase A	4.04	–	–	–	238
329	Insulin	4.06	–	–	–	55, 313
330	Hemoglobin, horse	4.09	–	–	–	464
331	α-Glycoprotein, fetal calf serum	4.1	–	0.702	47,000	465
332	Chloroperoxidase, *Caldariomyces fumago*	4.1	–	–	42,000	466
333	Pre-albumin	4.1	–	–	61,000	188, 350
334	Hemoglobin, *Salmo*	4.1	–	–	–	235, 317
335	Hemoglobin, *Anguilla*	4.1	–	–	–	235, 317
336	Acetylcholinesterase, *Electrophorus*	4.10	–	–	–	467

TABLE III: Incomplete data—globular proteins (Continued)

No.	Protein	$S_{20.w} \times 10^{13}$	$D_{20.w} \times 10^7$	V_{20}	Molecular Weight	Reference Number
337	α-Lipoprotein, human	4.11	4.7	–	75,000	188, 205
338	α-Lipoprotein, human serum	4.11	4.7	–	75,000	205
339	Hemoglobin, ox	4.11	–	–	–	464
340	Hemoglobin, human	4.13	–	–	–	464
341	Hemoglobin, sheep	4.13	–	–	–	464
342	Hemoglobin, pig	4.13	–	–	–	464
343	Hemoglobin, dog	4.19	–	–	–	464
344	Hemoglobin, mouse	4.19	–	–	–	464
345	Hemoglobin, dogfish	4.19	–	–	–	464
346	Albumin, rat serum	4.2	–	–	–	468
347	Pyrophosphatase, yeast	4.2	–	–	–	206
348	Hemoglobin, cat	4.2	–	–	–	235, 317
349	Hemoglobin, dog	4.2	–	–	–	235, 317
350	Hemoglobin, hen	4.2	–	–	–	235, 317
351	Hemoglobin, *Esox*	4.2	–	–	–	235, 317
352	Hemoglobin, *Tautoga*	4.2	–	–	–	235, 317
353	Hemoglobin, human	4.20	–	–	–	49
354	Hemoglobin, rabbit	4.21	–	–	–	464
355	Hemoglobin, turtle	4.21	–	–	–	464
356	Albumin, cow serum	4.22	–	–	–	55, 351
357	Albumin, dog serum	4.24	–	–	–	4
358	Albumin, cow serum	4.27	–	–	–	55, 348
359	Albumin, human serum	4.28	6.32	–	–	55, 351
360	Globulin, *Phaseolus* seed	4.29	–	–	–	43
361	Hemoglobin, cow	4.3	–	–	–	235, 317
362	Hemoglobin, *Syrnium*	4.3	–	–	–	235, 317
363	Hemoglobin, *Picus*	4.3	–	–	–	235, 317
364	Hemoglobin, *Parus*	4.3	–	–	–	235, 317
365	Hemoglobin, *Raja*	4.3	–	–	–	235, 317
366	Hemoglobin, *Protopterus*	4.3	–	–	–	235, 317
367	Hemoglobin, *Pleuronectes*	4.3	–	–	–	235, 317
368	Hemoglobin, *Opsanus*	4.3	–	–	–	235, 317
369	Malate dehydrogenase, bovine heart	4.3	6.45	–	62,000	217
370	Tyrosinase L, *Neurospora crassa*	4.3	11.9	–	33,000	469
371	Tyrosinase S, *Neurospora crassa*	4.3	10.7	–	33,000	469
372	Albumin, cow serum	4.30	–	–	–	55, 334
373	Hemoglobin, frog	4.31	–	–	–	464
374	Hemoglobin, human	4.31	–	–	–	55, 348
375	Albumin, cow serum	4.31	6.15	–	65,400	55, 352
376	Malate dehydrogenase, pig heart	4.32	–	–	–	248
377	Albumin, cow serum	4.32	–	–	–	55, 311
378	Hemoglobin, chicken	4.32	–	–	–	464
379	Hemoglobin, duck	4.32	–	–	–	464
380	Megacin	4.35	–	–	51,000	97
381	Malate dehydrogenase, horse heart	4.36	–	–	–	248
382	Hemoglobin, pigeon	4.37	–	–	–	464
383	α-Livetin	4.38	–	–	–	150
384	Pyrophosphatase	4.4	–	–	63,000	55, 206
385	Co-hemoglobin, horse	4.4	–	–	–	55, 287
386	Hemoglobin, rabbit	4.4	–	–	–	235, 317
387	Hemoglobin, pigeon	4.4	–	–	–	235, 317
388	Hemoglobin, duck	4.4	–	–	–	235, 317
389	Hemoglobin, *Corvus*	4.4	–	–	–	235, 317
390	Hemoglobin, *Cyprinus*	4.4	–	–	–	235, 317
391	Hemoglobin, *Prionotus*	4.4	–	–	–	235, 317
392	Albumin esterase, mouse	4.4	–	–	70,000	470
393	Acetyl-CoA synthetase, bovine heart	4.4	–	–	–	471
394	Albumin, bovine	4.41	5.9	–	67,000	188, 354
395	Hemoglobin, horse	4.41	–	0.749	–	235
396	Malate dehydrogenase, ox heart	4.44	–	–	–	248
397	Hemoglobin, human	4.46,	–	–	63,000	55
398	Albumin, horse serum	4.46	6.1	–	–	235, 356
399	Phosphoglyceric acid mutase, rabbit muscle	4.47	6.6	–	64,000	54
400	Hemoglobin, human	4.48	–	–	–	235
401	Albumin, cow serum	4.49	–	–	–	55, 351

TABLE III: Incomplete data—globular proteins (Continued)

No.	Protein	$S_{20.w} \times 10^{13}$	$D_{20.w} \times 10^{7}$	V_{20}	Molecular Weight	Reference Number
402	Lactotransferrin	4.5	–	–	–	16
403	Cobalamin protein B, hog gastric mucosa	4.5	4.3	–	100,000	262
404	Hemoglobin, *Rana*	4.5	–	–	–	235, 317
405	Hemoglobin II, *Chrysemys*	4.5	–	–	–	235, 317
406	Hemoglobin, hedgehog	4.5	–	–	–	235, 317
407	Hemoglobin, *Gasterosteus*	4.5	–	–	–	235, 317
408	Hemoglobin, *Lucioperca*	4.5	–	–	–	235, 317
409	Hemoglobin, human	4.5	–	–	–	55, 287
410	Albumin, horse serum	4.50	–	–	–	55, 336
411	Hemoglobin H, human (i)	4.55	–	–	–	10
412	Hemoglobin H, human (ii)	4.55	–	–	–	10
413	Hemoglobin A, human	4.56	–	–	64,450	472
414	Hemoglobin E, human	4.56	–	–	–	472
415	Luciferase, *Cypridina*	4.58	–	0.707	–	250
416	Hemoglobin, *Anadara (= Arca)*	4.6	6.3	–	71,000	272
417	Hemoglobin, *Chameleon*	4.6	–	–	–	235, 317
418	Hemoglobin, *Coluber*	4.6	–	–	–	235, 317
419	Hemoglobin II, *Lacerta*	4.6	–	–	–	235, 317
420	Co-hemoglobin, cow	4.6	–	–	–	55, 287
421	Met-hemoglobin, horse	4.6	–	–	–	55, 357
422	Malate-lactate transhydrogenase, *Micrococcus lactilyticus*	4.6	–	–	99,000	534
423	Choline acetyltransferase, human placenta	4.65	–	–	59,000	473
424	Lactotransferrin	4.66	4.6	–	89,000	160
425	α-Amylase, *Pseudomonas*	4.66	–	–	–	148
426	Hemoglobin, *Rana esculenta*	4.69	–	–	68,000	474
427	Laccase B, *Polyporus*	4.7	–	–	–	475
428	Albumin, bovine	4.73	–	–	–	185
429	Albumin, cow serum	4.73	–	0.730	–	55, 358
430	Cobalamin protein A, hog gastric mucosa	4.75	3.6	–	128,000	262
431	Hemoglobin F, human	4.76	–	–	–	472
432	Interferon	4.77	–	–	–	29
433	Galactose dehydrogenase, pseudomonad	4.78	7.0	–	64,000	476
434	Laccase A, *Polyporus*	4.8	–	–	62,000	475
435	Isocitric enzyme	4.8	6.73	–	64,000	163
436	Hemoglobin, *Anguis*	4.8	–	–	–	235, 317
437	Hemoglobin II, *Salamandra*	4.8	–	–	–	235, 317
438	Hemoglobin II, *Bufo*	4.8	–	–	–	235, 317
439	Hemoglobin III, *Bufo*	4.8	–	–	–	235, 317
440	Haemopexin	4.8	–	–	–	209
441	Arachin, *Arachis hypogaca* (ground nut)	4.8	–	–	47,000	108
442	Creatine kinase BB, rabbit	4.80	–	–	–	535
443	Globulin, *Phaseolus* seed	4.87	–	–	–	43
444	Dehydropeptidase II, bovine kidney	4.9	–	–	–	214
445	Creatine kinase, MM, rabbit	4.90	–	–	–	535
446	Transferrin, human	4.92	5.85	–	74,000	477
447	Albumin, carp	5.0	7.03	–	67,000	96
448	α-Globulin, human plasma	5.0	–	0.841	200,000	177
449	Transferrin, human	5.0	–	–	90,000	188, 350
450	L-Amino acid oxidase, rat kidney	5.0	4.0	–	120,000	161
451	Tryptophan synthetase B, *E. coli*	5.0	–	–	108,000	478
452	Thiogalactoside transacetylase, *E. coli*	5.0	–	–	65,300	479
453	Creatine kinase BB, chicken	5.09	–	–	–	535
454	Transferrin, human	5.1	–	–	68,000	480
455	Transferrin, rat	5.1	–	–	68,000	480
456	Iron-binding protein, cow milk	5.1	–	–	–	79
457	Malate dehydrogenase, beef heart	5.1	9.1	–	52,000	63
458	Choline acetyltransferase, rabbit brain	5.13	6.8	–	67,000	473
459	*p*-Hydroxybenzoate hydroxylase, *Pseudomonas putida*	5.13	–	–	83,600	481
460	Creatine kinase MM, chicken	5.18	–	–	–	535
461	Transferrin, monkey	5.2	–	–	68,000	480
462	Aspartate transaminase, ox heart (apo-enzyme)	5.2	–	–	96,000	536
463	Phosphoenolpyruvate carboxykinase, pig liver	5.21	–	–	73,300	537
464	Prothrombin, bovine	5.22	–	–	68,500	92
465	Polyphenol oxidase, *Camelia sinensis* (tea)	5.25	3.33	–	144,000	482
466	Aspartate transaminase, ox heart	5.3	–	–	–	536

TABLE III: Incomplete data—globular proteins (Continued)

No.	Protein	$S_{20.w} \times 10^{13}$	$D_{20.w} \times 10^{7}$	V_{20}	Molecular Weight	Reference Number
467	Ricin	5.3	6.0	–	85,000	114
468	Hemoglobin, human	5.3	6.7	–	76,000	55, 360
469	Phytohemagglutinin (lectin), *Phaseolus vulgaris*	5.37	–	–	132,000	538
470	Diaphorase, pig heart	5.38	6.08	–	81,000	204
471	Transferrin, human	5.38	–	–	–	483
472	Luteinizing hormone, pig	5.39	5.9	–	90,000	55, 361
473	Laccase	5.4	4.63	–	120,000	166
474	Collagenase	5.4	4.3	–	109,000	212
475	Glutamic-aspartic transaminase	5.45	4.6	–	110,000	107
476	Neuraminase, *Vibrio cholerae*	5.5	5.5	–	90,000	189
477	*Diphtheria* antitoxin	5.5	5.76	–	–	55, 362
478	Lactate dehydrogenase, ox heart	5.5	7.39	–	72,000	157
479	β-Globulin, human plasma	5.5	–	0.725	90,000	177
480	Transferrin, human	5.5	–	–	–	484
481	Acylase I (Hippuricase), hog kidney	5.5	7.02	–	76,500	485
482	Transamidinase, hog kidney	5.5	–	–	100,000	486
483	Transferrin, human plasma	5.505	–	–	–	484
484	Metapyrocatechase, *Pseudomonas*	5.54	3.92	–	140,000	487
485	D-Arabinose dehydrogenase, pseudomonad	5.60	–	–	104,000	476
486	Transferrin, human plasma	5.628	–	–	–	484
487	Ricin D	5.64	–	–	60,000	489
488	Red protein, bovine milk	5.65	–	–	–	47
489	apo-Aspartate transaminase, yeast	5.70	6.03	–	91,200	490
490	Ascorbate oxidase, *Cucurbita pepo* (reduced)	5.72	–	–	–	491
491	Old yellow enzyme	5.76	–	0.753	102,500	244
492	Ceruloplasmin, human	5.77	–	–	125,000	195
493	Ascorbate oxidase, *Cucurbita pepo* (inactivated)	5.78	–	–	–	491
494	Ascorbate oxidase, *Cucurbita pepo* (native)	5.79	–	–	–	491
495	Transferrin, pig	5.8	–	–	–	363
496	Transferrin, porcine	5.8	5.8	–	88,000	188, 363
497	Dihydrolipoic dehydrogenase, *Spinacea oleracea*	5.87	5.19	–	102,000	493
498	Procarboxypeptidase	5.87	–	–	96,000	123
499	Tyrosine transaminase, rat kidney	5.9	–	–	–	540
500	Hemocyanin, *Limulus*	5.9	–	–	–	235, 364
501	γ-Globulin, rabbit serum	6	–	–	–	55, 365
502	γ-Globulin, cow	6	–	–	–	55, 365
503	Lipoamide dehydrogenase, human liver	6.02	4.75	–	114,000	539
504	Transferrin, human	6.1	–	–	–	494
505	δ-Hemolysin, staphylococcal	6.1	–	–	74,000	495
506	Malate dehydrogenase, *B. subtilis*	6.15	–	–	148,000	496
507	Hemagglutinin, soya bean	6.15	–	–	–	256
508	Globulin, *Hordeum* seed	6.2	–	–	–	43
509	Alkaline phosphatase, calf	6.2	–	–	100,000	64
510	Arachin, *Arachis hypogaea* (ground nut)	6.2	–	–	68,000	108
511	Laccase	6.25	3.57	–	141,000	174
512	Alkaline phosphatase, *E. coli*	6.3	–	–	77,500	76
513	Ascorbate oxidase apoenzyme, *Cucurbita pepo*	6.3	–	–	–	491
514	Phosphoglyceric acid mutase, yeast	6.30	5.29	–	112,000	54
515	Hemagglutinin, castor bean	6.39	–	–	–	239
516	Hemagglutinin, soya bean	6.4	5.72	–	105,000	181
517	Tyrosinase, *Psalliota* (mushroom)	6.4	6.1	–	102,000	145
518	γ-Globulin, equine serum	6.4	4.81	–	127,000	188, 366
519	Denitrifying enzyme, bacterial (*Pseudomonas*?)	6.46	4.0	–	149,000	409
520	Laccase	6.5	3.9	–	130,000	174
521	Amino acid oxidase, *Crotalus*	6.54	–	–	130,000	261
522	Globulin, *Phaseolus* seed	6.55	–	–	–	43
523	Dihydrolipoic dehydrogenase, *E. coli*	6.6	6.7	–	88,000	126
524	20-β-Hydroxy steroid dehydrogenase, *Streptomyces*	6.64	5.51	–	118,400	497
525	Luteinizing hormone, pig	6.65	–	–	–	55, 367
526	γ-Globulin, rabbit	6.73	4.66	–	–	31
527	Globulin, *Medicago* seed	6.77	–	–	–	43
528	Glyceraldehyde phosphomutase, yeast	6.80	5.19	–	122,000	243
529	Ceruloplasmin, human	6.82	–	–	148,000	195
530	Tween hydrolyzing enzyme	6.83	–	–	–	257

TABLE III: Incomplete data—globular proteins (Continued)

No.	Protein	$S_{20.w} \times 10^{13}$	$D_{20.w} \times 10^7$	V_{20}	Molecular Weight	Reference Number
531	Ascorbate oxidase, *Cucurbita pepo condensa* (squash)	6.9	4.6	–	146,000	55, 368
532	T component, equine	6.9	4.87	–	135,000	188, 366
533	γ-Globulin, horse serum	6.90	–	–	–	55, 336
534	L-Amino acid oxidase, Moccasin snake	6.91	11.0	–	61,600	55, 369
535	Cytochrome *f*	6.91	6.1	–	110,000	44
536	Anticatalase	6.93	–	–	177,600	72
537	γ-Globulin, horse serum	7	–	–	–	55, 370
538	β₁-Globulin	7	–	0.74	–	177
539	γ-Globulin, cow	7	–	–	–	55, 370
540	Hemoglobin I, *Salamandra*	7.0	–	–	–	235, 317
541	Hemoglobin I, *Chrysemys*	7.0	–	–	–	235, 317
542	Aldose dehydrogenase, pseudomonad	7.03	5.4	–	140,000	476
543	γ-Globulin, rabbit serum	7.05	4.1	–	160,000	55, 394
544	Lactate dehydrogenase, ox heart	7.05	5.26	–	131,000	168
545	Globulin, *Vicia* seed	7.09	–	–	–	43
546	Globulin, horse serum	7.1	–	–	–	235
547	Glucose-6-phosphate dehydrogenase, human RBC	7.1	3.4	–	190,000	498
548	Hemoglobin I, *Lacerta*	7.1	–	–	–	235, 317
549	γ-Globulin, human serum	7.1	3.84	–	176,000	55, 307
550	Ceruloplasmin, human	7.1	–	–	151,000	188, 350
551	Globulin, *Vicia* seed	7.12	–	–	–	43
552	Globulin, *Lupinus angusbifolius* seed	7.15	3.86	–	170,000	112
553	γ-Globulin, human	7.2	–	0.739	156,000	55, 177
554	Globulin, *Ervum* seed	7.25	–	–	–	43
555	Globulin, *Phaseolus* seed	7.26	–	–	–	43
556	Globulin, *Trifolium* seed	7.27	–	–	–	43
557	γ-Globulin, pig serum	7.28	–	0.744	–	55, 371
558	Ceruloplasmin, human plasma	7.29	4.5	–	–	203
559	γ-Globulin, human	7.3	3.7	–	170,000	26
560	Triose-phosphate dehydrogenase, rabbit	7.31	–	–	–	499
561	Globulin, *Dolichos* seed	7.33	–	–	–	43
562	Triose-phosphate dehydrogenase, *E. coli*	7.36	–	–	–	499
563	Triose-phosphate dehydrogenase, pheasant	7.37	–	–	–	499
564	Triose-phosphate dehydrogenase, chicken	7.38	–	–	–	499
565	Triose-phosphate dehydrogenase, turkey	7.38	–	–	–	499
566	Globulin, *Acacia* seed	7.39	–	–	–	43
567	Globulin, *Phaseolus* seed	7.39	–	–	–	43
568	Ornithine transcarbamylase	7.4	–	–	–	197
569	Hemoglobin I, *Bufo*	7.4	–	–	–	235, 317
570	γ-Globulin, cow serum	7.4	–	–	–	55, 372
571	Triose-phosphate dehydrogenase, bovine	7.43	–	–	–	499
572	Triose-phosphate dehydrogenase, sturgeon	7.43	–	–	–	499
573	Triose-phosphate dehydrogenase, lobster	7.45	–	–	–	499
574	Globulin, *Lathyrus* seed	7.46	–	–	–	43
575	Triose-phosphate dehydrogenase, yeast	7.47	–	–	–	499
576	Globulin, *Lathyrus* seed	7.48	–	–	–	43
577	C-Reactive protein	7.5	–	–	–	269
578	Globulin, *Lathyrus* seed	7.55	–	–	–	43
579	Triose-phosphate dehydrogenase, human	7.57	–	–	–	499
580	Triose-phosphate dehydrogenase, halibut	7.59	–	–	–	499
581	Globulin, *Acacia* seed	7.59	–	–	–	43
582	Ceruloplasmin, pig blood	7.6	4.4	–	162,000	179
583	D-Amino acid oxidase, pig kidney	7.6	–	–	182,000	153
584	Alcohol dehydrogenase, yeast	7.61	–	–	–	245
585	Globulin, *Lathyrus* seed	7.64	–	–	–	43
586	Globulin, *Trifolium* seed	7.66	–	–	–	43
587	Globulin, *Trifolium* seed	7.69	–	–	–	43
588	Hemoglobin II, *Bufo*	7.7	–	–	–	235, 317
589	L-Iditol dehydrogenase	7.7	6.1	–	115,000	219
590	Globulin, *Acacia* seed	7.76	–	–	–	43
591	Globulin, *Acacia* seed	7.77	–	–	–	43
592	Globulin, *Lupinus angustifolius* seed	7.79	4.20	–	181,000	112
593	Aldolase, rabbit liver	7.8	4.8	–	151,000	500
594	Crotonase	7.84	–	–	–	228

TABLE III: Incomplete data—globular proteins (Continued)

No.	Protein	$S_{20,w} \times 10^{13}$	$D_{20,w} \times 10^7$	V_{20}	Molecular Weight	Reference Number
595	Glucose oxidase-microside protein, *Penicillium*	7.9	–	–	–	501
596	Globulin, *Acacia* seed	7.90	–	–	–	43
597	Phosphorylase, potato	7.94	3.76	–	207,000	134
598	Globulin, *Glycine* seed	7.97	–	–	–	43
599	Globulin, *Acacia* seed	8.02	–	–	–	43
600	Globulin, *Cytisus* seed	8.03	–	–	–	43
601	Globulin, *Acacia* seed	8.04	–	–	–	43
602	Globulin, *Cytisus* seed	8.08	–	–	–	43
603	Globulin, *Avena* seed	8.1	–	–	–	43
604	Globulin, *Pisum* seed	8.10	–	–	–	43
605	Cathepsin C	8.16	3.3	–	235,000	88
606	Phosphorylase, rabbit heart	8.2	–	–	–	276
607	Globulin, *Secale* seed	8.2	–	–	–	43
608	Globulin, *Triticum* seed	8.2	–	–	–	43
609	Globulin, *Phleum* seed	8.2	–	–	–	43
610	Thetin-homocysteinase	8.2	–	–	–	52
611	Globulin, *Lupinus* seed	8.20	–	–	–	43
612	Globulin, *Lupinus* seed	8.24	–	–	–	43
613	Carboxylesterase, pig kidney	8.25	–	–	170,000	557
614	Glucose oxidase (Notatin), *Penicillium*	8.27	5.13	–	152,000	33
615	Aldolase	8.27	4.29	–	180,000	55, 373
616	Globulin, *Hordeum vulgare* seed	8.3	–	–	–	43
617	Globulin, *Festuca* seed	8.3	–	–	–	43
618	Globulin, *Lupinus* seed	8.30	–	–	–	43
619	Globulin, *Lotus* seed	8.32	–	–	–	43
620	Globulin, *Astragalus* seed	8.33	–	–	–	43
621	Globulin, *Arachis* seed	8.40	–	–	–	43
622	Globulin, *Zea* seed	8.5	–	–	–	43
623	Globulin, *Panicum* seed	8.5	–	–	–	43
624	D-Glyceraldehyde-3-phosphate dehydrogenase	8.5	–	–	–	60
625	Fumarase, hog heart	8.51	4.05	–	204,000	55, 374
626	Globulin, *Genista* seed	8.54	–	–	–	43
627	Globulin, *Lupinus* seed	8.69	–	–	–	43
628	Conarachin	8.7	–	0.720	175,000	109
629	γ-Globulin, barley	8.7	3.6	–	210,000	43
630	Dextran saccharose, *Leuconostoc*	8.79	–	–	284,000	502
631	Alanine dehydrogenase, *B. subtilis*	8.8	–	–	228,000	503
632	Phosphorylase, rabbit muscle	8.8	–	–	–	276
633	β Amylase, sweet potato	8.9	5.77	–	152,000	55, 375
634	Monoamine oxidase, ox plasma	8.98	–	–	225,400	273
635	α_2-Globulin	9	–	0.693	300,000	177
636	Arachin, *Arachis hypogaea* (ground nut)	9.0	4.20	–	180,000	111
637	Tryptophanase, *E. coli*	9.0	–	–	490,000	504
638	Cytochrome b_2, yeast	9.17	3.80	–	186,400	7
639	Monoamine oxidase, plasma	9.23	–	0.76	261,000	505
640	Isocitrate lyase, *Pseudomonas*	9.49	3.87	–	222,000	506
641	Arachin, *A. hypogaea* (ground nut)	9.5	–	–	130,000	108
642	Tryptophanase, *E. coli*	9.65	–	–	281,000	507
643	Pseudocholinesterase, horse	9.9	–	–	–	106
644	γ-Globulin, human	10	–	–	300,000	185
645	Fluorokinase	10.04	3.96	–	237,000	258
646	Globulin, *Phaseolus* seed	10.10	–	–	–	43
647	L-Amino acid oxidase, rat kidney	10.5	–	–	88,900	541
648	Anthranilate synthetase, *E. coli*	10.7	–	–	–	542
649	Glycerokinase, *Candida*	10.87	4.2	–	251,000	11
650	Catalase, *Micrococcus*	11.0	–	–	–	34
651	Globulin, *Phaseolus* seed	11.02	–	–	–	43
652	Hemocyanin, *Loligo*	11.1	–	–	–	508
653	Catalase, pig blood	11.10	4.10	–	243,000	165
654	Catalase, bovine liver	11.15	4.1	–	244,000	202
655	Catalase, human blood	11.2	–	–	280,000	34
656	Carbamyl phosphate synthetase, frog liver	11.2	–	0.740	315,000	149
657	Globulin, *Trifolium* seed	11.22	–	–	–	43
658	Phycocyanin, *Ceramium*	11.4	–	–	270,000	55, 376
659	Pomelin	11.4	–	–	–	235, 326

TABLE III: Incomplete data—globular proteins (Continued)

No.	Protein	$S_{20.w} \times 10^{13}$	$D_{20.w} \times 10^7$	V_{20}	Molecular Weight	Reference Number
660	Globulin, *Medicago* seed	11.41	–	–	–	43
661	Globulin, *Lupinus angustifolius* seed	11.53	–	–	–	43
662	Protein, *Lupinus* seed	11.6	3.16	–	336,000	112
663	Globulin, *Acacia* seed	11.63	–	–	–	43
664	Globulin, *Dolichos* seed	11.66	–	–	–	43
665	Homogentisate oxygenase, *Pseudomonas fluorescens*	11.8	2.85	–	380,000	509
666	Hemoglobin, perienteric fluid, *Ascaris*	11.8	–	0.725	328,000	510
667	Globulin, *Vicia* seed	11.80	–	–	–	43
668	Globulin, *Vicia* seed	11.91	–	–	–	43
669	Cocosin	12	–	–	–	235, 377
670	Globulin, *Hordeum* seed	12.0	–	–	–	43
671	Phycoerythrin, *Ceramium*	12.0	–	0.746	–	235, 378
672	δ-Aminolevulinate dehydratase, mouse	12.0	4.2	–	270,000	511
673	Globulin, *Lathyrus* seed	12.00	–	–	–	43
674	Globulin, *Phaseolus* seed	12.16	–	–	–	43
675	Globulin, *Lupinus* seed	12.20	–	–	–	43
676	Globulin, *Lupinus* seed	12.29	–	–	–	43
677	*S*-Adenine deaminase	12.29	3.76	–	320,000	133
678	Amandin	12.5	–	0.746	–	235, 379
679	Hemoglobin I, *Bufo*	12.5	–	–	–	235, 317
680	Globulin, *Pisum* seed	12.64	–	–	–	43
681	Edestin	12.8	–	0.744	–	235, 380
682	Globulin, *Trifolium* seed	12.90	–	–	–	43
683	Globulin, *Lathyrus* seed	12.97	–	–	–	43
684	Globulin, *Lathyrus* seed	13.00	–	–	–	43
685	Globulin, *Lathyrus* seed	13.04	–	–	–	43
686	Globulin, *Arachis* seed	13.05	–	–	–	43
687	Globulin, *Lupinus* seed	13.05	–	–	–	43
688	Globulin, *Glycine* seed	13.06	–	–	–	43
689	Globulin, *Lotus* seed	13.07	–	–	–	43
690	Globulin, *Astragalus* seed	13.17	–	–	–	43
691	Globulin, *Ervum* seed	13.18	–	–	–	43
692	Phosphorylase, rabbit heart	13.2	–	–	–	276
693	Nerve protein, lobster	13.2	–	–	–	155
694	Excelsin	13.3	–	0.743	–	235, 379
695	Glutamate dehydrogenase, chicken liver	13.3	2.91	–	510,000	74
696	Globulin, *Genista* seed	13.34	–	–	–	43
697	Globulin, *Cytisus* seed	13.38	–	–	–	43
698	Citrate cleaving enzyme, rat liver	13.5	2.62	–	500,000	512
699	Phosphorylase, rabbit muscle	13.6	–	–	–	276
700	Globulin, *Acacia* seed	13.67	–	–	–	43
701	Phosphorylase a	13.7	3.3	–	400,000	84
702	Globulin, *Cytisus* seed	14.02	–	–	–	43
703	Glutamate dehydrogenase, chicken liver	15.4	–	–	500,000	513
704	Hemocyanin, *Pagurus*	16	–	–	–	235, 317
705	Hemocyanin, *Palaemon*	16	–	–	–	235, 317
706	Hemocyanin, *Achatina*	16	–	–	–	235, 317
707	Hemocyanin, *Chirodothea*	16	–	–	–	235, 317
708	Hemocyanin, *Limulus*	16.1	–	–	–	235, 364
709	β-Galactosidase, *E. coli* ML35	16.14	3.13	–	521,000	284
710	Citrate-oxalacetate lyase, *Aerobacter*	16.2	4.16	–	318,000	23, 514
711	Hemoglobin, *Daphnia*	16.3	–	–	–	235, 381
712	Hemocyanin, *Palinurus*	16.4	–	–	446,000	235, 364
713	Hemocyanin, *Cancer*	16.4	–	–	–	235, 364
714	Hemocyanin, *Carcinus*	16.7	–	–	–	235, 364
715	Pomelin	16.8	–	–	–	235, 326
716	Phenol oxidase, *Calliphora* larva	17	3.1	–	–	116
717	Hemocyanin, *Eupagurus*	17	–	–	–	235, 317
718	Hemocyanin, *Pandalus*	17.4	–	–	397,000	235, 364
719	Apoferritin, guinea pig	17.7	–	0.730	–	73
720	Hemagglutinin, cold	17.8	5.5	–	350,000	260
721	Globulin, pig	18.0	1.64	–	930,000	235, 307, 382
722	Globulin, *Acacia* seed	18.04	–	–	–	43
723	Globulin, bovine	18.1	1.69	–	910,000	235, 307, 382
724	Globulin, *Trifolium* seed	18.20	–	–	–	43

TABLE III: Incomplete data—globular proteins (Continued)

No.	Protein	$S_{20.w} \times 10^{13}$	$D_{20.w} \times 10^7$	V_{20}	Molecular Weight	Reference Number
725	α-Macroglobulin, rat serum	18.3	–	–	–	468
726	Globulin, *Acacia* seed	18.75	–	–	–	43
727	Hemocyanin, *Loligo*	19	–	–	–	508
728	Thyroglobulin, pig	19.2	–	0.72	–	235, 383
729	Hemoglobin, *Aethelges*	19.3	–	–	–	235, 317
730	Thyroglobulin, pig	19.4	2.61	–	–	48
731	Protein B, lobster nerve	19.6	4.5	–	422,000	155
732	Iso-hemagglutinin	19.8	–	0.73	–	188, 300
733	β-Globulin, human plasma	20	–	0.74	–	177
734	Cytochrome b_1, *E. coli*	20.3	–	–	700,000	516
735	Globulin, *Genista* seed	20.31	–	–	–	43
736	α-Glycoprotein, fetal calf serum	20.4	–	0.733	990,000	465
737	Hemocyanin, *Eupagurus*	22	–	–	–	235, 317
738	Cytochrome, *Rhodopseudomonas*	22.1	1.18	–	560,000	162
739	Mucoprotein, urinary	22.3	–	–	–	154
740	Hemocyanin, *Homarus*	22.6	–	–	752,000	235, 364
741	Hemocyanin, *Chirodothea*	23	–	–	–	235, 317
742	Hemocyanin, *Hyas*	23	–	–	–	235, 317
743	Hemocyanin, *Astacus*	23.3	–	–	–	235, 364
744	Hemocyanin, *Carcinus*	23.3	–	–	–	235, 364
745	Hemocyanin, *Cancer*	23.6	–	–	–	235, 364
746	Hemocyanin, *Squilla*	24	–	–	–	235, 317
747	Hemocyanin, *Nephrops*	24.5	–	–	812,000	235, 364
748	Hemocyanin, *Maia*	27	–	–	–	234, 317
749	α-Carboxylase, wheat germ	29.0	–	–	–	218
750	Mucoprotein, urinary	29.0	–	–	–	154
751	Hemoglobin, *Planorbis*	33.7	–	0.745	–	235, 314
752	Hemocyanin, *Euscorpius*	34	–	–	–	235, 317
753	Hemocyanin, *Calocaris*	34	–	–	1,329,000	235, 317
754	Hemocyanin, *Limulus*	34.6	–	–	–	235, 364
755	Hemoglobin, *Planorbis*	36.0	–	–	–	235, 317
756	Hemocyanin, *Eledone*	48	–	–	–	235, 317
757	Hemoglobin, *Tubifex*	48.9	1.57	–	3,010,000	207
758	Hemocyanin, *Eledone*	49.1	–	–	2,791,000	235, 364
759	Hemocyanin, Octopus	49.3	–	0.740	–	235, 364
760	Succinic dehydrogenase, bacterial	54	–	–	–	259
761	Hemoglobin, *Pectinaria*	54	–	–	–	235, 317
762	Hemocyanin, *Sepia*	55.9	–	–	–	235, 364
763	Hemocyanin, *Sepiola*	56	–	–	–	235, 317
764	Hemocyanin, *Rossia*	56.2	–	–	3,316,000	235, 364
765	Hemocyanin, *Limulus*	56'.6	–	–	–	235, 364
766	Hemocyanin, *Loligo*	56.7	–	–	–	235, 364
767	Hemoglobin, *Haemopsis*	57	–	–	–	235, 317
768	Hemoglobin, *Polymnia*	57	–	–	–	235, 317
769	Hemoglobin, *Arenicola*	57.4	–	–	3,000,000	235, 381
770	Chlorocruorin, *Sabella*	57.5	1.90	–	2,800,000	6
771	Hemoglobin, *Hirudo*	58	–	–	–	235, 317
772	Pyruvic acid oxidase	58.0	–	–	4,000,000	211
773	Hemoglobin, *Marphysa sanguinea*	58.2	–	–	2,400,000	518
774	Hemoglobin, *Neireis*	58.6	–	–	–	235, 317
775	Hemocyanin, *Loligo*	58.7	–	0.71	3,750,000	508
776	Hemoglobin, *Eumenia*	59	–	–	–	235, 317
777	Hemoglobin, *Lumbrinereis*	59	–	–	–	235, 317
778	Hemocyanin, *Limnea*	60.2	–	–	–	235, 317
779	Hemoglobin, *Lumbricus*	60.9	–	0.740	–	235, 317
780	Hemocyanin, *Arion*	61	–	–	–	235, 317
781	Hemocyanin, *Tonicella*	61	–	–	–	235, 317
782	Hemocyanin, *Eisenia*	63	–	–	–	235, 317
783	Hemocyanin, *Arion*	64	–	–	–	235, 317
784	Hemocyanin, *Achatina*	64	–	–	–	235, 317
785	Hemocyanin, *Paludina*	64.5	–	0.738	–	27
786	Ribonucleoprotein	80	–	0.664	3,600,000	90
787	Hemocyanin, *Helix*	91.2	–	–	–	235, 364
788	Hemoglobin, *Marphysa sanguinea*	97	–	–	–	518
789	Hemocyanin, *Paludina*	97	–	–	–	235, 317

TABLE III: Incomplete data—globular proteins (Continued)

No.	Protein	$S_{20.w} \times 10^{13}$	$D_{20.w} \times 10^7$	V_{20}	Molecular Weight	Reference Number
790	Hemocyanin, *Limax*	97.3	–	–	–	235, 364
791	Hemocyanin, *Limnea*	98	–	–	–	235, 317
792	Hemocyanin, *Helix*	98.9	–	0.738	–	235, 364
793	Hemocyanin, *Arion*	99	–	–	–	235, 317
794	Hemocyanin, *Littorina*	99.7	–	–	–	235, 364
795	Hemocyanin, *Paludina*	100	–	–	–	235, 317
796	Hemocyanin, *Agriolimax*	100.0	–	–	–	235, 317
797	Hemocyanin, *Helix*	100.0	–	–	–	235, 364
798	Hemocyanin, *Helix*	101.0	–	–	–	235, 364
799	Hemocyanin, *Busycon*	101.7	1.38	–	–	235, 364
800	Hemocyanin, *Achatina*	102	–	–	–	235, 317
801	Hemocyanin, *Buccinum*	102.1	–	–	–	235, 364
802	Hemocyanin, *Neptunea*	104.0	–	–	–	235, 364
803	Acetylcholinesterase, *Electrophorus*	109	8.1	–	13,400,000	519
804	Hemocyanin, *Busycon*	130	–	–	–	235, 364
805	Hemocyanin, *Buccinum*	132	–	–	–	235, 317
806	Hemocyanin, *Littorina*	132	–	–	–	235, 317
807	Hemoglobin, *Marphysa sanguinea*	150	–	–	–	518

Compiled by Malcolm H. Smith.

TABLE IV: Incomplete data–fibrous proteins

No.	Protein	$S_{20.w} \times 10^{13}$	$D_{20.w} \times 10^7$	V_{20}	Molecular Weight	Reference Number
808	Histone II, calf thymus	0.66	7.30	–	8,400	251
809	Silk fibroin	1.36	–	–	21,000	520
810	Zein	1.9	4.0	–	–	55, 384
811	β-Histone	2.0	3.29	–	57,000	40
812	Peptomyosin B	2.31	–	–	117,000	21
813	Sialoprotein, bovine cortical bone (EDTA extracted)	2.37	–	0.64	25,000	266
814	Glycoprotein ("ovoglycoprotein"), egg white	2.47	–	–	–	521
815	Tropomyosin, adult blowfly	2.53	–	–	65,600	127
816	Tropomyosin, rabbit	2.59	–	–	–	127
817	α-Glycoprotein, human	2.6	–	–	–	188, 385
818	γ Myosin	2.6	–	0.720	49,000	120
819	Tropomyosin, larval blowfly	2.62	–	–	84,400	127
820	β₁-Globulin, human plasma	2.9	–	0.950	1,300,000	177
821	β-Livetin, hen egg	2.9	7.0	–	37,000	264
822	γ-Histone	2.90	3.68	–	73,800	40
823	Tropocollagen, calf skin	3.0	–	0.706	290,000	522
824	Collagen, cod skin	3.05	–	0.710	280,000	275
825	Phosvitin, hen serum	3.17	–	–	42,000	159
826	G-Actin, cod	3.3	2.3	–	130,000	38
827	Collagen, cod swim bladder	3.39	–	–	320,000	275
828	α₁-Glycoprotein	3.5	–	–	54,000	188, 386
829	M₂-Glycoprotein, bovine	3.8	6.5	–	49,000	523
830	Mucoprotein, urinary	3.93	6.80	–	–	213
831	Collagen, cod swim bladder	4.03	–	–	480,000	275
832	Collagen A, earth worm cuticle	4.08	0.70	–	584,000	152
833	Haptoglobin, type 1-1, human	4.2	–	–	85,000	188, 387
834	Plasminogen, human plasma	4.28	2.92	–	143,000	216
835	Collagen B, earth worm cuticle	4.44	0.70	–	668,000	152
836	Mucin, pig submaxillary gland	4.6	–	–	830,000	524
837	β-Lipovitellin	4.6	1.36	–	390,000	129
838	Lipoprotein, human serum (HDL-3)	4.65	–	0.867	175,000	93
839	Mucoprotein, cow milk	4.8	3.8	–	123,000	104
840	α₁-Lipoprotein, human	5.01	–	–	195,000	177, 188, 388
841	Lipoprotein, human serum (HDL-2)	5.45	–	0.905	400,000	93
842	Chloroplast protein, spinach leaf	5.5	–	0.96	–	36
843	α₁-Lipoprotein, human	5.50	–	0.841	435,000	188, 338
844	Myosin, bovine	5.78	–	–	–	525
845	Myosin, dog heart	5.8	–	–	758,000	526
846	Haptoglobin II-methemoglobin complex	6.1	3.4	–	168,000	87
847	Myosin, cod	6.33	–	–	–	527
848	Myosin	6.43	–	0.725	540,000	110
849	Mucoprotein, cartilage	6.85	–	–	–	12
850	Myosin	7.2	–	0.74	–	55, 389
851	Fibrinogen, cow	7.9	2.02	–	–	55, 390
852	Fibrinogen, bovine	8.03	1.86	–	390,000	62
853	Lipoeuglobulin III, human	8.2	–	–	–	188, 391
854	Mucoprotein, sheep submaxillary gland	8.5	–	–	1,000,000	80
855	Fibrinogen, human	9	–	–	–	55, 177
856	Haptoglobin I-(methemoglobin-Hb)²	9.9	3.0	–	310,000	87
857	β-Crystallin, bovine lens	10	–	–	–	17
858	Lipovitellin	10.5	–	0.744	390,000	254
859	β-Histone, aggregated	10.75	1.87	–	540,000	40
860	Mucoprotein, human	14.2	–	–	–	188, 392
861	Globulin, human "cold-insoluble"	15.0	' –	–	–	188, 393
862	*Clostridium* toxin	17.3	2.14	–	–	55, 419
863	α-Crystallin, bovine lens cortex	19.47	2.3	–	770,000	182
864	α-Crystallin, bovine lens	19.5	–	–	–	17
865	α-Crystallin, bovine lens	19.57	2.0	–	960,000	182
866	α₂-Macroglobulin, human	19.6	2.41	–	820,000	188, 395
867	Mucoid, bovine estrous cervical	20	–	0.63	4,160,000	77
868	α-Glycoprotein, fetal calf serum	20.4	–	0.733	990,000	465
869	α-Crystallin, bovine lens	21.39	2.0	–	960,000	182
870	α-Crystallin, bovine lens cortex	21.58	1.7	α	1,150,000	182
871	Mucoprotein, urinary	22.3	–	α	–	154
872	Silk fibroin	22.3	–	–	1,200,000	520

TABLE IV: Incomplete data—fibrous proteins (Continued)

No.	Protein	$S_{20.w} \times 10^{13}$	$D_{20.w} \times 10^7$	V_{20}	Molecular Weight	Reference Number
873	Mucoid, bovine pregnancy cervical	25	–	0.64	3,930,000	77
874	Casein, mouse milk	27	2.34	–	1,130,000	198
875	Mucoprotein, human urinary	29.5	0.325	–	7,000,000	242
876	Myxomyosin	30	–	0.719	–	249
877	Mucoprotein, ovine urinary	30	–	–	–	528
878	F_1-Actin, polymerized	40	–	–	–	529
879	F_2-Actin, polymerized	98	–	–	–	529

Compiled by Malcolm H. Smith.

TABLE V: Sedimentation coefficients of vertebrate serum proteins

No.	Vertebrate Serum[a]	$S \times 10^{13}$
880	*Carcharhinus limbatus* (Black-tipped shark)	2.6
881	*Ameriurus nebulosus* (Bullhead)	3.1
882	*Ginglymostoma cirratum* (Nurse shark)	3.2
883	*Sphyrna tiburo* (Bonnet shark)	3.3
884	*Ancistrodon piscivorus* (Cottonmouth moccasin)	3.3
885	*Corvus brachyrhyncus* (Crow)	3.3
886	*Felis domesticus* (Cat)	3.3
887	*Rattus norvegicus* (Hooded rat)	3.3
888	*Ictalurus punctata* (Catfish)	3.4
889	*Sus scrofa* (Pig)	3.4
890	*Terrapene carolina* (Terrapin)	3.5
891	*Lampropeltis getulus* (King snake)	3.5
892	*Rhea rhea*	3.5
893	*Erinaceus europaeus* (European hedgehog)	3.5
894	*Iguana iguana*	3.5
895	*Petromyzon marinus* (Lamprey)	3.6
896	*Dasyatus americana* (Sting ray)	3.6
897	*Bufo marinus* (Marine toad)	3.6
898	*Deirochelys reticularia* (Chicken turtle)	3.6
899	*Masticopus flagellum* (Western coachwhip)	3.6
900	*Caiman sclerops*	3.6
901	*Tachyglossus aculeatus* (Echidna)	3.6
902	*Chelydra serpentina* (Snapping turtle)	3.7
903	*Crotalus viridis* (Prairie rattlesnake)	3.7
904	*Natrix gramhi* (Graham's watersnake)	3.7
905	*Electrophorus electricus* (Electriceel)	3.8
906	*Dromiceius novaehollandie* (Emu)	3.8
907	*Florida thula* (Snowy egret)	3.8
908	*Haliaetus leucoryphas* (Fishing eagle)	3.8
909	*Jabiru mycteria* (Jabiru stork)	3.9
910	*Macropus rufo* (Red kangaroo)	3.9
911	*Didelphis marsupialis* (Opossum)	3.9
912	*Homo sapiens* (Man)	3.9
913	*Lepisosteus osseus* (Gar)	4.0
914	*Terrapene carolina* (Terrapin)	4.0
915	*Sphenicus humboldti* (Humboldt's penguin)	4.0
916	*Eudocimus albus* (White ibis)	4.0
917	*Sylvilagus floridanus* (Cottontail rabbit)	4.0
918	*Rana catesbeiana* (Bullfrog)	4.1
919	*Siren lacertina* (Salamander)	4.2
920	*Xenopus laevi* (Clawed toad)	4.2
921	*Crotalus adamanteus* (Eastern diamond-back rattlesnake)	4.2
922	*Cyprinus carpio* (Carp)	4.3
923	*Crocodylus morleti* (Crocodile)	4.3
924	*Deirochelys reticularia* (Chicken turtle)	4.4
925	*Orycteropus afer* (Aardvark)	4.5
926	*Lepidosiren paradoxa* (Lungfish)	4.6
927	*Chrysemys picta* (Painted turtle)	4.7
928	*Erinaceus europaeus* (European hedgehog)	4.7
929	*Sylvilagus floridanus* (Cottontail rabbit)	4.8
930	*Crotalus viridis* (Prairie rattlesnake)	4.8
931	*Heterodontus francisci* (Horned shark)	4.9
932	*Didelphis marsupialis* (Opossum)	5.3
933	*Homo sapiens* (Man)	5.4
934	*Ameriurus nebulosus* (Bullhead)	5.5
935	*Orycteropus afer* (Aardvark)	5.5
936	*Petromyzon marinus* (Lamprey)	5.6
937	*Ancistrodon piscivorus* (Cottonmouth moccasin)	5.6
938	*Tachyglossus aculeatus* (Echidna)	5.7
939	*Iguana iguana*	5.8
940	*Sus scrofa* (Pig)	5.8
941	*Felis domesticus* (Cat)	5.9
942	*Siren lacertina* (Salamander)	~6
943	*Ginglymostoma cirratum* (Nurse shark)	6.0

TABLE V: Sedimentation coefficients of vertebrate serum proteins (Continued)

No.	Vertebrate Serum[a]	$S \times 10^{13}$
944	*Rhea rhea*	6.0
945	*Sphyrna tiburo* (Bonnet shark)	6.1
946	*Masticopus flagellum* (Western coachwhip)	6.2
947	*Lampropeltis getulus* (King snake)	6.3
948	*Corvus brachyrhyncus* (Crow)	6.3
949	*Macropus rufo* (Red kangaroo)	6.4
950	*Rattus norvegicus* (Hooded rat)	6.4
951	*Cyprinus carpio* (Carp)	6.5
952	*Xenopus laevi* (Clawed toad)	6.5
953	*Natrix gramhi* (Graham's watersnake)	6.5
954	*Haliaetus leucoryphas* (Fishing eagle)	6.5
955	*Electrophorus electricus* (Electric eel)	6.7
956	*Chrysemys picta* (Painted turtle)	6.7
957	*Crocodylus morleti* (Crocodile)	6.7
958	*Eudocimus albus* (White ibis)	6.7
959	*Bufo marinus* (Marine toad)	6.8
960	*Heterodontus francisci* (Horned shark)	7.1
961	*Ictalurus punctata* (Catfish)	7.1
962	*Crotalus adamanteus* (Eastern diamond-back rattlesnake)	7.1
963	*Jabiru mycteria* (Jabiru stork)	7.1
964	*Dromiceius novaehollandie* (Emu)	7.4
965	*Sphenicus humboldti* (Humboldt's penguin)	7.5
966	*Terrapene carolina* (Terrapin)	7.6
967	*Rana catesbeiana* (Bullfrog)	7.8
968	*Caiman sclerops*	7.8
969	*Carcharhinus limbatus* (Black-tipped shark)	7.9
970	*Lampropeltis getulus* (King snake)	~8
971	*Natrix gramhi* (Graham's watersnake)	8.1
972	*Dasyatus americana* (Sting ray)	8.8
973	*Chelydra serpentina* (Snapping turtle)	8.8
974	*Electrophorus electricus* (Electric eel)	8.8
975	*Ameriurus nebulosus* (Bullhead)	9.0
976	*Xenopus laevi* (Clawed toad)	9.2
977	*Masticopus flagellum* (Western coachwhip)	9.6
978	*Didelphis marsupialis* (Opossum)	9.6
979	*Sphenicus humboldti* (Humboldt's penguin)	10.0
980	*Rhea rhea*	10.3
981	*Sphyrna tiburo* (Bonnet shark)	10.4
982	*Cyprinus carpio* (Carp)	10.9
983	*Carcharhinus limbatus* (Black-tipped shark)	10.9
984	*Petromyzon marinus* (Lamprey)	11.6
985	*Heterodontus francisci* (Horned shark)	11.7
986	*Ameriurus nebulosus* (Bullhead)	12.3
987	*Chelydra serpentina* (Snapping turtle)	12.5
988	*Ancistrodon piscivorus* (Cottonmouth moccasin)	
989	*Orycteropus afer* (Aardvark)	12.7
990	*Electrophorus electricus* (Electric eel)	12.9
991	*Corvus brachyrhyncus* (Crow)	~13
992	*Terrapene carolina* (Terrapin)	13.0
993	*Ginglymostoma cirratum* (Nurse shark)	13.0
994	*Lepisosteus osseus* (Gar)	13.1
995	*Bufo marinus* (Marine toad)	13.3
996	*Caiman sclerops*	13.3
997	*Ictalurus punctata* (Catfish)	13.7
998	*Deirochelys reticularia* (Chicken turtle)	13.8
999	*Cyprinus carpio* (Carp)	13.8
1000	*Siren lacertina* (Salamander)	14.0
1001	*Ancistrodon piscivorus* (Cottonmouth moccasin)	14.0
1002	*Sphyrna tiburo* (Bonnet shark)	14.5
1003	*Rana catesbeiana* (Bullfrog)	14.5
1004	*Iguana iguana*	14.5
1005	*Erinaceus europaeus* (European hedgehog)	14.6
1006	*Rattus norvegicus* (Hooded rat)	14.8
1007	*Masticopus flagellum* (Western coachwhip)	14.9

TABLE V: Sedimentation coefficients of vertebrate serum proteins (Continued)

No.	Vertebrate Serum[a]	$S \times 10^{13}$
1008	*Lampropeltis getulus* (King snake)	14.9
1009	*Sus scofa* (Pig)	14.9
1010	*Chrysemys picta* (Painted turtle)	15.0
1011	*Rhea rhea*	15.0
1012	*Corvus brachyrhynchus* (Crow)	15.0
1013	*Homo sapiens* (Man)	15.0
1014	*Deirochelys reticularia* (Chicken turtle)	15.1
1015	*Sphenicus humboldti* (Humboldt's penguin)	15.1
1016	*Chelydra serpentina* (Snapping turtle)	15.2
1017	*Crotalus viridis* (Prairie rattlesnake)	15.3
1018	*Didelphis marsupialis* (Opossum)	15.4
1019	*Natrix gramhi* (Graham's watersnake)	15.5
1020	*Tachyglossus aculeatus* (Echidna)	15.5
1021	*Heterodontus francisci* (Horned shark)	15.6
1022	*Crocodylus morleti* (Crocodile)	15.7
1023	*Dasyatus americana* (Sting ray)	16.1
1024	*Crotalus adamanteus* (Eastern diamond-back rattlesnake)	16.2
1025	*Dromiceius novahollandie* (Emu)	16.4
1026	*Felis domesticus* (Cat)	16.5
1027	*Haliaetus leucoryphas* (Fishing eagle)	16.7
1028	*Sylvilagus floridanus* (Cottontail rabbit)	16.7
1029	*Rana catesbeiana* (Bullfrog)	16.8
1030	*Macropus rufo* (Red kangaroo)	16.9
1031	*Florida thula* (Snowy egret)	17.5
1032	*Xenopus laevi* (Clawed toad)	17.6
1033	*Lepidosiren paradoxa* (Lungfish)	18.0
1034	*Jabiru mycteria* (Jabiru stork)	18.2
1035	*Iguana iguana*	18.9
1036	*Eudocimus albus* (White ibis)	18.9
1037	*Chrysemys picta* (Painted turtle)	22.1

Compiled by Malcolm H. Smith.

[a] Unfractionated serum proteins. *S* values were obtained from the sedimentation patterns of serum itself, during centrifugation at ambient room temperature, "very close to 20°C and within the range 20–22°C" [530; Seal, personal communication].

TABLE VI: Miscellaneous data

No.	Protein	$S_{20.w} \times 10^{13}$	$D_{20.w} \times 10^{7}$	V_{20}	Molecular Weight	f/f_0	Reference Number
			GLOBULAR PROTEINS				
1038	Cytochrome *c*, horse heart	–	11.1	–	–	–	469
1039	Hemoglobin, *Lampetra*	–	10.65	–	–	–	235, 289
1040	Lactalbumin, cow	–	10.6	–	–	–	55, 289
1041	Cytochrome *c*, vertebrate heart	–	10.1	–	–	–	235, 289
1042	Pepsin	–	9.69	–	–	–	55, 396
1043	Pepsin	–	9.0	–	–	–	55, 289
1044	Carboxypeptidase	–	8.68	–	–	–	55, 397
1045	Lysozyme, chicken egg white	–	8.6	0.75	–	–	55, 316
1046	Penicillinase	–	7.80	–	–	–	89
1047	Ovalbumin	–	7.8	–	–	–	235, 398
1048	Lactoglobulin	–	7.3	–	–	–	235, 289
1049	Growth hormone, pituitary	–	7.15	0.76	49,000	–	55, 399
1050	Chymotrypsin, bovine pancreas	–	7.1	–	–	–	55, 400
1051	Hemoglobin, human	–	6.9	–	–	–	55, 235, 398
1052	Pyrophosphatase	–	6.8	–	–	–	55, 401
1053	Gliadin	–	6.72	–	–	–	235, 398
1054	Albumin, horse serum	–	6.5	–	–	–	55, 402
1055	Hemoglobin, horse	–	6.3	–	–	–	235, 376
1056	Prothrombin, bovine	–	6.24	–	–	–	92
1057	Albumin, horse serum	–	6.14	–	–	–	55, 403
1058	Albumin, horse serum	–	6.11	–	–	–	55, 404
1059	Albumin, cow serum	–	6.0	–	–	–	55, 405
1060	Excelsin	–	4.26	–	–	–	235, 289
1061	γ-Globulin, bovine	–	4.1	–	169,000	–	55, 406
1062	Phycocyanin, *Ceramium*	–	4.05	–	–	–	55, 376
1063	Globulin, horse serum	–	4.05	–	–	–	235, 289
1064	Phycoerythrin, *Ceramium*	–	4.00	–	–	–	235, 376
1065	Edestin	–	3.93	–	–	–	235, 289
1066	Amandin	–	3.62	–	–	–	235, 289
1067	Hemocyanin, *Palinurus*	–	3.4	–	–	–	235, 289
1068	Phosphorylase b	–	3.3	–	–	–	83
1069	Hemocyanin, *Nephrops*	–	2.79	–	–	–	235, 289
1070	Hemocyanin, *Homarus*	–	2.78	–	–	–	235, 289
1071	Thyroglobulin, pig	–	2.65	–	–	–	235, 289
1072	Hemoglobulin, *Planorbis*	–	1.96	–	–	–	235, 376
1073	Hemoglobulin, *Lumhricus*	–	1.81	–	–	–	235, 289
1074	Hemocyanin, octopus	–	1.65	–	–	–	235, 289
1075	Hemocyanin, *Eledone*	–	1.64	–	–	–	235, 289
1076	Hemocyanin, *Rossia*	–	1.58	–	–	–	235, 289
1077	Hemocyanin, *Helix*	–	1.38	–	–	–	235, 289
1078	Ribonuclease, bovine pancreas	–	–	0.693	–	–	515
1079	Trypsin inhibitor, soya bean	–	–	0.698	–	–	193
1080	Prothrombin, bovine	–	–	0.70	–	–	92
1081	Cytochrome *c*, vertebrate heart	–	–	0.707	–	–	235, 407
1082	γ-Globulin, cow	–	–	0.720	–	–	55, 408
1083	Thyroglobulin, pig	–	–	0.723	–	–	48
1084	Gliadin	–	–	0.724	–	–	70
1085	γ-Globulin, cow	–	–	0.725	–	–	55, 358
1086	Pepsin	–	–	0.725	–	–	515
1087	Albumin, human serum	–	–	0.729	–	–	55, 410
1088	Albumin, bovine serum	–	–	0.734	–	–	55, 188, 408
1089	γ-Globulin, horse	–	–	0.745	–	–	177, 188
1090	Globulin, horse serum	–	–	0.745	–	–	235, 411
1091	Albumin, horse serum	–	–	0.748	–	–	235, 411
1092	Ovalbumin	–	–	0.748	–	–	55, 408
1093	CO-hemoglobin, cow	–	–	0.749	–	–	55, 410
1094	Diphtheria anti-toxin	–	–	0.749	–	–	55, 412
1095	Insulin	–	–	0.749	–	–	55, 414
1096	Enolase, rabbit muscle, 1°C	3.46	3.418	0.728	84, 760	2.004	98
1097	Malate dehydrogenase, ox heart, 2°C	2.1	13.5	–	–	–	45
1098	Carbonic anhydrase, mammalian RBC, 25°C	3.80	–	–	–	–	55, 415
1098a	Transglutaminase, pig liver, 25°C	5.40	6.44	–	76,900	–	543
1099	Aldolase, bovine liver, 25°C	8.87	5.20	0.743	163,100	1.146	184

TABLE VI: Miscellaneous data (Continued)

No.	Protein	$S_{20.w} \times 10^{13}$	$D_{20.w} \times 10^7$	V_{20}	Molecular Weight	f/f_0	Reference Number
	FIBROUS PROTEINS						
1100	Myosin	–	0.87	–	–	–	55, 389, 416
1101	*Clostridium* toxin	–	2.10	0.755	–	–	55, 420
1102	Haptoglobin type *1-1*, human	–	4.8	–	85,000	–	188, 417
1103	Transferrin, human	–	5.30	0.72	92,000	–	139
1104	Fibrinogen, human	–	–	0.725	–	–	55, 418
1105	*Clostridium* toxin	–	–	0.736	–	–	55, 419
1106	Fibrinogen, cow	–	–	0.706	–	–	55, 358
1107	Zein	–	–	0.776	–	–	70
1108	Clupein sulfate	–	–	0.58	–	–	285
1109	Tropomyosin, rabbit muscle	–	–	0.71	–	–	55, 422
1110	Paramyosin, *Venus mercenaria*	–	–	0.730	220,000	–	545
	VIRUSES						
1111	Phage fd	40	–	0.71	11,800,000	–	151
1112	Tobacco necrosis virus	49	–	–	–	–	55, 423
1113	Phage fr	79	1.4	0.69	4,416,000	1.428	151
1114	Bromegrass mosaic virus	86.2	1.55	–	4,600,000	–	19
1115	Turnip yellow mosaic virus	106	1.55	0.666	4,970,000	1.255	147
1116	Southern bean mosaic virus	115	1.39	0.696	6,602,000	1.254	55, 424
1117	Potato latent mosaic virus	123.5	–	0.73	–	–	55, 425
1118	Tomato bushy stunt virus	132	–	–	10,600,000	–	55, 426
1119	Tomato bushy stunt virus	–	1.15	–	–	–	55, 427
1120	Tomato bushy stunt virus	146	–	0.739	7,600,000	–	235, 428
1121	Tobacco mosaic virus	174	0.3	–	–	–	55, 429
1122	Tobacco mosaic virus	–	–	0.727	–	–	55, 420
1123	Tobacco mosaic virus	185	0.53	0.73	31,340,000	1.927	131
1124	Tobacco mosaic virus TM 58	198	0.46	0.743	40,590,000	2.025	55, 431
1125	Horse encephalitis virus	253	–	–	–	–	55, 432
1126	Rabbit papilloma virus	280	0.585	0.754	47,140,000	1.507	55, 169
1127	Rabbit papilloma virus	297	–	0.761	–	–	55, 433
1128	*B. megaterium* G phage	321	0.26	0.667	89,990,000	2.848	164
1129	T_7 bacteriophage	487	0.90	–	37,500,000	–	554
1130	Chicken sarcoma virus	550	–	–	–	–	55, 434
1131	Influenza virus PR 8	660	–	–	–	–	55, 435
1132	Influenza virus PR 8	700	–	–	–	–	55, 436
1133	T2 phage	700	–	–	–	–	55, 437, 438
1134	Polyhedral silkworm virus	1871	0.215	0.770	916,200,000	1.515	55, 439
	PARTICLES AND ORGANELLES						
1135	Sodium taurodeoxycholate micelles	1.00	8.9	0.76	11,340	1.589	546
1136	Lysolecithin sol, egg	1.80	–	–	95,000	–	547
1137	Ganglioside micelles, ox brain	10.3	3.78	0.78	299,800	1.245	548
1138	Fatty acid synthetase particle, pigeon liver	14.7	2.50	0.744	566,600	1.556	549
1139	Bacterial ribosome particle	29.5	–	–	–	–	550
1140	Bacterial ribosome particle	37.5	–	–	–	–	550
1141	α-Ketoglutarate dehydrogenase system, *E. coli*	40	1.51	–	2,400,000	–	125
1142	Yeast ribosome	51.5	–	–	–	–	551
1143	Bacterial ribosome	56.3	–	–	–	–	550
1144	Pyruvate dehydrogenase system, *E. coli*	64.1	1.20	–	4,800,000	–	125
1145	Yeast ribosome	68.6	–	–	–	–	551
1146	Bacterial ribosome	76.7	–	–	–	–	550
1147	Yeast ribosome	86.7	–	–	–	–	551
1148	Bacterial ribosome	110.8	–	–	–	–	550
1148a	Lysosome, rat liver	9,400	–	–	–	–	353
1148b	Mitochondrion, rat liver	33,000	–	–	–	–	353
	NUCLEIC ACIDS						
1149	RNA, *E. coli*	16.7	–	–	500,000	–	552
1150	RNA, *E. coli*	23.0	–	–	1,120,000	–	552
1151	RNA, turnip yellow mosaic virus	28.4	–	–	2,000,000	–	553
1152	DNA, T7 bacteriophage	30.0	–	–	19,000,000	–	517

TABLE VI: Miscellaneous data (Continued)

No.	Protein	$S_{20.w} \times 10^{13}$	$D_{20.w} \times 10^7$	V_{20}	Molecular Weight	f/f_0	Reference Number
			CARBOHYDRATES				
1153	Glucosamino-glycan, bovine cornea	0.96	–	0.55	–	–	555
1154	Glucosamino-glycan, bovine cornea	1.16	6.9	0.53	8,696	2.525	555
1155	Glucosamino-glycan, bovine cornea	1.39	–	0.51	–	–	555
1156	Insulin	1.42	–	0.601	7,250	–	556
1157	Hemicellulose A, *Chlorella*	2.65	6.8	0.65	27,030	1.640	173
1158	Hyaluronic acid	3.1	1.254	0.66	177,100	4.743	255
1159	Fucan, *Fucus vesiculosus*	4.5	3.0	–	78,000	–	13
1160	Glucosamino-glycan, bovine cornea	1.47	5.6	0.49	12,520	2.828	555
1161	Glucosamino-glycan, bovine cornea	1.52	–	0.52	–	–	555
1162	Glucosamino-glycan, bovine cornea	1.59	–	0.49	–	–	555
1163	Glucosamino-glycan, bovine cornea	1.72	4.1	0.47	19,250	3.393	555
1164	Galactosamino-glycan, bovine cornea	1.8	–	–	–	–	555
1165	Galactosamino-glycan, bovine cornea	2.0	2.8	0.55	38,580	3.740	555
1166	Galactosamino-glycan, bovine cornea	2.0	–	0.52	43,000	–	555
1167	Galactosamino-glycan, bovine cornea	2.1	–	–	–	–	555
1168	Galactosamino-glycan, bovine cornea	2.1	–	–	–	–	555
1169	Galactosamino-glycan, bovine cornea	2.2	–	–	–	–	555
1170	Galactosamino-glycan, bovine cornea	2.3	–	–	–	–	555
			MISCELLANEOUS				
1171	Flavin mononucleotide (FMN), (dimer) 25°C	0.48	28.6	0.574	994.9	1.243	544
1172	Phosvitin calcium complex	38.8	2.38	0.475	755,200	1.714	113
1173	Phosvitin magnesium complex	62.5	1.71	0.403	1,490,000	2.010	113

Compiled by Malcolm H. Smith.

References

1. Abdel-Latif and Alivisatos, *J Biol Chem* **237**, 500 (1962).
2. Adair, Ogston and Johnston, *Biochem J* **40**, 867 (1946).
3. Agner, in Wyman, *Advanc Protein Chem* **4**, 407 (1948).
4. Allerton, Elwyn, Edsall, and Spahr, *J Biol Chem* **237**, 85 (1962).
5. Allison, Cecil, Charlwood, Gratzer, Jacobs, and Snow, *Biochim Biophys Acta* **42**, 43 (1960).
6. Antonini, Rossi-Fanelli, and Caputo, *Arch Biochem Biophys* **97**, 343 (1962).
7. Armstrong, Coates, and Morton, *Biochem J* **86**, 136 (1963).
8. Askonas, *Biochem J* **58**, 332 (1954).
9. Bartsh and Kamen, *J Biol Chem* **235**, 825 (1960).
10. Benesch, *Nature* **194**, 840 (1962).
11. Bergmeyer, Holz, Kauder, Mollering, and Wieland, *Biochem Z* **333**, 471 (1961).
12. Bernardi, *Nature* **180**, 93 (1957).
13. Bernardi and Springer, *J Biol Chem* **237**, 75 (1962).
14. Bezkorovainy and Doherty, *Arch Biochem Biophys* **96**, 491 (1962).
15. Birk, Gertler, and Khalef, *Biochem J* **87**, 281 (1963).
16. Blanc and Isliker, *Bull Soc Chim Biol* **43**, 929 (1961).
17. Bloemendal, Bont, Jongkind, and Wisse, *Nature* **193**, 437 (1962).
18. Boardman, *Biochim Biophys Acta* **62**, 63 (1962).
19. Bockstahler and Kaesberg, *Biophys J* **2**, I (1962).
20. Bomstein, Goldberger, and Tisdale, *Biochim Biophys Acta* **50**, 527 (1961).
21. Bourdillon, *J Am Chem Soc* **77**, 5308 (1955).
22. Bourrillon, Michon, and Got, *Biochim Biophys Acta* **47**, 243 (1961).
23. Bowen and Rogers, *Biochem J* **84**, 46 P (1962).
24. Bowen, *Biochem J* **55**, 766 (1953).
25. Brady and O'Connell, *Biochim Biophys Acta* **62**, 216 (1962).
26. Bridgman, *J Am Chem Soc* **68**, 857 (1946).
27. Brohult, *J Phys Chem* **51**, 206 (1947).
28. Bundy and Maehl, *J Biol Chem* **234**, 1124 (1959).
29. Burke, *Biochem J* **78**, 556 (1961).
30. Callaghan, *Biochem J* **67**, 651 (1957).
31. Cammack, *Nature* **194**, 745 (1962).
32. Caspary and Kekwick, *Biochem J* **67**, 41 (1957).
33. Cecil and Ogston, *Biochem J* **42**, 229 (1948).
34. Cecil and Ogston, *Biochem J* **43**, 205 (1948).
35. Cecil and Ogston, *Biochem J* **49**, 105 (1951).
36. Chiba, *Arch Biochem Biophys* **90**, 294 (1960).
37. Cohen, *Nature* **182**, 659 (1958).
38. Connell, *Biochem J* **70**, 81 (1958).
39. Creeth, *Biochem J* **53**, 41 (1958).
40. Cruft, Mauritzen, and Stedman, *Proc Roy Soc Ser B* **149**, 21 (1958).
41. Danielson, *Nature* **160**, 899 (1947).
42. Danielson, *Nature* **162**, 525 (1948).
43. Danielson, *Biochem J* **44**, 387 (1949).
44. Davenport and Hill, *Proc Roy Soc Ser B* **139**, 327 (1951–1952).
45. Davies and Kun, *Biochem J* **66**, 307 (1957).
46. Davies and Englert, *J Biol Chem* **235**, 1011 (1960).
47. Derechin and Johnson, *Nature* **194**, 473 (1962).
48. Derrien, Michel, Pedersen, and Roche, *Biochim Biophys Acta* **3**, 436 (1949).
49. Derrien and Reynaud, *Compt Rend Acad Sci (France)* **252**, 214 (1961).
50. Deutsch, *J Biol Chem* **216**, 97 (1955).
51. Dickie and Liener, *Biochim Biophys Acta* **64**, 41 (1962).
52. Durell, Anderson, and Cantoni, *Biochim Biophys Acta* **26**, 270 (1957).
53. Ebata and Yasunobu, *J Biol Chem* **237**, 1086 (1962).
54. Edelhoch, Rodwell, and Grisolia, *J Biol Chem* **228**, 891 (1957).
55. Edsall, in *The Proteins*, 1st ed. Neurath and Bailey ed., Academic, New York, (1953), p 549.
56. Ehrenberg, *Acta Chem Scand* **11**, 1257 (1957).
57. Ehrenberg and Agner, *Acta Chem Scand* **12**, 95 (1958).
58. Ehrenberg and Dalziel, *Acta Chem Scand* **12**, 465 (1958).
59. Ellfolk, *Acta Chem Scand* **14**, 1819 (1960).
60. Elödi, *Acta Physiol Acad Sci Hung* **13**, 199 (1958).
61. Elödi and Szorenyi, *Acta Physiol Acad Sci Hung* **9**, 367 (1956).
62. Ende, Meyerhoff, and Schulz, *Z Naturforsch B* **13**, 713 (1958).
63. Englard and Breiger, *Biochim Biophys Acta* **56**, 571 (1962).
64. Engström, *Biochim Biophys Acta* **52**, 36 (1961).
65. Esnouf and Williams, *Biochem J* **84**, 62 (1963).
66. Fedden and Chase, *Biochim Biophys Acta* **32**, 176 (1959).
67. Fischer, Sumerwell, Junge, and Stein, *Proc IV Biochem Congress* **VIII**, 124 (1958).
68. Fishkin and Berenson, *Arch Biochem Biophys* **95**, 130 (1961).
69. Folk, Piez, Carroll, and Gladner, *J Biol Chem* **235**, 2272 (1960).
70. Foster and French, *J Am Chem Soc* **67**, 687 (1964).
71. Fox and Dandliker, *J Biol Chem* **218**, 53 (1956).
72. Friedberg, *Experentia* **18**, 164 (1962).
73. Friedberg, *Can J Biochem* **40**, 983 (1962).
74. Frieden, *Biochim Biophys Acta* **62**, 421 (1962).
75. Fuller and Briggs, *J Am Chem Soc* **78**, 5253 (1956).
76. Garen and Levinthal, *Biochim Biophys Acta* **38**, 470 (1960).
77. Gibbons and Glover, *Biochem J* **73**, 217 (1959).
78. Gibson, *Biochem J* **79**, 151 (1961).
79. Gordon, Ziegler, and Basch, *Biochim Biophys Acta* **60**, 410 (1962).
80. Gottschalk and McKenzie, *Biochim Biophys Acta* **54**, 226 (1961).
81. Gralén, *Biochem J* **33**, 1342 (1939).
82. Gray, Priest, Blatt, Westphal, and Jensen, *J Biol Chem* **235**, 57 (1960).
83. Green, *J Biol Chem* **158**, 315 (1945).
84. Green and Cori, *J Biol Chem* **151**, 21 (1943).
85. Grisolia, Harmon, and Raijman, *Biochim Biophys Acta* **62**, 293 (1962).
86. Groves, *J Am Chem Soc* **82**, 3345 (1960).
87. Guinand, Tonnelat, Boussier, and Jayle, *Bull Soc Chim Biol* **38**, 329 (1956).
88. de la Haba, Cammarata, and Timasheff, *J Biol Chem* **234**, 316 (1959).
89. Hall and Ogston, *Biochem J* **62**, 401 (1956).
90. Hamilton, Cavalieri, and Peterman, *J Biol Chem* **237**, 1155 (1962).
91. Hammarsten, Agren, Hammarsten, and Wilander, *Biochem Z* **264**, 275 (1933).
92. Harmison and Seegers, *J Biol Chem* **237**, 3074 (1962).
93. Hazelwood, *J Am Chem Soc* **80**, 2152 (1958).
94. Helwig and Greenburg, *J Biol Chem* **198**, 695 (1952).
95. Henning, Helinski, Chao, and Yanofsky, *J Biol Chem* **237**, 1523 (1962).
96. Henrotte, *Arch Int Physiol Biochim* **62**, 294 (1954).
97. Holland, *Biochem J* **78**, 641 (1961).
98. Holt and Wold, *J Biol Chem* **236**, 3227 (1961).
99. Horio, Higashi, Yamanaka, Matsubara, and Okunuki, *J Biol Chem* **236**, 944 (1961).
100. Sumner and Gralén, *J Biol Chem* **125**, 33 (1935).
101. Huys, *Arch Int Physiol Biochim* **62**, 296 (1954).
102. Inoue, Nakagawa, and Morihara, *Biochim Biophys Acta* **73**, 125 (1963).
103. Isemura and Fujita, *J Biochem (Japan)* **44**, 443 (1957).
104. Jackson, Coulson, and Clark, *Arch Biochem Biophys* **97**, 373 (1962).
105. Jaenicke and Pfleiderer, *Biochim Biophys Acta* **60**, 615 (1962).
106. Jansz and Cohen, *Biochim Biophys Acta* **56**, 531 (1962).
107. Jenkins, Yphantis, and Sizer, *J Biol Chem* **234**, 51 (1959).
108. Johnson, *Trans Faraday Soc* **42**, 28 (1946).
109. Johnson and Naismith, *Discuss Faraday Soc* **13**, 98 (1953).
110. Johnson and Rowe, *Biochem J* **74**, 432 (I 60).
111. Johnson and Shooter, *Biochim Biophys Acta* **5**, 361 (1950).
112. Joubert, *Biochim Biophys Acta* **16**, 370 (1955).
113. Joubert and Cook, *Can J Biochem* **36**, 399 (1958).
114. Kabat, Heidelberger, and Bezer, *J Biol Chem* **168**, 629 (1947).
115. Kägi and Vallee, *J Biol Chem* **236**, 2435 (1961).
116. Karlson and Liebau, *Hoppe-Seyler's Z Physiol Chem* **326**, 135 (1961).
117. Kasper and Deutsch, *J Biol Chem* **238**, 2325 (1963).
118. Katoh, Shiratori, and Takamiya, *J Biochem (Japan)* **51**, 32 (1962).
119. Kay, *Biochim Biophys Acta* **27**, 469 (1958).
120. Kay and Pabst, *J Biol Chem* **237**, 727 (1962).
121. Keilin, *Biochem J* **64**, 663 (1956).
122. Kekwick, *Biochem J* **50**, 471 (1952).

123. Keller, Cohen, and Neurath, *J Biol Chem* **223**, 457 (1956).
124. Kimmel, Markowitz, and Brown, *J Biol Chem* **234**, 46 (1959).
125. Koike, Reed, and Carroll, *J Biol Chem* **235**, 1924 (1960).
126. Koike, Shah, and Reed, *J Biol Chem* **235**, 1939 (1960).
127. Kominz, Maruyama, Levenbrook, and Lewis, *Arch Biochem Biophys* **63**, 106 (1962).
128. Kraut, Korbel, Scholtan, and Schultz, *Hoppe-Seyler's Z Physiol Chem* **321**, 90 (1960).
129. Kratohvil, Martin, and Cook, *Can J Biochem* **40**, 877 (1962).
130. Kusai, Bekuzu, Hagihara, Okunuki, Yamauchi, and Nakai, *Biochim Biophys Acta* **40**, 555 (1960).
131. Lauffer, *J Am Chem Soc* **66**, 1188 (1944).
132. Laurent, *Arch Biochem Biophys* **92**, 224 (1961).
133. Lee, *J Biol Chem* **227**, 993 (1957).
134. Lee, *Biochim Biophys Acta* **43**, 18 (1960).
135. Legault-Démare, Clauser, and Jutisz, *Bull Soc Chim Biol* **43**, 897 (1961).
136. Lenhert, Love, and Carlson, *Biol Bull* **111**, 293 (1956).
137. Li, *Symposium on Protein Structure*, Neuberger, Ed, Methuen, London, 1958, p. 302.
138. Li, Cole, and Coval, *J Biol Chem* **229**, 153 (1957).
139. Bezkorovainy and Rafelson, *Arch Biochem Biophys* **107**, 302 (1964).
140. Lindskog, *Biochim Biophys Acta* **39**, 218 (1960).
141. Lindquist, *Biochim Biophys Acta* **10**, 443 (1953).
142. Lipke and Kearns, *J Biol Chem* **234**, 2123 (1959).
143. Lundgren, Gurin, Bachman, and Wilson, *J Biol Chem* **142**, 367 (1942).
144. Maeno and Kiyosawa, *Biochem J* **83**, 271 (1962).
145. Mallette and Dawson, *Arch Biochem Biophys* **23**, 29 (1949).
146. Manning, Campbell, and Foster, *J Biol Chem* **236**, 2958 (1961).
147. Markham, *Discuss Faraday Soc* **11**, 221 (1951).
148. Markovitz, Klein, and Fischer, *Biochim Biophys Acta* **19**, 267 (1956).
149. Marshall, Metzenberg, and Cohen, *J Biol Chem* **236**, 2229 (1961).
150. Martin, Vandegaer, and Cook, *Can J Biochem* **35**, 241 (1957).
151. Marvin and Hoffman-Berling, *Nature* **197**, 517 (1963).
152. Maser and Rice, *Biochim Biophys Acta* **63**, 255 (1962).
153. Massey, Palmer, and Bennett, *Biochim Biophys Acta* **48**, 1 (1961).
154. Maxfield, *Arch Biochem Biophys* **55**, 382 (1955).
155. Maxfield and Hartley, *J Biophys Biol Cytol* **1**, 279 (1955).
156. Mihashi, *Arch Biochem Biophys* **107**, 441 (1964).
157. Millar, *J Biol Chem* **237**, 2135 (1962).
158. Mills and Wilkins, *Biochim Biophys Acta* **30**, 63 (1958).
159. Mok, Martin, and Common, *Can J Biochem* **39**, 109 (1961).
160. Montreuil, Tonnelat, and Mullet, *Biochim Biophys Acta* **45**, 413 (1960).
161. Moore, *J Biol Chem* **161**, 597 (1945).
162. Morita, *J Biochem (Japan)* **48**, 870 (1960).
163. Moyle and Dixon, *Biochem J* **63**, 548 (1956).
164. Murphy and Philipson, *J Gen Physiol* **45**, 155 (1962).
165. Nagahisa, *J Biochem (Japan)* **51**, 216 (1962).
166. Nakamura, *Biochim Biophys Acta* **30**, 44 (1958).
167. Neilands, *J Biol Chem* **197**, 701 (1952).
168. Neilands, *J Biol Chem* **208**, 225 (1954).
169. Neurath, Cooper, Sharp, Taylor, Beard, and Beard, *J Biol Chem* **140**, 293 (1940).
170. Nomoto and Narahashi, *J Biochem (Japan)* **46**, 1645 (1959).
171. Nozaki, *J Biochem (Japan)* **47**, 592 (1960).
172. Nyman, *Biochim Biophys Acta* **52**, 1 (1961).
173. Olaitan and Northcote, *Biochem J* **82**, 509 (1962).
174. Omura, *J Biochem (Japan)* **50**, 264 (1961).
175. Omura, *J Biochem (Japan)* **50**, 394 (1961).
176. Omura, Fujita, Yamada, and Yamato, *J Biochem (Japan)* **50**, 400 (1961).
177. Oncley, Scatchard, and Brown, *J Phys Colloid Chem* **51**, 184 (1947).
178. Orlando, *Biochim Biophys Acta* **57**, 373 (1962).
179. Osaki, *J Biochem (Japan)* **48**, 190 (1960).
180. Pain, *Biochem J* **88**, 234 (1963).
181. Pallansch and Liener, *Arch Biochem Biophys* **45**, 366 (1953).
182. Papaconstantinou, Resnik, and Saito, *Biochim Biophys Acta* **60**, 205 (1962).
183. Papkoff, Li, and Liu, *Arch Biochem Biophys* **96**, 216 (1962).
184. Peanasky and Lardy, *J Biol Chem* **233**, 371 (1958).
185. Pedersen, in *Lés Protéines*, Stoops, ed. Neuvième Conseil de Chimie, Bruxelles, 1953.
186. Pedersen, *J Phys Chem* **51**, 164 (1947).
187. Pollock and Torriani, *Compt Rend Acad Sci (France)* **237**, 276 (1953).
188. Phelps and Putnam, in *Plasma Proteins*, **Vol. I**, Putnam, ed. Academic, New York, 1960, p 143.
189. Pyeand Curtain, *J Gen Microbiol* **24**, 423 (1961).
190. Raijman, Grisolia, and Edelhoch, *J Biol Chem* **235**, 2340 (1960).
191. Record and Grinstead, *Biochem J* **58**, 85 (1954).
192. Renard, *Arch Int Physiol Biochem* **61**, 466 (1953).
193. Wu and Scheraga, *Biochemistry* **1**, 698 (1962).
194. Reynaud, Rametta, Savary, and Derrien, *Biochim Biophys Acta* **77**, 521 (1963).
195. Richterich, Temperli, and Aebi, *Biochim Biophys Acta* **56**, 240 (1962).
196. Rothen, *J Biol Chem* **152**, 679 (1944).
197. Rogers and Novelli, *Arch Biochem Biophys* **96**, 398 (1962).
198. Ross and Moore, *Biochim Biophys Acta* **16**, 293 (1955).
199. Ross and Moore, *Biochim Biophys Acta* **15**, 50 (1954).
200. Rossi-Fanelli, Antonini, and Poveledo, in *Symposium on Protein Structure*, Neuberger, ed. Methuen, London, 1958, p 144.
201. Rumen and Appella, *Arch Biochem Biophys* **97**, 128 (1962).
202. Samejima, Kamata, and Shibata, *J Biochem (Japan)* **51**, 181 (1962).
203. Sanders, Miller, and Richard, *Arch Biochem Biophys* **84**, 60 (1959).
204. Savage, *Biochem J* **67**, 146 (1957).
205. Seanu, Lewis, and Bumpus, *Arch Biochem Biophys* **74**, 390 (1958).
206. Schachman, *J Gen Physiol* **35**, 451 (1952).
207. Scheler and Schneiderat, *Acta Biol Med Germ* **3**, 588 (1959).
208. Schultze, Heide, and Haupte, *Naturwiss* **48**, 719 (1961).
209. Schultze, Heide, and Haupte, *Naturwiss* **48**, 696 (1961).
210. Schultze, Schmidtberger, and Haupte, *Biochem Z* **329**, 490 (1958).
211. Schweet, Katchman, Bolk, and Jagannathan, *J Biol Chem* **196**, 563 (1952).
212. Seifter, Gallop, Klein, and Meilman, *J Biol Chem* **234**, 285 (1959).
213. Seppala, *Scand J Clin Lab Invest* **13**, 665 (1961).
214. Shack, *J Biol Chem* **180**, 411 (1949).
215. Shin and Nakamura, *J Biochem (Japan)* **50**, 500 (1961).
216. Shulman, Alkjaersig, and Sherry, *J Biol Chem* **233**, 91 (1958).
217. Siegel and Englard, *Biochim Biophys Acta* **54**, 67 (1961).
218. Singer and Pensky, *J Biol Chem* **196**, 375 (1952).
219. Smith, *Biochem J* **83**, 135 (1962).
220. Smith, *Biochem J* **89**, 45P (1963).
221. Smith, *J Theoret Biol* **13**, 261 (1966).
222. Smith, Brown, Weimer, and Winzler, *J Biol Chem* **185**, 569 (1950).
223. Smith, Brown, Ghosh, and Sayers, *J Biol Chem* **187**, 631 (1950).
224. Smith, Kimmel, Brown, and Thompson, *J Biol Chem* **215**, 67 (1955).
225. Smith, George, and Preer, *Arch Biochem Biophys* **99**, 313 (1962).
226. Smith, Hill, and Kimmel, in *Symposium on Protein Structure*, Neuberger, ed. Methuen, London, 1958, p. 182.
227. Sophianopoulos, Rhodes, Holcomb, and Van Holde, *J Biol Chem* **237**, 1107 (1962).
228. Stern, del Campillo, and Raw, *J Biol Chem* **218**, 971 (1956).
229. Sörbo, *Acta Chem Scand*, 7, 1129 (1953).
230. Spiro, *J Biol Chem*, **235**, 2860 (1960).
231. Squire and Li, *J Am Chem Soc*, **83**, 3521 (1961).
232. Stansell and Deutsch, *J Biol Chem* **240**, 4306 (1965).
233. Strittmatter, *J Biol Chem* **235**, 2492 (1960).
234. Suzuki and Iwasaki, *J Biochem (Japan)* **52**, 193 (1962).
235. Svedberg and Pedersen, in *The Ultracentrifuge*, Oxford University Press, London, 1940.
236. Sullivan, Fitzpatrick, Stanton, Annino, Kissel, and Palermiti, *Arch Biochem Biophys* **55**, 455 (1955).
237. Tagawa and Arnon, *Nature* **195**, 537 (1962).
238. Takagi and Toda, *J Biochem (Japan)* **52**, 16 (1962).
239. Takashi, Funatsu, and Funatsu, *J Biochem (Japan)* **52**, 50 (1962).
240. Takahashi and Schmid, *Biochim Biophys Acta* **63**, 343 (1962).
241. Takemori, Sekuzu, and Okunuki, *Biochim Biophys Acta* **51**, 464 (1961).

242. Tamm, Bugher, and Horsfall, *J Biol Chem* **212**, 125 (1955).
243. Taylor and Lowry, *Biochim Biophys Acta* **20**, 109 (1956).
244. Theorell and Åkeson, *Arch Biochem Biophys* **65**, 439 (1956).
245. Theorell and Bonnichsen, *Acta Chem Scand* **5**, 1105 (1951).
246. Theorell, Holman, and Åkeson, *Acta Chem Scand* **1**, 571 (1947).
247. Theorell and Pedersen, in Wyman, *Advanc Protein Chem* **4**, 407 (1948).
248. Thorne, *Biochim Biophys Acta* **59**, 624 (1962).
249. Ts'o, Eggman and Vinograd, *Biochim Biophys Acta* **25**, 532 (1957).
250. Tsuji and Sowinski, *J Cell Comp Physiol* **58**, 125 (1961).
251. Ui, *Biochim Biophys Acta* **25**, 493 (1957).
252. Ui and Tarutani, *J Biochem (Japan)* **49**(9) (1961).
253. Uspenskaya, Alekseenko, Rodionov, and Solov'eva, *Biokhimiya* **26**, 592 (1961).
254. Vandegaer, Reichmann, and Cook, *Arch Biochem Biophys* **62**, 328 (1956).
255. Varga, Pietruszkiewicz, and Ryan, *Biochim Biophys Acta* **32**, 155 (1959).
256. Wada, Pallansch, and Leiner, *J Biol Chem* **233**, 395 (1958).
257. Wallach, Ko, and Marshall, *Biochim Biophys Acta* **59**, 690 (1962).
258. Warner, *Arch Biochem Biophys* **78**, 494 (1958).
259. Warringa, Smith, Guiditta, and Singer, *J Biol Chem* **230**, 97 (1958).
260. Weber, *Vox Sanguin N.S.* **1**, 37 (1956).
261. Wellner and Meister, *J Biol Chem* **235**, 2013 (1960).
262. Wijmenga, Thompson, Stern, and O'Connell, *Biochim Biophys Acta* **13**, 144 (1954).
263. Wilcox, Kraut, Wade, and Neurath, *Biochim Biophys Acta* **24**, 72 (1957).
264. Williams, *Biochem J* **83**, 346 (1962).
265. Williams and Esnouf, *Biochem J* **84**, 52 (1963).
266. Williams and Peacocke, *Biochim Biophys Acta* **101**, 327 (1965).
267. Wolf and Briggs, *Arch Biochem Biophys* **85**, 186 (1959).
268. Wolfe and Nielands, *J Biol Chem* **221**, 61 (1956).
269. Wood, McCarty and Slater, *J Exp Med* **100**, 71 (1954).
270. Yagi and Ozawa, *Biochim Biophys Acta* **62**, 397 (1962).
271. Yagi, Ozawa, and Ooi, *Biochim Biophys Acta* **54**, 199 (1961).
272. Yagi, Mishima, Tsujimura, Sato, and Egami, *Compt Rend Soc Biol* **149**, 2283 (1955).
273. Yamada and Yasunobu, *J Biol Chem* **237**, 1511 (1962).
274. Yamashita and Okunuki, *J Biochem (Japan)* **52**, 117 (1962).
275. Young and Lorimer, *Arch Biochem Biophys* **92**, 183 (1961).
276. Yunis, Fischer, and Krebs, *J Biol Chem* **237**, 2109 (1962).
277. Chandon, Shahani, Hill, and Scholz, *Enzymologia* **26**, 87 (1963).
278. Seegers, Cole, Harrison, and Marciniak, *Can J Biochem* **41**, 1047 (1963).
279. Wasserman and Burris, *Phytochemistry* **4**, 413 (1965).
280. Jungblut and Turba, *Biochem Z* **337**, 88 (1963).
281. Markert and Appella, *Ann N Y Acad Sci* **94**, 678 (1961).
282. Pesce, McKay, Stolzenbach, Cahn, and Kaplan, *J Biol Chem* **239**, 1753 (1964).
283. Criddle, Bock, Green, and Tisdale, *Biochemistry* **1**, 827 (1962).
284. Sund and Weber, *Biochem Z* **337**, 24 (1963).
285. Gehatia and Hashimoto, *Biochim Biophys Acta* **69**, 212 (1963).
286. Seibert, Pedersen, and Tiselius, *J Exp Med* **68**, 413 (1938).
287. Pedersen, *Cold Spring Harbor Symp* **14**, 140 (1949).
288. Rothen, *J Gen Physiol* **24**, 203 (1940).
289. Polson, *Thesis*, University of Stellenbosch, 1937.
290. Theorell, *Biochem Z* **268**, 46 (1934).
291. Schwert and Koufman, *J Biol Chem* **190**, 807 (1951).
292. Tietze, *J Biol Chem* **204**, 1 (1953).
293. Schwert, *J Biol Chem* **190**, 799 (1951).
294. Gralén and Svedberg, *Biochem J* **32**, 1375 (1938).
295. Sumner, Gralén, and Eriksson-Quensel, *J Biol Chem* **125**, 45 (1938).
296. Schwert, *J Biol Chem* **179**, 655 (1949).
297. Bergold, *Z Naturforsch* **1**, 100 (1946).
298. Agrawal and Goldstein, *Biochim Biophys Acta* **133**, 376 (1967).
299. Petermann and Pappenheimer, *J Phys Chem* **45**(1) (1941); Tiselius and Dahl, *Ark Kemi* **14B**(31), 7 (1941).
300. Pedersen, *Ultracentrifugal Studies on Serum and Serum Fractions*, Almqvist and Wiksell, Boktryckeri AB, Uppsala, 1945.
301. Li and Pedersen, *J Gen Physiol* **35**, 629 (1952).
302. Kekwick and Pedersen, *Biochem J* **30**, 2201 (1936).
303. Sumner and Gralén, *Science* **87**, 284 (1938); Sumner and Gralén, *J Biol Chem* 125, 33 (1935).
304. Sumner, Gralén, and Eriksson-Quensel, *J Biol Chem* **125**, 37 (1938).
305. Olson and Anfinsen, *J Biol Chem* **197**, 67 (1952).
306. Pedersen, *J Phys Colloid Chem* **51**, 156 (1947).
307. Kabat, *J Exp Med* **69**, 103 (1939).
308. Fredericq and Neurath, *J Am Chem Soc* **72**, 2684 (1950).
309. Moody, PhD Thesis University of Wisconsin, 1944; quoted in Williams *Annu Rev Phys Chem* **2**, 412 (1951).
310. Gutfreund, *Biochem J* **50**, 564 (1952).
311. Taylor, *Arch Biochem Biophys* **36**, 357 (1952).
312. Abraham, *Biochem J* **33**, 622 (1939).
313. Oncley, Ellenbogen, Gitlin, and Gurd, *J Phys Chem* **56**, 85 (1952).
314. Svedberg and Eriksson-Quensel, *J Am Chem Soc* **56**, 1700 (1934).
315. Alderton, Ward, and Fevold, *J Biol Chem* **157**, 43 (1945).
316. Passynskii and Plaskeyev, *CR Acad Sci URSS* **48**, 579 (1945).
317. Svedberg and Hedenius, *Biol Bull* **66**, 191 (1934).
318. Quensel and Svedberg, *Compt Rend Lab Carlsberg* **22**, 441 (1938).
319. Li and Pedersen, *Arch Biochem Biophys* **36**, 462 (1952).
320. Sayers, White, and Long, *J Biol Chem* **149**, 425 (1943).
321. Atlas and Farber, *J Biol Chem* **219**, 31 (1956).
322. Krejci and Svedberg, *J Am Chem Soc* **57**, 946 (1935).
323. Li, Evans, and Simpson, *J Biol Chem* **149**, 413 (1943).
324. Wetter and Deutsch, *J Biol Chem* **192**, 237 (1951).
325. Vilbrandt, Tennent, and Hakala, Quoted in Bridgman and Williams, *Ann NY Acad Sci* **43**, 195 (1942).
326. Krejci and Svedberg, *J Am Chem Soc* **56**, 1706 (1934).
327. Smith, Brown, and Laskowski, *J Biol Chem* **191**, 639 (1951).
328. Peterman and Hakala, *J Biol Chem* **145**, 701 (1942).
329. Cunningham, Tietze, Green, and Neurath, *Discuss Faraday Soc* **58**(13) (1953).
330. Schwert and Kaufman, *J Biol Chem* **180**, 517 (1949).
331. Van Dyke, Chow, Greep, and Rothen, *J Pharmacol Exp Therap* **74**, 190 (1942).
332. Li, Lyons, and Evans, *J Biol Chem* **140**, 43 (1941).
333. Krejci, Stock, Sanigar, and Kraemer, *J Biol Chem* **142**, 785 (1942).
334. Miller and Golder, *Arch Biochem Biophys* **36**, 249 (1952).
335. Steinhardt, *J Biol Chem* **123**, 543 (1938).
336. Johnston and Ogston, *Trans Faraday Soc* **42**, 789 (1946).
337. Smith, Brown, and Hanson, *J Biol Chem* **180**, 33 (1949).
338. Hess and Williams, cited in Oncley *Ann NY Acad Sci* **41**, 121 (1942).
339. Pederson, *Biochem J* **30**, 948 (1936).
340. Bain and Deutsch, *Arch Biochem Biophys* **16**, 221 (1948).
341. Schwert, *J Biol Chem* **179**, 655 (1949).
342. Philpot, *Biochem J* **29**, 2458 (1935).
343. Wallenius, Trautman, Kunkel, and Franklin, *J Biol Chem* **225**, 253 (1957).
344. Gutfreund and Ogston, *Biochem J* **40**, 432 (1946).
345. Gutfreund, *Biochem J* **42**, 544 (1948).
346. Miller and Anderson, *J Biol Chem* **144**, 459 (1942).
347. Smith, Brown, Fishman, and Wilhelmi, *J Biol Chem* **177**, 305 (1949).
348. Kegeles and Gutter, *J Am Chem Soc* **73**, 3770 (1951).
349. Svedberg and Sjogren, *J Am Chem Soc* **51**, 3594 (1929).
350. Schultze and Schwick, *Clin Chim Acta* **4**, 15 (1959).
351. Charlwood, *Biochem J* **51**, 113 (1952).
352. Creeth, *Biochem J* **51**, 10 (1952).
353. Corbett, *Biochem J* **102**, 43P (1967).
354. Loeb and Scheraga, *J Phys Chem* **60**, 1066, 1633 (1956).
355. Ogston, *Proc Roy Soc A (London)* **196**, 272 (1949).
356. Kekwick, *Biochem J* **32**, 552 (1938).
357. Gutfreund, cited in Boyes-Watson, Davidson and Perutz, *Proc Roy Soc A (London)* **191**, 83 (1947).
358. Koenig and Pedersen, *Arch Biochem Biophys* **25**, 97, 241 (1950);.
359. Ikenaka, Gitlin, and Schmid, *J Biol Chem* **240**, 2868 (1965).
360. Moon and Reiner, *J Biol Chem* **156**, 411 (1944).
361. Meyer, Thompson, Palmer, and Khorazo, *J Biol Chem* **113**, 303 (1936).
362. Northrop and Rothen, *J Gen Physiol* **25**, 465–487 (1941–1942).

363. Laurell and Ingleman, *Acta Chem Scand* **1**, 770 (1947).
364. Eriksson-Quensel and Svedberg, *Biol Bull* **71**, 498 (1936).
365. Cann, Brown, Stringer, Shumaker, and Kirkwood, *Science* **114**, 30 (1951).
366. Largier, *Arch Biochem Biophys* 77, 350 (1958).
367. Shedlovsky, Rothen, Greep, Van Dyke, and Chow, *Science* **92**, 178 (1940).
368. Dunn and Dawson, *J Biol Chem* **189**, 485 (1951).
369. Singer and Kearney, *Arch Biochem* **29**, 190 (1950).
370. Smith and Brown, *J Biol Chem* **183**, 241 (1950).
371. Koenig, *Arch Biochem* **23**, 229 (1949).
372. Hess and Deutsch, *J Am Chem Soc* **70**, 84 (1948).
373. Glikina and Finogenov, *Biokhimiya* **15**, 457 (1950).
374. Massey, *Biochem J* **51**, 490 (1952).
375. England and Singer, *J Biol Chem* **187**, 213 (1950).
376. Tiselius and Gross, *Kolloid Z* **66**, 11 (1934).
377. Sjögren and Spychalski, *J Am Chem Soc* **52**, 4400 (1930).
378. Eriksson-Quensel, *Biochem J* **32**, 585 (1938).
379. Svedberg and Sjögren, *J Am Chem Soc* **52**, 279 (1930).
380. Svedberg and Stamm, *J Am Chem Soc* **51**, 2170 (1929).
381. Svedberg and Eriksson, *J Am Chem Soc* **55**, 2834 (1933).
382. Kabat and Pederson, *Science* **87**, 372 (1938).
383. Heidelberger and Pedersen, *J Gen Physiol* **19**, 95 (1935).
384. Watson, Arrhenius, and Williams, *Nature* **137**, 322 (1936).
385. Schmid, *Biochem Biophys Acta* **21**, 399 (1956).
386. Schultze, Göllner, Heide, Schönenberger, and Schwick, *Z Naturforsch* **10b**, 463 (1955).
387. Jayle and Boussier, *Exposés Annu Biochim Méd* **17**, 157 (1955).
388. Shore, *Arch Biochem Biophys* **71**, 1 (1957).
389. Snellman and Erdös, *Biochim Biophys Acta* **2**, 650 (1948).
390. Ehrlich, Shulman, and Ferry, *J Am Chem Soc* **74**, 2258 (1952).
391. Sandor and Slizewicz, *Bull Soc Chim Biol* **39**, 857 (1957).
392. Brown, Baker, Peterkofsky, and Kauffman, *J Am Chem Soc* **76**, 4244 (1954).
393. Edsall, Gilbert, and Scheraga, *J Am Chem Soc* **77**, 157 (1955).
394. Nichol and Deutsch, *J Am Chem Soc* **70**, 80 (1948).
395. Schönenberger, Schmidtberger, and Schultze, *Z Naturforsch* **13b**, 761 (1958).
396. Northrop, *J Gen Physiol* **13**, 739 (1930).
397. Putnam, Neurath, Elkins, and Segal, *J Biol Chem* **166**, 603 (1946).
398. Lamm and Polson, *Biochem J* **30**, 528 (1936).
399. Li, *J Phys Colloid Chem* **51**, 218 (1947).
400. Kunitz and Northrop, *J Gen Physiol* **18**, 433 (1935).
401. Kunitz, cited by Schachman, *J Gen Physiol* **35**, 451 (1952).
402. Champagne, *J Chim Phys* **48**, 627 (1951).
403. Kojiro and Wanatabe, *Rep Radiat Chem Res Inst Tokyo Univ* No. 4, 7–8 (1949).
404. Cooper and Neurath, cited in Neurath, *Chem Rev* **30**, 357 (1942).
405. Stern, Singer, and Davis, *J Biol Chem* **167**, 321 (1947).
406. Kahn and Polson, quoted in Hess and Deutsch, *J Am Chem Soc* **70**, 84 (1948).
407. Theorell, *Biochem Z* **285**, 207 (1936).
408. Dayhoff, Perlmann and MacInnes, *J Am Chem Soc* **74**, 2515 (1952).
409. Iwasaki, Shidara, Suzuki, and Nori, *J Biochem (Japan)* **53**, 299 (1963).
410. Adair and Adair, *Proc Roy Soc A London* **190**, 341 (1947).
411. Svedberg and Sjögren, *J Am Chem Soc* **50**, 3318 (1928).
412. Northrop and Polson, *J Gen Physiol* **25**, 465–487 (1941–1942).
413. Ichishima and Yoshida, *Nature* **207**, 525 (1965).
414. Sjögren and Svedberg, *J Am Chem Soc* **53**, 2657 (1931).
415. Eirich and Rideal, *Nature* **146**, 541 (1940).
416. Johnson and Landolt, *Discuss Faraday Soc* No. 11, 179 (1951).
417. Nyman, *Scand J Clin Lab Invest* **11**(Suppl 39) (1959).
418. Armstrong, Budka, Morrison, and Hasson, *J Am Chem Soc* **69**, 1747 (1947).
419. Putnam, Lamanna, and Sharp, *J Biol Chem* **176**, 401 (1948).
420. Kegeles, *J Am Chem Soc* **68**, 1670 (1946).
421. Tietze and Neurath, *J Am Chem Soc* **75**, 1758 (1953).
422. Bailey, Gutfreund, and Ogston, *Biochem J* **43**, 279 (1948).
423. Ogston, *Brit J Expt Pathol* **26**, 286 (1945).
424. Miller and Price, *Arch Biochem* **10**, 467 (1946).
425. Lauffer and Cartwright, *Arch Biochem Biophys* **38**, 371 (1952).
426. Stanley and Anderson, *J Biol Chem* **139**, 325 (1941).
427. Neurath and Cooper, *J Biol Chem* **135**, 455 (1940).
428. McFarlane and Kekwick, *Biochem J* **32**, 1607 (1938).
429. Neurath and Saum, *J Biol Chem* **126**, 435 (1938).
430. Cecil and Ogston, *Biochem J* **43**, 592 (1948).
431. Schramm and Bergold, *Z Naturforsch* **B2**, 108 (1947).
432. Taylor, Sharp, Beard, and Beard, *J Inf Dis* **71**, 110, 115 (1942).
433. Sharp, Taylor, and Beard, *J Biol Chem* **163**, 289 (1940).
434. Claude, *Science* **91**, 77 (1940); Pollard, *Brit J Exp Pathol* **20**, 429 (1939).
435. Gard and Magnus, *Arkiv Kemi* **24B**(8), 1 (1947).
436. Stanley and Lauffer, *J Phys Colloid Chem* **51**, 148 (1947).
437. Loring, Morton, and Schwerdt, *Proc Soc Exp Biol Med* **62**, 291 (1946).
438. Hook, Beard, Taylor, Sharp, and Beard, *J Biol Chem* **165**, 241 (1946).
439. Bergold, *Z Naturforsch* **B2**, 122 (1947).
440. Kuehl, *Biochim Biophys Acta* **71**, 531 (1962).
441. Schrier, Broomfield, and Scheraga, *Arch Biochem Biophys* Supp 1, 309 (1962).
442. Kassell, Radicevic, Barlow, Peanasky, and Laskowski, *J Biol Chem* **238**, 3274 (1963).
443. Busch, Hnilica, Chien, Davis, and Taylor, *Cancer Res* **22**, 637 (1962).
444. Hartley, Rushizky, Greco, and Sober, *Biochemistry* **2**, 794 (1963).
445. Gillespie, *Aust J Biol Sci* **16**, 241 (1963).
446. Ganno, *J Biochem (Japan)* **58**, 556 (1965).
447. Sutherland and Wilkinson, *J Gen Microbiol* **30**, 105 (1962).
448. Adams and Norton, *J Biol Chem* **239**, 1525 (1964).
449. Matsubara, Chu, and Yasunobu, *Arch Biochem Biophys* **101**, 209 (1963).
450. Rackis, Sasame, Mann, Anderson, and Smith, *Arch Biochem Biophys* **98**, 471 (1962).
451. Kickhöfen and Burger, *Biochim Biophys Acta* **65**, 190 (1962).
452. Shimomura, Johnson, and Saiga, *J Cell-Comp Physiol* **62**, 1 (1963).
453. Reisfeld, Williams, Cirillo, Tong, and Brink, *J Biol Chem* **239**, 1777 (1964).
454. Nickerson and Durand, *Biochim Biophys Acta* **77**, 87 (1963).
455. Squire, Li, and Anderson, *Biochemistry* **1**, 412 (1962).
456. Habeeb, *Can J Biochem* **42**, 545 (1964).
457. Williams and Rajagopalan, *J Biol Chem* **241**, 4951 (1966).
458. Siebert, Schmitt, and Traxler, *Hoppe-Seyler's Z Physiol Chem* **332**, 160 (1963).
459. Allen, Kellermeyer, Stjernholm, Jacobson, and Wood, *J Biol Chem* **238**, 1637 (1963).
460. Gosselin-Rey, *Arch Int Physiol Biochem* **73**, 313 (1965).
461. Balls and Ryan, *J Biol Chem* **238**, 2976 (1963).
462. Torralba and Grisolia, *J Biol Chem* **241**, 1713 (1966).
463. Green and Bodansky, *J Biol Chem* **240**, 2574 (1965).
464. Chiancone, Vecchini, Forlani, Antonini, and Wyman, *Biochim Biophys Acta* **127**, 549 (1966).
465. Turner, *Biochim Biophys Acta* **69**, 518 (1963).
466. Morris and Hagers, *J Biol Chem* **241**, 1763 (1966).
467. Hargreaves, Wanderley, Hargreaves, and Goncales, *Biochim Biophys Acta* **67**, 641 (1963).
468. Boffa, Jacquot-Armand, and Fine, *Biochim Biophys Acta* **86**, 514 (1964).
469. Fling, Horowitz, and Heinemann, *J Biol Chem* **238**, 2045 (1963).
470. Popp, Heddle, Canning, and Allen, *Biochim Biophys Acta* **115**, 113 (1966).
471. Campagnari and Webster, *J Biol Chem* **238**, 1628 (1963).
472. Ganguly, Gupta and Chatterjea, *Nature* **199**, 919 (1963).
473. Bull, Feinstein, and Morris, *Nature* **201**, 1326 (1964).
474. Tantori, Vivaldi, Corta, Salvati, Sorcini, and Velani, *Arch Biochem Biophys* **109**, 404 (1965).
475. Mosbach, *Biochim Biophys Acta* **73**, 204 (1963).
476. Cline and Hu, *J Biol Chem* **240**, 4498 (1965).
477. Roberts, Makey, and Seal, *J Biol Chem* **241**, 4907 (1966).
478. Wilson and Crawford, *J Biol Chem* **240**, 4801 (1965).
479. Goldwasser, *J Biol Chem* **238**, 3306 (1963).

480. Charlwood, *Biochem J* **88**, 394 (1963).
481. Hosokawa and Stanier, *J Biol Chem* **241**, 2453 (1966).
482. Gregory and Bendall, *Biochem J* **101**, 569 (1966).
483. Nagler, Kochwa, and Wasserman, *Proc Soc Exp Biol* **111**, 746 (1962).
484. Mahling, *Z Naturforsch* **18B**, 1 (1963).
485. Bruns and Schultze, *Biochem Z* **336**, 162 (1962).
486. Conconi and Grazi, *J Biol Chem* **240**, 2461 (1965).
487. Nozaki, Kagamiyama, and Hayaishi, *Biochem Biophys Res Commun* **11**, 65 (1963).
488. Saito and Hanahan, *Biochemistry* **1**, 521 (1962).
489. Ishiguro, Takahashi, Hayashi, and Funatsu, *J Biochem (Tokyo)* **56**, 325 (1964).
490. Schreiber, Eckstein, Maas, and Hoker, *Biochem Z* **340**, 21 (1964).
491. Clark, Poillon, and Dawson, *Biochim Biophys Acta* **118**, 82 (1966).
492. Hofmann and Shaw, *Biochim Biophys Acta* **92**, 543 (1964).
493. Matthews and Reed, *J Biol Chem* **238**, 1869 (1962).
494. Schultze, Schönenberger, and Schwick, *Biochem Z* **328**, 267 (1956).
495. Yoshida, *Biochim Biophys Acta* **71**, 544 (1963).
496. Yoshida, *J Biol Chem* **240**, 1113 (1965).
497. Gehatia, *Z Naturforsch* **B 17**, 432 (1962).
498. Chung and Langdon, *J Biol Chem* **238**, 2309 (1963).
499. Allison and Kaplan, *J Biol Chem* **239**, 2140 (1964).
500. Christen, Göschke, Lenthardt, and Schmid, *Helv Chim Acta* **48**, 1050 (1965).
501. Monakhov and Neifakh, *Biokhimia* **27**, 494 (1962).
502. Ebert and Schenk, *Z Naturforsch* **B 17**, 732 (1962).
503. Yoshida and Freese, *Biochim Biophys Acta* **92**, 33 (1964).
504. Burns and Demoss, *Biochim Biophys Acta* **65**, 233 (1962).
505. Yamada, Gee, Ebata, and Yasunobu, *Biochim Biophys Acta* **81**, 165 (1964).
506. Shiio, Shiio, and McFadden, *Biochim Biophys Acta* **96**, 114 (1965).
507. Newton, Morino, and Snell, *J Biol Chem* **240**, 1211 (1965).
508. Van Holde and Cohen, *Biochemistry* **3**, 1803 (1965).
509. Adachi, Iwayama, Tanioka, and Takeda, *Biochim Biophys Acta* **118**, 88 (1966).
510. Okazaki, Briehl, Wittenberg, and Wittenberg, *Biochim Biophys Acta* **111**, 496 (1965).
511. Coleman, *J Biol Chem* **24**, 5511 (1966).
512. Inoue, Adachi, Suzuki, Fukinish, and Takada, *Biochem Biophys Res Commun* **21**, 432 (1965).
513. Rogers, Geiger, Thompson, and Hellerman, *J Biol Chem* **238**, 481 (1963).
514. Bowen and Rogers, *Biochim Biophys Acta* **67**, 633 (1963).
515. McMeekin, Wilensky, and Groves, *Biochem Biophys Res Commun* **7**, 151 (1962).
516. Fujita, Itagak and Sato, *J Biochem (Japan)* **53**, 282 (1963).
517. Davison and Freifelder, *J Mol Biol* **5**, 643 (1962).
518. Chew, Scutt, Oliver and Lugg, *Biochem J* **94**, 378 (1965).
519. Lawler, *J Biol Chem,* **238**, 132 (1963).
520. Rao and Pandit, *Biochim Biophys Acta* **94**, 238 (1965).
521. Ketterer, *Life Sciences* **1**, 163 (1962).
522. Rice, Casassa, Kerwin, and Maser, *Arch Biochem Biophys* **105**, 409 (1964).
523. Bezkorovainy, *Biochemistry* **2**, 10 (1963).
524. Hashimoto, Hashimoto, and Pigman, *Arch Biochem Biophys* **104**, 282 (1964).
525. Fryar and Gibbs, *Experientia* **19**, 493 (1963).
526. Brahms and Kay, *J Mol Biol* **5**, 132 (1962).
527. Connell, *Biochim Biophys Acta* **74**, 374 (1963).
528. Cornelius, Pangborn, and Heckly, *Arch Biachem Biophys* **101**, 403 (1963).
529. Johnson, Napper, and Rowe, *Biochim Biophys Acta* **74**, 365 (1963).
530. Roberts and Seal, *Comp Biochem Physiol* **16**, 327 (1965).
531. Jutisz, Hermier, Colonge, and Courrier, *Ann Endocrinol (Paris)* **26**, 670 (1965).
532. Pardee, *J Biol Chem* **241**, 5886 (1966).
533. Ohta, Ogura, and Wada, *J Biol Chem* **241**, 5919 (1966).
534. Allen, *J Biol Chem* **241**, 5266 (1966).
535. Dawson, Eppenberger, and Kaplan, *J Biol Chem* **242**, 210 (1967).
536. Marino, Greco, Scardi, and Zito, *Biochem J* **99**, 589 (1966).
537. Chang and Lane, *J Biol Chem* **241**, 2413 (1966).
538. Takahashi, Ramachandramurthy, and Liener, *Biochem Biophys Acta* **133**, 123 (1967).
539. Ide, Huyakawa, Okabe, and Koike, *J Biol Chem* **242**, 54 (1967).
540. Nakano, *J Biol Chem* **242**, 73 (1967).
541. Nakano and Danowski, *J Biol Chem* **241**, 2075 (1966).
542. Baker and Crawford, *J Biol Chem* **241**, 5577 (1966).
543. Folk and Cole, *J Biol Chem* **241**, 5518 (1966).
544. Gibson, Massey, and Atherton, *Biochem J* **85**, 369 (1962).
545. Lowey, Kucera, and Holtzer, *J Mol Biol* **7**, 234 (1963).
546. Laurent and Person, *Biochim Biophys Acta* **106**, 616 (1965).
547. Perrin and Saunders, *Biochim Biophys Acta* **84**, 216 (1964).
548. Gammack, *Biochem J* **88**, 373 (1963).
549. Yang, Bock, Hsu, and Porter, *Biochim Biophys Acta* **110**, 608 (1965).
550. DeLey, *J Gen Microbiol* **34**, 219 (1964).
551. De Ley, *J Gen Microbiol* **37**, 153 (1964).
552. Bogdanova, Gavrilova, Dvorkin, Kiselev, and Spirin, *Biokhimia* **27**, 387 (1962).
553. Mitra and Kaesberg, *J Mol Biol* **14**, 558 (1965).
554. Davison and Freifelder, *J Mol Biol* **5**, 635 (1962).
555. Laurent and Anseth, *Exp Eye Res* **1**, 99 (1961).
556. Phelps, *Biochem J* **95**, 41 (1965).
557. Franz and Krisch, *Biochem Biophys Res Commun* **23**, 816 (1966).

This material first appeared in the 2nd edition of the *Handbook of Biochemistry: Selected Data for Molecular Biology* (ed. H.A. Sober), CRC Press, Cleveland, Ohio, 1970 and in the 3rd edition of the *Handbook of Biochemistry and Molecular Biology* (ed. G.D.Fasman), CRC Press, Boca Raton, Florida, 1976).

MOLAR ABSORPTIVITY AND $A^{1\%}_{1cm}$ VALUES FOR PROTEINS AT SELECTED WAVELENGTHS OF THE ULTRAVIOLET AND VISIBLE REGION

Protein	ϵ^a ($\times 10^{-4}$)	$A^{1\% \, b}_{1cm}$	nm[c]	Reference	Comments[d]
Acetoacetate decarboxylase (EC 4.1.1.4)	3.05	10.5	280	567	MW = 29,000/subunit [567]
C. acetobutylicum					
Acetolactate synthase (EC 4.1.3.18)	–	8.3	280	568	pH 6, 50 mM P$_i$; data from Figure 1 [568]
Aerobacter aerogenes					
Acetyl coenzyme A carboxylase (EC 6.4.1.2)	–	11.6	280	569	Calc. using OD$_{230}$ × 0.86 = mg/ml [569]
Chicken liver					
Acetylcholinesterase (EC 3.1.1.7)					
Electrophorus electricus	–	21.4	280	1322	Kjeldahl or Dumas[e]
	–	21.8	280	1322	Microninhydrin[e]
	–	18.8	280	1322	Nitrogen from amino acid analysis[e]
	–	17.6	280	1322	DR
	–	18.2	280	1322	Dry wt.
	52.7	22.9	280	1	pH 7.0, 0.1 M NaCl, 0.03 M NaP$_i$, MW = 230,000 [1]
	–	16.1	280	2	0.02 M AcONH$_4$
	–	19.0	280	877	–
β-N-acetyl-D-glucosaminidase (EC 3.2.1.30)					
Aspergillus oryzae	29.3	20.9	280	777	MW = 140,000 [777]
Beef spleen					
Enzyme A	–	12.8	278	1323	–
Enzyme B	–	12.7	278	1323	–
O-Acetylserine sulfhydrase A (cysteine synthase) (EC 4.2.99.8)					
Salmonella typhimurium	8.2	12.1	280	634	MW = 68,000 [634]
	0.76	1.12	412	634	MW = 68,000 [634]
Acetylserotonin methyltransferase (EC 2.1.1.4) (see hydroxyindole-O-methyltransferase)					
Acid deoxyribonuclease (deoxyribonuclease 11) (EC 3.1.4.6)					
Pig spleen	4.6	12.1	280	635	MW = 38,000 [635]
Aconitase (aconitate hydrase) (EC 4.2.1.3)					
Pig heart	–	13.7	280	778	–
Actin					
Muscle	–	11.08	280	1324	–
F-Actin					
Rabbit	–	11.08	280	1156	Kjeldahl
Rabbit muscle	–	9.65	280	3	0.1 M KCl
	–	11.49	280	4	–
	–	11.5	280	636	–
G-Actin					
Rabbit muscle	5.05	10.97	280	5	MW = 46,000 [5]
β-Actinin					
Rabbit muscle	–	9.8	278	878	
Acyl phosphatase (EC 3.6.1.7)					
Horse muscle	1.09	11.58	280	639	pH 5.3, 0.05 M; AcO$^-$, MW = 9,400 [639]

---

[a] ϵ is the molar absorption coefficient with units of M^{-1} cm^{-1} and is either the value reported in the reference cited or calculated from the $A^{1\%}_{1cm}$ value and the molecular weight.

[b] $A^{1\%}_{1cm}$ is the absorbance for a 1% solution in a 1-cm cuvette and is either the value reported in the reference cited or calculated from the ϵ and the molecular weight. The relationship between ϵ, $A^{1\%}_{1cm}$ and molecular weight, MW, is $10\epsilon = (A^{1\%}_{1cm})$ (MW).

[c] Refers to the wavelength cited and may not be the peak of the absorption band.

[d] *Abbreviations used*: SC, corrected for light scattering; P$_i$, phosphate; GdmCl, guanidinium chloride; PP$_i$, pyrophosphate; Gro-P, glycerophosphate; S$_2$ threitol, dithiothreitol; NaDodSO$_4$, sodium dodecyl sulfate; HSEtOH, 2-mercaptoethanol; Gly$_2$, glycyl-glycine; ImzAc, imidazoleacetate; Tes, N-Tris(hydroxymethyl)methyl-2-aminoethanesulfonic acid; SucNBr, N-bromosuccinimide; albumin, bovine serum albumin.

Methods of protein determination: Dry wt., dry weight; AA, amino acid analysis; Refr., refractometry; Biuret, colorimetric method; Folin, colorimetric method; N, nitrogen determination; UC, ultracentrifuge; FC, fringe counting (interferometry); DR, differential refractometry; Kjeldahl: Lowry.

[e] Methods for determining nitrogen concentration in order to determine protein concentration.

MOLAR ABSORPTIVITY AND $A_{1cm}^{1\%}$ VALUES FOR PROTEINS AT SELECTED WAVELENGTHS OF THE ULTRAVIOLET AND VISIBLE REGION (Continued)

Protein	ϵ^a ($\times 10^{-4}$)	$A_{1cm}^{1\%\,b}$	nm[c]	Reference	Comments[d]
Acyl-carrier-protein					
Escherichia coli	0.27	3.0[g]	275	637	MW = 9,100 [637]; pH 7.0, 0.01 M KP$_i$, data from Figure 2 [638]
	0.18	–	275	638	–
Acyl-CoA dehydrogenase (see fatty acyl-CoA dehydrogenase)					
Adenosine deaminase (EC 3.5.4.4)					
Calf spleen	2.7	8.15	278	6	Estimated from Figure 1 [6]; MW = 33,120 [6]
Aspergillus oryzae	27.8	13.0	280	879	MW = 214,000 [879]
Adenosine 5′-phosphate deaminase (EC 3.5.4.17)					
Rabbit muscle	–	9.13	280	880	Dry wt.
	–	9.3	280	881	–
Adenosine 5′-phosphate nucleosidase (EC 3.2.2.4)					
Azotobacter vinelandii	5.58	9.73	280	1325	pH 8, 0.05 M triethanolamine · HC1 containing 0.1 mM S$_2$ threitol and 1 mM EDTA; MW = 57,300 [1325]
Adenosine triphosphate sulfurylase (sulfate adenylyltransferase) (EC 2.7.7.4) (see also ATP-sulfurylase)					
Penicillium chrysogenum	–	8.71	278	882	–
Adenovirus					
Hexon	–	14.6	279	1326	pH 7, 0.01 M NaP$_i$
Adenylic acid deaminase (EC 3.5.4.6)					
Rat muscle	28.5	9.84	280	1327	Dry wt., MW = 290,000 [1327]
Adrenodoxin					
Beef	1.14	–	276	1157	–
Beef adrenals	1.3	–	276	779	–
	1.26	–	325	779	–
	1.26	–	340	779	–
	0.98	–	414	779	–
	0.84	–	455	779	–
Beef adrenal cortex	0.579	–	276	1328	
	0.641	–	320	1328	Values cited are per mole of Fe
	0.496	–	414	1328	
	0.421	–	455	1328	
	–	6.75	276	1328	
	–	5.78	414	1328	
Apo-	0.76	–	276	779	
	0.35	–	276	1157	
Aequorin					
Aequorea	8.65	27.0[h]	280	780	MW = 32,000 [780]; protein det. by dry wt.
Apoaequorin-SH	–	18.2	280	780	
Apoaequorin-SO	–	18.2	280	780	
Agglutinin					
Wheat germ	10.9		280	1329	pH 7.0, 0.01 M NaP$_i$
	12		272	1329	
Alanine dehydrogenase (EC 1.4.1.1)					
Bacillus subtilis	51.2	22.3	280	883	pH 8, Tris Cl, 0.05 M, MW = 230,000 [883]
Alanine racemase (EC 5.1.1.1)					
Pseudomonas putida	–	10.8	275	781	pH 7.4, 0.005 M KP$_i$, data from Figure 2 of Ref. [781]
Albocuprein					
Human, brain					
I	8.4	11.65	280	1158	pH 6, 0.05 M NaCl/0.05 M AcONa, dry wt., MW = 72.000 [1, 1581]
II	1.2	8.63	280	1158	pH 6, 0.05 M NaCl/0.05 M AcONa, dry wt., MW = 14,000 [1158]
Albumin	–	10.6	278	1159	
Beef serum	–	6.49	280	1160	6 M GdmCl
	–	6.62	278	1161	pH 2, 0.01 N HCl

[g] Optical density used for calculation corrected for light scattering by extrapolation from 350 nm.

[h] 1 mg of aequorin in 1 ml added to 10^{-4} EDTA gives an OD of 2.52 at 280 nm. After freeze-drying and redissolving, the OD is now 2.25 at 280 nm [780].

MOLAR ABSORPTIVITY AND $A_{1cm}^{1\%}$ VALUES FOR PROTEINS AT SELECTED WAVELENGTHS OF THE ULTRAVIOLET AND VISIBLE REGION (Continued)

Protein	ϵ^a ($\times 10^{-4}$)	$A_{1cm}^{1\%\,b}$	nm^c	Reference	Comments^d
	–	3.58	255	1162	}
	–	6.14	280	1162	} pH 7.0, 0.01 M P$_i$
	–	0.50	310	1162	}
	–	6.8	280	12	–
	–	6.67	279	13	–
	–	6.6	280	14	–
	–	6.6	279.5	15	–
	–	6.6	279	16	–
	3.96	–	280	17	pH 7
	4.36	6.61	280	11	MW = 66,000 [11]
	–	6.3	280	640	Water
	–	270	210	640	Water
	–	840	191	640	Water
	4.69	6.9	279	641	MW = 68,000 [641]
	–	6.7	278	642	–
	2.77	–	288	643	–
	4.24	–	279	643	–
	19.43	–	234	643	–
	–	6.75	278	644	–
	–	6.2	280	645	–
	–	3.7	253.7	645	–
Beef,					
Mercapto-	–	6.82	279	894	–
(see also mercaptoalbumin, beef)					
	–	3.03	253	1330	} pH 6.2
	–	6.54	278	1330	}
	–	6.67	277.5	884	–
	4.37	–	280	885	2°C, alcohol–water mixtures
	4.6	–	280	886	–
	–	8.2	280	887	–
	–	650	191.4	887	–
	4.2	6.2	280	888	pH 7.96, Tris Cl, MW = 68,000 [888], water [889]
Fragment F$_2$	–	5.51	278	890	Dry wt.
	1.71	5.51	278	647	MW = 31,000 [647]
Fragment F$_3$	2.74	7.55	278	647	MW = 36,300 [647]
	–	7.55	278	890	Dry wt.
S-Carboxymethyl-	–	5.96	278	891	pH 8, 6 M GdmCl–0.02 M EDTA
S-Cysteinyl-	–	5.96	278	891	pH 8, 6 M GdmCl–0.02 M EDTA
	–	6.14	278	892	6 M GdmCl
Polypeptidyl derivatives					
Gly-261^i	4.9	5.8	278	893	–
L-Phe-31	4.8	6.4	278	893	–
L-Phe-36	4.7	6.3	278	893	–
DL-Phe-48	4.9	6.3	278	893	–
L-Glu-13	4.8	6.8	278	893	–
L-Glu-41	4.8	6.4	278	893	–
L-Glu-73	4.7	5.9	278	893	–
L-Glu-218	4.6	4.7	278	893	–
L-Glu-275	4.9	4.7	278	893	–
L-Lys-2	4.9	7.0	278	893	–
L-Lys-14	5.0	7.1	278	893	–
Methylated	–	6.5	280	645	–
	–	3.7	253.7	645	–
Acetylated	–	6.9	280	645	80% acetylated on amino groups
	–	3.7	253.7	645	–
Diazotized	–	7.5	280	645	–
	–	7.3	253.7	645	–
Guanidinated	–	9.2	280	645	–

i Gly-261 means that 261 moles of glycine have been attached to albumin. Other derivatives have been prepared similarly using other amino acids and are so indicated.

MOLAR ABSORPTIVITY AND $A_{1cm}^{1\%}$ VALUES FOR PROTEINS AT SELECTED WAVELENGTHS OF THE ULTRAVIOLET AND VISIBLE REGION (Continued)

Protein	ϵ^a ($\times 10^{-4}$)	$A_{1cm}^{1\%\,b}$	nm^c	Reference	Comments^d
	–	11.0	253.7	645	45 groups
Iodinated	–	12.0	312	645	
	–	7.5	280	645	32 mol I/mol
	–	18.6	253.7	645	
Glutaraldehyde modified	–	26.2	280	646	pH 8, borate
S-β-Pyridylethyl-	–	12.0	274	1161	pH 2, 0.01 N HCl
Cow's milk	4.55	6.6	280	901	MW = 69,000 [901]
Human serum	–	193	210	648	–
	–	143	215	648	–
	–	4.3	254	648	–
	–	7.15	280	648	–
	–	3.92	255	1162	
	–	5.94	280	1162	pH 7.0, 0.01 M P$_i$
	–	0.90	310	1162	
	–	6	280	7	
	4.0	5.8	280	8	MW = 69,000 [8]
	3.6	5.31	280	9	MW = 68,000 [10]
	3.5	5.3	280	11	MW = 66,000 [11]
	3.52	5.03	277.5	895	pH 2
					MW = 70,000 [895]
	–	7.15	280	896	–
	–	193	210	896	–
	–	143	215	896	–
	–	4.3	254	896	–
N$_2$ ph-^{q}	–	30.8	290	897	0.1 M NaOH
	–	11.7	360	897	0.1 M NaOH
Human mercapto-					
Fraction I	–	5.7	280	898	–
Fraction II	–	5.61	280	898	–
Fraction III	–	5.31	280	898	–
Fraction IV	–	5.8	280	898	–
Pig serum	–	6.72	280	899	pH 8.6, 0.2 M Tris Cl, 22°C, dry wt.
Rabbit serum	–	6.6	280	900	–
Albuminoid (insoluble protein)					
Young rat lens	–	18.4	280	782	
Young rat X-rayed lens	–	18.6	280	782	
Old rat lens	–	17.7	280	782	pH 9.8, 0.05 M borate/8 M urea
Medium-aged dogfish lens	–	22.4	280	782	
Old dogfish lens	–	21.2	280	782	
Albuminoid sulfonated					
Rat lens	–	17.3	280	902	–
	–	18.0	280	903	–
Dogfish lens	–	25.1	280	903	–
Beef lens	–	9.8	280	903	–
Human lens					
0–10 years old	–	11.1	280	903	–
11–20 years old	–	15.0	280	903	–
40–49 years old	–	15.9	280	903	–
50–59 years old	–	15.0	280	903	–
60–69 years old	–	16.5	280	903	–
70–79 years old	–	17.1	280	903	–
80 years old	–	18.0	280	903	–
Alcohol dehydrogenase (EC 1.1.1.1)					
Horse liver	–	4.55	280	904	–
	–	4.2	280	905	Dilute neutral buffer
	–	4.26	280	906	pH 7.2, 3 M GdmCl

^{q} N$_2$ ph- = 2,4-dinitrophenyl.

MOLAR ABSORPTIVITY AND $A^{1\%}_{1cm}$ VALUES FOR PROTEINS AT SELECTED WAVELENGTHS OF THE ULTRAVIOLET AND VISIBLE REGION (Continued)

Protein	ϵ^a ($\times 10^{-4}$)	$A^{1\% \; b}_{1cm}$	nm^c	Reference	Comments^d
	3.59	–	280	907	MW = 79,000 [907]
	3.82	4.55	280	18	–
	–	4.5	280	19	–
	3.83	4.6	280	20	MW = 83,300 [20]
	3.54	4.2	280	22	MW = 84,000 [21]
Zn-	3.44	4.3	280	908	⎫
Co-	3.92	4.9	280	910	⎬ MW 80,000 [909]
Cd-	4.56	5.7	280	910	⎭
	1.02	1.25	245	910	
Human liver	–	4.6	280	911	pH 7.0, 0.03 MP$_i$, 0.07 M NaCl
	5.3	6.1	280	23	pH 7.0, 0.1 μM NaP$_i$, MW = 87,000 [23]
Yeast	–	12.1	280	912	MW = 140,000 [913]
	20.78	14.8	278	913	MW = 141,000 [914]
	–	14.6	280	914	
	18.9	–	280	24	pH 8.1, 0.08 M glycine
	–	12.6	280	25	–
Arachis hypogea (Peanuts)	7.2	6.4	278	915	MW = 112,000 [915]
Drosophila melanogaster	3.96	9.0	280	916	MW = 44,000 [916]
Aldehyde dehydrogenase (EC 1.2.1.3-.5)					
Horse liver	–	20.8	280	1163	pH 7, AcONH$_4$, dry wt.
Pseudomonas aeruginosa	19.5	10.4	280	783	pH 7.0, 1 mM KP$_i$, protein con. det. by dry wt., MW = 187,000 [783]
Yeast	13.4	6.7	280	26	Reference states: "1 mg enzyme … OD equals 0.67," no volume given, assumed 1 ml, MW = 200,000 [26]
Aldehyde oxidase (EC 1.2.3.1)					
Rabbit liver	6.3	–	450	27	–
	2.2	–	550	27	–
Aldolase (EC 4.1.2.13)					
Rabbit muscle	–	9.1	280	28	–
	–	12.1	280	29	–
	11.8	8.32	277	30	pH 2
	13.3	9.38	280	30	pH 5.7, MW = 142,000 [31]
	–	7.8	276	32	pH 2
	11.8	7.4	280	917	pH 7.5–13, MW = 160,000 [918]
	–	8.4	280	919	⎫ pH 12.5, 0.1 M borate
	–	9.6	289.5	919	⎭
	–	8.16^i	276	920	3 M GdmCl
	–	8.20^i	276	920	5 M GdmCl
	–	8.21^i	276	920	6 M GdmCl
	–	8.23^i	276	920	7 M GdmCl
Succinyl-	–	8.2	276.5	921	Dry wt./KN^k
Rabbit liver	13.09	8.5	280	33	MW = 154,000 [33]
	13.3	8.40	280	922	MW = 158,000 [922]
Gallus domesticus, muscle (chicken)	16	10.3	280	923	pH 6.5, MW = 158,000 [923]
Liver	13.7	8.6	280	924	pH 7.5, 2 mM Tris, 0.2 mM EDTA, MW = 160,000 [925]
Rat muscle	15.0	9.39	280	926	MW = 160,000 [926]
Gradus morhua (Codfish) muscle	15.2	9.5	280	927	pH 7.5, MW = 160,000 [927]
Spinach	20.76	17.3	280	34	pH 7.4, 0.05 MP$_i$, MW = 120,000 [34]
	–	13.3	280	930	pH 7.5, 0.1 MP$_i$, Lowry^i
	–	11.0	280	930	Dry wt.
Yeast	7.95	10.6	280	35	MW = 75,000 [35]
	8	10	280	928	MW = 80,000 [928], dry wt.
	8.15	10.2	280	929	MW = 80,000 [929]
	8.0	10.1	280	929	Dry wt.

^{i} Calculated from an equation in Ref. [920].
^{k} KN, protein concentration determined by Kjeldahl nitrogen.
^{l} Lowry, protein concentration determined by Lowry method using bovine serum albumin as standard.

MOLAR ABSORPTIVITY AND $A_{1cm}^{1\%}$ VALUES FOR PROTEINS AT SELECTED WAVELENGTHS OF THE ULTRAVIOLET AND VISIBLE REGION (Continued)

Protein	ϵ^a ($\times 10^{-4}$)	$A_{1cm}^{1\% \, b}$	nm^c	Reference	Comments^d
	8.5	10.6	280	929	DR^m
	7.9	9.9	280	929	FD^n
Lobster muscle					
Homarus americanus	17.9	11.2	280	1164	MW = 160,000 [1164]
Shark muscle					
Mustelus canis	–	8.64	278.4	1165	Dry wt., Kjeldahl
	–	8.60	280	1165	
Rabbit liver	–	8.9	280	1166	Dry wt.
Rabbit brain	–	8.8	280	1166	Refractometry
Aldolase, L-rhamnulose 1-phosphate					
(EC 4.1.2.19) *Escherichia coli*	23.4	17.3	280	1167	MW = 135,000 [1167]
Aldolase, 3-deoxy-2-keto-6-phosphogluconate (EC 4.1.2.14)					
Pseudomonas putida	–	8.63	280	1168	0.1 N NaOH
Aldose 1-epimerase (EC 5.1.3.3)					
Escherichia coli K12	–	10.8	280	1331	–
Allantoicase (EC 3.5.3.4), 0.9S					
Pseudomonas aeruginosa	–	27.3	280	1169	Calcd. from the data in Figure 4 [1169], pH 7.7
	–	26.0	280	1169	Calcd. from the data in Figure 4 [1169], pH 4.6
	–	24.3	280	1169	Calcd. from the data in Figure 4 [1169], pH 4.6, in the presence of 0.1 M glycolate
	–	31.7	280	1169	Lowry
Allergen					
Short ragweed pollen					
Antigen E	–	11.3	280	1170	pH 7.15
Antigen Ra.3	16.4	10.9	280	1171	pH 7.3, 0.005 M NH$_4$ HCO$_3$, MW = 15,000 [1171]
Atopic					
Rye grass pollen					
I-B	–	15.0	280	1332	pH 7, MW = 34,000 [1332]
	–	2.18	305	1332	
II-B	–	10.3	280	1332	pH 7, MW = 11,000 [1332]
	–	0.88	305	1332	
B	–	14.1	280	1332	pH 7
	–	3.10	305	1332	
D[IEP]	–	14.7	280	1332	
	–	4.75	305	1332	
K	–	14.8	280	1332	pH 7, MW = 38,200 [1332]
Pool Cc	–	7.63	280	1332	
	–	1.05	305	1332	
Trifid in A	–	4.1	280	1332	
	–	1.20	305	1332	
Ipecac IPC-D	–	10.5	280	1332	pH 7
	–	4.10	305	1332	
Liquorice SL-F	–	11.0	305	1332	
Pyrethrum					
Whole dialysate	–	76.8	280	1332	
	–	69.8	305	1332	
Kapok KP-E	–	76.2	280	1332	pH 7
	–	64.4	305	1332	
Cotton CL-E	–	20.6	280	1332	
	–	13.0	305	1332	
Cotton seed CS 60C	–	6.58	255	1162	–
	–	6.85	280	1162	–
	–	4.89	310	1162	–
Castor bean					
[CB-1A] SRI	–	3.38	280	1332	pH 7
Human dandruff HD-E	–	5.21	305	1332	

^{m} DR, protein concentration determined by differential refractometry.
^{n} FD, protein concentration determined by fringe displacement method.

MOLAR ABSORPTIVITY AND $A_{1cm}^{1\%}$ VALUES FOR PROTEINS AT SELECTED WAVELENGTHS OF THE ULTRAVIOLET AND VISIBLE REGION (Continued)

Protein	ϵ^a $(\times\,10^{-4})$	$A_{1cm}^{1\%\,b}$	nm^c	Reference	Comments^d
	–	9.32	255	1162	–
	–	10.02	280	1162	–
	–	4.36	310	1162	–
Horse dandruff	–	8.28	255	1162	–
	–	9.62	280	1162	–
	–	3.44	310	1162	–
Whole dialysate	–	6.40	280	1332	
	–	1.20	305	1332	
Feathers FE-B	–	58.0	280	1332	
	–	43.3	305	1332	
Caddis fly					pH 7
Pool 2	–	35.2	280	1332	
	–	15.5	305	1332	
Alternaria	–	8.00	280	1332	
	–	4.14	305	1332	
Trichophytin	–	5.10	305	1332	
	–	7.96	255	1162	–
	–	7.94	280	1162	–
	–	4.80	310	1162	–
House dust HE-E	–	8.1	305	1332	pH 7
	–	13.80	255	1162	–
	–	13.64	280	1162	–
	–	8.36	310	1162	–
Tomato TO-G	–	21.0	280	1332	pH 7
	–	12.5	305	1332	
	–	14.56	255	1162	–
	–	13.80	280	1162	–
	–	9.40	310	1162	–
Cow's milk VM-5	–	9.20	280	1332	pH 7, MW = 36,000 [1332]
	–	1.95	305	1332	
Egg white VE,	–	4.44	280	1332	pH 7, MW = 31,500 [1332]
	–	0.40	305	1332	
Hay HH-C	–	84.2	280	1332	pH 7
		67.0	305	1332	
Succus liquiritiae	–	15.80	255	1162	–
	–	14.02	280	1162	–
	–	10.58	310	1162	–
Radix ipecacuanhae	–	9.66	255	1162	–
	–	11.02	280	1162	–
	–	3.84	310	1162	–
Alliin lyase (EC 4.4.1.4), garlic					
Allium sativum	–	16.6	280	1172	Calcd. from the data in Figure 4 [1172], pH 7.5, 10% glycerol-0.02 M P_i
Amandin					
Almonds	–	7	280	1173	Calcd. from Figure 1 [1173], pH 5.7
Amidophosphoribosyltransferase (EC 2.4.2.14) (see glutamine phosphoribosylpyrophosphate-amidotransferase and phosphoribosyldiphosphate amido-transferase)					
Amine dehydrogenase (amine oxidase)					
Pseudomonas AM 1	11.3	8.46	280	1174	pH 7.5, 0.05 $M\,P_i$, Lowry, MW = 133,000 [1174]
Amine oxidase (EC 1.4.3.4)					
Aspergillus niger	–	11.8	280	1179	–
Beef plasma	–	9.8	280	1180	–
Amine oxidase (EC 1.4.3.6) (see diamine oxidase and monoamine oxidase)					
D-Amino acid oxidase (EC 1.4.3.3)					
Pig kidney	–	15.6	277	1175	–
	–	126	220	1175	–
	7.31	16.0	280	36	MW = 182,000 [36]
Batch I enzyme	–	23.0	274	37	–

MOLAR ABSORPTIVITY AND $A_{1cm}^{1\%}$ VALUES FOR PROTEINS AT SELECTED WAVELENGTHS OF THE ULTRAVIOLET AND VISIBLE REGION (Continued)

Protein	ϵ^a ($\times 10^{-4}$)	$A_{1cm}^{1\% \, b}$	nm^c	Reference	Comments^d
Apo-	–	15.4	278	37	pH 8.5. 0.1 M PP$_i$
Batch II enzyme	–	19.8	274	37	pH 8.5, 0.1 M PP$_i$
Apo-	15.1	15.1	280	38	pH 8.3, M/60 PP$_i$, MW = 100,000 [39]
Apo-	17.5	14.0	280	40	pH 8.3, 0.1 M PP$_i$, MW = 125,000 [40]
Apo-	–	14	280	1176	pH 8.3, 0.1 M PP$_i$
L-Amino acid oxidase (EC 1.4.3.2)					
Crotalus adamanteus	23.6	17.9	275	41	0.1 M KCl, MW = 132,000 [41]
	2.35	1.78	390	41	0.1 M KCl, MW = 132,000 [41]
	2.26	1.71	462	41	0.1 M KCl, MW = 132,000 [41]
Rat kidney	8.5	9.55	275	42	MW = 89,000 [42]
	1.07	1.20	358	42	MW = 89,000 [42]
	1.27	1.43	455	42	MW = 89,000 [42]
Amino-acid racemase (EC 5.1.1.10)					
Pseudomonas striata	–	8.3	280	1177	Data from Figure 3 [1177], pH 7.0, 0.01 M KP$_i$
Aminoacyl-tRNA: ribosome-binding enzyme					
Rabbit reticulocytes	17.9	9.6	280	1178	Calc. from the data in Figure 3 [1178], pH 7.5, 0.01 M KP$_i$, MW = 186,000 [1178]
Aminopeptidase (EC 3.4.11.1-.2) (see also leucine aminopeptidase)					
Pig kidney	–	16.3	280	43	pH 7.2, 0.06 M P$_i$
	–	12.28	266	43	pH 7.2, 0.06 M P$_i$
	–	125	225	43	pH 7.2, 0.06 M P$_i$
	–	168	215	43	pH 7.2, 0.06 M P$_i$
Pig kidney, particulate (EC 3.4.11.2)	–	16	280	1182	Estd. from figure in Ref. [1182]
	47.3	16.9	280	1183	MW = 280,000 [1183], Refr. and Lowry
Rat kidney	–	16.1	280	44	–
Aeromonas proteolytica	4.18	14.4	278.5	1181	MW = 29,000 [1181]
B. stearothermophilus	41	10.2	280	1184	pH 7.2, 0.05 M Tris Cl, 0.001 M Co$^+$, MW = 400,000 [1184]
Aminopeptidase (microsomal) (EC 3.4.11.2)					
Pig kidney	45.5	16.2	280	1186	MW = 280,000 [1186]
Aminopeptidase P (aminoacyl-proline aminopeptidase, EC 3.4.11.9)					
Escherichia coli B.	–	10.3	280	1187	Kjeldahl
Aminotransferase alanine^o (EC 2.6.1.2)					
Rat liver	–	6.85	278.7	1333	DR, pH 7.0, 50 mM KP$_i$ containing 0.5 mM S$_2$ threitol
Amylase (EC 3.2.1.1-.3)					
Human plasma	–	9	280	1188	Water, calcd. from the data in Figure 4 [1188]
Rat pancreas	–	20	280	1189	–
B. subtilis Takamine	–	25.2	280	1190	
B. subtilis Kalle	–	25.2	280	1190	
α-Amylase (EC 3.2.1.1)	–	24.4	290	1191	0.1 N NaOH
Human saliva	–	26	280	45	–
Pig pancreas	–	26	280	45	–
	12.8	25	280	46	Water, MW = 51,300 [47]
B. subtilis	–	25.3	280	45	–
A. oryzae	–	19.7	280	45	–
B. macerans	9.9	7.11	280	48	pH 6.2, 0.01 MP$_i$, MW = 139,000 [48]
Pirkka barley	8.55	15.0	280	1334	Dry wt., pH 7.0, 0.05 M NaP$_i$, MW = 57,200 [1334]
B. subtilis	9.35	19.8	280	1192	MW = 47,300 [1193]
	12.5	25.6	280	1195	MW = 49,000 [1195]
B. stearothermophilus	13.8	28.7	280	1194	MW = 48,000 [1194]
Rat pancreas	–	16.4	–^{p}	1196	
Pig pancreas	12.0	24	280	1197	MW = 50,000 [1197], pH 7.4, Tris
B. subtilis	8.3	19.8	280	1198	MW = 41,900 [1198]
B. subtilis var. saccharitikus Fukumoto	8.2	20.0	280	1199	MW = 41,000 [1199], pH 6.8, 0.01 M AcO$^-$
	7.9	19.3	280	1199	0.1 N NaOH
β-Amylase (EC 3.2.1.2),					
sweet potato	–	17.7	280	1201	–

^{o} Pyridoxal or pyridoxamine form.
^{p} Wavelength not cited.

MOLAR ABSORPTIVITY AND $A_{1cm}^{1\%}$ VALUES FOR PROTEINS AT SELECTED WAVELENGTHS OF THE ULTRAVIOLET AND VISIBLE REGION (Continued)

Protein	ϵ^a ($\times 10^{-4}$)	$A_{1cm}^{1\%\,b}$	nm^c	Reference	Comments^d
	26	17.1	280	49	pH 4.8, 0.016 M AcO$^-$
Iodosobenzoate oxidized		17.05	–	1202	
α-Amylase inhibitor, wheat					
I	2.7	15.0	280	1200	MW = 18,215 [1200]
II	2.6	10.0	280	1200	MW = 26,200 [1200]
Anaphylatoxin					
Rat serum		4.1	280	1335	pH 7.2
Anthranilate synthase (EC 4.1.3.27)					
Salmonella typhimurium					
Component I	3.3	5.2	278	1202	pH 7.4, 0.05 M Tris Cl, MW = 64,000 [1202]
Escherichia coli	2.18	3.64	280	1204	pH 7.0, 0.05 M KP$_i$, MW = 60,000 [1204], calcd. from the data in Figure 5 [1204]
	2.94	4.91	295	1204	0.1 N NaOH, MW = 60,000 [1204], calcd. from the data in Figure 5 [1204]
Anthranilate synthase: anthranilate phosphoribosyl-transferase complex (EC 4.1.3.27: 2.4.2.18)					
Salmonella typhimurium	16.1	5.75	280	1205	pH 7.4, 0.05 M KP$_i$, MW = 280,000 [1205]
Antibody					
Rabbit					
Anti-N$_2$ ph^q	–	15.7	279	1206	–
Anguilla rostrata (Eel)					
Anti-human blood group H[O]	–	12.696	278	1207	Water
Antigen					
Human					
Hepatitis associated (Australia)	–	9.42	260	1208	–
Blood group N active Erythrocyte, NN	65	10.90	274	1209	MW = 595,000 [1209]
Meconium	23.2	4.49	274	1209	MW = 520,000 [1209]
Paramecium aurelia					
Immobilization	–	11.9	277	1210	From Figure 1 [1210]
Apocytochrome c					
Horse heart	–	9.2	277	1336	–
Apolipoprotein Glu-II					
Human plasma	1.91	10.97	276	1337	pH 8.0, 0.01% EDTA, MW = 17,380 [1337]
	1.80	10.35	280	1337	
α-L-Arabinofuranosidase (EC 3.2.1.55)					pH 7.0, 0.02 M NaP$_i$, MW = 53,000 [1211], data from Figure 8 [1211]
Aspergillus niger	12.7	23.1	280	1211	
Arachin	–	7.98	278	50	8 M urea, 0.1 M sulfite
	–	7.85	278	50	6 M GdmCl, 0.1 M sulfite
Arachis hypogaea (Peanut)	–	8.8	281.5	1338	pH 10.5, 0.1 M P$_i$
Arginase (EC 3.5.3.1)					
Rat liver	–	10.9	280	51	
Beef liver	–	9.6	278	1212	Dry wt.
Pig liver	–	13.0	280	1213	
Chicken liver	–	260	210	1339	pH 7.5, 0.05 M Tris Cl
	–	22	340	1339	
Arginine decarboxylase (EC 4.1.1.19)					
Escherichia coli	133	15.7	280	1214	MW = 850,000 dry wt. and Refr.
Arginine kinase (EC 2.7.3.3)					
Sipunculus nudus (Marine worm)	8.4	9.8	280	1215	MW = 86,000 [1215]
Cancer pagurus (Crab)	2.9	7.35	278	1216	MW = 39,500 [1216]
Homarus vulgaris (Lobster)	2.9	7.35	278	1216	MW = 39,500 [1216]
	–	7.8	275	1217	
	–	8.1	280	1218	pH 8.0, 0.01 M P$_i$
	–	6.1	271	1219	Alkaline sol.
Arginine racemase (EC 5.1.1.9)					
Pseudomonas graveolens	15.5	9.3	280	1220	Dry wt., MW = 167,000 [1220]

^{q} N$_2$ ph = 2,4-dinitrophenyl-.

MOLAR ABSORPTIVITY AND $A_{1cm}^{1\%}$ VALUES FOR PROTEINS AT SELECTED WAVELENGTHS OF THE ULTRAVIOLET AND VISIBLE REGION (Continued)

Protein	ϵ^a ($\times$ 10^{-4})	$A_{1cm}^{1\% \, b}$	nm[c]	Reference	Comments[d]
Argininosuccinase (EC 4.3.2.1)					
Beef liver	25.8	13.0[r]	280	1221	
	–	7.1[r]	260	1221	pH 7.5, 0.05 M KP$_i$, MW = 202,000 [1221]
Beef kidney	25.0	12.5[r]	280	1221	
	–	6.8[r]	260	1221	
Aromatic α-ketoacid reductase (diiodophenyl pyruvate reductase, EC 1.1.1.96)					
Rat kidney	–	10	280	1222	pH 6.5, 0.005 M NaP$_i$
Ascorbate oxidase (EC 1.10.3.3)					
Cucumis sativus	1480[s]	1120[s]	280	1340	
	61.6[s]	46.8[s]	607	1340	pH 7.0, 0.1 M P$_i$, MW = 132,000 [1340]
Cucumber	0.53	–	330	1223	–
	0.97	–	607	1223	–
	0.36	–	760	1223	–
Corcubita pepo condensa (Yellow crookneck squash)	28.5	–	280	1224	Dry wt.
Corcubita pepo medullosa (Green zucchini)	28.5	–	280	1224	Dry wt.
Asparaginase (EC 3.5.1.1)					
Proteus vulgaris	–	6.6	280	1225	Dry wt., pH 7.0, 0.05 M NaP$_i$
Escherichia coli	9.9	7.46	280	1226	MW = 133,000 [1226]
	–	7.2	278	1342	pH 7
	–	9.9	292	1342	pH 13
E. coli HAP	8.83	6.26	278	1227	MW = 141,000 [1227]
E. coli B	9.2	7.1	278	649	MW = 130,000 [649]
					pH 7.3, P$_i$
	–	7.1	278	650	pH 5, 0.05 M AcONa
	–	7.1	278	650	pH 8.5, 0.05 M Tris
	–	6.5	276	650	7 M urea
	–	6.5	276	650	5 M guanidine
Succinylated monomer	–	6.7	276	1228	–
Erwinia carotovora	8.2	6.1	280	1341	pH 7.4
Asparaginase A	–	7.5	278	652	pH 7, P$_i$, calcd. from opt. factor of 1.325
	–	9.5	290.5	652	0.1 N NaOH, calcd. from opt. factor of 1.059
Escherichia coli ATCC 9637	–	7.9	277	651	pH 7, M/15 P$_i$, data from Figure 2 [651]
Deaminated	–	7.9	277	651	pH 7, M/15 P$_i$, data from Figure 2 [651]
Aspartate aminotransferase (EC 2.6.1.1)					
Pig heart muscle	11.1	14.1	280	1230	MW = 78,600 [1230]
Apo-	10.6	13.5	280	1231	pH 7.4, 0.1 M P$_i$
					MW = 78,600 [1230]
Pig heart	13.5	15	280	1232	
Apo-	12.8	14.2	280	1232	MW = 90,000 [1232]
Pig heart	–	12.6	280	1233	pH 5.3, 0.1 M AcO$^-$, data from Figure 1 [1233]
a form	–	14.8	278	1234	–
Chicken heart	–	14.0	280	1235	pH 7.4, 0.1 M Tris Cl, pH 7.5, 0.05 M KP$_i$
Soluble mixture	–	14.2	280	1235	–
		15	280	53	pH 7.5
α soluble	–	13.7	280	1235	–
β soluble	–	14.5	280	1235	–
γ soluble	–	14.0	280	1235	–
Mitochondrial	–	13.2	280	1235	–
Apo-	–	14.5	280	53	pH 7.5
Rat brain					
Cytoplasmic	10.8	13.5	280	1236	
Mitochondrial	8.65	10.8	280	1236	pH 7.5, MW = 80,000 [1236]
Ox heart	–	14.40	278	1237	–
Apo-	–	14.14	278	1238	–
Beef kidney	12.5	13.4	280	1343	pH 8, 10 mM P$_i$

[r] Amino acid analysis used for determining protein concentration.
[s] Values calculated from data and are for 8 Cu atoms per molecule.

MOLAR ABSORPTIVITY AND $A_{1cm}^{1\%}$ VALUES FOR PROTEINS AT SELECTED WAVELENGTHS OF THE ULTRAVIOLET AND VISIBLE REGION (Continued)

Protein	ϵ^a ($\times 10^{-4}$)	$A_{1cm}^{1\%\,b}$	nm[c]	Reference	Comments[d]
L-Aspartate (β-decarboxylase (EC 4.1.1.12)					
A. faecalis	88	11	278	52	pH 6.8, 0.1 M P$_i$, MW = 800,000 [52]
Pseudomonas dacunhae	–	10.0	280	1229	pH 6.8, 0.1 M KP$_i$
D-Aspartate oxidase (EC 1.4.3.1)					
Octopus vulgaris	–	18.25	275	1344	Dry wt.
Aspartate kinase (see aspartokinase)					
Aspartate transcarbamoylase (EC 2.1.3.2)					
Escherichia coli	18.2	5.9	280	54	MW = 310,000 [54]
	18.2	5.9	279	55	MW = 310,000 [54]
	18.4	5.9	284	56	MW = 310,000 [54]
Mercury derivative	–	7.6	280	1239	–
Regulatory subunit	–	8.0	280	1240	–
	–	7.2	280	1239	–
	–	12	284	57	In presence of HSEtOH, MW = 30,000 [56]
Mercury derivative	–	8.3	280	1239	–
Zinc derivative	–	3.2	280	1239	–
Apo-	–	3.2	280	1239	–
Catalytic subunit	–	7.0	280	1240	–
	7.2	7.2	284	56	MW = 100,000 [56]
Permanganate modified	–	7.0	280	1241	–
5-Thio-2-nitrobenzoate derivative	–	9.2	280	1242	–
Aspartokinase (EC 2.7.2.4)					
Bacillus polymyxa	7.74	6.7	280	1243	pH 6.5, 6 M GdmCl/0.02 M KP$_i$, MW = 116,000 [1243]
Escherichia coli					
Lysine sensitive	4.7	3.6	276	1244	MW = 130,000 [1244]
Aspartokinase I: homoserine dehydrogenase I (EC 2.7.2.4:1.1.1.3)					AA, pH 7.2, 20 mM KP$_i$ containing 0.15 M KC1, 2 mM Mg titriplex, 1 mM L-threonine, and 1 mM S$_2$ threitol, MW = 86,000 [1345]
Escherichia coli	5.4	6.3	278	1345	
Threonine-sensitive	–	4.6	280	1245	–
	–	4.7	280	1246	6 M GdmCl
Aspartokinase II: homoserine dehydrogenase II (EC 2.7.2.4:1.1.1.3)					–
Escherichia coli K12	–	8.7	280	1247	–
Aspergillopeptidase A (EC 3.4.23.6)					
A. saitoi	4.5	13.15	280	58	MW = 34,500 [58]
Aspergillopeptidase B (EC 3.4.21.15)					
A. oryzae	1.73	9.08	278	59	pH 5, 0.1 M AcO$^-$, MW = 18,000 [59]
	1.62	9.00	280	59	pH 5, 0.1 M AcO$^-$, MW = 18,000 [59]
ATP: AMP phosphotransferase (EC 2.7.4.3)					
Human	1.43	6.67	279	1346	Dry wt., MW = 22,000 [1346]
ATP citrate-lyase (EC 4.1.3.8)					
Rat liver	–	11.8	280	1248	Calcd. from the data in Figure 5 [1248]
ATP phosphoribosyltransferase (see phosphoribosyltransferase and phosphoribosy-ATP)	–	7.1	280	1248	Calcd. from the data in Figure 5 [1248], corrected for light scattering
ATP-sulfurylase (sulfate adenylyltransferase) (EC 2.7.7.4)					
Penicillium chrysogenum	–	8.71	278	1347	Kjeldahl[e]
Avidin					
Egg white	8.3	15.7	280	1249	MW = 53,000 [1249]
		53	233	1250	–
Avimanganin					
Chicken liver					
Mitochondria	0.0508	0.057	480	1251	MW = 89,000 [1251]
	0.0250	0.028	600	1251	
Azobacter flavoprotein					
Azobacter vinelandii,	1.06	–	452	60	pH 7.0, 25 mM KP$_i$
Oxidized	–	16.5	274	60	pH 7.0, 25 mM KP$_i$
Azurin					
Pseudomonas fluorescens	0.0285	–	459	1252	–
	0.350	–	625	1252	–
	0.032	–	781	1252	–

MOLAR ABSORPTIVITY AND $A_{1cm}^{1\%}$ VALUES FOR PROTEINS AT SELECTED WAVELENGTHS OF THE ULTRAVIOLET AND VISIBLE REGION (Continued)

Protein	ϵ^a ($\times 10^{-4}$)	$A_{1cm}^{1\% \, b}$	nm[c]	Reference	Comments[d]
Pseudomonas aeruginosa	0.027	–	467	1252	–
	0.350	–	625	1252	–
	0.039	–	820	1252	–
Bacteriochlorophyll–protein complex					
Chloropseudomonas ethylicum	–	90	371	61	MW = 37,940/subunit [61]
Bacteriocin DF 13					
Enterobacter cloacae DF 13	5.5	9.87	280	931	pH 7.0, 0.06 $M\,P_i$, MW = 56,000 [931]
Biotin carboxylase (EC 6.3.4.14)					
Escherichia coli	–	6.25	280	932	⌐
	–	6.25[u]	280	785	
Brain					pH 6.8, 0.05 $N\,P_i$, estd. from Figure 7 [439], no value
Pig, basic	–	4	280	439	cited for wavelength
Bromelain (EC 3.4.22.4-.5)	6.33	19.0	280	62	MW = 33,315 [62]
	6.68	20.1	280	63	MW = 33,000 [64]
C1 inactivator					
Human plasma	–	4.5	280	1253	–
C1q component of complement					
Human serum	26.4	6.8	278	1254	1% NaDodSO$_4$, MW = 388,000 [1254]
C2 component of complement					
Guinea pig	–	13.9	280	786	–
Caerulein					
Hyla caerulae	0.725	–	280	787	80% ethanol
Calcitonin					
Salmon	0.15	4.5	280	788	–
Calcium-binding phosphoprotein					
Pig brain	0.36	3.1	Not cited	1348	Kjeldahl[e], MW = 11,500 [1348]
Chicken intestinal mucosa	–	21.9	280	451	pH 8.1, 0.2% Tris Cl, 0.77% glycine, 0.1 mM glutathione, estd. from Figure 8 [451]
Carbamate kinase (EC 2.7.2.2)					
S. faecalis	1.798	5.8	280	789	pH 7.5, 50 mM NaP$_i$, MW = 31,000 [789]
Carbamoylphosphate synthase (EC 2.7.2.5-.9)					
Rat liver	–	8.4	280	1349	DR
Carbonic anhydrase (carbonate dehydratase, EC 4.2.1.1)					
Beef					
B	5.7	19.0	280	1255	MW = 30,000 [1255]
	5.6	18.0	280	66	MW = 31,000 [66]
Beef erythrocyte					
B	5.2	16.8	280	656	MW = 31,000 [656], pH 7.4
Ox, rumen					
Isozyme a	–	17	280	1256	–
Isozyme b	–	17	280	1256	–
Gallus domesticus (Chicken)	5.6	20	280	1257	MW = 28,000 [1258]
Carcharhinus leucas (Bull shark)	7.5	20.9	280	1259	MW = 36,000 [1259]
Galeocerdo cuvieri (Tiger shark)	6.3	16.0	280	1259	MW = 39,500 [1259]
Guinea pig Blood/mucosa					
GI tract High activity	–	17.1	280	1260	Dry wt.
	–	16.9[r]	280	1260	–
	–	16.7[v]	280	1260	–
	–	17.0	280	1260	Value used
Low activity	–	16.4	280	1260	Dry wt.
	–	16.5[r]	280	1260	–
	–	16.1[v]	280	1260	–
	–	16.5	280	1260	Value used
Human erythrocytes					

[t] OD$_{230}$ = (mg protein/ml)/1.6 OD$_{280}$.
[u] Calculated from equation: mg protein/ml = 1.6 × OD$_{280}$ Ref. [785].
[v] Calculated according to Wetlaufer [1838].

MOLAR ABSORPTIVITY AND $A_{1cm}^{1\%}$ VALUES FOR PROTEINS AT SELECTED WAVELENGTHS OF THE ULTRAVIOLET AND VISIBLE REGION (Continued)

Protein	ϵ^a ($\times 10^{-4}$)	$A_{1cm}^{1\% \, b}$	nm[c]	Reference	Comments[d]
A	4.67	16.3	280	653	MW = 28,600 [653]
A, generated from B in vitro	4.29	16.0	280	653	MW = 26,800 [653]
B	4.56	16.3	280	653	MW = 28,000 [653]
	4.9	16.3	280	65	pH 7.0, 0.1 ionic strength Na P_i, MW = 30,000 [65]
	4.89	16.3[w]	280	1262	MW = 30,000 [1262]
	2.05	–	250	1262	
B	5.74	–	240	1262	
	12.8	–	235	1262	
	24.5	–	230	1262	MW = 30,000 [1262]
	36.0	–	225	1262	
	45.5	–	220	1262	
	54.5	–	215	1262	
B, nitrated	–	17.5	280	654	pH 9
C	5.34	17.8	280	65	pH 7.0, 0.1 ionic strength Na P_i, MW = 30,000 [68]
	5.05	18.7	280	653	MW = 27,000 [653]
	–	17.8	280	655	–
	5.34	17.8[x]	280	1262	
	2.01	–	250	1262	
	5.47	–	240	1262	
	12.9	–	235	1262	
	25.0	–	230	1262	MW = 30,000 [1262]
	37.0	–	225	1262	
	48.0	–	220	1262	
	60.0	–	215	1262	
D	4.52	16.0	280	653	MW = 28,200 [653]
D, generated from B in vitro	4.14	16.1	280	653	MW = 25,700 [653]
G	4.9	18.5	280	653	MW = 26,500 [653]
H	5.14	18.5	280	653	MW = 27,800 [653]
O	3.98	15.4	280	653	MW = 25,800 [653]
P	4.21	15.4	280	653	MW = 27,300 [653]
Pmut	4.47	16	280	1261	MW = 28,000 [1261]
Horse erythrocyte	4.38	15.9	280	653	MW = 27,500 [653]
B	3.95	13.6	280	657	MW = 29,007 [657]
C	3.73	13.4	280	657	MW = 27,918 [657]
Rat erythrocyte					
1a	5.22	18	280	658	MW = 29,000 [658]
2	5.22	18	280	658	MW = 29,000 [658]
3	4.93	17	280	658	MW = 29,000 [658]
Prostate					
Ib	5.22	18	280	658	MW = 29,000 [658]
Parsley (*Petroselinum crispum* var. *latifolium*)	3.18	11.3	280	659	MW = 28,150 [659]
Apocarbonic anhydrase	5.7	–	280	660	–
Precursor of above	5.7	–	280	660	–
Pig erythrocytes					
B	5.3	17.4	280	1263	MW = 30,375 [1263]
	5.6	18.5	280	1264	MW = 30,000 [1264]
C	4.6	15.2	280	1264	MW = 30,000 [1264]
Spinach	–	8.6	280	1265	pH 7.2, 0.03 M P_i
Monkey					
B	4.88	–	280	67	–
C, *M. mulata*	5.35	17.8	280	67	MW = 30,000 [67]
Neisseria sicca	3.575	12.5	280	1350	Kjeldahl,[e] MW = 28,600 [1350]
Carboxylesterase (EC 3.1.1.1)					
Ox liver	20.1	13.40	280	1266	pH 7.92, 0.15 M Tris, MW = 150,000 [1267]
Pig kidney					
Microsomes	15.3	9.4	280	1268	MW = 163,000 [1268]
Liver	20.27	13.05	280	69	pH 8.16, 0.15 M Tris, MW = 172,000 [69]

[w] The value of $A_{1cm}^{1\%}$ of 16.3 and $\epsilon = 4.89 \times 10^4$ taken from Rickli et al.[64], and a MW of 30,000 assumed [1262].
[x] The value of A of 17.8 and an e of 5.34×10^4 taken from Nyman and Lindskog [1839].

MOLAR ABSORPTIVITY AND $A_{1cm}^{1\%}$ VALUES FOR PROTEINS AT SELECTED WAVELENGTHS OF THE ULTRAVIOLET AND VISIBLE REGION (Continued)

Protein	ϵ^a ($\times 10^{-4}$)	$A_{1cm}^{1\%\,b}$	nm[c]	Reference	Comments[d]
S-Carboxymethylalbumin, beef (see albumin, beef)					
Carboxypeptidase (EC 3.4.12.1-.3)					
Beef pancreas	–	19.4	278	70	10% LiCl
	6.32	18.1	278	71	–
	6.42	–	278	72	–
	6.45	–	278	73	–
	6.49	–	278	74	–
	6.67	–	278	75	–
	–	23	280	76	–
	7.9	–	280	77	–
	8.6	25	278	78	MW = 34,300 [78]
Carboxypeptidase A					
Ox					
Squalis acanthias	6.48	18.5	280	790	MW = 35,000 [790]
Co II	–	0.0205	530	1351	–
	–	0.0195	572	1351	–
Co III	–	0.0500	503	1351	–
A_1, Pig	6.72	19.6	278	79	MW = 34,800 [79]
A_2, Pig	6.72	19.6	278	79	–
A_α, Beef	6.49	18.8	278	80	pH 7.0, 0.5 M NaCl, 0.01 M Tris, MW = 34,600 [80]
A, Acetyl-, beef	6.17	–	280	72	In the absence of β-phenylpropionate
	6.01	–	278	73	In the absence of β-phenylpropionate
	5.9	–	280	72	In the presence of β-phenylpropionate
	5.78	–	278	73	In the presence of β-phenylpropionate
A, Arsonilazo-, beef	7.32	–	278	1353	–
A, Succinyl-, beef	–	18.3	280	81	–
	6.47	–	278	71	–
Carboxypeptidase B					
Pig	7.34	21.4	278	82	pH 8.0, 0.005 M Tris
Beef	7.35	21	280	83	MW = 34,600 [83]
Barley	–	16.5	280	791	Water
P. omnivorum	5.53	17.6	278	792	pH 6.5, MW = 31,400 [792]
Gossypium hirsutum	17.3	20.5	280	1352	MW = 84,500 [1352]
Carnitine acetyltransferase (EC 2.3.1.7)					
Pigeon breast muscle	4.8	8.25	280	1269	–
Carotenoid–protein complex					
Pecten maximus Ovary	–	9.7	280	1270	pH 7, 0.2 M P$_i$
Plesionika edwardsi	–	13	280	1270	pH 7, 0.2 M P$_i$, data from Figure 3 [1270]
Carotenoproteins[y]					
Aristeus antennatus					
Carapace					
α (+ salt)	12.3	–	593	1271	–
Stomach					
α (+ salt)	12.4	–	588	1271	–
Scyllarus arctus					
Carapace					
α (+ salt)	12.0	–	616	1271	–
Clibanarius erythropus					
Exoskeleton					
α (+ salt)	12.6	–	620	1271	–
Labidocera acutifrons	–	152	640	1354	pH 7, 0.02 M P$_i$
Casein	–	10.0	280	84	–
French Friesian cows	–	6.7	278	1272	–
Bovine					
βA	–	4.6	280	1273	–
βB	–	4.7	280	1273	–

---

[y] All species are decapods.

MOLAR ABSORPTIVITY AND $A_{1cm}^{1\%}$ VALUES FOR PROTEINS AT SELECTED WAVELENGTHS OF THE ULTRAVIOLET AND VISIBLE REGION (Continued)

Protein	ϵ^a ($\times 10^{-4}$)	$A_{1cm}^{1\%\,b}$	nm^c	Reference	Comments^d
βC	–	4.6	280	1273	–
30% acid prep.	–	8.4	278	85	–
2% acid prep.	–	8.6	278	85	–
3% Am. sulfate prep.	–	8.7	278	85	–
20% Am. sulfate prep.	–	8.7	278	85	–
Calcium gel prep.	–	8.1	278	85	–
α_s	2.73	10.1	280	86	MW = 27,000 [85]
α_{si}	2.73	10.1	280	87	MW = 27,000 [85]
β	1.15	4.6	280	88	MW = 25,000 [85]
k	2.44	12.2	280	89	MW = 29,000 [85]
Catalase (EC 1.11.16)					
Human erythrocyte	28	12.5	280	90	MW = 225,000 [90], $A_{1cm}^{1\%}$ = 16.9–18.7 at 405 nm [90]
	–	14.4	280	91	–
	–	17.8	405	91	–
	30.8	13.2	280	1355	MW = 232,400 [1355]
	39.7	17.1	405	1355	
Beef erythrocyte	43.1	16.8	405	661	MW = 257,000 [661]
Liver	82.2	36.5	276	662	MW = 225,000 [662], pH 7.3, 0.05 M P$_i$
	63.6	28.2	404	662	MW = 225,000 [662], pH 7.3, 0.05 M P$_i$
	31	–	405	92	pH 7.4
	38	–	280	92	pH 7.4
	32.4	13.5	405	93	MW = 240,000 [93]
	31.4	12.9	276	1274	MW = 240,000 [1274]
	16.6	6.9	405	1274	
Horse liver	67.5	27	275	663	pH 8, 0.004 M P$_i$, data from Figure 1 [663]
	8.3	–	623	664	
	9.4	–	536	664	–
	78.5	–	400	664	–
	85.0	–	280	664	–
	65	–	280	665	pH 7.15, P$_i$, MW = 225,000, data from Figure 4 [665]
Horse blood	65	–	280		pH 7.15, P$_i$, MW = 225,000, data from Figure 4 [665]
Rat liver	–	15.8	276	1356	From Figure 1 [1356]
	–	16	407	666	–
	39.7	15.5	276	667	MW = 256,000 [667]
	43.0	16.8	407	667	MW = 256,000 [667]
Spinach	–	1.97	502	668	pH 7.4, 0.1 M Tricene-NaOH
	–	1.38	620	668	
	–	14.8	278	94	pH 7.4, 0.1 M Tricene-NaOH
	–	14.9	404	94	pH 7.4, 0.1 M Tricene-NaOH
Commercial					
Crystalline	41	16.4	276	669	
	30	12.0	406	669	
Lyophilized-A	32	12.8	276	669	MW = 250,000 [669]
	20	8.0	406	669	
Lyophilized-B	34	13.6	276	669	
	7.3	2.9	406	669	
Cathepsin B (EC 3.4.22.1)					
Beef spleen	–	–^{z}	280	1357	pH 7.6, 50 mM P$_i$
Cellulase (EC 3.2.1.4)					
Trichoderma koningi					
I	5.73	22	280	95	MW = 26,000 [95]
II	12.5	25	280	95	MW = 50,000 [95]
Stereum sanguinolentum					
P 1 Fraction	8	38	280	670	pH 5.4, 0.1 M, AmAc, MW = 21,000 [670]
Penicillium notatum	–	26	280	671	–
	9.1	–	280	672	pH 5, 0.05 M AcO$^-$, MW = 35,500 [672]

^{z} Refs. [14,15].

MOLAR ABSORPTIVITY AND $A_{1cm}^{1\%}$ VALUES FOR PROTEINS AT SELECTED WAVELENGTHS OF THE ULTRAVIOLET AND VISIBLE REGION (Continued)

Protein	ϵ^a ($\times 10^{-4}$)	$A_{1cm}^{1\% \, b}$	nm^c	Reference	Comments^d
Cerebrocuprein					
Human brain	–	7.35	265	1275	–
	–	0.075	675	1275	–
Beef brain	–	0.18	660	1276	–
Ceruloplasmin					
Human	–	0.684	610	1277	–
	1.13	–	610	1278	–
	–	15.03	280	1277	–
	0.40	–	332	1278	–
	0.12	–	459	1278	–
	0.22	–	794	1278	–
	–	16.3	280	8	–
	23.7	14.9	280	97	MW = 159,000 [97]
	8.15	–	280	98	–
	10	–	605	98	–
	–	14.6	280	99	MW = 160,000 [99]
	–	14.4	279	100	–
	–	0.68	610	100	–
Form I	–	15.5	280	1279	–
IIa/IIb	–	16.2	280	1279	–
IIIb	–	16.0	280	1279	–
Asialoceruloplasmin	–	15.0	280	1277	–
	–	0.64	610	1277	–
Pig	1.01	0.63	610	1280	MW = 160,000 [1281]
2 days old	–	0.52	610	1282	–
	–	11.5	280	1282	–
10 weeks old	–	0.61	610	1282	–
	–	12.8	280	1282	–
Rat, copper deficient	–	0.64	610	1283	–
Rabbit	–	13.1	280	101	–
	–	0.618	610	101	–
Chitinase (EC 3.2.1.14)					
Streptomyces	–	15.0	280	1358	–
Chloride peroxidase (EC 1.11.1.10)					
Caldariomyces fumago	7.53	–	403	102	–
	1.15	–	515	102	–
	1.08	–	542	102	–
	0.42	–	650	102	–
Choleragen					
(Cholera enterotoxin)	9.6	11.41	280	1284	pH 7.5, 0.2 M Tris, MW = 84,000 [1284]
	8.75	10.39	280	1284	pH 8.0, 5 M GdmCl, MW = 84,000 [1284], dry wt.
Choleragenoid					
(Toxoid)	1.43	9.56	280	1284	pH 7.5, 0.2 M Tris, MW = 15,000 [1284], dry wt.
	1.36	9.09	280	1284	pH 8.0, 5 M GdmCl, MW = 15,000 [1284], dry wt.
Cholinesterase (EC 3.1.1.8)					
Amiarus nebulosus (a fish)	–	3.5	275	1285	pH 7, 0.02 M KP,/0.13 M KCl, data from Figure 4 [1285]
Chorionic gonadotropin, human	1.4	5.2	280	1286	MW = 27,000 [1286]
	–	3.88	278	1287	–
Chorismate mutase (EC 5.4.99.5): Prephenate dehydrogenase (EC 1.3.1.12)					
E. coli	7.8	9.5	280	1288	MW = 82,000 [1289]
Aerobacter aerogenes	7.2^{aa}	9.5^{aa}	278	1290	pH 8.0, 0.1 M Tris Cl, MW = 76,000 [1290]
Chymopapain (EC 3.4.22.6)					
I	6.16	18.40	280	104	pH 5.0, AcO$^-$, MW = 33,500 [104]
II	6.18	18.45	280	104	pH 5.0, AcO$^-$, MW = 33,500 [104]
III	6.23	18.60	280	104	pH 5.0, AcO$^-$, MW = 33,500 [104]
IV	6.16	18.40	280	104	pH 5.0, AcO$^-$, MW = 33,500 [104]
B	–	19.6	280	103	pH 7.2, 0.1 M cacodylate, estd. from Figure 3 [103]

^{aa} The same values used at 280 nm in Ref. [1291].

MOLAR ABSORPTIVITY AND $A_{1cm}^{1\%}$ VALUES FOR PROTEINS AT SELECTED WAVELENGTHS OF THE ULTRAVIOLET AND VISIBLE REGION (Continued)

Protein	ϵ^a ($\times 10^{-4}$)	$A_{1cm}^{1\% \, b}$	nm^c	Reference	Comments^d
Chymosin (see rennin)					
Chymotrypsin (EC 3.4.21.1)					
Purified, commercial	5.205	–	281	1292	–
Commercial					
Diazoacetyl derivative	2.77	–	250	1293	–
Above photolytically modified	1.75	–	250	1293	–
Chymotrypsin II					
Human	4.75	19.0	280	1299	MW = 25,000 [1299]
Chymotrypsin A (EC 3.4.21.1)					
Beef pancreas	–	20.2	280	110	0.001 M HCl
Chymotrypsin C (EC 3.4.21.2)					
Pig pancreas	5.95	25	278	111	MW = 23,800 [111]
Chymotrypsin, iPr$_2$P-^{bb}					
Beef pancreas	5.0	–	280	112	–
α-Chymotrypsin					
Commercial	–	20.8	280	1294	–
	–	300	210	1294	–
	–	920	191	1294	–
	–	19.95	280	1295	pH 6.2, P$_i$
Polyvalyl-	–	18.51	280	1295	
Trans-cinnamoyl-	1.78	–	292	1296	–
Denatured derivative	1.78	–	281	1296	–
Furylacryloyl-	1.98	–	320	1296	–
Denatured derivative	2.00	–	310	1296	–
Indolacryloyl-	1.78	–	360	1296	–
Denatured derivative	1.90	–	335	1296	–
Beef	–	18.7	280	1297	–
Pancreas	–	21.5	280	1298	–
	4.46	20.75	282	105	MW = 21,500 [105]
	–	20.7	282	106	–
	5.0	20	280	107	MW = 25,000 [107]
	–	20.4	282	108	–
	–	18.9	280	109	–
Chymotrypsinogen					
Commercial	–	19.7	282	1300	Dry wt.
Carbon disulfide derivative	6.0	–	285	1301	Data from Figure 4 [301]
Alkaline denatured	3.66	–	292.8	1302	–
	4.56	–	285.5	1302	–
	23.07	–	230	1302	–
Acid denatured	3.66	–	293	1302	–
	4.56	–	285.5	1302	–
	4.75	–	276	1302	–
	23.06	–	230.5	1302	–
Rat pancreas	4.0	16	280	1303	MW = 25,000 [1303]
Chymotrypsinogen A					
Commercial	–	20.3	282	1304	pH 2.0
Beef	–	20.3	282	1305	pH 9.3, glycine buffer, 0.1 μM, dry wt.
	5.15	20	280	115	MW = 25,761 [115]
Pig	4.43	18	280	116	MW = 24,600 [116]
Spiny Pacific dogfish	–	21.4^r	280	1306	–
(Squalus acanthias)	–	21.7	280	1306	Refractometry
Chymotrypsinogen B					
Beef	–	18.7	280	117	0.001 M HCl
	–	18.4	280	115	–
Pig, pancreas	6.0	23.8	278	1307	MW = 26,000 [1307]
Chymotrypsinogen C					
Pig	7.6	23.8	278	118	MW = 31,800 [118]

---

^{bb} iPr$_2$P, -diisopropylphospho.

MOLAR ABSORPTIVITY AND $A_{1cm}^{1\%}$ VALUES FOR PROTEINS AT SELECTED WAVELENGTHS OF THE ULTRAVIOLET AND VISIBLE REGION (Continued)

Protein	ϵ^a ($\times 10^{-4}$)	$A_{1cm}^{1\% \, b}$	nm^c	Reference	Comments^d
Chymotrypsinogen, S-sulfo					
Beef pancreas	–	17.9	280	119	–
α-Chymotrypsinogen					
Beef pancreas	–	20.6	282	113	–
	5.02	20.0	282	114	MW = 25,100 [114]
Citramalate hydrolase (citramalate lyase) (EC 4.1.3.22)					
Clostridium tetanomorphum					
Component I	–	9.0	280	673	–
Component II	–	9.5	280	673	–
Citrate condensing enzyme [citrate (re)-synthase] (EC 4.1.3.28)					
Pig heart	13.15	15.5	280	120	MW = 85,000 [120]
Citrate synthase (EC 4.1.3.7)					
Pig heart	17.1	17.8	280	1308	MW = 96,000 [1308]
	15	15	280	674	MW = 100,000 [674]
Cobratoxin					
Naja naja atra	1.45	13.2	280	675	MW = 11,000 [675]
	–	12.1	280	676	Data from Figure 1 [676]
Cocoonase (EC 3.4.21.4), Silkmoth					
Antherea polyphemus	–	11	280	1309	1 N NaOH
	–	13	280	1310	0.1 N NaOH
Bombyx mori	–	9.8	280	1310	0.1 N NaOH
Cocosin					
Coconuts	–	7.0	280	677	–
	–	2.7	255	677	–
Cocytotaxin					
Rat serum	–	2.90	280	1363	pH 7.2, 0.05 M NaKP$_i$
Colicin					
D, Escherichia coli K12	–	7.26	280	1359	Neutral sol
E$_1$, E. coli	–	7.36	280	1311	pH 7.0, 0.01 M KP$_i$
E$_2$, E. coli W 3110	5.84	9.73	280	121	MW = 60,000
E$_3$, E. coli W 3110	7.45	12.42	280	121	MW = 60,000
1$_a$, E. coli W 3110-r	–	10.3	280	678	–
1$_b$, E. coli W 3110-r	–	10.9	280	678	–
Colipase					
Pig pancreas	–	4.0	280	1360	–
Coliphage N4					
Phenolic subunits	1.29	7.0	280	679	pH 7.2, 0.1 M Tris, MW = 18,500 [680]
Collagen proline hydroxylase					
Rat skin, newborn	–	12.3	280	1313	pH 7.0
Collagenase (EC 3.4.24.3)					
Clostridium histolyticum					
A	–	14.7	280	1312	–
B	–	13.8	280	1312	–
C	–	16.8	280	1312	–
Complement system (see also C1, C1q, and C2)					
Guinea pig serum	–	13.2	280	1314	–
Conalbumin					
Hen	8.5	11.1	280	122	0.02 M HCl, MW = 76,600
Egg	–	12.0	280	681	–
Egg white	8.8	–	280	1315	–
Iron	12.2	–	280	1315	–
	–	0.62	470	1316	pH5–10
Copper	12.2	–	280	1315	–
Concanavalin A					
Canavalia ensiformis	7.98	11.4	280	933	pH 7.0, 1 N NaCl, MW = 70,000 [933]
	7.75	11.4	280	934	1 M NaCl, MW = 68,000 [935]
	–	13.7	280	936	pH 6.8, 0.05 M P$_i$, 0.2 M NaCl
	–	12.4	280	936	pH 5.2, 0.05 M AcONa, 0.2 M NaCl

MOLAR ABSORPTIVITY AND $A_{1cm}^{1\%}$ VALUES FOR PROTEINS AT SELECTED WAVELENGTHS OF THE ULTRAVIOLET AND VISIBLE REGION (Continued)

Protein	ϵ^a ($\times 10^{-4}$)	$A_{1cm}^{1\% \, b}$	nm^c	Reference	Comments^d
Copper, blue					
Pseudomonas	–	6.7	280	444	–
C-Reactive protein					
Human	–	20	280	123	–
	–	18	280	124	–
Creatine kinase (EC 2.7.3.2)					
Rabbit muscle	3.28	–	250	1317	0.1 *M* Tris, 0.02 *M* EDTA
	3.7	8.88	280	793	pH 7.0, 0.05 *M* P$_i$, MW = 41,300 [793]
	7.3	8.9	280	125	pH 7, MW = 81,000 [125]
	7.1	8.7	280	125	pH 9.8, MW = 81,000 [125]
Cyrrinus carpio L.	8.0	9.38	280	794	MW = 85,100 [794]
Calf brain	–	8.24	280	795	pH 7.0, 0.05 *M* NaP$_i$
Human muscle	7.1	8.8	280	796	pH 8.0, MW = 81,000 [796]
Crotonase (Enoyl-CoA hydratase, EC 4.2.1.17)					
Beef liver	–	5.76	280	797	–
	–	5.56	280	797	pH 7.4, 6 *M* GdmCl or 8 *M* urea
Clostridium acetobutylicum	–	8.90	280	1362	pH 8, 0.05 *M* TrisCl, 0.1 *M* KCl
Crotoxin					
Crotalus terrificus terrificus	–	19	280	798	Neutral sol.
Crustacyanin					
Homarus grammarus	–	11.5	278	937	pH 7
	–	37.2	633	937	pH 7
	–	35.6^{cc}	600	937	Water
	–	5.4^{cc}	320	937	pH 7
	–	5.3^{cc}	360	937	Water
	–	5.7^{cc}	370	937	pH 7
Cryoglobulin, 6.6S					
Human blood	–	13.3	280	938	Dry wt.
Cryptocytochrome *c*					
Pseudomonas denitrificans					
Aerobic cells					
Ferri form	16.0	–	–^{dd}	1371	
	1.97	–	500	1371	
	0.65	–	642	1371	
Ferro form	18.3	–	426	1371	
	17.3	–	438	1371	
	1.97	–	–^{ee}	1371	
CO-ferro form	44.1	–	419	1371	
	2.2	–	540	1371	
	1.86	–	570	1371	
NO-ferro form	17.2	–	396	1371	pH 7, dry wt.
	2.1	–	490	1371	
	2.0	–	–^{ff}	1371	
Anaerobic cells	1.9	–	570	1371	
Ferri form	16.0	–	–^{dd}	1371	
	1.8	–	500	1371	
	0.6	–	642	1371	
Ferro form	17.8	–	426	1371	
	17.1	–	438	1371	
	1.8	–	–^{ee}	1371	
Crystallin					
Beef					
α	–	9.6	280	1318	–
	–	8.85	280	126	Value drops to 8.0 after aging 7 months

^{cc} Data from Figure 1 of Ref. [937].
^{dd} 400–402 nm.
^{ee} 550–560 nm.
^{ff} 530–540 nm.

MOLAR ABSORPTIVITY AND $A_{1cm}^{1\%}$ VALUES FOR PROTEINS AT SELECTED WAVELENGTHS OF THE ULTRAVIOLET AND VISIBLE REGION (Continued)

Protein	ϵ^a ($\times 10^{-4}$)	$A_{1cm}^{1\%\ b}$	nm[c]	Reference	Comments[d]
	73.1	8.7	280	127	MW = 840,000 [127]
α'	–	8.0	280	129	–
α''	–	8.3	280	129	–
γ	–	21.0	280	1318	–
	–	21.0	280	130	–
B_s	5.28	18.6	278	131	pH 8.2, 0.0005 M P$_i$, MW = 28,402 [131]
	5.25	18.5	280	131	pH 8.2, 0.0005 M P$_i$, MW = 28,402 [131]
Calf					
α	–	9.9	280	1319	7 M urea
Dogfish					
α	–	8.5	280	1318	–
Medium age	–	8.80	280	939	pH 9.8, 0.05 M borate–8 M urea
Old	–	7.88	280	939	pH 9.8, 0.05 M borate–8 M urea
β					
Medium age	–	15.9	280	939	pH 9.8, 0.05 M borate–8 M urea
Old	–	15.9	280	939	pH 9.8, 0.05 M borate–8 M urea
γ		22.4	280	1318	–
Medium age	–	23.1	280	939	pH 9.8, 0.05 M borate–8 M urea
Old	–	22.2	280	939	pH 9.8, 0.05 M borate–8 M urea
Fox					
α	55.2	8.9	280	127	MW = 620,000 [127]
Horse					
α	103.8	9.6	280	127	MW = 1,050,000 [127]
Human					
α, 0–10 years old	–	10.2	280	1318	–
β, 0–10 years old	–	16.7	280	1318	–
γ, 0–10 years old	–	15.7	280	1318	–
α, 11–20 years old	–	11.6	280	1318	–
β, 11–20 years old	–	16.5	280	1318	–
γ, 11–20 years old	–	15.6	280	1318	–
α, 40–49 years old	–	16.2	280	1318	–
β, 40–49 years old	–	16.0	280	1318	–
γ, 40–49 years old	–	15.4	280	1318	–
α, 50–59 years old	–	16.0	280	1318	–
β, 50–59 years old	–	16.8	280	1318	–
γ, 50–59 years old	–	15.2	280	1318	–
α, 60–69 years old	–	17.3	280	1318	–
β, 60–69 years old	–	15.7	280	1318	–
γ, 60–69 years old	–	15.9	280	1318	–
α, 70–79 years old	–	15.7	280	1318	–
β, 70–79 years old	–	16.3	280	1318	–
γ, 70–79 years old	–	15.9	280	1318	–
α, 80–89 years old	–	15.6	280	1318	–
β, 80–89 years old	–	14.8	280	1318	–
γ, 80–89 years old	–	17.3	280	1318	–
Mink					
α	55.4	8.8	280	127	MW = 630,000 [127]
Pig					
α	70.6	8.5	280	127	MW = 830,000 [127]
Rabbit					
α	43.8	8.4	280	127	MW-575,000 [127]
	–	8.3	280	128	–
β	–	21.5	280	128	–
γ	–	17.6	280	128	–
Rat					
α	–	8.0	280	1318	–

MOLAR ABSORPTIVITY AND $A_{1cm}^{1\%}$ VALUES FOR PROTEINS AT SELECTED WAVELENGTHS OF THE ULTRAVIOLET AND VISIBLE REGION (Continued)

Protein	ϵ^a ($\times 10^{-4}$)	$A_{1cm}^{1\% \; b}$	nm^c	Reference	Comments^d
Young	–	7.73	280	939	pH 9.8, 0.05 M borate–8 M urea
X-rayed	–	7.49	280	939	
Old	–	7.88	280	939	
α					
Young	–	18.6	280	939	pH 9.8, 0.05 M borate–8 M urea
X-rayed	–	16.8	280	939	
Old	–	16.5	280	939	
γ	–	18.0	280	1318	–
Young	–	19.9	280	939	pH 9.8, 0.05 M borate–8 M urea
Young, X-rayed	–	19.8	280	939	
Old	–	16.6	280	939	
Sulfonated	–	17.1	280	132	–
Sheep					
α	100.1	8.4	280	127	MW = 840,000 [127]
Cyanocobalamin-protein, pig pyloric mucosa	–	9	278	1320	–
Cyanocobalamin-binding factor, pig pyloris	–	8	278	1321	Water, dry wt.
Cystathione γ-lyase (EC 4.4.1.1) (see homoserine deaminase)					
Cysteamine dioxygenase (EC 1.13.11.19)					
Horse kidney	11.2	13.5	280	940	–
Cysteine desulfyhydrase (cystathionine γ-lyase, EC 4.4.1.1)					
S. typhimurium	7.85	21.2	280	1503a	MW = 37,000 [1503a]
Cysteine synthase (EC 4.2.99.8)					
S. typhimurium	28.4	9.2	280	575	MW = 309,000 [575]
S-Cysteinyl albumin (see albumin, beef)					
Cytochrome b					
B. anitratum	–	9.5	280	570	pH 7, 0.06 M P_i, data from Figure 5 [570]
Beef heart	11.4^{gg}	–	429	1364	pH 7.4, 0.01 M P_i, 0.001 M NaDodSO$_4$, values based on pyridine hemechromogen value From Figure 2 [1364]
	2.07^{gg}	–	–^{hh}	1364	
	1.32^{ii}	–	562.5	1364	
	–	36.6	418	1364	
	–	7.2	562	1364	
	–	3.7	532	1364	
Cytochrome b_2					
Yeast, oxidized	0.92	–	560	571	pH 7.0, 0.2 M P_i, 0.2 mM EDTA
	1.13	–	530	571	
	12.95	–	413	571	
	3.44	–	–^{kk}	571	
	8.35	–	280	571	
Reduced with 19.5 mM lactate	3.09	–	557	571	
	1.56	–	528	571	
	18.3	–	424	571	
	3.9	–	328	571	
	8.8	–	269	571	
Yeast					
Fraction B	–	11.0	275	1365	10% AcOH
Fraction C	–	6.7	275	1365	
Core, ferri-form	12.0	–	413	1366	–
Apo-	4.81	2.05	278	1367	MW = 235,000 [1368]
Polypeptide, oxidized	2.3^{ii}	–	260	572	MW = 11,000 [572]
	2.2^{ii}	–	280	572	

---

^{gg} Absolute reduced.
^{hh} 562.5–600 nm.
^{ii} Reduced-oxidized.
^{kk} 360–365 nm.
^{ll} Per heme.

MOLAR ABSORPTIVITY AND $A^{1\%}_{1cm}$ VALUES FOR PROTEINS AT SELECTED WAVELENGTHS OF THE ULTRAVIOLET AND VISIBLE REGION (Continued)

Protein	ϵ^a ($\times 10^{-4}$)	$A^{1\% b}_{1cm}$	nm^c	Reference	Comments^d
	11.2^{II}	–	413	572	
Reduced	15.8^{II}	–	423	572	MW = 11,000 [572]
	13.4^{II}	–	528	572	
	2.68^{II}	–	557	572	
Cytochrome b_5					
Rat liver					
Oxidized	11.7	–	413	1369	–
Reduced	17.1	–	423	1369	–
	1.34	–	526	1369	–
	2.56	–	556	1369	–
Cytochrome b_{562}					
E. coli B					
Reduced	3.16	–	562	1370	–
	1.74	–	531.5	1370	–
	18.01	–	427	1370	–
Oxidized	0.97	–	564	1370	–
	1.06	–	530	1370	–
	11.74	–	418	1370	–
	2.1	–	280	1370	From OD$_{562}$/OD$_{280}$ = 1.5 [1370]
Cytochrome c	–	19.5	280	1372	
	–	290	210	1372	Dry wt.
	–	870	191	1372	
Beef heart	2.77	–	550	137	–
	2.42	–	280	138	Calcd. from OD$_{550}$/OD$_{280}$ = 1.26
	2.9	–	550	139	Reduced with dithionite
	3.053	23.94	550	138	MW = 12,750 [138]
Dithionite reduced	–	23.94	550	1373	pH 6.8, 40 mM NH$_4$ P$_i$
Horse heart	–	17.1	280	1374	–
	–	650	–^{mm}	1374	–
	1.12	–	528	1375	–
	–	9.05	528	1376	–
	2.77	–	550	140	pH 6.8, 0.1 M P$_i$, reduced
	3.18	–	–	140	pH 6.8, 0.1 M P$_i$, reduced, wavelength 268–272 nm
	–	1.12	528	140	pH 6.8, 0.1 M P$_i$, oxidized
	–	2.32	280	140	pH 6.8, 0.1 M P$_i$, oxidized
NO-ferro form	0.54	–	570	1377	
	0.65	–	540	1377	
NO-ferri form	0.56	–	571	1377	
	0.69	–	561	1377	Wavelength determined from frequency
	0.67	–	540	1377	
	0.67	–	527	1377	
Human heart	–	23.1	550	135	–
	2.77	21.9	550	136	Reduced, MW = 12,600 [136]
	2.33	18.5	280	136	Oxidized, MW = 12.600 [136]
Micrococcus denitrificans					
NaBH$_4$ reduced	2.68	–	550	1378	–
	2.23	–	280	1378	From OD$_{550}$/OD$_{280}$ = 1.2 [1378]
Camelus dromedarius (Camel)					
Reduced	2.4	–	550	1379	
	0.646	–	535	1379	pH 7.5
	1.382	–	520	1379	
	10.95	–	417	1379	
Oxidized	0.056	–	695	1379	
	0.946	–	530	1379	
	9.197	–	409	1379	pH 7.5
	2.440	–	360	1379	
	2.033	–	280	1379	

^{mm} 191–194 nm.

MOLAR ABSORPTIVITY AND $A_{1cm}^{1\%}$ VALUES FOR PROTEINS AT SELECTED WAVELENGTHS OF THE ULTRAVIOLET AND VISIBLE REGION (Continued)

Protein	ϵ^a ($\times 10^{-4}$)	$A_{1cm}^{1\%\ b}$	nm[c]	Reference	Comments[d]
Cytochrome c_1					
Beef heart	–	14	276	1380	–
Cytochrome c_2					
Rhodospirillum rubrum					
Reduced	2.81[nn]	–	550	1381	
	1.7[nn]	–	521	1381	
	14.3[nn]	–	415	1381	
	3.71[nn]	–	316	1381	
	3.38[nn]	–	272	1381	pH 6.90, 0.1 M NaP$_i$
Oxidized	1.05[nn]	–	525	1381	
	11.5[nn]	–	410	1381	
	2.95[nn]	–	357	1381	
	2.47[nn]	–	275	1381	
Cytochrome c_{550}					
Bacillus subtilis					
Reduced	2.55	–	550	1384	–
	1.31	–	520	1384	–
	12.75	–	414	1384	–
	3.14	–	316	1384	–
	3.94	–	279	1384	–
Oxidized	1.18	–	528	1384	–
	9.25	–	407	1384	–
	3.06	–	279	1384	–
Spirillum itersonii					
Reduced[oo]	2.76	26.4	550	1385	
	1.61	15.5	522	1385	MW = 10,411 [1385]
	14.6	14.0	416	1385	
Oxidized[oo]	11.9	11.4	412	1385	
Thiobacillus novellus					
Reduced	2.58	–	550	1386	
	13.4	–	414.5	1386	At 77°K
Oxidized	2.92	–	280	1386	
Cytochrome c_{551}					
Thiobacillus novellus					
Reduced	1.96	–	551	1386	–
	13.9	–	416	1386	–
Oxidized	15.1	–	280	1386	–
Cytochrome $c_{551.5}$					
Chloropseudomonas ethylica					
Reduced[pp]	19.91	–	418	1387	
	1.58	–	523	1387	pH 7.0, 0.05 M Tris Cl
	3.08	–	551.5	1387	
Oxidized[pp]	2.75	–	351	1387	
	12.44	–	408	1387	pH 7.0, 0.05 M Tris Cl
	1.03	–	528	1387	
Cytochrome c_{552}					
B *Chromatium* strain D					
Reduced α peak	3.12	4.35	550	1388	MW = 72,000 [1388]
Cytochrome c_{552} [I]					
P. stutzeri, reduced	3.1[qq]	–	552	573	–
	1.63[qq]	–	523	573	–
	15.08[qq]	–	418	573	–
Oxidized	1.05[qq]	–	530	573	–
	10.04[qq]	–	410	573	–
	2.51[qq]	–	284	573	–

[nn] The value given here is 1/1000 of the value cited in Ref. [1364]. "I believe that a concentration of moles/1000 ml was used rather than mole/liter, which resulted in a very large value." [1840].

[oo] Based on one atom of Fe per molecule.

[pp] All values per heme.

[qq] All ϵ values are based on heme content.

MOLAR ABSORPTIVITY AND $A_{1cm}^{1\%}$ VALUES FOR PROTEINS AT SELECTED WAVELENGTHS OF THE ULTRAVIOLET AND VISIBLE REGION (Continued)

Protein	ϵ^a ($\times 10^{-4}$)	$A_{1cm}^{1\%\,b}$	nm[c]	Reference	Comments[d]
Cytochrome c_{552}, [II]					
P. stutzeri, reduced	1.95[qq]	–	552	573	–
	1.66[qq]	–	523	573	–
	15.35[qq]	–	417	573	–
Oxidized	0.99[qq]	–	525	573	–
	12.21[qq]	–	410	573	–
	1.69[qq]	–	277	573	–
Cytochrome c_{553}					
Petalonia fascia (an alga)					
Ferro form	2.68	25.5	273	1389	
	2.19	20.9	293	1389	
	4.40	41.9	317.5	1389	
	19.71	187.5	415.5	1389	
	0.38	3.6	471	1389	
	1.86	17.8	521.5	1389	MW = 10,500 [1389]
	2.85	27.1	553	1389	
Ferri form	2.68	25.5	269	1389	
	2.21	21.0	292	1389	
	3.62	34.5	360	1389	
	13.53	129.0	409	1389	
	1.29	12.3	528	1389	
Monochrysis lutheri (an alga)					
Reduced	2.59		553	1390	
	15.65		416	1390	pH 7, P_i value based on iron determination
Cytochrome c_{554}					
Bacillus subtilis					
Reduced	3.39	–	279	1384	–
	2.0	–	554	1384	–
	1.45	–	550	1384	–
	1.48	–	521	1384	–
	14.36	–	417	1384	–
	4.0	–	316	1384	–
Oxidized	2.4	–	280	1384	–
	1.02	–	523	1384	–
	10.67	–	409	1384	–
Cytochrome c_{555}					
Crithidia fasciculata					
Reduced[pp]	2.97	24.8	555.5	1391	
	1.68	14.0	525	1391	
	15.4	128	420	1391	
Oxidized[pp]	11.2	93	413	1391	MW = 12,051 [1391]
	1.22	10.2	533	1391	
	0.9	7.5	555.5	1391	
	0.84	7.0	565	1391	
Cytochrome $c_{555(550)}$					
Chloropseudomonas ethylica					
Reduced[pp]	15.34	–	417.5	1387	
	1.71	–	523	1387	
	2.04	–	555	1387	
Oxidized[pp]	4.02	–	275	1387	pH 7.0, 0.05 *M* TrisCl
	3.01	–	358	1387	
	13.20	–	412	1387	
	1.13	–	525	1387	
Cytochrome $c_{557(551)}$, *Alcaligenes faecalis*					
Reduced[rr]	4.46	–	557	1383	Dry wt

[rr] As diheme derivative.

MOLAR ABSORPTIVITY AND $A_{1cm}^{1\%}$ VALUES FOR PROTEINS AT SELECTED WAVELENGTHS OF THE ULTRAVIOLET AND VISIBLE REGION (Continued)

Protein	ϵ^a ($\times 10^{-4}$)	$A_{1cm}^{1\% \ b}$	nm[c]	Reference	Comments[d]
	3.72	5.7	557	1383	
	2.89	4.44	525	1383	
	28.3	43	420	1383	
Reduced-CO[rr]	3.72	5.7	557	1383	pH 7, 0.05 M P$_i$, MW = 65.000 [1383]
	2.89	4.44	525	1383	
	40.0	61.4	416	1383	
Oxidized[rr]	2.16	3.32	530	1383	
	26.2	40.2	408	1383	
Cytochrome cc'					
Pseudomonas denitrificans					
Ferri form[pp]	0.37	–	635	1382	
	1.02	–	495	1382	
	8.0	–	400	1382	
	3.08	–	280	1382	
Ferro form[pp]	0.71	–	550	1382	pH 7.3, 0.02 M Tris, 0.5 M NaCl
	8.75	–	434	1382	
	9.70	–	426	1382	
CO-ferro form[pp]	1.05	–	564	1382	
	1.18	–	534	1382	
	21.0	–	418	1382	
Ferri form[pp]	0.63	–	575	1382	
	0.94	–	538	1382	
	9.90	–	413	1382	
	2.51	–	348	1382	3 N NaOH
Ferro form[pp]	2.49	–	550	1382	
	1.32	–	522	1382	
	15.62	–	416	1382	
Ferri form[pp]	0.245	–	635	1382	pH 5
	0.41	–	635	1382	pH 10
Cytochrome cd					
Alcaligenes faecalis					
Reduced[pp]	18.9	21.0	418	1383	
	4.45	4.95	460	1383	
	2.87	3.18	556	1383	
	2.65	2.94	525	1383	pH 7, 0.05 M P$_i$, MW = 90,000 [1383]
	1.85	2.06	625	1383	
Oxidized[pp]	15.1	16.8	412	1383	
	2.12	2.35	640	1383	
	13.8	15.3	280	1383	pH 7, 0.05 M P$_i$, MW = 90,000 [1383], value calcd. from A$_{412}$/A$_{280}$ = 1.2 [1383]
Cytochrome P-450					
Rat liver microsomes					
Males	7.96	–	450	1392	Biuret
Females	9.41	–	450	1392	Biuret
Cytochrome oxidase (EC 1.9.3.1-.2)					
Pseudomonas (EC 1.9.3.2)	17,600	–	280	574	Data from Figure 2 [574]
Reduced	18,200	–	418	574	
	3,600	–	625	574	pH 6.0, 0.1 M NaP$_i$
Oxidized	14,900	–	408	574	
	3,020	–	630	574	
Pseudomonas aeruginosa	22	18.5	280	1393	Dry wt.
Beef heart	–	17.4	280	133	–
Cytochrome c peroxidase (EC 1.11.1.5)					
Pseudomonas	6.48	12.1	280	1394	Dry wt., MW = 53,500 [1394]
Yeast	8.1	–	408	941	Dimethyl protoheme
	9.3	23.2	408	134	pH 6, MW = 40,000 [134]
	7.4	18.5	282	134	pH 6, MW = 40,000 [134]
Apo-	5.5	13.75	282	134	pH 6, MW = 40,000 [134]

MOLAR ABSORPTIVITY AND $A_{1cm}^{1\%}$ VALUES FOR PROTEINS AT SELECTED WAVELENGTHS OF THE ULTRAVIOLET AND VISIBLE REGION (Continued)

Protein	ϵ^a ($\times 10^{-4}$)	$A_{1cm}^{1\% \, b}$	nm^c	Reference	Comments^d
Cytocuprein					
Human	–	210	210	576	
	–	5.8	268	576	
	–	5.5	280	576	
	–	0.08	675	576	Data from Figure 5 [576]
Apocytocuprein					
Human	–	210	210	576	
	–	4.3	268	576	
	–	4.2	280	576	
3-Deoxy-2-keto-6-phosphogluconate aldolase (see aldolase)					
Deoxyribonuclease I (EC 3.1.4.5) (DNase)					
Beef pancreas	–	11.5	280	141	–
	–	12.8	280	942	–
	–	11.1	280	942	Nbs inactivated
	–	11.8	280	799	2.5 mM HCl
	3.72	12.0	–	577	pH 4.7, 0.2 M AcONa, MW = 31,000 [577]
	–	12.3	280	578	pH 7.6, 0.1 M KP$_i$
	–	13.9	280	578	pH 13, 0.1 N NaOH
	–	12.3	280	142	pH 7.6, 0.1 M KP$_i$
	–	13.9	280	142	pH 13, 0.1 N NaOH
Deoxyribonuclease inhibitor					
Calf spleen	6.05	10.2	280	579	pH 7.6, 0.1 M KP$_i$, MW = 59,400 [579]
	6.2	10.4	280	579	0.1 N NaOH, MW = 59,400 [579]
Deoxyribonucleic acid polymerase (DNA polymerase, EC 2.7.7.7)					
E. coli	9.26	8.5	280	580	10 mM NH$_4$HCO$_3$, MW = 109,000 [580]
	11.5	10.5	290	580	0.1 M NaOH–5 mM NH$_4$ HCO$_3$, data from Figure 3 [580]
Large fragment	–	9.3	278	1401	
Ehrlich ascites tumor		23.9	280	581	pH 7.0, 0.2 M KP$_i$–0.001 M EDTA, 0.01 M 2–HSEtOH, data from Figure 4 [581]
	–	19.2	290	581	
	–	20.4	280	581	pH 10, data from Figure 4 [581]
	–	17.5	290	581	
Dextranase (EC 3.2.1.11)					
Aspergillus carneus	–	17.8	280	1395	Dry wt.
Diamine oxidase (amine oxidase, EC 1.4.3.6)					
Pig kidney	10.6	12.8	280	143	MW = 87,000 [143]
Dihydrofolate reductase (tetrahydrofolate dehydrogenase) (EC 1.5.1.3)					
Streptomyces faecium	4.47	22.0	280	1396	DR, MW = 20,300 [1396]
Lactobacillus casei	2.15	–	278	1397	pH 7
	2.76	–	268	1397	+ NADPH^{ss}
	0.72	–	340	1397	
E. coli, Methotrexate resistant	4	23.8	280	1398	Microbiuret and dry wt., MW = 16,810 [1398]
E. coli	–	19.1	280	1399	pH 7.0, 0.04 M KP$_i$
T4 phage	–	12.0	280	1399	
Chicken liver	3.4	15.5	278	682	MW = 22,000 [682]
Streptococcus faecium	–	20	280	683	
Dihydrolipoyl transacetylase (lipoate acetyltransferase, EC 2.3.1.12)					
E. coli	–	4.5	280	684	pH 7.0, P$_i$
Dihydroorotic dehydrogenase (orotate reductase, EC 1.3.1.14)					
Zymobacterium oroticum	3.5	–	450	27	–
	0.59	–	550	27	–
3,4-Dihydroxy-9,10-secoandrosta-1,3,5[10]-triene-9,17-dione 4,5-dioxygenase (steroid 4,5-dioxygenase) (EC 1.13.11.25)					
Nocardia restrictus	26.8	9.3	280	800	MW = 286,000 [800]

---

ss NADPH, nicotinamide adenine dinucleotide phosphate, reduced.

MOLAR ABSORPTIVITY AND $A_{1cm}^{1\%}$ VALUES FOR PROTEINS AT SELECTED WAVELENGTHS OF THE ULTRAVIOLET AND VISIBLE REGION (Continued)

Protein	ϵ^a ($\times 10^{-4}$)	$A_{1cm}^{1\% \ b}$	nm^c	Reference	Comments^d
Dimethylglycine dehydrogenase (EC 1.5.99.2)					
Rat liver, mitochondria	–	17	280	685	pH 7.5, 0.0075 M KP$_i$, data from Figure 4 [685]
Dipeptidase (EC 3.4.13.11), Pig kidney	4.2	8.96	280	686	pH 8.0, 0.002 M Tris, MW = 47,200 [686]
p-Diphenol oxidase (monophenol monooxygenase) (EC 1.14.18.1)					
Polyporus versicolor	–	11.5	280	1400	–
Diphtheria toxin	–	7.69	278	145	pH 6.8, M/15 P$_i$, 0.175 M NaCl
	–	7.82	278	145	0.1 N HCl
	–	8.52	293	145	0.1 N NaOH
DPNase (NAD nucleosidase, EC 3.2.2.5)					
Pig brain	8.0	3.1	280	144	MW = 26,000 [144]
Edeine A					
B. brevis Vm 4	0.131	–	270	582	Water
Edeine B					
B. brevis Vm 4	0.131	–	270	582	Water
Elastase (EC 3.4.21.11)	–	11.0	280	943	
Pig	5.74	22.2	280	801	0.1 M NaOH
	5.23	20.2	280	801	pH 5.0, 0.05 M AcONa
	–	18.5	280	583	–
	4.85	–	280	944	$\epsilon = [M/2.06] \times 10^5$
	–	22.0	280	945	–
Elastase-like enzyme					
Streptomyces griseus					
I	2.94	10.5	280	946	MW = 28,000 [946]
II	0.85	12.1	280	946	MW = 7,000 [946]
III	1.58	11.3	280	946	MW = 14,000 [946]
Elastoidin, soluble					
Prionace glauca, pectoral fins (Great blue shark)	–	1.86	277	947	0.5 M AcOH, data from Figure 2 [947]
Elinin					
Human erythrocyte	4420	22.1	274	948	MW = 20 $\times 10^6$ [948]^{tt}
Elongation factor 2					
ADP ribosylated					
Rat liver					
Aminoethylated	9.7	–	276	959 ⎫	pH 7.8, 5 M GdmCl, 50 mM Tris
	9.4	–	280	959 ⎬	
	9.9	–	273	959 ⎫	pH 3.3, 50 mM
	8.9	–	280	959 ⎬	
Endopolygalacturonase					
Verticillium albo-atrum	–	12.7^{uu}	280	802	–
	–	11.2^{uu}	280	802	–
Aspergillus niger	–	1.29	280	1404	–
Enolase (2-phosphoglycerate hydro-lyase) (EC 4.2.1.11)					
Oncorhynchus kisutch (Coho salmon)	7.8	7.4	280	949	MW = 105,560 [949]
Oncorhynchus keta (Chun salmon)	8.6	8.7	280	949	MW = 99,260 [949]
Yeast	7.8	8.9	280	949	MW = 88,000 [949]
	–	9.0	280	584	–
Rabbit	–	9.0	280	949	–
Rabbit muscle	–	8.95	280	141	–
	7.65	9	280	146	MW = 85,000 [146]
	6.1	9	280	147	MW = 67,200 [148]
	–	8.85	280	1407	Kjeldahl^e
E. coli	–	5.7	280	1405 ⎫	DR
	–	6.1	277	1405 ⎬	
Rhesus monkey	7.2	8.8	280	1406	MW = 82,000 [1406]
Trout	–	7.9	280	949	–

^{tt} In Figure 3 of Ref. [948], OD = 0.375 for a 0.4% solution. This is equivalent to an $A_{1cm}^{1\%}$ of 9.35. The value cited in the paper was "$E_{1cm}^{1\%}$ = 0.221" from which $A_{1cm}^{1\%}$ was obtained.
^{uu} Two different preparations.

MOLAR ABSORPTIVITY AND $A_{1cm}^{1\%}$ VALUES FOR PROTEINS AT SELECTED WAVELENGTHS OF THE ULTRAVIOLET AND VISIBLE REGION (Continued)

Protein	ϵ^a ($\times 10^{-4}$)	$A_{1cm}^{1\% b}$	nm^c	Reference	Comments^d
Enterokinase (enteropeptidase) (EC 3.4.21.9)					
Pig duodena	–	17.8	280	1408	–
Enterotoxin A					
Staphylococcus aureus	4.09	14.6	277	1409	MW = 28,000 [1409]
Enterotoxin B					
Staphylococci	–	12.1	277	149	–
	–	15	277	149	N = 16.1% [149]
	–	14	277	150	–
Enterotoxin B, nitrated					
Staphylococcal	6.29	20.6	277	687	pH 8, MW = 30,500 [687]
	2.42	7.9	428	687	
	2.16	7.1	360	687	pH 6.2, MW = 30,500 [687]
Enterotoxin C					
Staphylococcus aureus	–	12.1	277	688	–
Enterotoxin E					
Staphylococcus aureus	–	11.9	280	1410	–
	–	12.5	277	1410	–
Enzyme, thrombin-like					
Crotalus adamanteus trans-Epoxysuccinate hydratase (see tartrate epoxidase)	4.84	14.8	280	1411	Dry wt., MW = 32,700 [1411]
Erabutoxin a					
Laticauda semifasciata	0.7	–	280	803	Water
Erythrocruorin					
Lumbricus terrestris	1.18	5.13	504	804	
	11.36	49.4	430	804	
Oxygenated	1.37	5.95	542	804	
	11.27	49.0	417	804	
	5.22	22.7	283	804	pH 7.0, 0.1 MP$_i$, MW = 23,230 [804]
Plus CO	1.374	5.97	538	804	
	18.83	81.9	420	804	
Ferric derivative	1.165	5.07	500	804	
	10.0	43.7	395	804	
Erythrocruorin, oxy					
Cirraformia grandis (Annelid worm)	4.09	22.1	280	1412	
	2.58	13.9	345	1412	
	9.68	52.2	415	1412	Dry wt., MW = 18,500 [1412]
	1.21	6.59	539	1412	
	1.18	6.38	574	1412	
Erythrocuprein (superoxide dismutase, EC 1.15.1.1)					
Beef	0.0313	–	680	1413	–
	0.984	–	259	1414	–
Apo-	0.241	–	252	1415	
	0.367	–	259	1415	
	0.330	–	262	1415	
	0.419	–	264	1415	pH 7.2, 10 mMP$_i$
	0.413	–	268	1415	
	0.383	–	275	1415	
	0.330	–	252	1415	
	0.420	–	259	1415	
	0.420	–	261	1415	
	0.540	–	269	1415	GdmCl, pH 5.9
	0.540	–	275	1415	
	0.460	–	281	1415	
	0.790	–	295	1415	pH 11.7, GdmCl
	3.81	–	246	1415	
Human	–	5.06	265	805	
	–	0.075	655	805	pH 6.5, 0.15 M NaCl
	–	0.077	675	805	
Human blood	0.0284	0.085	655	98	MW = 33,200 [432]
	1.84	5.5	265	98	MW = 33,200 [432]

MOLAR ABSORPTIVITY AND $A_{1cm}^{1\%}$ VALUES FOR PROTEINS AT SELECTED WAVELENGTHS OF THE ULTRAVIOLET AND VISIBLE REGION (Continued)

Protein	ϵ^a ($\times 10^{-4}$)	$A_{1cm}^{1\%\ b}$	nm^c	Reference	Comments^d
	0.0350	0.104	655	151	MW = 33,600 [151]
	1.87	5.58	265	151	MW = 33,600 [151]
Erythropoietin					
Human urine	–	9.26	279	1416	–
Esterase (carboxylesterase, EC 3.1.1.1)					
Pig liver	–	13.8	280	585	pH 8.0
Goat intestine	–	14.73	275	586	–
	–	13.75	280	586	–
Excelsin					
Brazil nuts	–	9	279	806	pH 5.5
	–	14	279	806	pH 12.2
Exo-1, 3-3-glucosidase (EC 3.2.1.58) (see glucanase)					
Factor					
Antihemorrhagic					
Trimcresurus flavoviridis (Snake)					
Serum	–	8.8	280	1417	–
Direct lytic (acetate)					
Haemachatus haemachates (Snake) venom	0.29	4.2	278	1418	MW = 7,000 [1418]
Epidermal growth					
Mice (adult male, albino), submaxillary gland	1.81	30.9	280	1419	pH 5.6, 0.1 M AcONa or water DR, MW = 6,045 [1419]
X					
Beef plasma	–	12.4	280	1420	–
X, activated					
Beef plasma	4.1	8.6	280	1421	Dry wt., MW = 48,000 [1421]
X, thrombokinase, activated Stuart factor					
Human	–	5.8	280	587	–
XIII					
Human plasma	–	13.8	280	1503b	Dry wt.
Fatty acid synthetase (EC 2.3.1.41) (see also 3-oxoacyl-[ACP] reductase)					
Chicken liver	48.3	9.65	279	588	MW = 500,000 [588]
Pigeon liver	46.4	8.35	279	589	MW = 545,000 [589]
	38.7	8.6	280	153	MW = 450,000 [153]
Fatty acyl-CoA dehydrogenase (acyl-CoA dehydrogenase) (EC 1.3.1.8 or .9 or EC 1.3.99.3)					
Pig liver	–	13.8	275	152	pH 7.5, 0.036 M P$_i$, estd. from Figure 3 [152]
Fenedoxin Alfalfa	0.95	–	277	154	Per mole iron
	1.83	16.6	277	154	MW = 11,000 [154]
	–	7.2	465	154	–
	–	7.9	422	154	–
	–	10.6	331	154	–
Scenedesmus	1.5	13.1	276	155	MW = 11,500 [155]
	1.33	–	330	155	–
	0.98	–	421	155	–
Apo-	0.855	15.8	280	156	pH 5.4, estd. from Figure 1 [156], apoprotein made with α,α'-dipyridyl
	0.765	14.2	280	156	pH 7.4, estd. from Figure 1 [156], apoprotein made with mersalyl
Azotobacter vinelandii, oxidized, Fdl	2.7	19.2	400	1425	MW = 14,140 [1425]
Bacillus polymyxa, oxidized	–	21	279	950	
	–	12.3	325	950	
	–	11.1	400	950	pH 7.3, 25 mM Tris Cl, data from Figure 2 [950]
	–	5.1	500	950	
Reduced with Na$_2$S$_2$O$_4$	–	6.9	400	950	
	–	3.1	500	950	
Chlorobium thiosulfatophilum	2.04	34	280	951	pH 7.3, 0.3 M Tris, 0.54 M NaCl, data from Figure 1 [951], MW = 6,000 [951]
E. coli	0.96	7.6	416	952	MW = 12,600 [952]
	1.78	13.3	277	952	

MOLAR ABSORPTIVITY AND $A_{1cm}^{1\%}$ VALUES FOR PROTEINS AT SELECTED WAVELENGTHS OF THE ULTRAVIOLET AND VISIBLE REGION (Continued)

Protein	ϵ^a ($\times 10^{-4}$)	$A_{1cm}^{1\% \ b}$	nm^c	Reference	Comments^d
Clostridium pasteurianum	2.16	41.5	285	952	
	2.16	41.5	300	952	
	1.73	33.2	390	952	MW = 5,200
	3.0	–	390	952	
	–	34.0	390	811	–
	2.1	35.0	390	812	MW = 6,000 [812]
Monomer	2.600	–	390	1428	Dry wt.
	3.126	–	390	1428	Kjeldahl^e
Dimer	1.600	–	390	1428	Dry wt.
	1.540	–	390	1428	Kjeldahl^e
Lyophilized	1.617	–	390	1428	Dry wt.
	1.260	–	390	1428	Kjeldahl^e
C. tartarivorum	3.106	–	280	810	–
	2.422	–	290	810	–
C. thermosaccharolyticum	3.09	–	280	810	–
	2.413	–	390	810	–
C. acidi urici	–	37.0	390	811	–
	3.06	–	390	813	–
	3.15	58.4	280	156	pH 7.4, 0.1 M Tris, estd. from Figure 1 of Ref. [156], MW = 5,400 [156]
	3.06^w	–	390	955	–
	2.98	–	390	955	Dry wt.^{ww}
	3.36^{xx}	–	390	955	–
	3.02^{yy}	–	390	955	–
C. tetanomorphum	–	35.0	390	811	–
C. butyricun	–	31.0	390	811	–
C. cylindrosporum	–	29.6	390	811	–
Cyperus rotundus L.	0.88	–	465	807	–
	0.98	–	420	807	–
	1.45	–	330	807	–
	2.42	–	275	807	–
Cotton, type I	0.655	–	460	808	–
	0.758	–	419	808	–
	1.082	–	325	808	–
Bacterial	2.45	–	390	809	–
Horsetail leaves	0.88	–	421	956	–
	1.17	–	276	956	From A_{421}/A_{276} = 0.75
Methanobacterium omelianskii	–	39	280	957	pH 7.3, 0.07 M Tris Cl, data from Figure 1 [957]
Pseudomonas oleovorans	–	3.36	497	958	pH 7.3, 0.1 M Tris, one atom Fe
	–	20.2	280	958	From A_{280}/A_{491} = 6.3
	–	5.74	495	958	pH 7.3, 0.1 M Tris, two atoms Fe
	–	21.2	280	958	
Apo-	–	18	277	958	From A_{280}/A_{495}—3.7, 50% AcOH
Rhodospirillum rubrum					
Type I	2.43	27.9	385	1426	MW = 8,700 [1426]
Type II	0.88	11.7	385	1426	MW = 7,500 [1426]
Parsley	1.24	11.47	255	1427	
	1.27	11.75	260	1427	
	1.5	13.9	277	1427	
	0.98	9.09	294	1427	
	1.22	11.34	330	1427	
	0.74	6.92	390	1427	MW = 10,800 [1427]
	0.92^{zz}	8.65	422	1427	
	0.82	7.59	448	1427	
	0.84	7.79	463	1427	
	0.97	0.90	690	1427	

^{w} Protein concentration determined by release of C-terminal amino acid by carboxypeptidase A.
^{ww} MW = 6232, 8 eq. Fe and 8 eq. S.
^{xx} Protein concentration determined by aspartic acid analysis.
^{yy} Protein concentration determined by glutamic acid analysis.
^{zz} This value cited in Ref. [1427]. "I calculated 9350 as e." [1840].

MOLAR ABSORPTIVITY AND $A^{1\%}_{1cm}$ VALUES FOR PROTEINS AT SELECTED WAVELENGTHS OF THE ULTRAVIOLET AND VISIBLE REGION (Continued)

Protein	ϵ^a ($\times 10^{-4}$)	$A^{1\%\,b}_{1cm}$	nm[c]	Reference	Comments[d]
	1.01	–	420	814	–
Spinach	0.88	–	420	812	–
	0.94	–	420	814	–
Urea–oxygen denat.	2.0	–	275	815	Contains Fe
	1.3	–	275	815	Lacks Fe
Ferredoxin: NADP reductase (EC 1.6.7.1)					
Spinach	1.074	–	456	1429	–
Ferritin					
Apo-, horse spleen	–	–	280	157	$A^{1\%}_{1cm} = 8.6 - 9.7$
Rat liver	–	2	320	1430	–
	–	302	260	1430	–
Fetuin					
Commercial	–	4.5	278	1431	This value is good for native, reduced and carboxymethylated, oxidized, and neuraminidase-treated fetuin
Calf serum	–	4.1	278	1432	Water
	–	5.3	278	1432	–
Calf spleen	–	4.5	278	158	Australian sample
	–	4.8	278	158	Colorado sample
Fibrin					
Beef	–	16.16	283	816	6 M alkaline urea
	–	16.19	290	816	
	–	16.84	282	1433	40% urea, 0.2 N NaOH
Human	–	15	280	1434	–
Fibrin stabilizing factor					
Beef plasma	–	14.15	283	1422	8 M urea, 0.2 M NaOH
Fibrinogen					
Beef					
α chain	–	11.8	280	1435	
β chain	–	17.4	280	1435	0.1 M NaOH
γ chain	–	20.4	280	1435	
Beef	–	16.51	282	1433	8 M urea, 0.2 N NaOH
	–	15.4	279	1433	pH 2, 0.3 M NaCl
	–	14.0	279	1433	pH 6, 0.3 M NaCl
	–	15.6	282	1433	pH 11, 0.3 M NaCl
	–	15.04[a*]	280	1436	0.3 M NaCl
	–	15.49[a*]	280	1436	pH 6.9, 0.05 M P,
	–	15.16[a*]	280	1436	2% AcOH
	–	15.29[a*]	280	1436	pH 5.3, 1 M NaBr
	–	15.45[a*]	280	1436	30% urea
	–	15.60[a*]	280	1436	pH 5.45, 6 N GdmCl
	–	15.94[a*]	280	1436	pH 5.8, 2 A/KCNS
	–	15.06	280	161	pH 7.1, ionic strength = 0.3
	–	16.01	282.5	161	pH 12.8, 0.1 M KOH
	–	15.92	289.5	161	pH 12.8, 0.1 M KOH
	–	15.17	278.5	161	pH 5.8, 5 M GdmCl
	–	15.06	279	161	pH 7.4, 5 M urea
	–	15.00	278	161	pH 7.6
	–	15.1	280	162	–
	–	15	280	689	–
	–	15.87	283	816	6 M alkaline urea
	–	15.88	290	816	
	–	15.04	280	816	3 M NaCl
	–	15.5	280	816	–
Fragment D	–	20.7	280	816	–
Fragment E	–	13.0	280	816	–

[a*] Read against value at 320 nm.

MOLAR ABSORPTIVITY AND $A_{1cm}^{1\%}$ VALUES FOR PROTEINS AT SELECTED WAVELENGTHS OF THE ULTRAVIOLET AND VISIBLE REGION (Continued)

Protein	ϵ^a ($\times 10^{-4}$)	$A_{1cm}^{1\% \, b}$	nm^c	Reference	Comments^d
Calf	–	15.9	280	1439	
Dog	–	15.8	280	1439	0.2 M KC1, corrected for scattering
Elephant	–	15.7	280	1439	
Goat	–	15.6	280	1439	
Human	–	13.9	280	1437	pH 7.1, 0.055 M Na$_3$Cit·2H$_2$O
	–	17.65	282	1437	Alkaline urea
	46.4	13.6	280	96	MW = 341,000 [159]
	45.3	15.1	280	690	MW = 300,000 [690]
Fraction 1–4	–	14.5	280	819	
Fraction 1–8	–	15.6	280	819	
Fragment X	34.1	14.2	280	690	MW = 240,000 [690]
Fragment Y	27.3	17.6	280	690	MW = 155,000 [690]
Fragment D	16.7	20.8	280	690	MW = 83,000 [690]
	–	20.8	280	1438	
Fragment E	5.1	10.2	280	690	MW = 50,000 [690]
	–	10.2	280	1438	
Knot	–	11.8	280	1438	
Human, high solubility	–	16.8	282	160	0.1 N NaOH–5 M urea
Low solubility	–	16.7	280	160	0.1 N NaOH–5 M urea
Panulirus interruptus	52.5	12.5	280	820	MW = 420,000 [820]
Sheep	–	15.5	280	1439	0.2 M KCl, corrected for scattering
Fibroin					
Bombyx mori L.	–	11.3	276	691	pH 4.3–7.3, 0.2 M NaCl
Ficin (EC 3.4.22.3)	5.8	22.4	280	163	MW = 26,000 [163]
	5.9	22.6	280	164	MW = 26,000 [163]
	4.6	–	280	821	
Fraction III	5.1	21	280	165	0.05 M NH$_4$HCO$_3$, MW = 24,500 [165]
Ficus glabrata					
Component G	5.4	–	280	1440	–
F. carica var. *kodata*	–	20.2	280	822	–
Flavodoxin					
Desulfovibrio gigas					
Oxidized	4.7	–	273	959	–
	0.82	–	374	959	–
	1.02	–	456.5	959	–
Semiquinone	0.87	–	349	959	–
	0.41	–	580	959	–
Desulfovibrio vulgaris					
Oxidized	4.8	–	273	959	–
	0.87	–	375.5	959	–
	1.07	–	456–7	959	–
Semiquinone	0.9	–	349	959	–
	0.47	–	580	959	–
Apo-	2.00	–	278	1442	–
E. coli	0.825	–	467	960	–
	0.382	–	580	960	–
	5.0	–	274	960	From $\epsilon_{274}/\epsilon_{467}$ = 6.67 [960], MW = 14,500 [960]
Clostridium MP					
Oxidized	4.68	–	272	961	–
	0.91	–	376	961	–
	1.04	–	445	961	–
Semiquinone	0.84	–	350	961	–
	0.485	–	376	961	–
	0.24	–	445	961	–
	0.462	–	575	961	–
Reduced	0.175	–	445	961	–
Clostridium pasteurianum	4	27.4	272	166	MW = 14,600 [166]
	0.79	5.3	372	166	MW = 14,600 [166]
	0.91	6.2	443	166	MW = 14,600 [166]

MOLAR ABSORPTIVITY AND $A_{1cm}^{1\%}$ VALUES FOR PROTEINS AT SELECTED WAVELENGTHS OF THE ULTRAVIOLET AND VISIBLE REGION (Continued)

Protein	ϵ^a ($\times 10^{-4}$)	$A_{1cm}^{1\%\,b}$	nm^c	Reference	Comments^d
Oxidized	4.58	–	272	961	–
	0.847	–	374	961	–
	1.04	–	443	961	–
Semiquinone	0.766	–	350	961	–
	0.465	–	374	961	–
	0.208	–	443	961	–
	0.455	–	575	961	–
Reduced	0.16	–	443	961	–
	–	36.8	274	167	pH 7.3, 0.02 M Tris Cl
Apo-	2.5	–	278	962	–
	2.52	–	282	962	–
Peptostreptococcus elsdenii					
Oxidized	4.76	–	272	963	pH 7.8, 0.002 M NaP$_i$
	0.63	–	350	963	–
	0.875	–	377	963	–
	1.02	–	445	963	–
Semiquinone	0.765	–	350	963	–
	0.5	–	377	963	–
	0.21	–	445	963	–
	0.45	–	580	963	–
Reduced	0.16–0.18	–	445	963	–
Apo-	2.67	–	278	962	–
Rhodospirillum rubrum					
Oxidized	1.12	–	460	1441	–
	1.13	–	376	1441	–
	5.42	–	272	1441	–
Semiquinone	0.5	–	627	1441	–
	0.45	–	588	1441	–
	1.09	–	353	1441	–
	6.07	–	273	1441	–
Apo-	3.50	–	276	1442	–
Chlorella fuscea	1.0	–	464	1443	–
	5.46	–	275	1443	–
	0.905	–	379	1443	–
Flavoprotein	7.65	–	276	964	
Egg yolk	1.0	–	375	964	pH 7.2, 0.1 M NaP$_i$
	1.32	–	458	964	
Azobacter vinelandii	–	13.4	280	445	Biuret
Apo-	–	13.4	280	445	Lowry
Follicle-stimulating hormone (FSH)					
Sheep	1.23	4.9	275	168	Neutral and acidic solutions, MW = 25,000 [168]
Human	2.3	9.2	276	169	MW = 25,000 [169]
Formiminoglutamase (EC 3.5.3.8)					
Pseudomonas ATCC 11,299b	–	14.7	280	1444	Dry wt., pH 7.4, 1 mM KP$_i$, 20 mM NaCl, 1 mM HSEtOH
Formylglycinamide ribonucleotide amidotransferase (phosphoribosylformyl glycinamidine synthetase, EC 6.3.5.3)					
Chicken liver	18.6	–	280	170	pH 6.5, 0.1 M P$_i$
Formyltetrahydrofolate synthetase (EC 6.3.4.3)					
Clostridium acidi-urici	–	3.70	280	1445	Dry wt. and DR
C. cylindrosporum	12.7	5.3	280	1446	–
	12.2	5.3	280	171	MW = 230,000 [171]
C. thermoaceticum	–	7.37	280	823	pH 8.1, Tris Cl
β-Fructofuranosidase (see invertase)					
Fructokinase Rat liver	–	20	280	1447	pH 7, 0.12 M P$_i$, data from Figure 9 [1447]
Fructose-1,6-bisphosphatase (hexose bisphosphatase) (EC 3.1.3.11) (see also aldolase)					
Chicken					
Muscle	–	7.4	280	1448	–
Liver	–	7.4	280	1448	–

MOLAR ABSORPTIVITY AND $A_{1cm}^{1\%}$ VALUES FOR PROTEINS AT SELECTED WAVELENGTHS OF THE ULTRAVIOLET AND VISIBLE REGION (Continued)

Protein	ϵ^a $(\times 10^{-4})$	$A_{1cm}^{1\%\ b}$	nm^c	Reference	Comments[d]
Pig kidney	–	8.9	280	1448	pH 8.0, 0.05 M Tris Cl
	–	7.55	280	172	–
Rabbit					
Liver	–	8.9	280	824	–
	–	5.3	260	824	–
	–	8.3	280	174	–
Liver (neutral)	5.18	3.70	280	1450	Dry wt., MW = 140,000 [1450]
Liver (alkaline)	11.6	8.9	280	1451	MW = 130,000 [1451]
Muscle	–	6.1	260	1451	
	–	9.4	280	173	–
Kidney	9.7	6.9	280	1452	Dry wt., MW = 140,000 [1452]
L-Fucose binding *Lotus tetragonolobus*					
A	21.4	17.8	280	452	MW = 120,000 [452]
B	12.2	20.9	280	452	MW = 58,000 [452]
C	20.4	17.4	280	452	MW = 117,000 [452]
Fumarase (fumarate hydratase) (EC 4.2.1.2)					
Pig heart	9.9	5.1	280	175	pH 7.3, MW = 194,000 [175]
Pig heart muscle	11.65	5.3	280	1334	pH 7.2, 0.005 M P$_i$, MW = 220,000 [1453]
α-Galactosidase (EC 3.2.1.22)					
Sweet almonds	8.32	25.5	276	176	MW = 33,000 [176]
	7.99	24.3	280	176	MW = 33,000 [176]
Vicia sativa	2.7	9	280	591	pH 7.2, Tris Cl 10 mM MW = 30,000 [591], data from Figure 4 [591]
α-Galactosidase I					
Vicia faba	37.6	18	280	590	MW = 209,000 [590]
α-Galactosidase II					
Vicia faba	7.6	20	280	590	MW = 38,000 [590]
	7.2	19	278	590	MW = 38,000 [590]
β-Galactosidase (EC 3.2.1.23)					
E. coli ML 309	143.3	19.1	280	177	MW = 750,000 [178]
E. coli K12		19.1	280	1454	–
Galactosyl transferase A protein (lactose synthase, EC 2.4.1.22)					
Milk	5.3	12	279	1455	MW = 44,000 [1455]
Galactothermin		7.4	280	1456	pH 6.8, 0.01 M P$_i$
Human milk	1.04	7.4	277	965	0.1 M HCl, MW = 14,000 [965]
	1.20	8.55	290	965 ⎫	
	1.13	8.15	283	965 ⎭	0.1 M NaOH, MW = 14,000 [965]
Gastricsin					
Human gastric juice	–	4.56	247	1457	–
(Pepsin C, EC 3.4.23.3)	–	12.83	278	1457	–
Gastrin					
Human	4.83	15.32	278	179	MW = 31,500 [179]
Pig	5.02	15.3	280	180	MW = 32,500 [180]
Gliadin					
α-, Wheat	2.9	5.8	276	181	pH 0.7, 6 M HCl, or pH 3.0, 0.001 M HCl, MW = 5 0,000 [181]
	4.45	8.9	290	181	0.1 N NaOH, MW = 50,000 [181]
Hard, red winter wheat	–	5.7	276	1458	Dry wt., corrected for light scattering
α$_{1b}^-$	–	5.6	276	1458	–
α$_{1c}^-$	–	5.6	276	1458	–
α$_2^-$	–	5.6	276	1458	–
Globin					
Human	–	8.75	280	182	–
	–	8.5	280	183	
	–	8.74	280	184	pH 4.8, ionic strength 0.05
	3.36	8.0	280	185	MW = 42,000 [185]
	–	10.62	280	1459	Dry wt.
Horse	–	8.5	280	1460	–
Beef	–	7.9	280	1460	–

MOLAR ABSORPTIVITY AND $A_{1cm}^{1\%}$ VALUES FOR PROTEINS AT SELECTED WAVELENGTHS OF THE ULTRAVIOLET AND VISIBLE REGION (Continued)

Protein	ϵ^a ($\times 10^{-4}$)	$A_{1cm}^{1\% \, b}$	nm^c	Reference	Comments^d
Dog	–	8.9	280	1460	–
Rabbit	–	8.5	280	1460	
Rat	–	8.7	280	1460	
Chironomus thummi thummi	–	7.23	282	1461	Dry wt.
Globulin					
α-, human hepatoma	–	5.26	278	1462	Dry wt.
α-, human	1.0		280	1463	–
β-, human	1.54		280	1463	–
$β_{1c}^-$, human	–	10.0	280	186	–
$β_2^-$, micro-, human	1.99	16.8	280	187	pH 7.0, 0.1 $M\,P_i$, MW = 11,815 [187]
γ-, low MW human	1.72	10.1	280	188	MW = 17,000 [188]
Corticosteroid binding					
Human	3.78	7.4	279	189	MW = 51,700 [189]
Rabbit	3.43	8.4	279	190	MW = 40,700 [190]
Rat	3.84	6.2	279	191	MW = 61,000 [191]
Thyroxine binding					
Human	5.1	8.9	280	192	MW = 58,000 [192]
Rabbit lens					
1	–	8.5	$-^{k\dagger}$	440	–
2	–	4.5	$-^{k\dagger}$	440	–
3	–	4.5	$-^{k\dagger}$	440	–
4	–	4.4	$-^{k\dagger}$	440	–
5	–	4.2	$-^{k\dagger}$	440	–
Globulin, 75, soybean	–	6.9	280	1464	Dry wt.
Globulin, 11 S (Glycinin)	9.85	5.47	280	446	MW = 180,000 [447]
Soybean seed (Glycine max)	–	8.04	280	1465	–
Globulin, cold-insoluble					
Human plasma	–	12.8	280	825	pH 7.0, 0.05 $M\,P_i$, 0.15 M NaCl
	–	14.8	282	825	0.1 N NaOH-5 M urea
Glucagon					
Commercial	–	23.0	280	1466 ⎫	
	0.72	–	260	1466 ⎬	pH 10.0, 0.2 $M\,P_i$
	1.1	–	250	1466 ⎭	
Pig	–	23.0	279	1467	0.1 M glycine/0.1 M NaCl/0.1 N NaOH, pH 10.4
Beef	0.83	23.8	278	193	pH 2, MW = 3647 [193]
Glucanase, exo-β-D-[1 →, 3] (EXO-1-β-glucosidase, EC 3.2.1.58)					
Basidomycete QM 806	9.2	18.1	280	194	MW = 51,000 [194]
Gluconolactonase (see lactonase)					
Glucose dehydrogenase (EC 1.1.1.47 or .118 or .119)					
Bacterium anitratum	–	9.1	280	966	pH 7.0, 0.06 $M\,P_i$, data from Figure 1 [966]
Soluble	1.56	–	350	195	Oxidized state
	3.89	–	339	195	Reduced state
Glucose isomerase (EC 5.3.1.18)					
Streptomyces	15.7	10	280	692	MW = 157,000 [692]
Bacillus coagulans	17.0	10.6	280	826	pH 6.0, 0.1 M AcONa, MW = 160,000 [826]
	17.0	10.6	280	826 ⎫	0.1 M NaOH, data from Figure 7 [826], MW = 160,000.
	23.8	14.9	290	826 ⎭	
Glucose oxidase (EC. 1.1.3.4)					
A. niger	31.1	16.7	280	196	MW = 186,000 [196]
Penicillium amagasukiense	18.8	11.9	278	967	MW = 158,000 [967]
Apo-	19.2	–	278	1468	–
Glucose-6-phosphate dehydrogenase (EC 1.1.1.49)					
Human erythrocyte	–	6.15	280	693	–
Leuconostoc mesenteroides	11.9	11.5	280.5	968	MW = 103,700 [968]
D-Glucose-6-phosphate ketol isomerase (EC 5.2.1.9)					
Pea	9.6	8.75	280	197	MW = 110,000 [197]

MOLAR ABSORPTIVITY AND $A_{1cm}^{1\%}$ VALUES FOR PROTEINS AT SELECTED WAVELENGTHS OF THE ULTRAVIOLET AND VISIBLE REGION (Continued)

Protein	ϵ^a ($\times 10^{-4}$)	$A_{1cm}^{1\%\,b}$	nm^c	Reference	Comments^d
α-Glucosidase (EC 3.2.1.20)					
Beef liver	14.35	13.4	280	694	MW = 107,000 [694]
	11.2	10.5	288	694	
β-Glucosidase (EC 3.2.1.21)					
Aspergillus wentii	33.8	19.1	278	1469	MW = 170,000 [1470]
Sweet almonds	–	21.8	278	696	–
A	–	18.8	278	695	–
B	–	18.2	278	695	–
β-Glucuronidase (EC 3.2.1.31)					
Beef liver	47.6	17	280	198	pH 5, MW = 280,000 [198]
Glutamate decarboxylase (EC 4.1.1.15)					
E. coli	51.0	17	280	827	pH 7.0, MW = 300,000 [827]
Glutamate dehydrogenase (EC 1.4.1.2–4)					
Commercial	46.5	–$^{b^*}$	279	1471	MW = 56,100 [1472]
Clostridium SB4	–	10.7	280	1473	DR
Beef liver	–	9.3	280	1474	Dry wt., pH 7.0, 0.11 M P$_i$
	–	8.9	280		
	–	9.5	280	1474 / 1475	Dry wt., pH 7.0, 0.11 M P$_i$, corrected for light scattering, pH 7.6, M/15 KNaP$_i$
Frog liver	–	9.5	280	828	–
Pig liver	–	9.7	279	829	–
Glutamate dehydrogenase, (NAD dependent) (EC 1.4.1.2)					
C1. SB$_4$	29.4	10.7	280	830	pH 7, 50 mM KP$_i$ or pH 7.4, 50 mM Tris Cl, MW = 275,000 [830]
Glutamate mutase (methylaspartate mutase, EC 5.4.99.1)					
C. tetanomorphum H 1					
Component E	7.94	6.2	280	831	MW = 128,000 [831]
Component S	1.1	6.44	280	199	MW = 17,000 [199]
Glutamic dehydrogenase (EC 1.4.1.4)					
E. coli	–	12.9	278	1476	Dry wt., Kjeldahl, and ash^e
Beef liver	–	10.0	280	200	–
	–	9.73	279	201	pH 7, 0.2 M P$_i$
	–	8.55	276	202	5.1 M GdmCl
	–	9.71	279	203	–
	–	8.20	279	203	6 M GdmCl
Frog, liver	23.8	9.5	280	204	pH 8.0, 0.1 M Tris-AcO$^-$, 0.0001 M EDTA, MW = 250,000 [204]
Glutamin-(asparagin-)ase (EC 3.5.1.38)					
Achromobacteracae	–	10.2	280	1477	pH 7.2, 0.01 M NaP$_i$
Glutaminy 1-peptide glutaminase (see peptidoglutaminase 11)					
Glutamine cyclotransferase (glutaminyl-tRNA cyclotransferase, EC 2.3.2.5)	3.6	14.3	280	205	MW = 25,000 [205]
Glutamine phosphoribosylpyro-phosphateamidotransferase (amidophosphoribosyl transferase, EC 2.4.2.14)					
Pigeon liver	1.02	–	415	206	–
	8.18	8.18	279	207	MW = 100,000 [207]
Glutamine synthetase (EC 6.3.1.2)					
Pig brain	51	13.8	279	1478	pH 7.2, MW = 370,000 [1478]
Sheep brain	–	10.0	280	208	–
	–	13.5	280	832	–
E. coli	52.4	7.7	280	209	pH 7.0, 0.01 M imidazole HCl, MW = 680,000 [210]
Glutamine transaminase (EC 2.6.1.15)					
Rat liver	–	6.5	280	1479	
	–	3.26	260	1479	Lowry^e, pH 7.2, 0.005 M KP$_i$
	–	0.78	415	1479	
γ-Glutamylcysteine synthetase (EC 6.3.2.2)					
Rat kidney	10.6	11.5	280	1480	Lowry^e, MW = 92,000 [1480]

$^{b^*}$ Duplicate analyses: 8.31 and 8.36.

MOLAR ABSORPTIVITY AND $A_{1cm}^{1\%}$ VALUES FOR PROTEINS AT SELECTED WAVELENGTHS OF THE ULTRAVIOLET AND VISIBLE REGION (Continued)

Protein	ϵ^a ($\times 10^{-4}$)	$A_{1cm}^{1\% \; b}$	nm^c	Reference	Comments^d
Glutathione peroxidase (EC 1.11.1.9)					
Beef blood	6.3	7.5	280	969	MW = 84,000 [969]
Glutathione reductase (EC 1.6.4.2)					
Yeast	12.0	10.5	280	211	MW = 118,000 [211], protein det. by dry wt.
	–	18.6	280	212	Used biuret method for protein det.
	–	14.5	280	212	Protein det. by dry wt.
	18.6	15.4	280	213	MW = 121,000 [213]
Human red blood cell	19.5	16.3	275	214	Estimated from Figure 8 [214], MW = 120,000 [214]
Penicillium chrysogenum	–	18.6	280	833	
Rice embryos	9.51	9.1	275	1481	
	18.3	17.6	280	1481	
	1.09	10.5	370	1481	MW = 104,000 [1481]
	1.10	10.6	379	1481	
	1.16	11.1	463	1481	
Gluten					
Wheat	–	6.20	276	1482	
S-β-(1-Pyridylethyl)-	–	7.07	275	1482	pH 2, 0.01 *N* HCl
Acrylonitrile derivative	–	6.58	276	1482	
Glyceraldehyde-3-phosphate dehydrogenase (EC 1.2.1.12)					
Pig	–	9.6	280	970	5 *M* GdmCl
	14	10	280	971	0.1 *M* NaOH, MW = 140,000 [971]
	–	9.6	280	972	
Apo-	12.7	9.1	280	971	0.1 *N* NaOH, MW = 140,000 [971]
Pig, skeletal	–	9	280	221	0.1 NaOH, coenzyme free
Rabbit	17.5	12.7	280	973	MW = 145,000 [973]
	–	10.6	276	974	–
	–	8.15	280	974	Charcoal-treated enzyme
Rabbit muscle	–	10.3	280	1483	–
Denatured	3.0	–	337	1484	–
Furylacryloyl-	3.0	–	344	1484	–
Chicken heart	14	10.2	280	1485	MW = 137,600 [1485]
Lobster	–	5.55	290	975	–
	14	10	280	976	MW = 140,000 [977]
	–	9.6	280	978	With 4 NAD$^+$
	–	8.0	280	979	Charcoal treated
Lobster, muscle	14.8	10.1	276	218	MW = 146,650 [219]
	–	9.6	280	220	pH 8.5, 0.05 *M*, Na PP$_i$
Yeast	–	8.94	280	215	–
	10.9	9.08	280	216	MW = 120,000 [216]
	12.4	8.6	280	217	MW = 144,700 [217]
	–	9.4	280	980	–
	–	8.6	280	981	–
Apo-	–	8.94	280	982	–
	–	8.2	280	1485	–
Human erythrocyte	13.6	9.9	280	983	pH 8.0, 0.05 *M* Tris Cl, MW = 137,000 [983]
Beef liver	13.0	9.13	280	984	MW = 142,000 [984]
E. coli	14.4	10	280	1486	pH 8, 20 m*M* Tris Cl, 2 m*M* EDTA
Rabbit muscle	11.5	9.8	280	222	MW = 118,000 [222]
	11.4	8.29	280	223	MW = 138,000 [223], charcoal treated
	14.9	10.3	280	217	pH 8, PP$_i$, MW = 144,000 [217]
Glycerol dehydrogenase (EC 1.1.1.6)					
Aspergillus niger	–	17	280	985	pH 7.2, P$_i$
Glycerol kinase (EC 2.7.1.30)					
E. coli	–	15.6	280	986	pH 6.5, 6 *M* GdmCl, data from Figure 7 [986]
	–	14.1	280	986	pH 12.5, data from Figure 7 [986]
	–	14.7	290	986	
Glycerol-3-phosphate dehydrogenase (EC 1.1.1.8, EC 1.1.99.5)					
Apis mellifera, thorax	–	3.3	280	226	pH 7.8

MOLAR ABSORPTIVITY AND $A_{1cm}^{1\%}$ VALUES FOR PROTEINS AT SELECTED WAVELENGTHS OF THE ULTRAVIOLET AND VISIBLE REGION (Continued)

Protein	ϵ^a ($\times 10^{-4}$)	$A_{1cm}^{1\% \ b}$	nm[c]	Reference	Comments[d]
	2.5	–	280	227	pH 7.5
Chicken					
Liver	3.59[d*]	–	280	1488	–
Muscle	2.83[d*]	–	280	1488	–
Rabbit muscle	4.2	7.0	280	987	
	4.4	7.3	280	988	MW = 60,000 [987]
	3.8	6.3	280	989	
	–	6.3	280	224	–
	–	5.3	280	224	Charcoal treated
	–	7.5	280	141	–
	3.8	6.5	280	225	pH 6.6, 0.02 MP$_i$, MW = 58,300 [225]
	3.52	6.0	280	225	pH 7.2, 0.1 MP$_i$, MW = 58,300 [225]
Rat liver					
Fraction 1 enzyme	11.0	18.3	280	1487	pH 7.2, 0.1 MP$_i$, MW = 60,000 [1487]
Fraction 2 enzyme	4.0	6.7	280	1487	
Glycinin					
Soybean flakes	32.2	9.2	280	990	MW = 350,000 [991]
Glycocyaminekinase (guanidinoacetate kinase, EC 2.7.3.1)					
Nephthys coeca	7.5	8.6	278	228	pH 8.1, Tris-AcO⁻ 0.1 M10⁻⁴ MEDTA, MW = 87,500 [228]
Glyco-α-lactalbumin					
Cow's milk	–	17.7	280	1489	–
Glycollate oxidase (EC 1.1.3.1)					
Spinach	–	7.7	280	1490	Calcd. from Figure 3 [1490], pH 8.3
Glycoprotein					
Envelope-specific, E. coli	–	11	278	229	–
Tamm-Horsfall					
Rabbit urine	–	6.7	277	1503e	Water and 6 MGdmCl
Human urine	–	13	277	1491	Calcd. from Figure 1 [1491]
	–	10.8	277	1492	–
	–	9.5	277	1493	6 MGdmCl
	–	9.4	277	1493	Water
Acceptor of glycosyl transferase					
Rat intestinal mucosa	–	4.8	278	1494	–
Glycoprotein (α-globulin)					
Mouse plasma	–	8.8	278	1495	–
Tumor	–	11.6	278	1495	–
α_1-Glycoprotein, human					
Easily precipitable	4.5	9.0	280	230	MW = 50,000 [230]
Tryptophan poor	–	6.0	280	231	–
Acid (Orosomucoid)	3.9	8.9	280	232	MW = 44,100 [233]
Liver	4.0	9.16	279	1497	MW = 43,600 [1497]
Blood					
Variant pi 3.0	–	9.38	278	1498	–
Variant pi 3.2	–	9.31	278	1498	–
Variant pi 3.4	–	9.32	278	1498	–
Pool	–	9.33	278	1498	–
Serum	–	18.2	280	1503c	pH 7.0, 1/15 MP$_i$
Anti-trypsin	2.3	5.3	280		MW = 45,000 [234]
Chimpanzee plasma	–	8.52	278	1496	–
α_2-Glycoprotein					
Neuramino	–	5.0	280	235	–
Zinc	–	18	280	236	–
Histidine-rich 3.8S human serum	–	5.85	280	1499	–
Macroglobulin heat labile	68.9	8.4	280	8	MW = 820,000 [238]

[d*] Average of values obtained for two different preparations.

MOLAR ABSORPTIVITY AND $A_{1cm}^{1\%}$ VALUES FOR PROTEINS AT SELECTED WAVELENGTHS OF THE ULTRAVIOLET AND VISIBLE REGION (Continued)

Protein	ϵ^a ($\times 10^{-4}$)	$A_{1cm}^{1\%}$ [b]	nm[c]	Reference	Comments[d]
α_{2HS}-Glycoprotein	2.7	5.6	280	230	MW = 49,000 [237]
α_2, -β_1-Glycoprotein human plasma	–	11.5	278	1500	pH 6, 0.1 M NaCl
α_3-Glycoprotein, 8S human serum	–	10.0	280	1501	–
α_{ix}-Glycoprotein	–	6.0	280	230	
β-Glycoprotein glycine-rich					
Human serum	–	6.2	280	1502	–
β_1-Glycoprotein sialic acid free					
Human plasma	–	11.2	278	1503	pH 7
γ-Glycoprotein glycine-rich					
Human serum	–	10.0	280	1503d	–
Glyoxylate reductase (EC 1.1.1.26)					
Spinach leaves	–	9.76	280	834	Protein det. by Lowry method
	–	10.7	280	834	Protein det. by dry wt. and N
Isozyme R_f 0.22	–	10.8	280	834	–
Isozyme R_f 0.19	–	14.5	280	834	–
Isozyme R_f 0.17	–	13.8	280	834	–
Gramicidin A, HO-NBzl[e*]	7.25[f*]	–	410	1503f	
	7.27[g*]	–	410	1503f	0.1 N Na$_2$CO$_3$
	3.58[f*]	–	270	1503f	
	3.73[g*]	–	270	1503f	
Gramicidin D, HO-NBzl[e*]	7.18	–	410	1503f	0.1 N Na$_2$CO$_3$
	4.17	–	270	1503f	
Growth hormone					
Beef	–	1	280	239	–
	–	6.5	280	835	–
Haptoglobin human, type I					
Plasma	–	11.0	278	697	0.1 N HCl, pH 1
	–	11.9	278	697	0.02 M HCO$_3^-$, pH 8.6
	–	11.1	278	697	0.1 M NaOH, pH 12
Urine	–	12.7	278	697	0.02 M HCO$_3^-$, pH 8.6
Type II	–	15.6	278	698	–
	–	11.2	280	697	0.1 N HCl, pH 1
	–	12.1	280	697	0.02 M HCO$_3^-$, pH 8.6
	–	11.5	280	697	0.1 NaOH, pH 12
Type II complex with hemoglobin	–	14.5	280	698	–
	–	29	408	698	–
Canine	9.4	11.6	–	699	MW = 81,000 [699]
Haptoglobin 1–1, human	10.5	–	280	1503g	–
Haptoglobulin					
Human	12.1	12.1	280	240	MW = 100,000 [240]
	–	11.6	278	241	–
Hemagglutinin					
P. lunatus	–	12.3	280	836	–
Agaricus campestris	10.5	16.4	280	837	MW = 64,000 [837]
Pisum sp. (Peas)		10	280	1504	From Figure 1 [1504]
Phascolus vulgaris	9.6	10.5[h*]	280	1505	pH 2, 0.01 M HCl
Lens culimris	5.6	12.5	280	1506	MW = 44,050 [1506]
L. culimris A	6.2	12.6	280	1507	MW = 49,000 [1507]
L. culimris B	6.2	12.6	280	1507	
Hemerythrin					
Phascolosoma gouidii					
Coelomic fluid					
Methemerythrin					

[e*] HO-NBzl, 2-hydroxy-5-nitrobenzyl group.
[f*] Same fraction of two fractions.
[g*] Same fraction of two fractions.
[h*] Calculated from the amino acid analysis.

MOLAR ABSORPTIVITY AND $A_{1cm}^{1\%}$ VALUES FOR PROTEINS AT SELECTED WAVELENGTHS OF THE ULTRAVIOLET AND VISIBLE REGION (Continued)

Protein	ϵ^a ($\times 10^{-4}$)	$A_{1cm}^{1\% \, b}$	nm^c	Reference	Comments^d
Azide	0.019	–	680	1508	
	0.370	–	446	1508	
	0.675	–	326	1508	
Bromide	0.0165	–	677	1508	
	0.540	–	387	1508	ϵ/dimeric iron unit
	0.650	–	331	1508	
Chloride	0.018	–	656	1508	
	0.600	–	380	1508	
	0.660	–	329	1508	
Cyanate	0.0166	–	650	1508	
	0.650	–	377	1508	
	0.655	–	334	1508	
Cyanide	0.014	–	695	1508	
	0.077	–	493	1508	
	0.530	–	374	1508	
	0.640	–	330	1508	
Fluoride	0.500	–	362	1508	ϵ/dimeric iron unit
	0.560	–	317	1508	
Hydroxide	0.016	–	597	1508	
	0.590	–	362	1508	
	0.680	–	320	1508	
Thiocyanate	0.020	–	674	1508	
	0.510	–	452	1508	
	0.720	–	327	1508	
Water	0.640	–	355	1508	
	0.630	–	340	1508	ϵ/dimeric iron unit, plus iodide
Oxyhemerythrin	0.220	–	500	1508	ϵ/dimeric iron unit
	0.680	–	330	1508	
Dendrostomum pyroides	–	30.3	280	838	Protein det. by Biuret method
	–	31.0	280	838	Protein det. by Lowry method
Golfingia gouldii	–	25.8	280	839	–
Hemocyanin					
Busycon canaliculatum	–	15.1	280	1512	
	–	3.28	345	1512	
Cancer borealis	–	14.0	280	1512	FC, pH 8.2 Tris cont. 0.01 A/MgCl$_2$;^{9} SC
	–	2.29	336	1512	
Cancer magister	–	15.0	280	1512	
25S particle	–	14.7	279	843	pH 7.0, Tris
5S particle	–	14.1	–	843	pH 10, Bicarbonate
Carcinus meanas	–	14.2	280	1512	FC, pH 8.2 Tris cont. 0.01 M MgClj, SC
	–	2.33	335	1512	
C. sapidus	–	12.4	278	243	–
Dolabella auricularia (Gastropod)	9.84	17.6	278	1509	MW = 55,800 [1509]
Eriphia spinifrons	–	12.07	278	1510	pH 7.2, 0.01
(Arthropod)	–	12.7	278	1510	pH 9.7, 0.05 M CO$_3^{2-}$
	–	16.1	278	243	–
E. moschata	–	14.9	278	243	–
Homarus americanus	–	14.3	280	1512	FC, pH 8.2 Tris cont. 0.01 M MgCl$_2$, SC
	–	2.69	335	1512	
	–	13.4	280	840	pH 9.6, 0.014 M Ca^{++}, glycine buffer, protein det. by dry wt.
H. vulgaris	–	14.4	278	243	–
Levantina hierosolima	–	4.0	345	846	pH 6.6, oxygenated
	–	3.4	348	846	pH 12
Limulus polyphemus	–	13.9	280	1512	FC, pH 8.2 Tris cont. 0.01 M MgCl$_2$, SC
	–	2.23	340	1512	
	–	11.2	278	243	–
Loligo pealii	–	2.79	345	1512	FC, pH 8.2 Tris cont. 0.01 M MgCl$_2$, SC

MOLAR ABSORPTIVITY AND $A_{1cm}^{1\%}$ VALUES FOR PROTEINS AT SELECTED WAVELENGTHS OF THE ULTRAVIOLET AND VISIBLE REGION (Continued)

Protein	ϵ^a ($\times 10^{-4}$)	$A_{1cm}^{1\% \, b}$	nm^c	Reference	Comments[d]
	–	15.8	278	243	–
Helix pomatia	–	16.1	278	841	pH 9.2, borate
α-	–	13.8	278	242	–
β-	–	14.1	278	242	–
Succinylated	–	14.16	278	842	pH 9.2, 0.1 M Na$_2$ B$_4$ O$_7$
Megathura crenulata	–	17.7	280	844	Protein det. by dry wt.
	–	15.5	280	845	
Mwex trunculus (Whelk)	–	13.9	280	1511	pH 9.2
	–	18.9	278	243	–
Apo-	–	13.9	280	1511	pH 9.2
M. brandacis	–	18.1	278	243	–
O. vulgaris	–	13.5	278	243	–
O. macropus	–	16.6	278	243	–
Pagarus pollicarus	–	15.6	280	1512 ⎫	FC, pH 8.2 Tris cont. 0.01 M MgCl$_2$, SC
	–	2.58	335	1512 ⎭	
P. vulgaris	–	13.8	278	243	–
Hemoglobin					
Aphrodite aculeata					
(Polychaet annelid)[i*] nerves/ganglia	12.6	–	425	1513	–
	1.41	–	549	1513	–
	1.48	–	566	1513	–
HbO$_2$	14.7	–	414	1513	–
	1.70	–	541	1513	–
	1.84	–	577	1513	–
HbCO	22.0	–	419	1513	–
	1.82	–	537	1513	–
	1.84	–	567	1513	–
HbCN	14.6	–	434	1513	–
	1.5	–	536	1513	–
	1.9	–	564	1513	–
Aplysia californica (Mollusc)[i*] nerves	12.0	–	435	1513	–
	1.3	–	560	1513	–
HbO$_2$	13.0	–	416	1513	–
	1.5	–	543	1513	–
	1.4	–	578	1513	–
HbCO	17.0	–	423	1513	–
	1.5	–	541	1513	–
	1.4	–	571	1513	–
HbCN	15.0	–	437	1513	–
	1.6	–	539	1513	–
	1.8	–	568	1513	–
Ascaris, bodywall					
Oxygenated	0.22		621	700 ⎫	
	1.11		578	700	
	1.25		543	700	
	11.7		412	700	
Deoxygenated	0.3		615	700	
	1.32		556	700 ⎬	0.1 M P$_i$, pH 7.0, ϵ_M values expressed per mole heme
	11.1		429	700	
Carbon monoxide	0.31		614	700	
	1.32		566	700	
	1.33		538	700	
	18.2		419	700 ⎭	

<hr>

[i*] ϵ/mole heme.

MOLAR ABSORPTIVITY AND $A_{1cm}^{1\%}$ VALUES FOR PROTEINS AT SELECTED WAVELENGTHS OF THE ULTRAVIOLET AND VISIBLE REGION (Continued)

Protein	ϵ^a ($\times 10^{-4}$)	$A_{1cm}^{1\%\,b}$	nm^c	Reference	Comments^d
Cyanide	0.31		614	700	
	2.1		562	700	
	1.47		532	700	
	14.7		429	700	
Methemoglobin, acid	0.23		635	700	0.1 $M\,P_i$, pH 7.0, ϵ_M values expressed per mole heme
	1.02		499	700	
	14.1		405	700	
Methemoglobin, cyanide	1.2		542	700	
	10.9		417	700	
Ascaris lumbricoides					
Perienteric fluid^{i*}	1.22	–	553.5	1515	
	10.9	–	429.5	1515	
HbO$_2$	1.04	–	576.5	1515	pH 7.0, 0.1 $M\,P_i$
	1.23	–	542	1515	
	10.95	–	412	1515	
HbO$_2$I*	11.0	–	412	1514	
	1.23	–	541	1514	
	1.04	–	575	1514	
Hb IV^{i*}	9.75	–	411	1514	At 27 3° K
	1.06	–	542	1514	
	0.87	–	576	1514	
HbCO	1.28	–	568	1515	
	1.27	–	538	1515	
	16.8	–	417.5	1515	
HbCN	2.02	–	564	1515	
	1.48	–	534	1515	
	14.9	–	431	1515	
MetHb					
Acid	0.36	–	632	1515	pH 7.0.0.1 $M\,P_i$
	1.06	–	501	1515	
	15.5	–	404	1515	
CN$^-$	1.22	–	540	1515	
	11.4	–	417	1515	
N$_3^-$	0.31	–	630	1515	
	1.08	–	540	1515	
	11.7	–	414	1515	
Biomphalaria glabrata (Mollusc)	–	23.8	280	1516	Lowry, dry wt.
Glycera dibranchiata (Common bloodworm)					
Fe^{2+}-O$_2$ (P)^{k*}	1.51	–	576	1517	
	1.47	–	540	1517	
	14.2	–	414	1517	
Fe^{2+}-O$_2$ (M)^{l*}	1.71	–	575	1517	
	1.65	–	540	1517	
	14.2	–	420	1517	
Fe^{2+}-CO (P)	1.46	–	569	1517	pH 7, 0.1 $M\,P_i$, ϵ/mole hematin
	1.51	–	538	1517	
	19.8	–	419	1517	
Fe^{2+}-CO (M)	1.62	–	569	1517	
	1.63	–	538	1517	
	23.2	–	422	1517	
Fe^{2+}-H$_2$O (P)	1.34	–	555	1517	
	13.5	–	428	1517	
Fe^{2+}-H$_2$O (M)	1.47	–	564	1517	pH 7, 0.1 $M\,P_i$, ϵ/mole hematin
	11.7	–	429	1517	
Fe^{3+}-H$_2$O (P)	0.32	–	632	1517	

^{i*} Prepared from deoxyhemoglobin.
^{k*} (P) = polymer.
^{l*} (M) = monomer.

MOLAR ABSORPTIVITY AND $A_{1cm}^{1\%}$ VALUES FOR PROTEINS AT SELECTED WAVELENGTHS OF THE ULTRAVIOLET AND VISIBLE REGION (Continued)

Protein	ϵ^a ($\times 10^{-4}$)	$A_{1cm}^{1\% \, b}$	nm^c	Reference	Comments[d]
	0.95	–	503	1517	
	15.0	–	408	1517	
Fe^{3+}-H_2O (M)	0.32	–	637	1517	
	1.48	–	505	1517	
	12.9	–	391	1517	
Fe^{3+}-CN^- (P)	1.11	–	536	1517	
	13.9	–	418	1517	
Fe^{3+}-CN^- (M)	1.20	–	545	1517	pH 7, 0.1 $M\,P_i$, ϵ/mole hematin
	14.3	–	420	1517	
Fe^{3+}-N_3^- (P)	0.89	–	573	1517	
	1.13	–	539	1517	
	12.5	–	416	1517	
Fe^{3+}-N_3^- (M)	1.14	–	575	1517	
	1.20	–	542	1517	
	13.1	–	419	1517	
Fe^{3+}-OH^- (P)	0.87	–	574	1517	
	0.97	–	537	1511	pH 10.5 glycine buffer, ϵ/hematin
	11.4	–	411	1517	
Fe^{3+}-OH^- (M)	0.76	–	576	1517	
	0.99	–	534	1517	pH 9.9, methylamine buffer, ϵ/hematin
	9.5	–	398	1517	
Fe^{3+}-F^- (M)	1.07	–	593	1517	pH 7, 0.1 $M\,P_i$, ϵ/hematin
	12.3	–	395	1517	
Cucumaria miniata Brandt (Echinoderm)					
HbCO	1.33	–	570	1518	
	1.31	–	539	1518	
	12.33	–	416	1518	
Cucumaria piperata Stimpson (Echinoderm)					
HbCO	1.66	–	570	1518	
	1.65	–	539	1518	AA
	14.89	–	417	1518	
Molpadia intermedia Ludwig (Echinoderm)					
HbCO[m]	1.31	–	570	1518	
	1.46	–	540	1518	
	14.69	–	418	1518	
Thunnus orientalis (Tuna)[n]					
	12.4	–	428–9	1519	–
	1.37	–	555	1519	–
HbO₂	13.3	–	411	1519	–
	1.49	–	540	1519	–
	1.53	–	575	1519	–
HbCO	20.3	–	418	1519	–
	1.51	–	538	1519	–
	1.44	–	568	1519	–
MetHb	14.4	–	405	1519	–
	0.98	–	500	1519	–
	0.42	–	630	1519	–
MetHbCN	11.5	–	418	1519	–
Anguilla japonica (Eel)[n] Component F					
	12.6	–	430–1	1519	–
	1.33	–	555	1519	–
HbO₂	11.5	–	415	1519	–
	1.39	–	540	1519	–
	1.42	–	575	1519	–
HbCO	17.8	–	420–1	1519	–
	1.46	–	537–9	1519	–
	1.34	–	568–70	1519	–

[m] Half-molecule of Hb-2.
[n] Hb concentration determined using the value of $\epsilon = 1.15 \times 10^4$ at 540 nm for MetHbCN.

MOLAR ABSORPTIVITY AND $A_{1cm}^{1\%}$ VALUES FOR PROTEINS AT SELECTED WAVELENGTHS OF THE ULTRAVIOLET AND VISIBLE REGION (Continued)

Protein	ϵ^a ($\times 10^{-4}$)	$A_{1cm}^{1\%\ b}$	nm^c	Reference	Comments^d
MetHb	9.3	–	408–9	1519	–
	0.9	–	520–2	1519	–
	0.3	–	630–2	1519	–
MetHbCN	8.S	–	421	1519	–
Component S					
	13.5	–	430–1	1519	–
	1.35	–	555	1519	–
HbO$_2$	13.2	–	410–2	1519	–
	1.39	–	540	1519	–
	1.43	–	575	1519	–
HbCO	17.5	–	418–9	1519	–
	1.43	–	538–9	1519	–
	1.38	–	567–9	1519	–
MetHb	15.3	–	404–5	1519	–
	0.99	–	500	1519	–
	0.44	–	630	1519	–
MetHbCN	10.1	–	419	1519	–
Misgurnus anguillicaudalus (Loach)^{n*}					
Component F					
	12.4	–	430	1520	–
	1.20	–	555	1520	–
HbO$_2$	13.2	–	413	1520	–
	1.48	–	540–1	1520	–
	1.53	–	576	1520	–
HbCO	20.6	–	418	1520	–
	1.53	–	538	1520	–
	1.46	–	568	1520	–
MetHb	19.4	–	404–5	1520	–
	0.43	–	630	1520	–
	0.96	–	–^{o*}	1520	–
MetHbCN	12.8	–	419	1520	–
Component S					
	12.2	–	430	1520	–
	1.18	–	555	1520	–
HbO$_2$	12.4	–	413	1520	–
	1.47	–	541	1520	–
	1.53	–	576–577	1520	–
HbCO	20.4	–	419	1520	–
	1.5	–	538	1520	–
	1.43	–	568	1520	–
MetHb	18.2	–	405	1520	–
	0.96	–	–^{p*}	1520	–
	0.43	–	630	1520	–
MetHbCN	11.7	–	419	1520	–
Oncorhynchus tshawytscha (Chinook salmon)					
HbCS-1					
MetHb	0.44	–	628	1521	
	0.88	–	498	1521	
	13.2	–	405	1521	Dry wt
	4.6	–	276	1521	
CarboxyHb	1.34	–	566	1521	
	1.38	–	537	1521	

^{o*} 499–502 nm.
^{p*} 499–503 nm.

MOLAR ABSORPTIVITY AND $A_{1cm}^{1\%}$ VALUES FOR PROTEINS AT SELECTED WAVELENGTHS OF THE ULTRAVIOLET AND VISIBLE REGION (Continued)

Protein	ϵ^a ($\times 10^{-4}$)	$A_{1cm}^{1\% \, b}$	nm^c	Reference	Comments^d
	16.4	–	419	1521	
HbCS-2					
MetHb	0.41	–	625	1521	
	0.89	–	499	1521	
	12.3	–	404	1521	Dry wt
	3.8	–	276	1521	
CarboxyHb	1.29	–	564	1521	
	1.36	–	534	1521	
	16.9	–	417	1521	
Salmo gairdneri (Rainbow trout)					
Hemoglobin RT-1					
MetHb	0.39	–	628	1521	
	0.71	–	497	1521	
	13.7	–	406	1521	
	4.5	–	276	1521	
CarboxyHb	1.32	–	567	1521	
	1.39	–	536	1521	
	17.5	–	419	1521	
Hemoglobin RT-3					Dry wt
MetHb	0.35	–	628	1521	
	0.79	–	500	1521	
	13.6	–	405	1521	
	4.2	–	277	1521	
CarboxyHb	1.28	–	566	1521	
	1.34	–	536	1521	
	16.2	–	419	1521	
Chironomus plumosus, Larvae haemolymph					
MetHbCN	1.28	4.0	540	1522	MW = 32,000 [1522]
Sheep					
Hb A, β chain	1.53	9.5	280	1523	MW = 16,134 [1523]
Hb B, β chain	1.46	9.0	280	1523	MW = 16,245 [1523]
Hb C, β chain	1.56	9.9	280	1523	MW = 15,788 [1523]
Beef					
MetHb	–	5.32	550	1524	FC
Horse					
Hb	13.5^{n*}	–	430–1	1519	–
	1.37^{n*}	–	555	1519	–
	59.6		406	1526	–
	–	16.8	280	1527	–
	–	630	191–4	1527	–
Apo-	–	8.5	280	1528	–
	4.95	–	280	1529	Corrected for scattering
HbO$_2$	12.4^{n*}	–	412–3	1519	
	1.52^{n*}	–	541	1519	–
	1.59^{n*}	–	576	1519	–
HbCO	20.6^{n*}	–	419–20	1519	See footnote^{q*}
	1.49^{n*}	–	538	1519	–
	1.50^{n*}	–	568	1519	–
MetHb	66	–	406	1525	–
	13.9^{n*}	–	405–6	1519	–
	0.97^{n*}	–	500	1519	–
	0.43^{n*}	–	630	1519	–
MetHbCN	9.5^{n*}	–	420	1519	–
Mouse					
Hb	–	17.5	280	1530	–
Human					
Hb A	12.7	–	430	709	pH 6.4, 0.1 MP$_i$

^{q*} $\epsilon = 18.5–19.0 \times 10^4$ at 419 nm; $1.25–1.43 \times 10^4$ at 538 nm; $1.22–1.37 \times 10^4$ at 569 nm (see Ref. 1534).

MOLAR ABSORPTIVITY AND $A_{1cm}^{1\%}$ VALUES FOR PROTEINS AT SELECTED WAVELENGTHS OF THE ULTRAVIOLET AND VISIBLE REGION (Continued)

Protein	ϵ^a ($\times 10^{-4}$)	$A_{1cm}^{1\%\,b}$	nm^c	Reference	Comments^d
Oxy	0.43	–	523	710	–
	1.57	–	542	710	–
	1.64	–	578	710	–
Deoxy	1.36	–	558	710	–
	0.27	–	583	710	–
Hb	3.14	–	275	1531	–
	11.8	–	430	1531	–
	1.29	–	552.5	1531	–
	0.0396	–	755	1531	–
Apo-	–	8.5	280	702	0.1 N NaOH
HbO$_2$	3.60	–	275	1531	
	2.88	–	350	1531	
	12.85	–	415	1531	
	1.42	–	541.5	1531	
	1.54	–	576	1531	
	–	8.5	541	703	–
	5.6	–	540	706	–
	5.9	–	576	706	–
Hb FII	–	22.0	280	1532	
Hb AII	–	21.8	280	1532	From Figure 5 [1532]
Hb β$_4$	–	22.2	280	1532	
Hb γ$_4$	–	23.9	280	1532	
HbCO	6.63	–	429	1533	–
	20.8	–	419	1533	–
	17.4	–	419	1534	–
	1.43	–	540	702	–
	–	8.4	540	703	–
Hb-BuNC^{r*}	18.75	–	429	1533	–
	9.65	–	419	1533	–
MesoHb	11.5	–	421	1535	–
	1.2	–	550	1535	–
MesoHbO$_2$	1.28	–	543	1535	–
	1.06	–	568	1535	–
MesoHbCO	21.0	–	410	1535	–
	1.39	–	532	1535	–
	1.26	–	560	1535	–
MesoHb$^+$	14.4	–	396	1535	
	0.89	–	495	1535	pH 7
	0.38	–	620	1535	
DeuteroHb	11.5	–	421	1535	–
	1.13	–	544	1535	–
DeuteroHbO$_2$	11.6	–	403	1535	–
	1.21	–	532	1535	–
	0.91	–	565	1535	–
DeuteroHbCO	20.0	–	408	1535	–
	1.22	–	528	1535	–
	0.93	–	556	1535	–
DeuteroHb$^+$	11.6	–	394	1535	
	0.71	–	500	1535	pH 7
	0.28	–	620	1535	
ChloroHb	13.0	–	443	1535	–
	1.85	–	567	1535	–
ChloroHbCo	14.0	–	432	1535	–
	1.70	–	550	1535	–
	2.00	–	590	1535	–

r* BuNC, butylisocyanide.

MOLAR ABSORPTIVITY AND $A_{1cm}^{1\%}$ VALUES FOR PROTEINS AT SELECTED WAVELENGTHS OF THE ULTRAVIOLET AND VISIBLE REGION (Continued)

Protein	ϵ^a ($\times 10^{-4}$)	$A_{1cm}^{1\% \, b}$	nm[c]	Reference	Comments[d]
ChloroHb[+]	13.0	–	421	1535	
	1.45	–	550	1535	pH 7
	1.30	–	598	1535	
HematoHb	11.3	–	423	1535	–
	1.33	–	552	1535	–
HematoHbCO	18.3	–	412	1535	–
	1.33	–	536	1535	–
	1.10	–	564	1535	–
HematoHb[+]	15.0	–	398	1535	
	1.00	–	501	1535	pH 7
	0.41	–	628	1535	
Fetal (7% adult)	–	9.87	576	1536	
	–	10.0	541	1536	
	–	18.8	290	1536	pH 7, 0.02 $M P_i$
	–	24.0	280	1536	
	–	24.8	270	1536	
Adult	–	10.2	576	1536	
	–	9.6	541	1536	
	–	18.8	290	1536	pH 7,0.02 $M P_i$
	–	23.3	280	1536	
	–	25.8	270	1536	
MetHbCn	4.350	–	540	1537	pH 7.4
	10.800	–	281	1537	
	4.388	–	540	1538	Fe det.
	4.284	–	540	1539	Fe det.
	4.360	–	540	1540	Nitrogen det.
Cyanmethemoglobin	1.1	–	540	702	–
	–	20	280	704	–
	–	80	416	704	–
	4.59	–	541	705	–
	12.02	–	280	705	–
MetHb	–	5.97	540	708	–
No source cited					
60% MetHb	–	15.6	280	701	–
	–	330	210	701	–
	–	910	191	701	–
Hemoglobin chains					
α-HgBzO[-s*]	11.1	–	428	709	
β-HgBzO[-]	11.2	–	428	709	
α-HgBzO[-] + β-HgBzO[-]	12.6	–	430	709	pH 6.4, 0.1 $M P_i$
α-SH[t*]	11.1	–	429	709	
β-SH[t*]	11.0	–	428	709	
α-SH + β-SH	12.4	–	430	709	
Hemoglobins, synthetic					
Proto Hb	14.0	–	430	1541	
	1.34	–	555	1541	
ProtoHbO$_2$	13.5	–	414	1541	pH 7.0, 0.1 $M P_i$
	1.48	–	541	1541	
	1.57	–	577	1541	
ProtometHb	15.4	–	406	1541	
	0.95	–	500	1541	pH 6.5, 0.1 $M P_i$
	0.38	–	630	1541	
DimethylprotoHb	14.0	–	430	1541	
	1.36	–	555	1541	
DimethylprotoHbO$_2$	13.3	–	414	1541	pH 7.0, 0.1 $M P_i$
	1.46	–	540	1541	
	1.53	–	577	1541	

[s*] -HgBzO[-], paramercuribenzoate.
[t*] SH, free sulfhydryl group.

MOLAR ABSORPTIVITY AND $A_{1cm}^{1\%}$ VALUES FOR PROTEINS AT SELECTED WAVELENGTHS OF THE ULTRAVIOLET AND VISIBLE REGION (Continued)

Protein	ϵ^a ($\times 10^{-4}$)	$A_{1cm}^{1\% \, b}$	nm^c	Reference	Comments^d
Dimethylproto MetHb	15.1	–	405	1541	
	0.94	–	500	1541	pH 6.5, 0.1 MP$_i$
	0.39	–	630	1541	
MesoHb	13.5	–	421	1541	
	1.33	–	546	1541	
MesoHbO$_2$	13.9	–	404	1541	pH 7.0, 0.1 MP$_i$
	1.38	–	534	1541	
	1.24	–	567	1541	
MesometHb	18.5	–	395	1541	pH 6.5, 0.1 MP$_i$
	0.73	–	620	1541	
Deoxy Hb	–	4.25	524.5	707	–
DimethylmesoHb	13.5	–	421	1541	
	1.37	–	545	1541	
DimethylmesoHbO$_3$	13.8	–	404	1541	
	1.40	–	534	1541	
	1.30	–	568	1541	
EtioHb	13.4	–	420	1541	pH 7.0, 0.1 MP$_i$
	1.20	–	540	1541	
EtioHbO$_2$	13.8	–	401	1541	
	1.33	–	532	1541	
	1.15	–	566	1541	
EtiometHb	18.1	–	395	1541	
	1.32	–	490	1541	pH 6.5, 0.1 MP$_i$
	0.65	–	620	1541	
HematoHb	13.7	–	426	1541	
	1.42	–	551	1541	
HematoHbO$_2$	13.4	–	409	1541	
	1.47	–	537	1541	
	1.28	–	572	1541	
DeuteroHb	11.9	–	420	1541	pH 7.0, 0.1 MP$_i$
	1.29	–	542	1541	
DeuteroHbO$_2$	11.5	–	402	1541	
	1.35	–	531	1541	
	0.94	–	564	1541	
Human Hb subunits					
αCO	–	8.4	540	1542	–
α-HgBzO$^-$-CO^{u*}	1.4	–	540	1543	–
Ferric α-HgBzO^{-u*}	11.65	–	410	1544	ϵ/mole heme
	1.04	–	533	1544	
α(Mn^{2+})	1.19	–	585	1545	–
	1.23	–	570	1545	–
	2.03	–	555	1545	–
	1.09	–	535	1545	–
	15.7	–	430	1545	–
	10.0	–	420	1545	–
Apo-α	1.62	–	280	1545	–
βCO	–	8.4	540	1542	–
β-Fe^{2+}-CO	0.55	–	585	1545	–
	1.52	–	570	1545	–
	1.30	–	555	1545	–
	1.54	–	535	1545	–
	6.78	–	430	1545	–
	20.9	–	420	1545	–
Apo-β	1.62	–	280	1545	–
Hemoglobin-reductase complex, Candida					
Mycoderma (Yeast)	12	–	278	1546	pH 6.0, 0.1 MKP$_i$
	14	–	415	1546	

^{u*} -HgBzO–, p-mercuribenzoate.

MOLAR ABSORPTIVITY AND $A_{1cm}^{1\%}$ VALUES FOR PROTEINS AT SELECTED WAVELENGTHS OF THE ULTRAVIOLET AND VISIBLE REGION (Continued)

Protein	ϵ^a ($\times 10^{-4}$)	$A_{1cm}^{1\% \, b}$	nm^c	Reference	Comments^d
	17	–	420	1546	+ $Na_2S_2O_4$ + CO
	11	–	423	1546	+ $Na_2S_2O_4$
Hemopexin	13.5	16.9	280	246	MW = 80,000 [246]
Rabbit	–	21.8	280	1547 }	pH 7.1, 0.05 M KP, 0.05 M KC1, dry wt
	–	19.2	414	1547 }	
Rabbit blood	–	23.9	280	992 }	
	–	26.4	280	992 }	Contains 1 heme
	–	23.2	413.5	992 }	
Apo-	–	19.7	280	1547	pH 7.1, 0.05 M KP, 0.05 M KCl, dry wt.
Human blood	–	23.8	280	992	–
		26.4	280	992 }	
	–	23.0	414	992 }	Contains 1 heme
Hemoprotein					
Chironomus thummi	–	71.5	415	244	Ferric form, calcd. from equation in Reference 244, mg = absorbance $\times f$ where $f = 0.14$
559, Beef heart	6.95	–	400	245	pH 9.5, oxidized
	8.84	–	266	245	pH 9.5, oxidized
	6.94	–	394	245	pH 12, oxidized
	1.37	–	559	245	pH 9.5, reduced
	0.958	–	530	245	pH 9.5, reduced
	8.95	–	423	245	pH 9.5, reduced
	2.5	–	557	245	pH 12, reduced
	1.48	–	528	245	pH 12, reduced
	1.33	–	422	245	pH 12, reduced, also data for oxidized and KCN and reduced and CO in Ref. [245]
Hepatocuprein					
Human liver	–	0.075	675	592	–
	–	5.87	265	592	–
	–	7.00	265	592	–
	–	5.6	278	593	pH 8.6
Hexokinase					
B, Yeast	–	9.16	280	247	pH 5.0, 5 mM, sodium succinate
	–	9.20	278	247	pH 5.0, 5 mM sodium succinate
Yeast	12.5	13	278	248	MW = 96,000 [248]
	10	9	280	1549	MW = 106,000 [1549], refractometry
Rat brain	5.1	–	280	1548	–
Hexosebisphosphatase (see fructose-1,6-bisphosphatase)					
High potential iron protein					
Chromatium, strain D	1.61	16.1	388	993	MW = 10,074 [993], reduced with HSEtOH
	1.86	18.6	450	993 }	
	2.0	20.0	375	993 }	MW = 10,074 [993], oxidized with ferricyanide, pH 7.0, 0.05 M P,
	2.18	21.8	325	993 }	
	41.3	4.1	283	443	Reduced, MW = 10,074 [443]
	39.3	3.9	283	443	Oxidized, MW = 10,074 [443]
Rhodopseudomonas gelatinosa	1.53	16	388	993	MW = 9,579, pH 7.0, 0.05 M P, reduced with HSEtOH
	1.69	17.6	450	993 }	
	1.88	19.6	375	993 }	MW = 9,579 pH 7.0, 0.05 M P,, oxidized with ferricyanide
	2.11	22.2	325	993 }	
	35.4	3.7	283	443	Reduced, MW = 9,579 [443]
	33.8	3.5	283	443	Oxidized, MW = 9,579 [443]
Histaminase					
Pig plasma	–	9.2	278	994 }	Data from Figure 4 [994]
	–	0.169	470	994 }	
Histidine ammonia lyase					
Pseudomonas ATCC 11299b	–	5.6	280	995	Data from Figure 7 [995]
	–	4.0	280	995	Data from Figure 7 [995], $NaBH_4$ added
	–	3.9	280	995	Data from Figure 7 [995], cysteine added
Pseudomonas	–	5.0	280	996	pH 7.2, 0.1 M KP =
	10.3	4.80	279	1550	MW = 215,000 [1550], dry wt.

MOLAR ABSORPTIVITY AND $A_{1cm}^{1\%}$ VALUES FOR PROTEINS AT SELECTED WAVELENGTHS OF THE ULTRAVIOLET AND VISIBLE REGION (Continued)

Protein	ϵ^a ($\times 10^{-4}$)	$A_{1cm}^{1\% \, b}$	nm^c	Reference	Comments^d
Histidine decarboxylase (EC 4.1.1.22)					
Lactobacillus 30a	–	16.1	280	249	pH 4.8, 0.2 M AcONH$_4$
	–	16.2	280	249	pH 8.0, 0.05 M NH$_4$HCO$_3$
	–	17.3	280	250	pH 4.8, 0.2 M AcONH$_4$
	6.3	16.1	280	997	MW = 38,800 [997]
Chain I	1.1	12.1	280	997	MW = 9,000 [997]
Chain II	5.1	17.2	280	997	MW = 29,700 [997]
Histidinol dehydrogenase (EC 1.1.1.23)					
S. typhimurium	3.6	4.8	280	251	pH 6, 0.05 M P$_i$, MW = 75,000 [251], data from Figure 3 [251]
S. typhimurium LT-2	3.8	4.78	280	252	pH 7.5, MW = 80,000 [253]
LT-7	–	4.63	280	254	pH 8.0, 0.01 M NH$_4$HCO$_3$
N. crassa	–	12.11	280	255	Water
Histidinol dehydrogenase–histidinolphosphate aminotransferase (EC 1.1.1.23, EC 2.6.1.9)					
Salmonella typhimurium LT 2					
Strain TM 220		15.3	279	998	pH 7.5, 0.1 M triethanol-amine HCl, data from Figure 9 [998]
Histone					
Chicken erythrocyte	2.9	18.6	275	999	MW = 15,714 HCl der. used
Calf thymus F-8$_{2a}$	–	1.5	276	1000	–
F-8$_{b[z]}$	–	4.0	276	1000	–
F-6$_{3bb}$	–	3.8	276	1000	–
P-4$_4$C$_b$	–	4.5	276	1000	–
P-8$_{a[z]}$	–	4.6	276	1000	–
Histone f2					
Calf thymus	–	12	276	1552	pH 6.5
Histone IV					
Calf thymus	0.0047	–	230	1551	ϵ /mole of residue/l
Homoserine deaminase (cystathione γ-lyase, EC 4.4.1.1)					
Rat liver	–	6.64	280	1001	pH 7.5, 0.2 M KP$_i$
Homoserine dehydrogenase (EC 1.1.1.3)					
Rhodospirillum rubrum	–	3.85^i	280	1002	pH 7.5, 0.05 M KP$_i$ 0.05 M KCl, 0.001 M EDTA
Homoserine dehydrogenase - Aspartokinase (EC 1.1.1.3, EC 2.7.2.4)					
E. coli K-12	15.8	4.4	278	256	pH 7.2, 20 mM KP$_i$, 0.15 M KC1, 2 mM Mg titriplex and 4 mM DL-threonine
	16.5	4.6	278	1003	MW = 360,000 [1003]
Hormone					–
Chorionic gonadotropin, human	–	5.47	276	1553	
	–	5.72	276	1553	Asialo der.
Chorionic somatomammotropin, human	–	8.22	277	1554	pH 8.2, 0.1 M Tris
Follicle-stimulating, human	–	4.40	250	1555	–
	–	5.09	260	1555	–
	–	6.54	270	1555	–
	–	7.17	277	1555	–
	–	7.10	280	1555	–
	–	4.96	290	1555	–
Growth					
Beef pituitary	–	7.30	277	1556	0.1 N AcOH
Human pituitary	2	9.31	277	1557	pH 2.0–8.5, MW = 21,500 [1557]
Sheep pituitary	–	7.30	277	1556	0.1 N AcOH
Lactogen (MPL-2), monkey placenta	1.92	9.12	277	1558	MW = 21,000 [1558]
Lactogenic, sheep pituitary	–	9.09	277	1559	pH 8.0–8.5, dil. NH$_4$OH
	–	8.94	278	1560	–
Interstitial cell stimulating, sheep	–	4.39	276	1561	–
α subunit	–	5.86	276	1560	–
β subunit	–	3.01	276	1561	–
Parathyroid					
Pig	0.53	5.6	280	1562	MW = 9423 [1562]
Beef	0.63	6.6	280	1562	MW = 9563, data from Figure 5 [562], 0.1 N AcOH

MOLAR ABSORPTIVITY AND $A_{1cm}^{1\%}$ VALUES FOR PROTEINS AT SELECTED WAVELENGTHS OF THE ULTRAVIOLET AND VISIBLE REGION (Continued)

Protein	ϵ^a ($\times 10^{-4}$)	$A_{1cm}^{1\%\ b}$	nm^c	Reference	Comments^d
Prolactin					
Sheep	–	9.71	278	1563	–
Hyaluronidase inhibitor					
Human blood	–	8.5	280	1005	–
Hyaluronoglucuronidase [EC 3.2.1.36]					
Beef, testicular	–	9.6	280	1004	–
L-α-Hydroxyacid oxidase [EC 1.1.3.15]					
Rat liver	...	2.3	330	257	pH 7.9, 0.005 M NaP$_i$
	–	14.7	280	257	pH 7.9, 0.005 M NaP$_i$
Hydroxybenzoate hydroxylase EC 1.14.99.13)					
Pseudomonas desmolytica	–	10.8	280	1008	Data from the figure on p. 331, Ref. [1008]
Pseudomonas putida	10.4		278	1009	pH 7.5, 0.05 M KP$_i$ data from Figure 1 [1969], 2°C
Hydrogenase (EC 1.12.2.1)					
Desulfovibrio vulgaris	4.1	9.1	277	1006	–
Clostridium pasteurianum	0.82	–	400	1007	MW = 45,000 [1006]
(EC 1.12.7.1)	2.45	–	280	1007	–
Hydroxyindole-O-methyltransferase (acetylserotonin methyltransferase, EC 2.1.1.4)					
Beef pineal gland					
Fraction A	6.2	7.68	280	1564	pH 7.7, 0.05 M Tris Cl, data from Figure 6 [1564], MW = 81,000 [1564], SC
Fraction B	5.8	7.68	280	1564	pH 7.7, 0.05 M Tris Cl, data from Figure 6 [1564], MW = 76,000 [1564], SC
L-6-Hydroxynicotine oxidase (EC 1.5.3.5)					
Arthrobacter oxidans	19.3	20.7	274	258	pH 7.5, 0.1 M P$_i$, wavelength estd. from Figure 3 [258], MW = 93,000 [258]
Hydroxynitrilase (oxynitrilase, mandelonitrite lyase, EC 4.1.2.10)					
Prunaceae	11.2	15	275	259	pH 7.5, 0.1 M PP$_i$.
Prunus communis Stokes	11.4	14.3	275	260	MW = 80,000 [260]
Prunoideae amygdalus	–	15.8	275	1565	pH 7.5, 0.1 M P$_i$, data from Figure 1 [1565]
Maloideae communis	–	18.3	275	1565	
Almonds	–	1.500	460	1010	–
	–	1.654	390	1010	–
Isoenzyme I	–	14.14	275	1010	–
Isoenzyme II	–	13.93	275	1010	–
Isoenzyme III	–	14.22	275	1010	–
Hydroxyproline 2-epimerase (EC 5.1.1.8)					
Pseudomonas putida	–	11.89	280	1011	Dry wt.
Hydroxypyruvate reductase (EC5.1.1.1.81)					
Pseudomonas acidovorans	6.6	8.8	280	261	pH 7.5, MW = 75,000 [261]
Imidazole acetate monooxygenase (EC 1.14.13.5)					
Pseudomonas ATCC 1 1299B	9.61	10.7	270	847	
	1.08	1.2	383	847	MW = 90,000 [847]
	1.07	1.19	442	847	
Imidazolylacetolphosphate: L-glutamate aminotransferase					
Salmonella typhimurium	–	9.54	279	1012	pH 6, 0.1 M TEA, pyridoxamine enzyme, data from Figure 3 [1012]
	6.49	11.8	295	262	0.1 N NaOH, estd. from Figure 9 [262], MW = 59,000 [262]
	5.78	9.86	280	262	pH 7.5, 0.01 M Tris, MW = 59,000 [262]
Immunoglobulins					
Human					
Bence Jones protein	6.4	14.2	280	1013	MW = 45,000 [1013]
	2.7	12.2	280	1014	MW = 22,000 [1014]
Hac	–	10.5	280	1567	Neutral pH
Sch	–	10.5	280	1567	Neutral pH
Nu	–	13.0	280	1567	Neutral pH
Mlg	–	14.5	280	1567	Neutral pH
λ chain	–	14.6	280	1568	–

MOLAR ABSORPTIVITY AND $A_{1cm}^{1\%}$ VALUES FOR PROTEINS AT SELECTED WAVELENGTHS OF THE ULTRAVIOLET AND VISIBLE REGION (Continued)

Protein	ϵ^a ($\times 10^{-4}$)	$A_{1cm}^{1\%\,b}$	nm[c]	Reference	Comments[d]
Normal light chain	–	14.3	280	1568	–
½ Normal light chain	–	14.5	280	1568	–
Constant half of λ chain	–	14.6	280	1568	–
Variable half of λ chain	–	14.6	280	1568	–
Variable fragment	1.3	11.6	280	1014	MW = 11,000 [1014]
L chain	–	9.8	280	1569	pH 6.8, 0.01 M P$_i$
J chain	–	6.5	280	1569	pH 6.8, 0.01 M P$_i$
H chain	–	10.7	280	1569	pH 6.8, 0.01 M P$_i$
IgG	–	13.3	278	1570	pH 7.4, 0.01 M NaP$_i$–0.15 M NaCl
γ chain	–	13.8	282	1570	0.1 N NaOH
Light chain	–	11.0	282	1570	0.1 N NaOH
Heavy chain	7	14	280	1014	MW = 50,000 [1014]
Doty, type γ$_1$, K	–	14.10	280	1019	Dry wt
Sackfield	–	10.69	280	1019	Dry wt
Atypical	–	10.52	280	1018	–
Serum	21.6	13.3	277.5	1017	pH 2, MW = 162,000 [1017]
	–	13.42	280	595	–
IgG	21.2	13.8	280	1571	MW = 153,000 [1571]
IgA	21.7	13.4	280	1571	MW = 162,000 [1571]
Serum	–	13.4	280	1015	–
Secretory	–	13.9	280	1016	–
Colostrum	48.3	12.37	280	595	0.01 N HCl, MW = 390,000 [595]
IgE(PS)	–	12.5	280	1572	–
IgE(ND)	–	15.33	780	1572	–
IgM	–	14.5	280	1573	–
Serum	–	13.3	280	1020	–
Waldenstrom	–	13.5	280	600	0.25 M AcOH
IgG	–	13.5	280	1574	–
γ chain	–	14.0	280	1574	–
Light chain	–	12.0	280	1574	–
IgND, Myeloma	–	14	280	1021	–
Kappa chain urine	1.8	10.7	280	594	MW = 17,000 [594]
Chicken					
Anti-N$_2$ ph^{v*}	–	17.7	280	1022	Neutral buffer
	–	24.6	290	1022	0.1 N NaOH
	–	13.0	290	1022	0.1 N NaOH, another sample
Pig					
Anti-N$_2$ ph-BGG^{w*} λ chain	–	11.3	280	1023	–
π chain	–	9.8	280	1023	–
ρ chain	–	12.6	280	1023	From antibody
ρ chain	–	12.2	280	1023	Non-specific
γ chain	–	14.2	280	1023	–
Light chain fraction	–	11.3	280	1023	From antibody
	–	11.0	280	1023	Non-specific
Epinephelus itaiva (Giant grouper)					
IgG 6.4S	–	16.57	280	1024	0.3 M KCl
	–	17.82	280	1024	0.1 M NaOH
	–	16.50	280	1024	5.0 M GdmCl
IgG 16S	–	13.78	280	1024	0.3 M KCl
	–	15.03	280	1024	0.1 N NaOH
	–	13.53	280	1024	5.0 M GdmCl
Lepisosteus osseus [Gar]					
IgG 14S	–	15	280	1025	0.85% NaCl
Rabbit	21.9	14.6	280	1026	pH 8, Tris, MW = 150,000 [1026]
	8.98	6.0	250	1026	
IgG	–	14.0	280	1027	–

MOLAR ABSORPTIVITY AND $A_{1cm}^{1\%}$ VALUES FOR PROTEINS AT SELECTED WAVELENGTHS OF THE ULTRAVIOLET AND VISIBLE REGION (Continued)

Protein	ϵ^a ($\times 10^{-4}$)	$A_{1cm}^{1\% \, b}$	nm[c]	Reference	Comments[d]
IgM	–	13.0	280	1029	–
Anti-N$_2$ ph^v*	23.4	14.6	279	1030	MW = 160,000 [1030]
Anti azobenzenearsonate					
IgG	–	14.6	280	1031	
IgM	–	13.4	280	1031	
Polyalanylated Ab	–	14.6	280	1032	–
Goat					
IgG	18.7	13.0	280	1033	pH 7.0, MW = 144,000 [1033]
	–	14	280	1034	
	20.2	13.1	280	1579	pH 7.2, 5 mM NaP$_i$, 0.2 M NaCl, MW = 146,000 [1579]
Heavy chain	6.4	12.0	280	1033	pH 3.0 0.1 M AcOH MW = 53,600 [1033]
Light chain	2.9	12.7	280	1033	MW = 23,000 [1033]
IgM	–	13	280	1034	
Horse	–	14.4	277	1580	
IgG [Anti-tick-borne encephalitis]	–	15.06	278	1034	–
	–	1.37	330	1035	–
	–	1.27	333	1035	–
	–	1.22	335	1035	–
	–	1.20	338	1035	–
	–	1.18	340	1035	–
Heavy chain, reduced and alkylated	–	14.3	280	1036	–
Light chain, reduced and alkylated	–	12.7	280	1036	–
Anti-polysaccharide	–	15.0	287	1566	0.1 N NaOH
Type II	–	14.6	280	1566	pH 8.0, borate-NaCl
Mouse, myeloma protein with antibody activity					
IgA, MOPC-315 tumor	–	13.5	275	1578	pH 7.4, 0.01 M KP$_i$–0.15 M NaCl
Fraction III	–	14	278	1037	–
7S Monomer	15	12.5	278	1037	MW = 120,000 [1037]
Fab fragment	7.7	14.0	278	1037	MW = 55,000 [1037]
Rabbit					
IgG	–	13.5	280	1574	–
γ chain	–	14.0	280	1574	–
Light chain	–	12.0	280	1574	–
IgA	–	13.5	280	1575	0.1 N NaOH
Anti-benzylpenicilloyl-	–	13.8	280	1576	Saline + 0.25 N AcOH
	–	15.4	294	1576	0.1 N NaOH
Anti-N$_2$ ph^v*	–	15.5	280	1577	Dry wt.
Heavy chain	–	15.4	280	1577 ⎫	Refractometry
Light chain	–	13.2	280	1577 ⎭	
Zebra	–	15.2	277	1580	–
Donkey	–	13.2	277	1580	–
Mule	–	14.7	277	1580	–
Hinny	–	14.1	277	1580	–
Dog					
Colostral IgA	–	11.80	280	1581	pH 7.4, phosphate-buffered saline, FC
α chain	–	10.07	280	1581	6 M GdmCl, FC
L chain	–	7.32	280	1581 ⎫	pH 7.4, phosphate-buffered saline, FC
Scrum IgA	–	14.08	280	1581 ⎭	
α chain	–	10.63	280	1581 ⎫	6 M GdmCl, FC
L chain	–	8.37	280	1581 ⎭	
Beef					
IgG	–	13.7	280	1582	–
Sheep					
IgA	–	12	280	596	
Rat					
IgG	–	14.6	280	599	
IgM	–	12.5	280	599	
Guinea pig					

MOLAR ABSORPTIVITY AND $A_{1cm}^{1\%}$ VALUES FOR PROTEINS AT SELECTED WAVELENGTHS OF THE ULTRAVIOLET AND VISIBLE REGION (Continued)

Protein	ϵ^a ($\times 10^{-4}$)	$A_{1cm}^{1\% \, b}$	nm^c	Reference	Comments[d]
γM	–	10.5	280	848	0.5% $(NH_4)_2 CO_3$
$γ_2$ G	–	12.3	280	848	
$γ_1$ G	–	13.0	280	848	
$γ_2$ chain	–	13.2	280	848	0.1 M AcOH
$γ_1$ chain	–	13.5	280	848	
μ chain	–	9.2	280	848	0.1 M AcOH
Light chain	–	12.0	280	848	
F ab [trypsin]	–	15	280	597	
F c [trypsin]	–	15	280	597	
IgGs, colostrum	–	13.68	278	598	P_i buffered saline
	–	13.70	278	598	0.1 N HCl
	–	14.77	290	598	0.1 N NaOH, after 10–20 min
	–	14.73	283	598	
IgG_1, serum	–	13.57	278	598	P_i buffered saline
	–	13.44	278	598	0.1 N HCl
	–	14.77	290	598	0.1 N NaOH, after 10–20 min
	–	14.65	283	598	
IgG_2, serum	–	13.52	278	598	P_i buffered saline
	–	13.32	278	598	0.1 N HCl
	–	14.87	290	598	0.1 N NaOH, after 10–20 min
	–	14.73	283	598	
Immunoglobulins, specific					
Rabbit anti-HGG[x*]	–	14.4	279	263	0.25 M acetic acid
Anti-BSA[y*]	–	15.0	279	263	0.25 M acetic acid
Anti-N_2 ph[v*]	–	15.8	278	263	pH 7.4, 0.15 M NaCl, 0.02 M P_i
Anti-N_2 ph[v*] pepsin frag.	–	16.9	278	263	pH 7.4, 0.15 M NaCl, 0.02 M KP_i
Anti-N_2 ph[v*]	–	16.8	278	263	pH 7.4, 0.15 M NaCl, 0.02 M KP_i
Anti-N_2 ph[v*] Fab	–	16.5	278	263	pH 7.4, 0.15 M NaCl, 0.02 M KP_i
Anti-N_2 ph,[v*] Fc	–	13.5	278	263	pH 7.4, 0.15 M NaCl, 0.02 M KP_i
Anti-N_2 ph,[v*] pepsin frag.	–	18.1	278	263	pH 7.4, 0.15 M NaCl, 0.02 M KP_i
Anti-N_2 ph,[v*]	–	15.4	278	263	pH 7.4, 0.04 M KP_i
	–	15.7	278	263	pH 7.4, 0.04 M KP_i
	–	15.5	278	263	pH 7.4, 0.04 M KP_i
	–	15.6	278	263	pH 7.4, 0.04 M KP_i
	–	16.4	278	263	pH 7.4, 0.04 M KP_i
	–	13.6	278	263	pH 7.4, 0.15 M NaCl, 0.01 M P_i
	–	5.3	251	263	pH 7.4, 0.15 M NaCl, 0.01 M P_i
γG-Anti-N_2 ph[v*]	–	16.2	278	263	pH 7.4, 0.04 M KP_i
	–	16.0	278	263	pH 7.4, 0.04 M KP_i
	–	15.9	278	263	pH 7.4, 0.02 M KP_i
γG-Anti-N_3 ph[z*]	–	15.8	278	263	pH 7.4, 0.15 M NaCl 0.02 M KP_i
	–	14.9	278	263	pH 7.4, 0.15 M NaCl, 0.02 M KP_i
	–	15.3	278	263	pH 7.4, 0.15 M NaCl, 0.02 M KP_i
Anti-p-azobenzenearsonate	–	14.8	278	263	pH 7.4, 0.04 M KP_i
Light chains	–	12.8	278	263	pH 8.0, 0.05 M, Na dodecyl sulfate
γG-Anti-phenyl[p-aminobenzoylamino] acetate	–	13.9	279	263	pH 7.4, 0.15 M NaCl, 0.02 M PN_2
Horse, γG-Anti-lac	–	14.7	280	263	Neutral solvent
γA-Anti-lac	–	14.7	280	263	Neutral solvent
Pepsin fragment	–	14.6	280	263	Neutral solvent
γG, human	–	14.3	280	263	pH 7.5, 0.2 M NaCl
$γ_1$-globulin, human	–	14.7	280	263	pH 6.0, 0.1 M NaCl
γM, human	–	11.85	280	263	pH 7.5, 0.2 M NaCl
γM, human, subunit	–	12.0	280	263	pH 7.5, 0.2 M NaCl
γG, horse	–	13.8	280	263	pH 6.5, 0.0175 M $NaPN_2$
	–	13.8	280	263	8 M urea, neutral solution

[x*] HGG, human gamma globulin.
[y*] Albumin, bovine serum albumin.
[z*] N_3 ph, trinitrophenyl.

MOLAR ABSORPTIVITY AND $A_{1cm}^{1\%}$ VALUES FOR PROTEINS AT SELECTED WAVELENGTHS OF THE ULTRAVIOLET AND VISIBLE REGION (Continued)

Protein	ϵ^a ($\times 10^{-4}$)	$A_{1cm}^{1\% \ b}$	nm^c	Reference	Comments^d
Heavy chains	–	15.4	280	263	0.04 M NaDodSO‹
	–	15.2	280	263	1 N propionic acid
Light chains	–	14.0	280	263	0.04 M NaDodSO$_4$
	–	13.6	280	263	1 N propionic acid
γG, rabbit	–	14.6	280	263	–
	–	15.0	278	263	pH 7.4, 0.04 M KP$_i$
	–	15.4	278	263	pH 7.4, 0.04 M KP$_i$
	–	14.5	278	263	pH 7.4, 0.04 M KP$_i$
	–	15.1	278	263	pH 7.4, 0.04 M KP$_i$
	–	14.7	278	263	pH 7.4, 0.04 M KP$_i$
	–	14.9	278	263	pH 7.4, 0.04 M KP$_i$
	–	14.6	278	263	pH 7.4, 0.15 M NaCl, 0.02 M P$_i$
	–	13.5	280	263	0.01 N HCl
Heavy chains	–	13.7	280	263	0.01 N HCl
Light chains	–	11.8	280	263	0.01 N HCl
Fd fragment	–	14.4	280	263	0.01 N HCl
Heavy chains, mildly reduced and alkylated	–	14.5	280	263	pH 7.2, 0.04 M DodSI$_4^-$ 0.01 M P$_i$
Light chains mildly reduced and alkylated	–	13.2	280	263	pH 7.2, 0.04 M DodSO$_4^-$ 0.01 M P$_i$
γG, rabbit	–	13.6	280	263	pH 7, 5 M GdmCl
Heavy chains	–	13.7	280	263	pH 7, 5 M GdmCl
Light chains	–	11.4	280	263	pH 7, 5 M GdmCl
Fab fragment	7.5	15.0	278	263	MW = 50,000 [263]
γG, rabbit	–	13.8	278	263	–
Fab fragment	–	15.3	278	263	–
Fc fragment	–	12.2	278	263	
Fab fragment	–	15.0	280	263	pH 7.5, 0.1 M P$_i$
5S pepsin fragment	–	14.8	280	263	–
γA, rabbit, colostrum	–	13.5	280	263	0.1 NaOH
	–	12.8	280	263	5 M GdmCl
α-chains	–	10.6	280	263	5 M GdmCl
γ_1, guinea pig	–	15	278	263	–
γ_2, guinea pig	–	13.2	278	263	–
γ-globulin fraction, chicken	–	13.5	280	263	–
γG, Lemon shark	–	13.85	280	263	0.3 M KCl
	–	14.04	280	263	0.1 M NaOH
	–	12.82	280	263	5 M GdmCl
γM, Lemon shark	–	13.39	280	263	0.3 M KCl
	–	13.75	280	263	0.1 M NaOH
	–	12.79	280	263	5 M GdmCl
γG heavy chains	–	11.74	280	263	5 M GdmCl
γG light chains	–	13.1	280	263	5 M GdmCl
Indole-3-glycerophosphate synthase (EC 4.1.1.48)	3.6	8	280	264	pH 7.0,5 mM P$_i$
	4.3	9.5	280	264	0.1 M NaOH, estd. from Figure 8 [264]
Inhibitor					
Amylase, *Colocasia esculenta*	–	10.7	280	1583	pH 7
Phospholipase A, *Bothrops neuwiedii*	–	9.09	280	1584	–
(Snake) venom	–	16.36	260	1584	–
	–	201.60	230	1584	–
Proteinase, potato	–	9.18	280	1585	–
Proteinase IIa, potato	–	10.03	278	1586	pH 6,0.1 M NaCl,
Proteinase IIb, potato	–	10.06	278	1586	dry wt
Trypsin, *Phaseolus aureus*					
Roxb. (Mungbean)					
Type A	–	3.7	280	1587	–
Type B	–	3.7	280	1587	–
Trypsin-chymotrypsin					
Arachis hypogaea (Groundnut)	0.1958	2.5	280	1038	MW = 7832 [1038]
Protease					
Barley	–	8.82	280	1039	–

MOLAR ABSORPTIVITY AND $A_{1cm}^{1\%}$ VALUES FOR PROTEINS AT SELECTED WAVELENGTHS OF THE ULTRAVIOLET AND VISIBLE REGION (Continued)

Protein	ϵ^a ($\times 10^{-4}$)	$A_{1cm}^{1\% \ b}$	nm^c	Reference	Comments^d
Insulin	–	10.4	276	711	–
	0.553		277.5	712	–
	–	10.3	275	713	0.01 N HCl
	–	10.52	276	714	pH 7.0, 0.03 M P$_i$
	0.608	–	277	849	
Beef	0.57	10	280	265	MW = 5733 [265]
	–	10.4	277	11	–
	0.61	10.6	278	266	pH 7.0, 0.025 M P$_i$, MW = 5734 [266]
	0.52	–	280	267	
	–	9.91	276	1588	pH 7.2, 0.01 M NaP$_i$–0.1 N NaCl
Crystalline	0.6740	–	276	1589	–^{a†}
N$^{\alpha A1}$-Acetyl-	0.6110	–	276	1589	–^{a†}
	0.5790	–	276	1589	–^{b†}
I$_{A\text{-}a}$	0.6480	–	276	1589	–^{a†}
Amorphous	0.6870	–	276	1589	–^{a†}
	0.6230	–	276	1589	–^{b†}
N$^{\epsilon B29}$-Acetyl-	0.6630	–	276	1589	–^{a†}
	0.6180	–	276	1589	–^{b†}
N$^{\alpha A1}$, N$^{\epsilon B29}$-Diacetyl-	0.6440	–	275	1589	–^{a†}
	0.6020	–	275	1589	–^{b†}
N$^{\alpha A1}$, N$^{\alpha B1}$, N$^{\epsilon B29}$-Triacetyl-	0.6390	–	275	1589	–^{a†}
	0.6270	–	275	1589	–^{b†}
Diacetyl-	0.3420	–	264	1589	–^{a†}
	0.3020	–	264	1589	–^{b†}
Triacetyl-	0.3460	–	264	1589	–^{a†}
	0.3480	–	264	1589	–^{b†}
β-chain	0.31	–	276	268	–
Interferon					
Chick embryo	–	8.6	280	269	–
Intrinsic factor, pig pylorus	–	9.2	278	1590	Dry wt.
Invertase (β-fructofuranosidase, EC 3.2.1.26)					
Neurospora crassa	–	18.6	280	850	–
	–	18.6	280	270	–
Yeast	62.1	23	280	271	MW = 270,000 [271]
Isoamylase (EC 3.2.1.68)					
Pseudomonas sp. str Sb-15	–	22.6	280	851	pH 4.5, 0.01 M AcO$^-$
Isocitrate dehydrogenase (EC 1.1.1.41-.42)					
Saccharomyces cerevisiae (Baker's yeast)	–	6.9	280	1591	–
	–	3.5	260	1591	–
Pig heart	5.3	9.1	280	272	MW = 58,000 [272]
Pig liver					
Cytoplasm	4.73	12.6	280	716	MW = 37,500 [716]
Acobacter vinelandii	7.12	8.9	280	715	MW = 80,000 [715]
Isocitrate lyase (EC 4.1.3.1)					
P. indigofera	38	17.1	280	852	MW = 222,000 [852]
Isomerase [N-(5-phospho-D-ribosylformimino)-5-amino-(5″-phosphoribosyl)-4-imidazolecarboxamide isomerase, EC 5.3.1.16)					
S. typhimurium	3.3	11.4	280	273	pH 8, 0.05 M Tris Cl
C$_{55}$-Isoprenoid alcohol phosphokinase	3.188	18.7	280	1592	MW = 17,000 [1592]
Staphylococcus aureus	2.200	12.9	288	1592	
β-Isopropylmalate dehydrogenase (EC 1.1.1.85)					
Salmonella typhimurium	5.34	7.63	278	853	MW = 70,000 [853]
Kallikrein (kininogenin, EC 3.4.21.8)	–	16.6	280	1593	pH 7 P$_i$ buffer, dry wt.
Pig pancreas	4.92	20.5	280	1594	MW = 24,000 [98]

---

^{a†} Concentration calculated from the optical density at 210 nm.
^{b†} Weighed sample used.

MOLAR ABSORPTIVITY AND $A_{1cm}^{1\%}$ VALUES FOR PROTEINS AT SELECTED WAVELENGTHS OF THE ULTRAVIOLET AND VISIBLE REGION (Continued)

Protein	ϵ^a ($\times 10^{-4}$)	$A_{1cm}^{1\% \, b}$	nm^c	Reference	Comments^d
Kallikrein A,					
Cinnamoyl-	1.80	–	298	1594 }	pH 8.8
Indoleacrylyl-	2.24	–	353	1594 }	
Kallikrein B					
Cinnamoyl-	1.80	–	298	1594 }	pH 8.8
Indoleacrylyl-	2.17	–	353	1594 }	
Kallikrein inactivator					
Lung	5.5	8.4	276	274	MW = 6511 [274]
Kerateine fractions					
Wool, S-carboxymethyl-					
SCMKA2	–	8.6	276	1595	–
SCMKB1	–	5.5	276	1595	–
SCMKB2	–	5.9	276	1595	–
Feather rachis,					
S-carboxymethyl-SCMK	–	7.0	276	1595	–
Keratinase	–	8.4	280	275	pH 8, 0.1 M Tris
S. fradiae (EC 3.4.99.8)	–	10.42	280	276	pH 5.0, AcO$^-$
Trichophyton mentagrophytes (EC 3.4.99.12)	–	13.2	280	854	–
Keratinase (EC 3.4.99.11) conjugate					
S. fradiae	–	58.1	280	277	–
Keratins, zinc precipitatable fractions					
Hair					
Lincoln sheep	–	6.6	277	1596	–
Pig	–	6.5	277	1596	–
Cattle	–	8.3	277	1596	–
Macaca irus (Monkey)	–	8.7	277	1596	–
Lama glauca (Hama)	–	9.8	277	1596	–
Guinea pig	–	9.9	277	1596	–
Merino sheep	–	10.2	277	1596	–
Rat	–	11.7	277	1596	–
Mouse	–	14.2	277	1596	–
Homy keratin					
Diceros bicornis (Rhinocerous) horn	–	6.4	277	1596	–
Fingernail	–	7.0	277	1596	–
Sheep horn	–	7.6	277	1596	–
Cattle horn	–	8.0	277	1596	–
Sheep hoof	–	8.8	277	1596	–
Erethizon dorsatum (Porcupine) quill	–	9.3	277	1596	–
Balaenoptera musculus (Whale) baleen	–	12.1	277	1596	–
Erimceus europaeus (Hedgehog) quill	–	12.3	277	1596	–
Histrix cristata (Porcupine) quill	–	15.3	277	1596	–
Tachyglossus aculeatus aculeatus (Echidna) quill	–	20.4	277	1596	–
α-Keto acid dehydrogenase complex					
Pig heart	–	5.1	280	278	pH 7, 0.05 M KP$_i$, estd. from Figure 6 in Reference 278,
3-Keto-Δ5-steroid isomerase					
P. testosteroni	–	4.13	280	279	–
Kininogenin (see Kallikrein)					
Lac repressor, E. coli	–	6.9	280	1569	pH 6.8, 0.01 M P$_i$
Laccase (monophenol monooxygenase, EC 1.14.18.1)					
Rhus vernicfera	0.26	–	330	856	–
	0.52	–	614	856	–
	0.09	–	788	856	–
Oxidized	9.35	–	280	717	–
Reduced	0.57	–	614	717	–
	0.28	–	333	717	–
	0.55	–	614	717	–
Polyporus versicolor	8.4	13.7	280	718	MW = 61,000 [718]
	0.41	–	610	718	–
	0.33	–	330	858	–

MOLAR ABSORPTIVITY AND $A_{1cm}^{1\%}$ VALUES FOR PROTEINS AT SELECTED WAVELENGTHS OF THE ULTRAVIOLET AND VISIBLE REGION (Continued)

Protein	ϵ^a ($\times 10^{-4}$)	$A_{1cm}^{1\% \ b}$	nm^c	Reference	Comments^d
	0.08	–	440	858	
	0.46	–	610	858	–
	0.2	–	720	858	–
Rhus succedanea	0.32	–	325	857	–
	0.45	–	610	857	–
	0.12	–	770	857	–
Fungal	7.4	11.6	280	859	MW = 64,000 [859]
	7.44	–	280	1040	–
α-Lactalbumin	–	20.9	280	280	
	–	20.1	280	281	–
Human	2.04	–	280	1041	
	–	16.2	280	1597	–
	–	19.0	–^{ct}	1598	–
American Indian	–	14.1	280	1042	–
Caucasian	–	15.3	280	1042	–
Negro	–	15.2	280	1042	–
Japanese	–	15.0	280	1042	–
Beef	–	20.1	280	1042	–
	–	20.5	280	601	–
A, Droughtmaster	–	20.2	281.5	1043	–
B, Droughtmaster	–	20.9	281.5	1043	–
Cow's milk	2.9	–	280	719	–
	–	20.9	280	720	20 mM Tris, pH 7.4
Carboxyl modified with glucineamide	3.0	–	280	719	–
Goat	–	17.3	280	1042	–
Sheep	–	16.7	280	1042	–
Pig	–	18.1	280	1042	–
Guinea pig	–	16.7	–^{ct}	1598	–
Camel	–	19.0	–^{ct}	1598	——
β-Lactamase II (cephalosporinase, EC 3.5.2.8)					
Bacillus cereus 569H	–	8.7	277	1044	MW = 22,500
Hp	2.41	10.7	–^{ct}	1599	MW = 22,500, refractometry
β-Lactamase I *B. cereus* 569/H	2.44	8.76	–^{ct}	1599	MW = 27,800 [1599], refractometry
Lactate dehydrogenase (EC 1.1.1.27 and/or .28)					
Beef					
Heart	–	14.55	280	1600	5 M GdmCl, Kj
	21	15	280	284	–
	20	–	280	285	–
	–	15	280	1050	–^{et}
	–	13.8	280	1051	–
	–	14.2	280	1052	–
	–	14.5	280	1053	–
	–	14.9	280	1054	–
H_1 [92%]	–	14.6	280	1048	–
$H_2 M_2$ [80%]	–	14.4	280	1048	–
Skeletal muscle	20	–	280	285	–
Muscle	18.1	12.9	280	284	–
Isozyme A	21	15.6	280	286	MW = 134,000 [286]
Isozyme B	19.6	14.5	280	286	MW = 134,000 [286]
Duck, M_4	18.9	13.5	280	287	MW = 140,000 [287]
Turkey, M_4	20.4	14.6	280	287	MW = 140,000 [287]
Pheasant, M_4	19.1	13.7	280	287	MW = 140,000 [287]
Ostrich, M_4	18.6	13.3	280	287	MW = 140,000 [287]
Rhea, M_4	18.1	13	280	287	MW = 140,000 [287]
Halibut, M_4	18.9	13.5	280	287	MW = 140,000 [287]
Skeletal muscle	20	–	280	285	–

^{ct} No wavelength cited.
^{dt} mg protein/ml = (1.13) (OD$_{280}$).
^{et} mg/ml = (0.67) (OD$_{280}$).

MOLAR ABSORPTIVITY AND $A_{1cm}^{1\%}$ VALUES FOR PROTEINS AT SELECTED WAVELENGTHS OF THE ULTRAVIOLET AND VISIBLE REGION (Continued)

Protein	ϵ^a ($\times 10^{-4}$)	$A_{1cm}^{1\%\,b}$	nm[c]	Reference	Comments[d]
Bullfrog, M_4	19.3	13.8	280	287	MW = 140,000 [287]
Tuna, M_4	17.5	12.5	280	287	MW = 140,000 [287]
Dogfish, M_4	20.8	14.8	280	287	MW = 140,000 [287]
	19.7	–	280	287	Using Kjeldahl N
Chicken heart muscle	18	–	280	285	–
	19	13.6	280	284	–
Skeletal muscle	22	–	280	285	–
	21.8	15.6	280	284	–
Rabbit	20	–	280	285	–
M_4	–	14.4	280	286	–
	20.1	–	280	287	–
Muscle	16.2	12.3	280	288	pH 7.6, 0.1 M NaP$_i$, MW = 132,000 [288]
	16.7	12.6	280	289	0.2 N NaOH, MW = 132,000 [289]
	–	14.0	280	141	
Skeletal muscle V[96%]	20.68	14.6	279	1049	IV [2%], II/III [0.5%], I [1.5%], MW = 142,000 [1049]
	–	8.9	280	1050	–^{d†}
Pig heart	–	12.9	280	1045	0.1 NaOH, coenzyme free
	–	14.5	280	1046	–
	–	151	215	1047	0.9% NaCl
M_4 [96%]	–	14.0	280	1048	–
I [97%]	19.59	13.8	279	1049	II [2.5%], III [0.5%], MW = 142,000 [1049]
Heart [H_4]	–	13.7	280	286	–
Human	–	14.6	280	290	pH 7.0, P$_i$
Heart	–	16.4	280	1055	–
Uterus	18.7	12.3	280	295	MW = 152,000 [295]
Uterine myoma	17.7	12.4	280	295	MW = 143,000 [295]
Rat liver	–	12.6	280	291	MW = 132,000 [292]
	–	12.8	280	1058	–
Jensen sarcoma	–	11.7	280	1059	pH 7.4
Yeast	23.2	–	424	293	–
	–	29	423	1056	–
E. coli B	–	0.727††	280	294	–
Homarus americanus	21.8	15.6	280	1057	MW = 140,000 [1057]
Lactate-malate dehydrogenase (see malate-lactate transhydrogenase)					
L-Lactate oxidase (lactate 2-monooxygenase, EC 1.13.12.4)					
M. smegmatis	–	21.9	280	282	pH 7.0, NaP$_i$
	–	2.62	452	282	–
M. phlei	81.5	20.4	280	283	pH 7.0, 0.1 M P$_i$, MW = 399,000 [283]
	–	2.26	454	283	pH 7.0, 0.1 M P$_i$
Lactoferrin					
Beef	–	14.5	280	1060	–
	–	11.3	280	1060	6 M GdmCl
Cow's milk	–	15.1	280	306	–
	–	0.547	450	307	–
	–	0.460	470	1603	pH 7
Apo-	–	12.7	280	1603	–
Human milk	–	0.540	465	602	pH 8.2
	11.096	–	280	1601	–
	–	14.6	280	1602	–
	–	0.510	470	1603	pH 7
Apo-	8.512		280	1601	–
	–	11.2	280	1602	–
	–	10.9	280	1603	–
β-Lactoglobulin					
Beef	–	9.5	280	296	–

---

†† This may be in error. Value should be 7.27.

MOLAR ABSORPTIVITY AND $A_{1cm}^{1\%}$ VALUES FOR PROTEINS AT SELECTED WAVELENGTHS OF THE ULTRAVIOLET AND VISIBLE REGION (Continued)

Protein	ϵ^a ($\times 10^{-4}$)	$A_{1cm}^{1\% \, b}$	nm^c	Reference	Comments^d
	–	9.66	278.5	297	–
	–	9.7	280	298	–
	3.66	–	280	299	–
	–	9.6	278	300	pH 5.3, ionic strength 0.1, AcO⁻
β-A, β-B	–	9.6	278	301	–
β-C	–	9.5	278	301	
β-A, β-B	–	9.4	278	302	–
β-1	–	9.5	290	303	0.1 N NaOH
	–	9.5	282	303	0.1 N NaOH
β-2	–	9.9	288	303	0.1 N NaOH
Sheep, β-A	–	9.2	278	304	0.1 M NaCl
β-B	–	8.35	278	304	0.1 M NaCl
Goat	–	9.4	278	305	–
Pig's milk	1.05	5.65	280	603	0.1 M NaOH
Buffalo	–	9.4	279	1061	–
Cow's milk	–	5.12	255	1604	
	–	10.80	280	1604	pH 7.0, 0.01 M P$_i$
β-Lactoglobulin-B	–	1.00	310	1604	
Cow's milk	3.5	10.0	280	1062	MW = 35,000 [1062]
MalNEt^{gt}	3.5	10.0	280	1062	–
ClHgBzO⁻^{ht}	3.7	10.56	280	1062	–
Lactollin					
Cow's milk	7.1	16.5	280	1063	MW = 43,000 [1063]
Lactonase (gluconolactonase) (EC 3.1.1.17)					
Actinoplanes missouriensis	–	4	280	1064	pH 7.0, 0.07 M KP$_i$, data from Figure 8 [1064]
Lactoperoxidase (peroxidase, EC 1.11.1.7)					
Cow's milk					
B-1	–	14.9	280	1065	–
B-2$_I$	–	15.0	280	1065	–
B-2$_{II}$	–	14.9	280	1065	–
B-3	–	14.9	280	1065	–
A	–	15.5	280	1065	–
Cow's milk	–	15.2	280	1066	–
	–	15.41	280	1067	–
	–	1.37	497	1067	–
Cow's milk	11.6	–	412	604	
+ hydrogen peroxide	8.89	–	425	604	Data from Figure 2 [604]
+ Na$_2$S$_2$O$_4$	7.26	–	437	604	
Cow's milk	16.1	–	280	604	
+ hydrogen peroxide	12.3	–	280	604	Calculated from $\epsilon_{412}/\epsilon_{280} = 0.72$
+ Na$_2$S$_2$O$_4$	10.1	–	280	604	
Lactose synthetase, A protein, (see also galactosyl transferase)					
Cow's milk	–	16.1	280	1605	Refractometry
Lactosiderophilin lactotransferrin					
Human milk	10.9	11.7	280	308	pH 7, sat. with iron, MW = 93,000 [308]
	–	0.500	452.5	308	–
Leghemoglobin					
Soybean	1.51	–	574	1068	
	1.5	–	541	1068	pH 6.4, 0.01 M P$_i$
	13.9	–	411	1068	
Lupinus luteus (Yellow lupine), root nodules	3.8	–	275	1606	–
Lb^{3+}H$_2$O/OH⁻	16.0	–	403.5	1607	
	1.03	–	498	1607	pH 6.0
	0.44	–	624	1607	

^{gt} MalNEt, N-ethylmaleimide.
^{ht} ClHgBzO⁻, p-chloromercuribenzoate.

MOLAR ABSORPTIVITY AND $A_{1cm}^{1\%}$ VALUES FOR PROTEINS AT SELECTED WAVELENGTHS OF THE ULTRAVIOLET AND VISIBLE REGION (Continued)

Protein	ϵ^a ($\times 10^{-4}$)	$A_{1cm}^{1\% \, b}$	nm^c	Reference	Comments^d
	14.3	–	404	1607	
	1.05	–	495	1607	
	0.98	–	535	1607	pH 8.5
	0.7	–	574	1607	
	0.35	–	622	1607	
	12.3	–	411	1607	
	1.35	–	544	1607	pH 10.5
	1.12	–	574	1607	
LL³⁺F⁻	15.1	–	402.5	1607	
	0.99	–	495	1607	
	0.47	–	615	1607	pH 6.0
	14.5	–	403	1607	
	1.4	–	490	1607	
	0.84	–	538	1607	pH 8.5
	0.75	–	575	1607	
Lb²⁺NCS⁻	12.4	–	410	1607	pH 6.0
	1.33	–	534	1607	
	12.3	–	410	1607	pH 8.5
	1.14	–	534	1607	
	12.3	–	410	1607	pH 10.5
	1.63	–	534	1607	
Lb²⁺N₂⁻	13.0	–	414	1607	pH 6.0
	1.28	–	545	1607	
	13.3	–	414	1607	pH 8.5
	1.37	–	545	1607	
Lb²⁺CN⁻	11.9	–	416	1607	pH 6.0
	1.38	–	545	1607	
	12.0	–	416	1607	pH 8.5
	1.56	–	544	1607	
	12.0	–	416	1607	pH 10.5
	1.65	–	543	1607	
Lb⁺² imidazole	13.2	–	407.5	1607	pH 6.0
	1.32	–	533	1607	
	13.0	–	408	1607	pH 8.5
	1.38	–	535	1607	
	12.6	–	410	1607	pH 10.5
	1.4	–	533	1607	
Lb²⁺ pyridine	13.5	–	406	1607	
	1.27	–	530	1607	pH 6.0
	1.1	–	562	1607	
	13.3	–	406.5	1607	
	1.26	–	537	1607	pH 8.5
	1.08	–	574	1607	
	12.9	–	408	1607	
	1.52	–	530	1607	pH 10.5
	1.22	–	558	1607	
Lb²⁺ (desoxy)	10.7	–	421	1607	
	10.5	–	428	1607	pH 6.0
	1.38	–	555	1607	
	10.5	–	421	1607	
	10.5	–	428	1607	pH 8.5
	1.4	–	555	1607	
	10.3	–	421	1607	
	10.3	–	428	1607	pH 10.5
	1.3	–	555	1607	
Lb²⁺NCS⁻	11.2	–	421	1607	
	10.7	–	427	1607	pH 6.0
	1.43	–	555	1607	
	10.8	–	421.5	1607	
	10.0	–	427	1607	pH 8.5
	1.23	–	555	1607	

MOLAR ABSORPTIVITY AND $A^{1\%}_{1cm}$ VALUES FOR PROTEINS AT SELECTED WAVELENGTHS OF THE ULTRAVIOLET AND VISIBLE REGION (Continued)

Protein	ϵ^a ($\times 10^{-4}$)	$A^{1\% \, b}_{1cm}$	nm^c	Reference	Comments^d
	11.3	–	421	1607	
	11.3	–	428	1607	pH 10.5
	1.43	–	555	1607	
$Lb^{2+}N_3^-$	13.2	–	416.5	1607	
	1.52	–	525	1607	pH 6.0
	1.47	–	561.5	1607	
	11.1	–	417.5	1607	pH 8.5
	1.39	–	550	1607	
	13.4	–	416.5	1607	
	1.35	–	525	1607	pH 10.5
	1.74	–	553	1607	
$Lb^{2+}CN^-$	11.3	–	421	1607	
	9.4	–	425	1607	
	1.18	–	535	1607	pH 6.0
	1.29	–	560	1607	
	1.13	–	561	1607	
	13.1	–	430	1607	
	1.47	–	535	1607	pH 8.5
	2.0	–	562.5	1607	
	16.6	–	431.5	1607	pH 10.5
	2.0	–	534	1607	pH 10.5
	2.43	–	562.5	1607	
Lb^{2+} imidazole	12.4	–	422	1607	
	1.09	–	527	1607	pH 6.0
	1.6	–	556.5	1607	
	16.0	–	422	1607	
	1.43	–	527	1607	pH 8.5
	2.62	–	556.5	1607	
	15.1	–	422	1607	
	1.46	–	527	1607	pH 10.5
	2.90	–	556.5	1607	
Lb^{2+} pyridine	19.6	–	419	1607	
	1.26	–	467	1607	
	2.2	–	523.5	1607	pH 6.0
	3.72	–	555	1607	
	18.5	–	420	1607	
	2.26	–	523.5	1607	pH 8.5
	3.68	–	555	1607	
	17.7	–	419.5	1607	
	1.98	–	523.5	1607	pH 10.5
	3.46	–	555	1607	
Lb^{2+} nicotinic acid	11.6	–	418	1607	
	1.46	–	524	1607	pH 6.0
	2.53	–	554.5	1607	
	9.4	–	420	1607	
	1.36	–	524	1607	pH 8.5
	1.7	–	554.5	1607	
	10.0	–	420	1607	
	1.1	–	524	1607	pH 10.5
	1.5	–	554.5	1607	
Lb^{2+} ethyl isocyanide	15.7	–	426	1607	
	1.78	–	526	1607	pH 6.0
	1.98	–	556	1607	
	14.0	–	426	1607	
	1.68	–	526	1607	pH 8.5
	1.98	–	556	1607	
	14.8	–	426	1607	
	1.5	–	526	1607	pH 10.5
	1.98	–	556	1607	

MOLAR ABSORPTIVITY AND $A_{1cm}^{1\%}$ VALUES FOR PROTEINS AT SELECTED WAVELENGTHS OF THE ULTRAVIOLET AND VISIBLE REGION (Continued)

Protein	ϵ^a ($\times 10^{-4}$)	$A_{1cm}^{1\%\,b}$	nm^c	Reference	Comments^d
Lb^{2+}CO	17.1	–	417.5	1607	
	1.34	–	540	1607	pH 6.0
	1.33	–	562	1607	
	19.0	–	417	1607	
	1.29	–	536	1607	pH 8.5
	1.24	–	562	1607	
	20.6	–	417	1607	
	1.7	–	537.5	1607	pH 10.5
	1.7	–	562	1607	
Legumin					
Vicia sativa	–	7.5	280	1069	pH 6.5 and pH 12.4
Leucine aminopeptidase (amino peptidase, EC 3.4.11.1-.2)					
Pig kidney	–	8.4	280	309	pH 8.0, 0.005 M Tris, 0.005 M MgCl$_2$, estd. from Figure 5 [309]
Beef lens	–	9.2	280	605	–
	–	10	280	606	pH 8.0, 0.1 M Tris
Leucine binding					
E. coli	–	6.5	280	453	pH 6.9
Leucine dehydrogenase (EC 1.4.1.9)					
B. subtilis SJ-2	103.5	45	280	1070	MW = 230,000 [1070]
Bacillus sphacricus		6.44	280	1608	–
Lipase (triacylglycerol lipase, EC 3.1.1.3)					
Pig pancreas	6.65	13.3	280	1071	MW = 50,000 [1071]
N$_3$ ph-^{it}	–	14.2	280	1071	–
		11	280	1609	–
Rat pancreas	–	12	280	1072	–
Lipoamide dehydrogenase					
C. krusei	6.2	11.76	273	310	pH 7.0, MW = 53,000 [310]
Lipoate acetyltransferase (EC 2.3.1.12) (see dihydrolipoyl transacetylase)					
Lipoprotein, HDL$_2$, human					
Apo-	–	18.2	280	1610	
Fraction III	–	12.2	280	1610	–
Fraction IV	–	9.2	280	1611	–
Carboxymethyl-low density	–	9.2	280	1611	–
Apo-	–	8.0	–^{ct}	1612	Dry wt., 7.5 M GdmCl
	–	7.7	–^{ct}	1612	
Lipoprotein, very low density					
Human, ApoLP-Val	–	9.1	280	1073	pH 7.5, 0.02 M KP$_i$
ApoLP-Ala	–	16.1	280	1073	
Low density					
Rat serum	–	11.7	280	1074	pH 8.6, data from Figure 6 [1074]
	–	8.0	290	1074	
	–	11.3	280	1074	pH 11.6, data from Figure 6 [1074]
	–	9.7	290	1074	
Apo-	–	10.0	280	1074	pH 8.6, data from Figure 6 [1074]
	–	7.3	290	1074	
	–	10.4	280	1074	pH 11.6, data from Figure 6 [1074]
High density	–	10.0	290	1074	
Rat serum	–	12.5	280	1074	pH 8.6, data from Figure 5 [1074]
	–	9.6	290	1074	
	–	12.3	280	1074	pH 11.6, data from Figure 5 [1074]
	–	11.0	290	1074	
Apo-	–	11.3	280	1074	pH 8.6, data from Figure 6 [1074]
	–	8.8	290	1074	
	–	11.7	280	1074	pH 11.6, data from Figure 6 [1074]
	–	11.2	290	1074	

^{it} N$_3$ ph, trinitrophenyl.

MOLAR ABSORPTIVITY AND $A_{1cm}^{1\%}$ VALUES FOR PROTEINS AT SELECTED WAVELENGTHS OF THE ULTRAVIOLET AND VISIBLE REGION (Continued)

Protein	ϵ^a ($\times 10^{-4}$)	$A_{1cm}^{1\% \, b}$	nm^c	Reference	Comments^d
Human skin, high density	–	10.8	278	1074	
Lipovitellin					
Leucophaea maderae (Cockroach)	–	8.3	280	1613	–
Lipoxygenase (EC 1.13.11.12)					
Soybean	18.8	17.4	280	721	MW = 108,000 [721]
Isoenzyme		14	280	1614	–
Peas (*Pisum sativum L.*)	9.5	13.2	278	722	0.05 *M* Tris Cl, pH 7.2, MW = 72,000 [722]
Lombricine kinase (EC 2.7.3.5)					
Lumbricus terrestris	–	11.4	280	607	–
Photinus pyralis	7.5	7.5	278	608	MW = 100,000 [608]
Renilla reniformis	–	10.4	280	860	pH 7.5, 100 m*M* KP$_i$ plus 1.4 m*M* HSEtOH, plus 2.2
	–	0.38	500	860	m*M* EDTA, data from Figure 4 [860]
Diplocardia longa (Earthworm)	54	18	278	1615	Biuret, MW = 300,000 [1615]
Bacterial	6.3	8.3	280	311	MW = 76,000 [311]
Lutenizing hormone-releasing factor Synthetic					
[Gly^2]LRF	1.22	–	244	1423	
	0.574	–	280	1423	
	0.561	–	288	1423	
	0.410	–	294	1423	
des-His^2-LRF	1.0465	–	244	1423	0.1 *N* NaOH
	0.5310	–	280	1423	
	0.5177	–	288	1423	
	0.3706	–	294	1423	
Lysin					
Tegula pfeifferi					
Egg, membrane	2.1	23.8	280	861	pH 6.0, 0.03 *M* P$_i$
ε-Lysine acylase (lysine acetyltransferase, EC 2.3.1.32)					
A. pestifer	–	12.0	280	862	–
Lysine decarboxylase (EC 4.1.1.18)					
E. coli B	–	11.3	280	724	Data from Figure 2 [724], pH 6
	–	15.2	290	724	Data from Figure 2 [724], 2 *N* NaOH
Bacterium cadaveris	–	10.1	280	725	pH 6.2, 0.01 *M* KP$_i$
L-Lysine 6-aminotransferase (EC 2.6.1.36)					
Achromobacter liquidum	8.5	7.35	280	723	pH 7.4, MW = 116,000 [723]
L-Lysine 2-monooxygenase (EC 1.13.12.2)					
Psuedomonas fluorescens	34.2	17.9	280	726	MW = 191,000 [726]
Lysozyme (EC 3.2.1.17)	–	22.8	280	1616	–
	–	320	210	1616	–
	–	910	191	1616	–
Egg white	3.79		–^{ct}	1617	–
	–	26.04	280	1618	–^{it}
	–	12.60	255	1604	–
	–	24.80	280	1604	–
	–	0.72	310	1604	–
	3.60	24.7	280	1619	MW = 14,600 [1620]
	–	25.5	277.5	1621	Neutral pH
	–	20.2	290	1621	
	–	27.4	281	1622	pH 5–6,0.1 *M* KCl, dry wt.
	–	27.2	280	1623	0.02 *N* HCl
	3.9		280	1624	0.2 *M* AcO$^-$, pH 4.75
	3.8		280	1624	Carboxyl modified with aminomethyl-sulfonic acid
	–	26	280	11	–
	–	25.32	280	312	–
	–	26.9	280	313	–
	3.88	–	281	314	0.1 *N* HCl, MW = 14,700 [314]
	–	23.05	281	315	–

---

^{it} Values given for photo-oxidation products in Ref. [1618].

MOLAR ABSORPTIVITY AND $A_{1cm}^{1\%}$ VALUES FOR PROTEINS AT SELECTED WAVELENGTHS OF THE ULTRAVIOLET AND VISIBLE REGION (Continued)

Protein	ϵ^a ($\times 10^{-4}$)	$A_{1cm}^{1\%\,b}$	nm^c	Reference	Comments^d
	–	27.3	282	316	–
	–	26.35	280	317	pH 5.4
	3.65	25.5	280	318	MW = 14,307 [318]
	–	26.5	280	319	pH 7.0, 0.2 M NaP$_i$
	390	–	281	320	pH 3.9
	–	23.3	290	321	4.8 M guanidine-0.01 M HCl
Oxidized, tryptophan-108 oxidized to oxindole	–	22.7	280	1625	
N-Bromosuccinimide					
Modified	3.37	–	280	1626	–
Reduced, carboxymethylated and N-bromosuccimide modified	3.37	–	280	1626	See Figure 1 of Ref. [1626]
Azophenyl-p-sulfonic acid modified					
S-1	1.85	12.6	500	1627 }	0.1 N NaOH
S-2	3.60	24.5	330	1627 }	
Azophenyl-p-carboxylic acid modified					
B-1	8.58	58.4	340	1627	pH 7
B-1	2.28	15.5	500	1627	0.1 N NaOH
B-2	8.54	58.1	330	1627	pH 6
	2.84	19.3	478	1627	0.1 N NaOH
Azotetrazole modified					
T-1-2	5.58	38.0	330	1627	pH 7
	2.87	19.6	510	1627 }	0.1 N NaOH
T-2	1.96	13.3	478	1627 }	
Azophenyldiethyl-methylammonium chloride modified					
A-1	4.09	27.8	330	1627	pH 7
A-2	1.36	9.25	330	1627	pH 6
Mouse	–	21.7	280	1628	pH 6.5, 0.2 M P$_i$, dry wt.
Human					
Milk	–	25.1	280	1629	–
	–	25.65	280	1633	pH 6.0, 0.1 M AcONa—0.1 M NaC1
	3.1	20.7	280	322	Estd. from Figure 3 [322], MW = 15,000
Tear	3.6	24.2	280	323	pH 5.5, estd. from Figure [323], MW = 14,900,
Urine	–	25.1	280	1629	–
	3.51	24.7	280	1630	MW = 14,200 [1631]
	–	24.6	281	1632	pH 5.8
Duck	–	26.6	–^{c}†	1634	–
Goose	–	14.8	–^{c}†	1634	–
Chalaropis sp.	–	24.8	280	1634	Dry wt.
Bacteriophage T4	2.4	12.8	280	324	MW = 19,000 [324]
Papaya	5.95	23.8	280	325	MW = 25,000 [325]
Bacteriophage λ	1.9	10.7	280	326	MW = 17,900 [326]
Lysyl-tRNA synthetase (EC 6.1.1.6)					
Yeast	–	6.4	280	1075	pH 7,0.1 M P$_i$, 0.1 M EDTA, data from Figure 4 [1075]
α_2-Macroglobulin					
Beef plasma	80	10	280	863	pH 8.0
					MW = 800,000 [863]
Human	66.5	8.1	280	864	MW = 820,000 [864]
Pig	98	10.2	280	865	MW = 960,000 [865]
Mouse	–	7.42	280	1635	Dry wt
Rabbit	–	9	277	1028	–
Malate dehydrogenase (EC 1.1.1.37)					
Pig heart	1.78	–	280	867	–
	–	4.6	280	327	–
	–	2.8	280	328	–
	–	3.8	280	329	–
Mitochondria	1.98	3.05	280	337	pH 8.0, 0.05 μM Tris-AcO$^-$, MW = 65,000 [337]
	–	2.5	280	1636	–
5S protein	1.97	2.9	280	868	MW = 68,000 [868]
9S protein	7.74	5.6	280	868	MW = 138,000 [868]
Supernatant	6.9	9.3	280	869	MW = 74,000 [869]

MOLAR ABSORPTIVITY AND $A_{1cm}^{1\%}$ VALUES FOR PROTEINS AT SELECTED WAVELENGTHS OF THE ULTRAVIOLET AND VISIBLE REGION (Continued)

Protein	ϵ^a ($\times 10^{-4}$)	$A_{1cm}^{1\%\,b}$	nm^c	Reference	Comments^d
Chicken					
Intramitochondrial	–	2.9	280	870	–
Extramitochondrial	–	13.1	280	870	–
Rat liver					
Mitochondrial	3.4	5.08	280	871	MW = 66,300 [871]
Horse heart	–	2.8	280	327	–
Ox heart	–	8.5	280	330	–
Beef heart	3.25	5.0	280	331	MW = 65,000 [331]
B. subtilis	2.44	6.6	280	332	pH 7.7, 0.05 M P$_i$, MW = 37,000 [332]
	7.8	6.67	280	333	MW = 117,000 [333]
B. stearothermophilus	–	5.82	280	333	–
E. coli	2.03	3.39	280	333	MW = 60,000 [333]
Ostrich heart	8.96	12.8	280	334	pH 7.5, 0.1 M P$_i$, MW = 70,000 [334]
Tuna heart	20.8	31	280	335	pH 7.5, 0.1 M P$_i$, MW = 67,000 [335]
P. acidovorans	3.4	8.0	–^{kt}	336	MW = 43,000 [336]
Malate-lactate transhydrogenase (EC 1.1.99.7) (lactate-malate dehydrogenase)					
Veillonelia alcalescens	–	12.7	280	1637	–
Malic enzyme [malate dehydrogenase (decarboxylating)] (EC 1.1.1.38-.40)					
Pigeon liver	25.8	9.2	278	338	pH 7.0, 0.042 M Tris, MW = 280,000 [338], protein contains NADP^{it}
	24.1	8.6	278	338	pH 7.0, 0.042 M Tris, MW = 280,000 [338]
E. coli K 10 [HfrC]	26.5	4.8	279	872	MW = 550,000 [872], protein con. det. from tyr/trp content
	28.1	5.1	279	872	MW = 550,000 [872], protein con. det. by Lowry
Malic enzyme, NAD-linked [malate dehydrogenase (decarboxylating)] (EC 1.1.1.38-.39)					
E. coli	–	10.2	278	1638	Dry wt.
Mandelonitrite lyase (see hydroxynitrilase)					
α-Mannosidase (EC 3.2.1.24)					
Vicia sativa	–	13.3	280	727	Data from Figure 3 [727], pH 7.2, Tris–0.01 N HCl
Soybeans	–	20	280	1639	
α-Melanotropin; 5-glutamine, nitrophenyl sulfenyl					
Synthetic	1.65	–	282	873 ⎫	0.001 N HCl
	0.4	–	365	873 ⎭	
Melilotate hydroxylase (melilotate 3-monooxygenase, EC 1.14.13.4)					
Arthrobacter, apoenzyme	–	11.1	277	339	pH 7.3, 0.15 M P$_i$, 0.1 M KCl, 1 mM cysteine, estd. from Figure 6 [339]
Holoenzyme	–	18.9	280	339	pH 7.3, 0.15 M P$_i$, 0.1 M KCl, 1 mM cysteine, estd. from Figure 6 [339]
Mercaptoalbumin, human (see albumin, human)					
Mercaptopyruvate sulfurtransferase (EC 2.8.1.2)					
E. coli	2.23	9.3	280	1640	pH 7.5, 0.05 M Tris, 0.8 M KCl, MW = 24,000 [1640]
Meromyosin, heavy	–	6	280	1641	Kjeldahl, absorption corrected for light scattering
Rabbit	–	–	–	1642	See footnote^{mt}
Metallothionein					
Chicken liver	8.06	–	205	1643	pH 6.6
Rat liver	8.06	–	205	1643	pH 6.6
Metapyrocatechase (catechol 2,3-dioxygenase, (EC 1.1.3.11.2)					
Pseudomonas arvilla	18.9	13.5	280	1076	MW = 140,000 [1076]
	–	13.2	280	1644	See footnote^{nt}

---

^{kt} No value cited for wavelength.
^{it} NADP, nicotinamide adenine dinucleotide phosphate.
^{mt} $\epsilon_{211} - \epsilon_{350}$ = 776 cm^2/g in 0.5 N NaOH.
^{nt} Absorption at 280 nm taking the value of 1.32 ml/cm mg.

MOLAR ABSORPTIVITY AND $A_{1cm}^{1\%}$ VALUES FOR PROTEINS AT SELECTED WAVELENGTHS OF THE ULTRAVIOLET AND VISIBLE REGION (Continued)

Protein	ϵ^a ($\times 10^{-4}$)	$A_{1cm}^{1\%\,b}$	nm[c]	Reference	Comments[d]
Methemoglobin (see hemoglobin)					
Methemoglobin, N_3^-	0.34	–	630	700	
	1.07	–	542	700	0.1 $M P_i$, pH 7.0, ϵ_M values expressed per mole heme
	11.7	–	414	700	
Methemoglobin reductase (EC 1.6.2.1.-2?)					
Human, erythrocytes	1.13	–	462	1645	Oxidized enzyme
Form I	–	7.45	278	728	–
Form II	–	17.9	268	728	–
Methionyl-tRNA synthetase (EC 6.1.1.10)					
E. coli K 12	–	13.9	283	1077	Native enzyme
	–	16.2	283	1077	Trypsin modified
	–	20	280	874	pH 7.4, 0.02 M KP$_i$
β-Methylaspartase (methylaspartate ammonia-lyase, EC 4.3.1.2)					
C. tetranomorphum	5.63	5.63	279	340	pH 7.0, 0.5 M Me$_4$ NCl, MW = 100,000 [340]
	–	6.60	280	341	pH 6.5, 0.005 $M P_i$
Methylaspartate mutase (EC 5.4.99.1) (see glutamate mutase)					
Metmyoglobins (see myoglobin)					
β-Microglobulin					
Human urine	1.985	17	280	866	pH 7.0, MW = 11,600 [866]
Mitogenic components					
Phaseolus vulgaris					
A	–	6	280	1646	pH 7.0, 5 mM NaP$_i$, 0.1 M NaCl
B	–	3.6	280	1646	
Molybdoferredoxin					
Clostridium pasteurianum	22.5	13.4	280	1078	pH 7.0, 0.1 M TES buffer, data from Figure 7 [1078], MW = 168,000 [1078]
Monellin					
Dioscoreophyllum cumminsil	1.47	13.7	277	1647	pH 7.2
	1.83	17	290	1647	pH 12.8
Monoamine oxidase (amine oxidase, EC 1.4.3.4)					
Beef kidney	53.9	18.6	280	342	pH 7.6, 0.05 $M P_i$, MW = 290,000 [342]
	4.7	1.62	455	342	pH 7.6, 0.05 $M P_i$, MW = 290,000 [342]
Plasma	25.0	9.8	280	343	MW = 255,000 [343]
Myeloperoxidase (peroxidase, EC 1.11.2.2)					
Canine uterine pus	22	–	280	875	Data from Figure 3 [875]
Human leukocyte	–	24	280	344	pH 7.0, 0.2 $M P_i$
Myoglobin	17.1	–	409	609	
	0.97	–	500	609	
Synthetic					
Proto-Mb$^+$	18.8	–	409	1648	
	1.16	–	502	1648	
	0.47	–	630	1648	
+CN$^-$	12.6	–	422	1648	
	1.30	–	540	1648	
+N$_3^-$	12.5	–	419	1648	pH 6, 0.1 $M P_i$
	1.22	–	540	1648	
	0.97	–	574	1648	
+F$^-$	16.0	–	406	1648	
	1.09	–	490	1648	
	0.98	–	605	1648	
+H$_2$O$_2$	12.3	–	421	1648	–
	1.25	–	546	1648	–
+OH$^-$	11.7	–	413	1648	–
	1.16	–	542	1648	–
	1.10	–	583	1648	–
+Na$_2$S$_2$O$_4$	13.5	–	434	1648	
	1.54	–	556	1648	
+Na$_2$S$_2$O$_4$ + CO	20.1	–	422	1648	pH 6, 0.1 $M P_i$
	1.78	–	541	1648	
	1.56	–	578	1648	

MOLAR ABSORPTIVITY AND $A_{1cm}^{1\%}$ VALUES FOR PROTEINS AT SELECTED WAVELENGTHS OF THE ULTRAVIOLET AND VISIBLE REGION (Continued)

Protein	ϵ^a ($\times 10^{-4}$)	$A_{1cm}^{1\%\,b}$	nm^c	Reference	Comments^d
Meso-Mb$^+$	17.2	–	395	1648	
	0.88	–	495	1648	
	0.41	–	622	1648	
+CN$^-$	12.4	–	411	1648	
	0.992	–	531	1648	
+N$_3^-$	12.0	–	409	1648	pH 6, 0.1 M P$_i$
	0.9	–	530	1648	
	0.68	–	564	1648	
+F$^-$	15.4	–	394	1648	
	0.83	–	486	1648	
	0.69	–	598	1648	
+H$_2$O$_2$	11.6	–	408	1648	–
	1.02	–	536	1648	–
+OH$^-$	11.4	–	398	1648	–
	0.91	–	531	1648	–
	0.82	–	569	1648	–
	0.85	–	587	1648	–
+Na$_2$S$_2$O$_4$	11.1	–	421	1648	
	1.27	–	544	1648	
+Na$_2$S$_2$O$_4$ + CO	20.6	–	409	1648	
	1.46	–	530	1648	
	1.16	–	558	1648	
Deutero-Mb$^+$	12.8	–	392	1648	
	0.67	–	495	1648	
	0.29	–	620	1648	
+CN$^-$	10.8	–	409	1648	
	0.83	–	532	1648	
+N$_3^-$	10.5	–	408	1648	pH 6, 0.1 M P$_i$
	0.84	–	530	1648	
	0.61	–	560	1648	
+F$^-$	10.5	–	392	1648	
	0.69	–	483	1648	
	0.54	–	595	1648	
+Na$_2$S$_2$O$_2$	9.76	–	419	1648	
	1.0	–	542	1648	
+Na$_2$S$_2$O$_4$ + CO	17.2	–	408	1648	
	1.21	–	528	1648	
	0.81	–	556	1648	
+H$_2$O$_2$	9.64	–	409	1648	–
	0.72	–	534	1648	–
+OH$^-$	8.87	–	400	1648	–
	0.67	–	532	1648	–
	0.53	–	568	1648	–
	0.53	–	587	1648	–
Hemato-Mb$^+$	14.5	–	400	1648	
	0.94	–	499	1648	
	0.39	–	627	1648	
+CN$^-$	10.8	–	415	1648	
	1.05	–	537	1648	
+N$_3^-$	10.3	–	412	1648	
	0.96	–	535	1648	
	0.74	–	566	1648	pH 6, 0.1 M P$_i$
+F$^-$	13.2	–	400	1648	
	0.88	–	489	1648	
	0.66	–	600	1648	
+Na$_2$S$_2$O$_4$	11.0	–	426	1648	
	1.30	–	550	1648	
+Na$_2$S$_2$O$_4$ + CO	16.3	–	413	1648	
	1.50	–	534	1648	

MOLAR ABSORPTIVITY AND $A_{1cm}^{1\%}$ VALUES FOR PROTEINS AT SELECTED WAVELENGTHS OF THE ULTRAVIOLET AND VISIBLE REGION (Continued)

Protein	ϵ^a ($\times 10^{-4}$)	$A_{1cm}^{1\% \, b}$	nm^c	Reference	Comments^d
+H$_2$O$_2$	10.2	–	413	1648	
	1.07	–	540	1648	
+OH$^-$	10.6	–	402	1648	
	0.92	–	536	1648	
	0.83	–	589	1648	
Proto monomethyl					
Mb$^+$	16.6	–	406	1648	
	1.05	–	501	1648	
	0.45	–	630	1648	
+CN$^-$	11.7	–	418	1648	pH 6, 0.1 M P$_i$
	1.18	–	540	1648	
+N$_3^-$	11.5	–	418	1648	
	1.11	–	540	1648	
	0.90	–	572	1648	
+F$^-$	13.9	–	404	1648	
	1.00	–	488	1648	
	0.95	–	604	1648	
+Na$_2$S$_2$O$_4$	12.7	–	431	1648	
	1.49	–	556	1648	
+Na$_2$S$_2$O$_4$ + CO	17.5	–	419	1648	pH 6, 0.1 M P$_i$
	1.64	–	539	1648	
	1.37	–	573	1648	
+H$_2$O$_2$	11.1	–	418	1648	
	1.08	–	544	1648	
OH$^-$	11.1	–	410	1648	
	1.03	–	540	1648	
	0.96	–	580	1648	
Proto dimethyl					
Mb$^+$	14.5	–	407	1648	
	0.88	–	502	1648	
	0.40	–	630	1648	
+CN$^-$	10.5	–	420	1648	
	1.00	–	541	1648	
+N$_3^-$	10.5	–	418	1648	pH 6, 0.1 M P$_i$
	1.01	–	541	1648	
	0.83	–	572	1648	
+F$^-$	11.7	–	405	1648	
	0.86	–	486	1648	
	0.83	–	605	1648	
+Na$_2$S$_2$O$_4$	10.5		432	1648	
	1.30		556	1648	
+Na$_2$S$_2$O$_4$ + CO	15.9		421	1648	pH 6, 0.1 M P$_i$
	1.41		540	1648	
	1.23		570	1648	
+H$_2$O$_2$	9.15		418	1648	
	0.94		545	1648	
+OH$^-$	7.88		410	1648	
	0.96		538	1648	
	0.86		578	1648	
Oxyforms					
Proto	14.5		417	1649	
	1.73		543	1649	
	1.79		581	1649	
Meso	13.9		404	1649	
	1.50		533	1649	
	1.32		568	1649	
Deutero	11.4		402	1649	
	1.27		532	1649	
	0.89		565	1649	

MOLAR ABSORPTIVITY AND $A_{1cm}^{1\%}$ VALUES FOR PROTEINS AT SELECTED WAVELENGTHS OF THE ULTRAVIOLET AND VISIBLE REGION (Continued)

Protein	ϵ^a ($\times 10^{-4}$)	$A_{1cm}^{1\%\,b}$	nm^c	Reference	Comments^d
Hemato	11.9		410	1649	
	1.40		538	1649	
	1.16		574	1649	
Protomonoester	11.4		415	1649	
	1.40		541	1649	
	1.35		579	1649	
Protodiester	9.65		416	1649	
	1.64		542	1649	
	1.68		579	1649	
Albacore tuna (*Thunnus germo*)	–	6.4	555	1081	–
	–	61	430	1081	–
MetMb	–	2.1	630	1081	–
	–	1.7	580	1081	–
	–	4.8	502	1081	–
	–	81	408	1081	–
	–	15.5	280	1081	–
Myoglobin, carboxy-	–	6.7	570	1081	–
	–	7.5	538	1081	–
	–	95	421	1081	–
Beef, MetMbCN	2.96	–	280	1086	pH 7.2, 0.01 M P$_i$ containing 0.01% KCN
	0.945	–	340	1086	
Bluefin tuna (*Thunnus thynnus*)	–	7.1	558	1081	–
	–	56	431	1081	–
MetMb	–	2.1	634	1081	–
	–	1.7	580	1081	–
	–	4.8	504	1081	–
	–	86	407	1081	–
	–	13.3	275	1081	–
Myoglobin, carboxy-	–	7.6	570	1081	–
	–	8.4	540	1081	–
	–	104	420	1081	–
Camel	3.13	–	280	615	
	17.2	–	409	615	
	0.796	–	470	615	Ferri form, acidic
	0.987	–	503	615	
	0.360	–	580	615	
	0.366	–	630	615	
	3.43	–	280	615	
	10.4	–	414	615	Basic
	0.948	–	542	615	
	0.93	–	587	615	
	3.33	–	280	615	
	2.87	–	360	615	Cyanide form
	11.5	–	423	615	
	1.132	–	542	615	
MetMbCN	2.90	–	280	1086	pH 7.2, 0.01 M P$_i$ containing 0.01% KCN
	0.915	–	340	1086	
Chicken (*Gallus gallus*)	3.1	–	280	1651	–
Muscle					
MetMbCN	0.96	–	534	1650	
	10.2	–	423	1650	
MetMb	0.32	–	632	1650	
	0.84	–	504	1650	
Muscle, distrophic					
MetMbCN	0.95	–	543	1650	
	10.0	–	423	1650	
	0.32	–	632	1650	
	0.84	–	504	1650	
Chinook salmon (*Oncorhynchus tschawtscha*)	–	7.0	558	1081	–
	–	50	428	1081	–

MOLAR ABSORPTIVITY AND $A_{1cm}^{1\%}$ VALUES FOR PROTEINS AT SELECTED WAVELENGTHS OF THE ULTRAVIOLET AND VISIBLE REGION (Continued)

Protein	ϵ^a ($\times 10^{-4}$)	$A_{1cm}^{1\%\,b}$	nm[c]	Reference	Comments[d]
MetMb	–	2.2	632	1081	–
	–	1.9	580	1081	–
	–	5.1	502	1081	–
	–	85	404	1081	–
	–	20.4	280	1081	–
Myoglobin, carboxy-	–	7.4	569	1081	–
	–	7.7	539	1081	–
	–	95	420	1081	–
Cormorant (*Phalacrocorax*)	–	6.4	558	1081	–
	–	64	435	1081	–
MetMb	–	1.8	634	1081	–
	–	1.4	580	1081	–
	–	4.8	504	1081	–
	–	90	409	1081	–
	–	17.1	280	1081	–
Myoglobin, carboxy-	–	6.5	579	1081	–
	–	7.7	542	1081	–
	–	99	432	1081	–
Fin whale, component VII	3.2	18.28	280	1083	MW = 17,504 [1083]
Goat					
MetMbCN	2.95	–	280	1086	
	1.01	–	340	1086	pH 7.2, 0.01 M P$_i$ containing 0.01% KCN
Hamster					
MetMbCN	–	53.9	420	1087	
Habor seal	2.99	–	280	614	Ferri form, pH 6.2
	16.2	–	409	614	
Horse	1.33	–	555	1082	–
	11.3	–	434	1082	–
MetMbCN	2.95	–	280	1086	pH 7.2, 0.01 M P$_i$ containing 0.01% KCN
	0.95	–	340	1086	
MetMb	–	17.9	280	1088	–
Myoglobin, carboxy-	1.18	–	578	1082	–
	1.4	–	540	1082	–
	17.8	–	423	1082	–
Mb$^+$	16.0	–	408	1082	–
	1.02	–	505	1082	–
	0.42	–	630	1082	–
Mb-OH	9.0	–	414	1082	–
	0.91	–	540	1082	–
	0.86	–	580	1082	–
Human	3.05	17.4	280	610	MW = 17,510 [610]
Apo-	1.55	9.2	280	610	MW = 16,900 [610]
MetMbCN	3.07	–	280	1086	pH 7.2, 0.01 M P$_2$ containing 0.01% KCN
	1.04	–	340	1086	
Humpback whale (*Megaptera nodosa*)	–	6.5	558	1081	–
	–	61	434	1081	–
MetMb	–	1.9	634	1081	–
	–	1.5	580	1081	–
	–	5.0	504	1081	–
	–	85	409	1081	–
	–	15.9	281	1081	–
Myoglobin, carboxy-	–	6.1	577	1081	–
	–	7.2	543	1081	–
	–	96	423	1081	–
Lamb					
MetMbCN	3.09	–	280	1086	pH 7.2, 0.01 M P$_i$ containing 0.01% KCN
	1.08	–	340	1086	
Molluscs (*Aplysia depilans* and *Aplysia limacina*)	1.3	–	555	1082	–
	11.3	–	438	1082	–
(*Acanthopleura granulata*)					

MOLAR ABSORPTIVITY AND $A_{1cm}^{1\%}$ VALUES FOR PROTEINS AT SELECTED WAVELENGTHS OF THE ULTRAVIOLET AND VISIBLE REGION (Continued)

Protein	ϵ^a ($\times 10^{-4}$)	$A_{1cm}^{1\%\ b}$	nm^c	Reference	Comments^d
Myoglobin, carboxy-					
Type 1'	1.22	–	570	1094	–
	1.38	–	538	1094	–
	14.94	–	419	1094	–
Type 2'	1.24	–	572	1094	–
	1.32	–	538	1094	–
	17.90	–	419	1094	–
Type 3'	1.30	–	572	1094	–
	1.33	–	538	1094	–
	17.93	–	419	1094	–
(*Buccinum undatum L.*)					
Myoglobin, carboxy-	1.35	–	570	1095	–
	1.42	–	538	1095	–
	18.44	–	418	1095	–
	3.4	–	280	1095	–
(*Aplysia depilans* and *Aplysia limacina*)					
Myoglobin, carboxy-	1.37	–	571	1082	–
	1.42	–	541	1082	–
	17.6	–	424	1082	–
Mb$^+$	9.9	–	400	1082	–
	1.31	–	505	1082	–
	0.38	–	640	1082	–
Mb-OH	9.1	–	412	1082	–
	0.9	–	543	1082	–
	0.87	–	580	1082	–
	0.87	–	600	1082	–
Mb-O$_2$	10.8	–	416	1082	–
	1.32	–	542	1082	–
	1.33	–	578	1082	–
Monkey					
MetMbCn	3.01	–	280	1086	pH 7.2, 0.01 MP$_i$ containing 0.01% KCN
	1.02	–	340	1086	
Pelican (*Pelecanus occidentalis*)	–	6.2	556	1081	–
	–	57	433	1081	–
MetMb	–	1.6	632	1081	–
	–	1.3	581	1081	–
	–	4.8	504	1081	–
	–	78	409	1081	–
	–	14.6	280	1081	–
Myoglobin, carboxy-	–	6.2	577	1081	–
	–	7.3	540	1081	–
	–	87	423	1081	–
Penguin (*Aptenodytes forsteri*)	3.2	–	280	1651	–
Porpoise	2.98	–	280	614	Ferri form, pH 6.2
	16.2	–	409	614	
Skip jack tuna (*Katsuwonus pelamis*)	–	6.4	556	1081	–
	–	62	431	1081	–
MetMb	–	2.0	632	1081	–
	–	1.5	578	1081	–
	–	4.7	502	1081	–
	–	89	406	1081	–
	–	12.2	275	1081	–
Myoglobin, carboxy-	–	6.7	569	1081	–
	–	7.3	539	1081	–
	–	102	421	1081	–
Sperm whale	10.5	–	434	1079	pH 9.1, 0.1 M borax, data from Figure 14 [1079], MW = 17,800 [1080]
	1.08	–	558	1079	
	17.9	100	408	1080	
	3.45	19	280	1080	

MOLAR ABSORPTIVITY AND $A_{1cm}^{1\%}$ VALUES FOR PROTEINS AT SELECTED WAVELENGTHS OF THE ULTRAVIOLET AND VISIBLE REGION (Continued)

Protein	ϵ^a ($\times 10^{-4}$)	$A_{1cm}^{1\% \; b}$	nm^c	Reference	Comments[d]
	3.79	–	280	611	Fe 0.31% [611]
	3.34	–	280	612 ⎫	
	16.8	–	409	612 ⎬	Ferri form
	0.367	–	634	612 ⎭	
	3.06	–	280	614 ⎫	Ferri form, pH 6.2
	16.4	–	409	614 ⎭	
	30.6	–	589	1652	–
	1.15	–	557	1652	–
	0.64	–	521	1652	–
Apo-	1.59	8.9	280	1080	MW = 17,800 [1080]
	1.54	–	280	1084	Dry wt., corrected for light scattering
	–	9.3	280	1085	Neutral
	–	9.2	280	1085	0.1 N NaOH
	1.58	–	280	613	pH 6.8, 0.1 M P$_i$
MbNO	0.7	–	583	1652	–
	1.0	–	546	1652	–
MetMbCN	0.2	–	583	1652	–
	0.95	–	539	1652	–
MbCO	0.65	–	582	1652	–
	0.78	–	572	1652	–
	1.36	–	544	1652	–
	0.4	–	522	1652	–
MbO$_2$	1.08	–	582	1652	–
	0.41	–	571	1652	–
	1.06	–	550	1652	–
	0.79	–	533	1652	–
MetMbNO	0.77	–	575	1652	–
	0.215	–	562	1652	–
MetMbN$_3^-$	0.36	–	587	1652	–
	0.38	–	570	1652	–
	0.62	–	546	1652	–
	0.38	–	514	1652	–
MetMb	–	93.4	410	1088	–
	14.4	–	407	1079 ⎫	pH 6.5, P$_i$ buffer containing 25 mM Na$_2$ S$_2$ O$_4$, data
	0.82	–	502	1079 ⎬	from Figure 14 [1079], water/0.1 N NaOH
	0.34	–	633	1079 ⎭	
	–	18.0	280	1089	Water/0.1 N NaOH
	0.35	–	630	1090	–
	0.93	–	505	1090	–
	16.0	–	409	1090	–
	3.1	–	280	1090	–
	0.35	–	630	1090 ⎫	
	0.91	–	505	1090 ⎬	Regenerated
	15.9	–	409	1090 ⎬	
	3.2	–	280	1090 ⎭	
	–	17.9	280	1085	0.1 N NaOH
Myoglobin, carboxy-	3.24	18.2	280	1091	pH 8.8, dry wt., MW = 17,800 [1092], data from Figure 2 [1091]
	1.21	6.8	578	1093 ⎫	
	1.38	7.2	540	1093 ⎬	MW = 17,816 [1093]
	18.6	104	423	1093 ⎭	
Mb-Fe^{3+}	0.9	5.05	503	1093	–
	16.8	94	409	1093	–
	3.42	19.3	280	1093	–
MbO$_2$	1.45	8.13	581	1093	–
	1.36	7.6	543	1093	–
	12.5	70	418	1093	–
Mb-Fe^{2+}	1.17	6.6	555	1093	–
	11.6	65	434	1093	–

MOLAR ABSORPTIVITY AND $A_{1cm}^{1\%}$ VALUES FOR PROTEINS AT SELECTED WAVELENGTHS OF THE ULTRAVIOLET AND VISIBLE REGION (Continued)

Protein	ϵ^a ($\times 10^{-4}$)	$A_{1cm}^{1\% \, b}$	nm^c	Reference	Comments^d
Mb-Fe^{3+}-N$_3$	11.1	62.1	421	1093	–
Yellowfin tuna (*Neothunnis macropterus*)	–	6.6	556	1081	–
	–	60	431	1081	–
MetMb	–	2.1	631	1081	–
	–	1.6	578	1081	–
	–	4.8	501	1081	–
	–	85	406	1081	–
	–	13.9	275	1081	–
Myoglobin, carboxy-	–	7.0	568	1081	–
	–	7.7	538	1081	–
	–	107	420	1081	–
Myokinase	1.15	5.38	277	876	pH 7.0, 0.15 *M* KCl–0.01 *M* KP$_i$, MW = 21,400 [876], protein con. det. by dry wt.
Rabbit muscle	–	5.2	280	141	
	1.1	5.3	279	345	pH 6.9, MW = 21,000 [345]
	–	11.8	279	346	pH 7.0, 0.01 *M* P$_i$
Myosin					
Rabbit muscle	–	5.2	280	347	pH 7.0, 0.5 *M* KCl, 20 m*M* Tris
	–	2.5	250	347	pH 7.0, 0.5 *M* KCl, 20 m*M* Tris
	–	6.47	280	348	–
	–	5.07	276	348	pH 7.5, 5 *M* GdmCl
	–	5.88	280	348	0.5 *M* KCl^{ot}
	–	4.83	280	348	5 *M* GdmCl^{ot}
	–	5.43	280	349	–
	–	5.9	280	350	pH 7, 0.3 *M* KCl, 0.01 *M* Tris
	–	5.87	277	351	Neutral KCl
	–	5.50	280	616	
	–	5.52	280	616	} pH 7.3, 0.5 *M* KCl–0.01 *M* EDTA + 0.05 *M* P$_i$ + 0.2 *M* P$_i$
	–	5.55	280	616	+ 0.5 *M* P$_i$
	–	5.58	280	616	
	–	5.35	280	1097	Free of low molecular weight protein
Light chains	0.7	3.5	280	1098	MW = 20.200 [1098]
Meromyosin, heavy	–	6.35	280	1099	–
Meromyosin, light	–	3.0	280	1100	–
Rabbit filament	–	2.00	278	1653	–
Skeletal muscle	–	5.6	280	1654	–
Heavy meromyosin	–	6.25	280	352	–
	–	6.47	279	353	–^{ct}
		6.47	280	1654	
Beef heart	–	5.7	280	618	–
Light meromyosin, fraction I	–	3.69	279	353	Trypsin digestion for 25 sec
	–	3.29	279	353	Trypsin digestion for 25 min
Light component	–	3.5	280	1654	
Light subfragment 1					
Beef heart	–	6.4	280	618	–
Meromyosin, light					
Rabbit	–	2.97	278	619	pH 3, 0.1 *M* NaCl–HCl
Light chain	–	4.03	280	1655	N
Slime mold	–	5.2	278	617	pH 7.4, 0.5 *M* KCl–0.01 *M* Tris, data from Figure 3 [617]
Human heart	–	5.1	280	1096	pH 6.8, 0.4 *M* KCl-borate, corrected for scattering
Paramyosin	–	3.04	277	354	–
Heavy alkali subunit	–	5.77	277	351	Neutral KCl
	–	5.19	277	351	6 *M* GdmCl
	–	5.29	277	351	5 *M* GdmCl
Light alkali subunit	–	4.34	277	351	Neutral KCl
	–	4.79	277	351	5 *M* GdmCl

---

^{ot} These values have been corrected for light scattering.

MOLAR ABSORPTIVITY AND $A_{1cm}^{1\%}$ VALUES FOR PROTEINS AT SELECTED WAVELENGTHS OF THE ULTRAVIOLET AND VISIBLE REGION (Continued)

Protein	ϵ^a ($\times 10^{-4}$)	$A_{1cm}^{1\% \; b}$	nm^c	Reference	Comments^d
S-I fragment	–	7.9	280	355	–
S-n fragment	–	8.0	280	355	–
Chicken					
Red/slow muscle	–	5.33	280	356	–
White/fast muscle	–	5.05	280	356	–
Pectoral muscle	–	5.25	280	1655	–
Pig muscle					
Chesterwhite	–	4.9	280	347	pH 7.0, 0.5 M KCl, 20 mM Tris
	–	2.4	250	347	pH 7.0, 0.5 M KCl, 20 mM Tris
Poland China	–	4.9	280	347	pH 7.0, 0.5 M KCl, 20 mM Tris
	–	2.5	250	347	pH 7.0, 0.5 M KCl, 20 mM Tris
Poland China [PSE]	–	5.2	280	347	pH 7.0, 0.5 M KCl, 20 mM Tris
Myrosinase (thioglucosidase) (EC 3.2.3.1)					
Sinapsis alba (White mustard seed)	–	15	278	1656	–
NAD nucleosidase (EC 3.2.2.5) (see DPNase)					
NADH-cytochrome b_3 reductase					
Rat liver, microsomes	–	23	280	729	pH 7.5, 0.01 M KP$_i$
NADH:FAD oxidoreductase					
E. coli B	16.4	13	272	1101	MW = 126,000 [1101], pH 7.0, 0.05 M KP$_i$, data from Figure 1 [1101]
	2.33	1.85	380	1101	–^{pt}
	2.24	1.78	448	1101	–^{pt}
NADPH-adrenodoxin reductase					
Beef adrenocortical mitochondria	–	18	272	1657	From Figure 2 [1657]
	–	2.0	378	1657	
NADPH oxidase					
Rabbit liver, microsomes	–	19.1	280	730	pH 7.4, 0.34 M P$_i$
NADPH-sulfite reductase (EC 3.2.2.5)					
Bull semen	–	10.9	278	1658	pH 7.4, 0.01 M NaP$_i$, dry wt.
NADPH-sulfite reductase (EC 1.8.1.2)					
E. coli B	–	4.60	386	1659	Dry wt.
Nagarse [BPN']	–	8.8	280	357	–
Nerve growth factor					
Mouse, 2.5S	2.2	16.4	280	1660	AA, MW = 13,259
Salivary gland	–	14.7	280	1661	pH 4, 0.1 M AcO$^-$ or pH 4, 0.1 M AcO$^-$ 8 M urea, from Figure 1 [1661]
Submaxillary gland	4.15	13.86	280	1102	pH 5.0, 0.05 M AcO$^-$, MW = 30,000 [1102]
Naja naja	–	11.8	280	1661	pH 4, 0.1 M AcO$^-$ from Figure 1 [1661]
	–	12.9	280	1661	pH 4, 0.1 M AcO$^-$ 8 M urea, from Figure 1 [1661]
Vipera russelli venom	–	9.9	282	1662	
Cobra venom	3.22	12.7	280	620	Water, MW = 25,300 [620]
Neurophysin-II					
Beef pituitary	0.395	–	260	621	–
Neurotoxin					
Naja naja siamensis (Thailand cobra)	0.83	10.6	279	1103	Neutral sol., MW = 7820 [1130]
Reduced and carboxymethylated	0.68	–	279	1103	10% AcOH
Toxin 3	–	10.6	279	1664	–
Toxin 3C	0.89	12.9	279	1103	MW = 6793 [1103]
Toxin 5	1.3	19.1	280	1103	MW = 6875 [1103]
Toxin 7C	0.9	12.9	279	1103	MW = 6985 [1103]
Naja naja naja (Indian cobra)					
Toxin 3	0.85	10.9	279	1103	MW = 7834 [1103]
	–	10.9	279	1664	–
Reduced and carboxymethylated	0.66	–	279	1103	–
Toxin 4	0.85	10.9	279	1103	MW = 7807 [1103]
Reduced and carboxymethylated	0.65	–	279	1103	–
Naja haje (Cobra)					

---

^{pt} Calculated from OD$_{272}$/OD$_{448}$ = 7.33, and OD$_{380}$/OD$_{448}$ = 1.04.

MOLAR ABSORPTIVITY AND $A_{1cm}^{1\%}$ VALUES FOR PROTEINS AT SELECTED WAVELENGTHS OF THE ULTRAVIOLET AND VISIBLE REGION (Continued)

Protein	ϵ^a ($\times 10^{-4}$)	$A_{1cm}^{1\%\ b}$	nm[c]	Reference	Comments[d]
Toxin I[qt]	0.917	13.28	280	1104	MW = 6843 [1104]
Toxin I[rt]	0.923	13.49	279	1104	MW = 6843 [1104]
Toxin II[qt]	0.828	12.07	280	1104	MW = 6857 [1104]
Toxin II[rt]	1.123	16.31	278	1104	MW = 6887 [1104]
Toxin III[rt]	0.898	11.48	280	1104	MW = 7806 [1104]
Naja nigricollis	0.87	12.8	279	731	pH 7.3, 0.03 M NaP$_i$, MW = 6787 [731]
	0.84	12.4	279	731	pH 2.3, MW = 6787 [731]
Carboxymethyl-	0.66	–	279	731	–
I	0.901	13.26	280	1663	MW = 6794
II	0.886	13.03	280	1663	MW = 6796
Notechis scutatus scutatus (Australian tiger snake)					
Venom[st]	2.8	20.6	278	1665	Acid pH
Androctonus australis Hector (Scorpion)					
Toxin I	1.071	15.75	275	1105	MW = 6808 [1105]
	1.03	15.12	280	1105	
Toxin II	1.801	24.80	276	1105	MW = 7249 [1105]
	1.67	23.08	280	1105	
Toxin III	1.191	17.45	277.5	1105	MW = 6826 [1105]
	1.169	17.13	280	1105	
Buthus occitanus tunetanus (Scorpion)					
Toxin I	1.888	–	278	1105	MW[tt]
	–	26.75	280	1105	–
Toxin II	2.126	28.20	278	1105	MW = 7539 [1105]
	2.079	27.58	280	1105	
Toxin III	1.915	26.34	278	1105	MW = 7270 [1105]
	1.857	25.55	280	1105	
Leirus quinquestriatus quinquestriatus (Scorpion)					
Toxin I	1.511	21.81	275	1105	MW = 6928 [1105]
	1.467	21.17	280	1105	
Toxin II	1.340	–	277	1105	MW[ut]
	–	19.86	280	1105	–
Toxin III	2.153	–	276.5	1105	MW[vt]
	–	30.53	280	1105	–
Toxin IV	2.002	27.38	278	1105	MW = 7313 [1105]
	1.966	26.89	280	1105	
Toxin V	2.135	28.61	275	1105	MW = 7462 [1105]
	2.082	27.90	280	1105	
Nicotin oxidase (nicotine dehydrogenase, EC 1.5.99.4)					
A. oxydans	–	23.6	280	358	pH 7.9, 0.1 M PyP$_i$, mM EDTA
Nicotinic acid hydroxylase (nicotinate dehydrogenase, EC 1.5.1.13)					
Clostridium	33	11	275	1106	MW = 300,000 [1106], data from Figure 6 [1106]
Nitrate reductase					
Micrococcus denitrificans	41.9	26	280	1107	pH 7.4, 0.2 M P$_i$, MW = 161, 129 [1107], data from Figure 3 [1107]
Nitrite reductase (EC 1.7.99.3)					
Achromobacter cycloclastes	0.16	–	400	1666	Dry wt.
	0.40	–	464	1666	
	0.20	–	590	1666	
	0.17	–	700	1666	
Achromobacter fisheri	1.49	–	525	1667	pH 7.0, oxidized
	16.6	–	409	1667	
	11.8	–	278–80	1667	

qt From Miami Serpentarium.
rt From Institute Pasteur.
st Protein called "Notexin," Ref. [1665].
tt MW = 6919–6933.
ut MW = 6511–6545.
vt MW = 6764–6792.

MOLAR ABSORPTIVITY AND $A_{1cm}^{1\%}$ VALUES FOR PROTEINS AT SELECTED WAVELENGTHS OF THE ULTRAVIOLET AND VISIBLE REGION (Continued)

Protein	ϵ^a ($\times 10^{-4}$)	$A_{1cm}^{1\%\,b}$	nm^c	Reference	Comments^d
	4.26	–	551	1667	
	2.6	–	523	1667	pH 7.0, reduced
	21.9	–	420	1667	
Chlorella fusca	2.2	–	384	1668	
Nitrogenase					
Azotobacter vinelandii	47.0	17.4	280	1108	MW = 270,000 [1108]
	8.5	3.15	412	1108	
Mo-Fe protein	47	17.4	280	1669	pH 7.4, 0.25 M NaCl, 0.01 M Tris Cl under N_2,
	8.5	3.2	418	1669	MW = 270,000 [1669]
Klebsiella pneumonia					
Kp 1	26	–	258.5	1670	
	30	–	269	1670	
	33	–	277.5	1670	
	32	–	282	1670	Reduced and oxidized
	25	–	289	1670	
	35	–	430	1670	
	50	–	430	1670	Oxidized
Kp 2	11	–	258	1670	Reduced and oxidized
	11.2	–	268	1670	
	0.4–0.5	–	460	1670	Reduced
	1.0	–	460	1670	Oxygen inactivated
Non-histone					
Rat liver	1.8	12.3	275	442	pH 8, 0.01 M Tris, 0.01% NaDodSO$_4$, estd. from Figure 1 [442]
Nuclease					
Bacteriophage T4	–	14.8	280	1109	pH 7.5^{wt}
Staphylococcal	–	9.7	277	1110	–
Performic acid oxidized	–	7.0	274	1110	–
Lightly acetylated	–	9.7	277	1110	–
Heavily acetylated	–	9.7	277	1110	–
Trifluoroacetylated	–	9.0	277	1110	–
S. aureus	–	11.6	280	359	pH 7.2, 0.15 N NaP$_i$
3-Nucleotidase (see phosphodiesterase, 2′:3′-cyclic)					
Nucleoside triphosphate–adenylate kinase (EC 2.7.4.10)					
Beef heart mitochondria	4.55	8.75	280	1111	pH 8.5, 0.05 M N(EtOH)$_3$ HCl, MW = 52,000 [1111], data from Figure 3 [1111]
Octopine dehydrogenase (EC 1.5.1.11)	4.33	–	280	1671	–
Pecten maximus	–	11.4	280	732	–
Ornithine-oxoacid aminotransferase (EC 2.6.1.13)					
Rat liver	–	10.6	280	736	
With added ornithine	–	11.0	280	736	Data from Figure 3 [736], pH 8, 0.2 M Tris Cl
Apo-	–	10.8	280	736	
Ornithine transcarbamylase (EC 2.1.3.3)					
S. faecalis	–	8.32	280	1672	pH 7.0, 50 mM NaP$_i$, dry wt. and nitrogen
Beef liver		12.3	280	1672	
Orosomucoid					
Rabbit serum	1.93	6.05	276	1673	
	1.94	6.06	277	1673	MW = 32,000
	1.93	6.04	278	1673	
	1.92	6.00	280	1673	
Orotate reductase (EC 1.3.1.14) (see dihydroorotic dehydrogenase)					
Ovalbumin	2.85	–	280	17	pH 4.9
	–	7.5	280	16	–
	–	7.35	280	361	–

^{wt} 14 mM Tris-HCl, 140 mM KCl, 1.4 mM β-mercaptocthanol (HSEtOH), and 7.1% glycerol. Protein determined by Lowry method and absorption corrected for scattering.

MOLAR ABSORPTIVITY AND $A_{1cm}^{1\%}$ VALUES FOR PROTEINS AT SELECTED WAVELENGTHS OF THE ULTRAVIOLET AND VISIBLE REGION (Continued)

Protein	ϵ^a ($\times 10^{-4}$)	$A_{1cm}^{1\% b}$	nm^c	Reference	Comments^d
	–	7.5	280	733	
	–	260	210	733	
	–	750	191	733	0.1 M NaOH
	–	7.15	280	734	
	2.94	7.35	280	1674	MW = 45,000
	–	3.40	255	1675	
	–	7.60	280	1675	pH 7.0, 0.01 M P$_i$
	–	0.48	310	1675	
	–	7.37	280	1676	Native and SDS denatured, Refr.
	–	7.54	280	1676	6 M GdmCl, Refr.
	1.579	–	293	1112	–
	2.792	–	287	1112	–
	21.42	–	232	1112	–
Chicken	3.15	7.01	280	1113	MW = 45,000 [1114]
Chicken egg	3.218	–	280	1677	–
	–	6.9	280	1678	–
	–	7.14	280	1679	–
Turkey	3.74	8.32	280	1113	MW = 45,000 [1114]
Duck	3.72	8.28	280	1113	MW = 45,000 [1114]
Ovoglycoprotein					
Chicken egg	0.93	3.8	280	1680	MW = 24,440 [1680]
Ovoinhibitor					
Chicken	–	7.1	280	1681	pH 6.8, 0.01 M P$_i$
Chicken egg white	–	6.5–6.9	278	1682	–
	–	7.4	278	1115	
Quail egg white	–	7.1	278	1116	
	–	7.1	278	1116	pH 8, 0.1 M Tris
Ovomacroglobulin					
Chicken egg white	–	8.6	278	1117	Dry wt.
Ovomucin					
Chicken egg white	–	10.3	290	1118	pH 13
	–	9.3	277.5	1118	
	–	5.6	290	1118	Neutral sol.
Ovomucoid	–	4.55	280	362	–
	1.19	4.13	280	363	MW = 28,800 [363]
Chicken		4.1	280	1681	pH 6.8, 0.01 M P$_i$
	1.17	4.3	277	1683	pH 7.5, water:glycerol, 1:1
Chicken egg white	1.1	4.10	278	1119	MW = 27,300 [1119]
Turkey	–	4.15	280	1684	pH 7.8, Tris
Ovorubin					
Pomacea canaliculata australis	–	10.5	280	735	Data from Figure 3 [735]
Ovotransferrin (conalbumin)					
Chicken	0.475	0.620	470	1685	pH 6–9 MW = 76,600
	8.5	11.1	280	1685	0.02 M HCl, MW = 76,600 [1685]
	–	11.6	280	1686	–
	7.96	–	280	1687	pH 6.5, 6 M Gdn 0.02 M P$_i$
	9.03	–	280	1687	pH 10.5, 0.1 M glycine-NaOH
	–	11.2	280	1688	–
Iodate oxidized, pH 8.5	9.2	–	280	1687	
Iodate oxidized at pH 5.0	9.5	–	280	1687	pH 6.5, 6 M Gdn 0.02 M P$_i$
Iron free, oxidized	7.96	–	280	1687	
Iodate oxidized at pH 8.5	9.33	–	280	1687	
Iodate oxidized at pH 5.0	9.80	–	280	1687	pH 10.5, 0.1 M glycine–NaOH
Iron free, oxidized	9.33	–	280	1687	
Oxaloglycolate reductase (decarboxylating) (EC 1.1.1.92)					
P. putida	7.2	11.8	280	364	MW = 61,000 [364]
3-Oxoacyl-[acyl-carrier-protein] reductase (EC 1.1.1.100) (see also fatty acid synthetase)					
Pig liver	46	–	279	1424	–

MOLAR ABSORPTIVITY AND $A_{1cm}^{1\%}$ VALUES FOR PROTEINS AT SELECTED WAVELENGTHS OF THE ULTRAVIOLET AND VISIBLE REGION (Continued)

Protein	ϵ^a ($\times 10^{-4}$)	$A_{1cm}^{1\%\,b}$	nm^c	Reference	Comments^d
3-Oxosteroid $\Delta^{4,5}$-isomerase (steroid Δ-isomerase) (EC 5.3.3.1) (see also 3-keto-Δ^5-steroid isomerase)		3.28	280	1689	Refr.
Beef adrenals	11.3	10.1	–	855	MW = 112,000 [855]
Oxynitrilase (see hydroxynitrilase)	–	3.72	277	1689	Refr.
Oxytyrosinase (monophenol monooxygenase or tyrosinase, EC 1.14.18.1, or tyrosine 3-monooxygenase, EC 1.14.16.2)					
Mushroom	0.9	–	345	1690	Value per mole Cu
	0.6	–	600	1690	
Papain (EC 3.4.22.2)	–	25.0	278	365	–
	4.9	–	280	367	MW = 20,700 [366]
	5.1	–	280	368	–
	1.2	–	295	365	pH 5–8
Papaya	–	21.5	280	1691	0.01 N HCl, from Figure 1 [1691]
	–	27	278	1692	–
Papaya latex					
Trans-cinnamoyl-	2.6	–	326	1120	–
Furylacryloyl-	3.0	–	360	1121	–
	3.0	–	337	1121	Denatured
Indolacryloyl-	4.3	–	398	1121	–
	4.3	–	373	1121	Denatured
Mercury derivative	5.1	–	280	1122	–
Paramyosin					
Venus mercenaria	–	3.24^{xt}	277	1123	pH 7.4, 1 M KCl, 0.1 M KP$_i$
Reduced and carboxymethylated	–	3.39^{yt}	277	1123	–
Crassostrea commercialis (Oyster)	5.95	2.86	276	1124	pH 7.0, 1.1 M NaCl – 25 mM NaP$_i$ MW = 208,000 [1124]
Aulacomya magellanica (Mollusc)	8.76	3.4	280	1125	pH 7.5, 1 M KCl MW = 258,000 [1125]
	9.55	3.7	276	1125	
Parathyroid hormone					
Beef	0.72	7.6	280	369	pH 4.7, AcONH$_4$ MW = 9,500 [369]
Parvalbumin					
Chondrostoma nasus	–	1.84	260	1693	Water, from Figure 7 [1693]
	–	1.57	260	1693	0.1 N NaOH, from Figure 7 [1693]
Merluccius merluccius (Hake)	0.202	1.8	259	1694	MW = 11,500 [1694] AA
	0.215	–	259	1695	–
Raja clavata (Thornback ray)	0.142	–	275	1695	–
Penicillinase (EC 3.5.2.6)					
Bacillus cereus 569	–	6.0^{zt}	280	1126	–
	3.2	10.5	280	1127	Biuret
Bacillus cereus 569/H	–	6.35^{zt}	280	1126	–
Bacillus cereus 5/B	–	7.35^{zt}	280	1126	–
B. licheniformis 6346/C	–	5.65^{zt}	280	1126	–
B. licheniformis 749/C[c]	–	5.45^{zt}	280	1126	–
B. licheniformis 749/C	–	4.75^{zt}	280	1126	–
Staphylococcus aureus PC 1	–	7.38^{zt}	280	1126	–
E. coli K 12	6.1	21.0	280	1128	pH 6.8, 0.01 M KP$_i$ MW = 29,000 [1128]
Penicillocarboxypeptidase-S (peptidase B)					
Penicillium janthinelium	–	26	280	1696	–
Penicillopepsin (EC 3.4.23.7)					
Penicillium janthinellum	4.32	13.5	280	1129	MW = 32,000 [1129]
Pepsin	–	5.38	255	1675	
	–	12.20	280	1675	pH 7.0, 0.01 M P$_i$
	–	0.28	310	1675	

^{xt} In GdmCl: $\epsilon_{277} = 0.035\,(M\,\text{GdmCl}) + 3.24$.
^{yt} In GdmCl: $\epsilon_{277} = 0.34\,(M\,\text{GdmCl}) + 3.39$.
^{zt} $A_{1cm}^{1\%}$/mg N.

MOLAR ABSORPTIVITY AND $A_{1cm}^{1\%}$ VALUES FOR PROTEINS AT SELECTED WAVELENGTHS OF THE ULTRAVIOLET AND VISIBLE REGION (Continued)

Protein	ϵ^a ($\times 10^{-4}$)	$A_{1cm}^{1\%\ b}$	nm^c	Reference	Comments^d
	1.94	–	292.8	1697	
	3.68	–	286	1697	Denatured at pH 1.45, 3 h, 39°C
	5.02	–	279	1697	
	23.87	–	230	1697	
	–	13.1	280	1698	
	–	290	210	1698	Water, dry wt.
	–	920	191	1698	
	5.247	–	278	1699	–
Beef	4.94	14.81	280	1700	MW = 33,367 [1700]
	5.17	14.3	280	370	
	5.09	–	278	371	–
Pig	–	14.1	280	1701	–
	–	780	191–4	1701	–
Chicken	5.34	15.2	276	1702	pH 7.5, 0.1 $M\,P_i$, MW = 35,000 [1702]
	–	150	220	1702	
Human	6.2	17.3	278	179	pH 5, MW = 34,000 [179]
Pepsinogen					
Beef	5.6	12.5	278	373	MW = 41,000 [373]
	5.1	13.05	280	374	MW = 39,000 [374]
Succinyl-	5.5	–	278	375	pH 7.7, 0.032 $M\,P_i$
Bovine 1	–	13.45	280	1703	–
2	–	13.05	280	1703	–
4	–	13.25	280	1703	–
Dog	–	12.79	280	1704	–
Chicken	5.59	13.0	278	1702	pH 1.83, 0.02 N HCl, MW = 43,000 [1702]
	–	12.66	280	1702	
	–	139.9	220	1702	–
Peptidoglutaminase 1 peptidyl-glutaminase, EC 3.5.1.43)	–	7.27	280	1705	–
Peptidoglutaminase 11 (glutaminyl-peptide glutaminase) (EC 3.5.1.44)	–	11.62	280	1705	–
Peroxidase (EC 1.11.1.7) (see also lactoperoxidase, myeloperoxidase)					
Raphanus sativus (Japanese radish)	1.175	–	500	739	
Isoenzyme 3	2.72	–	280	1130	–
	11.14	–	404	1130	–
	1.17	–	502	1130	–
	0.323	–	644	1130	–
Isoenzyme 5	3.82	–	280	1130	–
	11.66	–	405	1130	–
	1.156	–	502	1130	–
	0.338	–	644	1130	–
Isoenzyme 16	2.97	–	280	1130	–
	10.42	–	403	1130	–
	1.186	–	504	1130	–
	0.339	–	645	1130	–
Apo-	1.72	–	–	739	–
Brassica napus L.					
P_1	3.8	–	276	740	–
P_2	3.4	–	276	740	–
P_3	3.0	–	277	740	–
P_6	3.0	–	278	740	–
P_7	2.9	–	278	740	–
Japanese radish, a (see also peroxidase a, apo-)					
Oxidized	3.38	–	276	379	–
	11.10	–	405	379	–
	1.18	–	500	379	–
	0.33	–	645	379	–
Japanese radish, c					
Oxidized	3.0	–	280	379	–

MOLAR ABSORPTIVITY AND $A_{1cm}^{1\%}$ VALUES FOR PROTEINS AT SELECTED WAVELENGTHS OF THE ULTRAVIOLET AND VISIBLE REGION (Continued)

Protein	ϵ^a ($\times 10^{-4}$)	$A_{1cm}^{1\%\,b}$	nm^c	Reference	Comments^d
	10.64	–	420	379	–
	1.17	–	540	379	–
Reduced	10.38	–	425	379	–
	1.26	–	560	379	–
Horseradish	–	22	403	1706	–
	9.1	–	403	1707	–
	10.2	–	403	737	–
	9.1	–	403	376	–
	–	13.4	275	377	pH 7.0
	10.4	–	498	378	Ferric derivative
Nitroso-	11.0	–	420	378	–
Carbon monoxide	15.3	–	422	378	–
Apoenzyme-Al	0.92	–	276	738	pH 6.8, 50 mM NaP$_i$
Apoenzyme-C	1.3	–	277	738	
A$_1$	10.2	–	401	1708	
A$_2$	10.2	–	401	1708	
A$_3$	9.7	–	401	1708	MW = 40,000 [1708]
B	9.5	–	401	1708	
C	9.5	–	401	1708	
Component I	1.31^{a‡}	–	440	1709	–
	1.74^{a‡}	–	432	1709	–
	1.86^{a‡}	–	430	1709	–
	2.83^{a‡}	–	420	1709	–
	4.12^{a‡}	–	410	1709	–
	4.80^{a‡}	–	400	1709	–
	4.62^{a‡}	–	390	1709	–
	4.30^{a‡}	–	380	1709	–
	4.00^{a‡}	–	370	1709	–
	3.60^{a‡}	–	360	1709	–
	3.28^{a‡}	–	350	1709	–
Fraction Ib	2.78^{b‡}	–	280	1710	–
	11.5^{b‡}	–	403	1710	–
Fraction IIIb	2.87^{b‡}	–	280	1710	–
	9.98^{b‡}	–	403	1710	–
Fraction Vb	3.68^{b‡}	–	280	1710	–
	9.50^{b‡}	–	280	1710	–
Fraction VI	4.08^{b‡}	–	403	1710	–
	12.29^{b‡}	–	403	1710	–
Native, oxidized	0.323	–	641	1711	
	1.095	–	498	1711	pH 7.0, 10 mM NaP$_i$
	10.00	–	402	1711	
Protoperoxidase	0.289	–	641	1711	pH 7.0, 10 mM NaP$_i$, oxidized
	1.046	–	499	1711	
	9.43	–	402	1711	
Dipropenyldeuterohematinperoxidase	0.287	–	635	1711	
	1.122	–	500	1711	
	10.22	–	402	1711	
Dibutenyldeuterohematinperoxidase	0.298	–	636	1711	
	1.123	–	502	1711	pH 7.0, 10 mM NaP$_i$
	11.18	–	404	1711	
Deuterohematinperoxidase	0.272	–	627	1711	
	0.708	–	497	1711	
	11.26	–	393	1711	
Mesoperoxidase	0.275	–	634	1711	
	0.942	–	492	1711	
	8.80	–	395	1711	

^{a‡} All values based on $\epsilon_m = 9.14 \times 10^4$ at 430 nm.
^{b‡} Based on hemin content.

MOLAR ABSORPTIVITY AND $A_{1cm}^{1\%}$ VALUES FOR PROTEINS AT SELECTED WAVELENGTHS OF THE ULTRAVIOLET AND VISIBLE REGION (Continued)

Protein	ϵ^a ($\times 10^{-4}$)	$A_{1cm}^{1\% \; b}$	nm^c	Reference	Comments^d
Diacetyldeuterohematinperoxidase	0.226	–	642	1711	
	0.732	–	508	1711	
	8.01	–	412	1711	
Hematoperoxidase	0.299	–	633	1711	pH 7.0, 10 mM NaP$_i$
	0.850	–	497	1711	
	10.27	–	397	1711	
Native, reduced	1.260	–	556	1711	
	8.86	–	436	1711	
Protoperoxidase	1.255	–	555	1711	
	7.53	–	433	1711	
Dipropenyldeuterohematinperoxidase	1.213	–	555	1711	
	8.45	–	433	1711	
Dibutenyldeuterohematinperoxidase	1.251	–	556	1711	
	8.49	–	433	1711	pH 7.0, 10 mM NaP$_i$, reduction by dithionite
Deuterohematinperoxidase	1.000	–	546	1711	
	7.90	–	427	1711	
Mesoperoxidase	1.156	–	549	1711	
	8.80	–	428	1711	
Diacetyldeuterohematinperoxidase	1.037	–	562	1711	
	7.82	–	447	1711	
Hematoperoxidase	1.093	–	549	1711	
	8.91	–	431	1711	
Fig latex (*Ficus carica*)	10.1	–	403	1713	–
	1.16	–	500	1713	–
	0.33	–	640	1713	–
Reduced	9.21	–	438	1713	–
	1.26	–	556	1713	–
Reduced + CO	15.52	–	423	1713	–
	1.31	–	543	1713	–
	1.38	–	573	1713	–
+OH$^-$	10.6	–	417	1713	–
	1.02	–	544	1713	–
	0.79	–	574	1713	–
+NaN$_3$	11.9	–	415	1713	–
	0.93	–	535	1713	–
	0.23	–	637	1713	–
+NaF	15.55	–	404	1713	–
	0.93	–	490	1713	–
	0.57	–	561	1713	–
	0.78	–	613	1713	–
+NaCN	10.25	–	421	1713	–
	1.17	–	540	1713	–
Complex I	5.8	–	402	1713	–
	0.76	–	562	1713	–
	0.62	–	657	1713	–
Complex II	9.6	–	419	1713	–
	0.9	–	527	1713	–
	0.95	–	558	1713	–
Complex III	10.45	–	418	1713	–
	1.17	–	546	1713	–
	1.01	–	583	1713	–
FPO-A	3.78	–	280	1713	
FPO-B	3.31	–	280	1713	Calculated
FPO-C	3.45	–	280	1713	
Pig intestinal mucosa	–	15.5	280	1714	–
	–	14.07	417	1714	–
	–	1.54	490	1714	–
	–	1.27	543	1714	–
	–	1.59	596	1714	–

MOLAR ABSORPTIVITY AND $A_{1cm}^{1\%}$ VALUES FOR PROTEINS AT SELECTED WAVELENGTHS OF THE ULTRAVIOLET AND VISIBLE REGION (Continued)

Protein	ϵ^a ($\times 10^{-4}$)	$A_{1cm}^{1\% \, b}$	nm^c	Reference	Comments^d
	–	0.89	642	1714	–
Peroxidase II					
Horseradish, oxidized	3.27	–	270	279	–
	10.77	–	403	279	–
	1.19	–	497	379	–
	0.34	–	641.5	379	–
Reduced	9.17	–	437	379	–
	1.33	–	556	379	–
Peroxidase a, apo-Japanese radish roots (*Raphanus salivus*)	1.22	2.7	280		MW = 45,300 [77]
Phenolase, mushroom (monophenol monooxygenase, EC 1.14.18.1)	–	26.92	282	380	–
Phenolhydroxylase (phenol 2-monoxygenase) (EC 1.14.13.7)					
Trichosporon cutaneum	–	9.87	276	1715	pH 7.6, 0.1 *M* KP$_i$, from Figure 5 [1715]
Phenoloxidase, pre- (ct. pre-phenoloxidase)					
L-Phenylalanine ammonia lyase (EC 4.3.1.5)					
Maize (*Zea mays*)	–	8.9	280	1716	AA
Phenylalanine 4-monooxygenase (EC 1.14.16.1)					
Rat liver	–	5.6	280	1717	pH 8.6, 0.01 *M* Tris Cl, from Figure 3 [1717]
Phenylalanine monooxygenase-stimulating protein					
Rat liver	4.67	9.06	280	1718	Biuret MW = 51,500 [1718]
Phenylpyruvate tautomerase (EC 5.3.2.1)					
Pig thyroid	5.95	13.5	280	741	pH 6.2, 0.1 *M* P$_i$, MW = 44,000 [741]
Phosphatase, acid (EC 3.1.3.2)					
Human prostate	–	24	280	1746	–
Phaseolus mungo	8.75	16	278	1747	pH 5.6, MW = 55,000 [1747]
Rat, liver	4.7	4.7	278	387	MW = 100,000 [387]
	6.18	6.18	278	1724	MW = 100,000 [1725]
Sweet potato	–	9.1	280	1726	pH 6.0, 0.01 *M* KP$_i$, from Figure 2 [1726]
	–	0.21	555	1726	
N. crassa	9.18	10.8	280	1727	Water, MW = 85,000 [1727]
Phosphatase, alkaline (EC 3.1.3.1)					
Escherichia coli	6.4	7.2	278	742	MW = 89,000 [742]
	0.0260	–	640	1722	–
	0.0220	–	605	1722	–
	0.0378	–	555	1722	–
	0.0335	–	510	1722	–
	–	7.2	278	1721	–
E. coli C90	6.2	7.7	280	381	MW = 80,000 [381]
E. coli K 12	5.6	7.0	278	382	MW = 80,000 [382]
	6.6	7.7	280	743	
Azatryptophan substituted for tryptophan	11	12.8	280	743	MW = 86,000 [744]
Tryptazan substituted for tryptophan	9.6	11.1	280	743	
B. licheniformis	7.5^{ct}	6.2	278	1719	MW = 121,000 [1719]
B. subtilis	0.0305	–	620	1720	–
	0.0335	–	596	1720	–
	0.0500	–	567	1720	–
	0.0382	–	517	1720	–
Micrococcus sodonensis	13.7	17.3	280	1723	–
N. crassa	17.4	11.3	280	383	pH 8.3, 0.01 *M* Tris HCl, MW = 154,000 [383]
A. nidulans	–	10.2	278	384	pH 7.0
Intestinal	7.0	–	280	385	–
Placental, human	9.75	7.8	278	386	pH 7.0, 0.05 *M* P$_i$, MW = 125,000 [386]
Calf intestine	–	10	280	745	pH 7.7
Milk	–	11.5	280	745	–
Pig kidney	–	13.9	280	746	–

---

^{ct} On p. 1369 of Ref. [1719], value is given as 7.25×10^4.

MOLAR ABSORPTIVITY AND $A_{1cm}^{1\%}$ VALUES FOR PROTEINS AT SELECTED WAVELENGTHS OF THE ULTRAVIOLET AND VISIBLE REGION (Continued)

Protein	ϵ^a ($\times 10^{-4}$)	$A_{1cm}^{1\%\ b}$	nm^c	Reference	Comments^d
	–	12.0	260	746	–
Phosphodiesterase 2':3'-cyclic (2':3'-cyclic-nucleoside monophosphate phosphodiesterase, EC 3.1.4.16)					
B. subtilis	–	11	280	1728	pH 7.5, 0.05 M Tris Cl
Phosphoenolpyruvate carboxykinase (EC 4.1.1.32,.38,.49) Baker's yeast	32	12.7	280	1729	pH 7.0, 1 M EDTA—0.025 M Na-borate, MW = 252,000 [1724]
Phosphoenolpyruvate carboxylase (EC4.1.1.31)					
E. coli	63.4	15.5	280	1730	MW = 402,000 [1730], dry wt.
E. coli, str. B	–	10.9	280	1731	pH 8.5, 0.1 M Tris Cl, 10 mM MgCl$_2$, 10 mM KHCO$_3$, 0.01 N NaOH
S. typhimurium	–	15.5	280	1732	–
Phosphofructokinase					
Rabbit muscle	–	10.2	279	388	–
	–	9.4	279	389	pH 7
	–	8.7	283	389	0.1 N NaOH
	–	8.7	290	389	0.1 N NaOH
	–	10.9	290	390	0.1 N NaOH
Sheep heart	–	10.0	280	391	–
Yeast	72.4	12.4	279	392	MW = 584,000 [392]
	54.2	9.5	279	1733	pH 7.0, 0.1 M P$_i$, MW = 570,000 [1733]
Phosphoglucoisomerase					
Rabbit muscle	17.2	13.2	280	393	pH 7.0, 0.01 M P$_i$, MW = 130,000 [393]
Phosphoglucomutase (EC 2.7.5.1)					
Rabbit muscle	–	7.7	278	394	–
	5.98	7.8	278	395	MW = 77,000 [395]
	4.77	7.7	278	1734	MW = 62,000 [1735]
Yeast	8.2	11.8	280	1736	MW = 69,500 [1736], turbidimetric
6-Phosphogluconate dehydrogenase (EC 1.1.1.44)					
C. utilis, Type I	12.8	12.7	280	396	MW = 101,000 [396]
Type II	14.1	12.7	280	396	MW = 111,000 [396]
Sheep liver	–	10.3	280	622	–
	10.7	11.4	280	1737	MW = 94,000 [1737], dry wt.
Phosphoglucose isomerase (glucosephosphate isomerase, EC 5.3.19)					
Rabbit muscle	17.4	13.2	280	623	pH 7.0, 0.01 M P$_i$, MW = 132,000 [623]
Human muscle	–	12	280	624	pH 7.2
Human erythrocytes	–	13.1	280	1738	Neutral pH, Refr.
Phosphoglycerate dehydrogenase					
E. coli	11.2	6.7	280	397	MW = 165,000 [397]
3-Phosphoglycerate kinase (EC 2.7.2.3)					
Rabbit muscle	3.12	6.9	280	1739	MW = 45,200 [1739]
Yeast	2.24	4.9	280	1739	MW = 45,800 [1739]
	–	5.0	280	141	–
Rabbit muscle	2.16	5.7	280	1740	MW = 38,000 [1740]
Yeast	–	5.35^{d‡}	278	1741	Dry wt.
Phosphoglycerate phosphomutase (EC 5.4.2.1)					
Yeast, Component I	–	14.2	280	1742	–
Component II	–	14.9	280	1742	–
Phosphoglyceromutase (EC 2.7.5.3)					
Rabbit muscle	–	12.5	280	398	–
Yeast	–	14.2	280	399	–
Sheep muscle	–	7.1	280	1743	pH 7.0, 0.1 μm P$_i$
Phospholipase A$_2$ (EC 3.1.1.4)					
Agkistrodon halys blomhoffi (Snake)					
A-I	2.06^{e‡}	14.9	278.5	1744	pH 7.2, 0.1 M NaP$_i$, MW = 13,800 [1744]
A-II	2.06^{f‡}	15.1	278.5	1744	pH 7.2, 0.1 M NaP$_i$, MW = 13,700 [1744]
Pig pancreas	–	14.2	280	1745	pH 8, AA

---

^{d‡} Value may be in error by 10% [1741].

MOLAR ABSORPTIVITY AND $A_{1cm}^{1\%}$ VALUES FOR PROTEINS AT SELECTED WAVELENGTHS OF THE ULTRAVIOLET AND VISIBLE REGION (Continued)

Protein	ϵ^a ($\times 10^{-4}$)	$A_{1cm}^{1\%\,b}$	nm^c	Reference	Comments^d
Crotalus adamanteus	6.76	22.7	280	401	MW = 29,864 [401]
Phosphomonoesterase, acid (see phosphatase, acid)					
5-Phosphoriboisomerase (ribosephosphate isomerase, EC 5.3.1.6)					
Spinach	–	4.35	280	1748	Biuret
Phosphoribosyl-ATP pyrophosphorylase (ATP phosphoribosyl transferase, EC 2.4.2.17)					
S. typhimurium	16.0	7.45	280	400	MW = 215,000 [400]
Phosphoribosyldiphosphate amidotransferase					
Chicken liver	–	12.5	280	1749	pH 8.0, 0.05 *M* Tris Cl, from Figure 1 [1749]
N-(5′-Phospho-D-ribosyl formimino)-5-amino-(5″-phosphoribosyl)-4-imidazolecarboxamide isomerase (see isomerase)					
Phosphoribosyl formylglycinamidine synthetase (see formylglycinamide ribonucleotide amidotransferase)					
Phosphoribosyltransferase (ATP phosphoribosyltransferase, EC 2.4.2.17)					
S. typhimurium	–	10.7	280	1750	pH 7.5, 6 *M* GdmCl—0.025 *M* Tris Cl
Phosphorylase					
Rabbit muscle	–	11.8	277	405	pH 8.0, 0.1 *M* HCO$_3$
Pig liver	–	11.9	277	406	–
Frog muscle	–	12.8	288	407	–
Rabbit muscle	–	13.2	280	407	–
	–	12.3^{g‡}	280	408	pH 6.8, 5 mM P$_i$, dry wt.
	–	13.1	279	409	pH 7, 0.01 *M* NaP$_i$
	–	11.5	278	410	–
	–	11.9	278	411	–
	–	13.2^{h‡}	280	404	–
Apo-	–	12.0	278	411	–
Human	28.8	11.9	278	410	MW = 242,000 [410]
Potato	–	11.7	278	1757	pH 7.5, 0.005 *M* Tris Cl
Rat muscle	–	12.5	280	1751	–
Beef spleen	21.8	11.5	278	1752	pH 7.4, 0.01 *M* Tris Cl, 2 mM HSEtOH, MW = 190,000
	1.1	0.565	333	1752	[1752], dry wt.
Rabbit muscle	–	13.1	280	1753	pH 7, 50 mM P$_i$, 1.0 mM EDTA, 1.5 mM HSEtOH,
Pacific dogfish (*Squalus sucklii*)	25.8	12.9	280	1753	MW = 200,000 [1753]
Baker's yeast (*Saccharomyces cerevisiae*)					
a	15.3	14.9	280	1754	Refr. MW = 103,000 [1754]
b	15.3	14.9	280	1754	Refr. MW = 103,000 [1754]
Silky shark (*Carcharhinus falciformis*)					
b	'	13.0	280	1755	pH 7.5, 0.15 *M* Tris, 0.01 *M* EDTA, N
Lobster (*Homarus americanus*)					
b	–	13.5	280	1756	pH 6.9, 0.04 *M* Tris, 0.01 *M* EDTA
Phosphorylase kinase (EC 2.7.1.38)					
Rabbit muscle	–	12.4	280	1758	Refr.
	–	11.8	280	1759	pH 7.0, 5 mM P$_i$—0.2 mM EDTA, Biuret
Phosphorylase, purine-nucleoside					
Beef liver	–	16	280	402	–
Human erythrocyte	8.91	11	280	403	pH 7.5, MW = 81,000 [403]
Phosphotransacetylase (phosphate acetyltransferase, EC 2.3.1.8)					
C. kluyveri	–	4.2	280	415	Calculated from data
Phosphovitin					
Salmon	1.8	9.4^{i‡}	280	1760	pH 2, from Figure 2 [1760], MW = 19,000 [1760]

^{e‡} From Figure 12 of Ref. [1744], the following values were estimated: ϵ_M = 7500 (277 nm, pH 1.2, 0.1 *M* HCl); ϵ_M = 9500 (278.5 nm, pH 7.2, 0.1 *M* NaP$_i$); ϵ_M = 9800 (290 nm, pH 12.5, 0.1 *M* NaOH). The value at pH 7.2 does not agree with the value calculated from the molecular weight, 13,800, and the A1%/1 cm value of 14.9.
^{f‡} From Figure 13 of Ref. [1744], the following values were estimated: ϵ_M = 8800 (277 nm, pH 1.2, 0.1 *M* HCl); ϵ_M = 10,000 (278.5 nm, pH 7.2, 0.1 *M* NaP$_i$); ϵ_M = 11,200 (290 nm, pH 12.5, 0.1 *N* NaOH). The value at pH 7.2 does not agree with the value calculated from the molecular weight, 13,700, and the A1%/1 cm of 15.
^{g‡} A1%/1 cm by amino acid analysis, 13.2.
^{h‡} A1%/1 cm by Biuret and amino acid analysis, 13.5; by refractive index increment, 13.2.

MOLAR ABSORPTIVITY AND $A_{1cm}^{1\%}$ VALUES FOR PROTEINS AT SELECTED WAVELENGTHS OF THE ULTRAVIOLET AND VISIBLE REGION (Continued)

Protein	ϵ^a ($\times 10^{-4}$)	$A_{1cm}^{1\% \, b}$	nm^c	Reference	Comments^d
Trout	1.8	9.3‡	280	1760	pH 2, from Figure 2 [1760], MW = 19,350 [1760]
Phosphovitin kinase					
Calf brain	–	15.7	280	1761	Lowry
Phycocyanin					
Chroomonas sp.	–	114	645	1763	pH 6.0, dry wt.
Synechococcus sp.	10.40	–	352	1764	MW = 36,700 [1764]
	10.65	–	662.5	1764	
α-Subunit	3.26	–	352	1764	MW = 17,700 [1764]
	3.32	–	662.5	1764	
β-Subunit	6.63	–	352	1764	MW = 19,000 [1764]
	6.95	–	662.5	1764	
Allophycocyanin	3.17	–	352	1764	MW = 16,500 [1764]
	3.22	–	662.5	1764	
		72	610	1765	
Synechcococcus lividus	–	72	610	1765	pH 7.0, 0.01 M P$_i$, from Figure 1 [1765]
Plectonema calothricoides	–	72	620	1765	
Phormidium luridum	–	19	620	1765	pH 6.2 M urea, from Figure 2 [1765]
	–	9.2	620	1765	pH 6, 4 M urea
	–	10	620	1765	pH 6, 6 M and 8 M urea
Coccochloris elabens	–	60	620	1766	pH 6.0
Phycocyanin, anacystis	9.9	7.9	615	412	MW = 12,500 [412]
C-Phycocyanin					
Alga (*Anacystis nidulans*)					
Monomer	23	–	615	1762	pH 7.0, 0.05 M P$_i$
Hexamer	33	–	621	1762	pH 5.5, 0.2 M AcOH
α-Subunit	9.8	–	620	1762	
β-Subunit	14.3	–	608	1762	pH 7.0, 0.05 M P$_i$
Phycoerythrin					
Porphyridium cruentin	2.4	2.73	565	412	MW = 87,000 [412]
Phytochrome					
Oat seedlings	–	12.5	280	1767	–
	–	12.5	660	1767	–
Winter rye (*Secale cereale*)	9	–	280	1768	Red-absorbing
	9	–	280	1768	Far-red-absorbing
	7	–	665	1768	Red-absorbing
	4	–	730	1768	Far-red-absorbing
Phytohemagglutinin					
Robinia pseudoaccacia	–	9.65	278	1769	–
Pigeon droppings					
Old	–	27.5	280	1770	pH 7, dialyzed and lyophilized extracts
Fresh	–	30.5	280	1770	
Pigment					
Serum, Eel (*Anguilla japonica*)	4.41	–	279	1771	MW = 89,100 [1771]
	0.948	–	383–4	1771	
	0.222	–	704–5	1771	
Pinguinain (EC 3.4.99.18)	–	22.0	280	413	–
	4.72	24.6	280	414	pH 7.3 and pH 4.6, MW = 19,200 [414]
Plasma					
Human, basic B$_2$	0.299	3.32	278	438	pH 6.0, 0.1 M NaCl, MW = 9,000 [438]
Plasmin (EC 3.4.21.7)					
Human, urokinase activated	–	16.7	280	418	0.1 N NaOH
Streptokinase activated	–	17.3	280	418	0.1 N NaOH
Human	–	19.4	280	419	0.01 N HCl
	–	20.0	280	419	0.01 N HCl
Plasmin, iPr$_2$ P-human	–	16.8	280	1772	AA

---

‡ Same values at pH 7.

MOLAR ABSORPTIVITY AND $A_{1cm}^{1\%}$ VALUES FOR PROTEINS AT SELECTED WAVELENGTHS OF THE ULTRAVIOLET AND VISIBLE REGION (Continued)

Protein	ϵ^a ($\times 10^{-4}$)	$A_{1cm}^{1\%\ b}$	nm^c	Reference	Comments^d
Plasminogen					
Human	–	17.1	280	418	0.1 N NaOH
	–	18.4	280	419	0.01 N HCl
	–	21.7	280	419	0.01 N HCl, ascending portion of peak on DEAE-cellulose
	–	19.8	280	419	0.0 1 N HCl, descending portion of peak on DEAE-cellulose
	–	16.1	280	1773	–
Human, A	–	16.8	280	1772	AA
B	–	16.8	280	1772	AA
Plastocyanin					
Comfrey (*Symphytum officinale*)	0.45	–	597	1774	⎫
Elder (*Sambucus nigra*)	0.45	–	597	1774	⎪
Nettle (*Urtica dioica*)	0.45	–	597	1774	⎬ Extinction coefficient of copper chromophore
Dog's mercury (*Mercurialis perennis*)	0.45	–	597	1774	⎪
Goose grass (*Galium aparine*)	0.45	–	597	1774	⎪
Lettuce (*Lactuca sativa*)	4.5^{i‡}	–	597	1774	⎭
Spinach (*Spinacea oleracea*)	0.118	–	460	1775	–
	0.980	–	597	1775	–
	0.330	–	770	1775	–
French beau (*Phaseolus vulgaris*)	0.45	4.2	597	1776	⎫ MW = 10,690 [1776]
	0.45	4.2	278	1776	⎭
Pokeweed mitogen					
Phytolacca americana	5.9	18.5	280	416	pH 6 and water, MW = 32,000 [416]
Polymerase, DNA (EC 2.7.7.7)	92.7	8.5	280	417	10 mM NH$_4$ HCO$_3$, MW = 109,000 [417]
Polynucleotide phosphorylase (EC 2.7.7.8)					
M. luteus	–	4.30	280	1777	N: assumed 16.5%
Form I	–	5.30	280	1777	Lowry
Form T	–	4.40	280	1777	N: assumed 16.5%
	–	4.40	280	1777	Lowry
Polyphenol oxidase (monophenol monooxygenase, EC 1.14.18.1)					
Mushroom	–	26.92	280	420	–
Camellia sinensis L.	–	13.5	279	421	pH 6.8, 0.3 M NaP$_i$
	–	0.84	611	421	–
Polysaccharide depolymerase					
Aerobacter aerogenes	41	10.8	280	1778	MW = 379,000 [1778]
Porphyrenglobin					
Human, fast moving	13.3	–	403	1779	–
	1.01	–	506	1779	–
	0.91	–	542	1779	–
	0.57	–	568	1779	–
	0.37	–	621.5	1779	–
Slow moving	13.3	–	403	1779	–
	0.99	–	506	1779	–
	0.92	–	542	1779	–
	0.58	–	568	1779	–
	0.38	–	621.5	1779	–
Postalbumin, 4.6S					
Human serum	–	8.0	280	1781	–
Post-γ-globulin					
Human urine	–	9.1	280	1780	pH 7
Prealbumin					
Human serum	8.5	13.3	280	1782	MW = 64,000 [1782]
	–	14.4	280	1783	pH 7.0
	–	14.1	280	1784	Dry wt.
	–	12.2	280	1785	–

---

^{i‡} This is given as $45 \times 10^3\ M$ [1774]. It may be a typographical error.

MOLAR ABSORPTIVITY AND $A_{1cm}^{1\%}$ VALUES FOR PROTEINS AT SELECTED WAVELENGTHS OF THE ULTRAVIOLET AND VISIBLE REGION (Continued)

Protein	ϵ^a ($\times 10^{-4}$)	$A_{1cm}^{1\%\ b}$	nm^c	Reference	Comments^d
Tryptophan-rich	–	13.2	280	1786	–
Thyroxine-binding	–	12.3	280	1787	–
	9.93	13.6	280	1788	MW = 73,000 [1788]
Cynomolgus monkey					
(*Macaca irus*)	8.71	15	280	1789	MW = 58,000 [1789]
Rhesus monkey					
Pt-1-1	–	14.4	280	1790	–
Pt-2-2	–	14.4	280	1790	–
Chicken egg yolk	–	18.5	280	1791	pH 7.0, 0.05 M NaP$_i$
Mouse					
Urinary	–	6.0	280	422	–
Serum	–	8.0	280	422	–
Pre-phenoloxidase					
Bombyx mori	–	13.0	280	1792	–
	0.029	–	650	1792	Per atom copper
Principle, sweet					
Dioscoreophyllum cumminsii	–	16.2	278	1793	pH 5.6
	–	17.6	288	1793	pH 13
Procarboxypeptidase					
A					
Cobalt derivative	0.0110	–	500	1794	–
	0.0140	–	555	1794	–
	0.0140	–	570	1794	–
Shrimp (*Penaeus setiferus*)	–	25.8	280	1795	AA
Spiny Pacific dogfish (*Squalus acanthias*)	–	16.5	280	1796	pH 8.0, 0.1 M Tris, 0.01 M CoCl$_2$, Refr.
Beef pancreas	18.2	19	280	77	MW = 96,000 [77]
S$_5$	11.5	17.7	280	1797	Refr., MW = 63,000 [1791]
S$_6$	16.5	19	280	77	MW = 87,000 [77]
B					
Shrimp (*Penaeus setiferus*)	–	27.8	280	1795	UC
African lungfish (*Protopterus aethiopicus*)	7.3	16.2	280	1798	Refr., MW = 45,000 [1798]
Beef	9.2	16	280	83	MW = 57,400 [83]
Proelastase					
Pig pancreas	4.4	17.0	280	1799	MW = 25,840 [1799]
	–	15.8	280	1800	–
Progesterone-binding globulin					
Pregnant guinea pig serum	–	7.3	280	1801	–
Proinsulin					
Beef	–	7.0	276	1802	–
	–	5.9	276	1803	pH 7.2, 0.1 N NaCl, 10^{-5} M EDTA
Pig	–	6.67	276	423	pH 7.0, 0.03 M P$_i$
Prolactin					
Sheep	2.05	9.09^{k‡}	280	1804	–
Proline hydroxylase (EC 1.14.11.2), collagen (see collagen)					
Protease (proteinase)					
Chinese gooseberry (*Actinidia chinensis*)		21.2	280	1809	–
Acremonium Kiliense	2.73	10.1	280	1826	1 mM HCl, dry wt., MW = 27,000
Agkistrodonhalys blomhoffi					
a	4.54	9.08	280	424	Water, MW = 50,000 [424]
b	7.0	7.4	280	425	MW = 95,000 [425]
c	7.7	10.98	280	424	Water, MW = 70,000 [424]
Alternaria tenuissima	3.2	13	277	426	0.1 M AcONa, MW = 24,750 [426]
Aspergillus candidus		7.1	280	1827	Dry wt.
Aspergillus flavus	1.61	9.04	280	1828	pH 5, MW = 17,800 [1828]
Aspergillus sojae	2.03	8.98	280	1829	MW = 22,600 [1829]
I	6.96	16.7	280	1810	pH 7.3, 50 mM Tris Cl, dry wt., MW = 41,700 [1810]

^{k‡} Personal communication from Dr. Li. The value cited in Ref. [1804] is an error. The correct value is 9.09.

MOLAR ABSORPTIVITY AND $A_{1cm}^{1\%}$ VALUES FOR PROTEINS AT SELECTED WAVELENGTHS OF THE ULTRAVIOLET AND VISIBLE REGION (Continued)

Protein	ϵ^a ($\times 10^{-4}$)	$A_{1cm}^{1\% \; b}$	nm^c	Reference	Comments^d
II	1.78	9.0	280	1810	pH 7.3, 50 mM TrisCl, dry wt., MW = 19,800 [1810]
Bacillus natto	2.38	8.8	280	1811	–
B. subtilis	2.7	10	278	427	MW = 27,000 [427]
Neutral	–	13.6	280	428	–
B. subtilis NRRL B3411					
A	–	14.8	280	1825	–
B	–	14.7	280	1825	–
B. subtilis var. *amylosaccchariticus*	–	13.6–8	280	1812	–
B. thermoproteolyticus	6.63	17.65	280	429	pH 7.0, 0.05 M Tris, MW = 37,500 [429]
	7.34	19.6	280	429	0.1 N NaOH
Lotus seed (*Nelumbo nucifera Gaertn*)	–	10	278	1813	pH 4.0, 50 mM AcO⁻
Mouse, submaxillary					
A	7.5	24.9	280	1814	MW = 30,000 [1814]
B	7.25	25.9	280	1814	MW = 28,000 [1814]
Myxobacter, α-lytic	1.94		280	1815	–
Myxobacter, AL-1	2.2	15.8	280	430	0.1 M P$_i$, MW = 14,000 [430]
Rhizopus chinensis	–	12.6	280	431	–
S. fradiae	–	8.4	280	275	pH 8, 0.1 M Tris
Streptomyces griseus str. K		8.1	280	1820	Folin
Streptomyces naraensis	4.16	11.22	280	1824	pH 7.5, 0.005 M Tris Cl, MW = 37,000 [1824]
Streptomyces rectus var. *proteolyticus*	3.92	18.2	280	1830	MW = 21,500 [1830]
S. griseus K1					
I	–	16.2	278	433	–
III	–	11.5	278	433	–
IV	–	10.2	278	433	–
S. maraensis, neutral	–	9.15	280	434	pH 7.5, 0.005 M Tris, HCl, 0.005 M Ca(OH)$_2$
Tricophyton granulosum extracellular	7.6	22.15	274	435	pH 6.0, 0.1 M AcO⁻, MW = 34,300 [435]
Sorangium, α-lytic	1.94	–	280	1816	–
	–	9.7	280	1817	–
Worm (*Schistosoma mansoni*)	2.42^{l‡}	–	280	1818	pH 3.95
	3.75^{l‡}	–	280	1818	pH 13
Vibrio B-30	–	10	280	1819	–
Streptococcal	–	16.4	280	1821	–
Zymogen	–	13.7	280	1821	–
Yeast, A	–	11.9	280	1822	–
	–	11.9	280	436	pH 6.2, 0.01 M NaP$_i$
C	–	16.6	280	1822	
Yeast	–	16.6	280	436	pH 6.2, 0.01 M NaP$_i$
(*Saccharomyces cerevisiae*)	–	14.82	280	1823	pH 7.0, 0.01 M NaP$_i$, 0.1 M KCl, dry wt.
Protease, acid					
Cladosporium sp. 45-2	–	10.7	280	1805	Dry wt.
Rhizopus chimensis	–	12.1	280	1806	From Figure 1 [1806]
Rhodotorula glutinis K-24	–	12.9	280	1807	–
	–	14.0	280	1808	pH 4, 0.01 M citrate
Protease inhibitor, soybean	0.35	4.4	280	537	MW = 7975 [437]
Proteinase (see piotease)					
Proteolipid					
Beef brain white matter					
Crude	–	7.6	278	1831	–
Purified	–	14	278	1831	–
Prothrombin					
Beef	–	13.4	280	454	pH 6. Estd. from Figure 1 [454]
	–	10.8	280	455	0.1 N NaOH
	–	15.3	280	456	pH 6, P$_i$NaCl
	–	14.8	280	456	0.1 N NaOH
Prep. I	–	13.2	280	1832	–

^{l‡} MW = 28,000.

MOLAR ABSORPTIVITY AND $A_{1cm}^{1\%}$ VALUES FOR PROTEINS AT SELECTED WAVELENGTHS OF THE ULTRAVIOLET AND VISIBLE REGION (Continued)

Protein	ϵ^a ($\times 10^{-4}$)	$A_{1cm}^{1\% b}$	nm^c	Reference	Comments^d
Prep. II	–	14.4	280	1832	–
Human	–	15.2	280	457	–
	–	13.6	280	458	pH 6 and 7, 0.1 M P$_i$
A-DEAE purified	–	11.7	280	459	pH 7.4, 0.02 M Tris, 0.1 M NaCl
B-DEAE purified	–	12.6	280	459	pH 7.4, 0.02 M Tris, 0.1 M NaCl
C-Disc electrophoresis prep.	–	13.8	280	459	pH 7.4, 0.02 M Tris, 0.1 M NaCl
D,E-NIH-DEAE purified	–	13.3	280	459	pH 7.4, 0.02 M Tris, 0.1 M NaCl
F-NIH-DEAE purified	–	11.6	280	459	pH 7.4, 0.02 M Tris, 0.1 M NaCl
G-NIH=Disc electrophoresis prep.	–	12.9	280	459	pH 7.4, 0.02 M Tris, 0.1 M NaCl
Protocatechuate 3,4-dioxygenase (EC 1.13.11.3)					
Pseudomonas aeruginosa	–	13.2	280	1833	pH 8.5
	92.4	13.2	280	460	pH 8.5, 50 mM Tris Cl, MW = 700,000 [460]
Protocatechuate 4,5-dioxygenase (EC 1.13.11.8)					
Pseudomonad	11.15	7.45	280	1834	pH 75., 0.05 M KP$_i$ + 10% EtOH, MW = 150,000 [1834], from Figure 3 [1834]
Protocollagen hydroxylase (proline, 2-oxoglutarate dioxygenase, EC 1.14.11.2)					
Chicken embryo	–	49.5	230	1835	–
Protoheme, P-450 particle					
Rabbit liver	9.6	–	414	441	Reduced
	2.15	–	543	441	Reduced
	13.8	–	415–8	441	Oxidized
	1.9	–	532	441	Oxidized
	1.85	–	567	441	Oxidized
Putrescine oxidase (EC 1.4.3.10)					
Micrococcus rubens	1.08	–	458	1836	–
	11.45	–	275	1836	–
Apo-		10.0	280	1836	–
Pyocin R					
P. aeruginosa R	–	16.9	280	461	–
Sheath	–	18.1	280	1837	0.1 N NaOH—0.1 M NaCl
S-β-Pyridylethylalbumin (see albumin, beef)					
Pyridoxamine-pyruvate transaminase (EC 2.6.1.30)					
Pseudomonas MA-1	–	9.75	280	462	–
Pyrocatechase (catechol 1,2-dioxygenase, EC 1.13.11.1)					
P. arvilla	0.47	0.52	440	463	pH 8.0, 0.05 M Tris, MW = 90,000 [463]
	8.04	8.93	280	463	pH 8.0, 0.05 M Tris, MW = 90,000 [463]
Pyrophosphatase, inorganic					
Yeast	–	14.5	280	464	0.1 M HCl or water
Pyruvate dehydrogenase (EC 1.2.4.1)					
E. coli K-12	30	10	276	747	pH 7, 0.05 M KP$_i$, MW 3 × 10^6 [747], data from Figure 3A [747]
	1.07	0.40	355	465	MW = 265,000 [465]
	1.13	0.43	370	465	MW = 265,000 [465]
	1.05	0.40	415	465	MW = 265,000 [465]
	1.46	0.55	438	465	MW = 265,000 [465]
	1.27	0.47	460	465	MW = 265,000 [465]
Pyruvate kinase					
Rabbit muscle	–	5.4	280	466	–
Human	–	5.4	280	466	–
Rat	–	5.4	280	466	–
Yeast	10.8	6.53	280	748	MW = 166,000 [748]
Quinolinate phosphoribosyltransferase (nicotinatemononucleotide pyrophosphorylase, EC 2.4.2.19)					
Pseudomonad	6.04	3.4	278	467	pH 7, 0.05 M KP$_i$, MW = 178,000 [467]
RNA polymerase (EC 2.7.7.6)					

---

^{m‡} OD = 1 when con. = 1.65 mg/ml.

^{n‡} OD$_{412}$ = OD$_{278}$/2.9.

MOLAR ABSORPTIVITY AND $A_{1cm}^{1\%}$ VALUES FOR PROTEINS AT SELECTED WAVELENGTHS OF THE ULTRAVIOLET AND VISIBLE REGION (Continued)

Protein	ϵ^a ($\times 10^{-4}$)	$A_{1cm}^{1\% \, b}$	nm^c	Reference	Comments^d
E. coli	24.0	5.41	280	1135	MW = 440,000 [1135]
E. coli B	–	5.9	280	749	Con. by Biuret and Lowry [749]
	–	6.7	280	749	Con. det. by refract. incr. with BSA as standard [749]
	–	6.5	280	749	–
	–	11.8	278	750	Calc. from data in Figure 1 [750]
Relaxing protein					
Rabbit muscle	–	3.32	278	1131	–
Rennin (chymosin, EC 3.4.23.4)	–	14.3	278	468	–
Retinol-binding protein					
Human serum	3.91	18.5	280	1132	MW = 21,000 [1132]
Retinol-transporting protein					
Human urine	–	18.7	280	1133	–
Rhodanese (thiosulfate sulfur transferase, EC 2.8.1.1)					
Beef liver	–	17.5	280	469	–
Rhodopsin	4.2	–	498	470	pH 6.5 M/15 P$_i$, 1% Emulphogene BC720
	1.1	–	350	470	pH 6.5 M/15 P$_i$, 1% Emulphogene BC720
	7.4	–	280	470	pH 6.5 M/15 P$_i$, 1% Emulphogene BC720
	4.06	–	498	471	–
	–	9.8	278	471	–
Cattle	4.06	10.1	500	625	MW = 40,000 [626]
	8.12	20.2	278	625	Calc. from $\epsilon_{27x}/\epsilon_{500} = 2.0$
	7.17	–	279	627 ⎫	
	1.06	–	345	627 ⎬	In cetyltrimethylammonium bromide
	3.97	–	498	627 ⎭	
Ribitol dehydrogenase					
Aerobacter aerogenes	–	11.1	280	628	pH 7.4, data from Figure [628]
Ribonuclease	1.19	–	278	472	0.2 M NaCl, 99.85% D$_2$O
Beef pancreatic	0.88	6.95	280	473	–
	–	6.9	280	474	–
	0.98	7.2	227.5	475	–
	–	7.2	280	476	–
	0.98	7.2	278	477	pH 6.5, MW = 13,700 [477]
	1.13	8.3	278	478	MW = 13,683 [478]
	1.06	–	279.5	479	Ethylene glycol
	1.14	–	278	480	Ethylene glycol
Corn	4.32	18.8	280	485	MW = 23,000 [485]
Ribonuclease I (EC 3.1.4.22)					
Beef pancreatic	0.91	7.14	277.5	481	–
	–	6.95	280	482	–
41-N$_2$ ph	–	11.2	280	488	–
	–	6.7	280	484	–
Sheep pancreas	–	7.1	280	483	–
Ribonuclease II (T$_2$) (EC 3.1.4.23)					
A. oryzae	7.16	19.9	281	487	MW = 36,000 [487]
Ribonuclease P					
Pig pancreas	0.41	3	280	486	MW = 13,500 [486]
Ribonuclease S	–	6.95	280	482	–
S Protein	–	7.84	280	482	–
Ribonucleotide-diphosphate reductase (EC 1.17.4.1)					
E. coli B					
Protein B-1	8.2	10.5	280	751 ⎫	MW = 78,000 [751]
Protein B-2	11.5	14.8	280	751 ⎭	
	0.4	–	410	752 ⎱	G-200 prep.
	0.6	–	360	752 ⎰	
	0.33	–	410	752 ⎱	Gel electrophoresis prep.
	0.56	–	360	752 ⎰	
Ribosephosphate isomerase (see 5-phosphoriboisomerase)					
L-Ribulokinase, E. coli	–	15.1	280	489	–

MOLAR ABSORPTIVITY AND $A_{1cm}^{1\%}$ VALUES FOR PROTEINS AT SELECTED WAVELENGTHS OF THE ULTRAVIOLET AND VISIBLE REGION (Continued)

Protein	ϵ^a ($\times 10^{-4}$)	$A_{1cm}^{1\%\,b}$	nm^c	Reference	Comments^d
E. coli B/r	15.2	15.5	280	753	pH 7.6, MW = 98,000 [753]
Ribulosebisphosphate carboxylase (EC 4.1.1.39)					
Spinacea oleracea	–	16	280	490	–
Hydrogenomonas eutropha	80.0	15.51	280	1134	pH 8.0, 0.02 Tris SO$_4$, 0.1 M MgCl$_2$, MW = 515,000 [1134]
Hydrogenomonas facilis	62.6	12.28	280	1134	pH 8.0, 0.02 Tris SO$_4$, 0.01 M MgCl$_2$, MW = 551,000 [1134]
L-Ribulose phosphate 4-epimerase (EC 5.1.3.4)					
E. coli	16.2	15.7	280	491	pH 7.75, 10 mM NH$_4$ HCO$_3$, MW = 103,000 [491]
L-Rhamnulose-1-phosphate (see aldolase)					
Rubredoxin					
Desulfovibrio desulfurican	1.342	–	280	492	Oxidized
	0.596	–	380	492	Oxidized
	0.512	–	490	492	Oxidized
	1.413	–	277	492	Reduced
	0.543	–	312	492	Reduced
	0.219	–	335	492	Reduced
Peptostreptococcus elsdenii	1.83	–	280	493	–
	0.819	–	350	493	–
	0.94	–	378	493	–
	0.763	–	390	493	–
	0.38	–	566	493	–
M. lactilyticus	2.2	36.7	280	494	MW = 6,000 [494]
	0.91	15.3	490	494	–
M. aerogenes	1.83	30.5	280	495	MW = 6,000 [495]
	0.84	14	350	495	MW = 6,000 [495]
	0.92	15.3	378	495	MW = 6,000 [495]
	0.765	12.8	490	495	MW = 6,000 [495]
	0.35	5.8	570	495	MW = 6,000 [495]
P. oleovarans	1.11	8.7	495	496	MW = 12,800 [496]
	1.08	8.4	280	496	MW = 12,800 [496]
Rubredoxin, S-aminoethyl					
M. aerogenes	0.85	14.1	280	495	MW = 6,000 [495]
Rubredoxin, Apo					
C. pasteurianum	1.85	30.8	280	497	MW = 6,000 [497]
Rubredoxin reductase (EC 1.6.7.2)					
Pseudomonas oleovorans	7.3	–	272	1402	–
	1.0	–	378	1402	–
	1.1	–	450	1402	–
Serine dehydratase (EC 4.2.1.13,.14,.16)					
Rat liver	6.66	10.4	280	629 }	pH 7.2, 0.025 M KP$_i$, 0.001 M EDTA, 0.001 S$_2$ threitol, data from Figure 14 [629]
Aposerine dehydratase	6.02	9.4	280	629 }	
D-Serine dehydratase (EC 4.2.1.14)					
E. coli K 12	5.33	14.2	280	1136 }	MW = 37,300 [1136]
	0.533	1.42	415	1136 }	
E. coli	4.78	10.5	280	1137	pH 6.5–7.8, 0.1 M KP$_i$, dry wt./R, MW = 45,500 [1137]
	4.11	9.02	280	1137	pH 6.5, 0.4 M imidazolecitrate, MW = 45,500 [1137]
	4.35	9.56	280	1137	0.1 N NaOH, MW = 45,500 [1137]
Apo-	–	9.78	280	1137	pH 7.8, 0.1 M KP$_i$
	–	9.56	280	1137	0.1 N NaOH
Serine hydroxymethylase					
Rabbit liver, soluble	–	9	278	630 }	pH 7.1, 0.05 M KP$_i$, data from Figure 4 [630]
Mitochondrial	–	7	278	630 }	
Siderophilin					
Human	–	14	280	7	See transferrin
	–	10.9	280	8	–
	–	11.2	280	308	–
Pig	–	11.0	278	498	0.1 N HCl
	–	13.8	280	498	pH 7
	–	13.3	290	498	0.1 N NaOH

MOLAR ABSORPTIVITY AND $A_{1cm}^{1\%}$ VALUES FOR PROTEINS AT SELECTED WAVELENGTHS OF THE ULTRAVIOLET AND VISIBLE REGION (Continued)

Protein	ϵ^a ($\times 10^{-4}$)	$A_{1cm}^{1\%\,b}$	nm^c	Reference	Comments^d
Spectrin					
Human erythrocytes	–	8.8	280	631	–
Stellacyanin					
Rhus vernicifera	2.6	–	280	499	0.1 *N* NaOH
	2.8	–	290	499	0.1 *N* NaOH
Oxidized	2.32	–	280	717	–
	0.096	–	450	717	–
	0.48	–	604	717	–
	0.079	–	850	717	–
Reduced	0.088	–	450	717	–
	0.408	–	604	717	–
	0.079	–	850	717	–
Steroid 4,5-dioxygenase (EC 1.13.11.25) (see 3,4-dihydroxy-9,10-secoandrosta-1,3,5[10]-triene-9,17-dione 4,5-dioxygenase)					
Streptavidin					
S. avidinii	–	34	280	500	–
	–	31	282	501	–
Streptokinase, Streptococcus	–	9.49	280	502	–
Subtilisin (EC 3.4.21.14)	–	8.6	280	357	–
Subtilisin, Thiol-	3.31	–	278	506	–
Subtilisin BPN′	–	8.8	280	754	–
Subtilisin BPN′, iPr$_2$P^{bb}	3.23	11.7	278	504	pH 7.0, 0.05 *M* AcONa, MW = 27,600 [504]
Subtilisin Carlsberg, iPr$_2$P^{bb}	–	8.6	278.1	505	–
Subtilisin, Nova	3.11	–	278	506	–
Subtilopeptidase (subtilisin, EC 3.4.21.14)	–	10.7	280	507	–
Succinyl-Co A synthetase (EC 6.2.1.4, .5)					
E. coli	7.2	5.11	280	508	pH 7.2, 1 m*M* KP$_i$, MW = 141,000 [508]
Sulfate adenylyltransferase (see ATP-sulfurylase)					
Sulphatase (aryl sulfatase, EC 3.1.6.1)					
Beef liver					
A	7.5	7.0	280	509	pH 7.5, MW = 107,000 [509]
B	3.5	14.0	280	509	pH 7.5, MW = 25,000 [509]
B$_{\alpha 2}$	–	20	280	509	Protein det. by Folin method
	–	13.3	280	509	Refractometric method used to det. protein
B$_\beta$	–	19.9	280	509	Protein det. by Folin method
	–	13.8	280	509	Refractometric method used to det. protein
Tartrate dehydrogenase (EC 1.1.1.93)					
P. putida	20.9	14.4	280	510	MW = 145,000 [510]
Tartrate epoxidase (*trans*-epoxysuccinate hydratase, EC 4.2.1.37)					
Pseudomonas putida	–	14.0	280	632	–
Tartronic semialdehyde reductase (EC 1.1:1.60)					
P. putida	7.1	6.83	280	511	MW = 104,000 [511]
Taurocyamine kinase					
Arenicola marinae	–	9.7	280	607	–
Tetanus toxin					
C. tetani	–	7.8	280	512	–
Thermolysin (EC 3.4.24.4)					
B. thermoproteolyticus Rokko	6.63	17.6	280	1138	MW = 37,500 [1138]
Thioredoxin					
Bacteriophage T4	6.3	6.06^{m‡}	280	1139	MW = 104,000 [1139]
E. coli	1.37	11.4	280	513	MW = 12,000 [513]
Thioredoxin reductase (EC 1.6.4.5)					
E. coli	0.33	14.0	280	514	MW = 66,000 [515]
Threonine aldolase (EC 4.1.2.5)					
Candida humicola	11.6	4.17	280	755	pH 6.4, 0.03 *M* KP$_i$, 0.005 *M* HSEtOH, 0.001 *M* EDTA, MW = 277,000 [755], calc. from Figure 2 [755]

^{m‡} OD = 1 when con. = 1.65 mg/ml.

MOLAR ABSORPTIVITY AND $A_{1cm}^{1\%}$ VALUES FOR PROTEINS AT SELECTED WAVELENGTHS OF THE ULTRAVIOLET AND VISIBLE REGION (Continued)

Protein	ϵ^a ($\times 10^{-4}$)	$A_{1cm}^{1\% \, b}$	nm^c	Reference	Comments^d
Threonine deaminase (threonine dehydratase, EC 4.2.1.1.6)					
S. typhimurium	18.0	9.3	278	516	pH 7.4, 0.05 M KPh, 0.8 mM L-isoleucine, 0.5 mM EDTA, 0.5 mM S$_2$ threitol
E. coli	2.6	1.75	415	517	MW = 147,000 [517]
	8.1	5.5	277	517	MW = 147,000 [517]
Rhodospirillum rubrum	–	3.82	278	1140	pH 6.8, 25 mM KP$_i$, data from Figure 7 [1140]
	–	1.31^{n‡}	412	1140	
Bα_2	–	20	280	509	Protein det. by Folin method
	–	13.3	280	509	Refractometric method used to det. protein
Bβ	–	19.9	280	509	Protein det. by Folin method
	–	13.8	280	509	Refractometric method used to det. protein
Tartrate dehydrogenase (EC 1.1.1.93)					
P. putida	20.9	14.4	280	510	MW = 145,000 [510]
Tartrate epoxidase (trans-epoxysuccinate hydratase, EC 4.2.1.37)					
Pseudomonas putida	–	14.0	280	632	–
Tartronic semialdehyde reductase (EC 1.1:1.60)					
P. putida	7.1	6.83	280	511	MW = 104,000 [511]
Taurocyamine kinase					
Arenicola marinae	–	9.7	280	607	–
Tetanus toxin					
C. tetani	–	7.8	280	512	–
Thermolysin (EC 3.4.24.4)					
B. thermoproteolyticus Rokko	6.63	17.6	280	1138	MW = 37,500 [1138]
Thioredoxin					
Bacteriophage T4	6.3	6.06^{m‡}	280	1139	MW = 104,000 [1139]
E. coli	1.37	11.4	280	513	MW = 12,000 [513]
Thioredoxin reductase (EC 1.6.4.5)					
E. coli	0.33	14.0	280	514	MW = 66,000 [515]
Threonine aldolase (EC 4.1.2.5)					
Candida humicola	11.6	4.17	280	755	pH 6.4, 0.03 M KP$_i$, 0.005 M HSEtOH, 0.001 M EDTA, MW = 277,000 [755], calc. from Figure 2 [755]
Threonine deaminase (threonine dehydratase, EC 4.2.1.1.6)					
S. typhimurium	18.0	9.3	278	516	pH 7.4, 0.05 M KPh, 0.8 mM L-isoleucine, 0.5 mM EDTA, 0.5 mM S$_2$ threitol
E. coli	2.6	1.75	415	517	MW = 147,000 [517]
	8.1	5.5	277	517	MW = 147,000 [517]
Rhodospirillum rubrum	–	3.82	278	1140	pH 6.8, 25 mM KP$_i$, data from Figure 7 [1140]
	–	1.31^{n‡}	412	1140	
Thrombin (EC 3.4.21.5)					
Human	–	16.2	280	518	–
Beef	–	19.5	280	519	–
Thyrocalcitonin	0.76	21	280	520	MW = 3,604 [520]
Pig	0.757	21	280	756	0.1 M AcOH
Thyroid-stimulating hormone					
Beef	2.6	10.5	292	521	0.1 N NaOH, estd. from Figure 1 [521], MW = 25,000 [521]
Human	2.5	9.9	292	521	0.1 N NaOH, estd. from Figure 1 [521], MW = 25,000 [521]
Thyroglobulin, beef					
19S	–	10.0	280	503	pH 7.4, KCl-P$_i$
19S	–	10.5	280	96	–
19S	65	10	280	757	MW = 650,000
	1310	201	210	757	

---

^{n‡} OD$_{412}$ = OD$_{278}$/2.9.

MOLAR ABSORPTIVITY AND $A_{1cm}^{1\%}$ VALUES FOR PROTEINS AT SELECTED WAVELENGTHS OF THE ULTRAVIOLET AND VISIBLE REGION (Continued)

Protein	ϵ^a ($\times 10^{-4}$)	$A_{1cm}^{1\% \ b}$	nm^c	Reference	Comments^d
27S	132	10.8	280	757 }	MW = 1,220,000
	2700	221	210	757 }	
27S Iodoprotein	–	10.8	280	503	pH 7.4, KCl-P$_i$
Human	–	10.5	280	360	–
Lamprey, 12S	–	8.8	280	372	–
Transaldolase (EC 2.2.1.2), *C. utilis*	–	11	280	522	0.1 *N* NaOH
Transcortin, Human plasma	–	7.4	280	523	–
Transferrin, Human plasma	–	14.1	280	524	Iron saturated
	–	11.2	280	525	–
Human apoenzyme	–	11.4	280	524	–
Pig	–	14.1	280	526	Iron saturated
	–	0.6	470	526	–
Apoenzyme	–	11.4	280	526	
Transglutaminase					
Pig heart	–	15.8	280	527	–
Guinea pig liver	14.2	15.8	280	528	MW = 90,000 [528]
Tripeptide synthetase (glutathione synthetase, EC 6.3.2.3)					
Yeast	18.5	15	280	529	MW = 123,000 [529]
Tropomyosin B					
Rabbit muscle	–	3.3	277	530	pH 7.0, ionic strength 1.1
	–	3.1	276	530	8 *M* urea
Troponin					
Rabbit muscle	–	42	260	758	pH 7.5, 2 m*M* Tris Cl, data from Figure 1 [758]
Trypsin (see also cocoonase) (EC 3.4.21.4)					
Beef pancreas	0.154	–	280	531	–
	–	16.6	280	532	–
	–	15.6	280	533	–
	–	15.0	280	534	–
	–	17.1	280	535	Acid sol.
	–	14.4	280	536	–
	–	16	_^{kt}	537	1 m*M* HCl
	–	12.9	280	538	–
	–	17.24	280	539	–
	–	15.5	280	540	–
Acetyltrypsin B	–	14.4	280	541	pH 7.5
N$_2$ ph–trypsin	–	14.9	280	535	Acid sol.
Sheep pancreas	–	17.4	280	540	–
Pig pancreas	–	15.0	280	540	–
Trypsin inhibitor					
Inter-α, human	–	7.1	280	542	–
Beef pancreas	–	7.9	280	535	Acid sol.
	–	8.2	280	535	Neutral sol.
	–	8.25	280	543	Acid sol.
	–	8.35	280	543	Neutral sol.
	0.38	6.2	276.1	544	MW = 6,155 [544]
	0.36	5.9	280	544	MW = 6,155 [544]
Kazals	–	6.5	280	535	Neutral sol.
Pig pancreas					
I	–	5.18	280	545	pH 7.8
II	–	6.06	280	545	pH 7.8
Soybean	–	9.1	280	535	Acid sol.
	–	9.54	280	535	Neutral sol.
	–	10.5	280	546	–
	–	4.8	280	547	–
A$_2$	–	9.94	280	548	–
I	–	9.44	280	549	–
F$_1$	–	7.16	280	550	–
F$_2$	–	10.4	280	550	–

MOLAR ABSORPTIVITY AND $A_{1cm}^{1\%}$ VALUES FOR PROTEINS AT SELECTED WAVELENGTHS OF THE ULTRAVIOLET AND VISIBLE REGION (Continued)

Protein	ϵ^a ($\times 10^{-4}$)	$A_{1cm}^{1\% \, b}$	nm^c	Reference	Comments^d
F_3	–	6.34	280	550	–
Colostrum, beef	–	5.0	280	535	Acid sol.
Barley	1.78	12.7	280	759	MW = 14,000 [759]
Trypsin–trypsin inhibitor complex					
Pancreatic inhibitor, beef	–	12.3	280	535	Acid sol.
Soybean inhibitor	–	13.1	280	535	–
Colostrum inhibitor, beef	–	11.9	280	535	Acid sol.
Trypsinogen					
Beef pancreas	–	13.9	280	536	–
Pig pancreas	–	13.9	280	536	–
Sheep pancreas	–	14.1	280	551	–
Beef pancreas, S-Sulfo-	–	14.2	280	552	–
Tryptophan oxygenase (EC 1.13.11.11)					
Pseudomonas acidovorans	14.6	12.0	280	760 ⎫	MW = 121,000 [760]
	22.9	18.8	405	760 ⎬	
Tryptophan synthase (EC 4.2.1.20)					
E. coli					
A protein	1.37	4.05	278	761	pH 7.2, 0.01 M KP, MW = 29,500 [761]
	1.4	4.75	293	761	0.1 M NaOH, MW = 29,500 [761]
B protein	–	6.5	280	762	pH 7.3, 0.05 M KPh cone. 1γ/ml, pyridoxal-P and 0.001 M HSEtOH
	–	1.11	300	762 ⎫	
	–	0.71	335	762 ⎬ Calc. from ratios of ODs
	–	1.14	414	762	
	–	3.2	290	762 ⎭	
	6.2	–	278	763	pH 7.5, 0.01 M KP$_i$, 0.01 M HSEtOH
Apo B protein	–	5.8	280	762	
B component	–	5.7	278	554	–
Tryptophanase (EC 4.1.99.1)					
E. coli					
Apo-	1.74	7.95	278	553	pH 7.5, 0.1 M KP, 2 mM, EDTA, 2 mM mercaptoethanol, MW = 22,000 [553]
Reduced holoenzyme	0.34	1.5	336	553	MW = 22,000 [553]
	1.79	8.14	277	553	MW = 22,000 [553]
Tryptophanyl-tRNA synthetase (EC 6.1.1.2)					
Beef pancreas	9	8.4	280	764	pH 7.5, 0.2 M KCl, MW = 108,000 [764]
	–	8.0	280	764	8 M urea, pH 8
Tyramine oxidase (amine oxidase, EC 1.4.3.4)					
Sarcina lutea	34.8	27	280	555	MW = 129,000 [555]
β-Tyrosinase (tyrosine phenol-lyase) (EC 4.1.99.2)					
E. intermedia	–	83.7	280	556	–
Tyrosine aminotransferase (EC 2.6.1.5)					
Rat liver	9.1	10	277	557	pH 7.0, 0.1 M P$_i$, MW = 91,000 [557] est. from Figure 6 [557]
UDPG dehydrogenase (EC 1.1.1.22)					
Beef liver	–	9.8	277	633	–
Umecyanin					
Armoacia lapathiofolia (Horseradish root)	0.34	2.3	610	765 ⎫	
	0.012	0.083	400	765 ⎬ pH 5.75, 30 mM AcONa, MW = 14,600 [765]
	0.021	0.144	330	765	
	1.27	8.7	280	765 ⎭	
Urease (EC 3.5.1.5)					
Beans	–	5.5	280	766	
Cajanus indicus	–	20.1	280	767 ⎫	pH 7.0, 0.05 M Tris-AcO⁻
	–	20.6	277	767 ⎬	
Jack bean	28.4	5.89	280	768	MW = 483,000 [768]
Carboxymethyl-	–	7.2	—^{o‡}	769	–
Jack bean meal	37	7.7	272	558	MW = 480,000 [558]

^{o‡} Wavelength not cited; may be 277 nm.

MOLAR ABSORPTIVITY AND $A_{1cm}^{1\%}$ VALUES FOR PROTEINS AT SELECTED WAVELENGTHS OF THE ULTRAVIOLET AND VISIBLE REGION (Continued)

Protein	ϵ^a ($\times 10^{-4}$)	$A_{1cm}^{1\%\,b}$	nm^c	Reference	Comments^d
	–	7.71	272	559	–
	–	7.54	278	560	pH 7, 0.02 M P$_i$
	–	6.4	278	560	pH 7, 0.02 M P$_i$, HSEtOH added
Uricase, pig liver	–	11.3	276	561	1% sodium carbonate
Urocanase (EC 4.2.1.99)					
Pseudomonas putida	–	8.3	280	1141	pH 7.5, 0.2 M KP$_i$, data from Figure 6 [1141] and corrected for scattering
	–	8.03	280	770	Calc. from data in Figure 4 [770], corrected for scattering of light
Urokinase (EC 3.4.99.26)					
Human urine, S$_1$	4.23	13.2	280	1142	pH 6.5, MW = 32,000 [1142]
S$_2$	7.48	13.6	280	1142	pH 6.5, MW = 55,000 [1142]
Human placenta	–	10.7	280	771	–
Virus					
Barley stripe mosaic	–	34	240	562	
	–	26	260	562	
	–	25	280	562	
	–	17	280	449	–
	–	28	260	449	–
	–	17	280	1143	Dry wt., Lowry, and Biuret
Broad bean mottle	–	3.2	276.5	1144	Water
	–	5.5	292	1144	0.1 N NaOH, data from Figure 1 [1144]
Brome mosaic	–	36	240	562	
	–	48	260	562	
	–	31	280	562	
Bromegrass mosaic	–	4.6^{p‡}	260	1145	–
	–	7.6^{p‡}	280	1145	–
	2.0	5.0	260	1145 ⎱	pH 6.0, 1 M CaCl$_2$–0.05 M Na cacodylate, MW = 40,000 [1145], data from Figure 1 [1145]
	3.52	8.8	280	1145 ⎰	
Foot-and-mouth disease	–	11.1	276	1146	–
Mouse-Elberfeld (ME)	–	14.9	280	1147	0.002 M AcOH
Southern bean mosaic	–	48	240	562	
	–	58	260	562	
	–	37	280	562	–
	–	5.85	260	1148 ⎱	0.1 N NaOH
	–	12^{pt}	260	1148 ⎰	
Tobacco etch	–	9.5	280	1149	pH 6.5, 0.02 M P$_i$, 6 M GdmCl
Tobacco mosaic	–	57	240	562	–
	–	32.4	260	562	–
	–	27	280	562	–
	–	27	260	563	pH 7.5, 0.033 M P$_i$
	–	26	263	774	
	–	27	260	1150	
	–	13	281	1150	
	–	13	281	774	pH 7.1, 0.033 M NaP$_i$
	–	13	281	563	pH 7.5, 0.033 M P$_i$
PM 2					
Non-functioning	–	13.7	280	450	–
Tomato ringspot	–	10.3	260	1151	–
Turnip yellow mosaic Artificial top component	–	11.8	275	1152	pH 7.0, 0.01 M NaP$_i$
White clover mosaic, str. WCD-17	1.88	13.2	280	1153	Water, MW = 14,300 [1153]
Mengo					
L-	–	17.1	280	772	–
M-	–	16.8	280	772	–
S-	–	17.0	280	772	–
Alfalfa mosaic	–	52	260	773	–
Potato X	–	12.3	280	775	pH 7.5, 0.05 M P$_i$

---

^{pt} Calculated from the content of tyrosine, tryptophan, and phenylalanine.

MOLAR ABSORPTIVITY AND $A_{1cm}^{1\%}$ VALUES FOR PROTEINS AT SELECTED WAVELENGTHS OF THE ULTRAVIOLET AND VISIBLE REGION (Continued)

Protein	ϵ^a $(\times\ 10^{-4})$	$A_{1cm}^{1\%\ b}$	nm^c	Reference	Comments^d
Visual pigment, beef	3.7	13.7	280	564	MW = 27,000 [564]
	2.3	8.5	500	564	MW = 27,000 [564]
Vitellogenin					
Xenopus laevis	–	7.5	280	1154	Dry wt.
Wool, helix-rich fraction	–	5.9–6.5	277	776	–
Xanthine oxidase (EC 1.2.3.2)					
milk	–	2.3	450	565	pH 7.8, 0.05 $M\,P_i$
	–	11.5	280	565	–
	20.4	11.26	280	566	pH 8.0, 0.02 $M\,P_i$, MW = 181,000 [566]
	2.2	–	550	27	–
	–	2.41	450	1155	–
High mol. wt. fract.	–	0.87	450	1155	–

Compiled with the assistance of Waldo E. Cohn.

References

1. Kremzner and Wilson, *Biochemistry*, 3, 1902 (1964).
2. Leuzinger, Baker, and Cauvin, *Proc. Natl. Acad. Sci. U.S.A.*, 59, 620 (1968).
3. Nanninga, *Biochim. Biophys. Acta*, 82, 507 (1964).
4. Eisenberg and Moos, *J. Biol. Chem.*, 242, 2945 (1967).
5. Rees and Young, *J. Biol. Chem.*, 242, 4449 (1967).
6. Pfrogner, *Arch. Biochem. Biophys.*, 119, 147 (1967).
7. Tombs, Souter, and Maclagan, *Biochem. J.*, 73, 167 (1959).
8. Schonenberger, *Z. Naturforsch.*, 10b, 474 (1955).
9. Hunter and McDuffie, *J. Am. Chem. Soc.*, 81, 1400 (1959).
10. Phelps and Putnam, in *The Plasma Proteins*, Putnam, ed., Academic Press, New York, 1960, p. 143.
11. Wetlaufer, *Adv. Protein Chem.*, 17, 378 (1962).
12. Van Kley and Stahmann, *J. Am. Chem. Soc.*, 81, 4374 (1959).
13. Everett, *J. Biol. Chem.*, 238, 2676 (1963).
14. Tanford and Roberts, *J. Am. Chem. Soc.*, 74, 2509 (1952).
15. Kolthoff, Shore, Tan, and Matsuoka, *Anal. Biochem.*, 12, 497 (1965).
16. Foster and Yang, *J. Am. Chem. Soc.*, 76, 1015 (1954).
17. Weber, in *The Biochemists Handbook*, Long, ed., E. and F. N. Spon, Ltd., 1961, 82.
18. Bonnichsen, *Acta Chem. Scand.*, 4, 715 (1950).
19. Bonnichsen and Brink, *Methods Enzymol.*, 1, 495 (1955).
20. Theorell, Taniguchi, Akeson, and Skursky, *Biochem. Biophys. Res. Commun.*, 24, 603 (1966).
21. Sund and Theorell, *Enzymology*, 7, 25 (1963).
22. Rosenberg, Theorell, and Yonetani, *Arch. Biochem. Biophys.*, 110, 413 (1965).
23. Mourad and Woronick, *Arch. Biochem. Biophys.*, 121, 431 (1967).
24. Ohta and Ogura, *J. Biochem.* (Tokyo), 58, 73 (1965).
25. Hayes and Velick, *J. Biol. Chem.*, 207, 225 (1954).
26. Steinman and Jakoby, *J. Biol. Chem.*, 242, 5019 (1967).
27. Rajagopalan and Handler, *J. Biol. Chem.*, 239, 1509 (1964).
28. Baranowski and Niederland, *J. Biol. Chem.*, 180, 543 (1949).
29. Taylor, Green, and Cori, *J. Biol. Chem.*, 173, 591 (1948).
30. Donovan, *Biochemistry*, 3, 67 (1964).
31. Stellwagen and Schachman, *Biochemistry*, 1, 1056 (1962).
32. Sia and Horecker, *Arch. Biochem. Biophys.*, 123, 186 (1968).
33. Rajkumar, Woodfin, and Rutter, *Methods Enzymol.*, 9, 491 (1966).
34. Fluri, Ramasarma, and Horecker, *Eur. J. Biochem.*, 1, 117 (1967).
35. Rutter, Hunsley, Groves, Calder, Rajkumar, and Woodfin, *Methods Enzymol.*, 9, 479 (1966).
36. Massey, Palmer, and Bennett, *Biochim. Biophys. Acta*, 48, 1 (1961).
37. Antonini, Brunori, Bruzzesi, Chiancone, and Massey, *J. Biol. Chem.*, 241, 2358 (1960).
38. Yagi, Naoi, Harada, Okamura, Hidaka, Ozawa, and Kotaki, *J. Biochem.* (Tokyo), 61, 580 (1967).
39. Kotaki, Harada, and Yagi, *J. Biochem.* (Tokyo), 61, 598 (1967).
40. Miyake, Aki, Hashimoto, and Yamano, *Biochim. Biophys. Acta*, 105, 86 (1965).
41. Wellner and Meister, *J. Biol. Chem.*, 235, 2013 (1960).
42. Nakano and Danowski, *J. Biol. Chem.*, 241, 2075 (1966).
43. Wachsmuth, Fritze, and Pfleiderer, *Biochemistry*, 5, 169 (1966).
44. Hanson, Hutter, Mannsfeldt, Kretschmer, and Sohr, *Hoppe-Seyler's Z. Physiol. Chem.*, 348, 680 (1967).
45. Fischer and Stein, in *The Enzymes*, Vol. 4, 2nd ed., Bover, Lardy, and Myrbäck, eds., Academic Press, New York, 1960, p. 319.
46. Caldwell, Adams, Kung, and Toralballa, *J. Am. Chem. Soc.*, 74, 4033 (1952).
47. Caldwell, Dickey, Hanrahan, Kung, Kung, and Misko, *J. Am. Chem. Soc.*, 76, 143 (1954).
48. DePinto and Campbell, *Biochemistry*, 7, 114 (1968).
49. Englard and Singer, *J. Biol. Chem.*, 187, 213 (1950).
50. Tombs and Lowe, *Biochem. J.*, 105, 181 (1967).
51. Schmike, *J. Biol. Chem.*, 239, 3808 (1964).
52. Wilson and Meister, *Biochemistry*, 5, 1166 (1966).
53. Bertland and Kaplan, *Biochemistry*, 7, 134 (1968).
54. Gerhart and Schachman, *Biochemistry*, 4, 1054 (1965).
55. Dratz and Calvin, *Nature*, 211, 497 (1966).
56. Gerhart and Holoubek, *J. Biol. Chem.*, 242, 2886 (1967).
57. Gerhart and Schachman, *Biochemistry*, 7, 538 (1968).
58. Ichishima and Yoshida, *Biochim. Biophys. Acta*, 110, 155 (1965).
59. Subramanian and Kalnitsky, *Biochemistry*, 3, 1868 (1964).
60. Hinkson and Bulen, *J. Biol. Chem.*, 242, 3345 (1967).
61. Thornber and Molson, *Biochemistry*, 7, 2242 (1968).
62. Murachi and Yasui, *Biochemistry*, 4, 2275 (1965).
63. Murachi, Inagami, and Yasui, *Biochemistry*, 4, 2815 (1965).
64. Murachi, Yasui, and Yasuda, *Biochemistry*, 3, 48 (1964).
65. Rickli, Ghazanfar, Gibbons, and Edsall, *J. Biol. Chem.*, 239, 1065 (1964).
66. Lindskog, *Biochim. Biophys. Acta*, 39, 218 (1960).
67. Duff and Coleman, *Biochemistry*, 5, 2009 (1966).
68. Edsall, Mehta, Meyers, and Armstrong, *Biochem. Z.*, 345, 9 (1966).
69. Horgan, Webb, and Zerner, *Biochem. Biophys. Res. Commun.*, 23, 23, (1966).
70. Vallee, Rupley, Coombs, and Neurath, *J. Biol. Chem.*, 235, 64 (1960).
71. Bethune, Ulmer, and Vallee, *Biochemistry*, 6, 1955 (1967).

72. Simpson, Riordan, and Vallee, *Biochemistry*, 2, 616 (1963).
73. Riordan and Vallee, *Biochemistry*, 2, 1460 (1963).
74. McClure, Neurath, and Walsh, *Biochemistry*, 3, 1897 (1964).
75. Smith and Stockell, *J. Biol. Chem.*, 207, 501 (1954).
76. Blostein and Rutter, *J. Biol. Chem.*, 238, 3280 (1963).
77. Keller, Cohen, and Neurath, *J. Biol. Chem.*, 223, 457 (1956).
78. Neurath, *Methods Enzymol.*, 1, 77 (1955).
79. Folk and Schirmer, *J. Biol. Chem.*, 238, 3884 (1963).
80. Bargetzi, Sampathkumar, Cox, Walsh, and Neurath, *Biochemistry*, 2, 1468 (1963).
81. Freisheim, Walsh, and Neurath, *Biochemistry*, 6, 3010 (1967).
82. Folk, Piez, Carroll, and Gladner, *J. Biol. Chem.*, 235, 2272 (1960).
83. Cox, Wintersberger, and Neurath, *Biochemistry*, 1, 1078 (1962).
84. Herskovits, *Biochemistry*, 5, 1018 (1966).
85. McKenzie, *Adv. Protein Chem.*, 22, 55 (1967).
86. Herskovits, *J. Biol. Chem.*, 240, 628 (1965).
87. Thompson and Kiddy, *J. Dairy Sci.*, 47, 626 (1964).
88. Thompson and Pepper, *J. Dairy Sci.*, 47, 633 (1964).
89. Zittle and Custer, *J. Dairy Sci.*, 46, 1183 (1963).
90. Bonnichsen, *Methods Enzymol.*, 2, 781 (1955).
91. Stansell and Deutsch, *J. Biol. Chem.*, 240, 4299 (1965).
92. Hiraga, Anan, and Abe, *J. Biochem.* (Tokyo), 56, 416 (1964).
93. Samejima and Yang, *J. Biol. Chem.*, 238, 3256 (1963).
94. Gregory, *Biochim. Biophys. Acta*, 159, 429 (1968).
95. Iwasaki, Hayashi, and Funatsu, *J. Biochem.* (Tokyo), 55, 209 (1964).
96. Edelhoch, *J. Biol. Chem.*, 235, 1326 (1960).
97. Kasper and Deutsch, *J. Biol. Chem.*, 238, 2325 (1963).
98. Markowitz, Cartwright, and Wintrobe, *J. Biol. Chem.*, 234, 40 (1959).
99. Schwick and Heide, in *Protides of the Biological Fluids*, Vol. 14, Peeters, ed., Elsevier, Amsterdam, 1967, p. 55.
100. Sgouris, Coryell, Gallick, Storey, McCall, and Anderson, *Vox Sang.*, 7, 394 (1962).
101. Morell, Irvine, Stemlieb, Scheinberg, and Ashwell, *J. Biol. Chem.*, 243, 155 (1968).
102. Morris and Hager, *J. Biol. Chem.*, 241, 1763 (1966).
103. Tsunoda and Yasunobu, *J. Biol. Chem.*, 241, 4610 (1966).
104. Kunimitsu and Yasunobu, *Biochim. Biophys. Acta*, 139, 405 (1967).
105. Schwert and Kaufman, *J. Biol. Chem.*, 190, 807 (1951).
106. Narasinga, Rao, and Kegeles, *J. Am. Chem. Soc.*, 80, 5724 (1958).
107. Dixon and Neurath, *J. Biol. Chem.*, 225, 1049 (1957).
108. Morimoto and Kegeles, *Biochemistry*, 6, 3007 (1967).
109. Moon, Sturtevant, and Hess, *J. Biol. Chem.*, 240, 4204 (1965).
110. Laskowski, *Methods Enzymol.*, 2, 8 (1955).
111. Folk and Cole, *J. Biol. Chem.*, 240, 193 (1965).
112. Wootton and Hess, *J. Am. Chem. Soc.*, 84, 440 (1962).
113. Schwert, *J. Biol. Chem.*, 190, 799 (1951).
114. Wilcox, Cohen, and Tan, *J. Biol. Chem.*, 228, 999 (1957).
115. Guy, Gratecos, Rovery, and Desnuelle, *Biochim. Biophys. Acta*, 115, 404 (1966).
116. Charles, Gratecos, Rovery, and Desnuelle, *Biochim. Biophys. Acta*, 140, 395 (1967).
117. Smillie, Enenkel, and Kay, *J. Biol. Chem.*, 241, 2097 (1966).
118. Folk and Schirmer, *J. Biol. Chem.*, 240, 181 (1965).
119. Pechere, Dixon, Maybury, and Neurath, *J. Biol. Chem.*, 233, 1364 (1958).
120. Srere, *J. Biol. Chem.*, 241, 2157 (1966).
121. Herschman and Helinski, *J. Biol. Chem.*, 242, 5360 (1967).
122. Warner and Weber, *J. Am. Chem. Soc.*, 75, 5094 (1953).
123. Gotschlich and Edelman, *Proc. Natl. Acad. Sci. U.S.A.*, 54, 558 (1965).
124. Wood and McCarty, *J. Clin. Invest.*, 30, 616 (1951).
125. Noda, Kuby, and Lardy, *J. Biol. Chem.*, 209, 203 (1954).
126. Wisse, Zweers, Jongkind, Bont, and Bloemendal, *Biochem. J.*, 99, 179 (1966).
127. Bjork, *Exp. Eye Res.*, 7, 129 (1968).
128. Mason and Hines, *Invest. Ophthalmol.*, 5, 601 (1966).
129. Bjork, *Exp. Eye Res.*, 2, 339 (1963).
130. Bjork, *Exp. Eye Res.*, 3, 254 (1964).
131. Van Dam, *Exp. Eye Res.*, 5, 255 (1966).
132. Zigman and Lerman, *Biochim. Biophys. Acta*, 154, 423 (1968).

133. Yonetani, *J. Biol. Chem.*, 236, 1680 (1961).
134. Yonetani, *J. Biol. Chem.*, 242, 5008 (1967).
135. Paleus, *Arch. Biochem. Biophys.*, 96, 60 (1962).
136. Matsubara, Chu, and Yasunobu, *Arch. Biochem. Biophys.*, 101, 209 (1962).
137. Paul, *Acta Chem. Scand.*, 5, 389 (1951).
138. Flatmark, *Acta Chem. Scand.*, 18, 1517 (1964).
139. Flatmark, *Acta Chem. Scand.*, 20, 1476 (1966).
140. Margoliash and Frohwirt, *Biochem. J.*, 71, 570 (1959).
141. Jirgensons, *J. Biol. Chem.*, 240, 1064 (1965).
142. Linberg, *Biochemistry*, 6, 335 (1967).
143. Mondovi, Rotilio, Costa, Finazzi-Agro, Chiancone, Hansen, and Beinert, *J. Biol. Chem.*, 242, 1160 (1967).
144. Swislocki and Kaplan, *J. Biol. Chem.*, 242, 1083 (1967).
145. Raynaud, *Proc. 2nd Meet. Fed. Eur. Biochem. Soc.*, Vienna 1965, 1, 199 (1967).
146. Holt and Wold, *J. Biol. Chem.*, 236, 3227 (1961).
147. Bucher, *Methods Enzymol.*, 1, 427 (1955).
148. Malmstrom, Kimmel, and Smith, *J. Biol. Chem.*, 234, 1108 (1959).
149. Bergdoll, Chu, Huang, Rowe, and Shih, *Arch. Biochem. Biophys.*, 112, 104 (1965).
150. Schantz, Roessler, Wagman, Spero, Dunnery, and Bergdoll, *Biochemistry*, 4, 1011 (1965).
151. Stansell and Deutsch, *J. Biol. Chem.*, 240, 4306 (1965).
152. Crane, Mii, Hauge, Green, and Beinert, *J. Biol. Chem.*, 218, 701 (1956).
153. Yang, Butterworth, Bock, and Potter, *J. Biol. Chem.*, 242, 3501 (1967).
154. Keresztes-Nagy and Margoliash, *J. Biol. Chem.*, 241, 5955 (1966).
155. Matsubara, *J. Biol. Chem.*, 243, 370 (1968).
156. Malkin and Rabinowitz, *Biochemistry*, 5, 1262 (1966).
157. Hofmann and Harrison, *J. Mol. Biol.*, 6, 256 (1963).
158. Verpoorte, Green, and Kay, *J. Biol. Chem.*, 240, 1156 (1965).
159. Caspary and Kekwick, *Biochem. J.*, 56, 35 (1954).
160. Mosesson, Alkjaersig, Sweet, and Sherry, *Biochemistry*, 6, 3279 (1967).
161. Mihalyi, *Biochemistry*, 7, 208 (1968).
162. Mihalyi and Godfrey, *Biochim. Biophys. Acta*, 67, 73 (1963).
163. Gould and Liener, *Biochemistry*, 4, 90 (1965).
164. Hornby, Lilly, and Crook, *Biochem. J.*, 98, 420 (1966).
165. Englund, King, Craig, and Walti, *Biochemistry*, 7, 163 (1968).
166. Knight and Hardy, *J. Biol. Chem.*, 241, 2752 (1966).
167. Knight, D'Eustachio, and Hardy, *Biochim. Biophys. Acta*, 113, 626 (1966).
168. Papkoff, Gospodarowicz, and Li, *Arch. Biochem. Biophys.*, 120, 434 (1967).
169. Papkoff, Mahlmann, and Li, *Biochemistry*, 6, 3976 (1967).
170. Mizobuchi and Buchanan, *J. Biol. Chem.*, 243, 4842 (1968).
171. Himes and Cohn, *J. Biol. Chem.*, 242, 3628 (1967).
172. Marcus and Hubert, *J. Biol. Chem.*, 243, 4923 (1968).
173. Fernando, Enser, Pontremoli, and Horecker, *Arch. Biochem. Biophys.*, 126, 599 (1968).
174. Pontremoli, Grazi, and Accorsi, *Biochemistry*, 7, 3628 (1968).
175. Kanarek and Hill, *J. Biol. Chem.*, 239, 4202 (1964).
176. Malhotra and Dey, *Biochem. J.*, 103, 508 (1967).
177. Wallenfells and Golker, *Biochem. Z.*, 346, 1 (1966).
178. Wallenfells and Malhotra, in *The Enzymes*, Vol. 4, 2nd ed., Boyer, Lardy, and Myrback, eds., Academic Press, New York, 1960, 413.
179. Mills and Tang, *J. Biol. Chem.*, 242, 3093 (1967).
180. Chiang, Sanchez-Chiang, Mills, and Tang, *J. Biol. Chem.*, 242, 3098 (1967).
181. Bernardin, Kasarda, and Mecham, *J. Biol. Chem.*, 242, 445 (1967).
182. Vodrazka, Hrkal, Cejka, and Sipalova, *Collect. Czech. Chem. Commun.*, 32, 3250 (1967).
183. Gibson and Antonini, *J. Biol. Chem.*, 238, 1384 (1963).
184. Hrkal and Vodrazka, *Biochim. Biophys. Acta*, 133, 527 (1967).
185. Rossi-Fanelli, Antonini, and Caputo, *J. Biol. Chem.*, 234, 2906 (1959).
186. Schultze, Heide, and Haupt, *Klin. Wochenschr.*, 40, 729 (1962).
187. Berggard and Beam, *J. Biol. Chem.*, 243, 4095 (1968).
188. Deutsch, *Science*, 141, 435 (1963).

189. Muldoon and Westphal, *J. Biol. Chem.*, 242, 5636 (1967).
190. Chader and Westphal, *J. Biol. Chem.*, 243, 928 (1968).
191. Chader and Westphal, *Biochemistry*, 7, 4272 (1968).
192. Giorgio and Tabachnick, *J. Biol. Chem.*, 243, 2247 (1968).
193. Gratzer, Bailey, and Beaven, *Biochem. Biophys. Res. Commun.*, 28, 914 (1967).
194. Huotari, Nelson, Smith, and Kirkwood, *J. Biol. Chem.*, 243, 952 (1968).
195. Hauge, *Methods Enzymol.*, 9, 107 (1966).
196. Swoboda and Massey, *J. Biol. Chem.*, 240, 2209 (1965).
197. Takeda, Hizukuri, and Nikuni, *Biochim. Biophys. Acta*, 146, 568 (1967).
198. Plapp and Cole, *Arch. Biochem. Biophys.*, 116, 193 (1966).
199. Switzer and Barker, *J. Biol. Chem.*, 242, 2658 (1967).
200. Tomkins, Yielding, Curran, Summers, and Bitensky, *J. Biol. Chem.*, 240, 3793 (1965).
201. Eisenberg and Tomkins, *J. Mol. Biol.*, 31, 37 (1968).
202. Olson and Anfinsen, *J. Biol. Chem.*, 197, 67 (1952).
203. Reithel and Sakura, *J. Phys. Chem.*, 67, 2497 (1963).
204. Fahien, Wiggert, and Cohen, *J. Biol. Chem.*, 240, 1083 (1965).
205. Messer and Ottesen, *C. R. Trav. Lab. Carlsberg Ser. Chim.*, 35, 1 (1965).
206. Rowe and Wyngaarden, *Fed. Proc.*, 27(2), 340 (1968).
207. Rowe and Wyngaarden, *J. Biol. Chem.*, 243, 6373 (1968).
208. Pamiljans, Krishnaswamy, Dumville, and Meister, *Biochemistry*, 1, 153 (1962).
209. Shapiro and Stadtman, *J. Biol. Chem.*, 242, 5069 (1967).
210. Woolfolk, Shapiro, and Stadtman, *Arch. Biochem. Biophys.*, 116, 177 (1966).
211. Colman and Black, *J. Biol. Chem.*, 240, 1796 (1965).
212. Massey and Williams, *J. Biol. Chem.*, 240, 4470 (1965).
213. Mavis and Stellwagen, *J. Biol. Chem.*, 243, 809 (1968).
214. Icen, *Scand. J. Clin. Lab. Invest., Suppl.*, 20, 96 (1967).
215. Kirschner and Voigt, *Hoppe-Seyler's Z. Physiol. Chem.*, 349, 632 (1968).
216. Krebs, *Methods Enzymol.*, 1, 407 (1955).
217. Jaenicke, Schmid, and Knof, *Biochemistry*, 7, 919 (1968).
218. Trentham, *Biochem. J.*, 109, 603 (1968).
219. Davidson, Sajgo, Noller, and Harris, *Nature*, 216, 1181 (1967).
220. Allison, *Methods Enzymol.*, 9, 212 (1966).
221. Mora and Elodi, *Eur. J. Biochem.*, 5, 574 (1968).
222. Velick, Hayes, and Harting, *J. Biol. Chem.*, 203, 527 (1953).
223. Fox and Dandliker, *J. Biol. Chem.*, 221, 1005 (1958).
224. Ankel, Bucher, and Czok, *Biochem. Z.*, 332, 315 (1960).
225. Fondy, Levin, Sollohub, and Ross, *J. Biol. Chem.*, 243, 3148 (1968).
226. Marquardt and Brosemer, *Biochim. Biophys. Acta*, 128, 454 (1966).
227. Brosemer and Marquardt, *Biochim. Biophys. Acta*, 128, 464 (1966).
228. Pradel, Kassab, Conlay, and Thoai, *Biochim. Biophys. Acta*, 154, 305 (1968).
229. Okuda and Weinbaum, *Biochemistry*, 7, 2819 (1968).
230. Schultze and Heremans, in *Molecular Biology of Human Proteins*, Vol. 1, Elsevier, New York, 1966, p. 176.
231. Haupt and Heide, *Clin. Chim. Acta*, 10, 555 (1964).
232. Schmidt, *J. Am. Chem. Soc.*, 72, 2816 (1950).
233. Smith, Brown, Weimer, and Winzler, *J. Biol. Chem.*, 185, 569 (1950).
234. Bundy and Mehl, *J. Biol. Chem.*, 234, 1124 (1959).
235. Schultze, Heide, and Haupt, *Naturwissenschaften*, 49, 133 (1962).
236. Burgi and Schmid, *J. Biol. Chem.*, 236, 1067 (1961).
237. Schmid and Burgi, *Biochim. Biophys. Acta*, 47, 440 (1961).
238. Schonenberger, Schmidtberger, and Schultze, *Z. Naturforsch.*, 13b, 761 (1958).
239. Edelhoch, Condliffe, Lippoldt, and Burger, *J. Biol. Chem.*, 241, 5205 (1966).
240. Polonovski and Sayle, *Bull. Soc. Chim. Biol.*, 21, 661 (1939).
241. Lisowska and Dobryszycka, *Biochim. Biophys. Acta*, 133, 338 (1967).
242. Heirwegh, Borginon, and Lontie, *Biochim. Biophys. Acta*, 48, 517 (1961).
243. Ghiretti-Magaldi, Nuzzolo, and Ghiretti, *Biochemistry*, 5, 1943 (1966).
244. Formanek and Engel, *Biochim. Biophys. Acta*, 160, 151 (1968).
245. Schichi and Kuroda, *Arch. Biochem. Biophys.*, 118, 682 (1967).
246. Schultze, Heide, and Haupt, *Naturwissenschaften.*, 48, 696 (1961).
247. Derechin, Ramel, Lazarus, and Barnard, *Biochemistry*, 5, 4017 (1966).
248. McDonald, *Methods Enzymol.*, 1, 269 (1955).
249. Riley and Snell, *Biochemistry*, 7, 3520 (1968).
250. Chang and Snell, *Biochemistry*, 7, 2005 (1968).
251. Loper and Adams, *J. Biol. Chem.*, 240, 788 (1965).
252. Yourno and Ino, *J. Biol. Chem.*, 243, 3273 (1968).
253. Yourno, *J. Biol. Chem.*, 243, 3277 (1968).
254. Loper, *J. Biol. Chem.*, 243, 3264 (1968).
255. Bennett, Creaser, and McDonald, *Biochem. J.*, 109, 307 (1968).
256. Truffa-Bachi, Van Rapenbusch, Jannin, Gros, and Cohen, *Eur. J. Biochem.*, 5, 73 (1968).
257. Nakano, Ushijima, Saga, Tsutsumi, and Asami, *Biochim. Biophys. Acta*, 167, 9 (1968).
258. Dai, Decker, and Sund, *Eur. J. Biochem.*, 4, 95 (1968).
259. Becker and Pfeil, *Biochem. Z.*, 346, 301 (1966).
260. Becker, Benthin, Eschenhof, and Pfeil, *Biochem. Z.*, 337, 156 (1963).
261. Kohn and Jakoby, *J. Biol. Chem.*, 243, 2494 (1968).
262. Martin and Goldberger, *J. Biol. Chem.*, 242, 1168 (1967).
263. Little and Donahue, *Meth. Immunol. Immunochem.*, 2, 343 (1968).
264. Creighton and Yanofsky, *J. Biol. Chem.*, 241, 4616 (1966).
265. Porter, *Biochem. J.*, 53, 320 (1953).
266. Weil, Seibles, and Herskovits, *Arch. Biochem. Biophys.*, 111, 308 (1965).
267. Praissman and Rupley, *Biochemistry*, 7, 2431 (1968).
268. Nakaya, Horinishi, and Shibata, *J. Biochem. (Tokyo)*, 61, 345 (1967).
269. Lampson, Tytell, Nemes, and Hilleman, *Proc. Soc. Exp. Biol. Med.*, 112, 468 (1963).
270. Metzenberg, *Arch. Biochem. Biophys.*, 100, 503 (1963).
271. Neumann and Lampen, *Biochemistry*, 6, 468 (1967).
272. Colman, *J. Biol. Chem.*, 243, 2454 (1968).
273. Margolies and Goldberger, *J. Biol. Chem.*, 242, 256 (1967).
274. Anderer and Hornle, *J. Biol. Chem.*, 241, 1568 (1966).
275. Morihara, Oka, and Tsuzuki, *Biochim. Biophys. Acta*, 139, 382 (1967).
276. Nickerson and Durand, *Biochim. Biophys. Acta*, 77, 87 (1963).
277. Nickerson, Noval, and Robison, *Biochim. Biophys. Acta*, 77, 73 (1963).
278. Hirashima, Hayakawa, and Koike, *J. Biol. Chem.*, 242, 902 (1967).
279. Kawahara, Wang, and Talalay, *J. Biol. Chem.*, 237, 1500 (1962).
280. Wetlaufer, *C. R. Trav. Lab. Carlsberg Ser. Chim.*, 32, 125 (1960).
281. Kronman and Andreotti, *Biochemistry*, 3, 1145 (1964).
282. Sullivan, *Biochem. J.*, 110, 363 (1968).
283. Takemori, Nakazawa, Nakai, Suzuki, and Katagiri, *J. Biol. Chem.*, 243, 313 (1968).
284. Pesce, McKay, Stolzenbach, Cahn, and Kaplan, *J. Biol. Chem.*, 239, 1753 (1964).
285. DiSabato, Pesce, and Kaplan, *Biochim. Biophys. Acta*, 77, 135 (1963).
286. Markert and Appella, *Ann. N. Y. Acad. Sci.*, 94, 678 (1961).
287. Pesce, Fondy, Stolzenbach, Castillo, and Kaplan, *J. Biol. Chem.*, 242, 2151 (1967).
288. Fromm, *J. Biol. Chem.*, 238, 2938 (1963).
289. Schellenberg, *J. Biol. Chem.*, 242, 1815 (1967).
290. Jaenicka, *Biochem. Z.*, 338, 614 (1963).
291. Gibson, Davisson, Bachhawat, Ray, and Vestling, *J. Biol. Chem.*, 203, 397 (1961).
292. Wieland and Pfleiderer, *Ann. N. Y. Acad. Sci.*, 94, 691 (1961).
293. Appleby and Morton, *Biochem. J.*, 73, 539 (1969).
294. Tarmy and Kaplan, *J. Biol. Chem.*, 243, 2579 (1968).
295. Okabe, Hayakawa, Hamada, and Koike, *Biochemistry*, 7, 79 (1968).
296. Polis, Schmuckler, Custer, and McMeekin, *J. Am. Chem. Soc.*, 72, 4965 (1950).
297. Baker and Saroff, *Biochemistry*, 4, 1670 (1965).
298. Wetlaufer and Lovrien, *J. Biol. Chem.*, 239, 596 (1964).
299. Gordon, Basch, and Kalan, *J. Biol. Chem.*, 236, 2908 (1961).
300. Townend, Winterbottom, and Timasheff, *J. Am. Chem. Soc.*, 82, 3161 (1960).

301. Townend, Herskovits, Swaisgood, and Timasheff, *J. Biol. Chem.,* 239, 4196 (1964).
302. Tanford and Nozaki, *J. Biol. Chem.,* 234, 2874 (1959).
303. Ogston and Tombs, *Biochem. J.,* 66, 399 (1957).
304. Bell and McKenzie, *Biochim. Biophys. Acta,* 147, 123 (1967).
305. Ghose, Chaudhuri, and Sen, *Arch. Biochem. Biophys.,* 126, 232 (1968).
306. Groves, *J. Am. Chem. Soc.,* 82, 3345 (1960).
307. Masson and Heremans, in *Protides of the Biological Fluids,* Peeters, Ed., Vol. 14, Elsevier, Amsterdam, 1967, 115.
308. Montreuil, Tonnelat, and Mullet, *Biochim. Biophys. Acta,* 45, 413 (1960).
309. Spackman, Smith, and Brown, *J. Biol. Chem.,* 212, 255 (1955).
310. Kawahara, Misaka, and Nakanishi, *J. Biochem. (Tokyo),* 63, 77 (1968).
311. Hastings, Riley, and Massa, *J. Biol. Chem.,* 240, 1473 (1965).
312. Bruzzesi, Chiancone, and Antonini, *Biochemistry,* 4, 1796 (1965).
313. Hamaguchi and Kutono, *J. Biochem. (Tokyo),* 54, 111 (1963).
314. Fromageot and Schnek, *Biochim. Biophys. Acta,* 6, 113 (1950).
315. Chandan, Parry, and Shahani, *Biochim. Biophys. Acta,* 110, 389 (1965).
316. Glazer, *Aust. J. Chem.,* 12, 304 (1959).
317. Sophianopoulos, Rhodes, Holcomb, and Van Holde, *J. Biol. Chem.,* 237, 1107 (1962).
318. Praissman and Rupley, *Biochemistry,* 7, 2446 (1968).
319. Canfield, *J. Biol. Chem.,* 238, 2691 (1963).
320. Wetlaufer and Stahmann, *J. Am. Chem. Soc.,* 80, 1493 (1958).
321. Yutani, Yutani, Imanishi, and Isemura, *J. Biochem. (Tokyo),* 64, 449 (1968).
322. Jolles and Jolles, *Biochemistry,* 6, 411 (1967).
323. Bonavida, Sapse, and Sercarz, *J. Lab. Clin. Med.,* 70, 951 (1967).
324. Tsugita, Inouye, Terzaghi, and Streisinger, *J. Biol. Chem.,* 243, 391 (1968).
325. Howard and Glazer, *J. Biol. Chem.,* 242, 5715 (1967).
326. Black, Ph.D. thesis, Stanford University, 1967.
327. Wolfe and Neilands, *J. Biol. Chem.,* 221, 61 (1956).
328. Thorne, *Biochim. Biophys. Acta,* 59, 624 (1962).
329. Pfliederer and Hohnholz, *Biochem. Z.,* 331, 245 (1959).
330. Davies and Kun, *Biochem. J.,* 66, 307 (1957).
331. Grimm and Doherty, *J. Biol. Chem.,* 236, 1980 (1961).
332. Yoshida, *J. Biol. Chem.,* 240, 1113 (1965).
333. Murphey, Barnaby, Lin, and Kaplan, *J. Biol. Chem.,* 242, 1548 (1967).
334. Kitto, *Biochim. Biophys. Acta,* 139, 16 (1967).
335. Kitto and Lewis, *Biochim. Biophys. Acta,* 139, 1 (1967).
336. Kohn and Jakoby, *J. Biol. Chem.,* 243, 2472 (1968).
337. Harada and Wolfe, *J. Biol. Chem.,* 243, 4123 (1968).
338. Hsu and Lardy, *J. Biol. Chem.,* 242, 520 (1967).
339. Levy, *J. Biol. Chem.,* 242, 747 (1967).
340. Hsiang and Bright, *J. Biol. Chem.,* 242, 3079 (1967).
341. Barker, Smyth, Wilson, and Weissbach, *J. Biol. Chem.,* 234, 320 (1959).
342. Erwin and Hellerman, *J. Biol. Chem.,* 242, 4230 (1967).
343. Yamada and Yasunobu, *J. Biol. Chem.,* 237, 1511 (1962).
344. Rohrer, van Wartburg, and Aebi, *Biochem. Z.,* 344, 478 (1966).
345. Noda and Kuby, *J. Biol. Chem.,* 226, 551 (1957).
346. Callaghan and Weber, *Biochem. J.,* 73, 473 (1959).
347. Quass and Briskey, *J. Food Sci.,* 33, 180 (1968).
348. Kielley and Harrington, *Biochim. Biophys. Acta,* 41, 401 (1960).
349. Gellert and Englander, *Biochemistry,* 2, 39 (1963).
350. Nanninga, *Biochim. Biophys. Acta,* 82, 507 (1964).
351. Frederiksen and Holtzer, *Biochemistry,* 7, 3935 (1968).
352. Morita and Yagi, *Biochem. Biophys. Res. Commun.,* 22, 297 (1966).
353. Young, Himmelfarb, and Harrington, *J. Biol. Chem.,* 239, 2822 (1964).
354. Riddiford, *J. Biol. Chem.,* 241, 2792 (1966).
355. Yagi, Yazawa, and Yasui, *Biochem. Biophys. Res. Commun.,* 29, 331 (1967).
356. Wu, *Biochemistry,* 8, 39 (1969).
357. Hagihara, in *The Enzymes,* Vol. 4, 2nd ed., Boyer, Lardy, and Myrbäck, eds., Academic Press, New York, 1960, p. 193.
358. Hochstein and Dalton, *Biochim. Biophys. Acta,* 139, 56 (1967).
359. Taniuchi and Anfinsen, *J. Biol. Chem.,* 241, 4366 (1966).
360. Edelhoch and Lippoldt, *J. Biol. Chem.,* 237, 2788 (1962).
361. Cunningham and Nuenke, *J. Biol. Chem.,* 234, 1447 (1959).
362. Edelhoch and Steiner, *J. Biol. Chem.,* 240, 2877 (1965).
363. Chatterjee and Montgomery, *Arch. Biochem. Biophys.,* 99, 426 (1962).
364. Kohn and Jakoby, *J. Biol. Chem.,* 243, 2486 (1968).
365. Glazer and Smith, *J. Biol. Chem.,* 236, 2948 (1961).
366. Smith, Light, and Kimmel, *Biochem. Soc. Symp.,* 21, 88 (1962).
367. Finkle and Smith, *J. Biol. Chem.,* 230, 669 (1958).
368. Whitaker and Bender, *J. Am. Chem. Soc.,* 87, 2728 (1965).
369. Potts, Aurbach, and Sherwood, *Recent Prog. Horm. Res.,* 22, 114 (1966).
370. Edelhoch, *J. Am. Chem. Soc.,* 79, 6100 (1957).
371. Perlman, *J. Biol. Chem.,* 241, 153 (1966).
372. Aloj, Salvatore, and Roche, *J. Biol. Chem.,* 242, 3810 (1967).
373. Perlman, Oplatka, and Katchalsky, *J. Biol. Chem.,* 242, 5163 (1967).
374. Chow and Kassel, *J. Biol. Chem.,* 243, 1718 (1968).
375. Gounaris and Perlman, *J. Biol. Chem.,* 242, 2739 (1967).
376. Keilin and Hartree, *Biochem. J.,* 49, 88 (1951).
377. Maehly, *Methods Enzymol.,* 2, 801 (1955).
378. Wittenberg, Antonini, Brunori, Noble, Wittenberg, and Wyman, *Biochemistry,* 6, 1970 (1967).
379. Paul, in *The Enzymes,* Vol. 8, 2nd ed., Boyer, Lardy, and Myrbäck, eds., Academic Press, New York, 1963, p. 233.
380. Kertesz and Zito, in *Oxygenases,* Hayashi, ed., Academic Press, New York, 1962, p. 307.
381. Rothman and Byrne, *J. Mol. Biol.,* 6, 330 (1963).
382. Plocke, Levinthal, and Vallee, *Biochemistry,* 1, 373 (1962).
383. Kadner, Nye, and Brown, *J. Biol. Chem.,* 243, 3076 (1968).
384. Dom, *J. Biol. Chem.,* 243, 3500 (1968).
385. Neumann, *J. Biol. Chem.,* 243, 4671 (1968).
386. Harkness, *Arch. Biochem. Biophys.,* 126, 503 (1968).
387. Igarashi and Hollander, *J. Biol. Chem.,* 243, 6084 (1968).
388. Parmeggiani, Luft, Love, and Krebs, *J. Biol. Chem.,* 241, 4625 (1966).
389. Paetkau and Lardy, *J. Biol. Chem.,* 242, 2035 (1967).
390. Younathan, Paetkau, and Lardy, *J. Biol. Chem.,* 243, 1603 (1968).
391. Froede, Geraci, and Mansour, *J. Biol. Chem.,* 243, 6021 (1968).
392. Lindell and Stellwagen, *J. Biol. Chem.,* 243, 907 (1968).
393. Chatterjee and Noltman, *Eur. J. Biochem.,* 2, 9 (1967).
394. Najjar, *J. Biol. Chem.,* 175, 281 (1948).
395. Najjar, *Methods Enzymol.,* 1, 294 (1955).
396. Rippa, Signorini, and Pontremoli, *Eur. J. Biochem.,* 1, 170 (1967).
397. Sugimoto and Pizer, *J. Biol. Chem.,* 243, 2090 (1968).
398. Zwaig and Milstein, *Biochem. J.,* 98, 360 (1966).
399. Sugimoto, Sasaki, and Chiba, *Arch. Biochem. Biophys.,* 113, 444 (1966).
400. Voll, Appella, and Martin, *J. Biol. Chem.,* 242, 1760 (1967).
401. Wells and Hanahan, *Biochemistry,* 8, 414 (1969).
402. Korn and Buchanan, *J. Biol. Chem.,* 217, 183 (1955).
403. Agarwal and Parks, *Fed. Proc.,* 27, 585, Abstract No. 2072 (1968).
404. Buc and Buc, in *Symposium on Regulation of Enzyme Activity and Allosteric Interactions,* 4th Federation of European Biochemical Societies, Oslo, 1967. Academic Press, 1967, p. 109.
405. Velick and Wicks, *J. Biol. Chem.,* 190, 741 (1951).
406. Appleman, Krebs, and Fischer, *Biochemistry,* 5, 2101 (1966).
407. Metzger, Glaser, and Helmreich, *Biochemistry,* 7, 2021 (1968).
408. Kastenschmidt, Kastenschmidt, and Helmreich, *Biochemistry,* 7, 3590 (1968).
409. Gold, *Biochemistry,* 7, 2106 (1968).
410. Appleman, Yunis, Krebs, and Fischer, *J. Biol. Chem.,* 238, 1358 (1963).
411. Shaltiel, Hedrick, and Fischer, *Methods Enzymol.,* 11, 675 (1967).
412. Brody and Brody, *Biochim. Biophys. Acta,* 50, 348 (1961).
413. Toro-Goyco and Matos, *Nature,* 210, 527 (1966).
414. Toro-Goyco, Maretzki, and Matos, *Arch. Biochem. Biophys.,* 126, 91 (1968).
415. Bergmeyer, Holz, Klotzsch, and Lang, *Biochem. Z.,* 338, 114 (1963).
416. Reisfeld, Borjeson, Chessin, and Small, *Proc. Natl. Acad. Sci. U.S.A.,* 58, 2020 (1967).

417. Jovim, Englund, and Bertsch, *J. Biol. Chem.* (1969).
418. Robbins, Summaria, Elwyn, and Barlow, *J. Biol. Chem.*, 240, 541 (1965).
419. Robbins and Summaria, *J. Biol. Chem.*, 238, 952 (1963).
420. Kertesz and Zito, *Biochim. Biophys. Acta*, 96, 447 (1965).
421. Gregory and Bendall, *Biochem. J.*, 101, 569 (1966).
422. Reuter, Hamoir, Marchand, and Kennes, *Eur. J. Biochem.*, 5, 233 (1968).
423. Frank and Veros, *Biochem. Biophys. Res. Commun.*, 32, 155 (1968).
424. Oshima, Matsuo, Iwanaga, and Suzuki, *J. Biochem. (Tokyo)*, 64, 227 (1968).
425. Oshima, Iwanaga, and Suzuki, *J. Biochem. (Tokyo)*, 54, 215 (1968).
426. Jonsson, *Arch. Biochem. Biophys.*, 129, 62 (1969).
427. Ganno, *J. Biochem. (Tokyo)*, 58, 556 (1965).
428. McConn, Tsuru, and Yasunobu, *J. Biol. Chem.*, 239, 3706 (1964).
429. Ohta, Ogura, and Wada, *J. Biol. Chem.*, 241, 5919 (1966).
430. Jackson and Wolfe, *J. Biol. Chem.*, 243, 879 (1968).
431. Fukumoto, Tsuru, and Yamamoto, *Agric. Biol. Chem.*, 31, 710 (1967).
432. Kimmel, Markowitz, and Brown, *J. Biol. Chem.*, 234, 46 (1959).
433. Narahashi, Shibuya, and Yanagita, *J. Biochem. (Tokyo)*, 64, 427 (1968).
434. Hiramatsu, *J. Biochem. (Tokyo)*, 62, 353 (1967).
435. Day, Toncic, Stratman, Leeman, and Harmon, *Biochim. Biophys. Acta*, 167, 597 (1968).
436. Hata, Hayashi, and Doi, *Agr. Biol. Chem.*, 31, 357 (1967).
437. Frattali, *J. Biol. Chem.*, 244, 274 (1969).
438. Iwasaki and Schmid, *J. Biol. Chem.*, 242, 5247 (1967).
439. Tomasi and Komguth, *J. Biol. Chem.*, 242, 4933 (1967).
440. Wood, Massi, and Solomon, *J. Biol. Chem.*, 234, 329 (1959).
441. Miyake, Gaylor, and Mason, *J. Biol. Chem.*, 243, 5788 (1968).
442. Marushige, Britlag, and Bonner, *Biochemistry*, 7, 3149 (1968).
443. Dus, De Klerk, Sletten, and Bartsch, *Biochim. Biophys. Acta*, 140, 291 (1967).
444. Tang and Coleman, *J. Biol. Chem.*, 243, 4286 (1968).
445. Hinkson, *Biochemistry*, 7, 2666 (1968).
446. Koshiyama, *Cereal Chem.*, 45, 405 (1968).
447. Koshiyama, *Cereal Chem.*, 45, 394 (1968).
448. Shore and Shore, *Biochemistry*, 6, 1962 (1967).
449. Gumpf and Hamilton, *Virology*, 35, 87 (1968).
450. Zaitlin and McCaughey, *Virology*, 26, 500 (1965).
451. Wasserman, Corradino, and Taylor, *J. Biol. Chem.*, 243, 3978 (1968).
452. Kalb, *Biochim. Biophys. Acta*, 168, 532 (1968).
453. Penrose, Nicholalds, Piperno, and Oxender, *J. Biol. Chem.*, 243, 5921 (1968).
454. Lamy and Waugh, *J. Biol. Chem.*, 203, 489 (1953).
455. Shulman and Hearon, *J. Biol. Chem.*, 238, 155 (1963).
456. Tishkoff, Williams, and Brown, *J. Biol. Chem.*, 243, 4151 (1968).
457. Aronson, *Thromb. Diath. Haemorrh.*, 16, 491 (1966).
458. Shapiro and Waugh, *Thromb. Diath. Haemorrh.*, 16, 469 (1966).
459. Lanchantin, Hart, Friedman, Saavedra, and Mehl, *J. Biol. Chem.*, 243, 5479 (1968).
460. Fujisawa and Hayashi, *J. Biol. Chem.*, 243, 2673 (1968).
461. Yui, Ishii, and Egami, *J. Biochem. (Tokyo)*, 65, 37 (1969).
462. Ayling and Snell, *Biochemistry*, 7, 1616 (1968).
463. Kojima, Fujisawa, Nakazawa, *et al. J. Biol. Chem.*, 242, 3270 (1967).
464. Kunitz, *J. Gen. Physiol.*, 35, 423 (1952).
465. Williams and Hager, *Methods Enzymol.*, 9, 265 (1966).
466. Bucher and Pfleiderer, *Methods Enzymol.*, 1, 435 (1955).
467. Packman and Jakoby, *J. Biol. Chem.*, 240, PC4107 (1965).
468. Foltman, *C. R. Trav. Lab. Carlsberg Ser. Chim.*, 34, 319 (1964).
469. Wang and Volini, *J. Biol. Chem.*, 243, 5465 (1968).
470. Shichi, Lewis, Irreverre, and Stone, *J. Biol. Chem.*, 244, 529 (1969).
471. Shields, Dinovo, Henriksen, Kimbel, and Millar, *Biochim. Biophys. Acta*, 147, 238 (1967).
472. Meadows and Jardetzky, *Proc. Natl. Acad. Sci. U.S.A.*, 61, 406 (1968).
473. Hill and Schmidt, *J. Biol. Chem.*, 237, 389 (1962).
474. Taborsky, *J. Biol. Chem.*, 234, 2915 (1959).
475. Sela, Anfinsen, and Harrington, *Biochim. Biophys. Acta*, 26, 502 (1957).
476. Jaenicke, Schmid, and Knof, *Biochemistry*, 7, 919 (1968).
477. Tanford, Hauenstein, and Rands, *J. Am. Chem. Soc.*, 77, 6409 (1955).
478. Blumenfeld and Levy, *Arch. Biochem. Biophys.*, 76, 97 (1958).
479. Sage and Singer, *Biochim. Biophys. Acta*, 29, 663 (1958).
480. Sage and Singer, *Biochemistry*, 1, 305 (1962).
481. Bigelow, *J. Biol. Chem.*, 236, 1706 (1961).
482. Sherwood and Potts, *J. Biol. Chem.*, 240, 3799 (1965).
483. Keller, Cohen, and Neurath, *J. Biol. Chem.*, 233, 344 (1958).
484. Aqvist and Anfinsen, *J. Biol. Chem.*, 234, 1112 (1959).
485. Wilson, *J. Biol. Chem.*, 242, 2260 (1967).
486. Yamasaki, Murakami, Irie, and Ukita, *J. Biochem. (Tokyo)*, 63, 25 (1968).
487. Uchida, *J. Biochem. (Tokyo)*, 60, 115 (1966).
488. Ettinger and Hirs, *Biochemistry*, 7, 3374 (1968).
489. Lee and Bendet, *J. Biol. Chem.*, 242, 2043 (1967).
490. Akoyunoglou, Argyroudi-Akoyunoglou, and Methenitou, *Biochim. Biophys. Acta*, 132, 481 (1967).
491. Lee, Patrick, and Masson, *J. Biol. Chem.*, 243, 4700 (1968).
492. Newman and Postgate, *Eur. J. Biochem.*, 7, 45 (1968).
493. Bachmayer, Yasunobu, Peel, and Mayhew, *J. Biol. Chem.*, 243, 1022 (1968).
494. Lovenberg, in *Protides of the Biological Fluids*, Vol. 14, Peeters, ed., Elsevier, Amsterdam 1967, p. 165.
495. Bachmayer, Benson, Yasunobu, Garrard, and Whiteley, *Biochemistry*, 7, 986 (1968).
496. Peterson and Coon, *J. Biol. Chem.*, 243, 329 (1968).
497. Lovenberg and Williams, *Biochemistry*, 8, 141 (1969).
498. Laurell, *Acta Chem. Scand.*, 7, 1407 (1953).
499. Peisach, Levine, and Blumberg, *J. Biol. Chem.*, 242, 2841 (1967).
500. Green and Malamed, *Biochem. J.*, 100, 614 (1966).
501. Chaiet and Wolf, *Arch. Biochem. Biophys.*, 106, 1 (1964).
502. Taylor and Botts, *Biochemistry*, 7, 232 (1968).
503. Salvatore, Vecchio, Salvatore, Cahnman, and Robbins, *J. Biol. Chem.*, 240, 2935 (1965).
504. Matsubara, Kaspar, Brown, and Smith, *J. Biol. Chem.*, 240, 1125 (1965).
505. Landon, Evans, and Smith, *J. Biol. Chem.*, 243, 2165 (1968).
506. Neet, Nanci, and Koshland, *J. Biol. Chem.*, 243, 6392 (1968).
507. Gounaris and Ottesen, *C. R. Trav. Lab. Carlsberg Ser. Chim.*, 35, 37 (1965).
508. Ramaley, Bridger, Moyer, and Boyer, *J. Biol. Chem.*, 242, 4287 (1967).
509. Allen and Roy, *Biochim. Biophys. Acta*, 168, 243 (1968).
510. Kohn, Packman, Allen, and Jakoby, *J. Biol. Chem.*, 243, 2479 (1968).
511. Kohn, *J. Biol. Chem.*, 243, 4426 (1968).
512. Murphy, Plummer, and Miller, *Fed. Proc.*, 27, 268 Abstract No. 298 (1968).
513. Holmgren and Reichard, *Eur. J. Biochem.*, 2, 187 (1967).
514. Thelander, *J. Biol. Chem.*, 242, 852 (1967).
515. Thelander and Baldesten, *Eur. J. Biochem.*, 4, 420 (1968).
516. Burns and Zarlengo, *J. Biol. Chem.*, 243, 178 (1968).
517. Shizuta, Nakazawa, Tokushige, and Hayaishi, *J. Biol. Chem.*, 244, 1883 (1969).
518. Kezdy, Lorand, and Miller, *Biochemistry*, 2302 (1965).
519. Winzor and Scheraga, *Arch. Biochem. Biophys.*, 104, 202 (1964).
520. Brewer, Keutmann, Potts, Reisfeld, Schlueter, and Munson, *J. Biol. Chem.*, 243, 5739 (1968).
521. Shome, Brown, Howard, and Pierce, *Arch. Biochem. Biophys.*, 126, 456 (1968).
522. Lai, Chen, and Tsolas, *Arch. Biochem. Biophys.*, 121, 790 (1967).
523. Seal and Doe, *J. Biol. Chem.*, 237, 3136 (1962).
524. Aisen, Aasa, Malstrom, and Vanngard, *J. Biol. Chem.*, 242, 2484 (1967).
525. Koechlin, *J. Am. Chem. Soc.*, 74, 2649 (1952).
526. Leibman and Aisen, *Arch. Biochem. Biophys.*, 121, 717 (1967).
527. Folk, Mullooly, and Cole, *J. Biol. Chem.*, 242, 1838 (1967).
528. Folk and Cole, *J. Biol. Chem.*, 241, 5518 (1966).
529. Mooz and Meister, *Biochemistry*, 6, 1722 (1967).
530. Woods, *J. Biol. Chem.*, 242, 2859 (1967).
531. Mee, Navon, and Stein, *Biochim. Biophys. Acta*, 104, 151 (1965).

532. Mihalyi and Harrington, *Biochim. Biophys. Acta,* 36, 447 (1959).
533. Green, *Biochem. J.,* 66, 407 (1957).
534. Kassell, Radicevic, Berlow, Peanasky, and Laskowski, *J. Biol. Chem.,* 238, 3274 (1963).
535. Laskowski and Laskowski, *Adv. Protein Chem.,* 9, 203 (1954).
536. Davie and Neurath, *J. Biol. Chem.,* 212, 515 (1955).
537. Labeyrie, Groudinsky, Jacquot-Armand, and Naslin, *Biochim. Biophys. Acta,* 128, 492 (1966).
538. Shaw, Mares-Guia, and Cohen, *Biochemistry,* 4, 2219 (1965).
539. Meloun, Fric, and Sorm, *Eur. J. Biochem.,* 4, 112 (1968).
540. Buck, Vithayathil, Bier, and Nord, *Arch. Biochem. Biophys.,* 97, 417 (1962).
541. Labouesse and Gervais, *Eur. J. Biochem.,* 2, 215 (1967).
542. Heide, Heilburger, and Haupt, *Clin. Chim. Acta,* 11, 82 (1956).
543. Pharo, Sordahl, Edelhoch, and Sanadi, *Arch. Biochem. Biophys.,* 125, 416 (1968).
544. Greene, Rigbi, and Fackre, *J. Biol. Chem.,* 241, 5610 (1966).
545. Greene, DiCarlo, Sussman, Bartelt, and Roark, *J. Biol. Chem.,* 243, 1804 (1968).
546. Kunitz, *J. Gen. Physiol.,* 30, 291 (1947).
547. Birk, Gertler, and Khalef, *Biochem. J.,* 87, 281 (1963).
548. Rackis, Sasame, Mann, Anderson, and Smith, *Arch. Biochem. Biophys.,* 98, 471 (1962).
549. Wu and Scheraga, *Biochemistry,* 1, 698 (1962).
550. Frattali and Steiner, *Biochemistry,* 7, 521 (1968).
551. Schyns, Bricteux-Gregoire, and Florkin, *Biochim. Biophys. Acta,* 175, 97 (1969).
552. Pechere, Dixon, Maybury, and Neurath, *J. Biol. Chem.,* 233, 1364 (1958).
553. Morino and Snell, *J. Biol. Chem.,* 242, 2800 (1967).
554. Hathaway, Kida, and Crawford, *Biochemistry,* 8, 989 (1969).
555. Kumagai, Matsui, Ogata, and Yamada, *Biochim. Biophys. Acta,* 171, 1 (1968).
556. Yamada, Kumagi, Matsui, Ohgishi, and Ogata, *Biochem. Biophys. Res. Commun.,* 33, 10 (1968).
557. Hayashi, Granner, and Tomkins, *J. Biol. Chem.,* 242, 3998 (1967).
558. Gorin and Chin, *Biochim. Biophys. Acta,* 99, 418 (1965).
559. Gorin, Fuchs, Butler, Chopra, and Hersh, *Biochemistry,* 1, 911 (1962).
560. Gorin and Chin, *Anal. Biochem.,* 17, 49 (1966).
561. Mahler, Hubscher, and Baum, *J. Biol. Chem.,* 216, 625 (1955).
562. *Iscotables,* Instrumentation Specialities Co., Inc., Lincoln, Nebraska, 1967, p. 9.
563. Shalaby, Banerjee, and Lauffer, *Biochemistry,* 7, 955 (1968).
564. Heller, *Biochemistry,* 7, 2906 (1968).
565. Avis, Bergel, and Bray, *J. Chem. Soc. (Lond.),* 1219 (1956).
566. Massey, Brumby, Komai, and Palmer, *J. Biol. Chem.,* 224, 1682 (1969).
567. O'Leary and Westheimer, *Biochemistry,* 7, 913 (1968).
568. Stormer, *J. Biol. Chem.,* 243, 3740 (1968).
569. Gregolin, Ryder, and Lane, *J. Biol. Chem.,* 243, 4227 (1968).
570. Hauge, *Arch. Biochem. Biophys.,* 94, 308 (1961).
571. Pajot and Groudinsky, *Eur. J. Biochem.,* 12, 158 (1970).
572. Labeyrie, Groudinsky, Jacquot-Armand, and Naslin, *Biochim. Biophys. Acta,* 128, 492 (1966).
573. Kodama and Shidara, *J. Biochem. (Tokyo),* 65, 356 (1969).
574. Horio, Higashi, Yamanaka, Matabara, and Okunuki, *J. Biol. Chem.,* 23, 944 (1961).
575. Kredich, Becker, and Tomkin, *J. Biol. Chem.,* 244, 2428 (1969).
576. Carrico and Deutsch, *J. Biol. Chem.,* 245, 723 (1970).
577. Price, Liu, Stein, and Moore, *J. Biol. Chem.,* 244, 917 (1969).
578. Lindberg, *Biochemistry,* 6, 335 (1967).
579. Lindberg, *Biochemistry,* 6, 323 (1967).
580. Jovin, Englund, and Bertsch, *J. Biol. Chem.,* 244, 2996 (1969).
581. Roychoudhury and Bloch, *J. Biol. Chem.,* 244, 3359 (1969).
582. Roncari, Kurylo-Borowska, and Craig, *Biochemistry,* 5, 2153 (1966).
583. Bender, Begue-Canton, Blakeley, et al., *J. Am. Chem. Soc.,* 88, 5890 (1966).
584. Warburg and Christian, *Biochem. Z.,* 310, 384 (1941).
585. Barker and Jencks, *Biochemistry,* 8, 3879 (1969).
586. Malhotra and Philip, *Indian J. Biochem.,* 3, 7 (1966).
587. Lanchantin, Friedman, and Hart, *J. Biol. Chem.,* 244, 865 (1969).
588. Hsu and Yun, *Biochemistry,* 9, 239 (1970).
589. Hsu, Wasson, and Porter, *J. Biol. Chem.,* 240, 3736 (1965).
590. Dey and Pridham, *Biochem. J.,* 113, 49 (1969).
591. Petek, Villarroya, and Courtois, *Eur. J. Biochem.,* 8, 395 (1969).
592. Carrico and Deutsch, *J. Biol. Chem.,* 244, 6087 (1969).
593. Porter, Sweeney, and Porter, *Arch. Biochem. Biophys.,* 105, 319 (1964).
594. Deutsch, *Immunochemistry,* 2, 207 (1965).
595. Newcomb, Normansell, and Stanworth, *J. Immunol.,* 101, 905 (1968).
596. Heimer, Jones, and Maurer, *Biochemistry,* 8, 3937 (1969).
597. Doi and Jirgensons, *Biochemistry,* 9, 1066 (1970).
598. Kickhofen, Hammer, and Scheel, *Hoppe-Seylers Z. Physiol. Chem.,* 349, 1755 (1968).
599. Binaghi and Oriol, *Bull. Soc. Chim. Biol.,* 50, 1035 (1968).
600. Mihaesco and Mihaesco, *Biochem. Biophys. Res. Commun.,* 33, 869 (1968).
601. Krigbaum and Kugler, *Biochemistry,* 9, 1216 (1970).
602. Johansson, *Acta Chem. Scand.,* 23, 683 (1969).
603. Kessler and Brew, *Biochim. Biophys. Acta,* 200, 449 (1970).
604. Morrison, Hamilton, and Stotz, *J. Biol. Chem.,* 228, 767 (1957).
605. Frohne and Hanson, *Hoppe-Seylers Z. Physiol. Chem.,* 350, 207 (1969).
606. Kretschmer, *Hoppe-Seylers Z. Physiol. Chem.,* 349, 846 (1968).
607. Oriol-Audit, Landon, Robin, and van Thoai, *Biochim. Biophys. Acta,* 188 132 (1969).
608. Lee and McElroy, *Biochemistry,* 8, 130 (1969).
609. Antonini, *Physiol. Rev.,* 45, 123 (1965).
610. Harris and Hill, *J. Biol. Chem.,* 244, 2195 (1969).
611. Straus, Gordon, and Wallach, *Eur. J. Biochem.,* 11, 201 (1969).
612. Willick, Schonbaum, and Kay, *Biochemistry,* 8, 3729 (1969).
613. Stryer, *J. Mol. Biol.,* 13, 482 (1965).
614. Hapner, Bradshaw, Hartzell, and Gurd, *J. Biol. Chem.,* 243, 683 (1968).
615. Awad and Kotite, *Biochem. J.,* 98, 909 (1966).
616. Godfrey and Harrington, *Biochemistry,* 9, 886 (1970).
617. Adelman and Taylor, *Biochemistry,* 8, 4976 (1969).
618. Tada, Bailin, Barany, and Barany, *Biochemistry,* 8, 4842 (1969).
619. Woods, *Int. J. Protein Res.,* 1, 29 (1969).
620. Angeletti, *Proc. Natl. Acad. Sci., U.S.A.,* 65, 668 (1970).
621. Furth and Hope, *Biochem. J.,* 116, 545 (1970).
622. Villet and Dalziel, *Biochem. J.,* 115, 639 (1969).
623. Pon, Schnackerz, Blackburn, Chatterjee, and Noltmann, *Biochemistry,* 9, 1506 (1970).
624. Carter and Yoshida, *Biochim. Biophys. Acta,* 181, 12 (1969).
625. Wald and Brown, *J. Gen. Physiol.,* 37, 189 (1953–1954).
626. Hubbard, *J. Gen. Physiol.,* 37, 381 (1953–1954).
627. Schichi, *Biochemistry,* 9, 1973 (1970).
628. Nordlie and Fromm, *J. Biol. Chem.,* 234, 2522 (1959).
629. Nakagawa and Kinnura, *J. Biochem. (Tokyo),* 66, 669 (1969).
630. Fojioka, *Biochim. Biophys. Acta,* 185, 338 (1969).
631. Marchesi, Steers, Marchesi, and Tillack, *Biochemistry,* 9, 50 (1970).
632. Allen and Jakoby, *J. Biol. Chem.,* 244, 2078 (1968).
633. Zalitis and Feingold, *Arch. Biochem. Biophys.,* 132, 457 (1969).
634. Becker, Kredich, and Tomkins, *J. Biol. Chem.,* 244, 2418 (1969).
635. Bernardi, *Adv. Enzymol.,* 31, 1 (1968).
636. Eisenberg, Zobel, and Moos, *Biochemistry,* 7, 3186 (1968).
637. Pugh and Wakil, *J. Biol. Chem.,* 240, 4727 (1965).
638. Sauer, Pugh, Wakil, Delany, and Hill, *Proc. Natl. Acad. Sci., U.S.A.,* 52, 1360 (1964).
639. Ramponi, Guerritore, Treves, Nassi, and Baccari, *Arch. Biochem. Biophys.,* 130, 362 (1969).
640. Webster, *Biochim. Biophys. Acta,* 207, 371 (1970).
641. Koberstein, Weber, and Jaenicke, *Z. Naturforsch. B,* 23, 474 (1968).
642. Andersson, *Int. J. Protein Res.,* 1, 151 (1969).
643. Glazer and Smith, *J. Biol. Chem.,* 235, PC43 (1960).
644. Bonewell and Rossini, *Italian J. Biochem.,* 18, 457 (1969).
645. Kaldor, Saifer, and Westley, *Arch. Biochem. Biophys.,* 99, 275 (1962).

646. Habeeb and Hiramoto, *Arch. Biochem. Biophys.*, 126, 16 (1968).
647. Pederson and Foster, *Biochemistry*, 8, 2357 (1969).
648. Groulade, Chicault, and Waltzinger, *Bull. Soc. Chim. Biol.*, 48, 1609 (1967).
649. Frank and Veros, *Fed. Proc.*, 28, 728 (1969).
650. Frank, Peker, Veros, and Ho, *J. Biol. Chem.*, 245, 3716 (1970).
651. Wagner, Irion, Arens, and Bauer, *Biochem. Biophys. Res. Commun.*, 37, 383 (1969).
652. Arens, Rauenbusch, Irion, Wagner, Bauer, and Kaufmann, *Hoppe-Seylers Z. Physiol Chem.*, 351, 199 (1970).
653. Funakoshi and Deutsch, *J. Biol. Chem.*, 244, 3438 (1969).
654. Verpoorte and Linnblow, *J. Biol. Chem.*, 243, 5993 (1968).
655. Armstrong, Myers, Verpoorte, and Edsall, *J. Biol. Chem.*, 241, 5137 (1966).
656. Carpy, *Biochem. Biophys. Acta*, 151, 245 (1968).
657. Furth, *J. Biol. Chem.*, 243, 4832 (1968).
658. McIntosh, *Biochem. J.*, 114, 463 (1969).
659. Tobin, *J. Biol. Chem.*, 245, 2656 (1970).
660. Emery, *Biochemistry*, 8, 877 (1969).
661. Deisseroth and Dounce, *Arch. Biochem. Biophys.*, 131, 18 (1969).
662. Petit and Tauber, *J. Biol. Chem.*, 195, 703 (1952).
663. Stern and Lavin, *Science*, 88, 263 (1938).
664. Agner, *Biochem. J.*, 32, 1702 (1938).
665. Bonnichsen, *Arch. Biochem.*, 12, 83 (1947).
666. Ushijima and Nakano, *Biochim. Biophys. Acta*, 178, 429 (1969).
667. Greenfield and Price, *J. Biol. Chem.*, 220, 607 (1956).
668. Gregory, *Biochim. Biophys. Acta*, 159, 429 (1968).
669. Tanford and Lovrien, *J. Am. Chem. Soc.*, 84, 1892 (1962).
670. Bjorndal and Eriksson, *Arch. Biochem. Biophys.*, 124, 149 (1968).
671. Eriksson and Pettersson, *Arch. Biochem. Biophys.*, 124, 160 (1968).
672. Pettersson and Eaker, *Arch. Biochem. Biophys.*, 124, 154 (1968).
673. Wang and Barker, *Methods Enzymol.*, 13, 331 (1969).
674. Wu and Yang, *J. Biol. Chem.*, 245, 212 (1970).
675. Yang, *J. Biol. Chem.*, 240, 1616 (1965).
676. Chang and Hayashi, *Biochem. Biophys. Res. Commun.*, 37, 841 (1969).
677. Sjogren and Spychalski, *J. Am. Chem. Soc.*, 52, 4400 (1930).
678. Konisky and Richards, *J. Biol. Chem.*, 245, 2973 (1970).
679. Schito, *G. Microbiol.*, 14, 77 (1966).
680. Schito, Molina, and Pesce, *Biochem. Biophys. Res. Commun.*, 28, 611 (1967).
681. Tan and Woodworth, *Biochemistry*, 8, 3711 (1969).
682. Freisheim and Huennekens, *Biochemistry*, 8, 2271 (1969).
683. Nixon and Blakley, *J. Biol. Chem.*, 243, 4722 (1968).
684. Schwartz and Reed, *J. Biol. Chem.*, 243, 639 (1968).
685. Frisell and Mackenzie, *J. Biol. Chem.*, 237, 94 (1962).
686. Rene and Campbell, *J. Biol. Chem.*, 244, 1445 (1969).
687. Chu, *J. Biol. Chem.*, 243, 4342 (1968).
688. Borja, *Biochemistry*, 8, 71 (1969).
689. Huseby and Murray, *Biochem. Biophys. Res. Commun.*, 35, 169 (1969).
690. Marder, Shulman, and Carroll, *J. Biol. Chem.*, 244, 2111 (1969).
691. Iizuka and Yang, *Biochemistry*, 7, 2218 (1968).
692. Takasaki, Kosugi, and Kambayashi, *Agr. Biol. Chem.*, 33, 1527 (1969).
693. Rattazzi, *Biochim. Biophys. Acta*, 181, 1 (1969).
694. Bruni, Auricchio, and Covelli, *J. Biol. Chem.*, 244, 4735 (1969).
695. Legler, *Hoppe-Seylers Z. Physiol. Chem.*, 349, 1755 (1970).
696. Legler, *Hoppe-Seylers Z. Physiol. Chem.*, 348, 1359 (1967).
697. Herman-Boussier, Moretti, and Jayle, *Bull. Soc. Chim. Biol.*, 42, 837 (1960).
698. Guinand, Tonnelat, Boussier, and Jayle, *Bull. Soc. Chim. Biol.*, 38, 329 (1956).
699. Dobryszycka, Elwyn, and Kukral, *Biochim. Biophys. Acta*, 175, 220 (1969).
700. Okazaki, Wittenberg, Briehl, and Wittenberg, *Biochim. Biophys. Acta*, 140, 258 (1967).
701. Webster, *Biochim. Biophys. Acta*, 207, 371 (1970).
702. Bucci, Fronticelli, and Ragatz, *J. Biol. Chem.*, 243, 241 (1968).
703. Chiancone, Curell, Vecchini, Antonini, and Wyman, *J. Biol. Chem.*, 245, 4105 (1970).
704. Peacock, Pastewka, Reed, and Ness, *Biochemistry*, 9, 2275 (1970).
705. Atassi, Brown, and McEwan, *Immunochemistry*, 2, 379 (1965).
706. Benesch and Benesch, *J. Biol. Chem.*, 236, 405 (1961).
707. Bucci, Fronticelli, Bellelli, Antonini, Wyman, and Rossi-Fanelli, *Arch. Biochem. Biophys.*, 100, 364 (1963).
708. Li and Johnson, *Biochemistry*, 3, 2083 (1969).
709. Antonini, Bucci, Fronticelli, Chiancone, Wyman, and Rossi-Fanelli, *J. Mol. Biol.*, 17, 29 (1966).
710. Ueda, Shiga, and Tyuma, *Biochem. Biophys. Acta*, 207, 18 (1970).
711. Ozawa, *Biochemistry*, 9, 2158 (1970).
712. Harrison and Garratt, *Biochem. J.*, 113, 733 (1969).
713. Moller, Castleman, and Terhorst, *FEBS Lett.*, 8, 192 (1970).
714. Frank and Veros, *Biochem. Biophys. Res. Commun.*, 32, 155 (1968).
715. Chung and Franzen, *Biochemistry*, 8, 3175 (1969).
716. Illingworth and Tipton, *Biochem. J.*, 118, 253 (1970).
717. Malmstrom, Reinhammar, and Vanngard, *Biochim. Biophys. Acta*, 205, 48 (1970).
718. Tang, Coleman, and Myer, *J. Biol. Chem.*, 243, 4286 (1968).
719. Lin, *Biochemistry*, 9, 984 (1970).
720. Ebner, Denton, and Brodbeck, *Biochem. Biophys. Res. Commun.*, 22, 232 (1966).
721. Stevens, Brown, and Smith, *Arch. Biochem. Biophys.*, 136, 413 (1970).
722. Eriksson and Svensson, *Biochim. Biophys. Acta*, 198, 449 (1970).
723. Soda and Misone, *Biochemistry*, 7, 4110 (1968).
724. Sher and Mallette, *Arch. Biochem. Biophys.*, 53, 354 (1954).
725. Soda and Moriguchi, *Biochem. Biophys. Res. Comm.*, 34, 34 (1969).
726. Takeda, Yamamoto, Kojima, and Hayaishi, *J. Biol. Chem.*, 244, 2935 (1969).
727. Petek and Villarroya, *Bull. Soc. Chim. Biol.*, 50, 725 (1968).
728. Kajita, Kerwar, and Huennekens, *Arch. Biochem. Biophys.*, 130, 662 (1969).
729. Takesue and Omura, *J. Biochem. (Tokyo)*, 67, 267 (1970).
730. Nishibayashi-Yamashita and Sato, *J. Biochem. (Tokyo)*, 67, 199 (1970).
731. Karlsson, Eaker, and Porath, *Biochim. Biophys. Acta*, 127, 505 (1966).
732. Pho, Olomucki, Hue, and Thoai, *Biochim. Biophys. Acta*, 206, 46 (1970).
733. Webster, *Biochim. Biophys. Acta*, 207, 371 (1970).
734. Willumsen, *C. R. Trav. Lab. Carlsberg*, 37, 21 (1969).
735. Cheesman, *Proc. R. Soc. Lond. (Biol.)*, 149, 571 (1958).
736. Peraino, Bunville, and Tahmisian, *J. Biol. Chem.*, 244, 2241 (1969).
737. Willick, Schonbaum, and Kay, *Biochemistry*, 8, 3729 (1969).
738. Hardin Strickland, Kay, and Shannon, *J. Biol. Chem.*, 243, 3560 (1968).
739. Hamaguchi, Ikeda, Yoshida, and Morita, *J. Biochem. (Tokyo)*, 66, 191 (1969).
740. Mazza, Charles, Bouchet, Ricard, and Raynaud, *Biochim. Biophys. Acta*, 167, 89 (1968).
741. Blasi, Fragomele, and Corelli, *J. Biol. Chem.*, 244, 4866 (1969).
742. Simpson, Vallee, and Taft, *Biochemistry*, 7, 4336 (1968).
743. Schlesinger, *J. Biol. Chem.*, 243, 3877 (1968).
744. Rothman and Byrne, *J. Mol. Biol.*, 6, 330 (1963).
745. Morton, *Biochem. J.*, 60, 573 (1955).
746. Alvarez and Lora-Tamayo, *Biochem. J.*, 69, 312 (1958).
747. Dennert and Hoglund, *Eur. J. Biochem.*, 12, 502 (1970).
748. Hunsley and Suelter, *J. Biol. Chem.*, 244, 4185 (1969).
749. Richardson, *Proc. Natl. Acad. Sci., U.S.A.*, 55, 1616 (1966).
750. Neuhoff, Schill, and Sternbach, *Hoppe-Seylers Z. Physiol. Chem.*, 350, 767 (1969).
751. Brown, Canellakis, Lundin, Reichard, and Thelander, *Eur. J. Biochem.*, 9, 561 (1969).
752. Brown, Eliasson, Reichard, and Thelander, *Eur. J. Biochem.*, 9, 512 (1969).
753. Lee, Patrick, and Barnes, *J. Biol. Chem.*, 245, 1357 (1970).
754. Matsubara and Nishimura, *J. Biochem. (Tokyo)*, 45, 503 (1958).
755. Yamada, Kumagi, Nagate, and Yoshida, *Biochem. Biophys. Res. Commun.*, 39, 53 (1970).
756. Brewer and Edelhoch, *J. Biol. Chem.*, 245, 2402 (1970).
757. Salvatore, Vecchio, Salvatore, Cahnmann, and Robbins, *J. Biol. Chem.*, 240, 2935 (1965).

758. Han and Benson, *Biochem. Biophys. Res. Commun.*, 38, 378 (1970).
759. Mikola and Suolinna, *Eur. J. Biochem.*, 9, 555 (1969).
760. Poillon, Maeno, Koike, and Feigelson, *J. Biol. Chem.*, 244, 3447 (1968).
761. Henning, Helinski, Chao, and Yanofsky, *J. Biol. Chem.*, 237, 1523 (1962).
762. Hathaway and Crawford, *Biochemistry*, 9, 1801 (1970).
763. Wilson and Crawford, *J. Biol. Chem.*, 240, 4801 (1965).
764. Lemaire, van Rapenbusch, Gros, and Labouesse, *Eur. J. Biochem.*, 10, 334 (1969).
765. Paul and Stigbrand, *Biochim. Biophys. Acta*, 221, 255 (1970).
766. Haas, Lumfrom, and Goldblatt, *Arch. Biochem. Biophys.*, 44, 79 (1953).
767. Malhorta and Roni, *Indian J. Biochem.*, 6, 15 (1969).
768. Blakeley, Webb, and Zerner, *Biochemistry*, 8, 1984 (1969).
769. Bailey and Boulter, *Biochem. J.*, 112, 669 (1969).
770. George and Phillip, *J. Biol. Chem.*, 245, 529 (1970).
771. Kawano, Morimoto, and Uemura, *J. Biochem. (Tokyo)*, 67, 333 (1970).
772. Scraba, Hostvedt, and Colter, *Can. J. Biochem.*, 47, 165 (1969).
773. Hull, Hills, and Markham, *Virology*, 37, 416 (1969).
774. Stevens and Lauffer, *Biochemistry*, 4, 31 (1965).
775. Reichman, *J. Biol. Chem.*, 235, 2959 (1966).
776. Crewther and Harrap, *J. Biol. Chem.*, 242, 4310 (1967).
777. Mega, Ikenaka, and Matsushima, *J. Biochem. (Tokyo)*, 68, 109 (1970).
778. Villafranca and Mildvan, *J. Biol. Chem.*, 246, 772 (1971).
779. Kimura and Huang, *Arch. Biochem. Biophys.*, 137, 357 (1963).
780. Shimomura and Johnson, *Biochemistry*, 8, 3991 (1969).
781. Rosso, Takashima, and Adams, *Biochem. Biophys. Res. Commun.*, 34, 134 (1969).
782. Hamlin, *Exp. Gerontol.*, 4, 189 (1969).
783. Von Tigerstron and Razzell, *J. Biol. Chem.*, 243, 2691 (1968).
784. Von Tigerstron and Razzell, *J. Biol. Chem.*, 243, 6495 (1968).
785. Dimroth, Guchhait, Stoll, and Lane, *Proc. Natl. Acad. Sci., U.S.A.*, 67, 1353 (1970).
786. Mayer and Miller, *Anal. Biochem.*, 36, 91 (1970).
787. Anastasi, Erspamer, and Endean, *Arch. Biochem. Biophys.*, 125, 57 (1968).
788. Keutmann, Parsons, Potts, Jr., and Schlueter, *J. Biol. Chem.*, 245, 1491 (1970).
789. Marshall and Cohen, *J. Biol. Chem.*, 241, 4197 (1970).
790. Lacko and Neurath, *Biochemistry*, 9, 4680 (1970).
791. Visuri, Mikola, and Enari, *Eur. J. Biochem.*, 7, 193 (1969).
792. Boston and Prescott, *Arch. Biochem. Biophys.*, 128, 88 (1968).
793. Yue, Palmieri, Olson, and Kuby, *Biochemistry*, 6, 3204 (1967).
794. Gosselin-Rey and Gerday, *Biochim. Biophys. Acta*, 221, 241 (1970).
795. Yue, Jacobs, Okabe, Keutel, and Kuby, *Biochemistry*, 7, 4291 (1968).
796. Kumudavalli, Moreland, and Watts, *Biochem. J.*, 117, 513 (1970).
797. Hass and Hill, *J. Biol. Chem.*, 244, 6080 (1969).
798. Fraenkel-Conrat and Singer, *Arch. Biochem. Biophys.*, 60, 64 (1956).
799. Zimmerman and Coleman, *J. Biol. Chem.*, 246, 309 (1971).
800. Tai and Sih, *J. Biol. Chem.*, 245, 5062 (1970).
801. Shotton, *Methods Enzymol.*, 19, 113 (1970).
802. Wang and Keen, *Arch. Biochem. Biophys.*, 141, 749 (1970).
803. Seto, Sato, and Tamiya, *Biochim. Biophys. Acta*, 214, 483 (1970).
804. Fanelli, Chiancone, Vecchini, and Antonini, *Arch. Biochem. Biophys.*, 141, 278, (1970).
805. Hartz and Deutsch, *J. Biol. Chem.*, 244 4565 (1969).
806. Svedberg and Sjogren, *J. Am. Chem. Soc.*, 52, 279 (1930).
807. Lee, Travis, and Black, Jr., *Arch. Biochem. Biophys.*, 141, 676 (1970).
808. Newman, Ihle, and Dure, III, *Biochem. Biophys. Res. Commun.*, 36, 947 (1969).
809. Mayhew, Petering, Palmer, and Foust, *J. Biol. Chem.*, 244, 2830 (1969).
810. Devanathan, Akagi, Hersh, and Himes, *J. Biol. Chem.*, 244, 2846 (1969).
811. Lovenberg, Buchanan, and Rabinowitz, *J. Biol. Chem.*, 238, 3899 (1963).
812. Bayer, Eckstein, Hagenmaier, et al., *Eur. J. Biochem.*, 8, 33 (1969).
813. Hong and Rabinowitz, *J. Biol. Chem.*, 245, 4982 (1970).
814. Moss, Petering, and Palmer, *J. Biol. Chem.*, 244, 2275 (1969).
815. Petering, Fee, and Palmer, *J. Biol. Chem.*, 246, 643 (1971).
816. Hormann and Gollwitzer, *Z. Physiol. Chem.*, 346, 21 (1966).
817. Mihalyi, *Biochemistry*, 7, 208 (1968).
818. Budzynski, *Biochim. Biophys. Acta*, 229, 663 (1971).
819. Huseby, Mosesson, and Murray, *Physiol. Chem. Phys.*, 2, 374 (1970).
820. Fuller and Doolittle, *Biochemistry*, 10, 1305 (1971).
821. Holloway, Antonini, and Brunori, *FEBS Lett.*, 4, 299 (1969).
822. Kramer and Whitaker, *J. Biol. Chem.*, 239, 2178 (1964).
823. Brewer, Ljungdahl, Spencer, and Neece, *J. Biol. Chem.*, 245, 4798 (1970).
824. Pontremoli, *Methods Enzymol.*, 9, 625 (1966).
825. Mosesson and Umfleet, *J. Biol. Chem.*, 245, 5728 (1970).
826. Danno, *Agr. Biol. Chem.*, 34, 1795 (1970).
827. Strausbauch and Fischer, *Biochemistry*, 9, 226 (1970).
828. Fahien and Cohen, *Methods Enzymol.*, 17A, 839 (1970).
829. Dessen and Pantaloni, *Eur. J. Biochem.*, 8, 292 (1969).
830. Winnacker and Barker, *Biochim. Biophys. Acta*, 212, 225 (1970).
831. Barker, *Methods Enzymol.*, 13, 319 (1969).
832. Rowe, Ronzio, Wellner, and Meister, *Methods Enzymol.*, 17A, 900 (1970).
833. Woodin and Segel, *Biochim. Biophys. Acta*, 167, 64 (1968).
834. Kohn, Warner, and Carroll, *J. Biol. Chem.*, 245, 3820 (1970).
835. Edelhoch and Lippoldt, *J. Biol. Chem.*, 245, 4199 (1970).
836. Gould and Scheinberg, *Arch. Biochem. Biophys.*, 137, 1 (1970).
837. Sage and Connett, *J. Biol. Chem.*, 244, 4713 (1969).
838. Ferrell and Kitto, *Biochemistry*, 9, 3053 (1970).
839. Keresztes-Nagy, PhD thesis, Northwestern University, 1962: cited in Subramanian, Holleman, and Klotz, *Biochemistry*, 7, 2859 (1968).
840. Morimoto and Kegeles, *Arch. Biochem. Biophys.*, 142, 247 (1971).
841. Gruber, in *Physiology and Biochemistry of Hemocyanins*, Ghiretti, ed., Academic Press, New York, 1968, p. 49.
842. Konings, Dijk, Wichertjes, Beuvery, and Gruber, *Biochim. Biophys. Acta*, 188, 43 (1969).
843. Ellerton, Carpenter, and Van Holde, *Biochemistry*, 9, 2225 (1970).
844. Joniau, Grossberg, and Pressman, *Immunochemistry*, 7, 755 (1970).
845. Amkraut, personal communication.
846. Shaklai and Daniel, *Biochemistry*, 9, 564 (1970).
847. Maki, Yamamoto, Nozaki, and Hayaishi, *J. Biol. Chem.*, 244, 2942 (1969).
848. Leslie and Cohen, *Biochem. J.*, 120, 787 (1970).
849. Herskovits, *Arch. Biochem. Biophys.*, 130, 19 (1969).
850. Meachum, Jr., Colvin, Jr., and Braymer, *Biochemistry*, 10, 326 (1971).
851. Yokobayashi, Misaki, and Harada, *Biochim. Biophys. Acta*, 212, 458 (1970).
852. McFadden, *Methods Enzymol.*, 13, 163 (1969).
853. Parsons and Burns, *J. Biol. Chem.*, 244, 996 (1969).
854. Yu, Harmon, Wachter, and Blank, *Arch. Biochem. Biophys.*, 135, 363 (1969).
855. Alfsen, Baulieu, Claquin, and Falcoz-Kelly, *Proc. 2nd Int. Congr. Hormonal Steroids*, 1967, 508.
856. Malkin and Malmstrom, *Adv. Enzymol.*, 33, 178 (1970).
857. Nakamura and Ogura, *J. Biochem. (Tokyo)*, 59, 449 (1966).
858. Malkin, Malmstrom, and Vanngard, *Eur. J. Biochem.*, 10, 324 (1969).
859. Malkin, Malmstrom, and Vanngard, *Eur. J. Biochem.*, 7, 253 (1969).
860. Karkhanis and Cormier, *Biochemistry*, 10, 317 (1971).
861. Haino, *Biochim. Biophys. Acta*, 229, 459 (1971).
862. Chibata, Ishikawa, and Tosa, *Methods Enzymol.*, 19, 675 (1970).
863. Nagasawa, Sugihara, Han, and Suzuki, *J. Biochem. (Tokyo)*, 67, 809 (1970).
864. Schonenberger, Schmidtberger, and Schultze, *Z. Naturforsch.*, 136, 761 (1958).
865. Jacquot-Armand and Guinand, *Biochim. Biophys. Acta*, 133, 289 (1967).
866. Berggard and Bearn, *J. Biol. Chem.*, 243, 4095 (1968).
867. Gregory and Harrison, *Biochem. Biophys. Res. Commun.*, 40, 995 (1970).

868. Covelli, Consiglio, and Varrone, *Biochim. Biophys. Acta,* 184, 678 (1969).
869. Gerding and Wolfe, *J. Biol. Chem.,* 244, 1164 (1969).
870. Kitto, *Methods Enzymol.,* 13, 106 (1969).
871. Mann and Vestling, *Biochemistry,* 8, 1105 (1969).
872. Spina, Jr., Bright, and Rosenbloom, *Biochemistry,* 9, 3794 (1970).
873. Ramachandran, *Biochem. Biophys. Res. Commun.,* 41, 353 (1970).
874. Lawrence, *Eur. J. Biochem.,* 15, 436 (1970).
875. Agner, *Acta Chem. Scand.,* 12, 89 (1958).
876. Schirmer, Schirmer, Schulz, and Thuma, *FEBS Lett.,* 10, 333 (1970).
877. Leuzinger, *Biochem. J.,* 123, 139 (1971).
878. Muruyama, *J. Biochem. (Tokyo),* 69, 369 (1971).
879. Minato, *J. Biochem. (Tokyo),* 64, 813 (1969).
880. Zielke and Suelter, *J. Biol. Chem.,* 246, 2179 (1971).
881. Zielke and Suelter, *Fed. Proc.,* 28, 2624 (1969).
882. Tweedie and Segel, *J. Biol. Chem.,* 246, 2438 (1971).
883. Lebeault, Zevaco, and Hermier, *Bull. Soc. Chim. Biol.,* 52, 1073 (1970).
884. Sterman and Foster, *J. Am. Chem. Soc.,* 78, 3656 (1956).
885. Frigerio and Hettinger, *Biochim. Biophys. Acta,* 59, 228 (1962).
886. Emery, *Biochemistry,* 8, 877 (1969).
887. Mayer and Miller, *Anal. Biochem.,* 36, 91 (1970).
888. King and Spencer, *J. Biol. Chem.,* 245, 6134 (1970).
889. Webster, *Biochim. Biophys. Acta,* 207, 371 (1970).
890. Pederson and Foster, *Biochemistry,* 8, 2357 (1969).
891. Noelken, *Biochemistry,* 9, 4117 (1970).
892. Noelken, *Biochemistry,* 9, 4122 (1970).
893. Van Kley and Stahmann, *J. Am. Chem. Soc.,* 81, 4374 (1959).
894. Janatova, Fuller, and Hunter, *J. Biol. Chem.,* 243, 3612 (1968).
895. Lerner and Bamum, *Arch. Biochem. Biophys.,* 10, 417 (1946).
896. Groulade, Chicault, and Waltzinger, *Bull. Soc. Chim. Biol.,* 49, 1609 (1967).
897. Warner and Schumaker, *Biochemistry,* 9, 451 (1970).
898. Petersen and Foster, *J. Biol. Chem.,* 240, 3861 (1965).
899. Laggner, Kratky, Palm, and Holasek, *FEBS Lett.,* 15, 220 (1971).
900. Joniau, Grossberg, and Pressman, *Immunochemistry,* 7, 755 (1970).
901. Polis, Shmukler, and Custer, *J. Biol. Chem.,* 187, 349 (1950).
902. Zigman and Lerman, *Biochim. Biophys. Acta,* 154, 423 (1968).
903. Lerman, *Can. J. Biochem.,* 47, 1115 (1969).
904. Bonnichsen, *Acta Chem. Scand.,* 4, 715 (1950).
905. Ehrenberg and Dalziel, *Acta Chem. Scand.,* 12, 465 (1958).
906. Green and McKay, *J. Biol. Chem.,* 244, 5034 (1969).
907. Cannon and McKay, *Biochim. Biophys. Res. Commun.,* 35, 403 (1969).
908. Drum, Li, and Vallee, *Biochemistry,* 8, 3783 (1969).
909. Drum, Harrison, Li, Bethune, and Vallee, *Proc. Natl. Acad. Sci., U.S.A.,* 57, 1434 (1967).
910. Drum and Vallee, *Biochem. Biophys. Res. Commun.,* 41, 33 (1970).
911. Von Wartburg, Bethune, and Vallee, *Biochemistry,* 3, 1775 (1964).
912. Negelein and Wulff, *Biochem. Z.,* 293, 351 (1937).
913. Koberstein, Weber, and Jaenicke, *Z. Naturforsch. B,* 23, 474 (1968).
914. Buhner and Sund, *Eur. J. Biochem.,* 11, 73 (1969).
915. Swaisgood and Pattee, *J. Food Sci.,* 33, 400 (1968).
916. Sofer and Ursprung, *J. Biol. Chem.,* 243, 3110 (1968).
917. Biszku, Boross, and Szabolcsi, *Acta Physiol. Acad. Sci. Hung.,* 25, 161 (1964).
918. Kawahara and Tanford, *Biochemistry,* 5, 1578 (1966).
919. Sine and Hass, *J. Biol. Chem.,* 244, 430 (1969).
920. Reisler and Eisenberg, *Biochemistry,* 8, 4572 (1969).
921. Hass, *Biochemistry,* 3, 535 (1964).
922. Gracy, Lacko, and Horecker, *J. Biol. Chem.,* 244, 3913 (1969).
923. Marquardt, *Can. J. Biochem.,* 47, 517 (1969).
924. Marquardt, *Can. J. Biochem,* 49, 647 (1971).
925. Marquardt, *Can. J. Biochem.,* 49, 658 (1971).
926. Suh, *Fed. Proc.,* 30, 1157 (1971).
927. Lai and Chen, *Arch. Biochem. Biophys.,* 144, 467 (1971).
928. Kobes, Simpson, Vallee, and Rutter, *Biochemistry,* 8, 585 (1969).
929. Harris, Kobes, Teller, and Rutter, *Biochemistry,* 8, 2442 (1969).
930. Rapoport, Davis, and Horecker, *Arch. Biochem. Biophys.,* 132, 286 (1969).
931. DeGraaf, Goedvolk-DeGroot, and Stouthamer, *Biochem. Biophys. Acta,* 221, 566 (1971).

932. Dimroth, Guchhait, and Lane, *Hoppe-Seylers Z. Physiol. Chem.,* 352, 351 (1971).
933. Doyle, Pittz, and Woodside, *Carbohydr. Res.,* 8, 89 (1968).
934. Agrawal and Goldstein, *Biochim. Biophys. Acta,* 133, 376 (1967).
935. Olson and Liener, *Biochemistry,* 6, 105 (1967).
936. Yariv, Kalb, and Levitzki, *Biochim. Biophys. Acta,* 165, 303 (1968).
937. Cheesman, Zagalsky, and Ceccaldi, *Proc. Roy. Soc. Lond. (Biol.),* 164, 130 (1966).
938. Cummings, *Biochem. Biophys. Res. Commun.,* 33, 165 (1968).
939. Hamlin, *Exp. Gerentol.,* 4, 189 (1969).
940. Cavallini, Scandurra, and Dupre, in *Biological and Chemical Aspects of Oxygenases,* Bloch and Hayaishi, eds., Maruzen, Tokyo, 1966, p. 73.
941. Mochan, *Biochim. Biophys. Acta,* 216, 80 (1970).
942. Poulos and Price, *J. Biol. Chem.,* 246, 4041 (1971).
943. Jargenson, *J. Biol. Chem.,* 240, 1064 (1965).
944. Kaplan and Dugas, *Biochem. Biophys. Res. Commun.,* 34, 681 (1969).
945. Wasi and Hofmann, *Biochem. J.,* 106, 926 (1968).
946. Gertler and Trop, *Eur. J. Biochem.,* 19, 90 (1971).
947. Kimura and Kubata, *Bull. Jpn. Soc. Sci. Fish.,* 34, 535 (1968).
948. Vulpis, Vulpis, and Santoro, *Italian J. Biochem.,* 15, 189 (1966).
949. Ruth, Soja, and Wold, *Arch. Biochem. Biophys.,* 140, 1 (1970).
950. Shethna, Stombaugh, and Burris, *Biochem. Biophys. Res. Commun.,* 42, 1108 (1971).
951. Buchanan, Matsubara, and Evans, *Biochim. Biophys. Acta,* 189, 46 (1969).
952. Vetter and Knappe, *Hoppe-Seylers Z. Physiol. Chem.,* 352, 433 (1970).
953. Mortenson, *Biochim. Biophys. Acta,* 81, 71 (1964).
954. Sobel and Lovenberg, *Biochemistry,* 5, 6 (1966).
955. Hong and Rabinowitz, *J. Biol. Chem.,* 245, 4982 (1970).
956. Aggarwal, Rao, and Matsubara, *J. Biochem. (Tokyo),* 69, 601 (1971).
957. Buchanan and Rabinowitz, *J. Bacteriol.,* 88, 806 (1964).
958. Lode and Coon, *J. Biol. Chem.,* 246, 791 (1971).
959. Dubourdieu and Le Gall, *Biochem. Biophys. Res. Commun.,* 38, 965 (1970).
960. Vetter, Jr. and Knappe, *Hoppe-Seylers Z. Physiol. Chem.,* 352, 433 (1970).
961. Mayhew, *Biochim. Biophys. Acta,* 235, 276 (1971).
962. Mayhew, *Biochim. Biophys. Acta,* 235, 289 (1971).
963. Mayhew and Massey, *J. Biol. Chem.,* 244, 794 (1969).
964. Zak, Steczko, and Ostrowski, *Bull. Soc. Chim. Biol.,* 51, 1065 (1969).
965. Schade and Reinhart, *Biochem. J.,* 118, 181 (1970).
966. Hauge, *Arch. Biochem. Biophys.,* 94, 308 (1961).
967. Yoshimura and Isemura, *J. Biochem. (Tokyo),* 69, 839 (1971).
968. Olive and Levy, *J. Biol. Chem.,* 246, 2043 (1971).
969. Flohe, Eisele, and Wendel, *Hoppe-Seylers Z. Physiol. Chem.,* 352, 151 (1971).
970. Harrington and Karr, *J. Mol. Biol.,* 13, 885 (1965).
971. Cseke and Boross, *Acta Biochim. Biophys. Acad. Sci. Hung.,* 2, 39 (1967).
972. Parker and Allison, *J. Biol. Chem.,* 244, 180 (1969).
973. Koberstein, Weber, and Jaenicke, *Z. Naturforsch. (B),* 23, 474 (1968).
974. Murdock and Koeppe, *J. Biol. Chem.,* 239, 1983 (1964).
975. McMurray and Trentham, *Biochem. J.,* 115, 913 (1959).
976. Wassarman, Watson, and Major, *Biochim. Biophys. Acta.* 191, 1 (1969).
977. Davidson, Sajgo, Noller, and Harris, *Nature,* 216, 1181 (1962).
978. Allison, *Methods Enzymol.,* 9, 210 (1966).
979. Devijlder, Boers, and Slater, *Biochim. Biophys. Acta,* 191, 214 (1969).
980. Warburg and Christian, *Biochem. Z.,* 303, 40 (1939).
981. Jaenicke, in *Pyridine Nucleotide Dependent Dehydrogenases,* Sund, ed., Springer-Verlag, Berlin, 1970, p. 70.
982. Durchschlag, Puchwein, Kratky, Schuster, and Kirschner, *Eur. J. Biochem.,* 19, 9 (1971).
983. Oguchi, *J. Biochem. (Tokyo),* 68, 427 (1970).
984. Heinz and Kulbe, *Hoppe-Seylers Z. Physiol. Chem.,* 351, 249 (1970).
985. Baliga, Bhatnagar, and Jagannathan, *Indian J. Biochem.,* 1, 86 (1964).

986. Thorner and Paulus, *J. Biol. Chem.*, 246, 3385 (1971).
987. Fondy, Ross, and Sollohub, *J. Biol. Chem.*, 244, 1631 (1969).
988. Beisenherz, Bucher, and Gorbade, *Methods Enzymol.*, 1, 397 (1955).
989. Ankel, Bucher, and Czok, *Biochem. Z.*, 332, 315 (1960).
990. Catsimpoolas, Berg, and Meyer, *Int. J. Protein Res.*, 3, 63 (1971).
991. Wolf and Briggs, *Arch. Biochem. Biophys.*, 63, 40 (1959).
992. Hrkal and Muller-Eberhard, *Biochemistry*, 10, 1746 (1971).
993. Dus, DeKlerk, Sletten, and Bartsch, *Biochem. Biophys. Acta*, 140, 291 (1967).
994. Buffoni and Blaschko, *Proc. Roy. Soc. Lond. (Biol.)*, 161, 153 (1965).
995. Klee, *J. Biol. Chem.*, 245, 3143 (1970).
996. Rechler, *J. Biol. Chem.*, 244, 551 (1969).
997. Riley and Snell, *Biochemistry*, 9, 1485 (1970).
998. Rechler and Bruni, *J. Biol. Chem.*, 246, 1806 (1971).
999. Champagne, Pouyet, Ouellet, and Garel, *Bull. Soc. Chim. Biol.*, 52, 377 (1970).
1000. Oh, *J. Biol. Chem.*, 245, 6404 (1970).
1001. Matsuo and Greenberg, *J. Biol. Chem.*, 230, 545 (1958).
1002. Datta, *J. Biol. Chem.*, 245, 5779 (1970).
1003. Janin, van Rapenbusch, Truffa-Bachi, and Cohen, *Eur. J. Biochem.*, 8, 128 (1969).
1004. Rhodes, Dodgson, Olavesen, and Hogberg, *Biochem. J.*, 122, 575 (1971).
1005. Newman, Berenson, Mathews, Goldwasser, and Dorfman, *J. Biol. Chem.*, 217, 31 (1955).
1006. Haschke and Campbell, *J. Bacteriol.*, 105, 249 (1971).
1007. Nakos and Mortenson, *Biochemistry*, 10, 2442 (1971).
1008. Yano, Morimoto, Higashi, and Arima, in *Biological and Chemical Aspects of Oxygenases*, Bloch and Hayaishi, eds., Maruzen, Tokyo, 1966, p. 331.
1009. Hesp, Calvin, and Hosokawa, *J. Biol. Chem.*, 244, 5644 (1968).
1010. Aschhoff and Pfeil, *Hoppe-Seylers Z. Physiol. Chem.*, 351, 818 (1970).
1011. Finlay and Adams, *J. Biol. Chem.*, 245, 5248 (1970).
1012. Martin, *Arch. Biochem. Biophys.*, 138, 239 (1970).
1013. Hamaguichi and Migita, *J. Biochem. (Tokyo)*, 56, 512 (1964).
1014. Ruffilli and Givol, *Eur. J. Biochem.*, 2, 429 (1967).
1015. Heimburger, Heide, and Haupt, *Clin. Chim. Acta*, 10, 293 (1964).
1016. Tomasi and Bienenstock, *Adv. Immunol.*, 9, 1 (1968).
1017. Lerner and Barnum, *Arch. Biochem.*, 10, 417 (1946).
1018. Lewis, Bergsagel, Bruce-Robertson, Schachter, and Connell, *Blood*, 32, 189 (1968).
1019. Connell, Dorington, Lewis, and Parr, *Can. J. Biochem.*, 48, 784 (1970).
1020. Schultze and Heremans, *Molecular Biology of Human Protein*, Vol. I, Elsevier, Amsterdam, 1966, p. 234.
1021. Bennich and Johansson, in *Gamma Globulins, Nobel Symposium No. 3*, Killander, ed., Interscience, New York, 1967, p. 200.
1022. Orlans, *Immunology*, 14, 61 (1968).
1023. Yamashita, Franek, Skvaril, and Simek, *Eur. J. Biochem.*, 6, 34 (1968).
1024. Clem, *J. Biol. Chem.*, 246, 9 (1971).
1025. Acton, Weinheimer, Dupree, Evans, and Bennett, *Biochemistry*, 10, 2028 (1971).
1026. Freedman, Grossberg, and Pressman, *Biochemistry*, 7, 1941 (1968).
1027. Porter, *Biochem. J.*, 66, 677 (1957).
1028. Knight and Dray, *Biochemistry*, 7, 3830 (1968).
1029. Van Dalen, Seijen, and Gruber, *Biochim. Biophys. Acta*, 147, 421 (1967).
1030. Day, Sturtevant, and Singer, *Ann. N. Y. Acad. Sci.*, 103, 611 (1963).
1031. Onoue, Yagi, Grossberg, and Pressman, *Immunochemistry*, 2, 401 (1965).
1032. Freedman, Grossberg, and Pressman, *Immunochemistry*, 5, 367 (1968).
1033. Givol and Hurwitz, *Biochem. J.*, 115, 371 (1969).
1034. Haimovich, Schechter, and Sela, *Eur. J. Biochem.*, 4, 537 (1969).
1035. Sokol, Hana, and Albrecht, *Folia Microbiol. (Praha)*, 6, 145 (1961).
1036. Montgomery, Dorrington, and Rockey, *Biochemistry*, 8, 1247 (1969).
1037. Eisen, Simms, and Potter, *Biochemistry*, 7, 4126 (1968).
1038. Tur-Sinai, Birk, Gertler, and Rigbi, *Isr. J. Chem.*, 8, 176 (1970).
1039. Mikola and Suolinna, *Arch. Biochem. Biophys.*, 144, 566 (1971).
1040. Malmstrom, Agro, and Antonini, *Eur. J. Biochem.*, 9, 383 (1969).
1041. Phillips and Jenness, *Biochim. Biophys. Acta*, 229, 407 (1971).
1042. Schmidt and Ebner, *Biochim. Biophys. Acta*, 243, 273 (1971).
1043. Bell, Hopper, McKenzie, Murphy, and Shaw, *Biochim. Biophys. Acta*, 214, 437 (1970).
1044. Kuwabara and Lloyd, *Biochem. J.*, 124, 215 (1971).
1045. Möra and Elödi, *Eur. J. Biochem.*, 5, 574 (1968).
1046. Gutfreund, Cantwell, McMurray, Criddle, and Hathaway, *Biochem. J.*, 106, 683 (1968).
1047. Reeves and Fimognari, *Methods Enzymol.*, 9, 289 (1966).
1048. Jaenicke, in *Pyridine Dependent Dehydrogenases*, Sund, ed., Springer-Verlag, New York, 1970, p. 70.
1049. Koberstein, Weber, and Jaenicke, *Z. Naturforsch. (B)*, 23, 474 (1968).
1050. Foye and Solis, *J. Pharm. Sci.*, 58, 352 (1969).
1051. Pfleiderer and Jeckel, *Biochem. Z.*, 329, 370 (1957).
1052. Velick, *J. Biol. Chem.*, 233, 1455, (1958).
1053. Hakala, Glaid, and Schwert, *J. Biol. Chem.*, 221, 191 (1956).
1054. Neilands, *J. Biol. Chem.*, 199, 373 (1952).
1055. Nisselbaum and Bodansky, *J. Biol. Chem.*, 236, 323 (1961).
1056. Symons and Burgoyne, *Methods Enzymol.*, 9, 314 (1966).
1057. Kaloustian, Stolzenbach, Everse, and Kaplan, *J. Biol. Chem.*, 244, 2891 (1969).
1058. Vestling and Kunsch, *Arch. Biochem. Biophsy.*, 127, 568 (1968).
1059. Kubowitz and Ott, *Biochem. Z.*, 314, 94 (1943).
1060. Castellino, Fish, and Mann, *J. Biol. Chem.*, 245, 4269 (1970).
1061. Ghosh, Chaudhuri, Roy, Sinha, and Sen, *Arch. Biochem. Biophys.*, 144, 6 (1971).
1062. Joniau, Bloemmen, and Lontie, *Biochim. Biophys. Acta*, 214, 468 (1970).
1063. Groves, in *Milk Proteins, Chemistry and Molecular Biology*, McKenzie, ed., Vol. 2, Academic Press, New York, 1971, p. 367.
1064. Hou and Perlman, *J. Biol. Chem.*, 245, 1289 (1970).
1065. Carlstrom, *Acta Chem. Scand.*, 23, 185 (1969).
1066. Theorell and Pedersen, in *The Svedberg*, Tiselius and Pedersen, eds., Almqvist and Wiksells Boktryckeri, Uppsala and Stockholm, 1944, p. 523.
1067. Polis and Shmukler, *J. Biol. Chem.*, 201, 475 (1953).
1068. Appleby, *Biochim. Biophys. Acta*, 188, 222 (1969).
1069. Sjögren and Svedberg, *J. Am. Chem. Soc.*, 52, 3279 (1930).
1070. Hermier, Lebeault, and Zevaco, *Bull. Soc. Chim. Biol.*, 52, 1089 (1970).
1071. Verger, Sarda, and Desnuelle, *Biochim. Biophys. Acta*, 242, 580 (1971).
1072. Vandermeers and Christophe, *Biochim. Biophys. Acta*, 154, 110 (1968).
1073. Brown, Levy, and Fredrickson, *J. Biol. Chem.*, 245, 6588 (1970).
1074. Koga, Horwitz, and Scanu, *J. Lipid Res.*, 10, 577 (1969).
1075. Chlumecka, Tigerstrom, D'Obrenan, and Smith, *J. Biol. Chem.*, 245, 5481 (1969).
1076. Hayaishi, in *Oxidases and Related Systems*, King, Mason, and Morrison, eds., John Wiley & Sons, New York, 1965, p. 286.
1077. Cassio and Waller, *Eur. J. Biochem.*, 20, 283 (1971).
1078. Dalton, Morris, Ward, and Mortensen, *Biochemistry*, 10, 2066 (1971).
1079. Keilin and Hartree, *Biochem. J.*, 61, 153 (1953).
1080. Harrison and Blout, *J. Biol. Chem.*, 240, 299 (1965).
1081. Brown, Martinez, Johnstone, and Olcott, *J. Biol. Chem.*, 237, 81 (1962).
1082. Rossi-Fanelli, Antonini, and Povoledo, in *Symposium on Protein Structure*, Neuberger, ed., Methuen and Co., London, 1958, 144.
1083. Atassi and Saplin, *Biochem. J.*, 98, 82 (1966).
1084. Herskovits, *Arch. Biochem. Biophys.*, 130, 19 (1969).
1085. Crumpton and Wilkinson, *Biochem. J.*, 94, 545 (1965).
1086. Atassi, *Biochim. Biophys. Acta*, 221, 612 (1970).
1087. Cameron, Azzam, Kotite, and Awad, *J. Lab. Clin. Med.*, 65, 883 (1965).
1088. Crumpton and Polson, *J. Mol. Biol.*, 11, 722 (1965).
1089. Boegman and Crumpton, *Biochem. J.*, 120, 373 (1970).
1090. Breslow, *J. Biol. Chem.*, 239, 486 (1964).

1091. Hermans, Jr., *Biochemistry*, 1, 193 (1962).
1092. Edmundson and Hirs, *Nature*, 190, 663 (1961).
1093. Ray and Gurd, *J. Biol. Chem.*, 242, 2062 (1967).
1094. Terwilliger and Read, *Comp. Biochem. Physiol.*, 29, 551 (1969).
1095. Terwilliger and Read, *Comp. Biochem. Physiol.*, 31, 55 (1969).
1096. Kritcher, Thyrum, and Luchi, *Biochim. Biophys. Acta*, 221, 264 (1970).
1097. Gazith, Himmelfarb, and Harrington, *J. Biol. Chem.*, 245, 15 (1970).
1098. Gershman, Stracher, and Dreizen, *J. Biol. Chem.*, 244, 2726 (1969).
1099. Shimizu, Morita, and Yagi, *J. Biochem. (Tokyo)*, 69, 447 (1971).
1100. Young, Blanchard, and Brown, *Proc. Natl. Acad. Sci. U.S.A.*, 61, 1087 (1968).
1101. Otaiza and Jaenicke, *Hoppe-Seylers Z. Physiol. Chem.*, 352, 385 (1971).
1102. Bocchini, *Eur. J. Biochem.*, 15, 127 (1970).
1103. Karlsson, Amberg, and Eaker, *Eur. J. Biochem.*, 21, 1 (1971).
1104. Miranda, Kupeyan, Rochat, Rochat, and Lissitzky, *Eur. J. Biochem.*, 17, 477 (1970).
1105. Miranda, Kupeyan, Rochat, Rochat, and Lissitzky, *Eur. J. Biochem.*, 16, 514 (1970).
1106. Holcenberg and Stadtman, *J. Biol. Chem.*, 244, 1194 (1969).
1107. Forget, *Eur. J. Biochem.*, 18, 442 (1971).
1108. Burns, Holsten, and Hardy, *Biochem. Biophys. Res. Commun.*, 39, 90 (1970).
1109. Nossal and Hershfield, *J. Biol. Chem.*, 246, 541 (1971).
1110. Omenn, Onjes, and Anfinsen, *Biochemistry*, 9, 304 (1970).
1111. Albrecht, *Biochemistry*, 9, 2462 (1970).
1112. Glazer and Smith, *J. Biol. Chem.*, 235, PC43 (1960).
1113. Weintraub and Schlamowitz, *Comp. Biochem. Physiol.*, 38B, 513 (1971).
1114. Weintraub and Schlamowitz, *Comp. Biochem. Physiol.*, 37, 49 (1970).
1115. Tomimatsu, Clary, and Bartulovich, *Arch. Biochem. Biophys.*, 115, 536 (1966).
1116. Liu, Means, and Feeny, *Biochim. Biophys. Acta*, 229, 176 (1971).
1117. Donovan, Mapes, Davis, and Hamburg, *Biochemistry*, 8, 4190 (1969).
1118. Donovan, Davis, and White, *Biochim. Biophys. Acta*, 207, 190 (1970).
1119. Davis, Mapes, and Donovan, *Biochemistry*, 10, 39 (1971).
1120. Bender and Brubacher, *J. Am. Chem. Soc.*, 86, 5333 (1964).
1121. Hinkle and Kirsch, *Biochemistry*, 9, 4633 (1970).
1122. Arnon and Shapira, *J. Biol. Chem.*, 244, 1033 (1969).
1123. Olander, *Biochemistry*, 10, 601 (1971).
1124. Woods, *Biochem. J.*, 113, 39 (1969).
1125. Milstein, *Biochem. J.* 103, 634 (1967).
1126. Citri and Pollock, *Adv. Enzymol.*, 28, 237 (1966).
1127. Imsande, Gillin, Tanis, and Atherly, *J. Biol. Chem.*, 245, 2205 (1970).
1128. Lindstrom, Boman, and Steele, *J. Biol. Chem.*, 101, 218 (1970).
1129. Sodek and Hofmann, *Methods Enzymol.*, 19, 372 (1970).
1130. Morita, Toshida, and Maeda, *Agr. Biol. Chem.*, 35, 1074 (1971).
1131. Staprans and Watanabe, *J. Biol. Chem.*, 245, 5962 (1970).
1132. Peterson, *J. Biol. Chem.*, 246, 34 (1971).
1133. Peterson and Berggard, *J. Biol. Chem.*, 246, 25 (1971).
1134. Kuehn and McFadden, *Biochemistry*, 8, 2394 (1968).
1135. Nicholson, *Biochem. J.*, 123, 117 (1971).
1136. Labow and Robinson, *J. Biol. Chem.*, 241, 1239 (1966).
1137. Dowhan, Jr. and Snell, *J. Biol. Chem.* 245, 4618 (1970).
1138. Matsubara, *Methods Enzymol.*, 19, 642 (1970).
1139. Berglund and Sjöberg, *J. Biol Chem.*, 245, 6030 (1970).
1140. Fedberg and Datta, *Eur. J. Biochem.*, 21, 438 (1971).
1141. Hug and Roth, *Biochemistry*, 10, 1397 (1971).
1142. White and Barlow, *Methods Enzymol.*, 19, 665 (1970).
1143. Gumpf and Hamilton, *Virology*, 35, 87 (1968).
1144. Yamazaki and Kaesberg, *J. Mol. Biol.*, 6, 465 (1963).
1145. Stubbs and Kaesberg, *J. Mol. Biol.*, 8, 314 (1964).
1146. Bachrach and Van den Woude, *Virology*, 34, 282 (1968).
1147. Rueckert, *Virology*, 26, 345 (1965).
1148. Ghabrial, Shepherd, and Grogan, *Virology*, 33, 17 (1967).
1149. Damirdagh and Shepherd, *Virology*, 40, 84 (1970).
1150. Budzynski and Fraenkel-Conrat, *Biochemistry*, 9, 3300 (1970).
1151. Tremaine and Stace-Smith, *Virology*, 35, 102 (1968).
1152. Dorne, Jonard, Witz, and Hirth, *Virology*, 43, 279 (1971).
1153. Miki and Knight, *Virology*, 31, 55 (1967).
1154. Wallace, *Biochim. Biophys. Acta*, 215, 176 (1970).
1155. Bray, Chisholm, Hart, Meriwether, and Watts, in *Flavins and Flavoproteins*, Slater, ed., Elsevier, Amsterdam, 1966, p. 117.
1156. West, Nagy, and Gergely, in *Symposium on Fibrous Proteins*, Crewther, ed., Plenum Press, New York, 1968, p. 164.
1157. Kimura and Ting, *Biochem. Biophys. Res. Commun.*, 45, 1227 (1971).
1158. Fushimi, Hamison, and Ravin, *J. Biochem. (Tokyo)*, 69, 1041 (1971).
1159. Shinowara, in *Blood Platelets, Henry Ford International Symposium No. 10*, Johnson, Monto, Rebuck, and Horn, Jr., eds., Little Brown, Boston, MA, 1961, 347.
1160. Reynolds and Johnson, *Biochemistry*, 10, 2821 (1971).
1161. Wu, Cluskey, Krull, and Friedman, *Can. J. Biochem.*, 49, 1042 (1971).
1162. Berrens and Bleumink, *Int. Arch. Allergy*, 28, 150 (1965).
1163. Feldman and Weiner, *J. Biol. Chem.*, 247, 260 (1972).
1164. Guha, Lai, and Horecker, *Arch. Biochem. Biophys.*, 147, 692 (1971).
1165. Caban and Hass, *J. Biol. Chem.*, 246, 6807 (1971).
1166. Penhoet, Kochman and Rutter, *Biochemistry*, 8, 4396 (1969).
1167. Chiu and Feingold, *Biochemistry*, 8, 98 (1969).
1168. Robertson, Hammerstedt, and Wood, *J. Biol. Chem.*, 246, 2075 (1971).
1169. 'S-Gravenmade, Drift, Van Der, and Vogels, *Biochim. Biophys. Acta*, 251, 393 (1971).
1170. King and Norman, *Biochemistry*, 1, 709 (1962).
1171. Underdown and Goodfriend, *Biochemistry*, 8, 980 (1969).
1172. Mazelis and Crews, *Biochem. J.*, 108, 725 (1968).
1173. Svedberg and Sjögren, *J. Am. Chem. Soc.*, 52, 279 (1930).
1174. Eady and Large, *Biochem. J.*, 123, 757 (1971).
1175. Henn and Ackers, *J. Biol. Chem.*, 244, 465 (1969).
1176. Miyake and Yamano, *Biochim. Biophys. Acta*, 198, 438 (1970).
1177. Soda and Osumi, *Biochem. Biophys. Res. Commun.*, 35, 363 (1969).
1178. McKeehan and Hardesty, *J. Biol. Chem.*, 244, 4330 (1969).
1179. Yamada, Adachi, and Ogata, in *Pyridoxyl Catalysis: Enzymes and Model Systems*, Snell, Braunstein, Severin, and Torchinsky, eds., Interscience, New York, 1968, p. 347.
1180. Wang, Achee, and Yasunobu, *Arch. Biochem. Biophys.*, 128, 106 (1968).
1181. Prescott, Wilkes, Wagner, and Wilson, *J. Biol. Chem.*, 246, 1756 (1971).
1182. Hanson, Hutter, Mansfeldt, Kretschmer, and Sohr, *Hoppe-Seylers Z. Physiol. Chem.*, 348, 680 (1967).
1183. Wacker, Lehky, Fischer, and Stein, *Helv. Chim. Acta*, 54, 473 (1971).
1184. Roncari and Zuber, *Int. J. Protein Res.*, 1, 45 (1969).
1185. Pfleiderer and Femfert, *FEBS Lett.*, 4, 265 (1969).
1186. Auricchio and Bruni, *Biochem. Z.*, 340, 321 (1964).
1187. Yaron and Mlynar, *Biochem. Biophys. Res. Commun.*, 32, 658 (1968).
1188. Grszkiewicz, *Acta Biochem. Pol.*, 9, 301 (1962).
1189. Vandermeers and Christophe, *Biochim. Biophys. Acta*, 154, 110 (1968).
1190. Menzi, Stein, and Fischer, *Helv. Chim. Acta*, 40, 534 (1957).
1191. Yutani, Yutani, and Isemura, *J. Biochem. (Tokyo)*, 66, 823 (1969).
1192. Nishida, Fukumoto, and Yamamoto, *Agr. Biol. Chem.*, 31, 682 (1967).
1193. Nishida, PhD thesis; cited in Nishida, Fukumoto, and Yamamoto, *Agr. Biol. Chem.*, 31, 682 (1967).
1194. Ogasahara, Imanishi, and Isemura, *J. Biochem. (Tokyo)*, 67, 65 (1970).
1195. Junge, Stein, Neurath, and Fischer, *J. Biol. Chem.*, 234, 556 (1959).
1196. Sanders and Rutter, *Biochemistry*, 11, 130 (1972).
1197. Krysteva and Erodi, *Acta Biochim. Biophys. Acad. Sci. Hung.*, 3, 275 (1968).
1198. Yoshida, Hiroshi, and Ono, *J. Biochem. (Tokyo)*, 65, 741 (1969).
1199. Yutani, Yutani, and Isemura, *J. Biochem. (Tokyo)*, 65, 201 (1969).
1200. Shainkin and Berk, *Biochim. Biophys. Acta*, 221, 502 (1970).

1201. Takeda and Hizukuri, *Biochim. Biophys. Acta*, 185, 469 (1969).
1202. Englard, Sorof, and Singer, *J. Biol. Chem.*, 189, 217 (1951).
1203. Nagano and Zalkin, *J. Biol. Chem.*, 245, 3097 (1970).
1204. Ito, Cox, and Yanofsky, *J. Bacteriol.*, 97, 725 (1969).
1205. Henderson and Zalkin, *J. Biol. Chem.*, 246, 6891 (1971).
1206. Warner and Schumaker, *Biochemistry*, 9, 451 (1970).
1207. Bezkorovainy, Springer, and Dese, *Biochemistry*, 10, 3761 (1971).
1208. Kim, *Vox Sang*, 20, 461 (1971).
1209. Bezkorovainy, Springer, and Hotti, *Biochim. Biophys. Acta*, 115, 501 (1966).
1210. Preer, *J. Immunol.*, 33, 385 (1959).
1211. Kaji and Tagawa, *Biochim. Biophys. Acta*, 207, 456 (1970).
1212. Harell and Sokolovsky, *Eur. J. Biochem.*, 25, 102 (1972).
1213. Sakai and Murachi, *Physiol. Chem. Phys.*, 1, 31 (1969).
1214. Blethen, Boeker, and Snell, *J. Biol. Chem.*, 243, 1671 (1968).
1215. Regnouf, Pradel, Kassab, and Thoai, *Biochim. Biophys. Acta*, 194, 540 (1969).
1216. Oriol-Audit, Landon, Robin, and Thoai, *Biochim. Biophys. Acta*, 188, 132 (1969).
1217. Kassab, Fattoum, and Pradel, *Eur. J. Biochem.*, 12, 264 (1970).
1218. Kassab, Roustan, and Pradel, *Biochim. Biophys. Acta*, 167, 308 (1968).
1219. Landon, Oriol, and Thoai, *Biochim. Biophys. Acta*, 214, 168 (1970).
1220. Yorifuji, Ogata, and Soda, *J. Biol. Chem.*, 246, 5085 (1971).
1221. Bray and Ratner, *Arch. Biochem. Biophys.*, 146, 531 (1971).
1222. Nakano, Tsutsumi, and Danowski, *J. Biol. Chem.*, 245, 4443 (1974).
1223. Nakamura, Makino, and Ogura, *J. Biochem. (Tokyo)*, 64, 189 (1969).
1224. Penton and Dawson, in *Oxidases and Related Redox Systems*, King, Mason, and Morrison, eds., John Wiley and Sons, New York, 1965, p. 221.
1225. Tosa, Sano, Yamamoto, Nakamura, and Chibata, *Biochemistry*, 11, 21 (1972).
1226. Lu and Handschumacher, *J. Biol. Chem.*, 247, 66 (1972).
1227. Nishumara, Makino, Takenaka, and Inada, *Biochim. Biophys. Acta*, 227, 171 (1971).
1228. Shifrin and Grochowski, *J. Biol. Chem.*, 247, 1048 (1972).
1229. Kakimoto, Kato, Shibatani, Nishimura, and Chibata, *J. Biol. Chem.*, 244, 353 (1969).
1230. Banks, Doonan, Lawrence, and Vernon, *Eur. J. Biochem.*, 5, 528 (1968).
1231. Banks and Vernon, *J. Chem. Soc.*, p. 1968 (1961).
1232. Arrio-Dupont, Cournil, and Duie, *FEBS Lett.*, 11, 144 (1970).
1233. Martinez-Carrion, Kuczenski, Tiemeier, and Peterson, *J. Biol. Chem*, 245, 799 (1970).
1234. Bergami, Marino, and Scardi, *Biochem. J.*, 110, 471 (1968).
1235. Bertlund and Kaplan, *Biochemistry*, 9, 2653 (1970).
1236. Magee and Phillips, *Biochemistry*, 10, 3397 (1971).
1237. Marino, Greco, Scardi, and Zito, *Biochem. J.*, 99, 589 (1966).
1238. Scardi, in *Pyridoxal Catalysis: Enzymes and Model Systems*, Snell, Braunstein, Severin, and Torchinsky, Eds., Interscience, New York, 1968, p. 179.
1239. Nelbach, Pigiet, Gerhart, and Schachman, *Biochemistry*, 11, 315 (1972).
1240. Meighen, Pigiet, and Schachman, *Proc. Natl. Acad. Sci., U.S.A.*, 65, 234 (1970).
1241. Benisek, *J. Biol. Chem.*, 246, 3151 (1971).
1242. Vanaman and Stark, *J. Biol. Chem.*, 245, 3565 (1970).
1243. Biswas, Gray, and Paulus, *J. Biol. Chem.*, 245, 4900 (1970).
1244. Lafuma, Gros, and Patte, *Eur. J. Biochem.*, 15, 111 (1970).
1245. Janin, van Rapenbusch, Truffa-Bachi, Cohen, and Gros, *Eur. J. Biochem.*, 8, 128 (1969).
1246. Truffa-Bachi, van Rapenbusch, Janin, Gros, and Cohen, *Eur. J. Biochem.*, 7, 401 (1969).
1247. Falcoz-Kelly, van Rapenbusch, and Cohen, *Eur. J. Biochem.*, 8, 146 (1969).
1248. Inoue, Suzuki, Fukunishi, Adachi, and Takeda, *J. Biol. Chem.*, 60, 543 (1966).
1249. Melamed and Green, *Biochem. J.*, 89, 591 (1963).
1250. Green, *Biochem. J.*, 89, 599 (1963).
1251. Scrutton, *Biochemistry*, 10, 3897 (1971).
1252. Brill, Bryce, and Maria, *Biochim. Biophys. Acta*, 154, 342 (1968).
1253. Haupt, Heimburger, Krantz, and Schwick, *Eur. J. Biochem.*, 17, 254 (1970).
1254. Vonemasu, Stroud, Niedermeier, and Butler, *Biochem. Biophys. Res. Commun.*, 43, 1388 (1971).
1255. Nilsson and Lindskog, *Eur. J. Biochem.*, 2, 309 (1967).
1256. Carter, *Biochim. Biophys. Acta*, 235, 222 (1971).
1257. Bernstein and Schraer, *J. Biol. Chem.*, 247, 1306 (1972).
1258. Bernstein and Schraer, *Fed. Proc.*, Abstract 1387, 30 (1291).
1259. Maynard and Coleman, *J. Biol. Chem.*, 246, 4455 (1971).
1260. Carter and Parsons, *Biochem. J.*, 120, 797 (1970).
1261. Funakoshi and Deutsch, *J. Biol. Chem.*, 245, 4913 (1970).
1262. Edsall, Mehta, Myers, and Armstrong, *Biochem. Z.*, 345, 9 (1966).
1263. Ashworth, Spencer, and Brewer, *Arch. Biochem. Biophys.*, 142, 122 (1971).
1264. Tanis, Tashian, and Yu, *J. Biol. Chem.*, 245, 6003 (1970).
1265. Rossi, Chersi, and Cortivo, in CO_2: *Chemical, Biochemical and Physiological Aspects*, Forster, Edsall, Otis, and Roughton, eds., NASA SP-188, 1969, p. 131.
1266. Runnegar, Scott, Webb, and Zerner, *Biochemistry*, 8, 2013 (1969).
1267. Runnegar, Webb, and Zerner, *Biochemistry*, 8, 2018 (1969).
1268. Franz and Krisch, *Hoppe-Seylers Z. Physiol. Chem.*, 149, 575 (1968).
1269. Chase and Tubbs, *Biochem. J.*, 111, 225 (1969).
1270. Zagalsky, Cheesman, and Ceccaldi, *Comp. Biochem. Physiol.*, 22, 851 (1967).
1271. Zagalsky, Ceccaldi, and Daumas, *Comp. Biochem. Physiol.*, 34, 579 (1970).
1272. Dumas and Gamier, *J. Dairy Res.*, 37, 269 (1970).
1273. Thompson and Pepper, *J. Dairy Sci.*, 47, 633 (1964).
1274. Herskovits, *Arch. Biochem. Biophys.*, 130, 19 (1969).
1275. Carrico and Deutsch, *J. Biol. Chem.*, 244, 6087 (1969).
1276. Porter and Folch, *J. Neurochem.*, 1, 260 (1957).
1277. Ashwell and Morell, in *Red Cross Scientific Symposium on Glycoproteins of Blood Cells and Plasma*, Jamieson and Greenwalt, eds., J. B. Lippincott, Philadelphia, 1971, p. 173.
1278. Blumberg, Eisinger, Aisen, Morell, and Scheinberg, *J. Biol. Chem.*, 238, 1675 (1963).
1279. Ryden, *Int. J. Protein Res.*, 3, 131 (1971).
1280. Matsunaga and Nosoh, *Biochim. Biophys. Acta*, 215, 280 (1970).
1281. Osaki, *J. Biochem. (Tokyo)*, 48, 190 (1960).
1282. Milne and Matrone, *Biochim. Biophys. Acta*, 212, 43 (1970).
1283. Holtzman and Gaumnitz, *J. Biol. Chem.*, 245, 2350 (1970).
1284. Lospalluto and Finkelstein, *Biochim. Biophys. Acta*, 257, 158 (1972).
1285. Kover, Szaboic, and Csabal, *Arch. Biochem. Biophys.*, 106, 333 (1964).
1286. Schumberger, *Z. Naturforsch. (B)*, 23, 1412 (1968).
1287. Bahl, *J. Biol. Chem.*, 244, 567 (1969).
1288. Koch, Shaw, and Gibson, *Biochim. Biophys. Acta*, 229, 805 (1971).
1289. Koch, Shaw, and Gibson, *Biochim. Biophys. Acta*, 229, 795 (1971).
1290. Koch, Shaw, and Gibson, *Biochim. Biophys. Acta*, 212, 375 (1970).
1291. Koch, Shaw, and Gibson, *Biochim. Biophys. Acta*, 212, 387 (1970).
1292. Nakagawa and Bender, *Biochemistry*, 9, 259 (1970).
1293. Singh, Thornton, and Westheimer, *J. Biol. Chem.*, 237, PC3006 (1962).
1294. Webster, *Biochim. Biophys. Acta*, 207, 371 (1970).
1295. Krausz and Becker, *J. Biol. Chem.*, 243, 4606 (1968).
1296. Oliver, Viswanatha, and Whish, *Biochem. Biophys. Res. Commun.*, 27, 107 (1967).
1297. Babul and Stellwagen, *Anal. Biochem.*, 28, 216 (1969).
1298. Rovery, *Methods Enzymol.*, 11, 231 (1967).
1299. Coan, Roberts, and Travis, *Biochemistry*, 10, 2711 (1971).
1300. Jackson and Brandts, *Biochemistry*, 9, 2294 (1970).
1301. Chervenka and Wilcox, *J. Biol. Chem.*, 222, 621 (1956).
1302. Glazer and Smith, *J. Biol. Chem.*, 235, PC43 (1960).
1303. Vandermeers and Christophe, *Biochim. Biophys. Acta*, 188, 101 (1969).
1304. Brandts and Lumry, *J. Phys. Chem.*, 67, 1484 (1963).
1305. Nichol, *J. Biol. Chem.*, 243, 4065 (1968).
1306. Prahl and Neurath, *Biochemistry*, 5, 2131 (1966).
1307. Gratecos, Guy, Rovery, and Desnuelle, *Biochim. Biophys. Acta*, 175, 82 (1969).

1308. Singh, Brooks, and Srere, *J. Biol. Chem.*, 245, 4636 (1970).
1309. Berger, Kafatos, Felsted, and Law, *J. Biol. Chem.*, 246, 4131 (1971).
1310. Hruska and Law, *Methods Enzymol.*, 19, 221 (1970).
1311. Schwartz and Helinski, *J. Biol. Chem.*, 246, 6318 (1971).
1312. Grant and Album, *Arch. Biochem. Biophys.*, 82, 245 (1959).
1313. Rhoads and Udenfriend, *Arch. Biochem. Biophys.*, 139, 329 (1970).
1314. Shin and Mayer, *Biochemistry*, 7, 2991 (1968).
1315. Emery, *Biochemistry*, 8, 877 (1969).
1316. Ehrenpreis and Warner, *Arch. Biochem. Biophys.*, 61, 38 (1956).
1317. Grant-Greene and Friedberg, *Int. J. Protein Res.*, 2, 235 (1970).
1318. Lerman, *Can. J. Biochem.*, 47, 1115 (1969).
1319. Augusteyn and Spector, *Biochem. J.*, 124, 345 (1971).
1320. Gregory, Holdsworth, and Ottesen *C. R. Trav. Lab. Carlsberg Ser. Chim.*, 30, 147 (1957).
1321. Holdsworth, *Biochim. Biophys. Acta*, 51, 295 (1961).
1322. Rosenberry, Chang, and Chen, *J. Biol. Chem.*, 247, 1555 (1972).
1323. Verpoorte, *J. Biol. Chem.*, 247, 4787 (1972).
1324. West, Nagy, and Gergely, in *Symposium on Fibrous Proteins*, Crewther, ed., Plenum Press, New York, 1968, p. 164.
1325. Schramm and Hochstein, *Biochemistry*, 11, 2777 (1972).
1326. Day, Franklin, Pettersson, and Philipson, *Eur. J. Biochem.*, 29, 537 (1972).
1327. Ronca-Testoni, Ranieri, Raggi, and Ronca, *Ital. J. Biochem.*, 19, 262 (1970).
1328. Suhara, Takemori, and Katagiri, *Biochim. Biophys. Acta*, 263, 272 (1972).
1329. Levine, Kaplan, and Greenaway, *Biochem. J.*, 129, 847 (1972).
1330. Claesson, *Ark. Kem.*, 10, 4 (1956).
1331. Wallenfels and Herrmann, *Methods Enzymol.*, 9, 608 (1966).
1332. Berrens, in *The Chemistry of Atopic Allergens*, Karger, Basel, 1971, 205.
1333. Marsuzawa and Segal, *J. Biol. Chem.*, 243, 5929 (1968).
1334. Visuri and Nummi, *Eur. J. Biochem.*, 28, 555 (1972).
1335. Wissler, *Eur. J. Immunol.*, 2, 73 (1972).
1336. Stellwagen, Rysavy, and Babul, *J. Biol. Chem.*, 247, 8074 (1972).
1337. Lux, John, and Brewer, *J. Biol. Chem.*, 247, 7510 (1972).
1338. Tombs, *Biochem. J.*, 96, 119 (1965).
1339. Grazi and Magri, *Biochem. J.*, 126, 667 (1972).
1340. Nakamura, Makino and Ogura, *J. Biochem. (Tokyo)*, 64, 189 (1968).
1341. Cammack, Marlborough, and Miller, *Biochem. J.*, 126, 316 (1972).
1342. Laboureur, Langlois, Labrousse, et al., *Biochimie*, 53, 1147 (1971).
1343. Scandurra and Cannella, *Eur. J. Biochem.*, 27, 196 (1972).
1344. D'Aniello and Rocca, *Comp. Biochem. Physiol.*, B41, 625 (1972).
1345. Falcoz-Kelly, Janin, Saari, Veron, Truffa-Bachi, and Cohen, *Eur. J. Biochem.*, 28, 507 (1972).
1346. Thuma, Schirmer, and Schirmer, *Biochim. Biophys. Acta*, 268, 81 (1972).
1347. Tweedie and Segel, *Prep. Biochem.*, 1, 91 (1971).
1348. Wolff and Siegel, *J. Biol. Chem.*, 247, 4180 (1972).
1349. Virden, *Biochem. J.*, 127, 503 (1972).
1350. Brundell, Falkbring, and Nyman, *Biochim. Biophys. Acta*, 284, 311 (1972).
1351. Kang, Storm, and Carson, *Biochim. Biophys. Res. Commun.*, 49, 621 (1972).
1352. Ihle and Dure, III, *J. Biol. Chem.*, 247, 5034 (1972).
1353. Johansen, Livingston, and Vallee, *Biochemistry*, 11, 2584 (1972).
1354. Zagalsky and Herring, *Comp. Biochem. Physiol.*, B41, 397 (1972).
1355. Bonaventura, Schroeder, and Fang, *Arch. Biochem. Biophys.*, 150, 606 (1972).
1356. Price, Sterling, Tarantola, Hartley, and Rechcigl, *J. Biol. Chem.*, 237, 3468 (1962).
1357. Otto and Bhakdi, *Hoppe-Seyler's Z. Physiol. Chem.*, 350, 1577 (1969).
1358. Skujins, Pukite, and McLaren, *Enzymologia*, 39, 353 (1970).
1359. Timmis, *J. Bacteriol.*, 109, 12 (1972).
1360. Maylie, Charles, Gache, and Desnuelle, *Biochim. Biophys. Acta*, 229, 286 (1971).
1361. Barth, Bunnenberg, and Djerassi, *Anal. Biochem.*, 48, 471 (1972).
1362. Waterson, Castellino, Hass, and Hill, *J. Biol. Chem.*, 247, 5266 (1972).
1363. Wissler, *Eur. J. Immunol.*, 2, 84 (1972).
1364. Goldberger, Smith, Tisdale, and Bomstein, *J. Biol. Chem.*, 236, 2788 (1961).
1365. Lederer and Simon, *Eur. J. Biochem.*, 20, 469 (1971).
1366. Groudinsky, *Eur. J. Biochem.*, 18, 480 (1971).
1367. Mevel-Ninio, Pajot, and Labeyrie, *Biochimie*, 53, 35 (1971).
1368. Monteilhet and Risler, *Eur. J. Biochem.*, 12, 165 (1970).
1369. Strittmatter and Velick, *J. Biol. Chem.*, 221, 253 (1956).
1370. Itagaki and Hager, *J. Biol. Chem.*, 241, 3687 (1966).
1371. Iwasaki and Shidara, *Plant Cell Physiol.*, 10, 291 (1969).
1372. Webster, *Biochim. Biophys. Acta*, 207, 371 (1970).
1373. Flatmark and Sletten, *J. Biol. Chem.*, 243, 1623 (1968).
1374. Mayer and Miller, *Anal. Biochem.*, 36, 91 (1970).
1375. Herskovits, *Arch. Biochem. Biophys.*, 130, 19 (1969).
1376. Herskovits, Jaillet, and Gadegbeku, *J. Biol. Chem.*, 245, 4544 (1970).
1377. Bolard and Gamier, *Biochim. Biophys. Acta*, 263, 535 (1972).
1378. Scholes, McLain, and Smith, *Biochemistry*, 10, 2072 (1971).
1379. Schejter, Grosman, and Sokolovsky, *Isr. J. Chem.*, 10, 37 (1972).
1380. Yu, Yu, and King, *J. Biol. Chem.*, 247, 1012 (1972).
1381. Horio and Kamen, *Biochim. Biophys. Acta*, 48, 266 (1961).
1382. Cusanovich, Tedro, and Kamen, *Arch. Biochem. Biophys.*, 141, 557 (1970).
1383. Iwasaki and Matsubara, *J. Biochem. (Tokyo)*, 69, 847 (1971).
1384. Miki and Okunuki, *J. Biochem. (Tokyo)*, 66, 831 (1969).
1385. Clark-Walker and Lascelles, *Arch. Biochem. Biophys.*, 136, 153 (1970).
1386. Yamanaka, Takenami, Akijama, and Okunuki, *J. Biochem. (Tokyo)*, 70, 349 (1971).
1387. Shioi, Takamiya, and Nishimura, *J. Biochem. (Tokyo)*, 71, 285 (1972).
1388. Yongand King, *J. Biol. Chem.*, 245, 1331 (1970).
1389. Sugimura and Yakushiji, *J. Biochem. (Tokyo)*, 63, 281 (1968).
1390. Laycock and Craigie, *Can. J. Biochem.*, 49, 641 (1971).
1391. Kusel, Suriano, and Weber, *Arch. Biochem. Biophys.*, 133, 293 (1969).
1392. Stripp, Greene, and Gillette, *Pharmacology*, 6, 56 (1971).
1393. Kuronen and Ellfolk, *Biochim. Biophys. Acta*, 275, 308 (1972).
1394. Ellfolk and Soininen, *Acta Chem. Scand.*, 25, 1535 (1971).
1395. Hiraoka, Fukumoto, and Tsuru, *J. Biochem. (Tokyo)*, 71, 57 (1972).
1396. D'Souza, Warwick, and Freisheim, *Biochemistry*, 11, 1528 (1972).
1397. Gunderson, Dunlap, Harding, Freisheim, Otting, and Huennekens, *Biochemistry*, 11, 1018 (1972).
1398. Greenfield, Williams, Poe, and Hoogsteen, *Biochemistry*, 11, 4706 (1972).
1399. Erickson and Mathews, *Biochemistry*, 12, 372 (1973).
1400. Butzow, *Biochim. Biophys. Acta*, 168, 490 (1968).
1401. Setlow, Brutlag, and Kornberg, *J. Biol. Chem.*, 247, 224 (1972).
1402. Ueda, Lode, and Coon, *J. Biol. Chem.*, 247, 2109 (1972).
1403. Robinson and Maxwell, *J. Biol. Chem.*, 247, 7023 (1972).
1404. Rexova-Benkova and Slezarik, *Collect. Czech. Chem. Commun.*, 35, 1255 (1970).
1405. Spring and Wold, *J. Biol. Chem.*, 246, 6797 (1971).
1406. Winstead, *Biochemistry*, 11, 1046 (1972).
1407. Malmstrom, *Arch. Biochem. Biophys. Suppl.*, 1, 247 (1962).
1408. Maroux, Baratti, and Desnuelle, *J. Biol. Chem.*, 246, 5031 (1971).
1409. Schantz, Roessler, Woodburn, et al., *Biochemistry*, 11, 360 (1972).
1410. Borja, Fanning, Huang, and Bergdoll, *J. Biol. Chem.*, 247, 2456 (1972).
1411. Markland, and Damus, *J. Biol. Chem.*, 246, 6460 (1971).
1412. Swaney, and Klotz, *Arch. Biochem. Biophys.*, 147, 475 (1971).
1413. Weser, Bunnenberg, Cammack, et al., *Biochim. Biophys. Acta*, 243, 203 (1971).
1414. Weser and Hartmann, *Fed. Eur. Biochem. Soc. Lett.*, 17, 78 (1971).
1415. Weser, Barth, Djerassi, et al., *Biochem. Biophys. Acta*, 278, 28 (1972).
1416. Espada, Langton, and Dorado, *Biochim. Biophys. Acta*, 285, 427 (1972).
1417. Omori-Satoh, Sadahiro, Ohsaka, and Murata, *Biochim. Biophys. Acta*, 285, 414 (1972).
1418. Aloof-Hirsch, DeVries, and Berger, *Biochim. Biophys. Acta*, 154, 53 (1968).
1419. Taylor, Mitchell, and Cohen, *J. Biol. Chem.*, 247, 5928 (1972).

1420. Fujikawa, Legaz, and Davie, *Biochemistry*, 11, 4882 (1972).
1421. Radcliffe and Barton, *J. Biol. Chem.*, 247, 7735 (1972).
1422. Takagi and Konishi, *Biochim. Biophys. Acta*, 271, 363 (1972).
1423. Monahan, Rivier, Vale, Guillemin, and Burgus, *Biochim. Biophys. Res. Commun.*, 47, 551 (1972).
1424. Dutler, Coon, Kull, Vogel, Waldvogel, and Prelog, *Eur. J. Biochem.*, 22, 203 (1971).
1425. Yoch and Arnon, *J. Biol. Chem.*, 247, 4514 (1972).
1426. Shanmugam, Buchanan, and Arnon, *Biochim. Biophys. Acta*, 256, 477 (1972).
1427. Fee and Palmer, *Biochim. Biophys. Acta*, 245, 175 (1971).
1428. Gersonde, Trittelvitz, Schlaak, and Stabel, *Eur. J. Biochem.*, 22, 57 (1971).
1429. Nakamura and Kimura, *J. Biol. Chem.*, 245, 6235 (1971).
1430. Jackson, Munro, and Korner, *Biochim. Biophys. Acta*, 91, 666 (1964).
1431. Murray, Oikawa, and Kay, *Biochim. Biophys. Acta*, 175, 331 (1969).
1432. Graham, in *Glycoproteins*, Gottschalk, ed., Elsevier, Amsterdam, 1966, p. 361.
1433. Blomback, *Ark, Kem.*, 12, 99 (1958).
1434. Pisano, Finlayson, Peyton, and Nagai, *Proc. Natl. Acad. Sci. U.S.A.*, 68, 770 (1971).
1435. Gollwitzer, Timpl, Becker, and Furthmayr, *Eur. J. Biochem.*, 28, 497 (1972).
1436. Gollwitzer, Karges, Hormann, and Kuhn, *Biochim. Biophys. Acta*, 207, 445 (1970).
1437. Kazal, Amsel, Miller, and Tocantins, *Proc. Soc. Exp. Biol. Med.*, 113, 989 (1963).
1438. Marker, Budzynski, and James, *J. Biol. Chem.*, 247, 4775 (1972).
1439. Bion, Marguérie, Hudry, and Chagniel, *C.R. Acad. Sci. (D) (Paris)*, 273, 901 (1971).
1440. Whitaker, *Biochemistry*. 8, 1896 (1969).
1441. Cusanovich and Edmondson, *Biochem. Biophys. Res. Commun.*, 45, 327 (1971).
1442. D'Anna and Tollin, *Biochemistry*, 11, 1073 (1972).
1443. Zumft and Spiller, *Biochem. Biophys. Res. Commun.*, 45, 112 (1971).
1444. Wickner and Tabor, *J. Biol. Chem.*, 247, 1605 (1972).
1445. Curthoys and Rabinowitz, *J. Biol. Chem.*, 246, 6942 (1971).
1446. Welch, Buttlaire, Hersh, and Himes, *Biochim. Biophys. Acta*, 236, 599 (1971).
1447. Sanchez, Gonzalez, and Pontis, *Biochim. Biophys. Acta*, 227, 67 (1971).
1448. Olson and Marquardt, *Biochim. Biophys. Acta*, 268, 453 (1972).
1449. Mendicino, Kratowich, and Oliver, *J. Biol. Chem.*, 247, 6643 (1972).
1450. Traniello, Melloni, Pontremoli, Sia, and Horecker, *Arch. Biochem. Biophys.*, 149, 222 (1972).
1451. Fernando, Pontremoli, and Horecker, *Arch. Biochem. Biophys.*, 129, 370 (1969).
1452. Tashima, Tholey, Drummond, Bertrand, Rosenberg, and Horecker, *Arch. Biochem. Biophys.*, 149, 118 (1972).
1453. Frieden, Bock, and Alberty, *J. Am. Chem. Soc.*, 76, 2482 (1953).
1454. Loontiens, Wallenfels, and Weil, *Eur. J. Biochem.*, 14, 138 (1970).
1455. Klee and Klee, *J. Biol. Chem.*, 247, 2336 (1972).
1456. Barth, Bunnenberg, and Djerassi, *Anal. Biochem.*, 48, 471 (1972).
1457. Tang, Wolf, Caputto, and Trucco, *J. Biol. Chem.*, 234, 1174 (1959).
1458. Platt and Kasarda, *Biochim. Biophys. Acta*, 243, 407 (1971).
1459. Konieczny and Domanski, *Acta Biochim. Pol.*, 10, 325 (1963).
1460. Vodrazka, Hrkal, Kodicek, and Jandova, *Eur. J. Biochem.*, 31, 296 (1972).
1461. Amiconi, Antonini, Brunori, Formaneck, and Huber, *Eur. J. Biochem.*, 31, 52 (1972).
1462. Nashi, *Cancer Res.*, 30, 2507 (1970).
1463. Yip, Waks, and Beychok, *J. Biol. Chem.*, 247, 7237 (1972).
1464. Marshall and Pensky, *Arch. Biochem. Biophys.*, 146, 76 (1971).
1465. Kohsiyama, *Int. J. Pept. Protein Res.*, 4, 167 (1972).
1466. Swann and Hammes, *Biochemistry*, 8, 1 (1969).
1467. Kay and Marsh, *Biochim. Biophys. Acta*, 33, 251 (1959).
1468. D'Anna, Jr. and Tollin, *Biochemistry*, 11, 1073 (1972).
1469. Legler, von Radloff, and Kempfle, *Biochim. Biophys. Acta*, 257, 40 (1971).
1470. Legler, *Hoppe-Seyler's Z. Physiol. Chem.*, 348, 1359 (1967).

1471. Malcolm, *Hoppe-Seyler's Z. Physiol. Chem.*, 352, 883 (1971).
1472. Smith, Langdon, Piszkiewicz, Brattin, Langley, and Melamed, *Proc. Natl. Acad. Sci. U.S.A.*, 67, 724 (1970).
1473. Winnacker and Barker, *Biochim. Biophys. Acta*, 212, 225 (1970).
1474. Egan and Dalziel, *Biochim. Biophys. Acta*, 250, 47 (1971).
1475. Sund and Akeson, *Biochem. Z.*, 340, 421 (1964).
1476. Miller and Stadtman, *J. Biol. Chem.*, 247, 7407 (1972).
1477. Roberts, Holcenberg, and Dolowy., *J. Biol. Chem.*, 247, 84 (1972).
1478. Stahl and Jaenicke, *Eur. J. Biochem.*, 29, 401 (1972).
1479. Cooper and Meister, *Biochemistry*, 11, 661 (1972).
1480. Orlowski and Meister, *J. Biol. Chem.*, 246, 7095 (1971).
1481. Ida and Morita, *Agr. Biol. Chem.*, 35, 1542 (1971).
1482. Wu, Cluskey, Krull, and Friedman, *Can. J. Biochem.*, 49, 1042 (1971).
1483. Jaenicke, in *Pyridine Nucleotide-dependent Dehydrogenases*, Sund, ed., Springer-Verlag, Berlin, 1970, p. 70.
1484. Malhotra and Bernhard, *J. Biol. Chem.*, 243, 1243 (1968).
1485. Aune and Timasheff, *Biochemistry*, 9, 1481 (1970).
1486. D'Alessio and Josse, *J. Biol. Chem.*, 246, 4326 (1971).
1487. Ross, Curry, Schwartz, and Fondy, *Arch. Biochem. Biophys.*, 145, 591 (1971).
1488. White, III and Kaplan, *J. Biol. Chem.*, 244, 6031 (1969).
1489. Barel, Tumeer, and Dolmans, *Eur. J. Biochem.*, 30, 26 (1972).
1490. Frigerio and Harbury, *J. Biol. Chem.*, 231, 135 (1958).
1491. Tamm and Horsfall, *J. Exp. Med.*, 95, 71 (1952).
1492. Maxfield, *Arch. Biochem. Biophys.*, 85, 382 (1959).
1493. Fletcher, Neuberger, and Ratcliffe, *Biochem. J.*, 120, 417 (1970).
1494. Frot-Coutaz, Louisot, and Got, *Biochim. Biophys. Acta*, 264, 362 (1972).
1495. Nisselbaum and Bemfeld, *J. Am. Chem. Soc.*, 78, 687 (1965).
1496. Li and Li, *J. Biol. Chem., Soc.*, 245, 825 (1970).
1497. Patrito and Martin, *Hoppe-Seyler's Z. Physiol. Chem.*, 352, 89 (1971).
1498. Ryan and Westphal, *J. Biol. Chem.*, 247, 4050 (1972).
1499. Heimburger, Haupt, Kranz, and Baudner, *Hoppe-Seyler's Z. Physiol. Chem.*, 353, 1133 (1972).
1500. Iwasaki and Schmid, *J. Biol. Chem.*, 245, 1814 (1970).
1501. Haupt, Baudner, Kranz, and Heimburger, *Eur. J. Biochem.*, 23, 242 (1971).
1502. Boenisch and Alper, *Biochim. Biophys. Acta*, 221, 529 (1970).
1503. Labat, Ishiguro, Fujisaki, and Schmid, *J. Biol. Chem.*, 244, 4975 (1969).
1503a. Kredich, Keenan, and Foote, *J. Biol. Chem.*, 247, 7157 (1972).
1503b. Schwartz, Pizzo, Hill, and McKee, *J. Biol. Chem.*, 248, 1395 (1973).
1503c. Haupt, Heimburger, Kranz, and Boudner, *Hoppe-Seyler's Z. Physiol. Chem.*, 353, 1841 (1972).
1503d. Boenisch and Alper, *Biochim. Biophys. Acta*, 214, 135 (1970).
1503e. Marr, Neuberger, and Ratcliffe, *Biochem. J.*, 122, 623 (1971).
1503f. Rambhar and Ramachandran, *Indian J. Biochem. Biophys.*, 9, 21 (1972).
1503g. Waks, Kahn, and Beychok, *Biochem. Biophys. Res. Commun.*, 45, 1232 (1971).
1504. Huprikar and Sohonie, *Enzymologia*, 28, 333 (1965).
1505. Dahlgren, Porath, and Lindahl-Kiessling, *Arch. Biochem. Biophys.*, 37, 306 (1970).
1506. Howard and Sage, *Biochemistry*, 8, 2436 (1969).
1507. Howard, Sage, Stein, Yound, Leon, and Dyckes, *J. Biol. Chem.*, 246, 1590 (1971).
1508. Garbett, Darnall, Klotz, and Williams, *Arch. Biochem. Biophys.*, 135, 419 (1969).
1509. Makino, *J. Biochem. (Tokyo)*, 70, 149 (1971).
1510. Giamberardino, *Arch. Biochem. Biophys.*, 118, 273 (1967).
1511. Bannister and Wood, *Comp. Biochem. Physiol.*, B40, 7 (1971).
1512. Nickerson and Van Holde, *Comp. Biochem. Physiol.*, B39, 855 (1971).
1513. Wittenberg, Briehl, and Wittenberg, *Biochem. J.*, 96, 363 (1965).
1514. Wittenberg, Wittenberg, and Noble, *J. Biol. Chem.*, 247, 4008 (1971).
1515. Wittenberg, Ozazaki, and Wittenberg, *Biochim. Biophys. Acta*, 111, 485 (1965).
1516. Figueiredo, Gomez, Heneine, Santos, and Hargreaves, *Comp. Biochem. Physiol.*, B44, 481 (1973).

1517. Seamonds, Forster, and George, *J. Biol. Chem.*, 246, 5391 (1971).
1518. Terwilliger and Read, *Comp. Biochem. Physiol.*, 36, 339 (1970).
1519. Yamaguchi, Kochiyama, Hashimoto, and Matsuura, *Bull. Jpn. Soc. Sci. Fish.*, 28, 184 (1962).
1520. Yamaguchi, Kochiyama, Hashimoto, and Matsuura, *Bull. Jpn. Soc. Sci. Fish.*, 29, 174 (1963).
1521. Buhler, *J. Biol. Chem.*, 238, 1665 (1963).
1522. Mohr, Scheler, Schumann, and Muller, *Eur. J. Biochem.*, 3, 158 (1967).
1523. Boyer, Hathaway, Pascasio, Bordley, Orton, and Naughton, *J. Biol. Chem.*, 242, 2211 (1967).
1524. Babul and Stellwagen, *Anal. Biochem.*, 28, 216 (1969).
1525. Inada, Kurozumi, and Shibata, *Arch. Biochem. Biophys.*, 93, 30 (1961).
1526. Herskovits, Gabegbeku, and Jzillet, *J. Biol. Chem.*, 245, 2588 (1970).
1527. Mayer and Miller, *Anal. Biochem.*, 36, 91 (1970).
1528. Javahezian and Beychok, *J. Mol. Biol.*, 37, 1 (1968).
1529. Herskovits, *Arch. Biochem. Biophys.*, 130, 19 (1969).
1530. Malchy and Dixon, *Can. J. Biochem.*, 48, 192 (1970).
1531. Sidwell, Munch, Guzman Barron, and Hogness, *J. Biol. Chem.*, 123, 335 (1938).
1532. Jones and Schroeder, *Biochemistry*, 2, 1357 (1963).
1533. Olson and Gibson, *J. Biol. Chem.*, 246, 5241 (1971).
1534. Allis and Steinhardt, *Biochemistry*, 9, 2286 (1970).
1535. Antonini, Brunori, Caputo, Chiancone, Rossi-Fanelli, and Wyman, *Biochim. Biophys. Acta*, 79, 284 (1964).
1536. Beaven, Hoch, and Holiday, *Biochem. J.*, 49, 374 (1951).
1537. Itano, Fogarty, Jr., and Alford, *Am. J. Clin. Pathol.*, 55, 135 (1971).
1538. Morningstar, Williams, and Suutarinen, *Am. J. Clin. Pathol.*, 46, 603 (1966).
1539. Zettner and Mensch, *Am. J. Clin. Pathol.*, 49, 196 (1968).
1540. Tentori, Vivaldi, and Salvati, *Clin. Chim. Acta*, 14, 276 (1966).
1541. Sugita and Yoneyama, *J. Biol. Chem.*, 246, 389 (1971).
1542. Bucci and Fronticelli, *J. Biol. Chem.*, 240, PC 551 (1965).
1543. DeBruin and Bucci, *J. Biol. Chem.*, 246, 5228 (1971).
1544. Bucci and Fronticelli, *Biochim. Biophys. Acta*, 243, 170 (1971).
1545. Waterman and Yonetani, *J. Biol. Chem.*, 245, 5842 (1970).
1546. Oshino, Asakura, Tamura, Oshino, and Chance, *Biochem. Biophys. Res. Commun.*, 46, 1055 (1972).
1547. Seery, Hathaway, and Eberhard, *Arch. Biochem. Biophys.*, 150, 269 (1972).
1548. Chou and Wilson, *Arch. Biochem. Biophys.*, 151, 48 (1972).
1549. Easterby and Rosemeyer, *Eur. J. Biochem.*, 28, 241 (1972).
1550. Klee, *J. Biol. Chem.*, 247, 1398 (1972).
1551. Wickett, Li, and Isenberg, *Biochemistry*, 11, 2952 (1972).
1552. Pieri and Kergueris, *C. R. Acad. Sci., Paris*, 2740, 2366 (1973).
1553. Mori and Hollands, *J. Biol. Chem.*, 246, 7223 (1971).
1554. Bewley and Li, *Arch. Biochem. Biophys.*, 144, 589 (1971).
1555. Donini, Puzzuoli, D'Alessio, and Donini, in *Pharmacology of Hormonal Polypeptides and Proteins*, Beck, Martini, and Paoletti, eds., Plenum Press, New York, 1968, p. 229.
1556. Bewley and Li, *Biochemistry*, 11, 927 (1972).
1557. Bewley, Brovetto-Cruz, and Li, *Biochemistry*, 8, 4701 (1969).
1558. Shome and Friesen, *Endocrinology*, 89, 631 (1971).
1559. Bewley and Li, *Biochemistry*, 11, 884 (1972).
1560. Ma, Brovetto-Cruz, and Li, *Biochemistry*, 9, 2302 (1970).
1561. Bewley, Sairam, and Li, *Biochemistry*, 11, 932 (1971).
1562. Woodhead, O'Riordan, Keutmann, Stolz, Dawson, Niall, Robinson, and Potts, Jr., *Biochemistry*, 10, 2787 (1971).
1563. Bewley and Li, *Int. J. Protein Res.*, 1, 117 (1969).
1564. Jackson and Lovenberg, *J. Biol. Chem.*, 246, 4280 (1971).
1565. Gerstner and Pfeil, *Hoppe-Seyler's Z. Physiol. Chem.*, 353, 271 (1972).
1566. Comeil and Wofsy, *Immunochemistry*, 4, 183 (1967).
1567. PoUet, Rossi, and Edelhoch, *J. Biol. Chem.*, 247, 5921 (1972).
1568. Anders Karlsson, Peterson, and Berggard, *J. Biol. Chem.*, 247, 1065 (1972).
1569. Barth, Bunnenberg, and Djerassi, *Anal. Biochem.*, 48, 471 (1972).
1570. Evans, Herron, and Goldstein, *J. Immunol.*, 101, 915 (1968).
1571. Grey, Abel, and Zimmerman, *Ann. N.Y. Acad. Sci.*, 190, 37 (1972).
1572. Kochwa, Terry, Capra, and Yang, *Ann. N.Y. Acad. Sci.*, 190, 49 (1971).
1573. Kaygorodova and Kaversneva, *Mol. Biol. USSR*, 1, 224 (1967); cited in Egaroy, Chernyak, Dunaevsky, Gavrilova, and Moiseev, *Immunochemistry*, 8, 157 (1971).
1574. Stevenson and Dorrington, *Biochem. J.*, 118, 703 (1970).
1575. O'Daly and Cebra, in *Protides of the Biological Fluids*, Peeters, ed., Pergamon Press, New York, 1969, p. 205.
1576. Levine and Levytska, *J. Immunol.*, 102, 647 (1969).
1577. Painter, Sage, and Tanford, *Biochemistry*, 11, 1327 (1972).
1578. Underdown, Simms, and Eisen, *Biochemistry*, 10, 4359 (1971).
1579. Weintraub and Schlamowitz, *Comp. Biochem. Physiol.*, B38, 513 (1971).
1580. Helms and Allen, *Comp. Biochem. Physiol.*, B38, 439 (1971).
1581. Reynolds and Johnson, *Biochemistry*, 10, 2821 (1971).
1582. Butler, *Biochim Biophys. Acta*, 251, 435 (1971).
1583. Narayana, Shurpalekab, and Sundarvalli, *Indian J. Biochem.*, 7, 241 (1970).
1584. Vidal and Stoppani, *Arch. Biochim. Biophys.*, 147, 66 (1971).
1585. Kiyohara, Iwasaki, and Yoshikawa, *J. Biochem.* (Tokyo), 73, 89 (1972).
1586. Iwasaki, Kiyohara, and Yoshikawa, *J. Biochem.* (Tokyo), 70, 817 (1971).
1587. Chu and Chi, *Sci. Sin.*, 14, 1441 (1965).
1588. Markussen, *Int. J. Protein Res.*, 3, 201 (1971).
1589. Brandenberg, Gattner, and Wollmer, *Hoppe-Seyler's Z. Physiol. Chem.*, 353, 599 (1972).
1590. Holdsworth, *Biochim. Biophys. Acta*, 51, 295 (1961).
1591. Illingworth, *Biochem. J.*, 129, 1119 (1972).
1592. Sanderman, Jr., and Strominger, *J. Biol. Chem.*, 247, 5123 (1972).
1593. Kutzbach and Schmidt-Kastner, *Hoppe-Seyler's Z. Physiol. Chem.*, 353, 1099 (1972).
1594. Fielder, Muller, and Werle, *Fed. Eur. Biochem. Soc. Lett.*, 22, 1 (1972).
1595. Crewther, Fraser, Lennox, and Lindley, *Adv. Protein Chem.*, 20, 191 (1965).
1596. Gillespie, *Comp. Biochem. Physiol.*, B41, 723 (1972).
1597. Barel, Prieels, Maes, Looze, and Leonis, *Biochim. Biophys. Acta*, 257, 288 (1972).
1598. Cowbum, Brew, and Gratzer, *Biochemistry*, 11, 1228 (1972).
1599. Dagleish and Peacocke, *Biochem. J.*, 125, 155 (1971).
1600. Apella and Markert, *Biochem. Biophys. Res. Commun.*, 6, 171 (1961).
1601. Thuwissen, Masson, Osinski, and Heremans, *Eur. J. Biochem.*, 31, 239 (1972).
1602. Masson, *La Lactoferrine*, Arsica, Brussels, Paris, 1970.
1603. Aisen and Leibman, *Biochim. Biophys. Acta*, 257, 314 (1972).
1604. Berrens and Bleumink, *Int. Arch. Allergy*, 28, 150 (1965).
1605. Trayer and Hill, *J. Biol. Chem.*, 246, 6666 (1971).
1606. Peive, Atanasov, Zhiznevskaya, and Krasnobaeva, *Dokl. Akad. Nauk SSR Biochem. Sect. (Transl.)*, 202, 39 (1972).
1607. Atanasov, Bulgarian Academy of Sciences, Bulgaria, submitted.
1608. Soda, Misono, Mori, and Sakato, *Biochem. Biophys. Res. Commun.*, 44, 931 (1971).
1609. Garner, Jr. and Smith, *J. Biol. Chem.*, 247, 561 (1972).
1610. Edelstein, Lim, and Scanu, *J. Biol. Chem.*, 247, 5842 (1972).
1611. Scanu, Lim, and Edelstein, *J. Biol. Chem.*, 247, 5850 (1972).
1612. Smith, Dawson, and Tanford, *J. Biol. Chem.*, 247, 3376 (1972).
1613. Dejmal and Brookes, *J. Biol. Chem.*, 247, 869 (1972).
1614. Christopher, Pistorius, and Axelrod, *Biochim. Biophys. Acta*, 198, 12 (1970).
1615. Bellisario, Spencer, and Cormier, *Biochemistry*, 11, 2256 (1972).
1616. Webster, *Biochim. Biophys. Acta*, 207, 371 (1970).
1617. Bradshaw and Deranleau, *Biochemistry*, 9, 3310 (1970).
1618. Kravchenko and Lapuk, *Biokhimia*, 34, 832 (1969).
1619. Davies, Neuberger, and Wilson, *Biochim. Biophys. Acta*, 178, 294 (1969).
1620. Blake, Johnson, Mair, North, Phillips, and Sarma, *Proc Roy. Soc. Lond. (Biol.)*, 167, 378 (1967).
1621. Donovan, Davis, and White, *Biochim. Biophys. Acta*, 270, 190 (1970).
1622. Roxby and Tanford, *Biochemistry*, 10, 3348 (1971).

1623. Ehrenpreis and Warner, *Arch Biochem. Biophys.*, 61, 38 (1956).

1624. Lin and Koshland, *J. Biol. Chem.*, 244, 505 (1969).

1625. Teichberg, Kay, and Sharon, *Eur. J. Biochem.*, 16, 55 (1970).

1626. Hayashi, Imoto, Funatsu, and Funatsu, *J. Biochem.*, *(Tokyo)*, 58, 227 (1965).

1627. Franek and Pechan, *Scr. Fac. Sci. Nat. Ujep. Brunensis Chem.*, 1, 67 (1971).

1628. Riblet and Herzenberg, *Science*, 168, 45 (1970).

1629. Barel, Prieels, Maes, Looze, and Leonis, *Biochim. Biophys. Acta*, 257, 288 (1972).

1630. Fawcett, Limbird, Oliver, and Borders, *Can. J. Biochem.*, 49, 816 (1971).

1631. Latovitzki, Halper, and Beychok, *J. Biol. Chem.*, 246, 1457 (1971).

1632. Parry, Jr., Chandan, and Shahani, *Arch. Biochem. Biophys.*, 130, 59 (1969).

1633. Cowburn, Brew, and Gratzer, *Biochemistry*, 11, 1228 (1972).

1634. Mitchell and Hash, *J. Biol. Chem.*, 244, 17 (1969).

1635. Greene, Damian, and Hubbard, *Biochim. Biophys. Acta*, 236, 659 (1971).

1636. Humphries, Rohrbach, and Harrison, *Biochem. Biophys. Res. Commun.*, 50, 493 (1973).

1637. Allen, *Eur. J. Biochem.*, 35, 338 (1973).

1638. Yamaguchi, Tokushige, and Katsuki, *J. Biochem. (Tokyo)*, 73, 169 (1973).

1639. Saita, Ikenaka, and Mutsushima, *J. Biochem. (Tokyo)*, 70, 827 (1971).

1640. Vachek and Wood, *Biochim. Biophys. Acta*, 258, 133 (1972).

1641. Heazlitt, Conway, and Montag, *Biochim. Biophys. Acta.* 317, 316 (1973).

1642. Lymn and Taylor, *Biochemistry*, 10, 4617 (1971).

1643. Weser, Donay, and Rupp, *FEBS Lett.*, 32, 171 (1973).

1644. Hirata, Nakazawa, Nozaki, and Hayaishi, *J. Biol. Chem.*, 246, 5882 (1971).

1645. Kuma and Inomata, *J. Biol. Chem.*, 247, 556 (1972).

1646. Oh and Conrad, *Arch. Biochem. Biophys.*, 146, 525 (1971).

1647. Morris, Martenson, Deibler, and Cagan, *J. Biol. Chem.*, 248, 534 (1973).

1648. Tamura, Asakura, and Yonetani, *Biochim. Biophys. Acta*, 295, 467 (1973).

1649. Tamura, Woodrow, and Yonetani, *Biochim. Biophys. Acta*, 317, 34 (1973).

1650. Goldbloom and Brown, *Arch. Biochem. Biophys.*, 147, 367 (1971).

1651. Deconinck, Peiffer, Schnek, and Leonis, *Biochimie*, 54, 969 (1972).

1652. Bolard and Gamier, *Biochim. Biophys. Acta*, 263, 535 (1972).

1653. Harrington and Himmilfarb, *Biochemistry*, 11, 2945 (1972).

1654. Kakol, *Biochem. J.*, 125, 261 (1972).

1655. Katoh, Kubo, and Takahashi, *J. Biochem. (Tokyo)*, 74, 771 (1973).

1656. Bjorkman and Janson, *Biochim. Biophys. Acta*, 276, 508 (1972).

1657. Suhara, Ikeda, Takemori, and Katagiri, *FEBS Lett.*, 28, 45 (1972).

1658. Yuan, Barnett, and Anderson, *J. Biol. Chem.*, 247, 511 (1972).

1659. Siegel, Murphy, and Kamin, *J. Biol. Chem.*, 248, 251 (1973).

1660. Frazier, Hogue-Angeletti, Sherman, and Bradshaw, *Biochemistry*, 12, 328 (1973).

1661. Angeletti, *Biochim. Biophys. Acta*, 214, 478 (1970).

1662. Pearce, Banks, Banthorpe, Berry, Davies, and Vernon, *Eur. J. Biochem.*, 29, 417 (1972).

1663. Kopeyan, vanRietschoten, Martinez, Rochat, and Miranda, *Eur. J. Biochem.*, 35, 244 (1973).

1664. Karlsson, Eaker, and Ponterius, *Biochim. Biophys. Acta*, 257, 235 (1972).

1665. Karlsson, Eaker, and Ryden, *Toxicon*, 10, 405 (1972).

1666. Iwasaki and Matsubara, *J. Biochem. (Tokyo)*, 71, 645 (1972).

1667. Prakash and Sadana, *Arch. Biochem. Biophys.*, 148, 614 (1972).

1668. Zumft, *Biochim. Biophys. Acta*, 276, 363 (1972).

1669. Burns and Hardy, *Methods Enzymol.*, 24B, 480 (1972).

1670. Eady, Smith, Cook, and Postgate, *Biochem. J.*, 128, 655 (1972).

1671. Luisi, Olomucki, Baici, and Karlovic, *Biochemistry*, 12, 4100 (1973).

1672. Marshall and Cohen, *J. Biol. Chem.*, 247, 1641 (1972).

1673. Marcais, Nicot, and Moretti, *Bull. Soc. Chim. Biol.*, 52, 741 (1970).

1674. Joniau, Bloemmen, and Lontie, *Biochim. Biophys. Acta*, 214, 468 (1970).

1675. Berrens and Bleumink, *Int. Arch. Allergy*, 28, 150 (1965).

1676. Holt and Creeth, *Biochem. J.*, 129, 665 (1972).

1677. Willumsen, *C.R. Trav. Lab. Carlsberg*, 36, 247 (1967).

1678. Ifft, *C.R. Trav. Lab. Carlsberg*, 38, 315 (1971).

1679. Babul and Stellwagen, *Anal. Biochem.*, 28, 216 (1969).

1680. Ketterber, *Biochem. J.*, 96, 372 (1965).

1681. Barth, Bunnenberg, and Djerassi, *Anal. Biochem.*, 48, 471 (1972).

1682. Davis, Zahnley, and Donovan, *Biochemistry*, 8, 2044 (1966).

1683. Kay, Strickland, and Billups, *J. Biol. Chem.*, 249, 797 (1974).

1684. Sjoberg, and Feeney, *Biochim. Biophys. Acta*, 168, 79 (1968).

1685. Warner and Weber, *J. Biol. Chem.*, 191, 173 (1951).

1686. Rhodes, Azari, and Feeney, *J. Biol. Chem.*, 230, 399 (1958).

1687. Azari, and Phillips, *Arch. Biochem. Biophys.*, 138, 32 (1970).

1688. Azari, and Baugh, *Arch. Biochem. Biophys.*, 118, 138 (1967).

1689. Weintraub, Vincent, Baulieu, and Alfsen, *FEBS Lett.*, 37, 82 (1973).

1690. Jolley, Evans, Makino, and Mason, *J. Biol. Chem.*, 249, 335 (1974).

1691. Darby, *J. Biol. Chem.*, 139, 721 (1941).

1692. Lauwers, in *West European Symposium on Clininical Chemistry – Symposium on Enzymes in Clinical Chemistry*, Ruyssen and Vandendriessche, eds., Elsevier, New York, 1965, p. 19.

1693. Piront and Gerday, *Comp. Biochem. Physiol.*, 46B, 349 (1973).

1694. Pechere, Capony, and Ryden, *Eur. J. Biochem.*, 23, 421 (1971).

1695. Parello and Pechere, *Biochimie*, 53, 1079 (1971).

1696. Jones and Hofmann, *Can. J. Biochem.*, 50, 1297 (1972).

1697. Glazer and Smith, *J. Biol. Chem.*, 235, PC43 (1960).

1698. Webster, *Biochim. Biophys. Acta*, 207, 371 (1970).

1699. Blumenfeld and Perlmann, *J. Gen. Physiol.*, 42, 563 (1959).

1700. Lang and Kassell, *Biochemistry*, 10, 2296 (1971).

1701. Mayer and Miller, *Anal. Biochem.*, 36, 91 (1970).

1702. Bohak, *J. Biol. Chem.*, 244, 4638 (1969).

1703. Meitner and Kassell, *Biochem. J.*, 121, 249 (1971).

1704. Marcinszyn, and Kassell, *J. Biol. Chem.*, 246, 6560 (1971).

1705. Kikuchi and Sakaguchi, *Agr. Biol. Chem.*, 37, 827 (1973).

1706. Temynck and Avrameas, *FEBS Lett.*, 23, 24 (1972).

1707. Herskovits, *Arch. Biochem. Biophys.*, 130, 19 (1969).

1708. Shih, Shannon, Kay, and Lew, *J. Biol. Chem.*, 246, 4546 (1971).

1709. Roman and Dunford, *Biochemistry*, 11, 2076 (1972).

1710. Paul and Stigbrand, *Acta Chem. Scand.*, 24, 3607 (1970).

1711. Ohlsson and Paul, *Biochim. Biophys. Acta*, 315, 293 (1973).

1712. Morita and Yoshida, *Agr. Biol. Chem.*, 34, 590 (1970).

1713. Ex-Fekih and Kertesz, *Bull. Soc. Chim. Biol.*, 50, 547 (1968).

1714. Stelmaszynska and Zgliczynski, *Eur. J. Biochem.*, 19, 56 (1971).

1715. Neujahr and Gaal, *Eur. J. Biochem.*, 35, 386 (1973).

1716. Havir and Hanson, *Biochemistry*, 12, 1583 (1973).

1717. Fisher, Kirkwood, and Kaufman, *J. Biol. Chem.*, 247, 5161 (1972).

1718. Huang, Max, and Kaufman, *J. Biol. Chem.*, 248, 4235 (1973).

1719. Hulett-Cowling and Campbell, *Biochemistry*, 10, 1364 (1971).

1720. Yoshizumi and Coleman, *Arch. Biochem. Biophys.*, 160, 255 (1974).

1721. Halford, Benneti, Trentham, and Gutfreund, *Biochem. J.*, 114, 243 (1969).

1722. Taylor, Lau, Applebury, and Coleman, *J. Biol. Chem.*, 248, 6216 (1973).

1723. Glew and Heath, *J. Biol. Chem.*, 246, 1556 (1971).

1724. Igarashi, Takahashi, and Tsuyama, *Biochim. Biophys. Acta*, 220, 85 (1970).

1725. Igarashi and Hollander, *J. Biol. Chem.*, 243, 6084 (1968).

1726. Uehara, Fujimoto, and Taniguchi, *J. Biochem. (Tokyo)*, 70, 183 (1971).

1727. Jacobs, Nyc, and Brown, *J. Biol. Chem.*, 246, 1419 (1971).

1728. Shimada and Sugino, *Biochim. Biophys. Acta*, 185, 367 (1969).

1729. Cannata, *J. Biol. Chem.*, 245, 792 (1970).

1730. Smith, *J. Biol. Chem.*, 246, 4234 (1971).

1731. Wohl and Markus, *J. Biol. Chem.*, 237, 5785 (1972).

1732. Maeba and Sanwal, *J. Biol. Chem.*, 244, 2549 (1969).

1733. Kopperschlager, Lorenz, Diezel, Marquardt, and Hofmann, *Acta Biol. Med. Ger.*, 29, 561 (1972).

1734. Najjar, in *The Enzymes* Vol. 6, Boyer, Lardy, and Myrbach, eds., Academic Press, New York, 1962, p. 161.

1735. Filmer and Koshland, *Biochim. Biophys. Acta*, 77, 334 (1963).

1736. Hirose, Sugimoto, and Chiba, *Biochim. Biophys. Acta*, 250, 514 (1971).

1737. Silverberg and Dalziel, *Eur. J. Biochem.*, 38, 229 (1973).

1738. Tsuboi, Fukunaga, and Chervenka, *J. Biol. Chem.*, 246, 7586 (1971).
1739. Krietsch and Bucher, *Eur. J. Biochem.*, 17, 568 (1970).
1740. Scopes, *Biochem. J.*, 113, 551 (1969).
1741. Scopes, *Biochem. J.*, 122, 89 (1971).
1742. Sasaki, Sugimoto, and Chiba, *Biochim. Biophys. Acta*, 227, 584 (1971).
1743. James, Hurst, and Flynn, *Can. J. Biochem.*, 49, 1183 (1971).
1744. Kawauchi, Iwanaga, Samejima, and Suzuki, *Biochim. Biophys. Acta*, 236, 142 (1971).
1745. Janssen, deBruin, and Haas, *Eur. J. Biochem.*, 28, 156 (1972).
1746. Boman, *Ark. Kem.* 12, 453 (1958).
1747. Felenbok, *Eur. J. Biochem.*, 17, 165 (1970).
1748. Rutner, *Biochemistry*, 9, 178 (1970).
1749. Hartman, *J. Biol. Chem.*, 238, 3024 (1963).
1750. Blasi, Aloj, and Goldberger, *Biochemistry*, 10, 1409 (1971).
1751. Sevilla and Fischer, *Biochemistry*, 8, 2161 (1969).
1752. Kamogawa and Fukui, *Biochim. Biophys. Acta*, 242, 55 (1971).
1753. Cohen, Duewer, and Fischer, *Biochemistry*, 10, 2683 (1971).
1754. Fosset, Muir, Nielsen, and Fischer, *Biochemistry*, 10, 4105 (1971).
1755. Assaf and Yunis, *Biochemistry*, 12, 1423 (1973).
1756. Assaf and Graves, *J. Biol. Chem.*, 244, 5544 (1969).
1757. Kamogawa, Fukui, and Nikuni *J. Biochem. (Tokyo)*, 63, 361 (1968).
1758. Cohen, *Eur. J. Biochem.*, 34, 1 (1972).
1759. Hayakawa, Perkins, Walsh, and Krebs, *Biochemistry*, 12, 567 (1973).
1760. Mano and Yoshida, *J. Biochem. (Tokyo)*, 66, 105 (1969).
1761. Walinder, *Biochim. Biophys. Acta*, 258, 411 (1972).
1762. Glazer, Fang, and Brown, *J. Biol. Chem.*, 248, 5679 (1973).
1763. Maccoll, Habig, and Berns, *J. Biol. Chem.*, 248, 7080 (1973).
1764. Glazer and Fang, *J. Biol. Chem.*, 248, 659 (1973).
1765. Boucher, Crespi, and Katz, *Biochemistry*, 5, 3796 (1968).
1766. Kao, Berns, and Town, *Biochem. J.*, 131, 39 (1973).
1767. Anderson, Jenner, and Mumford, *Biochim. Biophys. Acta*, 221, 69 (1970).
1768. Tobin and Briggs, *Photochem. Photobiol.*, 18, 487 (1973).
1769. Bourrillon and Font, *Biochim. Biophys. Acta*, 154, 28 (1968).
1770. Berrens and Maesen, *Clin. Exp. Immunol.*, 10, 383 (1972).
1771. Kochiyama, Yamaguchi, Hashimoto, and Matsuura, *Bull. Jpn. Soc. Sci. Fish.*, 32, 867 (1966).
1772. Sjoholm, Wiman, and Wallen, *Eur. J. Biochem.*, 39, 471 (1973).
1773. Wallen and Wiman, *Biochim. Biophys. Acta*, 221, 20 (1970).
1774. Ramshaw, Brown, Scawen, and Boulter, *Biochim. Biophys. Acta*, 303, 269 (1973).
1775. Katoh, Shiratori, and Takamiya, *J. Biochem. (Tokyo)*, 51, 32 (1962).
1776. Milne and Wells, *J. Biol. Chem.*, 245, 1566 (1970).
1777. Klee, *J. Biol. Chem.*, 244, 2558 (1969).
1778. Yurewicz, Ghalambor, Duckworth, and Heath, *J. Biol. Chem.*, 246, 5607 (1971).
1779. Treffry and Ainsworth, *Biochem. J.*, 137, 319 (1974).
1780. Cejka and Fleischmann, *Arch. Biochem. Biophys.*, 157, 168 (1973).
1781. Heide, Haupt, and Schultze, *Nature*, 201, 1218 (1964).
1782. Peterson, *J. Biol. Chem.*, 246, 34 (1971).
1783. Schultze, Schonenberger, and Schwick, *Biochem. Z.*, 328, 267 (1956).
1784. Raz and Goodman, *J. Biol. Chem.*, 244, 3230 (1969).
1785. Seal and Doe, in *Proceedings of the 2nd Internatial Congress Endocrinology*, Vol. 19, Sect. 3, Part 1, Excerpta Medica, Amsterdam, 1964, p. 229.
1786. Schultze and Heremans, *Molecular Biology of Human Proteins*, Vol. 1, Elsevier, Amsterdam, 1966, p. 234.
1787. Tritsch, *J. Med. (Basel)*, 3, 129 (1972).
1788. Oppenheimer, Surks, Smith, and Squef, *J. Biol. Chem.*, 240, 173 (1965).
1789. Vahlquist and Peterson, *Biochemistry*, 11, 4526 (1972).
1790. Jaarsveld, Branch, Robbins, Morgan, Kanda, and Canfield, *J. Biol. Chem.*, 248, 7898 (1973).
1791. Stratil, *Animal Blood Groups Biochem. Genet.*, 3, 63 (1972).
1792. Ashida, *Arch. Biochem. Biophys.*, 144, 749 (1973).
1793. Van der Wei, *FEBS Lett.*, 21, 88 (1972).
1794. Behnke and Vallee, *Fed. Proc.*, 31, 435 (1972).
1795. Gates and Travis, *Biochemistry*, 12, 1867 (1973).
1796. Lacko and Neurath, *Biochemistry*, 9, 4680 (1970).
1797. Uren and Neurath, *Biochemistry*, 11, 4483 (1972).
1798. Reeck and Neurath, *Biochemistry*, 11, 3947 (1972).
1799. Gertler and Birk, *Eur. J. Biochem.*, 12, 170 (1970).
1800. Uram and Lamy, *Biochim. Biophys. Acta*, 194, 102 (1969).
1801. Lea, *Biochim. Biophys. Acta*, 317, 351 (1973).
1802. Frank, Veros, and Pekar, *Biochemistry*, 11, 4926 (1972).
1803. Markussen, *Int. J. Protein Res.*, 3, 201 (1971).
1804. Dixon, Schmidt, and Pankov, *Arch. Biochem. Biophys.*, 141, 705 (1970).
1805. Murao, Funakoshi, and Oda, *Agr. Biol. Chem.*, 36, 1327 (1972).
1806. Tsuru, Hattori, Tsuji, and Fukumoto, *J. Biochem. (Tokyo)*, 67, 15 (1970).
1807. Sodek and Hofmann, *Methods Enzymol.*, 19, 372 (1970).
1808. Oda, Kamada, and Murao, *Agr. Biol. Chem.*, 36, 1103 (1972).
1809. McDowell, *Eur. J. Biochem.*, 14, 214 (1970).
1810. Sekine, *Agr. Biol. Chem.*, 36, 198 (1972).
1811. Yoshimoto, Fukumoto, and Tsuru, *Int. J. Protein Res.*, 3, 285 (1971).
1812. Tsuru, Yoshimoto, Yoshida, Kira, and Fukumoto, *Int. J. Protein Res.*, 2, 75 (1970).
1813. Shinano and Fukushima, *Agr. Biol. Chem.*, 33, 1236 (1969).
1814. Levy, Fishman, and Schenkein, *Methods Enzymol.*, 19, 672 (1970).
1815. Jurasek and Whitaker, *Can. J. Biochem.*, 43, 1955 (1965).
1816. Kaplan and Whitaker, *Can. J. Biochem.*, 47, 305 (1969).
1817. Paterson and Whitaker, *Can. J. Biochem.*, 47, 317 (1969).
1818. Sauer and Senft, *Comp. Biochem. Physiol.*, 42B, 205 (1972).
1819. Merkel and Sipos, *Arch. Biochem. Biophys.*, 145, 126 (1971).
1820. Siegel, Brady, and Awad, *J. Biol. Chem.*, 247, 4155 (1972).
1821. Liu, Neumann, Elliott, Moore, and Stein, *J. Biol. Chem.*, 238, 251 (1963).
1822. Hata, Hayashi, and Doi, *Agr. Biol. Chem.*, 31, 357 (1967).
1823. Aibard, Hayashi, and Hata, *Agr. Biol. Chem.*, 35, 658 (1971).
1824. Hiramatsu and Ouchi, *J. Biochem. (Tokyo)*, 71, 676 (1972).
1825. Pangburn, Burstein, Morgan, Walsh, and Neurath, *Biochem. Biophys. Res. Commun.*, 54, 371 (1973).
1826. Van Heyningen, *Eur. J. Biochem.*, 27, 436 (1972).
1827. Nasuno and Ohara, *Agr. Biol. Chem.*, 36, 1791 (1972).
1828. Turkova, Mikes, Gancev, and Boublik, *Biochim. Biophys. Acta*, 178, 100 (1969).
1829. Gertler and Hayashi, *Biochim. Biophys. Acta*, 235, 378 (1971).
1830. Mizusawa and Yoshida, *J. Biol. Chem.*, 247, 6978 (1972).
1831. Lees, Leston, and Marfey, *J. Neurochem.*, 16, 1025 (1969).
1832. Cox and Hanahan, *Biochim. Biophys. Acta*, 207, 49 (1970).
1833. Fujisawa and Hayaishi, *J. Biol. Chem.*, 243, 2673 (1968).
1834. Ono, Nozaki, and Hayaishi, *Biochim. Biophys. Acta*, 220, 224 (1970).
1835. Berg and Prockop, *J. Biol. Chem.*, 248, 1175 (1973).
1836. DeSa, *J. Biol. Chem.*, 247, 5527 (1972).
1837. Yui, *J. Biochem. (Tokyo)*, 69, 101 (1971).
1838. Wetlaufer, *Adv. Protein Chem.*, 17, 362 (1962).
1839. Nyman and Lindskog, *Biochim. Biophys. Acta*, 85, 141 (1964).
1840. Kirschenbaum, *Anal. Biochem.*, 55, 166 (1973).

TEMPERATURE COEFFICIENTS OF APPARENT PARTIAL SPECIFIC VOLUMES OF PROTEINS EXPRESSED IN ml/g/deg (dV/dT)

Protein	Temperature Range (°C)	$dV/dT \times 10^4$	Reference
NATIVE PROTEINS			
Bovine ribonuclease	10–34	4.6	1
Bovine ribonuclease	14–30	4.64	2
Human mercaptalbumin	20–32	3.65	3
Bovine mercaptalbumin	20–32	3.65	3
Human apotransferrin	21–27.5	3.3	4
Bovine serum albumin	20–32	3.65	3
Bovine serum albumin	25–45	3.75	5
Chicken lysozyme	25–50	3.03	5
Chicken egg albumin	25–45	3.50	5
Chicken egg albumin (dry)	25–75	0.895	5
Bovine β-lactoglobulin	25–45	3.75	5
Bovine methemoglobin	25–50	3.05	5
HEAT COAGULATED PROTEINS			
Chicken egg albumin	83–30	4.04	5
Bovine serum albumin	83–30	4.12	5
Chicken lysozyme	83–35	3.00	5
Bovine methemoglobin	83–35	3.67	5
Bovine β-lactoglobulin	83–35	3.80	5

Compiled by Henry B. Bull.

References

1. Cox and Schumaker, *J. Am. Chem. Soc.*, 83, 2433 (1961).
2. Holcomb and Van Holde, *J. Phys. Chem.*, 66, 1999 (1962).
3. Hunter, *J. Phys. Chem.*, 70, 3285 (1966).
4. Hunter, *J. Phys. Chem.*, 71, 3717 (1967).
5. Bull and Breese, *Biopolymers*, 12, 2351 (1973).

Taken from the *Handbook of Biochemistry and Molecular Biology*, 3rd edn., ed. G.D. Fasman, CRC Press, Boca Raton, FL, 1976.

PROTEIN pK VALUES

Lynne H. Botelho and Frank R. N. Gurd

The general techniques for determining individual pK values in proteins usually depend on NMR,[1,2] absorption,[3] or kinetic[4] procedures. Effects of neighboring groups may be evident in chemical shift influences[5-7] or in electrostatic influences on the hydrogen ion equilibria proper.[8]

1. Markley, Finkenstadt, Dugas, Leduc, and Drapeau, *Biochemistry*, 14, 998 (1975).
2. Markley, *Acc. Chem. Res.*, 8, 70 (1975).
3. Tanford, Hanenstein, and Rands, *J. Am. Chem. Soc.*, 77, 6409 (1955).
4. Garner, Bogardt, and Gurd, *J. Biol. Chem.*, in press.
5. Sachs, Schechter, and Cohen, *J. Biol. Chem.*, 246, 6576 (1971).
6. Shrager, Cohen, Heller, Sachs, and Schechter, *Biochemistry*, 11, 541 (1972).
7. Deslauriers, McGregor, Sarantakis, and Smith, *Biochemistry*, 13, 3443 (1974).
8. Roxby and Tanford, *Biochemistry*, 10, 3348 (1971).

TABLE 1A: Specific His pK Assignments in Ribonuclease A

Protein	pK Values	Reference
Bovine		
His 12	6.3	1
His 48	5.8	1
His 73	6.4	1
His 105	6.7	1
Rat		
His 12	6.6	1
His 48	6.2	1
His 73	7.6	1
His 105	6.3	1
His 119	6.1	1

Reference

1. Migchelsen and Beintema, *J. Mol Biol.*, 79, 25 (1973).

TABLE 1B: Nonspecific His pK Values for Ribonuclease A

Protein	pK Values				Reference
Coypu	5.8	6.3	6.3	8.0	1
Chinchilla	4.9	6.0	6.1	7.2	1
Bovine	6.01	6.17	6.72	6.9	2

References

1. Migchelsen and Beintema, *J. Mol. Biol.*, 79, 25 (1973).
2. Markley, *Acc. Chem. Res.*, 8, 70 (1975).

TABLE 1C: pK Values for Histidine Residues in Myoglobin

Species	pK Observed		Reference
Sperm whale	5.37	5.33	1, 2
	5.53	5.39	
	6.34	6.21	
	6.44	6.31	
	6.65	6.55	
	6.83	6.72	
	8.05	7.97	
Horse	5.7	5.5	1, 2
	6.0	5.8	
	6.6	6.5	
	6.9	6.8	
	7.0	6.9	
	7.6	7.6	
California grey whale	5.7		2
	6.2		
	6.6		
	6.8		
	7.8		
Inia geoffrensis	5.53		2
	5.95		
	6.17		
	6.31		
	6.45		
	6.66		
	8.05		
Tursiops truncatns	5.50		2
	5.95		
	6.24		
	6.26		
	6.42		
	6.60		
	7.82		
Balaenoptera acutorostrata	5.46		2
	5.65		
	6.10		
	6.23		
	6.41		
	6.59		
	7.86		

References

1. Cohen, Hagenmaier, Pollard, and Schechter, *J. Mol. Biol.*, 71, 513 (1972).
2. Botelho, Hanania, and Gurd, unpublished observations.

TABLE 1D: Histidine pK Values in Human Hemoglobin

Hemoglobin	pK Values	Reference
Human	6.8	1, 2
	7.0	
	7.0	
	7.1	
	7.2	
	7.13	
	7.7	
	8.1	
	8.1	

References

1. Donovan, *Methods Enzymol.*, 27, 497 (1973).
2. Mandel, *Proc. Natl. Acad. Sci. U.S.A.*, 52, 736 (1964).

TABLE 1E: pK Value for Human Hb His 146 β

Protein	His 146 β pK Value	Reference
Human hemoglobin		
Deoxy, His 146 β	8.0	1
	8.1	2
	7.4	3
Human hemoglobin		
Carboxy, His 146 β	7.1	1
	6.8	2

References

1. Kilmartin, Breen, Roberts, and Ho, *Proc. Natl. Acad. Sci. U.S.A.*, 70, 1246 (1973).
2. Greenfield and Williams, *Biochim. Biophys. Acta*, 257, 187 (1972).
3. Huestis and Raftery, *Biochemistry*, 11, 1648 (1972).

TABLE 1F: Specific Histidine pK Value for Cytochrome c

Species	pK Values	Reference
Horse		
His 33	6.41	1
Yeast		
His 33	6.74	2
His 39	6.56	2

References

1. Cohen, Fisher, and Schechter, *J. Biol. Chem.*, 249, 1113 (1974).
2. Cohen and Hayes, *J. Biol. Chem.*, 249, 5472 (1974).

TABLE 1G: pK Values for Histidine Residues in Carbonic Anhydrase

Species		pK Values		Reference
Human, B	5.91	5.88	6	1–3
	6.04	6.09	6.98	
	7.00	6.93	7.23	
	7.23	7.23	8.2	
		8.2	8.24	
Human, C	5.87	5.74		2, 3
	5.96	6.43		
	6.10	6.49		
	6.20	6.5		
	6.63	6.57		
	7.20	6.63		
	7.28	7.25		

References

1. King and Roberts, *Biochemistry*, 10, 558 (1971).
2. Cohen, Yem, Kandel, Gornall, Kandell, and Friedman, *Biochemistry*, 11, 327 (1972).
3. Pesando, *Biochemistry*, 14, 675 (1975).

TABLE 1H: Histidine PK Values from Nuclease

Protein	pK Values		Reference
Staphylococcus aureus			
Foggi	5.46	5.37	1, 2
	5.76	5.71	
	5.66, 5.74, 6.54[a]	5.74	
	6.57	6.50	
Staphylococcus aureus			
V8	5.55		1
	5.80, 6.10[a]		
	6.50		

[a] pK values of one histidine existing in multiple conformational forms of the enzyme which slowly interconvert.

References

1. Markley, *Acc. Chem. Res.*, 8, 70 (1975).
2. Cohen, Shrager, McNeel, and Schechter, *Nature*, 228, 642 (1970).

TABLE 1I: Histidine pK Values in Various Proteins

Protein	Number of His resolved	pK	Specific Assignment	Reference
Adenylate kinase (pig)	2 of 2	<5.5		1
		6.3		
Chymotrypsin A$_\delta$ (cow)	1 of 2	7.2	His 57	2, 3
Chymotrypsinogen A (cow)	1 of 2	7.2	His 57	2, 3
Lysozyme				
chicken		5.8		4, 5
human		7.1		4, 6
Neurophysin II (cow)	1 of 1	6.87		7
Ovomucoid (chicken)	4 of 4	5.94		8
		6.71		
		6.75		
		8.07		
Protease				
α-Lyter (Myxobacter 495)	1 of 1	<4		9, 10
(Staphylococcus aureus, V8)	3 of 3	6.69		11
		6.85		
		7.19		
Ribonuclease T$_1$ (Aspergillus oryzae)	2 of 3	7.9		12
		8.0		
Serine esterase		6.5–7.5		13
Trypsin (pig, β form)	4 of 4	5.0		14
		6.54		
		6.66		
		7.20		
Trypsin inhibitor (soybean, Kunitz)	2 of 2	5.27		15
		7.00		

References

1. Cohn, Leigh, and Reed, *Cold Spring Harbor Symp. Quant. Biol.*, 36, 533 (1972).
2. Robillard and Shulman, *J. Mol. Biol.*, 71, 507 (1972).
3. Robillard and Shulman, *Ann. N.Y. Acad. Sci.*, 69, 599 (1972).
4. Meadows, Markley, Cohen, and Jardetsky, *Proc. Natl. Acad. Sci. U.S.A.*, 58, 1307 (1967).
5. Cohen, Hagenmaier, Pollard, and Schechter, *J. Mol. Biol.*, 71, 513 (1972).
6. Cohen, *Nature* (Lond.), 223, 43 (1969).
7. Cohen, Griffen, Camier, Caizergues, Fromageot, and Cohen, *FEBS Lett.*, 25, 282 (1972).
8. Markley, *Ann. N.Y. Acad. Sci.*, 222, 347 (1973).
9. Hunkapiller, Smallcombe, Whitaker, and Richards, *J. Biol. Chem.*, 248, 8306 (1973).
10. Hunkapiller, Smallcombe, Whitaker, and Richards, *Biochemistry*, 12, 4732 (1973).
11. Markley, Finkenstadt, Dugas, Leduc, and Drapeau, *Biochemistry*, 14, 998 (1975).
12. Riterjans and Pongs, *Eur. J. Biochem.*, 18, 313 (1971).
13. Polgar and Bender, *Proc. Natl. Acad. Sci. U.S.A.*, 69, 599 (1972).
14. Markley, *Acc. Chem. Res.*, 8, 70 (1975).
15. Markley, *Biochemistry*, 12, 2245 (1973).

TABLE 2: pK Values for α-Amino Groups in Proteins

Protein	pK' Value	Reference
Human hemoglobin		
Carboxy		
α chain	6.72	1
	6.95	2
β chain	7.05	2
Cyano		
α chain	6.74	2
β chain	6.93	2
Deoxy		
α chain	7.79	2
β chain	6.84	2
Myoglobin		
Sperm whale	7.77	2
	7.96	3
California grey whale	7.74	3
Pilot whale	7.43	3
Dall porpoise	7.22	3
Harbor seal	7.66	3
Bovine pancreatic ribonuclease A	8.14	4
Horse hemoglobin		
Oxy		
α chain	7.3	5
Deoxy		
α chain	7.7	5

References

1. Hill and Davis, *J. Biol. Chem.*, 242, 2005 (1967).
2. Garner, Bogardt, Jr., and Gurd, *J. Biol. Chem*, in press.
3. Garner, Garner, and Gurd, *J. Biol. Chem.*, 248, 5451 (1973).
4. Carty and Hirs, *J. Biol. Chem.*, 243, 5254 (1968).
5. Kilmartin and Rossi-Bernardi, *Biochem. J.*, 124, 31 (1971).

TABLE 3: pK Values for ε-Amino Groups in Proteins

Protein	pK' Value	Method	Reference
Bovine pancreatic ribonuclease A			
Lys-41	9.11	Kinetic	1
Other Lys	10.1	Kinetic	1
All Lys	10.2	Titration	2
Sperm whale myoglobin			
All Lys except one	10.6	Titration (intrinsic pK)	3
Hen egg white Lysozyme			
Lys 97	10.1	NMR	4
Lys 116	10.2		
Lys 13	10.3		
Lys 33	10.4		
Lys 1	10.6		
Lys 96	10.7		

References

1. Carty and Hirs, *J. Biol. Chem.*, 243, 5254 (1968).
2. Tanford and Hanenstein, *J. Am. Chem. Soc.*, 78, 5287 (1956).
3. Shire, Hanania, and Gurd, *Biochemistry*, 13, 2967 (1974).
4. Bradbury and Brown, *Eur. J. Biochem.*, 40, 565 (1973).

TABLE 4A: Tyrosine pK Values

Protein	No of Groups	pK	Reference
Ribonuclease A	3 of 6	9.9	1
Insulin		9.7	2
Pepsin		9.5	3
Serum albumin		10.35	3
Lysozyme		10.8	4
Trypsin inhibitor (BPTI)			
Bovine, tyrosines		10.6	5
		10.8	
		11.1	
		11.6	

References

1. Tanford, Hauenstein, and Rands, *J. Am. Chem. Soc.*, 77, 6409 (1955).
2. Tanford and Epstein, *J. Am. Chem. Soc.*, 76, 2163 (1954).
3. Tanford and Roberts, Jr., *J. Am. Chem. Soc.*, 74, 2509 (1952).
4. Fromageot and Schnek, *Biochem. Biophys. Acta*, 6, 113 (1950): Tanford and Wagner, *J. Am. Chem. Soc.*, 76, 2331 (1954).
5. Karplus, Snyder, and Sykes, *Biochemistry*, 12, 1323 (1973).

TABLE 4B: Tyrosine pK Values in Hb

Species	No. of Residues	pK	Specific Residue pK	Reference
Horse	8 of 12	10.6		1
	4 of 12	>12		
Human A	8 of 12	10.6		1
	4 of 12	>12		
Human A carboxy	8 of 12	10.60	β0145 10.6	2
			β3130 10.6	
	4 of 12	>10.6	β335 >10.6	
Human a deoxy	6 of 12	10.77		2
Human F carboxy	6 of 10	10.45		2
Human F deoxy	4 of 10	10.65		2

References

1. Hermans, Jr., *Biochemistry*, 1, 193 (1962).
2. Nagel, Ranney, and Kucinskis, *Biochemistry*, 5, 1934 (1966).

TABLE 4C: Tyrosine pK Values in Mb

Species	pK	Reference
Sperm whale	10.3	1
	11.5	
	>12.8	
Horse	10.3	1
	11.5	
	>12.8	

Reference

1. Hermans, Jr., *Biochemistry*, 1., 193 (1962).

TABLE 5: pK Values for Human Hb Cys β 93 SH

Human hemoglobin	pK	Reference
Deoxy, cys β 93 SH	>11	1
	>10	2
	>9.5	3
Carboxy, cys β 93 SH	>11	1

References

1. Janssen, Willekens, De Bruin, and van Os, *Eur. J. Biochem.*, 45, 53 (1974).
2. Snow, *Biochem. J.*, 84, 360 (1962).
3. Guidotti, *J. Biol. Chem.*, 242, 3673 (1967).

TABLE 6: Carboxyl Side Chain pK Values Estimated in Lysozymes

Residue	Range of pK Values[1]
Gin 35	6–6.5
Asp 101	4.2–4.7
Asp 66	1.5–2
Asp 52	3–4.6

Reference

1. Imoto, Johnson, North, Phillips, and Rupley, in *The Enzymes*, Vol. VII, 3rd ed. Bayer, Ed., Academic Press, New York, 1972, 665.

INTRINSIC VISCOSITY OF PROTEINS

Intrinsic viscosity of proteins in native and denatured states[a]

Protein	Native state (ml/g)	Denatured state in concentrated guanidine hydrochloride solution	
		S–S bond intact (ml/g)	S–S bond broken (ml/g)
Insulin	–	–	6.1
Ribonuclease	3.3	9.4	16.6 (16.3)
Lysozyme	2.7	6.5	17.1
Hemoglobin	3.6	–	18.9
Myoglobin	3.1	–	20.9
β-Lactoglobulin	3.4	19.1	22.8
Ovomucoid	5.5[2]	8.1[3]	16.0[3]
Ovalbumin A_1[4]	3.5	27.0	31.0
Papain[5]	3.5	–	24.5
Chymotrypsinogen	2.5	11.0	26.8
Phosphoribosyl transferase	–	–	31.9
Glyceraldehyde-3-phosphate dehydrogenase	–	–	34.5
Tropomyosin	4.5	–	33.0
Pepsinogen	–	27.2	31.5
Aldolase	4.0	–	33.5
Serum albumin	3.7	22.9	52.2
Thyroglobulin	4.7	–	82.0
Myosin	217	–	92.6
Paramyosin	103	–	65.6
Ovomucin[6]	210	–	78.0

Compiled by V.S. Ananthanarayanan.

[a] Unless otherwise indicated, the data have been taken from Tanford [1].

References

1. Tanford, *Adv. Protein Chem.*, 23, 121 (1968).
2. Donavan, *Biochemistry*, 6, 3918 (1967).
3. Ahmad and Salahuddin, *Int. J. Pept. Protein Res.*, 7, 417 (1975).
4. Ahmad and Salahuddin, *Biochim. Biophys. Acta*, 576, 333 (1979).
5. Ahmad and Salahuddin, *Biochemistry*, 13, 245 (1974).
6. Donavan, Davis, and White, *Biochim. Biophys. Acta*, 207, 190 (1970).

Taken from *Handbook of Biochemistry and Molecular Biology*, 3rd Edition, Ed. G.D.Faswan, CRC Press, Boca Raton, Florida, USA, 1976.

Intrinsic Viscosity of Some Proteins[a]

Protein	$[\eta]$ mL g^{-1}	Conditions	Reference
Bovine fibrinogen	25	50 mM sodium phosphate–0.4 M NaCl, pH 6.2, 25°C	1
Bovine prothrombin	3.4	0.1 M phosphate–0.65 M NaCl, pH 6.0, 25°C	2
Bovine prothrombin	12–14	0.1 M phosphate–0.65 M NaCl, pH 6.0, 25°C + 6 M GuCl[b]	2[a]
Bovine prothrombin	≤ 74	0.1 M phosphate–0.65 M NaCl, pH 6.0, 25°C	2
Human fibronectin[c]	10.2	Tris-NaCl, I = 0.15, pH 7.4, 20°C	3
Human fibronectin[c]	35	Tris-NaCl, I = 1.0, pH 7.4, 20°C	3
Human fibronectin[c]	44	Phosphate–NaCl, I = 0.15, pH 11.0, 20°C	3
Human fibronectin[c]	50	Phosphate–NaCl, I = 0.15, pH 11.0, 20°C	3
Native asparate Transcarbamylase[c]	4.5	0.1 M Tris, pH 8.0, 25°C	4
Catalytic subunit asparate transcarbamylase[e]	32	50 mM Tris, pH 7.5 with 6 M GuCl-0.1 BME[f], pH 7.5, 25°C	5
Regulatory subunit asparate transcarbamylase[g]	22.3	50 mM Tris, pH 7.5 with 6 M GuCl-0.1 BME, pH 7.5, 25°C	5
Bovine serum albumin	52.2	50 mM Tris, pH 7.5 with 6 M GuCl-0.1 BME, pH 7.5, 25°C	5
Rabbit muscle aldolase	33.5	6.0 M GuCl, 0.1 BME, 25°C	6
Poly-γ-benzyl-L-glutamate[h]	45	Dimethyl formamide	7
Poly-γ-benzyl-L-glutamate[i]	720	Dimethyl formamide	7
Poly-γ-benzyl-L-glutamate[h]	45	Dichloroacetic acid, 25°C	7
Poly-γ-benzyl-L-glutamate[j]	184	Dichloroacetic acid, 25°C	7
Tobacco mosaic virus	36.7	0.01 M phosphate, pH 7.1	8

Complied by Roger L. Lundblad.

[a] See Harding, S.E., The intrinsic viscosity of biological macromolecules. Progress in measurement, interpretation and application to structure in dilute solution, *Prog. Biophys. Mol. Biol.*, 68, 207–262, 1997; Tanford, C., Protein Denaturation, *Adv. Prot. Chem.* 23, 121–286, 1968.

[b] Guanidine hydrochloride

[c] Purified fibronectin characterized as dimer (M_r = 440 kDa) with trace amounts of fibronectin monomer and polymer.

[d] Subunit proteins, M_r = 200,000.

[e] Catalytic subunit, M_r = 34 kDa.

[f] BME, 2-mercaptoethanol, 2-sulfanylethan-1-ol.

[g] Catalytic subunit, M_r = 17.2 kDa

[h] M_r = 65,500.

[i] M_r = 340,000.

[j] M_r = 300,000.

References

1. Martínez, M.C.L., Rodes, V., and de al Torre, J.G., Estimation of the shape and size of fibrinogen in solution from its hydrodynamic properties using theories for bead models and cylinders, *Int. J. Biol. Macromol.*, 6, 261–265, 1984.

2. Ingwall, J.S., and Scheraga, H.A., Purification and properties of bovine prothrombin, *Biochemistry*, 8, 1860–1868, 1969.

3. Williams, E.C., Janmay, P.A., Ferry, J.D., and Mosher, D.F., Conformational states of fibronectin. Effect of pH, ionic strength, and collagen binding, *J. Biol. Chem.*, 257, 14973–14978, 1982.

4. Gerhart, J.C., and Schachman, H.K., Distinct subunits for the regulation and catalytic activity of aspartate transcarbamylase, *Biochemistry* 4, 1054–1062, 1965.

5. Rosenbusch, J.P., and Weber, K., Subunit structure of aspartate transcarbamylase, *J. Biol. Chem.*, 246, 1644–1651, 1971.

6. Kawahara, K., and Tanford, C., The number of polypeptide chains in rabbit muscle aldolase, *Biochemistry*, 5, 1578–1584, 1996.

7. Yang, J.T., The viscosity of macromolecules in relation to molecular conformation, *Adv. Prot. Chem.*, 16, 323–400, 1961.

8. Boedtker, H., and Simmons, N.S., The preparation of the preparation and characterization of essentially uniform tobacco mosaic virus particles, *J. Am. Chem. Soc.*, 80, 2550–2557, 1958.

INFRARED SPECTRA OF PROTEINS

H. Susi

The following tables summarize the frequencies and, for ordered solids, the polarization characteristics of conformation-sensitive infrared absorption bands of polypeptides and proteins. In the commonly used rock salt region of the spectra, there are two such bands, one at 1650 ± 40 cm^{-1} and a second one at 1530 ± 30 cm^{-1}. The precise frequency and polarization (for ordered solids) of these bands depends on the secondary structure (conformation) of the sample. Table 1 lists the calculated frequencies for unordered solids and for five different ordered conformations in the solid state. Note that each conformation gives rise to more than one component of each band, but some of these predicted components are very weak. The polarization is parallel ($\parallel$) or perpendicular ($\perp$) with respect to the direction of chain propagation.

Table 2 lists the prominent components of absorption bands for the unordered form and five different conformations. In practice, conformational information is usually deduced from the frequencies and polarization characteristics of these prominent components.

Table 3 gives comparative data for proteins and polypeptides in the solid state, in H$_2$O solution, and in D$_2$O solution. The data are limited to the amide I band because in aqueous solution the amide II band is extremely difficult to observe. Spectra are much easier to obtain in D$_2$O solution than in H$_2$O solution because H$_2$O is less transparent in this region of the infrared spectrum.

TABLE 1: Table of calculated characteristic polypeptide frequencies[a] cm^{-1}

Conformation	Amide I[b]	Amide II	Polarization
Unordered	1658	1520	–
Antiparallel-chain pleated sheet	1685 w	1530 s	$\parallel$
	1632 s	1510 w	$\perp$
	1668 vw	1550 w	$\perp$
Parallel-chain pleated sheet	1648 w	1530 s	$\parallel$
	1632 s	1550 w	$\perp$
Parallel-chain polar sheet	1648 s	1550 s	$\perp$, $\parallel$[c]
	1632 vw	1530 w	$\perp$
α-Helix	1650 s	1516 w	$\parallel$
	1646 w	1546 s	$\perp$
Triple helix (polyglycine II)	1624 vw	1558 s	$\parallel$
	1648 s	1531 w	$\perp$

Compiled by H. Susi.
[a] Based on Ref. [1].
[b] s, strong; w, weak; vw very weak.
[c] Amide I, $\perp$; amide II, $\parallel$.

Reference

1. Krimm, *J. Mol. Biol.*, 4, 528 (1962).

TABLE 2: Table of prominent amide I and amide II components[a] cm^{-1} (solid state)

Conformation	Strongest amide I component	Strongest amide II component	Weak amide I component
Unordered	1658	1520	–
Antiparallel-chain pleated sheet	1632 $\perp$	1530 $\parallel$	1685 $\parallel$
Parallel-chain pleated sheet	1632 $\perp$	1530 $\parallel$	–
Parallel-chain polar sheet	1648 $\perp$	1550 $\parallel$	–
α-Helix	1650 $\parallel$	1546 $\perp$	–
Triple helix (polyglycine II)	1648 $\perp$	1558 $\parallel$	–

Compiled by H. Susi.
[a] Based on Ref. [1].

Reference

1. Susi, in *Structure and Stability of Biological Macromolecules*, Timasheff and Fasman, eds., Marcel Dekker, New York, 1969, Chapter 7.

TABLE 3: Observed amide I frequencies of proteins in solid state and in solution[a]

	D$_2$O solution	H$_2$O solution	Solid	Example
Antiparallel-chain pleated sheet	1632	1632	1632	β-Lactoglobulin
	–	–	1630–34	Fibrous proteins
	1675	1690	1690	β-Lactoglobulin
	–	–	1695	Fibrous proteins
α-Helix	1649	–	–	β-Lactoglobulin
	1650	1652	1652	Myoglobin
	–	–	1652	Fibrous proteins
Unordered	1643	1656	–	β-Lactoglobulin (denatured)
	1643	1656	–	α_s-Casein
	–	–	1664	Fibrous proteins

Compiled by H. Susi.
[a] Based on Ref. [1].

Reference

1. Susi, in *Structure and Stability of Biological Macromolecules*, Timasheff and Fasman, eds., Marcel Dekker, New York, 1969, Chapter 7.

VOLUME CHANGES FOR SOME MACROMOLECULE ASSOCIATION REACTIONS

System	Molecular Weight Polymer	n, Degree of Polymerization	ΔV^a (ml/g)	Reference
Poly-L-valyl ribonuclease	Indefinite	Indefinite	1.5×10^{-2b}	1
S-Peptide + S-protein (ribonuclease)	13,700	A + B = C	2.3×10^{-3}	2
35 S + 56 S subunits (ribosomes)	2.8×10^6	A + B = C	1.8×10^{-4}	3
Collagen	$>10^8$	$>3 \times 10^2$	8×10^{-4}	4
Myosin	50×10^6	~100	6×10^{-4}	5
Lobster hemocyanin	9.4×10^5	6–12	6×10^{-5}	6
Tobacco mosaic virus	$>50 \times 10^6$	>500	5×10^{-3}	7
Actin	Indefinite	Indefinite	1.5×10^{-3}	8
Flagellin	Indefinite	Indefinite	3.8×10^{-3}	9
Sickle cell hemoglobin	Indefinite	Indefinite	5.9×10^{-3b} (<50 atm pressure)	10
β-Casein	1.25×10^6	52	>0	11
Serum albumin	Indefinite	Indefinite	1.2×10^{-3}	12
Lysozyme	28,800	2	-3×10^{-2}	13
tRNA synthetase and tRNA	125,000	A + B = C	<0	14
α-Chymotrypsin	72,000	3	>0	15
ANTIBODY-ANTIGEN				
DNP + DNP-lysine	155,000	A + nB = C	$2.3–5.2 \times 10^{-3c}$	16
DNP + DNP-B-γG	155,000	A + nB = C	$2.6–5.5 \times 10^{-3c}$	16
FAB (DNP) + DNP-lysine	52,000	A + nB = C	$3.1–3.8 \times 10^{-3c}$	16
Poly Glu^{56} Lys^{38} Tyr^6 + poly Glu^{56} Lys^{38} Tyr^6	155,000	A + B = C	4.2×10^{-3c}	16
Poly Glu^{66} Lys^{40} and poly Glu^{66} Lys^{40}	155,000	A + B = C	1.5×10^{-3}	16
ENZYME-INHIBITOR				
Lysozyme + N-acetyl-D-glucosamine	14,600	A + B = C	3.3×10^{-3}	17
Ribonuclease + cytidine 2'(3')-monophosphate	13,700	A + B = C	1.7×10^{-3}	18, 19

Source: From Harrington and Kegeles, *Methods Enzymol.,* 27, 324, 1973. With permission.

a   For the reaction n monomer = polymer.

b   Activation volume (ΔV^*) obtained from rate measurements.

c ΔV based on molecular weight of antibody. Most, if not all, molar volume change is associated with this particle.

References

1. Kettman, Nishikawa, Morita, and Becker, *Biochem. Biophys. Res. Commun.,* 22, 262 (1965).
2. Morita and Becker, in *High Pressure Effects on Cellular Processes,* Zimmerman, ed., Academic Press, New York, 1970, p. 71.
3. Infante and Baierlein, *Proc. Natl. Acad. Sci. U. S. A.,* 68, 1780 (1971).
4. Cassel and Christensen, *Biopolymers,* 5, 431 (1967).
5. Josephs and Harrington, *Biochemistry,* 7, 2834 (1968).
6. Saxena and Kegeles, personal communication, 1972.
7. Stevens and Lauffer, *Biochemistry,* 4, 31 (1965).
8. Ikkai and Ooi, *Biochemistry,* 5, 1551 (1966).
9. Gerber and Noguchi, *J. Mol. Biol.,* 26, 197 (1967).
10. Murayama and Hasegawa, *Fed. Proc.,* 28, 536 (1969).
11. Payens and Heremans, *Biopolymers,* 8, 335 (1969).
12. Jaenicke, *Eur. J. Biochem.,* 21, 110 (1971).
13. Howlett, Jeffrey, and Nichol, *J. Phys. Chem.,* 76, 777 (1972).
14. Knowles, Katze, Konigsberg, and Söll, *J. Biol. Chem.,* 245, 1407 (1970).
15. Kegeles and Johnson, *Arch. Biochem. Biophys.,* 141, 59 (1970).
16. Ohta, Gill, and Leung, *Biochemistry,* 9, 2708 (1970).
17. Chipman and Sharon, *Science,* 165, 454 (1969).
18. Hummel, Ver Ploeg, and Nelson, *J. Biol. Chem.,* 236, 3168 (1961).
19. Hammes and Schimmel, *J. Am. Chem. Soc.,* 87, 4665 (1965).
20. Harrington and Kegeles, *Methods Enzymol.,* 27, 324 (1973).

Taken from *Handbook of Biochemistry and Molecular Biology,* 3rd Edition, Ed. G.D.Fasman, CRC Press, Boca Raton, Florida, USA, 1976.

ASSAY OF SOLUTION PROTEIN CONCENTRATION

Roger L. Lundblad

The determination of protein concentration is a somewhat overlooked procedure that is critical for the determination of the specific biological/therapeutic activity of most biopharmaceuticals, the "standardization" or normalization of samples for proteomic analysis and the comparison of cell homogenates. As such, it is unfortunate that most investigators do not recognize the limitations of the various procedures. The reader is recommended to some recent reviews of protein assay methods.[1–3] The purpose of this short section is to describe some commonly used techniques for the determination of protein concentration. Care must be taken with the use of these techniques several of the more frequently used techniques depend on protein quality as well as quantity. Thus the technique which is facile might not be accurate. It is noted that accuracy is an attribute in assay validation while facile is not. There are two issues which are common to any of the below assays. The first is the standard and the second is the solvent. The standard should be representative of the sample; albumin might not be the best choice. The concentration of the standard protein cannot be verified by preparation but must be verified by analysis. In other words, accurate dispensing of the standard protein and subsequent dissolution to a given volume does not ensure an accurate standard. The final concentration of a standard solution must be verified by analysis. For well-characterized proteins it is possible to employ ultraviolet spectroscopy using the known extinction coefficient for the standard protein. Thus the A280 of a 1 mg/mL of bovine serum albumin is 0.66 in a cuvette of 1 cm pathlength [126]. It is important to correct for any light scattering due to aggregated material, dust, etc., by recording the baseline over the range 400 to 310 nm where the protein does not absorb. While this procedure may seem somewhat tedious, it is necessary. It is possible to prepare a standard solution which can be used for a substantial period of time. The standard solution is best stored frozen in small aliquots, each of which is used once to calibrate the assay. The precise storage conditions used would require validation.

Solvent can have an effect on the analytical response and should be selected for (1) lack of an effect on the signal and (2) the ability to be used for both standard and samples. The reader is directed to the List of Buffers (p. 695) for a discussion of the effect of various buffers on protein analysis.

Biuret assay

The biuret assay measures the formation of a purple complex between copper salts and two or more peptide bonds under alkaline conditions. The assay was developed by Gornall and coworkers[4] and modified to a microplate format by Jenzano and coworkers.[5] The biuret assay is not available in kit form and the preparation of the reagents requires some skill. The biuret assay also lacks the sensitivity of many of the other assays. The biuret assay is accurate as it is insensitive to protein quality.[2,3]

Selected references on the use of this method with various proteins are provided in Table 1.

Bicinchoninic acid (BCA) protein assay

This assay was developed by Smith and coworkers.[6] A modification for microplate use was developed by Jenzano and coworkers,[5] This procedure is a modification of the Lowry et al.[7] reaction, but it is significantly easier and somewhat more sensitive.[6] The reaction is based on the formation of a complex of BCA with cuprous ion (Brenner, A.J. and Harris, E.D., A quantitative test for copper using bicinchoninic acid, Anal.Biochem. 226, 80–84, 1995). The BCA reaction has the advantage of being able to measure protein bound to surfaces. This reaction is quite sensitive but it does reflect qualitative differences in proteins. As a reflection of the dependence on protein quality,[2] it is critical to select a standard that is qualitatively similar, if not identical, with the samples. This is obviously difficult when the assay is used with heterogeneous mixtures such as saliva or serum. Selected references to the use of this method are given in Table 2. Information on the use of the Lowry assay is presented in Table 3.

Dye-binding assay for protein using Coomassie Brilliant Blue G-250 (Bradford assay)

The dye-binding assay for proteins using Coomassie Brilliant Blue G-250 is likely the most sensitive and most extensively used protein assay at this time. It is also extremely easy to perform. The technique, as noted below, is extremely dependent on the quality of the protein. The procedure was developed by Bradford.[8] A modification for microplate technology is given by Jenzano and coworkers.[5] As noted above, this assay technique is likely the most sensitive and facile of the currently available procedures. Rigorous application of the dye-binding assay to the quantitative determination of a broad spectrum of proteins is difficult because of the marked influence of protein quality on the reaction. This is reflected by various studies attempting to modify the assay system to eliminate dependence on the quality of the protein.[9–14] Examples of the application of the Coomassie Blue dye-binding assay are presented in Table 4.

Kjeldahl assay

The Kjeldahl assay was developed in 1883[15] and is based on the determination of ammonia after hydrolysis of the sample in sulfuric acid. Most recent references to the use of this method relate to its use in food and environmental sciences.[16–20] It is our view that the Kjeldahl method remains a "gold" standard for protein assays[21] but we also appreciate the issues of technical complexity and lack of sensitivity which make routine use difficult for biopharmaceuticals. In addition, problems can arise in the analysis of proteins which contain impurities which themselves contain significant quantities of nitrogen, or in the analysis of proteins of unusual amino acid composition where the usual conversion factors may not apply. There are numerous commercial sources for support of the Kjeldahl assay.[22–27] Zellmer et al.,[28] have recently described an assay system which appears to have the accuracy of the Kjeldahl method with greatly improved sensitivity. Recent applications of the Kjeldahl assay are presented in Table 5.

Total amino acid analysis

Current technology for total amino acid analysis certainly has the various analytical attributes (sensitivity, accuracy, ruggedness) and is sufficiently rapid for use in the analysis of protein concentration[29-34] and has been suggested as a reference procedure for the determination of total protein concentration[35,36] With a characterized biopharmaceutical such as a growth factor, the concentration of the protein can be determined by measuring the amounts of specific stable and abundant amino acids such as alanine and lysine with reference to an added internal standard such as norleucine.[37] Application of amino acid analysis for total protein concentration are presented in Table 6.

Amido schwartz

The above approaches are certainly worth considering. However, it is somewhat remarkable that more attention has not been given to the amido black (Amidoschwarz 10B) assay developed by Schaeffner and Weissman.[38] This assay is based on the quantitative precipitation of protein from solution with trichloroacetic acid, the capture of the precipitated material by filtration followed by quantitative measurement of captured protein with amido schwarz dye (amido black is the preferred term). This study has been cited 2356 times (ISI) since its publication in 1973. The original assay used the addition of an equal amount of 60% trichloroacetic acid to a final concentration of 10%. The precipitate is capture by filtration and stained with amido black dye in methanol/glacial acetic acid/H_2O. The protein is visualized as a blue spot on an almost colorless background. The spot is excised from the filter, eluted with 25 mM NaOH-0.05 mM EDTA in 50% aqueous ethanol. The absorbance of the eluate at 630 nm is determined and concentration is determined by comparison with the results obtained with a standard protein. This assay has been used for the determination of protein concentration in grape juices and wines,[39] low concentration of protein in phospholipids,[40] and the *Escherichia coli* multidrug transporter EmrE[41] in the presence of detergents. Of direct relevance to proteomic analyses are the studies of Eliane[42] and coworkers on the determination of protein concentration of a *Medicago truncatula* root microsomal fraction with the amido black assay in a solution composed of 7.0 M urea-2.0 M thiourea-4% CHAPS (w/v)-0.1% (w/v) Triton X-100-2 mM tributylphosphine-2% ampholines. The reader is also commended to the study by Tate and coworkers[41] who validated the amido black assay with quantitative amino acid analysis which has been suggested as a method of choice for accurate determination of protein concentration.[34,35] A list of some other applications of amido black for protein assay is given in Table 7.

There has been limited application of fluorescent dyes for the determination of protein concentration (Table 8).

References

1. Dawnay, A. B. StJ., Hirst, A. D., Perry, D. E., and Chambers, R. E., A critical assessment of current analytical methods for the routine assay of serum total protein and recommendations for their improvement, *Ann. Clin. Biochem.*, 28, 556, 1991.
2. Sapan, C. V., Price, N. C., and Lundblad, R. L., Colorimetric protein assay techniques, *Biotechnol. Appl. Biochem.*, 29, 99-108, 1999.
3. Lundblad, R. L. and Price, N. C., Protein concentration determination. The Achilles' heel of cGMP, *Bioprocess International*, January, 2004, 1–7.
4. Gornall, A. G., Bardawill, C. J., and David, M. M., Determination of serum proteins by means of the biuret reaction, *J. Biol. Chem.*, 177, 751, 1949.
5. Jenzano, J. W., Hogan, S. L., Noyes, C. M., Featherstone, G. L., and Lundblad, R. L., Comparison of five techniques for the determination of protein content in mixed human saliva, *Anal. Biochem.*, 159, 370, 1986.
6. Smith, P. K., Krohn, R. I., Hermanson, G. T., Mallia, A. K., Gartner, F. H., Provenzano, M. D., Fujimoto, E. K., Goeke, N. M., Olson, B. J., and Klenk, D. C., Measurement of protein using bicinchoninic acid, *Anal. Biochem.*, 150, 76, 1985.
7. Lowry, O. H., Rosebrough, N. J., Farr, A. L., and Randall, R. J., Protein measurement with the folin phenol reagent, *J. Biol. Chem.*, 193, 265, 1951.
8. Bradford, M. M., A rapid and sensitive method for the determination of microgram quantities of protein utilizing the principle of protein-dye binding, *Anal. Biochem.*, 72, 248, 1976.
9. Wilmsatt, D. K. and Lott, J. A., Improved measurement of urinary total protein (including light-chain proteins) with a Coomassie Brilliant Blue G-250-sodium dodecyl sulfate reagent, *Clin. Chem.*, 33, 2100, 1987.
10. Tal, M., Silberstein, A., and Nusser, E., Why does Coomassie Brilliant Blue R interact differently with different proteins, *J. Biol. Chem.*, 260, 9976, 1985.
11. Pierce, J. and Suelter, C. H., An evaluation of the Coomassie Brilliant Blue G-250 dye-binding method for quantitative protein determination, *Anal. Biochem.*, 81, 478, 1977.
12. Read, S. M. and Northcote, D. H., Minization of variation in the response to different proteins of the coomassie blue G dye-binding assay for protein, *Anal. Biochem.*, 116, 53, 1981.
13. Sedmak, J. J. and Grossberg, S. F., A rapid, sensitive, and versatile assay for protein using coomassie brilliant blue G250, *Anal. Biochem.*, 79, 544, 1977.
14. Stoscheck, C. M., Increased uniformity in the response of the Coomassie blue G protein assay to different proteins, *Anal. Biochem.*, 184, 111, 1990.
15. Kjeldahl, J. Z., *Zeitschrift für Analytische Chemie*, 22, 366–382, 1883.
16. McPherson, T. N., Burian, S. J., Turin, H. J., Stenstrom, M. K. and Suffet, I. H., *Water Sci. Technol.* 45, 255–261, 2003.
17. Belloque, J. and Ramos, M., *J. Dairy Res.*, 69, 411–418, 2002, 2002.
18. Shan, S. B., Bhumbla, D. K., Basden, T. J. and Lawrence, L. D., *J. Environ. Sci. Hlth.*, B 37, 493–505, 2002.
19. Matttila, P., Salo-Vaananen, P., Konko, P., Aro, H. and Jalava, T. J., *Agricul. Food Chem.*, 50, 6419–6422, 2002.
20. Thompson, M., Owen, L., Wilkinson, K., Wood, R. and Damant, A., *Analyst* 127, 1666–1668, 2002.
21. Johnson, A. M., Rohlfs, E. M. and Silverman, L. M., (1999), Proteins, in *Teitz Textbook of Clinical Chemistry*, ed. C. A. Burhs and E. R. Ashwood, W. B. Saunders Co., Philadelphia, PA., Chapter 20, pp. 524–525.
22. http://www.calixo.net/braun/biochimie/kjeldahl.htm.
23. http://www.labconco.com/pdf/kjeldahl/index.shtml.
24. http://www.buchi-analytical.com/haupt.asp?nv=3759.
25. http://www.storesonline.com/site/251298.page/73181.
26. http://www.slrsystems.com/products.htm.
27. http://www.voigtglobal.com/kjeldahl_flasks.htm.
28. Zellmer, S., Kaltenborn, G., Rothe, U., Lehnich, H., Lasch, J., and Pauer, H.-D., *Anal. Biochem.*, 273, 163–167, 1999.
29. Anders, J. C., Parton, B. F., Petrie, G. E., Marlowe, R. L., and McEntire, J. E., *Biopharm International*, February, 30–37, 2003.
30. Weiss, M., Manneberg, M., Juranville, J.-F., Lahm, H.-W., and Fountaoulakis, M. Effect of the hydrolysis of method on the determination of the amino acid composition of proteins, *J. Chromatog. A.*, 795, 263–275, 1998.
31. Fountoulakis, M. and Lahm, H.-W., Hydrolysis and amino acid composition of proteins, *J. Chromatog. A.*, 826, 109–134, 1998.
32. Engelhart, W. G., Microwave hydrolysis of peptides and proteins for amino acid analysis, *Am. Biotechnol. Lab.*, 8, 30–34, 1990.
33. Chiou, S. H. and Wang, K. T., Peptide and protein hydrolysis by microwave irradiation, *J. Chromatog.*, 491, 424–431, 1989.
34. Bartolomeo, M. P. and Malsano, F., Validation of a reversed-phase method for quantitative amino acid analysis, *J. Biomol. Tech.*, 17, 131–137, 2006.
35. Sittampalam, G. S., Ellis, R. M., Miner, D. J., *et al.*, Evaluation of amino acid analysis as reference method to quantitate highly purified proteins, *J. Assoc. Off. Anal. Chem.*, 71, 833–838, 1988.

36. Henderson, L. O., Powell, M. R., Smith, S. J., *et al.*, Impact of protein measurements on standardization of assays of apolipoproteins A-I and B1, *Clin.Chem.*, 36, 1911–1917, 1990.

37. Price, N. C. (1996) The determination of protein concentration, in *Enzymology Labfax*, ed. P. C. Engel, Bios Scientific Publishers, Oxford, UK, pp. 34–41.

38. Schaeffner, W. and Weissman, C., A rapid, sensitive, and specific method for the determination of protein in dilute solutions, *Anal. Biochem.*, 56, 502–514, 1973.

39. Weiss, K. C. and Bisson, L. F., Optimisation of the Amido Black assay for the determination of protein content of grape juices and wines, *J. Science Food Agriculture*, 81, 583–589, 2001.

40. Bergo, H. O. and Christiansen, C., Determination of low levels of protein impurities in phospholipids samples, *Analyt. Biochem.*, 288, 225–227, 2001.

41. Butler, P. J. G., Ubarretxena-Belandia, I., Warne, T., and Tate, C. G., The *Escherichia coli* multidrug transporter EmrE is a dimer in the detergent solubilized state, *J. Mol. Biol.*, 340, 797–808, 2004.

42. Valot, B., Gianinazzi, S., and Elaine, D.-G., Sub-cellular proteomic analysis of a *Medicago truncatula* root microsomal fraction, *Phytochemistry*, 65, 1721–1732, 2004.

TABLE 1: Biuret Assay

Application	Reference
Dextran interferes with biuret assay of serum proteins	1
Interference of amino acids with the biuret reaction for urinary peptides. These investigators showed that, contrary to "conventional wisdom", the biuret assay showed cross-reaction with some amino acids and other compounds forming 5-membered and 6-membered complexes with copper.	2
Measurement of protein content of apple homogenates in an allergenicity study	3
Measurement of protein on surgical instruments	4
Measurement of protein concentration in serum and synovial fluid from human patients with arthropathies	5

TABLE 2: Bicinchoninic Acid Assay for Protein

Application	Reference
Protein concentration in synovial fluid	6
Measurement of protein concentration in liposomes	7
Measurement of cells attached to hyaluronic surfaces	8
Measurement of tear protein concentration	9
Proteins released by venom digestion	10

TABLE 3: Lowry Assay for Protein Concentration

Application	References
Determination of salivary protein concentration	11
Determination of protein concentration in aqueous humor	12
Determination of protein concentration in human milk	13
Determination of protein in human lens	14
Protein assay in cell-based toxicity studies	15

TABLE 4: Coomassie Blue Dye-Binding Assay (Bradford Assay)

Application	Reference
Measured soy protein extraction from various sources including soybean meal, soyprotein concentrate, and textured soy flake	16
Measured protein in aqueous phase from oil-water distribution. The amount of protein measured with Coomassie blue dye correlated ($r^2 = 0.91$) with protein concentration determined by tryptophan emission spectra (fourth derivative)	17
Measured glomalin extraction from soil	18
Automation of Coomassie dye-binding assay	19
Resonance light scattering with Bordeaux red correlates with Coomassie method for the determination of protein concentration in human serum, saliva, and urine	20
Measured protein concentration in phenol extracts of plant tissues after precipitation with ammonium acetate in methanol	21
Measured total protein concentration in rat tissue (pancreas, parotid gland, submandibular gland, lacrimal gland) extracts	22
Measure protein release from alginate-dextran microspheres	23
Protein release from *Candida albicans* secondary to microwave irradiation	24

TABLE 5: Kjeldahl Assay for Protein Concentration

Application	Reference
Measurement of protein concentration in therapeutic protein concentrate. Kjeldahl used as the "gold standard." The biuret assay gave comparable values while dye-binding was lower. Specific activity differed with the protein concentration	25
Measurement of crude microbial protein derived from carbohydrate fermentation	26
Measurement of polylysine coating on alginate beads	27
Measurement of IgG concentration in the presence of nonionic surfactants and glycine	28
Manure protein concentration	29
Whey protein concentration	30

TABLE 6: Amino Acid Analysis for Protein Concentration

Application	Reference
Use of amino acid analysis as a primary method for the determination of the concentration of poly ADP-ribose polymerase 1 (PARP-1)	31
Determination of the concentration of NADH:ubiquinone oxidoreductase and establishment of coenzyme (FMN) and iron-sulfur cluster stoichiometry	32
Determination of the concentration of immobilized protein	33
Determination of IgG protein concentration	34
Protein concentration of troponin in standard reference preparations	35

TABLE 7: Amido Black (Schwarz) Method for Protein Assay

Application	Reference
Measurement of protein concentration by binding to a nitrocellulose membrane by filtration followed by staining with amido black. Protein concentration determined by densitometry	36
Measurement of protein in antibody-polysaccharide complexes	37
Measurement of anchorage-dependent cells	38
Measurement of cell viability in an immortalized keratinocyte cell line	39
Determination of protein concentration after transfer to nitrocellulose from SDS-PAGE gel	40

TABLE 8: Fluorescent Dyes for Determination of Protein Concentration

Dye	References
NanoOrange	41–45

References

1. Delanghe, J.R., Hamers, N., Taes, Y.E., and Libeer, J.C., Interference of dextran in biuret-type assays of serum proteins, *Clin.Chem.Lab. Med.* 43, 71–74, 2005.
2. Hortin, G.L. and Meilinger, B., Cross-reactivity of amino acids and other compounds in the biuret reaction: interference with urinary peptide measurements, *Clin.Chem.* 51, 1411–1419, 2005.
3. Carnes, J., Ferrer, A., and Fernandez-Caldas, E., Allergenicity of 10 different apple varieties, *Ann.Allergy Asthma Immunol.* 96, 564–570, 2006.
4. Lipscomb, I.P., Pinchin, H.E., Collin, R., et al., The sensitivity of approved Ninhydrin and Biuret tests in the assessment of protein contamination on surgical steel as an aid to prevent iatrogenic prion transmission, *J.Hosp.Infect.* 64, 288–292, 2006.
5. Popko, J. Marciniak, J., Zalewska, A., et al., Activity of *N*-acetyl-β-hexosaminidase and its isoenzymes in serum and synovial fluid from patients with different arthropathies, *Clin.Exp.Rheumatol.* 24, 690–693, 2006.
6. Uehara, J., Kuboki, T, Fujisawa, T., et al., Soluble tumour necrosis factor receptors in synovial fluids from tempromandibular joints with painful anterior disc displacement without reduction and osteoarthritis, *Arch.Oral.Biol.* 49, 133–142, 2004.
7. Were, L.M., Bruce, B., Davidson, P.M., and Weiss, J., Encapsulation of nisin and lysozyme in liposomes enhances efficacy against *Listeria monocytogenes*, *J.Food Prot.* 67, 622–627, 2004.
8. Cen, L., Neoh, K.G., Li, Y., and Kang, E.T., Assessment of *in vitro* bioactivity of hyaluronic acid and sulfated hyaluronic acid functionalized electroactive polymer, *Biomacromolecules* 5, 2238–2246, 2004.
9. Yamada, M., Mochizuki, H., Kawai, M., et al., Decreased tear lipocalin concentration in patients with meibomian gland dysfunction, *Br.J.Ophthalmol.* 89, 803–805, 2005.
10. Nicholson, J., Mirtschin, P., Madaras, F., et al., Digestive properties of the venom of the Australian Costal Taipan, *Oxyranus scutellatus* (Peters, 1867), *Toxicon* 48, 422–428, 2006.
11. Yarat, A., Tunali, T., Pisiriciler, R., et al., *Clin.Oral Investig.* 8, 36–39, 2004.
12. Kawai, K., Sugiyama, K., and Kitazawa, Y., The effect of α2-agonist on IOP rise following Nd-YAG laser iridotomy, *Tokai J.Exp.Clin. Med.* 29, 23–26, 2004.
13. Milnewowicz, H. and Chmarek, M., Influence of smoking on metallothionein level and other proteins binding essential metals in human milk, *Acta Pediatr.* 94, 402–406, 2005.
14. Raitelaitiene, R., Paunksnis, A., Ivanov, L., and Kurapkiene, S., Ultrasound and biochemical evaluation of human diabetic lens, *Medicina (Kaunas)* 41, 641–648, 2005.
15. Dierickx, P., Prediction of human acute toxicity by the hep G2/24-hour/total protein assay, with protein measurement by the CBQCA method, *Altern.Lab.Anim.* 33, 207–213, 2005.
16. Koppelman, S.J., Lakemond, C.M., Vlooswijk, R., and Hefle, S.L., Detection of soy protein in processed foods: literature overview and new experimental work, *J.AOAC Int.* 87, 1398–1407, 2004.
17. Granger, C., Barey, P., Toutain, J., and Cansell, M., Direct quantification of protein partitioning in oil-to-water emulsion by frontface fluorescence: avoiding the need for centrifugation, *Colloids Surf. B Biointerfaces* 43, 158–162, 2005.
18. Wright, S.F., Nichols, K.A., and Schmidt, W.F., Comparison of efficacy of three extractants to solubilize glomalin on hyphae and in soil, *Chemosphere* 64, 1219–1224, 2006.
19. da Silva, M.A. and Arruda, M.A., Mechanization of the Bradford reaction for the spectrophotometric determination of total protein, *Anal.Biochem.* 351, 1551–157, 2006.
20. Feng, S., Pan, Z., and Pan, J., Determination of proteins at nanogram levels with Bordeaux red based on the enhancement of resonance light scattering, *Sprectrochim.Acta A Mol.Biomol. Spectrosc.* 64, 574–579, 2006.
21. Faurobert, M., Pelpoir, E., and Chaib, J., Phenol extraction of proteins for proteomic studies of recalcitrant plant tissues, *Methods Mol.Biol.* 359, 9–14, 2007.
22. Changrani, N.R., Chonkar, A., Adeghate, E., and Singh, J., Effects of streptoozotocin-induced type 1 diabetes mellitus on total protein concentrations and cation contents in the isolated pancreas, parotid, submandibular, and lacrimal glands of rats, *Ann.N.Y.Acad. Sci.* 1084, 503–519, 2006.
23. Reis, C.P., Ribeiro, A.J., Huong, S., et al., Nanoparticulate delivery system for insulin: design, characterization and in vitro/in vivo bioactivity, *Eur.J.Pharm.Sci.* 30, 392–397, 2007.
24. Campanha, N.H., Pavarina, A.C., Brunetti, I.L., et al., *Candida albicans* inactivation and cell membrane integrity damage by microwave irradiation, *Mycoses* 50, 140–147, 2007.
25. Lof, A.L., Gustafsson, G., Novak, V., et al., Determination of total protein in highly purified factor IX concentrates, *Vox Sang.* 63, 172–177, 1992.
26. Hall, M.B. and Herejk, C., Differences in yields of microbial crude protein from *in vitro* fermentation of carbohydrates, *J.Dairy Sci.* 84, 2486–2493, 2001.
27. Simsek-Ege, F.A., Bond, G.M., and Stringer, J., Matrix molecular weight cut-off for encapsulation of carbonic anhydrase in polyelectrolyte beads, *J.Biomater.Sci.Polym.Ed.* 13, 1175–1187, 2002.
28. Vidanovic, D., Milic Askrabic, J., Stankovic, M., and Poprzen, V., Effects of nonionic surfactants on the physical stability of immunoglobulin G in aqueous solution during mechanical agitation, *Pharmazie* 58, 399–404, 2003.
29. Leek, A.B., Hayes, E.T., Curran, T.F., et al., The influence of manure composition on emissions of odour and ammonia from finishing pigs fed different concentrations of dietary crude protein, *Bioresour.Technol.*, in press, 2006.
30. Cheison S.C., Wang, Z., and Xu, S.Y., Preparation of whey protein hydrolysates using a single- and two-stage enzymatic membrane reactor and their immunological and antioxidant properties: Characterization by multivariate data analysis, *J.Agric.Food Chem.*, in press, 2007.
31. Knight, M.I. and Chambers, P.J., Problems associated with determining protein concentration: a comparison of techniques for protein estimations, *Mol.Biotechnol.* 23, 19–28, 2003.
32. Albracht, S.P., van der Linden, E., and Faber, B.W., Quantitative amino acid analysis of bovine NADH:ubiquinone oxidoreductase (Complex I) and related enzymes. Consequences for the number of prosthetic groups, *Biochim.Biophys.Acta* 1557, 41–49, 2003.
33. Salchert, K., Pompe, T., Sperling, C., and Wenner, C., Quantitative analysis of immobilized proteins and protein mixtures by amino acid analysis, *J.Chromatog.A* 1005, 113–122, 2003.
34. Schauer, U., Stemberg, F., Rieger, C.H., et al., IgG subclass concentrations in certified reference material 470 and reference values for children and adults determined with the binding site reagents, *Clin.Chem.* 49, 1924–1929, 2003.
35. Bunk, D.M. and Welch, M.J., Characterization of a new certified reference material for human cardiac troponin I, *Clin.Chem.* 52, 212–219, 2006.
36. Nakamura, K., Tanaka, T., Kuwahara, A., and Takeo, K., Microassay for proteins on nitrocellulose filter using protein dye-staining procedure, *Anal.Biochem.* 148, 311–319, 1985.
37. Cabrera, M.M. and Lund, F.A., Determination of protein in polysaccharide-antibody complexes, *Ann.Inst.Pasteur Immunol.* 137C, 51–55, 1986.
38. Everitt, E. Wohlfart, C., Spectrophotometric quanitation of anchorage-dependent cell numbers using extraction of naphthol blue-black-stained cellular protein, *Anal.Biochem.* 162, 122–129, 1987.

39. White, P.J., Fogarty, R.D., Werther, G.A., and Wraight, C.J., Antisense inhibition of IGF receptor expression in HaCaT keratinocytes: a model for antisense strategies in keratinocytes, *Antisense Nucleic Acid Drug Dev.* 10, 195–203, 2000.

40. Himmelfarb, J. and McMonagle, E., Albumin is the major plasma protein target of oxidant stress in uremia, *Kidney Int.* 60, 358–363, 2001.

41. Liu, T., Foote, R.S., Jacobson, S.C., *et al.*, Electrophoretic separation of proteins on a microchip with noncovalent, postcolumn labeling, *Anal.Chem.* 72, 4608–4613, 2000.

42. Harvey, M.D., Bablekis, V., Banks, P.R., and Skinner, C.D., Utilization of the non-covalent fluorescent dye, NanoOrange, as a potential clinical diagnostic tool. Nanomolar human serum albumin quantitation, *J.Chromatog.B.Biomed.Sci.Appl.* 754, 345–356, 2001.

43. Jones, L.J, Haugland, R.P., and Singer, V.L., Development and characterization of the NanoOrange protein quantitation assay: a fluorescence-based assay of proteins in solution, *BioTechniques* 34, 850–854, 2003.

44. Stoyanov, A.V., Fan, Z.H., Das, C., *et al.*, On the possibility of applying noncovalent dyes for protein labeling in isoelectric focusing, *Anal.Biochem.* 350, 263–267, 2006.

45. Williams, J.C, Jr., Zarse, C.A., Jackson, M.E., *et al.*, Variability of protein content in calcium oxalate monohydrate stones, *J. Endourol.* 20, 560–564, 2006.

SPECTROPHOTOMETRIC DETERMINATION OF PROTEIN CONCENTRATION IN THE SHORT-WAVELENGTH ULTRAVIOLET

W. B. Gratzer

Whereas the extinction coefficients of proteins in the aromatic absorption band at 280 nm vary widely, the spectrum at shorter wavelengths is dominated by the absorption of the peptide bond and, therefore, has only a secondary dependence on amino acid composition and conformation. Measurements in this region can therefore serve for approximate concentration determinations of any protein. The following relations are available:

1. Scopes, *Anal. Biochem.*, 59, 277 (1974):
   a. E(1 mg/mL; 1 cm) at 205 nm = 31 with a stated error of 5%.
   b. This can be improved by applying a correction for the relatively strongly absorbing aromatic residues, by measuring the absorbance also at 280 nm. Two forms of this correction are

$$E(1 \text{ mg/ml}; 1 \text{ cm}) \text{ at } 205 \text{ nm} = 27.0 + 120 \times (A^{280}/A^{205})$$

or

$$E(1 \text{ mg/ml}; 1 \text{ cm}) \text{ at } 205 \text{ nm} = \frac{27.0}{1 - 3.85(A^{280}/A^{205})}$$

where the bracket term is the ratio of the absorbances measured at 280 and 205 nm; stated error, 2%.

2. Tombs, Soutar, and Maclagan, *Biochem. J.*, 73, 167 (1959):

$$E(1 \text{ mg/mL}; 1 \text{ cm}) \text{ at } 210 \text{ nm} = 20.5$$

3. Waddell, *J. Lab. Clin. Med.*, 48, 311 (1956): To avoid wavelength-setting error on steeply sloping curves, measurements are made at two wavelengths 10 nm apart and the absorbance difference is used to give the concentration:

$$C(\text{mg/ml}) = 0.144(A^{215} - A^{225})$$

where A^{215} and A^{225} are the absorbances read in 1 cm at 215 and 225 nm.

Note that the longer the wavelength, the lower the sensitivity of the spectrophotometric memethod method, but the hazard of interference from ultraviolet absorbing contaminants is less.

Section II
Enzymes

TURNOVER OF ENZYMES IN TISSUES

Molecular turnover of enzymes in animal tissues

Enzyme	E.C. No.	Animal	Tissue	Turnover[a] t1/2	kD	Reference
Ornithine decarboxylase	4.1.1.17	Rat	Liver	11 min[b]	3.78	1
δ-Aminolevulinate synthetase	–	Rat	Liver	67–72 min[c]	0.597	2
δ-Aminolerulinate synthetase	–	Rat	Liver (mitochondria)	68 min[d]	0.612	3
δ-Aminolevulinate synthetase	–	Rat	Liver (soluble fraction)	20 min[d]	2.08	3
Tyrosine transaminase	2.6.1.5.	Rat	Liver	3 h[e]	0.231	4
Tyrosine transaminase	–	Rat	Liver	3–4 h[j]	0.173–0.231	5
Tyrosine transaminase	–	Rat	Liver	2 h[e]	0.347	6
Tyrosine transaminase	–	Rat	Liver	2.5 h[k]	0.277	7
Tyrosine transaminase	–	Rat	Liver	1.7 h[e,uu]	0.408	7–9
Tyrosine transaminase	–	Rat	Liver	1.5 h[h]	0.462	9
Tyrosine transaminase	–	Rat	Hepatoma HTC culture cells	7 h[i]	0.099	10
Tyrosine transaminase	–	Rat	Hepatoma HTC culture cells	2–3 h[j]	0.231–0.347	11
Tyrosine transaminase	–	Rat	Hepatoma HTC culture cells	3–7 h	0.099–0.231	12
Tyrosine transaminase	–	Rat	Hepatoma HTC culture cells	2–3 h[j]	0.231–0.347	13
Histidine decarboxylase	–	Rat	Stomach	1.8–2.1 h[k]	0.330–0.385	14
Ribonucleotide reductase	–	Mouse	L cells in culture	2.0 h[i]	0.347	15
Tryptophan oxygenase	1.13.1.12	Rat	Liver	2.2–2.4 h[m]	0.301	16
Tryptophan oxygenase	–	Rat	Liver	2.5 h[n]	0.277	17
Tryptophan oxygenase	–	Rat	Liver	2–4 h[o]	0.231	18
Tryptophan oxygenase	–	Rat	Liver	2.5 h[p]	0.277	19
Tryptophan oxygenase	–	Rat	Liver	2.5 h[q]	0.277	20
Deoxythymidine kinase	–	Rat	Liver	2.6 h[r,s]	0.267	21
Deoxythymidine kinase	–	Rat	Liver (regenerating)	3.7 h[r,s]	0.187	21
Deoxythymidine kinase	–	Rat	Hepatoma Novikoff ascites cells	3.5 h[r,s]	0.198	22
Deoxythymidine kinase	–	Rat	Liver (neonatal)	3.8 h[r,s]	0.182	22
Aryl hydrocarbon hydroxylase	–	Hamster	Embryo cells	3–4 h[t]	0.198	23
Serine dehydratase	4.2.1.13	Rat	Liver	3 h[u]	0.231	24
Serine dehydratase	–	Rat	Liver	4.4 h[r,e]	0.157	25, 26
Serine dehydratase	–	Rat	Liver	9.3 h[r,w]	0.075	25, 26
Serine dehydratase	–	Rat	Liver	20.3 h[r,x]	0.034	25, 26
Aniline hydroxylase	–	Rat	Liver	5–7 h	0.099–0.139	27
Phosphoenolpyruvate carboxykinase	–	Rat	Liver	5.5 h	0.126	28
RNA polymerase	–	Rat (estrogen treated)	Uterus	1 h	0.693	29, 30
RNA polymerase	–	Rat	Liver (regenerating)	2.5–3 h[q]	0.231–0.277	31
RNA polymerase	–	Rat	Liver (sham operated)	12 h[q]	0.058	31
Glucokinase	–	Rat	Liver	11 h	0.063	32
Glucokinase	–	Rat	Liver	12–18 h	0.039–0.058	33
Glucokinase	–	Rat	Liver	30 h	0.023	34
Dihydroorotase	–	Rat	Liver	0.5 days[vv]	0.058	35
Arginine synthetase	–	Rat	Liver	14 h	0.049	36
Creatine transamidinase	–	Chicken	Liver	14 h	0.049	37
Creatine transamidinase	–	Rat	Kidney	38 h	0.018	37
Ornithine aminotransferase	2.6.1.13	Rat	Liver	19 h[y]	0.037	38
Ornithine aminotransferase	–	Rat	Liver	15 h	0.045	39
Thymidylate kinase	–	Rat	Liver	18 h[aa]	0.039	40
3-Phosphoglycerate dehydrogenase	–	Rat	Liver	14.6 h[bb]	0.047	41
3-Phosphoglycerate dehydrogenase	–	Rat	Liver	2.3 days[cc]	0.013	42
3-Phosphoglycerate dehydrogenase	–	Rat	Liver	1.9–2.3 days[dd]	0.013–0.015	43
Catalase	–	Rat	Liver	26–32 h[ee,ff,gg]	0.022–0.027	44–46
Catalase	–	Rat	Kidney	30 h[ee,gg]	0.023	44–46
Catalase	–	Rat (young male)	Liver	30 h	0.023[ee]	47
Catalase	–	Rat (young female)	Liver	31.5 h	0.022[ee]	47
Catalase	–	Rat (adult male)	Liver	23 h	0.030[ee]	47
Catalase	–	Rat (adult female)	Liver	23 h	0.030[ee]	47
Catalase	–	Rat (young male)	Kidney	30 h	0.023[ee]	47
Catalase	–	Rat (young female)	Kidney	30 h	0.023[ee]	47

Molecular turnover of enzymes in animal tissues (Continued)

Enzyme	E.C. No.	Animal	Tissue	Turnover[a] t1/2	kD	Reference
Catalase	–	Rat (adult male)	Kidney	43 h	0.016[ee]	47
Catalase	–	Rat (adult female)	Kidney	46 h	0.015[ee]	47
Catalase	–	Rat (casein-fed)	Liver	37 h	0.020[ee]	48
Catalase	–	Rat (protein-deficient)	Liver	33 h	0.021[ee]	48
Catalase	–	Rat (protein-deficient)	Liver	30 h	0.023[gg]	48
Catalase	–	Rat (starved)	Liver	35 h	0.02[gg]	49
Catalase	–	Rat (chow fed)	Liver	31 h	0.0225[ee]	49
Catalase	–	Rat (casein-fed)	Kidney	33 h	0.021[ee]	48
Catalase	–	Rat (starved)	Kidney	35 h	0.02[ee]	49
Catalase	–	Rat (chow fed)	Kidney	31 h	0.0227[ee]	49
Catalase	–	Rat (cycasin treated)	Liver	49.5 h	0.014[ee]	50
Catalase	–	Rat (Pair-fed controls)	Liver	23.9 h	0.029[ee]	50
Catalase	–	Rat (cycasin treated)	Kidney	38.5 h	0.018[ee]	50
Catalase	–	Rat (pair-fed controls)	Kidney	21 h	0.033[ee]	50
Catalase	–	Rat	Liver	1.5 days[ee]	0.019	51
Catalase	–	Rat	Liver	1.8 days[hh]	0.016	51
Catalase	–	Rat	Liver	2.5 days[ii]	0.012	51
Catalase	–	Rat	Liver	3.7 days[ii]	0.008	51
Catalase	–	Rat (tumor-bearing)	Liver	29–36 h	0.019–0.024	52
Catalase	–	Rat	Hepatoma (5123)	29 h	0.024	52
Catalase	–	Rat	Hepatoma (7316A)	26.7 h	0.026	52
Catalase	–	Rat (tumor-bearing)	Liver	35 h	0.02	53
Catalase	–	Mouse (B/He)	Liver	36 h[ee]	0.019	54
Catalase	–	Mouse (B/6)	Liver	15 h[ee]	0.045	54
Catalase	–	Mouse (DBA)	Liver	39 h[ee,tt]	0.018	55
Catalase	–	Mouse (B/6)	Liver	40 h[ee,tt]	0.017	55
Catalase	–	Mouse (B/Ha)	Liver	90 h[ee,tt]	0.008	55
Pyruvate kinase	–	Rat	Liver	1–2 days	0.014–0.029	56, 57
Dihydroxyacetone kinase	–	Rat	Liver	1–2 days	0.014–0.029	57
6-Phosphogluconate dehydrogenase	–	Rat	Liver	1–2 days	0.014–0.029	57
Phosphofructokinase	–	Rat	Liver	1–2 days	0.014–0.029	57
Malic enzyme	–	Rat	Liver	1–3 days	0.014–0.029	57
Aminopyrine demethylase	–	Rat	Liver	2 days[ii]	0.014	58
Barbiturate side-chain oxidation enzyme	–	Rat	Liver	2.2 days[kk]	0.013	59
Barbiturate side-chain oxidation enzyme	–	Rat	Liver	2.6 days[ii]	0.011	59
Barbiturate side-chain oxidation enzyme	–	Rat	Liver	—	—	60
Aspartic transcarbamylase	–	Rat	Liver	>24 h[r,s]	0.029	21
Aspartic transcarbamylase	–	Rat	Liver (regenerating)	>24 h[r,s]	0.029	21
Amino-azo dye N-demethylase	–	Rat	Liver	> 24 h[mm]	0.029	61
Alanine aminotransferase	–	Rat	Liver	1.2 days[nn]	0.024	62
Analine aminotransferase	–	Rat	Liver	3.5 days[oo]	0.008	62
Alanine aminotransferase	–	Rat	Liver	3–3.5 days[pp]	0.008–0.010	63
Alanine aminotransferase	–	Rat	Liver	40 h	0.017	64
Alanine aminotransferase	–	Rat	Muscle	20 days	0.001	65
Alanine aminotransferase	–	Rat	Liver	18 h[pp]	0.039	38
Alanine aminotransferase	–	Rat	Liver	18 h[y]	0.040	38
Glucose 6-phosphate dehydrogenase	–	Rat	Liver	10–12 h	0.058–0.069	66
Glucose 6-phosphate dehydrogenase	–	Rat	Liver	22 h	0.031	56
Glucose 6-phosphate dehydrogenase	–	Rat	Liver	1.5–2.5 days	0.012–0.019	57
Aspartate transcarbamylase	–	Rat	Liver	2.5 days[vv]	0.011	35
NADPH-cytochrome c reductase	–	Mouse	Liver	2.8 days[f]	0.010	67
NADPH-cytochrome c reductase	–	Rat	Liver	3.0–3.5 days[ii]	0.009	68
NADPH-cytochrome c reductase	–	Rat	Liver	2.5 days[ii]	0.011	69
NADPH-cytochrome c reductase	–	Rat	Liver	48–56 h	0.012–0.014	70
NADPH-cytochrome c reductase	–	Rat	Liver	2.5–3.0 days	0.010–0.011	60
α-Glycerophosphate dehydrogenase	–	Rat	Liver	4 days[qq]	0.008	71
α-Glycerophosphase dehydrogenase	–	Rat	Liver	24 h	0.029	56
Malate dehydrogenase	–	Rat	Liver	4 days[qq]	0.008	71
Arginase	3.5.3.1	Rat	Liver	4–5 days[r]	0.006–0.008	72
Xanthine oxidase	–	Rat	Liver	4 days[rr]	0.008	73
δ-Aminolerulinate dehydratase	–	Mouse	Liver	5–6 days	0.005–0.006	74
Lactate dehydrogenase-5	–	Rat	Heart	1.6 days	0.018	75

Molecular turnover of enzymes in animal tissues (Continued)

Enzyme	E.C. No.	Animal	Tissue	Turnover[a]		Reference
				$t1/2$	kD	
Lactate dehydrogenase-5	–	Rat	Liver	16.0 days	0.002	75
Lactate dehydrogenase-5	–	Rat	Muscle (skeletal)	31.0 days	0.0009	75
NAD glycohydrolase	–	Rat	Liver	~20 days[tt]	0.0015	76
Fructosediphosphate aldolase	–	Rat	Muscle	20 days	0.001	77
Fructosediphosphate aldolase	–	Rabbit	Muscle	50 days	0.0006	78
Fructosediphosphate aldolase	–	Rabbit	Serum	3.33 h[ss]	0.208	79
Glycogen phosphorylase	2.4.1.1	Rabbit	Muscle	50 days	0.006	78
Glyceraldehydephosphate dehydrogenase	1.2.1.12	Rabbit	Muscle	100 days	0.0003	78

Compiled by M. Rechcigl, Jr.

[a] Besides the conventional way of expression, that is, as a half-life ($t_{1/2}$), the turnover rates of specific enzymes are also given in terms of the first-order rate decay constant (kD), which can be derived from the former, using the following relationship: $t_{1/2} = 0.693/kD$, where 0.693 is the natural logarithm of 2 (ln 2).

[b] Determined by following a decay curve from normal as well as high levels induced in regenerating liver after the administration of either cycloheximide or puromycin.

[c] Determined by measuring the rate of decline of the enzyme from elevated levels, induced by allylisopropylacetamide after puromycin administration.

[d] Determined by following a decay curve of the enzyme from normal as well as high levels induced by allylisopropylacetamide after cycloheximide administration.

[e] Determined by following a decay curve from elevated levels induced by hydrocortisone.

[f] Determined by isotope decay under basal conditions.

[g] Determined by following a stress-induced decline (by tyrosine or celite) in the enzyme activity.

[h] Determined by a "label and chase" procedure under conditions where the amount of basal enzyme undergoes no change.

[i] Measured in control and dexamethasone treated cells after administering cycloheximide and then following decay of enzyme activity.

[j] Measured by the "label and chase" procedure in basal cultures and those induced by hydrocortisone or insulin.

[k] Determined both by the rate of decline of enzyme activity of freely feeding rats after cycloheximide administration as well as by following a decay curve from elevated levels induced by gastrin.

[l] Determined from fall in specific activity of enzyme after protein synthesis was stopped with cycloheximide, using partially synchronized or random cultures.

[m] Determined by following a decay curve of the enzyme from high levels induced with tryptophan or cortisone.

[n] Determined from decay curve following inhibition of protein synthesis.

[o] Determined by decay of basal, and high levels, induced with tryptophan after administering puromycin.

[p] Determined by following a decay curve from elevated levels induced with hydrocortisone after administration of puromycin.

[q] Using puromycin and p-fluorophenylalanine.

[r] Determined by following specific activity decay of prelabeled enzyme.

[s] Determined from the decay of the prelabeled enzyme after cycloheximide administration.

[t] Calculated from the rate of decay after the addition of cycloheximide to pre-induced cells.

[u] Determined by following a decay curve from high levels induced with casein hydrolysate.

[v] On normal diet and after glucose.

[w] After pyridoxine administration.

[x] After amino acid administration.

[y] Determined by decay method from induction by diet high in protein.

[z] Determined by the rate of isotope incorporation.

[aa] From decay of induced activity.

[bb] Determined by following a decay curve from normal as well as high levels induced by 2% casein after administration of cycloheximide.

[cc] Determined during the rise in the enzyme activity following the feeding of a 2% casein diet.

[dd] Determined from a fall in the enzyme activity after a return to 25% casein from a 2% casein diet induction of the enzyme.

[ee] Determined from the rate of reappearance of the enzyme activity after destruction with 3-amino-1,2,4-triazole.

[ff] Calculated from the rate of incorporation of radioiron into the enzyme after administration of 3-amino-1,2,4-triazole.

[gg] Determined by following a decay of normal levels after administration of allylisopropylacetamide.

[hh] Determined by isotope decay using δ-aminolevulinic acid-4-^{14}C.

[ii] Determined by isotope decay using guanidino-^{14}C-L-arginine.

[jj] Determined by isotope decay using l-^{14}C-DL-leucine.

[kk] Determined from the full time course of change in the basal enzyme level during the administration of phenobarbital.

[ll] Determined by following a decay curve from high levels induced with phenobarbital.

[mm] Determined by measuring the decline in enzyme activity from basal or induced levels after puromycin administration.

[nn] Determined from the full time course of change in the basal enzyme level during the administration of prednisolone.

[oo] Determined by following a decay curve from high levels induced with prednisolone.

[pp] Determined by decay method from prednisolone induction.

[qq] Determined by following a decay curve from elevated levels induced with L-thyroxine after administration of ethionine.

[rr] Determined from decay of elevated enzyme activity.

[ss] Determined by following specific activity decay of the enzyme labeled with I^{131}.

[tt] A rough estimate, based on a double-labeling isotope decay (using l-^{14}C-DL-leucine and ^{3}H-DL-leucine).

[uu] The value may represent "turnover" or inactivation of induced enzyme rather than that of basal enzyme.

[vv] Determined from the decay of induced enzyme after returning the orotic acid fed rats to normal diet.

References

1. Russell and Snyder, *Mol. Pharmacol.*, 5, 253 (1969).
2. Marver, Collins, Tschudy and Rechcigl, *J. Biol. Chem.*, 241, 4323 (1966).
3. Hayashi, Yoda and Kikuchi, *Arch. Biochem. Biophys.*, 131, 83 (1969).
4. Lin and Knox, *J. Biol. Chem.*, 233, 1186 (1958).
5. Kenney, *J. Biol. Chem.*, 237, 3495 (1962).
6. Berlin and Schimke, *Mol. Pharmacol.*, 1, 149 (1965).
7. Kenney and Albritton, *Proc. Natl. Acad. Sci. (US).*, 54, 1693 (1965)
8. Grossman and Mavrides, *J. Biol. Chem.*, 242, 1398 (1967).
9. Kenney, *Science*, 156, 525 (1967).
10. Peterkofsky and Tomkins, *J. Mol. Biol.*, 30, 49 (1967).
11. Reel and Kenney, *Proc. Natl. Acad. Sci. (US)*, 61, 200 (1968).
12. Thompson, E. B. and Granner, D. K., unpublished data.
13. Kenney, F. T., unpublished data.
14. Snyder and Epps, *Mol. Pharmacol.*, 4, 187 (1968).

15. Turner, Abrams and Lieberman, *J. Biol. Chem.*, 243, 3725 (1968).
16. Feigelson, Dashman and Margolis, *Arch. Biochem. Biophys.*, 85, 478 (1959).
17. Goldstein, Stella and Knox, *J. Biol. Chem.*, 237, 1723 (1962).
18. Nemeth, *J. Biol. Chem.* 237, 3703 (1962).
19. Garren, Howell, Tomkins and Crocco, *Proc. Natl. Acad. Sci. (US)*, 52, 1121 (1964).
20. Schimke, Sweeney and Berlin, *J. Biol. Chem.*, 240, 322 (1965).
21. Bresnick, Williams and Mosse, *Cancer Res.*, 27, 469 (1967).
22. Bresnick and Burleson, *Cancer Res.*, 30, 1060 (1970).
23. Nebert and Gelboin, *J. Biol. Chem.*, 243, 6250 (1968).
24. Pitot and Peraino, *J. Biol. Chem.*, 239, 1783 (1964).
25. Jost, Khairallah and Pitot, *J. Biol. Chem.*, 243, 3057 (1968).
26. Khairallah and Pitot, in *Symposium on Pyridoxile Enzymes*, Yamada, Katunuma and Wada, eds., Maruzen Co., Tokyo, 1968, p. 154.
27. Holtzman and Gillette, *J. Biol. Chem.*, 243, 3020 (1968).
28. Shrago, Lardy, Nordlie and Foster, *J. Biol. Chem.*, 238, 3188 (1963).
29. Gorski and Morgan, *Biochim. Biophys. Ada*, 149, 282 (1967).
30. Gorski and Notides, in *Biochemistry of Cell Division*, Baserga, ed., Thomas, Springfield, 1969, p. 57.
31. Tsukuda and Lieberman, *J. Biol. Chem.*, 240, 1731 (1965).
32. Sharma, Manjeshivar and Weinhouse, *J. Biol. Chem.*, 238, 3840 (1963).
33. Salas, Vinnuela and Sols, *J. Biol. Chem.*, 238, 3535 (1963).
34. Niemeyer, *National Cancer Institute Monograph* No. 27, p. 29 (1967).
35. Bresnick, Mayfield and Mosse, *Mol. Pharmacol.*, 4, 173 (1968).
36. Szepesi and Freedland, *Life Sci.*, 8, 1067 (1969).
37. Walker, *Advan. Enzym. Reg.*, 1, 151 (1963).
38. Swick, Rexroth and Stange, *J. Biol. Chem.*, 243, 3581 (1968).
39. Swick, R. W. and Peraino, C., unpublished data.
40. Hiatt and Bojarski, *Cold Spring Harbor Symp. Quant. Biol.*, 26, 367 (1961).
41. Fallon, Hackney and Byrne, *J. Biol. Chem.*, 241, 4157 (1966).
42. Fallon, *Advan. Enzym. Reg.*, 5, 107 (1967).
43. Fallon, H. J., unpublished data.
44. Price, Sterling, Tarantola, Hartley and Rechcigl, *J. Biol. Chem.*, 237, 3468 (1962).
45. Rechcigl and Price, in *Newer Methods of Nutritional Biochemistry*, Albanese, ed., Academic, New York, p. 185.
46. Rechcigl and Price, *Progr. Exp. Tumor Res.*, 10, 112 (1967).
47. Rechcigl, in *Regulatory Mechanisms for Protein Synthesis in Mammalian Celts*, Pietro, Ramborg and Kenney, eds., Academic Press, New York, 1968, p. 399.
48. Rechcigl, *Nutr. Diela.*, 11, 214 (1969).
49. Rechcigl, *Arch. Intern. Physiol. Biochim.*, 76, 693 (1968).
50. Rechcigl and Laqueur, *Enzymol. Biol. Clin.*, 9, 276 (1968).
51. Poole, Leighton and de Duve, *J. Cell. Biol.*, 41, 536 (1969).
52. Rechcigl, Hruban and Morris, *Enzymol. Biol. Clin.*, 10, 161 (1969).
53. Rechcigl, *Enzymologia*, 34, 23 (1968).
54. Rechcigl and Heston, *Biochem. Biophys. Res. Commun.*, 27, 119 (1967).
55. Ganschow and Schimke, *J. Biol. Chem.*, 244, 4649 (1969).
56. Szepesi and Freedland, *J. Nutr.*, 94, 37(1968).
57. Szepesi and Freedland, *Can. J. Biochem.*, 46, 1459 (1968).
58. Argyris and Magnus, *Develop. Biol.*, 17, 187 (1968).
59. Arias and DeLeon, *Mol. Pharmacol.*, 3, 216(1967).
60. Arias, Doyle and Schimke, *J. Biol. Chem.*, 244, 3303 (1969).
61. Conney and Gilman, *J. Biol. Chem.*, 238, 3682 (1963).
62. Segal and Kim, *Proc. Natl. Acad. Sci. (US)*, 50, 912 (1963).
63. Kim, *Mol. Pharmacol.*, 5, 105 (1969).
64. Nichol and Rosen, *Advan. Enzym. Reg.*, 1, 341 (1963).
65. Segal, *Biochem. Biophys. Res. Commun.*, 36, 764 (1969).
66. Tepperman and Tepperman, *Advan. Enzvm. Reg.*, 1, 121 (1963).
67. Jick and Shuster, *J. Biol. Chem.*, 241, 5366 (1966).
68. Omura, Siekevitz and Palade, *J. Biol. Chem.*, 242, 2389 (1967).
69. Kuriyama, Omura, Siekevitz and Palade, *J. Biol. Chem.*, 244, 2017 (1969).
70. Ernstcr and Orrenius, *Fed. Proc.*, 24, 1190 (1965).
71. Tarentino, Richert and Westerfeld, *Biochim. Biophys. Acta.*, 124, 309(1966).
72. Schimke, *J. Biol. Chem.*, 239, 3808 (1964).
73. Rowe and Wyngaarden, *J. Biol. Chem.*, 241, 557 (1966).
74. Doyle and Schimke, *J. Biol. Chem.*, 244, 5449 (1969).
75. Fritz, Vessell, White and Pruit, *Proc. Natl. Acad. Sci. (US)*, 62, 558 (1969).
76. Bock, K. W., Siekevitz, P. and Palade, G. E., unpublished data.
77. Schapira, Kruh, Dreyfus and Schapira, *J. Biol. Chem.*, 235, 1738 (1960).
78. Velick, *Biochim. Biophys. Acta.*, 20, 228 (1956).
79. Schapira, *Rev. Fr. Et. Clin. Biol.*, 7, 829 (1962).
80. Grossman, A., personal communication.

MOLECULAR TURNOVER OF CYTOCHROMES IN ANIMALS

Cytochrome	Animal	Tissue	Turnover		Reference
			$t_{1/2}$	kD	
Cytochrome P-450	Rat	Liver	50 h[a]	0.014	1
Cytochrome P-450	Rat	Liver	<12 h	>0.058	2
Cytochrome P-450	Rat	Liver			5
Cytochrome b_5	Rat	Liver	4.2 days[b]	0.007	3
Cytochrome b_5	Rat	Liver	4.9–5.1 days[c]	0.006	4
Cytochrome b_5	Rat	Liver	1.3–1.9 days	0.015–0.022	5
Cytochrome b_5	Rat	Liver (mitochondrial)	4.4 days[d]	0.007	6
Cytochrome b_5	Rat	Liver (microsomal)	2.3–2.4 days[d]	0.012–0.013	6
Cytochrome b_5	Rat	Liver (microsomal)	2.5 days[e]	0.011	6
Cytochrome b_5	Rat	Liver (mitochondrial)	5.5 days[d]	0.005	6
Cytochrome c	Rat	Liver (mitochondrial)	6.1 days[d]	0.0047	6
Cytochrome c	Rat	Liver	9.7 days[f]	0.003	7
Cytochrome c	Rat	Liver	8.56 days[g]	0.0034	8
Cytochrome c	Rat	Liver	5.0 days[h]	0.0058	9
Cytochrome c	Rat	Liver	13 days[i]	0.002	10
Cytochrome c	Rat	Liver (regenerating)	5.4 days	0.0053	11
Cytochrome c	Rat	Liver	10.5 days[j]	0.0027	12, 15
Cytochrome c	Rat	Liver	8,6 days	0.0034	14
Cytochrome c	Rat	Kidney	15.6 days[k]	0.0019	15
Cytochrome c	Rat	Kidney	11.5 days[l]	0.0025	15
Cytochrome c	Rat	Skeletal muscle	32 days[l]	0.0009	15
Cytochrome c	Rat	Heart	43 days[l]	0.0006	15

Compiled by M. Rechicigl, Jr.

[a] Determined from decay of induced activity.
[b] Determined by isotope decay under basal conditions (using ^{14}C-L-arginine).
[c] Determined by isotope decay under basal conditions (using 1-^{14}C-DL-leucine).
[d] Determined from biological decay *in vivo* after injection of 8-aminolevulinic acid-^3H.
[e] Determined from decay after labeling the protein moiety with arginine-^{14}C (guanido).
[f] Determined by isotope decay using ^{35} S-methionine.
[g] Determined by isotope decay using ^{35}C-leucine.
[h] Using^{17} $CaCO_3$ label. steady-state model. Values obtained over a 12-day interval.
[i] Calculated from turnover time (the time required for synthesis) of total rat liver cytochrome c.
[j] Calculated from degradation rate of cytochrome c.
[k] Using^{59} Fe as the label.
[l] Determined by isotope decay using ^{14}C-leucine.

References

1. Ernster and Orrenius, *Fed. Proc.*, 24, 1190 (1965).
2. Schmid, Marver, and Hammaker, *Biochem. Biophys. Res. Commun.*, 24, 319 (1966).
3. Kuriyama, Omura, Siekevitz, and Palade, *J. Biol. Chem.*, 244, 2017 (1969).
4. Omura, Siekevitz, and Palade, *J. Biol. Chem.*, 242, 2389 (1967).
5. Arias, Doyle, and Schimke, *J. Biol. Chem.*, 244, 3303 (1969).
6. Druyan, DeBemard, and Rabinowitz, *J. Biol. Chem.*, 244, 5874 (1969).
7. Fletcher and Sanadi, *Biochim. Biophys. Acta*, 51, 356 (1961).
8. Bailey, Tayloi, and Bartley, *Biochem. J.*, 104, 1026 (1967).
9. Swick, Rexroth, and Stange, *J. Biol. Chem.*, 243, 3581 (1968).
10. Kadenbach, *Eur. J. Biochem.*, 10, 312 (1969).
11. Drabkin, *Proc. Soc. Exp. Biol. Med.*, 76, 527 (1951).
12. Kadenbach, *Biochim. Biophys. Acta*, 186, 399 (1969).
13. Beattie, Basford, and Koritz, *J. Biol. Chem.*, 242, 4584 (1967).
14. Flatmark and Sletten, *J. Biol. Chem.*, 243, 1623 (1968).
15. Kadenbach, *Biochim. Biophys. Acta*, 186, 399 (1969).

MATRIX METALLOPROTEINASES

Roger L. Lundblad

MATRIX METALLOPROTEINASE (MMP) AND THEIR CHARACTERISTICS, SPECIFICITY, AND FUNCTION[a]

MMP-1 (Interstitial collagenase; tissue collagenase)

MMP-1 (interstitial collagenase) was one of the first matrix metalloproteinases[1] and has been purified from human skin fibroblasts.[2,3] Much of the work on MMP-1 was performed with the enzyme purified by tissue culture[4] (purification from the tissue was difficult[2]). MMP-1 differs from many of the matrix metalloproteinases described later in that (1) it was identified in tissue by biological activity and (2) it was purified from tissue culture media; early work described MMP-1 as tissue collagenase. Most of the later matrix metalloproteinases were identified by PCR cloning and only the recombinant form has been evaluated. A generic structure for MMP-1 is shown in Figure 1. A mutant enzyme missing in the C-terminal hemopexin domain is similar to the native purified enzymes in the hydrolysis of synthetic substrates but does not cleave collagen.[5] The hemopexin domain is thought to contribute to the specificity of MMP-1. MMP-1 degrades type-I, type-II, type-III, type-VII, and type-X collagens,[6,7] and IGFBP-3.[8] MMP-1 preferentially degrades type III collagen. The rate of fibrillar collagen cleavage is slow; cleavage of collagen III in solution is more rapid.[9,10] Application of a mechanical load to the collagen substrate increases the rate of cleavage.[11] MMP-1 is less active in the degradation of gelatin than collagen.[10] The cleavage of native collagen involves a conformational change in the substrate collagen induced by binding of MMP-1.[12] MMP-1 is produced in a wide variety of tissues[13] and the expression of MMP-1 is increased in tumors and thought to be involved, with other MMPs, in the metastatic process.[14] MMP-1 is inhibited by α_2-macroglobulin[15] and tissue inhibitor of metalloproteinase-1 (TIMP-1).[16] α_1-Protease inhibitor is degraded by MMP-1[17,18] yielding fragments[b,c] with proinflammatory activity with monocytes[19] and neutrophils.[20] There has been a therapeutic application of MMP-1 for muscle healing by degrading fibrous tissue and releases local growth factors.[21]

MMP-2 (Gelatinase A)

MMP-2 (gelatinase A)[22] is produced in a variety of normal tissues as well as by various tumors. MMP-2 is also known as the 72 kDa gelatinase/type-IV collagenase.[22,23] MMP-2 is a separate gene product from the 92 kDa gelatinase (gelatinase b; MMP-9).[22] However, MMP-9 expression is frequently concomitant with MMP-2 expression.[24–28] A gelatinase is defined as a proteolytic enzyme that will work on gelatin (denatured collagen). In the MMP-2, this means that it does not degrade types I–III collagen but is highly specific for the degradation of collagen IV, a major component of basement membranes.[29–31] The ability of MMP-2 to degrade collagen type IV in the basement membrane is considered critical to the process of tumor metastasis.[32] Degradation of collagen IV in the extracellular matrix by MMP-2 (and/or MMP-9) exposes a cryptic epitope important for angiogenesis.[33,34] Although TIMP-2 is a specific inhibitor of MMP-2,[31,35] TIMP-2 also functions as a "cofactor" in the activation of proMMP-2 by membrane type 1 matrix metalloproteinase (MT1-MMP; MMP-14).[36] The association between MMP-2 and TIMP-2 and the resulting activation on the cell surface by MMP-14 is thought to represent a unique regulatory mechanism.[37] MMP-2 is unique in that there is intracellular and extracellular expression of the active enzyme.[38,39] It is noted (see below) that MP-27 is confined to an intracellular site. MMP-2 contains three tandem fibronectin domains which are important in MMP-2 binding to collagen in extracellular matrix.[40–42] Endogenous MMP-2 in fibroblasts is activated by culturing on type I collagen.[43] MMP-2 cannot cleave native collagen I but can degrade collagen I fragments' product by MMP-14.[44] Angiostatin is produced from plasminogen by cleavage by MMP-2.[45,46] It is of interest that MMP-2 is inhibited by red wine providing an explanation for the protective effect of red wine in coronary disease.[47,48] MMP-2 acting with MMP-14 activates pro-MMP-13.[49] ProMMP-2 can be activated by a number of proteases including thrombin.[50–53] The activation of proMMP-2 by thrombin has been suggested to require the participation of MMP-14[30] or the presence of heparan sulfate.[43] Other work[54] suggests the participation of activated protein C in processing proMMP-2 to an intermediate form which is then activated by thrombin. There is earlier data to suggest that thrombin does not activate proMMP-2.[55] It does appear that the activation of proMMP-2 by thrombin is a complex process occurring on a cell surface. Genetic polymorphism of MMP-2 is associated with a number of disparate pathologies from ischemic stroke to cancer.[56–59]

MMP-3 (Stromelysin 1)[c1]

MMP-3 is a stromal cell-derived matrix metalloproteinase that degrades the extracellular matrix, hence the alternative designation as stromelysin-1.[60] MMP-3 was originally described as an enzyme that hydrolyzes proteoglycans and hence was referred to as proteoglycanase.[61–63] Approximately 20% of proMMP-3 is produced in a glycosylated form.[64] MMP-3 is also referred to as transin.[65] ProMMP-3 can be activated by thrombin,[66] cathepsin G,[67] neutrophil elastase,[67] plasma kallikrein,[64] trypsin,[64] plasmin,[64] and chymotrypsin.[64] MMP-3 activates KLK-4[68] (Table 8.2) as well as proMMP-9.[69] MMP-3 has broad pH dependence for both activity and reaction with inhibitors.[70] Digestion of fibronectin and gelatin was more extensive at pH 5.5, whereas the digestion of azocoll was more extensive at pH 6.2.[71] MMP-3 digestion of collagen IX was performed at pH 7.4[72] or pH 7.5[73] but it is not clear that this is optimum pH. MMP-3 has a broad specificity in degrading collagens II, IX, X, XI[73] as well as proteoglycans, casein, fibronectin, laminin type IV collagen and gelatin but not type I collagen.[74] MMP-3 also degrades IGF-BP,[75] substance P,[76] fetuin,[77] plasminogen activator inhibitor-1 (PAI-1),[78] and plasminogen with the generation of angiostatin.[79] MMP-3 is also inhibited by α_2-macroglobulin[75,80] and by tissue inhibitor of matrix metalloproteinase (TIMP).[60,81,82]

MMP-4 (Procollagen peptidase)

MMP-4 activity is reported to be identical with MMP-3 with possible contributions from MMP-13.

MMP-5 (3/4 collagenase)

MMP-5 is reported to be identical with MMP-2.

MMP-6[d]

MMP-6 is reported to be identical with MMP-3.

MATRIX METALLOPROTEINASES (Continued)

MMP-7 (Matrilysin)

MMP-7 (matrilysin)[83,84] is one of the better known matrix metalloproteinases and is also known as matrin,[85] uterine metalloproteinase (UPP), putative metalloproteinase I (Pump-1), or punctuated metalloproteinase. MMP-7 is unique among the matrix metalloproteinase in that it is small; zymogen form has a molecular mass of 28 kDa, the active enzyme approximately 20 kDa.[84,85] MMP-7 lacks the hemopexin domain which appears to confer specificity to other matrix metallproteinase.[86,87] As with other matrix metalloproteinases, pro-MMP-7 is activated by mercurials,[85,88] trypsin,[88] and heat.[89] Pro-MMP-7 can be activated[90] and inactivated by hypochlorite.[91] ProMMP-7 can also be activated by reaction with an electrophilic derivative of a fatty acid, nitrooleic acid.[92]

MMP-7 degrades a broad range of proteins in the interstitium including fibronectin, laminin, type IV collagen, and gelatins.[85,93] MMP-7 degrades fetuin.[77] MMP-7 also regulated β-catenin function in epithelial cell growth via degradation of the adherens junction protein E-cadherin.[85] As with other matrix metalloproteinases, MMP-7 is inhibited by TIMP-1[57] and α_2-macroglobulin.[94]

MMP-8 (Neutrophil collagenase)

MMP-8 is synthesized and secreted from neutrophils as a zymogen or latent form[95] which can be activated by limited proteolysis[95] by several enzymes including cathepsin G[96] or stromelysin (MMP-3).[97] Activation of MMP-8 by nitric oxide has also been reported.[98] Reversible activation of MMP-8 by hypochlorous acid (HOCl) has been reported.[99,100]

MMP-8 degrades collagen I, II, and III triple helical collagen; it also degrades other proteins including fibronectin, fibrinogen, and cartilage aggrecan.[95] There has been considerable work on the mechanism of collagen cleavage by MMP-8. As with other matrix metalloproteinases, the latent form of MMP-8 can be activated with mercuric chloride.[99,101] There has been work on the role the hemopexin domain of MMP-8 in the recognition of the substrate collagen molecule.[102,103] MMP-8 degrades α_1-antitrypsin.[101,104] Degradation of α_1-antitrypsin permits enhanced expression of neutrophil elastase.[105] As with other matrix metalloproteinases, MMP-8 can be inhibited by doxycycline[93,106] and α_2-macroglobulin and TIMPs (tissue inhibitors of metalloproteinases).[107,108] MMP-8 which is bound to the neutrophil membrane is protected from inhibition by TIMP-1 or TIMP-2.[109] MMP-8 stability is also increased when bound to the neutrophil membrane.[109]

MMP-9 (Gelatinase B)

MMP-9 (gelatinase B) was first described as a "gelatin-specific protease" from human leucocytes (neutrophils) in 1974.[110] Later work[111] reported that neutrophil gelatinase was secreted as a monomer (92 kDa), a dimer (220 kDa) which is reduced to a monomer (92 kDa), and a 130 kDa species which could also be converted to a monomer (92 kDa). In addition to the secretion by leukocytes, MMP-9 is produced in a variety of other tissues.[112] MMP-9 is also known as the 92 kDa/type IV collagenase and is a different gene product than MMP-2.[111] As with other matrix metalloproteinases, MMP-9 is activated as a zymogen (proMMP-9) and can be activated by reaction with an organic mercurials, cathepsin G, trypsin, α-chymotrypsin, and MMP-3.[113] ProMMP-9 can also be partially activated by hypochlorite[113,114] and by a protease from German cockroach frass.[115] Pro-MMP-9 derived from neutrophils occurs as heterodimer with lipocaliin.[116] Pro-MMP-9 derived from a macrophage cell line (THP-1) covalently links chondroitin sulfate proteoglycan.[117] Disulfide bonds have been suggested to be involved in heterodimer/oligomer formation[117] but other data suggest alternatives to disulfide bonds.[118] MMP-9 binds to CD44 and promotes cell migration.[119,120] CD44 is a receptor found on a number of hematopoietic and non-hematopoietic cells and is important for cell–cell and cell–matrix interactions[121,122] MMP-9 can cleave collagen IV and collagen V forming discrete fragments.[123] MMP-9 was able to specifically cleave soluble collagen type I and type III.[124] However, MMP-9 does not cleave native triple-helical collagen type I.[125,126] MMP-1 cleavage of triple helical collagen type I facilitates subsequent degradation by MMP-9.[125] MMP-9 has also been suggested to be important for the generation of active IL-1β being much more effective than either MMP-2 or MMP-3 in this process.[127] MMP-9 can degrade a number of other proteins in the interstitium[122,128] and is inhibited by TIMPs[129] and α_2-macroglobulin.[130] MMP-9 can form angiostatin from plasminogen.[131,132] As observed with other matrix metalloproteinases, MMP-9 can degrade α_1-protease inhibitors;[104,133,134] the degraded α_1-protease inhibitor is proinflammatory.[135] α_1-antichymotrypsin attenuates MMP-9 activation in skin during wound healing.[136,137] Increased expression of MMP-9 results in poor wound healing; a porcine matrix product used in the promotion of wound healing in periodontal disease, EMD(*), contains α_1-antichymotrypsin.[138]

MMP-10 (Stromelysin-2)

As with MMP-3 (stromelysin-1), MMP-10 (stromelysin-2) degrades various components of the extracellular matrix including collagens III,IV, V, and fibronectin.[139] MMP-3 and MMP-10 are not isoenzymes but do demonstrate approximately 80% homology based on analysis of cDNA sequences.[140,141] There are differences in the regulation of the expression of the two proteins.[141,142] MMP-10 together with other matrix metalloproteinases is suggested to be important for angiogenesis.[143] MMP-10 is inhibited by TIMP-1 and TIMP-2 but with less avidity than that observed with MMP-3.[144,145]

MMP-11 (Stromelysin-3)

Native MMP-11[146] has restricted substrate specificity with early studies showing only cleavage of α_1-antiprotease inhibitor.[147] Deletion of approximately 175 amino acids from the C-terminal (hemopexin domain) and substitution of proline for alanine235 resulted in a mutant enzyme which can now degrade casein, laminin, and type IV collagen.[148] More recent work with phage display suggests that there are unique substrates for MMP-11 in tumors that remain to be identified.[149] The degradation of IGF-BP by MMP-11 has been reported which would favor cellular proliferation.[150] The development of a novel FRET[e] substrate permitted the intracellular and extracellular localization of MMP-11 in tumor cells.[151] MMP-11 is found in tissues undergoing rapid remodeling as observed in tumor growth and wound healing as well as embryonic development.[152–154] Furin activates the zymogen form of MMP-11.[153,155]

MMP-12 (Macrophage elastase)f

MMP-12 is also known as macrophage metalloelastase.[156] Murine macrophage elastase was described in 1975,[157] whereas the human enzyme was not characterized until 1993.[158] The murine enzyme has a mass of 22 kDa[157] Subsequent isolation and characterization of the cDNA for the human protein showed a proenzyme (pro-MMP-12) of 54 kDa which is processed to a 45 kDa product with the removal of an N-terminal region resulting in an active enzyme containing a catalytic domain and a hemopexin domain.[158] The 45 kDa species is subjected to autolysis yielding a 22 kDa catalytic domain which can cleave a triple helical fluorescent peptide derived from collagen V.[159] MMP-12 degradation of human α_1-protease inhibitor by murine MMP-12[157] has been observed and the degradation product has been suggested to have chemotactic activity.[160] There are no studies with human MMP-12 nor are any other studies with the murine enzyme; there are a number of other studies on the activity of peptide fragments obtained from α_1-proteinase inhibitor.[b,c] MMP-12 is also efficient in generating angiostatin from plasminogen.[161] MMP-12 degrades a large number of extracellular matrix proteins including fibronectin, laminin, type IV collagen, and α_1-protease inhibitor.[162] Oxidation of α_1-antiprotease inhibitor resulting in the formation of methionine sulfoxide at Met358 changes the site of cleavage from Pro357-Met358 to Phe352-Leu353.[163] MMP-12 is less effective than neutrophil elastase in solubilizing elastin.[162] MMP-12 stimulates IL-9/CXCL8 release from alveolar epithelium by EGF receptor–mediated pathway.[164]

MATRIX METALLOPROTEINASES (Continued)

MMP-13 (Collagenase 3)

MMP-13 (collagenase 3) degrades type II collagen more rapidly than either type I or type III.[165] MMP-13 also has general protease activity degrading, for example, fibrinogen and fibronectin. MMP-13 was first described in breast tumor tissue and subsequently in chondrocytes.[166] α_1-Acid glycoprotein inhibits MMP-3 collagenolytic activity as well as the binding of MMP-3 to collagen.[167] As with other metalloproteinases, MMP-13 occurs as a precursor which can be activated by a variety of agents including MMP-10.[168] MMP-13-activated PAR1 receptors at an noncanonical site resulted in cellular activation via a tethered ligand.[169] Thrombin promotes MMP-13 expression in chondrocytes.[170] As with other matrix metalloproteinases, MMP-13 is inhibited by tissue inhibitors of metalloproteinases (TIMPs) and α_2-macroglobulin.[171]

MMP-14 (Membrane-type 1 matrix metalloproteinase)

MT1-MMP (membrane-type 1 matrix metalloproteinase) is an integral membrane protein[172] which was discovered by cloning technology[173] focused on identifying the factor(s) responsible for the activation of pro-MMP-2 (pro-gelatinase A). MT1-MMP is expressed as a proenzyme which is activated in a least a two-step process[174] involving furin, possibly in complex with Golgi reassembly stacking protein.[175] MT1-MMP initiates the degradation of collagen I followed by the action of MMP-2.[176,177] TIMP-2, TIMP-3, and TIMP-4 have been shown to inhibit the MT1-MMP[94] although the relationship of TIMP-2 and MT1-MMP is complex as both stimulation and inhibition of MT1-MMP activity are reported with this TIMP.[177–180] TIMP-2 forms a complex with MT1-MMP and pro-MMP-2 leading to the formation of MMP-2 and efficient degradation of collagen.[181] MT1-MMP is not inhibited by TIMP-1.[182] MT1-MMP also acts as a sheddase in releasing EMMPRIN (extracellular matrix metalloproteinase inducer)[183–185] from tumor cells.[186] There is considerable interest in the role of MT1-MMP in cancer biology[86,187] as well as in the etiology of rheumatoid arthritis.[188] MMP-14 is synthesized in a latent or zymogen form which is activated by furin or other convertases.[189] The activation of pro-MMP-14 and the subsequent production of a brain-specific angiogenesis inhibitor 1 (BAI1) is viewed as a proteolytic cascade.[190,g]

MMP-15 (Membrane-type 2 matrix metalloproteinase)

Membrane-type 2 matrix metalloproteinase (MMP-15, MT2-MMP)[191] was identified by PCR cloning of a human lung cDNA library.[192] MMP-15 shows extensive structural homology to MMP-14 and is bound by a transmembrane domain to the cell surface. MMP-15 activates pro-MMP-2 in a process not requiring the participation of TIMP-2. [193,194] As with MMP-14, MMP-15 is inhibited by TIMP-2, TIMP-3, and TIMP-4 but not by TIMP-1.[181,191] Despite the structural homology between MMP-14 and MMP-15, the two proteins show different expression profiles.[195–197]

MMP-16 (Membrane-type 3 matrix metalloproteinase)

Membrane-type 3 matrix metalloproteinases (MMP-16, MT3-MMP) was identified by PCR cloning of a cDNA library from human tissues.[198,199] MMP-16 is similar to MMP-14 and MMP-15 (and MMP-24) in that it is attached to the membrane though a stem from catalytic domain to a transmembrane domain with a cytoplasmic tail (Figure 7.3)[200] Although MMP-14 and MMP-15 are widely distributed, MMP-16 expression is restricted to brain, lung, heart, and placenta.[200] MMP-16, as with MMP-14 and MMP-15, is an activator of pro-MMP-2 in the presence of either TIMP-2 or TIMP-3; TIMP-3 is also a high affinity inhibitor of MMP-16 (K_i = 0.008 nM).[201] Inhibition of MMP-16 is observed with TIMP-2 (0.17 nM) and TIMP-4 (0.34 nM). MMP-16 can degrade fibronectin and type II collagen.[200] A soluble form of MMP-16 resulting from alternative splicing has been described and has been suggested to have direct role in degradation of extracellular matrix in addition to the activation of pro-MMP-2.[202] A recombinant soluble form of MMP-16 lacking the transmembrane and cytoplasmic domains degraded type III collagen but not type I collagen.[203] The truncated MMP-16 also degraded cartilage proteoglycan, gelatin, fibronectin, vitronectin, laminin-1, α_1-proteinase inhibitor, and α_2-macroglobulin yielding fragments identical to those obtained with a truncated MMP-14.

MMP-17 (Membrane-type 4 matrix metalloproteinase)

MMP-17 (membrane-type 4 matrix metalloproteinase) was identified by PCR cloning of a human breast carcinoma cDNA library.[204,205] It was not possible to express the first cDNA isolate,[205] and subsequent work[206] identified a novel transcript which could be expressed. Other work[207] showed that MMP-17 differed from the other membrane-type matrix metalloproteinases in that MMP-17 (and MMP-25) is linked to the membrane via linkage to glycosylphosphatylinositol (Figure 8.4).[208] The catalytic domain of MMP-17 (Figure 7.4) has been expressed as in an inclusion body and purified after solubilization in 8 M urea and renaturation.[209] The MMP-17 catalytic domain degrades gelatin and was a poor activator of pro-MMP-2 (pro-gelatinase A. The MMP-17 catalytic domain was inactive in the degradation of other extracellular matrix proteins such as type I collagen, type IV collagen, fibronectin, and laminin. It was suggested that the absence of the hemopexin domain might influence the observed activities. Another study[210] with the MMP-17 catalytic domain obtained similar results except it was not possible to show activation of pro-MMP-2. Both studies[209,210] showed that, differing from other membrane-type matrix metalloproteinases, the MMP-17 catalytic domain was inhibited by TIMP1; inhibition was also observed with TIMP. The recombinant murine MMP-17 catalytic domain was unable to activate pro-MMP-2 but did degrade fibrin and fibrinogen.[211] The murine MMP-17 catalytic domain was also inhibited by TIMP1, TIMP2, or TIMP3. This later study[211] also showed that MMP-17 has TNFα convertase activity and could shed pro-TNFα. MMP-17 also activates ADAMTS4 (aggrecanase-1).[212]

MMP-18 (Collagenase 4)

MMP-18 is a poorly described MMP which degrades type I,II, and III collagen.[213] It was first identified through PCR cloning of human mammary gland DNA and subsequent analysis of mRNA shows a wide tissue distribution but absent in brain, skeletal muscle, kidney, liver, or peripheral blood leukocytes.[214] Studies in *Xenopus* suggested a role of MMP-18 in amphibian development.[215] mRNA analysis identified the presence of MMP-18 in a variety of cultured human cell lines including mammary cell lines, prostate cell lines, and human fibroblasts,[216] as well as cartilage.[217] MMP-18 may also be important for macrophage migration through tissue.[218]

MMP-19

Matrix metalloproteinase-19 (MMP-19)[219] was identified by PCR cloning from a human liver cDNA library.[220] Northern blot analysis showed higher MMP-19 mRNA expression in placenta, lung, pancreas, ovary, spleen and intestine with lower expression in other tissues such as liver and prostate.[220] An identical matrix metalloproteinase designated RASI-1 was identified in a cDNA library from inflamed human synovium.[221] MMP-19 is also expressed in normal keratinocytes.[222,223] Recombinant pro-MMP-19 was expressed in *Escherichia coli* and purified from inclusion bodies.[224] The zymogen form of MMP-19 could be activated by trypsin and was inhibited by TIMP-2.[220] MMP-19 also cleaves several FRET[e] peptides[220] with sequences consistent with an enzyme with a close relationship to the stromelysin group[225–227] of matrix metalloproteinases. Intact MMP-19 has been reported to cleave IGF-BP-3[224], whereas the recombinant catalytic domain cleaves type IV collagen, fibronectin, laminin, and nidogen.[228] The recombinant MMP-19 hemopexin domain binds IGF-BP-3.[229] Other studies with the carboxyl-terminal deletion mutant (recombinant catalytic domain) which does not contain the hemopexin domain demonstrated cleavage of aggrecan at the canonical MMP cleavage site between Asn341 and Phe342.[230] Upregulation of MMP-19 is observed in melanoma metastasis.[231]

MATRIX METALLOPROTEINASES (Continued)

MMP-20 (Enamelysin)

Matrix metalloproteinase-20 (MMP-20, enamelysin)[232] was cloned (PCR cloning) from a porcine enamel organ cDNA library.[233] Human MMP-20 has a domain structure similar to other matrix metalloproteinases consisting a prosequence containing the conserved cysteine residue, a catalytic domain containing a zinc-binding site, and a carboxyl-terminal similar to the hemopexin domain observed with other matrix metalloproteinases.[234,235] Porcine MMP-20 did show 49% homology to porcine MMP-1.[234]

The recombinant pro-MMP-20 undergoes autocatalytic activation during refolding from inclusion bodies in urea. MMP-20 degrades amelogenin[234,235] and is inhibited by TIMP-2.[234] MMP-20 activates pro-KLK4.[236,237] Both MMP-20 and KLK4 are important in the process of enamel development in teeth.[238] MMP-20 also activates kallikrein-like peptidases other than KLK4.[238] Although most work has focused on the expression of MMP-20 in developing teeth, expression of MMP-20 in oral tumors has been reported.[239,240] MMP-20 degrades a number of proteins other than amelogenin and pro-kallikrein-like peptidases including fibronectin, type IV collagen, laminen-1 and laminen-5, and tenascin-C.[239]

MMP-21 (Xenopus matrix metalloproteinase, XMMP)

MMP-21 (Xenopus matrix metalloproteinase, XMMP)[241] was described in *Xenopus* embryos.[242] A human homologue/orthologue[243] to XMMP was identified in a cDNA library from human ovary.[244] Subsequent work has shown expression in macrophages and fibroblasts.[245] Recent interest has focused on MMP-21 expression in human tumors.[246]

MMP-22 (Chicken matrix metalloproteinase, CMMP)

MMP-22 (chicken metalloproteinase)[247] shows limited sequence identity with other matrix metalloproteinases.[248] There is a unique cysteine residue in catalytic domain; a similar cysteine residue has been reported in MMP-21 and MMP-18. A recombinant form missing the N-terminal region was observed to undergo autocatalytic activation and degraded gelatin and casein with a rate similar to that observed with recombinant MMP-1; however, the digestion products were different suggesting a difference in specificity between MMP-1 and MMP-22.
A human homologue for MMP-22 has not been reported.

MMP-23 (Cysteine array matrix metalloproteinase)

MMP-23 was identified by PCR cloning of a human ovary cDNA library.[249] Earlier work had identified several isoforms of a matrix metalloproteinase which were designated MMP 20/21.[250] A murine homologue, cysteine array matrix metalloproteinase (CA-MMP), was subsequently identified.[251,252] A rat MMP-23 has also been identified.[253] The recombinant human MMP-23 had low activity in the hydrolysis of one synthetic substrate but lacked activity against two other peptide substrates or gelatin.[249] The murine protein had efficient activity in the hydrolysis of gelatin.[251] It is noted that there are other examples of difference in the activity of orthologues.[254,255]

MMP-24 (Membrane-type 5 matrix metalloproteinase)

Membrane-type 5 matrix metalloproteinase (MMP-24)[256] was identified by PCR cloning of a cDNA library from human brain.[257] MMP-24 can activate pro-MMP-2 (progelatinase A).[258] Murine MMP-24 truncated in transmembrane domain has been expressed in MDCK cells.[259] The purified protein activates pro-MMP-2 in a process requiring TIMP2; this study[259] also demonstrated that recombinant MMP-24 could degrade gelatin and extracellular matrix proteoglycans (chondroitin sulfate proteoglycans, dermatan sulfate proteoglycans) and fibronectin but was not active in the degradation of laminin or type 1 collagen. The recombinant MMP-24 is subjected to rapid autolysis under physiological conditions perhaps representing a control mechanism. The convertase furin can remove MMP-25 from the membrane by cleavage in the stem region perhaps representing another control mechanism.[260]

MMP-25 (Membrane-type 6 matrix metalloproteinase)

Membrane-type 6 matrix metalloproteinase (leukolysin, MMP-25)[261] would seem as if MMP-25 was described as leukolysin in 1970.[262] However, the first unambiguous identification of MMP-25 in leukocytes was obtained by use of an EST (expressed sequence tag) library.[263] A C-terminal truncated form of the enzyme was expressed and was shown to have activity in the degradation of gelatin.[263] MMP-25 activates pro-MMP-2 (progelatinase A).[264,265] Although the expression of MMP-25 was originally considered to be confined to leukocytes, MMP-26 has been identified in lung, spleen, colon carcinoma, glioblastoma, and astrocytoma.[264,266,267] As with MMP-17, MMP-25 is attached to membrane via a glycosyl phosphatidylinositol linkage.[267–269] A homodimer form of MMP-25[267,269] has been identified on the surface of colon cancer cells and HL-60 cells. The homodimer is formed by a disulfide bond joining the stem domains of proximate MMP-25 monomers.[269] The dimer form is active and degrades α_1-proteinase inhibitor.[270] Studies with recombinant MMP-25 catalytic domain[271] demonstrated degradation of type IV collagen, gelatin, fibronectin, and fibrin but not laminin. The recombinant MMP-25 domain was unable to activate pro-MMP-2[271] differing with results obtained with the intact protein.[264,265] It has been suggested that MMP-25 is responsible for the degradation of myelin basic protein in the etiology of multiple sclerosis.[272,273]

MMP-26 (Matrilysin-2)

MMP-26 (matrilysin-2)[274] is also known as endometase stemming from its discovery in human endometrial tumor.[275] It is similar to matrilysin (MMP-7) in that it is smaller (28 kDa zymogen; 19 kDa active enzyme) than the other matrix metalloproteinases as a result of lack of the hemopexin domain.[276] MMP-26 degrades α_1-antiprotease inhibitor and certain extracellular matrix proteins.[275] Pro-MMP-26, differing from other matrix metalloproteinases, is not activated by organic mercurials.[277,278] Recombinant pro-MMP-26 underwent autocatalytic activation with a single peptide bond cleavage[278,279]; further proteolysis resulted in inactivation of the enzyme.[278] Auto-digestion of pro-MMP-26 has been observed during the folding process of the recombinant enzyme from inclusion bodies expressed in *Escherichia coli*.[279] MMP-26 cleaves a variety of protein with specificity determined by both P and P' sequences.[280] MMP-26 cleaves fibronectin, vitronectin, fibrinogen, IGF-BP, and α_1-antiproteinase inhibitor.[279]

MMP-27

MMP-27 is a poorly described matrix metalloproteinase. Studies in the mouse[281] show substantial mRNA expression in liver and spleen with lesser expression in other tissues. A later study in the rat[282] found low levels of MMP-27 mRNA expression in bone and kidney. We could not find an original citation for the identification of MMP-27. An earliest paper described the expression of MMP-27 (mRNA) in B lymphocytes.[283] A more recent paper[284] showed a C-terminal domain in MMP-27 provided for retention in the endoplasmic reticulum and prevented access to the secretion pathway; a mutant missing the C-terminal extension was secreted.

MATRIX METALLOPROTEINASES (Continued)

MMP-28 (Epilysin)

MMP-28 (epilysin)[285] was identified by PCR cloning of a cDNA library obtained from epithelial cells.[286] There has been particular interest in the expression of MMP-28 in keratinocytes and during wound healing.[287–289] MMP-28 is also expressed in macrophages.[290] Other work has suggested that MMP-28 is confined to action within the extracellular matrix.[291] MMP-28 is also expressed in tumors.[292,293]

---

a   Also known as matrix metallopeptidases. A group (clan) of proteolytic enzymes which use zinc in the catalytic process.[294,295] Matrix metalloproteinases are expressed as precursors of zymogen forms which can be activated by a variety of processes. Activation by non-enzymatic mechanisms with oxidizing agents such as hypochlorite or cysteine modification with mercuric chloride is thought to be based on the disruption of interaction between a cysteine residue in the propeptide and a zinc ion at the active site[296,297] although other mechanisms have been suggested.[298,299] One of the mechanisms involves the activation of matrix metalloproteinases by hypochlorite.[90,300] Hypochlorite can also cause the inactivation of MMP-7 by modification of a tryptophan adjacent to a glycine residue resulting in a unique condensation product.[91] The reader is directed to the review by Sternlicht and Werb.[301]

b   Although the primary function of α_1-antiproteinase inhibitor is the control of proteases in biological fluids, there are several studies which show that the intact and latent serpin has biological activities unrelated to the anti-protease function. Both native and latent α_1-antitrypsin inhibit the inflammatory response (LPS-stimulated synthesis and release of TNFα).[302] Native α_1-antitrypsin inhibited the proliferation of breast tumor cell line (MDA-MB 468), whereas a C-terminal fragment of α_1-antitrypsin increased the proliferation of the same cell line.[303]

c α_1-Proteinase inhibitor is also degraded by some exogenous proteases of interest regarding its function in the interstitial space, a protease from dust mite[304] and German cockroach frass.[115]

d   Matrix metalloproteinse 6 is identical with MMP-3.[305]

e   FRET peptide substrate (fluorescent resonance energy transfer peptide substrate) is an assay used extensively for matrix metalloproteinases. It is based on the presence of a fluorophore on (usually) the N-terminal of a peptide and a quencher at the C-terminus; hydrolysis of an internal peptide bond relieves quenching of the fluorophore with a concomitant increase in fluorescence.[306] This is not a sensitive assay but allows recognition of amino acid residues on both side of the scissile peptide bond.[307]

f   There is some confusion between macrophage elastase which is a matrix metalloproteinase and neutrophil elastase (Table 8.1).

g   The cascade concept is found in a number of biological systems possibly dating to the use of the term *cascade* to describe the process of blood coagulation.[308] Implicit in the coagulation hypothesis is the ability to use a cascade to amplify a biological signal.[309] It is not clear that amplification of MMP systems occurs with homeostasis but is amplified with the extravasation of tumors and in inflammation.[310]

References

1. Houck, J.C., Sharma, V.K.., Patel, Y.M., and Gladner, J.A., Induction of collagenolytic and proteolytic activities by anti-inflammatory drugs in the skin and fibroblast, *Biochem. Pharmacol.*, 17, 2081–2090, 1968.

2. Bauer, E.A., Eisen, A.Z., and Jeffrey, J.J., Immunologic relationship of a purified human skin collagenase to other human and animal collagenases, *Biochim. Biophys. Acta*, 206, 152–160, 1970.

3. Fields, G.B., Van Wart, H.E., and Birkedal-Hansen, H., Sequence specificity of human skin fibroblast collagenase. Evidence for the role of collagen structure in determining the collagenase cleavage site, *J. Biol. Chem.*, 262, 6221–6226, 1987.

4. Springman, E.B., Angleton, E.L., Birkedal-Hansen, H., and Van Wart, H.E., Multiple modes of activation of latent human fibroblast collagenase: Evidence for the role of a Cys73 active site zinc complex in latency and a "cysteine switch" mechanism for activation, *Proc. Natl. Acad. Sci. U. S. A.*, 87, 364–368, 1990.

5. Brownell, J., Earley, W., Kunec, E., et al., Comparison of native matrix metalloproteinases and their recombinant catalytic domains using a novel radiometric assay, *Arch. Biochem. Biophys.*, 314, 120–125, 1994.

6. Cawston, T.E., Matrix metallopeptidase-1/interstitial collagenase, in *Handbook of Proteolytic Enzymes*, 3rd edn., N.D. Rawlings and G. Salvesen, eds., pp. 718–725, Elsevier, Amsterdam, Netherlands, 2013.

7. Stetler-Stevenson, W.G., Talano, J.A., Gallagher, M.E., et al., Inhibition of human type IV collagenase by a highly conserved peptide sequence derived from its prosegment, *Am. J. Med. Sci.*, 302, 163–170, 1991.

8. Fowlkes, J.L., Enghild, J.J., Suzuki, K., and Nagase, H., Matrix metalloproteinases degrade insulin-like growth factor-binding protein-3 in dermal fibroblast cultures, *J. Biol. Chem.*, 269, 25742–25746, 1994.

9. Birkedal-Hansen, H., Taylor, R.E., Bhown, A.S., et al., Cleavage of bovine skin type III collagen by proteolytic enzymes. Relative resistance of the fibrillar form, *J. Biol. Chem.*, 260, 16411–16417, 1985.

10. Welgus, H.G., Jeffrey, J.J., Stricklin, G.P., and Eisen, A.Z., The gelatinolytic activity of human skin fibroblast collagenase, *J. Biol. Chem.*, 257, 11534–11539, 1982.

11. Adhikari, A.S., Chai, J., and Dunn, A.R., Mechanical load induces a 100-fold increase in the rate of collagen proteolysis by MMP-1, *J. Am. Chem. Soc.*, 133, 1686–1689, 2013.

12. Fasciglione, G.F., Magda, G., Tsukada, H., et al., The collagenolytic action of MMP-1 is regulated by the interaction between the catalytic domain and the hinge region, *J. Biol. Inorg. Chem.*, 17, 663–672, 2012.

13. Montfort, I., and Perez-Tamayo, R., Distribution of collagenases in normal rat tissues, *J. Histochem. Cytochem.*, 23, 910–920, 1975.

14. Casimiro, S., Mohammed, K.S., Pires, R., et al., RANKL/RANK/MMP-1 molecular triad contributes to the metastatic phenotype of breast and prostate cancer cells in vitro, *PLoS One*, 8, e63153, 2013.

15. Sottrup-Jensen, L., and Birkedal-Hansen, H.Y., Human fibroblast collagenase-α-macroglobulin interactions. Localization of cleavage sites in the bait regions of five mammalian α-macroglobulins, *J. Biol. Chem.*, 264, 393–401, 1989.

16. Sudbeck, B.D., Jeffrey, J.J, Welgus, H.G., et al., Purification and characterization of bovine interstitial collagenase and tissue inhibitor of metalloproteinases, *Arch. Biochem. Biophys.*, 293, 370–376, 1992.

17. Mast, A.E., Enghild, J.J., Nagase, H., et al., Kinetics and physiologic relevance of the inactivation of α_1-proteinase inhibitor, α_1-antichymotrypsin, and antithrombin III by matrix metalloproteinase-1 (tissue collagenase), -2(72 kDa gelatinase/Type IVcollagenase), and -3 (stromelysin), *J. Biol. Chem.*, 266, 15810–15816, 1991.

18. Desrochers, P.E., Jeffrey, J.J., and Weiss, S.J., Interstitial collagenase (matrix metalloproteinase-1) expresses serpinase activity, *J. Clin. Invest.*, 87, 2258–2265, 1991.

19. Janciauskiene, S., Zelvyte, I., Jansson, L., and Stevens, T., Divergent effects of α-1-antitrypsin on neutrophil activation, *in vitro*, *Biochem. Biophys. Res. Commun.*, 315, 288–296, 2004.

20. Moraga, F., Lindgren, S., and Janciauskiene, S., Effects of noninhibitory α-1-antitrypsin on primary human monocyte activation *in vitro*, *Arch. Biochem. Biophys.*, 386, 221–226, 2001.

21. Bedair, H., Liu, T.T., Kaar, J.L., et al., Matrix metalloproteinase-1 therapy improves muscle healing, *J. Appl. Physiol.*, 102, 2338–2345, 2007.

22. Murphy, G., Matrix metallopeptidase-2 (Gelatinase A), in *Handbook of Proteolytic Enzymes*, 3rd edn., N.D. Rawlings and G. Salvesen, eds., pp. 747–753, Elsevier, Amsterdam, Netherlands, 2013.

23. Fujimoto, N., Mouri, N., Iwata, K., et al., A one-step sandwich enzyme immunoassay for human matrix metalloproteinase 2 (72-kDa gelatinase/type IV collagenase) using monoclonal antibodies, *Clin. Chim. Acta*, 221, 91–103, 1993.

24. Florentini, C., Bodei, S., Bedussi, F., et al., GPNMB/OA protein increases the invasiveness of human metastatic prostate cancer cell lines DU145 and PC3 through MMP-2 and MMP-9 activity, *Exp. Cell Res.*, 323, 100–111, 2014.

25. Liu, W.H., Chen, Y.J., Chien, J.H., and Chang, L.S., Amsacrine suppresses matrix metalloproteinase-2 (MMP-2)/MMP-9 expression in human leukemia cells, *J. Cell. Physiol.*, 229, 588–598, 2014.

26. Uwafuji, S., Goi, T., Naruse, T., et al., Protein-bound polysaccharide K reduced the invasive ability of colon caner cell lines, *Anticancer Res.*, 33, 4841–4845, 2013.

27. Lipari, L., and Gerbino, A., Expression of gelatinases (MMP-2, MMP-9) in human articular cartilage, *Int. J. Immunopathol. Pharmacol.*, 26, 817–823, 2013.

28. Marbaix, E., Donnez, J., Courtoy, P.J., and Eeckhout, Y., Progesterone regulates the activity of collagenase and related gelatinases A and B in human endometrial explants, *Proc. Natl. Acad. Sci. U. S. A.*, 89, 11789–11793, 1992.

29. Li, Z., Li, L., Zielke, H.R., et al., Increased expression of 72-kd type IV collagenase (MMP-2) in human aortic atherosclerotic lesions, *Am. J. Pathol.*, 148, 121–128, 1996.

30. Nakoman, C., Resmi, H., Ay, O., et al., Effects of basic fibroblast factor (bFGF) on MMP-2, TIMP-2 and type-1 collagen in human lung carcinoma, *Biochimie*, 87, 343–351, 2005.

31. Maymon, E., Romero, R., Pacora, P., et al., A role for the 72 kDa gelatinase (MMP-2) and its inhibitor (TIMP-2) in human parturation, premature rupture of membranes and intraamniotic infection, *J. Perinatal Med.*, 29, 308–316, 2001.

32. Brinckerhoff, C.E., Rutter, J.L., and Benbow, U., Interstitial collagenases as markers of tumor progression, *Clin. Cancer Res.*, 6, 4823–4830, 2000.

33. Xu, J., Rodriguez, D., Petitclerc, E., et al., Proteolytic exposure of a cryptic site within collagen type IV is required for angiogenesis and tumor growth *in vivo*, *J. Cell Biol.*, 154, 1069–1079, 2001.

34. Pearce, W.H., and Shively, V.P., Abdominal aortic aneurysm as a complex multifactorial disease: Interactions of polymorphisms of inflammatory genes, features of autoimmmunity, and current status of MMPs, *Ann. N. Y. Acad.*, 1085, 117–132, 2006.

35. Willenbrock, F., Crabbe, T., Slocombe, P.M., et al., The activity of the tissue inhibitors of metalloproteinases is regulated by C-terminal domain interactions: A kinetic analysis of the inhibition of gelatinase A, *Biochemistry*, 32, 4330–4337, 1993.

36. Bernardo, M.M., and Fridman, R., TIMP-2 (tissue inhibitor of metalloproteinase-2) regulates MMP-2 (matrix metalloproteinase-2) activity in the extracellular environment after pro-MMP-2 activation by MT1 I(membrane type 1)-MMP, *Biochem. J.*, 374, 739–745, 2003.

37. Yu, A.E., Hewitt, R.E., Kleiner, D.E., and Stetler-Stevenson, W.G., Molecular regulation of cellular invasion—Role of gelatinase A and TIMP-2, *Biochem. Cell Biol.*, 74, 823–831, 1996.

38. Ali, M.A., Fan, X., and Schulz, R., Cardiac sarcomeric proteins: Novel intracellular targets of matrix metalloproteinase-2 in heart disease, *Trends Cardiovasc. Med.*, 21, 112–128, 2011.

39. Jacob-Ferreira, A.L., and Schulz, R., Activation of intracellular matrix metalloproteinase-2 by reactive oxygen-nitrogen species: Consequences and therapeutic strategies in heart, *Arch. Biochem. Biophys.*, 540, 82–93,. 2013.

40. Steffensen, B., Wallon, U.M., and Overall, C.M., Extracellular matrix binding properties of recombinant fibronectin tyep II-like modules of 72-KDa gelatinase/type IV collagenase. High affinity binding to matrix type I collagen but not native type IV collagen, *J. Biol. Chem.*, 270, 11555–11566, 1995.

41. Hornebeck, W., Bellon, G., and Emonard, H., Fibronectin type II (FnII)-like modules regulate gelatinase A activity, *Pathol. Biol.*, 53, 405–410, 2005.

42. Mikhailova, M., Xu, X., Robichaud, T.K., et al., Identification of collagen binding domain residues that govern catalytic activities of matrix metalloproteinase-2 (MMP-2), *Matrix Biol.*, 31, 380–388, 2012.

43. Azzam, H.S., and Thompson, E.W., Collagen-induced activation of M_r 72,000 type IV collagenase in normal and malignant human fibroblast cells, *Cancer Res.*, 52, 4540–4544, 1992.

44. Sato, H., and Takino, T., Coordinate action of membrane-type matrix metalloproteinase -1 (MT1-MMP) and MMP-2 enhances pericellular proteolysis and invasion, *Cancer Sci.*, 101, 843–847, 2010.

45. O'Reilly, M.S., Wiederschain, D., Stetler-Stevenson, W.G., et al., Regulation of angiostatin production by matrix metalloproteinase-2 in a model of concomitant resistance, *J. Biol. Chem.*, 274, 29568–29571, 2006.

46. Chung, A.W., Hsiang, Y.N., Matzke, L.A., et al., Reduced expression of vascular endothelial growth factor paralleled with the increased angiostatin expression resulting from the upregulated activities of matrix metalloproteinase-2 and -9 in human type 2 diabetic arterial vasculature, *Circ. Res.*, 99, 140–148, 2006.

47. Guo, H., Liu, L., Shi, Y., et al., Chinese yellow wine and red wine inhibit matrix metalloproteinase-2 and improve atherosclerotic plaque in LDL receptor knockout mice, *Cardiovasc. Ther.*, 28, 161–168, 2010.

48. Walter, A., Etienne-Swelloum, N., Sarz, M., et al., Angiotensis II induces the vascular expression of VEGF and MMP-2 *in vivo*: Preventive effect of red wine polyphenols, *J. Vasc. Res.*, 45, 386–394, 2008.

49. Knäuper, V., Will, H., López-Otin, C., et al., Cellular mechanisms for human procollagenase-3 (MMP-13) activation. Evidence that MT1-MMP(MMP-14) and gelatinase a (MMP-2) are able to generate active enzyme, *J. Biol. Chem.*, 271, 17124–17131, 1996.

50. Galis, Z.S., Krankhöfer, R., Fenton, J.W., 2nd., and Libby, P., Thrombin promotes activation of matrix metalloproteinase-2 produced by cultured vascular smooth muscle cells, *Arterioscler. Thromb. Vasc. Biol.*, 17, 483–489, 1997.

51. Lafleur, M.A., Hollenberg, M.D., Atkinson, S.J., et al., Activation of pro-(matrix metalloproteinase-2)(pro-MMP-2) by thrombin is membrane-type-MMP-dependent in human umbilical vein endothelial cells and generates a distinct 63 kDa active species, *Biochem. J.*, 357, 107–115, 2001.

52. Wang, Z., Kong, L., Kang, J., et al., Thrombin stimulates mitogenesis in pig cerebrovascular smooth muscle cells involving activation of pro-matrix metalloproteinase-2, *Neurosci. Let.*, 452, 199–203, 2009.

53. Koo, B.H., Han, J.H., Jeom, Y.I., et al., Thrombin-dependent MMP-2 activity is regulated by heparan sulfate, *J. Biol. Chem.*, 285, 41270–41279, 2010.

54. Pekovich, S.R., Bock, P.E., and Hoover, R.L., Thrombin-thrombomodulin activation of protein C faciltates the activation of progelatinase A, *FEBS Lett.*, 494, 129–132, 2001.

55. Okada, Y., Morodomi, T., Enghild, J.J., et al., Matrix metalloproteinase 2 from human rheumatoid synovial fibroblasts. Purification and activation of the precursor and enzymatic properties, *Eur. J. Biochem.*, 194, 721–739, 1990.

56. Guo, X.T., Wang, J.F., Zhang, L.Y., et al., Quantitative assessment of the effects of MMP-2 polymorphisms on lung carcinoma risk, *Asian Pac. J. Cancer Prev.*, 13, 2853–2856, 2012.

57. Ortak, H., Demir, S., Ates, Ö., et al., The role of MMP2 (-1306C>T and TIMP2 (-418 G>C) promoter variants in age-relaed macular degeneration, *Ophthalmic Genet.*, 34, 217–222, 2013.

58. Kaminska, A., Banas-Lezanska, P., Przybylowska, K., et al., The protective role of the735C/T and the -1306C/T polymorphisms of the MMP-2 gene in the development of primary open-angle glaucoma, *Ophthalmic Genet.*, 35, 41–46, 2014.

59. Nie, S.W., Wang, X.F., and Tang, Z.C., Correlations between MMP-2/MMP-9 promoter polymorphisms and ischemic stroke, *Int. J. Clin. Exp. Med.*, 7, 400–404, 2014.

60. Nagase, H., Matrix metalloproteinase 3/Stromelysin 1, in *Handbook of Proteolytic Enzymes*, 3rd edn., N.D. Rawlings and G. Salvesen, eds., pp. 763–774, Elsevier, Amsterdam, Netherlands, 2013.

61. Sapolsky, A.I., Malemud, C.J., Norby, D.P., et al., Neutral proteinases from articular chondrocytes in culture. 2. Metal-dependent latent neutral proteoglycanase, and inhibitory activity, *Biochim. Biophys. Acta*, 658, 138–147, 1981.

62. Galloway, W.A., Murphy, G., Sandy, J.D., et al., Purification and characterization of a rabbit bone metalloproteinase that degrades proteoglycan and other connective-tissue components, *Biochem. J.*, 209, 741–752, 1983.

63. Gowen, M., Wood, D.D., Ihrie, E.J., et al., Stimulation by human interleukin 1 of cartilage breakdown and production of collagenase and procollagenase and proteoglycanase by human chondrocytes but not by human osteoblasts *in vitro*, *Biochim. Biophys. Acta*, 797, 186–193, 1984.

64. Okada, Y., Harris, E.D., Jr., and Nagase, H., The precursor of a metallopeptidase from human rheumatoid synovial fibroblasts. Purification and mechanisms of activation by endopeptidases and 4-aminophenylmercuric acetate, *Biochem. J.*, 254, 731–741, 1988.

65. Machida, C.M., Scott, J.D., and Ciment, G., NGF-induction of the metalloproteinase-transin/stromelysin in PC12 cells: Involvement of multiple protein kinases, *J. Cell Biol.*, 114, 1037–1048, 1991.

66. Fang, Q., Liu, X., Al-Mugotir, M., et al., Thrombin and TNF-α/IL-1β synergistically induce fibroblast-mediated collagen gel degradation, *Am. J. Respir. Cell Mol. Biol.*, 35, 714–721, 2006.

67. Okada, Y., and Nakanishi, I., Activation of matrix metalloproteinase 3 (stromelysin) and matrix metalloproteinase 2 ("gelatinase") by human neutrophil elastase and cathepsin G, *FEBS Lett.*, 249, 353–356, 1989.

68. Beaufort, N., Plaza, K., Utzschneider, D., et al., Interdependence of kallikrein-related peptidases in proteolytic networks, *Biol. Chem.*, 391, 581–587, 2010.

69. Geurts, N., Martens, E., Van Aelst, I., et al., β-Hematin interaction with the hemopexin domain of gelatinase B/MMP-9 provokes autocatalytic processing of the propeptide, thereby priming activation by MMP-3, *Biochemistry*, 47, 2689–2699, 2008.

70. Johnson, L.L., Pavlovsky, A.G., Johnson, A.R., et al., A rationalization of the acidic pH dependence for stromelysin-1 (matrix metalloproteinase-3) catalysis and inhibition, *J. Biol. Chem.*, 275, 11026–11933, 2000.

71. Gunja-Smith, Z., Nagase, H., and Woessner, J.F., Jr., Purification of the neutral proteoglycan-degrading metalloproteinase from human articular cartilage and its identification as stromelysis matrix metalloproteinase-3, *Biochem. J.*, 258, 115–119, 1989.

72. Okada, Y., Konomi, H., Yada, T., et al., Degradation of type IX collagen by matrix metalloproteinase-3 (stromelysin) from human rheumatoid synovial cells, *FEBS Lett.*, 244, 473–476, 1989.

73. Wu, J.J., Lark, M.W., Chun, L.E., and Eyre, D.R., Sites of stromelysin cleavage in collagen type II, IX, X, and XI of cartilage, *J. Biol. Chem.*, 266, 5625–5628, 1991.

74. WIlhelm, S.M., Wunderlich, D., Maniglia, C.A., et al., Primary structure and function of stromelysin/transin in cartilage matrix, *Matrix Suppl.*, 1, 37–44, 1992.

75. Coppock, H.S., White, A., Aplin, J.D., and Westwood, M., Matrix metalloprotease-3 and -9 proteolyze insulin-like growth factor-binding protein-1, *Biol. Reprod.*, 71, 438–443, 2004.

76. Teahan, J., Harrison, R., Izquierdo, M., and Stein, R.L., Substrate specificity of human fibroblast stromelysin. Hydrolysis of substance P and and its analogues, *BIochemistry* 28, 8497–8501, 1989.

77. Schure, R., Costa, K.D., Rezaei, R., et al., Impact of matrix metalloproteinases on inhibition of mineralization by fetuin, *J. Periodont. Res.*, 46, 357–366, 2013.

78. Lijnen, H.R., Arza, B., Van Hoef, B., Collen, D., and Declerck, P.J., Inactivation of plasminogen activator inhibitor-1 by specific proteolysis with stromelysin-1 (MMP-3), *J. Biol. Chem.*, 275, 37645–37650, 2000.

79. Lijnen, H.R., Ugwu, F., Bini, A., and Collen, D., Generation of an angiostatin-like fragment from plasminogen by stromelysin-1(MMP-3), *Biochemistry*, 37, 4699–4702, 1998.

80. Enghild, J.J., Salvesen, G., Brew, K., and Nagase, H., Interaction of human rheumatoid synovial collagenase (matrix metalloproteinase-1) and stromelysin (matrix metalloproteinase 3) with human α$_2$-macroglobulin and chicken ovostatin. Binding kinetics and identification of matrix metalloproteinase cleavage sites, *J. Biol. Chem.*, 264, 8779–8785, 1989.

81. Willenbrock, F., and Murphy, G., Structure-function relationships in the tissue inhibitors of metalloproteinases, *Am. J. Respir. Crit. Care Med.*, 150, S165–S170, 1994.

82. Woessner, J.F., MMPs and TIMPs an historical perspective, in *Matrix Metalloproteinases Protocols (Methods in Molecular Biology)*, vol. 151, I. Clark, ed., pp. 1–23, Humana Press, Totowa, NJ, 2001.

83. Matrisian, L.M., Matrix metalloproteinase-7/matrilysin, in *Handbook of Proteolytic Enzymes*, 3rd ed., N.D. Rawlings and G. Salvesen, eds., pp. 785–795, Elsevier, Amsterdam, Netherlands, 2013.

84. Woessner, J.F., Jr., Matrilysin, *Methods Enzymol.*, 248, 485–495, 1995.

85. Miyazaki, K., Hattori, Y., Umenishi, F., et al., Purification and characterization of extracellular matrix-degrading metalloproteinase, matrin (Pump-1), secreted from human rectal carcinoma cell line, *Cancer Res.*, 50, 7758–7764, 1990.

86. Remacle, A.G., Golubkov, V.S., Shiryaev, S.A., et al., Novel MT1-MMP small-molecule inhibitors based on insights into hemopexin domain function in tumor growth, *Cancer Res.*, 72, 2339–2349, 2012.

87. Correia, A.L., Mori, H., Chen, E.I., et al., The hemopexin domain of MMP-3 is responsible for mammary epithelial invasion and morphogenesis through extracellular interaction with HSP90β, *Genes Dev.*, 27, 805–817, 2013.

88. Crabbe, T., Willenbrock, F., Eaton, D., et al., Biochemical characterization of matrilysin. Activation conforms to the stepwise mechanisms proposed for other matrix metalloproteinases, *Biochemistry*, 31, 8500–8507, 1992.

89. Rims, C.R., and McGuire, J.K., Matrilysin (MMP-7) catalytic activity regulates β-catenin localization and signaling activation in lung epithelial cells, *Exp. Lung Res.*, 40, 126–136, 2014.

90. Fu, X., Kassim, S.Y., Parks, W.C., and Heinecke, J.W., Hypochlorous acid oxygenates the cysteine switch domain of pro-matrilysin (MMP-7). A mechanism for matrix metalloproteinase activation and atherosclerotic plaque rupture by myeloperoxidase, *J. Biol. Chem.*, 276, 41279–41287, 2001.

91. Fu, X., Kao, J.L., Bergt, C., et al., Oxidative cross-linking of tryptophan to glycine restrains matrix metalloproteinase activity: Specific structural motifs control protein oxidation, *J. Biol. Chem.*, 279, 6209–6212, 2004.

92. Bonacci, G., Schopfer, F.J., Batthyany, C.I., et al., Electrophilic fatty acids regulate matrix metalloproteinase activity and expression, *J. Biol. Chem.*, 286, 16074–16081, 2011.

93. Wilson, C.L., and Matrisian, L.M., Matrilysin: An epithelial matrix metalloproteinase with potentially novel functions, *Int. J. Biochem. Cell Biol.*, 28, 123–136, 1996.

94. Baker, A.H., Edwards, D.R., and Murphy, G., Metalloprotease inhibitors: Biological actions and therapeutic opportunities, *J. Cell Sci.*, 115, 3719–3727, 2002.

95. Tscheche, H., and Wenzel, H., Neutrophil collagenase, in *Handbook of Proteolytic Enzymes*, 3rd edn., N.D. Rawlings and G. Salvesen, eds., pp. 725–738, Elsevier, Amsterdam, Netherlands, 2013.

96. Capodici, C., Muthukumaran, G., Amoruso, M.A., and Berg, R.A., Activation of neutrophill collagenase by cathepsin G, *Inflammation*, 13, 245–258, 1989.

97. Knäuper, V., Wilhelm, S.M., Seperack, P.K., et al., Direct activation of human neutrophil procollagenase by recombinant stromelysin, *Biochem. J.*, 295, 581–586, 1993.

98. Okamoto, T., Akaike, T., Nagano, T., et al., Activation of human neutrophil procollagenase by nitrogen dioxide and peroxynitrite: A novel mechanism for procollagenase activation involving nitric oxide, *Arch. Biochem. Biophys.*, 342, 262–274, 1997.

99. Saari, H., Suomalainen, K., Lindy, O., et al., Activation of latent human neutrophil collagenase by reactive oxygen species and serine proteases, *Biochem. Biophys. Res. Commun.*, 171, 979–987, 1990.

100. Chatham, W.W., Blackburn, W.D., Jr., and Heck, L.W., Additive enhancement of neutrophil collagenase activity by HOCl and cathepsin G, *Biochem. Biophys. Res. Commun.*, 184, 560–567, 1992.

101. Michaelis, J., Vissers, M.C., and Winterbourn, C.C., Human neutrophil collagenase cleaves α$_1$-antitrypsin, *Biochem. J.*, 270, 809–814, 1990.

102. Gioia, M., Fasciglione, G.F., Marini, S., et al., Modulation of the catalytic activity of neutrophil collagenase MMP-8 on bovine collagen I. Role of the activation cleavage and of the hemopexin-like domain, *J. Biol. Chem.*, 277, 23123–23130, 2002.

103. Brandstetter, H., Grams, F., Glitz, D., et al., The 1.8-A crystal structure of a matrix metalloproteinase 8-barbiturate inhibitor complex reveals a previously unobserved mechanism for collagenase substrate recognition, *J. Biol. Chem.*, 276, 17405–17412, 2001.

104. Desrochers, P.E., Mookhtiar, K., Van Wart, H.E., et al., Proteolytic inactivation of α$_1$-proteinase inhibitor and α$_1$-antichymotrypsin by oxidatively activated human neutrophil metalloproteinases, *J. Biol. Chem.*, 267, 5005–5012, 1992.

105. Sorsa, T., Lindy, O., Konttinen, Y.T., et al., Doxycycline in the protection of serum α$_1$-antitrypsin from human neutrophil collagenase and gelatinase, *Antimicrob. Agents Chemother.*, 37, 592–594, 1993.

106. Lee, H.M., Ciancio, S.G., Tüter, G., et al., Subantimicrobial dose doxycycline efficacy as a matrix metalloproteinase inhibitor in chronic periodontitis patients is enhanced when combined with a non-steroidal anti-inflammatory drug, *J. Periodontol.*, 75, 453–463, 2004.

107. Mäkitalo, L., Rintamäki, H., Tervahartinala, T., et al., Serum MMPs 7-9 and their inhibitors during glucocorticoid and anti-TNF-α therapy in pediatric inflammatory bowel disease, *Scand. J. Gastroenterol.*, 47, 785–794, 2012.

108. Farr, M., Pieper, M., Calvete, J., and Tschesche, H., The N-terminus of collagenase MMP-8 determines superactivity and inhibition: A relation of structure and function analyzed by biomolecular interaction analysis, *Biochemistry*, 38, 7332–7338, 1999.

109. Owen, C.A., Hu, Z., Lopez-Otin, C., and Shapiro, S.D., Membrane-bound matrix metalloproteinase-8 on activated polymorphonuclear cells is a potent tissue inhibitor of metalloproteinase-resistant collagenase and serpinase, *J. Immunol.*, 172, 7791–7803, 2004.

110. Sopata, I., and Dancewicz, A.M., Presence of a gelatin-specific proteinase and its latent form in human leucocytes, *Biochim. Biophys. Acta*, 370, 510–523, 1974.

111. Triebel, S., Bläser, J., Reinke, H., and Tschesche, H., A 25 kDa α-2-microglobulin-related protein is a component of the 125 kDa form of human gelatinase, *FEBS Lett.*, 314, 386–388, 1992.

112. Eisen, A.Z., Sarker, S.K., Newman, K.C., and Goldberg, G.I., Matrix metalloproteinase 9/gelatinase B, in *The Handbook of Proteolytic Enzymes*, 3rd edn., N.D. Rawlings and G. Salvesen, eds., pp. 754–763, Elsevier, Amsterdam, Netherlands, 2013.

113. Okada, Y., Gonoji, Y., Naka, K., et al., Matrix metalloproteinase 9 (93-kDa gelatinase/type IV collagenase) from HT 1080 human fibrosarcoma cells, *J. Biol. Chem.*, 267, 21712–21719, 1992.

114. Meli, D.N., Christen, S., and Lieb, S.L., Matrix metalloproteinase-9 in pneumococcal menigitis activation via an oxidative pathway, *J. Infect. Dis.*, 187, 1411–1415, 2003.

115. Hughes, V.S., and Page, K., German cockroach frass proteases cleave pro-matrix metalloproteinase-9, *Exp. Lung Res.*, 33, 135–150, 2007.

116. Kjeldsen, L., Johnson, A.H., Sengeløv, H., and Borregaard, N., Isolation and primary structure of NGAL, a novel protein associated with human neutrophil gelatinase, *J. Biol. Chem.*, 268, 10425–10432, 1993.

117. Winberg, J.-O., Kolset, S.O., Berg, E., and Uhlin-Hansen, L., Macrophage secrete matrix metalloproteinase 9 covalently linked to the core protein of chondroitin sulphate proteoglycans, *J. Mol. Biol.*, 304, 669–680, 2000.

118. Vandooren, J., Van den Steem, P.E., and Opdenakker, G., Biochemistry and molecular biology of gelatinase B or matrix metalloproteinase-9 (MMP-9): The next decade, *Crit. Rev. Biochem. Mol. Biol.*, 48, 222–272, 2013.

119. Yu, Q., and Stamenkovic, I., Cell surface-localized matrix metalloproteinase-9 proteolytically activated TGF-β and promotes tumor invasion and angiogenesis, *Genes Dev.*, 14, 163–176, 2000.

120. Chetty, C., Vanamala, S.K., Gondi, C.S., et al., MMP-9 induces CD44 cleavage and CD44 mediated cell migration in glioblastoma xenograft cells, *Cell Signal.*, 24, 549–559, 2012.

121. Naor, D., CD44, in *Encyclopedia of Immunology*, 2nd edn., P.J. Delves and I.M. Raitt, eds., vol. 1, pp. 488–491, Academic Press, San Diego, CA, 1998.

122. Schmidt, S., and Friedl, P., Interstitial cell migration: Integrin-dependent and alternative adhesion mechanisms, *Cell Tissue Res.*, 339, 92, 2010.

123. Niyibizi, C., Chan, R., Vu, J.-J., and Eyre, D., A 93 kDa gelatinase (MMP-9) cleavage site in native type V collagen, *Biochem. Biophys. Res. Commun.*, 202, 328–333, 1994.

124. Bigg, H.F., Rowan, A.D., Barker, M.D., and Cawston, T.E., Activity of matrix metalloproteinase 9 against native collagenase types I and III, *FEBS J.*, 274, 1246–1255, 2007.

125. Christiansen, V.J., Jackson, K.W., Lee, K.N., and McKee, P.A., Effect of fibroblast activation protein and α2-antiplasmin cleaving enzyme on collagen types I, III, and IV, *Arch. Biochem. Biophys.*, 457, 177–186, 2007.

126. Minond, D., Lauer-Fields, J.L., Cudic, M., et al., The roles of substrate thermal stability and P_2 and P_1' subsite identity on matrix metalloproteinase triple-helical peptidase activity and collagen specificity, *J. Biol. Chem.*, 281, 38302–38313, 2006.

127. Schönbeck, U., Mach, F., and Libby, P., Generation of biologically active IL-1β by matrix metalloproteinases: A novel caspace-1-independent pathway of IL-1β processing, *J. Immunol.*, 161, 3340–3346, 1998.

128. Yin, K.J., Cirrito, J.R., Yan, P., et al., Matrix metalloproteinases expressed by astrocytes mediate extracellular amyloid-β peptide catabolism, *J. Neurosci.*, 26, 10939–10948, 2006.

129. Senior, R.M., Griffin, G.L., Fliszar, C.J., et al., Human 92- and 72-kilodalton type IV collagenases are elastases, *J. Biol. Chem.*, 266, 7870–7875, 1991.

130. Opdenakker, G., Van den Steen, P.E., Dubois, B., et al., Gelatinase B functions as regulator and effector in leukocyte biology, *J. Leukocyte Biol.*, 69, 851–859, 2001.

131. Patterson, B.C., and Sang, Q.A., Angiostatin-converting enzyme activities of human matrilysin (MMP-7) and gelatinase B/type IV collagenase (MMP-9), *J. Biol. Chem.*, 272, 28823–28825, 1997.

132. Pozzi, A., LeVine, W.F., and Gardner, H.A., Low plasma levels of matrix metalloproteinase 9 permit increased tumor angiogenesis, *Oncogene*, 21, 272–281, 2002.

133. Lium, Z., Zhou, K, Shapiro, S.D., et al., The serpin α1-proteinase inhibitor is a critical substrate for gelatinase B/MMP-9 *in vivo*, *Cell*, 102, 647–655, 2000.

134. Muroski, M.E., Roycik, M.D., Newcomer, R.G., et al., Matrix metalloproteinase-9/gelatinase B is a putative therapeutic target of chronic obstructive pulmonary disease and multiple sclerosis, *Curr. Pharmaceut. Biotechnol.*, 9, 34–46, 2008.

135. Janciauskiene, S., Zelvyte, I., Jansson, L., et al., Divergent effects of α1-antitrypsin on neutrophil activation, in vitro, *Biochem. Biophys. Res. Commun.*, 315, 288–296, 2004.

136. Han, Y.-P., Yan, C., and Garner, W.L., Proteolytic activation of matrix metalloproteinase-9 in skin wound healing is inhibited by α-1-antichymotrypsin, *J. Invest. Derm.*, 128, 2334–2342, 2008.

137. Reiss, M.J., Han, Y.-P., and Garner, W.L., α1-Antichymotrypsin activity correlates with and may modulate matrix metalloproteinase-9 in human acute wounds, *Wound Rep. Reg.*, 17, 418–426, 2009.

138. Zilm, P.S., and Bartold, P.M., Proteomic identification of proteinase inhibitors in the porcine enamel matrix derivative, EMD®, *J. Periodontol. Res.*, 46, 111–117, 2011.

139. Fingleton, B., Matrix metallopeptidase-10/stromelysin 2, in *Handbook of Proteolytic Enzymes*, 3rd edn., N.D. Rawlings and G. Salvesen, eds., pp. 774–778, Elsevier, Amsterdam, Netherlands, 2013.

140. Sirum, K.L., and Brinckerhoff, C.E., Cloning of the gene for human stromelysin and stromelysin-2: Differential expression in rheumatoid synovial fibroblasts, *Biochemistry*, 28, 8691–8698, 1989.

141. Bord, S., Horner, A., Hembry, R.M., and Compton, J.E., Stromelysin-1 (MMP-3) and stromelysin-2 (MMP-10) expression in developing human bone: Potential roles in skeletal development, *Bone*, 23, 7–12, 1998.

142. Bodey, B., Bodey, B., Jr., Siegel, S.E., and Kaiser, H.E., Matrix metalloproteinases in neoplasm-induced extracellular matrix remodeling in breast carcinoma, *Anticancer Res.*, 21, 2021–2028, 2001.

143. Burbridge, M.F., Cogé, F., Galizzi, J.P., et al., The role of the matrix metalloproteinases during in vitro vessel formation, *Angiogenesis*, 5, 215–226, 2002.

144. Batra, J., Robinson, J., Soares, A.S., et al., Matrix metalloproteinase-10 (MMP-10) interaction with tissue inhibitors of metalloproteinases TIMP-1 and TIMP-2: Binding studies and crystal structure, *J. Biol. Chem.*, 287, 15935–15946, 2012.

145. Batra, J., Soares, A.S., Mehner, C., and Radisky, E.S., Matrix metalloproteinase-10/TIMP-2 structure and analyses define conserved core interactions and diverse exosite interactions in MMP/TIMP complexes, *PLoS One*, 8, e75836, 2013.

146. Rio, M.-C., Matrix metalloproteinase-11/stromelysin 3, in *Handbook of Proteolytic Enzymes*, 3rd edn., N.D. Rawlings and G. Salvesen, eds., pp. 779–786, Elsevier, Amsterdam, Netherlands, 2013.

147. Pei, D., Majmudar, G., and Weiss, S.J., Hydrolytic inactivation of a breast carcinoma cell-derived serpin by serpin stromelysin-3, *J. Biol. Chem.*, 269, 25849–25855, 1994.

148. Noël, A., Santavicca, M., Stoll, I., et al., Identification of structural determinants controlling human and mouse stromelysin-3 proteolytic activities, *J. Biol. Chem.*, 270, 22866–22872, 1995.

149. Pan, W., Arnone, M., Kendall, M., et al., Identification of peptide substrates for human MMP-11 (stromelysin-3) using phage display, *J. Biol. Chem.*, 278, 27820–27827, 2003.

150. Mañes, S., Mira, E., del Mar Barbarcid, M., et al., Identification of insulin-like growth factor-binding protein-1 as a potential physiological substrate for human stromelysin-3, *J. Biol. Chem.*, 272, 27506–25712, 1997.

151. Meyer, B.S., and Rademann, J., Extra- and intracellular imaging of human matrix metalloprotease 11(*h*MMP-11) with a cell-penetrating FRET substrate, *J. Biol. Chem.*, 287, 37857–37867, 2012.

152. Tan, J., Buache, E., Alpy, F., et al., Stromal matrix metalloproteinase-11 is involved in the mammary gland postnatal development, *Oncogene*, 33(31), 4050–4059, 2014.

153. Okada, A., Saez, S., Misumi, Y., et al., Rat stromelysin 3: cDNA cloning from healing skin wound, activation by furin and expression in rat tissues, *Gene*, 185, 187–193, 1997.

154. Asch, P.H., Basset, P., Roos, M., et al., Expression of stromelysin 3 in keratoarcanthoma and squamous cell carcinoma, *Am. J. Dermatopathol.*, 21, 146–150, 1999.

155. Pei, D., and Weiss, S.J., Furin-dependent intracellular activation of the human stromelysin-3 zymogen, *Nature*, 375, 244–247, 1995.

156. Kaynar, M., and Shapiro, S.D., Matrix metallopeptidase-12/macrophage elastase, in *Handbook of Proteolytic Enzymes*, 3rd edn., N.D. Rawlings and G. Salvesen, eds., pp. 800–864, Elsevier, Amsterdam, Netherlands, 2013.

157. Banda, M.J., and Werb, Z., Mouse macrophage elastase. Purification and characterization as a metalloproteinase, *Biochem. J.*, 193, 589–605, 1981.

158. Shapiro, S.D., Kobayashi, D.K., and Ley, T.J., Cloning and characterization of a unique elastolytic metalloproteinase produced by human alveolar macrophages, *J. Biol. Chem.*, 268, 23824–23829, 1993.

159. Bhaskaran, R., Palmier, M.O., Lauer-Fields, J.L., et al., MMP-12 catalytic domain recognizes triple helical peptide models of collagen V with exosites and high activity, *J. Biol. Chem.*, 283, 21779–21783, 2008.

160. Banda, M.J., Rice, A.G., Griffin, G.L., and Senior, R.M., α_1-Proteinase inhibitor is a neutrophil chemoattractant after proteolytic inactivation by macrophage elastase, *J. Biol. Chem.*, 263, 4481–4484, 1988.

161. Cornelius, L.A., Nehring, L.C., Harding, E., et al., Matrix metalloproteinases generate angiostatin: Effects on neovascularlization, *J. Immunol.*, 161, 6845–6852, 1998.

162. Gronski, T.J., Jr., Martin, R.L., Kobayashi, D.K., et al., Hydrolysis of a broad spectrum of extracellular matrix proteins by human macrophage elastase, *J. Biol. Chem.*, 272, 12189–12194, 1997.

163. Banda, M.J., Clark, E.J., Sinha, S., and Travis, J., Interaction of mouse macrophage elastase with native and oxidized human α_1-proteinase inhibitor, *J. Clin. Invest.*, 79, 1314–1317, 1987.

164. Le Quément, C., Guénon, I., Gillon, J.Y., et al., MMP-12 induces IL-8/CSCL8 secretion through EGFR and ERK1/2 activation in epithelial cells, *Am. J. Physiol. Lung Cell Mol. Physiol.*, 294, L1076–L1084, 2008.

165. Henriet, P., and Eeckhout, Y., Matrix metallopeptidase-13 (collagenase 3), in *Handbook of Proteolytic Enzymes*, 3rd edn., N.D. Rawlings and G. Salvesen, eds., pp 734–744, 2013.

166. Borden, P., Solymar, D., Sucharczuk, A., et al., Cytokine control of interstitial collagenase and collagenase-3 gene expression in human chondrocytes, *J. Biol. Chem.*, 271, 23577–23581, 1996.

167. Haston, J.L., FitzGerald, O., Kane, D., and Smith, K.D., The influence of α_1-acid glycoprotein on collagenase-3 activity in early rheumatoid arthritis, *Biomed. Chromatog.*, 17, 361–364, 2003.

168. Barksby, H.E., Milner, J.M., Patterson, A.M., et al., Matrix metalloproteinase 10 promotion of collagenolysis via procollagenase activation: Implications for cartilage degradation in arthritis, *Arthritis Rheum.*, 54, 3244–3253, 2006.

169. Austin, K.M., Covic, L., and Kuliopulos, A., Matrix metalloproteases and PAR1 activation, *Blood*, 121, 431–439, 2013.

170. Huang, C.-Y., Lin, H.-J., Chen, H.-S., et al., Thrombin promotes matrix metalloproteinase-13 expression through the PKCδ/c-Src/EGFR/P13K/Akt/AP-1 signaling pathway in human chondrocytes, *Mediators Inflamm.*, 2013, 326041, 2013.

171. Beekman, B., Drijfhout, J.W., Ronday, H.K., and TeKoppele, J.M., Fluorogenic MMP activity assay for plasma including MMPs complexed to α_2-macroglobulin, *Ann. N. Y. Acad. Sci.*, 878, 150–158, 1999.

172. Itoh, Y., and Selki, M., Membrane-type matrix metalloprotenase 1, in *Handbook of Proteolytic Enzymes*, 3rd edn., N.D. Rawlings and G.Salvesen, eds., pp. 804–814, Elsevier, Amsterdam, Netherlands, 2013.

173. Sato, H., Takino, T., Okada, Y., et al., A matrix metalloproteinase expressed on the surface of invasive tumor cells, *Nature*, 370, 61–65, 1994.

174. Golubkov, V.S., Chekanov, A.V., Shiryaev, S.A., et al., Proteolysis of the membrane type-1 matrix metalloproteinase prodomain: Implications for a two-step proteolytic processing and activation, *J. Biol. Chem.*, 282, 36283–36291, 2007.

175. Roghi, C., Jones, L., Gratian, M., et al., Golgi reassembly stacking protein 55 interacts with membrane-type (MT) 1-matrix metalloproteinase (MMP) and furin and plays a role in the activation of the MT1-MMP zymogen, *FEBS J.*, 277, 3158–3175, 2010.

176. Holmbeck, K., Bianco, P., Yamada, S., and Birkedal-Hanson, H., MT1-MMP, a tethered collagenase, *J. Cell Physiol.*, 200, 11–19, 2004.

177. Sato, H., and Takino, T., Coordinate action of membrane-type matrix metalloproteinase -1 (MT1-MMP) and MMP-2 enhances pericellular proteolysis and invasion, *Cancer Sci.*, 101, 843–847, 2010.

178. Ries, C., Egea, V., Karow, M., et al., MMP-2, MT1-MMP, and TIMP-2 are essential for the invasive capacity of human mesenchymal cells: Differential regulation by inflammatory cytokines, *Blood*, 109, 4055–4063, 2007.

179. Lafleur, M.A., Tester, A.M., and Thompson, E.W., Selective involvement of TIMP-2 in the second activational cleavage of pro-MMP-2: Refinement of the pro-MMP-2 activation mechanism, *FEBS Lett.*, 553, 457–463, 2003.

180. Hernandez-Barrantas, S., Toght, M., Bernardo, M.M., et al., Binding of active (57 kDa) membrane type 1-matrix metalloproteinase (MT1-MMP) to tissue inhibitor of metalloproteinase (TIMP)-2 regulates MT1-MPP processing and pro-MMP-2 activation, *J. Biol. Chem.*, 275, 12080–12089, 2008.

181. Strongin, A.Y., Collier, I., Bannikov, G., et al., Mechanism of cell surface activation of 72-kDa type IV collagenase. Isolation of the activated form of the membrane metalloprotease, *J. Biol. Chem.*, 270, 5331–5338, 1995.

182. Lambert, E., Dassé, E., Haye, B., and Petitfrère, E., TIMPs as multifacial proteins, *Crit. Rev. Oncology Hematol.*, 49, 287–198, 2004.

183. Toole, B.P., Emmprin (CD147), a cell surface regulator of matrix metalloproteinase production and function, *Curr. Top. Dev. Biol.*, 54, 371–389, 2003.

184. Schmidt, R., Redecke, V., Breitfeld, Y., et al., EMMPRIN (CD 147) is a central activator of extracellular matrix degradation by *Chlamydia pneumoniae*-infected monocytes. Implications for plaque rupture, *Thromb. Haemost.*, 95, 151–158, 2006.

185. Huet, E., Gabison, E.E., Mourah, S., and Menashi, S., Role of emprin/CD147 in tissue remodeling, *Connect. Tissue Res.*, 49, 175–179, 2008.

186. Egawa, N., Koshikawa, N., Tomari, T., et al., Membrane type 1 matrix metalloproteinase (MT1-MMP) cleaves and releases a 22-kDa extracellular matrix metalloproteinase inducer (EMMPRIN) from tumor cells, *J. Biol. Chem.*, 281, 37576–37586, 2006.

187. Polette, M., Nawrocki-Raby, B., Gilles, C., et al., Tumour invasion and matrix metalloproteinases, *Crit. Rev. Oncol. Hematol.*, 49, 179–186, 2004.

188. Remacle, A.G., Shiryaev, S.A., Golubkov, V.S., et al., Non-destructive and selective imaging of the functionally active, pro-invasvive membrane type-1 matrix metalloproteinase (MT1-MMP) enzyme in cancer cells, *J. Biol. Chem.*, 288, 20568–20580, 2013.

189. Miller, M.C., Manning, H.B., Jain, A., et al., Membrane type 1 matrix metalloproteinase is a crucial promoter of synovial invasion in human rheumatoid arthritis, *Arthritis Rheum.*, 60, 686–697, 2009.

190. Cork, S.M., Kaur, B., Devi, N.S., et al., A proprotein convertase (MMP-14) proteolytic cascase releases a novel 40 kDa vasculostatin from tumor suppressor BAI1, *Oncogene*, 31, 5144–5152, 2012.

191. Yama, I., and Seikli, M., Membrane-type-2 metalloproteinase, in *Handbook of Proteolytic Enzymes*, 3rd edn., N.D. Rawlings and G. Salvesen, eds., pp. 815–817, Elsevier, Amsterdam, Netherlands, 2013.

192. Will, H., and Hinzmann, B., cDNA sequence and mRNA tissue distribution of a novel human matrix metalloproteinase with a potential transmembrane segment, *Eur. J. Biochem.*, 231, 602–608, 1995.

193. Morrison, C.J., Butler, G.S., Biggs, H.F., et al., Cellular activation of MMP-2 (gelatinase A) by MT2-MMP occurs via a TIMP-2 independent pathway, *J. Biol. Chem.*, 276, 47402–47410, 2001.

194. Morrison, C.J., and Overall, C.M., TIMP independence of matrix metalloproteinase (MMP)-2 activation by membrane type 2 (MT2)-MMP is determined by contributions of both the MT2-MMP catalytic and hemopexin C domains, *J. Biol. Chem.*, 281, 26528–26539, 2006.

195. Kontinnen, Y.T., Ainola, M., Valleala, H., et al., Analysis of 16 different matrix metalloproteinases (MMP-1 to MMP-20) in the synovial membrane: Different profiles in trauma and rheumatoid arthritis, *Ann. Rheum. Dis.*, 58, 691–697, 1999.

196. Mohammaed, F.F., Pennington, C.J., Kassiri, Z., et al., Metalloproteinase inhibitor TIMP-1 affects hepatocyte cell cycle via HGF activation in murine liver regeneration, *Hepatology*, 41, 857–867, 2005.

197. Bodnar, M., Szylberg, L., Kazmierczak, W., and Marszalek, A., Differentiated expression of membrane type metalloproteinases (MMP-14, MMP-15) and pro-MMP2 in laryngeal squamous cell carcinoma. A novel mechanism, *J. Oral Pathol. Med.*, 42, 267–274, 2013.

198. Fu, H.-L., and Friedman, R., Membrane-type 3-matrix metalloproteinase (MMP-16), in *Handbook of Proteolytic Enzymes*, 3rd edn., N.D. Rawlings and G. Salvesen, eds., pp. 817–822, Elsevier, Amsterdam, Netherlands, 2013.

199. Shofuda, K.-I., Yasumistui, H., Nishihashi, A., et al., Expression of thee membrane-type matrix metalloproteinases (MT-MMPs) in rat vascular smooth muscle cells and characterization of MT3-MMPs with and without transmembrane domain, *J. Biol. Chem.*, 272, 9749–9754, 1997.

200. Zucker, S., Pei, D., Cao, J., and Lopez-Otin, C, Membrane type-matrix metalloproteinase, *Curr. Top. Dev. Biol.*, 54, 1–74, 2003.

201. Zhao, H., Bernardo, M.M., Osenkowski, P., et al., Differential inhibition of membrane type 3 (MT3-matrix metalloproteinase (MMP) and MT1-MMP by tissue inhibitor of metalloproteinase (TIMP)-2 and TIMP-3 regulates pro-MMP-2 activation, *J. Biol. Chem.*, 279, 8592–8601, 2004.

202. Matsumoto, S., Katoh, M., Saito, S., et al., Identification of soluble type of membrane-type matrix metalloproteinase-3 formed by alternative spliced mRNA, *Biochim. Biophys. Acta*, 1354, 159–170, 1997.

203. Shimada, T., Nakamura, H., Ohuchi, E., et al., Characterization of a truncated recombinant form of human membrane type 3 matrix metalloproteinase, *Eur. J. Biochem.*, 262, 907–914, 1999.

204. Itoh, Y., and Seikli, M., Membrane-type matrix metalloproteinase 4, in *Handbook of Proteolytic Enzymes*, 3rd edn., N.D. Rawlings and G. Salvesen, eds., pp. 823–826, Elsevier, Amsterdam, Netherlands, 2013.

205. Puente, X.S., Pendás, A.M., Llano, E., et al., Molecular cloning of a novel membrane-type matrix metalloproteinase from a human breast carcinoma, *Cancer Res.*, 56, 944–949, 1996.

206. Kajita, M., Kinoh, H., Ito, N., et al., Human membrane type-4 matrix metalloproteinase (*MT4-MMP*) is encoded by a novel major transcript: Isolation of complementary DNA clones for human and mouse mt4-mmp transcripts, *FEBS J.*, 457, 353–356, 1999.

207. Itoh, Y., Kajita, M., Kinoh, H., et al., Membrane type 4 matrix metalloproteinase (MT4-MMP, MMP-17) is a glycosylphosphatidylinositol-anchored proteinase, *J. Biol. Chem.*, 274, 34260–34266, 1999.

208. Paulick, M.G., Forstner, M.B., Groves, J.T., and Bertozzi, C.R., A chemical approach to unraveling the biological function of the glycosylphosphatidylinositol anchor, *Proc. Natl. Acad. Sci. U. S. A.*, 104, 20332–20337, 2007.

209. Wang, Y., Johnson, A.R., Ye, Q.-Z., et al., Catalytic activities and substrate specificity of the human membrane type 4 matrix metalloproteinase catalytic domain, *J. Biol. Chem.*, 274, 33043–33049, 1999.

210. Kolkenbrock, H., Essers, L., Ulrich, N., and Will, H., Biochemical characterization of the catalytic domain of membrane-type 4 matrix metalloproteinase, *Biol. Chem.*, 380, 1103–1108, 1999.

211. English, W.R., Puente, X.S., Freije, J.M.P., et al., Membrane type 4 matrix metalloproteinase (MMP17) has tumor necrosis factor-α convertase activity but does not activate pro-MMP2, *J. Biol. Chem.*, 275, 14046–14055, 2000.

212. Gao, G., Plaas, A., Thompson, V.P., et al., ADAMTS4 (aggreganase-I) activation on the cell surface involves C-terminal cleavage by glycosylphosphatidyl inositol-anchored membrane type-4 matrix metallproteinase and binding of the activated proteinase to chondroitin sulfate and heparan sulfate on syndecan-1, *J. Biol. Chem.*, 279, 10042–10051, 2004.

213. Sang, Q.A., and Shi, Y.-B., Matrix metallopeptidase-18 (collagenase 4), in *Handbook of Proteolytic Enzymes*, 3rd edn., N.D. Rawlings and G. Salvesen, eds., pp. 744–747, Elsevier, Amsterdam, Netherlands, 2013.

214. Cossins, J., Dudgeon, T.J., Catlin, G., et al., Identification of MMP-18, a putative novel human matrix metalloproteinase, *Biochem. Biophys. Res. Commun.*, 228, 494–498, 1996.

215. Stolow, M.A., Bauzon, D.D., Li, J., et al., Identification and characterization of a novel collagenase in *Xenopus* laevis: Possible roles during frog development, *Molec. Biol. Cell*, 7, 1471–1483, 1996.

216. Grant, G.M., Giambernardi, T.A., Grant, A.M., and Klebe, R.J., Overview of expression of matrix metalloproteinases (MMP-17, MMP-18, and MMP-20) in cultured human cells, *Matrix Biol.*, 18, 145–148, 1999.

217. Foos, M.J., HIckox, J.R., Mansour, P.G., et al., Expression of matrix metalloproteases and tissue inhibitor of metalloprotease genes in human anterior cruciate ligament, *J. Orthopaedic Res.*, 19, 642–649, 2001.

218. Tomlinson, M.L., Garcia-Morales, C., Abu-Elmagd, M., and Wheeler, G.N., Three main metalloproteinases are required *in vivo* for macrophage migration during embryonic development, *Mech. Dev.*, 125, 1059–1070, 2008.

219. Fanjul-Fernández, M., and López-Otín, C., Matrix metalloproteinase 19, in *Handbook of Proteolytic Enzymes*, 3rd edn., N.D. Rawlings and G. Salvesen, eds., pp. 830–835, Elsevier, Amsterdam, Netherlands, 2013.

220. Pendás, A.M., Knäuper, V., Puente, X.S., et al., Identification and characterization of a novel human matrix metalloproteinase with unique structural characteristics, chromosomal location, and tissue distribution, *J. Biol. Chem.*, 272, 4281–4286, 1997.

221. Kolb, C., Mauch, S., Peter, H.-H., et al., The matrix metalloproteinase RASI-1 is expressed in synovial blood vessels of a rheumatold arthritis patient, *Immunol.Lett.*, 57, 83–88, 1997.

222. Impola, U., Toriseva, M. Suomela, S., et al., Matrix metalloproteinase-19 is expressed by proliferating epithelium but disappears with neoplastic dedifferentiation, *Int. J. Cancer*, 103, 709–716, 2003.

223. Sadowski, T., Dietrich, S., Müller, M., et al., Matrix metalloproteinase-19 expression normal and diseased skin: Dysregulation by epidermal proliferation, *J. Invest. Derm.*, 121, 989–996, 2003.

224. Sadowski, T., Dietrich, S., Koschinsky, F., and Sedlacek, R., Matrix metalloproteinase 19 regulates insulin-like growth factor-mediated proliferation, migration, and adhesion in human keratinocytes through proteolysis of insulin-like growth factor binding protein-3, *Mol. Biol. Cell*, 14, 4569–4580, 2003.

225. Evans, C.H., The role of proteases in cartilage destruction, *Agents Actions Suppl.*, 32, 137–152, 1991.

226. Stockman, B.J., Waldon, D.J., Gates J.A., et al., Solution structures of stromelysin complexed to thiadiazole inhibitors, *Protein Sci.*, 7, 2291–2286, 1998.

227. Schache, M., and Baird, P.N., Assessment of the association of matrix metalloproteinases with myopia, refractive error and ocular biometric measures in an Australian cohort, *PLoS One*, 7, e47181, 2012.

228. Stracker, J.O., Hutton, M., Stewart, M., et al., Biochemical characterization of the catalytic domain of human matrix metalloproteinase 19, *J. Biol. Chem.*, 275, 14809–14816, 2000.

229. Mysliwy, J., Dingley, A.J., Sedlacek, R., and Grötzinger, J., Structural characterization and binding properties of the hemopexin-like domain of matrix metalloproteinase-19, *Protein Expr. Purif.*, 46, 406–413, 2006.

230. Stracke, J.O., Fosang, A.J., Last, K., et al., Matrix metalloproteinases 19 and 20 cleave aggrecan and cartilage oligomeric matrix protein (COMP), *FEBS Lett.*, 478, 53–56, 2000.

231. Müller, M., Beck, I.M., Gadesmann, J., et al., MMP19 is upregulated during melanoma progression and increases invasion of melanoma cells, *Mod. Pathol.*, 23, 511–521, 2010.

232. Bartlett, J.D., Matrix metalloproteinase-20/enamelysin, in *Handbook of Proteolytic Enzymes*, 3rd edn., N.D. Rawlings and G. Salvesen, eds., pp. 835–840, Elsevier, Amsterdam, Netherlands, 2013.

233. Yang, M., Murray, M.T., and Kurkinen, M., A novel matrix metalloproteinase gene (XMMP) encoding vitronectin-like motifs is transiently expressed in *Xeropus laevis* embryo development, *J. Biol. Chem.*, 272, 13527–13533, 1997.

234. Llano, E., Pendás, A.M., Knäuper, V., et al., identification and structural and functional characterization of human enamelysin (MMP-20), *Biochemistry*, 36, 15101–15108, 1997.

235. Ryu, O.H., Fincham, A.G., Hu, C.-C., et al., Characterization of recombinant pig enamelysin activity and cleavage of recombinant pig and mouse amelogenins, *J. Dent. Res.*, 78, 743–750, 1999.

236. Ryu, O.H., Hu, J.C.C., Yamakoshi, Y., et al., Porcine kallikrein-4 activation, glycosylation, activity and expression in prokaryotic and eukaryotic hosts, *Eur. J. Oral Sci.*, 110, 358–365, 2002.

237. Yamakoshi, Y., Simmer, J.P., Bartlett, J.D., et al., MMP20 and KLK4 activation and inactivation in vitro, *Arch. Oral. Biol.*, 58, 1569–1577, 2013.

238. Lu, Y., Papagerakis, P., Yamakoshi, Y., et al., Functions of KLK4 and MMP-20 in dental enamel formation, *Biol. Chem.*, 389, 695–700, 2008.

239. Väänänen, A., Srinivas, R., Parikka, M., et al., Expression and regulation of MMP-20 in human tongue carcinoma cells, *J. Dent. Res.*, 80, 1884–1889, 2001.

240. Liu, Y., Li, Y., Liu, Z., et al., Prognostic significance of matrix metalloproteinase-20 overexpression in laryngeal squamous cell carcinoma, *Acta Otolaryngol.*, 131, 769–773, 2011.

241. Yang, M., and Kurkinen, M., Matrix metalloproteinase 21, in *Handbook of Proteolytic Enzymes*, 3rd edn., N.D. Rawlings and G. Salvesen, eds., pp. 840–841, Elsevier, Amsterdam, Netherlands, 2013.

242. Yang, M., Murray, M.T., and Kurkinen, M., A novel matrix metalloproteinase gene (XMMP) encoding vitronectin-like motifs is transiently expressed in *Xenopus laevis* early embryo development, *J. Biol. Chem.*, 272, 13527–13533, 1997.

243. Dixon, K.H., Cowell, I.G., Xia, C.L., et al., Control of expression of the human glutathione S-transferse pi gene differs from its rat orthologue, *Biochem. Biophys. Res. Commun.*, 163, 815–822, 1989.

244. Ahokas, K., Lohi, J., Lohi, H., et al., Matrix metalloproteinase-21, the human orthologue for XMMP, is expressed during fetal development and in cancer, *Gene*, 301, 31–41, 2002.

245. Skoog, T., Ahokas, K., Oramark, C., et al., MMP-21 is expressed by macrophages and fibroblasts in vivo and in culture, *Exp. Dermatol.*, 15, 775–783, 2006.

246. Pu, Y., Wang, L., Wu, H., et al., High MMP-21 expression in metastatic lymph nodes predicts unfavorable overall survival for oral squamous cell carcinoma patients with lymphatic metastasis, *Oncol. Rep.*, 31, 2644–2650, 2014.

247. Yang, M., and Kurkinen, M., Chicken matrix metalloproteinase 22, in *Handbook of Proteolytic Enzymes*, 3rd edn., N.D. Rawlings and G. Salvesen, eds., pp. 842–843, Elsevier, Amsterdam, Netherlands, 2013.

248. Yang, M., and Kurkinen, M., Cloning and characterization of a novel matrix metalloproteinase (MMP), CMMP from chicken embryo fibroblasts, *J. Biol. Chem.*, 273, 17893–17900, 1998.

249. Velasco, G., Pendás, A.M., Fueyo, A., et al., Cloning and characterization of human MMP-23, a new matrix metalloproteinase predominantly expressed in reproductive tissues and lacking conserved domains in other family members, *J. Biol. Chem.*, 274, 4570–4576, 1999.

250. Guruajen, R., Grenet, J., Lahti, J.M., and Kidd, V.J., Isolation and characterization of two novel metalloproteinase genes linked to the *Cdc2L* locus on human chromosome 1p36.3, *Genomics*, 52, 101–106, 1998.

251. Pei, D., CA-MMP: A matrix metalloproteinase with a novel cysteine array, but without the classic cysteine switch, *FEBS Lett.*, 457, 262–270, 1999.

252. Pei, D., Kang, T., and Qi, H., Cysteine array matrix metalloproteinase (CA-MMP)/MMP-23 is a type II transmembrane matrix metalloproteinase regulated by a single cleavage for both secretion and activation, *J. Biol. Chem.*, 275, 33988–33997, 2000.

253. Ohnishi, J., Ohnishi, E., Jin, M., et al., Cloning and characterization of a rat ortholog of MMP-23 (matrix metalloproteinase-23), a unique type of membrane-anchored matrix metalloproteinase and conditioned switching of its expression during the ovarian follicular development, *Mol. Endocrinol.*, 15, 747–764, 2001.

254. Dixon, K.H., Cowell, I.G., Xia, C.L., et al., Control of expression of the human glutathione S-transferase pi gene differs from its rat orthologue, *Biochem. Biophys. Res. Commun.*, 163, 815–822, 1989.

255. Sesardic, D., Boobis, A.R., Murrya, B.P., et al., Furafylline is a potent and selective inhibitor of cytochrome P450IA2 in man, *Br. J. Clin. Pharmacol.*, 29, 651–663, 1990.

256. Pei, D., Membrane-type matrix metalloproteinase-5, in *Handbook of Proteolytic Enzymes*, 3rd edn., N.D. Rawlings and G. Salvesen, eds., pp. 826–828, Elsevier, Amsterdam, Netherlands, 2013.

257. Liano, E., Pendás, A.M., Freije, J.P., et al., Identification and characterization of human MT5-MMP, a new membrane-bound activator of progelatinase A overexpressed in brain tumors, *Cancer Res.*, 59, 2570–2576, 1999.

258. Pei, D., Identification and characterization of teh fifth membrane-type matrix metalloproteinase MT5-MMP, *J. Biol. Chem.*, 274, 8925–8932, 1999.

259. Wang, X., Yi, J., Lei, J., and Pei, D., Expression, purification and characterization of recombinant mouse MT5-MMP protein products, *FEBS Lett.*, 462, 261–266, 1999.

260. Wang, X., and Pei, D., Shedding of membrane type matrix metalloproteinase 5 by a furin-type convertase, *J. Biol. Chem.*, 276, 35953–35960, 2001.

261. Pei, D., Membrane-type matrix metalloproteinase-6, in *Handbook of Proteolytic Enzymes*, 3rd edn., N.D. Rawlings and G. Salvesen, eds., pp. 828–830, Elsevier, Amsterdam, Netherlands, 2013.

262. Wenk, K., and Blobel, H., Investigations on staphyllococcal leucocidins of varying origins, *Zentralbl. Bakteriol. Orig.*, 213, 479–487, 1972.

263. Pei, D., Leukolysin/MMP-25/MT6-MMP: A novel matrix metalloproteinase specifically expressed in the leukocyte linage, *Cell Res.*, 9, 291–303, 1999.

264. Velasco, G., Cal, S., Merios-Suarez, A., et al., Human MT6-matrix metalloproteinase: Identification, progelatinase A activation, and expression in brain tumors, *Cancer Res.*, 60, 877–882, 2000.

265. Nie, J., and Pei, D., Direct activation of pro-matrix metalloproteinase-2 by leukolysin/membrane-type 6 matrix metalloproteinase/matrix metalloproteinase 25 at the Asn[109]-Tyr bond, *Cancer Res.*, 63, 6758–6762, 2003.

266. Nuti, E., Casalini, F., Santamaria, S., et al., Synthesis and biological evaluation in U87MG glioma cells of (ethynylthiophene)sulfonamido-based hydroxamates as matrix metalloproteinase inhibitors, *Eur. J. Med. Chem.*, 46, 2617–2629, 2011.

267. Sun, Q., Weber, C.R. Sohail, A., et al., MMP25 (MT6-MMP) is highly expressed in human colon cancer, promotes tumor growth, and exhibits unique biochemical properties, *J. Biol. Chem.*, 282, 21998–22010, 2007.

268. Kojima, S.-I., Itoh, Y., Matsumoto, S.-I., et al., Membrane-type 6 matrix metalloproteinase (MT6-MMP, MMP-25) is the second glycosyl-phosphatidyl-inositol (GPI) anchored MMP, *FEBS Lett.*, 480, 142–146, 2000.

269. Zhao, H., Sohail, A., Sun, Q., et al., Identification and role of the homodimerization interface of the glycosylphosphatidylinositol-anchored membrane type 6 matrix metalloproteinase (MMP 25), *J. Biol. Chem.*, 283, 35023–35032, 2008.

270. Nie, J., and Pei, D., Rapid inactivation of α_1-proteinase inhibitor by neutrophil specific leukolysin/membrane -type matrix, *Exp. Cell Res.*, 296, 145–150, 2004.

271. English, W.R., Velasco, G., Stracke, J.O., et al., Catalytic acitivities of membrane-type 6 matrix metalloproteinase (MMP25), *FEBS Lett.*, 491, 137–142, 2001.

272. Shiryaev, S.A., Savinov, S.Y., Cieplak, P., et al., Major metalloproteinase proteolysis of the myelin basic protein isoforms is a source of immunogenic peptides in autoimmune multiple sclerosis, *PLoS One*, 4(3), e4952, 2009.

273. Shiryaev, S.A., Remacle, A.C., Savinov, A.Y., et al., Inflammatory proprotein convertase-matrix metalloproteinase proteolytic pathway in antigen-presenting cells as a step to autoimmune multiple sclerosis, *J. Biol. Chem.*, 284, 30615–30626, 2009.
274. Sang, Q.Y.A., Matrix metalloproteinase-26/matrilysin 2 (Homo sapiens), in *Handbook of Proteolytic Enyzmes*, 3rd edn., N.D. Rawlings and G. Salvesen, eds., pp. 795–800, Elsevier, Amsterdam, Netherlands, 2013.
275. Park, H.I., Ni, J., Gerkema, F.E., et al., Identification and characterization of human endometase (matrix metalloproetinase-26) from endometrial tumor, *J. Biol. Chem.*, 275, 20540–20544, 2000.
276. Benoit de Coignac, A., Elson, G., Delneste, Y., et al., Cloning of MMP-26. A novel matrilysin-like proteinase, *Eur. J. Biochem.*, 267, 3323–3329, 2000.
277. Marcenko, G.H., Ratnikov, B.I., Rozanov, D.V., et al., Characterization of matrix metalloproteinase-26, a novel metalloproteinase widely expressed in cancer cells of epithelial origin, *Biochem. J.*, 356, 705–718, 2001.
278. Marchenko, N.D., Marchenko, G.N., and Strongin, A.Y., Unconventional activation mechanisms of MMP-26, a human matrix metalloproteinase with a unique PHCGXXD cysteine switch motif, *J. Biol. Chem.*, 277, 18967–18972, 2002.
279. Park, H.L., Turk, B.E., Gerkema, F.E., et al., Peptide substrate specificities and protein cleavage sites of human endometase/matrilysin-2/matrix metalloproteinase-26, *J. Biol. Chem.*, 277, 35168–35175, 2002.
280. Schechter, I., and Berger, A., On the size of the active site in proteases. I. Papain, *Biochem. Biophys. Res. Commun.*, 27, 157–162, 1967.
281. Nuttad, R.K., Sampieri, C.L., Pennington, C.J., et al., Expression analysis of the entire MMP and TIMP gene families during mouse tissue development, *FEBS Lett.*, 563, 129–134, 2004.
282. Bernal, F., Hartung, H.-P., and Kieseier, B.C., Tissue mRNA expression in rat of newly described matrix metalloproteinases, *Biol. Res.*, 38, 267–271, 2005.
283. Bar-Or, A., Nuttall R.K., Duddy, M., et al., Analyses of all matrix metalloproteinase members in leukocytes emphasize monocytes as major inflammatory mediators in multiple sclerosis, *Brain*, 126, 2738–2749, 2003.
284. Cominelli, A., Halbout, M., N'Kuli, F., et al., A unique C-terminal domain allows retention of matrix metalloproteinase-27 in the endoplasmic reticulum, *Traffic*, 15, 401–417, 2014.
285. Lohi, J., Parks, W.C., and Manicone, M., Matrix metalloproteinase-28/epilysin, in *Handbook of Proteolytic Enzymes*, 3rd edn., N.D. Rawlings and G.Salvesen, eds., pp. 845–850, Elsevier, Amsterdam, Netherlands, 2013.
286. Lohi, J., Wilson, C.L., Roby, J.D., and Parks, W.C., Epilysin, a novel human matrix metalloproteinase (MMP-28) expressed in testes and keratinocytes and in response to injury, *J. Biol. Chem.*, 276, 10134–10144, 2001.
287. Saarialho, U., Kekelä, E., Jahkola, T., et al., Epilysin (MMP-28) expression is associated with cell proliferation during epithelial repair, *J. Invest. Dermatol.*, 139, 14–21, 2002.
288. Reno, F., Sabbatini, M., Stella, M.D., et al., Effect of in vitro mechanical compression on epilysin (matrix metalloproteinase-28) expression in hypertrophic scars, *Wound Rep. Reg.*, 13, 255–261, 2005.
289. Illman, S.A., Lohi, J., and Keski-Oja, J., Epilysin (MMP-28)--structure, expression and potential functions, *Exp. Dermatol.*, 17, 897–907, 2008.
290. Manicone, A.M., Birkland, T.P., Lin, M., et al., Epilysin (MMP-28) restrains early macrophage recruitment in *Pseudomonas aeruginosa* pneumonia, *J. Immunol.*, 182, 3866–3876, 2009.
291. Rodgers, U.R., Kevorkian, L., Surridge, A.K., et al., Expression and function of matrix metalloproteinase (MMP)-28, *Matrix Biol.*, 28, 263–272, 2009.
292. Marchenko, G.N., and Strongin, A.Y., MMP-28, a new human matrix metalloproteinase with an unusual cysteine-switch sequence is widely expressed in tumors, *Gene*, 265, 87–93, 2001.
293. Lin, M.H., Liu, S.Y., Su, H.J., and Liu, Y.C., Functional role of matrix metalloproteinase-28 in the oral squamous cell carcinoma, *Oral Oncol.*, 42, 907–913, 2006.
294. Tallant, C., Marrero, A., and Gomis-Rüth, F.S., Matrix metalloproteinases: Fold and function of their catalytic domains, *Biochim. Biophys. Acta*, 1803, 20–28, 2010.
295. Fanjul-Fernández, M., Folgueras, A.R., Cabrera, S., and López-Otín, C., Matrix metalloproteinases: Evolution, gene regulation and functional analysis in mouse models, *Biochim. Biophys. Acta*, 1803, 3–19, 2010.
296. Bläser, J., Knäuper, V., Osthues, A., et al., Mercurial activation of human polymorphonuclear leucocyte procollagenase, *Eur. J. Biochem.*, 202, 1223–1230, 1991.
297. Shetty, V., Spellman, D.S., and Neubert, T.A., Characterization by tandem mass spectrometry of stable cysteine sulfenic acid in a cysteie switch peptide of matrix metalloproteinases, *J. Am. Soc. Mass Spectrom.*, 18, 1544–1551, 2007.
298. Chen, L.-C., Noelken, M.E., and Nagase, H., Disruption of the cysteine-75 and zinc ion coordination is not sufficient to activate the precursor of human matrix metalloproteinase 3 (stromelysin 1), *Biochemistry*, 32, 10289–10295, 1993.
299. Rosenblum, G., Meroueh, S., Toth, M., et al., Molecular structures and dynamics of the stepwise activation mechanism of a matrix metalloproteinase zymogen: Challenging the cysteine switch dogma, *J. Am. Chem. Soc.*, 129, 13566–13574, 2007.
300. Michaelis, J., Vissers, M.C., and Winterbourne, C.C., Different effects of hypochlorous acid on human neutrophil metalloproteinases: Activation of collagenase and inactivation of collagenase and gelatinase, *Arch. Biochem. Biophys.*, 292, 555–562, 1992.
301. Sternlicht, M.D., and Werb, Z., How matrix metalloproteinases regulate cell behavior, *Annu. Rev. Cell Dev. Biol.*, 17, 463–516, 2001.
302. Janciauskiene, S., Larsson, S., Larsson, P., et al., Inhibition of lipopolysaccharide-mediated human monocyte activation, in vitro, by α1-antitrypsin, *Biochem. Biophys. Res. Commun.*, 321, 592–600, 2004.
303. Zelvyte, I., Sjögren, H.O., and Janciauskiene, S., Multiple effects of α_1-antitrypsin on breast carcinoma MDA-MB 468 cell growth and invasiveness, *Eur. J. Cancer Prev.*, 12, 117–124, 2003.
304. Kalsheker, N.A., Deam, S., Chambers, L., et al., The house dust mite allergen *Der* p1 catalytically inactivates α_1-antitrypsin by specific reactive centre loop cleavage: A mechanism that promotes airway inflammation and asthma, *Biochem. Biophys. Res. Commun.*, 221, 59–61, 1996.
305. Wilhelm, S.M., Shao, E.M., and Housley, T.J., Matrix metalloproteinase-3 (stromelysin-1). Identification as the cartilage acid metalloproteinase and effects of pH on catalytic properties and calcium affinity, *J. Biol. Chem.*, 268, 21906–21913, 1993.
306. Matayoshi, E.D., Wang, G.T., Krafft, G.A., and Erickson, J., Novel fluorogenic substrates for assaying retroviral proteases by resonance energy transfer, *Science*, 247, 954–958, 1990.
307. Schechter, I., and Berger, A., On the size of the active site of proteases. I. Papain, *Biochem. Biophys. Res. Commun.*, 27, 157–162, 1967.
308. MacFarlane, R.G., An enzyme cascade in the blood clotting mechanism and its function as a biological amplifier, *Nature*, 202, 498–499, 1964.
309. Teijaro, J.R, Walsh, K.G., Rice, S., et al., Mapping the innate signaling cascade essential for cytokine storm during influenza virus infection, *Proc. Natl. Acad. Sci. U. S. A.*, 111, 3799–3804, 2014.
310. Eberhardt, W., Huwiler, A., Beck, K.F., et al., Amplification of IL-1 β-induced matrix metalloproteinase-9 expression by superoxide in rat glomerular mesangial cells is mediated by increased activities of NF-κB and activating protein-1 and involves activation of the mitogen-activated protein kinase pathways, *J. Immunol.*, 165, 5788–5797, 2000.

PROTEASES IN THE INTERSTITIAL SPACE

Roger L. Lundblad

PROTEOLYTIC ACTIVITIES DESCRIBED IN THE INTERSTITIAL SPACE[a]

Enzyme	Comment
ADAM proteases (a disintegrin and metalloprotease domain)	ADAM proteases (a disintegrin and metalloprotease) are a group of metallproteinases[1,2] composed of a disintegrin domain and a metalloprotease domain.[1] ADAM proteases are members of the adamlysin family in the metzincin subfamily which also includes matrix metalloproteinases.[3] The disintegrin domain functions in binding to integrins on the cell membrane possibly positioning the protease to act as a sheddase.[4] Not all of the members of the ADAM family have proteolytic activity suggesting the importance of protein–ligand interactions in function.[5] ADAM proteases have a major role in development[6] and are of interest in oncology research.[7] The function of ADAM protease as a sheddase is of importance in inflammation as shown by the release of TNFα by ADAM17.[8] See Section 4.2 for more detail.
ADAMTS (a disintegrin and metalloprotease with a thrombospondin type 1 motif repeats)	ADAMTS is a protease with ADAM domain and thrombospondin 1 repeats.[9–11] Unlike the ADAM proteases which are membrane bound, the ADAMTS proteases are soluble proteins that are processed and secreted in a furin-mediated pathway.[12] Early work suggested that the thrombospondin domains in ADAMTS proteases enabled binding to the extracellular matrix.[13] ADAMTS proteases are best known for their degradation of proteoglycans such as aggrecan[14] and collagen processing.[15] One ADAMTS protease, ADAMTS13, is involved in the processing of von Willebrand factor in endothelial cells.[16] See Section 4.3 for more detail.
Chymase	Chymase is a chymotryptic-like serine protease which is a product of mast cells.[17,18] More specifically, chymase arising from mast cell degranulation in the arterial intimal fluid has been reported.[19–22] Chymase has biological activity in the interstitial space such as stimulation of angiotensin II formation,[19] degradation of HDL,[21,23] and activation of matrix metalloproteinases.[24–26] It is demonstrated to cleave nidogen but less effective than leucocyte elastase.[27] It is also shown to increase glomerular permeability by cleavage of PAR2 receptor.[28]
Factor VIIa	There is no direct measurement of factor Xa in interstitial fluid but indirect evidence supports the presence of this protease in interstitial fluid.[29,30] It is suggested that the formation of the thrombin in the interstitium occurs via the tissue factor pathway which would require the conversion of factor VII to factor VIIa.[23,31] Perivascular tissue factor binds factor VIIa.[32] See Chapter 8 for more detail.
Factor Xa	There is no direct measurement of factor Xa in interstitial fluid but indirect evidence supports the presence of this protease in interstitial fluid.[33,34] Factor Xa can activate cells via cleavage of the PAR2 receptor.[35] See Chapter 8 for more detail.
Hepsin	Hepsin is a hepatic enzyme of unclear function.[36] There are studies with *in vitro* substrates but *in vivo* substrates have not been described. Hepsin is a type II-transmembrane serine protease (TTSP)[37] as is matripase.[38,39] Hepsin has been shown to activate factor VII.[40] Hepsin is also involved in malignancy and is proposed as a therapeutic target.[41–45]
Hyaluronan-binding serine protease	Hyaluronan-binding serine protease was isolated from human plasma by affinity chromatography on hyaluronan conjugated to agarose.[46] Analysis of amino acid sequence derived from cDNA showed homology to hepatocyte growth factor activator. Further analysis of the gene for HABP showed some homology with coagulation factor XII, tPA, and urokinase.[47] HABP has been shown to undergo autocatalytic activation[48,49] which was stimulated by the presence of either positively charged (poly-lysine) or negatively charged (heparin) factors.[48] Heparan sulfate and chondroitin sulfate have also been shown to stimulate the action of hyaluronan-binding serine protease on kininogens forming kinins.[49] Although a substrate in plasma has not been clearly identified,[50]hyaluronan-binding serine protease has been shown to upregulate ERK1/2 and P13K/Akt signalling pathways in fibroblasts stimulating cell proliferation and migration.[51] The conditioned media from HABP-treated fibroblasts had a growth-stimulating effect on quiescent fibroblasts.
Insulin-like growth factor binding protein-3 protease (IGFBP-3 protease)	IGFBP-3 protease is described more as an activity[52,53] than as discrete molecular entity and the activity may be more a reflection of the susceptibility of IGFBP-3 to proteolysis by a wide variety of enzymes.[54–63] There is evidence to suggest that there is little proteolysis of IGFBP-3 in "normal" serum but there is a marked increase during pregancy.[64] Proteolysis of IGFBP-3 may increase IGF-1 bioavailability.[58,65] Proteolysis of IGFBP-3 occurs to a higher extent in interstitial fluid.[66–68]
Kallikrein-related peptidases[b]	These are a family of regulatory proteases related by structural homology and not by biological function[69,70] (see Chapter 6).
Mastin	Mastin is a soluble tryptase-like enzyme[71] secreted by canine mast cells.[72] Mastin has a tryptic like specificity with a preference for cleavage of arginine-containing peptide bonds.
Matriptase	Matriptase (MT-SP1, epitin, SNC19, TADG-15) was identified as a matrix-degrading serine protease in tumor cells.[73] Subsequent studies[74] demonstrated that matriptase was expressed on epithelial cells as a membrane-bound protease which could activate hepatocyte growth factor and urokinase plasminogen activator. Matriptase is inhibited by hepatocyte growth factor activator inhibitor-1 (HAI-1)[75] and antithrombin.[76,77] Matriptase can be detected by reaction with a biotinylated peptide chloromethyl ketone.[78] Matriptase occurs as surface-bound zymogen under autocatalytic transactivation.[79] Matriptase is considered to be part of a proteolytic cascade involving the activation of prostasin necessary for the functionality of the stratum corneum barrier function.[80]
Matrix metalloproteinase	Matrix metalloproteinases (MMP; matrixins)[81–83] are a group of proteolytic enzymes which are members of the metzincin superfamily[84,85] and involved in degradation of extracellular matrix components.[86] Matrix metalloproteinases vary considerably in structure and size but have a common mechanism involving a cysteine residue and a metal ion, usually zinc. Matrix metalloproteinases are synthesized as precursors or zymogen forms which require activation.[87–90] Glycosaminoglycans may modulate matrix metalloproteinase action.[91] Matrix metalloproteinases are discussed in detail in Chapter 7.

Enzyme	Comment
Meprin metalloproteases	Meprin A (meprin α) and Meprin B (meprin β) are zinc metalloproteinases which are astacins[92] in the metzincin superfamily[84,85] Meprin A and Meprin B are transmembrane proteases which can be released (shed) into interstitial space.[93,94] Merpin A may be secreted as a zymogen form. The functions of the meprin proteases are still being defined but a number of potential substrates[95] have been identified including amyloid protein,[96] procollagens,[97] and IL-6.[98]
Mesotrypsin[b]	Mesotrypsin was described as a minor form of pancreatic trypsin derived from mesotrypsinogen by the action of enterokinase.[99,100] As with trypsin IV, mesotrypsin is resistant to inactivation by protein protease inhibitors.[99,101] It has been suggested that mesotrypsin is important for the degradation of trypsin inhibitors such as soybean trypsin inhibitor permitting the digestion of food rich in natural trypsin inhibitors.[102] Mesotrypsin has been described in the upper epidermis as an enzyme responsible for the activation of epidermal kallikrein-like peptidases and for the degradation of lymphoepitelial Kazal-type-related inhibitor (LEKTI1), an inhibitor of the kallikrein-like peptidases.[103] As with the pancreatic proenzyme, epidermal mesotrypsinogen is activated by enterokinase, also found in the epidermis. These observations support a role for mesotrypsin in the desquamation process..
Neutrophil elastase	Neutrophil elastase has a chymotrypsin-like specificity and degrades elastin and collagen in the interstitial space.[104,105] Not to be confused with macrophage elastase (MMP-12, Chapter 8). The degradation of pulmonary elastin by neutrophil elastase is inhibited by hyaluronan.[106] Neutrophil elastase has been suggested to be important for the development of interstitial edema during pericardial inflammation.[107] Cleavage of E-cadherin by neutrophil elastase is suggested to result in loss of cell–cell contacts and adherens junctions in the development of experimental pancreatis.[108]
Neutrophil protease 3	A protease contained in neutrophils and expressed in the interstitial space after migration of the neutrophils from the vascular space.[109,110] Neutrophil protease 3, with other neutrophil proteases such as neutrophil elastase, is synthesized as zymogens, processed to mature enzymes by dipeptidyl peptidase I[111], and stored in azurophil granules.[110] A small amount of activated neutrophil 3 protease is expressed on the surface of resting neutrophils.[112] Neutrophil protease 3 cleaves the PAR-1 receptor at site different from the thrombin cleavage site.[113] However, the neutrophil proteinase 3 cleavage did activate MAP-kinase. Antibodies against neutrophil protease 3 are observed in anti-neutrophil cytoplasmic antigens.[114,115] The surface presentation of neutrophil protease 3 is important for its role as an anti-neutrophil cytoplasmic antigen.[92] Neutrophil migration from the vascular space into the interstitial space is critical for the normal immune response[116] and the expression of neutrophil proteinase 3 is critical for the defense response in the interstitial space.[117,118]
Plasma kallikrein	The presence of plasma kallikrein in the interstitial space can be inferred from the presence of bradykinin and other kinin products released by plasma kallikrein from high molecular weight kininogen.[119–122] Plasma prekallikrein and high molecular weight kininogen have been found in cerebrospinal fluid.[123] Plasma kallikrein activates vascular smooth muscle cells by action on PAR receptors.[124] There is more extensive information of plasma kallikrein in Chapter 6.
Plasmin	Plasmin is a serine protease derived from plasminogen which has a specificity for cleavage of peptide bonds where the carboxyl group is contributed by lysine.[125] Plasminogen is found in plasma and interstitial fluid[126,127]; plasmin can be found in serum,[128,129] urine,[130] and synovial fluid.[131–133] Plasmin is rapidly inhibited by α_2-antiplasmin, α_2-macroglobulin, and α_1-antitrypsin.[134–137] Cleavage of plasmin/plasminogen by a variety of proteolytic enzymes gives rise to angiostatin.[138–143] Although best recognized for fibrinolytic activity, plasmin can directly interact with cells within the interstitium[144–146] and can regulate extracellular matrix and function.[147–152] See Chapter 5 for more detail.
Reelin	Reelin is a large glycoprotein serine protease[153,154] associated with the extracellular matrix which is important for nervous system development and regulation of synaptic transmission in the adult brain.[155] Reelin was identified as a product of the reeler gene[156] which is a protein component of the extracellular matrix during early cortical development[157]
Thrombin	Thrombin is a serine protease derived from prothrombin[158,159] which has specificity for cleavage of peptide bonds where the carboxyl group is contributed by basic amino acids (arginine and lysine).[160,161] Thrombin is important in the development of interstitial fibrosis.[162–164] Although thrombin can form fibrin in the interstitial space,[165] the majority of interest is direct toward the interaction of thrombin with cells.[162,163,166] Thrombin may have direct role in extracellular matrix degradation through degradation of fibronectin[167] and proteoglycans[168] but also activates matrix metalloproteases.[169,170] There are data to suggest that antithrombin can inactivate thrombin in the interstitial space[171] but no direct evidence for formation of a thrombin–antithrombin complex. Thrombin can also activate hepatocyte growth factor activator.[172] See Chapter 8 for more detail.
Tissue kallikrein (KLK1)[b]	Tissue kallikrein (KLK1)[b] is a tryptic-like serine protease best known for the formation of kinins from kininogens.[173] It is suggested that tissue kallikrein is released into the interstitial space during inflammation[174,175] or secondary to tissue damage[176,177] (See Chapter 6).
Tissue plasminogen activator (tPA)	tPA is a specific activator of plasminogen that is found in a variety of tissues[178,179] with some emphasis on nervous tissue[180,181] and eye.[182] There is a major interest on tPA expression in endothelial cells.[183] tPA is thought to bind to endothelial cell surfaces following secretion, with such binding important for fibrinolytic activity.[184] tPA is present in interstitial fluid[185,186] but is rapidly inactivated by PAI-1.[187] tPA is also found on macrophage surfaces.[128] tPA is active in a bound phase but poorly active in free solution.[188,189] The formation of plasmin on melanoma cell surface mediated by tPA activation of plasminogen bound on the cell surface is considered important for invasiveness.[190]
Tryptase	Tryptase is a tryptic-like serine protease which is a product of mass cells.[18,191] There are several isoforms of tryptase[192] arising from variation in the tetramer structure of this protein.[193,194] Cleavage of PAR-2 on epithelial cells by tryptase may be of importance in the interstitium.[195,196] Tryptase activates TGFβ in airway smooth muscle cells in a PAR-2 independent mechanism.[197] Heparin and other macropolyanions are involved in the storage and modulations of tryptase activity.[198–202] Human tryptase loses activity via a process described as spontaneous inactivation; the process of spontaneous inactivation is slowed/reversed by sulfated polyanions such as heparin or dextran sulfate.[203–206]
Trypsin IV[b]	Trypsin IV is an extrapancreatic isoform of trypsin found in brain derived from trypsinogen IV which may be a splice variant of mesotrypsinogen.[207,208] Trypsin IV may also be secreted by other extrahepatic sources including certain epithelial cells.[209] Trypsin IV differs from classic pancreatic trypsin in being resistant to inhibition by protein trypsin inhibitors.[210] Trypsin IV has the ability to activate PAR receptors and may have a role in inflammation.[211]

Enzyme	Comment
Urokinase plasminogen activator (urokinase)	Urokinase plasminogen activator (uPA) is an enzyme synthesized in the kidney.[212,213] In addition to proteolysis, urokinase acts through binding to a specific cell surface receptor (urokinase plasminogen activator receptor, uPAR).[214] Urokinase and urokinase plasminogen activator receptor (uPAR) together with plasminogen activator inhibitor-1 (PAI-1) are important in inflammation[215] and VEGF-stimulated angiogenesis.[216] uPA is important in the programmed degradation of extracellular matrix during development.[217] uPA is different from tissue plasminogen activator (tPA).[218,219] See Chapter 5 for more detail.

a These proteins are not unique to interstitial space but are found in other fluid compartments including the vascular bed. See Chapter 1 for a discussion of the origin of proteins in the interstitium.

b There are some issues with the nomenclature in this area and there are studies where mesotrypsin and trypsin IV are considered interchangeable. Trypsin IV and mesotrypsin do appear to be different enzymes but share some unusual properties such as the resistance to inactivation by protein protease inhibitors.

References

1. Yamamoto, S., Higuchi, Y., Yoshiyama, K., et al., ADAM family proteins in the immune systems, *Immunol. Today*, 20, 278–284, 1999.
2. Kleiin, T., and Bischoff, R., Active metalloproteases of the A Disintegrin and Metalloproteinases (ADAM) family: Biological function and structure, *J. Proteome Res.*, 10, 17–33, 2011.
3. Rawlings, N.D., Protease families, evolution and mechanism of action, in *Proteases: Structure and Function*, K. Brix and W. Stöcker, eds., pp. 1–35, Springer, Vienna, Austria, 2013.
4. White, J.M., ADAMS: Modulators of cell-cell and cell-matrix interactions, *Curr. Opin. Cell Biol.*, 15, 598–606, 2003.
5. Edwards, D.R., Handsley, M.M., and Pennington, C.J., The ADAM metalloproteineases, *Mol. Aspects Med.*, 29, 258–289, 2008.
6. Christian, L., Bahudhanapati, H., and Wei, S., Extracellular metalloproteinases in neural crest development and craniofacial morphogenesis, *Crit. Rev. Biochem. Mol. Biol.*, 48, 544–560, 2013.
7. Moro, N., Mauch, C., and Zigrino, P., Metalloproteinases in melanoma, *Eur. J. Cell Biol.*, 93, 23–29, 2014.
8. Lisi, S., D'Amore, M., and Sisto, M., ADAM17 at the interface between inflammation and autoimmunity, *Immunol. Lett.*, 162, 159–169, 2014.
9. Kuno, K., Kanada, N., Nakashima, E., et al., Molecular cloning of a gene encoding a new type of metalloproteinase-disintegrin family protein with thrombospondin motifs as an inflammatory associated gene, *J. Biol. Chem.*, 272, 556–562, 1997.
10. Tang, B.L., and Hong, W., ADAMTS: A novel family of proteases with an ADAM protease domain and Thrombospondin 1 repeats, *FEBS Lett.*, 445, 223–225, 1999.
11. Apte, S.S., The ADAMTS endopeptideases, in *The Handbook of Proteolytic Enzymes*, N.D. Rawlings and G.S. Salvesen, eds., pp. 1149–1155, Academic Press/Elsevier, Amsterdam, Netherlands, 2013.
12. Kuno, K., Terashima, Y., and Matsushima, K., ADAMTS-1 is an active metalloproteinase associated with the extracellular matrix, *J. Biol. Chem.*, 274, 18821–18826, 1999.
13. Kuno, K., and Matsushima, K., ADAMTS-1 protein anchors at the extracellular matrix through the thrombospondin type I motifs and its spacing region, *J. Biol. Chem.*, 273, 13912–13917, 1998.
14. Stanton, H., Melrose, J. Little, C.B., and Fosang, A.J., Proteoglycan degradation by the ADAMTS family of proteinases, *Biochim. Biophys. Acta*, 1812, 1616–1629, 2011.
15. Bekhouche, M., and Colige, A., The procollagen N-proteinases ADAMTS2, 3 and 14 in pathophysiology, *Matrix Biol.*, 44–46, 46–53, 2015.
16. Shang, D., Zheng, X.W., Niiya, M., and Zheng, X.L., Apical sorting of ADAMTS13 in vascular endothelial cells and Madin-Darby canine kidney cells depends on the CUB domains and their association with lipid rafts, *Blood*, 108, 2207–2215, 2006.
17. Craig, S.S., and Schwartz, L.B., Tryptase and chymase, markers of distinct types of human mast cells, *Immunol. Res.*, 8, 130–148, 1989.
18. Caughey, G.H., Chymases, in *Handbook of Proteolytic Enzymes*, 3rd edn., N.D. Rawlings and G. Salvesen, eds., pp. 2675–2683, Elsevier, Amsterdam, Netherlands, 2013.
19. Wei, C.C., Meng, Q.C., Palmer, R., et al., Evidence for angiotensin-converting enzyme-and chymase-mediated angiotensin II formation in the interstitial fluid space of the dog heart *in vivo*, *Circulation* 99, 2583–2589, 1999.
20. Lindstedt, L., Lee, M., and Kovanen, P.T., Chymase bound to heparin is resistant to its natural inhibitors and capable of proteolyzing high density lipoproteins in aortic intimal fluid, *Atherosclerosis*, 155, 87–97, 2001.
21. Lee-Rueckert, M., and Kovanen, P.T., Extracellular modifications of HDL *in vivo* and the emerging concept of proteolytic inactivation of preβ-HDL, *Curr. Opin. Lipidol.*, 22, 394–402, 2011.
22. Wei, C.C., Chen. Y., Powell, L.C., et al., Cardiac kallikrein-kinin system is upregulated in chronic volume overload and mediates an inflammatory induced collagen loss, *PLoS One*, 7(6), e40110, 2012.
23. Zucker, S., Mirza, H., Conner, C.E., et al., Vascular endothelial growth factor induces tissue factor and matrix metalloproteinase production in endothelial cells: Conversion of prothrombin to thrombin results in progelatinase A activation and cell proliferation, *Int. J. Cancer*, 75, 780–786, 1998.
24. Suzuki, K., Lees, M., Newlands, G.F., et al., Activation of precursors for matrix metalloproteinase 1(interstitial collagenase) and 3 (stromelysin) by rat mast-cell proteinase I and II, *Biochem. J.*, 305, 301–306, 1995.
25. Lundequist, A., Aabrink, M., Pejler, G., Mass cell-dependent activation of pro matrix metalloprotease 2: A role forserglycin proteoglycan-dependent mass cell proteases, *Biol. Chem.*, 387, 1513–1519, 2006.
26. Saarinen, J., Kalkkinen, N., Welgus, H.G., and Kovanen, P.T., Activation of human interstitial procollagenase through direct cleavage of the Leu83-Thr84 bond by mast cell chymase, *J. Biol. Chem.*, 269, 18134–18140, 1994.
27. Mayer, U., Mann, K., Timpl, R., and Murphy, G., Sites of nidogen cleavage by proteases involved in tissue homeostasis, *Eur. J. Biochem.*, 217, 877–884, 1993.
28. Sharma, R., Prasad, V., McCarthy, E.T., et al., Chymase increases glomerular albumin permeability via protease-activated receptor-2, *Mol. Cell. Biochem.*, 297, 161–169, 2007.
29. Cella, G., Cipriani, A., Tommasini, A., et al., Tissue factor pathway inhibitor (TFPI) antigen plasma level in patients with interstitial lung disease before and after heparin administration, *Semin. Thromb. Hemost.*, 23, 45–49, 1998.
30. Wygrecka, M., Jablonska, E., Guenther, A., et al., Current view on alveolar coagulation and fibrinolysis in acute inflammatory and chronic interstitial lung diseases, *Thromb. Haemost.*, 99, 494–501, 2008.
31. Günther, A., Mosavi, P., Ruppert, C., et al., Enchanced tissue factor pathway activity and fibrin turnover in the alveolar compartment of patients with interstitial lung disease, *Thromb. Haemost.*, 83, 853–860, 2000.
32. Hoffman, M., Collina, C.M., McDonald, A.G., et al., Tissue factor around dermal vessels has bound factor VII in the absence of injury, *J. Thromb. Haemost.*, 5, 1403–1408, 2007.
33. Idell, S., Gonzalez, K., Bradford, H., et al., Procoagulant activity in bronchoalveolar lavage in the adult respiratory distress syndrome. Contribution of tissue factor associated with factor VII, *Am. Rev. Respir. Dis.*, 136, 1466–1474, 1987.

34. Uhicha, M., Okajima, K., Murakami, K., et al., Effect of human urinary thrombomodulin on endotoxin-induced intravascular coagulation and pulmonary vascular injury in rats, *Am. J. Hematol.*, 54, 118–123, 1997.

35. Grandaliano, G., Pontrelli, P., Cerullo, G., et al., Protease-activated receptor-2 expression in IgA nephropathy: A potential role in the pathogenesis of interstitial fibrosis, *J. Am. Soc. Nephrol.*, 14, 2072–2083, 2003.

36. Wu, Q., and Peng, J., Hepsin, in *Handbook of Proteolytic Enzymes*, 3rd edn., N.D. Rawlings and G. Salvesen, eds., pp. 2985–2989, Elsevier, Amsterdam, Netherlands, 2013.

37. Wu, Q., Type II transmembrane serine proteases, *Curr. Top. Dev. Biol.*, 54, 167–206, 2003.

38. Qiu, D., Owen, K., Gray, K., et al., Roles and regulation of membrane-associated serine proteases, *Biochem. Soc. Trans.*, 35, 583–587, 2007.

39. Owen, K.A., Qiu, D., Alves, J., et al., Pericellular activation of hepatocyte growth factor by the transmembrane proteases matriptase and hepsin, but not by the membrane-associated protease uPA, *Biochem. J.*, 426, 219–228, 2010.

40. Kazama, Y., Hamamoto, T., Foster, D.C., and Kisiel, W., Hepsin, a putative membrane-associated serine protease, activates human factor VII and initiates a pathway of blood coagulation on the cell surface leading to thrombin formation, *J. Biol. Chem.*, 270, 66–72, 1995.

41. Koschubs, T., Dengl, S., Dürr, H., et al., Allosteric antibody inhibition of human hepsin protease, *Biochem. J.*, 42, 483–494, 2012.

42. Kim, H.J., Han, J.H., Chang, I.H., et al., Variants in the HEPSIN gene are associated with susceptibility to prostate cancer, *Prostate Cancer Prostatic Dis.*, 15, 353–358, 2012.

43. Hemstreet, G.P., 3rd., Rossi, G.R., Pisarev, V.M., et al., Cellular immunotherapy study of prostate cancer patients and resulting IgG responses to peptide epitopes predicted from prostate tumor-associated autoantigens, *J. Immunother.*, 36, 57–65, 2013.

44. Guo, J., Li, G., Tang, J., et al., HLA-A2-restricted cytotoxic T lymphocyte epitopes from human hepsi as novel targets for prostate cancer immunotherapy, *Scand. J. Immunol.*, 78, 248–257, 2013.

45. Tang, X., Mahajan, S.S., Nguyen, L.T., et al., Targeted inhibition of cell-surface serine protease Hepsin blocks prostate cancer bone metastasis, *Oncotarget*, 5, 1352–1362, 2014.

46. Choi-Miura, N.-H., Tobe, T., Sumiya, J.-I., et al., Purification and characterization of a novel hyaluronan-binding protein (PHBP) from human plasma: It has three EGF, a kringle and a serine protease domain, similar to hepatocyte growth factor activator, *J. Biochem.*, 119, 1157–1165, 1996.

47. Sumiya, J.-I., Asakawa, S., Tobe, T., et al., Isolation and characterization of the plasma hyaluronan-binding protein (PHBP) gene (HABP2), *J. Biochem.*, 122, 983–990, 1997.

48. Etscheid, M., Hunfeld, A., König, H., Seitz, R., and Dodt, J., Activation of proPHBSP, the zymogen of a plasma hyaluronan binding serine protease, by an intermolecular autocatalytic mechanism, *Biol. Chem.*, 381, 1223–1231, 2000.

49. Etscheid, M., Beer, M., Fink, E., Seitz, R., and Johannes, D., The hyaluronan-binding serine protease from human plasma HMW and LMW kininogen and releases bradykinin, *Biol. Chem.*, 383, 1633–1643, 2002.

50. Factor VII activating protease: Does it do what it says on the tin? *J. Thromb. Haemost.*, 10, 857–858, 2012.

51. Estascheid, M., Beer, N., and Dodt, J., The hyaluronan-binding protease upregulates ERK1/2 and PI3K/Akt signalling pathways in fibroblasts and stimulates cell proliferation and migration, *Cell Signal.*, 17, 1486–1494, 2005.

52. Davenport, M.L., Pucilowska, J., Clemmons, D.R., et al., Tissue-specific expression of insulin-like growth factor binding protein-3 protease activity during rat pregnancy, *Endocrinology*, 130, 2505–2512, 1992.

53. Maile, L.A., and Holly, J.M.P., Insulin-like growth factor binding protein (IGFBP) proteolysis: Occurrence, identification, role and regulation, *Growth Hormone & IGF Res*, 9, 85–95, 1999.

54. Berg, U., Bang, P., and Carlsson-Skwirut, C., Calpain proteolysis of insulin-like growth factor binding protein (IGFBP)-2 and -3, but not of IGFBP-1, *Biol. Chem.*, 388, 859–863, 2007.

55. Nwosu, B.U., Soyka, L.A., Angelescu, A., and Lee, M.M., Evidence of insulin-like growth factor binding protein-3 proteolysis during growth hormone stimulation testing, *J. Pediatr. Endocrinol. Metab.*, 24, 163–167, 2011.

56. Elzi, D.J., Lai, Y., Song, M., et al., Plasminogen activator inhibitor 1-insulin-like growth factor binding protein 3 cascade regulates stress-induced senescence, *Proc. Natl. Acad. Sci. U. S. A.*, 109, 12052–12057, 2012.

57. Mitui, Y., Mochizuki, S., Kodama, T., et al., ADAM28 is overexpressed in human breast carcinomas: Implications for carcinoma cell proliferation through cleavage of insulin-like growth factor binding protein-3, *Cancer Res.*, 66, 9913–9920, 2006.

58. Miyamoto, S., Yano, K., Sugimoto, S., et al. Matrix metalloproteinase-7 facilitates insulin-like growth factor bioavailability through its proteinase activity on insulin-like growth factor binding protein 3, *Cancer Res.*, 64, 665–671, 2004.

59. Sadowski, T., Dietrich, S., Kochinsky, F., and Sedlacek, R., Matrix metalloproteinase 19 regulates insulin-like growth factor-mediated proliferation, migration, and adhesion in human keratinocytes through proteolysis of insulin-like growth factor binding protein-3, *Mol. Biol. Cell*, 14, 4569–4580, 2003.

60. Koistinen, H., Paju, A., Koistinen, R., et al., Prostate-specific antigen and other prostate-derived proteases cleave IGFBP-3, but prostate cancer is not associated with proteolytically cleaved circulating IGFBP-3, *Prostate*, 50, 112–118, 2002.

61. Loechel, F., Fox, J.W., Murphy, G., et al., ADAM 12-S cleaves IGFBP-3 and IGFBP-5 and is inhibited by TIMP-3, *Biochem. Biophys. Res. Commun.*, 278, 511–515, 2000.

62. Kübler, B., Draeger, C., John, H., et al., Isolation and characterization of circulating fragments of the insulin-like growth factor binding protein-3, *FEBS Lett.*, 518, 124–128, 2002.

63. Booth, B.A., Boes, M., Dake, B.L., et al., IGFBP-3 binding to endothelial cells inhibits plasmin adn thrombin proteolysis, *Am. J. Physiol. Endocrinol. Metab.*, 282, E52–E58, 2002.

64. Yan, X., Payet, L.D., Baxter, R.C., and Firth, S.M., Activity of human pregancy insulin-like growth factor binding protein-3: Determination by reconstituting recombinant complexes, *Endocrinology*, 150, 4968–4976, 2009.

65. Bhat, C., Villaudy, J., and Binoux, M., In vivo proteolysis of serum insulin-like growth factor (IGF) binding protein-3 results in increased availability of IGF to target cells, *J. Clin. Invest.*, 93, 2286–2290, 1994.

66. Lalou C., and Binoux, M., Evidence that limited proteolysis of insulin-like growth factor binding protein-3 (IGFBP-3) occurs in the normal state outside of the bloodstream, *Regul. Pept.*, 48, 179–188, 1993.

67. Hughes, S.C., Xu, S., Fernihough, J., et al., Tissue IGFBP-3 proteolysis: Contrasting pathophysiology to that in the circulation, *Prog. Growth Factor Res.*, 6, 293–299, 1995.

68. Xu, S., Savage, P., Burton, J.L., et al., Proteolysis of insulin-like growth factor-binding protein-3 by human skin keratinocytes in culture in comparison to that in skin interstitial fluid: The role and regulation of components of the plasmin system, *J. Clin. Endocrinol. Metab.*, 82, 1863–1868, 1997.

69. Clements, J.A., Reflections on the tissue kallikrein and kallikrein-related peptidase family – From mice to men – What have we learnt in the last two decades?, *Biol. Chem.*, 389, 1447–1454, 2008.

70. Pampakalis, G., and Sotiropoulou, G., Pharmacological targeting of human tissue kallikrein-related peptidases, in *Proteinases as Drug Targets*, B.M. Dunn, ed., pp. 199–228, RSC Publishing, Cambridge, United Kingdom, 2012.

71. Trivedi, N.N., Tong, Q., and Raman, K., Mast cell α and β tryptases changed rapidly during primate speciation and evolved from γ-like transmembrane peptidases in ancestral vertebrates, *J. Immunol.*, 179, 6072–6079, 2007.

72. Raymond, W.W., Sommerhoff, C.P., and Caughey, G.H., Mastin is a gelatinolytic mast cell peptidase resembling mini-proteosome, *Arch. Biochem. Biophys.*, 435, 311–322, 2005.

73. Lin, C.-Y., Anders, J., Johnson, M., et al., Molecular cloning of cDNA for matriptase, a maxtix-degrading serin protease with trypsin-like activity, *J. Biol. Chem.*, 274, 18231–18239, 1999.

74. Lee, S.L., Dickson, R.B., and Lin, C.Y., Activation of hepatocyte growth factor and urokinase/plasminogen activator by matriptase, an epithelial membrane serine protease, *J. Biol. Chem.*, 275, 36720–36725, 2000.

75. Miller, G.S., and List, K., The matriptase-prostasin proteolytic cascade in epithelial development and pathology, *Cell Tissue Res.*, 351, 245–253, 2013.

76. Chou, F.P., Xu, H., Lee, M.S., et al., Matriptase is inhibited by extravascular antithrombin in epithelial cells but not in most carcinoma cells, *Am. J. Physiol. Cell Physiol.*, 301, C1093–C1103, 2011.

77. Chen, Y.-W., Xu, Z., Baksh, A.N.H., et al., Antithrombin regulates matriptase activity involved in plasmin generation, syndecan shedding, and HGF activation in keratinocytes, *PLoS One*, 8(5), e62826, 2013.

78. Godiksen, S., Soendergaard, C., Friis, S., et al., Detection of active matriptase using a biotinylated chloromethyl ketone peptide, *PLoS One*, 8(10), e77146, 2013.

79. Oberst, M.D., Williams, C.A., Dickson, R.B., Johnson, M.D., and Lin, C.Y., The activation of matriptase requires its noncatalytic domains, serine protease domain, and its cognate inhibitor, *J. Biol. Chem.*, 278, 26773–26779, 2003.

80. Buzza, M.S., Martin, E.W., Driesbaugh, K.H., et al., Prostasin is required for matriptase activation in intestinal epithelial cells to regulate closure of the paracellular pathway, *J. Biol. Chem.*, 288, 10328–10337, 2013.

81. Woessner. J.F., Jr., Matrix metalloproteinases and their inhibitors in connective tissue remodeling, *FASEB J.*, 5, 2145–2154, 1991.

82. Woessner, J.F., Jr., Quantification of matrix metalloproteinase in tissue samples, *Methods Enzymol.*, 248, 510–528, 1995.

83. Chase, A.J., and Newby, A.C., Regulation of matrix metalloproteinase (matrixin) genes in blood vessels: A multi-step recruitment model for pathological remodelling, *J. Vasc. Res.*, 40, 329–343, 2003.

84. Yamamoto, K., Murphy, G., and Troeberg, L., Extracellular regulation of metalloproteinases, *Matrix Biol.*, 44–46, 255–263, 2015.

85. Ricard-Blum, S., and Vallet, S.D., Proteases decode the extracellular matrix cryptome, *Biochemie*, 122, 300–313, 2015.

86. Ugalde, A.P., Ordóñez, G.R., Quirós, P.M., et al., Metalloproteinases in the degradome, in *Matrix Metalloproteinases Protocols*, I.M. Clark, ed., pp. 2–29, Springer/Humana, New York, 2010.

87. Kleiner, D.E., Jr., and Stetler-Stevenson, W.G., Structural biochemistry and activation of matrix metalloproteases, *Curr. Opin. Cell Biol.*, 5, 891–897, 1993.

88. Ra, H.J., and Parks, W.C., Conrol of matrix metalloproteinase catalytic activity, *Matrix Biol.* 26, 587–596, 2007.

89. Piperi, C., and Papavasssiliou, A.G., Molecular mechanisms regulating matrix metalloproteases, *Curr. Top. Med. Chem.*, 12, 1095–1112, 2012.

90. Jacob-Ferreira, A.L., and Schulz, R., Activation of intracellular matrix metalloproteinase-2 by reactive oxygen-nitrogen species: Consequences and therapeutic strategies in the heart, *Arch. Biochem. Biophys.*, 540, 82–93, 2013.

91. Tocci, A., and Parks, W.C., Functional interactions between matrix metalloproteinase and glycosaminoglycans, *FEBS J.*, 280, 2332–2341, 2013.

92. von Vietinghoff, S., Eulenberg, C., Wellner, M., et al., Neutrophil surface presentation of the anti-neutrophil cytoplasmic antibody-antigen proteinase 3 depends on N-terminal processing, *Clin. Exp. Immunol.*, 152, 508–516, 2008.

93. Bond, J.S., and Beynon, R.J., Meprin: A membrane-bound metalloendopeptidase, *Curr. Top. Cell. Regul.*, 28, 263–290, 1986.

94. Villa, J.P., Bertenshaw, G.P., Bylander, J.E., and Bond, J.S., Meprin proteolytic complexes at the cell surfaces and in the extracellular spaces, *Biochem. Soc. Symp.*, 70, 53–63, 2003.

95. Jefferson, T., auf dem Keller, U., Bellac, C., et al., The substrate degradome of meprin metalloproteases reveals an unexpected proteolytic link between meprin β and ADAM10, *Cell. Mol. Life Sci.*, 70, 309–333, 2013.

96. Bien, J., Jefferson, T., Causević, M., et al., The metalloprotease meprin β generates amino terminal-truncated amyloid β peptide species, *J. Biol. Chem.*, 287, 33304–33313, 2012.

97. Prox, J., Arnold, P., and Becker-Pauly, C., Meprin α and meprin: Procollagen proteinases in health and disease, *Matrix Biol.*, 44–46, 7–13, 2015.

98. Keiffer, T.R., and Bond, J.S., Meprin metalloproteases inactivated interleukin-6, *J. Biol. Chem.*, 289, 7580–7588, 2014.

99. Rinderknecht, H., Renner, I.G., Abramson, S.B., and Carmack, C., Mesotrypsin: A new inhibitor-resistant protease from a zymogen in human pancreatic tissue and fluid, *Gastroenterology*, 86, 681–692, 1984.

100. Knecht, W., Cottrell, G.S., Amadesi, S., et al., Trypsin IV or mesotrypsin and 23 cleave protease-activated receptors 1 and 2 to induce inflammation and hyperalgesia, *J. Biol. Chem.* 282, 26089–26100, 2007.

101. Sabin-Tóth, M., Human mesotrypsin defies natural trypsin inhibitors: From passive resistanc to active destruction, *Protein Pept. Lett.*, 12, 457–464, 2005.

102. Szmola, R., Kukor, Z., and Sabin-Tóth, M., Human mesotrypsin is a unique digestive protease specialized for the degradation of trypsin inhibitors, *J. Biol. Chem.*, 278, 48580–48589, 2003.

103. Miyai, M., Matsumoto, Y., Yamanishi, H., et al., Keratinocyte-specific mesotrypsin conributes to the desquamation process via kallikrein activation an LEKTI degradation, *J. Invest. Dermatol.*, 134, 1665–1674, 2014.

104. Ohlsson, K., and Olsson, I., The extracellular release of granulocyte collagenase and elastase during phagocytosis and inflammatory processes, *Scand. J. Haematol.*, 19, 145–152, 1977.

105. Averhoff, P., Kolbe, M., Zychlinsky, A., and Weinrauch, Y., Single residue determies the specificity of neutrophil elastase for *Shigella* virulence factors, *J. Mol. Biol.*, 377, 1053–1066, 2008.

106. Cantor, J.O., Cerreta, J.M., Armand, G., et al., The pulmonary matrix glycosaminoglycans and pulmonary emphysema, *Connect. Tissue Res.*, 40, 97–104, 1999.

107. Zawieja, D.C., Garcia, C., and Granger, H.J., Oxygen radicals, enzymes, and fluid transport through periocardial interstitium, *Am. J. Physiol.*, 262, H136–H143, 1992.

108. Molayerle, J., Schnekenburger, J., Juergen, K., et al., Extracellular cleavage of E-cadherin by leukocyte elastase during acute experimental pancreatitis in rats, *Gastroenterology*, 129, 1251–1267, 2005.

109. Rao, N.V., Wehner, N.B., Marshall, B.C., et al., Characterization of proteinase-3 (PR-3), a neutrophil serine proteinase. Structural and functional properties, *J. Biol. Chem.*, 266, 9540–9548, 1991.

110. Rao, N.V., Rao, G.V., Marshall, B.C., and Hoidal, J.R., Biosynthesis and processing of proteinase 3 in U937 cells. Processing pathways are distinct from those of cathepsin G, *J. Biol. Chem.*, 271, 2972–2976, 1996.

111. Adkison, A.M., Raptis, S.Z., Kelley, D.G., and Pham, C.T, Dipeptidyl peptidase I activates neutrophil-derived serine proteases and regulates the development of acute experimental arthritis, *J. Clin. Invest.*, 109, 363–371, 2002.

112. Hinkofer, L.C., Seidel, S.A.I., Korkmaz, B., et al., A monoclonal antibody (MCPR3-7) interfering with the activity of proteinase 3 by an allosteric mechanism, *J. Biol. Chem.*, 288, 26635–26648, 2013.

113. Mihara, K., Ramachandran, R., Renaux, B., et al., Neutrophil elastase and proteinase-3 trigger G protein-biased signaling through proteinase-activated receptor-1 (PAR-1), *J. Biol. Chem.*, 288, 32979–32990, 2013.

114. Gaudin, P.B., Askin, F.B., Falk, R.J., and Jennette, J.C., The pathologic spectrum of pulmonary lesions in patients with anti-neutrophil cytoplasmic autoantibodies specific for anti-proteinase 3 and anti-myeloperoxidase, *Am. J. Clin. Pathol.*, 104, 7–16, 1995.

115. Korkmaz, B., Lesner, A., Letast, S., et al., Neutrophil proteinase 3 and dipeptidyl peptidase I (cathepsin C) as pharmacological targets in granulomatosis with polyangiitis (Wegener granulomatosis), *Semin. Immunopathol.*, 35, 411–421, 2013.

116. Weninger, W., Biro, M., and Jain, R., Leukocyte migration in the interstitial space of non-lymphoid organs, *Nat. Rev. Immunol.*, 14, 232–246, 2014.

117. Ley, K., Molecular mechanisms of leukocyte recruitment in the inflammatory process, *Cardiovasc. Res.*, 32, 733–742, 1996.

118. Ng, L.G., Qin, J.S., Roediger, B., et al., Visualizing the neutrophil response to sterile tissue injury in mouse dermis reveals a three-phase cascade of events, *J. Invest. Dermatol.*, 131, 2058–2068, 2011.

119. Orce, G.G., Carretero, O.A., Scicli, G., and Scicli, A.G., Kinins contribute to the contractile effects of rat glandular kallikrein on the isolated rat uterus, *J. Pharmacol. Exp. Ther.*, 249, 470–475, 1989.

120. Meini, S., Cucchi, P., Catalani, C., et al., Pharmacological characterization of the bradykinin B2 receptor antagonist MEN16132 in rat *in vitro* bioassays, *Eur. J. Pharmacol.*, 615, 10–16, 2009.

121. Garbe, G., and Vogt, W., Zur Natur der in menschlichem Plasma durch Pancreakallikrein, Glaskontakt under Säurebehandlung gebildeten Kinine, *Naunyn-Schmiedebergs Arch. Pharmak. u. exp. Path.* 256, 119–126, 1967.

122. Andreasson, S., Smith, L., Aasen, A.O., Saldeen, T., and Risberg, B., Local pulmonary activation after *Escherichia coli*-induced lung injury in sheep, *Eur. J. Surg.*, 20, 289–297, 1988.

123. Dellalibera-Joviliano, R., Dos Reis, M.L., Cunha Fde, Q., and Donadi, E.A., Kinins and cytokines in plasma and cerebrospinal fluid of patients with neuropsychiatric lupus, *J. Rheumatol.*, 30, 485–492, 2003.

124. Addallah, R.T., Keum, J.S., El-Shewy, H.M., et al., Plasma kallikrein promotes epidermal growth factor receptor transactivation and signaling in vascular smooth muslce through direct activation of protease-activated receptors, *J. Biol. Chem.*, 285, 35206–35215, 2010.

125. Castellino, F.J., and Ploplis, V.A., Structure and function of the plasminogen/plasmin system, *Thromb. Haemost.*, 93, 647–654, 2005.

126. Gonzalez, J., Klein, J., Chauhan, S.D., et al., Delayed treatment with plasminogen activator inhibitor-1 decoys reduces tubulointerstitial fibrosis, *Exp. Biol. Med.*, 234, 1511–1518, 2009.

127. Schuliga, M., Westall, F., Xia, Y., and Stewart, A.G., The plasminogen activation system: New targets in lung inflammation and remodeling, *Curr. Opin. Pharmacol.*, 13, 386–393, 2013.

128. Zhang, W.Y., Ishii, I., and Kruth, H.S., Plasmin-mediated macrophage reversal of low density lipoprotein aggregation, *J. Biol. Chem.*, 275, 33176–33183, 2000.

129. Ferreira, H.C., A simple rapid method for estimating serum plasmin activity with fibrin-coated latex particles, *Blood*, 25, 258–260, 1965.

130. Navarrete, M., Ho, J., Krokhin, O., et al., Proteomic characterization of serine hydrolase activity and composition in normal urine, *Clin. Proteomics*, 10(1), 17, 2013.

131. Inman, R.D., and Harpel, P.C., Alpha 2-plasmin inhibitor-plasmin complexes in synovial fluid, *J. Rheumatol.*, 13, 535–357, 1986.

132. Sakamaki, H., Ogura, N., Kujiraoka, H., et al., Activities of plasminogen activator, plasmin and kallikrein in synovial fluid from patients with tempromandibular joint disorders, *Int. J. Oral Maxillofac. Surg.*, 30, 323–328, 2001.

133. Sinz, A., Bantscheff, M., Mikkat, S., et al., Mass spectrometric proteome analyses of synovial fluids and plasmas from patients suffering from rheumatoid arthritis and comparison to reactive arthritis or osteoarthritis, *Electrophoresis*, 23, 3445–3456, 2002.

134. Idell, S., James, K.K., Levin, E.G., et al., Local abnormalities in coagultion and fibrinolytic pathways predispose to alveolar fibrin deposition in the adult respiratory distress syndrome, *J. Clin. Invest.*, 84, 695–705, 1989.

135. Favier, R., Aoki, N., and Moerloose, P., Congenital α_2-antiplasmin deficiencie: A review, *Br. J. Haematol.*, 114, 4–10, 2001.

136. Banbula, A., Zimmerman, T.P., and Novokhatny, V.V., Blood inhibitory capacity toward exogenous plasmin, *Blood Coagul. Fibrinolysis*, 18, 241–246, 2007.

137. Lee, K.N., Jackson, K.W., Christiansen, V.J., et al., Enhancement of fibrinolysis by inhibiting enzymatic cleavage of precursor α_2-antiplasmin, *J. Thromb. Haemost.*, 9, 987–996, 2011.

138. Patterson, B.C., and Sang, Q.A., Angiostatin-converting enzyme activities of human matrilysin (MMP-7) and gelatinase B/type IV collagenase (MMP-9), *J. Biol. Chem.*, 272, 28823–28825, 1997.

139. Falcone, D.J., Khan, K.M., Layne, T., and Fernandes, L., Macrophage formation of angiostatin during inflammation. A byproduct of the activation of plasminogen, *J. Biol. Chem.*, 273, 31480–31485, 1998.

140. Wareicka, D.J., Narayan, M., and Twining, S.S., Maspin increases extracellular plasminogen activator activity associated with corneal fibroblasts and myofibroblasts, *Exp. Eye Res.*, 93, 618–627, 2011.

141. Simard, B., Bouamrani, A., Jourdes, P., et al., Induction of the fibrinolytic system by cartilage extract mediates its antiangiogenic effect in mouse glioma, *Microvasc. Res.*, 82, 6–17, 2011.

142. Brauer, R., Beck, I.M., Roderfeld, M., et al., Matrix metalloproteinase-19 inhibits growth of endothelial cells by generating angiostatin-like fragments from plasminogen, *BMC Biochem.*, 12, 38, 2011.

143. Butera, D., Wind, T., Lay, A.J., et al., Characterization of a reduced form of plasma plasminogen as the precursor for angiostatin formation, *J. Biol. Chem.*, 289, 2992–3000, 2014.

144. Zhang, G., Kernan, K.A., Collins, S.J. et al., Plasmin(ogen) promotes renal interstitial fibrosis by promoting epithelial-to-mesenchymal transition: Role of plasmin-activated signals, *J. Am. Soc. Nephrol.*, 18, 846–859, 2007.

145. Deryugina, E.I., and Quigley, J.P., Surface remodeling by plasmin: A new function for an old enzyme, *J. Biomed. Biotechnol.*, 2012(September), 564259, 2012.

146. Stewart, A.G., Xia, Y.C., Harris, T., et al., Plasminogen-stimulated airway smooth muscle cell proliferation is mediated by urokinase and annexin A2, involving plasmin-activated cell signalling, *Br. J. Pharmacol.*, 170, 1421–1435, 2013.

147. Bogenmann, E., and Jones, P.A., Role of plasminogen in matrix breakdown by neoplastic cells, *J. Natl. Cancer Inst.*, 71, 1177–1182, 1983.

148. Rao, J.S., Kahler, C.G., Baker, J.B., and Festoff, B.W., Protease nexin I, a serpin, inhibits plasminogen-dependent degradation of muscle extracellular matrix, *Muscle Nerve*, 12, 640–646, 1989.

149. Chiangjong, W., and Thongboonkerd, V., A novel assay to evaluate promoting effects of proteins on calcium oxalate crystal invasion through extracellular matrix based on plasminogen/plasmin activity, *Talanta*, 101, 240–245, 2012.

150. Yamamoto, H., Okada, R., Iguchi, K., et al., Involvement of plasmin-mediated extracellular activation of proglanin in angiogenesis, *Biochem. Biophys. Res. Commun.*, 430, 990–1004, 2013.

151. Ingram, K.C., Curtis, C.D., Silasi-Mansat, R., et al., The NuRD chromatin-remodeling enzyme CHD4 promotes embryonic vascular intergrity by transcriptionally regulating extracellular matrix proteolysis, *PLoS Genet.*, 9(12), e1004031, 2013.

152. Atkinson, J.M., Pullen, N., and Johnson, T.S., An inhibitor of thrombin activated fibrinolysis inhibitor (TAFI) can reduce extracellular matrix accumulation in an *in vitro* model of glucose induced ECM expansion, *Matrix Biol.*, 32, 277–287, 2013.

153. Levenson, J.M., Qiu, S., and Weeber, E.J., The role of reelin in adult synaptic function and the genetic and epigenetic regulation of the reelin gene, *Biochim. Biophys. Acta*, 1779, 422–431, 2008.

154. Förster, E, Bock, H.H., Herz, J., et al., Emerging topics in Reelin function, *Eur. J. Neurosci.*, 31, 1511–1518, 2010.

155. Fatemi, S.H., Reelin glycoprotein: Structure, biology and roles in health and disease, *Mol. Psychiatry*, 10, 251–257, 2005.

156. Hirotsune, S., Takahara, T., Sasaki, N., et al., The reeler gene encodes a protein with an EGF-like motif expressed by pioneer neurons, *Nat. Genetics*, 10, 77–83, 1995.

157. Pearlman, A.L., and Sheppard, A.M., Extracellular matrix in early cortical development, *Prog. Brain Res.*, 108, 117–134, 1996.

158. Krishnaswamy, S., The transition of prothrombin to thrombin, *J. Thromb. Haemost.*, 11(Suppl. 1), 265–276, 2013.

159. Le Bonniec, B.F., Thrombin, in *Handbook of Proteolytic Enzymes*, 3rd edn., N.D. Rawlings and G. Salvesen, eds., pp. 2915–2932, Elsevier, Amsterdam, Netherlands, 2013.

160. Chang, J.-Y., Thrombin specificity. Requirement for apolar amino acids adjacent to the thrombin cleavage site of polypeptide substrate, *Eur. J. Biochem.*, 151, 217–224, 1985.

161. Violand, B.N., Takano, M., Curran, D.F., and Bentle, L.A., A novel concatenated dimer of recombinant bovine somatotropin, *J. Prot. Chem.*, 8, 619–628, 1989.

162. Tani, K., Yasuoka, S., Ogushi, F., et al., Thrombin enhances lung fibroblast proliferation in bleomycin-induced pulmonary fibrosis, *Am. J. Respir. Cell Mol. Biol.*, 5, 34–40, 1991.

163. Hewitson, T.D., Martic, M., Kelynack, K.J., et al., Thrombin is a pro-fibrotic factor for rat renal fibroblasts *in vitro.*, *Nephron Exp. Nephrol.*, 101, e42–e49, 2005.

164. Atanelishvili, I., Liang, J., Akter, T., et al., Thrombin increases lung fibroblast survival while promoting alveolar epithelial cell apoptosis via the ER stress marker CHOP, *Am. J. Respir. Cell Mol. Biol.*, 50(5), 893–902, 2014.

165. Idell, S. Garcia, J.G., Gonzalez, K., et al., Fibrinopeptide A reactive peptides and procoagulant activity in bronchoalveolar lavage: Relationship to rheumatoid interstitial lung disease, *J. Rheumatol.*, 16, 592–598, 1989.

166. Song, J.S., Kang, C.M., Park, C.K., and Yoon, H.K., Thrombin induces epithelial-mesenchymal transition via PAR-1, PKC, and ERK$_{1/2}$ pathways in A549 cells, *Exp. Lung Res.*, 39, 336–348, 2013.

167. Goldfarb, R.H., and Liotta, L.A., Thrombin cleavage of extracellular matrix proteins, *Ann. N. Y. Acad. Sci.*, 485, 288–292, 1986.

168. Richardson, M., Hatton, M.W.C., and Moore, S., The plasma proteinases, thrombin and plasmin, degrade the proteoglycan of rabbit aorta segments *in vitro*: An integrated ultrastructural and biochemical study, *Clin. Invest. Med.*, 11, 139–150, 1988.

169. Tamburro, A., Zanni, M., Mariani, B., et al., Thrombin induces the synthesis of stromelysin 1 (MMP-3): A novel effect of thrombin on extracellular matrix degradation, *Fibrinolyis & Proteolysis*, 11, 251–257, 1997.

170. Fang, Q., Llu, X., Al-Mugotir, M., et al., Thrombin and TNF-α/IL-1β synergistically induce fibroblast-mediated collagen gel degradation, *Am. J. Respir. Cell Mol. Biol.*, 35, 714–721, 2006.

171. Chappell, D., Jacob, M., Hofmann-Kiefer, K., et al., Antithrombin reduces shedding of the endothelial glycocalyx followng ischaemia/reperfusion, *Cardiovasc. Res.*, 83, 388–396, 2009.

172. Shimomura, T., Kondo, J., Ochiai, M., et al., Activation of the zymogen of hepatocyte growth factor activator by thrombin, *J. Biol. Chem.*, 268, 22927–22932, 1993.

173. Proud, D., and Kaplan, A.P., Kinin formation: Mechanisms and role in inflammatory disorders, *Annu. Rev. Immunol.*, 6, 49–83, 1988.

174. Wei, C.C., Chen, Y., Powell, L.C., et al., Cardiac kalikrein-kinin system is upregulated in chronic volume overload and mediates an inflammatory induced collagen loss, *PLoS One*, 7(6), e40110, 2012.

175. Standnicki, A., Intestinal tissue kallikrein-kinin system in inflammatory bowel disease, *Inflamm. Bowel Dis.*, 17, 645–654, 2011.

176. Gautvik, K.M., Hilton, S.M., and Torres, S.H., Consumption of the plasma substrate for glandular kallikrein on activation of the submandibular gland, *J. Physiol.*, 197, 22P–23P, 1968.

177. Maier, H., Adler, D., Menstell, S., and Lenarz, T., Glandular kallikrein in chronic recurrent parotitis, *Laryngol. Rhinol. Otol.*, 63, 633–635, 1984.

178. Astrup, T., Tissue activators of plasminogen, *Fed. Proc.*, 25, 42–51, 1966.

179. Lu, X.-G., Wu, X.-G., Xu, X.-H., et al., Novel distribution pattern of fibrinolytic components in rabbit tissue extracts: A preliminary study, *J. Zhejiang Univ. Sci. B*, 8, 570–574, 2007.

180. O'Rourke, J., Jiang, X., Hao, Z., et al., Distribution of sympathetic tissue plasminogen activator (tPA) to a distant microvasculature, *J. Neurosci. Res.*, 79, 727–733, 2005.

181. Parmer, R.J., and Miles, L.A., Targeting of tissue plasminogen activator to the regulated pathway of secretion, *Trends Cardiovasc. Med.*, 8, 306–312, 1998.

182. Tripathi, R.C., Tripathi, B.J., and Park, J.K., Localization of urokinase-type plasminogen activator in human eyes: An immunocytochemical study, *Exp. Eye Res.*, 51, 545–552, 1990.

183. van Hinsbergh, V.W., Regulation of the synthesis and secretion of plasminogen activators by endothelial cells, *Haemostasis* 18, 307–327, 1988.

184. Suzuki, Y., Yasui, H., Brzoska, T., et al., Surface-retained tPA is essential for effective fibrinolysis on vascular endothelial cells, *Blood*, 118, 3182–3185, 2011.

185. Kirsten, C.G., Tuttle, P.R., and Berger, H., Jr., Quantitative assessment of subcutaneous fibrinolysis in the rat, *J. Phamacol. Methods*, 16, 125–138, 1986.

186. Hatton, M.W.C., Southward, S.M.R., Ross, B.L., et al., Relationships among tumor burden, tumor size, and the changing concentrations of fibrin degradation products and fibrinolytic factors in the pleural effusions of rabbits with VX2 lung tumors, *J. Lab. Clin. Med.*, 147, 27–35, 2006.

187. Laschinger, C.A., Johnston, M.G., Hay, J.B., and Wasi, S., Production of plasminogen activator and plasminogen activator inhibitor by bovine lymphatic endothelial cells: Modulation by TNF-α, *Thromb. Res.*, 59, 567–579, 1990.

188. Silverstein, R.L., Nachman, R.L., Leung, L.L.K., and Harpel, P.C., Activation of immobilized plasminogen by tissue activator. Multimolecular complex formation, *J. Biol. Chem.*, 260, 10346–10352, 1985.

189. Suenson, E., and Petersen, L.C., Fibrin and plasminogen structures essential to stimulation of plasmin formation by tissue-type plasminogen activator, *Biochim. Biophys. Acta*, 870, 510–519, 1986.

190. Meissnauer, A., Kramer, M.D., Schirrmacher, V., and Brunner, G., Generation of cell surface-bound plasmin by cell-associated urokinase-type of secreted tissue-type plasminogen activator: A key event in melanoma cell invasiveness *in vitro*, *Exp. Cell Res.*, 199, 179–190, 1992.

191. Trivedi, N.N., and Caughey, G.H., Human α-, β-, and γ-tryptases, in *Handbook of Proteolytic Enzymes*, 3rd edn., N.D. Rawlings and G. Salvesen, eds., pp. 2683–2693, Elsevier, Amsterdam, Netherlands, 2013.

192. Selwood, T., Wang, Z.M., McCaslin, D.R., and Schechter, N.M., Diverse stability and catalytic properties of human tryptase: Alpha and beta isoforms and mediated by residue differences at the S1 pocket, *Biochemistry*, 41, 3329–3340, 2002.

193. Schwartz, L.B., Bradford, T.R., Lee, D.C., and Chlebowski, J.F., Immunologic and physicochemical evidence for conformational changes occuring on conversion of human mast cell tryptase from active tetramer to inactive monomer. Production of monoclonal antibodies recognizig active tryptase, *J. Immunol.*, 144, 2304–2311, 1990.

194. Sommerhoff, C.P., Bode, W., Pereira, P.J.B., et al., The structure of the human βII-tryptase tetramer: For (u)r better or worse, *Proc. Natl. Acad. Sci. U. S. A.*, 96, 10984–10991, 1999.

195. He, S., Aslam, A., Gaca, M.D., et al., Inhibitors of tryptase as mast cell-stabilizing agents in the human airways: Effects of tryptase and other agonists of proteinase-activated receptor 2 of histamine release, *J. Pharmacol. Exp. Ther.*, 309, 119–126, 2004.

196. Jacob, C., Yang, P.C., Darmoul, D., et al., Mast cell tryptase controls paracellular permeability of the intestine. Role of protease-activated receptor 2 and β-arrestins, *J. Biol. Chem.*, 280, 31936–31948, 2005.

197. Tatler, A.L. Porte, J., Knox, A., et al., Tryptase activates TGFβ in human airway smooth muscle cells via direct proteolysis, *Biochem. Biophys. Res. Commun.*, 370, 239–242, 2008.

198. Stevens, R.L., and Adachi, R., Protease-proteoglycan complexes of mouse and human mast cells and importance of their β-tryptase-heparin complexes in inflammation and innate immunity, *Immunol. Rev.*, 217, 155–167, 2007.

199. Fukuoka, Y., Xia, H.Z., Sanchez-Muñoz, L.B., et al., Generation of anaphylatoxins by human β-tryptase form C3, C4, and C5, *J. Immunol.*, 180, 6307–6316, 2008.

200. Shin, K., Nigrovic, P.A., Crish, J., et al., Mast cells contribute to autoimmune inflammatory arthritis via their tryptase/heparin complexes, *J. Immunol.*, 182, 647–656, 2009.

201. Nagyeri, G., Radacs, M., Ghassemi-Nejad, S., et al., TSG-6 protein, a negative regulator of inflammatory arthritis, forms a ternary complex with murine mast cell tryptases and heparin, *J. Biol. Chem.*, 286, 23559–23569, 2011.

202. Anower-E-Khuda, M.R., Habuchi, H., Nagai, N., et al., Heparan sulfate 6-O-sulfotransferase isoform-dependent regulatory effects of heparin on the activities of various proteases in mast cells and the biosynthesis of 6-O-sulfated heparin, *J. Biol. Chem.*, 288, 3705–3717, 2013.

203. Schechter, N.M., Eng, G.Y., Selwood, T., and McCaslin, D.R., Structural changes associated with the spontaneous inactivation of the serine proteinase human tryptase, *Biochemistry*, 34, 10628–10638, 1995.

204. Selwood, T., McCaslin, D.R., and Schechter, N.M., Spontaneous inactivation of human tryptase involves conformational changes consistent with conversion of the active site to a zymogen-like structure, *Biochemistry*, 37, 13174–13183, 1998.

205. Selwood, T., Smolensky, H., McCaslin, D.R., and Schechter, N.M., The interaction of tryptase-β with small molecule inhibitors provides new insights into the unusual functional instability and quaternary structure of the protease, *Biochemistry*, 44, 3580–3590, 2005.

206. Schechter, N.M., Choi, E.J., Selwood, T., and McCaslin, D.R., Characterization of three distinct catalytic forms of human tryptase-β: Their interrelationships and relevance, *Biochemistry*, 46, 9615–9629, 2007.

207. Wiegand, U., Corbach, S., Minn, A., Kang, J., and Müller-Hill, B., Cloning of the cDNA encoding human brain trypsinogen and characterization of its product, *Gene*, 136, 167–175, 1993.

208. Tóth, J., Siklódi, E., Medveczky, P., et al., Regional distribution of human trypsinogen 4 in human brain at mRNA and protein level, *Neurochem. Res.*, 32, 1423–1433, 2007.

209. Cottrell, G.S., Adamesi, S., Grady, E.F., and Bunnett, N.W., Trypsin IV, a novel agonist of protease-activated receptors 2 and 4, *J. Biol. Chem.*, 279, 13532–13539, 2004.

210. Katona, G., Berglund, G.I., Hajdu, J., Graf, L., and Szilagyi, L., Crystal structure reveals basis for inhibitor resistance of human brain trypsin, *J. Mol. Biol.*, 315, 1209–1218, 2002.

211. Fu, Q., Cheng, J., Gao, Y., et al., Protease-activated receptor 4: A critical participator in inflammatory response, *Inflammation* 38, 886–895, 2014.

212. White, W.F., and Barlow, G., Urinary plasminogen activator (urokinase), *Methods Enzymol.*, 19, 665–672, 1970.

213. Barlow, G.H., Urinary and kidney cell plasminogen activator (urokinase), *Methods Enzymol.* 45, 239–244, 1976.

214. Eden, G., Archinti, M., Furlan, F., et al., The urokinase receptor interactome, *Curr. Pharm. Des.*, 17, 1874–1889, 2011.

215. Schuliga, M., Westall, G., Xia, Y., and Stewart, A.G., The plasminogen activation system: New targets in lung inflammation and remodeling, *Curr. Opin. Pharmacol.*, 13, 386–393, 2013.

216. Breuss, J.M., and Uhrin, P., VEGF-initiated angiogenesis and the uPA/uPAR system, *Cell Adh. Migr.*, 6, 535–615, 2012.

217. Liu, Y.X., Regulation of the plasminogen activator system in the ovary, *Biol. Signals Recept.*, 8, 160–177, 1999.

218. Thorsen, S., and Astrup, T., Biphasic inhibition of urokinase-induced fibrinolysis by epsilon-aminocaproic acid; distinction from tissue plasminogen activator, *Proc. Soc. Exp. Biol. Med.*, 130, 811–813, 1969.

219. Thorsen, S., and Astrup, T., Differences in the reactivities of human urokinase and the porcine tissue plasminogen activator, *Haemstasis*, 5, 295–305, 1976.

ENZYMES IN SYNTHETIC ORGANIC CHEMISTRY[a,b]

Roger L. Lundblad

The specificity of enzymes has proved useful in organic synthesis where stereochemistry is critical for success.

Aldolase/Aldol Condensation   **Catalysis of Aldol Condensation**

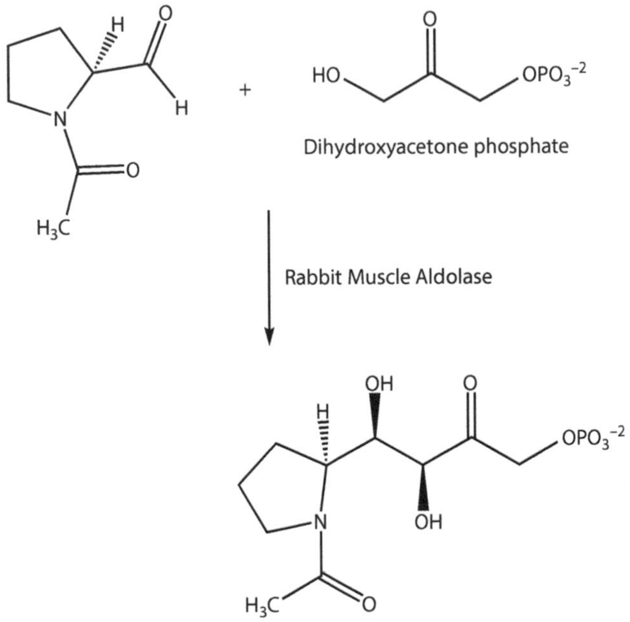

Dihydroxyacetone phosphate

Rabbit Muscle Aldolase

Austin, M.B., Izumikawa, M., Bowman, M.E., Crystal structure of a bacterial type III polyketide synthase and enzymatic control of reactive polyketide intermediates, *J.Biol.Chem.* 279, 45162–45174, 2004; Xiang, L., Kokaitzis, J.A, and Moore, B.S., EncM, a versatile enterocin biosynthetic enzyme involved in Favorskii oxidative rearrangement, aldol condensation, and heterocyclic-forming reactions, *Proc.Nat.Acad.Sci.* 101, 15609-15614, 2004; Suzuki, H., Ohnishi, Y. Fursho, Y., *et al.*, Novel benzene ring biosynthesis from C(3) and C(4) primary metabolites by two enzymes, *J.Biol.Chem.* 281, 36944–36951, 2006; Zhang, W., Watanabe, K., Wang, C.C., and Tang, Y., Heterologous biosynthesis of amidated polyketides with novel cyclization regioselectivity from oxytetracycline polyketide synthase, *J.Natl.Prod.* 69, 1633–1636, 2006; Williams, G.J., Woodhall, T., Farnsworth, L.M., *et al.*, Creation of a pair of stereochemically complementary biocatalysts, *J.Am.Chem.Soc.* 128, 16238–16247, 2006; Schetter, B. and Mahrwald, R., Model aldol methods for the total synthesis of polyketides, *Angewandte Chem. Int.Ed.* 45, 7506–7535, 2006; Suzuki, H., Ohnishi, Y., Furusho, Y., *et al.*, Novel benzene ring biosynthesis from C_3 and C_4 primary metabolites by two enzymes, *J.Biol.Chem.* 281, 36944–39511, 2007.

---

[a] *Handbook of Enzyme Biotechnology*, 2nd edn., ed. A. Wiseman, Ellis Horwood, Ltd., Chichester, UK, 1985; Laskin, A.T., *Enzymes and Immobilized Cells in Biotechnology*, Benjamin Cummings, Menlo Park, CA, USA, 1985; *Biocatalysis in Organic Media*, ed. C. Laane and J. Trayser, Elsevier, Amsterdam, Nethelands, 1987; Halgaš, J. *Biocatalysis in Organic Synthesis*, Elsevier, Amsterdam, Netherlands, 1992; Holland, H.L., *Organic Synthesis with Oxidative Enzymes*, VCH Publishers, New York, NY, USA, 1992; *Enzyme Catalysis in Organic Synthesis. A Comprehensive Handbook*, ed. K. Drauz and H. Waldman, VCH Verlagesellschaft, Weinheim, Germany, 1995; *Bioorganic Chemistry Peptides and Proteins*, ed S.M. Hecht, Oxford University Press, New York, NY, USA, 1998; Faber, K., *Biotransformations in Organic Chemistry*, 5th edn., Springer-Verlag, Berlin, Germany, 2005.
[b] Ribozymes have been used for chiral synthesis – See Schlatterer, J.C., Stuhlman, F., and Jäschke, A., Stereoselective synthesis using immobilized Diels-Alderase ribozymes, *ChemBioChem.* 4, 1089-1092, 2003

Enzymes in Synthetic Organic Chemistry[a,b] (Continued)

Hydrolases (Esterases)   A group of enzymes which catalyze the cleavage of ester and amide bonds with addition of water. Esterases, of which lipases are a singularly important group, are important in synthetic organic chemistry. Of particular importance is the stereoselectivity of the reaction[c]. A racemic mixture of an ester can be resolved can be resolved into enantiomeric pairs by stereospecific hydrolysis. Butyrylcholine esterase and cocaine esterase are listed with the therapeutic enzymes.

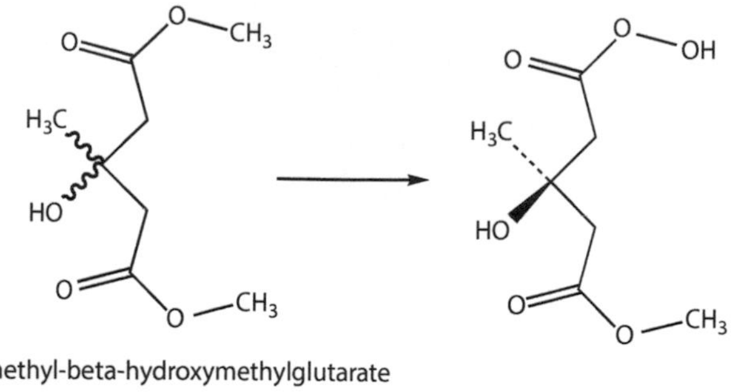

dimethyl-beta-hydroxymethylglutarate

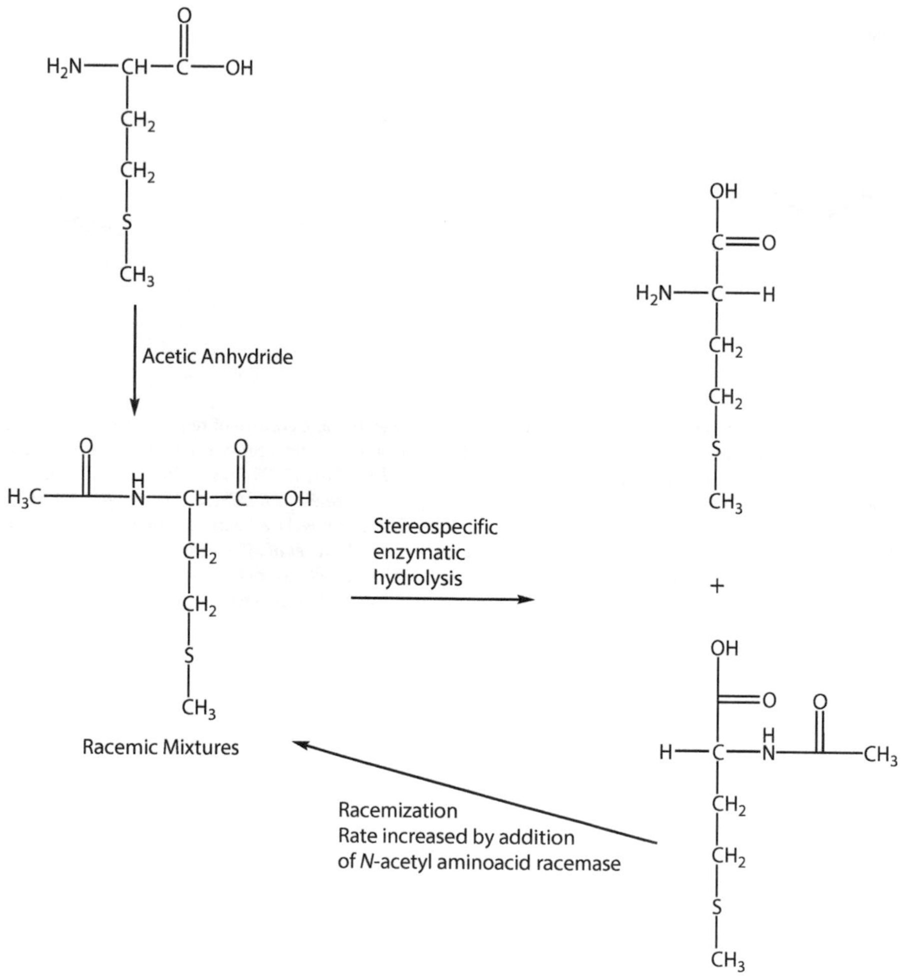

Acetic Anhydride

Racemic Mixtures

Stereospecific enzymatic hydrolysis

+

Racemization
Rate increased by addition
of *N*-acetyl aminoacid racemase

---

[c] A carbon center may be asymmetric in having four different substituents (other atoms such as sulfur can also be asymmetric centers). In the case of carbon, this can be result in a mixture of the two optical isomers resulting in a racemic mixture. Generally there is no driving force for the formation of a racemic mixture so there are equal forms of the D and L isomers. With an enzyme stereoselectivity can be achieved and the quality of an asymmetric mixture may be expressed as enantiomeric excess (enantiomeric excess = (moles of major enantiomer - moles of other enantiomer / Total moles of both enantiomers) × 100 and is usually expressed as a percentage.

Enzymes in Synthetic Organic Chemistry[a,b] (Continued)

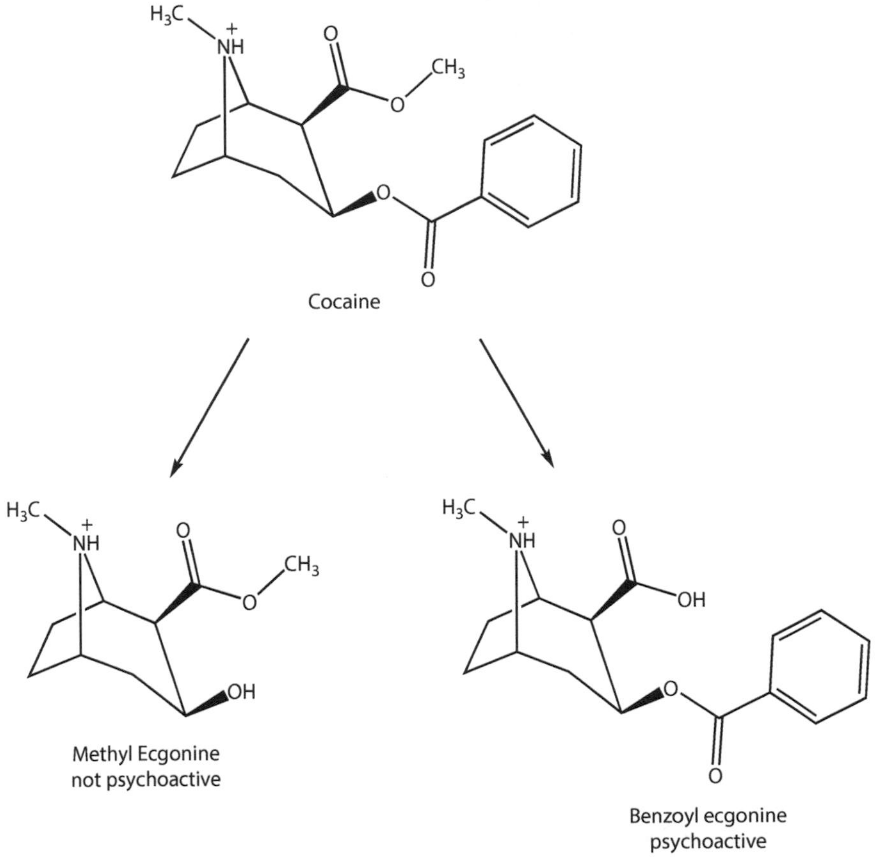
H3C
+
NH
O
CH3
O
O
O
Cocaine
H3C
+
NH
O
CH3
O
OH
Methyl Ecgonine
not psychoactive
H3C
+
NH
O
OH
O
O
Benzoyl ecgonine
psychoactive

Venkatachalam, T.K., Samuel, P., Li, G., *et al.*, Lipase-mediated stereoselective hydrolysis of stampidine and other phosphoroamidate derivatives of stavudine, *Bioorg.Med.Chem.* 12, 3371–3381, 2004; Li, Y., Aubert, S.D., Maes, E.G., and Raushel, F.M., Enzymatic resolution of chiral phosphinate esters, *J.Am.Chem.Soc.* 126, 8888–8889, 2004; Kim, S. and Lee, S.B., Thermostable esterase from a thermoacidophilic archaeon: purification and characterization for enzymatic resolution of a chiral compound, *Biosci.Biotechnol.Biochem.* 68, 2289–2298, 2004; Molinari, F., Romano, D., Gandolfi, R., *et al.*, Newly isolated *Streptomyces* spp. As enantioselective biocatalysts: hydrolysis of 1,2-O-isopropylidene glycerol racemic esters, *J.Appl.Microbiol.* 99, 960–967, 2005; Hu, S., Martinez, C.A., Yazbeck, D.R., and Tao, J., An efficient and practical chemoenzymatic preparation of optically active secondary amines, *Org.Lett.* 7, 4329–4331, 2005; Nowlan, C., Li, Y., Hermann, J.C., *et al.*, Resolution of chiral phosphate, phosphonate, and phosphinate esters by an enantioselective enzyme library, *J.Am.Chem.Soc.* 128, 15892–15902, 2006; Gadler, P. and Faber, K., New enzymes for biotransformations: microbial alkyl sulfatases displaying stereo- and enantioselectivity, *Trends Biotechnol.* 25, 83–88, 2007.

Enzymes in Synthetic Organic Chemistry[a,b] (Continued)

Lipases   A group of hydrolytic enzymes that catalyze the release of fatty acids from triglycerides; more specifically the catalysis of the hydrolysis of ester bonds between alkanoic acids and glycerol. Phospholipases are a subclass which uses phospholipids as substrates. The ability to use alcohols and amines as acceptors of the fatty acid hydrolytic product permits the synthesis of chiral products. There has been recent interest in the use of lipases for the synthesis of combinatorial libraries.[d]

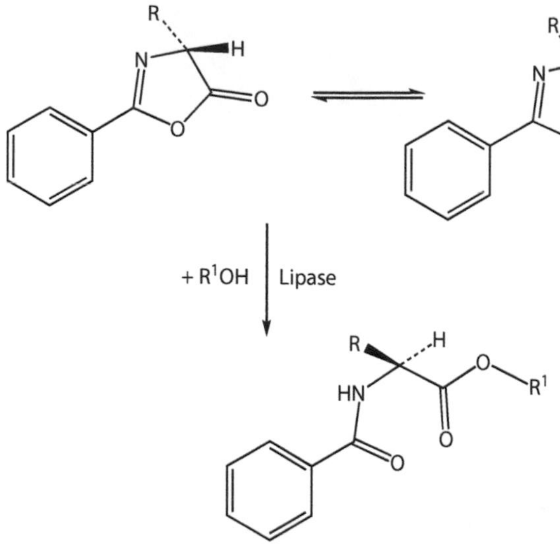

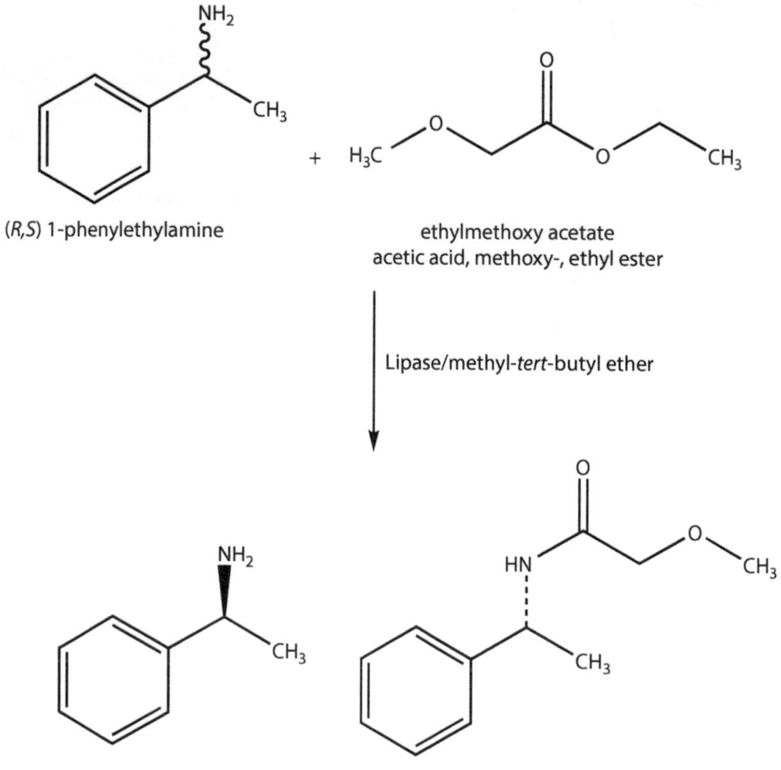

(R,S) 1-phenylethylamine

ethylmethoxy acetate
acetic acid, methoxy-, ethyl ester

Lipase/methyl-*tert*-butyl ether

(S)1-phenylethylamine   (R)-phenylethylmethoxyamide

---

[d] Use of lipases in the manufacture of combinatorial libraries: Liu, K.-C., Clark, D.S., and Dordick, J.S., Chemoenzymatic construction of a four-component Ugi combinatorial library, *Biotechnol.Bioeng.* 69, 457–460, 2000; Reetz, M.T., Lipases as practical biocatalysts, *Curr.Opin.Chem.Biol.* 6, 145–150, 2002; Rich, J.G., Michels, P.C., and Khmeinitsky, Y.L., Lipases as practical biocatalysts, *Curr.Opin.Chem.Biol.* 6, 161–167, 2002; Secundo, F., Garrea, G., De Amici, M., *et al.*, A combinatorial biocatalysis approach to an array of cholic acid derivatives, *Biotechnol.Bioeng.* 81, 392–396, 2003; Kumar, R., Bruno, F., Parmar, V.S., *et al.*, "Green"-enzymatic synthesis of pegylated phenolic macromer and polymer, *Chem.Commun.* (7), 862–863, 2004; Rege, K., Hu. S., Moore, J.A., Chemoenzymatic synthesis and high-throughput screening of high-affinity displacers and DNA-binding ligands, *J.Am.Chem.Soc.* 126, 12306–12315, 2004; Vongvilal, P., Angelin, M., Larsson, R., and Ramstrom, O., Dynamic combinatorial resolution: direct asymmetric lipase-mediated screening of a dynamic nitroaldol library, *Angew.Chem.Int.Ed.Engl.* 46, 948–950, 2007.

Enzymes in Synthetic Organic Chemistry[a,b] (Continued)

Tuomi, W.V., and Kazlauskas, R.J., Molecular basis for enantioselectivity of lipase from *Pseudomonas cepacia* towards primary alcohols. Modeling, kinetics, and chemical modification of tyr29 to increase or decrease enantioselectivity, *J.Org.Chem.* 64, 2638–2647, 1999; Ghorpade, S.R., Khani, R.K., Ioshi, R.R., *et al.*, Desymmetrization of *meso*-cyclopentene-*cis*-1, 4-diol to 4-(R)-hydroxycyclopent-2-en-1-(S)-acetate by irreversible transesterification using Chirazyme˙, *Tetrahedron Asymm.* 10, 891–899, 1999; Chen, J.-W. and Wu, W.-T., Regeneration of immobilized *Candida anartica* lipase for transesterification, *J.Biosci.Bioeng.* 95, 466–469, 2003; Gupta, R., Gupta, N., and Rathi, P., Bacterial lipases: an overview of production, purification and biochemical properties, *Appl.Microbiol.Biotechnol.* 64, 763–781, 2004; Kijima, T., Sato, N., Izumi, T., Lipase-catalyzed enantioselective esterification of mono-aza-benzo-15-crown-5-ether derivatives in organic media, *Biotechnol.Lett.* 26, 1505–1509, 2004; Domínguez de Maria, P., Carboni-Oerlemans, C., Tuin, B., *et al.*, Biotechnological applications of *Candida antartica* lipase A: state-of-the-art, *J.Molec.Catal.B:Enzymatic* 37, 36–46, 2005; Sharma, J., Batovska, D., Kuwamori, Y., and Asano, Y., Enzymatic chemoselective synthesis of secondary-amide surfactant from *N*-methylethanol amine, *J.Biosci. Bioeng.* 100, 662–666, 2005; Patel, R.N., Banerjee, A., Pendri, Y.R., *et al.*, Preparation of a chiral synthon for an HBV inhibitor: enzymatic asymmetric hydrolysis of (1α, 2β, 3α)-2-(benzyloxymethyl)cyclopent-4-ene-1,3-diol diacetate and enzymatic asymmetric acctylation of (1α, 2β, 3α)-2-(benzyloxymethyl)cyclopent-4-ene-1,3-diol, *Tetrahedron Asymm.* 17, 175–175, 2006; Otero, C., Lopez-Herandez, A, Garcia, H.S., *et al.*, Continuous enzymatic transesterification of sesame oil and a fully hydrogenated fat: effects of reaction conditions on product characterization, *Biotechnol.Bioeng.* 94, 877–887, 2006.

Enzymes in Synthetic Organic Chemistry[a,b] (Continued)

Monooxygenase

Insertion of oxygen into organic frameworks such as the oxidation of olefins (Baeyer-Villiger Reaction); hydroxylation of alkanes and aromatics. The cytochrome P-450-dependent monooxygenase is one of the better-known examples. Monooxygenases also oxidize organic sulfur

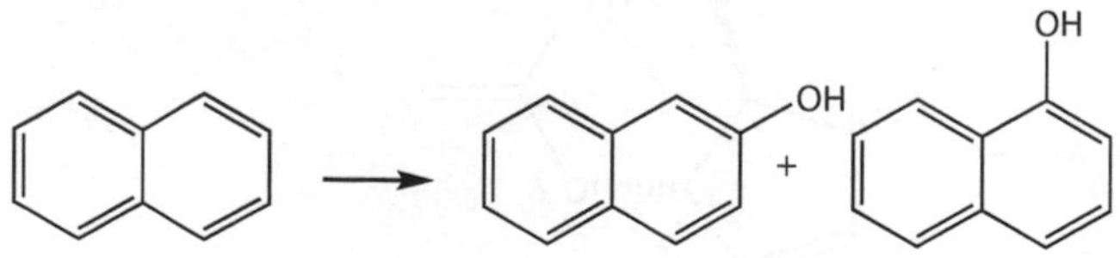
OH
+
OH

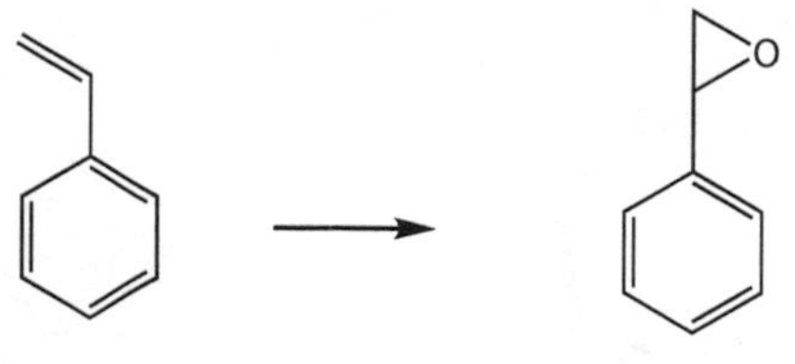
O

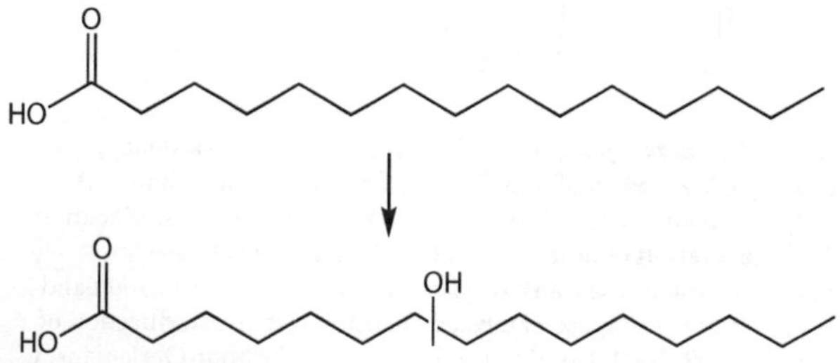
O
HO
O
OH
HO

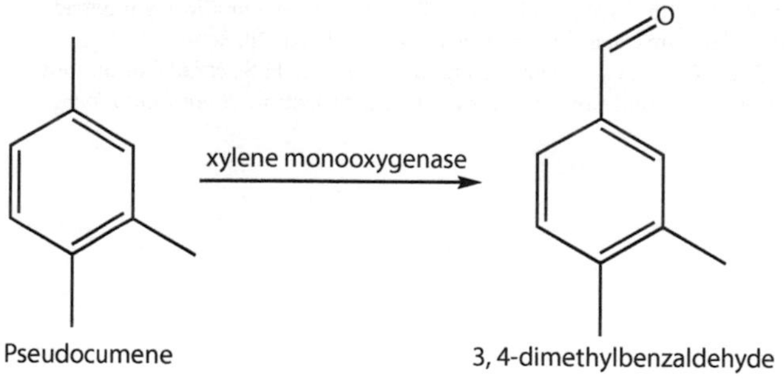
xylene monooxygenase
O
Pseudocumene
3, 4-dimethylbenzaldehyde

Enzymes in Synthetic Organic Chemistry[a,b] (Continued)

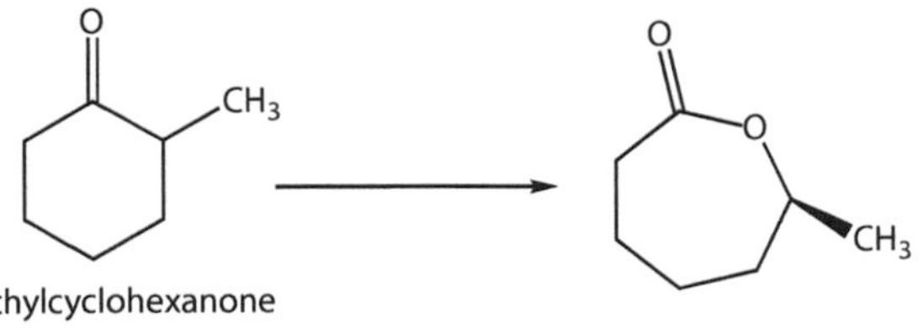

2-methylcyclohexanone

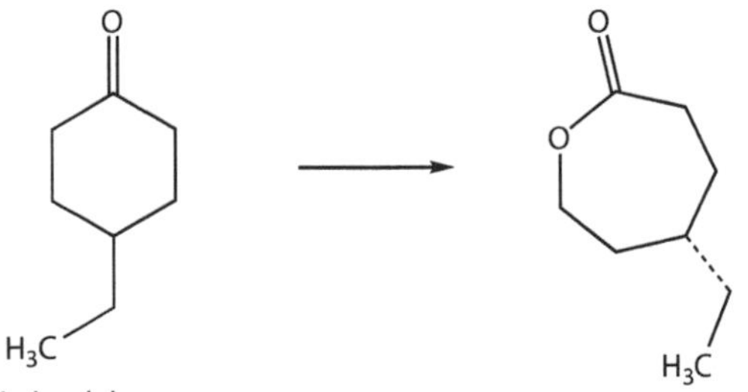

4-ethylcyclohexanone

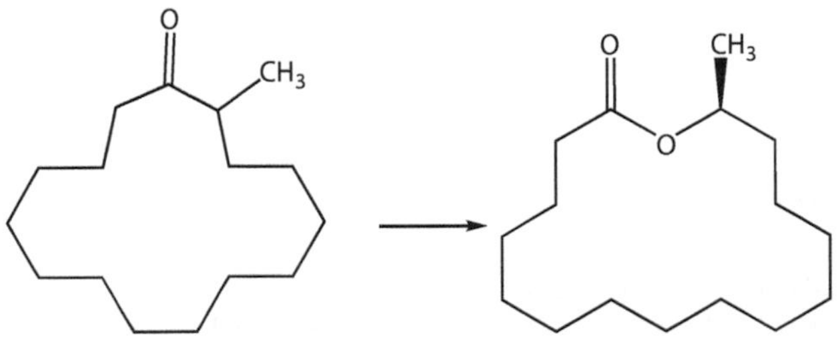

2-methylcyclopentadecanone

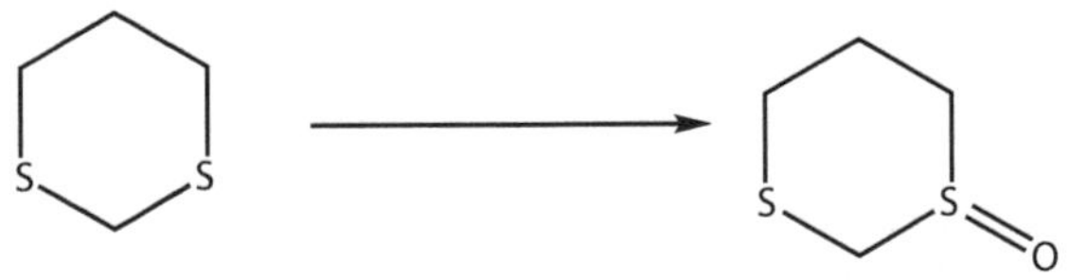

(R) 81%

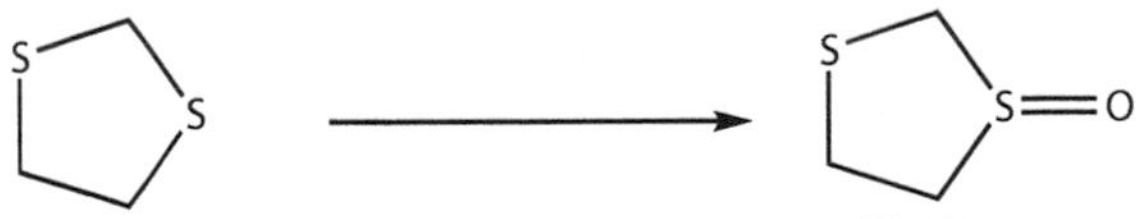

(R) 94%

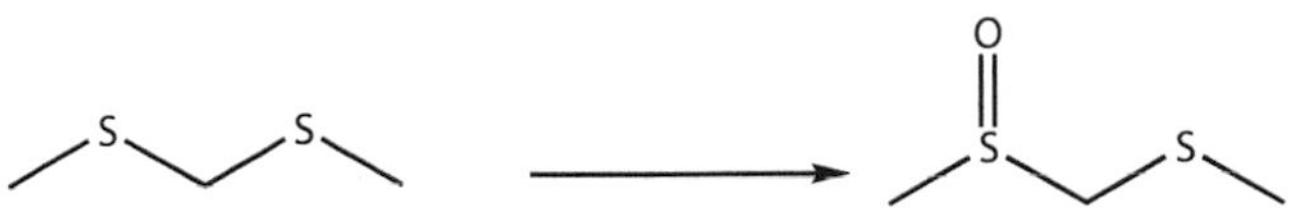

(R) 92%

Enzymes in Synthetic Organic Chemistry[a,b] (Continued)

(R-2)   OR   (S-2)

Sphingomonas sp.; 40% enantioselective   *Beauuveria bassiana*; 99% enantioselective

Ogawa, J. and Shimizu, S., Microbial enzymes: new industrial applications from traditional screening methods, *Trends Biotechnol.* 17, 13-21, 1999; Stewart, J.D., Organic transformations catalyzed by engineered yeast cells and related systems, *Curr.Opin.Biotechnol.* 11, 363-368, 2000; Mihovilovic, M.D., Muller, B., and Stanetty, P., Monooxygenase-mediated Baeyer-Villiger oxidations, *Eur.J.Org.Chem.* (22), 3711-3730, 2002; Lee, W.H., Park, Y.C., Lee, D.H., Simultaneous biocatalyst production and Baeyer-Villiger oxidation for bioconversion of cyclohexanone by recombinant *Escherichia coli* expressing cyclohexanone monooxygenase, *Appl.Biochem.Biotechnol.* 121-124, 827-836, 2005; Han, J.H., Yoo, S.K., Seo, J.S., *et al.,* Biomimetic alcohol oxidations by an iron (III) porphyrin complex: relevance to cytochrome P-450 catalytic oxidation and involvement of the two-state radical rebound mechanism, *Dalton Trans.* (2), 402–406, 2005; Kagawa, H., Tatkahashi, T., Ohta, S., and Harigaya, Y., Oxidation and rearrangements of flavanones by mammalian cytochrome P450, *Xenobiotica* 34, 797–810, 2004; Gillam, E.M., Exploring the potential of xenobiotic-metabolising enzymes as biocatalysts: evolving designer catalysts from polyfunctional cytochrome P450 enzymes, *Clin.Exp.Pharmacol.Physiol.* 32, 147–152, 2005; Bocola, M., Schultz, F., Leca, F., *et al.,* Converting phenylacetone monooxygenase into phenylcyclohexanone monooxygenase by rational design: towards practical Baeyer-Villiger monooxygenases, *Adv.Synth.Catal.* 347, 979–986, 2005; Urlacher, V.B. and Eiben, S., Cytochrome P450 monooxygenases: perspectives for synthetic application, *Trends Biotechnol.* 24, 324–330, 2006; Iwaki, H., Wang, S. ,Grosse, S., *et al.,* Pseudomonad cyclopentadecanone monooxygenase displaying an uncommon spectrum of Baeyer-Villiger oxidations of cyclic ketones, *Appl.Environ.Microbiol.* 72, 2707–2720, 2006; Mihovilovic, M.D., Enzyme mediated Baeyer-Villiger oxidations, *Curr.Org.Chem.* 10, 1265–1287, 2006.Application to the stereospecific oxidation of organic sulfur: Dodson, R.M., Newman, N., and Tsuchiya, H.M., Microbiological transformations. XI. The properties of optically active sulfoxides, *J.Am.Chem.Soc.* 27, 2707–2708, 1962; Light, D.R., Waxman, D.J., and Walsh, C., Studies on the chirality of sulfoxidation catalyzed by bacterial flavoenzyme cyclohexanone monooxygenase and hog liver flavin adenine dinucleotide containing monooxygenase, *Biochemistry* 21, 2490–2498, 1982; Waxman, D.J., Light, D.R., and Walsh, C., Chiral sulfoxidation catalyzed by rat live cytochrome P-450, *Biochemistry* 21, 2499–2507, 1982; Colonna, S., Gaggero, N., Pasta, P., and Ottolina, G., Enantioselective oxidation of sulfides to sulfoxides catalyzed by bacterial cyclohexanone monooxygenase, *Chem.Commun.* (20), 2303–2307, 1996; Mata, E.G., Recent advances in the synthesis of sulfoxides from sulfides, *Phosphorus, Sulfur and Silicon and the Related Elements* 117, 231–286, 1996; Hamman, M.A., Haehner-Daniels, B.D., Wrighton, S.A., *et al.,* Stereoselective sulfoxidation of sulindac sulfide by flavin-containing monooxygenase-Comparison of human liver and kidney microsomes and mammalian enzymes, *Biochem.Pharmacol.* 60, 7–17, 2000; Reetz, M.T., Daligault, F., Brunner, B., *et al.,* Directed evolution of cyclohexanone monooxygenases: enantioselective biocatalysts for the oxidation of prochiral thioethers, *Angewandte Chem.Int.* 43, 4078–4081, 2005; Legros, J., Dehli, J.R., and Bolm, C., Applications of catalytic asymmetric sulfide oxidations to the syntheses of biologically active sulfoxides, *Adv.Synthes.& Catal.* 19–31, 2005; Olivo, H.F., Osorio-Lozada, A., and Peeples, T.L., Microbial oxidation/ amidation of benzhydrylsulfanyl acetic acid. Synthesis of (+)-modafinil, *Tetrahedron Asymmetry* 16, 3507–3511, 2005.

Enzymes in Synthetic Organic Chemistry[a,b] (Continued)

Dioxygenase
An enzyme activity which inserts an oxygen molecule into an organic substrate. Where hydroxyl function(s) is the terminal reaction product, the overall reaction is the sum of two separate enzymatic reactions; an oxidation followed by a reduction.

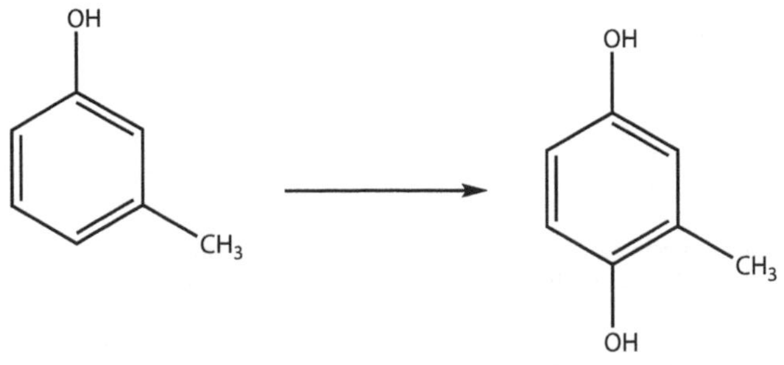

m-cresol → methyl hydroquinone

(1)

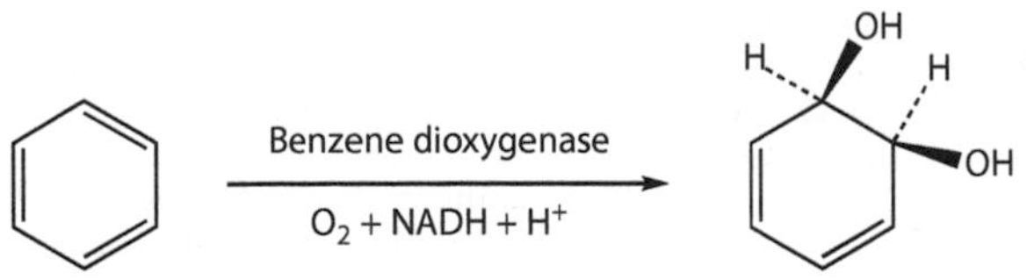

Benzene dioxygenase

$O_2 + NADH + H^+$

(2)

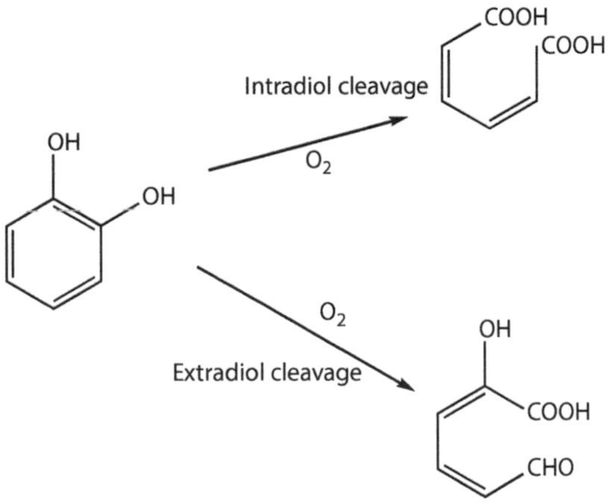

Intradiol cleavage

O_2

O_2

Extradiol cleavage

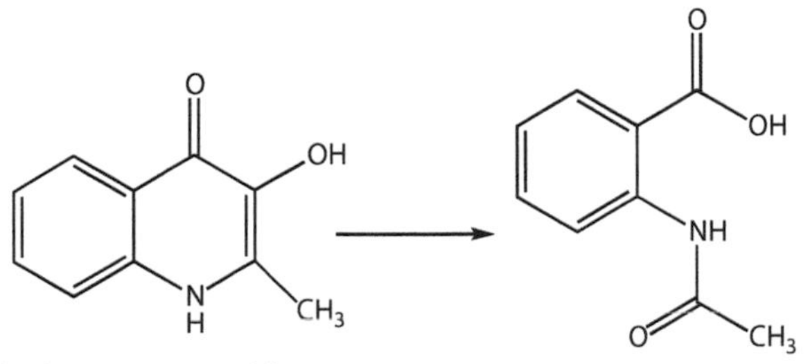

1H-3-hydroxy-4-oxoquinaldine → N-acetylanthranilic acid

ENZYMES IN SYNTHETIC ORGANIC CHEMISTRY[a,b] (Continued)

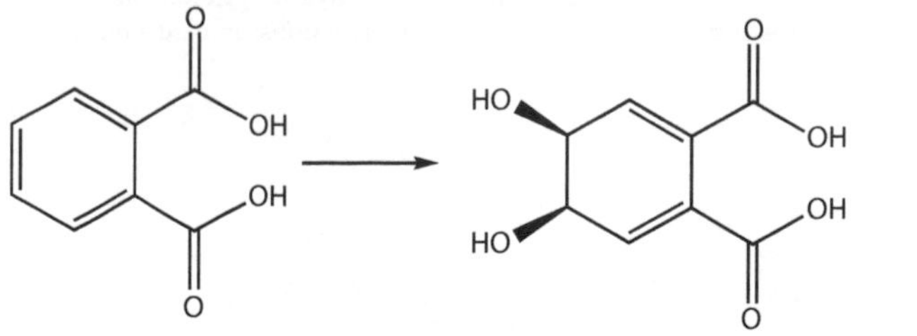

Phthalic Acid   cis-4,5-dihydro-4,5-dihydroxyphthalic acid

Nakata, H., Yamuchi, T., and Fujisawa, H., Studies on the reaction intermediate of protocatechuate 3,4-dioxygenase. Formation of enzyme-product complex, *Biochim.Biophys.Acta* 527, 171–181, 1978; Gassner, G.T., Ludwig, M.L., Gatti, D.L., *et al.*, Structure and mechanism of the iron-sulfur flavoprotein phthalate dioxygenase reductase, *FASEB J.* 9, 1411–1418, 1995; Miyauchi, K., Adachi, Y, Nagata, T., and Takagi, M., Cloning and sequencing of a novel *meta*-cleavage dioxygenase gene whose product is involved in degradation of γ-hexachlorocyclohexane in *Sphingomonas paucimobilis*, *J.Bacteriol.* 181, 6712–6719, 1999; Calderone, V., Trabucco, M., Menin, V. *et al.*, Cloning of human 3-hydroxyanthranilic acid dioxygenase in *Escherichia coli*: characterization of the purified enzyme in its *in vitro* inhibition by Zn^{2+}, *Biochim.Biophys.Acta* 1596, 283–292, 2002; Johnson-Winters, K., Purpero, V.M., Kavana, M., *et al.*, (4-Hydroxyphenyl)pyruvate dioxygenase from *Streptomyces avermitilis*: the basis for ordered substrate addition, *Biochemistry* 42, 2072–2080, 2003; Frerichs-Deeken, U., Ranguelova, K., Kappl, R., *et al.*, Dioxygenases without requirement for cofactors and their chemical model reaction: compulsory order ternary complex mechanism of 1H-3-hydroxy-4-oxyquinaldine 2,4-dioxygenase involving general base catalysis by histidine 251 and single-electron oxidation of the substrate dianion, *Biochemistry* 43, 14485–14499, 2004; Yin, C.X. and Finke, R.G., It is true dioxygenase or classic autoxidation catalysis? Re-investigation of a claimed dioxygenase catalyst based on a Ru(2)-incorporated, polyoxometalate precatalyst, *Inorg.Chem.* 44, 4175–4188, 2005; Matsumura, E., Ooi, S., Murakami, S., *et al.*, Constitutive synthesis, purification, and characterization of catechol 1,2-dioxygenase from the aniline-assimilating bacterium *Rhodococcus* sp. An-22, *J.Biosci.Bioeng.* 98, 71–76, 2004; Lee, K., *p*-Hydroxylation reactions catalyzed by naphthalene dioxygenase, *FEMS Microbiol.Lett.* 255, 316–320, 2006; Suvorova, M.M., Solyanikova, I.P., and Gobovleva, L.A., Specificity of catechol *ortho*-cleavage during *para*-toluate degradation by *Rhodococcus opacus* 1cp, *Biochemistry*(Mosc) 71, 1316–1323, 2006.

Ketone Reductases; engineered   Enantiomeric and diastereoisomeric reductions of ketones and β-keto esters
yeast cells; alcohol dehydrogenases

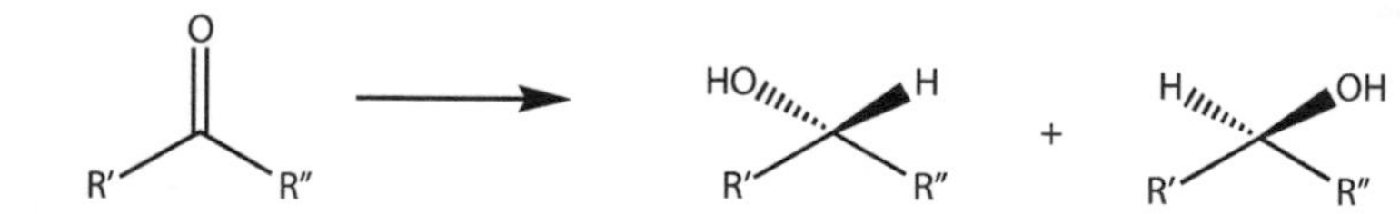

Enantioselective reactions

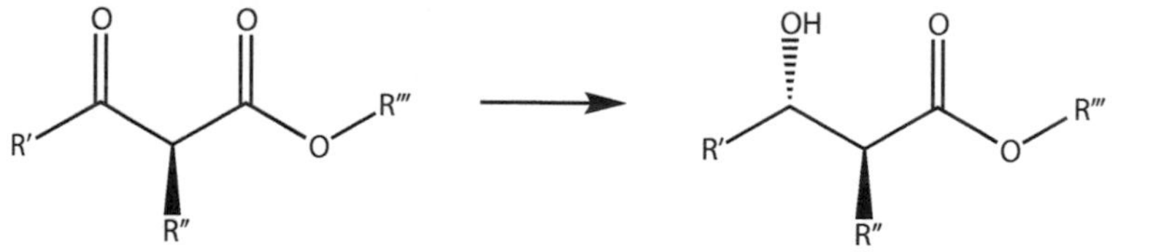

Diastereoselective reactions

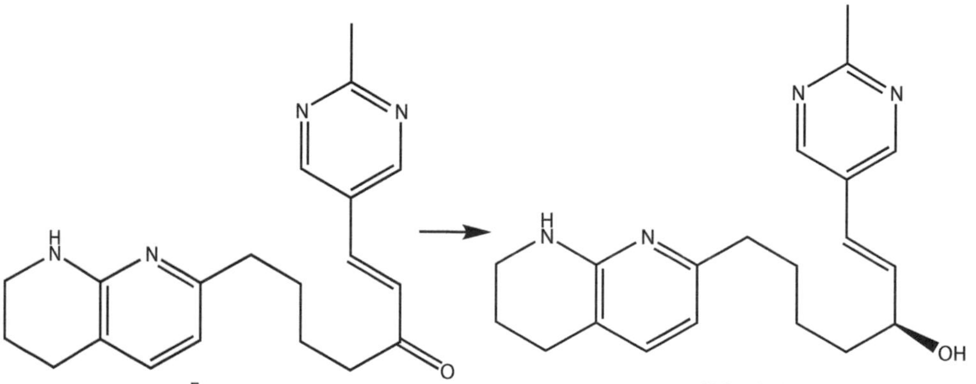

Enone   (*R*)allylic alcohol

Stewart, J.D., Organic transformations catalyzed by engineered yeast cells and related systems, *Curr.Opin.Biotechnol.* 11, 363–368, 2000; Habrych, M., Rodriguez, S., and Stewart, J.D., Purification and identification of an *Escherichia coli* β-keto ester reductase as 2,5-diketo-D-gluconate reductase YquE, *Biotechnol.Progress* 18, 257–261, 2002; Katz, M., Sarvary, I., Frejd, T., *et al.*, An improved stereoselective reduction of a bicyclic diketone by *Saccharomyces cerevisiae* combining process optimization and strain engineering, *Appl.Microbiol.Biotechnol.* 59, 641–648, 2002; Ravot, G., Wahler, D., Favre-Bulle, O., *et al.*, High throughput discovery of alcohol dehydrogenase for industrial biocatalysis, *Adv.Synthesis Catalysis* 345, 691–694, 2003; Lou, W.Y., Zong, M.H., Zhang, Y.Y. and Wu, H., Efficient synthesis of optically active organosilyl alcohol via asymmetric reduction of acyl silane with immobilized yeast, *Enzyme Microb.Technol.* 35, 190–196, 2004; Rodrigues, J.A.R., Moran, P.J.S., Conceicao, G.J.A., and Fardelone, L.C., Recent advances in the biocatalytic asymmetric reduction of acetophenones and α,β-unsaturated carbonyl compounds, *Food Technol.Biotechnol.* 42, 295–303, 2004; Pollard, D.J., Telari, K., Lane, J., *et al.*, Asymmetric reduction of α,β-unsaturated ketone to (R) allylic alcohol by *Candida chilenis*, *Biotechnol.Bioengineer.* 93, 674–686, 2006.

Enzymes in Synthetic Organic Chemistry[a,b] (Continued)

Cephalosporin Acylase   Conversion of cephalosporin C or adipyl-7-aminodesacetoxycephalosporonic acid to derivatives useful in the synthesis of semi-synthetic β-lactam antibiotics.

Sio, C.F., Otten,L.G., Cool, R.H., and Quax, W.M., Analysis of substrate specificity switch residue of cephalosporin acylase, *Biochem.Biophys.Res.Commun.* 312, 755–760, 2003; Sio, C.F., and Quax. W., Improved β-lactam acylases and their use as biocatalysts, *Curr.Opin.Biotechnol.* 15, 349–355, 2004; Sonawane, V.C., Enzymatic modifications of cephalosporins by cephalosporin acylase and other enzymes, *Crit.Rev.Biotechnol.* 26, 95–120, 2006.

Penicillin Acylase   Catalyzes the conversion of benzylpenicillin (penicillin G) to 6-aminopenicillinic acid for the production of β-lactam antibiotics. Penicillin acylase also converts cephalosporin C to 6-aminopenicillinic acid. There has been considerable work on the engineering and stabilization of the enzyme. Penicillin acylase can catalyze the reverse reaction resulting in a condensation.

Penicillin G

Penicillin Acylase

Phenylacetic Acid   +   6-aminopenicillanic acid

Mahajan, P.B., Penicillin acylases. an update, *Appl.Biochem.Biotechnol.* 9, 538-554, 1984; Andersson, E. and Hahn-Hagerdal, B., Bioconversion in aqueous two-phase systems, *Enzyme Microb.Technol.* 12, 242–254, 1990; Valle, F., Balbas, P., Merino, E., and Bolivar, F., *Trends Biotechnol.* 16, 36–40, 1991; Zaks, A., Industrial biocatalysis, *Curr.Opin.Chem.Biol.* 5, 130–136, 2001; Arroyo, M. de la Mata, I., Acebal, C, and Castillon, M.P., Biotechnological application of penicillin acylases: state-of-the-art, *Appl.Microbiol.Biotechnol.* 60, 507–514, 2003; Albian, O., Mateo, C., Fernandez-Lorente, G., *et al.*, Improving the industrial production of 6-APA: enzymatic hydrolysis of penicillin G in the presence of organic solvents, *Biotechnol.Prog.* 19, 1639–1642, 2003; Calleri, E., Temporini, C., Massolini, G., and Caccilanza, G., Penicillin G acylase-based stationary phases: analytical applications, *J.Pharm.Biomed. Anal.* 35, 243–258, 2004; Sio, C.F. and Quzx, W.J., Improved beta-lactam acylases and their use as industrial biocatalysts, *Curr.Opin.Biotechnol.* 15, 349–355, 2004; Guranda, D.T., Volovik, T.S., and Svedas, V.K., pH stability of penicillin acylase from *Escherichia coli, Biochemistry* 69, 1386–1390, 2004; Girelli, A.M. and Maltei, E., Application of immobilized enzyme reactor in on-line high performance liquid chromatography: a review, *J.Chromatog B. Analyt.Technol.Biomed.Life Sci.* 819, 3–16, 2005; Torres, R., Pessela, B., Fuentes, M., *et al.*, Stabilization of enzymes by multipoint attachment via reversible immobilization on phenylboronic activated supports, *J.Biotechnol.* 120, 396–401, 2005; Nigam, V.K., Kundu, S., and Ghosh, P., Single-step conversion of cephalosporin-C to 7-aminocephalosporonic acid by free and immobilized cells of *Pseudomonas diminuta, Appl.Biochem.Biotechnol.* 126, 13–21, 2005; van Roon, J.L., Boom, R.M., Paasman, M.A., *et al.*, Enzyme distribution and matrix characteristics in biocatalytic particles, *J.Biotechnol.* 119, 400–415, 2005; Giorando, R.C., Ribeiro, M.P., and Giordano, R.L., Kinetics of beta-lactam antibiotic synthesis by penicillin G acylase (PGA) from the view of the industrial enzyme reactor optimization, *Biotechnol.Adv.* 24, 27–41, 2006. Narayanan, N. Xu, Y., and Chou, G.P., High-level gene expression for recombinant penicillin acylase production using the *araB* promoter system in *Escherichia coli, Biotechnol.Prog.* 22, 1518–1523, 2006; De Leon-Rodriguez, A., Rivera-Pastrana, D., Medina-Rivero, E., *et al.*, Production of penicillin Acylase by a recombinant *Escherichia coli* using cheese whey as substrate and inducer, *Biomol.Eng.* 23, 299–305, 2006; Wang, L., Wang, Z., Xu., J.H., *et al.*, An eco-friendly and sustainable process for enzymatic hydrolysis of penicillin G in cloud point system, *Bioprocess Biosyst.Eng.* 29, 157–162, 2006; Aguilar, O., Albiter, V., Serrano-Carreon, L., and Rito-Palomares, M., Direct comparison between ion-exchange chromatography and aqueous two-phase processes for the partial purification of penicillin acylase produced by *E.coli, J.Chromatog.B. Analyt.Techol.Biomed.Life Sci.* 835, 77–83, 2006; Shah, S. ,Sharma, A. and Gupta, M.N., Preparation of cross-linked enzyme aggregates by using bovine serum albumin as a proteic feeder, *Anal.Biochem.* 351, 207–213, 2006.

Synthetic reaction: Nam, D.H. and Ryu, D.D., Biochemical properties of penicillin amidohydrolase from *Micrococcus luteus, Appl.Environ.Microbiol.* 38, 35–38, 1979; Youshko, M.I., van Langen, L.M., de Vroom, E., *et al.*, Highly efficient synthesis of ampicillin in an "aqueous solution-precipitate" system; repetitive addition of substrates in a semicontinuous process, *Biotechnol.Bioengineer.* 73, 4260430, 2001; Youshko, M.I., van Langen, L.M., de Vroom, E., *et al.*, Penicillin acylase-catalyzed ampicillin synthesis using a pH gradient: a new approach to optimization, *Biotechnol.Bioeng.* 78, 589–593, 2002; Goncalves, L.R., Fernandez-Lafuente, R., Guisan, J.M., *et al.*, Inhibitory effects in the side reactions occurring during the enzymic synthesis of amoxicillin: *p*-hydroxyphenylglycine methyl ester and amoxicillin hydrolysis, *Biotechnol. App..Biochem.* 38, 77–85, 2003; Alkema, W.B., de Vries, E., Floris, R., and Janssen, D.B., Kinetics of enzyme acylation and deacylation in the penicillin acylase-catalyzed synthesis of beta-lactam antibiotics, *Eur.J.Biochem.* 270, 3675–3683, 2003; Alfonso, I. and Gotor, V., Biocatalytic and biomimetic aminolysis reactions: useful tools for selective transformations or polyfunctional substrates, *Chem.Soc.Rev.* 33, 201–209,. 2004' Gabor, E.M. and Janssen, D.B., Increasing the synthetic performance of penicillin acylase PAS2 by structure-inspired semi-random mutagenesis, *Eng.Des.Sci.* 17, 571579, 2004. An unusual synthetic application was removal blocking groups from synthetic insulin; Svoboda, I., Brandenburg, D., Barth, T., *et al.*, Semisynthetic insulin analogues modified in positions B24, B25 and B29, *Biol.Chem.Hoppe Seyler* 375, 373–378, 1994.

THERAPEUTIC ENZYMES[a]

Roger L. Lundblad

Asparaginase

Catalyzes the hydrolysis of asparagine to aspartic acid; used for the treatment of acute lymphoblastic leukemia. Normal cells can synthesize asparagine while tumor cells in acute lymphoblastic leukemia cannot synthesize asparagine

Hill, J.M., Roberts, J., Loeb, E., *et al.*, L-Asparaginase therapy for leukemia and other malignant neoplasms. Remission in human leukemia, *JAMA* 202, 882–888, 1967; Broome, J.D., Studies on the mechanism of tumor inhibition by L-asparaginase. Effects of the enzyme on asparaginase levels in the blood, normal tissue, and 6C3HED lymphomas of mice: differences in asparagine formation and utilization in asparaginase-sensitive and –resistant lymphoma cells, *J.Exp.Med.* 127, 1055–1072, 1968; Adamson, R.H. and Fabro, S., Antitumor activity and other biologic properties of L-asparaginase (NSC-109229)-a review, *Cancer Chemother.Rep.* 52, 617–626, 1968; Keating, M.J., Holmes, R., Lerner, R., and Ho, D.H., L-Asparaginase and PEG asparaginase –past, present, and future, *Leuk.Lymphoma* 10(Suppl) 153–157, 1993; Davis, F.F., PEG-adenosine deaminase and PEG-asparaginase, *Adv. Exp.Med.Biol.* 519, 51–58, 2003; Pinheiro, J.P. and Boos, J., The best way to use asparaginase in childhood acute lymphatic leukemia—still to be defined?, *Br.J.Haematol.* 125, 119–127, 2004

Blood Coagulation Factor VIIa

Treatment of Blood Coagulation factor VIII inhibitors, potentially a general intravascular hemostatic agent

Siddiqui, M.A. and Scott, L.J., Recombinant factor VIIa (Eptacog Alfa): A review of its use in congenital or acquired haemophilia and other congenital bleeding disorders, *Drugs* 65, 1161–1177, 2005; Franchini, M., Zaffanello, M., and Veneri, D., Recombinant factor VIIa. An update on its clinical use, *Thromb.Haemostas.* 93, 1027–1035, 2005; Margaritis, P. and High, K.A., Advances in gene therapy using factor VIIa in hemophilia, *Semin.Hematol.* 43(Suppl 1), S101–S104, 2006; Farrugia, A., Assessing efficacy and therapeutic claims in emerging indications for recombinant Factor VIIa: regulatory perspectives, *Semin.Hematol.* 43(1 Suppl 1), S64–S69, 2006; Bosinski, T.J. and El Solh, A.A., Recombinant factor VIIa, its clinical properties, and the tissue factor pathway of coagulation, *Mini Rev.Med.Chem.* 6, 1111–1117, 2006

Butyryl cholinesterase

Detoxification of neurotoxic agents related to DFP; bioscavenger of anticholinesterase agents; Also used for treatment of cocaine overdoses

Doctor, B.P., Raveh, L., Wolfe, A.D., *et al.*, Enzymes as pretreatment drugs for organophosphate toxicity, *Neurosci.Biobehav.Rev.* 15, 123–128, 1991; Broomfield, C.A., Maxwell, D.M., Solana, R.P., *et al.*, Protection by butyrylcholinesterase against organophosphorus poisoning in nonhuman primates, *J.Pharmacol.Exp.Ther.* 259, 633–638, 1991; Grunwald, J., Marcus, D., Papier, Y., *et al.*, Large-scale purification and long-term stability of human butyrylcholinesterase: a potential bioscavenger drug, *J.Biochem.Biophys.Methods* 34, 123–135, 1997; Lynch, T.J., Mattes, C.E., Singh, A., *et al.*, Cocaine detoxification by human plasma butyrylcholinesterase, *Toxicol.Appl.Pharmacol.* 145, 363–371, 1997; Mattes, C.E., Lynch, T.J., Singh, A., *et al.*, Therapeutic use of butyrylcholinesterase for cocaine intoxication, *Toxicol.Appl. Pharmacol.* 145, 372–380, 1997; Browne, S.P., Slaughter, E.A., Couch, R.A., *et al.*, The influence of plasma butyrylcholinesterase concentration on the in vitro hydrolysis of cocaine in human plasma, *Biopharm.Drug. Dispos.* 19, 309–314, 1998; Yuan, H.J., Yu, W.Y., Shi, C.H., and Sun, M.J., Characteristics of recombinant human butyrylcholinesterase, *Zhongguo Yao Li Xue Bao* 20, 74–80, 1999; Chambers, J. and Oppenheimer, S.F., Organophosphates, serine esterase inhibition, and modeling of organophosphate toxicity, *Toxicol.Sci.* 77, 185–187, 2004; Guven, M., Sungur, M., Eser, B. *et al.*, The effects of fresh frozen plasma on cholinesterase levels and outcomes in patients with organophosphate poisoning, *J.Toxicol.Clin.Toxicol.* 42, 617–623, 2004; Fischer, S., Arad, A., and Margalit, R., Liposome-formulated enzymes for organophosphate scavenging: butyrylcholinesterase and Demeton-S, *Arch.Biochem.Biophys.* 434, 108–115, 2005; Saez-Valero, J., de Gracia, J.A., and Lockridge, O. Intraperitoneal administration of 340 kDa human plasma butyrylcholinesterase increases the level of the enzyme in the cerebrospinal fluid of rats, *Neurosci.Lett.* 383, 93–98, 2005; Lockridge, O., Schopfer, L.M., Winger, G., and Woods, J.H., Large scale purification of butyrylcholinesterase from human plasma suitable for injection into monkeys: A potential new therapeutic for protection against cocaine and nerve agent toxicity, *J.Med. Chem.Biol.Radiol.Def.* 3:nihms5095, 2005; Gardiner, S.J. and Begg, E.J., Pharmacogenetics, drug-metabolizing enzymes, and clinical practice, *Pharmacol. Rev.* 58, 521–590, 2006; Lucic Vrdoljak, A., Calic, M., Radic, B., *et al.*, Pretreatment with pyridinium oximes improves antidotal therapy against tabun poisoning, *Toxicology* 228, 41–50, 2006

Cocaine Esterase

Cocaine Detoxification

Brzezinski, M.R., Abraham, T.L., Stone, C.L., *et al.*, Purification and characterization of a human liver cocaine carboxylesterase that catalyzes the production of benzoylecgonine and the formation of cocaethylene from alcohol and cocaine, *Biochem.Pharmacol.* 48, 1747–1755, 1994; Turner, J.M., Larsen, N.A., Basran, A., *et al.*, Biochemical characterization and structural analysis of a highly proficient cocaine esterase, *Biochemistry* 41, 12297–12307, 2002; Ascenzi, P., Clementi, E., and Polticelli, F., The *Rhodococcus* sp. cocaine esterase: a bacterial candidate for novel pharmacokinetic-based therapies for cocaine abuse, *IUBMB Life* 55, 397–402, 2003; Rogers, C.J., Mee, J.M., Kaufmann, G.F., *et al.*, Toward cocaine esterase therapeutics, *J.Am.Chem.Soc.* 127, 10016–10017, 2005; Rogers, C.J., Eubanks, L.M., Dickerson, T.J., and Janda, K.D., Unexpected acetylcholinesterase activity of cocaine esterase, *J.Am.Chem.Soc.* 128, 15364–15365, 20006; Cooper, Z.D., Narasimhan, D., Sunahara, R.K., *et al.*, Rapid and robust protection against cocaine-induced lethality in rates by bacterial cocaine esterase, *Mol.Pharmacol.* 70, 1885–1891, 2006

---

[a] Targeting of therapeutic enzymes is a challenge and is the subject of current study. See Ribeiro, C.C. Barrias, C.C., and Barbosa, M.A., Calcium phosphate-alginate microspheres as enzyme delivery matrices, *Biomaterial* 25, 4363–4373, 2004; Vogler, C., Levy, B., Grubb, J.H., *et al.*, Overcoming the blood-brain barrier with high-dose enzyme replacement therapy in murine mucopolysaccharidosis VII, *Proc.Nat.Acad.Sci.USA* 102, 14777–14782, 2005; Fukudo, T., Ahearn, M., Roberts, A., *et al.*, Autophagy and mistargeting of therapeutic enzymes in skeletal muscle in Pompe disease, *Mol.Ther.* 14, 831–839, 2006; Lee, S., Yang, S.C., Hefferman, M.J., *et al.*, Polyketal microparticles: a new delivery vehicle for superoxide dismutase, *Bioconjug.Chem.* 18, 4–7, 2007.

Therapeutic Enzymes (Continued)

DNAse

Originally used for the resolution of localized abscesses by viscosity reduction due to hydrolysis of high-molecular weight DNA arising from tissue damage. There is more recent use in the treatment of cystic fibrosis as Dornase™ alpha. A combination of streptokinase and streptodornase was developed as well and is still used as Varidase[b]

Sherry, S., Johnson, A., and Tillett, W.R., The action of streptococcal desoxyribose nuclease (Streptodornase): *In vitro and* on purulent pleural exudations of patients, *J.Clin.Invest.* 29, 1094–1104, 1949; Johnson, A.J., Cytological studies in association with local injections of streptokinase-streptodornase into patients, *J.Clin.Invest.* 29, 1376–1386, 1950; Bryson, H.M. and Borkin, E.M., Dornase alpha. A review of its pharmacological properties and therapeutic potential in cystic fibrosis, *Drugs* 48, 894–906, 1994; Thomson, A.H., Human recombinant DNAse in cystic fibrosis, *J.R.Soc.Med.* 88 (suppl 25), 24–29, 1995; Davies, J. ,Trindale, M., Wallis, C. et al., The clinical use of rhDNAse, *Pediatr.Pulmonol.Suppl.* 16, 273–274, 1997; Goa, K.L. and Lamb, H., Dornase alpha. A review of pharmacoeconomic and quality-of-life aspects of its use in cystic fibrosis, *Pharmacoeconomics* 12, 409–422, 1997; Jones, A.F. and Wallis, C.E., Recombinant human deoxyribonuclease for cystic fibrosis, *Cochrane Database Syst.Rev.* (3), CD001127, 2000; Suri, R., The use of human deoxyribonuclease (rhDNAse) in the management of cystic fibrosis, *BioDrugs* 19, 135–144, 2005; Fayon, M., CF-emerging therapies: Modulation inflammation, *Pediatr.Respir.Rev.* 7 Suppl 1, S170–S174, 2006

Digestive Enzymes

Usually a crude homogenate of pancreas using to treatment pancreatic disease. Lipase is an individual enzyme which is used to treat steatorrhea[c]. An artificial saliva is available to treat salivary gland dysfunction[d].

Gullo, L., Indication for pancreatic enzyme treatment in non-pancreatic digestive diseases, *Digestion* 54(suppl 2), 43–47, 1993; Kitagawa, M., Naruse, S., Ishiguro, H., and Hayakawa, T., Pharmaceutical development for treating pancreatic disease, *Pancreas* 16, 427–431, 1998; Nakamura, T., Takeuchi, T., and Tando, Y., Pancreatic dysfunction and treatment options, *Pancreas* 16, 329–336, 1998; Divisi, D., Di Tomaso, S., Salvemini, S., *et al.*, Diet and cancer, *Acta Biomed.* 77, 118–123, 2006

Glucocerebrosidase (Acid β-glucosidase/lysosomal β-glucosidase) (Ceredase*/Cerezyme*)

Replacement of a lysosomal enzyme deficiency which results in Gaucher's Disease

Wiltink, E.H. and Hollak, C.E., Alglucerase (ceredase), *Pharm.World Sci.* 18, 16–19, 1996; Bijsterbosch, M.K., Donker, W., van de Bilt, H., *et al.*, Quantitative analysis of the targeting of mannose-terminal glucocerebrosidase. Predominant uptake by liver endothelial cells, *Eur.J.Biochem.* 237, 344–349, 1996; Grabowski, G.A., Leslie, N., and Wenstrup, R., Enzyme therapy for Gaucher disease: the first 5 years, *Blood Rev.* 12, 115–133, 1998; Barranger, J.A. and O'Rourke, E., Lessons learned from the development of enzyme therapy for Gaucher disease, *J.Inherit.Metab.Dis.* 24(suppl 2), 89–96, 2001; Charrow, J., Anderson, H.C., Kaplan, P., *et al.*, *J.Pediatr.* 144, 112–120, 2004; Beutler, E., Enzyme replacement in Gaucher disease, *PLoS Med.* 1, e21, 2004; Connock, M., Burls, A., Frew, E., *et al.*, The clinical effectiveness and cost-effectiveness of enzyme replacement therapy for Gaucher's disease: a systemic review, *Health Technol.Assess.* 10, iii–iv, ix–134, 2006; vom Dahl, S., Poll, L., di Rocco, M., *et al.*, Evidence-based recommendations for monitoring bone disease and the response to enzyme replacement therapy in Gaucher's patients, *Curr.Med.Res.Opin.* 22, 1045–1064, 2006

Lactase

Used as an oral formulation for the treatment of lactose intolerance

Ramirez, F.C., Lee, K., and Graham, D.Y., All lactase preparations are not the same: results of a prospective, randomized placebo-controlled trial, *Am.J.Gastroenterol.* 89, 566–570, 1994; Gao, K.P., Mitsui, T., Fujiki, K., *et al.*, Effect of lactase preparations in asymptomatic individuals with lactase deficiency—gastric digestion of lactose and breath hydrogen analysis, *Nagoya J.Med.Sci.* 65, 21–28, 2002; Erasmus, H.D., Ludwig-Auser, H.M., Paterson, P.G., *et al.*, Enhanced weight gain in preterm infants receiving lactose-treated feeds: a randomized, double-blinded, controlled trial, *J.Pediatr.* 141, 532–537, 2002; Tan-Dy, C.R. and Ohlsson, A., Lactase treated feeds to promote growth and feeding tolerance in preterm infants, *Cochrane Database Syst.Rev.* 18, CD004591, 2005; Montalto, M., Curigliano, V., Santoro, L., *et al.*, Management and treatment of lactose malabsorption, *World J.Gastroenterol.* 12, 187–191, 2006; O'Connell, S. and Walsh, G., Physicochemical characteristics of commercial lactases relevant to their application in the alleviation of lactose intolerance, *Appl.Biochem.Biotechnol.* 134, 179–191, 2006

---

[b] Tillett, W.S. and Sherry, S., The effect in patients of streptococcal fibrinolysin (streptokinase) and streptococcal deoxyribonuclease on fibrinous, purulent, and sanguinous pleural exudations, *J.Clin.Invest.* 28, 173–190, 1949; Tillett, W.E., Sherry, S., and Read, C.T., The use of streptokinase-streptodornase in the treatment of postneumonic empyema, *J.Thorac. Surg.* 21, 275–297, 1951; Miller, J.M., Ginsberg, M., Lipin, R.J., and Long, P.H., Clinical experience with streptokinase and streptodornase, *J.Am.Med.Assoc.* 145, 620–624, 1951; Nemoto, K., Hirota, K., Ono, T., *et al.*, Effect of varidase (streptokinase) on biofilm formed by *Staphylococcus aureus*, *Chemotherapy* 46, 111–115, 2000; Light, R.W., Nguyen, T., Mulligan, M.E., and Sasse, S.A., The in vitro efficacy of varidase versus streptokinase or urokinase for liquefying thick purulent exudative material from loculated empyema, *Lung* 178, 13–18, 2000; Rutter, P.M., Carpenter, B., Hill, S.S., and Locke, I.C., Varidase: the science behind the medicament, *J.Wound Care* 9, 223–226, 2000; Zhu, E., Hawthorne, M.L, Guo, Y., *et al.*, Tissue plasminogen activator combined with human recombinant deoxyribonuclease is effective therapy for empyema in a rabbit model, *Chest* 129, 1577–1583, 2006.

[c] Greenberger, N.J., Enzymatic therapy in patients with chronic pancreatitis, *Gastroenterol.Clin.North Am.* 28, 687–693, 1999; Layer, P., Keller, J., and Lankisch, P.G., Pancreatic enzyme replacement therapy, *Curr.Gastroenterol.Rep.* 3, 101–108, 2001; DiMagno, E.P., Gastric acid suppression and treatment of severe exocrine pancreatic insufficiency, *Best Pract.Res.Clin.Gastroenterol.* 15, 477–486, 2001; Layer, P. and Keller, J., Lipase supplementation therapy: standards, alternatives, and perspectives, *Pancreas* 26, 1–7, 2003.

[d] Gaffar, A., Hunter, C.M., and Mirajkar, Y.R., Applications of polymers in dentifrices and mouthrinses, *J.Clin.Dent.*13, 138–148, 2002; Brennan, M.T., Shariff, G., Lockart, P.B., and Fox, F.C., Treatment of xerostomia: a systematic review of the therapeutic trials, *Dent.Clin.North Am.* 46, 847–856, 2002; Guggenheimer, J. and Moore, P.A., Xerostomia: etiology, recognition and treatment, *J.Am.Dent.Assoc.* 134, 61–69, 2003; Porter, S.R., Scully, C., and Hegarty, A.M., An update of the etiology and management of xerostomia, *Oral.Surg. Oral.Med.Oral.Pathol.Radiol.Endod.* 97, 28–46, 2004; Urquhart, D. and Fowler, C.E., Review of the use of polymers in saliva substitutes for symptomatic relief of xerostomia, *J.Clin.Dent.* 17, 29–33, 2006.

Therapeutic Enzymes (Continued)

Superoxide Dismutase

Superoxide toxicity; treatment of inflammatory disorders; Also gene therapy[e] target in amyelotropic lateral sclerosis[f]

Omar, B.A., Flores, S.C., and McCord, J.M., Superoxide dismutase, in *Therapeutic Proteins. Pharmacokinetics and Pharmacodynamics*, ed. A.H.C. King, R.A. Baughman, and J.W. Larrick, W.H. Freeman and Company, New York, New York, Chapter 14, pps. 295–315, 1993; di Napoli, M. and Papa, F., M-40403 Metaphore Pharmaceuticals, *IDrugs* 8, 67–76, 2005; Leite, P.F., Liberman, M., Sandoli de Brito, F., and Laurindo, F.R., Redox processes underlying the vascular repair reaction, *World J.Surg.* 28, 331–336, 2004; Hernanez-Savedra, D., Zhou, H., and McCord, J.M., Anti-inflammatory properties of a chimeric recombinant superoxide dismutase: SOD2/3, *Biomed.Pharmacother.* 59, 204–206, 2005; St. Clair, D., Zhao, Y., Chaiswing, L., and Oberly, T., Modulation of skin tumorigenesis by SOD, *Biomed.Pharmacol.* 59, 209–214, 2005; Emerit, J., Samuel, D., and Pavio, N., Cu-Zn superoxide dismutase as a potential antifibrotic drug for hepatitis C related fibrosis, *Biomed.Pharmacother.* 60, 1–4, 2006; Yasui, K. and Baba, A., Therapeutic potential of superoxide dismutase (SOD) for resolution of inflammation, *Inflamm.Res.* 55, 359–363, 2006

Streptokinase

Plasminogen activator derived from β-hemolytic *Streptococcus* (groups A,C, and G); approximately 40–50 kD; streptokinase does not have any known catalytic activity but functions by formation of a complex with plasminogen which results in plasminogen activation. Now available as a recombinant product. Streptokinase is used in combination with DNAse(streptodornase) to treat abscesses and empyema[b].

de la Fuente Garcia, J. and Estrade, M.P., Experimental studies with recombinant streptokinase, in *Therapeutic Proteins. Pharmacokinetics and Pharmacodynamics*, ed. A.H.C. King, R.A. Baughman, and J.W. Larrick, W.H. Freeman and Company, New York, New York, Chapter 13, pps. 283–293, 1993; Konstantinides, S., Should thrombolytic therapy be used in patients with pulmonary embolism?, *Am.J.Cardiovasc.Drugs.* 4, 69–74, 2004; Capstick, T. and Henry, M.T., Efficacy of thrombolytic agents in the treatment of pulmonary embolism, *Eur.Respir.J.* 26, 664–674, 2005; Ueshima, S. and Matsuo, O., Development of new fibrinolytic agents, *Curr.Pharm.Des.* 12, 849–857, 2006; Caceres-Loriga, P.M., Perez-Lopez, H., Morlana-Herandez, K., Facundo-Sanchez, H., Thrombolysis as first choice therapy in prosthetic heart valve thrombosis. A study of 68 patients, *J.Thromb.Thrombolysis* 21, 185–190, 2006

Tissue Plasminogen Activator (tPA)

A serine protease which activate plasminogen resulting in fibrinolysis. tPA is used for the treatment of myocardial infarction and stroke. The first recombinant protein was manufactured in CHO cells; more recently an engineered form (Reteplase®) has been developed in *Escherichia coli* and is seeing clinical use.

Collen, D. and Lijnen, H.R., Tissue-type Plasminogen activator. Mechanisms of action and thrombolytic properties, *Haemostasis* 16(Suppl 3), 25–32, 1986; Anderson, J.L. Recent clinical developments in thrombolysis in acute myocardial infarction, *Drugs* 33(Suppl 3), 22–32, 1987; Hollander, J.J., Plasminogen activators and their potential in therapy, *Crit.Rev.Biotechnol.* 6, 253–271, 1987; Grossbard, E.B., Recombinant tissue plasminogen activators: a brief review, *Pharm.Res.* 4, 375–378, 1987; Montaner, J., Stroke biomarkers: Can they help us to guide stroke thrombolysis?, *Drug News Perspect.* 19, 523–532, 2006; Khaja, A.M. and Grotta, J.C., Established treatments for acute ischaemic stroke, *Lancet* 369, 319–330, 2007; Simpson, D., Siddiqui, M.A, Scott, L.J., and Hilleman, D.E., Spotlight on reteplase in thrombotic occlusive disorders, *BioDrugs* 21, 65–68, 2007

Thrombin

Therapeutic action based on the clotting of fibrinogen and aggregation of blood platelets. Thrombin is a component in fibrin sealant which is used as a tissue adhesive and is used as free-standing product as a suture support and for the treatment of vascular pseudoaneurysms.

Lundblad, R.L., Bradshaw, R.A., Gabriel, D., *et al.*, A review of the therapeutic uses of thrombin, *Thromb.Haemost.* 91, 851–860, 2004; Hagberg, R.C., Safi, H.J., Sabik, J., *et al.*, Improved intraoperative management of anastomotic bleeding during aortic reconstruction: results of a randomized controlled trial, *Am.Surg.* 70, 307–311, 2004; Aziz, O., Athanasiou, T., and Darzi, A., Haemostasis using a ready-to-use collagen sponge coated with activated thrombin and fibrinogen, *Surg.Technol.Int.* 14, 35–40, 2005; Valbonesi, M., Fibrin glues of human origin, *Best Pract.Res.Clin.Haematol.* 19, 191–203, 2006; Evans, L.A. and Morey, A.F., Hemostatic agents and tissue glues in urologic injuries and wound healing, *Urol.Clin.North Am.* 33, 1–12, 2006; Stone, P.A., AbuRhama, A.F., Flaherty, S.K., and Bates, M.C., Femoral pseudoaneurysms, *Vasc.Endovascular Surg.* 40, 109–117, 2006; Gabay, M., Absorbable hemostatic agents, *Am.J.Health Syst.Pharm.* 63, 1244–1253, 2006; Drobnic, M., Radosavljevic, D., Ravnik, D., *et al.*, Comparison of four techniques for the fixation of a collagen scaffold in the human cadaveric knee, *Osteoarthritis Cartilage* 14, 337–344, 2006

Urate oxidase (Rasburicase)

Catalyzes the oxidation of urate to 5-hydroxyisourate. Used for the treatment of hyperuricemia (excess uric acid). Specifically for tumor lysis syndrome, gout.

Bessmertny, O., Robitaille, L.M., and Cairo, M.S., Rasburicase: a new approach for preventing and/or treating tumor lysis syndrome, *Curr.Pharm.Des.* 11, 4177–4185, 2005; Oldfield, V. and Perry, C.M., Rasburicase: a review of its use in the management of anticancer therapy-induced hyperuricaemia, *Drugs* 66, 529–545, 2006; Oldfield, V. and Perry, C.M., Spotlight on rasburicase in anticancer therapy-induced hyperuricemia, *BioDrugs* 20, 197–199, 2006; Lee, S.J. and Terkeltaub, R.A., New developments in clinically relevant mechanisms and treatment of hyperuricemia, *Curr.Rheumatol.Rep.* 8, 224–230, 2006; Teng, G.G., Nair, R., and Saag, K.G., Pathophysiology, clinical presentation and treatment of gout, *Drugs* 66, 1547–1563, 2006; Higdon, M.L. and Higdon, J.A., Treatment of oncologic emergencies, *Am.Fam.Physician* 74, 1873–1880, 2006; Sood, A.R., Burry, L.D., and Cheng, D.K., Clarifying the role of rasburicase in tumor lysis syndrome, *Pharmacotherapy* 27, 111–121, 2007

[e] In this context, gene therapy can refer to gene augmentation therapy, gene correction therapy, and RNA silencing.
[f] Xu, Z. and Xia, X.G., RNAi therapy: dominant disease gene gets silenced, *Gene Ther.* 12, 1159–1160, 2005; Hino, T., Yokota, T., Ito, S., *et al.*, *In vivo* delivery of small interfering RNA targeting brain capillary endothelial cells, *Biochem.Biophys.Res. Commun.* 340, 263-267, 2006; Zemlyak, I., Nimon, V., Brooke, S., *et al.*, Gene therapy in the nervous system with superoxide dismutase, *Brain Res.* 1088, 12–18, 2006; Azzouz, M., Gene therapy for ALS: progress and prospects, *Biochim.Biophys.Acta* 1762, 1122–1127, 2006; Xia, X., Zhou, H., Huang, T., and Zu, Z., Allele-specific RNAi selectively silences mutant SOD1 and achieves significant therapeutic benefit *in vivo*, *Neurobiol.Dis.* 23, 578–586, 2006; Miller, T.M., Smith, R.A., and Cleveland, D.W., Amyelotropic lateral sclerosis and gene therapy, *Nat.Clin.Pract.Neurol.* 2, 462–463, 2006; Davis, A.S., Zhao, H., Sun, G.H. *et al.*, Gene therapy using SOD1 protects striatal neurons from experimental stroke, *Neurosci.Lett.* 411, 32–36, 2007; Qi, X., Nauswirth, W.W., and Guy, J., Dual gene therapy with extracellular superoxide dismutase and catalase attenuates experimental optic neuritis, *Mol.Vis.* 13, 1–11, 2007; Epperly, M.W., Wegner, R., Kanai, A.J., Effects of MnSOD-plasmid liposome gene therapy on antioxidant levels in irradiated murine oral cavity orthotopic tumors, *Radiat.Res.* 167, 289–297, 2007.

Therapeutic Enzymes (Continued)

Urokinase Originally isolated from urine, urokinase is now available a recombinant protein and is used for the treatment of thrombosis in myocardial infarction and stroke; tPA is more often used for stroke. Urokinase acts by converting plasminogen to plasmin[g].

Maksimenko, A.V. and Tischenko, E.G., New thrombolytic strategy: bolus administration of tPA and urokinase-fibrinogen conjugate, *J.Thromb. Thrombolysis* 7, 307–312, 1999; Stepanova, V.V., and Tkachuk, V.A., Urokinase as a multidomain protein and polyfunctional cell regulation, *Biochemistry* 67, 109–118, 2002; Bourekas, E.C., Slivka, A.F., and Casavant, M.J., Intra-arterial thrombolysis of a distal internal carotid artery occlusion in an adolescent, *Neurocrit.Care* 2, 179–182, 2005; Roychoudhury, P.K., Khaparde, S.S., Mattisson, R., and Kumar, A., Synthesis, regulation and production of urokinase using mammalian cell culture: a comprehensive review, *Biotechnol.Adv.* 24, 514–526, 2006; Bansal, V. and Roychoudhury, P.K., Production and purification of urokinase: a comprehensive review, *Protein Expr.Purif.* 45, 1–14, 2006; Juttler, E., Kohrmann, M., and Schellinger, P.D., Therapy for early reperfusion after stroke, *Nat.Clin.Pract.Cardiovasc.Med.* 3, 656–663, 2006; Mullen, M.T., McGarvey, M.L., and Kasner, S.E., Safety and efficacy of thrombolytic therapy in postoperative cerebral infarctions, *Neurol.Clin.* 24, 783–793, 2006.

---

[g] Plasmin is a serine protease which digests fibrin. An acyl-plasmin was developed for therapeutic use – Smith, R.A., Dupe, R.J., English, P.D., and Green, J., Fibrinolysis with acyl-enzymes: a new approach to thrombolytic therapy, *Nature* 290, 505–508, 1981; Dupe, R.J., English, P.D., Smith, R.A., and Green, D.J., Acyl-enzymes as thrombolytic agents in dog models of venous thrombosis and pulmonary embolism, *Thromb.Haemost.* 51, 249–253, 1984; Tomiya, N., Watanabe, K., Awaya, J., *et al.*, Modification of acyl-plasmin-streptokinase complex with polyethylene glycol. Reduction of sensitivity to neutralizing antibody, *FEBS Lett.* 193, 44–48, 1985; Kalindjian, S.B. and Smith, R.A., Reagents for reversible coupling of proteins to the active centres of trypsin-like serine proteinases, *Biochem.J.* 249, 409–413, 1987; Teuten, A.J., Cooper, A., Smith, R.A., and Dobson, C.M., Binding of a substrate analogue can induce co-operative structure in the plasmin-serine proteinase domain, *Biochem.J.* 293, 567–572, 1993; Lijnen, H.R., van Hoef, B., Smith, R.A., and Collen, D., Functional properties of *p*-anisolylated plasmin-staphylokinase complex, *Thromb.Haemost.* 70, 326–331, 1993.

PROTEASE INHIBITORS AND PROTEASE INHIBITOR COCKTAILS

Roger L. Lundblad

While protease inhibitor cocktails have been in use for some time,[1] there are few rigorous studies examining their effect on proteolysis and very few concerned with proteolytic degradation during the processing of material for analysis or during purification.[2] It is usually assumed that proteolysis can be a problem and protease inhibitors or protease inhibitor cocktails are usually included as part of a protocol without the provision of justification. There are several excellent review articles in this area. Salveson and Nagase[3] discuss the inhibition of proteolytic enzymes in great detail including much practical information that should be considered in experimental design. The discussion of the relationship between inhibitor concentration, inhibitor/enzyme binding constants (association constants, binding constants, $t_{1/2}$, inhibition constants, etc.), and enzyme inhibition is of particular importance. For example, with a reversible enzyme inhibitor (such as benzamidine), if the K_i value is 100 nM, a 100 μM concentration of inhibitor would be required to decrease protease activity by 99.9%. Salveson and Nagase[3] also note the well-known differences in the reaction rates of inhibitors such as DFP and PMSF with the active site of serine proteases. DFP is much faster than PMSF with trypsin but equivalent rates are seen with chymotrypsin. PMSF is included in commercial protease inhibitor cocktails because of its lack of toxicity compared to DFP; 3, 4-dichloroisocoumarin (3, 4-DCI), as described by Powers and colleagues,[4] is faster than either DFP or PMSF. Also enzyme inhibition occurs in the presence of substrate (proteins), which will influence the effectiveness of both irreversible and reversible enzyme inhibitors. In addition, some protease inhibitor cocktails include both PMSF and benzamidine. Benzamidine is a competitive inhibitor of trypticlike serine proteases and slows the rate of inactivation of such enzymes by reagents such as PMSF.[5] The investigator is also advised to consider the modification of proteins and other biological compounds by protease inhibitors in reactions not associated with proteases such as the modification of tyrosine by DFP or PMSF.[6] In addition, some of the protease inhibitors such as DFP and PMSF are subject to hydrolysis under conditions (pH ≥ 7.0) used for modification. For those unfamiliar with the history of DFP, DFP is a potent neurotoxin (inhibitor of acetyl cholinesterase) and should be treated with considerable care; a prudent investigator has a DFP repair kit in close proximity (weak base and pralidoxime-2-chloride [2-PAM]). Given these various issues, it is critical to validate that, in fact, the sample is being protected against proteolysis.

References

1. Takei, Y., Marzi, I., Kauffman, F.C. et al., Increase in survival time of liver transplants by protease inhibitors and a calcium channel blocker, nisoldipine. *Transplantation* 50, 14–20, 1990.
2. Pyle, L.E., Barton, P., Fujiwara, Y., Mitchell, A., and Fidge, N., Secretion of biologically active human proapolipoprotein A-1 in a baculovirus-insect cell system: protection from degradation by protease inhibitors, *J. Lipid Res.* 36, 2355–2361, 1995.
3. Salveson, G. and Nagase, H., Inhibition of proteolytic enzymes, in *Proteolytic Enzymes: Practical Approaches,* 2nd ed., R. Benyon and J.S. Bond, Eds., Oxford University Press, Oxford, UK, pp. 105–130, 2001.
4. Harper, J.W., Hemmi, K., and Powers, J.C., Reaction of serine proteases with substituted isocoumarins: discovery of 3,4-dichloroisocoumarin, a new general mechanism-based serine protease inhibitor, *Biochemistry* 24, 1831–1841, 1985.
5. Lundblad, R.L., A rapid method for the purification of bovine thrombin and the inhibition of the purified enzyme with phenylmethylsulfonyl fluoride, *Biochemistry* 10, 2501–2506, 1971.
6. Lundblad, R.L., *Chemical Reagents for Protein Modification,* CRC Press, Boca Raton, FL, 2004.

Characteristics of Selected Protease Inhibitors, Which Can be Used in Protease Inhibitor Cocktails[a]

Common Name	Other Nomenclature	M.W.	Primary Design
Amastatin	N-[(2S,3R)-3-amino-2-hydroxy-5-methyl hexanoyl]-L-valyl-L-valyl-L-aspartic acid	529.0	Inhibitor of some aminopeptidases.

Amastatin

Characteristics of Selected Protease Inhibitors, Which Can be Used in Protease Inhibitor Cocktails
(Continued)

Common Name	Other Nomenclature	M.W.	Primary Design

Amastatin is a complex peptidelike inhibitor of aminopeptidases obtained from *Actinoycetes* culture. Amastatin is a competitive inhibitor of aminopeptidase A, aminopeptidase M, and other aminopeptidases. Amastatin has been used for the affinity purification of aminopeptidases. Amastatin has been shown to inhibit amino acid iosomerases. Amastatin is structurally related to bestatin and has been described as an immunomodulatory factor. See Aoyagi, T., Tobe, H., Kojima, F. et al., Amastatin, an inhibitor of aminopeptidase A, produced by actinomycetes, *J. Antibiot.* 31, 636–638, 1978; Tobe, H., Kojima, F., Aoyagi, T., and Umezawa, H., Purification by affinity chromatography using amastatin and properties of he aminopeptidase A from pig kidney, *Biochim. Biophys. Acta* 613, 459–468, 1980; Rich, D.H., Moon, B.J., and Harbeson, S., Inhibition of aminopeptidases by amastatin and bestatin derivatives. Effect of inhibitor structure on slow-binding processes, *J. Med. Chem.* 27, 417–422 , 1984; Meisenberg, G. and Simmons, W.H., Amastatin potentiates the behavioral effects of vasopressin and oxytocin in mice, *Peptides* 5, 535–539, 1984; Wilkes, S.H. and Prescott, J.M., The slow, tight binding of bestatin and amastatin to aminopeptidases, *J. Biol. Chem.* 260, 13154–13162, 1985; Matsuda, N., Katsuragi, Y., Saiga, Y. et al., Effects of aminopeptidase inhibitors actinonin and amastatin on chemotactic and phagocytic responses of human neutrophils, *Biochem. Int.* 16, 383–390, 1988; Orawski, A.T. and Simmons, W.H., Dipeptidase activities in rat brain synaptosomes can be distinguished on the basis of inhibition by bestatin and amastatin: identification of a kyotrophin (Tyr-Arg)-degrading enzyme, *Neurochem. Res.* 17, 817–820, 1992; Kim, H. and Lipscomb, W.N., X-ray crystallographic determination of the structure of bovine lens leucine aminopeptidase complexed with amastatin: formation of a catalytic mechanism, featuring a gem-diolate transition state, *Biochemistry* 32, 8365–8378, 1993; Bernkop-Schnurch, A., The use of inhibitory agents to overcome the enzymatic barrier to perorally administered therapeutic peptides and proteins, *J. Control. Release* 52, 1–16, 1998; Fortin, J.P., Gera, L., Bouthillier, J. et al., Endogenous aminopeptidase N decreases the potency of peptide agonists and antagonists of the kinin B1 receptors in the rabbit aorta, *J. Pharmacol. Exp. Ther.* 312, 1169–1176, 2005; Olivo Rdo, A., Teixeira Cde, R., and Silveira, P.F., Representative aminopeptidases and prolyl endopeptidase from murin macrophages; comparative activity levels in resident and elicited cells, *Biochem. Pharmacol.* 69, 1441–1450, 2005; Gera. L., Fortin, J.P., Adam, A. et al., Discovery of a dual-function peptide that combines aminopeptidase N inhibition and kinin B1 receptor antagonism, *J. Pharmacol. Exp. Ther.* 317, 300–308, 2006; Krsyanovic, M., Brgles, M., Halassy, B. et al., Purification and characterization of the *l*,(*l*/*d*)-aminopeptidase from guinea pig serum, *Prep. Biochem. Biotechnol.* 36, 175–195, 2006; Torres, A.M., Tsampazi, M., Tsampazi, C. et al., Mammalian *l* to *d*-amino-acid-residue isomerase from platypus venom, *FEBS Lett.* 580, 1587–1591, 2006.

Aprotinin   6512   Protein protease inhibitor.

Basic pancreatic trypsin inhibitor; Kunitz pancreatic trypsin inhibitor; Trasylol°. This protein inhibits some but not all trypticlike serine proteinases and is included in some protease inhibitor cocktails. See Hulsemann, A.R., Jongejan, R.C., Rolien Raatgeep, H. et al., Epithelium removal and peptidase inhibition enhance relaxation of human airways to vasoactive intestinal peptide, *Am. Rev. Respir. Dis.* 147, 1483–1486, 1993; Cornelius, R.M. and Brash, J.L., Adsorption from plasma and buffer of single- and two-chain high molecular weight kininogen to glass and sulfonated polyurethane surfaces, *Biomaterials* 20, 341–350, 1999; Lafleur, M.A., Handsley, M.M., Knauper, V. et al., Endothelial tubulogenesis with fibrin gels specifically requires the activity of membrane-type-matrix metalloproteinases (MT-MMPs), *J. Cell Sci.* 115, 3427–3438, 2002; Shah, R.B., Palamakula, A., and Khan, M.A., Cytotoxicity evaluation of enzyme inhibitors and absorption enhancers in Caco-2 cells for oral delivery of salmon calcitonin, *J. Pharm. Sci.* 93, 1070–1982; Spens, E. and Häggerström, L., Protease activity in protein-free (NS) myeloma cell cultures, In Vitro *Cell Dev. Biol.* 41, 330–336, 2005. As it is a potent inhibitor of plasmin, aprotinin is frequently included in fibrin gel-based cultures to preserve the fibrin gel structure. See Ye, Q., Zund, G., Benedikt, P. et al., Fibrin gel as a three-dimensional matrix in cardiovascular tissue engineering, *Eur. J. Cardiothorac. Surg.* 17, 587–591, 2000; Krasna, M., Planinsek, F., Knezevic, M. et al., Evaluation of a fibrin-based skin substitute prepared in a defined keratinocyte medium, *Int. J. Pharm.* 291, 31–37, 2005; Sun, X.T., Ding, Y.T., Yan, X.G. et al., Antiangiogenic synergistic effect of basic fibroblast growth factor and vascular endothelial growth factor in an *in vitro* quantitative microcarrier-based three-dimensional fibrin angiogenesis system, *World J. Gastroenterol.* 10, 2524–2528, 2004; Gille, J., Meisner, U., Ehlers, E.M. et al., Migration pattern, morphology and viability of cells suspended in or sealed with fibrin glue: a histomorphology study, *Tissue Cell* 37, 339–348, 2005; Yao, L., Swartz, D.D., Gugino, S.F. et al., Fibrin-based tissue-engineered blood vessels: differential effects of biomaterial and culture parameters on mechanical strength and vascular reactivity, *Tissue Eng.* 11, 991–1003, 2005. Aprotinin is used therapeutically in the inhibition of plasmin activity both as a freestanding product and as a component of fibrin sealant products.

Benzamidine HCI   156.61   Inhibitor of trypticlike
                                                                                                            serine proteases.

Benzamidine

An aromatic amidine derivative (Markwardt, F., Landmann, H., and Walsmann, P., Comparative studies on the inhibition of trypsin, plasmin, and thrombin by derivatives of benzylamine and benzamidine, *Eur. J. Biochem.* 6, 502–506, 1968; Guvench, O., Price, D.J., and Brooks, C.L., III, Receptor rigidity and ligand mobility in trypsin-ligand complexes, *Proteins* 58, 407–417, 2005), which is used as a competitive inhibitor of trypticlike serine proteases. It is not a particularly tight-binding inhibitor and is usually used at millimolar concentrations. Ensinck, J.W., Shepard, C., Dudl, R.J., and Williams, R.H., Use of benzamidine as a proteolytic inhibitor in the radioimmunoassay of glucagon in plasma, *J. Clin. Endocrinol. Metab.* 35, 463–467, 1972; Bode, W. and Schwager, P., The refined crystal structure of bovine beta-trypsin at 1.8 Å resolution. II. Crystallographic refinement, calcium-binding site, benzamidine-binding site, and active site at pH 7.0., *J. Mol. Biol.* 98, 693–717, 1975; Nastruzzi, C., Feriotto, G., Barbieri, R. et al., Differential effects of benzamidine derivatives on the expression of *c-myc* and HLA-DR alpha genes in a human B-lymphoid tumor cell line, *Cancer Lett.* 38, 297–305, 1988; Clement, B., Schmitt, S., and Zimmerman, M., Enzymatic reduction of benzamidoxime to benzamidine, *Arch. Pharm.* 321, 955–956, 1988; Clement, B., Immel, M., Schmitt, S., and Steinman, U., Biotransformation of benzamidine and benzamidoxime *in vivo*, *Arch. Pharm.* 326, 807–812, 1993; Renatus, M., Bode, W., Huber, R. et al., Structural and functional analysis of benzamidine-based inhibitors in complex with trypsin: implications for the inhibition of factor Xa, tPA, and urokinase, *J. Med. Chem.* 41, 5445–5456, 1998; Henriques, R.S., Fonseca, N., and Ramos, M.J., On the modeling of snake venom serine proteinase interactions with benzamidine-based thrombin inhibitors, *Protein Sci.* 13, 2355–2369, 2004; Gustavsson, J., Farenmark, J., and Johansson, B.L., Quantitative determination of the ligand content in Benzamidine Sepharose° 4 Fast Flow media with ion-pair chromatography, *J. Chromatog. A* 1070, 103–109, 2005. Concentrated solutions of benzamidine will require pH adjustment prior to use.

Characteristics of Selected Protease Inhibitors, Which Can be Used in Protease Inhibitor Cocktails (Continued)

Common Name	Other Nomenclature	M.W.	Primary Design
Bestatin	*N*-[(2*S*,3*R*)-3-amino-2-hydroxy-L-oxo-4-phenylbutyl]-L-leucine	344.8	Aminopeptidase inhibitor; also described as a metalloproteinase inhibitor.

Bestatin

Bestatin is an inhibitor of some aminopeptidases and it was isolated from *Actinomycetes* culture. Bestatin was subsuently shown to have immunomodulatory activity and induces apoptosis in tumor cells. Bestatin is included in some proteaseinhibitor cocktails and has been demonstrated to inhibit intracellular protein degradation. See Umezawa, H., Aoyagi, T., Suda, H. et al., Bestatin, an inhibitor of aminopeptidase B, produced by actinomycetes, *J. Antibiot.* 29, 97–99, 1976; Suda, H., Takita, T., Aoyagi, T., and Umezawa, H., The structure of bestatin, *J. Antibiot.* 29, 100–101, 1976; Saito, M., Aoyagi, T., Umezawa, H., and Nagai, Y., Bestatin, a new specific inhibitor of aminopeptidases, enhances activation of small lymphocytes by concanavalin A, *Biochem. Biophys. Res. Commun.* 76, 526–533, 1976; Botbot, V. and Scornik, O.A., Degradation of abnormal proteins in intact mouse reticulocytes: accumulation of intermediates in the presence of bestatin, *Proc. Natl. Acad. Sci. USA* 76, 710–713, 1979; Botbol, V. and Scornik, O.A., Peptide intermediates in the degradation of cellular proteins. Bestatin permits their accumulation in mouse liver *in vivo, J. Biol. Chem.* 258, 1942–1949, 1983; Rich, D.H., Moon, B.J., and Harbeson, S., Inhibition of aminopeptidases by amastatin and bestatin derivatives. Effect of inhibitor structure on slow-binding processes, *J. Med. Chem.* 27, 417–422, 1984; Wilkes, S.H. and Prescott, J.M., The slow, tight binding of bestatin and amastatin to aminopeptidases, *J. Biol. Chem.* 260, 13154–13160, 1985; Patterson, E.K., Inhibition by bestatin of a mouse ascites tumor dipeptidase. Reversal by certain substrates, *J. Biol. Chem.* 264, 8004–8011, 1989; Botbol, V. and Scornik, O.A., Measurement of instant rates of protein degradation in the livers of intact mice by the accumulation of bestatin-induced peptides, *J. Biol. Chem.* 266, 2151–2157, 1991; Tieku, S. and Hooper, N.M., Inhibition of aminopeptidases N, A, and W. A re-evaluation of the actions of bestatin and inhibitors of angiotensin converting enzyme, *Biochem. Pharmacol.* 44, 1725–1730, 1992; Taylor, A., Peltier, C.Z., Torre, F.J., and Hakamian, N., Inhibition of bovine lens leucine aminopeptidase by bestatin: number of binding sites and slow binding of this inhibitor, *Biochemistry* 32, 784–790, 1993; Schaller, A., Bergey, D.R., and Ryan, C.A., Induction of wound response genes in tomato leaves by bestatin, an inhibitor of aminopeptidases, *Plant Cell* 7, 1893–1898, 1995; Nemoto, H., Ma, R., Suzuki, I.I., and Shibuya, M., A new one-pot method for the synthesis of alpha-siloxyamides from aldehydes or ketones and its application to the synthesis of (-)bestatin, *Org. Lett.* 2, 4245–4247, 2000; van Hensbergen, Y., Brfoxterman, H.J., Peters, E. et al., Aminopeptidase inhibitor bestatin stimulates microvascular endothelial cell invasion in a fibrin matrix, *Thromb. Haemost.* 90, 921–929, 2003; Stamper, C.C., Bienvenue, D.L., Bennett, B. et al., Spectroscopic and X-ray crystallographic characterization of bestatin bound to the aminopeptidase from *Aeromonas(Vibrio)proteolytica, Biochemistry* 43, 9620–9628, 2004; Zheng, W., Zhai, Q., Sun, J. et al., Bestatin, an inhibitor of aminopeptidases, provides a chemical genetics approach to dissect jasmonate signaling in *Aribidopsis, Plant Physiol.* 141, 1400–1413, 2006; Hui, M. and Hui, K.S., A novel aminopeptidase with highest preference for lysine, *Neurochem. Res.* 31, 95–102, 2006.

Cystatins

Protein Inhibitors of Cysteine Proteases

Inhibitors of cysteine proteinases.

Cystatin refers to a diverse family of protein cysteine protease inhibitors. There are three general types of cystatins: Type 1 (stefens), which are primarily found in the cytoplasm but can appear in extracellular fluids; Type 2, which are secreted and found in most extracellular fluids; and Type 3, which are multidomain protease inhibitors containing carbohydrates and that include the kininogens. Cystatin 3 is used to measure renal function in clinical chemistry. See Barrett, A.J., The cystatins: a diverse superfamily of cysteine peptidase inhibitors, *Biomed. Biochim. Acta* 45, 1363–1374, 1986; Katunuma, N., Mechanisms and regulation of lysosomal proteolysis, *Revis. Biol. Cellular* 20, 35–61, 1989; Gauthier, F., Lalmanach, G., Moeau, T. et al., Cystatin mimicry by synthetic peptides, *Biol. Chem. Hoppe Seyler* 373, 465–470, 1992; Bobek, L.A. and Levine, M.J., Cystatins — inhibitors of cysteine proteineases, *Crit. Rev. Oral Biol. Med.* 3, 307–332, 1992; Calkins, C.C., and Sloane, B.F., Mammalian cysteine protease inhibitors: biochemical properties and possible roles in tumor progression, *Biol. Chem. Hoppe Seyler* 376, 71–80, 1995; Turk, B., Turk, V., and Turk, D., Structural and functional aspects of papainlike cysteine proteinases and their protein inhibitors, *Biol. Chem.* 378, 141–150, 1997; Kos, J., Stabuc, B., Cimerman, N., and Brunner, N., Serum cystatin C, a new marker of glomerular filtration rate, is increased during malignant progression, *Clin. Chem.* 44, 2556–2557, 1998; Vray, B., Hartman, S., and Hoebeke, J., Immunomodulatory properties of cystatins, *Cell. Mol. Life Sci.* 59, 1503–1512, 2002; Arai, S., Matsumoto, I., Emori, Y., and Abe, K., Plant seed cystatins and their target enzymes of endogenous and exogenous origin, *J. Agric. Food Chem.* 50, 6612–6617, 2002; Abrahamson, M., Alvarez-Fernandez, M., and Nathanson, C.M., Cystatins, *Biochem. Soc. Symp.* 70, 179–199, 2003; Dubin, G., Proteinaceous cysteine protease inhibitors, *Cell. Mol. Life Sci.* 62, 653–669, 2005; Righetti, P.G., Castagna, A., Antonucci, F. et al., Proteome analysis in the clinical chemistry laboratory: myth or reality? *Clin. Chim. Acta* 357, 123–139, 2005; Overall, C.M. and Dean, R.A., Degradomics: systems biology of the protease web. Pleiotropic roles of MMPs in cancer, *Cancer Metastasis Rev.* 25, 69–75, 2006; Kotsylfakis, M., Sá-Nunes, A., Francischetti, I.M.B. et al., Anti-inflammatory and immunosuppressive activity of sialostatin L, a salivary cystatin from Tick *Ixodes scapularis, J. Biol. Chem.* 281, 26298–26307, 2006.

DCI was developed by James C. Powers and coworkers at Georgia Institute of Technology (Harper, J.W., Hemmi, K., and Powers, J.C., Reaction of serine proteases with substituted isocoumarins: discovery of 3,4-dichloroisocoumarin, a new general mechanism-based serine protease inhibitor, *Biochemistry* 24, 1831–1841, 1985). This inhibitor is reasonably specific, although side reactions have been described. As with the sulfonyl fluorides and DFP, the modification is slowly reversible and enhanced by basic solvent conditions and/or nucleophiles. DCI has been used as a proteosome inhibitor. See Rusbridge, N.M. and Benyon, R.J., 3,4-dichloroisocoumarin, a serine protease inhibitor, inactivates glycogen phosphorylase b, *FEBS Lett.* 30, 133–136, 1990; Weaver,

Characteristics of Selected Protease Inhibitors, Which Can be Used in Protease Inhibitor Cocktails (Continued)

Common Name		Other Nomenclature	M.W.	Primary Design
3, 4-Dichloroisocoumarin		DCI	215	Mechanism-based inhibitor of serine proteases.

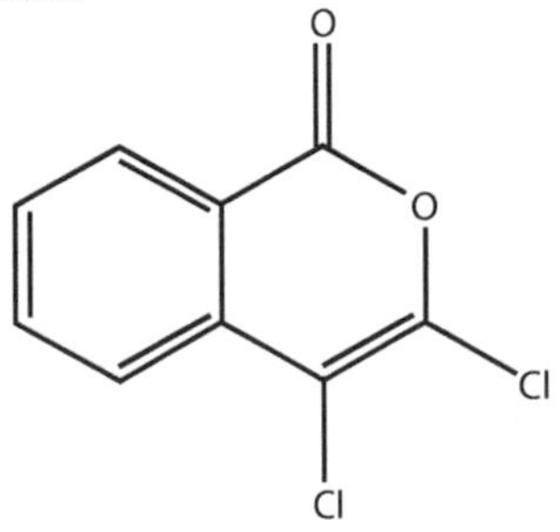

3, 4-dichloroisocoumarin

V.M., Lach, B., Walker, P.R., and Sikorska, M., Role of proteolysis in apoptosis: involvement of serine proteases in internucleosomal DNA fragmentation in immature thymocytes, *Biochem. Cell Biol.* 71, 488–500, 1993; Garder, A.M., Aviel, S., and Argon, Y., Rapid degradation of an unassembled immunoglobulin light chain is mediated by a serine protease and occurs in a pre-Golgi compartment, *J. Biol. Chem.* 268, 25940–25947, 1993; Lu, Q. and Mellgren, R.L., Calpain inhibitors and serine protease inhibitors can produce apoptosis in HL-60 cells, *Arch. Biochem. Biophys.* 334, 175–181, 1996; Adams, J. and Stein, R., Novel inhibitors of the proteosome and their therapeutic use in inflammation, *Annu. Rep. Med. Chem.* 31, 279–288, 1996; Olson, S.T., Swanson, R., Patston, P.A., and Bjork, I., Apparent formation of sodium dodecyl sulfate-stable complexes between serpins and 3, 4-dichloroisocoumarin-inactivated proteinases is due to regeneration of active proteinase from the inactivated enzyme, *J. Biol. Chem.* 272, 13338–13342, 1997; Mesner, P.W., Bible, K.C., Martins, L.M. et al., Characterization of caspase processing and activation in HL-60 cell cytosol under cell-free conditions — nucleotide requirement and inhibitor profile, *J. Biol. Chem.* 274, 22635–22645, 1999; Kam, C.M., Hudig, D., and Powers, J.C., Granzymes (lymphocyte serine proteases): characterization with natural and synthetic substrates and inhibitors, *Biochim. Biophys. Acta* 1477, 307–323, 2000; Rivett, A.J. and Gardner, R.C., Proteosome inhibitors: from *in vitro* uses to clinical trials, *J. Pep. Sci.* 6, 478–488, 2000; Bogyo, M. and Wang, E.W., Proteosome inhibitors: complex tools for a complex enzyme, *Curr. Top. Microbiol. Immunol.* 268, 185–208, 2002; Powers, J.C., Asgian, J.L., Ekici, O.D., and James, K.E., Irreversible inhibitors of serine, cysteine, and threonine proteases, *Chem. Rev.* 102, 4639–4740, 2002; Pochet, L., Frederick, R., and Masereei, B., Coumarin and isocoumarin as serine protease inhibitors, *Curr. Pharm. Des.* 10, 3781–3796, 2004.

| **Diisopropyl Phosphorofluoridate** | | DFP; Diisopropyl Fluorophosphate | 184 | Reaction at active site serine. |

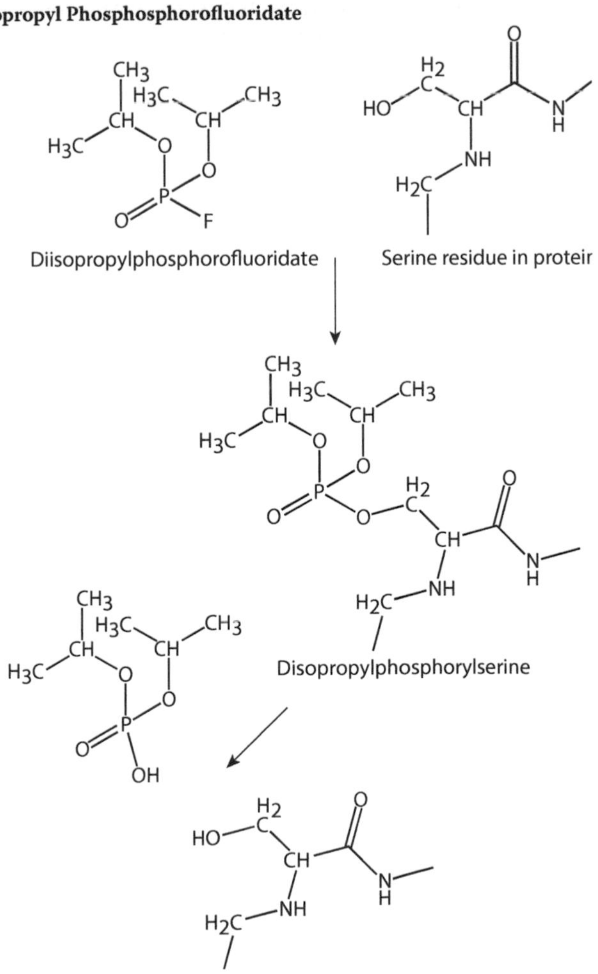

Diisopropylphosphorofluoridate   Serine residue in protein

Disopropylphosphorylserine

Characteristics of Selected Protease Inhibitors, Which Can be Used in Protease Inhibitor Cocktails (Continued)

Common Name	Other Nomenclature	M.W.	Primary Design

DFP was developed during World War II as a neurotoxin. DFP reacts with the active serine of serine proteases and was used to define the presence of this amino acid at the active sites of trypsin and chymotrypsin. DFP has been replaced by PMSF as a general reagent for inhibition of proteases although it is still used on occasion because of the ease of identification of the phosphoserine derivative. See Jansen, E.F., Jang, R., and Balls, A.K., The inhibition of purified, human plasma cholinesesterase with diisopropylfluorophosphate, *J. Biol. Chem.* 196, 247–253, 1952; Gladner, J.A. and Neurath, H.A., C-terminal groups in chymotrypsinogen and DFP-alpha-chymotrypsin in relation to the activation process, *Biochim. Biophys. Acta* 9, 335–336, 1952; Schaffer, N.K., May, S.C., Jr., and Summerson, W.H., Serine phosphoric acid from diisopropylphosphoryl chymotrypsin, *J. Biol. Chem.* 202, 67–76, 1953; Oosterbaan, R.A., Kunst, P., and Cohen, J.A., The nature of the reaction between diisopropylfluorophosphate and chymotrypsin, *Biochim. Biophys. Acta.* 16, 299–300, 1955; Wahlby, S., Studies on *Streptomyces griseus* protease. I. Separation of DFP-reacting enzymes and purification of one of the enzymes, *Biochim. Biophys. Acta* 151, 394–401, 1968; Hoskin, R.J. and Long, R.J., Purification of a DFP-hydrolyzing enzyme from squid head ganglion, *Arch. Biochem. Biophys.* 150, 548–555, 1972; Craik, C.S., Roczniak, S., Largman, C., and Rutter, W.J., The catalytic role of the active aspartic acid in serine proteases, *Science* 237, 909–913, 1987; D'Souza, C.A., Wood, D.D., She, Y.M., and Moscarello, M.A., Autocatalytic cleavage of myelin basic protein: an alternative to molecular mimicry, *Biochemistry* 44, 12905–12913, 2005. DFP is a potent neurotoxin and attention should be given to antidotes to organophosphates (Tuovinen, K., Kaliste-Korhonen, E., Raushel, F.M., and Hanninen, O., Phosphotriesterase, pralidoxime-2-chloride (2-PAM), and eptastigmine treatments and their combinations in DFP intoxication, *Toxicol. Appl. Pharmacol.* 141, 555–560, 1996; Auta, J., Costa, E., Davis, J., and Guidotti, A., Imidazenil: a potent and safe protective agent against diisopropyl fluorophosphate toxicity, *Neuropharmacology* 46, 397–403, 2004; Tuovinen, K., Organophosphate- induced convulsions and prevention of neuropathological damages, *Toxicology* 196, 31–39, 2004).

E-64

E-64 from *Aspergillus japonicus*

	L-*trans*-epoxysuccinyl-leucylamide-(4-guanido) butane or *N*-[*N*-(L- *trans*-carboxyoxiran-2-carbonyl)-L-leucyl]-agmatine	357.4	Inhibitor of sulfhydryl proteases.

E-64 is a reasonably specific inhibitor of sulfhydryl proteases and it functions by forming a thioether linkage with the active site cysteine. E-64 is frequently referred to as an inhibitor of lysosomal proteases and antigen processing. See Hashida, S., Towatari, T., Kominami, E., and Katunuma, N., Inhibition by E-64 derivatives of rat liver cathepsins B and cathepsin L *in vitro* and *in vivo*, *J. Biochem.* 88, 1805–1811, 1980; Grinde, B., Selective inhibition of lysosomal protein degradation by the thiol proteinase inhibitors E-64, Ep-459, and Ep-457 in isolated rat hepatocytes, *Biochim. Biophys. Acta* 701, 328–333, 1982; Barrett, A.J., Kembhavi, A.A., Brown, A.A. et al., L-*trans*-epoxysuccinyl-leucylamiodo (4-guanidino) butane (E-64) and its analogues as inhibitors of cysteine proteinases including cathepsins B, H, and L, *Biochem. J.* 201, 189–198, 1982; Ko, Y.M., Yamanaka, T., Umeda, M., and Suzuki, Y., Effects of thiol protease inhibitors on intracellular degradation of exogenous β-galactosidase in cultured human skin fibroblasts, *Exp. Cell Res.* 148, 525–529, 1983; Tamai, M., Matsumoto, K., Omura, S. et al., *In vitro* and *in vivo* inhibition of cysteine proteinases by EST, a new analog of E-64, *J. Pharmacobiodyn.* 9, 672–677, 1986; Shaw, E., Cysteinyl proteinases and their selective inactivation, *Adv. Enzymol. Relat. Areas Mol. Biol.* 63, 271–347, 1990; Mehdi, S., Cell-penetrating inhibitors of calpain, *Trends Biochem. Sci.* 16, 150–153, 1991; Min, K.S., Nakatsubo, T., Fujita, Y. et al., Degradation of cadmium metallothionein *in vitro* by lysosomal proteases, *Toxicol. Appl. Pharmacol.* 113 299–305, 1992; Schirmeister, T. and Klackow, A., Cysteine protease inhibitors containing small rings, *Mini Rev. Med. Chem.* 3, 585–596, 2003.

EACA

Epsilon-aminocaproic acid
6-aminohexanoic acid   Lysine

	ε-aminocaproic acid; 6-aminocaproic acid; 6-aminohexanoic acid; Amicar™	131.2	Analogue of lysine; inhibitor of trypsinlike enzymes such as plasmin.

EACA is an inhibitor of trypticlike serine proteases. It has been used as a hemostatic agent that functions by inhibiting fibrinolysis. It is included in some protease inhibitor cocktails. See Soter, N.A., Austen, K.F., and Gigli, I., Inhibition by epsilon-aminocaproic acid of the activation of the first component of the complement system, *J. Immunol.* 114, 928–932, 1975; Burden, A.C., Stacey, R., Wood, R.F., and Bell, P.R., Why do protease inhibitors enhance leukocyte migration inhibition to the antigen PPD? *Immunology* 35, 959–962, 1978; Nakagawa, H., Watanabe, K., and Sato, K., Inhibitory action of synthetic proteinase inhibitors and substrates on the chemotaxis of rat polymorphonuclear leukocytes *in vitro*, *J. Pharmacobiodyn.* 11, 674–678, 1988; Hill, G.E., Taylor, J.A., and Robbins, R.A., Differing effects of aprotinin and ε-aminocaproic acid on cytokine-induced inducible nitric oxide synthase expression, *Ann. Thorac. Surg.* 63, 74–77, 1997; Stonelake, P.S., Jones, C.E., Neoptolemos, J.P., and Baker, P.R., Proteinase inhibitors reduce basement membrane degradation by human breast cancer cell lines, *Br. J. Cancer* 75, 951–959, 1997; Sun, Z., Chen, Y.H., Wang, P. et al., The blockage of the high-affinity lysine-binding sites of plasminogen by EACA significantly inhibits prourokinase-induced plasminogen activation, *Biochim. Biophys. Acta* 1596, 182–192, 2002.

Characteristics of Selected Protease Inhibitors, Which Can be Used in Protease Inhibitor Cocktails
(Continued)

Common Name	Other Nomenclature	M.W.	Primary Design
Ecotin			Broad-spectrum protease inhibitor derived from *Escherichia coli*.

Ecotin is a broad-spectrum inhibitor of serine proteases that can be engineered to enhance inhibition of specific enzymes. See McGrath, M.E., Hines, W.M., Sakanari, J.A. et al., The sequence and reactive site of ecotin. A general inhibitor of pancreatic serine proteases from *Escherichia coli*, *J. Biol. Chem.* 266, 6620–6625, 1991; Erpel, T., Hwang, P., Craik, C.S. et al., Physical map location of the new *Escherichia coli* gene eco, encoding the serin protease inhibitor ecotin, *J. Bacteriol.* 174, 1704, 1992; Wang, C.I., Yang, Q., and Craik, C.S., Isolation of a high affinity inhibitor of urokinase-type plasminogen activator by phage display of ecotin, *J. Biol. Chem.* 270, 12250–12256, 1995; Yang, S.Q., Wang, C.T., Gilmor, S.A. et al., Ecotin: a serine protease inhibitor with two distinct and interacting binding sites, *J. Mol. Biol.* 279, 945–957, 1998; Gilmor, S.A., Takeuchi, T., Yang, S.Q. et al., Compromise and accommodation in ecotin, a dimeric macromolecular inhibitor of serine proteases, *J. Mol. Biol.* 299, 993–1003, 2000; Eggers, C.T., Wang, S.X., Fletterick, R.J., and Craik, C.S., The role of ecotin dimerization in protease inhibition, *J. Mol. Biol.* 308, 975–991, 2001; Wang, B., Brown, K.C., Lodder, M. et al., Chemical-mediated site-specific proteolysis. Alteration of protein–protein interaction, *Biochemistry* 41, 2805–2813, 2002; Stoop, A.A. and Craik, C.S., Engineering of a macromolecular scaffold to develop specific protease inhibitors, *Nat. Biotechnol.* 21, 1063–1068, 2003; Eggers, C.T., Murray, I.A., Delmar, V.A. et al., The periplasmic serine protease inhibitor ecotin protects bacteria against neutrophil elastase, *Biochem. J.* 379, 107–118, 2004.

Ethylenediamine Tetraacetic Acid	EDTA	292.2	Metal ion chelator; inhibitor of metalloenzymes.

Edetic acid; EDTA; ethylenediaminetetraacetic acid;
N, *N*′-1, 2-ethanediaminediylbis[*N*-(carboxymethylglycine)]

(Ethylenedinitrilo)tetraacetic acid (ethylenediamine tetraacetic acid) chelates metal ions with a preference for divalent cations. EDTA functions as an inhibitor of metalloproteinases. See Manna, S.K., Bhattacharya, C., Gupta, S.K., and Samanta, A.K., Regulation of interleukin-8 receptor expression in human polymorphonuclear neutrophils, *Mol. Immunol.* 32, 883–893, 1995; Martin-Valmaseda, E.M., Sanchez-Yague, Y., Marcos, R., and Lianillo, M., Decrease in platelet, erythrocyte, and lymphocyte acetylcholinesterase activities due to the presence of protease inhibitors in the storage buffers, *Biochem. Mol. Biol. Int.* 41, 83–91, 1997; Oh-Ishi, M., Satoh, M., and Maeda, T., Preparative two-dimensional gel electrophoresis with agarose gels in the first dimension for high molecular mass proteins, *Electrophoresis* 21, 1653–1669, 2000; Shah, R.B., Palamakula, A., and Khan, M.A., Cytotoxicity evaluation of enzyme inhibitors and absorption enhancers in Caco-2 cells for oral delivery of salmon calcitonin, *J. Pharm. Sci.* 93, 1070–1082, 2004; Pagano, M.R., Paredi, M.E., and Crupkin, M., Cytoskeletal ultrastructure and lipid composition of I-Z-I fraction in muscle from pre- and post-spawned female hake (*Meriluccius hubbsi*), *Comp. Biochem. Physiol. B Biochem. Mol. Biol.* 141, 13–21, 2005; Wei, G.X. and Bobek, L.A., Human salivary mucin MUC7 12-mer-L and 12-mer-D peptides: antifungal activity in saliva, enhancement of activity with protease inhibitor cocktail or EDTA, and cytotoxicity to human cells, *Antimicrob. Agents Chemother.* 49, 2336–2342, 2005.

Iodoacetamide		185	Primary reaction with sulfhydryl groups and slower reaction with other protein nucleophiles.

Iodoacetamide Iodoacetic acid

Iodoacetic acid and iodoacetamide can both be used to modify nucleophiles in proteins. The chloro- and bromo-derivatives can be used as well but the rate of modification is slower. The haloacetyl function can also be used as the reactive function for more complex derivatives. Iodoacetamide is neutral compared to iodoacetic acid and is less influenced by the local environment of the reactive nucleophile. See Janatova, J., Lorenz, P.E., and Schechter, A.N., Third component of human complement: appearance of a sulfhydryl group following chemical or enzymatic inactivation, *Biochemistry* 19, 4471–4478, 1980; Haas, A.L., Murphey, K.E., and Bright, P.M., The inactivation of ubiquitin accounts for the inability to demonstrate ATP, ubiquitin-dependent proteolysis in liver extracts, *J. Biol. Chem.* 260, 4694–4703, 1985; Molla, A., Yamamoto, T., and Maeda, H., Characterization of 73 kDa thiol protease from *Serratia marcescens* and its effect on plasma proteins, *J. Biochem.* 104, 616–621, 1988; Wingfield, P., Graber, P., Turcatti, G. et al., Purification and characterization of a methionine-specific aminopeptidase from *Salmonella tyrphimurium*, *Eur. J. Biochem.* 180, 23–32, 1989; Kembhavi, A.A., Buttle, D.J., Rauber, P., and Barrett, A.J., Clostripain: characterization of the active site, *FEBS Lett.* 283, 277–280, 1991; Jagels, M.A., Travis, J., Potempa, J. et al., Proteolytic inactivation of the leukocyte C5a receptor by proteinases derived from *Porphyromas gingivalis*, *Infect. Immun.* 64, 1984–1991, 1996; Tanksale, A.M., Vernekar, J.V., Ghatge, M.S., and Deshpande, V.V., Evidence for tryptophan in proximity to histidine and cysteine as essential to the active site of an alkaline protease, *Biochem. Biophys. Res. Commun.* 270, 910–917, 2000; Karki, P., Lee, J., Shin, S.Y. et al., Kinetic comparison of procapase-3 and caspases-3, *Arch. Biochem. Biophys.* 442, 125–132, 2005. The haloalkyl derivatives do react with thiourea and are perhaps less reliable than maleimides.

Characteristics of Selected Protease Inhibitors, Which Can be Used in Protease Inhibitor Cocktails (Continued)

Common Name	Other Nomenclature	M.W.	Primary Design
LBTI	Lima Bean Trypsin Inhibitor	6500	Protein protease inhibitor.

Lima bean trypsin inhibitor is a protein/peptide with unusual stability. It is stable to heat (90°C for 15 minutes at pH 7 with no loss of activity) and acid (the original purification uses extraction with ethanol and dilute sulfuric acid). This is a reflection of the high content of cystine resulting in a "tight" structure. As a Bowman–Birk inhibitor, LBTI has seven disulfide bonds (Weder, J.K.P. and Hinkers, S.C., Complete amino acid sequence of the Lentil trypsin-chymotrypin inhibitor LCI-1.7 and a discussion of atypical binding sites of Bowman–Birk inhibitors, *J. Agric. Food Chem.* 52, 4219–4226, 2004). LBTI also inhibits both trypsin and chymotrypsin (Krahn, J. and Stevens, F.C., Lima bean trypsin inhibitor. Limited proteolysis by trypsin and chymotrypsin, *Biochemistry* 27, 1330–1335, 1970) as well as various other serine proteases. For additional information, see Fraenkel-Conrat, H., Bean, R.C., Ducay, E.D., and Olcott, H.S., Isolation and characterization of a trypsin inhibitor from lima beans, *Arch. Biochem. Biophys.* 37, 393–407, 1952; Stevens, F.C. and Doskoch, E., Lima bean protease inhibitor: reduction and reoxidation of the disulfide bonds and their reactivity in the trypsin-inhibitor complex, *Can. J. Biochem.* 51, 1021–1028, 1973; Nordlund, T.M., Liu, X.Y., and Sommer, J.H., Fluorescence polarization decay of tyrosine in lima bean trypsin inhibitor, *Proc. Natl. Acad. Sci. USA* 83, 8977–8981, 1986; Hanlon, M.H. and Liener, I.E., A kinetic analysis of the inhibition of rat and bovine trypsins by naturally occurring protease inhibitors, *Comp. Biochem. Physiol. B* 84, 53–57, 1986; Xiong, W., Chen, L.M., Woodley-Miller, C. et al., Identification, purification, and localization of tissue kallikrein in rat heart, *Biochem. J.* 267, 639–646, 1990; Briseid, K., Hoem, N.O., and Johannesen, S., Part of prekallikrein removed from human plasma together with IgG-immunoblot and functional tests, *Scand. J. Clin. Lab. Invest.* 59, 55–63, 1999; Yamasaki, Y., Satomi, S., Murai, N. et al., Inhibition of membrane-type serine protease 1/matriptase by natural and synthetic protease inhibitors, *J. Nutr. Sci. Vitaminol.* 49, 27–32, 2003.

Leupeptin	(ac/pr-LeuLeuArginal)		Transition-state inhibitor of proteinase.

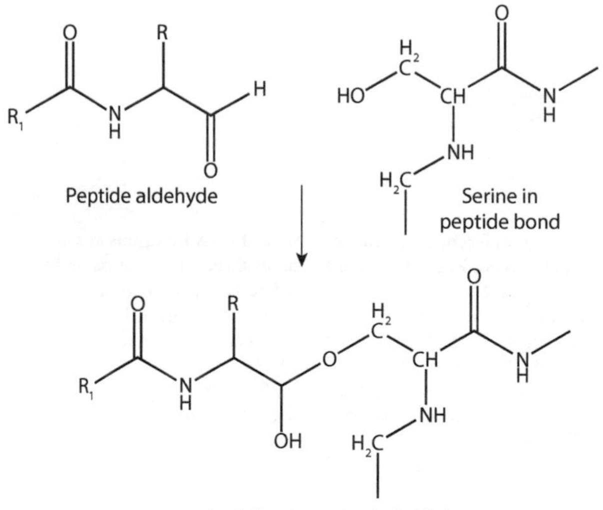

Peptide aldehyde

Serine in peptide bond

Stabilized tetrahedral aldol

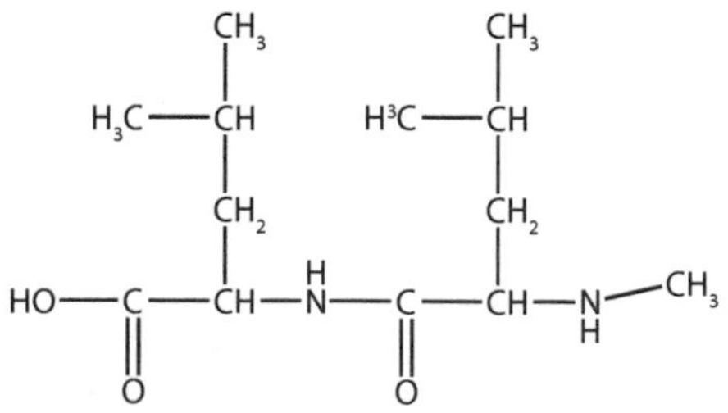

Leupeptide A

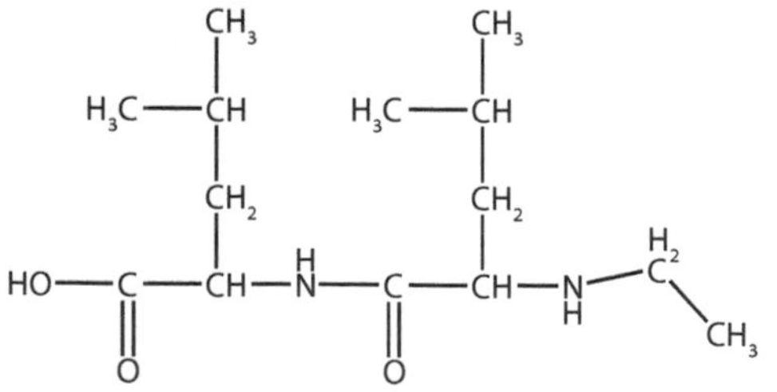

Leupeptin B

Characteristics of Selected Protease Inhibitors, Which Can be Used in Protease Inhibitor Cocktails
(Continued)

Common Name	Other Nomenclature	M.W.	Primary Design

A tripeptide aldehyde (ac/pr-LeuLeuArginal) proteinase inhibitor isolated from *Actinomycetes*. It is a relatively common component of protease inhibitor cocktails used to preserve proteins during storage and purification. See Alpi, A. and Beevers, H., Proteinases and enzyme stability in crude extracts of castor bean endosperm, *Plant Physiol.* 67, 499–502, 1981; Ratajzak, T., Luc, T., Samec, A.M., and Hahnel, R., The influence of leupeptin, molybdate, and calcium ions on estrogen receptor stability, *FEBS Lett.* 136, 115–118, 1981; Takei, Y., Marzi, I., Kauffman, F.C. et al., Increase in survival time of liver transplants by protease inhibitors and a calcium channel blocker, nisoldipine, *Transplantation* 50, 14–20, 1990; Satoh, M., Hosoi, S., Miyaji, M. et al., Stable production of recombinant pro-urokinase by human lymphoblastoid Namalwa KJM-1 cells: host-cell dependency of the expressed-protein stability, *Cytotechnology* 13, 79–88, 1993; Hutchesson, A.C., Hughes, C.V., Bowden, S.J., and Ratcliffe, W.A., *In vitro* stability of endogenous parathyroid hormone-related protein in blood and plasma, *Ann. Clin. Biochem.* 31, 35–39, 1994; Agarwal, S. and Sohal, R.S., Aging and proteolysis of oxidized proteins, *Arch. Biochem. Biophys.* 309, 24–28, 1994; Yamada, T., Shinnoh, N., and Kobayashi, T., Proteinase inhibitors suppress the degradation of mutant adrenoleukodytrophy proteins but do not correct impairment of very long chain fatty acid metabolism in adrenoleukodystrophy fibroblasts, *Neurochem. Res.* 22, 233–237, 1997; Bi, M. and Singh, J., Effect of buffer pH, buffer concentration, and skin with or without enzyme inhibitors on the stability of [Arg(9)]-vasopressin, *Int. J. Pharm.* 197, 87–93, 2000; Bi, M. and Singh, J., Stability of luteinizing hormone-releasing hormone: effects of pH, temperature, pig skin, and enzyme inhibitors, *Pharm. Dev. Technol.* 5, 417–422, 2000; Ratnala, V.R., Swarts, H.G., VanOostrum, J. et al., Large-scale overproduction, functional purification, and ligand affinities of the His-tagged human histamine H1 receptor, *Eur. J. Biochem.* 271, 2636–2646, 2004.

Common Name	Other Nomenclature	M.W.	Primary Design
(*p*-Amidinophenyl) Methanesulfonyl Fluoride	aPMSF	163	Reaction at active site serine.

(*p*-amidinophenyl) methanesulfonyl fluoride

(*p*-Amidinophenyl) methanesulfonyl fluoride was developed by Bing and coworkers (Laura, R., Robison, D.J., and Bing, D.H., [*p*-Amidinophenyl] methanesulfonyl fluoride, an irreversible inhibitor of serine proteases, *Biochemistry* 19, 4859–4864, 1980) to improve the specificity of PMSF for trypticlike enzymes. aPMSF readily reacts with trypsin but is only poorly reactive with chymotrypsin. See Katz, I.R., Thorbecke, G.J., Bell, M.K. et al., Protease-induced immunoregulatory activity of platelet factor 4, *Proc. Natl. Acad. Sci. USA* 83, 3491–3495, 1986; Unson, C.G. and Merrifield, R.B., Identification of an essential serine residue in glucagon: implications for an active site triad, *Proc. Natl. Acad. Sci. USA* 91, 454–458, 1994; Nikai, T., Komori, Y., Kato, S., and Sugihara, I.I., Bioloical properties of kinin-releasing enzyme from *Trimeresurus okinavensis(himehabu)* venom, *J. Nat. Toxins* 7, 23–35, 1998; Ishidoh, K., Takeda-Ezaki, M., Watanabe, S. et al., Analysis of where and which types of proteinases participate in lysosomal proteinase processing using balifomycin A1 and *Helicobacter pylori* Vac A toxin, *J. Biochem.* 125, 770–779, 1999; Komori, Y., Tatematsu, R., Tanida, S., and Nikai, T., Thrombin-like enzyme, flavovilase, with kinin-releasing activity from *Trimesurus flavoviridis(habu)* venom, *J. Nat. Toxins* 10, 239–248, 2001; Luo, L.Y., Shan, S.J., Elliott, M.B. et al., Purification and characterization of human kallikrein 11, a candidate prostate and ovarian cancer biomarker, from seminal plasma, *Clin. Cancer Res.* 12, 742–750, 2006. Reaction at a residue other than a serine has not been demonstrated although it is not unlikely that, as with DFP and PMSF, reaction could occur at a serine residue.

Common Name	Other Nomenclature	M.W.	Primary Design
p-(Aminoethyl) Benzene Sulfonyl Fluoride	AEBSF; 4-(2-aminoethyl)-benzenesulfonyl fluoride (Pefabloc™ SC)	165	Reaction at active site serine.

4-(2-aminoethyl)benzenesulfonyl fluoride

This reagent was developed to improve the reactivity of PMSF. It was originally considered to be somewhat more effective than PMSF; however, AEBSF has been shown to be somewhat promiscuous in its reaction pattern and care is suggested in its use during sample preparation. See Su, B., Bochan, M.R., Hanna, W.L. et al., Human granzyme B is essential for DNA fragmentation of susceptible target cells, *Eur. J. Immunol.* 24, 2073–2080, 1994; Helser, A., Ulrichs, K., and Muller-Ruchholtz, W., Isolation of porcine pancreatic islets: low trypsin activity during the isolation procedure guarantees reproducible high islet yields, *J. Clin. Lab. Anal.* 8, 407–411, 1994; Dentan, C., Tselepis, A.D., Chapman, M.J., and Ninio, E., Pefabloc, 4-[2-aminoethyl'benzenesulfonyl fluoride, is a new potent nontoxic and irreversible inhibitor of PAF-degrading acetylhydrolase, *Biochim. Biophys. Acta* 1299, 353–357, 1996; Sweeney, B., Proudfoot, K., Parton, A.H. et al., Purification of the T-cell receptor zeta-chain: covalent modification by 4-(2-aminoethyl)-benzenesulfonyl fluoride, *Anal. Biochem.* 245, 107–109, 1997; Diatchuk, V., Lotan, O., Koshkin, V. et al., Inhibition of NADPH oxidase activation by 4-(2-aminoethyl)benzenesulfonyl fluoride and related compounds, *J. Biol. Chem.* 272, 13292–13301, 1997; Chu, T.M. and Kawinski, E., Plasmin, subtilisin-like endoproteases, tissue plasminogen activator, and urokinase plasminogen activator are involved in activation of latent TGF-beta 1 in human seminal plasma, *Biochem. Biophys. Res. Commun.* 253, 128–134, 1998; Guo, Z.J., Lamb, C., and Dixon, R.A., A serine protease from suspension-cultured soybean cells, *Phytochemistry* 47, 547–553, 1998; Wechuck, J.B., Goins, W.F., Glorioso, J.C., and Ataai, M.M., Effect of protease inhibitors on yield of HSV-1-based viral vectors, *Biotechnol. Prog.* 16, 493–496, 2000; Baszk, S., Stewart, N.A., Chrétien, M., and Basak, A., Aminoethyl benzenesulfonyl fluoride and its hexapeptide (AC-VFRSLK) conjugate are both *in vitro* inhibitors of subtilisin kexin isozyme-1, *FEBS Lett.* 573, 186–194, 2004; King, M.A., Halicka, H.D., and Dzrzynkiewicz, Z., Pro- and anti-apoptotic effects of an inhibitor of chymotrypsin-like serine proteases, *Cell Cycle* 3, 1566–1571, 2004; Odintsova, E.S., Buneva, V.N, and Nevinsky, G.A., Casein-hydrolyzing activity of sIGA antibodies from human milk, *J. Mol. Recog.* 18, 413–421, 2005; Solovyan, V.T. and Keski-Oja, J., Proteolytic activation of latent TGF-beta precedes caspase-3 activation and enhances apoptotic death of lung epithelial cells, *J. Cell Physiol.* 207, 445–453, 2006.

Characteristics of Selected Protease Inhibitors, Which Can be Used in Protease Inhibitor Cocktails (Continued)

Common Name	Other Nomenclature	M.W.	Primary Design
Pepstatin		685.9	Acid protease inhibitor.

Pepstatin

A group of pentapeptide acid protease inhibitors isolated from *Streptomeyces* (Umezawa, H., Aoyagi, T., Morishima, H. et al., Pepstatin, a new pepsin inhibitor produced by *Actinomycetes*, *J. Antibiot.* 23, 259–262, 1970; Aoyagi, T., Kunimoto, S., Morichima, H. et al., Effect of pepstatin on acid proteases, *J. Antibiot.* 24, 687–694, 1971). Pepstatins are frequently included in protease inhibitor cocktails and used for the stabilization of proteins during extraction, storage, and purification. See Takei, Y., Marzi, I., Kaufmann, F.C. et al., Increase in survival time of liver transplants by protease inhibitors and a calcium channel blocker, nisoldipine, *Transplantation* 50, 14–20, 1990; Liang, M.N., Witt, S.N., and McConnell, H.M., Inhibition of class II MHC-peptide complex formation by protease inhibitors, *J. Immunol. Methods* 173, 127–131, 1994; Deng, J., Rudick, V., and Dory, L., Lysosomal degradation and sorting of apolipoprotein E in macrophages, *J. Lipid Res.* 36, 2129–2140, 1995; Wang, Y.K., Lin, H.H., and Tang, M.J., Collagen gel overlay induces two phases of apoptosis in MDCK cells, *Am. J. Physiol. Cell Physiol.* 280, C1440–C1448, 2001; Lafleur, M.A., Handsley, M.M., Knaupper, V. et al., Endothelial tubulogenesis within fibrin gels specifically requires the activity of membrane-type-matrix-metalloproteinases (MT-MMPs), *J. Cell Sci.* 155, 3427–3438, 2002.

Phenanthroline Monohydrate	1, 10-phenanthroline	198.2	Metal ion chelator; inhibitor of metalloenzymes; specificity for zinc-metalloenzymes.

o-Phenanthroline
1,10-Phenanthroline

Characteristics of Selected Protease Inhibitors, Which Can be Used in Protease Inhibitor Cocktails
(Continued)

Common Name	Other Nomenclature	M.W.	Primary Design

1, 10-phenanthroline, *o*-phenanthroline: an inhibitor of metalloproteinases and a reagent for the detection of ferrous ions. See Felber, J.P., Cooobes, T.L., and Vallee, B.L., The mechanism of inhibition of carboxypeptidase A by 1,10-phenanthroline, *Biochemistry* 1, 231–238, 1962; Hakala, M.T. and Suolinna, E.M., Specific protection of folate reductase against chemical and proteolytic inactivation, *Mol. Pharmacol.* 2, 465–480, 1966; Latt, S.A., Holmquist, B., and Vallee, B.L., Thermolysin: a zinc metalloenzyme, *Biochem. Biophys. Res. Commun.* 37, 333–339, 1969; Berman, M.B. and Manabe, R., Corneal collagenases: evidence for zinc metalloenzymes, *Ann. Ophthalmol.* 5, 1993–1995, 1973; Seltzer, J.L., Jeffrey, J.J., and Eisen, A.Z., Evidence for mammalian collagenases as zinc ion metalloenzymes, *Biochim. Biophys. Acta* 485, 179–187, 1977; Krogdahl, A. and Holm, H., Inhibition of human and rat pancreatic proteinases by crude and purified soybean trypsin inhibitor, *J. Nutr.* 109, 551–558, 1979; St. John, A.C., Schroer, D.W., and Cannavacciuolo, L., Relative stability of intracellular proteins in bacterial cells, *Acta. Biol. Med. Ger.* 40, 1375–1384, 1981; Kitjaroentham, A., Suthiphongchai, T., and Wilairat, P., Effect of metalloprotease inhibitors on invasion of red blood cells by *Plasmodium falciparum*, *Acta Trop.* 97, 5–9, 2006; Thwaite, J.E., Hibbs, S., Tritall, R.W., and Atkins, T.P., Proteolytic degradation of human antimicrobioal peptide LL-37 by *Bacillus anthracis* may contribute to virulence, *Antimicrob. Agents Chemother.* 50, 2316–2322, 2006.

Phenylmethylsulfonyl Fluoride	PMSF	174	Reaction at active site serine.

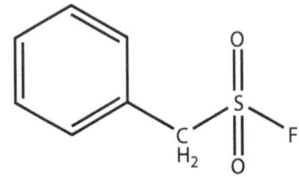

Phenylmethylsulfonyl fluoride (PMSF)

Phenylmethylsulfonyl fluoride was developed by David Fahrney and Allen Gold and inhibits serine proteases such as trypsin and chymotrypsin in a manner similar to DFP. The rate of modification of trypsin and chymotrypsin with PMSF is similar to that observed with DFP; however, the reaction with acetylcholinesterase with PMSF is much less than that of DFP ($>6.1 \times 10^{-2}$ $M^{-1}min^{-1}$ vs. 1.3×10^4 $M^{-1}min^{-1}$)(Fahrney, D.E. and Gold, A.M., Sulfonyl fluorides as inhibitors of esterases. I. Rates of reaction with acetylcholinesterase, α-chymotrypsin, and trypsin, *J. Amer. Chem. Soc.* 85, 997–1000, 1963). For other applications see Lundblad, R.L., A rapid method for the purification of bovine thrombin and the inhibition of the purified enzyme with phenylmethylsulfonyl fluoride, *Biochemistry* 10, 2501–2506, 1971; Pringle, J.R., Methods for avoiding proteolytic artefacts in studies of enzymes and other proteins from yeasts, *Methods Cell Biol.* 12, 149–184, 1975; Bendtzen, K., Human leukocyte migration inhibitory factor (LIF). I. Effect of synthetic and naturally occurring esterase and protease inhibitors, *Scand. J. Immunol.* 6, 125–131, 1977; Carter, D.B., Efird, P.H., and Chae, C.B., Chromatin-bound proteases and their inhibitors, *Methods Cell Biol.* 19, 175–190, 1978; Hubbard, J.R. and Kalimi, M., Influence of proteinase inhibitors on glucocorticoid receptor properties: recent progress and future perspectives, *Mol. Cell. Biochem.* 66, 101–109, 1985; Kato, T., Sakamoto, E., Kutsana, H. et al., Proteolytic conversion of STAT3alpha to STAT3gamma in human neutrophils: role of granule-derived serine proteases, *J. Biol. Chem.* 279, 31076–31080, 2004; Cho, I.H., Choi, E.S., Lim, H.G., and Lee, H.H., Purification and characterization of six fibrinolytic serine proteases from earthworm *Lumbricus rubellus*, *J. Biochem. Mol. Biol.* 37, 199–205, 2004; Khosravi, J., Diamandi, A., Bodani, U. et al., Pitfalls of immunoassay and sample for IGF-1: comparison of different assay methodologies using fresh and stored serum samples, *Clin. Biochem.* 38, 659–666, 2005; Shao, B., Belaaouaj, A., Velinde, C.L. et al., Methionine sulfoxide and proteolytic cleavage contribute to the inactivation of cathepsin G by hypochlorous acid: an oxidative mechanism for regulation of serine proteinases by myeloperoxidase, *J. Biol. Chem.* 260, 29311–29321, 2005; Pagano, M.R., Paredi, M.E., and Crupkin, M., Cytoskeletal ultrastructural and lipid composition of 1-Z-1 fraction in muscle from pre- and post-spawned female hake (*Merluccius hubbsi*), *Comp. Biochem. Physiol. B Biochem. Mol. Biol.* 141, 13–21, 2005. Although PMSF is reasonably specific for reaction with the serine residue at the active site of serine proteinases, as with DFP, reaction at tyrosine has been reported (De Vendittis, E., Ursby, T., Rullo, R. et al., Phenylmethanesulfonyl fluoride inactivates an archeael superoxide dismutase by chemical modification of a specific tyrosine residue. Cloning, sequencing, and expression of the gene coding for *Sulfolobus solfataricus* dismutase, *Eur. J. Biochem.* 268, 1794–1801, 2001). PMSF does have solubility issues and usually ethanol or another suitable water-miscible organic solvent is used to introduce this reagent. On occasion, the volume of ethanol required influences the reaction (see Bramley, T.A., Menzies, G.S., and McPhie, C.A., Effects of alcohol on the human placental GnRH receptor system, *Mol. Hum. Reprod.* 5, 777–783, 1999).

SBTI	Soybean Trypsin Inhibitor	21,500	Protein protease inhibitor.

Soybean trypsin inhibitor (SBTI, STI) usually refers to the inhibitor first isolated by Kunitz (Kunitz, M., Crystalline soybean trypsin inhibitor, *J. Gen. Physiol.* 29, 149–154, 1946; Kunitz, M., Crystalline soybean trypsin inhibitor. II. General properties, *J. Gen. Physiol.* 30, 291–310, 1947). This material is described as the Kunitz inhibitor and is reasonably specific for trypticlike enzymes. There are other protease inhibitors derived from soybeans; the Bowman–Birk inhibitor (Birk, Y., The Bowman–Birk inhibitor. Trypsin and chymotrypsin-inhibitor from soybeans, *Int. J. Pept. Protein Res.* 25, 113–131, 1985; Birk, Y., Protein proteinase inhibitors in legume seeds — overview, *Arch. Latinoam. Nutr.* 44 (4 Suppl. 1), 26S–30S, 1996) is the best known and, unlike the Kunitz inhibitor, inhibits both trypsin and chymotrypsin; the Bowman–Birk inhibitor is also a double-headed inhibitor having two reactive sites (see Frattali, V. and Steiner, R.F., Soybean inhibitors. I. Separation and some properties of three inhibitors from commercial crude soybean trypsin inhibitor, *Biochemistry* 7, 521–530, 1968; Frattali, V. and Steiner, R.F., Interaction of trypsin and chymotrypsin with a soybean proteinase inhibitor, *Biochem. Biophys. Res. Commun.* 34, 480–487, 1969; Krogdahl, A. and Holm, H., Inhibition of human and rat pancreatic proteinases by crude and purified soybean trypsin inhibitor, *J. Nutr.* 109, 551–558, 1979). Soybean trypsin inhibitor (Kunitz) is used as a model protein (Liu, C.L., Kamei, D.T., King, J.A. et al., Separation of proteins and viruses using two-phase aqueous micellar systems, *J. Chromatog. B* 711, 127–138, 1998; Higgs, R.E., Knierman, M.D., Gelfanova, Y. et al., Comprehensive label-free method for the relative quantification of proteins from biological samples, *J. Proteome Res.* 4, 1442–1450, 2005). The broad specificity of the Kunitz inhibitor for trypticlike serine proteases provides the basis for its use in the demonstration of protease processing steps (Hansen, K.K., Sherman, P.M., Cellars, L. et al., A major role for proteolytic and proteinase-activated receptor-3 in the pathogenesis of infectious colitis, *Proc. Natl. Acad. Sci. USA* 102, 8363–8368, 2005).

Characteristics of Selected Protease Inhibitors, Which Can be Used in Protease Inhibitor Cocktails (Continued)

Common Name	Other Nomenclature	M.W.	Primary Design
Tosyl-lysine Chloromethyl Ketone	TLCK; 1-chloro-3-tosylamido-7-amino-2-heptanone	369.2 (HCl)	Reaction at active site histidine residues of trypsinlike serine proteases.

Tosyl-lysine chloromethyl ketone

Tosyl-lysine chloromethyl ketone (TLCK) was developed by Elliott Shaw and colleagues (Shaw, E., Mares-Guia, M., and Cohen, W., Evidence of an active center histidine in trypsin through use of a specific reagent, 1-chloro-3-tosylamido-7-amido-2-heptanone, the chloromethyl ketone derived from N-α tosyl-L-lysine, *Biochemistry* 4, 2219–2224, 1965). As with TPCK, reaction is not absolutely specific for trypticlike serine proteases (Earp, H.S., Austin, K.S., Gillespie, G.Y. et al., Characterization of distinct tyrosine-specific protein kinases in B and T lymphocytes, *J. Biol. Chem.* 260, 4351–4356, 1985; Needham, L. and Houslay, M.D., Tosyl-lysyl chloromethylketone detects conformational changes in the catalytic unit of adenylate cyclase induced by receptor and G-protein stimulation, *Biochem. Biophys. Res. Commun.* 156, 855–859, 1988). Reaction of this chloroalkyl compound with sulfydryl groups would be expected and it is possible that other protein nucleophilic centers would react, although this has not been unequivocally demonstrated. Attempts to synthesize the direct arginine analogue were unsuccessful; it was possible to make more complex arginine derivatives such as Ala-Phe-Arg-CMK, which was more effective with human plasma Kallikrein than the corresponding lysine derivatives (Ki = 0.078 µM vs. M vs. 4.9 µM) (Kettner, C. and Shaw, E., Synthesis of peptides of arginine chloromethyl ketone. Selective inactivation of human plasma kallikrein, *Biochemistry* 17, 4778–4784, 1978).

Tosyl-phenylalanine Chloromethyl Ketone	TPCK; L-1-tosylamido-2-phenylethyl chloromethyl ketone)	351.9	Reaction at active site histidine residues of chymotrypsinlike serine proteases.

Tosyl phenylalanine chloromethylketone

Tosyl-phenylalanine chloromethyl ketone (TPCK) was developed by Guenther Schoellmann and Elliott Shaw (Schoellmann, G. and Shaw, E., Direct evidence for the presence of histidine in the active center of chymotrypsin, *Biochemistry* 2, 252–255, 1963). TPCK was developed as an affinity label (Plapp, B.V., Application of affinity labeling for studying structure and function of enzymes, *Methods Enzymol.* 87, 469–499, 1982) where binding to chymotrypsin is driven by the phenyl function with subsequent alkylation of the active site histidine. The chloroalkyl function was selected to reduce reactivity with other protein nucleophiles such as cysteine. TPCK does undergo a slow rate of hydrolysis to form the corresponding alcohol. TPCK inactivates proteases with chymotrypsinlike specificity. The rate of inactivation is relatively slow but is irreversible; reaction rates can be enhanced by a more elaborate peptide chloromethyl ketone structure. In the case of cucumisin, a plant serine proteinase, TPCK did not result in inactivation while inactivation was achieved with Z-Ala-Ala-Pro-Phe-chloromethyl ketone (Yonezawa, H., Uchikoba, T., and Kaneda, M., Identification of the reactive histidine of cucumisin, a plant serine protease: modification with peptidyl chloromethyl ketone derivative of peptide substrate, *J. Biochem.* 118, 917–920, 1995). There is, however, significant reaction of TPCK with other proteins at residues other than histidine (see Rychlik, I., Jonak, J., and Sdelacek, J., Inhibition of the EF-Tu factor by L-1-tosylamido-2-phenylethyl chloromethyl ketone, *Acta Biol. Med. Ger.* 33, 867–876, 1974); TPCK has been described as an inhibitor of cysteine proteinases (Bennett, M.J., Van Leeuwen, E.M., and Kearse, K.P., Calnexin association is not sufficient to protect T cell receptor proteins from rapid degradation in CD4⁺CD8⁺ thymocytes, *J. Biol. Chem.* 273, 23674–23680, 1998). TPCK has been suggested to react with a lysine residue in aminoacylase (Frey, J., Kordel, W., and Schneider, F., The reaction of aminoacylase with chloromethylketone analogs of amino acids, *Z. Naturforsch.* 32, 769–776, 1966). Other reactions continue to be described (McCray, J.W. and Weil, R., Inactivation of interferons: halomethyl ketone derivatives of phenylalanine as affinity labels, *Proc. Natl. Acad. Sci. USA* 79, 4829–4833, 1982; Conseiller, E.C. and Lederer, F., Inhibition of NADPH oxidase by aminoacyl chloromethane protease inhibitors in phorbol-ester-stimulated human neutrophils: A reinvestigation. Are proteases really involved? *Eur. J. Biochem.* 183, 107–114, 1989; Borukhov, S.I. and Strongin, A.Y., Chemical modification of the recombinant human α-interferons and β-interferons, *Biochem. Biophys. Res. Commun.* 167, 74–80, 1990; Gillibert, M., Dehry, Z., Terrier, M. et al., Another biological effect of tosylphenylalanylchloromethane (TPCK): it prevents p47(phox) phosphorylation and translocation upon neutrophil stimulation, *Biochem. J.* 386, 549–556, 2005).

Characteristics of Selected Protease Inhibitors, Which Can be Used in Protease Inhibitor Cocktails (Continued)

Common Name	Other Nomenclature	M.W.	Primary Design

Peptide Halomethyl Ketones: While TPCK and TLCK represented a major advance in modifying active site residues in serine proteases, slow and relatively nonspecific reaction was a problem. The development of tripeptide halomethyl ketones provided a major advance in the value of such derivatives as presented in some specific examples below. However, even with these derivatives, reactions occur with "unexpected" enzymes. More general information can be obtained from the following references: Poulos, T.L., Alden, R.A., Freer, S.T. et al., Polypeptide halomethyl ketones bind to serine proteases as analogs of the tetrahedral intermediate. X-ray crystallographic comparison of lysine- and phenylalanine-polypeptide chloromethyl ketone-inhibited subtilisin, *J. Biol. Chem.* 251, 1097–1103, 1976; Powers, J.C., Reaction of serine proteases with halomethyl ketones, *Methods Enzymol.* 46, 197–208, 1977; Navarro, J., Abdel Ghany, M., and Racker, E., Inhibition of tyrosine protein kinases by halomethyl ketones, *Biochemistry* 21, 6138–6144, 1982; Conde, S., Perez, D.I., Martinez, A. et al., Thienyl and phenyl α-halomethyl ketones: new inhibitors of glycogen synthase kinase (GSK-3β) from a library of compound searching, *J. Med. Chem.* 46, 4631–4633, 2003.

Peptide Fluoromethyl Ketones: Fluoroalkyl derivatives of the peptide chloromethyl ketones have been prepared in an attempt to improve specificity by reducing nonspecific alkylation at cysteine residues (Rasnick, D., Synthesis of peptide fluoromethyl ketones and the inhibition of human cathepsin B, *Anal. Biochem.* 149, 461–465, 1985). Nonspecific reaction with sulfydryl groups such as those in glutathione was reduced; there was still reaction with active site cysteine although at a slower rate than with the chloroalkyl derivative (16,200 $M^{-1}s^{-1}$ vs. 45,300 $M^{-1}s^{-1}$; $t_{1/2}$ 21.9 min. vs. 5.1 min.). Reaction also occurred with serine proteases (Shaw, E., Angliker, H., Rauber, P. et al., Peptidyl fluoromethyl ketones as thiol protease inhibitors, *Biomed. Biochim. Acta* 45, 1397–1403, 1986) where the modification occurred at a histidine residue (Imperiali, B. and Abeles, R.H., Inhibition of serine proteases by peptide fluoromethyl ketones, *Biochemistry* 25, 3760–3767, 1986). The trifluoromethyl derivative was also an inhibitor but formed a hemiacetal derivative. The peptide fluoromethyl ketone, z-VAD-FMK, has proved to be a useful inhibitor of caspases

Common Name	Other Nomenclature	M.W.	Primary Design
D-Phe-Pro-Arg-chloromethyl Ketone	PPACK		Reaction at active site histidine residues of trypsinlike serine proteases.

D-Phe-Pro-Arg-chloromethyl ketone was one of the first complex peptide halomethyl ketones synthesized. These derivatives have the advantage of increased reaction rate and specificity (see Williams, E.B. and Mann, K.G., Peptide chloromethyl ketones as labeling reagents, *Methods Enzymol.* 222, 503–513, 1993; Odake, S., Kam, C.M., and Powers, J.C., Inhibition of thrombin by arginine-containing peptide chloromethyl ketones and bis chloromethyl ketone-albumin conjugates, *J. Enzyme Inhib.* 9, 17–27, 1995; Lundblad, R.L., Bergstrom, J., De Vreker, R. et al., Measurement of active coagulation factors in Autoplex®-T with colorimetric active site-specific assay technology, *Thromb. Haemostas.* 80, 811–815, 1998). With chymotrypsin, CHO-PheCH$_2$Cl, k_{obsv}/[I] = 0.55 $M^{-1}s^{-1}$ and Boc-Ala-Gly-Phe-CH$_2$Cl, k_{obsv}/[I] = 3.34 $M^{-1}s^{-1}$ (Kurachi, K., Powers, J.C., and Wilcox, P.E., Kinetics of the reaction of chymotrypsin A α with peptide chloromethyl ketones in relation to subsite specificity, *Biochemistry* 12, 771–777, 1973. See also Ketter, C. and Shaw, E., The selective affinity labeling of factor Xa by peptides of arginine chloromethyl ketone, *Thromb. Res.* 22, 645–652, 1981; Shaw, E., Synthetic inactivators of kallikrein, *Adv. Exp. Med. Biol.* 156, 339–345, 1983; McMurray, J.S. and Dyckes, D.F., Evidence for hemiketals as intermediates in the inactivation of serine proteinases with halomethyl ketones, *Biochemistry* 25, 2298–2301, 1986). There is a similar peptide chloromethyl ketone, PPACK II (D-Phe-Phe-Arg-CMK), which has been used to stabilize B-type natriuretic peptide (BNP) in plasma samples (Belenky, A., Smith, A., Zhang, B. et al., The effect of class-specific protease inhibitors on the stabilization of B-type natriuretic peptide in human plasma, *Clin. Chim. Acta* 340, 163–172, 2004).

Common Name	Other Nomenclature	M.W.	Primary Design
z-VAD-FMK	Benzyloxycarbonyl-Val-Ala-Asp(OMe) fluoromethyl ketone		Inhibitor of caspases.

z-VADFMK

Benzyloxycarbonyl-Val-Ala-Asp(OMe) fluoromethyl ketone (z-VAD-FMK) is a peptide halomethyl ketone used for the inhibition of caspases and related enzymes. Because z-VAD-FMK is neutral, it passes the cell membrane and can inhibit intracellular proteolysis and is useful in understanding the role of caspases and related enzymes in cellular function. See Zhu, H., Fearnhead, H.O., and Cohen, G.M., An ICE-like protease is a common mediator of apoptosis induced by diverse stimuli in human monocytes THP.1 cells, *FEBS Lett.* 374, 303–308, 1995; Mirzoeva, O.K., Yaqoob, P., Knox, K.A., and Calder, P.C., Inhibition of ICE-family cysteine proteases rescues murine lymphocytes from lipoxygenase inhibitor-induced apoptosis, *FEBS Lett.* 396, 266–270, 1996; Slee, E.A., Zhu, H., Chow, S.C. et al., Benzyloxycarbonyl-Val-Ala-Asp(OMe) fluoromethylketone (z-VAD.FMK) inhibits apoptosis by blocking the processing of CPP32, *Biochem. J.* 315, 21–24, 1996; Gottron, F.J., Ying, H.S., and Choi, D.W., Caspase inhibition selectively reduces the apoptotic component of oxygen-glucose deprivation-induced cortical neuronal cell death, *Mol. Cell. Neurosci.* 9, 159–169, 1997; Longthorne, V.L. and Williams, G.T., Caspase activity is required for commitment to Fas-mediated apoptosis, *EMBO J.* 16, 3805–3812, 1997; Hallan, E., Blomhoff, H.K., Smeland, E.B., and Long, J., Involvement of ICE (Caspase) family in gamma-radiation-induced apoptosis of normal B lymphocytes, *Scand. J. Immunol.* 46, 601–608, 1997; Polverino, A.J. and Patterson, S.D., Selective activation of caspases during apoptotic induction in HL-60 cells. Effects of a tetrapeptide inhibitor, *J. Biol. Chem.* 272, 7013–7021, 1997; Cohen, G.M., Caspases: the executioners of apoptosis, *Biochem. J.* 328, 1–16, 1997; Sarin, A., Haddad, E.K., and Henkart, P.A., Caspase dependence of target cell damage induced by cytotoxic lymphocytes, *J. Immunol.* 161, 2810–2816, 1998; Nicotera, P., Leist, M., Single, B., and Volbracht, C., Execution of apoptosis: converging or diverging pathway? *Biol. Chem.* 380, 1035–1040, 1999; Grfaczyk, P.P., Caspase inhibitors as anti-inflammatory and antiapoptotic agents, *Prog. Med. Chem.* 39, 1–72, 2002; Blankenberg, F., Mari, C., and Strauss, H.W., Imaging cell death *in vivo*, *Q. J. Nucl. Med.* 47, 337–348, 2003; Srivastava, A., Henneke, P., Visintin, A. et al., The apoptotic response to pneumolysin in Toll-like receptor 4 dependent and protects against pneumococcal disease, *Infect. Immun.* 73, 6479–6489, 2005; Clements, K.M., Burton-Wurster, N., Nuttall, M.E., and Lust, G., Caspase-3/7 inhibition alters cell morphology in mitomycin-C treated chondrocytes, *J. Cell Physiol.* 205, 133–140, 2005; Coward, W.R., Marie, A., Yang, A. et al., Statin-induced proinflammatory response in mitogen-activated peripheral blood mononuclear cells through the activation of caspases-1 and IL-18 secretion in monocytes, *J. Immunol.* 176, 5284–5292, 2006.

---

[a] The protease inhibitor cocktails referred to herein are not to be confused with the protease inhibitor cocktails that are used for therapy for patients who have Acquired Immune Deficiency Syndrome (AIDS).

General References for Inhibitors of Proteolytic Enzymes

Albeck, A. and Kliper, S., Mechanism of cysteine protease inactivation by peptidyl epoxides, *Biochem. J.* 322, 879–884, 1997.

Banner, C.D. and Nixon, R.A., Eds., *Proteases and Protease Inhibitors in Alzheimer's Disease Pathogenesis*, New York Academy of Sciences, New York, 1992.

Barrett, A.J. and Salvesen, G., Eds., *Protease Inhibitors*, Elsevier, Amsterdam, NL, 1986.

Bernstein, N.K. and James, M.N., Novel ways to prevent proteolysis — prophytepsin and proplasmepsin II, *Curr. Opin. Struct. Biol.* 9, 684–689, 1999.

Birk, Y., Ed., *Plant Protease Inhibitors: Significance in Nutrition, Plant Protection, Cancer Prevention, and Genetic Engineering*, Springer, Berlin, 2003.

Cheronis, J.C.D. and Repine, J.E., *Proteases, Protease Inhibitors, and Protease-Derived Peptides: Importance in Human Pathophysiology and Therapeutics*, Birkhäuser Verlag, Basel, Switzerland, 1993.

Church, F.C., Ed., *Chemistry and Biology of Serpins*, Plenum Press, New York, 1997.

Frlan, R. and Gobec, S., Inhibitors of cathepsin B, *Curr. Med. Chem.* 13, 2309–2327, 2006.

Giglione, C., Boularot, A., and Meinnel, T., Protein N-terminal excision, *Cell. Mol. Life Sci.* 61, 1455–1474, 2004.

Johnson, S.L. and Pellechhia, M., Structure- and fragment-based approaches to protease inhibition, *Curr. Top. Med. Chem.* 6, 317–329, 2006.

Kim, D.H., Chemistry-based design of inhibitors for carboxypeptidase A, *Curr. Top. Med. Chem.* 4, 1217–1226, 2004.

Lowther, W.T., and Matthews, B.W., Structure and function of the methionine aminopeptidases, *Biochim. Biophys. Acta* 1477, 157–167, 2000.

Magnusson, S., Ed., *Regulatory Proteolytic Enzymes and Their Inhibitors*, Pergamon Press, Oxford, UK, 1986.

Powers, J.C. and Harper, J.W., Inhibition of serine proteinases, in *Proteinase Inhibitors*, Barrett, A.J. and Salvesen, G., Eds., Elsevier, Amsterdam, NL, chapter 3, pp. 55–152.

Saklatvala, J., and Nagase, H., Eds., *Proteases and the Regulation of Biological Processes*, Portland Press, London, UK, 2003.

Shaw, E., Cysteinyl proteinases and their selective inactivation, *Adv. Enzymol. Relat. Areas Mol. Biol.* 63, 271–347, 1990.

Stennicke, H.R. and Salvesen, G.S, Chemical ligation — an unusual paradigm in protease inhibition, *Mol. Cell.* 21, 727–728, 2006.

Tam, T.F., Leung-Toung, R., Li, W. et al., Medicinal chemistry and properties of 1,2,4-thiadiazoles, *Mini Rev. Med. Chem.* 5, 367–379, 2005.

Vogel, R., Trautschold, I., and Werle, E., *Natural Proteinase Inhibitors*, Academic Press, New York, 1968.

Section III
Lipidomics and Lipidomes

EVOLUTION OF THE CLASSIFICATION AND NOMENCLATURE OF LIPIDS

Roger L. Lundblad

Bloor, W.R., *Biochemistry of the Fatty Acids and Their Compounds, the Lipids*, American Chemical Society/Reinhold Publishing, New York, 1943.

"Lipids may be defined as a group of naturally occurring substances consisting of higher fatty acids, their naturally occurring compounds, and substances found naturally in chemical association with them."

"The group is characterized in general by insolubility in water and solubility in "fat solvents.""

Classification of Lipids

Simple lipids: Esters of fatty acids with various alcohols.

- *Fats*: Defined as esters of fatty acids with glycerol; fats which are liquid at room temperature are defined as oils.
- *Waxes*: Defined as esters of fatty acids with alcohols other than glycerol.

Compound lipids: Compounds of fatty acids with alcohols but containing other groups in addition to the alcohol.

- *Phospholipids (phosphatides)*: Defined as substituted fats containing phosphoric acid and a nitrogen compound (e.g. lecithin, cephalin, sphingomyelin).
- *Phosphatidates*: Defined as phospholipids minus the organic bases.
- *Glycolipids*: Defined as compounds of fatty acids with a carbohydrate and a nitrogen compound but no phosphoric acids (e.g. cerebrosides)
- *Sulfolipids*: Defined as lipids containing sulfuric acid.
- *Aminolipids*: Not well characterized as of this writing (1943).

Derived lipids: Substances from the preceding groups which have the general properties of lipids.

Fatty acids

- Alcohols (e.g., cetyl alcohol $C_{16}H_{33}OH$), myricyl alcohol ($C_{30}H_{61}OH$), and cholesterol ($C_{27}H_{45}OH$)
- *Hydrocarbons*: Compounds such as squalene.
- *Bases*: Choline, aminoethyl alcohol, sphingosine.

The last IUPAC recommendation on the nomenclature of lipids was published in 1976.

IUPAC-IUB Committee on Biochemical Nomenclature

http://www.chem.qmul.ac.uk/iupac/lipid/

From IUPAC Goldbook

http://goldbook.iupac.org/L03571.html

IUPAC/IUBMB Recommendations for Nomenclature of Glycolipids

http://www.chem.qmul.ac.uk/iupacmisc/glylp.html

Fahy, E., Subramaniam, S., Brown, H.A., et al., A comprehensive classification system for lipids, *J. Lipid Res.*, 46, 839–861, 2005 (in 4th edition of *Handbook of Biochemistry and Biophysics*).

Other References for Lipid Nomenclature

Fahy, E., Lipid classification, structures and tools, *Biochim. Biophys. Acta*, 1811, 637–647, 2011.

Fahy, E., Subramaniam, S., Murphy, R.C., et al., Update of the LIPID MAPS comprehensive classification system for lipids, *J. Lipid Res.*, 50, S9–S14, 2009.

Taylor, R., Miller, R.H., Miller, R.D., et al., Automated structural classification of lipids by machine learning, *Bioinformatics*, 31, 621–625, 2015.

There are some literature on arachidonic acid metabolites:

Jahn, U., Galano, J.-M., and Durand, T., A cautionary note on the correct structure assignment of phytoprostanes and the emergence of a new prostane ring system, *Prostaglandins Leukot. Essent. Fatty Acids*, 82, 83–86, 2010.

Kühn, H., and Borngräber, S., Eicosanoids and related compounds: structures, nomenclatuture and biosynthetic pathways, in *Eicosnoids and Related Compounds in Plants and Animals*, A.F. Rowley, H. Kühn, and T. Schewe, eds., pp. 3–24, Princeton University Press, Princeton, NJ, 2015.

Mueller, M.J., Isoprotane nomenclature: Inherent problems may cause setbacks for the development of the isoprostanoid field, *Prostaglandins Leukot. Essent. Fatty Acids*, 82, 71–81, 2010.

Murphy, R.C., and Fahy, E., Isoprostane nomenclature: More suggestions, *Prostanglandins Leukot. Essent. Fatty Acids*, 82, 69–70, 2010.

A BRIEF GLOSSARY FOR LIPIDOMICS

Roger L. Lundblad

Glossary for Fatty Acids

Iodine number: Also known as iodine value. A measurement of the degree of unsaturation of fatty acids. Defined as the percentage by weight of iodine absorbed by a sample. The iodine number is used extensively in the biodiesel and food industry.

Essential fatty acids: Two fatty acids are essential and they must be supplied from an exogenous source. These are linoleic acid ((9Z,12Z)-octadeca-9,12-dienoic acid) and α-linolenic acid ((9Z,12Z,15Z)-octadeca-9,12,15-trienoic acid). Both of these are found in plants and are converted to other critical lipid metabolites such as arachidonic acid in the ω6 (linoleic) series by the liver (Lagarde, M., Bernound-Hubac, N., Calzada, C., Véricel, E., and Guichardant, M., Lipidomics of essential fatty acids and oxygenated metabolites, *Mol. Nutr. Food Res.*, 57, 1347–1358, 2013; Spector, A.A., and Kim, H.Y., Discovery of essential fatty acids, *J. Lipid Res.*, 56, 11–21, 2015).

Saponification: The alkaline hydrolysis of acyl lipids such as glycerol to yield free fatty acids.

Saponification number: Amount of KOH in milligrams required to saponify 1 g of fat under specified conditions.

Transesterification: The process by which alcohol is exchanged for another. Early work refers to this process as interesterification. This process is used most often in the analysis of total fatty acids in blood and tissues where methanol is exchanged for a glycerol in triglycerides. This process is very important in the processing of oils for biodiesel production (Lerin, L.A., Loss, R.A., Remonatto, D., et al., A review on lipase-catalyzed reaction in ultrasound-assisted systems, *Bioprocess Biosys. Eng.*, 37, 2381–2394, 2014; Lee, A.F., Bennett, J.A., Manayil, J.C., and Wilson, K., Heterogeneous catalysis for sustainable biodiesel production via esterification and transesterification, *Chem. Soc. Res.*, 43, 7887–7916, 2014).

A COMPREHENSIVE CLASSIFICATION SYSTEM FOR LIPIDS[1]

Eoin Fahy,* Shankar Subramaniam,[†] H. Alex Brown,[§] Christopher K. Glass,[**]
Alfred H. Merrill Jr., [††]Robert C. Murphy,[§§] Christian R. H. Raetz,[***] David W. Russell,[†††]
Yousuke Seyama,[§§§] Walter Shaw,[****] Takao Shimizu,[††††] Friedrich Spener,[§§§§] Gerrit van Meer,[*****]
Michael S. Van Nieuwenhze,[†††††] Stephen H. White,[§§§§§] Joseph L. Witztum,[******] and Edward A. Dennis[2,††††††]

San Diego Supercomputer Center,* University of California, San Diego, 9500 Gilman Drive, La Jolla, CA 92093-0505; Department of Bioengineering,[†] University of California, San Diego, 9500 Gilman Drive, La Jolla, CA 92093-0412; Department of Pharmacology,[§] Vanderbilt University Medical Center, Nashville, TN 37232-6600; Department of Cellular and Molecular Medicine,[**] University of California, San Diego, 9500 Gilman Drive, La Jolla, CA 92093-0651; School of Biology,[††] Georgia Institute of Technology, Atlanta, GA 30332-0230; Department of Pharmacology,[§§] University of Colorado Health Sciences Center, Aurora, CO 80045-0508; Department of Biochemistry,[***] Duke University Medical Center, Durham, NC 27710; Department of Molecular Genetics,[†††] University of Texas Southwestern Medical Center, Dallas, TX 75390-9046; Faculty of Human Life and Environmental Sciences,[§§§] Ochanomizu University, Tokyo 112-8610, Japan; Avanti Polar Lipids, Inc.,[****] Alabaster, AL 35007; Department of Biochemistry and Molecular Biology,[††††] Faculty of Medicine, University of Tokyo, Tokyo 113-0033, Japan; Department of Molecular Biosciences,[§§§§] University of Graz, 8010 Graz, Austria; Department of Membrane Enzymology,[*****]Institute of Biomembranes, Utrecht University, 3584 CH Utrecht, The Netherlands; Department of Chemistry and Biochemistry,[†††††] University of California, San Diego, 9500 Gilman Drive, La Jolla, CA 92093-0358; Department of Physiology and Biophysics,[§§§§§] University of California at Irvine, Irvine, CA 92697-4560; Department of Medicine,[******] University of California, San Diego, 9500 Gilman Drive, La Jolla, CA 92093-0682; and Department of Chemistry and Biochemistry and Department of Pharmacology,[††††††] University of California, San Diego, La Jolla, CA 92093-0601

Abstract Lipids are produced, transported, and recognized by the concerted actions of numerous enzymes, binding proteins, and receptors. A comprehensive analysis of lipid molecules, "lipidomics," in the context of genomics and proteomics is crucial to understanding cellular physiology and pathology; consequently, lipid biology has become a major research target of the postgenomic revolution and systems biology. To facilitate international communication about lipids, a comprehensive classification of lipids with a common platform that is compatible with informatics requirements has been developed to deal with the massive amounts of data that will be generated by our lipid community. As an initial step in this development, we divide lipids into eight categories (fatty acyls, glycerolipids, glycerophospholipids, sphingolipids, sterol lipids, prenol lipids, saccharolipids, and polyketides) containing distinct classes and subclasses of molecules, devise a common manner of representing the chemical structures of individual lipids and their derivatives, and provide a 12 digit identifier for each unique lipid molecule. The lipid classification scheme is chemically based and driven by the distinct hydrophobic and hydrophilic elements that compose the lipid.[jlr] This structured vocabulary will facilitate the systematization of lipid biology and enable the cataloging of lipids and their properties in a way that is compatible with other macromolecular databases.—Fahy, E., S. Subramaniam, H. A. Brown, C. K. Glass, A. H. Merrill, Jr., R. C. Murphy, C. R. H. Raetz, D. W. Russell, Y. Seyama, W. Shaw, T. Shimizu, F. Spener,

G. van Meer, M. S. VanNieuwenhze, S. H. White, J. L. Witztum, and E. A. Dennis. **A comprehensive classification system for lipids.** *J. Lipid Res.* 2005. 46: 839–861.

Supplementary key words lipidomics • informatics • nomenclature • chemical representation • fatty acyls • glycerolipids • glycerophospholipids • sphingolipids • sterol lipids • prenol lipids • saccharolipids • polyketides

The goal of collecting data on lipids using a "systems biology" approach to lipidomics requires the development of a comprehensive classification, nomenclature, and chemical representation system to accommodate the myriad lipids that exist in nature. Lipids have been loosely defined as biological substances that are generally hydrophobic in nature and in many cases soluble in organic solvents (1). These chemical properties cover a broad range of molecules, such as fatty acids, phospholipids, sterols, sphingolipids, terpenes, and others (2). The LIPID MAPS (LIPID Metabolites And Pathways Strategy; http://www.lipidmaps.org), Lipid Library (http://lipidlibrary.co.uk), Lipid Bank (http://lipidbank.jp), LIPIDAT (http://www.lipidat.chemistry.ohiostate.edu), and Cyberlipids (http://www.cyberlipid.org) websites provide useful online resources for an overview of these molecules and their structures. More accurate definitions are possible when lipids are considered from a structural and biosynthetic perspective, and many different classification schemes have been used over the years. However, for the purpose of comprehensive classification, we define lipids as hydrophobic or amphipathic small molecules that may originate entirely or in part by carbanion-based

Manuscript received 22 December 2004 and in revised form 4 February 2005.

Published, JLR Papers in Press, February 16, 2005. DOI 10.1194/jlr. E400004-JLR200.

---

[1] The evaluation of this manuscript was handled by the former Editor-in-Chief Trudy Forte.

[2] To whom correspondence should be addressed.
E-mail: edennis@ucsd.edu

TABLE 1: Lipid Categories and Examples

Category	Abbreviation	Example
Fatty acyls	FA	dodecanoic acid
Glycerolipids	GL	1-hexadecanoyl-2-(9 Z-octadecenoyl)-sn-glycerol
Glycerophospholipids	GP	1-hexadecanoyl-2-(9 Z-octadecenoyl)-sn-glycero-3-phosphocholine
Sphingolipids	SP	N-(tetradecanoyl)-sphing-4-enine
Sterol lipids	ST	cholest-5-en-3β-ol
Prenol lipids	PR	2E,6E-farnesol
Saccharolipids	SL	UDP-3-O-(3R-hydroxy-tetradecanoyl)-αD-N-acetylglucosamine
Polyketides	PK	aflatoxin B$_1$

condensations of thioesters (fatty acids, polyketides, etc.) and/or by carbocation-based condensations of isoprene units (prenols, sterols, etc.). Additionally, lipids have been broadly subdivided into "simple" and "complex" groups, with simple lipids being those yielding at most two types of products on hydrolysis (e.g., fatty acids, sterols, and acylglycerols) and complex lipids (e.g., glycerophospholipids and glycosphingolipids) yielding three or more products on hydrolysis. The classification scheme presented here organizes lipids into well-defined categories that cover eukaryotic and prokaryotic sources and that is equally applicable to archaea and synthetic (man-made) lipids.

Lipids may be categorized based on their chemically functional backbone as polyketides, acylglycerols, sphingolipids, prenols, or saccharolipids. However, for historical and bioinformatics advantages, we chose to separate fatty acyls from other polyketides, the glycerophospholipids from the other glycerolipids, and sterol lipids from other prenols, resulting in a total of eight primary categories. An important aspect of this scheme is that it allows for subdivision of the main categories into classes and subclasses to handle the existing and emerging arrays of lipid structures. Although any classification scheme is in part subjective as a result of the structural and biosynthetic complexity of lipids, it is an essential prerequisite for the organization of lipid research and the development of systematic methods of data management. The classification scheme presented here is chemically based and driven by the distinct hydrophobic and hydrophilic elements that constitute the lipid. Biosynthetically related compounds that are not technically lipids because of their water solubility are included for completeness in this classification scheme.

The proposed lipid categories listed in **Table 1** have names that are, for the most part, well accepted in the literature. The fatty acyls (FA) are a diverse group of molecules synthesized by chain elongation of an acetyl-CoA primer with malonyl-CoA (or methylmalonyl-CoA) groups that may contain a cyclic functionality and/or are substituted with heteroatoms. Structures with a glycerol group are represented by two distinct categories: the glycerolipids (GL), which include acylglycerols but also encompass alkyl and 1 Z-alkenyl variants, and the glycerophospholipids (GP), which are defined by the presence of a phosphate (or phosphonate) group esterified to one of the glycerol hydroxyl groups. The sterol lipids (ST) and prenol lipids (PR) share a common biosynthetic pathway via the polymerization of dimethylallyl pyrophosphate/isopentenyl pyrophosphate but have obvious differences in terms of their eventual structure and function. Another well-defined category is the sphingolipids (SP), which contain a long-chain base as their core structure. This classification does not have a glycolipids category per se but rather places glycosylated lipids in appropriate categories based on the identity of their core lipids. It also was necessary to define a category with the term "saccharolipids" (SL) to account for lipids in which

fatty acyl groups are linked directly to a sugar backbone. This SL group is distinct from the term "glycolipid" that was defined by the International Union of Pure and Applied Chemists (IUPAC) as a lipid in which the fatty acyl portion of the molecule is present in a glycosidic linkage. The final category is the polyketides (PK), which are a diverse group of metabolites from plant and microbial sources. Protein modification by lipids (e.g., fatty acyl, prenyl, cholesterol) occurs in nature; however, these proteins are not included in this database but are listed in protein databases such as GenBank (http://www.ncbi.nlm.nih.gov) and SwissProt (http://www.ebi.ac.uk/swissprot/).

Lipid Nomenclature

A naming scheme must unambiguously define a lipid structure in a manner that is amenable to chemists, biologists, and biomedical researchers. The issue of lipid nomenclature was last addressed in detail by the International Union of Pure and Applied Chemists and the International Union of Biochemistry and Molecular Biology (IUPAC-IUBMB) Commission on Biochemical Nomenclature in 1976, which subsequently published its recommendations (3). Since then, a number of additional documents relating to the naming of glycolipids (4), prenols (5), and steroids (6) have been released by this commission and placed on the IUPAC website (http://www.chem.qmul.ac.uk/iupac/). A large number of novel lipid classes have been discovered during the last three decades that have not yet been systematically named. The present classification includes these new lipids and incorporates a consistent nomenclature.

In conjunction with our proposed classification scheme, we provide examples of systematic (or semisystematic) names for the various classes and subclasses of lipids. The nomenclature proposal follows existing IUPAC-IUBMB rules closely and should not be viewed as a competing format. The main differences involve *a*) clarification of the use of core structures to simplify systematic naming of some of the more complex lipids, and *b*) provision of systematic names for recently discovered lipid classes.

Key features of our lipid nomenclature scheme are as follows:

a) The use of the stereospecific numbering (*sn*) method to describe glycerolipids and glycerophospholipids (3). The glycerol group is typically acylated or alkylated at the *sn*-1 and/or *sn*-2 position, with the exception of some lipids that contain more than one glycerol group and archaebacterial lipids in which *sn*-2 and/or *sn*-3 modification occurs.

b) Definition of sphinganine and sphing-4-enine as core structures for the sphingolipid category, where the D-*erythro* or 2S,3R configuration and 4E geometry (in the case of sphing-4-enine) are implied. In molecules containing stereochemistries other than the 2*S*,3*R* configuration, the full systematic names are to be used instead (e.g., 2*R*-amino-1,3*R*-octadecanediol).

c) The use of core names such as cholestane, androstane, and estrane for sterols.

d) Adherence to the names for fatty acids and acyl chains (formyl, acetyl, propionyl, butyryl, etc.) defined in Appendices A and B of the IUPAC-IUBMB recommendations (3).

e) The adoption of a condensed text nomenclature for the glycan portions of lipids, where sugar residues are represented by standard IUPAC abbreviations and where the anomeric carbon locants and stereochemistry are included but the parentheses are omitted. This system has also been proposed by the Consortium for Functional Glycomics (http://web.mit.edu/glycomics/consortium/main.shtml).

f) The use of *E/Z* designations (as opposed to *trans/cis*) to define double bond geometry.

g) The use of *R/S* designations (as opposed to α/β or D/L) to define stereochemistries. The exceptions are those describing substituents on glycerol (*sn*) and sterol core structures and anomeric carbons on sugar residues. In these latter special cases, the α/β format is firmly established.

h) The common term "lyso," denoting the position lacking a radyl group in glycerolipids and glycerophospholipids, will not be used in systematic names but will be included as a synonym.

i) The proposal for a single nomenclature scheme to cover the prostaglandins, isoprostanes, neuroprostanes, and related compounds, where the carbons participating in the cyclopentane ring closure are defined and where a consistent chain-numbering scheme is used.

j) The "d" and "t" designations used in shorthand notation of sphingolipids refer to 1,3-dihydroxy and 1,3,4-trihydroxy long-chain bases, respectively.

Lipid Structure Representation

In addition to having rules for lipid classification and nomenclature, it is important to establish clear guidelines for drawing lipid structures. Large and complex lipids are difficult to draw, which leads to the use of shorthand and unique formats that often generate more confusion than clarity among lipidologists. We propose a more consistent format for representing lipid structures in which, in the simplest case of the fatty acid derivatives, the acid group (or equivalent) is drawn on the right and the hydrophobic hydrocarbon chain is on the left (**Figure 1**). Notable exceptions are found in the eicosanoid class, in which the hydrocarbon chain wraps around in a counterclockwise direction to produce a more condensed structure. Similarly, with regard to the glycerolipids and glycerophospholipids, the radyl chains are drawn with the hydrocarbon chains to the left and the glycerol group depicted horizontally with stereochemistry at the *sn* carbons defined (if known). The general term "radyl" is used to denote either acyl, alkyl, or 1-alkenyl substituents (http://www.chem.qmul.ac.uk/iupac/lipid/lip1n2.html), allowing for coverage of alkyl and 1 *Z*-alkenylglycerols. The sphingolipids, although they do not contain a glycerol group, have a similar structural relationship to the glycerophospholipids in many cases and may be drawn with the C1 hydroxyl group of the long-chain base to the right and the alkyl portion to the left. This methodology places the head groups of both sphingolipids and glycerophospholipids on the right side. Although the structures of sterols do not conform to these general rules of representation, the sterol esters may conveniently be

drawn with the acyl group oriented according to these guidelines. In addition, the linear prenols or isoprenoids are drawn in a manner analogous to the fatty acids, with the terminal functional group on the right side. Inevitably, a number of structurally complex lipids, such as acylaminosugar glycans, polycyclic isoprenoids, and polyketides, do not lend themselves to these simplified drawing rules. Nevertheless, we believe that the adoption of the guidelines proposed here will unify chemical representation and make it more comprehensible.

Databasing Lipids, Annotation, and Function

A number of repositories, such as GenBank, SwissProt, and ENSEMBL (http://www.ensembl.org), support nucleic acid and protein databases; however, there are only a few specialized databases [e.g., LIPIDAT (7) and Lipid Bank (8)] that provide a catalog, annotation, and functional classification of lipids. Given the importance of these molecules in cellular function and pathology, there is an imminent need for the creation of a well-organized database of lipids. The first step toward this goal is the establishment of an ontology of lipids that is extensible, flexible, and scalable. Before establishing an ontology, a structured vocabulary is needed, and the IUPAC nomenclature of the 1970s was an initial step in this direction.

The ontology of lipids must contain definitions, meanings, and interrelationships of all objects stored in the database. This ontology is then transformed into a well-defined schema that forms the foundation for a relational database of lipids. The LIPID MAPS project is building a robust database of lipids based on the proposed ontology.

Our database will provide structural and functional annotations and have links to relevant protein and gene data. In addition, a universal data format (XML) will be provided to facilitate exportation of the data into other repositories. This database will enable the storage of curated information on lipids in a web-accessible format and will provide a community standard for lipids.

An important database field will be the LIPID ID, a unique 12 character identifier based on the classification scheme described here. The format of the LIPID ID, outlined in **Table 2**, provides a systematic means of assigning unique IDs to lipid molecules and allows for the addition of large numbers of new categories, classes, and subclasses in the future, because a maximum of 100 classes/subclasses (00 to 99) may be specified. The last four characters of the ID constitute a unique identifier within a particular subclass and are randomly assigned. By initially using numeric characters, this allows 9,999 unique IDs per subclass, but with the additional use of 26 uppercase alphabetic characters, a total of 1.68 million possible combinations can be generated, providing ample scalability within each subclass. In cases in which lipid structures are obtained from other sources such as LipidBank or LIPIDAT, the corresponding IDs for those databases will be included to enable cross-referencing. The first two characters of the ID contain the database identifier (e.g., LM for LIPID MAPS), although other databases may choose to use their own two character identifier (at present, LB for Lipid Bank and LD for LIPIDAT) and assign the last four or more characters uniquely while retaining characters 3 to 8, which pertain to classification. The corresponding IDs of the other databases will always be included to enable cross-referencing. Further details regarding the numbering system will be decided by the International Lipids Classification and Nomenclature Committee (see below). In addition to the LIPID ID, each lipid in the database will be searchable

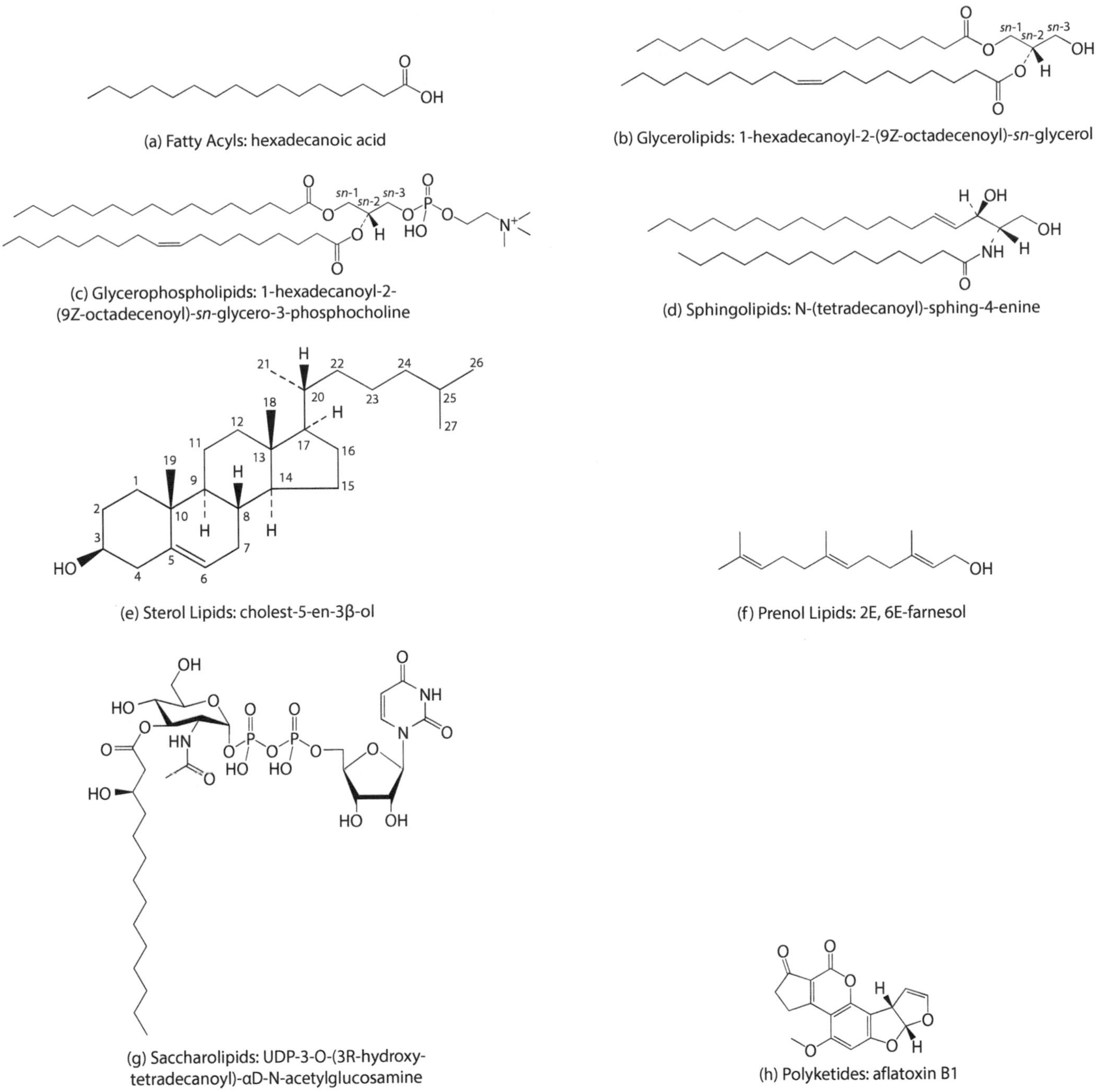

(a) Fatty Acyls: hexadecanoic acid

(b) Glycerolipids: 1-hexadecanoyl-2-(9Z-octadecenoyl)-*sn*-glycerol

(c) Glycerophospholipids: 1-hexadecanoyl-2-(9Z-octadecenoyl)-*sn*-glycero-3-phosphocholine

(d) Sphingolipids: N-(tetradecanoyl)-sphing-4-enine

(e) Sterol Lipids: cholest-5-en-3β-ol

(f) Prenol Lipids: 2E, 6E-farnesol

(g) Saccharolipids: UDP-3-O-(3R-hydroxy-tetradecanoyl)-αD-N-acetylglucosamine

(h) Polyketides: aflatoxin B1

FIGURE 1 Representative structures for each lipid category.

TABLE 2: Format of 12 Character LIPID ID

Characters	Description	Example
1–2	Fixed database designation	LM
3–4	Two letter category code	FA
5–6	Two digit class code	03
7–8	Two digit subclass code	02
9–12	Unique four character identifier within subclass	7312

TABLE 3: Shorthand Notation for Selected Lipid Categories

Category	Abbreviation	Class or Subclass	Example[a]
GP	GPCho	Glycerophosphocholines	GPCho (16:0/9Z,12Z-18:2)
GP	GPnCho	Glycerophosphonocholines	
GP	GPEtn	Glycerophosphoethanolamines	
GP	GPnEtn	Glycerophosphonoethanolamines	
GP	GPSer	Glycerophosphoserines	
GP	GPGro	Glycerophosphoglycerols	
GP	GPGroP	Glycerophosphoglycerophosphates	
GP	GPIns	Glycerophosphoinositols	
GP	GPInsP	Glycerophosphoinositol monophosphates	
GP	GPInsP$_2$	Glycerophosphoinositol bis-phosphates	
GP	GPInsP$_3$	Glycerophosphoinositol tris-phosphates	
GP	GPA	Glycerophosphates	
GP	GPP	Glyceropyrophosphates	
GP	CL	Glycerophosphoglycerophosphoglycerols	
GP	CDP-DG	CDP-glycerols	
GP	[glycan] GP	Glycerophosphoglucose lipids	
GP	[glycan] GPIns	Glycerophosphoinositolglycans	EtN-P-6Manα1–2Manα1–6 Manα1–4GlcNα1–6GPIns (14:0/14:0)
SP	Cer	Ceramides	Cer (d18:1/9E-16:1)
SP	SM	Phosphosphingolipids	SM (d18:1/24:0)
SP	[glycan]Cer	Glycosphingolipids	NeuAcα2–3Galβ1–4Glcβ-Cer (d18:1/16:0)
GL	MG	Monoradyl glycerols	MG (16:0/0:0/0:0)
GL	DG	Diradyl glycerols	DG (18:0/16:0/0:0)
GL	TG	Triradyl glycerols	TG (12:0/14:0/18:0)

[a] Shorthand notation for radyl substituents in categories GP and GL are presented in the order of sn-1 to sn-3. Shorthand notation for category SP is presented in the order of long-chain base and N-acyl substituent. Numbers separated by colons refer to carbon chain length and number of double bonds, respectively.

by classification (category, class, subclass), systematic name, synonym(s), molecular formula, molecular weight, and many other parameters that are part of its ontology. An important feature will be the databasing of molecular structures, allowing the user to perform web-based substructure searches and structure retrieval across the database. This aim will be accomplished with a chemistry cartridge software component that will enable structures in formats such as MDL molfile and Chemdraw CDX to be imported directly into Oracle database tables.

Furthermore, many lipids, in particular the glycerolipids, glycerophospholipids, and sphingolipids, may be conveniently described in terms of a shorthand name in which abbreviations are used to define backbones, head groups, and sugar units and the radyl substituents are defined by a descriptor indicating carbon chain length and number of double bonds. These shorthand names lend themselves to fast, efficient text-based searches and are used widely in lipid research as compact alternatives to systematic names. The glycerophospholipids in the LIPIDAT database, for example, may be conveniently searched with a shorthand notation that has been extended to handle side chains with acyl, ether, branched-chain, and other functional groups (7). We propose the use of a shorthand notation for selected lipid categories (**Table 3**) that incorporates a condensed text nomenclature for glycan substituents. The abbreviations for the sugar units follow the current IUPAC-IUBMB recommendations (4).

Lipid Classes and Subclasses

Fatty Acyls [FA]

The fatty acyl structure represents the major lipid building block of complex lipids and therefore is one of the most fundamental categories of biological lipids. The fatty acyl group in the fatty acids and conjugates class (**Table 4**) is characterized by a repeating series of methylene groups that impart hydrophobic character to this category of lipids. The first subclass includes the straight-chain saturated fatty acids containing a terminal carboxylic acid. It could also be considered the most reduced end product of the polyketide pathway. Variants of this structure have one or more methyl substituents and encompass quite complex branched-chain fatty acids, such as the mycolic acids. The longest chain in branched-chain fatty acids defines the chain length of these compounds. A considerable number of variations on this basic structure occur in all kingdoms of life (9–12), including fatty acids with one or more double bonds and even acetylenic (triple) bonds. Heteroatoms of oxygen, halogen, nitrogen, and sulfur are also linked to the carbon chains in specific subclasses. Cyclic fatty acids containing three to six carbon atoms as well as heterocyclic rings containing oxygen or nitrogen are found in nature. The cyclopentenyl fatty acids are an example of this latter subclass. The thia fatty acid subclass contains sulfur atom(s) in the fatty acid structure and is exemplified by lipoic acid and biotin. Thiols and thioethers are in this class, but the thioesters are placed in the ester class because of the involvement of these and similar esters in fatty acid metabolism and synthesis.

Separate classes for more complex fatty acids with multiple functional groups (but nonbranched) are designated by the total number of carbon atoms found in the critical biosynthetic precursor. These include octadecanoids and lipids in the jasmonic acid pathway of plant hormone biosynthesis, even though jasmonic acids have lost some of their carbon atoms from the biochemical precursor, 12-oxophytodienoic acid (13). Eicosanoids derived from arachidonic acid include prostaglandins, leukotrienes, and other structural derivatives (14). The docosanoids contain 22 carbon atoms and derive from a common precursor, docosahexaenoic acid (15). Many members of these separate subclasses of more complex fatty acids have distinct biological activities.

TABLE 4: Fatty acyls [FA] Classes and Subclasses

Fatty acids and conjugates [FA01]
   Straight-chain fatty acids [FA0101]
   Methyl branched fatty acids [FA0102]
   Unsaturated fatty acids [FA0103]
   Hydroperoxy fatty acids [FA0104]
   Hydroxy fatty acids [FA0105]
   Oxo fatty acids [FA0106]
   Epoxy fatty acids [FA0107]
   Methoxy fatty acids [FA0108]
   Halogenated fatty acids [FA0109]
   Amino fatty acids [FA0110]
   Cyano fatty acids [FA0111]
   Nitro fatty acids [FA0112]
   Thia fatty acids [FA0113]
   Carbocyclic fatty acids [FA0114]
   Heterocyclic fatty acids [FA0115]
   Mycolic acids [FA0116]
   Dicarboxylic acids [FA0117]
Octadecanoids [FA02]
   12-Oxophytodienoic acid metabolites [FA0201]
   Jasmonic acids [FA0202]
Eicosanoids [FA03]
   Prostaglandins [FA0301]
   Leukotrienes [FA0302]
   Thromboxanes [FA0303]
   Lipoxins [FA0304]
   Hydroxyeicosatrienoic acids [FA0305]
   Hydroxyeicosatetraenoic acids [FA0306]
   Hydroxyeicosapentaenoic acids [FA0307]
   Epoxyeicosatrienoic acids [FA0308]
   Hepoxilins [FA0309]
   Levuglandins [FA0310]
   Isoprostanes [FA0311]
   Clavulones [FA0312]
Docosanoids [FA04]
Fatty alcohols [FA05]
Fatty aldehydes [FA06]
Fatty esters [FA07]
   Wax monoesters [FA0701]
   Wax diesters [FA0702]
   Cyano esters [FA0703]
   Lactones [FA0704]
   Fatty acyl-CoAs [FA0705]
   Fatty acyl-acyl carrier proteins (ACPs) [FA0706]
   Fatty acyl carnitines [FA0707]
   Fatty acyl adenylates [FA0708]
Fatty amides [FA08]
   Primary amides [FA0801]
   N-Acyl amides [FA0802]
   Fatty acyl homoserine lactones [FA0803]
   N-Acyl ethanolamines (endocannabinoids) [FA0804]
Fatty nitriles [FA09]
Fatty ethers [FA10]
Hydrocarbons [FA11]
Oxygenated hydrocarbons [FA12]
Other [FA00]

TABLE 5: Glycerolipids [GL] Classes and Subclasses

Monoradylglycerols [GL01]
   Monoacylglycerols [GL0101]
   Monoalkylglycerols [GL0102]
   Mono-(1 *Z*-alkenyl)-glycerols [GL0103]
   Monoacylglycerolglycosides [GL0104]
   Monoalkylglycerolglycosides [GL0105]
Diradylglycerols [GL02]
   Diacylglycerols [GL0201]
   Alkylacylglycerols [GL0202]
   Dialkylglycerols [GL0203]
   1 *Z*-Alkenylacylglycerols [GL0204]
   Diacylglycerolglycosides [GL0205]
   Alkylacylglycerolglycosides [GL0206]
   Dialkylglycerolglycosides [GL0207]
   Di-glycerol tetraethers [GL0208]
   Di-glycerol tetraether glycans [GL0209]
Triradylglycerols [GL03]
   Triacylglycerols [GL0301]
   Alkyldiacylglycerols [GL0302]
   Dialkylmonoacylglycerols [GL0303]
   1 *Z*-Alkenyldiacylglycerols [GL0304]
   Estolides [GL0305]
Other [GL00]

adenylates, which are mixed anhydrides. The fatty alcohols and fatty aldehydes are typified by terminal hydroxy and oxo groups, respectively. The fatty amides are also *N*-fatty acylated amines and unsubstituted amides, and many simple amides have interesting biological activities in various organisms. Fatty acyl homoserine lactones are fatty amides involved in bacterial quorum sensing (16).

Hydrocarbons are included as a class of fatty acid derivatives because they correspond to six electron reduction products of fatty acids that may have been generated by loss of the carboxylic acid from a fatty acid or fatty acyl moiety during the process of diagenesis in geological samples. Long-chain ethers also have been observed in nature. Chemical structures of the fatty acyls are shown in **Figure 2**.

Glycerolipids [GL]

The glycerolipids essentially encompass all glycerol-containing lipids. We have purposely made glycerophospholipids a separate category because of their abundance and importance as membrane constituents, metabolic fuels, and signaling molecules. The glycerolipid category (**Table 5**) is dominated by the mono-, di- and tri-substituted glycerols, the most well-known being the fatty acid esters of glycerol (acylglycerols) (17, 18). Additional subclasses are represented by the glycerolglycans, which are characterized by the presence of one or more sugar residues attached to glycerol via a glycosidic linkage (19). Examples of structures in this category are shown in **Figure 3**. Macrocyclic ether lipids also occur as glycerolipids in the membranes of archaebacteria (20).

Glycerophospholipids [GP]

The glycerophospholipids are ubiquitous in nature and are key components of the lipid bilayer of cells. Phospholipids may be subdivided into distinct classes (**Table 6**) based on the nature of the polar "head group" at the *sn*-3 position of the glycerol backbone in eukaryotes and eu-bacteria or the *sn*-1 position in the case of archaebacteria (21). In the case of the glycerophosphoglycerols and glycerophosphoglycerophosphates, a second glycerol unit constitutes part of the head group, whereas for the

Other major lipid classes in the fatty acyl category include fatty acid esters such as wax monoesters and diesters and the lactones. The fatty ester class also has subclasses that include important biochemical intermediates such as fatty acyl thioester-CoA derivatives, fatty acyl thioester-acyl carrier protein (ACP) derivatives, fatty acyl carnitines (esters of carnitine), and fatty

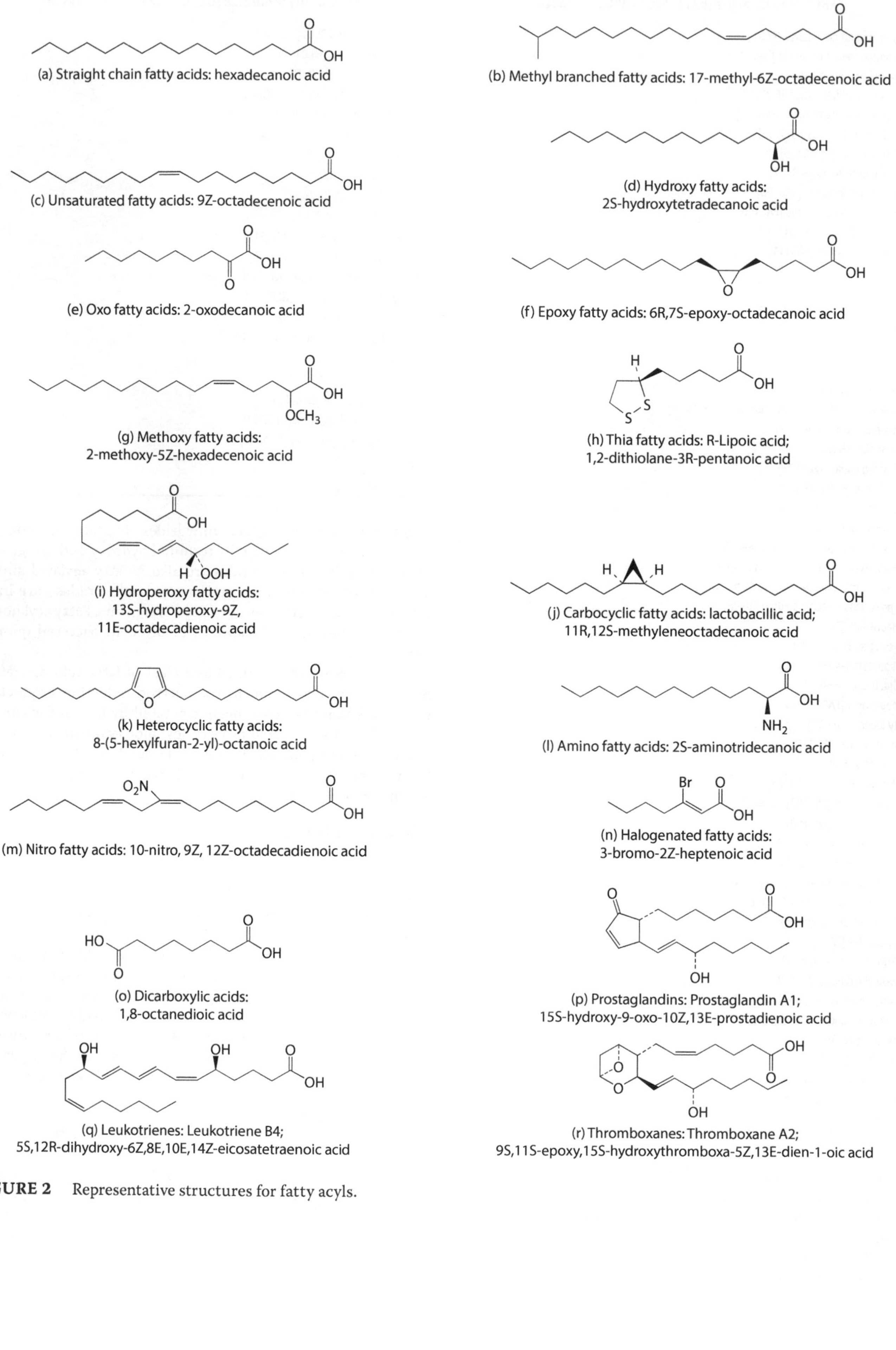

(a) Straight chain fatty acids: hexadecanoic acid

(b) Methyl branched fatty acids: 17-methyl-6Z-octadecenoic acid

(c) Unsaturated fatty acids: 9Z-octadecenoic acid

(d) Hydroxy fatty acids:
2S-hydroxytetradecanoic acid

(e) Oxo fatty acids: 2-oxodecanoic acid

(f) Epoxy fatty acids: 6R,7S-epoxy-octadecanoic acid

(g) Methoxy fatty acids:
2-methoxy-5Z-hexadecenoic acid

(h) Thia fatty acids: R-Lipoic acid;
1,2-dithiolane-3R-pentanoic acid

(i) Hydroperoxy fatty acids:
13S-hydroperoxy-9Z,
11E-octadecadienoic acid

(j) Carbocyclic fatty acids: lactobacillic acid;
11R,12S-methyleneoctadecanoic acid

(k) Heterocyclic fatty acids:
8-(5-hexylfuran-2-yl)-octanoic acid

(l) Amino fatty acids: 2S-aminotridecanoic acid

(m) Nitro fatty acids: 10-nitro, 9Z, 12Z-octadecadienoic acid

(n) Halogenated fatty acids:
3-bromo-2Z-heptenoic acid

(o) Dicarboxylic acids:
1,8-octanedioic acid

(p) Prostaglandins: Prostaglandin A1;
15S-hydroxy-9-oxo-10Z,13E-prostadienoic acid

(q) Leukotrienes: Leukotriene B4;
5S,12R-dihydroxy-6Z,8E,10E,14Z-eicosatetraenoic acid

(r) Thromboxanes: Thromboxane A2;
9S,11S-epoxy,15S-hydroxythromboxa-5Z,13E-dien-1-oic acid

FIGURE 2   Representative structures for fatty acyls.

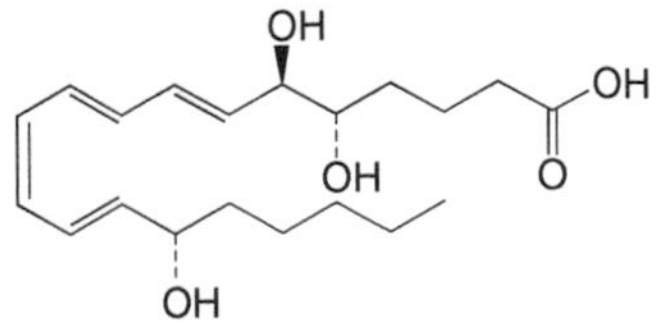

(s) Lipoxins: Lipoxin A4;
5S,6R,15S-trihydroxy-7E,9E,11Z,13E-eicosatetraenoic acid

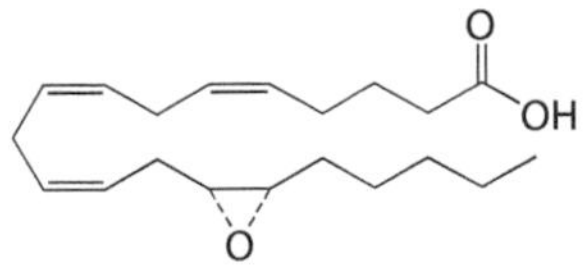

(t) Epoxyeicosatrienoic acids:
14R,15S-epoxy-5Z,8Z,11Z-eicosatrienoic acid

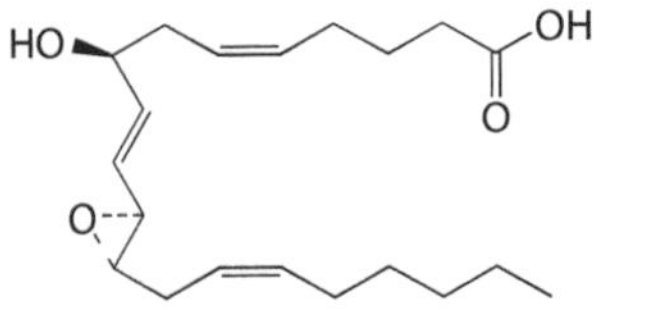

(u) Hepoxilins: Hepoxilin A3;
8R-hydroxy-11R,12S-epoxy-5Z,9E,14Z-eicosatrienoic acid

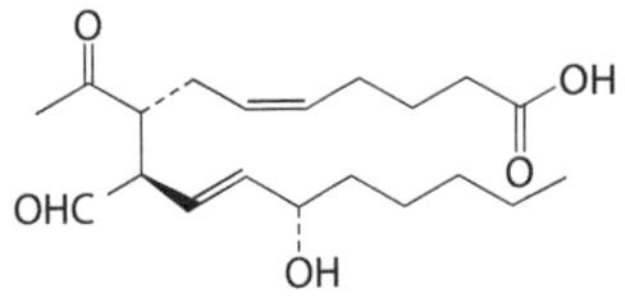

(v) Levuglandins: LGE2;
10,11-seco-9,11-dioxo-15S-hydroxy-5Z,13E-prostadienoic acid

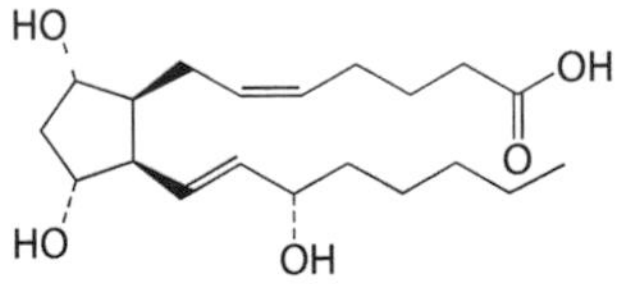

(w) Isoprostanes: 9S,11S,15S-trihydroxy-5Z,
13E-prostadienoic acid-cyclo[8S,12R]

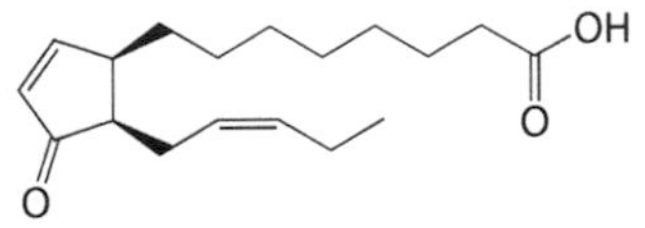

(x) Octadecanoids: 12-oxophytodienoic acid metabolites;
(9R,13R)-12-oxo-phyto-10Z,15Z-dienoic acid

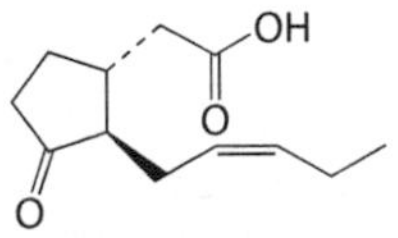

(y) Octadecanoids: Jasmonic acids: jasmonic acid;
(1R,2R)-3-oxo-2-(pent-2Z-enyl)-cyclopentaneacetic acid

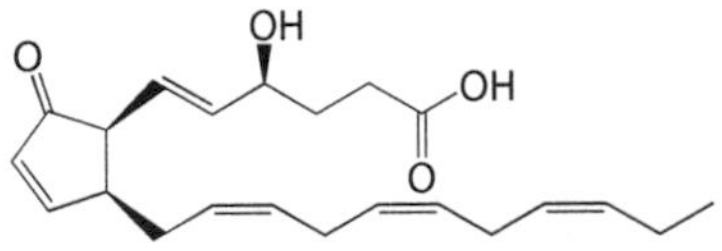

(z) Docosanoids: Neuroprostanes; 4S-hydroxy-8-oxo-
(5E,9Z,13Z,16Z,19Z)-neuroprostapentaenoic acid-cyclo[7S,11S]

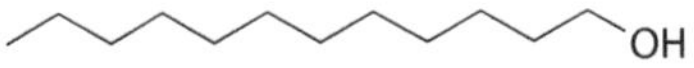

(aa) Fatty alcohols: dodecanol

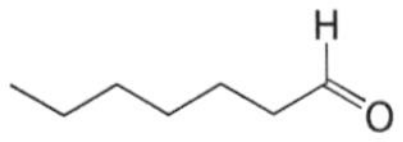

(ab) Fatty aldehydes: heptanal

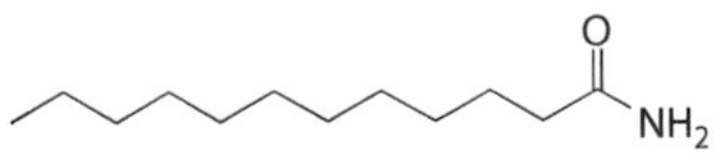

(ac) Fatty amides: N-acyl amides: dodecanamide

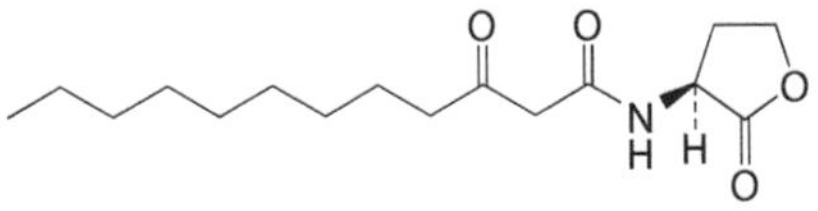

(ad) Fatty amides: Fatty acyl homoserine lactones:
N-(3-oxodecanoyl) homoserine lactone

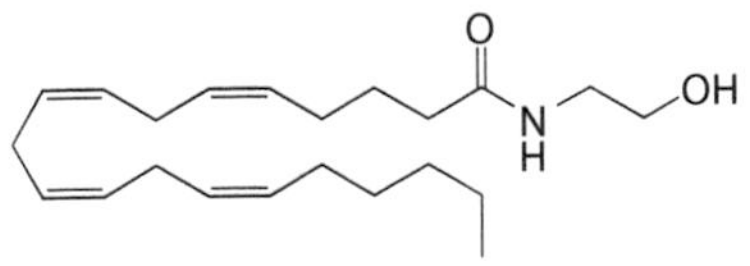

(ae) Fatty amides: N-acyl ethanolamides (endocannabinoids):
Anandamide; N-(5Z,8Z,11Z,14Z-eicosatetraenoyl)-ethanolamine

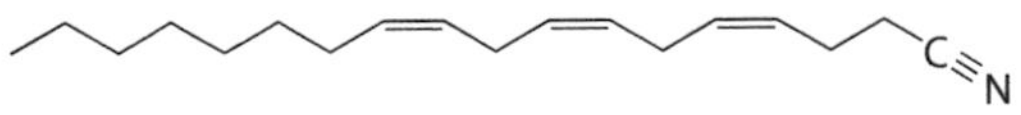

(af) Fatty nitriles: 4Z,7Z,10Z-octadecatrienenitrile

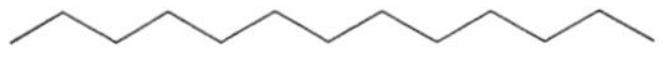

(ag) Hydrocarbons: tridecane

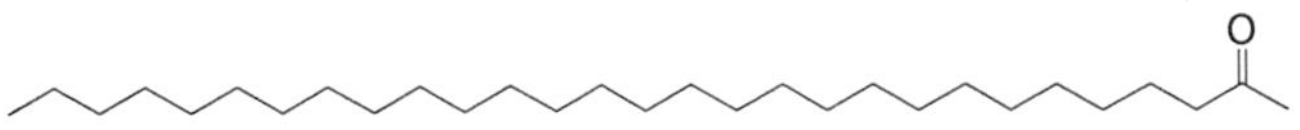

(ah) Oxygenated hydrocarbons: nonacosan-2-one

FIGURE 2 Representative structures for fatty acyls (Continued).

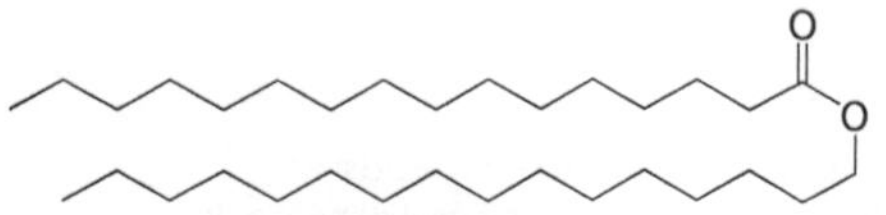

(ai) Wax monoesters:
1-hexadecyl hexadecanoate

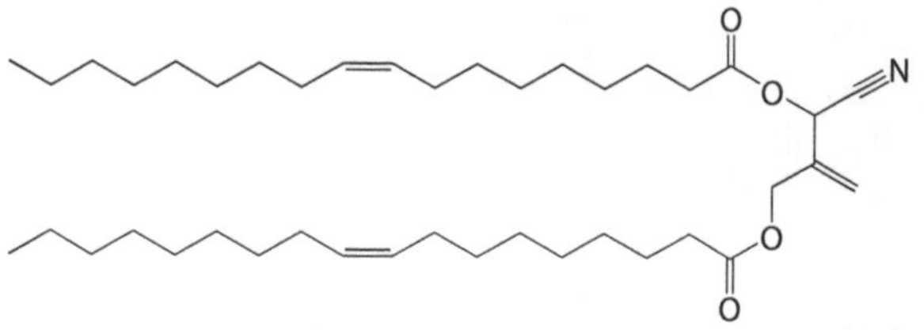

(aj) Cyano esters: 1,3-di-(octadec-9Z-enoyl)-1-cyano-2-
methylene-propane-1,3-diol

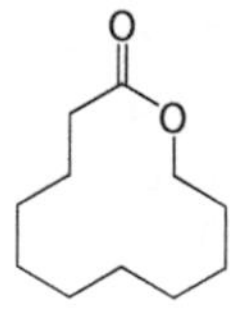

(ak) Lactones:
11-undecanolactone

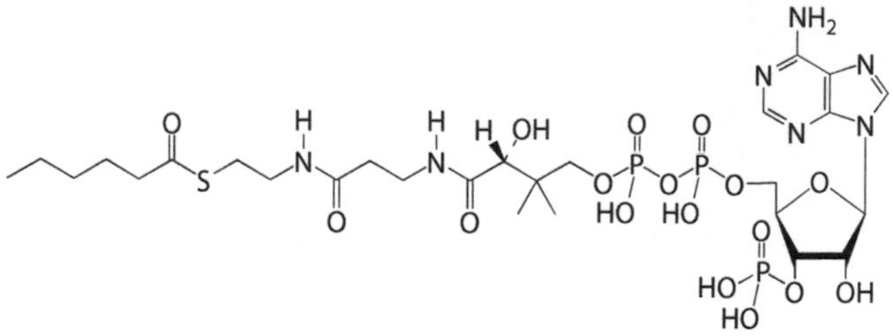

(al) Fatty acyl CoAs: R-hexanoyl CoA

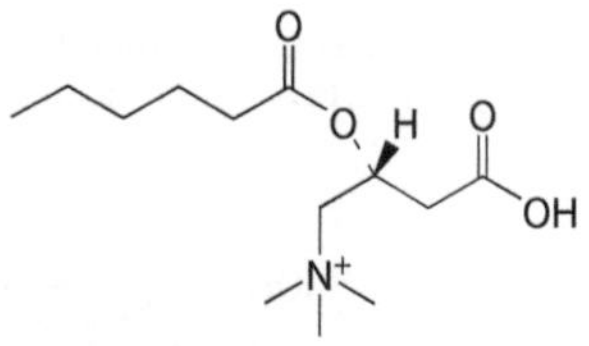

(am) Fatty acyl carnitines:
O-hexanoyl-R-carnitine

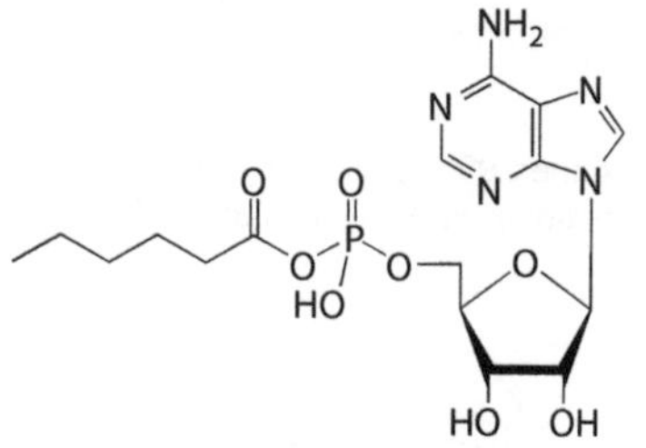

(an) Fatty acyl adenylates:
O-hexanoyladenosine monophosphate

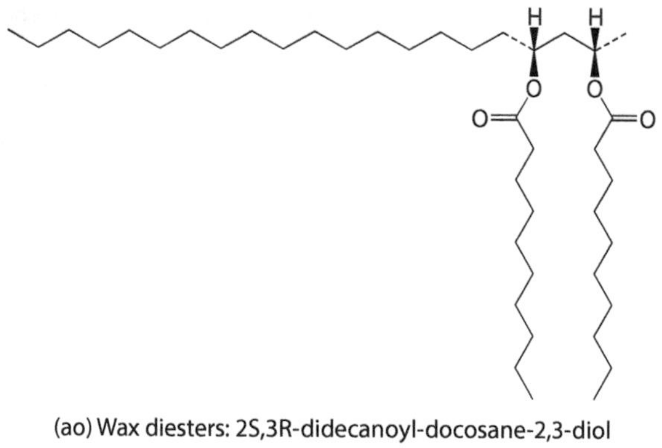

(ao) Wax diesters: 2S,3R-didecanoyl-docosane-2,3-diol

FIGURE 2   Representative structures for fatty acyls (Continued).

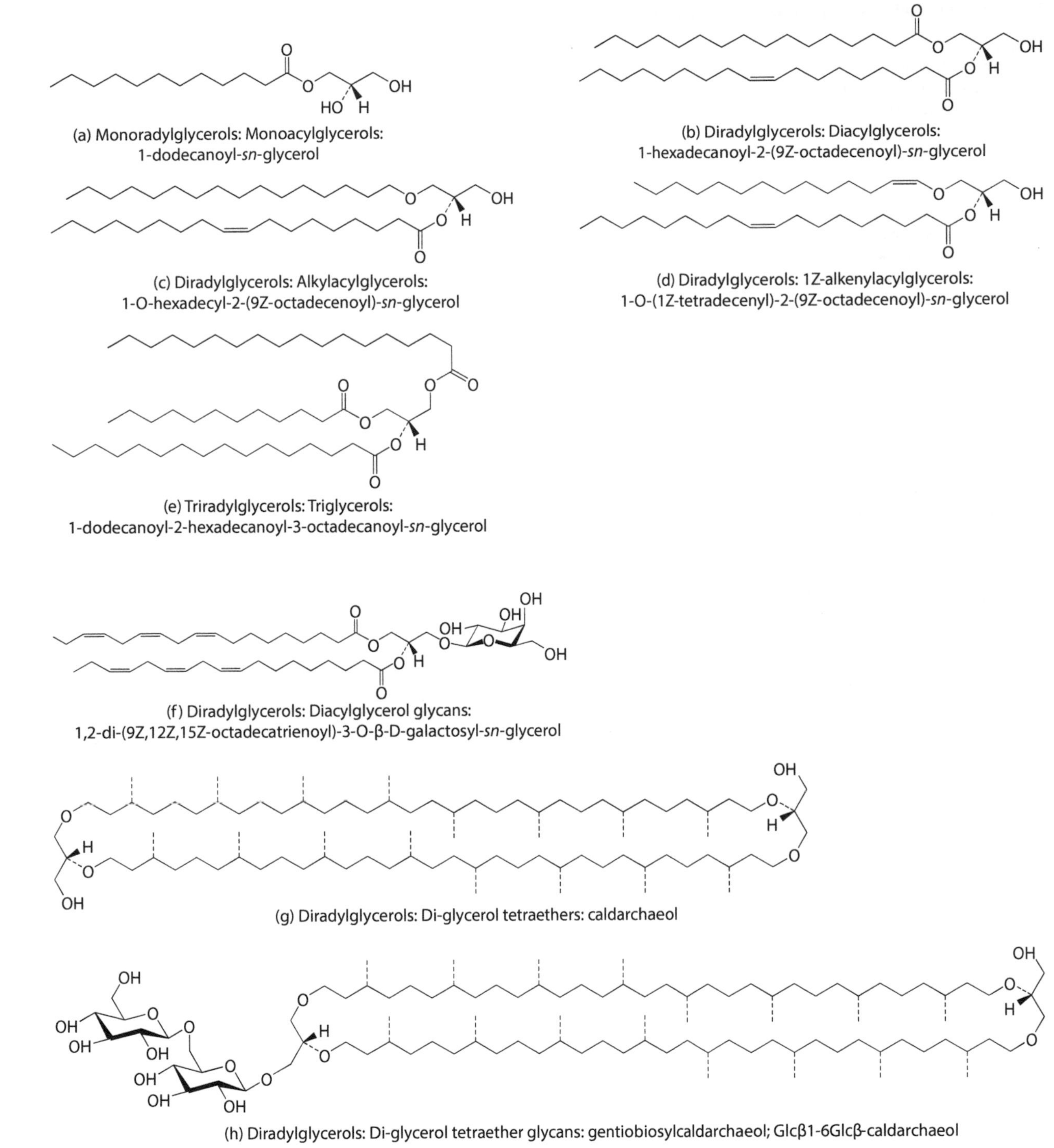

(a) Monoradylglycerols: Monoacylglycerols:
1-dodecanoyl-*sn*-glycerol

(b) Diradylglycerols: Diacylglycerols:
1-hexadecanoyl-2-(9Z-octadecenoyl)-*sn*-glycerol

(c) Diradylglycerols: Alkylacylglycerols:
1-O-hexadecyl-2-(9Z-octadecenoyl)-*sn*-glycerol

(d) Diradylglycerols: 1Z-alkenylacylglycerols:
1-O-(1Z-tetradecenyl)-2-(9Z-octadecenoyl)-*sn*-glycerol

(e) Triradylglycerols: Triglycerols:
1-dodecanoyl-2-hexadecanoyl-3-octadecanoyl-*sn*-glycerol

(f) Diradylglycerols: Diacylglycerol glycans:
1,2-di-(9Z,12Z,15Z-octadecatrienoyl)-3-O-β-D-galactosyl-*sn*-glycerol

(g) Diradylglycerols: Di-glycerol tetraethers: caldarchaeol

(h) Diradylglycerols: Di-glycerol tetraether glycans: gentiobiosylcaldarchaeol; Glcβ1-6Glcβ-caldarchaeol

FIGURE 3   Representative structures for glycerolipids.

TABLE 6:Glycerophospholipids [GP] Classes and Subclasses

Glycerophosphocholines [GP01]
   Diacylglycerophosphocholines [GP0101]
   1-Alkyl,2-acylglycerophosphocholines [GP0102]
   1 Z-Alkenyl,2-acylglycerophosphocholines [GP0103]
   Dialkylglycerophosphocholines [GP0104]
   Monoacylglycerophosphocholines [GP0105]
   1-Alkyl glycerophosphocholines [GP0106]
   1 Z-Alkenylglycerophosphocholines [GP0107]
Glycerophosphoethanolamines [GP02]
   Diacylglycerophosphoethanolamines [GP0201]
   1-Alkyl,2-acylglycerophosphoethanolamines [GP0202]
   1 Z-Alkenyl,2-acylglycerophosphoethanolamines [GP0203]
   Dialkylglycerophosphoethanolamines [GP0204]
   Monoacylglycerophosphoethanolamines [GP0205]
   1-Alkyl glycerophosphoethanolamines [GP0206]
   1 Z-Alkenylglycerophosphoethanolamines [GP0207]
Glycerophosphoserines [GP03]
   Diacylglycerophosphoserines [GP0301]
   1-Alkyl,2-acylglycerophosphoserines [GP0302]
   1 Z-Alkenyl,2-acylglycerophosphoserines [GP0303]
   Dialkylglycerophosphoserines [GP0304]
   Monoacylglycerophosphoserines [GP0305]
   1-Alkyl glycerophosphoserines [GP0306]
   1 Z-Alkenylglycerophosphoserines [GP0307]
Glycerophosphoglycerols [GP04]
   Diacylglycerophosphoglycerols [GP0401]
   1-Alkyl,2-acylglycerophosphoglycerols [GP0402]
   1 Z-Alkenyl,2-acylglycerophosphoglycerols [GP0403]
   Dialkylglycerophosphoglycerols [GP0404]
   Monoacylglycerophosphoglycerols [GP0405]
   1-Alkyl glycerophosphoglycerols [GP0406]
   1 Z-Alkenylglycerophosphoglycerols [GP0407]
   Diacylglycerophosphodiradylglycerols [GP0408]
   Diacylglycerophosphomonoradylglycerols [GP0409]
   Monoacylglycerophosphomonoradylglycerols [GP0410]
Glycerophosphoglycerophosphates [GP05]
   Diacylglycerophosphoglycerophosphates [GP0501]
   1-Alkyl,2-acylglycerophosphoglycerophosphates [GP0502]
   1 Z-Alkenyl,2-acylglycerophosphoglycerophosphates [GP0503]
   Dialkylglycerophosphoglycerophosphates [GP0504]
   Monoacylglycerophosphoglycerophosphates [GP0505]
   1-Alkyl glycerophosphoglycerophosphates [GP0506]
   1 Z-Alkenylglycerophosphoglycerophosphates [GP0507]
Glycerophosphoinositols [GP06]
   Diacylglycerophosphoinositols [GP0601]
   1-Alkyl,2-acylglycerophosphoinositols [GP0602]
   1 Z-Alkenyl,2-acylglycerophosphoinositols [GP0603]
   Dialkylglycerophosphoinositols [GP0604]
   Monoacylglycerophosphoinositols [GP0605]
   1-Alkyl glycerophosphoinositols [GP0606]
   1 Z-Alkenylglycerophosphoinositols [GP0607]
Glycerophosphoinositol monophosphates [GP07]
   Diacylglycerophosphoinositol monophosphates [GP0701]
   1-Alkyl,2-acylglycerophosphoinositol monophosphates [GP0702]
   1 Z-Alkenyl,2-acylglycerophosphoinositol monophosphates [GP0703]
   Dialkylglycerophosphoinositol monophosphates [GP0704]
   Monoacylglycerophosphoinositol monophosphates [GP0705]
   1-Alkyl glycerophosphoinositol monophosphates [GP0706]
   1 Z-Alkenylglycerophosphoinositol monophosphates [GP0707]
Glycerophosphoinositol bisphosphates [GP08]
   Diacylglycerophosphoinositol bisphosphates [GP0801]
   1-Alkyl,2-acylglycerophosphoinositol bisphosphates [GP0802]
   1 Z-Alkenyl,2-acylglycerophosphoinositol bisphosphates [GP0803]
   Monoacylglycerophosphoinositol bisphosphates [GP0804]
   1-Alkyl glycerophosphoinositol bisphosphates [GP0805]
   1 Z-Alkenylglycerophosphoinositol bisphosphates [GP0806]
Glycerophosphoinositol trisphosphates [GP09]
   Diacylglycerophosphoinositol trisphosphates [GP0901]

TABLE 6: Glycerophospholipids [GP] Classes and Subclasses (Continued)

   1-Alkyl,2-acylglycerophosphoinositol trisphosphates [GP0902]
   1 Z-Alkenyl,2-acylglycerophosphoinositol trisphosphates [GP0903]
   Monoacylglycerophosphoinositol trisphosphates [GP0904]
   1-Alkyl glycerophosphoinositol trisphosphates [GP0905]
   1 Z-Alkenylglycerophosphoinositol trisphosphates [GP0906]
Glycerophosphates [GP10]
   Diacylglycerophosphates [GP1001]
   1-Alkyl,2-acylglycerophosphates [GP 1002]
   1 Z-Alkenyl,2-acylglycerophosphates [GP1003]
   Dialkylglycerophosphates [GP 1004]
   Monoacylglycerophosphates [GP1005]
   1-Alkyl glycerophosphates [GP1006]
   1 Z-Alkenylglycerophosphates [GP1007]
Glyceropyrophosphates [GP11]
   Diacylglyceropyrophosphates [GP 1101]
   Monoacylglyceropyrophosphates [GP1102]
Glycerophosphoglycerophosphoglycerols (cardiolipins) [GP12]
   Diacylglycerophosphoglycerophosphodiradylglycerols [GP1201]
   Diacylglycerophosphoglycerophosphomonoradylglycerols [GP1202]
   1-Alkyl,2-acylglycerophosphoglycerophosphodiradylglycerols [GP1203]
   1-Alkyl,2-acylglycerophosphoglycerophosphomonoradylglycerols [GP1204]
   1 Z-Alkenyl,2-acylglycerophosphoglycerophosphodiradylglycerols [GP1205]
   1 Z-Alkenyl,2-acylglycerophosphoglycerophosphomonoradylglycerols [GP1206]
   Monoacylglycerophosphoglycerophosphomonoradylglycerols [GP1207]
   1-Alkyl glycerophosphoglycerophosphodiradylglycerols [GP1208]
   1-Alkyl glycerophosphoglycerophosphomonoradylglycerols [GP1209]
   1 Z-Alkenylglycerophosphoglycerophosphodiradylglycerols [GP1210]
   1 Z-Alkenylglycerophosphoglycerophosphomonoradylglycerols [GP1211]
CDP-glycerols [GP13]
   CDP-diacylglycerols [GP1301]
   CDP-1-alkyl,2-acylglycerols [GP1302]
   CDP-1 Z-alkenyl,2-acylglycerols [GP1303]
   CDP-dialkylglycerols [GP1304]
   CDP-monoacylglycerols [GP1305]
   CDP-1-alkyl glycerols [GP1306]
   CDP-1 Z-alkenylglycerols [GP1307]
Glycerophosphoglucose lipids [GP14]
   Diacylglycerophosphoglucose lipids [GP1401]
   1-Alkyl,2-acylglycerophosphoglucose lipids [GP1402]
   1 Z-Alkenyl,2-acylglycerophosphoglucose lipids [GP1403]
   Monoacylglycerophosphoglucose lipids [GP1404]
   1-Alkyl glycerophosphoglucose lipids [GP1405]
   1 Z-Alkenylglycerophosphoglucose lipids [GP1406]
Glycerophosphoinositolglycans [GP15]
   Diacylglycerophosphoinositolglycans [GP 1501]
   1-Alkyl,2-acylglycerophosphoinositolglycans [GP1502]
   1 Z-Alkenyl,2-acylglycerophosphoinositolglycans [GP1503]
   Monoacylglycerophosphoinositolglycans [GP1504]
   1-Alkyl glycerophosphoinositolglycans [GP1505]
   1 Z-Alkenylglycerophosphoinositolglycans [GP1506]
Glycerophosphonocholines [GP16]
   Diacylglycerophosphonocholines [GP 1601]
   1-Alkyl,2-acylglycerophosphonocholines [GP1602]
   1 Z-Alkenyl,2-acylglycerophosphonocholines [GP1603]
   Dialkylglycerophosphonocholines [GP1604]
   Monoacylglycerophosphonocholines [GP1605]
   1-Alkyl glycerophosphonocholines [GP1606]
   1 Z-Alkenylglycerophosphonocholines [GP1607]
Glycerophosphonoethanolamines [GP 17]
   Diacylglycerophosphonoethanolamines [GP1701]
   1-Alkyl,2-acylglycerophosphonoethanolamines [GP1702]
   1 Z-Alkenyl,2-acylglycerophosphonoethanolamines [GP1703]
   Dialkylglycerophosphonoethanolamines [GP 1704]
   Monoacylglycerophosphonoethanolamines [GP1705]
   1-Alkyl glycerophosphonoethanolamines [GP1706]
   1 Z-Alkenylglycerophosphonoethanolamines [GP1707]
Di-glycerol tetraether phospholipids (caldarchaeols) [GP18]
Glycerol-nonitol tetraether phospholipids [GP19]
Oxidized glycerophospholipids [GP20]
Other [GP00]

glycerophosphoglycerophosphoglycerols (cardiolipins), a third glycerol unit is typically acylated at the *sn*-1' and *sn*-2' positions to create a pseudosymmetrical molecule. Each head group class is further differentiated on the basis of the *sn*-1 and *sn*-2 substituents on the glycerol backbone. Although the glycerol backbone is symmetrical, the second carbon becomes a chiral center when the *sn*-1 and *sn*-3 carbons have different substituents. A large number of trivial names are associated with phospholipids. In the systematic nomenclature, mono/di-radylglycerophospholipids with different acyl or alkyl substituents are designated by similar conventions for naming of classes (see below) and are grouped according to the common polar moieties (i.e., head groups).

Typically, one or both of these hydroxyl groups are acylated with long-chain fatty acids, but there are also alkyl-linked and 1 Z-alkenyl-linked (plasmalogen) glycerophospholipids, as well as dialkylether variants in prokaryotes. The main biosynthetic pathways for the formation of GPCho and GPEtn (see Table 3 for shorthand notation) were elucidated through the efforts of Kennedy and co-workers (22) in the 1950s and 1960s, and more detailed interconversion pathways to form additional classes of phospholipids were described more recently. In addition to serving as a primary component of cellular membranes and binding sites for intracellular and intercellular proteins, some glycerophospholipids in eukaryotic cells are either precursors of, or are themselves, membrane-derived second messengers. A separate class, called oxidized glycerophospholipids, is composed of molecules in which one or more of the side chains have been oxidized. Several overviews are available on the classification, nomenclature, metabolism, and profiling of glycerophospholipids (18, 23–26). Structures from this category are shown in **Figure 4**.

Sphingolipids [SP]

Sphingolipids are a complex family of compounds that share a common structural feature, a sphingoid base backbone that is synthesized de novo from serine and a long-chain fatty acyl-CoA, then converted into ceramides, phosphosphingolipids, glycosphingolipids, and other species, including protein adducts (27, 28). A number of organisms also produce sphingoid base analogs that have many of the same features as sphingolipids (such as long-chain alkyl and vicinal amino and hydroxyl groups) but differ in other features. These have been included in this category because some are known to function as inhibitors or antagonists of sphingolipids, and in some organisms, these types of compounds may serve as surrogates for sphingolipids.

Sphingolipids can be divided into several major classes (**Table 7**): the sphingoid bases and their simple derivatives (such as the 1-phosphate), the sphingoid bases with an amide-linked fatty acid (e.g., ceramides), and more complex sphingolipids with head groups that are attached via phosphodiester linkages (the phosphosphingolipids), via glycosidic bonds (the simple and complex glycosphingolipids such as cerebrosides and gangliosides), and other groups (such as phosphono- and arseno-sphingolipids). The IUPAC has recommended a systematic nomenclature for sphingolipids (3).

The major sphingoid base of mammals is commonly referred to as "sphingosine," because that name was affixed by the first scientist to isolate this compound (29). Sphingosine is (2S,3R,4E)-2-aminooctadec-4-ene-1,3-diol (it is also called D-*erythro*-sphingosine and sphing-4-enine). This is only one of many sphingoid bases found in nature, which vary in alkyl chain length and branching, the number and positions of double bonds, the presence of additional hydroxyl groups, and other features. The structural variation has functional significance; for

example, sphingoid bases in the dermis have additional hydroxyls at position 4 (phytoceramides) and/or 6 that can interact with neighboring molecules, thereby strengthening the permeability barrier of skin. Sphingoid bases are found in a variety of derivatives, including the 1-phosphates, lyso-sphingolipids (such as sphingosine 1-phosphocholine as well as sphingosine 1-glycosides), and N-methyl derivatives (N-methyl, N,N-dimethyl, and N,N,N-trimethyl). In addition, a large number of organisms, such as fungi and sponges, produce compounds with structural similarity to sphingoid bases, some of which (such as myriocin and the fumonisins) are potent inhibitors of enzymes of sphingolipid metabolism.

Ceramides (N-acyl-sphingoid bases) are a major subclass of sphingoid base derivatives with an amide-linked fatty acid. The fatty acids are typically saturated or monounsaturated with chain lengths from 14 to 26 carbon atoms; the presence of a hydroxyl group on carbon 2 is fairly common. Ceramides sometimes have specialized fatty acids, as illustrated by the skin ceramide in **Figure 5i**, which has a 30 carbon fatty acid with a hydroxyl group on the terminal (ω) carbon. Ceramides are generally precursors of more complex sphingolipids. The major phosphosphingolipids of mammals are sphingomyelins (ceramide phosphocholines), whereas insects contain mainly ceramide phosphoethanolamines and fungi have phytoceramidephosphoinositols and mannose-containing head groups.

Glycosphingolipids (4) are classified on the basis of carbohydrate composition: 1) neutral glycosphingolipids contain one or more uncharged sugars such as glucose (Glu), galactose (Gal), N-acetylglucosamine (GlcNAc), N-acetylgalactosamine (GalNAc), and fucose (Fuc), which are grouped into families based on the nature of the glyco-substituents as shown in the listing; 2) acidic glycosphingolipids contain ionized functional groups (phosphate or sulfate) attached to neutral sugars or charged sugar residues such as sialic acid (N-acetyl or N-glycoloyl neuraminic acid). The latter are called gangliosides, and the number of sialic acid residues is usually denoted with a subscript letter (i.e., mono-, di- or tri-) plus a number reflecting the subspecies within that category; 3) basic glycosphingolipids; 4) amphoteric glycosphingolipids. For a few glycosphingolipids, historically assigned names as antigens and blood group structures are still in common use (e.g., Lewis x and sialyl Lewis x). Some aquatic organisms contain sphingolipids in which the phosphate is replaced by a phosphono or arsenate group. The other category includes sphingolipids that are covalently attached to proteins; for example, ω-hydroxyceramides and ω-glucosylceramides are attached to surface proteins of skin, and inositol-phosphoceramides are used as membrane anchors for some fungal proteins in a manner analogous to the glycosylphosphatidylinositol anchors that are attached to proteins in other eukaryotes. Some examples of sphingolipid structures are shown in Figure 5.

Sterol Lipids [ST]

The sterol category is subdivided primarily on the basis of biological function. The sterols, of which cholesterol and its derivatives are the most widely studied in mammalian systems, constitute an important component of membrane lipids, along with the glycerophospholipids and sphingomyelins (30). There are many examples of unique sterols from plant, fungal, and marine sources that are designated as distinct subclasses in this schema (**Table 8**). The steroids, which also contain the same fused four ring core structure, have different biological roles as hormones and signaling molecules (31). These are subdivided on the basis of the number of carbons in the core skeleton. The C_{18} steroids

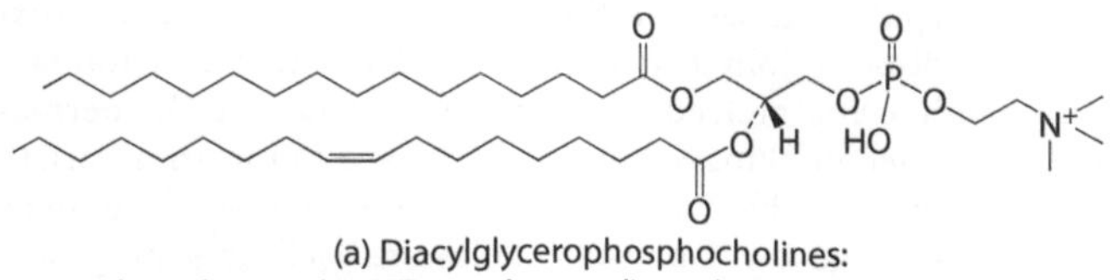

FIGURE 4   Representative structures for glycerophospholipids.

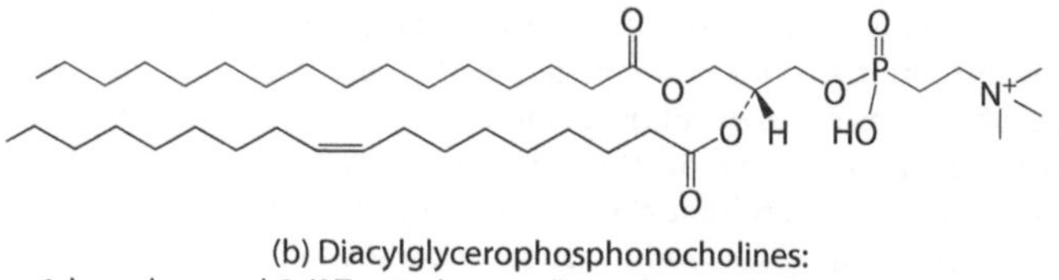

include the estrogen family, whereas the C_{19} steroids comprise the androgens such as testosterone and androsterone. The C_{21} subclass, containing a two carbon side chain at the C_{17} position, includes the progestogens as well as the glucocorticoids and mineralocorticoids. The secosteroids, comprising various forms of vitamin D, are characterized by cleavage of the B ring of the core structure, hence the "seco" prefix (32). Additional classes within the sterols category are the bile acids (33), which in mammals are primarily derivatives of cholan-24-oic acid synthesized from cholesterol in the liver and their conjugates (sulfuric acid, taurine, glycine, glucuronic acid, and others). Sterol lipid structures are shown in **Figure 6**.

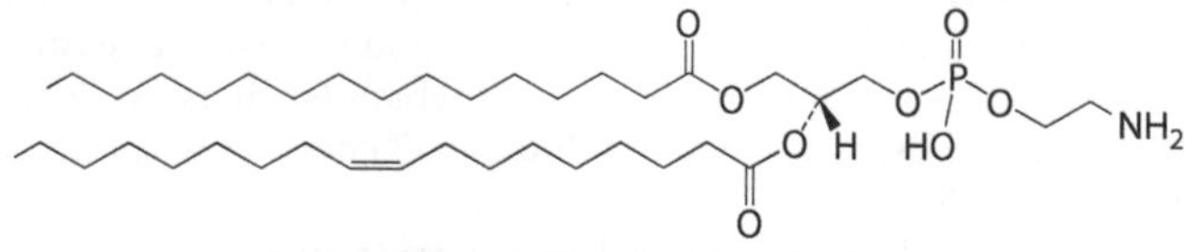

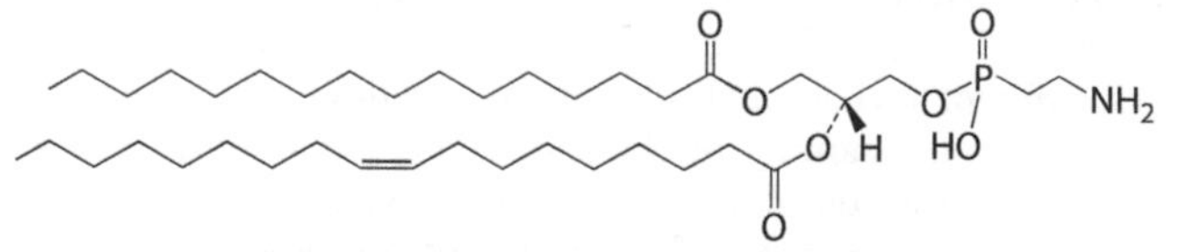

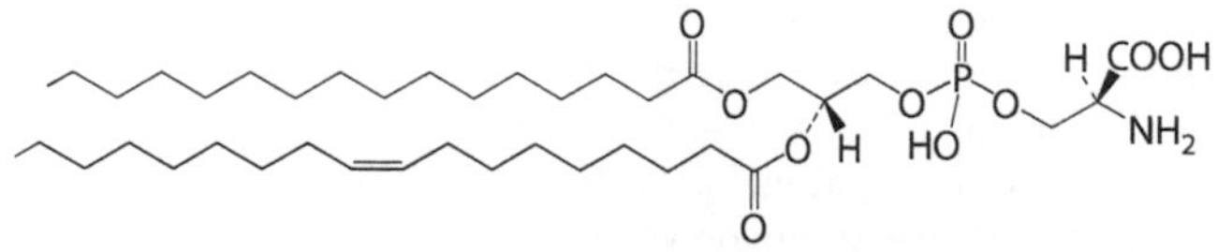

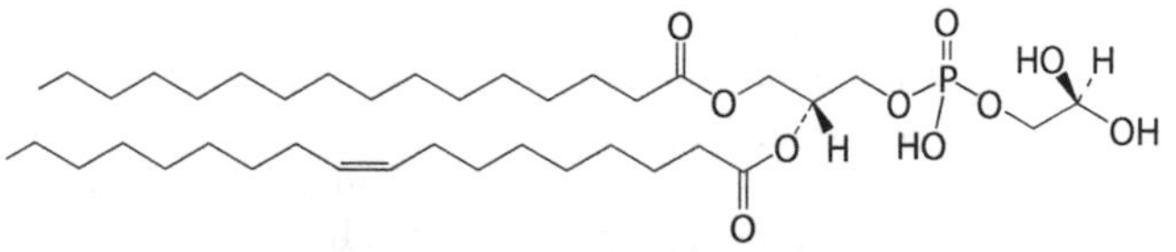

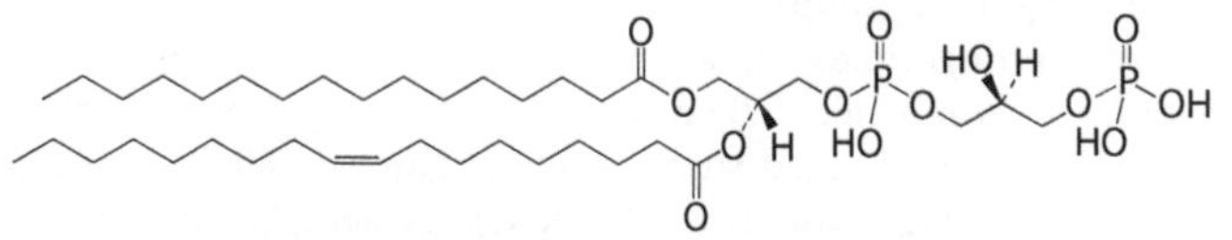

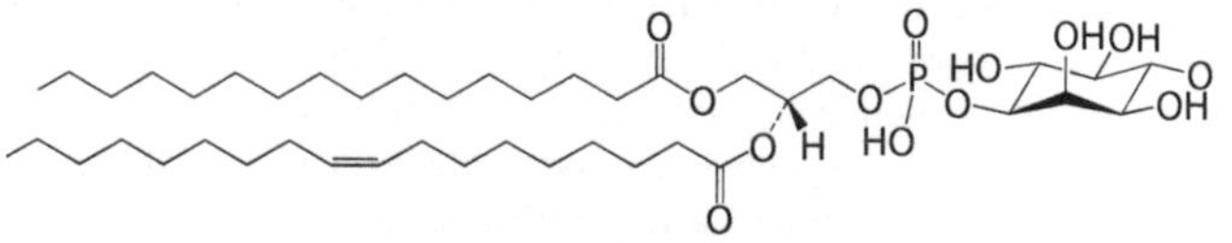

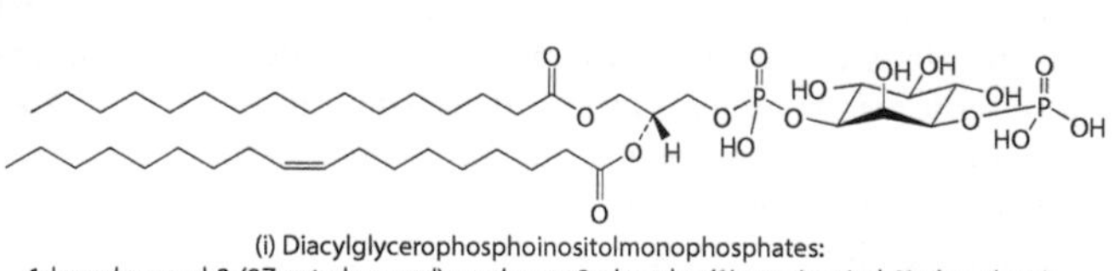

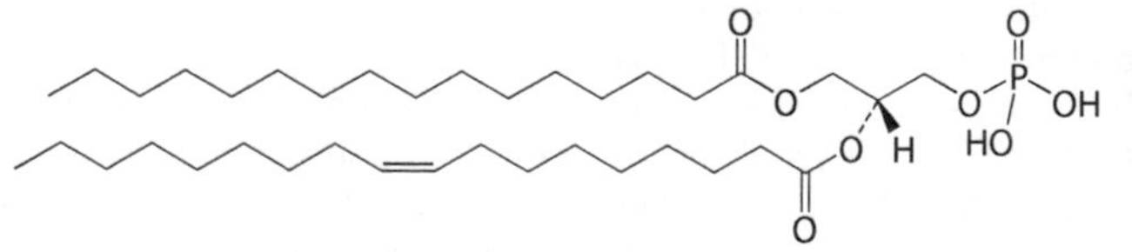

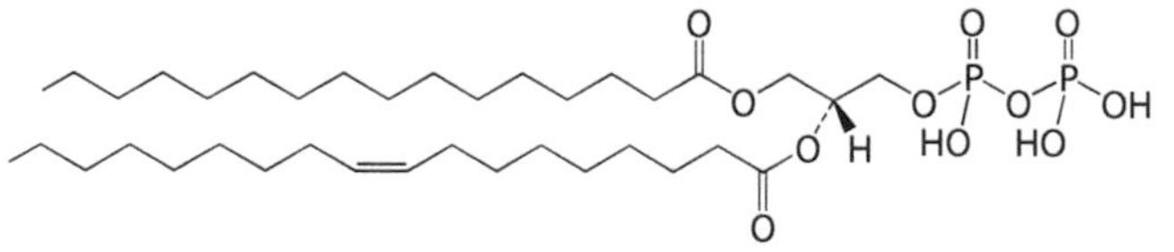

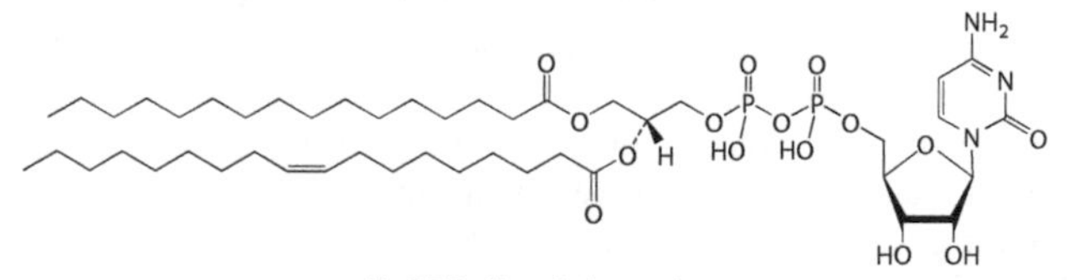

Prenol Lipids [PR]

Prenols are synthesized from the five carbon precursors isopentenyl diphosphate and dimethylallyl diphosphate that are produced mainly via the mevalonic acid pathway (34). In some bacteria (e.g., *Escherichia coli*) and plants, isoprenoid precursors are made by the methylerythritol phosphate pathway (35). Because the simple isoprenoids (linear alcohols, diphosphates, etc.) are formed by the successive addition of C_5 units, it is convenient to classify them in this manner (**Table 9**), with a polyterpene subclass for those structures containing more than 40 carbons (i.e., >8 isoprenoid units) (36). Note that vitamin A and its derivatives and phytanic acid and its oxidation product

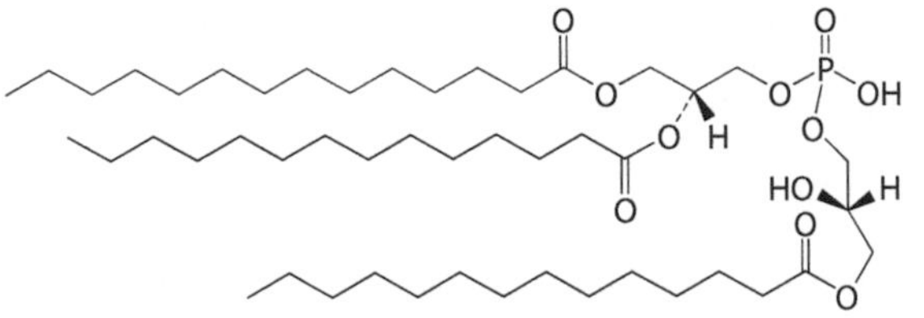

(m) Diacylglycerophosphomonoradylglycerols:
1,2-ditetradecanoyl-*sn*-glycero-3-phospho-
(3'-tetradecanoyl-1'-*sn*-glycerol)

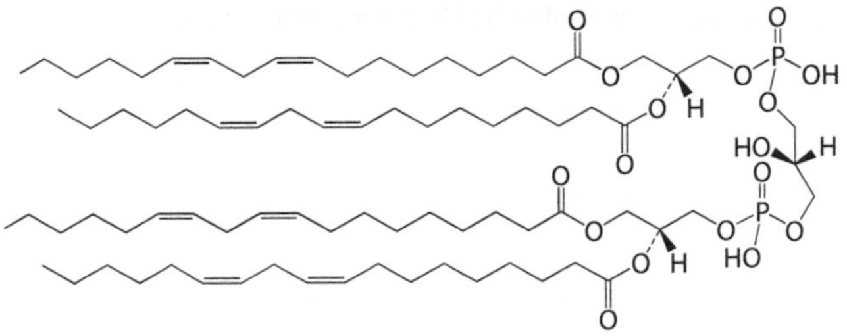

(n) Diacylglycerophosphoglycerophosphodiradylglycerols:
1',3'-Bis[1,2-Di-(9Z,12Z-octadecadienoyl)-
sn-glycero-3-phospho]-*sn*-glycerol

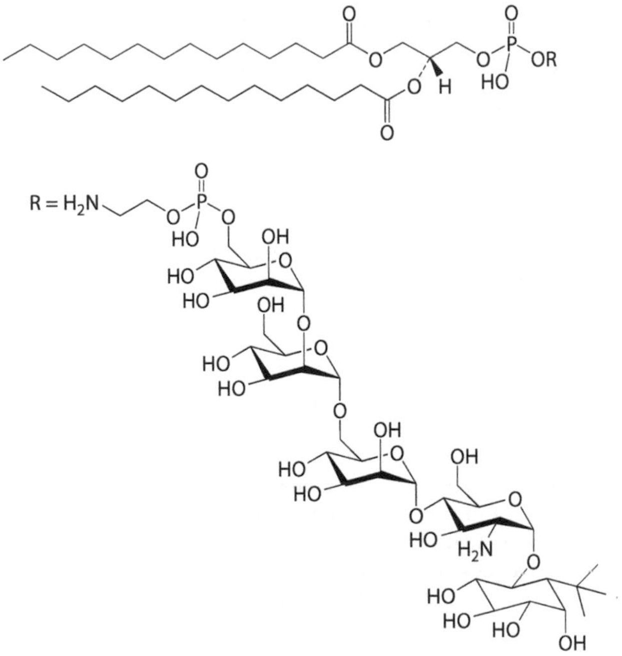

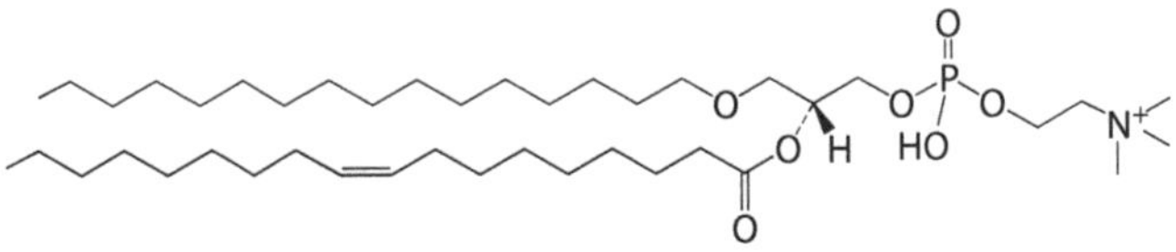

(p) 1-alkyl, 2-acylglycerophosphocholines:
1-O-hexadecyl-2-(9Z-octadecenoyl)-*sn*-glycero-3-phosphocholine

(o) Diacylglycerophosphoinositolglycans:
EtN-P-6Manα1-2Manα1-6Manα1-4GlcNα1-6GPIns(14:0/14:0)

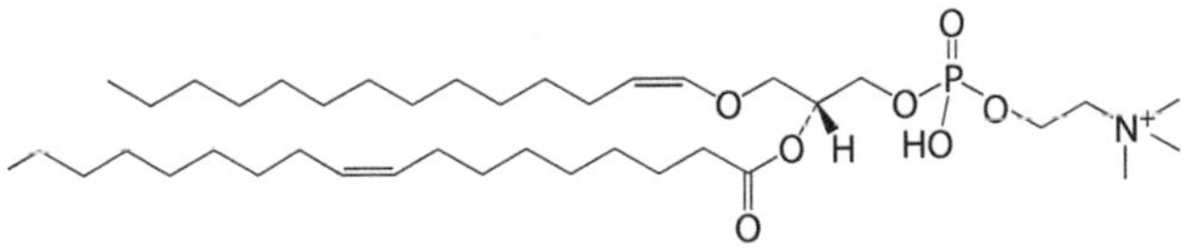

(q) 1Z-alkenyl, 2-acylglycerophosphocholines:
1-O-(1Z-tetradecenyl)-2-(9Z-octadecenoyl
-*sn*-glycero-3-phosphocholine

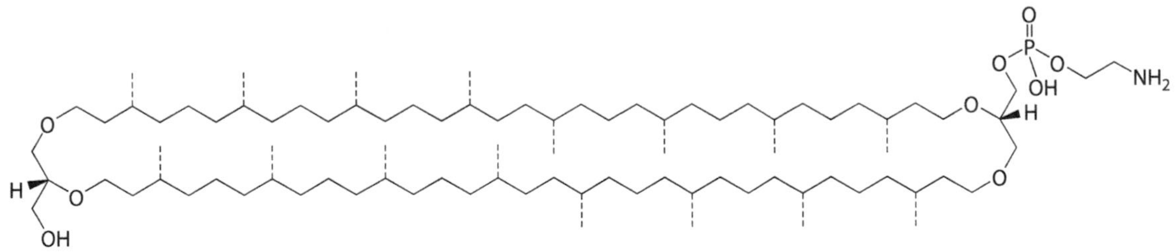

(r) Di-glycerol tetraether phospholipids (caldarchaeols): *sn*-caldarchaeo-1-phosphoethanolamine

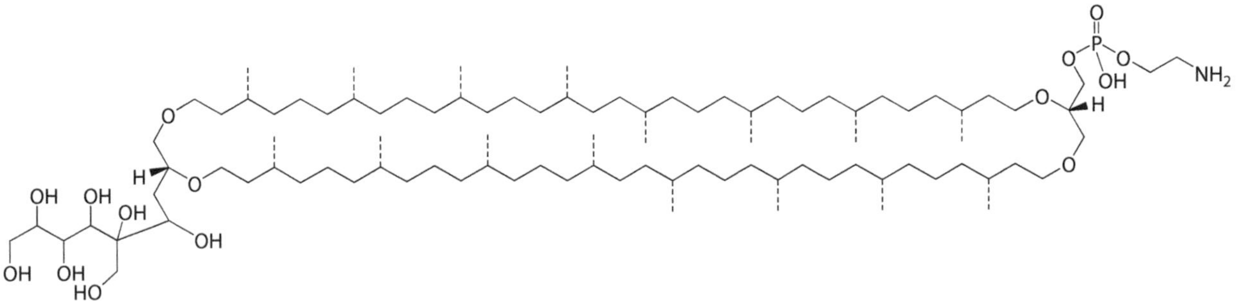

(s) Glycerol-nonitol tetraether phospholipids: *sn*-caldito-1-phosphoethanolamine

FIGURE 4 Representative structures for glycerophospholipids (Continued).

TABLE 7: Sphingolipids [SP] Classes and Subclasses

Sphingoid bases [SP01]

  Sphing-4-enines (sphingosines) [SP0101]

  Sphinganines [SP0102]

  4-Hydroxysphinganines (phytosphingosines) [SP0103]

  Sphingoid base homologs and variants [SP0104]

  Sphingoid base 1-phosphates [SP0105]

  Lysosphingomyelins and lysoglycosphingolipids [SP0106]

  N-Methylated sphingoid bases [SP0107]

  Sphingoid base analogs [SP0108]

Ceramides [SP02]

  N-Acylsphingosines (ceramides) [SP0201]

  N-Acylsphinganines (dihydroceramides) [SP0202]

  N-Acyl-4-hydroxysphinganines (phytoceramides) [SP0203]

  Acylceramides [SP0204]

  Ceramide 1-phosphates [SP0205]

Phosphosphingolipids [SP03]

  Ceramide phosphocholines (sphingomyelins) [SP0301]

  Ceramide phosphoethanolamines [SP0302]

  Ceramide phosphoinositols [SP0303]

Phosphonosphingolipids [SP04]

Neutral glycosphingolipids [SP05]

  Simple Glc series (GlcCer, LacCer, etc.) [SP0501]

  GalNAcβ1-3Galα1-4Galβ1-4Glc- (globo series) [SP0502]

  GalNAcβ1-4Galβ1-4Glc- (ganglio series) [SP0503]

  Galβ1-3GlcNAcβ1-3Galβ1-4Glc- (lacto series) [SP0504]

  Galβ1–4GlcNAcβ1-3Galβ1-4Glc- (neolacto series) [SP0505]

  GalNAcβ1-3Galα1-3Galβ1-4Glc- (isoglobo series) [SP0506]

  GlcNAcβ1-2Manα1-3Manβ1-4Glc- (mollu series) [SP0507]

  GalNAcβ1-4GlcNAcβ1-3Manβ1-4Glc- (arthro series) [SP0508]

  Gal- (gala series) [SP0509]

  Other [SP0510]

Acidic glycosphingolipids [SP06]

  Gangliosides [SP0601]

  Sulfoglycosphingolipids (sulfatides) [SP0602]

  Glucuronosphingolipids [SP0603]

  Phosphoglycosphingolipids [SP0604]

  Other [SP0600]

Basic glycosphingolipids [SP07]

Amphoteric glycosphingolipids [SP08]

Arsenosphingolipids [SP09]

Other [SP00]

pristanic acid are grouped under C_{20} isoprenoids. Carotenoids are important simple isoprenoids that function as antioxidants and as precursors of vitamin A (37). Another biologically important class of molecules is exemplified by the quinones and hydroquinones, which contain an isoprenoid tail attached to a quinonoid core of nonisoprenoid origin. Vitamins E and K (38, 39) as well as the ubiquinones (40) are examples of this class.

Polyprenols and their phosphorylated derivatives play important roles in the transport of oligosaccharides across membranes. Polyprenol phosphate sugars and polyprenol diphosphate sugars function in extracytoplasmic glycosylation reactions (41), in extracellular polysaccharide biosynthesis [for instance, peptidoglycan polymerization in bacteria (42)], and in eukaryotic protein N-glycosylation (43, 44). The biosynthesis and function of polyprenol phosphate sugars differ significantly from those of the polyprenol diphosphate sugars; therefore, we have placed them in separate subclasses. Bacteria synthesize polyprenols (called bactoprenols) in which the terminal isoprenoid unit attached to oxygen remains unsaturated, whereas in animal polyprenols

(dolichols) the terminal isoprenoid is reduced. Bacterial polyprenols are typically 10 to 12 units long (40), whereas dolichols usually consist of 18 to 22 isoprene units. In the phytoprenols of plants, the three distal units are reduced. Several examples of prenol lipid structures are shown in **Figure 7.**

Saccharolipids [SL]

We have avoided the term "glycolipid" in the classification scheme to maintain a focus on lipid structures. In fact, all eight lipid categories in the present scheme include important glycan derivatives, making the term glycolipid incompatible with the overall goal of lipid categorization. We have, in addition, coined the term "saccharolipids" to describe compounds in which fatty acids are linked directly to a sugar backbone, forming structures that are compatible with membrane bilayers. In the saccharolipids (**Table 10**), a sugar substitutes for the glycerol backbone that is present in glycerolipids and glycerophospholipids. Saccharolipids can occur as glycan or as phosphorylated derivatives. The most familiar saccharolipids are the acylated glucosamine precursors of the lipid A component of the lipopolysaccharides in Gram-negative bacteria (41). Typical lipid A molecules are disaccharides of glucosamine, which are derivatized with as many as seven fatty acyl chains (41, 45). Note that in naming these compounds, the total number of fatty acyl groups are counted regardless of the nature of the linkage (i.e., amide or ester). The minimal lipopolysaccharide required for growth in *E. coli* is a hexa-acylated lipid A that is glycosylated with two 3-deoxy-D-mannooctulosonic acid residues (see below). In some bacteria, the glucosamine backbone of lipid A is replaced by 2,3-diamino-2,3-dideoxyglucose (46); therefore, the class has been designated "Acylaminosugars." Included also in this class are the Nod factors of nitrogen-fixing bacteria (47), such as *Sinorhizobium meliloti*. The Nod factors are oligosaccharides of glucosamine that are usually derivatized with a single fatty acyl chain. Additional saccharolipids include fatty acylated derivatives of glucose, which are best exemplified by the acylated trehalose units of certain mycobacterial lipids (11). Acylated forms of glucose and sucrose also have been reported in plants (48). Some saccharolipid structures are shown in **Figure 8.**

Polyketides [PK]

Polyketides are synthesized by classic enzymes as well as iterative and multimodular enzymes with semiautonomous active sites that share mechanistic features with the fatty acid synthases, including the involvement of specialized acyl carrier proteins (49, 50); however, polyketide synthases generate a much greater diversity of natural product structures, many of which have the character of lipids. The class I polyketide synthases form constrained macrocyclic lactones, typically ranging in size from 14 to 40 atoms, whereas class II and III polyketide synthases generate complex aromatic ring systems (**Table 11**). Polyketide backbones are often further modified by glycosylation, methylation, hydroxylation, oxidation, and/or other processes. Some polyketides are linked with nonribosomally synthesized peptides to form hybrid scaffolds. Examples of the three polyketide classes are shown in **Figure 9.** Many commonly used antimicrobial, antiparasitic, and anticancer agents are polyketides or polyketide derivatives. Important examples of these drugs include erythromycins, tetracylines, nystatins, avermectins, and antitumor epothilones. Other polyketides are potent toxins. The possibility of recombining and reengineering the enzymatic modules that assemble polyketides has recently stimulated the search for novel "unnatural" natural products, especially in the antibiotic arena (51, 52).

We consider this minimal classification of polyketides as the first step in a more elaborate scheme. It will be important

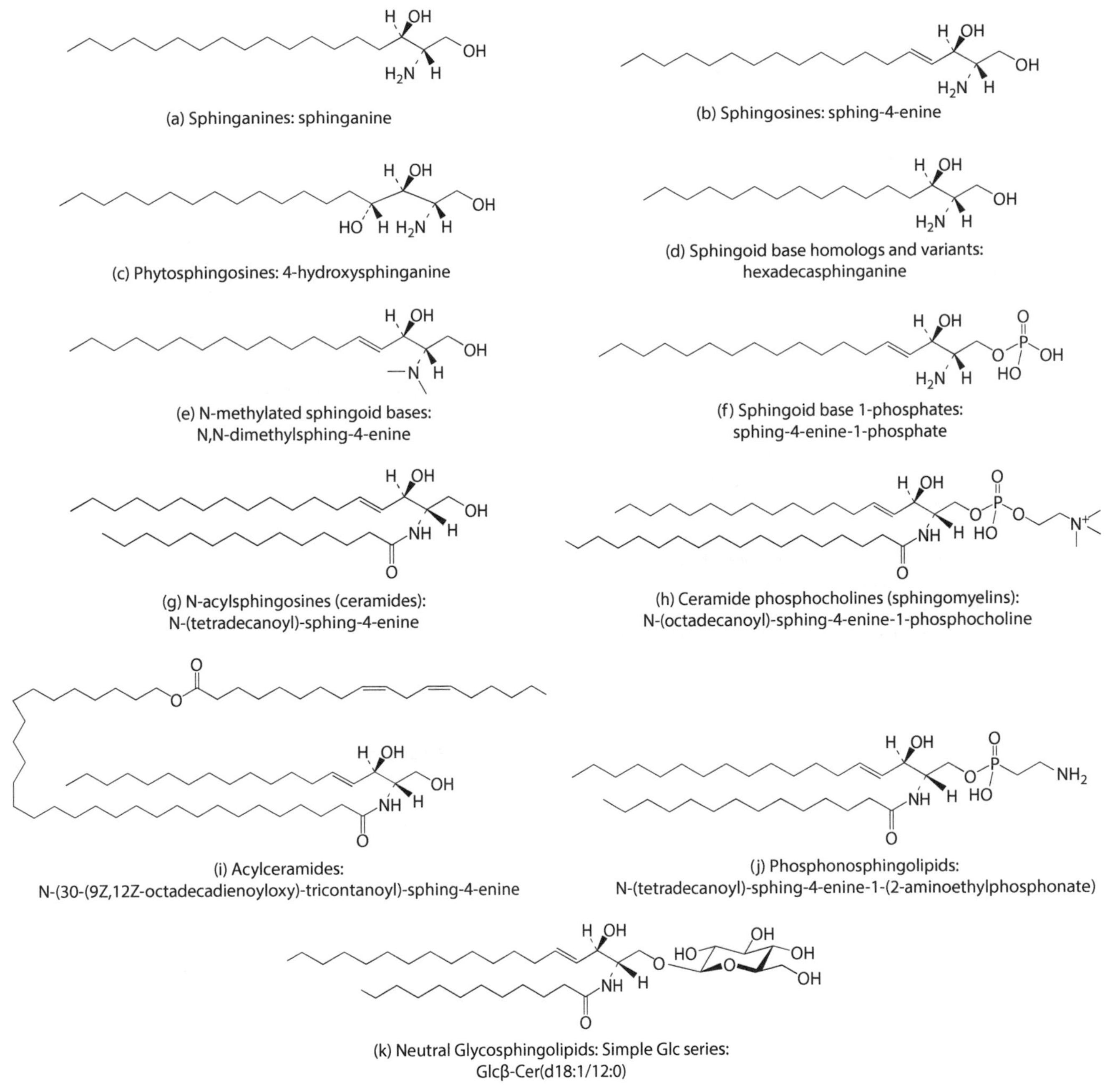

(a) Sphinganines: sphinganine

(b) Sphingosines: sphing-4-enine

(c) Phytosphingosines: 4-hydroxysphinganine

(d) Sphingoid base homologs and variants:
hexadecasphinganine

(e) N-methylated sphingoid bases:
N,N-dimethylsphing-4-enine

(f) Sphingoid base 1-phosphates:
sphing-4-enine-1-phosphate

(g) N-acylsphingosines (ceramides):
N-(tetradecanoyl)-sphing-4-enine

(h) Ceramide phosphocholines (sphingomyelins):
N-(octadecanoyl)-sphing-4-enine-1-phosphocholine

(i) Acylceramides:
N-(30-(9Z,12Z-octadecadienoyloxy)-tricontanoyl)-sphing-4-enine

(j) Phosphonosphingolipids:
N-(tetradecanoyl)-sphing-4-enine-1-(2-aminoethylphosphonate)

(k) Neutral Glycosphingolipids: Simple Glc series:
Glcβ-Cer(d18:1/12:0)

FIGURE 5 Representative structures for sphingolipids.

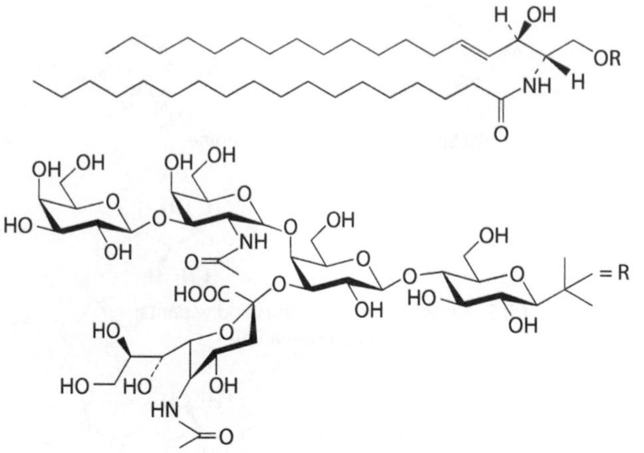

(l) Acidic Glycosphingolipids: Gangliosides:
Galβ1–3GalNAcβ1–4(NeuAcα2–3)Galβ1–4Glcβ-Cer(d18:1/18:0)

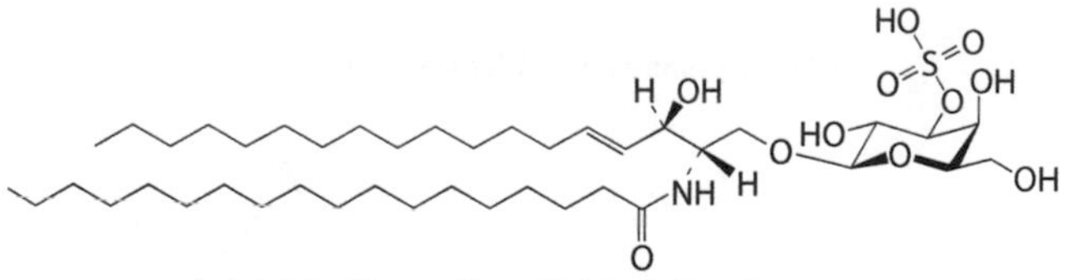

(m) Acidic Glycosphingolipids: Sulfosphingolipids:
(3'-sulfo)Galβ-Cer(d18:1/18:0)

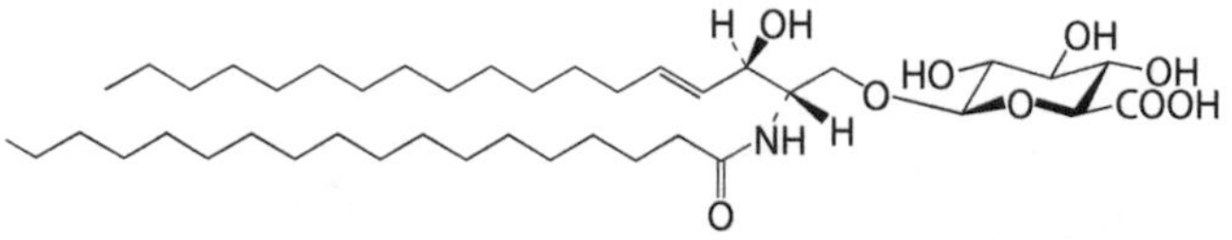

(n) Acidic Glycosphingolipids: Glucuronosphingolipids:
GlcUAβ-Cer(d18:1/18:0)

FIGURE 5　Representative structures for sphingolipids (Continued).

TABLE 8: Sterol Lipids [ST] Classes and Subclasses

Sterols [ST01]
Cholesterol and derivatives [ST0101]
　Cholesteryl esters [ST0102]
　Phytosterols and derivatives [ST0103]
　Marine sterols and derivatives [ST0104]
　Fungal sterols and derivatives [ST0105]
Steroids [ST02]
　C_{18} steroids (estrogens) and derivatives [ST0201]
　C_{19} steroids (androgens) and derivatives [ST0202]
　C_{21} steroids (gluco/mineralocorticoids, progestogins) and derivatives [ST0203]
Secosteroids [ST03]
　Vitamin D_2 and derivatives [ST0301]
　Vitamin D_3 and derivatives [ST0302]
Bile acids and derivatives [ST04]
　C_{24} bile acids, alcohols, and derivatives [ST0401]
　C_{26} bile acids, alcohols, and derivatives [ST0402]
　C_{27} bile acids, alcohols, and derivatives [ST0403]
　C_{28} bile acids, alcohols, and derivatives [ST0404]
Steroid conjugates [ST05]
　Glucuronides [ST0501]
　Sulfates [ST0502]
　Glycine conjugates [ST0503]
　Taurine conjugates [ST0504]
Hopanoids [ST06]
Other [ST00]

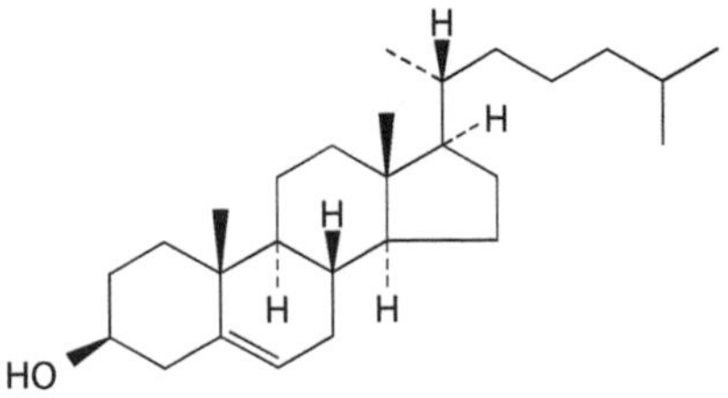

(a) Cholesterol and derivatives:
cholesterol; cholest-5-en-3β-ol

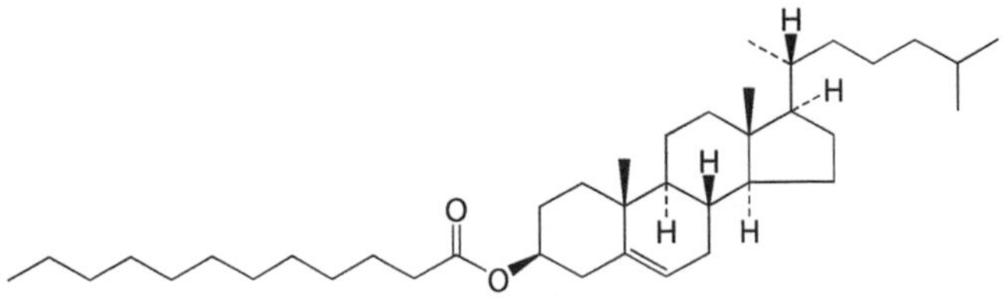

(b) Cholesteryl esters:
cholest-5-en-3β-yl dodecanoate

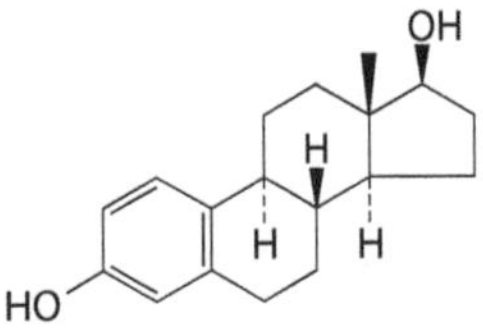

(c) C$_{18}$ steroids (estrogens) and derivatives:
β-estradiol; 1,3,5[10]-estratriene-3,17β-diol

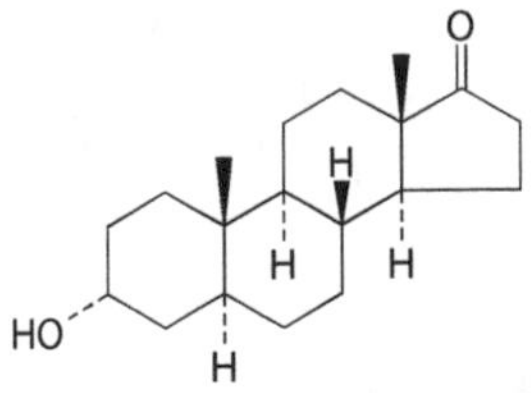

(d) C$_{19}$ steroids (androgens) and derivatives:
androsterone; 3α-hydroxy-5α-androstan-17-one

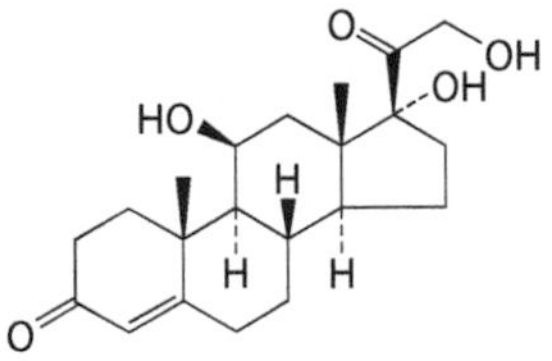

(e) C$_{21}$ steroids and derivatives:
cortisol;11β,17α,21-trihydroxypregn-4-ene-3,20-dione

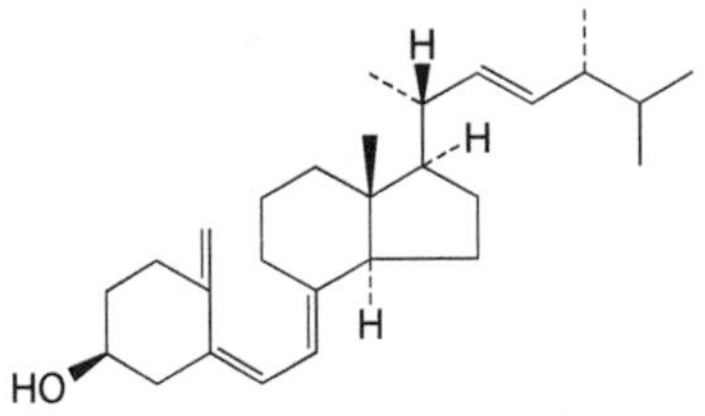

(f) Secosteroids: Vitamin D$_2$ and derivatives:
vitamin D$_2$; (5Z,7E,22E)-(3S)-9,10-seco-5,7,10(19),
22-ergostatetraen-3-ol

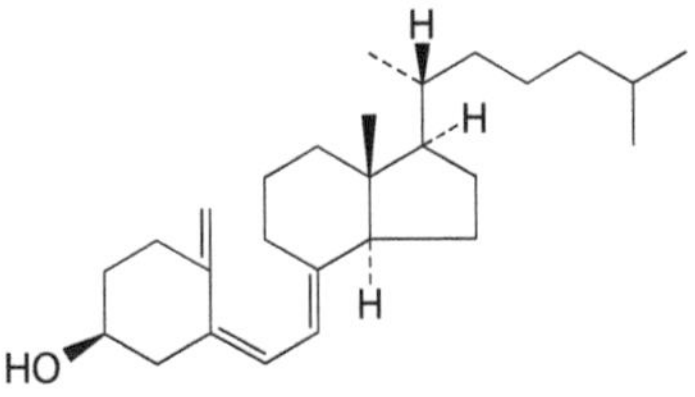

(g) Secosteroids: Vitamin D$_3$ and derivatives: vitamin D$_3$;
(5Z,7E)-(3S)-9,10-seco-5,7,10(19)-cholestatrien-3-ol

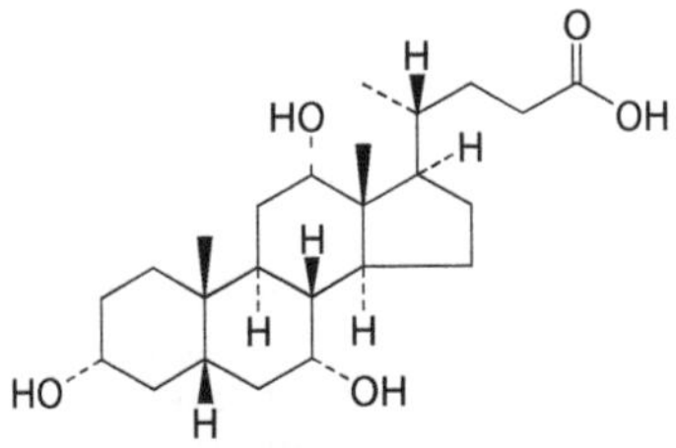

(h) C$_{24}$ bile acids, alcohols, and derivatives:
cholic acid; 3α,7α,12α-trihydroxy-5β-cholan-24-oic acid

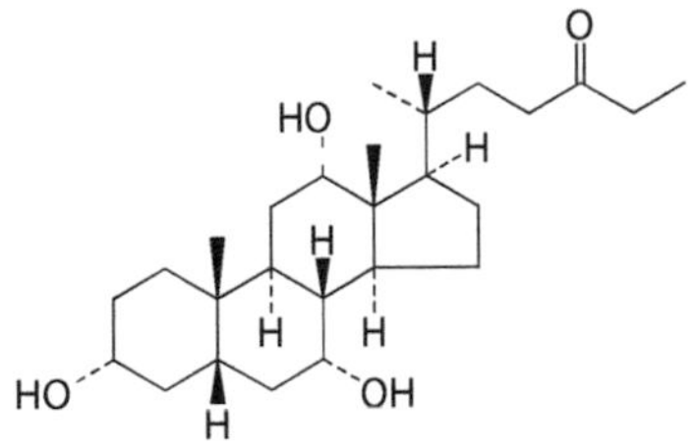

(i) C$_{26}$ bile acids, alcohols, and derivatives:
3α,7α,12α-trihydroxy-27-nor-5β-cholestan-24-one

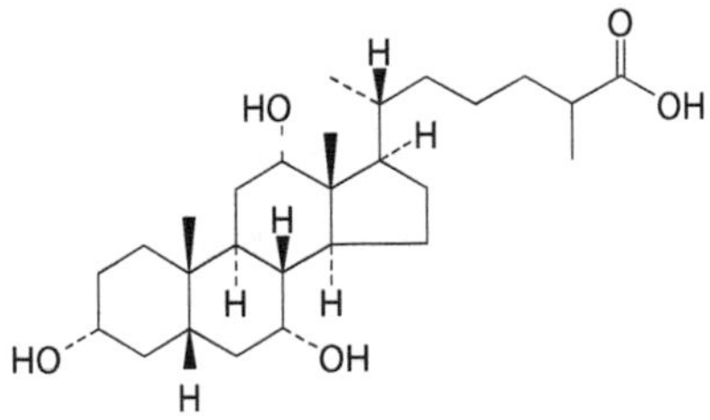

(j) C$_{27}$ bile acids, alcohols, and derivatives:
3α,7α,12α-trihydroxy-5β-cholestan-26-oic acid

FIGURE 6   Representative structures for sterol lipids.

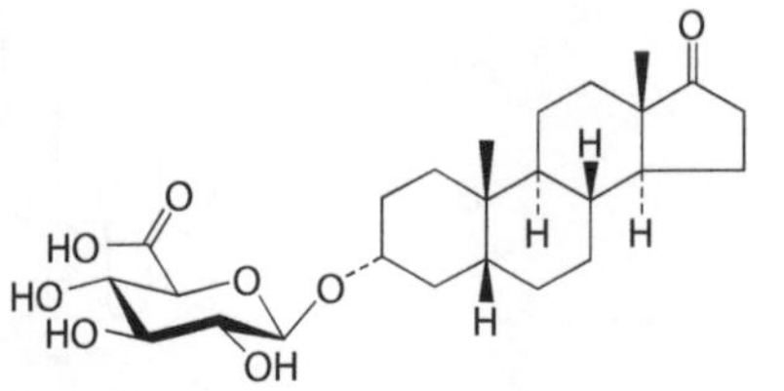

(k) Steroid conjugates: Glucuronides:
5α-androstane-3α-ol-17-one glucuronide

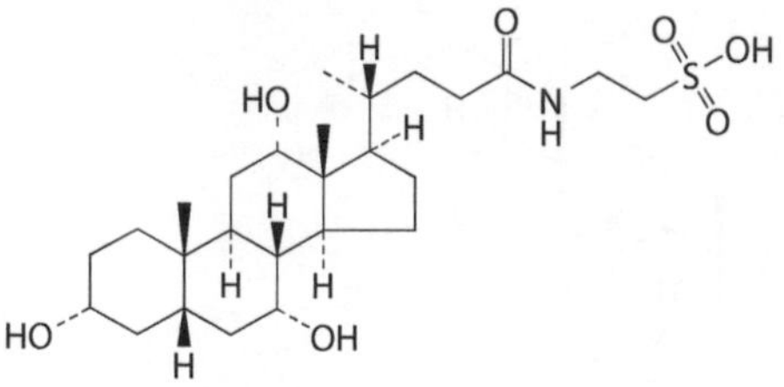

(l) Steroid conjugates: Taurine conjugates: taurocholic acid;
N-(3α,7α,12α-trihydroxy-5β-cholan-24-oyl)-taurine

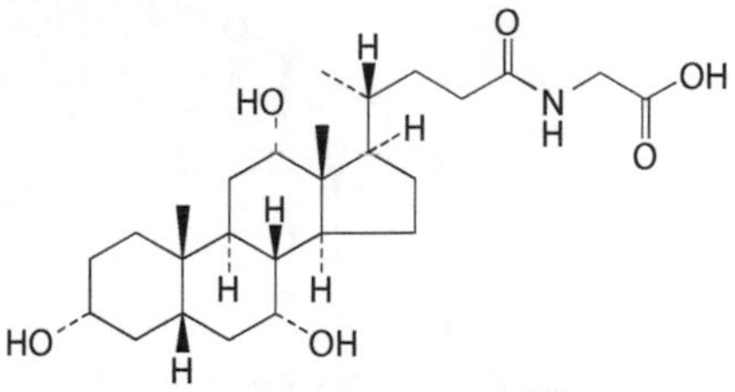

(m) Steroid conjugates: Glycine conjugates:
glycocholic acid; N-(3α,7α,12α-trihydroxy-5β-
cholan-24-oyl)-glycine

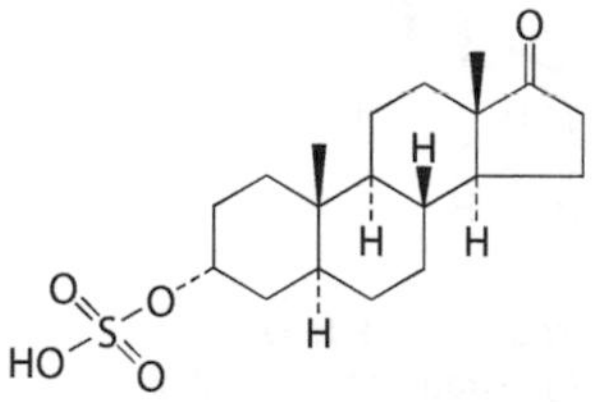

(n) Steroid conjugates: Sulfates:
5α-androstane-3α-ol-17-one sulfate

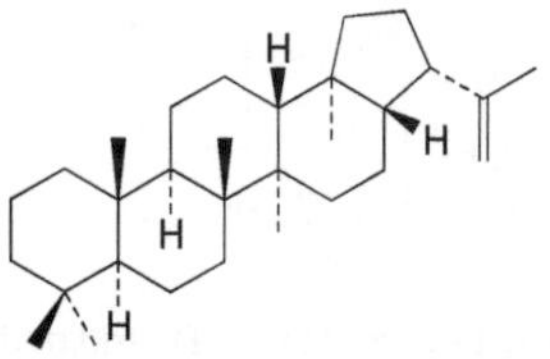

(o) Hopanoids: diploptene; hop-22(29)-ene

FIGURE 6   Representative structures for sterol lipids (Continued).

TABLE 9: Prenol Lipids [PR] Classes and Subclasses

Isoprenoids [PR01]
 C$_5$ isoprenoids [PR0101]
 C$_{10}$ isoprenoids (monoterpenes) [PR0102]
 C$_{15}$ isoprenoids (sesquiterpenes) [PR0103]
 C$_{20}$ isoprenoids (diterpenes) [PR0104]
 C$_{25}$ isoprenoids (sesterterpenes) [PR0105]
 C$_{30}$ isoprenoids (triterpenes) [PR0106]
 C$_{40}$ isoprenoids (tetraterpenes) [PR0107]
 Polyterpenes [PR0108]
Quinones and hydroquinones [PR02]
 Ubiquinones [PR0201]
 Vitamin E [PR0202]
 Vitamin K [PR0203]
Polyprenols [PR03]
 Bactoprenols [PR0301]
 Bactoprenol monophosphates [PR0302]
 Bactoprenol diphosphates [PR0303]
 Phytoprenols [PR0304]
 Phytoprenol monophosphates [PR0305]
 Phytoprenol diphosphates [PR0306]
 Dolichols [PR0307]
 Dolichol monophosphates [PR0308]
 Dolichol diphosphates [PR0309]
Other [PR00]

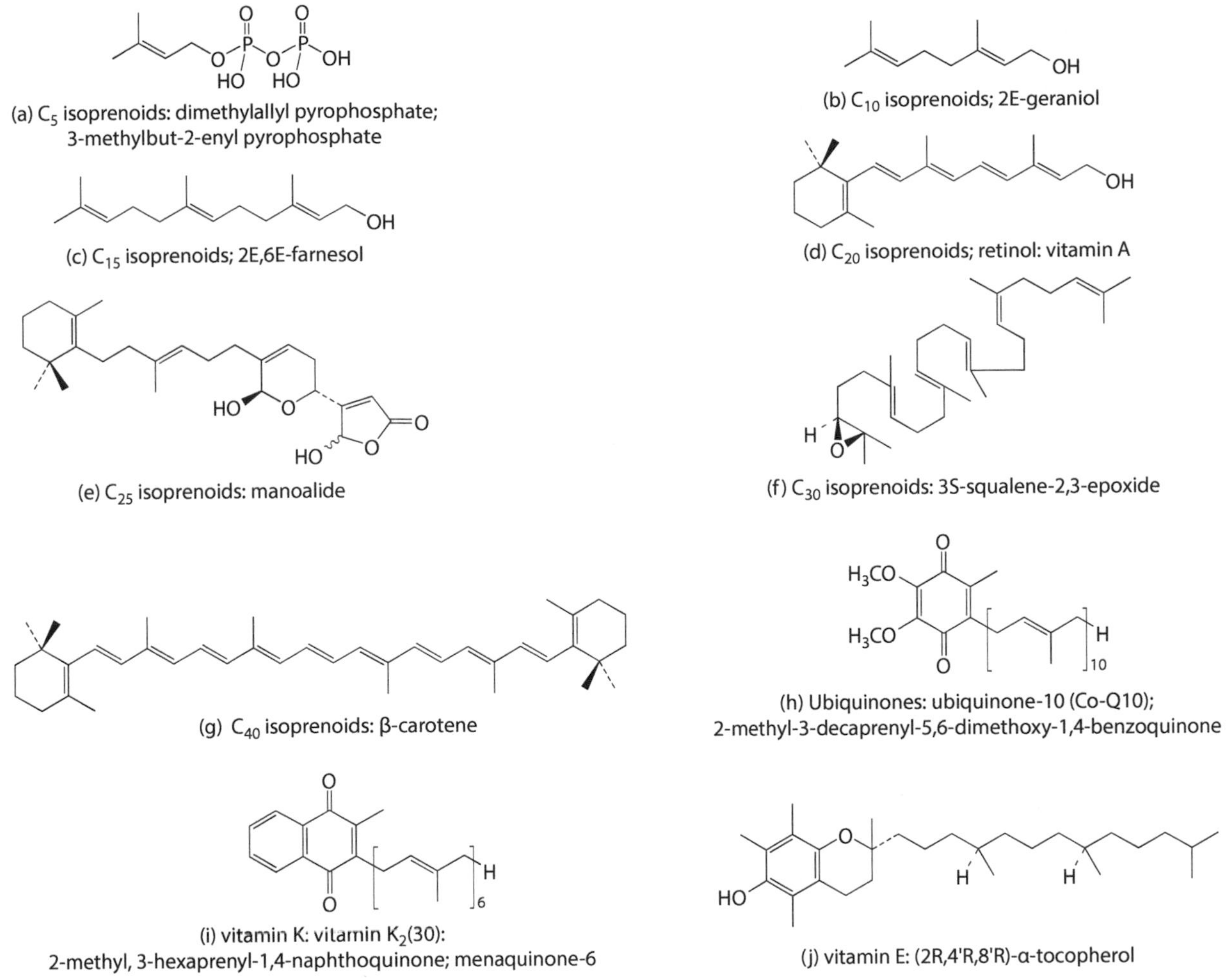

(a) C$_5$ isoprenoids: dimethylallyl pyrophosphate; 3-methylbut-2-enyl pyrophosphate

(b) C$_{10}$ isoprenoids; 2E-geraniol

(c) C$_{15}$ isoprenoids; 2E,6E-farnesol

(d) C$_{20}$ isoprenoids; retinol: vitamin A

(e) C$_{25}$ isoprenoids: manoalide

(f) C$_{30}$ isoprenoids: 3S-squalene-2,3-epoxide

(g) C$_{40}$ isoprenoids: β-carotene

(h) Ubiquinones: ubiquinone-10 (Co-Q10); 2-methyl-3-decaprenyl-5,6-dimethoxy-1,4-benzoquinone

(i) vitamin K: vitamin K$_2$(30): 2-methyl, 3-hexaprenyl-1,4-naphthoquinone; menaquinone-6

(j) vitamin E: (2R,4'R,8'R)-α-tocopherol

FIGURE 7   Representative structures for prenol lipids.

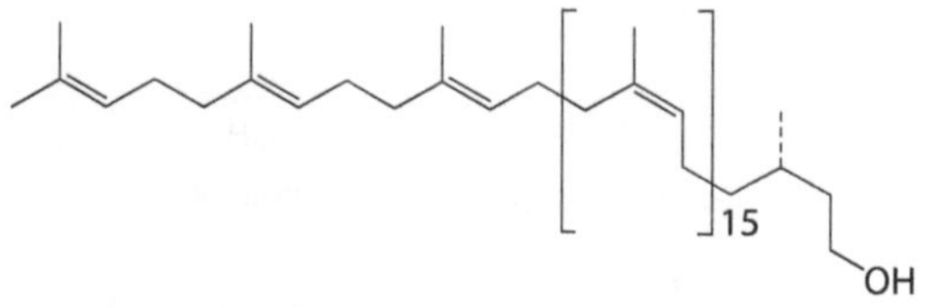

(k) Dolichols: Dol-19; α-dihydrononadecaprenol

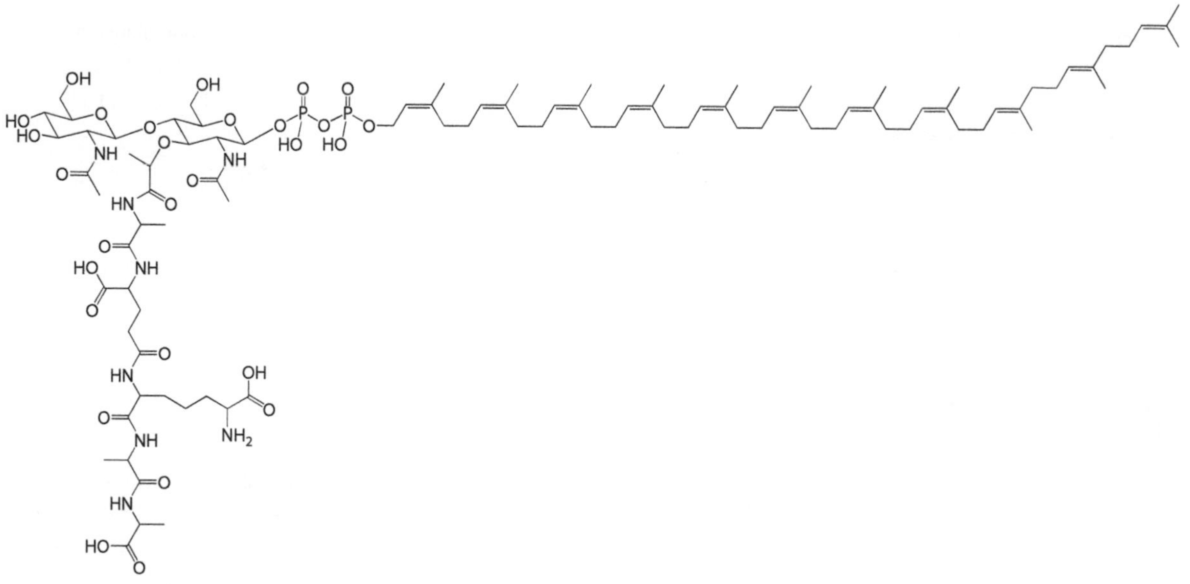

(l) Bactoprenol diphosphates: The Lipid II peptidoglycan precursor in *E. coli*; undecaprenyl diphosphate glycan

FIGURE 7   Representative structures for prenol lipids (Continued).

TABLE 10: Saccharolipids [SL]Classes and Subclasses

Acylaminosugars [SL01]
   Monoacylaminosugars [SL0101]
   Diacylaminosugars [SL0102]
   Triacylaminosugars [SL0103]
   Tetraacylaminosugars [SL0104]
   Pentaacylaminosugars [SL0105]
   Hexaacylaminosugars [SL0106]
   Heptaacylaminosugars [SL0107]
Acylaminosugar glycans [SL02]
Acyltrehaloses [SL03]
Acyltrehalose glycans [SL04]
Other [SL00]

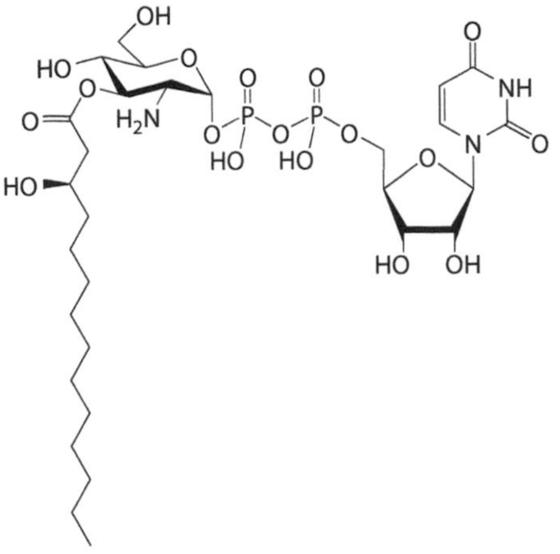

(a) Acylaminosugars: Monoacylaminosugars: UDP-3-O-(3R-hydroxy-tetradecanoyl)-GlcN

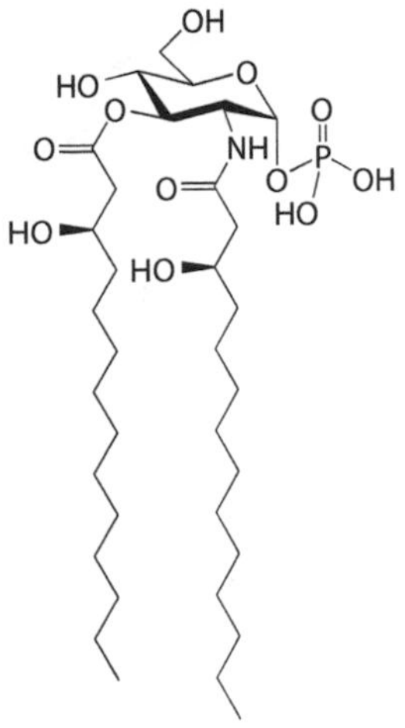

(b) Acylaminosugars: Diacylaminosugars: lipid X

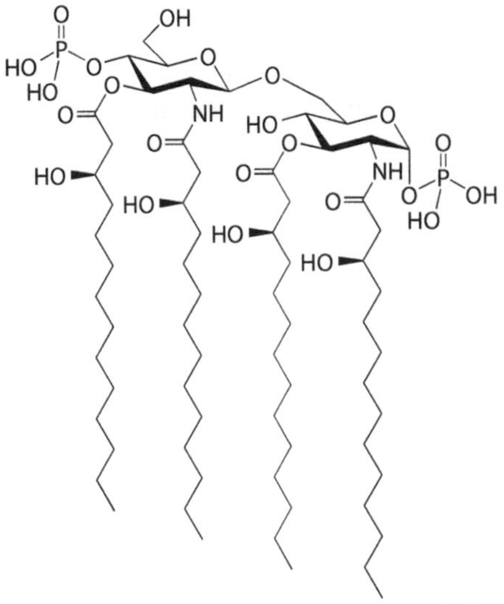

(c) Acylaminosugars: Tetraacylaminosugars: lipid IV$_A$

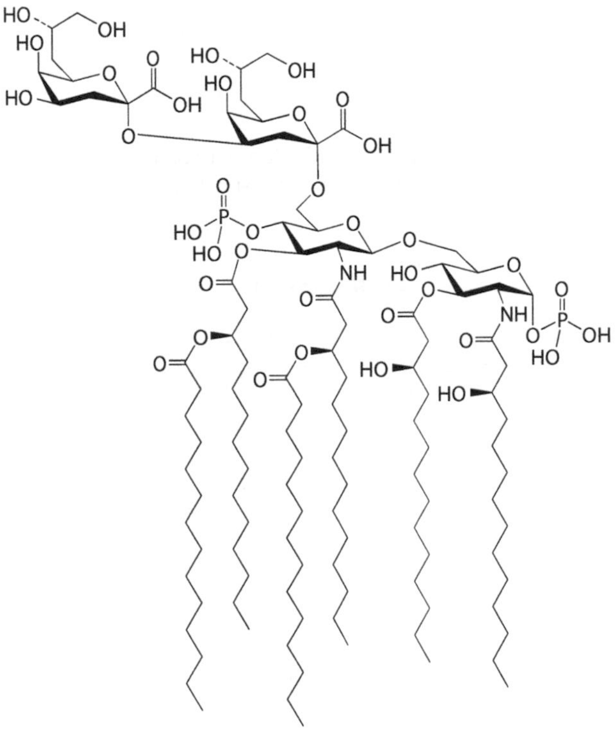

(d) Acylaminosugar glycans: Kdo$_2$ lipid A

FIGURE 8 Representative structures for saccharolipids.

TABLE 11: Polyketides [PK] Classes and Subclasses

Macrolide polyketides [PK01]
Aromatic polyketides [PK02]
Nonribosomal peptide/polyketide hybrids [PK03]
Other [PK00]

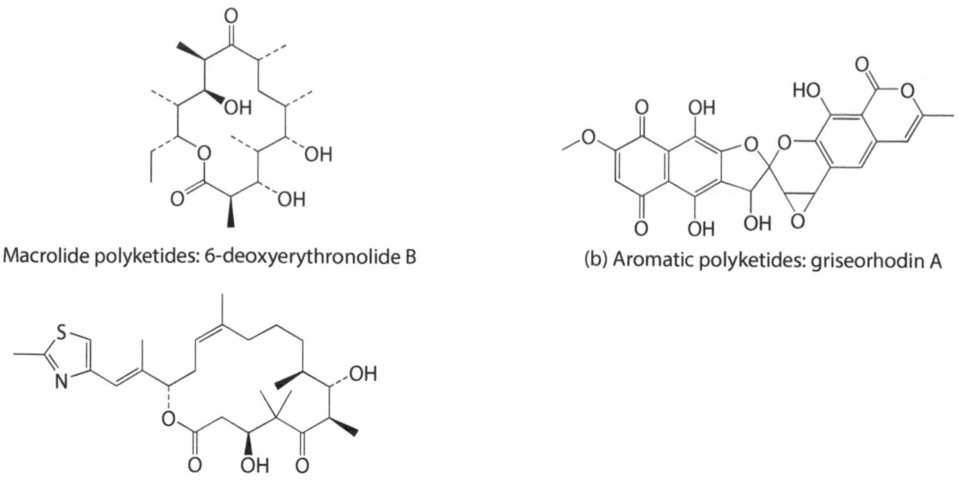

(a) Macrolide polyketides: 6-deoxyerythronolide B

(b) Aromatic polyketides: griseorhodin A

(c) Polyketide hybrids: epothilone D

FIGURE 9   Representative structures for polyketides.

ultimately to include as many polyketide structures as possible in a lipid database that can be searched for substructure and chemical similarity.

Discussion

The goals of the LIPID MAPS initiative are to characterize known lipids and identify new ones, to quantitate temporal and spatial changes in lipids that occur with cellular metabolism, and to develop bioinformatics approaches that establish dynamic lipid networks; the goals of Lipid Bank (Japan) are to annotate and curate lipid structures and the literature associated with them; and the goals of the European Lipidomics Initiative are to coordinate and organize scientific interactions and workshops associated with lipid research. To coordinate the independent efforts from three continents and to facilitate collaborative work, a comprehensive classification of lipids with a common platform that is compatible with informatics requirements must be developed to deal with the massive amounts of data that will be generated by the lipid community. The proposed classification, nomenclature, and chemical representation system was initially designed to accommodate the massive data that will result from the LIPID MAPS effort, but it has been expanded to accommodate as many lipids as possible. We also have attempted to make the system compatible with existing lipid databases and the lipids currently annotated in them. It is designed to be expandable should new categories, classes, or subclasses be required in the future, and updates will be maintained on the LIPID MAPS website. The development of this system has been enriched by interaction with lipidologists across the world in the hopes that this system will be internationally accepted and used.[jlr]

The authors appreciate the agreement of the International Lipids Classification and Nomenclature Committee to advise on future issues involving the maintenance of these recommendations. This committee currently includes Edward A. Dennis (chair), Christian Raetz and Robert Murphy representing LIPID MAPS, Friedrich Spener representing the International Conference on the Biosciences of Lipids, Gerrit van Meer representing the European Lipidomics Initiative, and Yousuke Seyama and Takao Shimizu representing the LipidBank of the Japanese

Conference on the Biochemistry of Lipids. The authors are most appreciative of informative discussions and encouragement of this effort with Professor Richard Cammack, King's College, London, who is the Chairman of the Nomenclature Committee of IUBMB and the IUPAC/IUBMB Joint Commission on Biochemical Nomenclature. The authors thank the Consortium for Functional Glycomics (headed by Ram Sasisekharan at the Massachusetts Institute of Technology) for providing us with their text nomenclature for glycosylated structures. We are grateful to Dr. Jean Chin, Program Director at the National Institutes of General Medical Sciences, for her valuable input to this effort. This work was supported by the LIPID MAPS Large-Scale Collaborative Grant GM-069338 from the National Institutes of Health.

References

1. Smith, A. 2000. Oxford Dictionary of Biochemistry and Molecular Biology. 2nd edition. Oxford University Press, Oxford, UK.
2. Christie, W. W. 2003. Lipid Analysis. 3rd edition. Oily Press, Bridge-water, UK.
3. IUPAC-IUB Commission on Biochemical Nomenclature (CBN). The nomenclature of lipids (recommendations 1976). 1977. *Eur. J. Biochem.* **79:** 11–21; 1977. *Hoppe-Seylers Z. Physiol. Chem.* **358:** 617–631; 1977. *Lipids.* **12:** 455–468; 1977. *Mol. Cell. Biochem.* **17:** 157–171; 1978. *Chem. Phys. Lipids.* **21:** 159–173; 1978. *J. Lipid Res.* **19:** 114–128; 1978. *Biochem. J.* **171:** 21–35 (http://www.chem.qmul.ac.uk/iupac/lipid/).
4. IUPAC-IUB Joint Commission on Biochemical Nomenclature (JCBN). Nomenclature of glycolipids (recommendations 1997). 2000. *Adv. Carbohydr. Chem. Biochem.* **55:** 311–326; 1988. *Carbohydr. Res.* **312:** 167–175; 1998. *Eur. J. Biochem.* **257:** 293–298; 1999. *Glycoconjugate J.* **16:** 1–6; 1999. *J. Mol. Biol.* **286:** 963–970; 1997. *Pure Appl. Chem.* **69:** 2475–2487 (http://www.chem.qmul.ac.uk/iupac/misc/glylp.html).
5. IUPAC-IUB Joint Commission on Biochemical Nomenclature (JCBN). 1987. Nomenclature of prenols (recommendations 1987). *Eur. J. Biochem.* **167:** 181–184 (http://www.chem.qmul.ac.uk/iupac/misc/prenol.html).
6. IUPAC-IUB Joint Commission on Biochemical Nomenclature (JCBN). 1989. Nomenclature of steroids (recommendations 1989). *Eur. J. Biochem.* **186:** 429–458 (http://www.chem.qmul.ac.uk/iupac/steroid/).

7. Caffrey, M., and J. Hogan. 1992. LIPIDAT: a database of lipid phase transition temperatures and enthalpy changes. *Chem. Phys. Lipids.* **61:** 1–109 (http://www.lipidat.chemistry.ohio-state.edu).

8. Watanabe, K., E. Yasugi, and M. Ohshima. 2000. How to search the glycolipid data in "Lipidbank for web," the newly-developed lipid database in Japan. *Trends Gycosci. Glycotechnol.* **12:** 175–184.

9. Vance, D. E., and J. E.Vance, editors. 2002. *Biochemistry of Lipids, Lipoproteins and Membranes.* 4th edition. Elsevier Science, New York.

10. Small, D. M. 1986. The Physical Chemistry of Lipids. Handbook of Lipid Research. Vol. 4. D. J. Hanahan, editor. Plenum Press, New York.

11. Brennan, P. J., and H. Nikaido. 1995. The envelope of mycobacteria. *Annu. Rev. Biochem.* **64:** 29–63.

12. Ohlrogge, J. B. 1997. Regulation of fatty acid synthesis. *Annu. Rev. Plant Physiol. Plant Mol. Biol.* **48:** 109–136.

13. Agrawal, G. K., S. Tamogami, O. Han, H. Iwahasi, and R. Rakwal. 2004. Rice octadecanoid pathway. *Biochem. Biophys. Res. Commun.* **317:** 1–15.

14. Murphy, R. C., and W. L. Smith. 2002. The eicosanoids: cyclooxygenase, lipoxygenase, and epoxygenase pathways. *In* Biochemistry of Lipids, Lipoproteins and Membranes. 4th edition. D. E. Vance and J. E. Vance, editors. Elsevier Science, New York. 341–371.

15. Bazan, N. G. 1989. The metabolism of omega-3 polyunsaturated fatty acids in the eye: the possible role of docosahexaenoic acid and docosanoids in retinal physiology and ocular pathology. *Prog. Clin. Biol. Res.* **312:** 95–112.

16. Roche, D. M., J. T. Byers, D. S. Smith, F. G. Glansdorp, D. R. Spring, and M. Welch. 2004. Communications blackout? Do N-acylhomoserine-lactone-degrading enzymes have any role in quorum sensing? *Microbiology.* **150:** 2023–2028.

17. Stam, H., K. Schoonderwoerd, and W. C. Hulsmann. 1987. Synthesis, storage and degradation of myocardial triglycerides. *Basic Res. Cardiol.* **82 (Suppl. 1):** 19–28.

18. Coleman, R. A., and D. P. Lee. 2004. Enzymes of triacylglycerol synthesis and their regulation. *Prog. Lipid Res.* **43:** 134–176.

19. Pahlsson, P., S. L. Spitalnik, P. F. Spitalnik, J. Fantini, O. Rakotonirainy, S. Ghardashkhani, J. Lindberg, P. Konradsson, and G. Larson. 1998. Characterization of galactosyl glycerolipids in the HT29 human colon carcinoma cell line. *Arch. Biochem. Biophys.* **396:** 187–198.

20. Koga, Y., M. Nishihara, H. Morii, and M. Akagawa-Matsushita. 1983. Ether polar lipids of methanogenic bacteria: structures, comparative aspects and biosyntheses. *Microbiol. Rev.* **57:** 164–182.

21. Pereto, J., P. Lopez-Garcia, and D. Moreira. 2004. Ancestral lipid biosynthesis and early membrane evolution. *Trends Biochem. Sci.* **29:** 469–477.

22. Kennedy, E. P. 1962. The metabolism and function of complex lipids. *Harvey Lecture Series.* **57:** 143–171.

23. G. Cevc, editor. 1993. Phospholipids Handbook. Marcel Dekker Inc., New York.

24. Forrester, J. S., S. B. Milne, P. T. Ivanova, and H. A. Brown. 2004. Computational lipidomics: a multiplexed analysis of dynamic changes in membrane lipid composition during signal transduction. *Mol. Pharmacol.* **65:** 813–821.

25. Ivanova, P. T., S. B. Milne, J. S. Forrester, and H. A. Brown. 2004. Lipid arrays: new tools in the understanding of membrane dynamics and lipid signaling. *Mol. Interventions.* **4:** 86–96.

26. Cronan, J. E. 2003. Bacterial membrane lipids: where do we stand? *Annu. Rev. Microbiol.* **57:** 203–224.

27. Merrill, A. H., Jr., and K. Sandhoff. 2002. Sphingolipids: metabolism and cell signaling. *In* New Comprehensive Biochemistry: Biochemistry of Lipids, Lipoproteins, and Membranes. D. E. Vance and J. E. Vance, editors. Elsevier Science, New York. 373–407.

28. Taniguchi, N., K. Honke, and M. Fukuda. 2002. Handbook of Glycosyltransferases and Related Genes. Springer-Verlag, Tokyo.

29. Thudichum, J. L. W. 1884. A Treatise on the Chemical Constitution of Brain. Bailliere, Tindall, and Cox, London.

30. Bach, D., and E. Wachtel. 2003. Phospholipid/cholesterol model membranes: formation of cholesterol crystallites. *Biochim. Biophys. Acta.* **1610:** 187–197.

31. Tsai, M. J., and B. W. O'Malley. 1994. Molecular mechanisms of action of steroid/thyroid receptor superfamily members. *Annu. Rev. Biochem.* **63:** 451–486.

32. Jones, G., S. A. Strugnell, and H. F. DeLuca. 1998. Current understanding of the molecular actions of vitamin D. *Physiol. Rev.* **78:** 1193–1231.

33. Russell, D. W. 2003. The enzymes, regulation, and genetics of bile acid synthesis. *Annu. Rev. Biochem.* **72:** 137–174.

34. Kuzuyama, T., and H. Seto. 2003. Diversity of the biosynthesis of the isoprene units. *Nat. Prod. Rep.* **20:** 171–183.

35. Rodriguez-Concepcion, M. 2004. The MEP pathway: a new target for the development of herbicides, antibiotics and antimalarial drugs. *Curr. Pharm. Res.* **10:** 2391–2400.

36. Porter, J. W., and S. L. Spurgeon. 1981. Biosynthesis of Isoprenoid Compounds. Vol. 1. John Wiley & Sons, New York.

37. Demming-Adams, B., and W. W. Adams. 2002. Antioxidants in photosynthesis and human nutrition. *Science.* **298:** 2149–2153.

38. Ricciarelli, R., J. M. Zingg, and A. AzziI. 2001. Vitamin E: protective role of a Janus molecule. *FASEBJ.* **15:** 2314–2325.

39. Meganathan, R. 2001. Biosynthesis of menaquinone (vitamin K2) and ubiquinone (coenzyme Q): a perspective on enzymatic mechanisms. *Vitam. Horm.* **61:** 173–218.

40. Meganathan, R. 2001. Ubiquinone biosynthesis in microorganisms. *FEMS Microbiol. Lett.* **203:** 131–139.

41. Raetz, C. R. H., and C. Whitfield. 2002. Lipopolysaccharide endotoxins. *Annu. Rev. Biochem.* **71:** 635–700.

42. Lazar, K., and S. Walker. 2002. Substrate analogues to study cell-wall biosynthesis and its inhibition. *Curr. Opin. Chem. Biol.* **6:** 786–793.

43. Schenk, B., F. Fernandez, and C. J. Waechter. 2001. The ins(ide) and out(side) of dolichyl phosphate biosynthesis and recycling in the endoplasmic reticulum. *Glycobiology.* 11: 61R–71R.

44. Helenius, J., and M. Aebi. 2001. Intracellular functions of N-linked glycans. *Science.* **291:** 2364–2369.

45. Zähringer, U., B. Lindner, and E. T. Rietschel. 1999. Chemical structure of Lipid A: recent advances in structural analysis of biologically active molecules. *In Endotoxin in Health and Disease.* H. Brade, S. M. Opal, S. N. Vogel, and D. C. Morrison, editors. Marcel Dekker, New York. 93–114.

46. Sweet, C. R., A. A. Ribeiro, and C. R. Raetz. 2004. Oxidation and transamination of the 3'-position of UDP-N-acetylglucosamine by enzymes from *Acidithiobacillus ferrooxidans*. Role in the formation of lipid A molecules with four amide-linked acyl chains. *J. Biol. Chem.* **279:** 25400–25410.

47. Spaink, H. P. 2000. Root nodulation and infection factors produced by rhizobial bacteria. *Annu. Rev. Microbiol.* **54:** 257–288.

48. Ghangas, G. S., and J. C. Steffens. 1993. UDP glucose: fatty acid transglucosylation and transacylation in triacylglucose biosynthesis. *Proc. Natl. Acad. Sci. USA.* **90:** 9911–9915.

49. Walsh, C. T. 2004. Polyketide and nonribosomal peptide antibiotics: modularity and versatility. *Science.* **303:** 1805–1810.

50. Khosla, C., R. Gokhale, J. R. Jacobsen, and D. E. Cane. 1999. Tolerance and specificity of polyketide synthases. *Annu. Rev. Biochem.* **68:** 219–253.

51. Reeves, C. D. 2003. The enzymology of combinatorial biosynthesis. *Crit. Rev. Biotechnol.* **23:** 95–147.

52. Moore, B. S., and C. Hartweck. 2002. Biosynthesis and attachment of novel bacterial polyketide synthase starter units. *Nat. Prod. Rep.* 19: 70–99.

PROPERTIES OF FATTY ACIDS AND THEIR METHYL ESTERS

This table gives the names and selected properties of some important fatty acids and their methyl esters. It includes most of the acids that are significant constituents of naturally occurring oils and fats. Compounds are listed first by number of carbon atoms and, secondly, by the degree of unsaturation. Both the systematic name and the common or trivial name are given, as well as the Chemical Abstracts Service Registry Number and the shorthand acid code that is frequently used. The first number in this code gives the number of carbon atoms; the number following the colon is the number of unsaturated centers (mainly double bonds). The location and orientation of the unsaturated centers follow. The symbols used are: c = *cis*; t = *trans*; a = acetylenic center; e = ethylenic center at end of chain; ep = *epoxy*. Thus 9c,11t indicates a double bond with *cis* orientation at the No. 9 carbon and another with *trans* orientation at the No. 11 carbon. More details on the codes can be found in Reference 1.

The table gives the molecular weight and melting point of the acid and the melting and boiling points of the methyl ester of the acid when available. A superscript on the boiling point indicates the pressure in mmHg (torr); if there is no superscript, the value refers to one atmosphere (760 mmHg). The references cover many

other fatty acids beyond those listed here and give additional properties.

We are indebted to Frank D. Gunstone for advice on the content of the table.

References

1. Gunstone, F. D., Harwood, J. L., and Dijkstra, A. J., eds., *The Lipid Handbook*, Third Edition, CRC Press, Boca Raton, FL, 2006.
2. Gunstone, F. D., and Adlof, R. O., *Common (non-systematic) Names for Fatty Acids*, www.aocs.org/member/division/analytic/fanames.asp, 2003.
3. Firestone, D., *Physical and Chemical Characteristics of Oils, Fats, and Waxes*, Second Edition, AOCS Press, Urbana, IL, 2006.
4. Dawson, R. M. C., Elliott, D. C., Elliott, W. H., and Jones, K. M., *Data for Biochemical Research*, Third Edition, Clarendon Press, Oxford, 1986.
5. Altman, P. L., and Dittmer, D. S., eds., *Biology Data Book*, Second Edition, Vol. 1, Federation of American Societies for Experimental Biology, Bethesda, MD, 1972.
6. Fasman, G. D., Ed., *Practical Handbook of Biochemistry and Molecular Biology*, CRC Press, Boca Raton, FL, 1989.

Systematic Name	Common Name	Mol. Form.	Acid Code	CAS RN	Mol. Weight	mp/°C	Methyl Ester	
							mp/°C	bp/°C
Butanoic acid	Butyric acid	$C_4H_8O_2$	4:0	107-92-6	88.106	−5.1	−85.8	102.8
Pentanoic acid	Valeric acid	$C_5H_{10}O_2$	5:0	109-52-4	102.132	−33.6		127.4
3-Methylbutanoic acid	Isovaleric acid	$C_5H_{10}O_2$	4:0 3-Me	503-74-2	102.132	−29.3		116.5
Hexanoic acid	Caproic acid	$C_6H_{12}O_2$	6:0	142-62-1	116.158	−3	−71	149.5
Heptanoic acid	Enanthic acid	$C_7H_{14}O_2$	7:0	111-14-8	130.185	−7.2	−56	174
Octanoic acid	Caprylic acid	$C_8H_{16}O_2$	8:0	124-07-2	144.212	16.5	−40	192.9
Nonanoic acid	Pelargonic acid	$C_9H_{18}O_2$	9:0	112-05-0	158.238	12.4		213.5
Decanoic acid	Capric acid	$C_{10}H_{20}O_2$	10:0	334-48-5	172.265	31.4	−18	224
9-Decenoic acid	Caproleic acid	$C_{10}H_{18}O_2$	10:1 9e	14436-32-9	170.249	26.5		120[20]
Undecanoic acid		$C_{11}H_{22}O_2$	11:0	112-37-8	186.292	28.6		123[10]
Dodecanoic acid	Lauric acid	$C_{12}H_{24}O_2$	12:0	143-07-7	200.318	43.8	5.2	267
cis-9-Dodecenoic acid	Lauroleic acid	$C_{12}H_{22}O_2$	12:1 9c	2382-40-3	198.302			
Tridecanoic acid		$C_{13}H_{26}O_2$	13:0	638-53-9	214.344	41.5	6.5	92[1]
Tetradecanoic acid	Myristic acid	$C_{14}H_{28}O_2$	14:0	544-63-8	228.371	54.2	19	295
cis-9-Tetradecenoic acid	Myristoleic acid	$C_{14}H_{26}O_2$	14:1 9c	13147-06-3	226.355	−4		
Pentadecanoic acid		$C_{15}H_{30}O_2$	15:0	1002-84-2	242.398	52.3	18.5	153.5
Hexadecanoic acid	Palmitic acid	$C_{16}H_{32}O_2$	16:0	57-10-3	256.424	62.5	30	417
cis-9-Hexadecenoic acid	Palmitoleic acid	$C_{16}H_{30}O_2$	16:1 9c	373-49-9	254.408	0.5		140[5]
Heptadecanoic acid	Margaric acid	$C_{17}H_{34}O_2$	17:0	506-12-7	270.451	61.3	30	185[9]
Octadecanoic acid	Stearic acid	$C_{18}H_{36}O_2$	18:0	57-11-4	284.478	69.3	39.1	443
cis-6-Octadecenoic acid	Petroselinic acid	$C_{18}H_{34}O_2$	18:1 6c	593-39-5	282.462	29.8		
cis-9-Octadecenoic acid	Oleic acid	$C_{18}H_{34}O_2$	18:1 9c	112-80-1	282.462	13.4	−19.9	218.5[20]
trans-9-Octadecenoic acid	Elaidic acid	$C_{18}H_{34}O_2$	18:1 9t	112-79-8	282.462	45	13.5	218[24]
cis-11-Octadecenoic acid	*cis*-Vaccenic acid	$C_{18}H_{34}O_2$	18:1 11c	506-17-2	282.462	15		163[0.1]
trans-11-Octadecenoic acid	Vaccenic acid	$C_{18}H_{34}O_2$	18:1 11t	693-72-1	282.462	44		172[3]
cis-12,13-Epoxy-*cis*-9-octadecenoic acid	Vernolic acid	$C_{18}H_{32}O_3$	18:1 12,13-ep,9c	503-07-1	296.445	32.5		
12-Hydroxy-*cis*-9-octadecenoic acid	Ricinoleic acid	$C_{18}H_{34}O_3$	18:1 12-OH,9c	141-22-0	298.461	5.5		226[15]

Systematic Name	Common Name	Mol. Form.	Acid Code	CAS RN	Mol. Weight	mp/°C	Methyl Ester mp/°C	bp/°C
cis,trans-9,11-Octadecadienoic acid	Rumenic (CLA)	$C_{18}H_{32}O_2$	18:2 9c,11t	1839-11-8	280.446	20		
cis,cis-9,12-Octadecadienoic acid	Linoleic acid	$C_{18}H_{32}O_2$	18:2 9c,12c	60-33-3	280.446	−7	−35	215[20]
trans,cis-10,12-Octadecadienoic acid	(CLA)	$C_{18}H_{32}O_2$	18:2 10t,12c	22880-03-1	280.446	23	−12	
cis-9-Octadecen-12-ynoic acid	Crepenynic acid	$C_{18}H_{30}O_2$	18:2 9c,12a	2277-31-8	278.430			
cis,cis,cis-5,9,12-Octadecatrienoic acid	Pinolenic acid	$C_{18}H_{30}O_2$	18:3 5c,9c,12c	27213-43-0	278.430			
trans,cis,cis-5,9,12-Octadecatrienoic acid	Columbinic acid	$C_{18}H_{30}O_2$	18:3 5t,9c,12c	2441-53-4	278.430			
cis,cis,cis-6,9,12-Octadecatrienoic acid	γ-Linolenic acid	$C_{18}H_{30}O_2$	18:3 6c,9c,12c	506-26-3	278.430			162[0.5]
trans,trans,cis-8,10,12-Octadecatrienoic acid	Calendic acid	$C_{18}H_{30}O_2$	18:3 8t,10t,12c	28872-28-8	278.430	40		
cis,trans,cis-9,11,13-Octadecatrienoic acid	Punicic acid	$C_{18}H_{30}O_2$	18:3 9c,11t,13c	544-72-9	278.430	45		
cis,trans,trans-9,11,13-Octadecatrienoic acid	α-Eleostearic acid	$C_{18}H_{30}O_2$	18:3 9c,11t,13t	506-23-0	278.430	49		148[1]
trans,trans,cis-9,11,13-Octadecatrienoic acid	Catalpic acid	$C_{18}H_{30}O_2$	18:3 9t,11t,13c	4337-71-7	278.430	32		
trans,trans,trans-9,11,13-Octadecatrienoic acid	β-Eleostearic acid	$C_{18}H_{30}O_2$	18:3 9t,11t,13t	544-73-0	278.430	71.5	13	162[1]
cis,cis,cis-9,12,15-Octadecatrienoic acid	α-Linolenic acid	$C_{18}H_{30}O_2$	18:3 9c,12c,15c	463-40-1	278.430	−11.3	−52	109[0.018]
6,9,12,15-Octadecatetraenoic acid, all *cis*	Stearidonic acid	$C_{18}H_{28}O_2$	18:4 6c,9c,12c,15c	20290-75-9	276.414	−57		
cis,trans,trans,cis-9,11,13,15-Octadecatetraenoic acid	Parinaric acid	$C_{18}H_{28}O_2$	18:4 9c,11t,13t,15c	593-38-4	276.414	86		
Nonadecanoic acid		$C_{19}H_{38}O_2$	19:0	646-30-0	298.504	69.4	41.3	190[4]
Eicosanoic acid	Arachidic acid	$C_{20}H_{40}O_2$	20:0	506-30-9	312.531	76.5	54.5	215[10]
3,7,11,15-Tetramethylhexadecanoic acid	Phytanic acid	$C_{20}H_{40}O_2$	16:0 3,7,11,15-tetramethyl	14721-66-5	312.531	−65		
cis-5-Eicosenoic acid		$C_{20}H_{38}O_2$	20:1 5c	7050-07-9	310.515	27		
cis-9-Eicosenoic acid	Gadoleic acid	$C_{20}H_{38}O_2$	20:1 9c	29204-02-2	310.515	24.5		
cis-11-Eicosenoic acid	Gondoic acid	$C_{20}H_{38}O_2$	20:1 11c	2462-94-4	310.515	24		
cis,cis,cis-8,11,14-Eicosatrienoic acid	Dihomo-γ-linolenic acid	$C_{20}H_{34}O_2$	20:3 8c,11c,14c	1783-84-2				
5,8,11,14-Eicosatetraenoic acid, all *cis*	Arachidonic acid	$C_{20}H_{32}O_2$	20:4 5c,8c,11c,14c	506-32-1	304.467	−49.5		195[0.7]
5,8,11,14,17-Eicosapentaenoic acid, all *cis*	Timnodonic acid, EPA	$C_{20}H_{30}O_2$	20:5 5c,8c,11c,14c,17c	10417-94-4	302.451	−54		
Heneicosanoic acid		$C_{21}H_{42}O_2$	21:0	2363-71-5	326.557	82	49	207[4]
Docosanoic acid	Behenic acid	$C_{22}H_{44}O_2$	22:0	112-85-6	340.583	81.5	54	
cis-11-Docosenoic acid	Cetolic acid	$C_{22}H_{42}O_2$	22:1 11c	506-36-5	338.567	33		
cis-13-Docosenoic acid	Erucic acid	$C_{22}H_{42}O_2$	22:1 13c	112-86-7	338.567	34.7		221[5]
trans-13-Docosenoic acid	Brassidic acid	$C_{22}H_{42}O_2$	22:1 13t	506-33-2	338.567	61.9	35	
cis,cis-5,13-Docosadienoic acid		$C_{22}H_{40}O_2$	22:2 5c,13c	676-39-1	336.552	−4		
7,10,13,16,19-Docosapentaenoic acid, all *cis*		$C_{22}H_{34}O_2$	22:5 7c,10c,13c,16c, 19c					
4,7,10,13,16,19-Docosahexaenoic acid, all *cis*	Cervonic acid, DHA	$C_{22}H_{32}O_2$	22:6 4c,7c,10c,13c, 16c,19c	2091-24-9		−45		
Tricosanoic acid		$C_{23}H_{46}O_2$	23:0	2433-96-7		79.6	53.4	
Tetracosanoic acid	Lignoceric acid	$C_{24}H_{48}O_2$	24:0	557-59-5	368.637	87.5	60	
cis-15-Tetracosenoic acid	Nervonic acid	$C_{24}H_{46}O_2$	24:1 15c	506-37-6	366.621	43	15	165[0.02]
Pentacosanoic acid		$C_{25}H_{50}O_2$	25:0	506-38-7	382.664	77.5	62	
Hexacosanoic acid	Cerotic acid	$C_{26}H_{52}O_2$	26:0	506-46-7	396.690	88.5	63.8	286[15]
Heptacosanoic acid		$C_{27}H_{54}O_2$	27:0	7138-40-1		87.6	64	
Octacosanoic acid	Montanic acid	$C_{28}H_{56}O_2$	28:0	506-48-9	424.744	90.9	67	
Nonacosanoic acid		$C_{29}H_{58}O_2$	29:0	4250-38-8	438.770	90.3	69	
Triacontanoic acid	Melissic acid	$C_{30}H_{60}O_2$	30:0	506-50-3	452.796	93.6	72	
Hentriacontanoic acid		$C_{31}H_{62}O_2$	31:0	38232-01-8	466.823	93.1		
Dotriacontanoic acid	Lacceric acid	$C_{32}H_{64}O_2$	32:0	3625-52-3	480.849	96.2		192[0.01]

DENSITIES, SPECIFIC VOLUMES, AND TEMPERATURE COEFFICIENTS OF FATTY ACIDS FROM C_8 TO C_{12}

Acid	Temperature, °C	Density,[a] g/cc	Specific Volume, l/d	Temp. Coeff. per °C
Caprylic	10.0	1.0326	0.9685	0.00098
	15	1.0274	0.9733	—
	20	0.9109	1.0979	0.00046
	20.02	0.9101[b]	—	—
	25	0.9090	1.1002	—
	50.27	0.8862[b]	—	0.00099
Nonanoic	5.0	0.9952	1.0048	0.00074
	10	0.9916	1.0085	—
	15	0.9097	1.0993	0.00104
	15.00	0.9087[b]	—	—
	25	0.9011	1.1097	—
Capric	15.0	1.0266	0.9741	0.00085
	25	1.0176	0.9827	—
	35	0.8927	1.1202	0.00128
	35.05	0.8884[b]	—	—
	40	0.8876	1.1266	—
Hendecanoic	0.12	1.0431	0.9587	0.00054
	10.0	1.0373	0.9640	—
	20	0.9948	1.0052	0.00079
	25	0.9905	1.0096	—
	30	0.8907	1.1227	0.00093
	30.00	0.8889[b]	—	—
	35	0.8871	1.1273	—
	50.15	0.8741[b]	—	0.00095
Lauric	35.0	1.0099	0.9902	0.00087
	40	1.0055	0.9945	—
	45	0.8767	1.1406	0.00142
	45.10	0.8744[b]	—	0.00095
	50	0.8713	1.1477	—
	50.25	0.8707[b]	—	0.00095

[a] By air thermometer method unless specified otherwise.
[b] By pycnometer method.
From Markley, Klare S., *Fatty Acids*, 2nd ed., Part 1, Interscience Publishers, Inc., New York, 1960, 535. With permission of copyright owners.

COMPOSITION AND PROPERTIES OF COMMON OILS AND FATS

This table lists some of the most common naturally occurring oils and fats. The list is separated into those of plant origin, fish and other marine life origin, and land animal origin. The oils and fats consist mainly of esters of glycerol (i.e., triglycerides) with fatty acids of 10 to 22 carbon atoms. The four fatty acids with the highest concentration are given for each oil; concentrations are given in weight percent. Because there is often a wide variation in composition depending on the source of the oil sample, a range (or sometimes an average) is generally given. More complete data on composition, including minor fatty acids, sterols, and tocopherols, can be found in the references.

The acids are labeled by the codes described in the previous table, "Properties of Fatty Acids and Their Methyl Esters," which gives the systematic and common names of the acids. Thus 18:2 9c,12c indicates a C_{18} acid with two double bonds in the 9 and 12 positions, both with a *cis* configuration (*cis,cis*-9,12-octadecadienoic acid, or linoleic acid).

The density and refractive index of the oils are typical values; superscripts indicate the temperature in °C.

Notes:

- The composition figure given for oleic acid (18:1 9c) often includes low levels of other 18:1 isomers.

- In some oils where a concentration is given for 18:2 9c,12c (linoleic acid), other isomers of 18:2 may be included.
- Likewise, where a concentration is given for 18:3 9c,12c,15c (α-linolenic acid), other isomers of 18:3 may be included.
- The acid 20:5 6c,9c,12c,15c,17c, which is prevalent in many fish oils, is often abbreviated as 20:5 ω-3 or 20:5 n-3.

The assistance of Frank D. Gunstone in preparing this table is gratefully acknowledged.

References

1. Firestone, D., *Physical and Chemical Characteristics of Oils, Fats, and Waxes,* Second Edition, AOCS Press, Urbana, IL, 2006.
2. Gunstone, F. D., Harwood, J. L., and Dijkstra, A. J., eds., *The Lipid Handbook,* Third Edition, CRC Press, Boca Raton, FL, 2006.
3. Dawson, R. M. C., Elliott, D. C., Elliott, W. H., and Jones, K. M., *Data for Biochemical Research,* Third Edition, Clarendon Press, Oxford, 1986.
4. Altman, P. L., and Dittmer, D. S., eds., *Biology Data Book,* Second Edition, Vol. 1, Federation of American Societies for Experimental Biology, Bethesda, MD, 1972.

Type of Oil	Principal Fatty Acid Components in Weight %				mp/ °C	Density/ g cm⁻³	Refractive Index	Iodine Value	Saponification Value
			PLANTS						
Almond kernel oil	18:1 9c	43–70%	18:2 9c,12c	24–30%		0.910[25]	1.467[26]	89–101	188–200
	16:0	4–13%	18:0	1–10%					
Apricot kernel oil	18:1 9c	58–66%	18:2 9c,12c	29–33%		0.910[25]	1.469[25]	97–110	185–199
	16:0	4.6–6%	18:0	1%					
Argan seed oil	18:1 9c	42–55%	18:2 9c,12c	30–34%		0.912[20]	1.467[20]	92–102	189–195
	16:0	12–16%	18:0	2–7%					
Avocado pulp oil	18:1 9c	56–74%	18:2 9c,12c	10–17%		0.912[25]	1.466[25]	85–90	177–198
	16:0	9–18%	16:1 9c	3–9%					
Babassu palm oil	12:0	40–55%	14:0	11–27%	24	0.914[25]	1.450[40]	10–18	245–256
	18:1 9c	9–20%	16:0	5.2–11%					
Blackcurrant oil	18:2 9c,12c	45–50%	18:3 6c,9c,12c	14–20%		0.923[20]	1.480[20]	173–182	185–195
	18:3 9c,12c,15c	12–15%	18:1 9c	9–13%					
Borage (star-flower) oil	18:2 9c,12c	36–40%	18:3 6c,9c,12c	17–25%				141–160	189–192
	18:1 9c	14–21%	16:0	9.4–12%					
Borneo tallow	18:0	39–43%	18:1 9c	34–37%	38	0.855[100]	1.456[40]	29–38	189–200
	16:0	18–21%	20:0	1.0%					
Cameline oil	18:3 9c,12c,15c	33–38%	18:2 9c,12c	15–16%		0.924[15]	1.477[20]	127–155	180–190
	20:1 total	14–16%	18:1 9c	12–24%					
Canola (rapeseed) oil (low linolenic)	18:1 9c	59–66%	18:2 9c,12c	24–29%	−10			91	
	16:0	4–5%	18:3 9c,12c,15c	2–3%					
Canola (rapeseed) oil (low erucic)	18:1 9c	52–67%	18:2 9c,12c	16–25%	−10	0.915[20]	1.466[40]	110–126	182–193
	18:3 9c,12c,15c	6–14%	16:0	3.3–6.0%					
Caraway seed oil	18:1 9c	40%	18:2 9c,12c	30%			1.471[35]	128	178
	18:1 6c	26%	16:0	3%					
Cashew nut oil	18:1 9c	57–80%	18:2 9c,12c	16–22%		0.914[15]	1.463[40]	79–89	180–196
	16:0	4–17%	18:0	2–12%					
Castor oil	18:1 12-OH,9c	88%	18:2 9c,12c	3–5%	−18	0.952[25]	1.475[25]	81–91	176–187
	18:1 9c	2.9–6%	22:0	2.1%					
Cherry kernel oil	18:2 9c,12c	42–45%	18:1 9c	35–49%		0.918[25]	1.468[40]	110–118	190–198
	16:0	4–9%	18:3 9c,11t,13t	3–10%					
Chinese vegetable tallow	16:0	58–72%	18:1 9c	20–35%	44	0.887[25]	1.456[40]	16–29	200–218
	18:0	1–8%	14:0	0.5–3.7%					
Cocoa butter	18:0	31–37%	18:1 9c	31–35%	34	0.974[25]	1.457[40]	32–40	192–200
	16:0	25–27%	18:2 9c,12c	2.8–4.0%					
Coconut oil	12:0	45–51%	14:0	17–21%	25	0.913[40]	1.449[40]	5–13	248–265

Composition and Properties of Common Oils and Fats (Continued)

Type of Oil	Principal Fatty Acid Components in Weight %				mp/ °C	Density/ g cm⁻³	Refractive Index	Iodine Value	Saponification Value

PLANTS (Continued)

Type of Oil	Principal Fatty Acid Components in Weight %				mp/ °C	Density/ g cm⁻³	Refractive Index	Iodine Value	Saponification Value
	16:0	7.7–10.2%	18:1 9c	5.4–9.9%					
Cohune nut oil	12:0	44–48%	14:0	16–17%		0.914^{25}	1.450^{40}	9–14	251–260
	18:1 9c	8–10%	16:0	7–10%					
Coriander seed oil	18:1 6c	53%	18:1 9c	32%		0.908^{25}	1.464^{25}	86–100	182–191
	18:2 9c,12c	7–14%	16:0	3–8%					
Corn oil	18:2 9c,12c	40–66%	18:1 9c	20–42%	−20	0.919^{20}	1.472^{25}	107–135	187–195
	16:0	9–16%	18:0	0–3%					
Cottonseed oil	18:2 9c,12c	47–58%	16:0	18–26%	−1	0.920^{20}	1.462^{40}	96–115	189–198
	18:1 9c	14–22%	18:0	2.1–3.3%					
Crambe oil	22:1 13c	55–60%	18:1 9c	12–15%		0.906^{25}	1.470^{25}	87–113	
	18:2 9c,12c	8–10%	18:3 9c,12c,15c	6–7%					
Cuphea seed oil (caprylic acid rich)	8:0	65–78%	10:0	19–24%					
	18:2 9c,12c	1–4%	16:0	0.6–3%					
Euphorbia lagascae seed oil	18:1 12,13-ep,9c	64%	18:1 other	19%		0.952^{25}	1.473^{25}	102	
	18:2 9c,12c	9%	16:0	4%					
Evening primrose oil	18:2 9c,12c	65–80%	18:3 6c,9c,12c	8–14%			1.479^{20}	147–155	193–198
	16:0	6–10%	18:1 9c	5–12%					
Grape seed oil	18:2 9c,12c	58–78%	18:1 9c	12–28%		0.923^{20}	1.475^{40}	130–138	188–194
	16:0	5.5–11%	18:0	3–6%					
Hazelnut oil (Chilean)	18:1 9c	39%	16:1 11c	22.7%					
	20:1 total	9.7%	22:1 total	9.5%					
Hazelnut oil (Filbert)	18:1 9c	72–84%	18:2 9c,12c	5.7–22%		0.909^{25}	1.473^{25}	83–90	188–197
	16:0	4.1–7.2%	18:0	1.5–2.4%					
Hempseed oil	18:2 9c,12c	45–60%	18:3 9c,12c,15c	15–30%		0.921^{25}	1.472^{40}	145–166	190–195
	18:1 9c	11–16%	16:0	6–12%					
Illipe (mowrah) butter	18:1 9c	34%	16:0	23%	27	0.862^{100}	1.460^{40}	53–70	188–207
	18:0	23%	18:2 9c,12c	14%					
Jojoba oil[a]	20:1 total	66–74%	22:1 undefined	9–19%					
	18:1 9c	5–12%	24:1 15c	1–5%					
Kapok seed oil[b]	18:1 9c	45–65%	16:0	10–28%	30	0.926^{15}	1.469^{25}	86–110	189–197
	18:2 9c,12c	7–35%	18:0	2–9%					
Kokum butter	18:0	49–56%	18:1 9c	39–49%	41		1.456^{40}	33–37	192
	16:0	2–5%	18:2 9c,12c	1–2%					
Kusum oil	18:1 9c	57–62%	20:0	20–25%			1.461^{40}	48–58	220–230
	16:0	5–8%	18:0	2–6%					
Linola oil	18:2 9c,12c	72%	18:1 9c	16%				142	
	16:0	5.6%	18:0	4.0%					
Linseed oil	18:3 9c,12c,15c	52–58%	18:1 9c	18–20%	−24	0.924^{25}	1.480^{25}	170–203	188–196
	18:2 9c,12c	17%	18:2 9c,12c	16%					
Macadamia nut oil	18:1 9c	56–59%	16:1 9c	21–22%					
	16:0	8–9%	18:0	2–4%					
Mango seed oil	18:1 9c	38–50%	18:0	31–49%		0.912^{15}	1.461^{25}	39–48	188–195
	18:2 9c,12c	3–6%	20:0	2–6%					
Meadowfoam seed oil	20:1 5c	58–77%	22:1 total	8–24%			1.464^{40}	86–91	168
	22:2 5c,13c	7–15%	18:1 9c	1–3%					
Melon oil	18:2 9c,12c	67% (av.)	18:1 9c	12% (av.)					
	16:0	11% (av.)	18:0	9% (av.)					
Moringa peregrina seed oil	18:1 9c	70%	16:0	9%		0.903^{24}	1.460^{40}	70	185
	18:0	3.8%	22:0	2.4%					
Mustard seed oil	22:1 13c	43%	22:1 13c	22–50%		0.913^{20}	1.465^{40}	92–125	170–184
	18:3 9c,12c,15c	12%	18:2 9c,12c	10–24%					
Neem oil	18:1 9c	49–62%	18:0	14–24%	−3	0.912^{30}	1.462^{40}	68–71	195–205
	16:0	13–18%	18:2 9c,12c	7–15%					
Niger seed oil	18:2 9c,12c	52–78%	16:0	5–12%		0.924^{15}	1.468^{40}	126–135	188–193
	18:1 9c	4–10%	18:0	2–12%					
Nutmeg butter	14:0	76–83%	18:1 9c	5–11%	45		1.468^{40}	48–85	170–190
	16:0	4–10%	12:0	3–6%					
Oat oil	18:2 9c,12c	24–48%	18:1 9c	18–53%		0.917^{25}	1.467^{40}	105–116	190–199
	16:0	13–39%	18:0	0.5–4%					
Oiticica oil	18:3 9c,11t,13t, 4-oxo	70–80%	16:0	7%		0.972^{20}	1.514^{25}	140–150	188–193
	18:0	5%	18:1 9c	4–7%					

Composition and Properties of Common Oils and Fats (Continued)

Type of Oil	Principal Fatty Acid Components in Weight %				mp/ °C	Density/ g cm⁻³	Refractive Index	Iodine Value	Saponification Value
			PLANTS **(Continued)**						
Olive oil	18:1 9c	55–83%	18:2 9c,12c	9%	-6	0.911^{20}	1.469^{20}	75–94	184–196
	16:0	7.5–20%	18:2 9c,12c	3.5–21%					
Palm kernel oil	12:0	40–55%	14:0	14–18%	24	0.922^{15}	1.450^{40}	14–21	230–250
	18:1 9c	12–21%	16:0	6.5–10%					
Palm oil	16:0	40–48%	18:1 9c	36–44%	35	0.914^{15}	1.455^{40}	49–55	190–209
	18:2 9c,12c	6.5–12%	18:0	3.5–6.5%					
Palm olein	18:1 9c	40–44%	16:0	38–43%		0.914^{0}	1.459^{40}	>56	194–202
	18:2 9c,12c	10–13%	18:0	3.7–4.8%					
Palm stearin	16:0	48–74%	18:1 9c	16–36%		0.884^{60}	1.449^{40}	<48	193–205
	18:0	3.9–5.6%	18:2 9c,12c	3.2–9.8%					
Parsley seed oil	18:1 6c	69–76%	18:1 9c	12–15%			1.4800^{40}	110–120	
	18:2 9c,12c	6–14%	16:0	2%					
Peanut oil	18:1 9c	36–67%	18:2 9c,12c	14–43%	3	0.914^{20}	1.463^{40}	86–107	187–196
	16:0	8.3–14%	22:0	2.1–4.4%					
Perilla oil	18:3 9c,12c,15c	59%	18:2 9c,12c	14–18%		0.924^{25}	1.477^{25}	192–208	188–197
	18:1 9c	11–13%	16:0	6–9%					
Phulwara butter	16:0	57–61%	18:1 9c	30–36%	43	0.862^{100}	1.458^{40}	40–51	188–200
	18:2 9c,12c	3–4%	18:0	3–4%					
Pine nut oil	18:2 9c,12c	47–51%	18:1 9c	36–39%		0.919^{15}		118–121	193–197
	16:0	6–8%	18:0	2–3%					
Poppy seed oil	18:2 9c,12c	62–73%	18:1 9c	16–30%	-15	0.916^{25}	1.469^{40}	132–146	188–196
	16:0	7–11%	18:0	1–4%					
Rice bran oil	18:1 9c	38–48%	18:2 9c,12c	16–36%		0.916^{25}	1.472^{25}	92–108	181–189
	16:0	16–28%	18:0	2–4%					
Safflower seed oil	18:2 9c,12c	68–83%	18:1 9c	8.4–30%		0.924^{15}	1.474^{25}	136–148	186–198
	16:0	5.3–8.0%	18:0	1.9–2.9%					
Safflower seed oil	18:1 9c	74–80%	18:2 9c,12c	13–18%		0.921^{20}	1.470^{25}	91–95	
(high oleic)	16:0	5–6%	18:0	1.5–2.0%					
Sal fat	18:0	33–57%	18:1 9c	31–52%	33		1.456^{40}	31–45	175–192
	16:0	6–23%	20:0	1–8%					
Sesame seed oil	18:2 9c,12c	40–51%	18:1 9c	33–44%	-6	0.917^{20}	1.467^{40}	104–120	187–195
	16:0	7.9–10.2%	18:0	4.4–6.7%					
Sheanut butter	18:1 9c	45–50%	18:0	36–41%	38	0.863^{100}	1.465^{40}	52–66	178–198
	16:0	4–8%	18:2 9c,12c	4–8%					
Soybean oil	18:2 9c,12c	50–57%	18:1 9c	18–28%	-16	0.920^{20}	1.468^{40}	118–139	189–195
	16:0	9–13%	18:3 9c,12c,15c	5.5–9.5%					
Stillingia seed kernel oil[c]	18:3 total	41–54%	18:2 9c,12c	24–30%		0.937^{25}	1.483^{25}	169–191	202–212
	18:1 9c	7–10%	16:0	6–9%					
Sunflower seed oil	18:2 9c,12c	48–74%	18:1 9c	13–40%	-17	0.919^{20}	1.474^{25}	118–145	188–194
	16:0	5–8%	18:0	2.5–7.0%					
Sunflower oil, high-oleic	18:1 9c	80%	18:2 9c,12c	10%					
(HO)	18:0	4.4%	16:0	3.5%		0.911^{25}	1.468^{25}	81	
Sunflower oil, mid-Oleic	18:1 9c	65%	18:2, 18:3	25%					
(NuSun oil)	16:0, 18:0	10%							
Tall oil	18:2 9c,12c	41–52%	18:1 9c	41–48%		0.969^{25}	1.494^{25}	140–180	154–180
	16:0	5–6%	18:0	2–3%					
Tung oil	18:3 9c,11t,13t	71–82%	18:2 9c,12c	8–15%	-2	0.912^{25}	1.517^{25}	160–175	189–195
	18:1 9c	4–10%	18:0	3%					
Ucuhuba butter oil	14:0	64–73%	12:0	13–15%		0.870^{100}	1.451^{50}	11–17	221–229
	18:1 9c	6–8%	16:0	3–9%					
Vernonia seed oil	18:1 12,13-ep,9c	62–72%	18:2 9c,12c	9–17%		0.901^{30}	1.486^{32}	55	176
	16:0	3–7%	18:0	2–6%					
Walnut oil	18:2 9c,12c	56–60%	18:1 9c	17–19%		0.921^{25}	1.474^{25}	138–162	189–197
	18:3 9c,12c,15c	13–14%	16:0	6–8%					
Wheatgerm oil	18:2 9c,12c	50–59%	18:1 9c	13–23%		0.926^{25}	1.479^{25}	100–128	179–217
	16:0	12–20%	18:3 9c,12c,15c	2–9%					
			MARINE ANIMALS						
Anchovy oil	20:5 6c,9c,12c,15c,17c	22%	16:0	17%				163–169	191–194
	16:1 undefined	13%	18:1 undefined	10%					
Capelin oil[d]	20:1 undefined	17%	22:1 undefined	15%			1.463^{50}	94–164	185–202
	18:1 undefined	14%	16:0	10%					

Composition and Properties of Common Oils and Fats (Continued)

Type of Oil	Principal Fatty Acid Components in Weight %				mp/ °C	Density/ g cm⁻³	Refractive Index	Iodine Value	Saponification Value
MARINE ANIMALS (Continued)									
Cod liver oil	18:1 undefined	24%	20:1 undefined	13%		0.924^{15}	1.482^{25}	142–176	180–192
	22:6 4c,7c,10c,13c, 16c,19c	11%	16:0	10%					
Herring oil	22:1 undefined	19%	16:0	17%		0.914^{20}	1.474^{25}	115–160	161–192
	20:1 undefined	15%	18:1 undefined	14%					
Mackerel oil	22:1 undefined	15%	16:0	14%		0.929^{15}	1.481^{20}	136–167	
	18:1 undefined	13%	20:1 undefined	12%					
Menhaden oil	16:0	19%	20:5 6c,9c,12c,15c,17c	14%		0.920^{15}		150–200	192–199
	16:1 undefined	12%	18:1 undefined	11%					
Salmon oil	22:6 4c,7c,10c,13c, 16c,19c	18%	20:5 6c,9c,12c,15c,17c	13%		0.924^{15}	1.475^{25}	130–160	183–186
	16:0	9.8%	16:1	4.8%					
Sardine oil	16:0	18%	20:5 6c,9c,12c,15c,17c	16%		0.915^{25}	1.464^{65}	159–192	188–199
	18:1 undefined	13%	16:1 undefined	10%					
Seal blubber oil, harp	18:1 9c	21%	20:1	12%					
	22:6 4c,7c,10c,13c, 16c,19c	7.6%	20:5 6c,9c,12c,15c,17c	6.4%					
Shark liver oil	18:1 undefined	45%	16:0	21%		0.917^{25}	1.476^{25}	150–300	170–190
	20:1	12%	22:1	9%					
Tuna oil	22:6 4c,7c,10c,13c, 16c,19c	22%	16:0	22%					
	18:1 undefined	21%	20:5 6c,9c,12c,15c,17c	6%					
Trout lipids	16:0	21–24%	18:1 undefined	18–31%					
	18:2	7–16%	16:1	4–10%					
Whale oil, minke	18:1 undefined	18%	20:1	17%					
	22:1	11%	16:1	9%					
LAND ANIMALS									
Beef tallow	18:1 undefined	31–50%	18:0	25–40%	47	0.902^{25}	1.454^{40}	33–47	190–200
	16:0	20–37%	14:0	1–6%					
Butterfat	16:0	28.1% (av.)	18:1 9c	20.8% (av.)	32	0.934^{15}	1.455^{40}	26–40	210–232
	14:0	10.8% (av.)	18:0	10.6% (av.)					
Chicken egg lipids, yolk	16:0	28%	18:1 9c	25%					
	18:0	17%	18:2 9c,12c	16%					
Chicken fat	18:1 undefined	37%	16:0	22%		0.918^{15}	1.456^{40}	76–80	
	18:2	20%	18:0	6%					
Milk fats, cow	16:0	28.2% (av.)	18:1 9c	21.4% (av.)					
	18:0	12.6% (av.)	14:0	10.6% (av.)					
Milk fats, human	18:1 9c	31.1% (av.)	16:0	21.6% (av.)					
	18:2 9c,12c	11.7% (av.)	14:0	6.6% (av.)					
Mutton tallow	18:1 undefined	30–42%	18:0	22–34%	48	0.946^{15}	1.455^{40}	35–46	
	16:0	20–27%	14:0	2–4%					
Pork lard	18:1 undefined	35–62%	16:0	20–32%	30	0.898^{20}			
	18:0	5–24%	18:2	3–16%					

[a] Jojoba oil consists primarily of wax esters of the acids listed here and long-chain alcohols.
[b] Kapok oil also contains up to 15% cyclopropene acids.
[c] Stillingia oil also contains 5–10% trans, cis-2,4-decadienoic acid (stillingic acid, 10:2 2t,4c).
[d] Capelin oil also contains about 10% 16:1.

SPECTRAL PROPERTIES OF FATTY ACIDS

Roger L. Lundblad

Most lipids including fatty acids lack the chromophores necessary for ultraviolet-visible spectrophotometry, but there are some studies of unsaturated fatty acids. Raman spectroscopy and infrared (IR) spectrophotometry do have considerable application in the study of lipids.

UV-Vis Spectral Properties of Fatty Acids

TABLE 1: UV-Vis spectra of some chromophoric groups important in fatty acids

Chromophore	Example	Λ_{max} (nm)	ε	Solvent
–C=C–	Octene	177	12,600	Heptane
–C=C–C=C–	Butadiene	217	20,900	Heptane
–C=C–C=C–C=C	1,3,5-*trans*-hexatriene[a]	247	68,000	Chloroform
–HC=O	Acetaldehyde	290	17	Hexane
C=O	Acetone	275	17	Ethanol
–C=C–CO–C	Methyl vinyl ketone	213	7,100	Ethanol
–COOH	Acetic acid	208	32	Ethanol
–COOH	Palmitic acid	210	50	Ethanol
–CO₂R	Ethyl acetate	211	50	Ethanol
CH₃CO–CH₂–COOR	Ethyl acetoacetate	245	6,700	Hexane
CH₃CH=CH–CH=CHCOOH	Sorbic acid	251	27,000	Ethanol

Source: Kates, M., *Techniques of Lipidology Isolation, Analysis and Identification of Lipids,* Elseveir, Amsterdam, Netherlands, 1986, p. 170.

[a] There are differences in the electronic spectra of the *cis*- and *trans*-isomers; *trans*-hexatriene does not exhibit fluorescence, whereas *cis*-hexatriene has weak fluorescence (Komainda, A., Zech, A., and Köppel, H., Ab initio quantum study of UV absorption spectra of *cis*- and *trans*-hexatriene, *J. Mol. Spectrosc.* 311, 25–35, 2015).

The principles of UV-Vis spectroscopy are discussed elsewhere.[1,2] Although fatty acids lack distinctive chromophores such as the indole ring of tryptophan or the purine/pyrimidine ring of nucleic acids, there are interesting structures that have absorbance in the UV-Visible region (Table 1). The presence of double bonds (alkenes) can provide UV absorbance.[1,2] The wavelengths of absorbance increase (bathochromic shift) with the increasing length of conjugation.[1] Most unsaturated fatty acids contain double bonds separated by a methylene group and are not conjugated[3,4] (Figure 1) and do not absorb above 220 nm and usually at lower wavelengths (there is absorbance in the near infrared [NIR]). α,β-unsaturated aliphatic carboxylic acids can absorb about 220 nm [5] reflecting conjugation with the carbonyl oxygen.

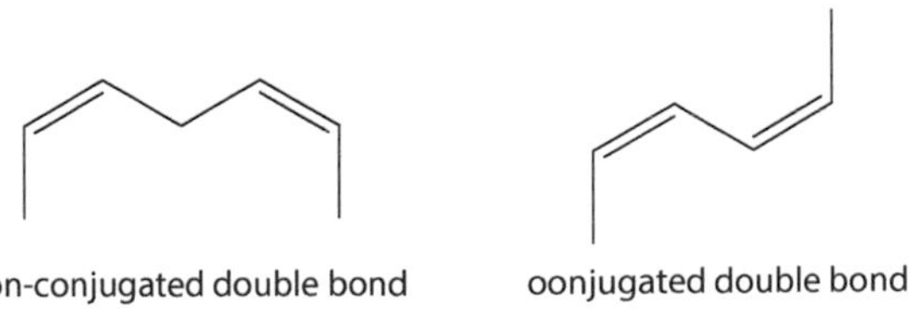

The lipoxygenase pathway can generate a compound absorbing at 282 nm from arachidonic acid.[6] There are several unsaturated fatty acids with conjugated double bonds which does absorb at wavelengths above 230 nm[7,8] such as α-eleostearic acid which absorbs at 270 nm[9] and *cis*-parinaric acid which absorbs at 303 nm[10] (Figure 2). The absorbance of these fatty acids increases on release from glycerides.

Providing an assay for phospholipase A,[11,12] linoleic acid does not contain conjugated double bonds but isomerization results in the formation of conjugated linoleic acid, a collection of linoleic isomers with conjugated double bonds (Figure 3).[13,14] Rumenic (bovinic acid) is found in dairy products and has been suggested to have health effects.[15] The presence of conjugated linoleic acid isomers was responsible for the UV absorbance of early commercial preparations of linoleic acid.[16]

The infrared spectrum can be divided into three regions (Table 2). Although there is use of far-infrared spectrometry in the study of proteins,[17] we could find only one study on the use of far-infrared spectroscopy in the study of liposomes.[18] The mid-infrared (MIR) region is quite useful in the study of fatty acids. Absorbance of foods and oils at 966 cm⁻¹ is used to determine the concentration of *trans*-fatty acid (*trans fats*).[19,20] MIR spectroscopy has been useful for the study of phase transition of fatty acids.[21-23] Some mid-infrared absorption bands useful for lipids are shown in Table 3. Near-infrared spectroscopy (NIR) (Table 4) can distinguish fatty acids based on the absorbance of carbon–hydrogen bonds.[24] NIR has considerable application in the analysis of the composition of food oils such as olive oil.[25,26]

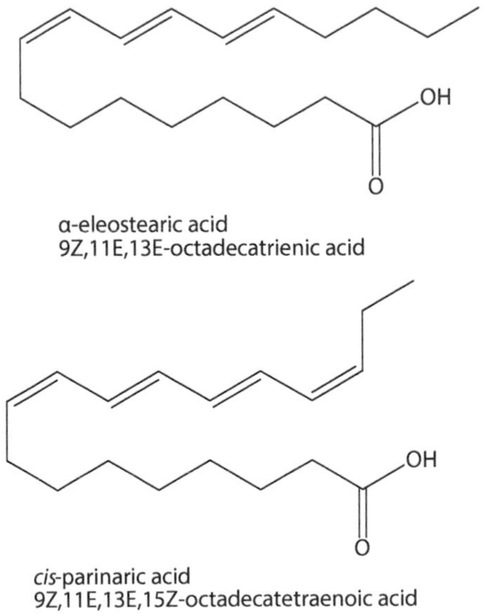

α-eleostearic acid
9Z,11E,13E-octadecatrienic acid

cis-parinaric acid
9Z,11E,13E,15Z-octadecatetraenoic acid

FIGURE 2 Eleostearic acid and parinaric acid.

Non-conjugated double bond   oonjugated double bond

FIGURE 1 Non-conjugated and conjugated double bonds.

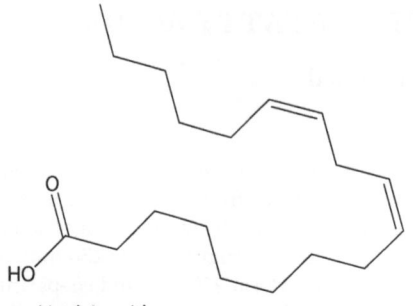

Linoleic acid
(9Z,12Z)-octadeca-9,12-dienoic acid

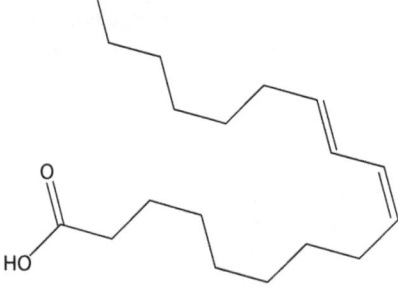

Rumenic acid (Bovinic acid)
(9Z,11E)-octadeca-9,11-dienoic acid

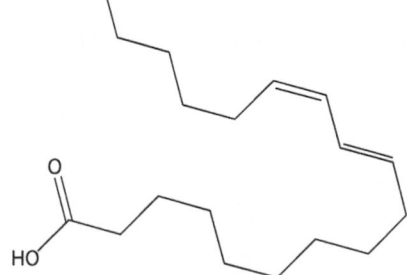

10,12-octadecadienoic acid
(10E,12Z)-octadeca-10,12-dienoic acid

FIGURE 3 Linoleic acid, rumenic acid, and 10,12-octadecadienoic acid.

TABLE 2: Classification of Infrared spectra

Classification	Wavelength/Wavenumber[a]
Near infrared (NIR)	800–2500 nm/12,500–4,000 cm⁻¹
Mid-infrared (MIR)	2.5–25 μm/4000–400 cm⁻¹
Far infrared (THz)[b]	25–300 μm/400–33.3 cm⁻¹

[a] The wavenumber is the reciprocal of the wavelength. The SI unit is m⁻¹ but the convention is cm⁻¹. σ (wave number, cm⁻¹ = 10000/λ (μm)).
[b] Far infrared is also referred as terahertz (https://www.nist.gov/programs-projects/far-infrared-spectroscopy-biomolecules).

TABLE 3: Some near-infrared absorbance bands useful in the analysis of fatty acids

Wavelength (nm)	Group	Absorbing bond
1090–1180	–CH₂	C–H
1100–1200	–CH₃	C–H
1150–1200	–CH=CH–	C–H
1350–1430	–CH₂	C–H
1360–1420	–CH₃	C–H
1390–1450	H₂O	O–H
1650–1780	–CH₃	C–H
1880–1930	H₂O	O–H
2010–2020	–CH=CH–	C–H
2100–2200	–CH=CH–	C–H
2240–2360	–CH₃	C–H
2290–2470	–CH₂	C–H

Source: Hourant, P., Baeten, V., Morales, M.T., Meurens, M., and Aparico, R., Appld. Spectroscopy, 54, 1168–1174, 2000.

Raman spectroscopy

Raman spectroscopy is an application of vibrational spectroscopy similar to infrared spectroscopy[27,28] It has the advantage of being substantially independent of the physical state of the sample permitting use on both fluid and solid samples[29,30] including tissue samples.[31] Raman spectroscopy can also be applied to samples containing water.[32] Raman spectroscopy can be used to determine the presence of conjugated linoleic acids (CLA) and *trans*-fatty acids in milk.[33] There are several excellent review on the application of Raman spectroscopy to the study of fatty acids and other lipids.[34-36] Some Raman band assignments important for the spectral analysis of lipids are shown in Tables 4 and 5.

TABLE 4: Raman spectral bands for isomers of octadecenoic and octadecynoic acid[a]

| Molecule/functional group | *cis*-Methyl ester | | | *trans* acid | |
	ν(C=C)[b]	ν(C=O)	ν(C–H)	ν(C=C)	ν(C–H)
Octa-2-decenoic acid	1648[c]	1729	3–40	1660	3023
Octa-3-decenoic acid	1660	1745	3028	1671	3000
Octa-4-decenoic acid	1656	1745	3011	1671	3000
Octa-15-decenoic acid	1656	1743	3015	1671	3000
Octa-16-decenoic acid	1657	1743	-	-	-
Octa-17-decenoic acid	1642	1745	-	--	-

| | Octadecynoic acid | | |
	ν(C≡C)		ν(C=O)
Octa-2-decynoic acid	2245[d]		1648
Octa-4-14-decynoic acid	2232 ± 1	2291 ± 2	1663 ± 1
Octa-15-decynoic acid	2233	2294	
Octa-16-decynoic acid	2234	2296	
Octa-17-decynoic acid		2120	

Source: Davies, J.E.D., Hodge, P., Barve, J.A., Gunstone, F.D., and Ismail, I.A., *J. Chem. Soc. Perkin II*, 1557–1561, 1972.
[a] The reader is directed to an excellent general reference for Raman spectroscopy (Vandenabeele, P., *Practical Raman Spectroscopy*, John Wiley and Sons, Chichester, West Sussex, England, 2013).
[b] Characterization of Raman bands.
  nu ν Stretching vibration
  delta δ Bending vibration
  rho ρ Rotational vibration
[c] Data are shown in cm⁻¹ (wavenumbers).
[d] The observed Raman spectra for a carbon–carbon triple bond usually provides a doublet except when in combination with a carbonyl group or in a terminal position.

TABLE 5: The vibrational Raman spectra for *cis,cis* and *trans,trans* isomers of a di-unsaturated fatty acid

Isomer	ν(C=C) *cis,cis* (Z,Z)	ν(C=C) *trans,trans* (E,E)
Octa-6,12-dienoic acid	1657[a]	1670
Octa-7,12-dienoic acid	1656	1670
Octa-8,12-dienoic acid	1655	1669
Octa-9,12-dienoic acid	1661	1670
Octa-10,12-dienoic acid	1646	1660
	ν(C=C)	
Octa-6,8-diynoic acid[b]	2258	
Octa-6,10-diynoic acid	2231,2296	
Octa-6,11-diynoic acid	2231/2290	
Octa-6,12-diynoic acid	2230/2291	
Octa-7,12-diynoic acid	2230/2290	
Octa-8,12-diynoic acid	2231/2296	
Octa-9,12-diynoic acid	2216/2263	
Octa-10,12-diynoic acid	2257[b]	

Source: Davies, J.E.D., Hodge, P., Gunstone, F.D., and Lie Ken Jie, M.S.F., *Chem. Phys. Lipids*, 15, 48–52, 1975.
[a] Data are reported as cm⁻¹ (wavenumbers).
[b] Methyl ester.

Nuclear magnetic resonance

Nuclear magnetic resonance (NMR) is another technique which has found wide application in the study of fatty acids and other lipids.[37-40] As with other spectral techniques, NMR is a nondestructive method but has relative low sensitivity and poor quantitation.[40] A listing of proton NMR signals is shown in Table 6, whereas a listing of ^{13}C NMR signals is shown in Table 7.

TABLE 6: Assignments of Proton Signals in the ^1H–NMR Spectra of Fatty Compounds; All Values Relative to Tetramethylsilane (TMS) = 0 ppm

Structure	Shift Values[a]
— CH_2 — (cyclopropane)	(−0.3) – 0.6
— CH_2 — (cyclopropene)	0.6 (singlet)
— CH_3, (terminal methyl in alkyl chain)	0.85–0.90 (triplet)
— CH_3, (branched, saturated isoprenoid)	0.85–0.90 (singlet or doublet)
— $C(CH_3)_2$ isopropyl methyl	1.2–1.3
$(\omega l)(col)CH_2$, saturated alkyl chain	1.21.3
— CH_2 — , acyl C-3, saturated chains	1.58
— CH_2 — , acyl C-4 to C–(ω3). saturated chains; (ω2)CH_2, saturated chain	1.2–1.3
RSH (sulfhydryl)	1.1–1.5b
RNH_2 (amino)	1.1–1.5 (1.8)[b]
R_2NH(imino)	0.4–1.6 (2.2)[b]
R_3C-H (saturated)	1.4–1.7
— C=C — CH_3 (allylic methyl)	1.6–1.9 (doublet)
— C=C — CH_2 — (allylic methylene)	2.04 (doublet)
— C=C — CH_2 — C=C — (diallylic methylene)	2.8 (triplet)
— CH_2 — COOR, acyl C2	2.1–2.3 (triplet)
— CH_2 — CO — (α-metbylene in ketone)	2.2–2.5
COOR–CH_3 (methyl in acetoxy)	1.9–2.6 (singlet)
Ar — CH_3	2.1–2.5
— C–C — H (terminal acetylene, nonconjugated)	2.5–2.7
— O — CH_2 (methoxy ether, aliphatic)	3.3–3.8 (singlet)
— O — CH_3, (methyl ester, aliphatic)	3.6–3.8 (singlet)
— CH — OH, sn-2 in glycerol	3.75 (multiplet)
— CH_2 — OH, sn-1 or sn-1 in glycerol	3.6 (doublet)
— O — CH_2 — (aliphatic saturated alcohol or ether)	3.4–3.7
— CH_2 — O — CO — R (sn-1 or sn-3 esterified glycerol)	4.2–4.4
— CH — O — CO — R (sn-2 esterified glycerol)	5.1–5.2 (quintet)
— CH_2 — O — R (O- or 5/7–3–O–alkylglycerol)	3.5–3.6
— CH — O — R (sn-2-O-alkylated glycerol)	3.6–3.7
— CH — O — P (O-acylglycerol; sn-1 or sn-3)	3.9
— CH_2 — O — P (O-alkylglycerol; sn-1 or sn-3)	3.9
— CH_2 — O — P (choline or sulfocholine)	4.3–4.4
R — OH (hydroxyl proton)	3.0–5.3
R — CH = CH — O (vinyl ether)	5.8 (cis), 6.0 (trans)
C=CH_2 (terminal vinyl, nonconjugated)	4.6–5.0
H — C = C — H (olefinic or cyclic; nonconjugated)	5.1–5.9 (multiplet)
— CH = CH — R, cis–Δ^2 in fatty acid chain	7.0.(-), 5.8 (-)
cis–Δ^3 in fatty acid chain	5.6
cis–Δ^4 in fatty acid chain	5.5
cis–Δ^5 in fatty acid chain	5.4
cis–Δ^6 in fatty acid chain	5.4
cis–Δ^9 in fatty acid chain	5.3
cis–Δ^{12} in fatty acid chain	5.3
— (CH_3)C=C — H (olefmic isbprenoid)	5.0–5.1
— C = CH_2 (terminal vinyl, conjugated)	5.3–5.7 (6.2)
H — C = C — H (olefinic, conjugated; diene or triene)	5.8–6.5 (7.1)
— CO — N — H (amide NH and CO)	5.5–8.5
Ar-H (benzenoid)	7.3–8.5
RCHO (aldehyde proton aliphatic saturated)	(9.5) 9.7–9.8
aliphatic, α,β-unsaturated	9.5–9.7
R–COOH (carboxyl)	10.5–12.0

[a] Values in parentheses apply to compounds that may absorb outside this range.
[b] Concentration–dependent; higher δ when diluted.
Source: Gunstone, F.D., Harwood. J.L., and Padley, F.B. (1994) *The Lipid Handbook*, 2nd ed., Chapman & Hall, London. With permission.

TABLE 7: Assignments of Carbon Signals in the ^{13}C-NMR Spectra of Fatty Compounds (CDCl$_3$)

Acids and Esters	Assignment
HOOC – (CH$_2$)$_x$	179–181
HOOC–CHCH$_3$–(CH$_2$)$_x$	183–184
CH$_3$O – CO – ; other alkyl esters	172–175
CH$_3$O – CO	51–52
Glycerol Esters	
Triacylglycerols	
Glyc-O-CO-(CH$_2$)$_x$ – CH$_3$	173–173.2 (-chain); 172.7–172.9 (-chain)
Glyc-O-CO-(CH$_2$)$_x$ – CH = CH-R	172.5–172.9 (-chain); 172.1–172.5 (-chain)
CH$_2$ – O – CO – R	62–62.5
|	
CH – O – CO – R	68.5–69
|	
CH$_2$ – O – CO – R	62–62.5
Diacylglycerols	
CH$_2$ – O – CO – R	ca. 61.5–62
|	
CH – O – CO – R	72–72.5
|	
CH$_2$OH	ca. 62
CH$_2$ – O – CO – R	ca. 65
|	
CH$_2$	68–68.5
|	
CH$_2$ – O – CO – R	ca. 65
Monoacylglycerols	
CH$_2$ – O – CO – R	63–63.5
|	
CHOH	70–70.5
|	
CH$_2$OH	65.65.5
CH$_2$OH	61.5–62
|	
CH – O – CO – R	74.5–75
|	
CH$_2$OH	61.5–62
Methyl Esters	
– (CH$_2$)$_x$ – CH$_3$; x > 1	13.5–14.5
Methylene in Saturated Chains	
(CH$_2$)$_x$	29–30
HOOC – CH$_2$ – (CH$_2$)$_x$ – or CH$_3$O – CO – CH$_2$ – (CH$_2$)$_x$ –	34–35
HOOC – CH$_2$ – CH$_2$ – (CH$_2$)$_x$ – or CH$_3$ O – CO – CH$_2$ – CH$_2$ (CH$_2$)$_x$ –	23–26
– (CH$_2$)$_x$ – CH$_2$ – CH$_3$	22–23
– (CH$_2$)$_x$ – CH$_2$ – CH$_2$ – CH$_3$	31.5–32.5
Double Bonds	
– CH = CH –	125–135 (exceptions given below)
(CH$_2$)$_x$ – CH = CH$_2$	114–115
(CH$_2$)$_x$ – CH = CH$_2$	139–140
(CH$_2$)$_x$ – CH$_2$ – CH = CH$_2$	33–35
(CH$_2$)$_x$ – CH$_2$ – C = C – CH$_2$ – (CH$_2$)$_y$	27–28 (*cis*); 32–33 (*trans*)
HOOC – CH$_2$ – C = C	33–34 (*cis*)
HOOC – CH_2 – CH$_2$ – C = C	22–23 (*cis*)
– CH=CH – CH$_2$ – CH$_3$	20–21(*cis*); 25–26 (*trans*)
– CH=CH – CH$_2$ – CH$_2$ – CH$_3$	29–30 (*cis*); 34–35 (*trans*)
– C = C – CH$_2$ – CH = CH –	25–26 (all *cis*); 35–36 (all *trans*); 30–31 (*cis, trans*)
– CH = C = CH –	200–205
– CH = C = CH –	90–92
Triple Bonds	
(CH$_2$)$_x$ – C ≡ C – (CH$_2$)$_y$	79–81
(CH$_2$)$_x$ – CH$_2$ – C ≡ C – CH$_2$ – (CH$_2$)$_y$	18–19
– C ≡ C – CH$_2$–C ≡ C –	74–75
– C ≡ C – CH$_2$ – C ≡ C –	9–10
– C ≡ C – CH$_2$ – CH$_2$ – C = C –	19–20
– C ≡ C – C = C	77–78
– C ≡ C – C = C –	65–66
– CH$_2$ – C ≡ C –	18–20
Hydroxy Groups	
(CH$_2$)$_x$ – CHOH – (CH$_2$)$_y$	71–73
(CH$_2$)$_x$ – CH$_2$ – CHOH – CH$_2$ – (CH$_2$)$_y$	37–38
(CH$_2$)$_x$ – CH = CH – CHOH – (CH$_2$)$_y$	67–68 (*cis*); 73–74 (trans)

(Continued)

TABLE 7: Assignments of carbon signals in the ^{13}C–NMR spectra of fatty compounds ($CDCl_3$) (Continued)

Acids and Esters	Assignment
$(CH_2)_x - CH = CH - CHOH - (CH_2)_y$	131–134; (*trans*; CH adjacent to CHOH downfield)
$(CH_2)_x - CH = CH - CH_2 - CHOH - (CH_2)_y$	133–134 (*cis*)
$(CH_2)_x - CH = CH - CH_2 - CHOH - (CH_2)_y$	125–126 (cis)
$(CH_2)_x - CH = CH - CH_2 - CHOH - (CH_2)_y$	35–36 (*cis*)
$(CH_2)_x - CH = CH - CH_2 - CH_2 - CHOH - (CH_2)_y$	130–131 (*cis*)
$(CH_2)_x - CH = CH - CH_2 - CH_2 - CHOH - (CH_2)_y$	129–130 (*cis*)
$(CH_2)_x - CH = CH - CH_2 - CH_2 - CHOH - (CH_2)_y$	23–24 (*cis*)
$(CH_2)_x - CH = CH - CH_2 - CH_2 - CHOH - (CH_2)_y$	37–38 (*cis*)
$(CH_2)_x - CHOH - CHOH - (CH_2)_y$	74–75 (erythro slightly > threo)
$(CH_2)_x - CH_2 - CHOH - CHOH - CH_2 - (CH_2)_y$	31–32 (erythro), 33–34 (threo)
$(CH_2)_x - CHOH - CH_2 - CH_2 - CHOH - (CH_2)_y$	32–33 (erythro), 33–34 (threo)
$(CH_2)_x - CH_2 - CHOH - CH_2 - CH_2 - CHOH - CH_2 - (CH_2)_y$	37–38 (threo slightly > erythro)
$(CH_2)_x - CHOH - CH = CH - CHOH - (CH_2)_y$	133–134; (trans; threo slightly > erythro)

Hydroperoxy Compounds	
$(CH_2)_x - CH_2 - CH(OOH) - CH = CH - CH = CH - (CH_2)_y$	86–88
$(CH_2)_x - CH_2 - CH(OOH) - CH = CH - CH = CH - (CH_2)_y$	25–26

Oxo Compounds	
$(CH_2)_x - CO - (CH_2)_y$	209–213
$(CH_2)_x - CH_2 - CO - (CH_2)_y$	42–43
$(CH_2)_x CH = CH - CH_2 - CO - (CH_2)_y$	41–42
$(CH_2)_x CH = CH - CH_2 - CO - (CH_2)_y$	133–134
$(CH_2)_x CH = CH - CH_2 - CO - (CH_2)_v$	121–122
$(CH_2)_x - CO - CH_2 - CH_2 - CO - (CH_2)_y$	36–37
$(CH_2)_x - CO - CH = CH - CO - (CH_2)_y$	203–204 *cis*; 200–201 *trans*
$(CH_2)_x - CO - CH = CH - CO - (CH_2)_y$	135–136 *cis*; 136–137 *trans*

Epoxy and Furanoid Compounds	
$(CH_2)_x - CH - CH - (CH_2)_y$ (epoxide)	56–57 (*cis*); 58–59 (*trans*)
$(CH_2)_x - CH_2 - CH - CH - CH_2 - (CH_2)_y$ (epoxide)	27–28 (*cis*); 31–32 (*trans*)
$(CH_2)_x - CH = CH - CH_2 - CH - CH - CH_2 - (CH_2)_y$ (epoxide)	25–26 (*cis*; *cis*–epoxy)
$(CH_2)_x - CH = CH - CH_2 - CH - CH - CH_2 - (CH_2)_y$ (epoxide)	132–133 (*cis*; *cis*–epoxy)
$(CH_2)_x - CH = CH - CH_2 - CH - CH - CH_2 - (CH_2)_y$ (epoxide)	123–124 (*cis*; *cis*–epoxy)
$- (CH_2)_2 - C - C - (CH_2) -$ (furanoid, C–C)	104–105
	154–155

Acetoxy	
$(CH_2)_x - CO(COCH_3) - (CH_2)_y$	73–75
$(CH_2)_x - CO(COCH_3) - (CH_2)_y$	170–171
$(CH_2)_x - CO(COCH_3) - (CH_2)_y$	20–22
$CH_3 - O - CO - CO(COCH_3) - (CH_2)_y$	72–73
$CH_3 - O - CO - CO(COCH_3) - (CH_2)_y$	70–71
$(CH_2)_x - CH_2 - COCH_3$	64–65

Cyclic Compounds (Cyclopropene Fatty Acids)	
$(CH_2)_x - CH = CH - (CH_2)_y$ (cyclopropene CH_2)	7–8
	109–110
$(CH_2)_x - CH_2 - CH = CH - CH_2 - (CH_2)_y$ (cyclopropene CH_2)	25.5–26.5
$HOOC - (CH_2)_x - CH_2 - CH = CH - CH_2 - (CH_2)_y$; x=2–3 (cyclopropene CH_2)	107–109
$HOOC - (CH_2)_x - CH_2 - CH = CH - CH_2 - (CH_2)_y$; x=2–3 (cyclopropene CH_2)	110–112

Branched Compounds	
$(CH_2)_x - CH(CH_3) - (CH_2)_y$	19–20
$(CH_2)_x - CH(CH_3) - (CH_2)_y$	32–33
$(CH_2)_x - CH_2 - CH(CH_3) - CH_2 - (CH_2)_y$	3637
$HOOC - CH(CH_3)_3 - (CH_2)_x -$ or $CH_3 - O - CO - CH(CH_3)_3 - (CH_2)_x$	39–40
$HOOC - CH(CH_3)_3 - (CH_2)_x -$ or $CH_3 - O - CO - CH(CH_3)_3 - (CH_2)_x$	16.5–17.5
$CH_3 - O - CO - CH_2 - CH(CH_3) - (CH_2)_x$	30–31
$CH_3 - O - CO - CH_2 - CH(CH_3)_3 - (CH_2)_x$	19–20
$CH_3 - O - CO - CH_2 - CH(CH_3) - (CH_2)_x$	41–42
$CH_3 - O - CO - CH_2 - CH_2 - CH(CH_3)_3 - (CH_2)_x$	31–32
$CH_3 - O - CO - CH_2 - CH_2 - CH(CH_3)_3 - (CH_2)_x$	19–20

Source: Gunstone, F.D., Harwood. J.L., and Padley, F.B. (1994) *The Lipid Handbook*, 2nd ed., Chapman & Hall, London. With permission.

References

1. Stewart, K.K. and Ebel, R.E., Ultraviolet and visible absorption spectrophotometry and photometry, in *Chemical Measurements in Biological Systems*, Chapter3, pp. 39-63, John Wiley & Sons, New York, New York, 2000.
2. Anderson, R.J., Bendell, D.J., and Groundwater, P.W., Ultraviolet-visible (UV-Vis) spectroscopy in organic spectroscopic analysis, Chapter 2, pp. 7–23, Royal Society of Chemistry, Cambridge, United Kingdom, 2004.
3. Gunstone, J.D. and Harwood, J.L., Occurrence and characterization of oils and fats, in *The Lipid Handbook*, 3rd edn., ed. F.D. Gunstone, J.L. Harwood, and A.J. Dijkstra, Chapter 2, pp. 37–141, CRC Press, Boca Raton, Florida, USA, 2007.
4. Carroll, K.K., Dietary fat and the fatty composition of tissue lipids, *J. Am. Oil Chem. Soc.* 42, 516–527, 1965.
5. Ungnade, H.E. and Ortega, I., The ultraviolet absorption spectra of acrylic acids and esters, *J. Am. Chem. Soc.* 73, 1564–1567, 1951.
5a. Pullanagari, R.R., Yule, I.J., and Agnew, M., On-line prediction of lamb fatty acid composition of visible near-infrared spectroscopy, *Meat Science* 100, 156–163, 2015.
6. Feltenmark, S., Bautam, N., Brunström, A., et al., Eoxins are proinflammatory arachidonic acid metabolites produced by 15-lipoxygenase-1 pathway in human eosinophils and mast cells, *Proc. Natl. Acad. Sci. USA* 105, 680–685, 2008.
7. Ōmura,, S., Iami, H., Takeshimae, H., and Nakagawa. A., Structure of a new antimicrobial unsaturated fatty acid from *Sm. kitasatoensis* NU-23-1, *Chem. Pharm. Bull.* 24, 3139–3143, 1976.
8. Smyk, B., Wieczorek, P., and Zadernowski, R., A method of concentration estimation of trienes, tetraenes and pentaenes in evening primrose oil, *Eur. J. Lipid Sci. Technol.* 113, 592–596, 2011.
9. Hoffmann, J.S., O'Connor, R.T., Heinzelman, D.C., and Bickford, W.G., A simplified method for the preparation of α- and β-eleostearic acids and a revised spectrophotometric procedure for their determination, *J. Am. Oil Chem. Soc.* 34, 338–342, 1957.
10. Sklar, L.A., Hudson, B.S., Petersen, M., and Diamond, J., Conjugated polyene fatty acids on fluorescent probes: Spectroscopic characterization, *Biochemistry* 16, 813–818, 1977.
11. El Alaoui, M., Noirel, A., Soulère, L., et al., Development of a high-throughput assay for measuring phospholipase A activity using synthetic 1,2-α-eleostearoyl-sn-glycero-3-phosphocholine coated on microtiter plates, *Anal. Chem.* 86, 10576–10583, 2014.
12. Ülker, S., Placidi, C., Point, V., et al., New lipase assay using Pomegranate oil coating in microtiter plates, *Biochimie* 120, 110–118, 2016.
13. Banni, S., Petroni, A., Blaevich, M., et al., Conjugated linoleic acids (CLA) as precursors of a distinct family of PUFA, *Lipids* 39, 1143–1146, 2004.
14. Wang, T. and Lee, H.G., Advances in research on *cis*-9, *trans*-11 conjugated linoleic acid: a major functional conjugated linoleic acid isomer, *Crit.Rev.Food Sci.Nutr.* 55, 720–731, 2015.
15. McCrorie, T.A., Keaveney, E.M., Wallace, J.M., Binns, N., and Livingstone, M.B., Human health effect of conjugated linoleic acid from mild and supplements, *Nutr. Res. Rev.* 24, 206–227, 2011.
16. Arudi, R.L., Sutherland , M.W., and Bielski, B.H.J., Purification of oleic and linoleic acid, *J. Lipid Res.* 24, 485–488, 1983.
17. Falconer, R.J., Zakaria, H.A., Fan, Y.Y., Bradley, A.P., and Middelberg, A.P., Far infrared spectroscopy of protein higher-order structures, *Appld.Spectrosc.* 64, 1259–1264, 2010.
18. Srour, B. Erhard, B., Süss, R., and Hellwig, P., Monitoring the pH triggered collapse of liposomes in the far-IR hydrogen bonding continuum, *J. Phys. Chem. B* 120, 4047–4052, 2016.
19. Mossoba, M.M., Moss, J., and Kramer, J.K.G., Trans fat labeling and levels in U.S. foods: assessment of gas chromatographic and infrared spectroscopic techniques for regulatory compliance, *J. AOAC Int.* 92, 1284–1300, 2009.
20. Tyburczy, C., Mossoba, M.M., and Rader, J.I., Determination of *trans* fat in edible oils: current official methods and overview of recent developments, *Anal. Bioanal. Chem.* 405, 5759–5772, 2013.
21. Micham, D., Bailey, A.V., and Tripp, V.W., Identification of fatty acid polymorphic modifications by infrared spectroscopy, *J.Am.Oil Chem. Soc.* 50, 446–449, 1973.
22. Kaneko, F., Tahiro, K., and Kobayashi, K., Polymorphic transformations during crystallization processes of fatty acids studied with FT-IR spectroscopy, *J.Crystal Growth* 199, 1352–1359, 1993.
23. Inoue, T., Hisatsugu, Y., Ishikawa, R., and Susuki, M., Solid-liquid phase behavior of binary fatty acid mixtures 2. Mixtures of oleic acid with lauric acid, myristic acid, and palmitic acid, *Chem. Phys. Lipids* 127, 161–173, 2004,
24. Hourant, P., Baeten, V., Morales, M.T., Meurens, M., and Aparico, R., Oil and fat classification by selected bands of near-infrared spectroscopy, *Appld. Spectroscopy* 54, 1168–1174, 2000.
25. Dupuy, N., Galtier, O., Le Dréau, Y., et al., Chemometric analysis of combined NIR and MIR spectra to characterize French olives, *Eur. J. Lipid Sci. Technol.* 112, 463–475, 2010.
26. Sánchez, J.A.C., Moreda, W., and García, J.M., Rapid determination of olive oil oxidative stability and its major quality parameters using Vis/NIR transmittance spectroscopy, *J. Argr. Food Chem.* 61, 8056–8062, 2013.
27. Gremlich, H.-V., Infrared and Raman spectroscopy, in *Handbook of Analytical Techniques*, ed. H. Guenzler and A. Williams, Chapter 17, pp. 465–507, 2001.
28. Schultz, Z.D. and Levin, A.W., Vibrational spectroscopy of biomembranes, *Annu. Rev. Anal. Chem.* 4, 343–366, 2011.
29. Beattie, J.R., Bell, S.E.J., and Moss, B.W., A critical evaluation of Raman spectroscopy for the analysis of lipids: Fatty acid methyl esters, *Lipids* 39, 407–419, 2004.
30. Mendes, T.O., Junqueira, G.M.A., Parto, B.L.S., et al., Vibrational spectroscopy for milk fat quantification: line shape analysis of the Raman and infrared spectra, *J. Raman Spectroscopy,* 47, 692–698, 2016.
31. Silveira, L., Jr., Leite, K.R., Silveiera, F.L., et al., Discrimination of prostate carcinoma from benign prostate tissue fragments in vitro by estimating the gross biochemical alterations through Raman spectroscopy, *Lasers Med. Sci.*, 1469–1477, 2014.
32. Campbell, T.D. and Dwek, R.A., Raman Spectroscopy, in *Biological Spectroscopy*, Chapter 9, pp. 239–254, Benjamin/Cummings Publishing, Menlo Park, California, USA, 1984.
33. Stefenov, I., Baeten, V.,Abbas, O., et al., Determining milk isolated and conjugated trans-unsaturated fatty acids using Fourier transform Raman spectroscopy, *J. Agric. Food Chem.* 59, 12771–12783, 2011.
34. Chapman, D., Goni, F.M., and F.D. Gunstone, Physical properties: Optical and spectral characteristics, in *The Lipid Handbook*, 2nd edn., ed. F.D. Gunstone, J.L. Harwood, and F.B. Padley, Chapter 9, Section 9.2, pp. 505–510, Chapman and Hall, London, England, 1984.
35. Beattie, J.R., Bell, S.E.J., and Moss, B.W., A critical evaluation of Raman spectroscopy for the analysis of lipids: fatty acid methyl esters, *Lipids* 39, 407–419, 2004.
36. Czamara, K., Majzner, K., Pacia, M.Z., et al., Raman spectroscopy of lipids: a review, *J. Raman Spectroscopy* 46, 4–20, 2015.
37. Knothe, G., Quantitative analysis of mixtures of fatty acids by 1H-NMR, *Lipid Technology* 15, 111–114, 2003.
38. Dijkstra, A.J., Christie, W.W., and Knothe, G., Analysis, in *The Lipid Handbook*, 3rd edn., F.D. Gunstone, J.L. Harwood, and A.J. Dijkstra, Chapter 6, pp. 415–470, CRC/Taylor and Francis, Boca Raton, Florida, USA, 2007.
39. Hamilton, J.A., NMR reveals molecular interactions and dynamics of fatty acid binding to albumin, *Biochim. Biophys. Acta* 1830, 5418–5426, 2013.
40. Wu, Z., Zhang, Q., Li, N., et al., Comparison of critical methods developed for fatty acid analysis, *J. Sep. Sci.*, in press, 20157.

IR ACTIVE BANDS OF PHOSPHATIDYLETHANOLAMINES (PE)

Optical and Spectral Characteristics

Table 1: Infrared-active bands (cm⁻¹) of various phosphatidylcholines (PC) and phosphatidylethanolamines (PE)[a].

Band	DPPC (dry)	DPPC (monohydrate)	DLPC (dry)	Egg PC (dry)	DPPE (dry)	DPPE (monohydrate)	Egg PE (dry)
$\nu_{symmetric}(CH_2)$	2848	2849	2848	2853	2848	2848	2848
$\nu_{asymmetric}(CH_2)$	2915	2918	2915	2920	2918	2915	2918
$\nu_{asymmetric}(CH_3)$	2957	2958	2953	2959	2958	2956	2958
$\delta(CH_2)$	1461	1466	1467	1469	1462	1469	1462
					1471		
$\nu(C=O)$	1724	1733	1734	1740	1739	1720	1740
	1734					1730	
$\nu(P=O)$	1254	1248	1252	1260	1222	1215	1224
					1241s		
Terminal CH$_2$rock	722	721	720	720	715	720	720
					725		
$\nu(NH^+_3)$					2128	2108	2558
					2328	2328	2638
					2558	2548	2708
					2646		
					2688		
					2728	2728	
$\delta(NH^+_3)$					1550	1580	1559
					1625	1620	1638
$\nu(CH_2)$ of N$^+$CH$_3$	3028	3028	3028	3013			
$\nu(OH)$		3373					
$\delta(OH)$		1645					

Source: Adapted from *The Lipid Handbook*, 2nd edn., ed. F.D. Gunstone, J.L Harwood, and F.B. Padley, Chapman and Hall, London, United Kingdom, 1994 and Wallach, D.F., Verma, S.P., and Fookson, J. Application of laser Raman and infrared spectroscopy to membrane strucrure, *Biochim.Biophys.Acta* 559, 153–208, 1979.

[a] All films were prepared from solutions in chloroform/methanol (2:1, v/v), except for DPPE films, which were prepared from a chloroform solution. DPPC, dipalmitoylphosphatidylcholine; DLPC, dilauroylphosphatidylcholine; DPPE, dipalmitoylphosphatidylethanolamine; s, shoulder.

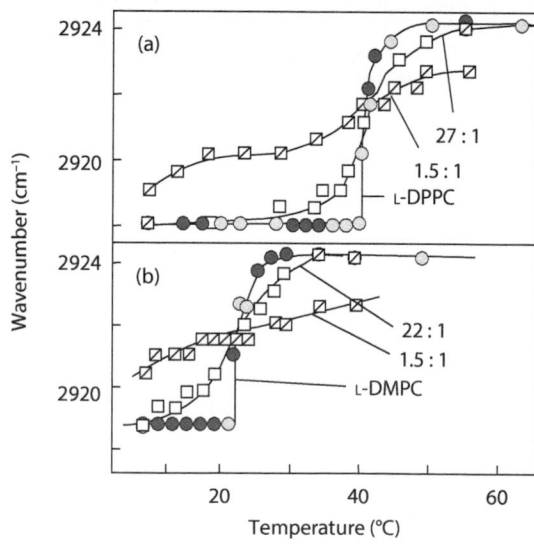

Temperature dependence of the maximum wave number of the CH$_2$ asymmetric stretching vibrations in (i) dipalmitoylphosphatidyl-choline (DPPC)-cholesterol and (ii) dimyristoylphosphatidylcholine (DMPC)-cholesterol at the molar ratios indicated. The temperature dependence for pure lipids (full circles) is also given. (Cortijo, M., Alonso, A., Gomez-Fernandez, J.C., and Chapman, D., Intrinsic protein-lipid interactions. Infrared spectroscopic studies of gramicidin A, bacteriorhodopsin and Ca^{2+}-ATPase in biomembranes and reconstituted systems, *J.Mol.Biol.* 157, 597–618, 1982.)

Table 2: Major infrared absorption bands in spectra of various lipids in chloroform or carbon tetrachloride or as oils

Functional group	Absorption mode	Frequency (cm^{-1})	Intensity[a]
—CH$_3$	CH stretch	2962; 2872 ± 10	s
	CH bend asymm.	1450 ± 20	m
	CH bend symm.	1375 ± 5	m
—OCH$_3$	CH bend	1430	m
N(CH$_3$)$_3$	CH stretch (asymm.)	3040	w
	CH$_3$ deformation (asymm.)	1470	w
		960–975	w
S(CH$_3$)$_2$	CH stretch (asymm.)	3023	w
	CH$_3$ deformation (asymm.)	1435	w
—CH$_2$	CH stretch	2926; 2853 ± 10	s
	CH bend	1465 ± 10	m
	[CH$_2$]$_4$ skeletal	750–720	m
	—CH$_2$ in cyclopropane CH stretch skeletal	3100–3000	m
		1025–1000	m
—C(CH$_3$)$_2$ (isopropyl)	CH bend	1385; 1365 ± 5	m (db)
	skeletal	1170 ± 5; 1150 ± 5	m (db)
—C(CH$_3$)$_3$ (t-butyl)	CH bend	1395–1385 (m); 1365	s
	skeletal	1250–1200	s
—CH (tertiary)	CH stretch	2890 ± 10	w
	CH bend	1340 ± 20	w
C=C (aliphatic)	C=C stretch, nonconjugated	1680–1620	v
	C=C stretch, phenyl conjugated	1625 ± 20	v
	C=C stretch, C=O or C=C conjugated	1600 ± 20	v
	CH stretch	3040–3010	m
—CH=CH (*trans*)	CH out-of-plane deformation	970–960	s
	CH in-plane deformation	1310–1295	s–w
—CH=CH (*cis*)	CH out-of-plane deformation	*ca* 690	m
—CH=CH$_2$ (vinyl)	CH stretch	3095–3075	m
	CH out-of-plane deformation	995–985	s
	CH$_2$ out-of-plane deformation	915–905	s
	CH$_2$ in-plane deformation	1420–1410	s
R$_1$R$_2$C=CH$_2$	CH stretch	3095–3075	m
	CH$_2$ out-of-plane deformation	895–885	s
	CH$_2$ in-plane deformation	1420–1410	s
R$_1$R$_2$C=CHR$_3$	CH out-of-plane deformation	840–790	s
—C(CH$_3$)=CH— (isoprenoid)	CH out-of-plane deformation	835	s
C=C (aromatic)	=C—H stretch	3030	sharp
	=C—H out-of-plane:		
	5 H atoms	770–730; 710–690 (2 bands)	vs
	4 H atoms	770–735 (1 band)	vs
	3 H atoms	810–750	vs
	2 H atoms	860–800	vs
	C=C skeletal	1600; 1500	v
RC≡CR	C≡C stretch	2260–2190	m
RC≡CH	C≡C stretch	2140–2100	m
	C—H stretch	3300	m
—C—OH	O—H stretch; free OH	3650–3590 (sharp)	v
	O—H stretch; associated OH (hydrogen bonded)	3400–3200 (broad)	
—C—OH	C—O stretch	1150–1140 (tertiary)	s
		1120–1100 (secondary)	s
		1075–1010 (primary)	s
—C—F	alkyl, stretch	1400–1000	s
—C—Cl	alkyl, stretch	800–600	s
	aryl, stretch	1100–1050	s
—C—Br	alkyl, stretch	600–500	s
—C—I	alkyl, stretch	*ca* 500	v
—C—O—C—alkyl ether	C—O stretch	1150–1060	vs
—C—O—C aryl ether	C—O stretch	1270–1230	vs
—C=C—O—C (*cis*-vinyl ether) H H	C—O stretch	1270–1230	s
	C=C stretch	1670	m
	CH deformation	732–730	m
—C—O—C—	C—C stretch	1250	s

Table 2: Major infrared absorption bands in spectra of various lipids in chloroform or carbon tetrachloride or as oils (Continued)

Functional group	Absorption mode	Frequency (cm^{-1})	Intensity[a]
	cis	830	m
	trans	890	m
Alkyl peroxides	C—O stretch	890–820	v–w
Acyl peroxides	C=O vibrations	1820–1810; 1800–1780	s
Aldehyde C=O	C=O vibrations: saturated aldehyde	1740–1720	s
	α,β-unsaturated aldehyde	1705–1680	s
Ketone C=O	C=O stretch: saturated ketone	1725–1705	s
	α,β-unsaturated ketone	1685–1665	s
Carboxyl, RCOOH	C=O stretch: saturated fatty acid	1725–1700	s
	α,β-unsaturated acid	1715–1690	s
	C—O stretch	1320–1210	s
R—COO⁻	C=O stretch (asymm.)	1610–1550	s
	C—O stretch (symm.)	1400–1300	s
Ester, RCOOR	C=O stretch: saturated ester	1750–1730	s
	α,β-unsaturated ester	1730–1717	s
	β-keto ester (enol)	1650–1540	s
	C—O stretch:		
	formates	1200–1180	m
	acetates	1250–1230	m
	propionates and higher	1200–1150	m
Primary amide, RCONH$_2$	NH stretch (free NH)	3500;3400	m
	NH stretch (bonded NH)	3350;3180	m
	C=O stretch	1690–1650	s
	NH$_2$ deformation	1620–1590	s
	C—N stretch	1420–1400	v
Secondary amide, RCONHR	NH stretch (free NH)	3440–3400	m
	NH stretch (bonded NH)	3320–3140	m
	C=O stretch	1680–1630	s
	NH deformation	1550–1510	s
Tertiary amide, RCONR$_2$	C=O stretch	1670–1630	s
Anhydride, CO—O—CO	C=O stretch	1850–1800; 1790–1740	s
	C—O stretch	1170–1050	
Primary amine, —NH$_2$	NH stretch	3500–3300 (2 bands)	m
	NH deformation	1650–1590	s–m
Secondary amine, —NH	NH stretch	3500–3300 (1 band)	m
	NH deformation	1650–1550	vw
Phosphates			
R—O—PO—O⁻	P=O stretch (free)	1300–1250	s
│	P=O stretch (bonded)	1250–1200	vs
O⁻	P—O—C (aliphatic)	1050–1000	vs
	P—O—C (aromatic)	1240–1190	s
		995–850	s
	P—O⁻	1110–1090	s
		2700–2560	w
R—O—PO(OH)$_2$ (free acid)	P—OH	2700–2560	w
	P=O stretch	1240–1180	m
	P—O—C	1070–1000	s
R—O—PO—(OCH$_3$)$_2$	P=O stretch	1275–1180	s
	P—O—CH$_3$	1190	w
		1040	s
Phosphonates			
R—O—PO—C⁻	P=O stretch (bonded)	*ca* 1200	s
│	P—C stretch	750–650	v
O⁻			
Sulfates			
R—O—SO$_2$—O⁻	S=O stretch	1265–1200	s
		1080–1040	v
	C—O stretch	1040–990 (primary)	m
		990–930 (secondary)	v
	S—O stretch	840–760	w
R—O—SO$_2$—O—R′	S=O stretch	1440–1350	s
		1230–1150	v
	C—O stretch	1040–930	m

Table 2: Major infrared absorption bands in spectra of various lipids in chloroform or carbon tetrachloride or as oils (Continued)

Functional group	Absorption mode	Frequency (cm^{-1})	Intensity[a]
	S—O stretch	850–760	m
Sulfonates			
R—SO$_2$—O$^-$	S=O stretch	1220–1210	s
		1055–1050	v
	C—S stretch	800–600	w
R—SO$_2$—O—R'	S=O stretch	1420–1330	s
		1200–1145	v
	S—O stretch	900–860	m
	C—S stretch	800–600	w
	C—O stretch	1000	w
R—SO$_2$—OH	S=O stretch	1200; 1050	s
	S—O stretch	650	s

Source: From Kates, M. (1986), *Techniques of Lipidology*, 2nd edn., North-Holland, Amsterdam.

[a] *Abbreviations*: w, weak; m, moderate; s, strong; v, variable; vs, very strong; db, doublet.

This material was taken from *The Lipid Handbook*, 2nd edn., ed. F.D. Gunstone, J.L. Harwood, and F.B. Padley, Chapman and Hall, London, United Kingdom, 1994.

Table 3: Maximum wavenumbers of the main bands appearing in the 1000–1300 cm^{-1} region of FTIR spectra of phosphate-containing molecules[a]

Compound	Maximum wavenumbers (cm^{-1})	Assignment
Inorganic phosphate KBr disc	1046 (intense, broad)	PO$_2^-$ stretch
Inorganic phosphate (buffer)	1077 (intense)	Symmetric PO$_2^-$ stretch
	1160	Asymmetric PO$_2^-$ stretch
l-α-Glycerophosphate	1085	Symmetric PO$_2^-$ stretch
	1102 (shoulder)	Asymmetric PO$_2^-$ stretch
Phosphorylcholine	1095	Symmetric PO$_2^-$ stretch
	1117 (shoulder)	Asymmetric PO$_2^-$ stretch
Glycerophosphorylcholine	1054 (shoulder)	R—O—P—O—R'
	1085	Symmetric PO$_2^-$ stretch
	1217	Asymmetric PO$_2^-$ stretch
Phosphatidic acid	1076	Symmetric PO$_2^-$ stretch
	1181	Asymmetric PO$_2^-$ stretch
DPPC KBr disc	1069 (shoulder)	R—O—P—O—R'
	1093	Symmetric PO$_2^-$ stretch
	1245	Asymmetric PO$_2^-$ stretch
DPPC (slurry)	1064 (shoulder)	R—O—P—O—R'
	1089	Symmetric PO$_2^-$ stretch
	1168	
	1230	Asymmetric PO$_2^-$ stretch
DPPC (buffer)	1060 (shoulder)	R—O—P—O—R'
	1086	Symmetric PO$_2^-$ stretch
	1180 (shoulder)	
	1222	Asymmetric PO$_2^-$ stretch

Source: From Arrondo, J.L.R., *et al.*, (1984), *Biochim. Biophys. Acta.*, 794, 165.

[a] All spectra were recorded in buffer except when otherwise stated.

CONCENTRATION OF SOME FATTY ACIDS IN HUMAN BLOOD, BLOOD PLASMA OR BLOOD SERUM

Roger L. Lundblad

Concentration of Fatty Acids in Blood and Blood Plasma

There are two major sources of fatty acids in blood, non-esterified fatty acids (NEFA) which are also referred to as free fatty acids (FFA) and fatty acids present in acyl linkage such triacyl glycerides. It is thought that NEFA in blood are derived from the hydrolysis of stored triacyl glycerols[1] but there can be some contribution from diet.[2,3] So, most of the studies are performed in fasting subjects. It has been reported that there is a small increase in free fatty acids in human serum following fasting.[4,5] Free fatty acids in blood are proposed as biomarkers.[6,7] Plasma free fatty acids are considered to be a major source of energy[8] and have physiological function.[9] Short-chain fatty acids (C2,C4,C6) are derived from carbohydrates by intestinal microbiota.[10] There are three steps in the process of determining the concentration of free fatty acids and total fatty acids in blood. First, blood is obtained by venipuncture in the form of whole blood, plasma, or serum. Blood and plasma both require the use of an anticoagulant such as EDTA, citrate, or heparin, whereas serum is obtained from the coagulation of blood. The choice of anticoagulant does not seem to make a difference[11] although studies are limited. There are differences between serum and plasma.[12] The processing of blood samples is more critical for oxygenated polyunsaturated fatty acids (PUFA) such as eicosanoids, and the levels of these lipid mediators are higher in serum than in plasma.[13,14] There are also gender differences[14,15] and age differences[15] in various lipids including lysophosphatidyl choline, diacyl glycerol, diHETrE (5,6-dihydroxyeicosatrienoic acid), and 8-HETE (8-hydroxyeicosatetraenoic acid).

Although plasma or serum can be processed for analysis immediately following venipuncture, most samples are frozen prior to subsequent processing. The long-term storage of serum has been reported to result in an increase in FFA.[16] The thawing of the sample has also been shown to be critical with the use of ultrasound found to be useful.[17] More recent work on human serum has shown a decrease in FFA.[18] The decrease is temperature dependent and is stabilized at 80% of initial value. The presence of lipoprotein lipase in plasma or serum could influence the concentration of free fatty acids[18] and phenylmethanesulfonyl fluoride, an inhibitor of lipoprotein is included in the plasma/serum in some studies.[10,19] Some studies include an antioxidant such as butylated hydroxyltoluene.[20] The quality of the sample container has been shown to affect total fatty acid measurement.[21]

Free fatty acids in plasma are bound to albumin[22] but are extracted with chloroform/methanol as in the Folch[23] extraction or by other organic solvents such as t-butyl methyl ether.[24–26] There have been several studies comparing extractions with varying effects on various lipid classes.[27–30] Free fatty acids can be obtained by solid-phase extraction.[31,32]

Fatty acids must be converted to a volatile form for GC analysis with the methyl ester being the most common derivative. Esterification refers to the conversion of NEFA to methyl esters, whereas transesterification (or interesterification) refers to conversion of acyl glyceride (and other fatty acid acyl derivatives) to methyl esters. Esterification of NEFA occurs at a lower temperature than transesterification.[2,33,34] Transesterification occurs at 90°C–100°C, whereas esterification occurs at 25°C.[3] One study has shown that fatty acid chain length and lipid class (e.g., cholesterol ester and acylglycerol) affect fatty acid methyl ester yield. Acid catalysts (e.g., HCl and acetyl chloride) can promote esterification and transesterification, whereas base catalysts (e.g., sodium methoxide) are only effective with transesterification.[26] There are other ester derivatives of fatty acids which are useful including pentafluorobenzyl bromide.[29] Fatty acids can be derivatized in plasma without extraction by the use of acetyl chloride in methanol and n-hexane at 95°C with the fatty acid methyl esters partitioned into the hexane layer.[35] The use of microwave irradiation seems to be increasing for the transesterification step in the determination of total fatty acids.[36,37]

Most early analytic methods for fatty acids in plasma used gas chromatography with flame ionization (FID) as the detection method of choice. The majority of current work in lipidomics uses mass spectrometry for detection.[38–42] Methods have been developed for the HPLC analysis of NEFA without derivatization.[43,44]

References

1. Yli-Jama, P., Haugen, T.S., Rebnord, H.M., Ringstad, J., and Pedersen, J.I., Selective mobilization of fatty acids from human adipose tissue, *Eur. J. Intern. Med.*, 12, 107–113, 2001.
2. Heimberg, M., Dunn, G.D., and Wilcox, H.G., The derivation of plasma-free fatty acids from dietary neutral fat in man, *J. Lab. Clin. Med.*, 83, 393–402, 1974.
3. Liebich, H.M., Wirth, C., and Jakober, B., Analysis of polyunsaturated fatty acids in blood serum after fish oil administration, *J. Chromatog.*, 572, 1–9, 1991.
4. Richieri, G.V., and Kleinfeld, A.M., Unbound free fatty acid levels in human serum, *J. Lipid Res.*, 36(2), 229–250, 1995.
5. Browning, J.D., Baxter, J., Satapati, S., and Burgess, S.C., The effect of short-term fasting on liver and skeletal muscle lipid, glucose, and energy metabolism in healthy women and men, *J. Lipid Res.*, 53, 577–586, 2012.
6. Choi, J.Y., Jung, J.M., Kwon, D.Y., et al., Free fatty acid as an outcome predictor of atrial fibrillation-associated stroke, *Ann. Neurol.*, 79, 317–325, 2016.
7. Li, X., Xy, Z., Lu, X., et al., Comprehensive two-dimensional gas chromatography/time-of-flight mass spectrometry for metabolomics: Biomarker discovery for diabetes mellitus, *Anal. Chim. Acta*, 633, 257–262, 2009.
8. Wolfe, R.R., Fat metabolism in exercise, *Adv. Exp. Med. Biol.*, 441, 147–156, 1998.
9. Barden, A.E., Mas, E., and Mori, T.A., n-e Fatty acid supplementation and proresolving mediators of inflammation, *Curr. Opin. Lipidol.*, 27, 26–32, 2016.
10. Clarke, G., Stilling, R.M., Kennedy, P.J., et al., Gut microbiota: The neglected endocrine organ, *Mol. Endocrinol.*, 28, 1221–1238, 2014.
11. Surma, M.A., Herzog, R., Vasilj, A., et al., An automated shotgun lipidomics platform for high throughput, comprehensive, and quantitative analysis of blood plasma intact lipids, *Eur. J. Lipid Sci. Technol.*, 117, 1540–1549, 2015.

12. Sőderberg, B., and Sőderberg, U., An effect of coagulation on the distribution of free fatty acids in human blood, *Life Sci.*, 6, 1013–1021, 1967.

13. Astarita, G., Kendall, A.C., Dennis, E.A., and Nicolaou, A., Targeted lipidomic strategies for oxygenated metabolites of polyunsaturated fatty acids, *Biochim. Biophys. Acta*, 1851, 456–468, 2015.

14. Ishikawa, M., Tajima, Y., Murayama, M., et al., Plasma and serum from nonfasting men and women differ in their lipidomic profiles, *Biol. Pharm. Bull.*, 36, 682–685, 2013.

15. Ishikawa, M., Maekawa, K., Saito, K., et al., Plasma and serum lipidomics of healthy white adults shows characteristic profiles by subjects' gender and age, *PLoS One*, 9(3), e91806, 2014.

16. Høstmark, A.T., Glattre, E., and Jellum, E., Effect of long-term storage on the concentration of albumin and free fatty acids in human sera, *Scand. J. Clin. Lab. Invest.*, 61, 443–448, 2001.

17. Pizaro, C., Arenzana-Rámila, I., Pérez-del Notario, N., Pérez-Matute, P., and Gonález-Sáiz, J.M., Thawing as a critical pre-analytical step in the lipidomic profiling of plasma samples: New standardized protocol, *Anal. Chim. Acta*, 912, 1–9, 2016.

18. Jansenm, H.J.M., Bookhof, P.K., and Schenk, E., Long term stability of parameters of lipid metabolism in frozen human serum: Triglycerides, free fatty acids, total HDL- and LDL-cholesterol, Apoliprotein-A1 and B, *Mol. Biomark. Diagn.*, 5, 4, 2014.

19. Wang, X., Gu, X., Song, H., et al., Phenylmethanesulfonyl fluoride pretreatment stabilizes plasma lipidome in lipodomic and metabolomic analysis, *Anal. Chim. Acta*, 893, 77–83, 2015.

20. Martorell, M., Capó, X., Sureda, A., Tur, J.A., and Pons, A., Chromatographic and enzymatic method to quantify individual plasma free and triacylglycerol fatty acids, *Chromatgraphia*, 78, 259–266, 2015.

21. Bowen, R.A.R., Vu, C., Remaley, A.T., Hortin, G.I., and Csako, G., Differential effect of blood collection tubes on total fatty acids (FFA) and total triiodothyronine (TT3) concentration: A model for studying interference from tube constituents, *Clin. Chim. Acta*, 378, 181–193, 2007.

22. Burczynski, F.J., Pond, S.M., Davis, C.K., Johnson, L.P., and Weisiger, R.A., Calibration of albumin-fatty acid binding constants measured by heptane-water partition, *Am. J. Physiol. Gastrintest. Liver Physiol.*, 285, G555–G563, 1993.

23. Folch, J., Lees, M., and Stanley, G.H.S., A simple method for the isolation and purification of total lipids from animal tissues, *J. Biol. Chem.*, 226, 497–510, 1957.

24. Matyash, V., Liebisch, G., Kurzchalia, T.V., Shevchenko, A., and Schwudke, D., Lipid extraction by methyl-tert-butyl ether for high-throughput lipidomics, *J. Lipid Res.*, 49, 1137–1146, 2008.

25. Ostermann, A.J., Müller, M., Willenberg, I., and Schebb, N.H., Determining the fatty acid composition in plasma and tissues as fatty acid methyl esters using gas chromatography-a comparison of different derivatization and extraction procedures, *Prostaglandins Leukot. Essent. Fatty Acids*, 91, 235–241, 2014.

26. Dijkstra, A.J., Christie, W.W., and Knothe, G., Analysis, in *The Lipid Handbook*, F.D. Gunstone, J.L. Harwood, and A.J. Dijkstra, eds., pp. 415–469, CRC Press, Boca Raton, FL, 2007.

27. Reis, A., Rudnitskaya, A., Blackburn, G.J., et al., A comparison of five lipid extraction solvent systems for lipidomic studies of human LDL, *J. Lipid Res.*, 54, 1812–1824, 2013.

28. Le, D.Y., Kind, T., Yoon, Y.-R., Fichn, O., and Liu, K.-H., Comarative evaluation of extraction methods for simultaneous mass-spectrometric analysis of complex lipids and primary metabolites

from human blood plasma, *Anal. Bioanal. Chem.*, 406, 7275–7286, 2014.

29. Quehenberger, O., Armando, A.M., Brown, A.H., et al., Lipidomics reveals a remarkable diversity of lipids in human plasma, *J. Lipid Res.*, 51, 3299–3305, 2010.

30. Patterson, R.E., Ducrocq, A.J., McDougall, D.J., Garrett, T.J., and Yost, R.A., Comparison of blood plasma sample preparation methods for combined LC-MS lipidomics and metabolomics, *J. Chromtog. B.*, 1002, 260–268, 2015.

31. Kaluzny, M.A., Duncan, L.A., Merritt, M.V., and Epps, D.E., Rapid separation of lipid classes in high yield and purity using bonded phase columns, *J. Lipid Res.*, 26, 135–140, 1985.

32. Christie, W.W., Solid-phase extraction columns in the analysis of lipids, in *Advances in Lipid Methodology-One*, W.W. Christie, ed., pp. 1–17, The Oily Press, Ayr, Scotland, 1992.

33. Lepage, G., and Roy, C.C., Direct transesterification of all classes of lipids in a one-step reaction, *J. Lipid Res.*, 27, 114–120, 1986.

34. Lepage, G., and Roy, C.C., Specific methylation of plasma nonesterified fatty acids in a one-step reaction, *J. Lipid. Res.*, 29, 227–235, 1988.

35. Ecker, J., Scherer, M., Schmitz, G., and Liebisch, G., A rapid GC-MS method for quantification of positional and geometric isomers of fatty acid methyl esters, *J. Chromatog. B*, 897, 98–104, 2012.

36. Lin, Y.H., Loewke, J.D., Hyun, D.Y., Leaszer, J., and Hibbein, J.R., Fast transmethylation of serum lipids using microwave irradiation, *Lipids*, 47, 1109–1117, 2012.

37. Teo, C.L., and Idris, A., Evaluation of direct transesterification of microalgae using microwave irradiation, *Bioresour. Technol.*, 174, 281–286, 2014.

38. Chiu, H.-H., Tsai, S.-J., Tseng, Y.J., et al., An efficient and robust fatty acid profiling method for plasma metabolomic studies by gas chromatography-mass spectrometry, *Clin. Chim. Acta*, 451, 183–190, 2015.

39. de Souza, V., Schantz, M., Mateus, V.L., et al., Using the L/O ratio to determine blend composition in biodiesel by EASI-MS corroborated by GC-FID and GC-MS, *Anal. Methods*, 8, 682–687, 2015.

40. Sobradoi, L.A., Freije-Carrelo, L., Moldovan, M., Encinar, J.R., and Garcia Alonzo, J.I., Comparison of gas chromatography-combustion-mass spectrometry and gas chromatography-flame ionization detector for the determination of fatty acid methyl esters in biodiesel without specific standards, *J. Chromatog. A.*, 1457, 134–143, 2016.

41. Hsu, W.Y., Lin, W.-D., Hwu, W.-L., Lai, C.-C., and Tsai, F.-J., Screening assay of very long chain fatty acids in human plasma with multiwalled carbon nanotube based surface-assisted laser desorption/ionization mass spectrometry, *Anal. Chem.*, 89, 6814–6820, 2010.

42. Fuchs, B., and Schiller, J., Application of MALDI-TOF mass spectrometry in lipidomics, *Eur. J. Lipid Sci.*, 111, 83–98, 2009.

43. Hellmuth, C., Weber, M., Koletzko, B., and Peissner, W., Nonesterified fatty acid determination for functional lipidomics: Comprehensive ultrahigh performance liquid chromatography-tandem mass spectrometry quantification, qualification, and parameter prediction, *Anal. Chem.*, 84, 1483–1490, 2012.

44. Rigano, F., Albergamo, A., Sciarrone, D., et al., Nanoliquid chromatography directly coupled to electron ionization mass spectrometry for free fatty acid elucidation in mussel, *Anal. Chem.*, 88, 4021–4028, 2016.

TABLE 1: Concentration of Some Saturated Fatty Acids in Human Plasma or Serum[a]

Fatty acid	Common name	Plasma[1] μg/mL[b]	μg/mL[c]	Serum[2] g/100 g[d]	Serum[3] μmol/dL[e]	Serum[3] μmol/dL[f]	Plasma[4] μg/mL[g]	Plasma[5] μg/dL[h]	Plasma[5] nmol/mL[h]	Plasma[6] μM[i]
Decanoic acid	Capric acid (10:0)									1.32
Hendecanoic acid	Undecanoic acid (11:0)									
Dodecanoic acid	Lauric acid (12:0)				0.31	0.52		14.4	0.719	3.72
Tridecanoic acid	(13:0)									
Tetradecanoic acid	Myristic acid (14:0)	20	25	2.26	2.74	1.95	21.8	138	6.06	12.12
Pentadecanoic acid	(15:0)			0.39				15.8	0.653	2.12
Hexadecanoic acid	Palmitic acid (16:0)	444	522	26.98	28.66	25.29	532.5	1634	63.8	83.18
Heptadecanoic acid	Margaric acid (17:0)							32.3		1.95
Octadecanoic acid	Stearic acid (18:0)	158	186	10.50	4.84	8.37	191.3	628	1.20	31.38
Nonadecanoic acid	(19:0)			0.11						0.21
Eicosanoic acid	Arachidonic acid (20:0)			0.11			6.0	7.43	0.238	0.29
Docosanoic acid	Behenic acid (22:0)						20.7	5.45	0.160	
Tetracosanoic acid	Lignoceric acid (24:0)	Trace	20				18.4	9.65	0.262	0.24
Hexacosanoic acid	Ceric acid (26:0)							4.38	0.110	

TABLE 2: Concentration of Some Saturated Fatty Acids in Biological Fluids[a]

Fatty acid	Common name	Plasma[10] μM[j]	Plasma[10] μM[k]	Plasma[10] μM[l]	Plasma[11] μM[m]	Plasma[11] μM[o]	Serum[12] μg/mL[p]	Serum[12] μg/mL[q]	Blood[13] %[r]	Plasma[14] μM[t]	Blood[15] Mol%[u]
Dodecanoic acid	Lauric acid (12:0)				2.015	1.048	31.1	13.65	0.04	5.6	
Tridecanoic acid	(13:0)				<LLOQ[n]		ND	ND			
Tetradecanoic acid	Myristic acid (14:0)	5.24	20.6	28.4	16.955	6.985	135.2	52.7	0.38	13.8	0.62
Pentadecanoic acid	(15:0)				1.754	0.782	ND	ND	0.07[s]		
Hexadecanoic acid	Palmitic acid (16:0)	123	438	649	99.957	96.505	367	163.5	16.32[s]	15.2	19.6
Heptadecanoic acid	Margaric acid (17:0)				1.616	1.115	69.1	32.5	0.33[s]		
Octadecanoic acid	Stearic acid (18:0)	99.3	306	622	55.351	20.585	310.2	144	9.45[s]	36.9	10.9
Nonadecanoic acid	(19:0)				-	-	ND	ND	0.05		
Eicosanoic acid	Arachidonic acid (20:0)	1.96	8.36	10.9	0.198	-	31.1	8.95	0.32	6.1	0.66
Docosanoic acid	Behenic acid (22:0)	3.52	42.3	52.5	-	-	156.4	67.4	0.97		1.77
Tetracosanoic acid	Lignoceric acid (24:0)				-	-	ND	ND	0.07		2.68
Hexacosanoic acid	Ceric acid (26:0)						95.6	37.1	0.08		

[a] There are some differences in the extraction and derivatization methods used in several studies. The analysis of fatty acid methyl esters was performed by gas liquid chromatography (GLC).

[b] Plasma from a single individual. Fatty acid methyl esters were obtained by transesterification of a Folch extract of plasma. A Folch extract of plasma uses chloroform/methanol (2/1).[7] The lipid is contained in the lower phase. There has been consistent use of the Folch method and a recent evaluation suggests that the Folch method is a valid method for the extraction of lipid from plasma.[8]

[c] Plasma from a single individual. Fatty acid methyl esters were obtained by direct transesterification of plasma.

[d] The average value was obtained from the serum samples of 104 individuals. The lipid fraction was obtained from serum by the Folch extraction and the free fatty acids were obtained by solid-phase extraction using aminopropyl-bonded silica[9] and converted to methyl esters by acid (HCl) catalyzed esterification with methanol.

[e] Average of free fatty acid (FFA) concentration in serum samples was obtained from 27 normal individuals. The fatty acids were extracted from serum with chloroform after addition of phosphate buffer, pH 6.4. The chloroform extract was taken to dryness and esterified with 9-anthryldiazomethane in methanol.

[f] Average of total fatty acid (TFA) concentration in serum samples was obtained from 27 normal individuals. Total fatty acids were obtained by the Folch extraction of serum, concentrated under reduced pressure, saponification with ethanolic KOH, extraction with n-hexane and derivatization with 9-anthryldiazomethane in methanol.

[g] Total fatty acids in normal human plasma (96 subjects) were determined by transesterification with acetyl chloride in MeOH/toluene followed by MeOH/H_2O with extraction of FAME in decane/pentane. Analysis was performed by GC with flame ionization detection (FID). A robotic system was used for processing the plasma samples.

[h] The sample was a standard plasma prepared by the National Institute of Standards and Technology (NIST) in cooperation with the National Institutes of Health (NIH). The standard plasma was obtained from 100 normal individuals under fasting conditions using heparin as an anticoagulant. The plasma was extracted with methanol-HCl/isooctane to obtain the FFA (also referred to as the non-esterified fatty acid; NEFA) fraction which was esterified with pentafluorobenzyl bromide and analyzed by GC/MS.

[i] The average value was obtained from the analysis of EDTA plasma obtained from eight individuals under fasting conditions. The plasma samples were precipitated with isopropanol containing a labeled internal standard (^{13}C-palmitic acid) and the supernatant fraction analyzed by LC/MS.

[j] The average value was obtained for FFA (NEFA) from the analysis of EDTA plasma obtained from 24 individuals (male) under fasting conditions. The anticoagulant also contained p-toluenesulfonyl fluoride as a lipase inhibitor and butylated hydroxyanisole as an antioxidant to prevent hydroxylation of unsaturated fatty acids. The plasma was diluted with MeOH/H_2O, subjected to solid-phase extraction to obtain the FFA fraction and converted to methyl esters with m-trifluoromethylphenyl trimethylammonium hydroxide in methanol prior to GLC analysis.

[k] The average value was obtained for triacylglyceride fatty acids (TGFA) from the analysis of EDTA plasma obtained from 24 individuals (male) under fasting conditions. The anticoagulant contained butylated hydroxyanisole as an antioxidant to prevent oxidation of unsaturated fatty acids. The plasma was treated with lipoprotein lipase to obtain fatty acids bound to triglyceride. The samples were subsequently treated as with the FFA fraction (footnote j).

[l] The average value was obtained for total plasma fatty acid (TPFA) from the analysis of EDTA plasma obtained from 24 individuals (male) under fasting conditions. A Folch fraction was obtained from the plasma samples, taken to dryness and converted to methyl esters with m-trifluoromethylphenyl trimethylammonium hydroxide in methanol prior to GLC analysis.

[m] NEFA in human adult plasma. NEFA were determined by HPLC analysis of the supernatant fraction from 2-propanol-precipitated human plasma.

[n] LLOQ, lower lever of quantitation.

[o] NEFA in human pediatric plasma. NEFA were determined by HPLC analysis of the supernatant fraction from 2-propanol-precipitated human plasma.

[p] Blood from 20 subjects was used to obtain serum (clotting in the cold). The serum was used as a source for the determination of esterified fatty acids (EFA) (KOH/MeOH) which were then removed in a hexane extraction. Analysis of the fatty acid methyl esters was accomplished with GC/MS. Although KOH/MeOH results in transesterification of fatty acid esters such as glycerol, these conditions do not result in the esterification of NEFA.

[q] Blood from 20 subjects was used to obtain serum (clotting in the cold). The serum was used as a source for the determination of free fatty acids NEFA. NEFA were obtained as methyl esters by H_2SO_4/MeOH. Analysis of the fatty acid methyl esters was accomplished with GC/MS.

[r] The data are expressed as relative abundance (%). A whole blood sample was obtained by finger stick and FAME obtained by transesterification with acetyl chloride in MeOH (90°C/30 minutes) followed by hexane extraction. Analysis of FAME was accomplished with capillary GC/MS. This group did show that acetyl chloride/MeOH was more effective in obtaining FAME from cholesterol esters than either H_2SO_4/MeOH or HCl/MeOH.

[s] Only clearly identified species are included. The reader is directed to the original work for more information for the minor species observed.

[t] Human plasma (fasting) was taken with 2-propanol/hexane/H_3PO_4 followed by the addition of hexane. The supernatant phase was taken for HPLC analysis (C_{18} bond phase) with detection by mass spectrometry.

[u] Total fatty acids were measured in dried blood samples. Data are expressed as mol% from the analysis of dried blood samples obtained from military personnel. The capillary blood samples were collected by fingertip prick taken onto filter paper impregnated with butylated hydroxytoluene, allowed to air dry, and stored for subsequent analysis. Transesterification was accomplished with acetyl chloride in MeOH/hexane in a microwave and the FAME extracted in the hexane phase, a completion of the reaction.

References

1. Lepage, G., and Roy, C.C., Direct transesterification of all classes of lipids in a one-step reaction, *J. Lipid Res.*, 27, 114–120, 1986.
2. Yli-Jama, P., Haugen, T.S., Rebnord, H.M., Ringstad, J., and Pedersen, J.J., Selective mobilization of fatty acids from human adipose tissue, *Europ. J. Int. Med.*, 12, 107–115, 2001.
3. Shinomura, Y., Sugiyama, S., and Takamura, T., Quantitative determination of the fatty acid composition of human serum by high-performance liquid chromatography, *J. Chromatog.*, 383, 9–17, 1986.
4. Lin, Y.H., Salem, N., Jr., Wells, E.M., et al., Automated high-throughput fatty acid analysis of umbilical cord serum and application to an epidemiological study, *Lipids*, 47, 527–539, 2012.
5. Quehenberger, O., Armando, A.M., Brown, A.H., et al., Lipidomics reveals a remarkable diversity of lipids in human plasma, *J. Lipid Res.*, 51, 3299–3305, 2010.
6. Hellmuth, C., Weber, M., Kolekzko, B., and Peissner, W., Nonesterified fatty acid determination for functional lipidomics. Comprehensive ultrahigh performance liquid chromatography-tandem mass spectrometry quantitation, qualification and parameter prediction, *Anal. Chem.*, 84, 1483–1490, 2012.
7. Folch, J., Lees, M., and Stanley, G.H.S., A simple method for the isolation and purification of total lipids from animal tissues, *J. Biol. Chem.*, 226, 497–510, 1957.
8. Lee, D.Y., Kind, T., Yoon, R.-Y., Fichn, O., and Liu, K.-H., Comparative evaluation of extraction methods for simultaneous mass-spectrometric analysis of complex lipids and primary metabolites from human blood plasma, *Anal. Bioanal. Chem.*, 406, 7275–7286, 2014.
9. Kaluzny, M.A., Duncan, L.A., Merritt, M.V., and Epps, D.E., Rapid separation of lipid classes in high yield and purity using bonded phase columns, *J. Lipid Res.*, 26, 135–140, 1985.
10. Matorell, M., Capó, X., Sureda, A., Tur, J.A., and Pons, A., Chromatographic and enzymatic method to quantify individual plasma free and triacylglycerol fatty acids, *Chromatographia*, 78, 259–266, 2015.
11. Christnat, N., Morin-Rivron, D., and Masoodi, M., High-throughput quantitative lipidomics analysis of nonesterified fatty acids in human plasma, *J. Proteome Res.*, 15, 2228–2235, 2016.
12. Sánchez-Ávila, N., Mata-Granadox, J.M., Ruiz-Jiménez, J., and Luque de Castro, M.D., Fast, sensitive and highly discriminant gas chromatography=mass spectrometry method for profiling analysis of fatty acids in serum, *J. Chromatog. A.*, 1216, 6864–6872, 2009.
13. Bicalho, B., David, F., Rumplel, K., Kindt, E., and Sandra, P., Creating a fatty acid methyl ester database for lipid profiling in a single drop of human blood using high resolution capillary gas chromatography and mass spectrometry, *J. Chromatog. A.*, 1211, 120–128, 2008.
14. Trufelli, H., Famiglini, G., Termopoli, V., and Cappiello, A., Profiling of non-esterified fatty acids in human plasma using liquid chromatography-electron ionization mass spectrometry, *Anal. Bioanal. Chem.*, 400, 2933–2941, 2011.
15. Lin, Y.H., Hanson, J.A., Strandjord, S.E., et al., Fast transmethylation of total lipids in dried blood by microwave irradiation and its application to a population study, *Lipids*, 49, 839–851, 2014.

TABLE 3: Concentration of Some Unsaturated Fatty Acids in Human Plasma or Serum[a]

#	Fatty Acid	Name	Plasma[d,1] ng/mL	Plasma[e,2] μg/mL	Serum[3] μmol/dL[f]	Serum[3] mmol/dL[g]	Serum[4] Mol%[h]	Plasma[5] nmol/mL[i]	Plasma[5] μg/dL[j]	Plasma[6] μM[l]	Plasma[6] μM[m]
1	C16:1 ω-7[b]	Palmitoleic acid;(Z)-hexadec-9-enoic acid[c]		39.5	4.96	3.04	4.27[i]	14.7[k]	372	21.819	13,869
2	C18:1ω-9	Oleic acid; (Z)-octadec-9-enoic acid		399.8	28.29	19.90	35.46[i]	80.3	2267	174.248	147.855
3	C18:1ω-7	cis-Vaccenic acid; (Z)-octadec-11-enoic acid		25.6			0.31[i]			8.962	8.553
4	C18:2ω-6	Linoleic acid; (9E,12E)-octadeca-9,12-dienoic acid		654.6	21.67	29.39	13.74	15.2	427	44.899	79.436
5	C18:3ω-6	γ-Linolenic acid; (6Z,9Z,12Z)-octadeca-6,9,12-trienoic acid		14.3	2.07	0.99	0.05	1.03	28.7	0.587	0.827
6	C18:4ω-3	Stearidonic acid; (6Z,9Z,12Z,15Z)-octadeca-6,9,12,15-tetraenoic acid					0.02	0.016	0.44	0.344	0.384
7	C20:1ω-9	Gondoic acid; (Z)-icos-11-enoic acid		3.7			0.38			2.098	0.762
8	C20:2ω-6	11,14-icosadienoic acid; icosa-11,14-dienoic acid		4.8			0.15	0.352	10.9	0.782	1.2
9	C20:3ω-6	Bishomo-γ-linolenic acid; Dihomo-γ-linolenic acid; (8Z,11Z,14Z)-icosa-8,11,14-trienoic acid		42.2	0.20	0.96	0.12	0.542	16.6	1.058	1.44
10	C20:4ω-6	Arachidonic acid; 5Z,8Z,11Z,14Z)-icosa-5,8,11,14-tetraenoic acid	472–574	130.3	3.0	5.74	0.86	2.94	89.4	2.999	5,781
11	C20:5ω-3	Eicosapentaenoic acid (EPA); (5Z,8Z,11Z,14Z,17Z)-icosa-5,8,11,14,17-pentaenoic acid	42.8–52.1	19.0	0.76	1.43	0.34	0.435	13.1	0.580	0.387
12	C22:4ω-6	Adrenic acid; (7Z,10Z,13Z,16Z)-docosa-7,10,13,16-tetraenoic acid		7.2			0.02	0.364	12.1	0.384	0.695
13	C22:5ω-6	4,7,10,13,16-Docosapentaenoic acid; (4E,7E,10E,13E,16E)-docosa-4,7,10,13,16-pentaenoic acid		3.2			0.10	0.400	13.2	0.260	0.588
14	C22:5ω-3	7,10,13,16,19-Docosapentaenoic acid; (7E,10E,13E,16E,19E)-docosa-7,10,13,16,19-pentaenoic acid		16.7			0.10			0.916	0.934
15	C22:6ω-3	Docosahexaenoic acids (DHA); (4E,7E,10Z,13E,16E,19E)-docosa-4,7,10,13,16,19-hexaenoic acid (other isomers exist)	328–388	27.1	2.80	2.45	0.04			3.016	2.979

TABLE 4: Concentration of Some Unsaturated Fatty Acids in Human Plasma, Serum or Whole Blood[a]

#	Fatty acid	Name	Blood[8] %[n]	Plasma[9] μM[p]	Serum[10] μg/mL[r]	Serum[10] μg/mL[t]	Plasma[11] μg/mL[u]	Blood[12] Mol%[v]
1	C16:1 ω-7[b]	Palmitoleic acid;(Z)-hexadec-9-enoic acid[c]	0.72[o]	18.83	96.8[s]	42.25[s]	0.23–23.67	1.15
2	C18:1ω-9	Oleic acid; (Z)-octadec-9-enoic acid	13.34	149.26[q]	535.6	228	9.27–179.44	18.0
3	C18:1ω-7	cis-Vaccenic acid; (Z)-octadec-11-enoic acid	1.06		151.2	67.45		1.74
4	C18:2ω-6	Linoleic acid; (9Z,12Z)-octadeca-9,12-dienoic acid	15.95	42.83	432.6[s]	186.4[s]	21-96–162.93	22.6
5	C18:3ω-6	γ-Linolenic acid; (6Z,9Z,12Z)-octadeca-6,9,12-trienoic acid		5.56				0.39
6	C18:4ω-3	Stearidonic acid; (6Z,9Z,12Z,15Z)-octadeca-6,9,12,15-tetraenoic acid		0.11				
7	C20:1ω-9	Gondoic acid; (Z)-icos-11-enoic acid	0.23	1.69	10.3	0.4	0.32–1.30	0.19
8	C20:2ω-6	11,14-icosadienoic acid; 11E,14E)-icosa-11,14-dienoic acid	0.22	1.01	40.1	14.65	0	0.33
9	C20:3ω-6	Bishomo-γ-linolenic acid; Dihomo-γ-linolenic acid; (8Z,11Z,14Z)-icosa-8,11,14-trienoic acid	1.39	1.47	61	27.05		1.52
10	C20:4ω-6	Arachidonic acid; 5Z,8Z,11Z,14Z)-icosa-5,8,11,14-tetraenoic acid	8.16	3.66	287.5	165.1	1.69–3.80	9.49
11	C20:5ω-3	Eicosapentaenoic acid (EPA); (5Z,8Z,11Z,14Z,17Z)-icosa-5,8,11,14,17-pentaenoic acid	0.87	0.66	66.4	21.35	0.22–2.13	0.42
12	C22:4ω-6	Adrenic acid; (7Z,10Z,13Z,16Z)-docosa-7,10,13,16-tetraenoic acid	0.93	0.5	29.5	8,15		1.50
13	C22:5ω-6	4,7,10,13,16-Docosapentaenoic acid; (4Z,7Z,10Z,13Z,16Z)-docosa-4,7,10,13,16-pentaenoic acid	0.25	1.27[q]				0.58
14	C22:5ω-3	7,10,13,16,19-Docosapentaenoic acid; (7E,10E,13E,16E,19E)-docosa-7,10,13,16,19-pentaenoic acid (other isomers exist)	0.25		32.3	14.95		1.18
15	C22:6ω-3	Docosahexaenoic acids (DHA); (4Z,7Z,10Z,13Z,16Z,19Z)-docosa-4,7,10,13,16,19-hexaenoic acid (other isomers exist)	2.25	3.58	120.3	57.4		1.67
16	C24:ω-9	Nervonic acid; (Z)-tetracos-15-enoic acid						

[a] There is some differences in the extraction and derivatization methods used in several studies. The analysis of fatty acid methyl esters (FAME) was performed by gas-liquid chromatography (GLC), whereas HPLC is used for non-esterified fatty acids (NEFA, also known as FFA, free fatty acids). Although internal standards are used in many studies, it is not clear that the concentrations given in the table represent blood/plasma concentrations. Both NEFA and total fatty acids are reported in this table, and the reader is directed to the appropriate footnote for the specific study.

[b] The shorthand gives the number of carbon atoms in the chain (e.g., C16 for hexadecenoic acid [palmitic acid]). With unsaturation, the number of double bonds is given after the number of carbon atoms followed by the position of the double bond closest to the terminal methyl group (designated by ω, omega, is given. The chemical term gives the placement of the double bond relative to the carboxyl carbon. Thus, for linoleic acid (9E,12E-octadeca-9,12-dienoic acid; IUPAC nomenclature), the shorthand is C18:2 ω-6. An alternative nomenclature for the location of the double bond is the use of n instead of ω; ω may be preferable as it is less ambiguous than n.[7] E is used to designate a *trans* double bond and Z is used to designate a *cis* double bond.

[c] IUPAC nomenclature.

[d] Free fatty acids obtained from plasma by a modified Folch extraction and analyzed by HPLC (cyanopropyl bonded phase). The data are from 9 female subjects (age range 18–35). This study contains data on collection and storage of plasma for use in the study of endocannabinoids including several bioactive polyunsaturated fatty acids.

[e] Total fatty acids in normal human plasma (96 subjects) were determined by transesterification with acetyl chloride in MeOH/toluene followed by MeOH/H₂O with extraction of FAME in decane/pentane. Analysis was performed by GC with flame ionization detection (FID). A robotic system was used for processing the plasma samples.

[f] NEFA were obtained in a chloroform extract of serum and converted to methyl esters by reaction with 8-anthryldiazomethane.

[g] Total fatty acid methyl esters were obtained by reaction with 8-anthryldiazomethane following saponification of the sample with KOH/EtOH (alkaline ethanol).

[h] NEFA concentration in human serum expressed as mol% (moles per 100 moles of similar species, in this case total NEFA). NEFA were obtained by solid-phase extraction (aminopropyl bonded phase) of a Folch extract of human serum. The data are the average value from 104 normal subjects. NEFA were converted to methyl esters by HCl/MeOH/Ci²⁻/CHCl₃ at 23°C/30 minutes) and subjected to GC analysis.

[i] cis (Z) and trans (E) combined.

[j] Free fatty acids were extracted from plasma with methanol/HCl:isooctane, converted to volatile derivatives by reaction with pentafluorobenzyl bromide and analyzed by GC/MS.

[k] Data are for the Z (cis) form [(Z)-hexadec-9-enoic acid].

[l] NEFA in human adult plasma. NEFA were determined by HPLC analysis of the supernatant fraction from 2-propanol-precipitated human plasma.

[m] NEFA in human pediatric plasma. NEFA were determined by HPLC analysis of the supernatant fraction from 2-propanol-precipitated human plasma.

[n] The data are expressed as relative abundance (%). A whole blood sample was obtained by finger stick and FAME obtained by transesterification with acetyl chloride in MeOH (90°C/30 minutes) followed by hexane extraction. Analysis of FAME was accomplished with capillary GC/MS. This group did show that acetyl chloride/MeOH was more effective in obtaining FAME from cholesterol esters than either H₂SO₄/MeOH or HCl/MeOH.

[o] Only clearly identified species are included. The reader is directed to the original work for more information for the minor species observed.

[p] Concentration of NEFA in plasma. DTA plasma was obtained from eight subjects (fasting) and mixed with 50% acetonitrile in water containing internal standards. The supernatant fraction was taken for uHPLC analysis (diphenyl bonded matrix) with detection by mass spectrometry.

[q] This study did not distinguish between C18:1 and C20:5 isomers. In the case of C18:1, it is assumed here that the C18:1 isomer is oleic acid.

[r] Blood from 20 subjects was used to obtain serum (clotting in the cold). The serum was used as a source for the determination of esterified fatty acids (EFA) (KOH/MeOH) which were then removed in a hexane extraction. Analysis of fatty acid methyl esters was accomplished with GC/MS. Although KOH/MeOH results in transesterification of fatty acid esters such as glycerol, these conditions do not result in the esterification of NEFA.

[s] Combined isomers.

[t] Blood from 20 subjects was used to obtain serum (clotting in the cold). The serum was used as a source for the determination of free fatty acids NEFA. NEFA were obtained as methyl esters by H₂SO₄/MeOH. Analysis of fatty acid methyl esters was accomplished with GC/MS.

[u] NEFA were determined by a process described as reductive alkylation. Iodomethane was added to plasma (diluted with phosphate, pH 8.0, containing tetrabutylammonium hydroxide) in dichloromethane. The bottom organic layer was taken for analysis by GG/MS. The results are reported as a range from an unknown number of subjects.

[v] Total fatty acids were measured in dried blood samples. Data are expressed as mol% from the analysis of dried blood samples obtained from military personnel. The capillary blood samples were collected by fingertip prick taken onto filter paper impregnated with butylated hydroxytoluene, allowed to air dry, and stored for subsequent analysis. Transesterification was accomplished with acetyl chloride in MeOH/hexane in a microwave and the FAME extracted in the hexane phase, a completion of the reaction.

References

1. Wood, J.T., Williams, J.S., Pandarinathan, L., et al., Comprehensive profiling of the human circulating endocannabinoid metabolome: Clinical sampling and sample storage parameters, *Clin. Chem. Lab. Med.*, 46, 1289–1295, 2008.
2. Lin, Y.H., Salem, N., Jr., Wells, E.M., et al., Automated high-throughput fatty acid analysis of umbilical cord serum and application to an epidemiological study, *Lipids*, 47, 527–539, 2012.
3. Shimomura, Y., Sugiyama, S., and Takamura, T., Quantitative determination of the fatty acid composition of human serum lipids by high-performance liquid chromatography, *J. Chromatog.*, 389, 9–17, 1986.
4. Yli-Jama, P., Meyer, H.E., Ringsted, J., and Pedersen, J.F., Serum free fatty acid pattern and risk of myocardial infarction: A case control study, *J. Intern. Med.*, 251, 19–28, 2002.
5. Quehenberger, O., Armando, A.M., Brown, A.H., et al., Lipidomics reveals a remarkable diversity of lipids in human plasma, *J. Lipid Res.*, 51, 3299–3305, 2010.
6. Christinat, N., Morin-Rivron, D., and Masoodi, M., High-throughput quantitative lipidomics analysis of nonesterified fatty acids in human plasma, *J. Proteome Res.*, 15, 2228–2235, 2016.
7. Daviid, B.G., and Cantril, R.C., Fatty acid nomenclature, *South Afr. Med. J.*, 67, 633–634, 1985.
8. Bicalho, B., David, F., Rumplel, K., Kindt, E., and Sandra, P., Creating a fatty acid methyl ester database for lipid profiling in a single drop of human blood using high resolution capillary gas chromatography and mass spectrometry, *J. Chromatog. A.*, 1211, 120–128, 2008.
9. Hellmuth, C., Weber, M., Koletzko, B., and Peissner, W., Nonesterified fatty acid determination for functional lipidomics: Comprehensive ultrahigh performance liquid chromatography-tandem mass spectrometry quantitation, qualification, and parameter prediction, *Anal. Chem.*, 84, 1483–1490, 2012.
10. Sánchez-Ávila, N., Mata-Granadox, J.M., Ruiz-Jiménez, J., and Luque de Castro, M.D., Fast, sensitive and highly discriminant gas chromatography=mass spectrometry method for profiling analysis of fatty acids in serum, *J. Chromatog. A.*, 1216, 6864–6872, 2009.
11. Ukolov, A.I., Orlova, T.I., Savel'eva, E.I., and Radilov, A.S., Chromatographic-mass spectrometric determination of free fatty acids in blood plasma and urine using extractive alkylation, *J. Anal. Chem.*, 70, 1123–1130, 2015.
12. Lin, Y.H., Hanson, J.A., Strandjord, S.E., et al., Fast transmethylation of total lipids in dried blood by microwave irradiation and its application to a population study, *Lipids*, 49, 839–851, 2014.

SOME UNUSUAL FATTY ACID STRUCTURES

Roger L. Lundblad

Stearic acid
octadecanoic acid

Oleic acid
Z-9-octadecaenoic

Linoleic acid (LA)
Z,Z-9,12-octadecadienoic acid

α-Linolenic acid
Z,Z,Z-9,12,15-octadecatrienoic acid

γ-Linolenic acid
Z,Z,Z-6,9,12,-octadecatrienoic acid

Pinolenic acid
5*Z*,9*Z*,12*Z*-octadecatrienoic acid

Rumenic acid, a conjugated linoleic acid (CLA)
Z,E-9,11-octadecadienoic acid

(R)-Laballenic acid
octa-5,6-dienoic acid

Tariric acid
octadec-6-ynoic acid

Tuberculostearic acid
10-methyloctadecanoic acid

Stearic acid: **Octadecanoic acid,**[a] a C18 saturated fatty acid.

Oleic acid: **(Z)-octadec-9-enoic acid**. A monounsaturated C18 fatty acid; a C18 fatty acid containing a single bond.

Linoleic acid: Also known as telfairic acid, **(9Z,12Z)-octadeca-9,12-dienoic acid**. A C18 polyunsaturated fatty acid (PUFA) containing two double bonds separated by a methylene group (methylene bridge). Linoleic acid is the major PUFA in the human diet (Whelan, J., and Fritsche, K., Linoleic acid, *Adv. Nutr.*, 4, 311–312, 2013). Linoleic acid can be converted to a

---

[a] IUPAC nomenclature.

form containing a conjugated double bond (CLA, conjugated linoleic acid) (Kepler, C.R., Hirons, K.P., McNeill, J.J., and Tove, S.B., Intermediates and products of the biohydrogenation of linoleic acid by *Butyrivibrio fibrisolvens, J. Biol. Chem.,* 241, 1350–1354, 1966) with a variety of biological activities (Gholami, Z., and Khosravi-Darani, K., An overview of conjugated linoleic acid: Microbial product and application, *Mini Rev. Med. Chem.,* 14, 734–746, 2014; Kim, J.H., Kim, Y., Kim, Y.J., and Park, Y., Conjugated linoleic acid: Potential health benefits as a functional food ingredient, *Annu. Rev. Food Sci. Technol.,* 7, 221–244, 2016).

α-Linolenic acid (ALA): **(9Z,12Z,15Z)-octadeca-9,12,15-trienoic acid.** A C18 PUFA containing three double bonds separated by methylene groups (methylene bridges). ALA is essential in the diet of human serving as a precursor for longer chain PUFAs (Burdge, G.C., Metabolism of alpha-linolenic acid in humans, *Prostaglandins Leukot. Essent. Fatty Acids,* 75, 161–168, 2006). ALA has been shown to have a positive effect on human health (Stark, A.H., Crawford, M.A., and Reifen, R., Update on alpha-linolenic acid, *Nutr. Rev.,* 66, 326–332, 2008; Kim, K.B., Nam Y.A., Kim, H.S., Hayes, A.W., and Lee, B.M.,α,-Linolenic acid: Nutraceutical, pharmacological and toxicological evaluation, *Food Chem. Toxicol.,* 70, 163–178, 2014; Piermartiri, T., Pan, H., Figueiredo, T.H., and Marini, A.M., α-Linolenic acid, a nutraceutical with pleiotropic properties that targets endogenous neuroprotective pathways to protect against organophosphate nerve agent-induced neuropathology, *Molecules,* 20, 20355–20380, 2015).

γ-Linolenic acid (GLA): **(6Z,9Z,12Z)-octadeca-6,9,12-trienoic acid.** A C18 PUFA containing three double bonds separated by methylene groups (methylene bridges). GLA is a ω-6 PUFA, whereas ALA is a ω-3 PUFA. GLA is one of a family of ω-6 fatty acids and is derived from linoleic acid serving as a precursor for arachidonic acid (Gunstone, F.D., Gamma-linolenic acid – occurrence and physical and chemical properties, *Prog. Lipid Res.,* 31, 145–161, 1992). GLA has been suggested to have a variety of positive effect on human health (Horrobin, D.F., Nutritional and medical importance of gamma-linolenic acid, *Prog. Lipid Res.,* 31, 163–194, 1992; Fan, Y.Y., and Chapkin, R.S., Importance of dietary γ-linolenic acid in human health and nutrition, *J. Nutr.,* 128, 1411–1414, 1998; Kapoor, R., and Huang, Y.A., Gamma linolenic acid: An antiinflammatory omega-6 fatty acid, *Curr. Pharm. Biotechnol.,* 7, 531–534, 2006).

Pinolenic acid: **(5Z,9Z,12Z)-octadeca-5,9,12-trienoic acid.** Pinolenic acid is an isomer of GLA and has different physiological effects (Matsuo, N., Osada, K., Kodama, T., et al., Effects of γ-linolenic acid and its positional isomer pinolenic acid on immune parameters of brown-Norway rats, *Prostaglandins Leukot. Essent. Fatty Acids,* 55, 223–229, 1996). Pinolenic acid was isolated from Finnish tall oil fatty acid distillates (Hase, A., Harva, O., and Pakkanen, T., Origin of bicyclic fatty acids in tall oil, *J. Am. Oil Chem. Soc.,* 51, 181–183, 1974). Finnish (Scandinavian) tall oil has been shown to contain more that 10% pinolenic acid (Hase, A., Ala-Peijari, M., Kaltia, S., and Matikainen, J., Separation and purification of pinolenic acid by the iodolactonization, *J. Am. Oil Chem. Soc.,* 69, 832–834, 1992). The current major source of pinolenic acid is found in pine nut oil (No, D.S., and In-Hwan, K., Pinolenic acid as a new source of phyto-polyunsaturated fatty acid, *Lipid Technol.,* 25, 135–138, 2013; Xie, K., Miles, E.A., and Calder, P.C., A review of the potential health benefits of pine nut oil and its characteristic fatty acid pinolenic acid, *J. Functional Foods,* 23, 464–473, 2016).

Bovinic acid (rumenic acid): **(9Z,11E)-octadeca-9,11-dienoic acid.** Rumenic acid is a conjugated linoleic acid (CLA). Rumenic acid is a *trans*-fatty acid formed from linoleic acid in the rumen of ruminant animals such as cows and pigs (Wallace, R.J., McKain, N., Shingfield, K.J., and Devillard, E., Isomers of conjugated linoleic acids are synthesized via different mechanisms in ruminal digesta and bacteria, *J. Lipid Res.,* 48, 2247–2254, 2007). Rumenic acid is of interest as a functional lipid (Gebauer, S.K., Chardigny, J.M., Jakobsen, M.U., et al., Effects of ruminant trans fatty acids on cardiovascular disease and cancer: A comprehensive review of epidemiological, clinical, and mechanistic studies, *Adv. Nutr.,* 2, 332–354, 2011; Jenkins, N.D., Housh, T.J., Miramonti, A.A., et al., Effects of rumenic acid rich conjugated linoleic acid supplementation on cognitive function and handgrip performance in older men and women, *Exp. Gerontol.,* 84, 1–11, 2016). *trans*-Vaccenic acid [(E)-octadec-11-enoic acid] is converted to rumenic acid by Δ^9-desaturase activity (Soyeurt, H., Dehareng, F., Mayeres, P., Bertozzi, C., and Gengler, N., Variation of Δ^9-desaturase activity in dairy cattle, *J. Dairy Sci.,* 91, 3211–3224, 2008; Toral, P.G., Chilliard, Y., and Bernard, L., In vivo deposition of [1-^{13}C]vaccenic acid and the product of its Δ^9-desaturation, [1-^{13}C] rumenic acid in the body tissues of lactating goats fed oils, *J. Dairy Sci.,* 95, 6755–6759, 2012).

Laballenic acid: **octadeca-5,6-dienoic acid.** Labellenic acid is an allenic compound with a chiral center and thus can exist in R and S configurations (Bagby, M.O., Smith, C.R., Jr., and Wolff, A., Laballenic acid: A new allenic acid from *Leonotis nepetaefolia* seed oil, *J. Org. Chem.,* 30, 4227–4229, 1965). Naturally occurring laballenic acid has been shown to possess R configuration (Landor., S.R., and Punja, N., Synthesis and absolute configuration of laballenic acid, *Tetrahedron Lett.,* 40, 4905–4907, 1966). Labellenic acid has been shown to be the precursor of phlomic acid (icosa-7,8-dienoic acid) (Aitzmuller, K., Tsevegsuren, N., and Vosmann, K., A new allenic fatty acid in *Phlomis* seed, *Fett/Lipid,* 99, 74–78, 1997).

Tariric acid: **octadec-6-ynoic acid.** Tariric acid contains a triple bond and is referred to as an acetylenic acid. Tariric acid was modified with iodine to form diododerivative with the tradename of Iodostarin which was used as a pharmaceutical source of iodine (Baur, E., Velhalten des Jodostarins im Licht, *Helv. Chim. Acta,* 18, 1149–1150, 1935). Tariric acid, present in triglyceride, is incorporated into depot fat and hepatic fat (Bernhard, K., Yekundi, K., and Kaempf, E., Das biologische Verhalten von Fettsäuren mit Dreifachbindung: III. Der abbau der Taririnsäure, *Helv. Chim. Acta,* 51, 373–376, 1968).

Tuberculostearic acid: **10-methyloctadecanoic acid.** Tuberculostearic acid is a branched chain fatty acid with an asymmetric center first described in 1929 (Anderson, R.J., and Chargaff, E., The chemistry of the lipoids of tubercle bacilli. V. Analysis of the acetone-soluble fat, *J. Biol. Chem.,* 84, 703–717, 1929). Subsequent work demonstrated the presence of tuberculostearic acid in tuberculous lung tissue (Anderson, R.J., Reeves, R.E., Creighton, M.M., and Lothrup, W.C., The chemistry of the lipids of tubercle bacilli. LXV. Investigation of tuberculous lung tissue, *Am. Rev. Tuberculosis,* 48, 65–75, 1943). The native form is the R isomer (Wallace, P.A., Minnikin, D.E., McCrudden, K., and Pizzarello, A., Synthesis of (R,S)-10-methyloctadecanoic acid (tuberculostearic acid) and key chiral 2-methyl branched intermediates, *Chem. Phys. Lipids,* 71, 145–162, 1994). The detection of tuberculostearic acid in human sputum is useful for the diagnosis of pulmonary tuberculosis (Odham, G., Larsson, L., and Mardh, P.A., Demonstration of tuberculostearic acid in sputum from patients with pulmonary tuberculosis by selected ion monitoring, *J. Clin. Invest.,* 63, 813–819, 1979; Dang, N.A., Mourão, M.,

Kuijper, S., et al., Direct detection of *Mycobacterium tuberculosis* in sputum using combined solid phase extraction-gas chromatography-mass spectrometry, *J. Chromatog. B. Analyt. Technol. Biomed. Life Sci.*, 986–987, 115–122, 2015).

Some cyclic fatty acids

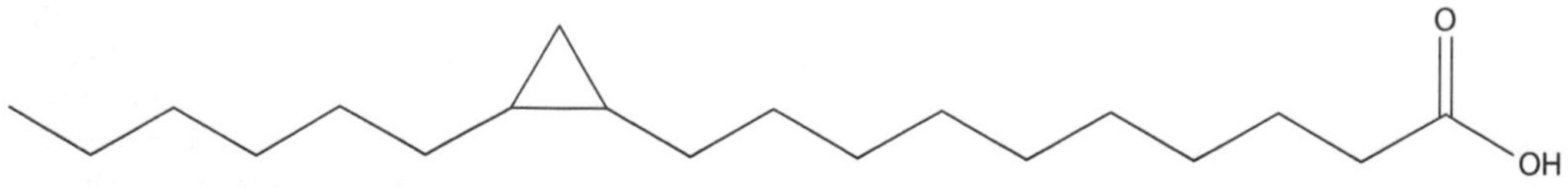

Lactobacillic acid
10-[(1R,2S)-2-hexylcyclopropyl]decanoic acid

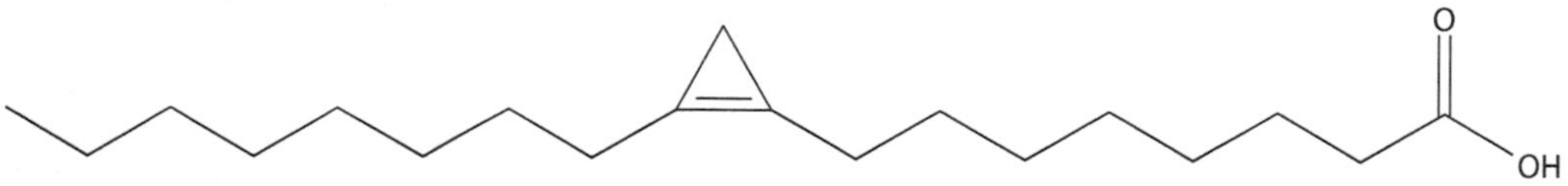

Sterculic acid
8-(2-octylcyclopropen-1-yl)octanoic acid

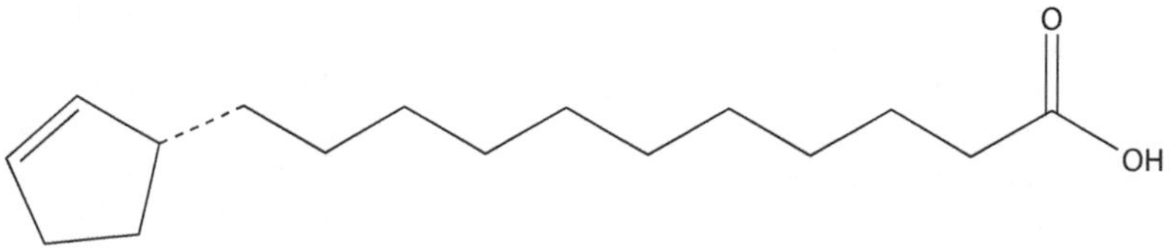

Hydnocarpic acid
11-[(1R)-cyclopent-2-en-1-yl]undecanoic acid

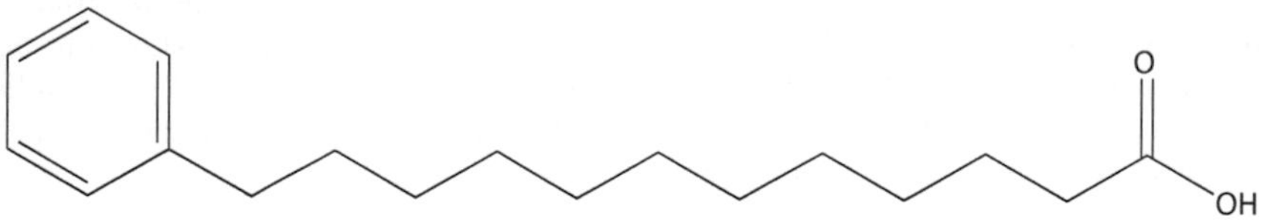

13-phenyltridecanoic acid

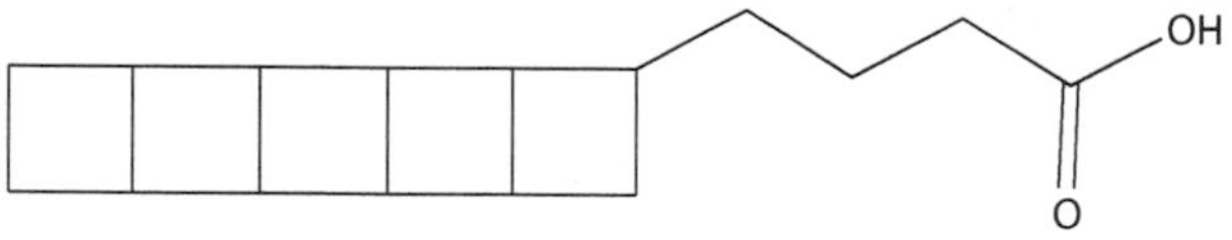

4-[5]-ladderane-butanoic acid;

Lactobacillic acid: **10-[(1R,2S)-2-hexylcyclopropyl]decanoic acid.**[a] Lactobacillic acid contains a cyclopropane ring. The naturally occurring form has been assigned the configuration of (11*R*, 12*S*) (Coxon, G.D., Al-Dulayymi, J.R., and Baird, M.S., The synthesis of (11*R*,12*S*)-lactobacillic acid and its enantiomer, *Tetrahedron Asymmetry*, 14, 1211–1222, 2003). Lactobacillic acid was originally described in *Lactobacillus casei* (Hoffman, K., and Lucas, R.A., The chemical nature of a unique fatty acid, *J. Am. Chem. Soc.*, 72, 4328–4329, 1950). Lactobacillic acid is found in a number of other bacteria including *Oenococcus oeni* (Teixeira, H., Goncalves, M.G., Rozès, A., Ramos, A., and San Romäno, M.V., Lactobacillis acid accumulation in the plasma membrane of *Oenococcus oeni*. A response to ethanol stress?, *Microbiol. Ecol.*, 43, 146–153, 2002). Lactobacillic acid has been recently used as biomarker for silage feeding in authentication of regional cheeses (Caligiani, A., Nocetti, M., Lolli, V., Marseglia, A., and Palla, G.,

Development of a quantitative GC-MS method for the deduction of cyclopropane fatty acids in cheese as new molecular markers for Parmaigiano Reggiano authentication, *J. Ag. Food Chem.*, 64, 4158–4164, 2016).

Sterculic acid: **8-(2-octylcyclopropen-1-yl)octanoic acid.** Sterculic acid is a fatty acid that contains a cyclopropane ring. Sterculic acid is found in seeds from a number of different plants and has been shown to inhibit the biosynthesis of unsaturated fatty acids (James, A.T., Harris, P., and Bezard, J., The inhibition of unsaturated fatty acid biosynthesis in plants by stercuic acid, *Eur. J. Biochem.*, 3, 318–325, 1968) by desaturases (Jeffcoat, R., and Pollard, M.R., Studies on the inhibition of the desaturases by cyclopropenoid fatty acids, *Lipids*, 12, 480–485, 1977).

Hydnocarpic acid: **11-[(1R)-cyclopent-2-en-1-yl]undecanoic acid.** Hydnocarpic acid is derived from a plant oil and was used for the treatment of leprosy (Anon, The treatment of leprosy by chaulmoogra oil, *Lancet*, 187, 790, 1916; Norton, S.A.,

---

[a] IUPAC nomenclature.

Useful plants of dermatology. I. *Hydnocarpus* and chaulmoogra, *J. Am. Acad. Dermatol.*, 31, 683–686, 1994). A commercial product, Alepol (Bhandari, A.D., Several commercial products were developed including Alepol for the treatment of leprosy, *Indian Med. J.*, 67, 244–246, 1932) was developed by Burroughs-Welcome.

13-Phenyltridecanoic acid: 13-Phenyltridecanoic acid is found in the seeds of Araceae (Aroideae subfamily, aroids) (Meija, J., and Soukup, V.G., Phenyl-terminated fatty acids in seeds of various aroids, *Phytochemistry*, 65, 2229–2237, 2004). 13-phenyltridecanoic acid and other ω-phenyl fatty acids have been found in butter fat (Schroeder, M., Abdurahman, H., Ruoff, T., Lehnert, K., and Vetter, W., Identification of aromatic fatty acids in butter fat, *J. Am. Oil Chem. Soc.*, 91, 1695–1702, 2014). It is not apparent as to whether this reflects endogenous or exogenous synthesis.

4-[5]-ladderane butanoic acid: Ladderane fatty acids are found in the membrane lipids of anammox (anaerobic ammonia-oxidizing) bacteria (Javidpour, P., Deutsch, S., Mutalik, V.K., et al., Investigation of proposed ladderane biosynthetic genes from anammox bacteria by heterologous expression in *E.coli.*, *PLoS One*, 11(3), e0151087, 2014).

Section IV
Vitamins and Coenzymes

VITAMIN A

Compound	Formula	Properties	Solubility (g/100 ml)	Stability
Retinol Vitamin A alcohol Vitamin A$_1$ Axeropthol Anti-infective vitamin Antixerophthalmia factor Lard factor Biosterol Oleovitamin A 3,7-Dimethyl-9-(2,6,6-trimethyl-1-cyclohexen-1-yl)-2,4,6,8-nonatetraen-1-ol 2,6,6-Trimethyl-1-8'-hydroxy-3',7'-dimethylnona-1',3',5',7'-tetraenyl)cyclohex-1-ene	OH $C_{20}H_{30}O$ mol wt 286.44	Pale yellow prism crystals; mp 62 to 64°C (all *trans*); λ_{max} = 325 nm (ethanol); $E_{1cm}^{1\%}$ = 1,835; optically inactive; 1 mg = 3,333 IU or USP units	Sol in most organic solvents; sol in fats and oils; insol in water and glycerol — —	Unstable to oxygen, air, and UV light; esters relatively more stable — —
Dehydroretinol Retinol$_2$ Vitamin A$_2$ 3-Dehydroretinol	OH $C_{20}H_{28}O$ mol wt 284.42	Yellow crystals or oil; mp 17 to 19°C (all *trans*); λ_{max} = 288, 352 nm (ethanol); $E_{1cm}^{1\%}$ = 820, 1,450; optically inactive; 1 mg = 1,333 IU or USP units	Sol in most organic solvents; sol in fats and oils; insol in water and glycerol	Unstable to oxygen
Retinaldehyde[a,b] Retinal[a] Vitamin A aldehyde Retinene Axerophthal	CHO $C_{20}H_{28}O$ mol wt 284.42	Orange crystals; mp 61 to 64°C (all *trans*); λ_{max} = 373 nm (cyclohexane); $E_{1cm}^{1\%}$ = 1,548; all *trans* retinal has about 90% of the biopotency of all *trans* vitamin A acetate	Sol in most organic solvents; sol in fats and oils; practically insol in water	Unstable to oxygen
Retinoic acid Vitamin A acid Tretinoin 3,7-Dimethyl-9-(2,6,6-trimethyl-1-cyclohexen-1-yl)-2,4,6,8-nonatetraenoic acid	COOH $C_{20}H_{28}O_2$ mol wt 300.44	Crystals; mp 180 to 182°C (all *trans*); λ_{max} = 350 nm (ethanol); $E_{1cm}^{1\%}$ = 1,510; fully active for growth but not for visual function or reproduction	Sol in most organic solvents and oils	Unstable and subject to oxidation but more stable than alcohol or esters
Retinyl acetate Vitamin A acetate	OCOCH$_3$ $C_{22}H_{32}O_2$ mol wt 328.5	Yellow prismatic crystals; mp 57 to 60°C (all *trans*); λ_{max} = 326 nm (ethanol) $E_{1cm}^{1\%}$ = 1,550; 1 mg = 2,907 IU or USP units	Like retinol; insol in water	Unstable but more stable than alcohol; can be stabilized
Retinyl palmitate Vitamin A palmitate	OCO(CH$_2$)$_{14}$CH$_3$ $C_{36}H_{60}O_2$ mol wt 524.8	Yellow amorphous or crystalline; mp 27 to 29°C (all *trans*) λ_{max} = 325 to 328 nm (ethanol); $E_{1cm}^{1\%}$ = 940 to 975; 1 mg = 1,820 IU or USP units	Like retinol; insol in water	Unstable but more stable than alcohol or acetate; can be stabilized

PROPERTIES OF VITAMINS (Continued)

Compound	Formula	Properties	Solubility (g/100 ml)	Stability
PROVITAMIN A CAROTENOIDS				
β-Carotene	$C_{40}H_{56}$ mol wt 536.89	Deep purple prisms or red leaflet crystals; mp 180 to 182°C (all *trans*); λ_{max} = 273, 453, 481 (petroleum ether); $E_{1cm}^{1\%}$ = 383, 2,592, 2,268; optically inactive; 1 mg = 1,667 to 333 IU (depending on species fed)	Slightly sol in most organic solvents; very slightly sol in alcohol and oils; insol in glycerol and water	Unstable to oxygen; oxidizes to colorless products; can be used, however, as food color
β-Apo-8'-carotenal	$C_{30}H_{40}O$ mol wt 416.65	Dark violet crystals; mp 136 to 140°C (all *trans*); λ_{max} = 461 and 488 nm (cyclohexane); $E_{1cm}^{1\%}$ = 2,640 at 461; 1 mg = 1,220 IU (rat)	Sol in most organic solvents; slightly sol in alcohol; insol in glycerol and water	Unstable to oxygen; can be used, however, as food color
VITAMIN D				
Ergocalciferol Vitamin D₂ Activated ergosterol Calciferol Oleovitamin D₂ Viosterol 9,10-Seccoergosta-5,7,10(19),-22-tetraen-3-ol Irradiated ergosta-5,7,22-trien-3β-ol	$C_{28}H_{44}O$ mol wt 396.66	White prism crystals; mp 115 to 118°C; λ_{max} = 264 nm (hexane); $E_{1cm}^{1\%}$ = 459; $[\alpha]_D^{25}$ = +103 to 106 (alcohol); 1 mg = 40,000 IU or USP units	Sol in most organic solvents; slightly sol in oils; insol in water	Crystals relatively unstable to air, accelerated by unsaturated fat and trace mineral contact; can be stabilized
Cholecalciferol Vitamin D₃ Activated 7-dehydrocholesterol Oleovitamin D₃ 22,23-Dihydro-24-demethylcalciferol Activated 5,7-cholestadien-3β-ol	$C_{27}H_{44}O$ mol wt 384.65	White, fine needle crystals; mp 84 to 88°C; λ_{max} = 264 nm (hexane); = 450 490; $[\alpha]_D^{25}$ = +105 to 112° (alcohol); 1 mg = 40,000 IU or USP units; E_{mol} = 18,300 (ethanol)	Like D₂	Similar to D₂

PROPERTIES OF VITAMINS (Continued)

Compound	Formula	Properties	Solubility (g/100 ml)	Stability

VITAMIN D (Continued)

25-Hydroxycholecalciferol

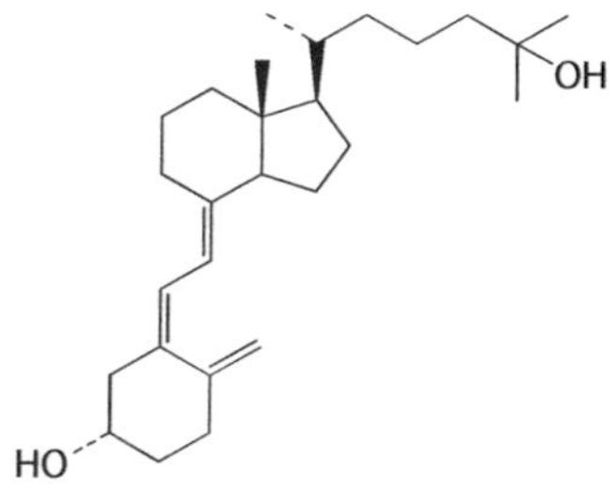

$C_{27}H_{44}O_2$
mol wt 416.65

Colorless, fine, needlelike crystals; mp 97 to 108°C; $[\alpha]_{D589} = +78$ (dioxane); $\lambda_{max} = 264$ nm $E_{1\,mol} = 17,400$ (ethanol)

Similar to D_3

Similar to D_3

1α,25-Dihydroxycholecalciferol

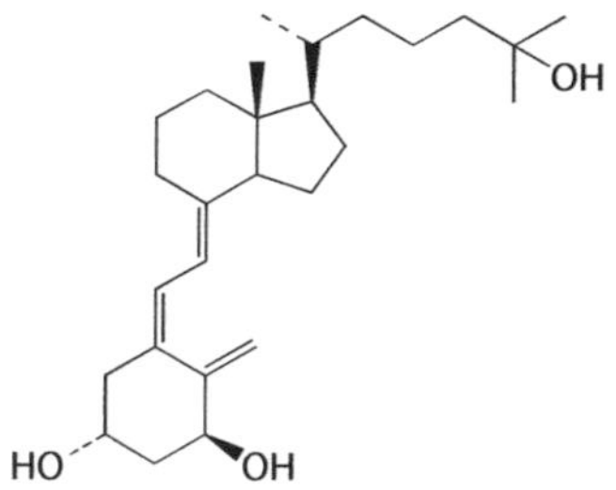

$C_{27}H_{44}O_2$
mol wt 400.65

Colorless, fine, needlelike crystals; mp 113 to 114°C; $[\alpha]_D^{25} = +48$ (ethanol); $\lambda_{max} = 264$ nm; $E_{1mol} = 14,270$ (ethanol)

Sol in esters, ethers, and alcohols

Similar to D_3

VITAMIN E

d-α-Tocopherol
2D,4'D,8'D-α-Tocopherol
2R,4'R,8'R-α-Tocopherol
Antisterility factor
5,7,8-Trimethyltocol
2,5,7,8-Tetramethyl-2-(4',8',12'-trimethyltridecyl)-6-chromanol
Abbreviation: α-T

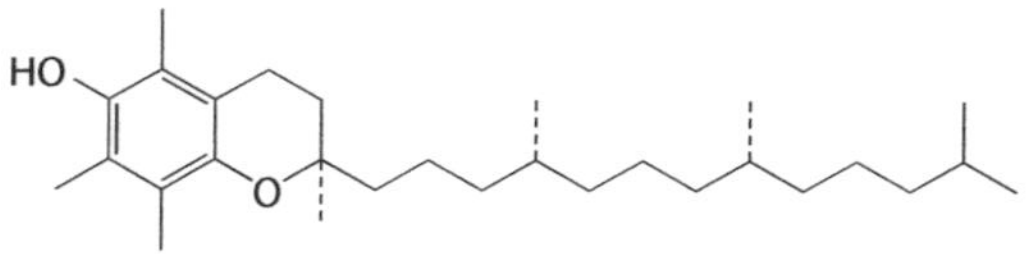

$C_{29}H_{50}O_2$
mol wt 430.69

Pale yellow viscous oil; mp 2.5 to 3.5°C; bp 200 to 220°C; (0.1 mm); $\lambda_{max} = 292$ (ethanol); $E_{1\,cm}^{1\%} = 74$ to 76; $[\alpha]_D^{25} = 0.32°$ (ethanol), K_3Fe $(CN)_6$ oxidation product: $[\alpha]_D^{25} = +26°$ (isooctane); 1 mg = 1.49 IU

Very sol in oils, fats, and many organic solvents; insol in water

Free tocopherol very unstable to air, iron salts, and bleaching agents; can be stabilized; esters quite stable

dl-α-Tocopherol
2DL,4'DL,8'DL-α-Tocopherol
2RS,4'RS,8'RS-α-Tocopherol
all-rac-α-Tocopherol

Pale yellow viscous oil; $\lambda_{max} = 292$ (ethanol); $E_{1\,cm}^{1\%} = 72$ to 76; 1 mg = 1.10 IU

Very sol in oils, fats, and many organic solvents; insol in water

Free tocopherol very unstable to air, iron salts, and bleaching agents; can be stabilized; esters quite stable

d-α-Tocopheryl acetate
d,α-Tocopheryl acetate
d,α-Tocopherol acetate
2,5,7,8-Tetramethyl-2-(4'8',12'-trimethyltridecyl) 6-chromanol acetate
2D,4'D,8'D-α-tocopheryl acetate
2R,4'R,8'R-α-tocopheryl acetate

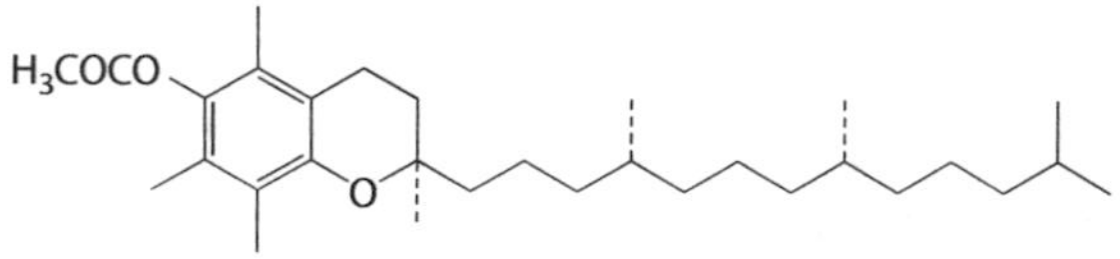

$C_{31}H_{52}O_3$
mol wt 472.73

Pale yellow crystals; mp 28°C; $\lambda_{max} = 284$ nm (ethanol); $E_{1\,cm}^{1\%} = 43.6$; $[\alpha]_D^{25} = +3.2°$ (ethanol); 1 mg = 1.36 IU

Like α-tocopherol

Relatively stable

PROPERTIES OF VITAMINS (Continued)

Compound	Formula	Properties	Solubility (g/100 ml)	Stability
VITAMIN E (Continued)				
dl-α-Tocopheryl acetate 2DL,4′DL,8′DL-α-tocopheryl acetate 2RS,4′RS,8′RS-α-tocopheryl acetate all-rac-α-Tocopheryl acetate		Yellow viscous oil; bp 184°C (0.01 mm), 194°C (0.025 mm), 224°C (0.3 mm); λ_{max} = 284 nm (ethanol); $E_{1cm}^{1\%}$ = 43.6; 1 mg = 1.00 IU	Less sol than acetate	Relatively stable
d-α-Tocopheryl acid succinate 2D,4′D,8′D-s,q		White crystals; mp 73 to 78°C; λ_{max}=286 nm (ethanol); $E_{1cm}^{1\%}$ =38.5; 1 mg=1.21 IU	Less sol than acetate	Relatively stable
dl-α-Tocopheryl acid succinate 2DL,4′DL,8′DL,-α-Tocopheryl acid succinate 2RS,4′RS,8′RS-α- Tocopheryl acid succinate all-rac-α-Tocopheryl acid succinate	HOOCH$_2$CH$_2$COCO C$_{33}$H$_{54}$O$_5$ mol wt 530.80	White crystals; λ_{max}=284 nm; $E_{1cm}^{1\%}$ =38.5; 1 mg=0.89 IU	Less sol than acetate	
VITAMIN K				
Phytylmenaquinone Vitamin K$_1$ Antihemorrhagic vitamin Phylloquinone Phytylmenadione Phytonadione Coagulation vitamin Prothrombin factor 2-Methyl-3-phytyl-1,4-naphthoquinone Abbreviation: K^a or PMQ^b	 C$_{31}$H$_{46}$O$_2$ mol wt 450.71	Yellow viscous oil; mp−20°C; λ_{max}=243, 248, 261, 269, 325 nm (isooctane); $E_{1cm}^{1\%}$=425, 428, 424,424, 350; $[\alpha]_D^{25}$ =−0.4° (benzene)	Sol in many organic solvents; insol in water	Fairly stable to heat decomposed by sunlight and alkali; can be stabilized
Prenylmenaquinone-6 Vitamin K$_2$ K$_2$ (30) Farnoquinone Menaquinone-6 2-Methyl-2-difarnesyl-1,-4-naphthoquinone Abbreviation: MQ-6	 n=6 C$_{41}$H$_{56}$O$_2$ mol wt 530.89	Yellow crystals; mp 53.5 to 54.5°C; λ_{max}=243, 248, 261, 270, 325 nm (petroleum ether); $E_{1cm}^{1\%}$ =304, 320, 290, 292, 53	Slightly less sol than K$_1$	Similar to K$_1$
Prenylmenaquinone-7 K$_2$ (35) Menaquinone-7 2-Methyl-3-all trans-farnesylgeranylgeranyl-1,4-naphthoquinone Abbreviation: MQ-7	 n=7 C$_{46}$H$_{64}$O$_2$ mol wt 649.02	Yellow crystals; mp 57°C; λ_{max}=243, 248, 261, 270, 325 nm (petroleum ether); $E_{1cm}^{1\%}$ =278, 295, 266, 267, 48	—	Similar to K$_1$

PROPERTIES OF VITAMINS (Continued)

Compound	Formula	Properties	Solubility (g/100 ml)	Stability
VITAMIN K (Continued)				
Menaquinone Vitamin K_3 Menadione Menaphthone 2-Methyl-1,4-naphthoquinone Abbreviation: MK	$C_{11}H_8O_2$ mol wt 172.19	Bright yellow crystals; mp 105 to 107°C; λ_{max}=244, 253, 264, 325, 328 nm (hexane); $E_{1cm}^{1\%}$ =1,150 (at 244 nm)	Sol in many organic solvents; insol in water; water sol forms are available	Fairly stable in air; decomposed by sun light
VITAMIN K WATER SOLUBLE COMPOUNDS				
Menadione sodium bisulfite 2-Methyl-1,4-naphthoquinone sodium bisulfite Abbreviation: MSB	$C_{11}H_8O_2HaHSO_3 \cdot 3H_2O$ mol wt 330.29	White hygroscopic crystals; λ_{max}=229, 267 nm (aqueous solution); $E_{1cm}^{1\%}$ = 868, 290	50, water; sol in alcohol; almost insol in benzene and water	—
Menadiol diphosphate (tetrasodium salt) 2-Methyl-1,4-naphthalenediol diphosphoric acid ester tetrasodium salt	$C_{11}H_8Na_4O_8P_2$ mol wt 422.09 (anhydrous) 530.18 (hexahydrate)	Hexahydrate, white to pinkish crystals; hygroscopic	Very sol in water; insol in ether and acetane	
Menadione dimethyl-pyrimidinol bisulphate Abbreviation: MPB	$C_{17}H_{18}O_6N_2S$ mol wt 378.41	White crystals; mp 215 to 217°C; λ_{max}=229, 267, 297 nm (water); $E_{1cm}^{1\%}$ =810, 285, 234	1, water	—
VITAMIN C				
Ascorbic acid L-Ascorbic acid Vitamin C Antiscorbutic factor Cevitamic acid Hexuronic acid Antiskorbutin L-Threo-3-ketohexonic acid-eno-lactone L-Threo-2,3,4,5,6-pentahydroxy-2-hexene-γ-lactone L-3-Ketothreo-hexuronic acid lactone	$C_6H_8O_6$ mol wt 176.13	Colorless or white crystals; mp 190 to 192°C; (decomposes); λ_{max}=245 nm (aqueous solution); $E_{1cm}^{1\%}$ =560; $[\alpha]_D^{25}$ =+20.5 to 21.5° (aqueous solution); 1 mg = 20 IU or USP units; characteristic acid taste	33, water; 3.5, alcohol; 1, glycerol; insol in oils and most organic solvents	Stable to air when dry; oxidizes in solution; catalyzed by metals, copper and iron, and by alkali

PROPERTIES OF VITAMINS (Continued)

Compound	Formula	Properties	Solubility (g/100 ml)	Stability
PABA				
p-Aminobenzoic acid PABA 4-Aminobenzoic acid Achromotrichia factor Antigray hair factor	COOH — NH$_2$ $C_7H_7NO_2$ mol wt 137.13	Monoclinic prisms; mp 187°C; λ_{max}=266 nm (water); $E_{1\,cm}^{1\%}$ -1,070; optically inactive	0.5, water; very sol in alcohol, ether and glacial acetic acid; slightly sol in benzene	Stable in dry form; unstable in presence of ferric salts and oxidizing agents
BIOTIN				
d-Biotin Vitamin H Coenzyme R Factor X Bios 11 or 11 B Egg white injury preventative or factor β-Hexahydro-2-oxo-1 H-thiene [3,4]-Imidazole-4-valeric acid 3,4-(2'-Ketoimidazolido)-2-(ω-carboxybutyl)-thiophane	(biotin structure) COOH $C_{10}H_{16}N_2O_3S$ mol wt 244.31	Colorless needle crystals; mp 230 to 233°C (decomposes); $[\alpha]_D^{25}$ =+91° (0.1 N NaOH)	0.020, water; 0.080 alcohol; more sol in hot water or dilute alkali	Stable, dry, in air and heat; stable in acid solution; less stable in alkali solution
CHOLINE				
Choline Bilineurine, amantine, gossypine, vidine (β-Hydroxyethyl) trimethylammonium hydroxide	$(H_3C)_3N(OH)CH_2CH_2OH$ $C_5H_{15}NO_2$ mol wt 121.18	Viscous hydroscopic liquid or colorless crystals; optically inactive	Very sol in water and alcohol; insol in ether	Stable in aqueous solution; decomposed by hot alkali
Chloride salt Choline chloride (β-Hydroxyethyl) trimethylammonium chloride (2-Hydroxyethyl) trimethylammonium chloride	$[(H_3C)_3NCH_2CH_2OH]Cl^-$ $C_5H_{14}ClNO$ mol wt 139.63	Deliquescent hydroscopic white crystals; optically inactive	Like choline	Similar to choline

PROPERTIES OF VITAMINS (Continued)

Compound	Formula	Properties	Solubility (g/100 ml)	Stability

VITAMIN B₁₂

Cyanobalamin
Vitamin B₁₂
Antipernicious anemia factor
Lactobacillus lactis-Dorner factor
Animal protein factor
Extrinsic factor
Zoopherin
5,6-Dimethylbenzimidazolyl
cyanocobamide

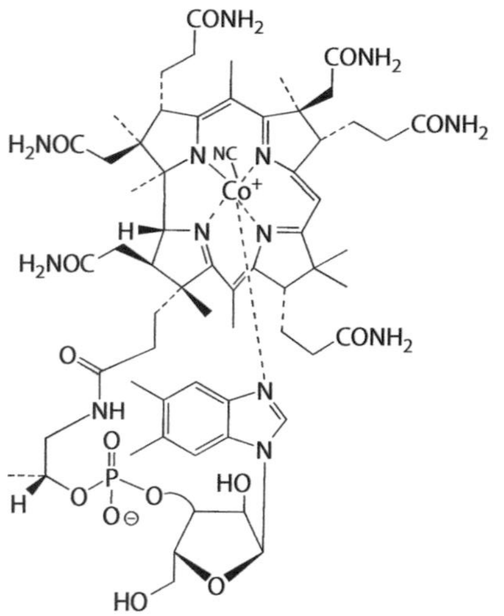

$C_{63}H_{88}N_{14}O_{14}PCo$
mol wt 1,355.42

Properties: Dark red crystals; mp > 212°C (decomposes); λ_{max}=278, 361, 550 nm (aqueous solution); $E_{1\,cm}^{1\%}$ =115,204, 63; $[\alpha]_{656}^{25}$ =−59±9° (aqueous solution)

Solubility: 1.25, water; sol in alcohol, insol in chloroform, acetone, and ether

Stability: Most stable in aqueous solution at pH 4.5 to 5; decomposes slowly in weak acid or alkali; decomposition accelerated by oxidizing and reducing agents, ferrous salts, etc.

FOLIC ACID[a] OR FOLACIN[a]

Pteroylglutamic acid
Folic acid+
Folacin
Vitamin M
Lactobacillus casei factor
Vitamin Bc; B₁₀ or B₁₁
Norite eluate factor
Factor U or R
Abbreviation: PGA+ or PteGlu[a]
N-[4-{(2-Amino-4-hydroxy-6-pteridyl) methyl]amino)-benzoyl] glutamic acid

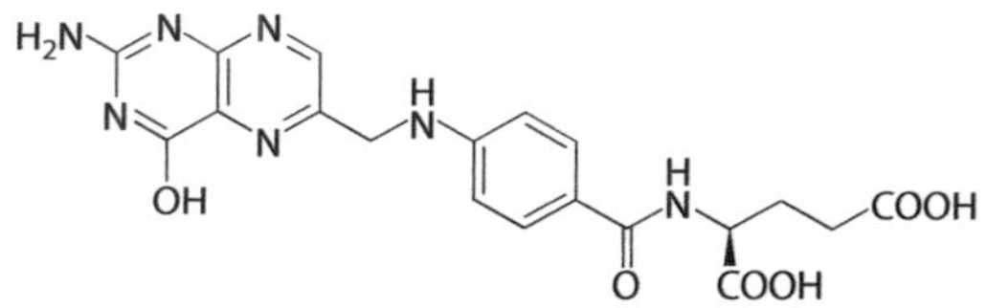

$C_{19}H_{19}N_7O_6$
mol wt 441.40

Properties: Yellowish-orange crystals; mp > 250°C (decomposes); λ_{max}=256, 283, 265 nm (alkaline solution); $E_{1\,cm}^{1\%}$ = 603, 600, 215

Solubility: Sol in acetic acid, alkaline solution; very sol in acetone; insol in chloroform, ether and benzene

Stability: Relatively stable dry; unstable in acid medium; decomposed by sunlight and heat

PROPERTIES OF VITAMINS (Continued)

FOLIC ACID[a] OR FOLACIN[a] (Continued)

Compound	Formula	Properties	Solubility (g/100 ml)	Stability
5-Formyltetrahydrofolic acid Folinic acid [N-[p-[(2-Amino-5-formyl-5,6,7,8-tetrahydro-4-hydroxy-6-pteridinyl) methyl] amino]benzoyl]glutamic acid Citrovorum factor Leucovorin Abbreviation: N⁵-formyl THFA or N⁵-F-PGAH₄ or 5-HCO-H₄PteGlu	$C_{20}H_{23}N_7O_7$ mol wt 473.44	Colorless crystals; mp 240 to 250°C (decomposes); λ_{max}=282 nm (alkaline solution); = +14.26°	Very slightly sol in water	More stable at neutral or mild alkaline pH

INOSITOL

Compound	Formula	Properties	Solubility (g/100 ml)	Stability
Myo-inositol Inositol meso-Inositol i-Inositol Bios 1 Inosite Mouse antialopecia factor Rat antispectacle eye factor Hexahydroxycyclohexane Cyclohexanehexol, cyclohexitol	$C_6H_{12}O_6$ mol wt 180.16	White crystals; mp 225 to 227°C (anhydrous); mp 218°C (dihydrate); optically inactive; sweet taste	15, water; insol in absolute alcohol and ether	Relatively stable

NIACIN

Compound	Formula	Properties	Solubility (g/100 ml)	Stability
Nicotinic acid Niacin Antiblacktongue factor Pellagra preventive (PP) factor Vitamin PP Pyridine-3-carboxylic acid Pyridine-β-carboxylic acid	$C_6H_5NO_2$ mol wt 123.11	Colorless or white needles; mp 235 to 237°C; λ_{max}=261 nm (0.1 N HCl), 263 nm (pH 11); $E_{1\ cm}^{1\%}$=435, 260; optically inactive	1.6, water; 0.73 alcohol; insol in ether	Stable to air, light, and PH
Nicotinamide Niacinamide Nicotinic acid amide Vitamin PP Vitamin B₃ 3-Pyridinecarboxylic acid amide	$C_6H_6N_2O$ mol wt 122.13	Colorless or white needles; mp129 to 131°C; λ_{max}=261 nm (0.1 N HCl), 262 nm (pH 11); $E_{1\ cm}^{1\%}$=432, 250; optically inactive	100, water; 66.6, alcohol; 10 glycerol; slightly sol in ether	Stable in air and heat, light, and pH (may hydrolyze to nicotinic acid)

PANTOTHENIC ACID

Compound	Formula	Properties	Solubility (g/100 ml)	Stability
Pantothenic acid, D-(+) Chick antidermatitis factor Liver filtrate factor Antidermatosis vitamin Vitamin B₅ D-(+)-N-(2,4-Dihydroxy-3,3-dimethylbutyryl)-β-alanine Pantoyl-β-alanine	$C_9H_{17}NO_5$ mol wt 219.23	Colorless, hydroscopic, viscous oil; $[\alpha]_D^{25}$ =+37.5° (aqueous) solution); only d-form is biologically active	Freely sol in water and acetic acid; moderately sol in alcohol; insol in benzene and chloroform	Stable at near neutral pH (5 to 7); unstable in acid or alkali; labile to prolonged heat

PROPERTIES OF VITAMINS (Continued)

PANTOTHENIC ACID (Continued)

Compound	Formula	Properties	Solubility (g/100 ml)	Stability
Calcium salt Calcium pantothenate	$C_{18}H_{32}CaN_2O_{10}$ mol wt 476.55	Colorless or white needles; mp 195 to 196°C (decomposes); $[\alpha]_D^{25} = +28.2°$ (aqueous solution); 1 g=70,000 to 75,000 chick units	35, water; very sol in glycerol and glacial acetic acid; slightly sol in ether, insol in benzene and chloroform	—
Pantothenyl alcohol Panthenol Provitamin for pantothenic acid N-(2,4-Dihydroxy-3,3-dimethylbutyryl-β-aminopropanol Pantoyl-β-aminopropanol	$C_9H_{19}NO_4$ mol wt 205.39	Viscous liquid (d); white crystals (dl); mp 64.5 to 67.5°C (dl); $[\alpha]_D^{20} = +29.7°$ (in water) (d)	Very sol in water and glycerol	More stable in solution than pantothenic acid or salts

VITAMIN B$_6$

Compound	Formula	Properties	Solubility (g/100 ml)	Stability
Pyridoxine · HCl Pyridoxol hydrochloride Adermine hydrochloride Antiacrodynia factor Yeast eluate factor 5-Hydroxy-6-methyl-3,4-pyridinedimethanol hydrochloride 2-Methyl-3-hydroxy-4,5-bis(hydroxymethyl)pyridine hydrochloride	$C_8H_{11}NO_3 \cdot HCl$ mol wt 205.64	Platelets or rods, white crystals; mp 206°C (decomposes); $\lambda_{max}=291$ nm (0.17 N HCl); $E^{1\%}_{cm}=422$; optically inactive	22, water; 1.1, ethanol; slightly sol in acetone; insol in ether	Stable, dry to air, light, and heat; sol in acid solution
Pyridoxal · HCl 3-Hydroxy-5-(hydroxymethyl)-2-methylisonicotinaldehyde	$C_8H_9NO_3$ mol wt 167.16 $C_8H_9NO_3 \cdot HCl$ mol wt 203.62	—	—	—
Pyridoxamine Dihydrochloride 2-Methyl-3-hydroxy-4-aminomethyl-5-hydroxymethylpyridine dihydrochloride	$C_8H_{12}N_2O_2$ mol wt 168.19 $C_8H_{12}N_2O_2 \cdot 2HCl$ mol wt 241.12	Colorless rhombic crystals; mp 165°C (decomposes); $\lambda_{max}=292.5$ nm; $E_{mol}=7,600$ Colorless crystals; mp 193 to 193.5°C Colorless platelets; mp 226 to 227°C (decomposes); $\lambda_{max}=287.5$ nm (at pH 1.94); $E_{mol}=9,100$	—	—

PROPERTIES OF VITAMINS (Continued)

VITAMIN B₂

Compound	Formula	Properties	Solubility (g/100 ml)	Stability
Riboflavin Riboflavine Vitamin B₂ Vitamin G Lactoflavin Ovoflavin Hepatoflavin Lyochrome 7,8-Dimethyl-10-(D-ribo-2,3,4,5-tetrahydroxypentyl) isoalloxazine 7,8-Dimethyl-10-ribitylisoalloxazine	$C_{17}H_{20}N_4O_6$ mol wt 376.37	Yellow to orange-yellow; polymorphic crystals; mp 280 to 290°C (decomposes); λ_{max}=223, 266, 271, 444 nm(0.1 NHCl); $E^{1\%}_{1cm}$ = 800, 870, 288, 310; $[\alpha]_D^{25}$ =−112 to 122° (dilute alcoholic NaOH); strong green fluorescence when irradiated by UV light	0.013, water; 0.040, alcohol; insol in ether, acetone, chloroform, and benzene; riboflavin phosphate, sodium salt quite water soluble	Unstable in alkali solution especially in light; stable in acid solution dark; reversibly reduced by sodium hydrosulfite and other reducing agents to dehydroriboflavin (leucoflavin); relatively stable in dry form
Vitamin B₂ phosphate sodium Riboflavin 5′-phosphate sodium Flavin mononucleotide Riboflavin 5′-phosphate ester monosodium salt	$C_{17}H_{20}N_4O_9PNa \cdot 2H_2O$ mol wt 514.37	Orange-yellow crystals; $[\alpha]_D^{25}$ =+38 to 42° (20% HCl)	4 to 11, water (depending on pH)	Similar to riboflavin

VITAMIN B₁

Compound	Formula	Properties	Solubility (g/100 ml)	Stability
Thiamine · HCl Thiamine chloride hydrochloride Vitamin B₁ hydrochloride Aneurine (hydrochloride) Oryzamin Antiberiberi vitamin 3-(4-Amino-2-methylpyrimidyl-5-methyl-4-methyl-5-(β-hydroxyethyl) thiazolium chloride hydrochloride	$C_{12}H_{17}ClN_4OS \cdot HCl$ mol wt 337.28	White monoclinic crystals; mp 246 to 250°C (decomposes); λ_{max}= 246 nm (0.1 N HCl); $E^{1\%}_{1cm}$ = 410; optically inactive; 1 mg=333 IU	100, water; 1, alcohol; insol in organic solvents	Stable when dry, stable in acid, unstable at alkaline pH, to prolonged heating, presence of bisulfite or thiaminase; very hygroscopic
Thiamine mononitrate Aneurine mononitrate Vitamin B₁ mononitrate	$C_{12}H_{17}N_5O_4S$ mol wt 327.36	White crystals; mp 196 to 200°C (decomposes); less hygroscopic than chloride hydrochloride; 1 mg=343 IU	2.7, water; insol in organic solvents	More stable than chloride salt in dry products; not hygroscopic

Compiled by J. C. Bauernfeind and E. De Ritter.

a Approved by IUPAC-IUB.
b Approved by IUNS.

BIOLOGICAL CHARACTERISTICS OF VITAMINS

Compound	Function	Deficiency Symptoms	Hyper-Use Symptoms	Coenzyme and Enzyme Involved	Remarks
Vitamin A	Primary role in vision as 11-cis retinal; synthesis of mucopolysaccharides; maintenance of mucous membranes and skin; bone development and growth; maintenance of cerebrospinal fluid pressure; production of corticosterone	Retarded growth, xerophthalmia, nyctalopia, hemeralopia, ataxia, tissue keratinization, cornification, desquamation, emaciation, lachrymation, impaired reproduction or hatchability (eggs), increased susceptibility to infection, optic nerve degeneration, odontoblast atrophy	Weight loss, bone abnormalities, inflammations, exfoliated epithelium, liver enlargement, pain, loss of hair, facial pigmentation	None identified	Other carotenes, α-, β-, γ-, and β-zeacarotene, cryptoxanthin, echinenone, certain apocarotenals, cis isomers of retinol, and dehydroretinol have fractional vitamin A activity, differing for various animal species; retinoic acid may be metabolically active form for certain functions
Vitamin D	Absorption and transport of calcium and phosphorus; synthesis of calcium protein carrier; interrelationship with parathyroid hormone; maintains alkaline phosphatase levels at bone site	Rickets, enlarged joints, softened bones, stilted gait, arched back, thin-shelled eggs, disturbed reproduction and hatchability, osteomalacia, faulty calcification of teeth, tetany, convulsions, raised plasma phosphatase, parturient paresis (dairy cattle)	Abnormal calcium deposition in bones and tissues, brittle or deformed bones, vomiting, abdominal discomfort, renal damage, weight loss	None identified	D_3 is the most effective form for the avian species; for man D_2 and D_3 are fully active; $1\alpha,25$ dihydroxycholecalciferol is the active metabolic form of D_3 and is considered by some, a hormone
Vitamin E	Biological antioxidant, interrelated with Se; metabolism of nucleic and sulfur amino acids; ubiquinone synthesis; detoxicant and oxidation-reduction action; stabilizes biological membranes against oxidative attack	Muscular dystrophy, encephalomalacia, hepatic necrosis, erythrocyte hemolysis, hock disorders, steatitis, reduced reproduction and hatchability, exudative diathesis, liver dystrophy, anemia, degeneration of testicular germinal epithelium, creatinuria	None identified; relatively nontoxic	None identified	Other tocols (β-, γ-, δ-tocopherol) and trienols (α-, β-, γ-, δ-tocotrienol) exist differing in ring substituents and in the side chain and having fractional vitamin activity; presence of unsaturated fat in the diet increases dietary vitamin E requirements
Vitamin K	Hepatic synthesis of prothrombin; synthesis of thromboplastin; needed in RNA formation and electron transport	Hemorrhage, impaired coagulation (low prothrombin levels), increased blood clotting time	Vomiting, albuminuria, porphyrinuria, polycythemia, splenomegaly, kidney and liver damage	None identified	K_1 is plant form of the vitamin; K_2 the microbiologically synthesized form; K_1 and K_2 are metabolically active forms; they also occur with longer or shorter side chain (isoprene) units; coumarin compounds and excess sulfa drugs are dietary stress agents for vitamin K
Ascorbic acid	Required for collagen formation; protects enzymes, hydrogen carriers, and adrenal steroids; functions in incorporation of iron into liver ferritin, folic acid into folinic acid; prevents scurvy, increases phagocytic activity	Scurvy, fragile capillaries, bleeding gums, loose teeth, anemia, follicular keratosis, sore muscles, weak bones, decreased egg shell strength, poor wound healing	None identified; relatively nontoxic	None identified	Dietary essential for man, monkey, guinea pig, fish, Indian pipistrel, Indian fruit bat, and flying fox, most other species synthesize it; glucoascorbic acid is an antagonist
p-Aminobenzoic acid	Function or need not well understood or accepted; a microbial factor involved in melanin formation and pigmentation; inhibits oxidation of adrenaline; influences activity of tyrosinase; involved in microbial synthesis of folic acid	Nutritional achromotrichia (animals), retarded growth (chicks), disturbed lactation (mice)	Rash, nausea, fever, acidosis, vomiting, pruritis	None identified	Sulfa drugs, carbarzones, and others are antagonists; PAB and sulfa drugs have a common point of attack on certain enzyme systems; PAB has some chemotherapeutic uses

BIOLOGICAL CHARACTERISTICS OF VITAMINS (Continued)

Compound	Function	Deficiency Symptoms	Hyper-Use Symptoms	Coenzyme and Enzyme Involved	Remarks
Choline	Source of methyl group, a methyl donor; for acetylcholine and phospholipid formation; essential for liver functioning	Fatty liver, hemorrhagic degeneration of kidneys, cirrhosis of liver, involution of thymus, enlarged spleen, retarded growth, impaired production (eggs) lactation and reproduction, perosis, muscle weakness or paralysis	Diarrhea and edema, erythrocyte formation inhibition	None identified	Choline occurs widespread in nature and is synthesized within the body to a limited extent; triethylcholine and others are choline antimetabolites
Cyanocobalamin	Cofactor for methyl malonyl CoA isomerase; involved in isomerizations; dehydrogenations, methylations; interrelated in choline, folic acid, ascorbic acid, pantothenic acid, biotin, and S-amino acid metabolism; synthesis of nucleoproteins	Retarded growth, perosis, poor feathering, megaloblastic anemia, anorexia, degenerative changes in spinal cord, posterior incoordination, impaired hatchability	Polycythemia	Cyanocobalamin coenzyme	Other B_{12} molecule variations exist wherein cyanide is replaced by chlorine, bromine, hydroxylcyanate, nitrite thiocyanate, etc; 5,6-dichlorobenzimidazole is an antimetabolite
Folic acid	Concerned with single carbon metabolism; for methyl, hydroxyl, and formyl transfers; for purine synthesis and normal histidine metabolism; interconversion of serine and glycine; a growth and hematopoietic factor; interrelationship with cyanocobalamin, ascorbic acid, iron, etc.	Retarded growth, sprue, diarrhea, macrocytic anemia, cervicular paralysis, reduction and abnormalities in white cells, dermatitis, impaired reproduction and lactation, perosis, poor feathering and lowered hatchability (poultry)	Obstruction of renal tubules	Tetrahydrofolic acid enzyme	The compound is a chelate, binding Co; certain molecular modifications of folic and tetrahydrofolic acid yield antagonists such as aminopterin, tetrahydroaminopterin, and others; the active forms of folic acid may have additional group such as formyl or methyl on the nitrogen in the molecule; thus, N^5-formyltetrahydrofolic acid is folinic acid and N^5-methyltetrahydrofolic acid is the form in blood
Inositol	Function or need not well understood or accepted; believed to be a lipotropic factor; a supply of methyl group functioning with cyanocobalamin; needed for acetyl choline production, functions in some microbial metabolic role	Fatty liver, hair loss, impaired reproduction and lactation, reduced growth (animal)	None identified; relatively nontoxic	None identified	Hexachlorocyclohexane (lindane) is an antimetabolite; while inositol can exist in eight cis-trans isomeric forms, only the optically inactive, i- or $meso$-inositol, is active; it occurs in animal tissues in free and phosphate ester form; inositol concentration is high in heart muscle, brain, and skeletal muscle
Nicotinic acid	Involved in enzyme mechanisms in carbohydrate, fat, and protein metabolism; functions as hydrogen transfer agent; interrelated with pyridoxine and tryptophan metabolism	Retarded growth, poor feathering or hair coat, black tongue (dog), pellagra, necrotic enteritis, impaired reproduction and hatchability, bowed legs (ducks and turkeys), enlarged hocks, perosis, stomatitis, diarrhea, headache, depression, paralysis, dermatitis	Vasodilation, flushing, tingling, pruritis, hyperhidrosis, nausea, abdominal cramps	NAD (DPN) NADP (TPN) dehydrogenases, coenzymes such as lactate dehydrogenase	In addition to vitamin need, niacin has pharmacological activity as a vasodilator; possessed to a markedly less degree by the amide; 3-acetyl-pyridine-6-aminonicotinamide and pyridine-3-sulfonic acid or amide are antagonists
Pantothenic acid	A component of coenzyme A; functions in acetylation (or 2 carbon) reactions in amino acid, carbohydrate, and fat metabolism; involved in biosynthesis of acetyl choline, steroids, triglycerides, phospholipids, and ascorbic acid; interrelationship with cyanocobalamin, folic acid, and biotin mechanisms	Retarded growth, dermatitis, anorexia, weakness, spastic abnormalities or gait, scours, achromotrichia (animals), adrenal hemorrhagic necrosis, burning sensation in hands and feet, impaired reproduction and hatchability	None identified; relatively nontoxic	Coenzyme A, acetylases	d-Form is the one in nature; the dl- and d-forms are also manufactured as calcium salts; ω-methyl pantothenic acid and other compounds are antagonists

BIOLOGICAL CHARACTERISTICS OF VITAMINS (Continued)

Compound	Function	Deficiency Symptoms	Hyper-Use Symptoms	Coenzyme and Enzyme Involved	Remarks
Pyridoxine	Functions in amino acid metabolism, decarboxylation, transamination, and desulfhydration; oxidation of amines and amino acid transport; phosphorylase activity of muscle; conversion of tryptophan to nicotinic acid and amino acids to biogenic amines	Retarded growth, hyperexcitability, myelin degeneration, convulsions, heart changes, spastic gait, nervousness, anorexia, insomnia, acrodynia, microcytic anemia, impaired production (eggs), reproduction and hatchability, tryptophan metabolites in urine	Convulsions and abnormal encephalograms	Pyridoxal phosphate, pyridoxamine phosphate, transaminases, amino acid decarboxylases	The term vitamin B_6 refers to the 3 compounds, pyridoxine (ol), pyridoxal, and pyridoxamine, the latter 2 being important metabolic forms; isonicotinic acid hydrazide, toxopyrimidine, deoxypyridoxine, and 1-amino-D-proline are antagonists; high tryptophan and/or methionine diets increase need for pyridoxine
Riboflavin	Functions as coenzyme; needed in cellular respiration, hydrogen and electron transfer; growth and tissue maintenance; role in visual mechanism	Retarded growth, ocular and orogenital disturbances, greasy scaling of nasolabial folds, cheeks, and chin, angular stomatitis, myelin degeneration, poor feathering or hair growth, impaired reproduction and hatchability, muscle weakness, curled toe paralysis, scours	Itching, paresthesia, anuria	Flavin mono- and dinucleotide, amino acid oxidase, cytochrome c reductase, succinic dehydrogenase, xanthine oxidase, others	Irradiation of alkaline solution produces lumiflavin of acid solution, lumichrome; riboflavin in solution is one of the most photosensitive compounds of the vitamin class; 5-deoxyriboflavin and several other compounds act as antimetabolites
Thiamine	Functions as a coenzyme; activation and transfer of active acetaldehyde, glycoaldehyde, and succinic semialdehyde; functions in carbohydrate metabolism	Polyneuritis, beriberi, convulsions, muscle paralysis, anorexia, bradycardia, heart dilation, myocardial lesions, retarded growth, edema, pyruvic acid accumulation in blood and tissues	Analgesic effect on peripheral nerves, vascular hypertension	Cocarboxylase, transketolase, carboxylases	Like most water-soluble vitamins, there is no significant tissue storage; amprolium, pyrithiamine, oxythiamine, and others are antimetabolites; the two important forms in production are the hydrochloride and the mononitrate

VITAMERS

A vitamer is one of several chemical compounds, most often of closely related structure, which can fulfill the function of a given vitamin. One of the more prominent examples is Vitamin B_6 where the vitamers include pyridoxal, pyridoxine, 4-pyridoxic acid, and pyridoxal 5'-phosphate. Other examples include Vitamin B2 (flavin Vitamers), folic acid, vitamin K, biotin, Vitamin A, Vitamin D and vitamin E. Vitamers are not pseudovitamins. There are also phytonutrients which have been considered to have vitamin-like status. For example, the bioflavonoids are plant derivatives with antioxidant and anti-inflammatory properties; derived from citrus fruit rinds, berries, grains, and wines. Some are considered to have anticancer activity. Bioflavonoids/flavonoids are considered to be polyphenols (Albert, A., Manach, C., Morand, C., Rémésy, C., and Jimémez, L., Dietary polyphenols and the prevention of diseases, *Crit.Rev.Food Sci.Nutr.* 45, 287–306, 2005).

Vitamin A: β-Carotene and retinaldehyde and other retinol derivatives can be considered vitamers of vitamin A. Retinoic acid, although derived from β-Carotene via retinaldehyde or by the oxidation of retinol, is suggested to have a totally different function in growth and development unrelated to vision.[1-6] In addition, there is considerable interest in the use of vitamin A in cosmeceuticals/skin therapy.[7-9]

Vitamin D: Vitamin D_2 and D_3 are derived from 7-dehydrocholesterol. Early work identified ergocalciferol (vitamin D_2) as an active component obtained from the irradiation of ergosterol. Later work established vitamin D_3 (cholecalciferol) as the major active component. Either must be converted to the 1α-hydroxylderivative (e.g. 1α,25-dihydroxyvitamin D_3 (1α,25-dihydroxyvitamin D).[10-13]

Vitamin E: There are a number of vitamin E (tocopherols/tocotrienols) vitamers[14-22] as well as the water-soluble derivative, Trolox[23-31] which is used as a standard for antioxidant measurements.

Vitamin K: Several vitamers[32-41] which have different activities in the support of γ-carboxylation reactions.

Thiamin (Vitamin B_1): Thiamine and several phosphate esters comprise the vitamers of thiamine[42-44] as well as some analogues.[45-47]

Niacin (Vitamin B_3): Niacin is also referred to as nicotinic acid. Nicotinic acid and nicotinamide have equivalent activity and are incorporated into a coenzyme, nicotinamide adenine dinucleotide (NAD) and nicotinamide adenine dinucleotide phosphate (NADP). Nicotinic acid and nicotinamide are the major niacin vitamers.[48-54]

Pyridoxine (Vitamin B_6): Multiple vitamers including pyridoxine, pyridoxal, pyridoxamine and the corresponding phosphates and precursors.[55-61]

Biotin (Vitamin B_7; also Vitamin H): Biotin and precursors and precursors including 7-oxo-8-aminopelargonic acid[62-68]

Folic Acid (Vitamin B_9): Several vitamers[69-74] which are derivatives of the parent pteroyl glutamate.

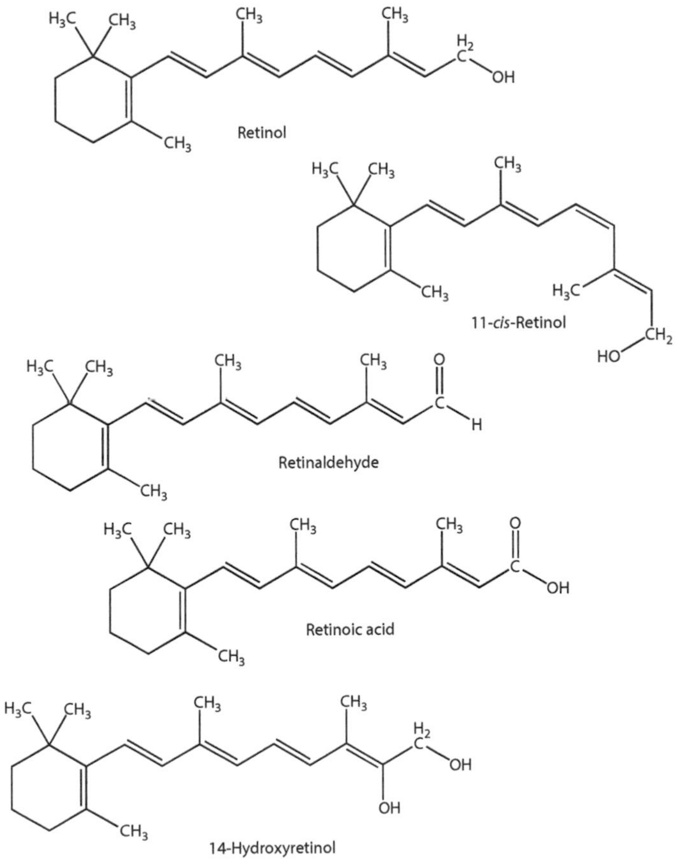

FIGURE 1 Structures of Vitamin A vitamers (retinol and retinol derivatives). See Sommer, A., Vitamin a Deficiency and Clinical Diseases: An Historical Overview, *J.Nutr.* 138, 1835–1839, 2008; Dragsted, L.O., Biomarkers of Exposure to Vitamins A, C, and E their Relation to Lipid and Protein Oxidation Markers, *Eur.J.Nutr.* 47 (suppl 2), 3–18, 2008.

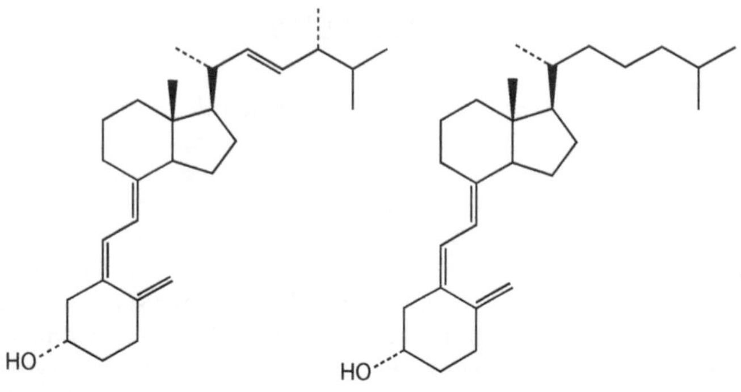

Vitamin D₂
Ergocalciferol

Vitamin D₃
Cholecalciferol

FIGURE 2 Structures of Vitamin D vitamers (Calciferol derivatives). See Holden, J.M., Lemar, L.E., and Exler, J., Vitamin D in Foods: Development of the US Department of Agriculture Database, *Am.J.Clin.Nutr.* 87, 1092S–1096S, 2008.

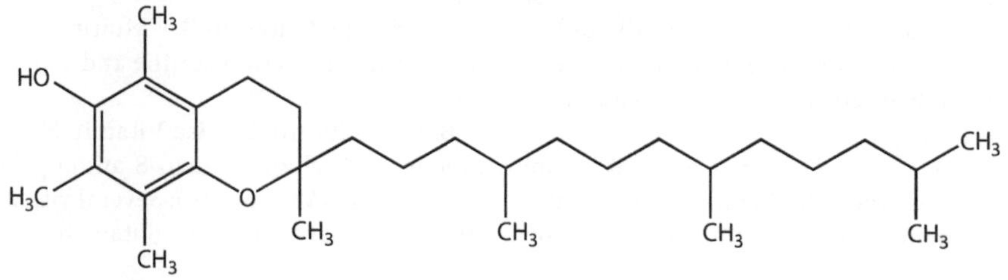

alpha-tocopherol

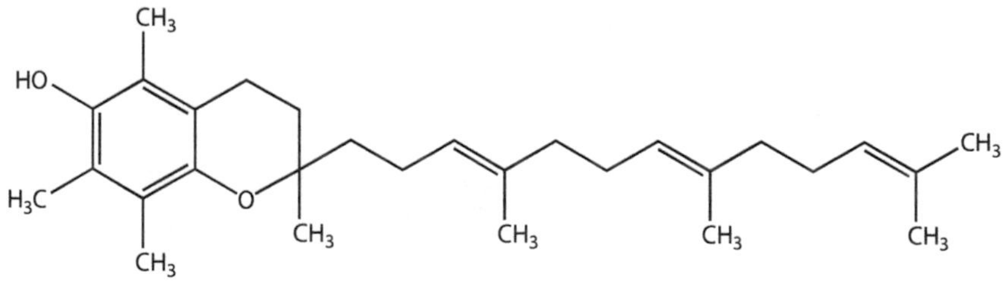

alpha-tocotrienol

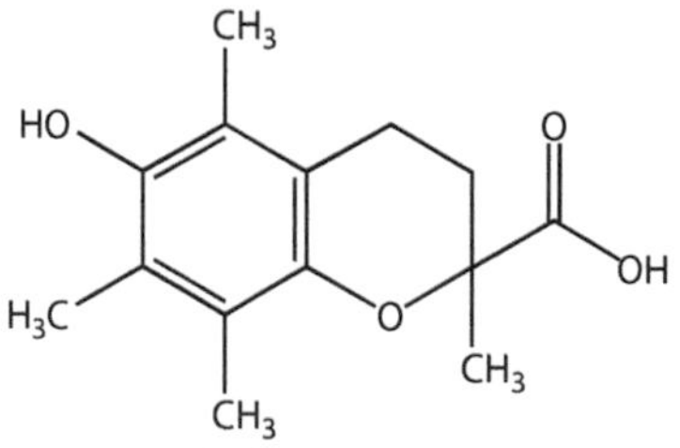

Trolox

FIGURE 3 Structures of Vitamin E vitamers (Tocopherol derivatives). See Yoshida, Y., Saito, Y., Jones, L.S., and Shigeri, Y., Chemical Reactivities and Physical Effects in Comparison between Tocopherols and Tocotrienols: Physiological Significance and Prospects as Antioxidants, *J.Biosci.Bioeng.* 104, 439–445, 2007; Clarke, M.W., Burnett, J.R., and Croft, K.D., Vitamin E in Human Health and Disease, *Crit.Rev.Clin.Lab.Sci.* 45, 417–450, 2008.

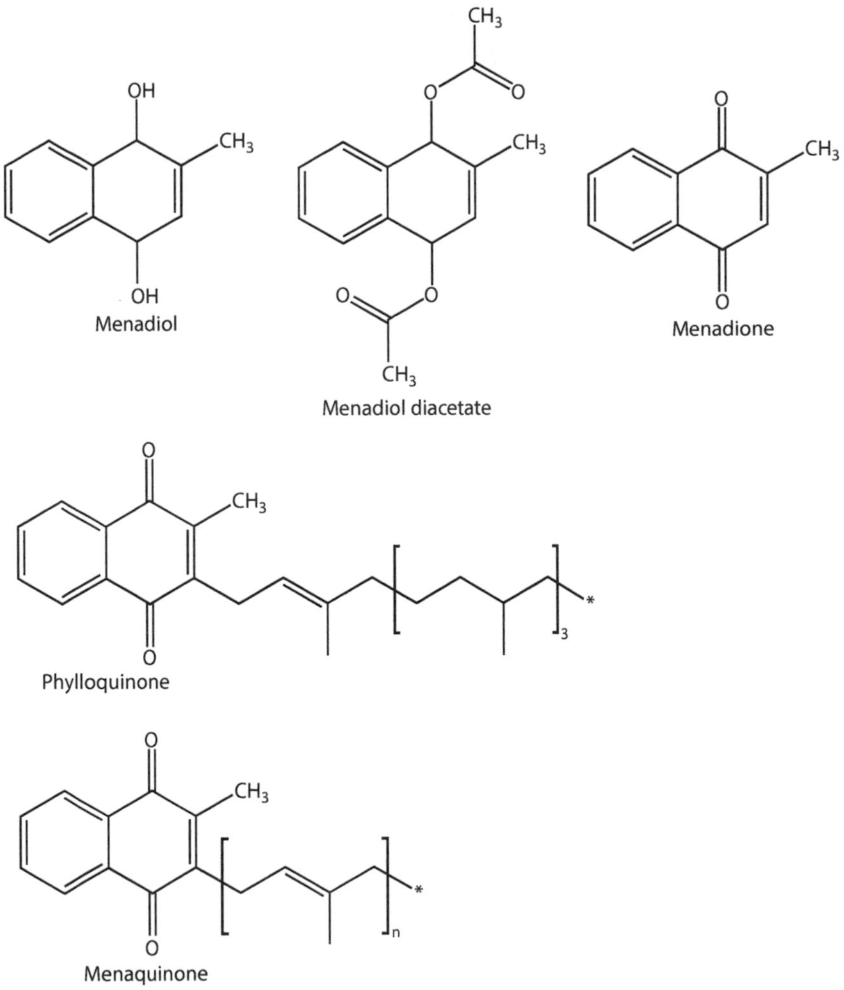

FIGURE 4 The structures of Vitamin K vitamers (Naphthoquinone derivatives). The K is derived from the German "koagulationvitamin." See Doisey, E.A., Brinkley, S.B., Thayer, S.A., and McKee, R.W., Vitamin K, Science 9, 58–62, 1940; Wolff, I.L. and Babior, B.M., Vitamin K and Warfarin. Metabolism, Function and Interaction, *Am.J.Med.* 53, 261–267, 1972; Sadowski, J.A. and Suttie, J.W., Mechanism of Action of Coumarins. Significance of Vitamin K epoxide, *Biochemistry* 13, 3696–3699, 1974; Yamada, Y., Inouye, G., Tahara, Y., and Kondo, K., The Structure of the Menaquinones with a Tetrahydrogenated Isoprenoid Side-Chain, *Biochim.Biophys. Acta* 488, 280–284, 1977; Bell, R.G., Vitamin K Activity and Metabolism of Vitamin K-1 Epoxide-1,4-diol, J.Nutr. 112, 287–292, 1982.

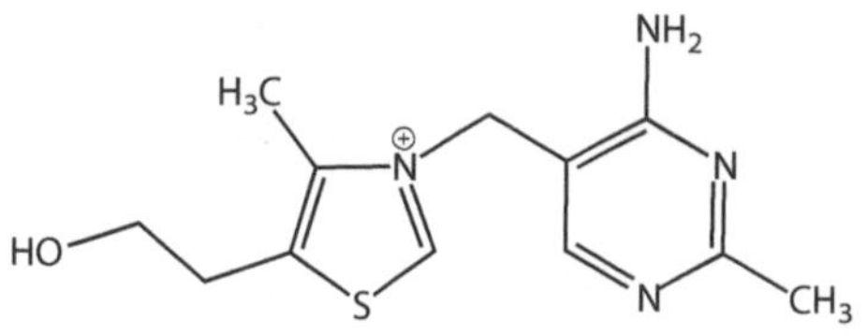

Thiamine

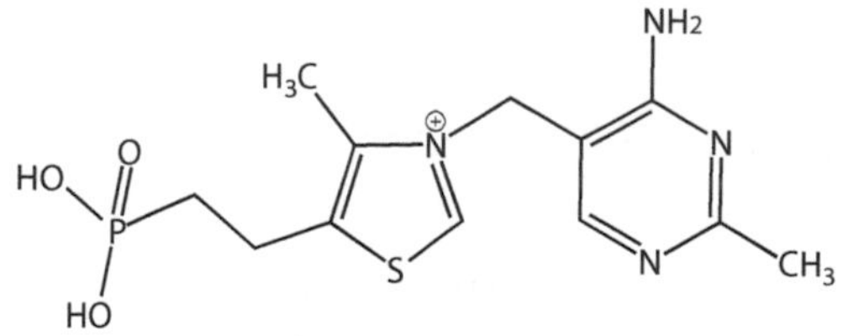

Thiamine monophosphate

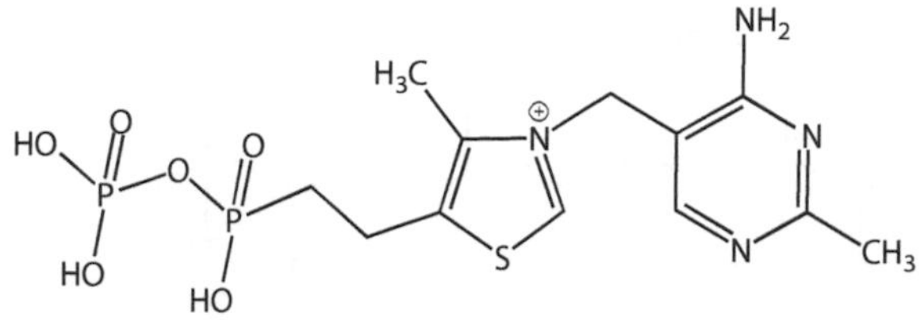

Thiamine diphosphate

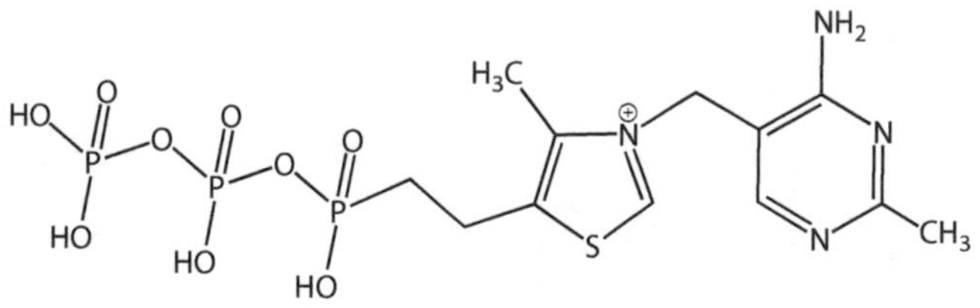

Thiamine triphosphate

FIGURE 5 The structures of Vitamin B1 vitamers (Thiamine and derivatives). See Maladrinos, G., Louloudi, M, and Hadjiliadis, N., Thiamine Models and Perspectives on the Mechanism of Action of Thiamine-Dependent Enzymes, *Chem.Soc.Rev.* 35, 684–692, 2006; Kowalska, E. and Kozik, A., The Genes and Enzymes Involved in the Biosynthesis of Thiamin and Thiamin Diphosphate in Yeasts, Cell *Mot.Biol.Lett.* 13, 271–282, 2008.

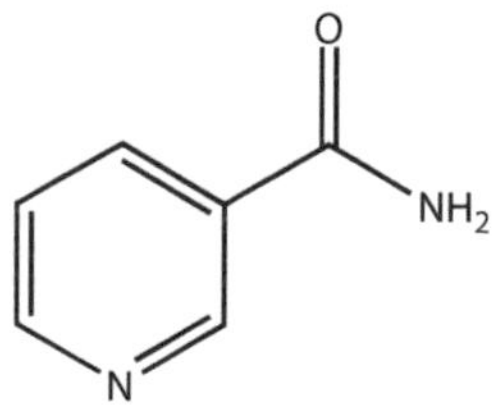

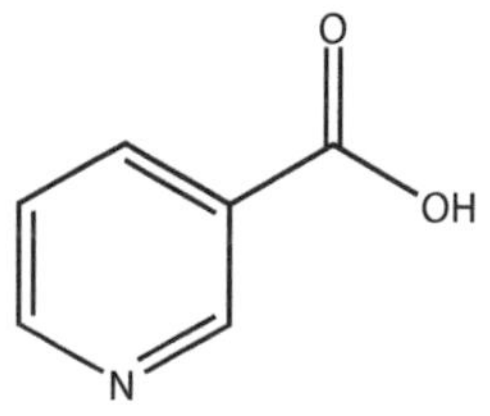

Nicotinamide   Nicotinic acid

FIGURE 6 The structures of Vitamin B3 (Niacin) vitamers (Nicotinic acid and derivatives). See Skinner, P.J., Cherrier, M.C., Webb, P.J., *et al.*, 3-Nitro-4-Amino Benzoic Acids and 6-Amino Nicotinic Acids are Highly Selective Agonists for GPR109b, *Bioorg.Med.Chem.Lett.* 17, 6619–6622, 2007; Boovanahalli, S.K., Jin, X., Jin, Y. *et al.*, Synthesis of (Aryloxyacetylamino)-isonicotinic Acid Analogues as Potent Hypoxia-inducible factor (HIF)-1α Inhibitors, *Bioorg.Med.Chem.Lett.* 17, 6305–6310, 2007; Deng, Q., Frie, J.L., Marley, D.M. *et al.*, Molecular Modeling Aided Design of Nicotinic acid Receptor GPR109A *Agonists, Bioorg.Med.Chem.Lett.* 18, 4963–4967, 2008.

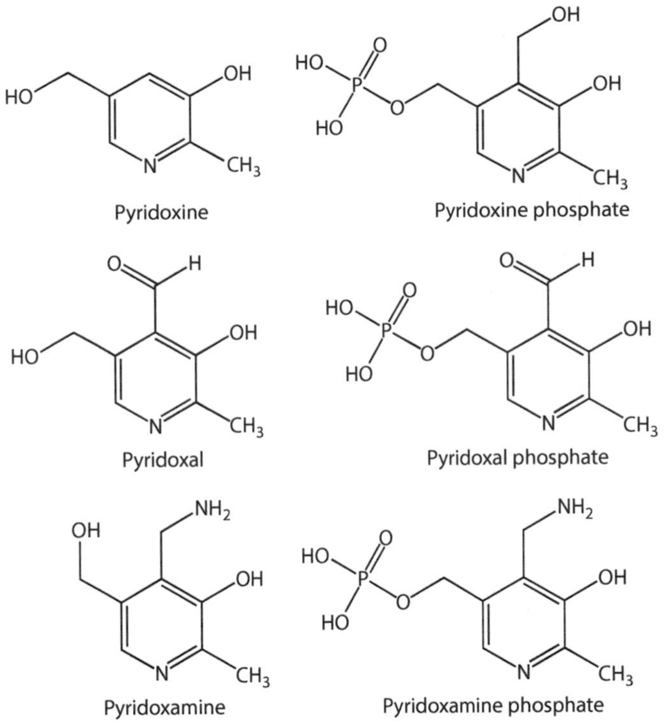

FIGURE 7 The structure of Pyridoxine (Vitamin B6) vitamers. See Snell, E.E., Analogs of Pyridoxal or Pyridoxal Phosphate: Relation of Structure to Binding with Apoenzymes and to Catalytic Activity, *Vitam.Horm.* 28, 265–290, 1970; Drewke, C. and Leistner, E., Biosynthesis of Vitamin B6 and Structurally Related Derivatives, *Vitam.Horm.* 61, 121–155, 2001; Garrido-Franco, M., Pyridoxine 5-Phosphate Synthase: *De novo* Synthesis of Vitamin B6 and *Beyond, Biochim.*Biophys.Acta 1647, 92–97, 2003.

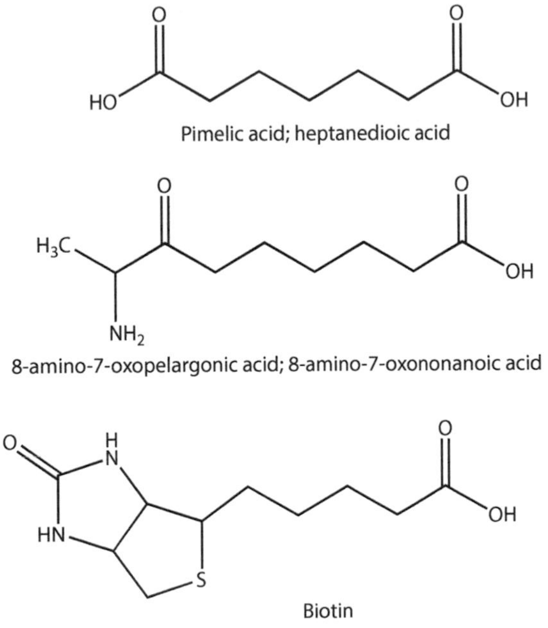

FIGURE 8 The structure of Biotin (Vitamin H) vitamers.

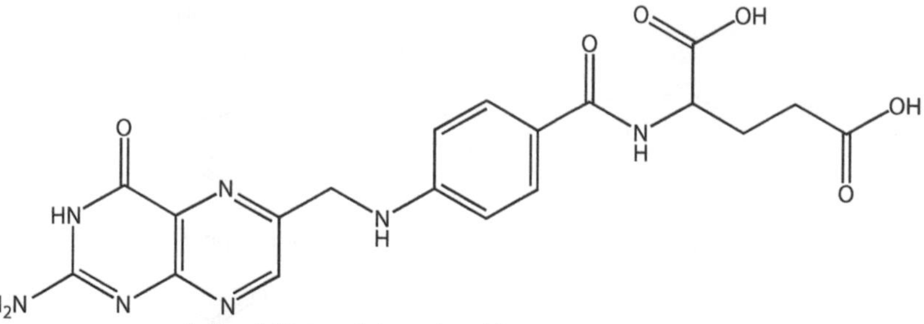

Folic acid (pteroylglutamic acid)

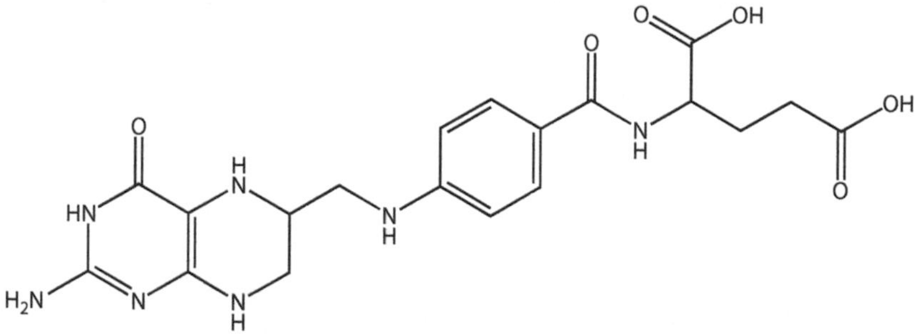

Tetrahydrofolic acid

FIGURE 9 The structure of Folic acid vitamers.

References

1. Pitt, G.A., Chemical structure and the changing concept of vitamin A activity, *Proc.Nutr.Soc.* 42, 43–51, 1983.
2. Wolf, G., The regulation of retinoic acid formation, *Nutr.Rev.* 54, 182–184, 1996.
3. Clagett-Dame, M. and DeLuca, H.F., The role of vitamin A in mammalian reproduction and embryonic development, *Annu.Rev. Nutr.* 22, 347–381, 2002.
4. Matt, N, Dupe, V., Garnier, J.M., Retinoic acid-dependent eye morphogenesis is orchestrated by neural crest cells, *Development* 132, 4789–4800, 2005.
5. Moise, A.R., Isken, A., Dominguez, M., et al., Specificity of zebrafish retinol saturase: formation of all-trans-13,14-dihydroretinol and all-trans-7,8-dihydroretinol, *Biochemistry* 46, 1811–1820, 2007.
6. Reichrath, J., Lebmann, B., Carlberg, C., et al., Vitamins as hormones, *Horm.Metab.Res.* 39, 71–84, 2007.
7. Mayer, H., Bollag, W., Hanni, R., and Ruegg, R., Retinoids, a new class of compounds with prophylactic and therapeutic activities in oncology and dermatology, *Experientia* 34, 1105–1119, 1978.
8. Zoubloulis, C.C., Retinoids—which dermatological indications will benefit in the near future?, *Skin Pharmacol.Appl.Skin Physiol.* 14, 303–315, 2001.
9. Borg, O., Antille, C., Kaya, G., and Saurat, J.H., Retinoids in cosmeceuticals, *Dermatol.Ther.* 19, 289–296, 2006.
10. Holick, M.F., The use and interpretation of assays for vitamin D and its metabolites, *J.Nutr.* 120, 1464–1469, 1990.
11. Coburn, J.W., Tan, A.U., Jr., Levine, B.S., et al., 1α-Hydroxy-vitamin D: a new look at an "old compound", *Nephrol.Dial.Transplant.* 11(supp 3), 153–157, 1996.
12. Wikvall, K., Cytochrome P450 enzymes in the bioactivation of vitamin D to its hormonal form, *Int.J.Mol.Med.* 7, 201–209, 2001.
13. Wu-Wong, J.R., Tian, J., and Goltzman, D., Vitamin D analogs as therapeutic agents: a clinical study update, *Curr.Opin.Investig. Drugs* 5, 32–326, 2004.
14. Panfili, G., Fratianni, A., and Irano, M., Normal phase high-performance liquid chromatography method for the determination of tocopherols and tocotrienols in cereals, *J.Agric.Food Chem.* 51, 3940–3944, 2003.

15. McCormick, C.C. and Parker, R.S., The cytotoxicity of vitamin E is both vitamer- and cell-specific and involves a selectable trait, *J Nutr.* 124, 3335–3342, 2004.
16. Sontag, T.J. and Parker, R.S., Vitamin E exhibits concentration- and vitamer-dependent impairment of microsomal enzyme activities, *Ann.N.Y.Acad.Sci.* 1031, 376–377, 2004.
17. Amaral, J.S., Casal, S., Torres, D., et al., Simultaneous determinations of tocopherols and tocotrienols in hazelnuts by a normal phase liquid chromatographic method, *Anal.Sci.* 21, 1545–1548, 2005.
18. Cunha, S.C., Amaral, J.S. Ferandes, J.O., and Oliviera, B.P., Quantification of tocopherols and tocotrienols in Portuguese olive oils using HPLC with three different detection systems, *J.Agric. Food Chem.* 54, 3351–3356, 2006.
19. Sookwong, P., Nakagawa, K., Murata, K., et al., Quantitation of tocotrienols and tocopherol in various rice brans, *J.Agric.Food Chem.* 55, 461–466, 2007.
20. Bustamante-Rangel, M. Delgado-Zamrreno, M.M., Sanchez-Perez A., and Carabias-Martinez, R., Determination of tocopherols and tocotrienols in cereals by pressurized liquid extraction-liquid chromatography-mass spectrometry, *Anal.Chim.Acta* 587, 216–221, 2007.
21. Hunter, S.C. and Cahoon, E.B., Enhancing vitamin e in oilseeds: unraveling tocopherol and tocotrienol biosynthesis, *Lipids* 41, 97–108, 2007.
22. Tsuzuki, W., Yunoki, R., and Yoshimura, H., Intestinal epithelial cell absorb γ-tocopherol faster than α-tocopherol, *Lipids* 42, 163–170, 2007.
23. Kralli, A. and Moss, S.H., The sensitivity of an actinic reticuloid cell strain to near-ultraviolet radiation and its modification by trolox-C, a vitamin E analogue, *Br.J.Dermatol.* 116, 761–772, 1987.
24. Nakamura, M., One-electron oxidation of Trolox C and vitamin E by peroxidase, *J.Biochem.* 110, 595–597, 1991.
25. Miura, T., Muraoka, S., and Ogiso, T., Inhibition of hydroxyl radical-induced protein damages by trolox, *Biochem.Mol.Biol.Int.* 31, 125–133, 1993.
26. Forrest, V.J., Kang, Y.H., McClain, D.E., et al., Oxidative stress-induced apoptosis prevented by Trolox, *Free Radic.Biol.Med.* 16, 675–684, 1994.

27. Albertini, R. and Abuja, P.M., Prooxidant and antioxidant properties of Trolox C, analogue of vitamin E, in oxidation of low-density lipoprotein, *Free Radic.Res.* 30, 181–188, 1999.

28. Wang, C.C., Chu, C.Y., Chu, K.O., *et al.*, Trolox-equivalent antioxidant capacity assay versus oxygen radical absorbance capacity assay in plasma, *Clin.Chem.* 50, 952–954, 2004.

29. Raspor, P., Plesnicar, S., Gazdag, Z., *et al.*, Prevention of intracellular oxidation in yeast: the role of vitamin E analogue, Trolox (6-hydroxy-2,5,7.8-tetramethylkorman-2-carboxyl acid), *Cell Biol. Int.* 29, 57–63, 2005.

30. Abudu, N., Miller, J.J., and Levinson, S.S., Fibrinogen is a co-antioxidant that supplements the vitamin E analog trolox in a model system, *Free Radic Res.* 40, 321–331, 2005.

31. Castro, I.A., Rogero, M.M., Junqueira, R.M., and Carrapeiro, M.M., Free radical scavenger and antioxidant capacity correlation of α-tocopherol and Trolox measured by three *in vitro* methodologies, *Int.J.Food Sci.Nutr.* 57, 75–82, 2006.

32. Lefevere, M.F., De Lennheer, A.P., and Claeys, A.E., High-performance liquid chromatography assay of vitamin K in human serum, *J.Chromatog.* 186, 749–762, 1979.

33. Lowenthan, J. and Vergel Rivera, G.M., Comparison of the activity of the *cis* and *trans* isomer of vitamin K1 in vitamin K-deficient and coumarin anticoagulant-pretreated rats, *J.Pharmacol.Exp. Ther.* 209, 330–333, 1979.

34. Preusch, P.C. and Suttie, J.W., Stereospecificity of vitamin K-epoxide reductase, *J.Biol.Chem.* 258, 714–716, 1983.

35. Hwang, S.M., Liquid chromatographic determination of vitamin K1 trans- and cis-isomers in infant formula, *J.Assoc.Off.Anal. Chem.* 68, 684–689, 1985.

36. Will, B.H., Usui, Y., and Suttie, J.W., Comparative metabolism and requirement of vitamin K in chicks and rats, *J.Nutr.* 122, 2354–2360, 1992.

37. Vermeer, C., Gijsbers, B.L., Craciun, A.M. *et al.*, Effects of vitamin K on bone mass and bone metabolism, *J.Nutr.* 126(4 suppl), 1187S–1191S, 1996.

38. Gijsbers, B.L., Jie, K.S., and Vermeer, C., Effect of food composition on vitamin K absorption in human volunteers, *Br.J.Nutr.* 76, 223–229, 1996.

39. Woolard, D.C., Indyk, H.E., Fong, B.Y., and Cook, K.K., Determination of vitamin K1 isomers in food by liquid chromatography with C$_{30}$ bonded phase column, *J. AOAC Int.* 85, 682–691, 2002.

40. Cook, K.K., Grundel, E., Jenkins, M.Y. and Mitchell, G.V., Measurement of *cis* and *trans* isomers of vitamin K1 in rat tissues by liquid chromatography with a C$_{30}$ column, *J.AOAC Int.* 85, 832–840, 2002.

41. Carrie, I., Pertoukalian, J., Vicaretti, R., *et al.*, Menequinone-4 concentration is correlated with sphingolipid concentration in rat brain, *J.Nutr.* 134, 167–172, 2004.

42. Botticher, B. and Botticher, D., A new HPLC-method for the simultaneous determination of B$_1$-, B$_2$- and B$_6$-vitamers in serum and whole blood, *Int.J.Vitam.Nutr.Res.* 57, 273–278, 1987.

43. Batifoulier, F., Verny, M.A., Bessom, C. *et al.*, Determination of thiamine and its phosphate esters in rat tissues analyzed as thiochromes on a RP-amide C$_{16}$ column, *J.Chromatog.B.Analyt. Technol.Biomed.Life Sci.* 816, 67–72, 2005.

44. Konings, E.J., Water-soluble vitamins, *J.AOAC Int.* 89, 285–288, 2006.

45. Lowe, P.N., Leeper. F.J., and Perham, R.N., Stereoisomers of tetrahydrothiamine pyrophosphate, potent inhibitors of the pyruvate dehydrogenase multienzyme complex from *Escherichia coli*, *Biochemistry* 22, 150–157, 1983.

46. Klein, E., Nghiem, H.O., Valleix, A., *et al.*, Synthesis of stable analogues of thiamine di- and triphosphate as tools for probing a new phosphorylation pathway, *Chemistry* 8, 4649–4655, 2002.

47. Erixon, K.M., Dabalos, C.L., and Leeper, F.J., Inhibition of pyruvate decarboxylase from *E.mobilis* by novel analogues of thiamine pyrophosphate: investigating pyrophosphate mimics, *Chem. Commun.* (9), 960–962, 2007.

48. Sauberlich, H.E., Newer laboratory methods for assessing nutriculture of selected B-complex vitamins, *Annu.Rev.Nutr.* 4, 377–407, 1984.

49. Stein, J., Hahn, A., and Rehner, G., High-performance liquid chromatographic determination of nicotinic acid and nicotinamide in biological samples applying post-column derivatization resulting in bathochrome absorption shifts, *J.Chromatog.B.Biomed.Appl.* 665, 71–78, 1995.

50. Gillmor, H.A., Bolton, C.H., Hopton, M., *et al.*, Measurement of nicotinamide and *N*-methyl-2-pyridone-5-carboxamide in plasma by high performance liquid chromatography, *Biomed.Chromatog.* 13, 360–362, 1999.

51. Khan, A.R., Khan, K.M, Perveen, S., and Butt, N., Determination of nicotinamide and 4-aminobenzoic acid in pharmaceutical preparations by LC, *J.Pharm.Biomed.Anal.* 29, 723–727, 2002.

52. Chatzimichalakis, P.F., Samanidou, V.F., Verpoorte, R., and Papadoyannis, I.N., Development of a validated HPLC method for the determination of B-complex vitamins in pharmaceuticals and biological fluids after solid phase extraction, *J.Sep.Sci.* 27, 1181–1188, 2004.

53. Hsieh, Y. and Chen, J., Simultaneous determination of nicotinic acid and its metabolites using hydrophilic interaction chromatography with tandem mass spectrometry, *Rapid Commun.Mass Spectrom.* 19, 3031–3036, 2005.

54. Marszall, M.P., Markuszewski, M.J., and Kaliszan, R., Separation of nicotinic acid and its structural isomers using 1-ethyl-3-methylimidazolium ionic liquid as a buffer additive by capillary electrophoresis, *J.Pharm.Biomed.Anal.* 41, 329–332, 2006.

55. Vanderslice, J.T., Maire, C.E., and Beecher, G.R., B$_6$ Vitamer analysis in human plasma by high performance liquid chromatography: a preliminary report, *Am.J.Clin.Nutr.* 34, 947–950, 1981.

56. Hachey, D.L. Coburn, S.P., Brown, L.T., *et al.*, Quantitation of vitamin B6 in biological samples by isotope dilution mass spectrometry, *Anal.Biochem.* 151, 159–168, 1985.

57. Driskell, J.A. and Chrisley, B.M., Plasma B-6 vitamer and plasma and urinary 4-pyridoxic acid concentrations in young women as determined using high performance liquid chromatography, *Biomed.Chromatogr.* 5, 198–201, 1991.

58. Sharma, S.K. and Dakshinamurti, K., Determination of vitamin B6 vitamers and pyridoxic acid in biological samples, *J.Chromatogr.* 578, 45–51, 1992.

59. Schaeffer, M.C., Gretz, D., Mahuren, J.D., and Coburn, S.P., Tissue B-6 vitamer concentrations in rats fed excess vitamin B-6, *J.Nutr.* 125, 2370–2378, 1995.

60. Fu, T.F., di Salvo, M., and Schirch, V., Distribution of B6 vitamers in *Escherichia coli* as determined by enzymatic assay, *Anal. Biochem.* 298, 314–321, 2001.

61. Bisp, M.R., Bor, M.V., Heinsvig, E.M., *et al.*, Determination of vitamin B6 vitamers and pyridoxic acid in plasma: development and evaluation of a high-performance liquid chromatography assay, *Anal.Biochem.* 305, 82–89, 2002.

62. Eisenberg, M.A., The biosynthesis of biotin in growing yeast cells: The formation of biotin from an early intermediate, *Biochem.J.* 101, 598–600, 1966.

63. Birnbaum, J., Pai, C.H., and Lichstein, H.C., Biosynthesis of biotin in microorganisms. V. Control of vitamer production, *J.Bacteriol.* 94, 1846–1853, 1967.

64. Eisenberg, M.A. and Star, C., Synthesis of 7-oxo-8-aminopelargonic acid, a biotin vitamer, in cell-free extracts of *Escherichia coli* biotin auxotrophs, *J.Bacteriol.* 96, 1846–1843, 1967.

65. Eisenberg, M.A. and Star, C., Synthesis of 7-oxo-8-aminopelargonic acid, a biotin vitamer, in cell-free extracts of *Escherichia coli* biotin autotrophs, *J.Bacteriol.* 96, 1291–1297, 1968.

66. Ohsugi, M., Miyauchi, K., and Inoue, Y., Biosynthesis of biotin-vitamers from unsaturated higher fatty acids by bacteria, *J.Nutr. Sci.Vitaminol.* 31, 253–263, 1985.

67. Sabatie, J., Speck, D., Reymund, J., *et al.*, Biotin formation by recombinant strains of *Escherichia coli*; influence of host physiology, *J.Biotechnol.* 20, 29–49, 1991.

68. Phalip, V., Kuhn, I., Lemoine, Y., and Jeltsch, J.M., Characterization of the biotin biosynthesis pathway in *Saccharomyces cerevisiae* and evidence for a cluster containing B105, a novel gene involved in vitamer uptake, *Gene* 232, 43–51, 1999.

69. Wegner, C., Trotz, M., and Nau, H., Direct determination of folate monoglutamates in plasma by high-performance liquid chromatography using an automatic precolumn-switching system as sample clean up procedure, *J.Chromatog.* 378, 55–65, 1986.

70. Freisleben, A., Schieberle, P., and Rychlik, M., Syntheses of labeled vitamers of folic acid to be used as internal standards in stable isotope dilution assays, *J.Agric.Food Chem.* 50, 4760–4768, 2002.

71. Freisleben, A., Schieberle, P., and Rychlik, M., Specific and sensitive quantification of folate vitamers in food by stable isotope dilution assay high-performance liquid chromatography-tandem mass spectrometry, *Anal.Bioanal.Chem.* 376, 149–156, 2003.

72. Pfeiffer, C.M., Fazili, Z., McCoy, L., *et al.*, Determination of folate vitamers in human serum by stable-isotope-dilution tandem mass spectrometry and comparison with radioassay and microbiological assay, *Clin.Chem.* 50, 423–432, 2004.

73. Smulders, Y.M., Smith, D.E, Kok, E.M., *et al.*, Cellular folate vitamer distribution during and after correction of vitamin B12 deficiency: a case for the methylfolate trap, *Br.J.Haematol.* 132, 623–629, 2006.

74. Smith, D.E., Kok, R.M., Teerlink, T., *et al.*, Quantitative determination of erythrocyte folate vitamer distribution by liquid chromatography-tandem mass spectrometry, *Clin.Chem.Lab. Med.* 44, 450–459, 2006.

VITAMIN NAMES DISCARDED

- Vitamins B_c, B_{10}, B_{11}, and B_x (these mostly have been used to refer to folic acid or folic acid precursors such p-aminobenzoic acid although it would appear that these terms were also used to refer to mixtures of vitamins).

- Vitamin M is a term that has recently been used to describe delta(Δ)-1-tetrahydrocannabinol Earlier the term vitamin M was used to describe a mixture of B-complex vitamins.

- Vitamin B_4 (mostly used to describe adenine but occasionally for choline) Lecoq, R., The role of adenine (vitamin B4 in the metabolism of organic compounds and its repercussions on acid-base equilibrium, *J.Physiol.* 46, 406–410, 1954; Whelan, W.J., Vitamin B4, *IUBMB Life* 57, 125. 2005; Hartmann, J. and Getoff, N., Radiation-induced effect of adenine (vitamin B4) on mitomycin C activity. *In vitro* experiments, *Anticancer Res.* 26, 3005–3010, 2006.

- Vitamin L (anthranilic acid; o-aminobenzoic acid).

- Vitamin Bc – folate although earlier used to describe the B complex vitamins.

- Vitamin B_{10} –folate, precursors of folate such as p-aminobenzoic acid; R factor; also used to refer to vitamin A/retinoic acid; Wang, Y. and Okabe, N., Crystal structures and spectroscopic properties of Zinc(II) ternary complexes of Vitamin L, H' and their isomer m-aminobenzoic acid with bipyridine, *Chem.Pharm.Bull.* 53, 645–652, 2005.

- Vitamin B_{11} – folic acid: Getoff, N., Transient absorption spectra and kinetics of folic acid (vitamin B11) and some kinetic data of folinic acid and methotrexate, *Oncol.Res.* 15, 295–300, 2005.

Pseudovitamins (also described as "fake" vitamins; Young, V.R. and Newberne, P.M., Vitamins and cancer prevention: Issues and dilemmas, *Cancer* 47, 1226-1240, 1981).

Vitamin B_{17} (Laetrile®; amygdalin; 1-mandelonitrile-β-glucuronic acid)

Vitamin B_{15} (pangamic acid; not a chemically defined entity)

Vitamin B_{13} (Orotic acid)

H_3 (Gerovital)

U (methionine sulfonium salts)

General References for Vitamins

Handbook of Vitamins, 2nd edn., ed. L.J. Machlin, Marcel Dekker, Inc., New York, NY, USA, 1991.

Coumbs, G.F., *The Vitamins. Fundamental Aspects in Nutrition and Health*, 2nd edn., Academic Press, San Diego, CA, USA, 1998.

Stipanuk, M.H., *Biochemical and Physical Aspects of Human Nutrition*, W.B. Saunders, Philadelphia, PA, USA, 2000.

Bender, D.A., *Nutritional Biochemistry of the Vitamins*, 2nd Edn., Cambridge University Press, Cambridge, United Kingdom, 2003.

Section V
Nucleic Acids

SOME DEFINITIONS FOR NUCLEIC ACIDS

Roger L. Lundblad

An *adaptor* is an oligonucleotide that is ligated to a nucleic acid polymer to add additional function. One function of an adaptor is to provide a primer for PCR amplification of a DNA fragment obtained from the genome (Saunders, R.D.C., Glover, D.M., Ashburner, M., et al., PCR amplification of DNA microdissected from a single polythene chromosome band: A comparison with conventional microcloning, *Nucleic Acids Res.*, 17, 9027–9037, 1981; O'Malley, R.C., Alonso, J.M., Kim, K.J., Leisse, T.J., and Ecker, J.R., An adaptor ligation-mediated PCR method for high-throughput mapping of T-DNA inserts in the *Arabidopsis* genome, *Nat. Protocols*, 2, 2910–2917, 2007). An adaptor may also be used to provide an additional function to a nucleic acid as shown by the ligation of a DNA to an siRNA providing enhanced therapeutic efficacy (Heissig, P., Klein, P.M., Hadwiger, P., and Wagner, E., DNA as tunable adaptor for siRNA polyplex stabilization and functionalization, *Mol. Ther. Nucleic Acids*, 5, 3288, 2016).

An *allele* is a variable form of a gene which can be inherited. *Allele-specific PCR* is used to identify the polymorphism defining the allele (Wu, D.Y., Ugozzoli, L., Pal, B.K., and Wallace, R.B., Allele-specific enzymatic amplification of β-globulin genomic DNA for diagnosis of sickle cell anemia, *Proc. Natl. Acad. Sci. U. S. A.*, 86, 2757–2760, 1989; Suciu, B.A., Pap, Z., Dénes, L., et al., Allele-specific PCR method for identification of EGFR mutations in non-small cell lung cancer: Formalin-fixed paraffin-embedded tissue versus fresh tissue, *Rom. J. Morphol. Embryol.*, 57, 495–500, 2016).

An *anchor primer* is a *primer* complementary [poly(dC)] to an oligodeoxyribonucleotide [e.g., poly(dG)] ligated to the 3'-terminus of a cDNA transcript from an mRNA (Loh, E.Y., Elliott, J.F., Cwirla, S., Lanier, L.L., and Davis, M.M., Polymerase chain reaction with single-sided specificity: Analysis of the T cell receptor δ chain, *Science*, 243, 217–220, 1989). The oligodeoxyribonucleotide linked to the 3' terminus is designated as the *anchor* and the technique designated as anchored PCR (Nielsen, C.R., Berdal, K.G., and Holst-Jensen, A., Anchored PCR for possible detection and characterisation of foreign integrated DNA near single nucleotide level, *Eur. Food Res. Technol.*, 226, 949–956, 2008) or ligation-anchored technology (Troutt, A.B., McHeyzer-Williams, M.G., Pullendran, B., and Nossal, G.J.V., Ligation-anchored PCR: A simple amplification technique with single-sided specificity, *Proc. Natl. Acad. Sci. U. S. A.*, 89, 9823–9825, 1992). An *anchor primer* can be considered to be an *adaptor*.

Although there is occasional use of the term *anchor sequence* to refer to a sequence in genomic DNA cleaved by an *anchor enzyme*, the predominant use of the term *anchor sequence* refers to a sequence in a protein which binds a protein to a membrane by insertion into the membrane (Steenaart, N.A., and Shore, G.C., Alteration of a mitochondrial outer membrane signal anchor sequence that permits its insertion into the inner membrane. Contribution of hydrophobic residues, *J. Biol. Chem.*, 272, 12057–12061, 1997; Sakaguchi, M., Autonomous and heteronomous positioning of transmembrane segments in multispanning membrane protein, *Biochem. Biophys. Res. Commun.*, 296, 1–4, 2002).

The term *anchoring enzyme* refers to a restriction enzyme, usually NlaIII, used in *SAGE* to prepare "tags." An *anchoring enzyme* is used to make the initial cleavage in cDNA closest the poly(dA) tail establishing one end of the tag. The *anchoring enzyme* is used again to remove the tag from the linker. The *anchoring enzyme* is a restriction endonuclease with greatest use of NlaIII, a restriction endonuclease from *Neisseria lactamica* (Qiang, B.Q., and Schildkraut, I., Two unique restriction endonucleases from *Neisseria lactamica*, *Nucleic Acids Res.*, 14, 1991–1999, 1986). Other restriction endonucleases have been used as *anchoring enzymes* (Pleasance, E.D., Marra, M.A., and Jones, S.J.M., Assessment of SAGE in transcript identification, *Genome Res.*, 13, 1205–1213, 2003; Matsumura, H., Reich, S., Ito, A., et al., Gene expression analysis of plant host-pathogen interactions by SuperSAGE, *Proc. Natl. Acad. Sci. U. S. A.*, 100, 15718–15723, 2003).

Antisense RNA is small noncoding RNA molecule that acts to regulate posttranscriptional gene expression (Green, P.J., Pines, O., and Inouye, M., The role of antisense RNA in gene regulation, *Annu. Rev. Biochem.*, 55, 569–597, 1986; Wagner, E.G., and Simons, R.W., Antisense RNA control in bacteria, phages, and plasmids, *Annu. Rev. Microbiol.*, 48, 713–742, 1994). *Antisense RNA* also regulates *plasmid* function (Brantl, S., Antisense RNA mediated control of plasmid replication, *Plasmid*, 78, 4–16, 2015).

An *antisense primer*, also referred to as the *reverse primer*, is the oligonucleotide which is used to initiate the DNA polymerase catalyzed synthesis of a DNA strand complementary to the *antisense strand* or *template strand* of duplex DNA.

The *antisense strand* is the non-coding strand of duplex DNA; the DNA strand of a duplex that is complementary to the strand encoding a polypeptide is the *template strand* which directly codes for mRNA through Watson–Crick base pairing.

The *blunt end* is the end of a duplex DNA molecule that terminates with a base pair (no overhang) unlike a *sticky end* which contains unpaired bases. The *blunt end* may be ligated non-specifically to the *blunt end* on another DNA duplex since there is no guidance such as provided by a *sticky end*. The efficiency of *blunt end* ligation is greatly increased by the presence of polyethylene glycol (Hayashi, K., Nakazawa, M., Ishizaki, Y., and Obayashi, A., Influence of monovalent cations on the activity of T4 DNA ligase in the presence of polyethylene glycol, *Nucleic Acids Res.*, 13, 61–71, 1985; Upcroft, P., and Healey, A., Rapid and efficient method for cloning of blunt-ended DNA fragments, *Gene*, 51, 69–75, 1985).

An *expression vector* is a vehicle for production of a polypeptide in a host cell, such as bacteria (*Escherichia coli*) (Peti, W., and Page, R., Strategies to maximize heterologous protein expression in *Escherichia* coli with minimal cost, *Protein Expr. Purif.*, 51, 1–10, 2007) or mammalian cells (Chinese Hamster Ovary [CHO]) (Dyson, M.R., Fundamentals of expression in mammalian cells, *Adv. Exp. Med. Biol.*, 896, 217–224, 2016).

Genome walking/chromosome walking is a technique involving the sequential isolation of clones carrying overlapping sequences of DNA permitting the determination of the DNA sequence. This technique uses PCR for the generation of material for DNA sequence analysis (Howell, M.D., Resner, J., Austin, R.K., and Kagnoff, M.F., Rapid identification of hybridization probes for chromosomal walking, *Gene*, 55, 41–45, 1987; Tonooka, Y., and Fujishima, M., Comparison and critical evaluation of PCR-mediated methods to walk along the sequence of genomic DNA,

Appl. Microbiol. Biotechnol., 85, 37–43, 2009; Fraiture, M.A., Herman, P., Lefèvre, L., et al., Integrated DNA walking system to characterize a broad spectrum of GMOs in food/feed matrices, *BMC Biotechnol.*, 15, 76, 2015).

A cis-*acting* element refers to a region on a polynucleotide (DNA or RNA)/chromosome that effects another element on the same polynucleotide/chromosome (Sgana, S.M., Chahal, J., and Sarnow, P., *cis*-Acting RNA elements in the hepatitis C virus RNA genome, *Virus Res.*, 206, 90–98, 2015; Spitz, F., Gene regulation at a distance: From remote enhances to 3D regulatory ensembles, *Semin. Cell Devel. Biol.*, 57, 57–67, 2016).

Concatenate is to link things (in this case, oligonucleotide fragments) together in chains (Hanage, W.P., Fraser, C., and Spratt, B.G., Sequences, sequence clusters and bacterial species, *Philos. Trans. R. Soc. Lond. B Biol. Sci.*, 361, 1917–1927, 2006; Haering, C.H., Farcas, A.M., Arumugam, P., Metson, J., and Nasmyth, K., The cohesion ring concatenates sister DNA molecules, *Nature*, 454, 297–301, 2008).

Cloning is the process of making a copy of a clone. In molecular biology, *cloning* is the process of making multiple copies of a DNA fragment which has been inserted into a *plasmid*, a *cosmid*, or a *virus* (including *bacteriophage*). The process of copying takes place in a suitable host cells such as bacteria or yeast (*Oxford English Dictionary*, Oxford University Press, Oxford, United Kingdom, 2016).

A *cosmid* is a genetically engineered plasmid containing bacteriophage *cos* sequence (Catalano, C.E., Cue, D., and Feiss, M., Virus DNAS packaging: The strategy used by phage lambda, *Mol. Microbiol.*, 16, 1075–1086, 1995; Morino, T., and Takahashi, H., Transduction of a cosmid with the R4 phage cos sequence by heterogeneous actinophages, SPA10 and SPA38, *Biosci. Biotechnol. Biochem.*, 60, 2076–2077, 1999). A cosmid is used as a cloning vector (Lam, K.N., Hall, M.W., Engel, K., et al., Evaluation of a pooled strategy for high-throughput sequencing of cosmid clones from metagenomics libraries, *PLoS One*, 9(6), e98968, 2014).

A *degenerate primer* may have several bases at a given position in the sequence to improve amplification. The degree of degeneracy is established by the number of possible sequence combinations (Telenius, H., Carter, N.P., Bebb, C.E., et al., Degenerate oligonucleotide-primed PCR: General amplification of target DNA by a single degenerate primer, *Genomics*, 13, 718–725, 1992; Linhart, C., and Shamir, R., The degenerate primer design problem, *Bioinformatics*, 18(Suppl 1), S172–S181, 2002).

DNA barcodes can refer to an amplifiable deoxyribooligonucleotide which can be attached to a fragment (chemical building block) which can serve as a tag for a chemical compound during high-throughput screening (Zimmerman, G., and Neri, D., DNA-encoded chemical libraries: Foundations and applications in lead discovery, *Drug Discovery Today*, 21(11), 1828–1834. doi:10.1016/j.drudis.2016.07.013, 2016). The term *DNA barcode* is also used in taxonomy, a specific sequence that can be used to identify an organism (Arnot, D.E., Roper, C., and Bayoumi, R.A., Digital codes from hypervariable tandemly repeated DNA sequences in the *Plasmodium falciparum* circumsporozoite gene can genetically barcode isolates, *Mol. Biochem. Parasitol.*, 61, 15–24, 1993). The gene for mitochondrial cytochrome C oxidase I is used as a barcode for identifying species (Herbert, P.D., Czwinska, A., Ball, S.L., and deWaard, J.R., Biological identifications through DNA barcodes, *Proc. Biol. Sci.*, 270, 313–321, 2000; Staats, M., Arulandhu, A.J., Gravendeel, B., et al., Advances in DNA metabarcoding for food and wildlife forensic species identification, *Anal. Bioanal. Chem.*, 408, 4615–4630, 2016).

DNA ligase is an enzyme (EC 6.5.1.1) that joins two DNA fragments forming a phosphodiester bond in a reaction requiring ATP (bacteriophage T4 enzyme) or NAD (*Escherichia coli* enzymes) (Higgins, N.P., and Cozzarelli, N.R., DNA-joining enzymes: A review, *Methods Enzymol.*, 68, 50–71, 1979; Pascal, J.M., DNA and RNA ligases: Structural variations and shared mechanisms, *Curr. Opin. Struct. Biol.*, 18, 96–105, 2008).

Duplex DNA is double-stranded DNA composed of complementary strands of DNA.

An *exome* is that region of the genome (exon) that codes for an expressed protein. An exon remains in the mature RNA after the removal of introns by splicing (Ng, P.C., Levy, S., Huang, J., et al., Genetic variation in an individual human exome, *PLoS One*, 4(8), e1000160, 2008; Biesecker, L.G., Exome sequencing makes medical genetics a reality, *Nat. Genet.*, 42, 13–14, 2010).

Gateway® cloning or Gateway® recombinational cloning (Reece-Hayes, J.S., and Walhout, A.J.M., Gateway recombinational cloning, in *Molecular Cloning A Laboratory Manual*, 4th edn., ed M.R. Green and J. Sambrook, Cold Spring Harbor Laboratory Press, Cold Spring Harbor, New York, 2012, pp. 261–276) is a proprietary process (Invitrogen/ThermoFisher Scientific) for high-throughput cloning of DNA fragments such as *open reading frames* (Walhout, A.J.M., Sardella, R., and Vidal, M., Protein interaction mapping in *C.elegans* using proteins involved in vulval development, *Science*, 287, 116–122, 2000; Walhout, A.J.M., Temple, G.F., Brasch, M.A., et al., GATEWAY recombinational cloning: Application to the cloning of large numbers of open reading frames of ORFeomes, *Methods Enzymol.*, 238, 575–592, 2000). The *Gateway®* system is based on the integration of λ bacteriophage into the *Escherichia coli* genome and subsequent excision yield vectors with different properties can be expressed in other hosts (Earley, K.W., Haag, J.R., Pontes, O., et al., Gateway-compatible vectors for plant functional genomics and proteomics, *Plant J.*, 45, 616–629, 2006).

Gene targeting is a method that uses homologous recombination to delete genetic information (*knockout*) or add genetic information (*knockin*). The classic approach used homologous recombination in a mouse embryonic stem cell. The engineered embryonic stem cell is injected into a mouse blastocyst which is then implanted in a foster parent, and offspring are selected for chimeras, usually on the basis of coat color. Gene editing can be considered a more efficient method of gene targeting for the generation of knockout gene modification (Hendriks, W.T., Warren, C.R., and Cowan, C.A., Genome editing in human pluripotent stem cells: Approaches, pitfalls, and solutions, *Cell Stem Cell*, 18, 53–65, 2016) or knockin gene modification (Zhu, Z., Verma, N., González, F., Shi, Z.D., and Huangfu, D., A CRISPR/Cas-mediated selection-free knockin strategy in human embryonic stem cells, *Stem Cell Reports*, 4, 1103–1111, 2015). It should be mentioned that a *knockdown* uses a different mechanism based on RNA interference (Fellmann, C., and Lowe, S.W., Stable RNA interference rules for silencing, *Nat. Cell Biol.*, 16, 10–18, 2014).

Heteroduplex DNA is a double-stranded DNA or DNA/RNA generated by base pairing between complementary single strands derived from *different* parental duplex DNA molecules (Tabone, T., Sallmann, G., Chiotis, M., Law, M., and Cotton, R., Chemical cleavage of mismatch (CCM) to locate base mismatches in heteroduplex DNA, *Nat. Protoc.*, 1, 2297–2304, 2006) or by association of a single-stranded DNA oligomer with an RNA oligomer (NIshina, K., Piao, W., Yoshida-Tanaka, K., et al., DNA/RNA heteroduplex oligonucleotide for highly efficient gene silencing, *Nat. Commun.*, 6, 7969, 2015).

Homologous recombination is mechanism in the cell where DNA sequence is exchanged between two similar or identical DNA molecules which serve as templates. This process is greatly facilitated by double-stranded DNA cleavage (Rovet, P., Smith, F., and Jasin, M., Expression of a site-specific nuclease stimulates homologous recombination in mammalian cells, *Proc. Natl. Acad. Sci. U. S. A.*, 91, 6064–6068, 1994).

An *intron* (intervening sequence) is removed from RNA during processing by the spliceosome to mature mRNA (Papsaikas, P., and Valcárcel, J., The spliceosome: The ultimate RNA chaperone and sculptor, *Trends Biochem. Sci.*, 41, 33–45, 2016).

The *Oxford English Dictionary* defines *ligation* as the action or process of binding. In nucleic acid chemistry, *ligation* refers to the process of binding two nucleic acid chains together by forming a phosphodiester bond (Conze, R., Shelye, A., Tanaka, Y., et al., Analysis of genes, transcripts, and proteins via DNA ligation, *Annu. Rev. Anal. Chem.*, 2, 215–239, 2009). A *proximal ligation assay* is a technique which uses the ligation of DNA probes to identify spatially related sites on proteins (Gustarfsdottir, S.M., Schallmeiner, E., Fredriksson, S., et al., Proximity ligation assays for sensitive and specific protein analyses, *Anal. Biochem.*, 345, 2–9, 2005). The term *ligation* has been used to describe other intermolecular reactions of nucleic acids (Sun, H., Fan, H., Ecom, H., and Peng, X., Coumarin-induced DNA ligation, rearrangement to DNA interstrand cross links and photo-release of coumarin moiety, *Chembiochem.*, 17(21), 2046–2053, 2016). *Adaptor ligation PCR* is a technique where a short DNA duplex oligonucleotide with an overhang which will hybridize to a site in, for example, genomic DNA which has been digested with a restriction enzyme to yield "sticky ends" (O'Malley, R.C., Alonso, J.M., Kim, C.J., Leisse, T.J., and Ecker, J.R., An adaptor ligation mediated PCR method for high-throughput mapping of T-DNA inserts in the *Arabidopsis* genome, *Nat. Protocols*, 2, 2910–2917, 2007).

Non-homologous end-to-end joining is a DNA repair process where strand breakage is repaired by ligation of DNA termini without the use of a template. This is a normal repair process but can result in translocation. It can be a complex process with the involvement of phosphodiesterases, nucleases, and polymerases (Barlett, E.J., Brissett, N.C., Plocinski, P., Carlberg, T., and Doherty, A.J., Molecular basis for DNA strand displacement by NHEJ repair polymerases, *Nucleic Acids Res.*, 44, 2173–2186, 2016; Menon, V., and Povrik, L.F., End-processing nucleases and phosphodiesterases: An elite supporting cast for the non-homologous end joining pathway of DNA double-strand break repair, *DNA Repair*, 43, 57–68, 2016).

An *open reading frame* is a DNA or RNA sequence of non-overlapping triplet bases (*reading frame*) which has the capability of coding for the expression of a protein (Contreras, R., Volckaert, G., Thys, F., Van de Voorde, A., and Fiers, W., Nucleotide sequence of the restriction fragment Hind F-Eco R12 of SV40 DNA, *Nucleic Acids Res.*, 4, 1001–1014, 1977; Volckaert, G., Van de Voorde, A., and Fiers, W., Nucleotide sequence of the simian virus 40 small t-gene, *Proc. Natl. Acad. Sci. U. S. A.*, 75, 2160–2164, 19787).

A *plasmid* is an extranuclear (extrachromosomal) genetic element mostly found in bacteria. A *plasmid* can replicate independently from its host and is used as an *expression vector* (Funnell, B.E., and Phillips, G.J., ed., *Plasmid Biology*, ASM Press, Washington, DC, 2004). A *plasmid* contains a promoter region, a site for antibiotic resistance, and an origin of replication in addition to the gene of interest (Durant, V., Sullivan, B.J., and Magliery, T.J., Simplifying protein expression with ligation-free, traceless and tag-switching plasmids, *Protein Expr. Purif.*, 85, 9–17, 2012).

RACE (rapid amplification of cDNA end) is a form of *anchored PCR* (Wang, G., and Fang, J., RLM-RACE, PPM-RACE, and qRT-PCR: An integrated strategy to accurately validate miRNA target gene, *Methods Mol. Biol.*, 1296, 175–186, 2015).

Restriction nucleases (restriction endonucleases) are a group of bacterial enzymes characterized by their ability to specifically cleave palindromic sequences in double-stranded DNA. Cleaved can result in blunt ends or strands with either 3'- or 5-prime overhangs. The name of a specific restriction endonuclease is derived from the first letter of the genus and the first two letters of the species; other letters can be added to further describe the source. Thus, the name for the widely used type II restriction endonuclease from *Escherichia coli* is *EcoR1*. The restriction endonuclease Fok1 is used in designer nucleases (Miller, J.C., Tan, S., Qiao, G., et al., A TALE nuclease architecture for efficient genome editing, *Nat. Biotechnol.*, 29, 143–148, 2011).

RNA-seq is the abbreviation for total RNA sequencing. Although it is possible to directly sequence RNA, the preferred approach uses next-generation sequencing of cDNA (Wilhelm, B.T., and Landry, J.R., Jr., RNA-seq-quantitative measurement of expression through massively parallel RNA-sequencing, *Methods*, 48, 249–257, 2009; Creecy, J.P., and Conway, T., Quantitative bacterial transcriptomics with RNA-seq, *Curr. Opin. Microbiol.*, 23, 133–140, 2015). The challenge is in data analysis (Capobianco, E., RNA-seq data: A complexity journey, *Comput. Struct. Biotechnol. J.*, 11, 123–130, 2014; Finotello, F., and Di Camillo, B., Measuring differential gene expression with RNA-seq: Challenges and strategies for data analysis, *Brief Funct. Genomics*, 14, 130–142, 2015). RNA-seq has been applied to the analysis of transcriptomics of single cells *(Marr, C., Zhou, J.X., and Huang, S., Single-cell gene expression profiling and cell state dynamics: Collecting data, correlating data points and connecting the dots, *Curr. Opin. Biotechnol.*, 39, 207–214, 2016). Quality control issue for RNA-seq has been discussed (Li, X., Nair, A., Wang, S., and Wang, L., Quality control of RNA-seq experiments, *Methods Mol. Biol.*, 1269, 137–146, 2015).

The *sense strand* of duplex DNA is also referred to as the coding strand and is complementary to the *antisense* or *non-coding strand*. There are *sense* and *antisense strand* in *siRNA*.

A *sense primer* is a PCR primer for the *sense strand* of duplex DNA. It is also called a *forward primer*.

Serial analysis of gene expression (SAGE) is a technique for the analysis of gene expression. *SAGE* is based on the analysis of tags obtained from cDNA. Tags are obtained from the cDNA by the action of an *anchoring enzyme* which cleaves the cDNA and a *tagging enzyme* which determines the length of tag. The tag is expected to be unique to a specific transcript with that probability increasing with increasing tag length (Velculescu, V.E., Zhang, L., Vogelstein, B., and Kinzier, K.W., Serial analysis of gene expression, *Science* 270, 484–487, 1995; Yamamoto, M., Wakasuki, T., Hada, A., and Ryo, A., Use of serial analysis of gene expression (SAGE) technology, *J. Immunol. Methods*, 250, 45–66, 2001; Gilchrist, M.A., Qin, H., and Zaretzki, R., Modeling SAGE tag formation and its effect on data interpretation with a Bayesian framework, *BMC Bioinformatics*, 8, 403, 2007).

Sticky ends are formed by the asymmetric cleavage of double-stranded DNA by some *restriction enzymes* resulting in a 5'-overhang or a 3'-overhang producing an unpaired nucleotide sequence which can selectively bind an asymmetric double-stranded DNA during *recombination* (Ban, E., and Pico, C.R., Strength of DNA sticky end links, *Biomacromolecules*, 15, 143–149, 2014). *Sticky ends* are important for the efficient ligation of DNA fragments via their complementary *sticky ends* (Graf, H., Optimization of conditions for the *in vitro* formation of hybrid DNA molecules by DNA ligase, *Biochim. Biophys. Acta,* 564, 225–234, 1979).

A *tagging enzyme* is used in *SAGE* to cleave the tag from the linker-oligodeoxyribonucleotide fragment derived from the 5-terminus of cDNA sequence obtained by cleavage with the *anchoring enzyme* (Velculescu, V.E., Vogelstein, B., and Kinzier, K.W., Analyzing uncharted transcriptomes with SAGE, *Trends Genet.,* 16, 423–425, 2000).

A trans-*acting element* encodes a protein that acts at a different site such as a cis-*acting element* (Jose-Estanyel, M., Poliard, A., Foiret, D., and Danan, J.L., A common liver-specific factor binds to the rat albumin and α-foetoprotein promoters *in vitro* and acts as a positive *trans*-acting factor *in vivo, Eur. J. Biochem.,* 181, 761–766, 1989; Xiao, W., Pelcher, L.E., and Rank, G.H., Evidence for *cis*- and *trans*-acting element coevolution of the 2-microns circle genome in *Saccharomyces cerevisiae, J. Mol. Evol.,* 32, 145–152, 1991; Goetstouwers, T., Van Poucke, M., Coppieters, W., et al., Refined candidate region for F4ab/ac enterotoxigenic *Escherichia coli* susceptibility situated proximal to MUC13 in pigs, *PLoS One,* 9(8), e105013, 2014).

Transcriptome: In the broadest sense, it is the ribonucleic acid product from the transcription of genomic DNA which would include mRNA, tRNA, microRNA, long noncoding RNA and ribosomal RNA (https://www.genome.gov/13014330/). Analysis of the transcriptome can be accomplished by microarray analysis (Touzot, M., Dahirel, A., Cappuccio, A., et al., Using transcriptional signatures to assess immune cell function: From basic mechanisms to immune-related disease, *J. Mol. Biol.,* 427, 3356–3367, 2015) or RNA-seq (de Klerk, E., and 't Hoen, P.A., Alternative mRNA transcription, processing and translation: Insights from RNA sequencing, *Trends Genet.,* 31, 128–139, 2015).

A *therapeutic transgene* is a therapeutic gene transferred from one organism to another organism for the purpose of augmentation gene therapy (Chao, H., Liu, Y., Rabinowitz, J., et al., Several log increase in therapeutic transgene delivery by distinct adeno-associated viral serotype vectors, *Mol. Ther.,* 2, 619–623, 2000; Miagkov, A.V., Varley, A.W., Mumford, R.S., and Makarov, S.S., Endogenous regulation of a therapeutic transgene restores homeostasis in arthritic joints, *J. Clin. Invest.,* 109, 1223–1229, 2002; VanderVeen, N., Raja, N., Yi, E., et al., Preclinical efficacy

and safety profile of allometrically scaled doses of doxycycline used to turn "on" therapeutic transgene expression from high-capacity adenoviral vectors in a glioma model, *Hum. Gene Ther. Methods,* 27, 98–111, 2016).

Translatome: This is a category of the *transcriptome* which consists of mRNA bound to ribosomes (King, H.A., and Gerber, A.P., Translatome profiling: Methods for genome-scale analysis of mRNA translation, *Brief. Funct. Genomics,* 15, 22–31, 2016). Elucidation of the translatome is closely related to the concept of ribosome profiling (Janich, P., Arpat, A.B., Castelo-Szekely, V., Lopes, M., and Garfield, D., Ribosome profiling reveals the rhythmic liver translatome and circadian clock regulation by upstream open reading frames, *Genome Res.,* 25, 1848–1859, 2015; Wahba, A., Rath, B.H., Kheem, Bisht, K., Camphausen, K., and Tofilon, P.J., Polysome profiling links translational control to the radioresponse of glioblastoma stem-like cells, *Cancer Res.,* 76, 3078–3087, 2016).

A Universal Primer

The phrase *variable number of tandem repeats (VNTR)* refers to the presence of repeating short nucleotide sequences in the genome. This is an inherited *allele* which can be used for personal identification (DNA "fingerprinting") (Jeffreys, A.J., Wilson, V., and Thein, S.L., Individual-specific "fingerprints" of human DNA, *Nature,* 316, 76–79, 1985; Chakraborty, R., Srinivasan, M.R., and de Andrade, M., Intraclass and interclass correlations of allele sizes within and between loci in DNA typing data, *Genetics,* 133, 411–419, 1993). Early work used Southern blot analysis (Cerrone, G.E., Caputo, M., Lopez, A.P., et al., Variable number of tandem repeats of the insulin gene determines susceptibility to latent autoimmune diabetes in adults, *Mol. Diagn.,* 8, 43–49, 2004), but more recent work uses PCR technology (Taylor, M., Cieslak, M., Rees, G.S., et al., Comparison of germ line minisatellite mutation detection at the CEG1 locus by Southern blotting and PCR amplification, *Mutagenesis,* 25, 343–349, 2010; Nikolayevskyy, V., Trovato, A., Broda, A., et al., MIRU-VNTR genotyping of *Mycobacterium turberculosis* strains using QIAxcel technology: A multicenter evaluation study, *PLoS One,* 11(3), e0149435, 2016).

UV SPECTRAL CHARACTERISTICS AND ACIDIC DISSOCIATION CONSTANTS OF 280 ALKYL BASES, NUCLEOSIDES, AND NUCLEOTIDES

B. Singer

The λ_{max} (nm), in those cases where more than one value has been reported, are either the most frequent value or an average of several values, the range being ± 1 to 2 nm for the λ_{max}. Since the λ_{min} is more sensitive than the λ_{max} to impurities in the sample, the values of λ_{min} in the table are generally the lowest reported. Values in parentheses are shoulders or inflexions. The cationic and anionic forms are either so stated by the authors or are arbitrarily taken at pH 1 and pH 13. Individual values are given for pK_a except when there are more than two values. In that case, a range is given.

Complete spectra representing a range of derivatives are shown in the figures, and reference to these is made in the table with an asterisk and number preceding the name of the compound.

All spectra were obtained in the author's laboratory from samples isolated from paper chromatograms. It is recognized that pH 1 or pH 13 is not ideal for obtaining the cationic or anionic forms when these pHs are close to a pK. Nevertheless, these conditions are useful for purposes of identification since the spectra are reproducible.

Additional data not quoted here are available in many of the references. These data include spectral characteristics in other solvents than H_2O and at other pH values, extinction coefficients, R_F values in various paper chromatographic systems, column chromatographic systems, methods of synthesis or preparation of alkyl derivatives, mass spectra, and NMR, optical rotatory dispersion and infrared spectra.

	Acidic		Basic			
	λ_{max}(nm)	λ_{min}(nm)	λ_{max}(nm)	λ_{min}(nm)	pKₐ	References
*1ADENINE						
MONOALKYLATED						
*21-Methyl-	259	228	270	234	7.2	1–7
1-Ethyl-	260	233	271	242	6.9, 7.0	5, 8, 9
1-Isopropyl-	259		269			10
1-Benzyl-	260		271		7.0	11, 12
1-(2-Hydroxypropyl)-	259		271		7.2	13
1-(2-Hydroxyethylthioethyl)-	262		271		7.2	6
2-Methyl-	267	228	270 (280)	239	~5.1	3, 4
*33-Methyl-	274	235	273	244	6.1, 6.1	2, 5, 6, 13–15
3-Ethyl-	274	240	273	247	6.5	5, 8, 16
3-Isopropyl-	274		273			10
3-Benzyl-	275		272		5.1	17, 18
3-(2-Hydroxypropyl)-	274		273		6.0	13
3-(2-Diethylaminoethyl)-	275	236	274	245		19
*4N^6-Methyl-	267	231	273 (280)	238	4.2, 4.2	1–4, 7, 15, 20, 21
N^6-Ethyl-	268	231	274 (281)	241		8, 21
N^6-Butyl-	270		275			21
N^6-(2-Hydroxyethyl)-	272	233	273	236	3. 7	72
N^6-(2-Diethylaminoethyl)-	275	233	274	239		19
*57-Methyl-	273	237	270 (280)	230	~3.5, 3.6	8, 15, 18, 23, 24
7-Ethyl-	272	239	270 (280)	234		8, 16
7-Isopropyl-	272		272			10
9-Methyl-	261	230	262	228	3.9	5, 13, 15
9-Ethyl-	258	230	262	228	4.1	5, 13, 25
9-Isopropyl-	260		262			10
9-(2-Hydroxypropyl)-	259		261			13
9-(2-Diethylaminoethyl)	258	227	261	229		19
9-Benzyl-	259		261			18
DIALKYLATED						
1,N^6-Dimethyl-	261	230	273	245		1, 8, 20
1,7-Dimethyl-	270					26
1-Butyl, 7-methyl-	268					26
1,9-Dimethyl-	260	235	260 (265)	235	9.08	13, 20, 27
1,9-Di(2-hydroxypropyl)-	260		260			13
1,9-Di(2-diethylaminoethyl)-	257	233	261	232		19
1-Ethyl-9-methyl-	261		261		9.16	27
1-Propyl-9-methyl-	261		261		9.15	27
3,N^6-Dimethyl-	281		287			28
3,N^6-Di(2-diethylaminoethyl)-	282	243	282	249		19

UV SPECTRAL CHARACTERISTICS AND ACIDIC DISSOCIATION CONSTANTS OF 280 ALKYL BASES, NUCLEOSIDES, AND NUCLEOTIDES[a] (Continued)

	Acidic		Basic			
	λ_{max}(nm)	λ_{min}(nm)	λ_{max}(nm)	λ_{min}(nm)	pK$_a$	References
[*1]*ADENINE* (Continued)						
3,7-Dimethyl-	276	246	225, 280	221, 247	11	2, 13, 20
3,7-Dibenzyl-	278		281		9.6	18
3,7-Di(2-hydroxypropyl)-	278		281			13
3,7-Di(2-diethylaminoethyl)-	276	237	279	245		19
N^6,N^6-Dimethyl-	276	236	282	245		7, 21
N^6,N^6-Diethyl-	278		282			21, 29
N^6,7-Dimethyl-	279		275			24, 26
[*6]N^6-Methyl-7-ethyl-	277 (285)	241	276	244		8
N^6-Propyl-7-methyl-	281		277			24
N^6-Butyl-7-methyl-	279					26
N^6,9-Dimethyl-	265		268		4.02	27, 29
N^6,9-Di-2-diethylaminoethyl)-	266	229	270	233		19
N^6-Ethyl-9-methyl-	265		268		4.08	27, 29
N^6-Propyl-9-methyl-	266		270		4.14	27
N^6-Butyl-9-ethyl-	266		269			27
TRIALKYLATED						
1,N^6,N^6-Trimethyl-	221, 293	246	232, 301	262		30
3,$N^6,N^{6'}$-Trimethyl-	290	243	293	250		30
N^6,N^6,7-Trimethyl-	233, 293	250	291	246		30
N^6,N^6,9-Trimethyl-	269	234	276	237		29, 30
N^6,N^6-Dimethyl-9-ethyl-	270		277			25
3,N^6,7-Tribenzyl-	289		Unstable		9.4	18
[*7]*GUANINE*						
MONOALKYLATED						
1-Methyl-	250 (270)	228	277 (262)	242	3.1	4, 7, 15, 23, 31–34
[*8]1-Ethyl-	251 (274)	229	278 (260)	243		35, 36
1-Isopropyl-	253					10
1-(2-Diethylaminoethyl)-	255, 275		257, 268			19
N^2-Methyl-[b]	251, 279	228	245–255, 278	238	3.3	4, 7, 23, 33, 34, 37, 38
[*9]N^2-Ethyl-	253 (280)	229	245, 279	263		37, 39
N^2-Isopropyl-	252		277			10
3-Methyl-	263 (244)	227	273	246		15, 33, 40, 41
[*10]3-Ethyl-	263 (244)	233	273	248		39
3-Isopropyl-	263		273			10
3-Benzyl-	263 (243)		274		4.00	42
O^6-Methyl-	286		246, 284			43, 44
[*11]O^6-Ethyl-	286	253	284 (246)	259		35, 44
O^6-Propyl-	286		246, 283			44
O^6-Isopropyl-	285 (230)		283 (245)			10, 45
O^6-Butyl-	286		246, 285			44
O^6-Isobutenyl-	286 (232)		283 (245)			45
7-Methyl-	249 (272)	226	281 (240)	255	3.5	4, 23, 31, 32, 46
[*12]7-Ethyl-	249 (274)	233	280	258	3.7	5, 35
7-Isopropyl-	249 (274)		278 (240)			10, 45
7-Benzyl-	250		281		3.2	11
7-(2-Hydroxyethyl)-	250	229	281	261		47
7-(2-Hydroxypropyl)-	250, 272	229	280	257		13
7-(2-Diethylaminoethyl)-	253, 270		275 (250)			19
7-(β-Hydroxyethylthioethyl)-	250		281			48
8-Propyl-	249, 276		276			45
8-Isobutyl-	249, 278		276			45
8-(3-Methylbutyl)-	249, 277		275			45
9-Methyl	251, 276		268 (258)		2.9	33
[*13]9-Ethyl-	252, 277	230	253, 268	238		35
9-Isopropyl-	253, 276		256, 258			10, 45
DIALKYLATED						
1,7-Dimethyl-	252 (272)	230	284 (251)	262		23, 33, 35
[*14]1,7-Diethyl-	252 (275)	232	285 (250)	263		49
1,9-Dimethyl-	254 (277)	229				33
N^2,N^2-Dimethyl-[b]	255 (289)	229	277–283			4, 34, 37, 38

UV SPECTRAL CHARACTERISTICS AND ACIDIC DISSOCIATION CONSTANTS OF 280 ALKYL BASES, NUCLEOSIDES, AND NUCLEOTIDES[a] (Continued)

	Acidic		Basic			
	λ_{max}(nm)	λ_{min}(nm)	λ_{max}(nm)	λ_{min}(nm)	pK_a	References
[7]*GUANINE* (Continued)						
7,8-Dimethyl-	249, 277		280 (235)		4.4	50
7,9-Dimethyl	254 (278)	229	c			28, 33
7,9-Di(2-diethylaminoethyl)-	257, 278		c			19
7-Methyl-9-ethyl-	254, 281		c		7.3	14
8,9-Dimethyl-	252, 277 (289)		280 (252)		4.11	50
TRIALKYLATED						
1,7,9-Trimethyl-	254, 280		c			33
[15]*CYTOSINE*						
MONOALKYLATED						
1-Methyl-	213, 283	241	274	250	4.55–4.61	51–53
O^2-Methyl-	260	241	270	246	5.41	53
3-Methyl-	273	240	294	251	7.4, 7.49	4, 53, 54
[16]3-Ethyl-	275	241	296	257		55
N^4-Methyl-	278	240	286 (230)	256	4.55	4, 56, 57
N^4-Ethyl-	277	244	284	253	4.58	55, 57
5-Methyl-	211, 284	242	288	254	4.6	58
6-Methyl-					5.13	59
DIALKYLATED						
1,3-Dimethyl-	281	243	272	247	9.29–9.4	51, 53, 54
1,N^4-Dimethyl-	218, 285	244	274 (235)	250	4.38–4.47	51, 53, 56
N^4,N^4-Dimethyl-	283	242	290 (235)	259	4.15, 4.25	56, 57
1,5-Dimethyl-	291	244			4.76	60
TRIALKYLATED						
1,3,N^4-Trimethyl-	212, 287	248	280	247	9.65	19, 51, 53
1,N^4,N^4-Trimethyl-	220, 288	248	283	242	4.2	56
5-HYDROXYMETHYLCYTOSINE						
Unmodified	279		284			7
3-Methyl-	278		296		7.1	14
[17]*XANTHINE*						
[18]1-Methyl-d	260–265, (235)	239	283 (245)	257	1.3	35, 61, 62
3-Methyl-d	266		275 (232)		0.8	61, 62
[19]7-Methyl-d	267	233	289 (237)	255	0.8	32, 35, 61
9-Methyl-d	260		245, 278		2.0	61, 62
1,3-Dimethyl-	266		275		0.7	61, 62
1,7-Dimethyl-	–260		233, 289		0.5	61, 62
1,9-Dimethyl-	262		248, 277		2.5	61, 62
3,7-Dimethyl-	265		234, 274		0.3	61, 62
3,9-Dimethyl-	265		270 (240)		1.0	61, 62
7,9-Dimethyl-	239, 262		c			63
8,9-Dimethyl-	238, 265		245, 278			63
1,3,7-Trimethyl-	266				0.5	61
1,3,9-Trimethyl-	266				0.6	61
1.7,9-Trimethyl-	232, 262		c			63
[20]*URACIL*						
1-Methyl-	208, 268	241	265	242	–1.8	58, 64
O^2-Ethyl-	218, 260		221, 265			58
[21]3-Methyl-	258	230	218, 283	245		4, 58, 65
O^4-Methyl-	267		276			65a
O^4-Ethyl-	269		220, 278			58
1,3-Dimethyl-	266	234	266	234		58
1,6-Dimethyl-	208, 268	234	266	241		65
O^2,3-Dimethyl-	213, 269					65 b
3,6-Dimethyl-	205, 259	231	281	245		65
5,6-Dimethyl-	267	236	275	245		65
1,5,6-Trimethyl-	206, 276	240	273	245		65

UV SPECTRAL CHARACTERISTICS AND ACIDIC DISSOCIATION CONSTANTS OF 280 ALKYL BASES, NUCLEOSIDES, AND NUCLEOTIDES[a] (Continued)

	Acidic		Basic		pK$_a$	References
	λ_{max}(nm)	λ_{min}(nm)	λ_{max}(nm)	λ_{min}(nm)		
[*22]THYMINE						
1-Methyl-			269	244		66
1-(2-Diethylaminoethyl)-			265	248		19
3-Methyl-	266	237	290	248		31, 35, 66
[*23]3-Ethyl-	265	237	289	247		35
3-(2-Diethylaminoethyl)-			288	244		19
1,3-Di(2-diethylaminoethyl)-			269	245		19
1,0^4-Di(2-diethylaminoethyl)-			274	245		19
O^2,3-Dimethyl-	217, 272					65b
HYPOXANTHINE						
1-Methyl-	249		260			15, 66a
3-Methyl-	253		265		2.61	15, 66a, 67
3-Ethyl-	254		266			68
3-Benzyl-	254		264 (277)			69
3-(2-Diethylaminoethyl)-	260	234	262	243		19
O^6-(3-Methyl-2-butenyl)-	247		262			45
7-Methyl-	250		262		2.12	15
9-Methyl-	250		254			15
1,7-Dimethyl-	252	232	267	237		70
1,7-Dibenzyl-	255		256			69
1,9-Dibenzyl-	263		259			69
3,7-Dimethyl-			267			20
3,7-Dibenzyl-	256		267			69
N^6,7-Dimethyl-	256		258			24
7,9-Dimethyl-	251		c			28
[*24]ADENOSINE						
[*25]1-Methyl-	257	231	258 (265)	233	8.8, 8.3	3, 4, 8, 16, 71
1-Methyldeoxy-	257	239	258	242		8, 72
[*26]1-Ethyl-	259	235	261, (268, 300)	237		8
1-Ethyldeoxy-	259	231	260 (268)	236		8
1-Benzyedeoxy-	259		259			11
2-Methyl-	258	230	264	227		3, 4, 73
[*27]N^6-Methyl-	262	231	266	223	4.0	1–4, 8, 74, 74a
N^6-Methyldeoxy-	262	231	266	226		4, 8, 72, 74
N^6-Ethyl-	264	239	268	243		8
N^6-Ethyldeoxy-	263	237	268	241		8
N^6-Benzyl-	265	235	268	236		69, 75
N^6-Benzyldeoxy-	264		268			11
N^6-Butyl-	263		267			76
N^6-(2-Hydroxyethyl)-	263	233	267	232	3.1	22
[*28]7-Ethyl-	268	239	c			8
[*29]1,N^6-Dimethyl-	261	234	263 (300)	234		1, 8, 20
N^6,N^6-Dimethyl-	268	233	276	237	4.5	3, 4, 30
[*30]N^6,7-Dimethyl-	276	241	c			8
N^6-Methyl-7-ethyl-	276	242	c			8
[*31]GUANOSINE						
[*32]1-Methyl-	258 (280)	230	255 (270)	228	2.6	4, 7, 20, 34
1-Methyldeoxy-	257 (278)	232	255 (270)	229		20, 31, 77
1-Ethyl-	261 (272)	232	258 (270)	239	2.8	49
1-Ethyldeoxy-	256		257			77
1-Butyldeoxy-	258 (282)		257 (280)			77
N^2-Methyl-[b]	251–258 (280–290)	222–234	248–258 (270–275)	227–238		4, 34, 38
O^6-Methyl-	284 (243)	259	243, 277	239, 261	2.4	49
O^6-Methyldeoxy-	284 (230)	252	243, 278	233, 261		31, 78
[*33]O^6-Ethyl-	244, 286	239, 260	247, 278	233, 261	2 5	49
O^6-Ethyldeoxy-	286	252	248, 280	261		77
O^6-Butyldeoxy-	246, 287	260	248, 280	261		77
7-Methyl-	257 (275)	230	c		6.7–7.3	4, 14, 46, 49, 74
7-Methyldeoxy-	256 (275)	229	c			31, 32, 74, 77

UV SPECTRAL CHARACTERISTICS AND ACIDIC DISSOCIATION CONSTANTS OF 280 ALKYL BASES, NUCLEOSIDES, AND NUCLEOTIDES[a] (Continued)

	Acidic		Basic			
	λ_{max}(nm)	λ_{min}(nm)	λ_{max}(nm)	λ_{min}(nm)	pK$_a$	References
[34]*GUANOSINE* (Continued)						
[34]7-Ethyl-	258 (277)	238	c		7.2, 7.4	14, 49
7-Isopropyl-	256 (275)		c			45
7-Benzyl-	258		c		7.2	11
7-Butyldeoxy-	257 (280)		c			77
8-Methyl-	260 (273)		256		3.01	50
1,7-Dimethyl-	260 (270)	236	c			20, 49
[35]1,7-Diethyl-	263 (270)	237	c			49
1-Methyl-7-ethyl-	259 (277)	233	c			49
1-Ethyl-7-methyl-	261 (275)	235	c			49
N^2,N^2-Dimethyl-	265 (290)	237	262 (283)	240		4, 7, 34, 38
N^2,O^6-Dimethyldeoxy-	288		249, 284			77
[36]N^2,O^6-Diethyl-	246, 292	239, 267	252, 281	237, 268		35, 49
N^2,N^2,7-Trimethyl-	267, 300	239, 286	c			79
[37]*CYTIDINE*						
O^2-Methyl-	233, 262	221, 243	Unstable		>8.6	35
[37a]O^2-Ethyl-	233, 262	221, 243	Unstable		>8.6	35
3-Methyl-	278	243	225, 267	212, 244	8.3–8.9	4, 54–56, 71
[38]3-Ethyl-	280	247	267	248	8.4	55
3-Ethyldeoxy-	280	245	268	247	8.6	55
3-Benzyl-	281		266		7.7	11
3-(2-Diethylaminoethyl)deoxy-	284	243	271			19
N^4-Methyl-	217, 281	207, 243	237, 273	250	3.85, 3.92	56, 57
N^4-Methyldeoxy-	282	242	236, 270	229, 248	4.01	57
[39]N^4-Ethyl-	281	244	272	253	4.2	55
N^4-Ethyldeoxy-	279	247	272	253	4.2	55
2'-O N^4-Dimethyl-[e]	281	242	271	250		80
2',3',5'-Tri-O-methyl-N^4-methyl-[e]	281	242	271	247		81
5-Methyl-	288	245	278	255	4.28	60
5-Methyldeoxy-	287	246	278	255	4.40	60, 82
5-Ethyldeoxy-			278	255		83
6-Methyl	278	241	273	252	4.42	59, 84
6-Methyldeoxy-	278	241	273	252		84
3,N^4-Dimethyl-	286	249	277	249		55
[40]3,N^4-Diethyl-	287	252	277	253		55
3,N^4Di(2-diethylaminoethyl)deoxy-	284	245				19
N^4, N^4-Dimethyl-	219, 285	245	279	238	3.7, 3.62	56, 57
N^4, N^4-Dimethyldeoxy-	287	245	278	238	3.79	57
[41]N^4,N^4-Diethyl-	286	249	276	249		55
2'-O,N^4,N^4-Trimethyl-[e]	287	246	278	238		80
N^4,5-Dimethyl-			275 (234)	252		60
N^4,5-Dimethyldeoxy-	218, 287	246	275 (235)		4.04	60
[42]3,N^4,N^4-Triethyl-	287	252	289	253		55
[43]*URIDINE*						
O^2-Methyl-	229, 251	213, 238				35, 86, 87
O^2-Ethyl-	228, 253	213, 237				87
3-Methyl-	263	233	262	233		4, 14, 55, 85
[44]3-Ethyl-	262	235	264	237		35, 55
3-Benzyl-			264	235		83
3-(2-Hydroxyethyl)-	261	235	262			88
[44a]O^4-Methyl-	271	235	274	239		80
6-Methyl-	261	230	264	242		65, 84
5,6-Dimethyl-	206, 269	236	270	248		65
[45]*THYMIDINE (DEOXY-)*						
3-Methyl-	266	238	267	239		31, 35
[46]3-Ethyl-	269	239	270	240		35
3-(2-Diethylaminoethyl)-			270	242		19
O^4-Methyl-(α)	279	245	279	243		89
O^4-Methyl-(β)	279	241	280	243		89

UV SPECTRAL CHARACTERISTICS AND ACIDIC DISSOCIATION CONSTANTS OF 280 ALKYL BASES, NUCLEOSIDES, AND NUCLEOTIDES[a] (Continued)

	Acidic		Basic			
	λ_{max}(nm)	λ_{min}(nm)	λ_{max}(nm)	λ_{min}(nm)	pK$_a$	References
[*47]INOSINE						
1-Methyl-	250	223	249			4
1-Methyldeoxy-	250		250 (265)			31
1-Benzyl-	251		249			69
1-(2-Hydroxyethyl)-	250	226	250	226		88
O^6-Methyl-	250		250			66a, 74a
[*48]7-Methyl-	252	221	c		6.4	35, 70
7-Ethyl-	252		c			68
1,7-Dimethyl-	265		c			70
XANTHOSINE						
7-Methyl-	262	237	c			32, 35
ADENYLIC ACID OR ADP[e,f]						
1-Methyl-	258	232	259 (268)	230		6, 35, 90
1-(2-Hydroxyethylthioethyl)-	261		261			6
2-Methyl-	259		263			73
N^6-Methyl-	261	231	265	229		6, 90
N^6-(2-Hydroxyethylthioethyl)-			268			6
N^6-(2-Hydroxyethyl)-	263	233	266	230		91
2,N^6-Dimethyl	263		269			92
GUANYLIC ACID OR GDP[e,f]						
1-Methyl-	258 (280)	230	256 (273)	230	<3	7, 93
7-Methyl-	259, 279	230	c		6.9–7.2	46, 94
O^6-Methyl-	245, 288	262	249, 281	263		95
N^2-Methyl-	263	237	263	240		96
N^2,N^2-Dimethyl-	265	232	263	237	~3	7, 96
N^2,N^2,7-Trimethyl-	262 (290)	237	c		7.4	96
CYTIDYLIC ACID OR CDP[e,f]						
3-Methyl-	276	242	223, 266	243	9.0, 9.2	97–99
N^4-Methyl-	217, 281	242	271	249	4.25	98, 99
N^4,N^4-Dimethyl-	219, 287	245	225, 278	238	4.0	98, 99
5-Methyl-	284		279			100
5-Methyldeoxy-	287	243	277	254	4.5	101
URIDYLIC ACID OR UDP[e,f]						
3-Methyl-	261	235	262	235		35, 91
3-Ethyl-	261		263			35
THYMIDYLIC ACID (DEOXY-)[f]						
[*49]3-Methyl-	267	240	268	241		35
3-Ethyl-	267	241	268	242		35

[a] Much of the data and some of the spectra were published in a review by B. Singer in *Prog. Nucleic Acids Res. Mol. Biol.*, 15, 219–284, 330–332 (1975).

[b] N^2-Alkyl guanines and guanosines do not exhibit sharp maxima or minima, particularly in basic solution, as shown in the spectra published by Hall,[4] Smith and Dunn,[34] and Singer and Fraenkel-Conrat.[39] Therefore, some of the data are given as a range of values.

[c] All 7-alkyl purine nucleosides and nucleotides and 7,9-dialkyl purines are unstable in alkali and the imidazole ring opens at varying rates. For this reason spectral data obtained in alkaline solution do not represent the original compound and thus such data are omitted. The opening of the imidazole ring in alkali can be used as a means of identifying this class of alkyl compounds. Ring opening can lead to a number of derivatives.[39]

[d] Basic values are those of the dianion (pH 14).

[e] Alkylation of ribose does not cause any change in spectrum.

[f] Alkylated nucleoside diphosphates have the same spectral characteristics as alkylated nucleotides and the data are not separated. Alkylation of the phosphate group does not cause any change in spectrum.

References

1. Wacker and Ebert, *Z. Naturforsch.*, 14b, 709 (1959).
2. Brookes and Lawley, *J. Chem. Soc., (Lond.)*, p. 539 (1960).
3. Garrett and Mehta, *J. Am. Chem. Soc.*, 94, 8532 (1972).
4. Hall, *The Modified Nucleosides in Nucleic Acids.* Columbia University Press, New York, 1971.
5. Pal, *Biochemistry*, 1, 558 (1962).
6. Shooter, Edwards, and Lawley, *Biochem. J.*, 125, 829 (1971).
7. Venkstern and Baer, *Absorption Spectra of Minor Bases.*, Plenum Press, New York, 1965.
8. Singer, Sun, and Fraenkel-Conrat, *Biochemistry*, 13, 1913 (1974).
9. Ludlum, *Biochim. Biophys. Acta*, 174, 773 (1969).
10. Lawley, Orr, and Jarman, *Biochem. J.*, 145, 73 (1975).
11. Brookes, Dipple, and Lawley, *J. Chem. Soc. C*, p. 2026 (1968).
12. Leonard and Fujii, *Proc. Natl. Acad. Sci. U.S.A.*, 51, 73 (1964).
13. Lawley and Jarman, *Biochem. J.*, 126, 893 (1972).
14. Lawley and Brookes, *Biochem. J.*, 89, 127 (1963).
15. Elion, *J. Org. Chem.*, 27, 2478 (1962).

16. Lawley and Brookes, *Biochem. J.*, 92, 19c (1964).
17. Montgomery and Thomas, *J. Am. Chem. Soc.*, 85, 2672 (1963).
18. Montgomery and Thomas, *J. Heterocycl. Chem.*, 1, 115 (1964).
19. Price, Gaucher, Koneru, Shibakawa, Sowa, and Yamaguchi, *Biochim. Biophys. Acta*, 166, 327 (1968).
20. Broom, Townsend, Jones, and Robins, *Biochemistry*, 3, 494 (1964).
21. Elion, Burgi, and Hitchings, *J. Am. Chem., Soc.*, 74, 411 (1952).
22. Windmueller and Kaplan, *J. Biol. Chem.*, 236, 2716 (1961).
23. Reiner and Zamenhof, *J. Biol Chem.*, 228, 475 (1957).
24. Prasad and Robins, *J. Am. Chem. Soc.*, 79, 6401 (1957).
25. Montgomery and Temple, *J. Am. Chem. Soc.*, 79, 5238 (1957).
26. Taylor and Loeffler, *J. Am. Chem. Soc.*, 82, 3147 (1960).
27. Itaya, Tanaka, and Fujii, *Tetrahedron*, 28, 535 (1972).
28. Jones and Robins, *J. Am. Chem. Soc.*, 84, 1914 (1962).
29. Robins and Lin, *J. Am. Chem. Soc.*, 79, 490 (1957).
30. Townsend, Robins, Loeppky, and Leonard, *J. Chem. Soc. (Lond.)*, p. 5320 (1964).
31. Friedman, Mahapatra, Dash, and Stevenson, *Biochim. Biophys. Acta*, 103, 286 (1965).
32. Haines, Reese, and Todd, *J. Chem. Soc. (Lond.)*, p. 5281 (1962).
33. Shapiro, *Prog. Nucleic Acid Res. Mol. Biol*, 8, 73 (1968).
34. Smith and Dunn, *Biochem. J.*, 72, 294 (1959).
35. Singer, *unpublished*.
36. Kriek and Emmelot, *Biochemistry*, 2, 733 (1963).
37. Elion, Lange, and Hitchings, *J. Am. Chem. Soc*, 78, 217 (1956).
38. Gerster and Robins, *J. Am. Chem. Soc.*, 87, 3752 (1965).
39. Singer and Fraenkel-Conrat, *Biochemistry*, 14, 772 (1975).
40. Lawley, Orr, and Shah, *Chem. Biol. Interact.*, 4, 431 (1971/72).
41. Townsend and Robins, *J. Chem. Soc. (Lond.)*, p. 3008 (1962).
42. Miyaki and Shimizu, *Chem. Pharm. Bull. (Tokyo)*, 18, 1446 (1970).
43. Lawley and Thatcher, *Biochem. J.*, 116, 693 (1970).
44. Balsiger and Montgomery, *J. Am. Chem. Soc.*, 25, 1573 (1960).
45. Leonard and Frihart, *J. Am. Chem. Soc.*, 96, 5894 (1974).
46. Hendler, Furer, and Srinivasan, *Biochemistry*, 9, 4141 (1970).
47. Brookes and Lawley, *J. Chem. Soc. (Lond.)*, p. 3923 (1961).
48. Brookes and Lawley, *Biochem. J.*, 77, 478 (1960).
49. Singer, *Biochemistry*, 11, 3939 (1972).
50. Pfleiderer, Shanshal, and Eistetter, *Chem. Ber.*, 105, 1497 (1972).
51. Kenner, Reese, and Todd, *J. Chem. Soc. (Lond.)*, p. 855 (1955).
52. Fox and Shugar, *Biochim. Biophys. Acta*, 9, 369 (1952).
53. Sukhorukov, Gukovskaya, Sukhoruchkina, and Lavrrenova, *Biophysica*, 17, 5 (1972).
54. Brookes and Lawley, *J. Chem. Soc. (Lond.)*, p. 1348 (1962).
55. Sun and Singer, *Biochemistry*, 13, 1905 (1974).
56. Szer and Shugar, *Acta Biochim. Pol.*, 13, 177 (1966).
57. Wempen, Duschinsky, Kaplan, and Fox, *J. Am. Chem. Soc.*, 83, 4755 (1961).
58. Shugar and Fox, *Biochim. Biophys. Acta*, 9, 199 (1952).
59. Notari, Witiak, DeYoung, and Lin, *J. Med Chem.*, 15, 1207 (1972).
60. Fox, Praag, Wempen, Doerr, Cheong, Knoll, Eidinoff, Bendich, and Brown, *J. Am. Chem. Soc.*, 81, 178 (1959).
61. Lichtenberg, Bergmann, and Neiman, *J. Chem. Soc. C*, p. 1676 (1971).
62. Pfleiderer and Nubel, *Justus Liebigs Ann. Chem.*, 647, 155 (1961).
63. Pfleiderer, *Justus Liebigs Ann. Chem.*, 647, 161 (1961).
64. Brown, Hoerger, and Mason, *J. Chem. Soc., (Lond.)*, p. 211 (1955).
65. Wittenburg, *Collect. Czech. Chem. Commun.*, 36, 246 (1971).
65a. Wong and Fuchs, *J. Org. Chem.*, 35, 3786 (1970).
65b. Wong and Fuchs, *J. Org. Chem.*, 36, 848 (1971).
66. Wierzchowski, Litonska, and Shugar, *J. Am. Chem. Soc.*, 87, 4621 (1965).
66a. Miles, *J. Org. Chem.*, 26, 4761 (1961).
67. Bergmann, Levin, Kalmus, and Kwietny-Govrin, *J. Am. Chem. Soc.*, 26, 1504 (1961).
68. Rajabalee and Hanessian, *Can. J. Chem.*, 49, 1981 (1971).
69. Montgomery and Thomas, *J. Am. Chem. Soc.*, 28, 2304 (1963).
70. Michelson and Pochon, *Biochim. Biophys. Acta*, 114, 469 (1966).
71. Haines, Reese, and Todd, *J. Chem. Soc. (Lond.)*, p. 1406 (1964).
72. Coddington, *Biochim. Biophys. Acta*, 59, 472 (1962).
73. Saneyoshi, Ohashi, Harada, and Nishimura, *Biochim. Biophys. Acta*, 262, 1 (1972).
74. Jones and Robins, *J. Am. Chem. Soc.*, 85, 193 (1963).
74a. Johnson, Thomas, and Schaeffer, *J. Am. Chem. Soc.*, 80, 699 (1958).
75. Kissman and Weiss, *J. Am. Chem. Soc.*, 21, 1053 (1956).
76. Fleysher, *J. Med. Chem.*, 15, 187 (1972).
77. Fanner, Foster, Jarman, and Tisdale, *Biochem. J.*, 135, 203 (1973).
78. Loveless, *Nature*, 223, 206 (1969).
79. Saponara and Enger, *Nature*, 223, 1365 (1969).
80. Robins and Naik, *Biochemistry*, 10, 3591 (1971).
81. Kusmierek, Giziewica, and Shugar, *Biochemistry*, 12, 194 (1973).
82. Dekker and Elmore, *J. Chem. Soc. (Lond.)*, p. 2864 (1951).
83. Imura, Tsuruo, and Ukita, *Chem. Pharm. Bull.*, 16, 1105 (1968).
84. Winkley and Robins, *J. Org. Chem.*, 33, 2822 (1968).
85. Miles, *Biochim. Biophys. Acta*, 22, 247 (1956).
86. Brown, Todd, and Varadarajan, *J. Chem. Soc. (Lond.)*, p. 868 (1957).
87. Kimura, Fujisawa, Sawada, and Mitsunobu, *Chem. Lett.*, 691 (1974).
88. Holy, Bald, and Hong, *Collect. Czech. Chem. Commun.*, 36, 2658 (1971).
89. Lawley, Orr, Shah, Farmer, and Jarman, *Biochem. J.*, 135, 193 (1973).
90. Griffin and Reese, *Biochim. Biophys. Acta*, 68, 185 (1963).
91. Michelson and Grunberg-Manago, *Biochim. Biophys. Acta*, 91, 92 (1964).
92. Hattori, Ikehara, and Miles, *Biochim. Biophys. Acta*, 13, 2754 (1974).
93. Pochon and Michelson, *Biochim. Biophys. Acta*, 145, 321 (1967).
94. Lawley and Shah, *Biochem. J.*, 128, 117 (1972).
95. Gerchman, Dombrowski, and Ludlum, *Biochim. Biophys. Acta*, 272, 672 (1972).
96. Pochon and Michelson, *Biochim. Biophys. Acta*, 182, 17 (1969).
97. Ludlum and Wilhelm, *J. Biol Chem.*, 243, 2750 (1968).
98. Brimacombe and Reese, *J. Chem. Soc. C*, p. 588 (1966).
99. Brimacombe, *Biochim. Biophys. Acta*, 142, 24 (1967).
100. Szer, *Biochem. Biophys. Res. Commun.*, 20, 182 (1965).
101. Cohn, *J. Am. Chem. Soc.*, 73, 1539 (1951).

ULTRAVIOLET ABSORBANCE OF OLIGONUCLEOTIDES CONTAINING 2′-O-METHYLPENTOSE[a] RESIDUES

Compound	Min	Max	Absorbance ratios[b]				
			240	250	270	280	290
pH 7							
Am-Cp	225	256	0.46	0.88	0.63	0.17	0.02
Am-Gp	227	261	0.59	0.81	0.83	0.42	0.12
Am-Up	225	256	0.54	0.93	0.70	0.38	0.14
AM-Up	228	260	0.41	0.79	0.72	0.26	0.03
CM-Cp	249	268	0.95	0.85	1.17	0.87	0.32
Cm-Ap	227	261	0.62	0.83	0.81	0.42	0.13
Cm-Gp	224	254	0.87	1.04	0.92	0.74	0.33
Gm-Ap	225	256	0.57	0.93	0.72	0.40	0.16
Gm-Cp	225	255	0.82	1.00	0.93	0.69	0.28
Gm-Up	226	255	0.63	0.97	0.81	0.52	0.19
Um-Ap	228	258	0.46	0.83	0.71	0.25	0.03
Um-Gp	226	255	0.62	0.98	0.79	0.51	0.18
Um-Up	229	260	0.43	0.78	0.79	0.35	0.04
Am-Am-Up	228	258	0.44	0.83	0.70	0.25	0.04
Am-Gm-Cp	225	257	0.65	0.94	0.79	0.45	0.17
Am-Um-Gp	227	257	0.53	0.86	0.76	0.39	0.13
pH 2							
Am-Ap	229	257	0.44	0.84	0.70	0.23	0.05
Am-Cp	234	264	0.40	0.74	0.97	0.75	0.45
Am-Gp	227	256	0.54	0.93	0.71	0.42	0.23
Am-Up	229	258	0.44	0.82	0.72	0.27	0.05
Cm-Cp	239	278	0.28	0.47	1.67	1.96	1.39
Cm-Ap	234	264	0.39	0.73	0.98	0.76	0.48
Cm-Gp	232	276	0.48	0.79	1.06	1.08	0.73
Gm-Ap	227	256	0.54	0.92	0.70	0.42	0.22
Gm-Cp	230	274	0.53	0.83	1.07	1.04	0.67
Gm-Up	228	257	0.53	0.89	0.77	0.50	0.26
Um-Ap	229	257	0.48	0.86	0.72	0.27	0.05
Um-Gp	228	258	0.49	0.86	0.78	0.52	0.28
Um-Up	230	260	0.44	0.80	0.76	0.31	0.03
Am-Am-Up	230	257	0.48	0.86	0.71	0.27	0.05
Am-Gm-Cp	230	258	0.53	0.86	0.88	0.69	0.42
Am-Um-Gp	228	258	0.48	0.86	0.74	0.40	0.19
pH 12							
Am-Ap	227	257	0.42	0.84	0.68	0.19	0.03
Am-Cp	226	261	0.59	0.83	0.81	0.41	0.12
Am-Gp	228	258	0.50	0.86	0.76	0.36	0.06
Am-Up	230	260	0.55	0.83	0.69	0.18	0.03
Cm-Cp	249	268	0.94	0.86	1.15	0.88	0.34
Cm-Ap	228	262	0.60	0.81	0.83	0.43	0.13
Cm-Gp	230	268	0.71	0.87	1.03	0.73	0.22
Gm-Ap	228	259	0.50	0.85	0.80	0.38	0.06
Gm-Cp	230	268	0.74	0.89	1.02	0.71	0.20
Gm-Up	226	255	0.63	0.97	0.81	0.52	0.19
Um-Ap	230	258	0.56	0.84	0.69	0.21	0.04
Um-Gp	233	260	0.65	0.87	0.87	0.48	0.09
Um-Up	241	260	0.79	0.86	0.79	0.29	0.04
Am-Am-Up	229	258	0.53	0.86	0.71	0.24	0.04
Am-Gm-Cp	228	261	0.59	0.86	0.83	0.46	0.12
Am-Um-Gp	230	259	0.55	0.85	0.79	0.36	0.14

Compiled by A. R. Trim.

[a] The pentose is presumed to be 2'-O-methylribose since the dinucleotides were obtained from yeast ribonucleic acid. Evidence for the chemical constitution of the modified pentose is given in Howlett et al.[1] and Trim and Parker.[2]

[b] Absorbance ratios were calculated from optical densities at 240, 250, 270, 280, and 290 nm relative to that at 260 nm.

Values for trinucleotides are from Trim and Parker.[3] Data on dinucleotides are from Trim and Parker, *Biochem*, J., 116, 589 (1970). With permission. Copyright by the Biochemical Society.

References

1. Howlett, Johnson, Trim, Eagles, and Self, *Anal. Biochem.*, 39, 429 (1971).

2. Trim and Parker, *Anal. Biochem.*, 46, 482 (1972).
3. Trim and Parker, unpublished data.

SPECTROPHOTOMETRIC CONSTANTS OF RIBONUCLEOTIDES

TABLE 1: Ultraviolet Absorbance of Mono- and Oligonucleotides

Compound	pH 7		Absorbance Ratios[a]					pH 1		Absorbance Ratios[a]					pH 12		Absorbance Ratios[a]					Slack[b] pct.
	λ_{min}	λ_{max}	240	250	270	280	290	λ_{min}	λ_{max}	240	250	270	280t	290	λ_{min}	λ_{max}	240	250	270	280	290	
Ap	226	259	0.41	0.79	0.65	0.14	0.00	226	257	0.46	0.87	0.67	0.22	0.00	227	259	0.40	0.79	0.66	0.14	0.00	cat.[c]
Cp	250	271	0.94	0.85	1.17	0.90	0.28	241	278	0.27	0.47	1.65	1.91	1.34	225	228	0.95	0.85	1.18	0.90	0.29	cat.
Gp	231	264	0.81	1.17	0.82	0.68	0.26	227	256	0.52	0.93	0.75	0.69	0.48	225	260	0.55	0.88	0.96	0.58	0.00	cat.
Up	230	261	0.39	0.75	0.82	0.33	0.00	229	261	0.41	0.78	0.79	0.30	0.00	242	261	0.75	0.83	0.79	0.27	0.00	cat.
pApA	227	258	0.41	0.83	0.66	0.19	0.00	229	256	0.45	0.86	0.67	0.21	0.00	229	258	0.42	0.82	0.66	0.18	0.00	1.0
ApCp	227	261	0.57	0.81	0.81	0.40	0.12	228	265	0.39	0.73	0.98	0.75	0.45	228	261	0.59	0.81	0.82	0.41	0.12	2.3
ApGp	225	256	0.58	0.97	0.71	0.37	0.13	229	257	0.47	0.88	0.71	0.42	0.24	229	259	0.46	0.83	0.79	0.35	0.00	0.9
ApUp	228	259	0.40	0.80	0.73	0.24	0.00	230	258	0.43	0.82	0.72	0.26	0.00	232	259	0.53	0.81	0.71	0.20	0.00	1.8
CpCp	250	269	0.94	0.85	1.17	0.90	0.30	241	278	0.24	0.44	1.69	1.96	1.37	250	270	0.95	0.85	1.19	0.92	0.33	1.3
CpGp	224	254	0.84	1.04	0.93	0.73	0.30	233	277	0.39	0.74	1.08	1.12	0.79	231	250	0.69	0.86	1.04	0.72	0.20	1.8
GpCp	224	255	0.83	1.01	0.94	0.70	0.27	233	276	0.43	0.76	1.08	1.10	0.76	231	267	0.71	0.88	1.04	0.70	0.17	1.7
GpUp	226	255	0.62	0.98	0.81	0.51	0.17	229	258	0.46	0.86	0.76	0.50	0.28	233	261	0.64	0.87	0.90	0.47	0.00	2.8
UpAp	228	259	0.42	0.81	0.70	0.24	0.00	228	257	0.45	0.85	0.72	0.27	0.00	231	259	0.54	0.83	0.70	0.21	0.00	2.9
UpGp	226	256	0.60	0.98	0.79	0.50	0.18	226	258	0.43	0.83	0.78	0.50	0.28	234	261	0.61	0.85	0.89	0.48	0.00	2.9
UpUp	229	260	0.41	0.78	0.80	0.33	0.00	229	260	0.42	0.79	0.78	0.31	0.00	242	260	0.79	0.85	0.78	0.29	0.00	0.4
pApApA	228	258	0.44	0.85	0.67	0.24	0.00	230	257	0.47	0.86	0.68	0.22	0.00	230	258	0.40	0.82	0.68	0.24	0.00	1.6
ApApCp	228	258	0.55	0.85	0.76	0.39	0.11	230	259	0.44	0.79	0.86	0.55	0.31	232	259	0.54	0.82	0.77	0.39	0.11	1.5
ApApGp	226	256	0.54	0.94	0.70	0.33	0.11	229	257	0.47	0.88	0.70	0.35	0.17	230	258	0.46	0.84	0.75	0.32	0.00	1.0
ApApUp	228	258	0.41	0.82	0.70	0.25	0.00	229	257	0.44	0.84	0.70	0.24	0.00	230	258	0.49	0.83	0.70	0.22	0.00	2.1
ApCpCp	229	262	0.66	0.82	0.89	0.52	0.18	236	270	0.37	0.67	1.16	1.04	0.69	234	263	0.67	0.81	0.91	0.54	0.20	2.6
ApCpGp	225	257	0.65	0.94	0.89	0.49	0.19	231	260	0.42	0.79	0.91	0.74	0.48	231	261	0.56	0.83	0.81	0.48	0.12	1.5
ApGpCp	226	257	0.65	0.94	0.81	0.47	0.18	231	260	0.43	0.79	0.89	0.70	0.45	230	261	0.56	0.83	0.87	0.47	0.12	1.8
ApGpUp	227	257	0.53	0.91	0.73	0.36	0.11	229	257	0.45	0.85	0.73	0.39	0.18	232	259	0.52	0.83	0.79	0.34	0.00	1.7
ApUpGp	227	257	0.51	0.90	0.73	0.36	0.11	229	258	0.43	0.83	0.74	0.40	0.19	231	259	0.51	0.82	0.80	0.34	0.00	1.9
CpApGp	226	257	0.67	0.93	0.82	0.53	0.21	231	260	0.42	0.79	0.91	0.74	0.48	230	260	0.58	0.84	0.87	0.51	0.12	0.9
CpCpGp	225	257	0.85	0.98	0.99	0.77	0.33	235	278	0.36	0.66	1.23	1.33	0.95	232	268	0.75	0.85	1.08	0.76	0.23	1.6
GpApCp	226	258	0.63	0.91	0.79	0.50	0.19	231	259	0.44	0.80	0.89	0.71	0.46	230	260	0.56	0.83	0.87	0.50	0.12	1.7
GpApUp	227	257	0.52	0.89	0.74	0.38	0.11	229	258	0.46	0.86	0.73	0.39	0.18	231	259	0.53	0.83	0.80	0.36	0.00	1.8
GpGpCp	224	254	0.79	1.06	0.87	0.65	0.27	230	260	0.45	0.82	0.92	0.87	0.61	231	266	0.61	0.87	1.00	0.65	0.14	2.6
GpGpUp	225	254	0.68	1.05	0.80	0.55	0.21	228	257	0.47	0.88	0.76	0.56	0.35	233	261	0.57	0.86	0.92	0.51	0.00	2.4
UpApUp	226	257	0.53	0.92	0.73	0.38	0.12	229	258	0.44	0.85	0.74	0.40	0.19	231	259	0.52	0.83	0.79	0.35	0.00	2.0
UpCpCp	230	264	0.72	0.83	0.99	0.65	0.20	236	273	0.32	0.59	1.28	1.22	0.79	248	266	0.92	0.88	1.02	0.67	0.22	2.3
UpUpGp	228	257	0.54	0.91	0.79	0.45	0.14	229	259	0.43	0.82	0.77	0.45	0.21	235	260	0.67	0.86	0.87	0.43	0.00	2.5
pApApApA	229	257	0.43	0.85	0.68	0.25	0.00	229	257	0.45	0.86	0.69	0.22	0.00	230	257	0.42	0.84	0.67	0.25	0.00	0.7
ApApApCp	230	258	0.50	0.84	0.72	0.34	0.00	232	258	0.44	0.82	0.79	0.43	0.00	231	258	0.51	0.83	0.73	0.35	0.00	2.1
ApApApGp	227	256	0.51	0.92	0.69	0.32	0.00	229	257	0.46	0.87	0.69	0.31	0.13	230	258	0.45	0.86	0.74	0.31	0.00	0.5
CpCpCpGp	227	267	0.86	0.95	1.01	0.78	0.34	236	278	0.34	0.62	1.31	1.44	1.03	235	268	0.78	0.86	1.09	0.79	0.27	1.3
UpUpUpGp	228	258	0.49	0.85	0.80	0.41	0.00	230	260	0.41	0.80	0.80	0.43	0.16	237	260	0.69	0.85	0.84	0.38	0.00	2.3

Contributed by Jane N. Toal.

a Absorbance ratios were calculated from optical densities at 240, 250, 270, 280, and 290 mμ relative to that at 260 mμ. Ratios not calculated where optical density was less than 0.1.

b Slack = the absolute sum of the catalog mismatch at every wavelength.

c cat. = catalog.

From data in Toal, Rushizky, Pratt, and Sober, Anal. Biochem., 23, 60 (1968). With permission of the copyright owners, Academic Press, New York.

TABLE 2: Hyperchromicity Ratios of Oligonucleotides at Different Wavelengths (mμ)[a]

Compound	pH 7						pH 1						pH 12					
	240	250	260	270	280	290	240	250	260	270	280	290	240	250	260	270	280	290
pApA	1.11	1.11	1.16	1.13	0.81	0.00	1.03	1.02	1.02	1.02	1.00	0.00	1.09	1.10	1.15	1.12	0.84	0.00
ApCp	1.10	1.09	1.08	1.11	1.05	0.88	1.02	1.02	1.02	1.02	1.03	1.01	1.09	1.10	1.08	1.10	1.04	0.91
ApGp	1.08	1.06	1.07	1.09	1.07	0.96	1.06	1.04	1.02	1.02	1.04	1.00	1.04	1.03	1.03	1.03	0.98	0.00
ApUp	1.08	1.09	1.09	1.07	0.97	0.00	1.06	1.05	1.04	1.03	1.01	0.00	1.01	1.03	1.04	1.03	0.95	0.00
CpCp	1.09	1.08	1.08	1.10	1.10	0.96	1.05	1.04	1.02	1.02	1.02	1.01	1.10	1.10	1.10	1.10	1.09	0.94
CpGp	1.08	1.06	1.05	1.09	1.10	0.94	1.08	1.04	1.02	1.02	1.03	1.01	1.07	1.05	1.04	1.05	1.03	0.88
GpCp	1.11	1.09	1.05	1.08	1.16	1.05	1.04	1.05	1.05	1.06	1.08	1.10	1.04	1.03	1.04	1.05	1.05	0.95
GpUp	1.07	1.05	1.05	1.07	1.08	0.99	1.12	1.09	1.08	1.10	1.12	1.09	1.02	1.02	1.02	1.02	1.01	0.00
UpAp	1.07	1.05	1.08	1.10	0.99	0.00	1.06	1.05	1.06	1.05	0.99	0.00	1.06	1.06	1.06	1.05	0.95	0.00
UpGp	1.05	1.02	1.02	1.07	1.06	0.91	1.08	1.05	1.01	1.01	1.03	1.00	1.01	1.01	1.00	1.01	0.97	0.00
UpUp	0.98	1.00	1.04	1.07	1.05	0.00	1.01	1.02	1.03	1.03	0.98	0.00	0.96	0.98	1.01	1.01	0.94	0.00
pApApA	1.20	1.20	1.27	1.23	0.78	0.00	1.05	1.05	1.04	1.03	1.01	0.00	1.33	1.25	1.29	1.24	0.79	0.00
ApApCp	1.20	1.19	1.22	1.22	0.99	0.85	1.04	1.04	1.04	1.04	1.04	1.02	1.21	1.21	1.23	1.22	1.00	0.90
ApApGp	1.11	1.11	1.15	1.16	1.01	0.85	1.01	1.01	1.00	1.00	1.01	0.98	1.07	1.07	1.11	1.10	0.92	0.00
ApApUp	1.18	1.16	1.21	1.18	0.88	0.00	1.06	1.05	1.05	1.04	0.99	0.00	1.14	1.14	1.18	1.14	0.86	0.00
ApCpCp	1.22	1.20	1.18	1.20	1.16	0.91	1.09	1.08	1.06	1.05	1.05	1.02	1.25	1.24	1.20	1.19	1.17	0.95
ApCpGp	1.14	1.11	1.12	1.16	1.13	0.90	1.06	1.06	1.05	1.05	1.05	1.01	1.11	1.10	1.09	1.10	1.05	0.85
ApGpCp	1.14	1.11	1.12	1.13	1.16	1.00	1.04	1.05	1.03	1.04	1.07	1.06	1.07	1.06	1.07	1.08	1.04	0.89
ApGpUp	1.10	1.08	1.10	1.12	1.09	0.93	1.09	1.07	1.05	1.05	1.05	1.01	1.05	1.04	1.04	1.04	0.97	0.00
ApUpGp	1.11	1.09	1.10	1.12	1.10	0.93	1.10	1.08	1.05	1.04	1.04	1.00	1.04	1.04	1.04	1.04	0.97	0.00
CpApGp	1.16	1.16	1.16	1.18	1.10	0.87	1.06	1.04	1.03	1.04	1.05	1.01	1.10	1.09	1.10	1.11	1.02	0.88
CpCpGp	1.15	1.12	1.10	1.15	1.15	0.89	1.05	1.05	1.03	1.03	1.04	1.01	1.09	1.08	1.07	1.08	1.08	0.89
GpApCp	1.19	1.17	1.13	1.18	1.11	0.94	1.04	1.06	1.05	1.06	1.08	1.04	1.11	1.11	1.10	1.11	1.02	0.90
GpApUp	1.14	1.13	1.12	1.13	1.05	0.92	1.07	1.07	1.07	1.07	1.09	1.06	1.04	1.06	1.06	1.05	0.96	0.00
GpGpCp	1.13	1.11	1.07	1.12	1.19	1.05	1.08	1.07	1.06	1.08	1.12	1.11	1.07	1.04	1.03	1.04	1.02	0.89
GpGpUp	1.09	1.08	1.07	1.11	1.11	0.97	1.12	1.09	1.08	1.09	1.11	1.07	1.07	1.03	1.02	1.01	0.99	0.00
UpApGp	1.13	1.10	1.12	1.15	1.08	0.94	1.10	1.06	1.05	1.05	1.05	1.01	1.08	1.07	1.07	1.07	1.00	0.00
UpCpCp	1.09	1.07	1.09	1.14	1.14	0.91	0.99	1.02	1.03	1.04	1.05	1.02	1.02	1.03	1.07	1.11	1.10	0.90
UpUpGp	1.06	1.04	1.04	1.08	1.07	0.89	1.09	1.07	1.04	1.05	1.03	0.98	1.00	1.01	1.00	1.00	0.97	0.00
pApApApA	1.29	1.28	1.36	1.31	0.76	0.00	1.09	1.07	1.06	1.03	1.01	0.00	1.32	1.29	1.38	1.36	0.80	0.00
ApApApCp	1.23	1.23	1.07	1.25	0.92	0.00	1.02	1.03	1.03	1.03	1.02	0.00	1.22	1.25	1.29	1.26	0.96	0.00
ApApApGp	1.18	1.18	1.25	1.24	0.95	0.00	1.03	1.03	1.02	1.01	1.01	0.97	1.15	1.14	1.22	1.19	0.88	0.00
CpCpCpGp	1.21	1.16	1.15	1.20	1.22	0.93	1.07	1.06	1.04	1.04	1.05	1.02	1.16	1.12	1.12	1.14	1.14	0.92
UpUpUpGp	1.08	1.06	1.07	1.10	1.07	0.00	1.10	1.06	1.05	1.05	1.03	0.97	1.00	1.02	1.03	1.02	0.98	0.00

Contributed by Jane N. Toal.

[a] Hyperchromicity ratios were calculated as the optical density of a hydrolyzed compound divided by the optical density of the corresponding intact compound at the same wavelength. Ratios are calculated where optical density was less than 0.1.

From data in Toal, Rushizky, Pratt, and Sober, *Anal. Biochem.*, 23, 60 (1968). With permission of the copyright owners, Academic Press, New York.

TABLE 3: Ultraviolet Absorbance of Mononucleotides in 7 M Urea

Compound	pH 7.0 (0.05 M Phosphate)		Absorbance Ratios					pH 1 (0.1 M HCl)		Absorbance Ratios					pH 12 (0.01 M NaOH)		Absorbance Ratios				
	λ_{min}	λ_{max}	240	250	270	280	290	λ_{min}	λ_{max}	240	250	270	280	290	λ_{min}	λ_{max}	240	250	270	280	290
pA	228	261	0.357	0.739	0.727	0.206	–	232	258	0.395	0.795	0.762	0.277	–	228	260	0.371	0.742	0.730	0.205	–
pC	251	272.5	0.998	0.881	1.240	1.068	0.424	243	281	0.342	0.456	1.795	2.333	1.949	251	272.5	1.004	0.877	1.237	1.078	0.438
pG	225	254	0.718	1.098	0.810	0.662	0.297	229	258	0.458	0.868	0.741	0.665	0.538	232	258	0.513	0.863	0.969	0.650	0.133
pU	231	263	0.353	0.706	0.898	0.438	–	231	262	0.361	0.718	0.879	0.423	–	242	262	0.704	0.801	0.855	0.355	–

TABLE 4: Ultraviolet Absorbance of Mononucleotides in 97% D_2O

Compound	pH 7.0 (0.05 M Phosphate)		Absorbance Ratios					pH 1 (0.1 M HCl)		Absorbance Ratios					pH 12 (0.01 M NaOH)		Absorbance Ratios				
	λ_{min}	λ_{max}	240	250	270	280	290	λ_{min}	λ_{max}	240	250	270	280	290	λ_{min}	λ_{max}	240	250	270	280	290
pA	226	258	0.414	0.817	0.618	0.136	–	229	257	0.473	0.875	0.650	0.206	–	227	258	0.418	0.814	0.608	0.135	–
pC	249	271	0.931	0.822	1.231	0.970	0.308	240	279	0.220	0.430	1.706	2.028	1.482	250	271	0.948	0.828	1.242	0.995	0.327
pG	223	252.5	0.589	1.181	0.829	0.664	0.248	227	256	0.535	0.957	0.740	0.705	0.505	230	264	0.543	0.883	0.951	0.549	–
pU	230	262	0.386	0.747	0.845	0.372	–	229	261	0.398	0.757	0.822	0.343	–	242	261	0.712	0.821	0.793	0.276	–

TABLE 5: Ultraviolet Absorbance of Mononucleotides in 90% V/V Ethylene Glycol

Compound	pH 7.0 (0.05 M Phosphate)		Absorbance Ratios					pH 1 (0.1 M HCl)		Absorbance Ratios					pH 12 (0.01 M NaOH)		Absorbance Ratios				
	λ_{min}	λ_{max}	240	250	270	280	290	λ_{min}	λ_{max}	240	250	270	280	290	λ_{min}	λ_{max}	240	250	270	280	290
pA	229	260	0.374	0.743	0.743	0.251	–	233	263	0.472	0.816	0.744	0.282	–	228	259	0.405	0.775	0.726	0.237	–
pC	253	279	1.082	0.937	1.253	1.162	0.518	243	283	0.372	0.443	1.838	2.480	2.210	252	274	1.040	0.909	1.267	1.165	0.560
pG	224	251	0.768	1.131	0.781	0.650	0.339	230	257.5	0.463	0.852	0.704	0.595	0.479	226	254	0.699	1.069	0.768	0.651	0.329
pU	232	263	0.344	0.687	0.932	0.486	–	232	262	0.366	0.712	0.897	0.445	–	232	263	0.353	0.698	0.931	0.481	–

From data of Hoffman, J. L., and Bock, R. M. Mononucleoside 5'-phosphates obtained from P-L Biochemicals, Milwaukee, Wisconsin, were used. The spectra were determined using a Cary 15 spectrometer. These tables originally appeared in Sober, H., *Handbook of Biochemistry and selected data for Molecular Biology*, 2nd ed., Chemical Rubber Co., Cleveland, 1970.

PURINES, PYRIMIDINES, NUCLEOSIDES, AND NUCLEOTIDES: PHYSICAL CONSTANTS AND SPECTRAL PROPERTIES

David B. Dunn, and Ross H. Hall

Data are included for most modified components of nucleic acids, for some naturally occurring purine and pyrimidine compounds, and for some related synthetic compounds. An index to the 246 compounds is provided (arranged as free bases, nucleosides, and nucleotides).

It is recommended that, where possible, compounds be referred to by the trivial names given in bold type. (Some of these, such as "wye", "wyosine" and "zeatosine", are new proposals made by W. E. Cohn and D. B. Dunn.) Systematic and other trivial names are given, particularly where these already occur in the literature. Compounds are arranged as: purines and pyrimidines, ribonucleosides (including arabinonucleosides), deoxyribonucleosides, ribonucleotides and deoxyribonucleotides. The principal compounds are arranged alphabetically, with derivatives grouped

after each, the position of the latter depending first on the locant of the substituent and second on its initial letter. Compounds with a modified, or more than one substituent group, follow the simpler compounds.

The symbols are in accord with the examples and principles set out by the IUPAC-IUB Commission on Biochemical Nomenclature. A summary of these rules is found elsewhere in the Handbook. The "3-letter" symbols are proposed for use in tables, figures, equations involving the monomeric units themselves, the "1-letter" symbols for sequences. For deoxyribonucleosides in sequences, d may precede the sequence and thus be eliminated from each residue. Symbols that have been proposed or used, but are not now recommended are marked by an asterisk. The following symbols for substituents are used:

		Symbols	
Substituent	Structure	3-Letter	1-Letter
acetyl-	CH_3CO-	Ac	ac
(-)amino-, imino-	NH_2^-, $-NH-$, $NH=$	NH_2, NH	n
-α-aminobutyric acid (3-carboxy-3-aminopropyl-)	$HOOC-C(NH_2)-(CH_2)_2-$	(NH_2Bto) (NH_2CxPr)	nbt
arabinosyl-		Ara	a
		a	
butyl-	$CH_3(CH_2)_3^-$	Bu	b
-butyramide (3-carbamoylpropyl-)	$NH_2CO(CH_2)_3^-$	Btn NcPr	
-butyric acid (3-carboxypropyl-)	$HOOC(CH_2)_3^-$	Bto CxPr	bt
dihydro		H_2	h
carbamoyl-	NH_2CO-	Nc	nc
carbamoylmethyl- (-acetamide)	$NH_2COCH_2^-$	Ncm NcMe	ncm
-carbonyl-	$-CO-$	CO	c
carboxy- (-oxycarbonyl-)	$HOOC-$, $-OOC-$	Cx	c
carboxymethyl- (-acetic acid)	$HOOC-CH_2^-$	Cm	cm
		CxMe	
cis		*cis*	
formamido-	$HCONH-$	Fn	fn
glycino-	$HOOC-CH_2NH-$	Gly	g
hydroperoxy-	$HOO-$	O_2	o_2
methoxy-	CH_3O-	MeO	mo
-oxy-	$-O-$	O	o
pentyl-	$CH_3(CH_2)_4^-$	Pe	
putrescino- (aminobutylamino-)	$NH_2(CH_2)_4NH-$	Put (NH_2BuNH)	nbn
propyl-	$CH_3(CH_2)_2^-$	Pr	
ribosyl-		Rib	r
(-)thio (mercapto-)	$-S-$, $S=$	S	s
threonino-	$CH_3-CHOH-C(COOH)NH-$	Thr	t
threoninocarbonyl-	$CH_3-CHOH-C(COOH)NH-CO-$	(ThrCO)	tc
trans		*tr*	
hydroxy-	$HO-$	HO	o
hydroxymethyl- (-methanol)	$HOCH_2^-$	HOMe Hm	om hm*
isopropeno-methyl-		im*	
iso		*iso*	
isopentenyl- (3-methyl-2-butenyl-)	$(CH_3)_2C=CHCH_2^-$	iPe Pe^i	i
methoxycarbonylmethyl- (-acetic acid methyl ester)	$CH_3O-CO-CH_2^-$	MeCm	mcm
3-methoxycarbonyl-3- methoxyformamidopropyl-	$CH_3O-CO-C(NHCOOCH_3)-(CH_2)_2^-$	Y (MeO)$_2$ FnBto	y m$_2$ fnbt
methyl-	CH_3^-	Me	m

Data were taken where possible on chemically synthesized material.

The first reference cited in the origin and synthesis column gives the origin of the compound used to obtain the principal spectral data. C = chemical synthesis; E = prepared enzymically; R = isolated from RNA; D = isolated from DNA; N = isolated from natural product other than nucleic acids.

The melting points were taken from the first reference to chemical synthesis except where otherwise indicated by footnote (*a*); dec. signifies decomposition.

For $[\alpha]_D^t$ the temperature is given as a superscript and the concentration and solvent used in obtaining the value in parenthesis; H_2O = in water; EtOH = in ethanol; MeOH = in methanol; Me_2SO = in dimethylsulfoxide.

pK values were taken from the first reference quoted except where values differed by only 0.2 pH units when a mean value was used. References that give values deviating from those quoted by more than ±0.1 pH units are marked with an asterisk (*). The pK values involved are similarly marked. The pK values for nucleotides are only those for the nucleoside moiety, not phosphate ionizations. Where pK values were determined from electrophoretic mobilities (footnote *p*) values were obtained from mobilities relative to the parent compounds and pK values of these given by Jordan (1955) in *The Nucleic Acids*, Chargaff and Davidson, Eds., Academic Press, New York I, p 447.

Where possible, all spectral values are given at pH values away from pK values; exceptions to this are indicated by a footnote. Data obtained at a pH value where the compound was unstable were obtained soon after subjecting the material to this pH and differ from those of the decomposition products. The reference giving the maximum amount of spectral data is cited first; other references giving additional data are marked by footnotes. (These, *c* to *e*, indicate that some but not necessarily all the data mentioned come from this reference.) The ratio columns give ratio of absorption at the wavelength given to that at 260 nm. In the pH column of spectral data. H_2O=in water; EtOH=in ethanol; MeOH=in methanol. References that give spectral data differing from the values quoted are marked with an asterisk as are also the values involved. For this, deviations were marked only where they were more than ±1 nm for λ_{max} or λ_{min}, ±5 per cent for ε_{max}, and ±10 per cent for spectral ratios. (The latter applies to all instances where spectral ratios are quoted in the additional reference but not necessarily to all references giving spectra.)

PURINES, PYRIMIDINES, NUCLEOSIDES AND NUCLEOTIDES: PHYSICAL CONSTANTS AND SPECTRAL PROPERTIES

PURINES AND PYRIMIDINES

No.	Compound	Symbol (3-Letter)	Symbol (1-Letter)	Structure	Formula (Mol Wt)	Melting Point °C	$[\alpha]_D^t$	pK Basic	pK Acidic
1	Adenine	Ade		(structure, NH_2)	$C_5H_5N_5$ (135.13)	360° (dec) (sublimes 220°)	–	<1,4,15	9.8
2	1-(Δ²-Isopentenyl)adenine / 1-(γγ-Dimethylallyl)adenine	1iPeAde / 1PeAde		(structure, NH)	$C_{10}H_{13}N_5$ (203.24)	237–238°	–	7.1*	11.6^b
3	1-Methyladenine	1MeAde		(structure, NH)	$C_6H_7N_5$ (149.16)	296–299° (dec)	–	7.2	11.0
4	1,N⁶-Dimethyladenine / 1-Methyl-6-methylaminopurine	1,6Me₂ Ade		(structure)	$C_7H_9N_5$ (163.18)	236° (picrate)	–	–	–

Acidic Spectral Data

No.	pH	λ_{max}	ε_{max} (×10⁻³)	λ_{min}	230	240	250	270	280	290
1	1	262.5	13.2	229	0.22	0.42	0.76	0.85	0.38	0.04
2	1	260	13.4	233	–	–	0.80	–	–	–
3	4	259	11.7	228*	0.20	0.41	0.80	0.73	0.23*	0.02*
4	1	261	12.9	230*	–	–	–	–	–	–

Neutral Spectral Data

No.	pH	λ_{max}	ε_{max} (×10⁻³)	λ_{min}	230	240	250	270	280	290
1	7	260.5	13.4	226	0.21	0.43	0.76	0.67	0.13	0.01
2	(EtOH)	273	12.3	246	1.43	0.39	0.52	1.34	0.87	0.14
3	8.8	270	11.9	242	–	–	–	–	–	–
4		–		–	–	–	–	–	–	–

Alkaline Spectral Data

No.	pH	λ_{max}	ε_{max} (×10⁻³)	λ_{min}	230	240	250	270	280	290
1	12	269	12.3	237	0.60	0.36	0.57	1.15	0.60	0.03
2	13	274*	15.2*	242	–	–	–	–	–	–
3	13	270*	14.4	239*	0.64	0.29	0.55*	1.27	0.85	0.35*
4	11	274	12.7	245	–	–	–	–	–	–

REFERENCES

No.	Origin and Synthesis	$[\alpha]_D^t$	pK	Spectral Data	Mass Spectra	R_f
1	C: 231,256ᵃ,257,337,357,358	–	56,22,220,51,336	232ᵇ,242ᵇᵉ,205,317ᵇ,358	–	258,21,18,242,291,292,402
2	C: 14,15	–	15,16*	14,15*	15	14,32,15
3	C: 8,10ᵃ,16,R: 9	–	8	8ᵇ,9ᵇ,10,11*,12*,265*ᵇ,317ᵇ	–	8-13,15
4	C: 24,12,30	–	–	24,12*	–	12,24

PURINES, PYRIMIDINES, NUCLEOSIDES AND NUCLEOTIDES: PHYSICAL CONSTANTS AND SPECTRAL PROPERTIES (Continued)

No.	Compound	Symbol (3-Letter)	1-Letter	Structure	Formula (Mol Wt)	Melting Point °C	$[\alpha]_D^t$	pK Basic	pK Acidic
5	2-Hydroxyadenine Isoguanine	2HOAde *isoGua**			$C_5H_5N_5O$ (151.13)	>360°	—	4.5	9.0
6	2-Methyladenine	2MeAde			$C_6H_7N_5$ (149.16)	>340°	—	*5.1[1]	—
7	3-(Δ^2-Isopentenyl)adenine Triacanthine	3iPeAde 3PeAde			$C_{10}H_{13}N_5$ (203.24)	231–232	—	—	5.4
8	N^6-Glycinocarbonyladenine N-(Purin-6-ylcarbamoyl)glycine	6(Gly C O) Ade			$C_8H_8N_6O_3$ (236.19)	233–234° (dec)	—	—	—

Acidic Spectral Data

No.	pH	λ_{max}	ε_{max} (×10⁻³)	λ_{min}	230	240	250	270	280	290
5	2	284*	11.7*	248	—	—	0.45	—	3.16	—
6	1	266	12.9	229	0.26	0.48	0.79	1.03	0.56	0.04
7	1	277	18.3	239	—	—	—	—	—	—
8	1.4	276.5	18.6	235	0.46	0.44	0.61	1.62	1.82	0.92

Neutral Spectral Data

No.	pH	λ_{max}	ε_{max} (×10⁻³)	λ_{min}	230	240	250	270	280	290
5	7	240	7.8	210	—	—	—	—	—	—
		286	8.0*	255						
6	7	263	12.7	226	—	0.46	0.89	0.83	0.16	—
7	7	273	12.5	247	—	—	—	—	—	—
8	6.2	269	17.4	231	0.40	0.49	0.68	1.43	0.98	0.17
		276	16.9							

Alkaline Spectral Data

No.	pH	λ_{max}	ε_{max} (×10⁻³)	λ_{min}	230	240	250	270	280	290
5	12	284	12.3	253	—	—	0.80	—	3.47	—
6	13	271	10.7	238	0.77	0.40	0.61	1.28	0.84	0.04
8	12.3	278	16.2	240	1.34	0.37	0.54	1.76	2.10	1.23

REFERENCES

No.	Origin and Synthesis	$[\alpha]_D^t$	pK	Spectral Data	Mass Spectra	R_f
5	C: 282,340ᵃ,358,111	—	22	28,283ᵃᵇᶜ,223*ᵉ,282ᵇ,284ᵇ,340,358*	—	340
6	C: 17ᵍ,257ᵃ,340,111 R: 18	—	19	18ᵇ,317ᵇᶜᵈᵉ,20ᵈ,21,257	—	18,21,291,340
7	C: 287,1	—	1	1	—	—
8	C: 408,R: 295	—	—	408	408	408

PURINES, PYRIMIDINES, NUCLEOSIDES AND NUCLEOTIDES: PHYSICAL CONSTANTS AND SPECTRAL PROPERTIES (Continued)

No.	Compound	Symbol 3-Letter	Symbol 1-Letter	Structure	Formula (Mol Wt)	Melting Point °C	$[\alpha]_D^t$	pK Basic	pK Acidic
9	N^6-Threoninocarbonyladenine N-(Purin-6-ylcarbamoyl)threonine	6(ThrCO)Ade			$C_{10}H_{12}N_6O_4$ (280.24)	215–220°	$+30^{25}$ (0.4, H_2O)	<2^p	~3
10	N^6-(Δ^2-Isopentenyl)adenine (N^6-(γ,γ-Dimethylallyl)adenine; 6-(3-Methyl-2-butenylamino)purine	6iPeAde 6PeAd			$C_{10}H_{13}N_5$ (203.24)	213–215°	–	3.4*	10.4*
11	N^6-(Δ^2-Isopentenyl)-2-methylthioadenine 6-(3-Methyl-2-butenylamino)-2-methylthiopurine	2MeS6PeAde 2MeS6iPeAde			$C_{11}H_{15}N_5S$ (249.32)	259–260°	–	–	–
12	N^6-Methyladenine 6-Methylaminopurine	6MeAde			$C_6H_7N_5$ (149.16)	319–320°	–	<1,4,2	10.0

Acidic Spectral Data

No.	pH	λ_{max}	ε_{max} (×10⁻³)	λ_{min}	230	240	250	270	280	290
9	1.6^a	277*	20.6	234*	0.42	0.41	0.60	1.63	1.76*	0.86*
10	1	273*	18.6	235	0.14	0.22	0.57	1.27	1.11	0.64
11	1	253	21.7	217	–	–	–	–	–	–
	(EtOH)	292	15.9	277						
12	1	267	15.3*	232*	0.22	0.31	0.64	1.06	0.70	0.32*

Neutral Spectral Data

No.	pH	λ_{max}	ε_{max} (×10⁻³)	λ_{min}	230	240	250	270	280	290
9	5	269 276*	19.2 18.9	232*	0.28	0.40	0.62	1.51*	1.13*	0.20*
10	7	269	19.4	225	0.06	0.17	0.38	1.31	0.95	0.26
11	7	242	25.2	220	–	–	–	–	0.55	–
	(EtOH)	279	15.9	257						
12	7	266	16.2	231*	0.13	0.24	0.55	0.98	0.55	0.07

Alkaline Spectral Data

No.	pH	λ_{max}	ε_{max} (×10⁻³)	λ_{min}	230	240	250	270	280	290
9	12	278	18.1	240	1.33*	0.32*	0.52	1.81	2.18*	1.32*
10	13	275	18.1	240	0.86	0.28	0.49	1.70	1.60	0.54
11	10 (EtOH)	287	14.8	256	–	–	–	–	–	–
12	13	273	15.9*	239*	0.77	0.39	0.55	1.48	1.19	0.25

REFERENCES

No.	Origin and Synthesis	pK	$[\alpha]_D^t$	Spectral Data	Mass Spectra	R_f
9	C: 408,290,409,4 R: 3	4,90	408	290^b,3*,408	4,404,408	290
10	C: 32,16^a,15	16	–	32,317^{be},14*,15	15,406	32,15
11	C: 293,274	–	–	293	–	–
12	C: 22,23,24,12 D: 21 R: 18	22	–	21^b,18^b,25^{be},317*^{be},28^d,8,23,12*,24*,265*^{b}	–	9,10,12,13,18,21,22,24–27,291,292

PURINES, PYRIMIDINES, NUCLEOSIDES AND NUCLEOTIDES: PHYSICAL CONSTANTS AND SPECTRAL PROPERTIES (Continued)

No.	Compound	Symbol 3-Letter	Symbol 1-Letter	Structure	Formula (Mol Wt)	Melting Point °C	$[\alpha]_D$	pK Basic	pK Acidic
13	N^6,N^6-Dimethyladenine / 6-Dimethylaminopurine	6Me$_2$Ade			$C_7H_9N_5$ (163.18)	257–258°	–	<1,3.9	10.5
14	7-Methyladenine	7MeAde			$C_6H_7N_5$ (149.16)	336° (dec)	–	4.2	–
15	Cytosine	Cyt			$C_4H_5N_3O$ (111.10)	312° (dec)	–	4.6*	12.2
16	3-Methylcytosine	3MeCyt			$C_5H_7N_3O$ (125.13)	242–245° (HCl salt)	–	7.4	>13

Acidic Spectral Data

No.	pH	λ_{max}	ε_{max} (×10⁻³)	λ_{min}	230	240	250	270	280	290
13	1	277	15.6	236	0.29	0.27	0.57	1.33	1.36	0.94
14	1	273*	14.0*	237	0.58*	0.35	0.60	1.35	1.06*	0.21*
15	1	276	10.0	239	0.37	0.22	0.48	1.53	1.53	0.78
16	4	274	9.4	240	0.52	0.27	0.50	1.47	1.33	0.56

(Spectral Ratios: 230, 240, 250, 270, 280, 290)

Neutral Spectral Data

No.	pH	λ_{max}	ε_{max} (×10⁻³)	λ_{min}	230	240	250	270	280	290
13	7	275	17.8	–	–	–	–	–	–	–
14	–	–	–	–	–	–	–	–	–	–
15	7	267	6.1	247	1.13	0.86	0.78	1.05	0.58	0.08
16	–	–	–	–	–	–	–	–	–	–

(Spectral Ratios: 230, 240, 250, 270, 280, 290)

Alkaline Spectral Data

No.	pH	λ_{max}	ε_{max} (×10⁻³)	λ_{min}	230	240	250	270	280	290
13	13	281	17.8	245	1.62	0.54	0.53	1.86	2.61	2.09*
14	12	270*	10.6*	231	0.40	0.48	0.70	1.21	0.80	0.06
15	13q	281.5	7.1	251	2.26	1.12	0.66	1.68	2.13	1.4
	14	282	7.9	251			0.60		3.28	2.6
16	12	294	11.9	250	5.10	1.60	0.53	2.60	5.90	9.30

(Spectral Ratios: 230, 240, 250, 270, 280, 290)

REFERENCES

No.	Origin and Synthesis	$[\alpha]_D$	pK	Spectral Data	Mass Spectra	R_f
13	C: 23,338,29a,22,R: 18	–	22	18b,23d,28c,d,21,265*,b,317b,338	–	18,22,32
14	C: 33,34	–	35	36b,33*,d,35b,37*b	–	26,33,36
15	C: 64,233,352,396	–	59,66*,80	66b,242be,232b,317b,205,64	–	258,21,242,402
16	C: 57,30	–	58,57	57,58b,317b	–	13,57

PURINES, PYRIMIDINES, NUCLEOSIDES AND NUCLEOTIDES: PHYSICAL CONSTANTS AND SPECTRAL PROPERTIES (Continued)

No.	Compound	Symbol (3-Letter)	Symbol (1-Letter)	Structure	Formula (Mol Wt)	Melting Point °C	$[\alpha]_D^t$	pK Basic	pK Acidic
17	N^4-Acetylcytosine 4-Acetylamino-2-pyrimidinone	4AcCyt			$C_6H_7N_3O_2$ (153.14)	326–328°	–	–	–
18	N^4-Methylcytosine 4-Methylamino-2-pyrimidinone	4MeCyt			$C_5H_7N_3O$ (125.13)	277–280° (dec)	–	4.5	12.7
19	5-Methylcytosine	5MeCyt			$C_5H_7N_3O$ (125.13)	270°	–	4.6	12.4
20	5-Hydroxymethylcytosine	5HmCyt 5HOMeCyt			$C_5H_7N_3O_2$ (141.13)	>200° (dec)	–	4.3	~13

Acidic Spectral Data

No.	pH	λ_{max}	ε_{max} (×10⁻³)	λ_{min}	230	240	250	270	280	290
17	7	–	–	–	–	–	–	–	–	–
18	1	277	10.5*	240	0.60	0.29	0.50	1.56	1.66	1.03
19	1	283	9.8	242	0.97	0.26	0.40	1.90	2.62	2.43
20	1	279	9.7	241	0.63	0.25	0.45	1.68	1.97	1.37

Neutral Spectral Data

No.	pH	λ_{max}	ε_{max} (×10⁻³)	λ_{min}	230	240	250	270	280	290
17	7	244.5 293	14.2 4.9	226 270	–	–	–	–	–	–
18	7	267	7.2*	248	1.07	0.89	0.79	1.07	0.66	0.14
19	7	273	6.2	252	1.60	1.10	0.80	1.35	1.21	0.54
20	7	269	5.7	251	0.59	0.93	0.80	1.14	0.80	0.15

Alkaline Spectral Data

No.	pH	λ_{max}	ε_{max} (×10⁻³)	λ_{min}	230	240	250	270	280	290
17	–	–	–	–	–	–	–	–	–	–
18	14	286	8.0*	256	3.18	2.02	0.96	2.02	3.27	3.23
19	14	289	8.1	254	5.05	1.97	0.84	2.02	3.64	4.71
20	13	283	7.6	254	3.91	2.59	0.83*	1.97	2.98	2.50

REFERENCES

No.	Origin and Synthesis	pK	$[\alpha]_D^t$	Spectral Data	Mass Spectra	R_f
17	C: 280,281,396	–	–	281	–	–
18	C: 59,60ᵃ,61,62 R: 353	59,63	–	59ᵇ,60*,317ᵇ	–	59
19	C: 64,65ᵃ	66	–	66ᵇ,67ᵇ,64ᵇ,68ᵇ,265ᵇ,317ᵇ,	–	67,69,70
20	C: 71	72	–	73ᵇ,72ᵇ,71,74,265*ᵇ,317ᵇ	74	69,70,73,75,74,402

PURINES, PYRIMIDINES, NUCLEOSIDES AND NUCLEOTIDES: PHYSICAL CONSTANTS AND SPECTRAL PROPERTIES (Continued)

No.	Compound	Symbol 3-Letter	Symbol 1-Letter	Structure	Formula (Mol Wt)	Melting Point °C	$[\alpha]_D^t$	pK Basic	pK Acidic
21	6-Amino-5-N-methylformamidoisocytosine / 2,6-Diamino-4-hydroxy-5-N-methylformamidopyrimidine	6NH₂5(M⁴eFn)isoCyt			$C_6H_9N_5O_2$ (183.17)	–	–	3.8	9.9ᵏ
22	Guanine	Gua			$C_5H_5N_5O$ (151.13)	>350°	–	<0, 3.2	9.6*, 12.4
23	1-Methylguanine	1MeGua			$C_6H_7N_5O$ (165.16)	None (dec)	–	⁻0, 3.1	10.5
24	N²-Methylguanine / 6-Hydroxy-2-methylaminopurine	2MeGua			$C_6H_7N_5O$ (165.16)	–	–	3.3	8.9, 12.8

Acidic Spectral Data

No.	pH	λ_{max}	ε_{max} (×10⁻³)	λ_{min}	230	240	250	270	280	290
21	1	263	17.8	232*	0.37	0.39	0.59	0.92	0.34	0.04
22	1	248	11.4	224	0.71	1.18	1.37	0.85	0.84*	0.50*
		276	7.35	267						
23	1	250	10.2	227	0.47	0.93	1.28	0.87	0.81	0.50
		272	7.1	–						
24	1	250*	13.9*	228*	0.51	0.95	1.34*	0.62*	0.64	0.54*
		279	6.2*	–						

Neutral Spectral Data

No.	pH	λ_{max}	ε_{max} (×10⁻³)	λ_{min}	230	240	250	270	280	290
21	7	264	13.8	242	–	–	–	–	–	–
22	7	246	10.7*	225	0.73	1.26	1.42	0.99	1.04	0.54
		276	8.15*	262						
23	7	248	10.0	227	0.54	1.01	1.24	0.96	0.93	0.46
		272	7.9	264						
24	7	249	14.1	227	0.56	0.86	1.18	0.72	0.72	0.49
		277	8.3	266						

Alkaline Spectral Data

No.	pH	λ_{max}	ε_{max} (×10⁻³)	λ_{min}	230	240	250	270	280	290
21	13	262	9.8	242	0.72	0.67	0.71	0.78	0.31	0.09
22	11	274	8.0	255	–	–	0.99	–	1.14	0.59
23	14	274	9.9	238	–	–	0.81	1.12	1.24	0.61
24	13	277	8.7	241*	1.49	0.64	0.80	–	1.19	0.81
	11	244	9.5*	263*						
		278*	7.2							

REFERENCES

No.	Origin and Synthesis	pK	$[\alpha]_D^t$	Spectral Data	Mass Spectra	Rf
21	C: 41	41,76	–	90,41*ᶜ,ᵈ	–	41
22	C: 234,257,354	170,56*,232	–	232ᵇ,242*ᵇᵉ,317ᵇ,205,257*	–	21,40,258,242,402
23	C: 33ᵃ,38ᵃ	39,27	–	40ᵇ,41ᶜ,ᵈ,27ᵇ,ᵉ,39ᵇ,ᶜ,ᵉ,25,33,42,265*ᵇ,317ᵇ	–	24,25,27,33,40,42
24	C: 43ᵇ,44,355	2	–	40ᵇ,44ᶜᵈ,317ᵈᵉ,43*,2*,27*,265*ᵇ,25	–	25,27,33,40

PURINES, PYRIMIDINES, NUCLEOSIDES AND NUCLEOTIDES: PHYSICAL CONSTANTS AND SPECTRAL PROPERTIES (Continued)

No.	Compound	Symbol 3-Letter	Symbol 1-Letter	Structure	Formula (Mol Wt)	Melting Point °C	$[\alpha]_D^t$	pK Basic	pK Acidic
25	N^2,N^2-Dimethylguanine 2-Dimethylamino-6-hydroxypurine	2Me₂Gua			$C_7H_9N_5O$ (179.18)	—	—	—	—
26	7-Methylguanine	7MeGua			$C_6H_7N_5O$ (165.16)	>390° (dec)	—	~0, 3.5	9.9*
27	Hypoxanthine	Hyp			$C_5H_4N_4O$ (136.11)	>350° (dec)	—	2.0	8.9*, 12.1
28	1-Methylhypoxanthine	1MeHyp			$C_6H_6N_4O$ (150.14)	311–312°	—	~2	8.9*, ~13

Acidic Spectral Data

No.	pH	λ_{max}	ε_{max} (×10⁻³)	λ_{min}	230	240	250	270	280	290
25	1	256*	19.0*	233*	0.36	0.48	0.92	0.52	0.37*	0.39
26	1	250 / 272	10.6* / 6.9*	228*	0.55	0.99	1.30	0.84	0.79	0.52
27	0	248	10.8	215	—	—	1.45	—	0.04	0.00
28	1	249	9.4	219	0.59	1.11	1.37	0.43	0.10	0.01

Neutral Spectral Data

No.	pH	λ_{max}	ε_{max} (×10⁻³)	λ_{min}	230	240	250	270	280	290
25	7	250 / 283	17.0 / 9.3	229	0.55	0.87	1.20	0.61	0.62	0.59
26	7	248 / 283	5.7* / 7.4*	235 / 261	1.54	1.42	1.46	1.35	1.87	1.73
27	6	249.5	10.7	222	0.53	1.05	1.32	0.57	0.09*	0.01*
28	5	251	9.4	223	0.51	0.95	1.31	0.53	0.16	0.02

Alkaline Spectral Data

No.	pH	λ_{max}	ε_{max} (×10⁻³)	λ_{min}	230	240	250	270	280	290
25	12	282*	9.2*	265	—	1.26	1.15	0.95	1.05	0.95
26	12	280*	7.4*	257	1.92	1.50	1.013	1.50	1.89	1.47
27	11	259	11.1	232	0.48	0.46	0.84	0.84	0.12	0.01
27	14	263	11.5	233			0.71		0.19*	0.01*
28	11	260	9.7	242	—	—	—	—	—	—

REFERENCES

No.	Origin and Synthesis	pK	$[\alpha]_D^t$	Spectral Data	Mass Spectra	Rf
25	C: 43⁹,44	—	—	317ᵇ,40ᵇᶜᵉ,44ᶜᵈ,265*,ᵇ,43	—	40
26	C: 45,10	39,27*	—	46ᵇ,47ᵇ,42*,ᵇ,35ᵇ,39,41,48	—	10,13,24,27,41,42,46,334
27	C: 257,337,358,359,377	22,170,253,51*	—	232ᵇ,242*,ᵉ,334*,317ᵇ,205,257,358	—	258,242,278
28	C: 33,26,360	33,27*	—	49,33ᶜᵈ,317ᵇᶜ,27,121,360	—	24,26,27,49,33,121

PURINES, PYRIMIDINES, NUCLEOSIDES AND NUCLEOTIDES: PHYSICAL CONSTANTS AND SPECTRAL PROPERTIES (Continued)

No.	Compound	Symbol 3-Letter	Symbol 1-Letter	Structure	Formula (Mol Wt)	Melting Point °C	$[\alpha]_D^1$	pK Basic	pK Acidic
29	3-Methylhypoxanthine	3MeHyp			$C_6H_6N_4O$ (150.14)	>280° (dec)	–	2.6	8.3
30	7-Methylhypoxanthine	7MeHyp			$C_6H_6N_4O$ (150.14)	355° (dec)	–	2.1	8.9
31	Uracil	Ura			$C_4H_4N_2O_2$ (112.09)	315° (dec)	–	–	9.5, >13
32	1-Methyluracil	1MeUra			$C_5H_6N_2O_2$ (126.11)	232–233°	–	–	9.7

Acidic Spectral Data

No.	pH	λ_{max}	ε_{max} (×10⁻³)	λ_{min}	230	240	250	270	280	290
29	0	253	11.0	–	–	–	–	–	–	–
30	0	250	10.2	224	–	–	–	–	–	–
31	0*	260	7.8	229	0.23	0.48	0.80	0.68	0.30	0.05
	4	259.5	8.2	227	–	–	0.84	–	0.17	0.01
32	2	272	–	–	–	–	0.60	–	0.64	0.08

Neutral Spectral Data

No.	pH	λ_{max}	ε_{max} (×10⁻³)	λ_{min}	230	240	250	270	280	290
29	5	264	14.0	–	–	–	–	–	–	–
30	5	256	9.5	229	0.42	0.81	0.97	0.55	0.07	0.00
31	7	259.5	8.2	227	0.21	0.47	0.84	0.68	0.17	0.01
32	7	267	9.8	232	0.17	0.25	0.59	1.12	0.70	0.12

Alkaline Spectral Data

No.	pH	λ_{max}	ε_{max} (×10⁻³)	λ_{min}	230	240	250	270	280	290
29	11	265	10.9	–	–	–	–	–	–	–
30	11	262	10.6	230	0.36	0.49	0.76	0.83	0.21	0.00
31	12	284	6.2	241	1.09	0.56	0.71	1.25	1.40	1.27
32	12	265*	7.0	241	0.92	0.53	0.68	1.00	0.44	0.03

REFERENCES

No.	Origin and Synthesis	$[\alpha]_D^1$	pK	Spectral Data	Mass Spectra	R_f
29	C: 26,50a	–	33	33,121	–	26,33,121
30	C: 45	–	33,51	52,33c,d	–	10,26,27,33
31	C: 364,362a,84,395	–	66,80	66b 242be 232bcde,317b	–	258,40,242,402
32	C: 79,78,362,	–	66,80	66b,81 *b,c,e	–	69,81

PURINES, PYRIMIDINES, NUCLEOSIDES AND NUCLEOTIDES: PHYSICAL CONSTANTS AND SPECTRAL PROPERTIES (Continued)

No.	Compound	Symbol (3-Letter)	Symbol (1-Letter)	Structure	Formula (Mol Wt)	Melting Point °C	$[\alpha]_D^t$	pK Basic	pK Acidic
33	2-Thiouracil	2SUra 2Sra			$C_4H_4N_2OS$ (128.15)	340° (dec)	—	—	—
34	2-Methylthiouracil S-Methyl-2-thiouracil	2(MeS)Ura 2MeSra			$C_5H_6N_2OS$ (142.18)	196–198°	—	—	—
35	5-Carboxymethyl-2-thiouracil 2-Thiouracil-5-acetic acid	5Cm2SUra 5Cm2Sra 5(CxMe)2SUra			$C_6H_6N_2O_3S$ (186.19)	275–279° (dec)	—	—	4.15, 8.4, ~13.5
36	5-Carbamoylmethyl-2-thiouracil 2-Thiouracil-5-acetamide	5Ncm2Sra 5(NcMe)2SUra 5(NcMe)2Sra 5Ncm2SUra			$C_6H_7N_3O_2S$ (185.21)	269–270° (dec)	—	—	—

Acidic Spectral Data

No.	pH	λ_{max}	ε_{max} (×10⁻³)	λ_{min}	230	240	250	270	280	290
33	1.5	270*	13.9*	241						
34	1 (MeOH)	221 248	10.0 7.9	242						
35	1	276	15.6	242						
36	1	214 274	13.9 14.9	240						

Neutral Spectral Data

No.	pH	λ_{max}	ε_{max} (×10⁻³)	λ_{min}	230	240	250	270	280	290
33	7.4	268*	11.8	240						
34	(MeOH)	228 286	7.9 7.9							

Alkaline Spectral Data

No.	pH	λ_{max}	ε_{max} (×10⁻³)	λ_{min}	230	240	250	270	280	290
33	11	259 307*	10.7 6.8	243* 291*						
34	13 (MeOH)	222 243	15.9 7.9	244						
35	13q	236 259 313	9.9 11.1 8.3	288						
36		234	—	244						

REFERENCES

No.	Origin and Synthesis	$[\alpha]_D^t$	pK	Spectral Data	Mass Spectra	R_f
33	C: 84	—	—	277b, 331bc, 86*bd	—	—
34	C: 301	—	—	301	—	301
35	C: 302	—	302	302	—	302
36	C: 302	—	—	302	—	302

PURINES, PYRIMIDINES, NUCLEOSIDES AND NUCLEOTIDES: PHYSICAL CONSTANTS AND SPECTRAL PROPERTIES (Continued)

No.	Compound	Symbol (3-Letter)	Structure	Formula (Mol Wt)	Melting Point °C	$[\alpha]_D^t$	pK Basic	pK Acidic
37	5-(Methoxycarbonylmethyl)-2-thiouracil / 2-Thio-5-carboxymethyluracil methyl ester	5(MeCm)2Sura / 5MeCm2Sra / 5(MeCxMe)2Sra		$C_7H_8N_2O_3S$ (200.22)	218–220°	–	–	–
38	5-Methoxy-2-thiouracil / 4-Hydroxy-2-mercapto-5-methoxypyrimidine	5Me02SUra / 5Me02Sra		$C_5H_6N_2O_2S$ (158.18)	280–281° (dec)	–	–	–
39	2-Thiothymine 5-Methyl-2-thiouracil	2Sthy / 5Me2SUra / 5Me2Sra		$C_5H_6N_2OS$ (142.18)	265–267°	–	–	–
40	3-Methyluracil	3MeUra		$C_5H_6N_2O_2$ (126.12)	179°	–	–	10.0

Acidic Spectral Data

No.	pH	λ_{max}	ε_{max} (×10⁻³)	λ_{min}	230	240	250	270	280	290
37	1.5	214 / 276	15.6 / 16.6	240	0.49	0.31	0.47	1.48	1.52	1.44
38										
39	1	276	19.5							
40	3	259	7.3	–	–	–	0.86	–	0.14	0.02

Neutral Spectral Data

No.	pH	λ_{max}	ε_{max} (×10⁻³)	λ_{min}	230	240	250	270	280	290
37	7	215 / 275	– / 16.6	240	0.47	0.32	0.47	1.45	1.49	1.41
38										
39	7	274	16.9							
40	7	259	7.3	230	0.29	0.46	0.84	0.66	0.14	0.00

Alkaline Spectral Data

No.	pH	λ_{max}	ε_{max} (×10⁻³)	λ_{min}	$[\alpha]_D^t$	230	240	250	270	280	290
37	12	260	12.0	290	–	0.91	0.83	0.85	0.80	0.59	0.51
38		313	8.6								
39	11	260 / 309	16.6 / 7.3								
40	12	283	10.7	243	–	1.43	0.34	0.37	2.23	3.47	3.01

REFERENCES

No.	Origin and Synthesis	$[\alpha]_D^t$	pK	Spectral Data	Mass Spectra	R_f
37	C: 5,302	–	–	317[b],302[ad],5[c]	–	302
38	C: 397	–	–	–	–	–
39	C: 301	–	–	86	–	–
40	C: 82,79[a],83	–	66,80	66[b],81[b,e]	–	13,69,81

PURINES, PYRIMIDINES, NUCLEOSIDES AND NUCLEOTIDES: PHYSICAL CONSTANTS AND SPECTRAL PROPERTIES (Continued)

No.	Compound	Symbol 3-Letter	Symbol 1-Letter	Structure	Formula (Mol Wt)	Melting Point °C	$[\alpha]_D^t$	pK Basic	pK Acidic
41	4-Thiouracil	4Sura / 4Sra			$C_4H_4N_2OS$ (128.15)	289–290° (dec)	–	–	–
42	5-Carboxymethyluracil Uracil-5-acetic acid	5CmUra / 5CxMeUra			$C_6H_6N_2O_4$ (170.12)	316–318° (dec)	–	–	4.3, 10.0
43	5-(Methoxycarbonylmethyl)uracil / 5-Carboxymethyluracil methyl ester / Uracil-5-acetic acid methyl ester	5MeCmUra / 5(MeCxMe)Ura			$C_7H_8N_2O_4$ (184.15)	236–237°	–	–	–
44	5-Hydroxyuracil	5HOUra			$C_4H_4N_2O_3$ (128.09)	>300° (dec)	–	–	8.0

Acidic Spectral Data

No.	pH	λ_{max}	ε_{max} (×10⁻³)	λ_{min}	230	240	250	270	280	290
41	1	327	17.5	277	–	–	–	–	–	–
42	1	262	8.1	231	0.23	0.37	0.71	0.89	0.42	0.05
43	1	262	8.2	232	–	–	–	–	–	–
44	2	278*	6.4	244	1.16	0.58	0.56	1.52	1.63	1.26

Neutral Spectral Data

No.	pH	λ_{max}	ε_{max} (×10⁻³)	λ_{min}	230	240	250	270	280	290
41	7	328	16.6	275	–	–	–	–	–	–
42	7	264	7.6	234	0.33	0.33	0.66	0.98	0.56	0.13
44	6	278*	6.4	244	1.08	0.53	0.54	1.45	1.55	1.18

Alkaline Spectral Data

No.	pH	λ_{max}	ε_{max} (×10⁻³)	λ_{min}	230	240	250	270	280	290
41	11	335	17.6	278	–	–	0.63	1.40	1.77	2.00
42	13	290	5.5	246	1.95	0.78	–	–	–	–
44	12	239	6.5*	270	–	–	1.65	0.69	0.83	1.13

REFERENCES

No.	Origin and Synthesis	$[\alpha]_D^t$	pK	Spectral Data	Mass Spectra	R_f
41	C: 85,84	–	–	86[b],317[b]	–	–
42	C: 279,278,302[a]	–	302	278[b],302[d]	278	278,302,402
43	C: 302	–	–	302	–	302
44	C: 87,88[a],89	–	90	87[b],317[bcde],91*[b]	–	–

PURINES, PYRIMIDINES, NUCLEOSIDES AND NUCLEOTIDES: PHYSICAL CONSTANTS AND SPECTRAL PROPERTIES (Continued)

No.	Compound	Symbol (3-Letter)	Symbol (1-Letter)	Structure	Formula (Mol Wt)	Melting Point °C	$[\alpha]_D^t$	pK Basic	pK Acidic
45	5-Methoxyuracil 2,4-Dihydroxy-5-methoxy-pyrimidine	5MeOUra			$C_5H_6N_2O_3$ (142.12)	341–345° (dec)	–	–	–
46	Thymine 5-Methyluracil	Thy 5MeUra			$C_5H_6N_2O_2$ (126.11)	310° (dec)	–	–	9.9 >13
47	5-(Putrescinomethyl)uracil 5-(4-Aminobutylaminomethyl) uracil; N-Thyminylputrescine	5(PutMe)Ura 5(NH₂BuNHMe)Ura 5PutThy*			$C_9H_{16}N_4O_2$ (212.25)	255° (dec) (HCl salt)	–	–	–
48	5-(Methylaminomethyl)uracil	5(MeNHMe)Ura			$C_6H_9N_3O_2$ (155.16)	230–232°	–	–	–

Acidic Spectral Data

No.	pH	λ_{max}	ε_{max} (×10⁻³)	λ_{min}	230	240	250	270	280	290
45	–									
46	4	264.5	7.9	233	–	–	0.67	0.97	0.53	0.09
47	1	261	7.8	230	–	–	–	–	–	–
48	1	262	–	230	0.01	0.07	0.70	0.85	0.39	0.13

Neutral Spectral Data

No.	pH	λ_{max}	ε_{max} (×10⁻³)	λ_{min}	230	240	250	270	280	290
45	–									
46	7	264.5	7.9	233	0.28	0.35	0.67	0.96	0.53	0.09
47	7	262	–	230.5	–	–	–	–	–	–
48	7.5	262	–	230	0.01	0.07	0.70	0.85	0.39	0.13

Alkaline Spectral Data

No.	pH	λ_{max}	ε_{max} (×10⁻³)	λ_{min}	230	240	250	270	280	290
45	12	305*	5.7	244	1.53	0.68	0.65	1.24	1.31	1.41
46	13	291	5.4	246	–	–	–	–	–	–
47		288.5	–	–	–	–	–	–	–	–
48	10.1	287	–	244	3.88	0.42	0.39	1.69	2.18	2.32

REFERENCES

No.	Origin and Synthesis	Spectral Data	$[\alpha]_D^t$	pK	Mass Spectra	R_f
45	C: 397	–	–	–	–	–
46	C: 263,361,254,101,348,356,395	66ᵇ,232ᵇ,317ᵇ	–	66,80	–	258,21,18,402
47	C: 402 D: 402	402	–	–	402	402
48	C: 270	270	–	–	270	270

PURINES, PYRIMIDINES, NUCLEOSIDES AND NUCLEOTIDES: PHYSICAL CONSTANTS AND SPECTRAL PROPERTIES (Continued)

No.	Compound	Symbol 3-Letter	Symbol 1-Letter	Structure	Formula (Mol Wt)	Melting Point °C	$[\alpha]_D^t$	pK Basic	pK Acidic
49	5-Hydroxymethyluracil	5HmUra 5HOMeUra		(structure)	$C_5H_6N_2O_3$ (142.11)	260–300° (dec)	–	–	9.4* ~14
50	S(+)5-(4,5-Dihydroxypentyl)uracil	5(HO)₂PeUra		(structure)	$C_9H_{14}N_2O_4$ (214.22)	255–226°	–	–	9.7
51	Dihydrouracil 5,6-Dihydrouracil	H₂Ura		(structure)	$C_4H_6N_2O_2$ (114.10)	275–276°	–	–	–
52	5,6-Dihydrothymine 5,6-Dihydro-5-methyluracil	H₂Thy		(structure)	$C_5H_8N_2O_2$ (128.13)	264–265°	–	–	–

Acidic Spectral Data

No.	pH	λ_{max}	ε_{max} (×10⁻³)	λ_{min}	230	240	250	270	280	290
49	2	261	8.0	231	–	–	0.77	–	0.32	–
		206	9.55							
50	2.8	264	7.05	–	–	–	–	–	–	–
51	–	–	–	–	–	–	–	–	–	–
52	–	–	–	–	–	–	–	–	–	–

Neutral Spectral Data

No.	pH	λ_{max}	ε_{max} (×10⁻³)	λ_{min}	230	240	250	270	280	290
49	7	261	8.1	231	0.27	0.43	0.77	0.80	0.33	0.05
	H₂O	207	9.5							
50		265	7.7	–	–	–	–	–	–	–
51	–	–	–	–	–	–	–	–	–	–
52	–	–	–	–	–	–	–	–	–	–

Alkaline Spectral Data

No.	pH	λ_{max}	ε_{max} (×10⁻³)	λ_{min}	230	240	250	270	280	290
49	12	286	7.4	245	1.77	0.75	0.67	1.39	1.80	1.75
50	12	291	5.9	–	–	–	–	–	–	–
51	13°	230	8.2	224*	–	–	–	–	–	–
52	13°	230	8.1	–	–	–	–	–	–	–

REFERENCES

No.	Origin and Synthesis	$[\alpha]_D^t$	pK	Spectral Data	Mass Spectra	R_f
49	C: 69,92,93 D: 96	–	72,94*	94b,69cde,317bd,72b,95b,74	–	69,96,97,74,402
50	C: 326 D: 325,326	–	325	326,325	326,325	401,325
51	C: 98,85,99–102	–	–	103b,317bc,383*b	–	383
52	C: 101,99	–	–	103b,383	–	383

PURINES, PYRIMIDINES, NUCLEOSIDES AND NUCLEOTIDES: PHYSICAL CONSTANTS AND SPECTRAL PROPERTIES (Continued)

No.	Compound	Symbol 3-Letter	Symbol 1-Letter	Structure	Formula (Mol Wt)	Melting Point °C	$[\alpha]_D^t$	pK Basic	pK Acidic
53	Orotic acid; Uracil-6-carboxylic acid; 6-Carboxyuracil	Oro	6CxUra		$C_5H_4N_2O_4$ (156.10)	345° (dec)	–	–	2.4, 9.5, >13
54	Wye; (Formerly "Yt base" or "Yt+") 4,9-Dihydro-4,6-dimethyl-9-oxo-1H-imidazo[1,2-a]purine; 1,N^2-isopropeno-3-methylguanine	Wye	ImGua*		$C_9H_9N_5O$ (203.20)	–	–	3.66	8.52
55	Wybutine; 7-[3-(Methoxycarbonyl)-3-(methoxyformamido)propyl] wye (Formerly "Y base" or "Yt"); α-(Carboxyamino)-4,9-dihydro-4,6-dimethyl-9-oxo-1H-imidazo[1,2-a]purine-7-butyric acid dimethyl ester	Y-Wye (MeO)₂ FnBtoWye	Y-imGua*		$C_{16}H_{20}N_6O_5$ (376.38)	204–206°	–	3.7*	8.6*

Acidic Spectral Data

No.	pH	λmax	εmax (×10⁻³)	λmin	230	240	250	270	280	290
53	1	280	7.5	241	0.61	0.41	0.54	1.54	1.82	1.56
54	1.5	227 / 284	36.0 / 8.7	244	7.55	1.17	0.89	1.34	1.96	1.87
55	2	233 / 286	35.6 / 7.6	254*	–	3.45	1.04*	1.03	1.12*	1.12

Neutral Spectral Data

No.	pH	λmax	εmax (×10⁻³)	λmin	230	240	250	270	280	290
53	7	279	7.7	241	0.68	0.43	0.57	1.49	1.71	1.36
54	6.0	230 / 264 / 307	31.5 / 5.3 / 5.9	249	6.73	2.30	0.67	1.01	0.54	0.74
55	6.5	235 / 263 / 313	32.0 / 5.8 / 5.0	258* / 288*	–	5.35	1.25	0.85	0.54*	0.50

Alkaline Spectral Data

No.	pH	λmax	εmax (×10⁻³)	λmin	230	240	250	270	280	290
53	12	286 / 240	6.0 / 8.9	244 / 222	1.36	0.80	0.80	1.38	1.71	1.72
54	11.0	231 / 275 / 301	33.4 / 6.6 / 8.05	252 / 284	8.11	3.64	0.80	1.39	1.36	1.44
55	10	236 / 265* / 304	32.8 / 6.8 / 7.2	262* / 287	–	4.95	1.35	1.01	0.91	0.86

REFERENCES

No.	Origin and Synthesis	$[\alpha]_D^t$	pK	Spectral Data	Mass Spectra	Rf
53	C: 104–106	–	66,105	66b,104b	–	69
54	C: 312 R: 312	–	312	312p,403b	312	312
55	C: 320 R: 316,310	–	320,310*	320,310,316*b	310,311	324,316,310,311

PURINES, PYRIMIDINES, NUCLEOSIDES AND NUCLEOTIDES: PHYSICAL CONSTANTS AND SPECTRAL PROPERTIES (Continued)

No.	Compound	Symbol: 3-Letter	Symbol: 1-Letter	Structure	Formula (Mol Wt)	Melting Point °C	$[\alpha]_D^t$	pK: Basic	pK: Acidic
56	Peroxywybutine[j] 7-[2-(Hydroperoxy)-3-(methoxycarbonyl)-3-(methoxyformamide)propyl] wye[j] (Formerly "Yw base, Yr base, Peroxy Y base" or "Yw+") α-(Carboxyamino)-4,9-dihydro-β-hydroperoxy-4,6-dimethyl-9-oxo-1*H*-imidazo[1,2-*a*]purine-7-butyric acid dimethyl ester	O_2 Y-Wye O_2 $(MeO)_2$ FnBto Wye[j] O_2 Y-imGua*		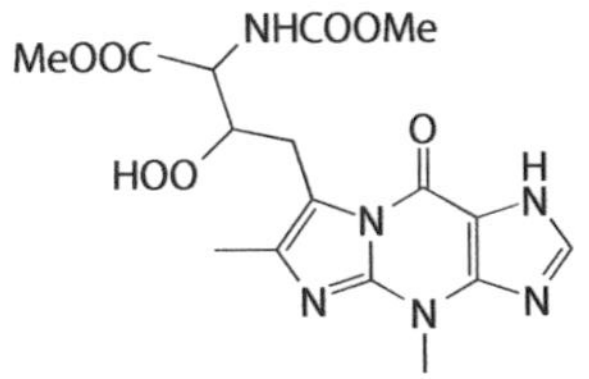	$C_{16}H_{20}N_6O_7$ (408.37)	–	–	~3.3[p]	~9[p]
57	Xanthine	Xan		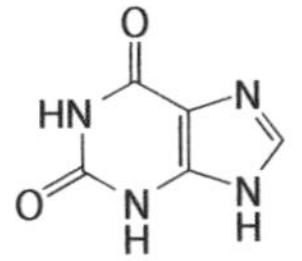	$C_5H_4N_4O_2$ (152.11)	None (dec)	–	~0.8	7.5*, 11.1*
58	7-Methylxanthine	7MeXan		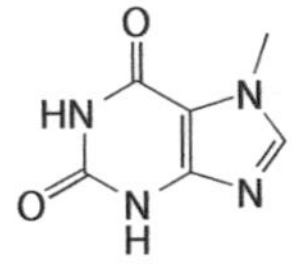	$C_6H_6N_4O_2$ (166.14)	~380° (dec)	–	–	8.4, ~13

Acidic Spectral Data

No.	pH	λ_{max}	ε_{max} (×10⁻³)	λ_{min}	230	240	250	270	280	290
56										
57	0[q]	260	9.15	242	–	–	0.77	–	0.15	0.01
	1[q]	–	–	–	0.53	0.42	0.66	0.94	0.40	0.04
58	2	268	9.3	241	–	0.38	–	–	0.75	–

Neutral Spectral Data

No.	pH	λ_{max}	ε_{max} (×10⁻³)	λ_{min}	230	240	250	270	280	290
56		236	32.0	211						
	H_2O	260*	6.0	256	5.02	4.07	1.16	0.81	0.56	0.69
		308	5.2	281						
57	6	267	10.25	239	–	–	0.57	–	0.61	0.07
	7[q]	–	–	–	0.45	0.42	0.62	1.16	0.69	0.14
58	6	269	10.0	240	–	–	–	–	–	–

Alkaline Spectral Data

No.	pH	λ_{max}	ε_{max} (×10⁻³)	λ_{min}	230	240	250	270	280	290
56										
57	10	240 277	8.9 9.3	222 257	–	–	1.29	–	1.71	0.92
	13	–	–	–	1.81	1.33	1.12	1.63	2.28	2.07
58	14	284	9.4	257	–	–	1.11	–	2.39	2.27

REFERENCES

No.	Origin and Synthesis	$[\alpha]_D^t$	pK	Spectral Data	Mass Spectra	R_f
56	R: 327,321,324	–	324	327[b],321*[b]	321,327	324,321,327
57	C: 231,377	–	22,248,170*,53*,55*,253*	232[b],242[e],205	–	258,242
58	C: 45	–	53–56	53[b],41[c,d],27[e],54*	–	10,27

PURINES, PYRIMIDINES, NUCLEOSIDES AND NUCLEOTIDES: PHYSICAL CONSTANTS AND SPECTRAL PROPERTIES (Continued)

No.	Compound	Symbol (3-Letter)	Symbol (1-Letter)	Structure	Formula (Mol Wt)	Melting Point °C	$[\alpha]_D$	pK Basic	pK Acidic
59	Zeatin; 6-(trans-4-Hydroxy-3-methyl-2-butenylamino)purine; N^6-(trans-4-Hydroxy isopentenyl)adenine	Zea, 6(tr HoIPe) Ade			$C_{10}H_{13}N_5O$ (219.24)	207–208°	–	–	–
	RIBONUCLEOSIDES								
60	Adenosine	Ado	A		$C_{10}H_{13}N_5O_4$ (267.24)	235–236°	-61^{25} (1.0, H_2O)	3.5*	12.5
61	1-(Δ²-Isopentenyl)adenosine 1-(γγ-Dimethylallyl)adenosine 1-(3-Methyl-2-butenyl)adenosine	1PelAdo 1PelA	i¹ A		$C_{15}H_{21}N_5O_4$ (355.36)	131–133° (HBr salt)	–	8.5	–

Acidic Spectral Data

No.	pH	λ_{max}	ε_{max} (×10⁻³)	λ_{min}	230	240	250	270	280	290
59	1	207	14.5	235	–	–	–	–	–	–
		275	14.65							
60	1	257	14.6	230	0.23	0.44	0.84	–	0.22	0.03
61	1	257.5	13.9	235	–	–	–	–	–	–

Neutral Spectral Data

No.	pH	λ_{max}	ε_{max} (×10⁻³)	λ_{min}	230	240	250	270	280	290
59	7	212	17.1	233	–	–	–	–	–	–
		270	16.2							
60	6	260	14.9	227	0.18	0.42	0.78	–	0.14	0.00
61	7	258	13.6	235	–	–	–	–	–	–

Alkaline Spectral Data

No.	pH	λ_{max}	ε_{max} (×10⁻³)	λ_{min}	230	240	250	270	280	290
59	13	220	15.9	242	–	–	–	–	–	–
		276	14.65							
60	11	259	15.4	227	0.24	0.40	0.79	–	0.15	0.00
61	13°	259*	14.25*	236	–	–	–	–	–	0.31

REFERENCES

No.	Origin and Synthesis	$[\alpha]_D$	pK	Spectral Data	Mass Spectra	R_f
59	C: 227 N: 228	–	–	227		32,227
60	C: 111,235,363,350,351,379	363,235,350	250,255*,336,371,51,220	232b,212cde,242e,183b,317b,205	315,341,317,405	258,110,18,242,291,292
61	C: 319,15*,14	–	15	319,15*	15	15,32,319

PURINES, PYRIMIDINES, NUCLEOSIDES AND NUCLEOTIDES: PHYSICAL CONSTANTS AND SPECTRAL PROPERTIES (Continued)

No.	Compound	Symbol 3-Letter	Symbol 1-Letter	Structure	Formula (Mol Wt)	Melting Point °C	$[\alpha]_D^t$	pK Basic	pK Acidic
62	1-Methyladenosine	1MeAdo	$m^1 A$		$C_{11}H_{15}N_5O_4$ (281.27)	214–217° (dec)	-59^{26} (2.0, H_2O)	8.8*	–
63	1,N^6-Dimethyladenosine 1-Methyl-6-methylamino-9-β-D-ribofuranosylpurine	1,6Me$_2$, Ado	m^1_2,^6A $m^1 m^6 A$		$C_{12}H_{17}N_5O_4$ (295.30)	206°	–	–	–
64	2-Hydroxyadenosine Crotonoside; Isoguanosine	2HOAdo; isoGuo*	0^2A isoG*		$C_{10}H_{13}N_5O_5$ (283.25)	237–252° (dec)	-71^{26} (1.06, 0.1 N NaOH)	–	–

Acidic Spectral Data

No.	pH	λ_{max}	ε_{max} (×10⁻³)	λ_{min}	230	240	250	270	280	290
62	2	258	13.7	232*	0.28*	0.41	0.81	0.70	0.23*	0.04
63	1	261	14.2	234	0.26	0.31	0.68	0.81	0.47	0.18
64	1.2	235	6.14	–	–	–	–	–	–	–
		283*	12.7*							

Neutral Spectral Data

No.	pH	λ_{max}	ε_{max} (×10⁻³)	λ_{min}	230	240	250	270	280	290
62	7	258	13.9*	232*	0.29	0.41	0.81	0.70	0.23	0.05
64	H_2O	247*	8.9	–	–	–	–	–	–	–
		293*	11.1*							

Alkaline Spectral Data

No.	pH	λ_{max}	ε_{max} (×10⁻³)	λ_{min}	230	240	250	270	280	290
62	10.5°	259*	14.6	231*	0.25	0.38	0.76	0.76	0.35	0.30
63	14	262	14.9	234	–	–	–	–	–	–
64	12.8	251*	6.9*	–	–	–	–	–	–	–
		285*	10.55*							

REFERENCES

No.	Origin and Synthesis	$[\alpha]_D^t$	pK	Spectral Data	Mass Spectra	R_f
62	C: 10,30	10	15,318*	90,10*^{d},317*^{bd},318*^{b},109,12^b	314,317	10,12,314,291
63	C: 24,12	–	–	24,90^e 12	–	24,12
64	C: 269,N: 268	269	–	269^b,268*^{b}	–	269

PURINES, PYRIMIDINES, NUCLEOSIDES AND NUCLEOTIDES: PHYSICAL CONSTANTS AND SPECTRAL PROPERTIES (Continued)

No.	Compound	Symbol (3-Letter)	Symbol (1-Letter)	Structure	Formula (Mol Wt)	Melting Point °C	$[\alpha]_D^t$	pK (Basic)	pK (Acidic)
65	2-Methyladenosine	2MeAdo	m²A		$C_{11}H_{15}N_5O_4$(281.27)	>200° (dec) (picrate)	-66.6^{25} (1.0, H₂O)	–	–
66	2-Methylthioadenosine	2MeSAdo	ms²A		$C_{11}H_{15}N_5O_4S$ (313.33)	227°	$+4^{29}$ (1.0, 0.1N HCl)	–	–
67	N⁶-Glycinocarbonyladenosine N-[(9-β-D-Ribofuranosylpurin-6-yl)carbamoyl]glycine	6(GlyCO)Ado	gc⁶A		$C_{13}H_{14}N_6O_7$ (368.31)	214–216°	–	–	–

Acidic Spectral Data

No.	pH	λmax	εmax (×10⁻³)	λmin	230	240	250	270	280	290
65	1	258*	14.0	230	0.22	0.44	0.84	0.86	0.40	0.05
	1	270	15.2							
66	1.2	271	18.2	238	0.58	0.37	0.59	1.58	1.58	0.57
		276	19.1							

Neutral Spectral Data

No.	pH	λmax	εmax (×10⁻³)	λmin	230	240	250	270	280	290
65	6	264	14.5	228	0.24	0.41	0.75	0.84	0.17	0.01
	7	235	17.7							
		274	13.5							
66	5.0	269	20.9	230	0.12	0.28	0.59	1.37	0.78	0.00
		276	17.1							

Alkaline Spectral Data

No.	pH	λmax	εmax (×10⁻³)	λmin	230	240	250	270	280	290
65	13	263	15.2	230	0.24	0.41	0.75	0.84	0.17	0.01
66	13	235	17.8*	236	0.37	0.32	0.57	1.41	1.00	0.60
		274*	13.5*							
		270ᵐ	13.5ᵐ							
67	12.1°	277	13.8							
		298	12.8							

REFERENCES

No.	Origin and Synthesis	$[\alpha]_D^t$	Spectral Data	pK
65	E: 18 C: 111,342 R: 18,291	342	18[b],342*[cd],317[bce],291[b]	–
66	C: 399,111[a]	111	399,111*,299	–
67	C: 408,295 R: 295	–	408,295[b],330	–

No.	Mass Spectra	R_f
65	317	18,291
66	–	299
67	295,408,330	295,408,330

PURINES, PYRIMIDINES, NUCLEOSIDES AND NUCLEOTIDES: PHYSICAL CONSTANTS AND SPECTRAL PROPERTIES (Continued)

No.	Compound	Symbol 3-Letter	Symbol 1-Letter	Structure	Formula (Mol Wt)	Melting Point °C	$[\alpha]_D^t$	pK Basic	pK Acidic
68	N^6-Methyl-N^6-glycinocarbonyladenosine N-[9-β-D-Ribofuranosylpurin-6-yl)-N-methylcarbamoyl]glycine	6Me6(GlyCO) Ado	m^6 gc^6 A		$C_{14}H_{18}N_6O_7$ (382.33)	173–174[o]	33.09[23] (0.55 H$_2$O)	–	–
69	N^6-Threoninocarbonyladenosine N-[9-β-D-Ribofuranosylpurin-6-yl)carbamoyl]-L-threonine; N-(Nebularin-6-ylcarbamoyl)-L-threonine	6(ThrCO)Ado	tc^6 A		$C_{15}H_{20}N_6O_8$ (412.36)	204–207[o]	-13.9^{25} (1.0, Me$_2$SO)	<2[p]	~3.0[p]

Acidic Spectral Data

No.	pH	λ_{max}	ε_{max} (×10⁻³)	λ_{min}	Spectral Ratios 230	240	250	270	280	290
68	1.0	283	16.7	239	0.75	0.44	0.62	1.70	2.39	1.83
69	1.6[i]	277	21.6	238	0.59	0.39	0.57	1.54	1.51	0.56

Neutral Spectral Data

No.	pH	λ_{max}	ε_{max} (×10⁻³)	λ_{min}	Spectral Ratios 230	240	250	270	280	290
68	5.5	277 / 284	17.1 / 16.7	236	0.49	0.35	0.60	1.68	2.14	1.28
69	6.5	269 / 276	22.9 / 19.4	231	0.17	0.30	0.59	1.40	0.93	0.00

Alkaline Spectral Data

No.	pH	λ_{max}	ε_{max} (×10⁻³)	λ_{min}	Spectral Ratios 230	240	250	270	280	290
68	13[o]	277 / 284	15.4 / 15.8	245	1.36	0.79	0.76	1.38	1.85	1.33
69	12.4[o]	270[m] / 277 / 299	16.3[m] / 16.0 / 11.1	236	0.40	0.34	0.59	1.44	1.16	0.42

REFERENCES

No.	Origin and Synthesis	$[\alpha]_D^t$	pK	Spectral Data	Mass Spectra	R$_f$
68	C: 330	330	–	330	–	330
69	C: 408,290,R: 4,296,407	408	407,90	290[p],6,296[p],297[b],317[b],313[b],330	408,330	290,295–297,407,408,330

PURINES, PYRIMIDINES, NUCLEOSIDES AND NUCLEOTIDES: PHYSICAL CONSTANTS AND SPECTRAL PROPERTIES (Continued)

No.	Compound	Symbol 3-Letter	Symbol 1-Letter	Structure	Formula (Mol Wt)	Melting Point °C	$[\alpha]_D$	pK Basic	pK Acidic
70	N^6-Methyl-N^6-threoninocarbonyladenosine N-[(9-β-D-Ribofuranosylpurin-6-yl)-N-methylcarbamoyl]threonine	6Me6(ThrCO)Ado			$C_{16}H_{22}N_6O_8$ (426.39)	159–160°	5.31^{23} (0.49, H_2O)	$<2^p$	$^{\sim}2.8^p$
71	N^6-(Δ²-Isopentenyl)adenosine N^6-(3-Methyl-2-butenyl)adenosine; 6-(γγ-Dimethylallylamino)-9-β-D-ribofuranosyl purine	6iPeAdo 6PeAdo	i⁶A		$C_{15}H_{21}N_5O_4$ (335.36)	145–147°	-103^{28} (0.14, EtOH)	3.8	–

Acidic Spectral Data

No.	pH	λ_{max}	ε_{max} (×10⁻³)	λ_{min}	230	240	250	270	280	290
70	1.0^u	277 283	22.3 22.3	237	0.54	0.40	0.62	1.62	2.10	1.36
71	1	265	20.4	232	0.27	0.30	0.57	1.05	0.69*	0.18*

Neutral Spectral Data

pH	λ_{max}	ε_{max} (×10⁻³)	λ_{min}	230	240	250	270	280	290
5.5	278 284	23.5 23.1	237	0.53	0.39	0.61	1.64	2.36	1.69
7	269	20.0	234*	0.24	0.29	0.52	1.17	0.94*	0.36*

Alkaline Spectral Data

pH	λ_{max}	ε_{max} (×10⁻³)	λ_{min}	230	240	250	270	280	290
13^p	277 283	22.5 21.5	249	1.57	1.01	0.91	1.23	1.44	1.01
12	269	20.0	234			0.52*	1.17	0.94	0.36

REFERENCES

No.	Origin and Synthesis	$[\alpha]_D$	pK	Spectral Data	Mass Spectra	R_f
70	C: 330 R: 297,407	330	407	$300^p,297^b,313^b$	297	297,407,330
71	C: 32,31,15,319,14 R: 32,116	319	15	$32^b,116*^b,317*^b,14,31,15,265*^b$	32,317,365,405	32,116,117,15,293,319

PURINES, PYRIMIDINES, NUCLEOSIDES AND NUCLEOTIDES: PHYSICAL CONSTANTS AND SPECTRAL PROPERTIES (Continued)

No.	Compound	Symbol 3-Letter	Symbol 1-Letter	Structure	Formula (Mol Wt)	Melting Point °C	$[\alpha]_D^t$	pK Basic	pK Acidic
72	N^6-(Δ^2-Isopentenyl)-2-methylthioadenosine; 6-(3-Methyl-2-butenyl-amino)-2-methylthio-9-β-D-ribofuranosylpurine	2MeS6iPeAdo 2MeS6PeAdo	ms²i⁶A		$C_{16}H_{23}N_5O_4S$ (381.147)	194–195°	–	–	–
73	N^6-(4-Hydroxyisopentenyl)adenosine N^6-(cis-4-Hydroxy-3-methyl-2-butenyl)adenosine cisZeatosine	6(HOiPe)Ado 6(HOPe)Ado 6(cisHOiPe)Ado	oi⁶A		$C_{15}H_{21}N_5O_5$ (351.36)	206°	-98^{27}_{546} (0.02, H₂O)	–	–

Acidic Spectral Data

No.	pH	λ_{max}	ε_{max} (×10⁻³)	λ_{min}	230	240	250	270	280	290
72	1 (EtOH)	246	18.6	265	0.83	1.12	1.27	1.00	1.12	1.13
		286	16.1							
73	1	265	20.4	–	0.53	0.42	0.68	1.01	0.65	0.21

Neutral Spectral Data

No.	pH	λ_{max}	ε_{max} (×10⁻³)	λ_{min}	230	240	250	270	280	290
72	(EtOH)	244	25.3	258	1.39	2.39	1.78	1.39	1.85	1.67
		283	18.1							
73	7	268	20.0		0.36	0.27	0.53	1.16	0.79	0.27

Alkaline Spectral Data

No.	pH	λ_{max}	ε_{max} (×10⁻³)	λ_{min}	230	240	250	270	280	290
72	10 (EtOH)	243	24.9	259	1.39	2.40	1.79	1.40	1.85	1.68
		283	18.0							
73	12	268	20.0		0.43	0.29	0.50	1.23	0.85	0.29

REFERENCES

No.	Origin and Synthesis	$[\alpha]_D^t$	pK	Spectral Data	Mass Spectra	R_f
72	C: 293,274 R: 274,288,299,335	–	–	293,288b,299b,317b,335b	293,299,274,317,332	274,288,293,299,335
73	R: 117a,332	117	–	117	117,332,317,366	117,332

PURINES, PYRIMIDINES, NUCLEOSIDES AND NUCLEOTIDES: PHYSICAL CONSTANTS AND SPECTRAL PROPERTIES (Continued)

No.	Compound	Symbol 3-Letter	Symbol 1-Letter	Structure	Formula (Mol Wt)	Melting Point °C	$[\alpha]_D^t$	pK Basic	pK Acidic
74	N^6-(4-Hydroxyisopentenyl)-2-methylthioadenosine N^6-(4-Hydroxy-3-methyl-2-butenyl)-2-methylthioadenosine Methylthio-*ciszeatosine*	2MeS6(HOiPe)Ado2MeS6(HOPe')Ado	ms² oi⁶ A		$C_{16}H_{23}N_5O_5S$ (397.46)	155–156°	–	–	–
75	N^6-Methyladenosine 6-Methylaminopurine ribonucleoside	6MeAdo	m⁶A		$C_{11}H_{15}N_5O_4$ (281.27)	219–221°	-54^{26}(0.6, H₂O)	4.0	–
76	N^6-Methyl-2-methylthioadenosine	2MeS6MeAdo	ms²m⁶A		$C_{12}H_{17}N_5O_3S$ (327.36)	–	–	–	–

Acidic Spectral Data

No.	pH	λ_{max}	ε_{max} (×10⁻³)	λ_{min}	230	240	250	270	280	290
74	1 (EtOH)	245	18.5	223	0.20	0.31	0.66	0.88	0.41	0.13
		285	15.5	263						
	1	262	16.6	231						

Neutral Spectral Data

No.	pH	λ_{max}	ε_{max} (×10⁻³)	λ_{min}	230	240	250	270	280	290
74	7 (EtOH)	243	24.3	223	0.17	0.22	0.57	1.09	0.68	0.24
		282	17.2	258						
	7	266	15.9	229						
	7	241.5								
		280.5								

Alkaline Spectral Data

No.	pH	λ_{max}	ε_{max} (×10⁻³)	λ_{min}	230	240	250	270	280	290	R_f
	12 (EtOH)	243	24.7	226	0.17	0.22	0.57	1.09	0.68	0.24	332
	13	282	17.3	258							
		266	15.9*	232*							299,288,335

REFERENCES

No.	Origin and Synthesis	$[\alpha]_D^t$	pK	Spectral Data	Mass Spectra	R_f
74	C: 332 R: 332,294	–	–	332	332	
75	E: 18 C: 10,112,166,30 R: 18,292	112	15	18b,112cd,10c,317be,292b,8,12	292,314,317,405	10,12,18,110,291,292,297,314
76	–	–	–	299	–	

PURINES, PYRIMIDINES, NUCLEOSIDES AND NUCLEOTIDES: PHYSICAL CONSTANTS AND SPECTRAL PROPERTIES (Continued)

No.	Compound	Symbol 3-Letter	Symbol 1-Letter	Structure	Formula (Mol Wt)	Melting Point °C	$[\alpha]_D^t$	pK Basic	pK Acidic
77	N^6,N^6-Dimethyladenosine 6-Dimethylamino-9-β-D-ribofuranosylpurine	6Me$_2$Ado	m$^6_2$A		$C_{12}H_{17}N_5O_4$ (295.30)	183–184°	-62.6^{25} (2.6, H$_2$O)	4.5	—
78	$O^{2'}$-Methyladenosine 2'-O-Methyladenosine	2'MeAdo	Am		$C_{11}H_{15}N_5O_4$ (281.27)	201–202°	-57.9^{23} (1.0, H$_2$O)	—	—
79	$O^{2'}$-Ribosyladenosine 2'-O-Ribosyladenosine	ORibAdo			$C_{15}H_{21}N_5O_8$ (399.36)	—	—	—	—

Acidic Spectral Data

No.	pH	λ_{max}	ε_{max} (×10^{-3})	λ_{min}	230	240	250	270	280	290
77	1	268	18.4	234	0.24	0.27	0.60	1.20	0.94	0.42
78	1	257	13.8	229	0.24	0.47	0.86	0.71	0.21	–
79	1.5	257	–	230	0.36	0.47	0.84	0.72	0.32	0.12

Neutral Spectral Data

No.	pH	λ_{max}	ε_{max} (×10^{-3})	λ_{min}	230	240	250	270	280	290
77	7	275	18.8	236	0.27	0.19	0.46	1.52	1.54	0.96
78	7	259	13.9*	228	0.17	0.40	0.80	0.70	0.15	–
79	7	259	–	227	0.35	0.47	0.82	0.67	0.21	0.04

Alkaline Spectral Data

No.	pH	λ_{max}	ε_{max} (×10^{-3})	λ_{min}	230	240	250	270	280	290
77	13	276	19.2	237	0.17	0.09	0.37	1.57	1.68	1.01
78	12	259	13.9	227	0.20	0.39	0.79	0.70	0.15	–
79	11	259	–	227	0.34	0.47	0.79	0.66	0.20	0.05

REFERENCES

No.	Origin and Synthesis	$[\alpha]_D^t$	pK	Spectral Data	Mass Spectra	R$_f$
77	E: 18 C: 114,113,115,339	113	15	18,32,117,291,314	314,405	18,114[cd],317[be],113
78	C: 107,108[a],369,370	108,370	–	107,109,110,369	315,317,367	317[b],107[d],369*
79	C: 286 R: 110	–	–	110	–	110,317[b]

PURINES, PYRIMIDINES, NUCLEOSIDES AND NUCLEOTIDES: PHYSICAL CONSTANTS AND SPECTRAL PROPERTIES (Continued)

No.	Compound	Symbol (3-Letter)	Symbol (1-Letter)	Structure	Formula (Mol Wt)	Melting Point °C	$[\alpha]_D$	pK Basic	pK Acidic
80	7-α-D-Ribofuranosyladenine Pseudovitamin B₁₂ nucleoside	7αDAdo		structure	$C_{10}H_{13}N_5O_4$ (267.24)	220–222° (0.4, H₂O)	0^{25} (0.4, H₂O)	3.9	—
81	2-Methyl-7-α-ribofuranosyladenine Factor A nucleoside	2Me7αDAdo		structure	$C_{11}H_{15}N_5O_4$ (281.27)	219–220°	—	4.8	—
82	Cytidine	Cyd	C	structure	$C_9H_{13}N_3O_5$ (243.22)	224–225° (dec) (sulfate)	$+34.2^{16}$ (2.0, H₂O)	4.15	12.5*

Acidic Spectral Data

No.	pH	λ_{max}	ε_{max} (×10⁻³)	λ_{min}	230	240	250	270	280	290
80	1	273	13.6	239	0.86	0.50	0.66	1.39	1.19	0.33
81	1	273	13.2	238	0.95	0.55	0.70	1.42	1.24	0.35
82	1	280	13.4	242	0.63	0.28	0.45	1.70	2.10	1.55

Neutral Spectral Data

No.	pH	λ_{max}	ε_{max} (×10⁻³)	λ_{min}	230	240	250	270	280	290
80	H₂O	271	9.8	233	0.59	0.65	0.78	1.26	0.97	0.25
81	7	276	9.1	233	0.85	0.90	0.89	1.40	1.35	0.51
82	7	229.5 / 271	8.3 / 9.1	226 / 250	0.98	0.82	0.86	1.28	0.93*	0.28*

Alkaline Spectral Data

pH	λ_{max}	ε_{max} (×10⁻³)	λ_{min}	230	240	250	270	280	290
13	271	9.8	—	—	—	—	—	—	—
12	244 / 276	5.7 / 9.1	—	—	—	—	—	—	—
13ᵃ	272.5	9.15	251	1.14	1.00	0.87	1.23	1.02	0.38
14	273	9.2	252						

REFERENCES

No.	Origin and Synthesis	$[\alpha]_D$	pK	Spectral Data	Mass Spectra	Rf
80	N: 119 C: 120	120	119	119ᵇ,120	—	119,120
81	N: 121ᵃ	—	121	121ᵇ	—	18
82	R: 236,181,C: 251,128,252,272,386,379	236,147	163*,231	163ᵇ,232ᵇᵉ,242*ᵉ,181ᵇ,212,183ᵇ,317ᵇ,205	315,317	258,110,298,242

PURINES, PYRIMIDINES, NUCLEOSIDES, AND NUCLEOTIDES: PHYSICAL CONSTANTS AND SPECTRAL PROPERTIES (Continued)

No.	Compound	Symbol (3-Letter)	Symbol (1-Letter)	Structure	Formula (Mol Wt)	Melting Point °C	$[\alpha]_D^t$	pK Basic	pK Acidic
83	2-Thiocytidine	2Syd, 2SCyd	s^2C		$C_9H_{13}N_3O_4S$ (259.28)	208–209°	$+64.2^{25}$ (1.8, H_2O)	–	–
84	3-Methylcytidine	3MeCyd	m^3C		$C_{10}H_{15}N_3O_5$ (257.24)	193–194° (methosulfate)	–	8.7*	>12
85	N^4-Acetylcytidine / 4-Acetylamino-1-β-D-ribofuranosyl-2-pyrimidinone	4AcCyd	ac^4C		$C_{11}H_{15}N_3O_6$ (285.25)	208–209°	$+60.1^{23}$ (1.0, H_2O)	<1.5	–

Acidic Spectral Data

No.	pH	λ_{max}	ε_{max} (×10⁻³)	λ_{min}	230	240	250	270	280	290
83	0	229	17.0	213	1.44*	1.14	0.86	1.33*	1.30*	1.11
		276	17.4	250						
84	4	278*	11.8	243*	0.75	0.33	0.47	1.67	1.89*	1.21
85	1^α,q	241	12.4	267	2.4	2.2*	1.7*	0.78	1.4	2.4*
		308	13.8							

Neutral Spectral Data

No.	pH	λ_{max}	ε_{max} (×10⁻³)	λ_{min}	230	240	250	270	280	290
83	7	249*	22.3	220	0.59	0.95	1.08	0.78	0.50*	0.42
84	7	278	11.6	243	0.55	0.36	0.48	1.63	1.82	1.18
85	7	247*	15.2	226	0.77	1.65	1.80	0.46	0.61*	0.95
		297*	8.7	271*						

Alkaline Spectral Data

No.	pH	λ_{max}	ε_{max} (×10⁻³)	λ_{min}	230	240	250	270	280	290
83	13	252	–	229	0.68	0.70	1.04	0.91	0.72	0.39
84	12°	266	9.0	243*	1.12	0.68	0.73	1.01	0.69*	0.26
85	13°	302	14.0	241	0.88	0.97	0.72	1.34	1.57	1.84

REFERENCES

No.	Origin and Synthesis	$[\alpha]_D^t$	pK	Spectral Data	Mass Spectra	R_f
83	C: 272,271ª,285,301 R: 270,329	285,301	–	271*,270ª,317ᵇᶜ,301*,329ᵇ	–	272,329
84	C: 57,30,125	–	58,57,59*	57,317ᵇᶜᵈᵉ,58ᵇ,59*,125*,126	317	57,59,110,125
85	C: 127,244,245,328 R: 116,298	127	127	127,116*ᵇᵉ,317ᵇᵈ,244*,245,265*ᵇ,298ᵇ	314,317,298	116,298,304,314

PURINES, PYRIMIDINES, NUCLEOSIDES AND NUCLEOTIDES: PHYSICAL CONSTANTS AND SPECTRAL PROPERTIES (Continued)

No.	Compound	Symbol		Structure	Formula (Mol Wt)	Melting Point °C	$[\alpha]_D^t$	pK	
		3-Letter	1-Letter					Basic	Acidic
86	N^4-Methylcytidine 4-Methylamino-1-β-D-ribofuranosyl-2-pyrimidinone	4MeCyd	m⁴C	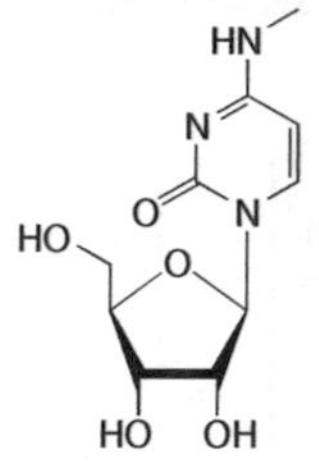	$C_{10}H_{15}N_3O_5$ (257.24)	237° (dec)	–	3.9	–
87	N^4-Methyl-2-thiocytidine	4Me2Syd 4Me2Scyd	m⁴s²C	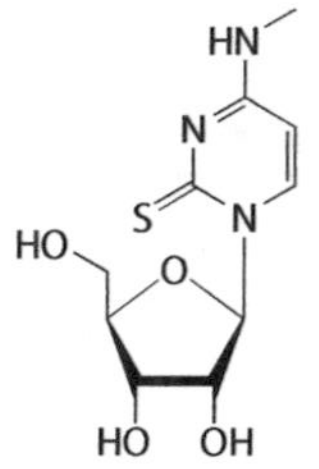	$C_{10}H_{15}N_3O_4S$ (273.32)	189–190°	–		
88	5-Methylcytidine	5MeCyd	m⁵C	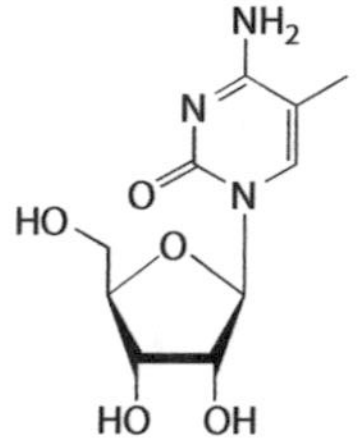	$C_{10}H_{15}N_3O_5$ (257.24)	210–211° (dec)	-3^{23} (2.5, 1 N NaOH)	4.3	>13

Acidic Spectral Data

No.	pH	λ_{max}	ε_{max} ($\times10^{-3}$)	λ_{min}	Spectral Ratios					
					230	240	250	270	280	290
86	1	281	14.3	243	0.85	0.37	0.49	1.72	2.13	1.73
87	0	238 276	18.5 18.1	216 257	1.31	1.50	1.05	1.39	1.40	0.86
88	0	287	12.6	245	1.72	0.42	0.33	2.24	3.59	3.96

Neutral Spectral Data

No.	pH	λ_{max}	ε_{max} ($\times10^{-3}$)	λ_{min}	Spectral Ratios					
					230	240	250	270	280	290
86	7	237 271	9.2 11.6	227 250	0.88	0.91	0.84	1.15	0.92	0.38
87	H₂O	224 262	14.9 27.4	236	0.49	0.51	0.64	0.92	0.65	0.37
88	7	277	8.9	255	1.53	1.34	1.03	1.33	1.45	0.96

Alkaline Spectral Data

No.	pH	λ_{max}	ε_{max} ($\times10^{-3}$)	λ_{min}	Spectral Ratios					
					230	240	250	270	280	290
86	14	236 273	8.9 11.6	251	0.93	0.93	0.84	1.22	1.06	0.51
87	–	–	–	–	–	–	–	–	–	–
88	14ᵃ	279	9.0	256	1.58	1.35	1.05	1.37	1.58	1.19

REFERENCES

No.	Origin and Synthesis	$[\alpha]_D^t$	pK	Spectral Data	Mass Spectra	R_f
86	C: 59,128	–	128,59	59ᵇ,128,317ᵇ	–	59,129,130,353
87	C: 271	–	–	271	–	–
88	C: 128	128	128	128ᵇ,132ᵇ,317ᵇ	314,317	110,132,314

PURINES, PYRIMIDINES, NUCLEOSIDES AND NUCLEOTIDES: PHYSICAL CONSTANTS AND SPECTRAL PROPERTIES (Continued)

No.	Compound	Symbol 3-Letter	Symbol 1-Letter	Formula (Mol Wt)	Melting Point °C	$[\alpha]_D^t$	pK Basic	pK Acidic
89	$O^{2'}$-Methylcytidine 2'-O-Methylcytidine	2'MeCyd	Cm	$C_{10}H_{15}N_3O_5$ (257.24)	252–253°	+54[21] (1.1, H_2O)	4.2[p]	–
90	$N^4,O^{2'}$-Dimethylcytidine	2',4Me₂Cyd	m⁴Cm	$C_{11}H_{17}N_3O_5$ (271.27)	–	–	3.9	–
91	5-N-Methylformamido-6-ribosylamino isocytosine[l] / 2-Amino-4-hydroxy-5-N-methylformamido-6-ribosylaminopyrimidine	5MeFn6(RibNH)isoCyt		$C_{11}H_{17}N_5O_6$ (315.29)	>180° (dec)	+32.5[25] (1, H_2O)	⁻0.6	9.6

Acidic Spectral Data

No.	pH	λ_{max}	ε_{max} (×10⁻³)	λ_{min}	230	240	250	270	280	290
89	1	281	12.9*	241	0.62	0.03	0.43	1.75	2.13	1.61
90	1	281	–	243	0.79	0.37	0.49	1.65	1.99	1.66
91	0.1[o]	270	25.1[n]	239	0.49	0.44	0.54	1.41	0.85	0.14
	1[o,q]	271	22.3	246						

Neutral Spectral Data

No.	pH	λ_{max}	ε_{max} (×10⁻³)	λ_{min}	230	240	250	270	280	290
89	(EtOH)	273	8.2	252	–	–	–	–	–	–
90	7	238, 270	–	227, 250	0.87	0.88	0.83	1.15	0.92	0.34
91	7	273	–	247	0.96	0.51	0.46	1.76	1.27	0.24

Alkaline Spectral Data

No.	pH	λ_{max}	ε_{max} (×10⁻³)	λ_{min}	230	240	250	270	280	290
89	11	272	8.9	251	1.46	0.96	0.85	1.18	0.94	0.31
90	–	–	–	–	–	–	–	–	–	–
91	12	265	16.3	244	0.74	0.57	0.59	0.99	0.24	0.02
	11.3	256–266	11.3	230	–	–	0.89	–	0.61	0.13

REFERENCES

No.	Origin and Synthesis	pK	$[\alpha]_D^t$	Spectral Data	Mass Spectra	R_f
89	C: 124,369[a]	124	124	124,369*[d],317[b]	315,317	109,110,124,369
90	R: 131	–	–	131[b]	–	131
91	C: 137,41	52	137	52,137[d],13[b],41	–	41

PURINES, PYRIMIDINES, NUCLEOSIDES AND NUCLEOTIDES: PHYSICAL CONSTANTS AND SPECTRAL PROPERTIES (Continued)

No.	Compound	Symbol 3-Letter	Symbol 1-Letter	Structure	Formula (Mol Wt)	Melting Point °C	$[\alpha]_D^t$	pK Basic	pK Acidic
92	Guanosine	Guo	G	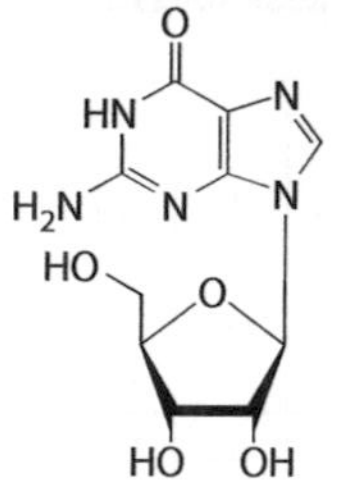	$C_{10}H_{13}N_5O_5$ (283.24)	>35° (dec)	-72^{26} (1.4, 0.1 N NaOH)	1.6*	9.2*, 12.4
93	1-Methylguanosine	1MeGuo	m¹G	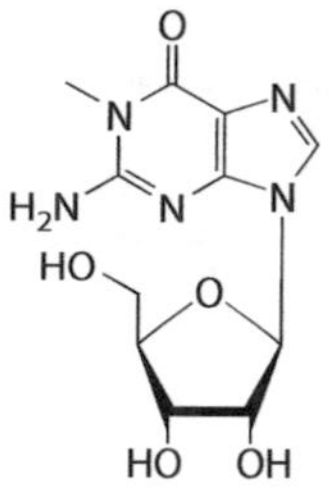	$C_{11}H_{15}N_5O_5$ (297.27)	225–227° (dec)	–	$^-2.4^1$	–
94	N^2-Methylguanosine 2-Methylamino-9-β-ribofuranosyl-purin-6-one	2MeGuo	m²G	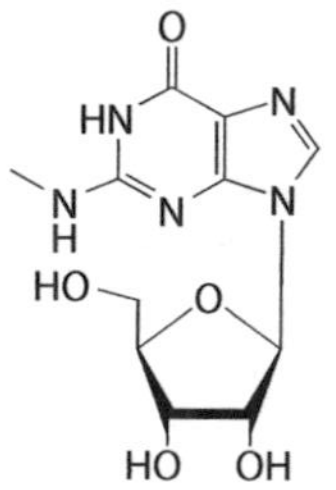	$C_{11}H_{15}N_5O_5$ (297.27)	>200° (dec)	-34.6^{26} (1.0 Me_2SO_4/EtOH)	2.3^p	9.7^p

Acidic Spectral Data

No.	pH	λ_{max}	ε_{max} (×10⁻³)	λ_{min}	230	240	250	270	280	290
92	0.7^q	256	12.3	228	0.26	0.56	0.94	0.75	0.70	0.50
93	1	258	11.4*	232*	0.28	0.45	0.85	0.77	0.71	0.53
94	1	259	14.2	231	0.52	0.49	0.85	0.73	0.56	0.52

Neutral Spectral Data

No.	pH	λ_{max}	ε_{max} (×10⁻³)	λ_{min}	230	240	250	270	280	290
92	6	253	13.6	223	0.36	0.79	1.15	0.83	0.67	0.28*
93	6	256	13.1*	225	0.28	0.61	1.00	0.84	0.63	0.21
94	7	253	15.9	225	0.35	0.70	1.18	0.68	0.58	0.52

Alkaline Spectral Data

No.	pH	λ_{max}	ε_{max} (×10⁻³)	λ_{min}	230	240	250	270	280	290
92	13	–	–	–	0.43	0.56	0.88	0.97	0.60	0.09
93	13	256*	12.9*	231	0.39	0.61	0.99	0.83	0.63	0.22*
94	13	258*	12.0*	237*	0.98	0.70	0.93	0.91	0.82	0.48

REFERENCES

No.	Origin and Synthesis	$[\alpha]_D^t$	pK	Mass Spectra	R_f
92	C: 237,231,351,372,373,111	237,351	231,170*,334*	314,315,374,317	258,110,40,189,314,242
93	E: 40 C: 24,400	–	–	314,317	24,40,110,314
94	E: 40 C: 44,372,381	44,381	40	314,317	40,44,110,314

No.	Spectral Data
92	$232^b,242*^e,183^b,317^b,212,205,111$
93	$40*,375^{c,d},317*^{b,c,e},24*,265*^b,400$
94	$40*,375^{c,d},317*^{b,c,d,e},381,44*$

PURINES, PYRIMIDINES, NUCLEOSIDES AND NUCLEOTIDES: PHYSICAL CONSTANTS AND SPECTRAL PROPERTIES (Continued)

No.	Compound	Symbol 3-Letter	Symbol 1-Letter	Structure	Formula (Mol Wt)	Melting Point °C	$[\alpha]_D^t$	pK Basic	pK Acidic
95	N^2,N^2-2-Dimethylguanosine; 2-Dimethylamino-9-β-ribofuranosyl-purin-6-one	2Me$_2$Guo	m$_2^2$G	(structure)	$C_{12}H_{17}N_5O_5$ (311.30)	242° (dec)	-35.6^{26} (1.1 Me$_2$SO$_4$/EtOH)	2.5^p	9.7^p
96	7-Methylguanosine	7MeGuo	m^{7}G	(structure)	$C_{11}H_{15}N_5O_5$ (297.27)	165° (hemihydrate)	-35.5^{27} (0.4, H$_2$O)	r	7.0*
97	N^2,N^2,7-Trimethylguanosine; 2-Dimethylamino-7-methyl-9-β-d-ribofuranosylpurin-6-one	2,2,7Me$_3$Guo	M$^2_{2}$$^{3\,7}G / m_2^2$m^{7}G	(structure)	$C_{13}H_{19}N_5O_5$ (325.33)	–	–	r	–

Acidic Spectral Data

No.	pH	λmax	εmax (×10⁻³)	λmin	230	240	250	270	280	290
95	1	265	17.7*	236*	0.45	0.32	0.63	0.92	0.56	0.48
96	3	257	10.7*	230	0.27	0.47	0.88	0.73	0.68	0.53
97	1	266 / 295	–	240	0.67	0.32	0.57	1.06	0.59	0.49

Neutral Spectral Data

No.	pH	λmax	εmax (×10⁻³)	λmin	230	240	250	270	280	290
95	7	260	18.9*^{n}	228	0.18	0.40	0.78	0.76	0.57	0.50
96	7^q	258 / 281	8.5 / 7.4	238*	–	–	0.89	–	1.04	0.90
97	5	266	10.3	239	0.67	0.32	0.57	1.08	0.63	0.51

Alkaline Spectral Data

No.	pH	λmax	εmax (×10⁻³)	λmin	230	240	250	270	280	290
95	11	262	12.2	240	–	–	–	–	–	–
96	13	263	14.3*	242*	1.37	0.75	0.85	0.88	0.78	0.65
97	9^q	282	8.0	242	2.10	0.84	0.90	1.16	1.46	1.30
97	10^q	234 / 302	–	280	2.04	1.93	1.31	0.84	0.62	0.73

REFERENCES

No.	Origin and Synthesis	$[\alpha]_D^t$	pK	Spectral Data	Mass Spectra	R$_f$
95	E: 40 C: 44,372,381	44,381	40	40^p,375^{cd},317*^{bcde},44*^{cd},265*^{b},381*	314,317	40,44,110,314
96	C: 13,41,10	10	41,13,334*	52,13^{bd},41*^{cd},10*^{s},334	314,317	10,41,314,334
97	C: 7,376	–	–	7^b	376	–

PURINES, PYRIMIDINES, NUCLEOSIDES AND NUCLEOTIDES: PHYSICAL CONSTANTS AND SPECTRAL PROPERTIES (Continued)

No.	Compound	Symbol (3-Letter)	Symbol (1-Letter)	Structure	Formula (Mol Wt)	Melting Point °C	$[\alpha]_D$	pK Basic	pK Acidic
98	O2'-Methylguanosine / 2'-O-Methyl guanosine	2'MeGuo	Gm	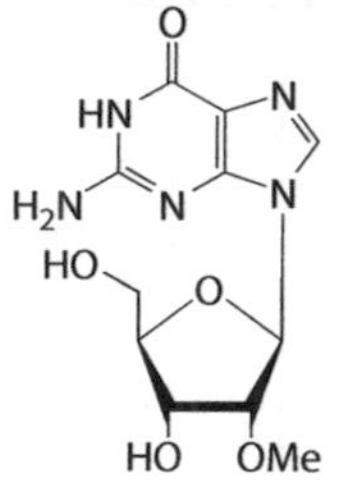 (structure)	$C_{11}H_{15}N_5O_5$ (297.27)	218–220°	-38.4^{22} (0.6, H_2O)	–	–
99	Inosine	Ino	I	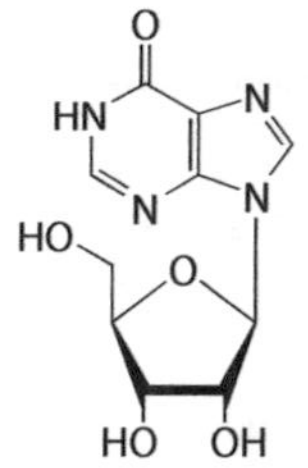 (structure)	$C_{10}H_{12}N_4O_5$ (268.23)	218°	-58.8 (2.5, H_2O)	1.2	8.8,12.
100	1-Methylinosine	1MeIno	m¹I	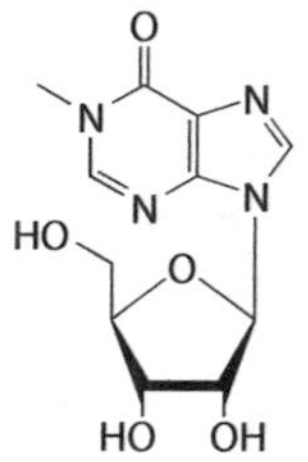 (structure)	$C_{11}H_{14}N_4O_5$ (282.25)	210–212°	-49.2^{28} (0.5, H_2O)	–	–

Acidic Spectral Data

No.	pH	λ_{max}	ε_{max} (×10⁻³)	λ_{min}	230	240	250	270	280	290
98	1	256	10.7	–	–	–	–	–	–	–
99	0	251	10.9	221	–	–	1.21	–	0.11	0.00
99	3	248	12.2	223	–	–	1.68	–	0.25	0.03
100	2t	250	10.4	223	0.59	1.14	1.42	0.57	0.23	0.03

Neutral Spectral Data

No.	pH	λ_{max}	ε_{max} (×10⁻³)	λ_{min}	230	240	250	270	280	290
98	6	248.5	12.3	223	–	–	1.68	–	0.25	0.03
99	6	249	10.4	223*	0.64	1.35	1.69	0.71	0.40	0.07

Alkaline Spectral Data

No.	pH	λ_{max}	ε_{max} (×10⁻³)	λ_{min}	230	240	250	270	280	290
98	11	258	9.8	–	–	–	–	–	–	–
99	11	253	13.1	224	–	–	1.05	–	0.18	0.01
100	12	249	10.7	–	0.86	1.28	1.6	0.67	0.35	0.07

REFERENCES

No.	Origin and Synthesis	$[\alpha]_D$	pK	Spectral Data	Mass Spectra	R_f
98	C: 108	108	–	108	315	109,110
99	R: 231ᵃ C: 377,378	255	170,231,51,250	232ᵇ,205,317ᵇ	314,317	110,314,378
100	C: 10,122	10	–	49,10*6,410ᵒˢ,122	314,317	10,49,110,122,314

PURINES, PYRIMIDINES, NUCLEOSIDES AND NUCLEOTIDES: PHYSICAL CONSTANTS AND SPECTRAL PROPERTIES (Continued)

No.	Compound	Symbol 3-Letter	Symbol 1-Letter	Structure	Formula (Mol Wt)	Melting Point °C	$[\alpha]_D^t$	pK Basic	pK Acidic
101	2-Methylinosine	2MeIno	m^2I		$C_{11}H_{14}N_4O_5$ (282.25)	165–166°	-50.0^{26} (1.0, H_2O)	–	–
102	Nebularine 9-β-Ribofuranosylpurine	Neb			$C_{10}H_{12}N_4O_4$ (252.33)	181–182°	-48.6^{25} (1.0, H_2O)	2.1	–
103	Uridine	Urd	U		$C_9H_{12}N_2O_6$ (244.20)	165–166°	$+9.6^{16}$ (2.0, H_2O)	–	9.2, 12.5

Acidic Spectral Data

No.	pH	λ_{max}	ε_{max} (×10⁻³)	λ_{min}	230	240	250	270	280	290
101	1	253	11.9	235	0.51	0.49	0.74	0.85	0.29	0.07
102	1	262	5.9	230	–	–	0.74	–	0.35	0.03
103	1	262	10.1	230						

Neutral Spectral Data

No.	pH	λ_{max}	ε_{max} (×10⁻³)	λ_{min}	230	240	250	270	280	290
101	7	251.5	12.7	222	0.35	0.54	0.71	0.68	0.11	0.04
102	H_2O	262	7.1							
103	7	262	10.1	230	–	–	0.74	–	0.35	0.03

Alkaline Spectral Data

No.	pH	λ_{max}	ε_{max} (×10⁻³)	λ_{min}	230	240	250	270	280	290
101	13	258	13.1	234	0.45	0.48	0.71	0.75	0.22	0.11
102	13	262	7.1	243	–	–	0.83	–	0.29	0.02
103	12	262	7.45	243						
103	14	264.5	7.5	243						

REFERENCES

No.	Origin and Synthesis	$[\alpha]_D^t$	pK	Spectral Data
101	C: 377	377	–	377
102	C: 123,363,391	123,363	123	123ᵇ,391
103	R: 236,181 C: 379,276ᵃ,380	236,276	163,231	163ᵇ,232*ᵇᵉ,181ᵇ,212,183ᵇ,

No.	Mass Spectra	R_f
101	–	377
102	405	–
103	341,315,317	258,110,40

PURINES, PYRIMIDINES, NUCLEOSIDES AND NUCLEOTIDES: PHYSICAL CONSTANTS AND SPECTRAL PROPERTIES (Continued)

No.	Compound	Symbol (3-Letter)	Symbol (1-Letter)	Structure	Formula (Mol Wt)	Melting Point °C	$[\alpha]_D$	pK Basic	pK Acidic
104	2-Thiouridine	2Srd / 2SUrd	s^2U	(structure)	$C_9H_{12}N_2O_5S$ (260.26)	214°	$+39^0$ (1.2, H_2O)	–	8.8
105	2,4-Dithiouridine	2,4Srd / 2,4S_2 Urd	$s_2^{2,4}U$ / s^2s^4U	(structure)	$C_9H_{12}N_2O_4S_2$ (276.33)	166–167°	–	–	7.4
106	5-Carboxymethyl-2-Thiouridine-5-acetic acid	5Cm2SUrd / 5Cm2Srd / 5(CxMe)2SUrd	cm^5s^2U / cm^5S	(structure)	$C_{11}H_{14}N_2O_7S$ (318.31)	–	–	–	–

Acidic Spectral Data

No.	pH	λ_{max}	ε_{max} (×10⁻³)	λ_{min}	230	240	250	270	280	290
104	2	279	16.4	247	1.32	0.63	0.53	1.66	1.86	1.66
105	–	–	–	–	–	–	–	–	–	–
106	1	274.5	–	–	–	–	–	–	–	–

Neutral Spectral Data

No.	pH	λ_{max}	ε_{max} (×10⁻³)	λ_{min}	230	240	250	270	280	290
104	7	218* / 275*	16.2 / 13.6*	247	1.16	0.70	0.62	1.47	1.57	1.40
105	5.8	283	22.5	–	–	–	–	–	–	–
106	7	277.5	–	–	–	–	–	–	–	–

Alkaline Spectral Data

No.	pH	λ_{max}	ε_{max} (×10⁻³)	λ_{min}	230	240	250	270	280	290
104	9i / 12	241 / 239 / 271	21.8 / 21.0 / 13.4	261	1.07	1.43	1.22	1.02	0.88	0.59
105	9	280 / 320	16.9 / 24.8	–	–	–	–	–	–	–
106	–	–	–	–	–	–	–	–	–	–

REFERENCES

No.	$[\alpha]_D$	pK	Spectral Data
104	276,301	285	276*b,277b,301*cd,306b,305b
105	–	271	271
106	–	–	303

No.	Mass Spectra	Origin and Synthesis	R_f
104	–	C: 276,285,301 E: 277	276,306,307,305
105	–	C: 271	271
106	–	R: 303	303

Purines, Pyrimidines, Nucleosides, and Nucleotides

PURINES, PYRIMIDINES, NUCLEOSIDES AND NUCLEOTIDES: PHYSICAL CONSTANTS AND SPECTRAL PROPERTIES (Continued)

No.	Compound	Symbol 3-Letter	Symbol 1-Letter	Structure	Formula (Mol Wt)	Melting Point °C	$[\alpha]_D^t$	pK Basic	pK Acidic
107	5-Carbamoylmethyl-2-thiouridine / 2-Thiouridine-5-acetamide	5Ncm2Srd / 5Ncm2SUrd / 5(NcMe)2Srd	ncm5s2U / ncm5S	(structure)	$C_{11}H_{15}N_3O_6S$ (317.32)	217–218°	–	–	–
108	5-(Methoxycarbonylmethyl)-2-thiouridine / 5-Carboxymethyl-2-thiouridine methyl ester	5(MeCm)2SUrd / 5(MeCm)2Srd	mcm5s2U / mcm5S	(structure)	$C_{12}H_{16}N_2O_7S$ (332.33)	199°	+19.8^{20} (0.5, H_2O)	–	–
109	5-Methoxy-2-thiouridine	5MeO2SUrd / 5MeO2Srd	mo5S / mo5s2U	(structure)	$C_{10}H_{14}N_2O_6S$ (290.30)	221–222°	+18.2^{24} (0.5, H_2O)	–	–

Acidic Spectral Data

No.	pH	λ_{max}	ε_{max} (×10⁻³)	λ_{min}	230	240	250	270	280	290
108	1	277*	15.6	244	1.22	0.73	0.68	1.49	1.54	1.41

Spectral Ratios columns: 230, 240, 250, 270, 280, 290

Neutral Spectral Data

No.	pH	λ_{max}	ε_{max} (×10⁻³)	λ_{min}	230	240	250	270	280	290
107	(MeOH)	221 / 276	12.9 / 13.7							
108	7	220 / 277*	15.3 / 15.8	244	1.18	0.84	0.76	1.42	1.45	1.24
109	(MeOH)	227 / 285	10.0 / 12.6							

Spectral Ratios columns: 230, 240, 250, 270, 280, 290

Alkaline Spectral Data

No.	pH	λ_{max}	ε_{max} (×10⁻³)	λ_{min}	230	240	250	270	280	290
108	13 (MeOH)	242 / 272	18.2 / 15.6							
109	12	242 / 271	22.4 / 15.8	261	1.06	1.37	1.16	1.02	0.86	0.46
109	13 (MeOH)	248 / 272	20.0 / 12.6							

Spectral Ratios columns: 230, 240, 250, 270, 280, 290

REFERENCES

No.	Origin and Synthesis	$[\alpha]_D^t$	pK	Spectral Data	Mass Spectra	R_f
107	C: 301	–	–	301	–	301
108	C: 5,310 R: 275,306	301	–	5,301[cd],31[bc],275*[b]	317,5,301,275	275,301,303,306,307
109	C: 301	301	–	301	–	–

PURINES, PYRIMIDINES, NUCLEOSIDES AND NUCLEOTIDES: PHYSICAL CONSTANTS AND SPECTRAL PROPERTIES (Continued)

No.	Compound	Symbol 3-Letter	Symbol 1-Letter	Structure	Formula (Mol Wt)	Melting Point °C	$[\alpha]_D^t$	pK Basic	pK Acidic
110	5-Methyl-2-thiouridine / 2-Thio-1-ribosylthymine	5Me2Surd / 5MeSrd	m5s2U / s2T	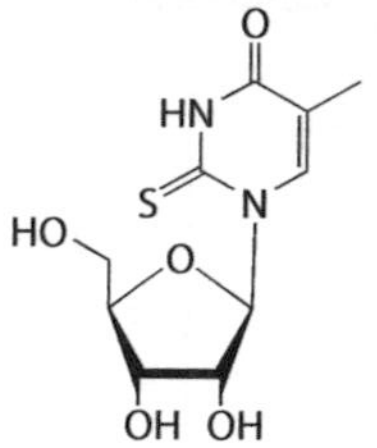	$C_{10}H_{14}N_2O_5S$ (274.30)	217°	$+31^{28}$ (1.23, H2O)	—	—
111	5-(Methylaminomethyl)-2-thiouridine / 5-(N-Methylaminomethyl)-2-thiouridine	5(MeNHMe)Srd / 5(MeNHMe)2Surd	mnm5s2U / mnm5S	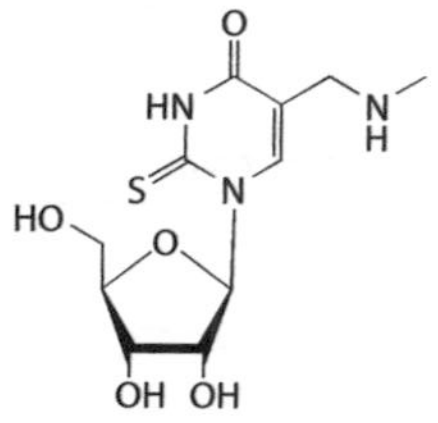	$C_{11}H_{17}N_3O_5S$ (303.33)	—	—	—	—
112	3-Methyluridine	3MeUrd	m3U	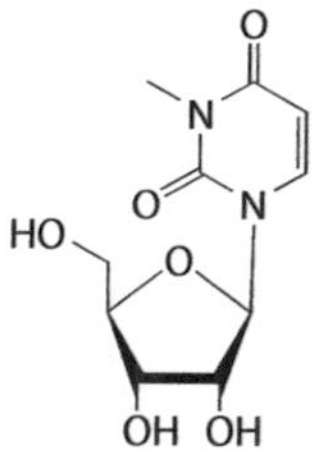	$C_{10}H_{14}N_2O_6$ (258.23)	119–120°	$+20.1^{26}$ (H2O)	—	—

Acidic Spectral Data

No.	pH	λ_{max}	ε_{max} (×10⁻³)	λ_{min}	230	240	250	270	280	290
110	2	218 / 273	17.4 / 14.8	243	1.05	0.53	0.58	1.41	1.43	1.22
111	1	220 / 273	–	242	0.84	0.56	0.66	1.31	1.29	1.20
112	2ʸ	262*	9.5	232	0.31	0.39	0.74	0.90	0.35*	0.04*

Neutral Spectral Data

No.	pH	λ_{max}	ε_{max} (×10⁻³)	λ_{min}	230	240	250	270	280	290
110	7	219 / 272	16.2 / 14.1	247	1.06	0.77	0.69	1.40	1.39	1.15
111	7	220 / 273	–	242	0.84	0.56	0.66	1.33	1.31	1.22
112	7	262	9.5*	232	0.31	0.39	0.74	0.90	0.35	0.04

Alkaline Spectral Data

No.	pH	λ_{max}	ε_{max} (×10⁻³)	λ_{min}	230	240	250	270	280	290
110	9ᵃ	239	21.0	259	1.35	1.64	1.20	1.10	1.04	0.60
111	13	243	–	227	1.00	1.33	1.21	1.01	0.87	0.49
112	12	263*	9.4	232	0.32	0.38	0.70	0.91	0.46*	0.10

REFERENCES

No.	Origin and Synthesis	$[\alpha]_D^t$	pK	Spectral Data	Mass Spectra	R_f
110	C: 276,307 R: 307	276	–	276ᵇ,307ᵇ	–	276,307,306
111	R: 270,305	–	–	270,317ᵇ,305ᵇ	270,317	270,305
112	C: 139,125,140–142,81	139	–	317ᵇ,142*,13*,81*,139,126*	314,317	13,57,81,110,125,126,142,143,173,314

PURINES, PYRIMIDINES, NUCLEOSIDES AND NUCLEOTIDES: PHYSICAL CONSTANTS AND SPECTRAL PROPERTIES (Continued)

No.	Compound	Symbol 3-Letter	Symbol 1-Letter	Structure	Formula (Mol Wt)	Melting Point °C	$[\alpha]_D^t$	pK Basic	pK Acidic
113	3-(3-Amino-3-carboxypropyl)uridine / Uridine-3-(α-aminobutyric acid)	3NH₂,BtoUrd / 3(NH₂,CxPr)Urd	nbt3U		$C_{13}H_{19}N_3O_8$ (345.31)	161–163° (2HCl salt)	–	–	–
114	4-Thiouridine	4Srd / 4SUrd	s4U		$C_9H_{12}N_2O_5S$ (260.26)	135–138° (dec)	–	–	8.2
115	4-Thiouridine disulfide bis(4-4'-Dithiouridine)	(4SUrd)₂			$C_{18}H_{22}N_4O_{10}S_2$ (518.51)	188–190°	–	–	–

Acidic Spectral Data

No.	pH	λ_{max}	ε_{max} (×10⁻³)	λ_{min}	230	240	250	270	280	290
113	2	263	8.5	233	0.41	0.45	0.76	0.89	0.43	0.05
114	2	245	5.2*	275*	–	–	–	–	–	–
		331	17.0*	–						
115	–	–	–	–						

Neutral Spectral Data

No.	pH	λ_{max}	ε_{max} (×10⁻³)	λ_{min}	230	240	250	270	280	290
113	6	263	8.5	233	0.41	0.45	0.76	0.89	0.43	0.05
114	6.5	245	4.0*	225	–	–	–	–	–	–
		331	21.2*	274						
115	7	261	–	236	–	–	–	–	–	–
		309	–	278						

Alkaline Spectral Data

No.	pH	λ_{max}	ε_{max} (×10⁻³)	λ_{min}	230	240	250	270	280	290
113	12	263	8.5	234	0.46	0.52	0.77	0.89	0.44	0.08
114	12	316	19.7*	268*	–	–	–	–	–	–
115	–	–	–	–	–	–	–	–	–	–

REFERENCES

No.	Origin and Synthesis	pK	$[\alpha]_D^t$	Spectral Data	Mass Spectra	R_f
113	C: 300 R: 300,345	–	–	300ᵇ	300	300,345
114	C: 344,128 R: 144	144	–	344*,144*ᵇᶜᵈ,317*ᵇ,128	–	144,344
115	C: 128	–	–	128,208ᵇ	–	144

PURINES, PYRIMIDINES, NUCLEOSIDES AND NUCLEOTIDES: PHYSICAL CONSTANTS AND SPECTRAL PROPERTIES (Continued)

No.	Compound	Symbol 1-Letter	Symbol 3-Letter	Structure	Formula (Mol Wt)	Melting Point °C	$[\alpha]_D^t$	pK Basic	pK Acidic
116	5-Carboxymethyluridine Uridine-5-acetic acid	cm5U	5CmUrd 5(CxMe)Urd	(structure: COOH)	$C_{11}H_{14}N_2O_8$ (302.24)	242–244°	-24.3^{25} (1N NaOH)	–	4.2, 9.8
117	5-Carbamoylmethyluridine Uridine-5-acetamide	ncm5U	5NcmUrd 5(NcMe)Urd	(structure: CONH$_2$)	$C_{11}H_{15}N_3O_7$ (301.26)	227–230°	–	–	–
118	5-(Methoxycarbonylmethyl)uridine 5-Carboxymethyluridine methyl ester Uridine-5-acetic acid methyl ester	mcm5U	5MeCmUrd 5(MeCxMe)Urd	(structure: COOMe)	$C_{12}H_{16}N_2O_8$ (316.27)	163–165°	–	–	–

Acidic Spectral Data

No.	pH	λ_{max}	ε_{max} (×10⁻³)	λ_{min}	230	240	250	270	280	290
116	1	265	9.7	234*	0.39	0.40	0.69	1.02	0.64	0.19
117	1	265	10.0	232*	–	–	–	–	–	–
118	1	265	5.2	232						

Neutral Spectral Data

No.	pH	λ_{max}	ε_{max} (×10⁻³)	λ_{min}	230	240	250	270	280	290
116	7	266.5	–	236	0.50	0.41	0.68	1.07	0.75	0.27
117	H$_2$O	266	–	233	0.24	0.34	0.67	1.05	0.66	0.17

Alkaline Spectral Data

No.	pH	λ_{max}	ε_{max} (×10⁻³)	λ_{min}	230	240	250	270	280	290
116	13	266.5*	7.1	245	1.29	0.84	0.80	1.05	0.71	0.25
117	13	267*	7.0	244	1.10	0.78	0.79	0.98	0.54	0.11

REFERENCES

No.	Origin and Synthesis	$[\alpha]_D^t$	pK	Spectral Data	Mass Spectra	R_f
116	R: 278 C: 302,322[a]	322	302	278[b],302*[d],317[b]	–	278,302,303,304
117	C: 302 R: 398	–	–	302*,398*[cs]	–	302
118	C: 302,304 R: 304	–	–	302,414[b]	414	302,303,304

PURINES, PYRIMIDINES, NUCLEOSIDES AND NUCLEOTIDES: PHYSICAL CONSTANTS AND SPECTRAL PROPERTIES (Continued)

No.	Compound	Symbol 3-Letter	Symbol 1-Letter	Structure	Formula (Mol Wt)	Melting Point °C	$[\alpha]_D^t$	pK Basic	pK Acidic
119	5-Hydroxyuridine	5HOUrd	o5U		$C_9H_{12}N_2O_7$ (260.20)	242–245°	–	–	7.8
120	5-Carboxymethoxyuridine Uridine-5-oxyacetic acid	5CmOUrd 5(CxMeO)Urd	cmo5U		$C_{11}H_{14}N_2O_9$ (318.24)	–	–	–	2.9
121	5-Methyluridine 1-β-Ribofuranosylthymine Ribosylthymine	5MeUrd rThd* Thd	m5UT		$C_{10}H_{14}N_2O_6$ (258.23)	183–185°	-10^{31} (2.0, H$_2$O)	–	9.7

Acidic Spectral Data

No.	pH	λ_{max}	ε_{max} (×10^{-3})	λ_{min}	230	240	250	270	280	290
119	2	280	–	245	0.92	0.50	0.56	1.52	1.76	1.46
120	2a	277	8.4	243	0.44	0.39	0.67	1.07	0.74	0.27
121	1	267	9.9*	235*						

Neutral Spectral Data

No.	pH	λ_{max}	ε_{max} (×10^{-3})	λ_{min}	230	240	250	270	280	290
119	7a	280*	8.2	–	–	–	–	–	–	–
120	7.5	280	7.6	247	–	–	–	–	–	–
121	7	267	9.8	236	0.44	0.39	0.67	1.07	0.74	0.27

Alkaline Spectral Data

No.	pH	λ_{max}	ε_{max} (×10^{-3})	λ_{min}	230	240	250	270	280	290
119	12	306	–	267	–	1.60	1.29	0.70	0.89	1.16
120	13	278	6.7	252	1.31	0.91	0.83	1.08	0.75	0.31*
121	13	268	7.5	246						

REFERENCES

No.	Origin and Synthesis	$[\alpha]_D^t$	pK	Spectral Data	Mass Spectra	R$_f$
119	C: 145-147 R: 148	–	382	148b, 145d, 146*	317	148
120	C: 308 R: 308,309	–	308	308b, 309i, 313b	308	308,309
121	E: 18,149 C: 150,69,380,386,379	150,322,379	150	18b,150bd,149bcd,317be,69*,265*b,379	314,317	18,69,110,142,149,314,304

PURINES, PYRIMIDINES, NUCLEOSIDES AND NUCLEOTIDES: PHYSICAL CONSTANTS AND SPECTRAL PROPERTIES (Continued)

No.	Compound	Structure	Symbol (3-Letter)	Symbol (1-Letter)	Formula (Mol Wt)	Melting Point °C	$[\alpha]_D^t$	pK Basic	pK Acidic
122	5-Hydroxymethyluridine		5HmUrd, 5HOMeUrd	om5U, hm5U*	$C_{10}H_{14}N_2O_7$ (274.23)	167–168°	–	–	–
123	Dihydrouridine 5,6-Dihydrouridine		H₂Urd	hU, D	$C_9H_{14}N_2O_6$ (246.22)	106–108°	-36.8^{20} (2.1, H_2O)	–	–
124	5-Methyl-5,6-dihydrouridine 5,6-Dihydroribosylthymine		5MeH₂ Urd	m5D, m5hU	$C_{10}H_{16}N_2O_6$ (260.25)	–		–	–

Acidic Spectral Data

No.	pH	λ_{max}	ε_{max} (×10⁻³)	λ_{min}	230	240	250	270	280	290
122	2	264	9.5	233	–	–	0.70	–	0.52	–
123	–	–	–	–	–	–	–	–	–	–
124										

Neutral Spectral Data

No.	pH	λ_{max}	ε_{max} (×10⁻³)	λ_{min}	230	240	250	270	280	290
122	7	263	–	–	–	–	–	–	–	–
123	H_2O	208	6.6	–	–	–	–	–	0.53	–
124										

Alkaline Spectral Data

No.	pH	λ_{max}	ε_{max} (×10⁻³)	λ_{min}	230	240	250	270	280	290
122	12	263	7.0	243	–	–	0.79	–	0.45	–
123	13°	235*	10.1	–	–	–	–	–	–	–
124										

REFERENCES

No.	Origin and Synthesis	$[\alpha]_D^t$	pK	Spectral Data	Mass Spectra	Rf
122	C: 69,151	–	–	69,94[co]		69
123	C: 266,384,99,147	384,412	–	266,283[cd],375*,265[b]	314,317	314,383,333
124	C: 333 R: 333	–	–	–	–	333

PURINES, PYRIMIDINES, NUCLEOSIDES AND NUCLEOTIDES: PHYSICAL CONSTANTS AND SPECTRAL PROPERTIES (Continued)

No.	Compound	Symbol 3-Letter	Symbol 1-Letter	Structure	Formula (Mol Wt)	Melting Point °C	$[\alpha]_D^t$	pK Basic	pK Acidic
125	O²′-Methyluridine / 2′-O-Methyluridine	2′MeUrd	Um		$C_{10}H_{14}N_2O_6$ (258.23)	159°	+41²⁰ (1.6, H₂O)	–	⁻9.3ᵖ
126	5,O²′-Dimethyluridine / O²′-Methylribothymidine	2′,5Me₂ Urd	m⁵Um / Tm		$C_{11}H_{16}N_2O_6$ (272.26)	–	–	–	–
127	Orotidine Uridine-6-carboxylic acid / 6-Carboxyuridine	Ord / 6CxUrd	O		$C_{10}H_{12}N_2O_8$ (288.21)	183–184° (CHA salt)ᵍ	–	–	–

Acidic Spectral Data

No.	pH	λ_{max}	ε_{max} (×10⁻³)	λ_{min}	230	240	250	270	280	290
							Spectral Ratios			
125	2	263*	10.0	231	0.23	0.39	0.75	0.86	0.38	0.04
126	1	268	–	237	0.52	0.37	0.66	1.10	0.76	0.26
127	1	267	9.8	234	0.39	0.41	0.66	1.12	0.81	0.37

Neutral Spectral Data

No.	pH	λ_{max}	ε_{max} (×10⁻³)	λ_{min}	230	240	250	270	280	290
							Spectral Ratios			
125	7	263	10.1	231	0.23	0.39	0.75	0.86	0.38	0.04
126	7	267	–	237	0.51	0.36	0.64	1.09	0.74	0.26
127	–	–	–	–	–	–	–	–	–	–

Alkaline Spectral Data

No.	pH	λ_{max}	ε_{max} (×10⁻³)	λ_{min}	230	240	250	270	280	290
							Spectral Ratios			
125	12	262	7.4	243	0.98	0.76	0.83	0.82	0.3	0.03
126	13	267	–	247	–	0.88	0.78	1.05	0.67	0.15
127	13	266	7.8	245	1.07	0.83	0.83	1.04	0.71	0.29

No.	Origin and Synthesis	$[\alpha]_D^t$	pK	Spectral Data	Mass Spectra	R_f
125	C: 124,369	124	124,138	124*,317ᵃᶜᵈᵉ,369	315,317	109,110,124,369
126	C: 323 R: 323	–	–	323	–	323
127	N: 160	–	–	160ᵇ	–	–

REFERENCES

PURINES, PYRIMIDINES, NUCLEOSIDES AND NUCLEOTIDES: PHYSICAL CONSTANTS AND SPECTRAL PROPERTIES (Continued)

No.	Compound	Symbol 3-Letter	Symbol 1-Letter	Structure	Formula (Mol Wt)	Melting Point °C	$[\alpha]_D^t$	pK Basic	pK Acidic
128	Spongouridine 1-β-D-Arabinofuranosyluracil	AraUrd aUrd	aU	(structure)	$C_9H_{12}N_2O_6$ (244.20)	222–224°	$+131^{20}$ (0.63, H_2O)	–	9.3
129	Spongothymidine 1-β-D-Arabinofuranosylthymine	AraThd aThd 5MeaUrd	aT m^5 aU	(structure)	$C_{10}H_{14}N_2O_6$ (258.23)	238–242°	$93^{24}{}_{589}$ (0.5, H_2O);	–	9.8
130	Pseudouridine β f-Pseudouridine Pseudouridine C; 5-β-D-Ribofuranosyluracil 5-Ribosyluracil	Ψrd βΨrd ΨrdC*	Ψ	(structure)	$C_9H_{12}N_2O_6$ (244.20)	223–224°	–3.0 (1.0, H_2O)	–	9.0*, >13

Acidic Spectral Data

No.	pH	λ_{max}	ε_{max} (×10⁻³)	λ_{min}	230	240	250	270	280	290
128	1	264	9.3	232	–	–	–	–	–	–
129	1	268	10.0	236	0.36	0.31	0.61	1.15	0.85	0.36
130	2ʸ	262	7.9*	233	–	–	0.74	–	0.42*	0.06*

Neutral Spectral Data

No.	pH	λ_{max}	ε_{max} (×10⁻³)	λ_{min}	230	240	250	270	280	290
128	H_2O	263	10.5*	231	–	–	–	–	–	–
129	7	268	10.0	236	0.36	0.31	0.61	1.15	0.85	0.36
130	7	263	8.1*	233	0.33	0.42	0.74	0.90	0.44	0.08

Alkaline Spectral Data

No.	pH	λ_{max}	ε_{max} (×10⁻³)	λ_{min}	230	240	250	270	280	290
128	11.5	263	7.2	242	–	–	–	–	–	–
128	14	265	7.9	241						
129	12	269	7.9	245	1.17	0.70	0.69	1.15	0.77	0.22
130	12	286	7.7*	245	2.06	0.73	0.62	1.51	2.06	2.16
130	14ᵍ	279	5.7ʰ	248	2.31	1.11	0.61	1.67	2.09	1.51

REFERENCES

No.	pK	$[\alpha]_D^t$	Spectral Data
128	392	392	393*ᵇ,392ᶜᵈ
129	163	162	163ᵇ,161ᵇ
130	155,156,94*,95*	95	155,94*ᵇᵈᵉ,154ᶜᵈ,95*ᵇᵉ,156ᵇ,157,265*ᵇ,317ᵇ

No.	Origin and Synthesis	Mass Spectra	R_f
128	N: 393 C: 394,392	–	392,393
129	N: 161 C: 162	–	393
130	N: 153 C: 154,387 R: 388	314,317	110,157–159,314

PURINES, PYRIMIDINES, NUCLEOSIDES AND NUCLEOTIDES: PHYSICAL CONSTANTS AND SPECTRAL PROPERTIES (Continued)

No.	Compound	Symbol (3-Letter)	Symbol (1-Letter)	Structure	Formula (Mol Wt)	Melting Point °C	$[\alpha]_D^t$	pK Basic	pK Acidic
131	α-f-Pseudouridine Pseudouridine B5-α-D-Ribofuranosyluracil	αfΨrd Ψrd B*	Ψ_B*		$C_9H_{12}N_2O_6$ (244.20)	–	–	–	9.2*, >13
132	β-p-Pseudouridine Pseudouridine A_s;5-β-D-Ribopyranosyluracil	βpΨrd Ψrd A_s*	Ψ_{AS}*		$C_9H_{12}N_2O_6$ (244.20)	–	–	–	9.6, >13

Acidic Spectral Data

No.	pH	λ_{max}	ε_{max} (×10⁻³)	λ_{min}	230	240	250	270	280	290
131	v	–	–	–	–	–	–	–	–	–
132	v	–	–	–	–	–	–	–	–	–

Neutral Spectral Data

No.	pH	λ_{max}	ε_{max} (×10⁻³)	λ_{min}	230	240	250	270	280	290
131	7	264	–	234	0.33	0.38	0.70	0.95	0.51	0.09
132	7	262	8.3	231	0.25	0.41	0.75	0.83	0.34	0.04

Alkaline Spectral Data

No.	pH	λ_{max}	ε_{max} (×10⁻³)	λ_{min}	230	240	250	270	280	290
131	12	288	–	245	1.88	0.76	0.70	1.26	1.46	1.56
131	14[a]	279	–	248	2.20	1.02	0.61	1.56	1.81	1.37
132	12	286	9.2	244	2.10	0.60	0.56	1.69	2.50	2.66
132	14[a]	281	7.5[n]	247	2.24	0.81	0.54	1.73	2.28	1.93

REFERENCES

No.	Origin and Synthesis	$[\alpha]_D^t$	pK	Spectral Data	Mass Spectra	R_f
131	C: 154 R: 94,388	–	156,94*	155,94[bca],156[b]	–	158
132	R: 94,388 C: 154	–	94	155,94[bcde]	–	97

PURINES, PYRIMIDINES, NUCLEOSIDES AND NUCLEOTIDES: PHYSICAL CONSTANTS AND SPECTRAL PROPERTIES (Continued)

No.	Compound	Symbol 3-Letter	Symbol 1-Letter	Structure	Formula (Mol Wt)	Melting Point °C	$[\alpha]_D^t$	pK Basic	pK Acidic
133	α-ρ-Pseudouridine Pseudouridine A_r; 5-α-D-Ribopyranosyluracil	αρΨrd, Ψrd A_r*	Ψ_{AF}*		$C_9H_{12}N_2O_6$ (244.20)	–	–	–	9.6, >13
134	1-Methylpseudouridine 1-Methyl-5-ribosyluracil	1MeΨrd	m¹ψ		$C_{10}H_{14}N_2O_6$ (258.23)				–
135	O²'-Methylpseudouridine 2'-O-Methylpseudouridine	2'MeΨrd	ψm		$C_{10}H_{14}N_2O_6$ (258.23)	–	–	–	–

Acidic Spectral Data

No.	pH	λ_{max}	ε_{max} (×10⁻³)	λ_{min}	230	240	250	270	280	290
133	v	–	–	–	–	–	–	–	–	–
134	2	–	–	–	–	–	0.54	–	1.03*	0.38
135	1	261	–	–	–	–	–	–	–	–

Neutral Spectral Data

No.	pH	λ_{max}	ε_{max} (×10⁻³)	λ_{min}	230	240	250	270	280	290
133	7	263	–	233	0.27	0.37	0.71	0.90	0.42*	0.05
134	7	265	–	–	–	–	–	–	0.66	–
135	7	261	–	–	–	–	–	–	–	–

Alkaline Spectral Data

No.	pH	λ_{max}	ε_{max} (×10⁻³)	λ_{min}	230	240	250	270	280	290
133	12	287	–	244*	1.59	0.62	0.67	1.26	1.49	1.58
	14ᵍ	278	–	248	2.09	1.04	0.65	1.52	1.75	1.32
134	12	269	–	246	–	–	0.62	–	0.69*	0.08
	14	272	–	–	–	–	–	–	1.05	–
135	13	281	–	–	–	–	–	–	–	–

REFERENCES

No.	Origin and Synthesis	$[\alpha]_D^t$	pK	Spectral Data	Mass Spectra	R_f
133	R: 94,388 C: 154	–	94	155,94ᵇᶜᵉ	–	97
134	C: 94,81	–	–	94*ᵇ,81ᵇᵉ,345ᶜ	–	81,345
135	R: 118,415	–	–	118ᵇ	–	118,415

PURINES, PYRIMIDINES, NUCLEOSIDES AND NUCLEOTIDES: PHYSICAL CONSTANTS AND SPECTRAL PROPERTIES (Continued)

No.	Compound	Symbol 3-Letter	Symbol 1-Letter	Structure	Formula (Mol Wt)	Melting Point °C	$[\alpha]_D^t$	pK Basic	pK Acidic
136	Wyosine (Formerly "Yt") 1-N^2-Isopropeno-3-methylguanosine; 4,9-Dihydro-4,6-dimethyl-9-oxo-3-β-D-ribofuranosyl 1H-imidazo[1,2-a]purine	Wyo, imGuo*	W		$C_{14}H_{17}N_5O_5$ (335.32)	—	—	—	—
137	Wybutosine (Formerly "Y") 7-[3-(Methoxycarbonyl)-3-(methoxyformamido)propyl] wyosine; α-(Carboxyamino)-4,9-dihydro-4,6-dimethyl-9-oxo-3-β-D-ribofuranosyl-1H-imidazo[1,2-a]purine-7-butyric acid dimethyl ester	Y-Wyo, (MeO)₂ FnBto-Wyo, Y-imGuo*	yW, m₂, fnbtW		$C_{21}H_{28}N_6O_9$ (508.49)	—	—	—	—

Acidic Spectral Data

No.	pH	λ_{max}	ε_{max} ($\times 10^{-3}$)	λ_{min}	230	240	250	270	280	290
136										
137										

Neutral Spectral Data

No.	pH	λ_{max}	ε_{max} ($\times 10^{-3}$)	λ_{min}	230	240	250	270	280	290
136	8.5	236 / 295		257	4.14	4.63	1.31	1.01	1.14	1.37
137	7	240 / 295		213 / 283	3.58	4.70	2.40	0.93	0.88	0.89

Alkaline Spectral Data

No.	pH	λ_{max}	ε_{max} ($\times 10^{-3}$)	λ_{min}	230	240	250	270	280	290
136	12	236 / 295		257	4.14	4.63	1.31	1.01	1.14	1.37
137	13°	236 / 269 / 303		255 / 288						

REFERENCES

No.	Origin and Synthesis	$[\alpha]_D^t$	pK	Spectral Data	Mass Spectra	R_f
136	R: 403	—	—	403ᵇ	—	—
137	R: 346	—	—	346ᵇ	—	—

PURINES, PYRIMIDINES, NUCLEOSIDES AND NUCLEOTIDES: PHYSICAL CONSTANTS AND SPECTRAL PROPERTIES (Continued)

No.	Compound	Symbol 3-Letter	Symbol 1-Letter	Structure	Formula (Mol Wt)	Melting Point °C	$[\alpha]_D^t$	pK Basic	pK Acidic
138	Xanthosine	Xao	X		$C_{10}H_{12}N_4O_6$ (284.23)	–	-51.2^{30} (8, 0.3N NaOH)	<2.5	5.7**13.0
139	Zeatosine Ribosylzeatin:N^6-(trans-4-Hydroxy-3-methyl-2-butenyl)adenosineN^6-(trans-4-Hydroxy isopentenyl)adenosine	Zeo 6(trHOiPe)Ado	Z		$C_{15}H_{21}N_5O_5$ (351.36)	180–182°	–	–	–

Acidic Spectral Data

No.	pH	λ_{max}	ε_{max} (×10⁻³)	λ_{min}	230	240	250	270	280	290
138	3	235	8.4	248	–	–	0.75	–	0.28	0.03
		263	8.95							
139	1	208	19.8	235	–	–	–	–	–	–
		266	18.5							

Neutral Spectral Data

No.	pH	λ_{max}	ε_{max} (×10⁻³)	λ_{min}	230	240	250	270	280	290
138	8	248	10.2	223	–	–	1.30	–	1.13	0.61
		278	8.9							
139	7	211	19.3	233	–	–	–	–	–	–
		270	17.8							

Alkaline Spectral Data

No.	pH	λ_{max}	ε_{max} (×10⁻³)	λ_{min}	230	240	250	270	280	290
138	14	252	8.6	230	–	–	1.12	–	1.16	0.59
		276	9.3	262						
139	11	215	18.1	235	–	–	–	–	–	–
		270	18.3							

REFERENCES

No.	Origin and Synthesis	$[\alpha]_D^t$	pK	Spectral Data	Mass Spectra	R_f
138	C: 224,377	224	150,53*,55*,170	232b,205	–	–
139	C: 277	–	–	227	–	32,227

PURINES, PYRIMIDINES, NUCLEOSIDES AND NUCLEOTIDES: PHYSICAL CONSTANTS AND SPECTRAL PROPERTIES (Continued)

No.	Compound	Symbol (3-Letter)	Symbol (1-Letter)	Structure	Formula (Mol Wt)	Melting Point °C	$[\alpha]_D^t$	pK Basic	pK Acidic
				DEOXYRIBONUCLEOSIDES					
140	Deoxyadenosine	dAdo	dA	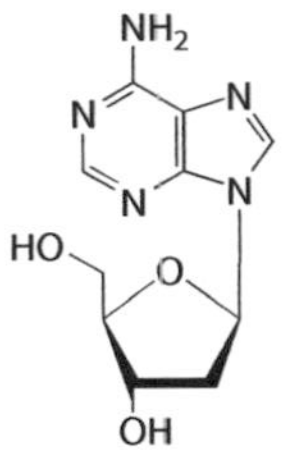	$C_{10}H_{13}N_5O_3$ (251.24)	187–189°	-26.0^{21} (1.0, H_2O)	3.8	–
141	N^6-Methyldeoxyadenosine / 6-Methylaminopurinedeoxyribonucleoside	6MedAdo / d6MeAdo	m6dA	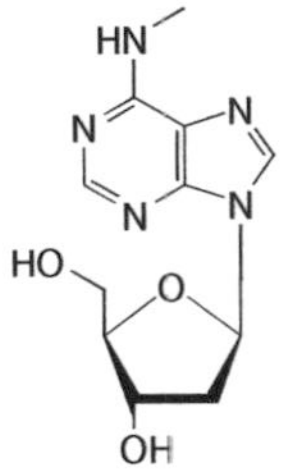	$C_{11}H_{15}N_5O_3$ (265.27)	206–208°	-23.5^{26} (1.0, H_2O)	–	–
142	Deoxycytidine	dCyd	dC	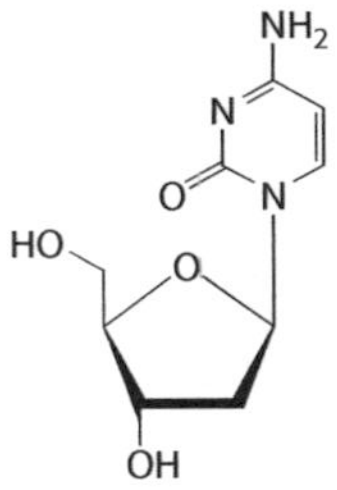	$C_9H_{13}N_3O_4$ (227.22)	200–201°	$+82.4^{19}$ (1.31, 1N NaOH)	4.3	>13

Acidic Spectral Data

No.	pH	λ_{max}	ε_{max} ($\times10^{-3}$)	λ_{min}	230	240	250	270	280	290
140	2	258	14.5	228	–	–	0.83	–	0.24	–
141	1.5	261	16.6*	232*	0.21	0.30	0.65	0.88	0.40	0.11
142	1	280	13.2	241	–	–	0.42	–	2.15	1.61

Neutral Spectral Data

No.	pH	λ_{max}	ε_{max} ($\times10^{-3}$)	λ_{min}	230	240	250	270	280	290
140	7	260	15.2	225	–	–	0.79	–	0.15	<0.01
141	7	265	15.4	229*	0.29	0.35	0.61	1.07	0.65	0.22
142	7	271	9.0	250	–	–	0.83	–	0.97	0.31

Alkaline Spectral Data

No.	pH	λ_{max}	ε_{max} ($\times10^{-3}$)	λ_{min}	230	240	250	270	280	290
140	13^q	261	14.9	–						
141	11	265	15.4	226*	0.17	0.30	0.58	1.08	0.63	0.11
142	11	271	9.0	250	–	–	0.83	–	0.97	0.31
	13^q	271.5	9.1	250						

REFERENCES

No.	Origin and Synthesis	$[\alpha]_D^t$	pK	Spectral Data	Mass Spectra	R_f
140	D: 238 C: 249,267,390,389	239,249,389	246,223	246,389^{cd},390^d,317^b,267^b,223,240,249	341,317	21,389
141	C: 10 D: 21	10	–	10*,21*,be,317*bcde	–	10,18,21
142	D: 238,241 C: 247,129	241	163	163^b,232^a,317^b	–	201

PURINES, PYRIMIDINES, NUCLEOSIDES AND NUCLEOTIDES: PHYSICAL CONSTANTS AND SPECTRAL PROPERTIES (Continued)

No.	Compound	Symbol (3-Letter)	Symbol (1-Letter)	Structure	Formula (Mol Wt)	Melting Point °C	$[\alpha]_D$	pK Basic	pK Acidic
143	N^4-Methyldeoxycytidine 1-β-2'-Deoxyribofuranosyl-4-methylamino-2-pyrimidinone	4MedCyd d4MeCyd	m⁴dC	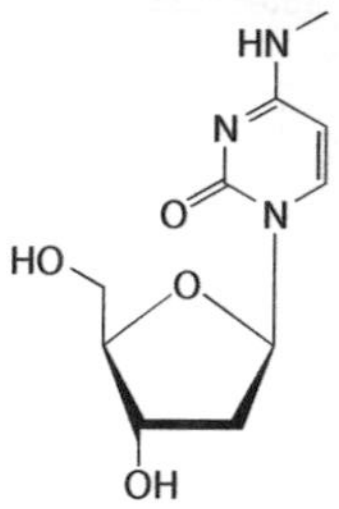	$C_{10}H_{15}N_3O_4$ (241.24)	191–193°	$+48^{28}$ (1.2, H_2O)	4.0	–
144	5-Methyldeoxycytidine	5MedCyd d5MeCyd	m⁵dC	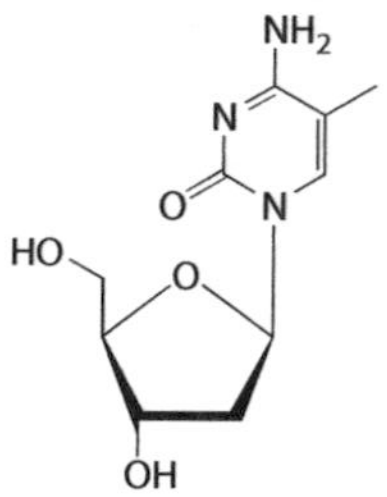	$C_{10}H_{15}N_3O_4$ (241.24)	211–212°	$+43^{22}$ (1.4, H_2O)	4.4	>13
145	5-Hydroxymethyldeoxycytidine	5HmdCyd d5HmCyd 5(HOMe)dCyd	om⁵dC hm⁵dC*	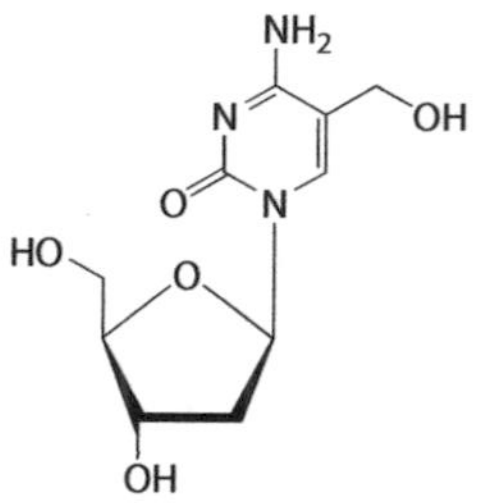	$C_{10}H_{15}N_3O_5$ (257.24)	203° (dec)	$+51^{20}$ (H_2O)	3.5	–

Acidic Spectral Data

No.	pH	λ_{max}	ε_{max} (×10⁻³)	λ_{min}	230	240	250	270	280	290
143	1	282	14.6	242	-	-	-	-	1.98	-
144	1	287	12.4*	245	1.34	0.43	0.42	1.93	2.93	3.12
145	1	283	12.6	243	0.16	0.21*	0.64*	1.88*	2.47*	2.27*

Neutral Spectral Data

No.	pH	λ_{max}	ε_{max} (×10⁻³)	λ_{min}	230	240	250	270	280	290
143	7	236 / 270	9.1 / 11.7	229	-	-	-	-	-	-
144	7	277	8.5	255	1.47	1.29	1.00	1.37	1.54	1.01
145	7	272	-	247	-	0.88	0.97	1.19	1.17	0.58*

Alkaline Spectral Data

No.	pH	λ_{max}	ε_{max} (×10⁻³)	λ_{min}	230	240	250	270	280	290
143	12	236 / 270	9.1 / 11.7	229	-	-	-	-	-	-
144	14	279	8.8	255	1.57	1.27	0.98	1.43	1.67	1.13
145	13	274	-	252	-	1.21	0.97	1.26	1.17*	0.68*

REFERENCES

No.	Origin and Synthesis	$[\alpha]_D$	pK	Spectral Data	Mass Spectra	R_f
143	C: 129	129	129	129	–	129
144	C: 128,391ᵃ D: 133,134	391	128	128ᵇ,133*ᵇ,134ᵇ,391,317ᵇ	–	70
145	D: 75,135 C: 136,385	136	75	75ᵇ,135*ᵇᶜᵈ136*ᵈ,317ᵇ	–	70,75

PURINES, PYRIMIDINES, NUCLEOSIDES AND NUCLEOTIDES: PHYSICAL CONSTANTS AND SPECTRAL PROPERTIES (Continued)

No.	Compound	Symbol 3-Letter	Symbol 1-Letter	Structure	Formula (Mol Wt)	Melting Point °C	$[\alpha]_D^t$	pK Basic	pK Acidic
146	Deoxyguanosine	dGuo	dG		$C_{10}H_{13}N_5O_4$ (267.24)	250°	$-30.2^{23.5}$ (0.2, H_2O)	2.5	–
147	1-Methyldeoxyguanosine	1MedGuo / d1MeGuo	m1dG		$C_{11}H_{15}N_5O_4$ (281.27)	249–250° (dec)	–	–	–
148	7-Methyldeoxyguanosine	7MedGuo / d7MeGuo	m7dG		$C_{11}H_{15}N_5O_4$ (281.27)	None (dec)	–	–	–

Acidic Spectral Data

No.	pH	λ_{max}	ε_{max} (×10⁻³)	λ_{min}	230	240	250	270	280	290
146	1°	255	12.1	232	0.26	0.60	1.0	0.84	0.69	0.47
147	1°	257	12.1	–	–	–	–	–	–	–
148	1°	256	10.8	229	–	–	–	–	–	–

Neutral Spectral Data

No.	pH	λ_{max}	ε_{max} (×10⁻³)	λ_{min}	230	240	250	270	280	290
146	H_2O	254	13.0	223	0.38	0.81	1.16	0.75	0.68	0.27
148	6	257	–	235	–	–	–	–	–	–

Alkaline Spectral Data

No.	pH	λ_{max}	ε_{max} (×10⁻³)	λ_{min}	230	240	250	270	280	290
146	12	260	9.2	230	0.40	0.55	0.87*	0.98	0.61	0.09
147	11	254	13.6	–	–	–	–	–	–	–
148	9°	–	–	–	–	–	–	–	–	–

REFERENCES

No.	Origin and Synthesis	$[\alpha]_D^t$	pK	Spectral Data	Mass Spectra	R_f
146	C: 267 D: 238	267	246	317b,242e,267*bcd	317	242
147	C: 24	–	–	24	–	24
148	C: 10,41	–	–	10c,41c	–	10

PURINES, PYRIMIDINES, NUCLEOSIDES AND NUCLEOTIDES: PHYSICAL CONSTANTS AND SPECTRAL PROPERTIES (Continued)

No.	Compound	Symbol 1-Letter	Symbol 3-Letter	Structure	Formula (Mol Wt)	Melting Point °C	$[\alpha]_D$	pK Basic	pK Acidic
149	Deoxyuridine	dU	dUrd		$C_9H_{12}N_2O_5$ (228.20)	163°	$+50.0^{22}$ (1.1 1N NaOH)	–	9.3, >13
150	Thymidine 5-Methyldeoxyuridine	dT	dThd		$C_{10}H_{14}N_2O_5$ (242.23)	183–184°	$+32.8^{16}$ (1.04, 1N NaOH)	–	9.8, >13
151	5-Hydroxymethyldeoxyuridine	om5dU hm5dU*	5HmdUrd 5(HOMe)dUrd d5HmUrd		$C_{10}H_{14}N_2O_6$ (258.23)	180–182°	$+19^{20}$ (H_2O)	–	–

Acidic Spectral Data

No.	pH	λ_{max}	ε_{max} (×10⁻³)	λ_{min}	230	240	250	270	280	290
149	1	262	10.2	231	0.20	0.40	0.74	0.83	0.32*	–
150	1	267	9.65	235	0.33	0.34	0.65	1.06	0.70	0.22
151	2	264	9.6	233	0.27	0.37	0.70	0.97	0.51	0.10

Neutral Spectral Data

No.	pH	λ_{max}	ε_{max} (×10⁻³)	λ_{min}	230	240	250	270	280	290
149	7	262	10.2	231	0.20	0.40	0.74	0.83	0.32*	–
150	7	267	9.65	235	0.32	0.33	0.65	1.06	0.70	0.21*
151	7	264	9.6^l	233	0.27	0.37	0.70	0.97	0.51	0.10

Alkaline Spectral Data

No.	pH	λ_{max}	ε_{max} (×10⁻³)	λ_{min}	230	240	250	270	280	290
149	12	262	7.6	242	0.95	0.70	0.80	0.80	0.27*	–
150	13	267	7.4	246	1.18	0.76	0.74	1.05	0.65	0.16
151	12	264	7.0	243	1.13	0.72	0.75	0.95	0.54*	0.18

REFERENCES

No.	Origin and Synthesis	$[\alpha]_D$	pK	Spectral Data	Mass Spectra	R_f
149	D: 238,243[a]	243	163	163[b],317[be],232*	341,317	243
150	D: 238 C: 128,356,69	241	163	163[b],242[b],232*,[b],317[b]	317	21,18,69,242
151	C: 69,152[a]	152	–	317[b],69*,[cd]	–	69

PURINES, PYRIMIDINES, NUCLEOSIDES AND NUCLEOTIDES: PHYSICAL CONSTANTS AND SPECTRAL PROPERTIES (Continued)

No.	Compound	Symbol 3-Letter	1-Letter	Structure	Formula (Mol Wt)	Melting Point °C	$[\alpha]_D$	pK Basic	pK Acidic
152	2-Thiothymidine 5-Methyl-2-thiodeoxyuridine	2SdThd	s²dT		$C_{10}H_{14}N_2O_4S$ (258.30)	182–183°	$+16^{20}$ (0.5 MeOH)	–	–
	RIBONUCLEOTIDES								
153	Adenosine 2'-phosphate	Ado-2'-P / 2'-AMP			$C_{10}H_{14}N_5O_7P$ (347.22)	183° (dec)	-65.4^{22} (0.5, 0.5M, Na₂HPO₄)	3.8	–
154	Adenosine 3'-phosphate	Ado-3'-P / 3'-AMP	ApA-		$C_{10}H_{14}N_5O_7P$ (347.22)	195° (dec)	-45.4^{22} (0.5, 0.5M Na₂HPO₄)	3.65	–

Acidic Spectral Data

No.	pH	λmax	εmax (×10⁻³)	λmin	230	240	250	270	280	290
152										
153	2	257[z]	14.4[z]	229[z]	–	–	0.85	–	0.23	0.04
154	1	257	15.1	230	–	–	0.85	0.71	0.22*	0.04*

Neutral Spectral Data

No.	pH	λmax	εmax (×10⁻³)	λmin	230	240	250	270	280	290
152	(MeOH)	221 / 276	15.2 / 16.3							
153	7	259[z]	15.4[z]	–	–	–	0.80	–	0.15	0.01
154	7	–	–	–	–	–	0.80	–	0.15	0.01

Alkaline Spectral Data

No.	pH	λmax	εmax (×10⁻³)	λmin	230	240	250	270	280	290
152	13 (MeOH)	242 / 264	22.8 / 16.6							
153	12	259[z]	15.4[z]	–	–	–	0.80	–	0.15	–
154	13	259	15.4	227	–	–	0.78	0.73	0.22	0.05

REFERENCES

No.	Origin and Synthesis	$[\alpha]_D$	pK	Spectral Data	Mass Spectra	R_f
152	C: 301			301	–	–
153	C: 191,193,219 R: 182,221	221	220,170,218	179[e],223[z]	–	258,219,263
154	C: 193,190,219 R: 182,221,194[z]	221	220,170,218	265*[b],179[e]	–	258,219,263,292

PURINES, PYRIMIDINES, NUCLEOSIDES AND NUCLEOTIDES: PHYSICAL CONSTANTS AND SPECTRAL PROPERTIES (Continued)

No.	Compound	Symbol 3-Letter	Symbol 1-Letter	Structure	Formula (Mol Wt)	Melting Point °C	$[\alpha]_D^t$	pK Basic	pK Acidic
155	Adenosine 5'-phosphate	Ado-5'-P / AMP	PA-A		$C_{10}H_{14}N_5O_7P$ (347.22)	192° (dec)	-46.3^{24} (H_2O)	3.8	–
156	Adenosine 5'-diphosphate	Ado-5'-P$_2$ / ADP	ppA		$C_{10}H_{15}N_5O_{10}P_2$ (427.21)	–	–	3.9	–
157	Adenosine 5'-triphosphate	Ado-5'-P$_3$ / ATP	pppA		$C_{10}H_{16}N_5O_{13}P_3$ (507.19)	–	–	4.1	–

Acidic Spectral Data

No.	pH	λ_{max}	ε_{max} (×10⁻³)	λ_{min}	230	240	250	270	280	290
155	2	257	15.0	230	0.23	0.43	0.84	0.68	0.22	0.44
156	2	257	15.0	230	–	–	0.85	–	0.21	–
157	2	257	14.7	230	–	–	0.85	–	0.22	–

Neutral Spectral Data

No.	pH	λ_{max}	ε_{max} (×10⁻³)	λ_{min}	230	240	250	270	280	290
155	7	259	15.4	227*	0.18	0.39	0.79	0.66	0.16	0.01
156	7	259	15.4	227	–	–	0.78	–	0.16	–
157	7	259	15.4	227	–	–	0.80	–	0.15	–

Alkaline Spectral Data

No.	pH	λ_{max}	ε_{max} (×10⁻³)	λ_{min}	230	240	250	270	280	290
155	11	259	15.4	227	–	–	0.79	–	0.15	–
156	11	259	15.4	227	–	–	0.78	–	0.15	–
157	11	259	15.4	227	–	–	0.80	–	0.15	–

REFERENCES

No.	Origin and Synthesis	$[\alpha]_D^t$	pK	Spectral Data	Mass Spectra	R_f
155	C: 191,197,368 R: 195 N: 198	368	220,170,212	212,179[a],184[b],183[b],368*	374	188,219,263,368
156	C: 255,211,188,196 E: 226 N: 198	–	212	212,183[b],206	–	188
157	C: 211,214,188 N: 198	–	212	212[b],206,183[b]	–	188

PURINES, PYRIMIDINES, NUCLEOSIDES AND NUCLEOTIDES: PHYSICAL CONSTANTS AND SPECTRAL PROPERTIES (Continued)

No.	Compound	Symbol 3-Letter	Symbol 1-Letter	Structure	Formula (Mol Wt)	Melting Point °C	$[\alpha]_D^t$	pK Basic	pK Acidic
158	1-Methyladenosine 3'(2')-phosphate	1MeAdo-3'(2')-P	m¹Ap, m¹A- for 3'		$C_{11}H_{16}N_5O_7P$ (361.25)	—	—	8.8[t]	—
159	1-Methyladenosine 5'-phosphate	1MeAdo-5'-P, 1MeAMP	pm¹A, -m¹A		$C_{11}H_{16}N_5O_7P$ (361.25)	—	—	8.8[t]	—

Acidic Spectral Data

No.	pH	λ_{max}	ε_{max} (×10⁻³)	230	240	250	270	280	290	λ_{min}
				Spectral Ratios						
158	2	258	13.2w	0.24	0.44	0.83	0.67	0.26	0.07	230
159	2	258	—	0.34	0.46	0.81	0.74	0.32	0.10	232

Neutral Spectral Data

No.	pH	λ_{max}	ε_{max} (×10⁻³)	230	240	250	270	280	290	λ_{min}
				Spectral Ratios						
158	—	—	—	—	—	—	—	—	0.07	—
159	H₂O⁰	259	—	0.22	0.34	0.77	0.74	0.27	0.10	233

Alkaline Spectral Data

No.	pH	λ_{max}	ε_{max} (×10⁻³)	λ_{min}	230	240	250	270	280	290
					Spectral Ratios					
158	13⁰	259	12.9w	230*	—	—	0.77	0.76	0.4	0.32
159	12⁰	259	13.1w	230*	0.22*	0.36*	0.75	0.71	0.36	0.3

REFERENCES

No.	Origin and Synthesis	$[\alpha]_D^t$	pK	Spectral Data	Mass Spectra	R_f
158	C: 90,292 R: 77	—	—	90	—	143,291,292
159	C: 164,8	—	—	164,8*bd	—	8,164

PURINES, PYRIMIDINES, NUCLEOSIDES AND NUCLEOTIDES: PHYSICAL CONSTANTS AND SPECTRAL PROPERTIES (Continued)

No.	Compound	Symbol (3-Letter)	Symbol (1-Letter)	Structure	Formula (Mol Wt)	Melting Point °C	$[\alpha]_D^t$	pK Basic	pK Acidic
160	1-Methyladenosine 5'-diphosphate	1MeAdo-5'-P, 1MeADP$_2$	ppm^1 A		$C_{11}H_{17}N_5O_{10}P_2$ (441.23)	–	–	–	–
161	2-Methyladenosine 3'-phosphate	2MeAdo-3'-P	m^2 Ap		$C_{11}H_{16}N_5O_7P$ (361.25)	–	–	–	–
162	2-Methyladenosine 5'-phosphate	2MeAdo-5'-P, 2MeAMP	pm^2 A		$C_{11}H_{16}N_5O_7P$ (361.25)	260° (dec) (Ba salt)	–	–	–

Acidic Spectral Data

No.	pH	λ_{max}	ε_{max} (×10^{-3})	λ_{min}	230	240	250	270	280	290
160	2	257	11.9	234	0.37	0.44	0.84	0.66	0.23	0.04
161	1	259	10.8	–	–	–	–	–	–	–
162	1	259	10.9	–	–	–	–	–	–	–

Spectral Ratios columns: 230, 240, 250, 270, 280, 290

Neutral Spectral Data

No.	pH	λ_{max}	ε_{max} (×10^{-3})	λ_{min}	230	240	250	270	280	290
160	H$_2$O	264	12.9	–	–	–	–	–	–	–
161	6	264	13.2	–	–	–	–	–	–	–
162										

Spectral Ratios columns: 230, 240, 250, 270, 280, 290

Alkaline Spectral Data

No.	pH	λ_{max}	ε_{max} (×10^{-3})	λ_{min}	230	240	250	270	280	290
160	12°	259	12.5	232	0.32	0.40	0.75	0.74	0.36	0.31
161	13	263	13.1	–	–	–	–	–	–	–
162	13	264	13.4	–	–	–	–	–	–	–

Spectral Ratios columns: 230, 240, 250, 270, 280, 290

REFERENCES

No.	Origin and Synthesis	$[\alpha]_D^t$	pK	Spectral Data	Mass Spectra	R$_f$
160	C: 164	–	–	164^b	–	164
161	C: 291 R: 291	–	–	291^b	–	291
162	C: 342	–	–	342	–	–

PURINES, PYRIMIDINES, NUCLEOSIDES AND NUCLEOTIDES: PHYSICAL CONSTANTS AND SPECTRAL PROPERTIES (Continued)

No.	Compound	Symbol 3-Letter	Symbol 1-Letter	Structure	Formula (Mol Wt)	Melting Point °C	$[\alpha]_D^t$	pK Basic	pK Acidic
163	N^6-(Δ²-Isopentenyl)adenosine 5'-phosphate: 6-(γγ-Dimethylallylamino)-9-β-D-ribofuranosylpurine 5'-phosphate	6Pe¹Ado-5'-P 6iPeAdo-5'-P 6iPeAMP	pi⁶ A		$C_{15}H_{22}N_5O_7P$ (415.35)	—	—	—	—
164	N^6-Methyladenosine 3'(2')-phosphate	6MeAdo-3'(2')-P	m6 Ap m6 A- for 3'		$C_{11}H_{16}N_5O_7P$ (361.25)	—	—	—	—
165	N^6-Methyladenosine 5'-phosphate	6MeAdo-5'-P 6MeAMP	pm⁶ A -m⁶ A		$C_{11}H_{16}N_5O_7P$ (361.25)	—	—	~3.7ᵇ	—

Acidic Spectral Data

No.	pH	λ_{max}	ε_{max} (×10⁻³)	λ_{min}	230	240	250	270	280	290
163	1	264	20.9	232.5			0.64	0.91	0.45	0.14
164	1	262	18.3	231*						
165	2	261	16.3	231	0.28	0.39	0.73	0.85	0.36*	0.13

Neutral Spectral Data

No.	pH	λ_{max}	ε_{max} (×10⁻³)	λ_{min}	230	240	250	270	280	290
163	7	267	19.2	233						
164	H₂O	264	13.4	229	0.17	0.29	0.63	0.97	0.56	0.17

Alkaline Spectral Data

No.	pH	λ_{max}	ε_{max} (×10⁻³)	λ_{min}	230	240	250	270	280	290
163	13	268	19.0	232						
164	12	266*		230*	0.20		0.58	1.05	0.67	0.22
165	12	266*	15.2ʰ	231*		0.32*	0.60	1.08	0.66*	0.26*

REFERENCES

No.	pK	$[\alpha]_D^t$	Origin and Synthesis	Spectral Data	Mass Spectra	Rf
163	—	—	C: 319	319	—	319
164	—	—	R: 165,292 C: 292	265*ᵇ,292*ᶜ,165*ᶜ,90ᵉ	—	143,165,291,292
165	164	—	C: 164,166	164*,8*ᵇᶜᵈᵉ	—	164,166,407

PURINES, PYRIMIDINES, NUCLEOSIDES AND NUCLEOTIDES: PHYSICAL CONSTANTS AND SPECTRAL PROPERTIES (Continued)

No.	Compound	Structure	Symbol 1-Letter	Symbol 3-Letter	Formula (Mol Wt)	Melting Point °C	$[\alpha]_D^t$	pK Basic	pK Acidic
166	N^6-Methyladenosine 5′-diphosphate		ppm^6 A	6MeAdo-5′-P$_2$ 6MeADP	$C_{11}H_{17}N_5O_{10}P_2$ (441.23)	—	—	⁻3.7^b	—
167	N^6,N^6-Dimethyladenosine 5′-phosphate		$pm_2^{6}A$ $-m_2^{6}A$	6Me$_2$Ado-5′-P 6Me$_2$AMP	$C_{12}H_{18}N_5O_7P$ (375.28)	225° (dec)	-51^{20} (2.0, H$_2$O)	—	—
168	N^6,N^6-Dimethyladenosine 5′-diphosphate		ppm^6 A	6Me$_2$Ado-5′P$_2$ 6Me$_2$ ADP	$C_{12}H_{19}N_5O_{10}P_2$ (455.26)	—	—	—	—

Acidic Spectral Data

No.	pH	λ_{max}	ε_{max} (×10⁻³)	λ_{min}	230	240	250	270	280	290
166	2	262	15.7	231	0.18	0.32	0.69	0.84	0.29	0.08
167	H₂O	268	18.3	—	—	—	—	—	—	—
168	—	—	—	—	—	—	—	—	—	—

Neutral Spectral Data

No.	pH	λ_{max}	ε_{max} (×10⁻³)	λ_{min}	230	240	250	270	280	290
166	—	—	—	—	—	—	—	—	—	—
167	7	274	—	—	—	—	—	—	—	—
168	—	—	—	—	—	—	—	—	—	—

Alkaline Spectral Data

No.	pH	λ_{max}	ε_{max} (×10⁻³)	λ_{min}	230	240	250	270	280	290
166	12	265	15.4	229	0.14	0.26	0.60	0.99	0.57	0.18
167	—	—	—	—	—	—	—	—	—	—
168	—	—	—	—	—	—	—	—	—	—

REFERENCES

No.	Origin and Synthesis	$[\alpha]_D^t$	pK	Spectral Data	Mass Spectra	R_f
166	C: 164	—	164	164^b	—	164
167	C: 115,166	115	—	115,166^c	—	115,166,167
168	C: 167	—	—	—	—	167

PURINES, PYRIMIDINES, NUCLEOSIDES AND NUCLEOTIDES: PHYSICAL CONSTANTS AND SPECTRAL PROPERTIES (Continued)

No.	Compound	Symbol 3-Letter	Symbol 1-Letter	Structure	Formula (Mol Wt)	Melting Point °C	$[\alpha]_D^t$	pK Basic	pK Acidic
169	N^6-Threoninocarbonyladenosine 3'(2')-phosphate N-[(9-β-D-Ribofuranosylpurin-6-yl)- N-carbamoyl]threonine 3'(2')-phosphate	6(ThrCO) Ado-3'(2')-P	tc6 AP for 3'		$C_{15}N_{21}N_6O_{11}P$ (492.34)	–	–	2.1p	–
170	N^6-Threoninocarbonyladenosine 5'-phosphate N-[(9-β-D-Ribofuranosylpurin-6-yl)- N-carbamoyl]threonine 3'(2')-phosphate	6(ThrCO)Ado-5'-P 6(ThrCO) AMP	ptc6 A		$C_{15}H_{21}N_6O_{11}P$ (492.34)	–	–	–	~3.0p

Acidic Spectral Data

No.	pH	λ_{max}	ε_{max} (×10⁻³)	λ_{min}	230	240	250	270	280	290
169	–	–	–	–	–	–	–	–	–	–
170	1	276	–	237	0.49	0.41	0.61	1.53	1.45	0.48

Neutral Spectral Data

No.	pH	λ_{max}	ε_{max} (×10⁻³)	λ_{min}	230	240	250	270	280	290
169	5	269 275	–	231	0.2	0.33	0.62	1.38	0.87	0.03
170	6.8	269 276	–	231	0.28	0.37	0.63	1.29	0.69	0.03

Alkaline Spectral Data

No.	pH	λ_{max}	ε_{max} (×10⁻³)	λ_{min}	230	240	250	270	280	290
169	–	–	–	–	–	–	–	–	–	–
170	13o	269 277 297		239 273 287	0.73	0.48	0.65	1.37	1.07	0.71

REFERENCES

No.	Origin and Synthesis	$[\alpha]_D^t$	pK	Spectral Data	Mass Spectra	R_f
169	R: 90,410	–	90	90	–	–
170	R: 407	–	407	407b	–	407

PURINES, PYRIMIDINES, NUCLEOSIDES AND NUCLEOTIDES: PHYSICAL CONSTANTS AND SPECTRAL PROPERTIES (Continued)

No.	Compound	Symbol 3-Letter	Symbol 1-Letter	Structure	Formula (Mol Wt)	Melting Point °C	$[\alpha]_D$	pK Basic	pK Acidic
171	N^6-Methyl-N^6-threoninocarbonyladenosine 5'-phosphate N-[(9-β-D-Ribofuranosylpurin-6-yl)-N-methylcarbamoyl] threonine 5'-phosphate	6Me6(ThrCO)Ado-5'-P 6Me6(ThrCO)AMP	pm6tc6A		$C_{16}H_{23}N_6O_{11}P$ (506.37)	–	–	–	~3.0p
172	Cytidine 2'-phosphate	Cyd-2'-P 2'CMP	Cp		$C_9H_{14}N_3O_8P$ (323.21)	238–240° (dec)	$+20.7^{20}$ (1.0, H_2O)	4.4	–
173	Cytidine 3'-phosphate	Cyd-3'-P 3'-CMP	C-		$C_9H_{14}N_3O_8P$ (323.21)	232–234° (dec)	$+49.4^{20}$ (1.0, H_2O)	4.3	–

Acidic Spectral Data

No.	pH	λ_{max}	ε_{max} (×10⁻³)	λ_{min}	230	240	250	270	280	290
171	1	283		240	0.82	0.58	0.68	1.41	1.89	1.68
172	2	278	12.7	240	–	–	0.48	–	1.80	1.22
173	2	279	13.0	240	–	–	0.45*	1.51	2.00*	1.43*

Neutral Spectral Data

No.	pH	λ_{max}	ε_{max} (×10⁻³)	λ_{min}	230	240	250	270	280	290
171	6.8	278 285		239	0.83	0.63	0.73	1.47	1.87	1.25
172	7	–	–	–	–	–	0.90	–	0.85	0.26
173	7	270ᶜ	9.0ᶜ	250ᶜ	–	–	0.86	–	0.93	0.30

Alkaline Spectral Data

No.	pH	λ_{max}	ε_{max} (×10⁻³)	λ_{min}	230	240	250	270	280	290
171	13	278		238	0.73	0.54	0.68	1.47	1.89	1.29
172	12	272	8.6	250	–	–	0.9	–	0.85	0.26
173	12	272	8.9	250	–	–	0.86	1.16	0.93	0.30*

REFERENCES

No.	Origin and Synthesis	$[\alpha]_D$	pK	Spectral Data	Mass Spectra	R_f
171	R: 407	–	407	407b	–	407
172	R:215a,192,178	215	218,170,192	223,179be	–	258
173	R: 215a,192,178	215	218,170,192	223,179be,181zbcd,251,265*be	–	258

PURINES, PYRIMIDINES, NUCLEOSIDES AND NUCLEOTIDES: PHYSICAL CONSTANTS AND SPECTRAL PROPERTIES (Continued)

No.	Compound	Symbol (1-Letter)	Symbol (3-Letter)	Structure	Formula (Mol Wt)	Melting Point °C	$[\alpha]_D^t$	pK Basic	pK Acidic
174	Cytidine 5'-phosphate	pC -C	Cyd-5'-P CMP		$C_9H_{14}N_3O_8P$ (323.21)	233° (dec)	+27.1[14] (0.54, H₂O)	4.5	–
175	Cytidine 5'-diphosphate	ppC	Cyd-5'-P₂ CDP		$C_9H_{15}N_3O_{11}P_2$ (403.18)	–	–	4.6	–
176	Cytidine 5'-triphosphate	pppC	Cyd-5'-P₃ CTP		$C_9H_{16}N_3O_{14}P_3$ (483.16)	–	–	4.8	–

Acidic Spectral Data

No.	pH	λ_{max}	ε_{max} (×10⁻³)	λ_{min}	230	240	250	270	280	290
174	2	280*	13.2	241*	0.56	0.25	0.44	1.73	2.09	1.55
175	2	280	12.8	241	–	–	0.46	–	2.07	1.48
176	2	280	12.8	241	–	–	0.45	–	2.12	–

Neutral Spectral Data

No.	pH	λ_{max}	ε_{max} (×10⁻³)	λ_{min}	230	240	250	270	280	290
174	7	271	9.1	249	1.07	0.92	0.84	1.21	0.98	0.33
175	7	271	9.1	249	–	–	0.83	–	0.98	0.32
176	7	271	9.0	249	–	–	0.84	–	0.97	–

Alkaline Spectral Data

pH	λ_{max}	ε_{max} (×10⁻³)	λ_{min}	230	240	250	270	280	290
11	271	9.1	249	–	–	0.84	–	0.98	0.33
11	271	9.1	249	–	–	0.83	–	0.98	–
11	271	9.0	249	–	–	0.84	–	0.97	–

REFERENCES

No.	Origin and Synthesis	pK	$[\alpha]_D^t$	Spectral Data	Mass Spectra	R_f
174	C: 190,196,368 R: 195 N: 198	212	190	212,183bc;184b,179,205,368*	–	74
175	C: 196 N: 198	212	–	212,179e,183b	–	–
176	N: 198	212	–	212b,183b	–	–

PURINES, PYRIMIDINES, NUCLEOSIDES AND NUCLEOTIDES: PHYSICAL CONSTANTS AND SPECTRAL PROPERTIES (Continued)

No.	Compound	Symbol 3-Letter	Symbol 1-Letter	Structure	Formula (Mol Wt)	Melting Point °C	$[\alpha]_D^t$	pK Basic	pK Acidic
177	2-Thiocytidine 3'(2')-phosphate	2Syd-3'(2')-P 2SCyd-3'(2')-P	S2Cp for 3'		$C_9H_{14}N_3O_7SP$ (339.27)	–	–	3.6p	–
178	3-Methylcytidine 3'(2')-phosphate	3MeCyd-3'(2')-P	m3CP m3C - for 3'		$C_{10}H_{16}N_3O_8P$ (337.22)	–	–	~9.0p	–
179	3-Methylcytidine 5'-phosphate	3MeCyd-5'-P 3MeCMP	pm3C -m3C		$C_{10}H_{16}N_3O_8P$ (337.22)	–	–	–	–

Acidic Spectral Data

No.	pH	λ_{max}	ε_{max} (×10⁻³)	λ_{min}	230	240	250	270	280	290
177	1	227 276	– 11.5	247	1.24	0.91	0.75	1.24	1.28	0.83
178	1	276	11.5	242	–	–	–	–	–	–
179	–	–	–	–	–	–	–	–	–	–

Neutral Spectral Data

No.	pH	λ_{max}	ε_{max} (×10⁻³)	λ_{min}	230	240	250	270	280	290
177	H_2O	248	–	220	0.64	0.94	1.08	0.88	0.69	0.39
178	7	276	11.2	242	0.66	0.34	0.50	1.56	1.64	0.98
179	–	–	–	–	–	–	–	–	–	–

Alkaline Spectral Data

No.	pH	λ_{max}	ε_{max} (×10⁻³)	λ_{min}	230	240	250	270	280	290
177	13	249	–	228	0.71	0.93	1.08	0.89	0.71	0.4
178	–	–	–	–	–	–	–	–	–	–
179	–	–	–	–	–	–	–	–	–	–

REFERENCES

No.	Origin and Synthesis	Spectral Data	pK	$[\alpha]_D^t$	Mass Spectra	R_f
177	R: 270,329 C: 329	270p,329p	329	–	–	270,329
178	C: 130 R: 413	130,413e	130	–	–	13,130,143
179	C: 125	–	–	–	–	125

PURINES, PYRIMIDINES, NUCLEOSIDES AND NUCLEOTIDES: PHYSICAL CONSTANTS AND SPECTRAL PROPERTIES (Continued)

No.	Compound	Symbol 3-Letter	Symbol 1-Letter	Structure	Formula (Mol Wt)	Melting Point °C	$[\alpha]_D^t$	pK Basic	pK Acidic
180	3-Methylcytidine 5'-diphosphate	3MeCyd-5'-P$_2$ / 3MeCDP	ppm3C		$C_{10}H_{17}N_3O_{11}P_2$ (417.21)	—	—	~9.0p	—
181	N^4-Methylcytidine 3'(2')-phosphate	4MeCyd-3'(2')-P	m4Cp / m4C- for 3'		$C_{10}H_{16}N_3O_8P$ (337.22)	—	—	—	—
182	N^4-Methylcytidine 5'-phosphate	4MeCyd-5'-P / 4MeCMP	pm4C / -m4C		$C_{10}H_{16}N_3O_8P$ (337.22)	—	—	—	—

Acidic Spectral Data

No.	pH	λ_{max}	ε_{max} ($\times10^{-3}$)	λ_{min}	230	240	250	270	280	290
180	1	278	11.0	241	—	—	—	—	—	—
181	1	281	12.9	242	—	—	—	—	—	—
182	1	280	14.8	242	—	—	—	—	—	—

Neutral Spectral Data

No.	pH	λ_{max}	ε_{max} ($\times10^{-3}$)	λ_{min}	230	240	250	270	280	290
180	7	277	11.0	241	—	—	—	—	—	—
181	H$_2$O	237 / 272	—	227 / 248	—	—	—	—	—	—

Alkaline Spectral Data

No.	pH	λ_{max}	ε_{max} ($\times10^{-3}$)	λ_{min}	230	240	250	270	280	290
180	—	—	—	—	—	—	—	—	—	—
181	—	—	—	—	—	—	—	—	—	—
182	—	—	—	—	—	—	—	—	—	—

REFERENCES

No.	Origin and Synthesis	$[\alpha]_D^t$	pK	Spectral Data	Mass Spectra	R$_f$
180	C: 130	—	130	130	—	130
181	C: 130	—	—	130	—	130
182	C: 130,59,168	—	—	130,168c	—	130,59

PURINES, PYRIMIDINES, NUCLEOSIDES AND NUCLEOTIDES: PHYSICAL CONSTANTS AND SPECTRAL PROPERTIES (Continued)

No.	Compound	Symbol 3-Letter	Symbol 1-Letter	Structure	Formula (Mol Wt)	Melting Point °C	$[\alpha]_D^t$	pK Basic	pK Acidic
183	N^4-Methylcytidine 5′-diphosphate	4MeCyd-5′-P$_2$ / 4MeCDP	ppm^{4}C		$C_{10}H_{17}N_3O_{11}P_2$ (417.21)	–	–	–	–
184	5-Methylcytidine 5′-phosphate	5MeCyd-5′-P / 5MeCMP	pm^{5}C / -m^{5}C		$C_{10}H_{16}N_3O_8P$ (337.22)	–	–	–	–
185	5-Methylcytidine 5′-diphosphate	5MeCyd-5′-P$_2$ / 5MeCDP	ppm^{5}C		$C_{10}H_{17}N_3O_{11}P_2$ (417.21)	–	–	–	–

Acidic Spectral Data

No.	pH	λ_{max}	ε_{max} (×10⁻³)	λ_{min}	230	240	250	270	280	290
183	1	280	12.9	241	–	–	–	–	–	–
	4^a	284	10.7	–	–	–	–	–	–	–
184	–	–	–	–	–	–	–	–	–	–
185	–	–	–	–	–	–	–	–	–	–

Neutral Spectral Data

No.	pH	λ_{max}	ε_{max} (×10⁻³)	λ_{min}	230	240	250	270	280	290
183	–	8	278	8.8	–	–	–	–	–	–
184	–	–	–	–	–	–	–	–	–	–
185	–	–	–	–	–	–	–	–	–	–

Alkaline Spectral Data

No.	pH	λ_{max}	ε_{max} (×10⁻³)	λ_{min}	230	240	250	270	280	290
183	–	–	–	–	–	–	–	–	–	–
184	–	–	–	–	–	–	–	–	–	–
185	–	–	–	–	–	–	–	–	–	–

REFERENCES

No.	Origin and Synthesis	$[\alpha]_D^t$	pK	Spectral Data	Mass Spectra	R_f
183	C: 130,59	–	–	130	–	130,59
184	C: 59	–	–	169	–	59
185	C: 59	–	–	–	–	59

PURINES, PYRIMIDINES, NUCLEOSIDES AND NUCLEOTIDES: PHYSICAL CONSTANTS AND SPECTRAL PROPERTIES (Continued)

No.	Compound	Structure	Symbol 3-Letter	Symbol 1-Letter	Formula (Mol Wt)	Melting Point °C	$[\alpha]_D$	pK Basic	pK Acidic
186	Guanosine 2'-phosphate	(structure)	Guo-2'-P / 2'-GMP		$C_{10}H_{14}N_5O_8P$ (363.22)	175–180° (dec) (dihydrate)	-57.0^{25z} (1.0, 2% NaOH)	–	–
187	Guanosine 3'-phosphate	(structure)	Guo-3'-P / 3'-GMP	Gp / G-	$C_{10}H_{14}N_5O_8P$ (363.22)	175–180° (dec) (dihydrate)	-57.0^{25z} (1.0, 2% NaOH)	2.3	9.7
188	Guanosine 5'-phosphate	(structure)	Guo-5'-P / GMP	pG / -G	$C_{10}H_{14}N_5O_8P$ (363.22)	190–200° (dec)	–	2.4	9.4

Acidic Spectral Data

No.	pH	λ_{max}	ε_{max} (×10⁻³)	λ_{min}	230	240	250	270	280	290
186	1	257	–	228*	–	–	0.9	–	0.68	0.48
187	1	257	12.2	228*	–	–	0.93	0.77	0.69	0.49
188	1	256	12.2	228	0.22	0.55	0.96	0.74	0.67	0.29

Neutral Spectral Data

pH	λ_{max}	ε_{max} (×10⁻³)	λ_{min}	230	240	250	270	280	290
7	–	–	–	–	–	–	–	–	–
7	252	13.4*	227*	–	–	1.15	0.86	0.68	0.29
7	252	13.7	224	0.36	0.81	1.16	0.81	0.66	0.29

Alkaline Spectral Data

pH	λ_{max}	ε_{max} (×10⁻³)	λ_{min}	230	240	250	270	280	290
12	–	–	230*	–	–	0.89	–	0.60	0.11
10.8^q	257	11.25	230*	–	–	0.92	1.00	0.64	0.15
11	258	11.6	230	0.38	0.82	0.90	0.97	0.61	0.29

REFERENCES

No.	Origin and Synthesis	$[\alpha]_D$	pK	Spectral Data	Mass Spectra	R_f
186	R: 222,170	222^z	–	179	–	334
187	R: 222,170	222^z	231	232^b,179^e,265^be,400*^be	–	258,334
188	C: 190,199,189 N: 198 R: 195	–	212	212,183^b,184^b,198	–	189,213,334

PURINES, PYRIMIDINES, NUCLEOSIDES AND NUCLEOTIDES: PHYSICAL CONSTANTS AND SPECTRAL PROPERTIES (Continued)

No.	Compound	Symbol (3-Letter)	Symbol (1-Letter)	Structure	Formula (Mol Wt)	Melting Point °C	$[\alpha]_D^t$	pK Basic	pK Acidic
189	Guanosine 5'-diphosphate	Guo-5'-P$_2$ / GDP	ppG	(structure)	$C_{10}H_{15}N_5O_{11}P_2$ (443.21)	–	–	2.9	9.6
190	Guanosine 5'-triphosphate	Guo-5'-P$_3$ / GTP	pppG	(structure)	$C_{10}H_{16}N_5O_{14}P_3$ (523.19)	–	–	3.3	9.3
191	1-Methylguanosine 3'(2')-phosphate	1MeGuo-3'(2')-P	m^1 GP / m^1 G- for 3'	(structure)	$C_{11}H_{16}N_5O_8P$ (377.25)	–	–	2.4^p	–

Acidic Spectral Data

No.	pH	λ_{max}	ε_{max} (×10^{-3})	λ_{min}	230	240	250	270	280	290
189	1	256	12.3	228	–	–	0.95	–	0.67	–
190	1	256	12.4	228	–	–	0.96	–	0.67	–
191	1	258	11.4^h	230*	0.21	0.45	0.86	0.8	0.72	0.51*

Neutral Spectral Data

No.	pH	λ_{max}	ε_{max} (×10^{-3})	λ_{min}	230	240	250	270	280	290
189	7	253	13.7	224	–	–	1.15	–	0.66	–
190	7	253	13.7	223	–	–	1.17	–	0.66	–
191	H$_2$O	255	12.4^h	222	0.23	0.67	1.04	0.86	0.63	0.20

Alkaline Spectral Data

No.	pH	λ_{max}	ε_{max} (×10^{-3})	λ_{min}	230	240	250	270	280	290
189	11	258	11.7	230	–	–	0.91	–	0.61	–
190	11	257	11.9	230	–	–	0.92	–	0.59	–
191	13	256	13.0^h	227*	0.3	0.66	1.02	0.84	0.63	0.20*

REFERENCES

No.	Origin and Synthesis	$[\alpha]_D^t$	pK	Spectral Data	Mass Spectra	R$_f$
189	C: 213,196 N: 198	–	212	212,183^b	–	213,334
190	C: 213 N: 198	–	212	212^b,183^b	–	213,334
191	R: 165,40	–	40	90,265*^{b},165	–	165

PURINES, PYRIMIDINES, NUCLEOSIDES AND NUCLEOTIDES: PHYSICAL CONSTANTS AND SPECTRAL PROPERTIES (Continued)

No.	Compound	Symbol (3-Letter)	Symbol (1-Letter)	Structure	Formula (Mol Wt)	Melting Point °C	$[\alpha]_D^t$	pK Basic	pK Acidic
192	N^2-Methylguanosine 3'(2')-phosphate	2MeGuo-3'(2')-P	m^2 Gp / m^2 G- for 3'		$C_{11}H_{16}N_5O_8P$ (377.25)	–	–	2.4^p	–
193	N^2,N^2-Dimethylguanosine 3'(2')-phosphate	2Me$_2$ Guo-3'(2')-P	$m_2{}^2$Gp / $m_2{}^2$G-; for 3'		$C_{12}H_{18}N_5O_8P$ (391.28)	–	–	2.6^p	–

Acidic Spectral Data

No.	pH	λ_{max}	ε_{max} (×10⁻³)	λ_{min}	230	240	250	270	280	290
192	1	259	14.2^n	232	0.29	0.44	0.81	0.77	0.60	0.53
193	1	265	17.7^n	237*	0.42	0.29	0.62	0.97	0.58*	0.57

Neutral Spectral Data

pH	λ_{max}	ε_{max} (×10⁻³)	λ_{min}	230	240	250	270	280	290
H_2O	253	15.7^n	224	0.4	0.78	1.12	0.71	0.69	0.45
H_2O	259	19.2^n	228	0.25	0.47	0.84	0.72	0.58	0.50

Alkaline Spectral Data

pH	λ_{max}	ε_{max} (×10⁻³)	λ_{min}	230	240	250	270	280	290
13	258	13.3^n	236	0.72	0.59	0.89	0.91	0.78	0.41
13	263	14.9^n	241*	1.18	0.54	0.77	0.93	0.83	0.60*

REFERENCES

No.	Origin and Synthesis	$[\alpha]_D^t$	pK	Spectral Data	Mass Spectra	R_f
192	R: 40	–	40	90	–	–
193	R: 165,40	–	40	90,265*^b,165	–	165

PURINES, PYRIMIDINES, NUCLEOSIDES AND NUCLEOTIDES: PHYSICAL CONSTANTS AND SPECTRAL PROPERTIES (Continued)

No.	Compound	Symbol 3-Letter	Symbol 1-Letter	Structure	Formula (Mol Wt)	Melting Point °C	$[\alpha]_D^t$	pK Basic	pK Acidic
194	7-Methylguanosine 2'-phosphate	7MeGuo-2'-P			$C_{11}H_{16}N_5O_8P$ (377.25)	—	—	r	7.0
195	7-Methylguanosine 3'-phosphate	7MeGuo-3'-P	m^7Gp m^7G-		$C_{11}H_{16}N_5O_8P$ (377.25)	—	—	r	6.9

Acidic Spectral Data

No.	pH	λ_{max}	ε_{max} (×10⁻³)	λ_{min}	230	240	250	270	280	290
194	2	257	12.6	230	-	-	-	-	-	-
195	2	257	13.2	230	0.26	0.51	0.89	0.74	0.68	0.52

Neutral Spectral Data

No.	pH	λ_{max}	ε_{max} (×10⁻³)	λ_{min}	230	240	250	270	280	290
194	7.4q	258 / 280	9.6 / 9.0	239 / 271	-	-	-	-	-	-
195	7.4q	258 / 282	9.8 / 9.6	240 / 270	-	-	-	-	-	-

Alkaline Spectral Data

No.	pH	λ_{max}	ε_{max} (×10⁻³)	λ_{min}	230	240	250	270	280	290
194	12at	268	9.6	245	-	-	-	-	-	-
195	8.9q / 12at	258 / 282 / 266	-9.9 / 9.9	241 / 245 / 245	-	0.84	0.92	1.09	1.4	1.26

REFERENCES

No.	pK	Spectral Data	Origin and Synthesis	$[\alpha]_D^t$	Mass Spectra	R_f
194	334	334	C: 334 R: 77	—	—	334
195	334	334b,90e	C: 334,90 R: 77	—	—	334

PURINES, PYRIMIDINES, NUCLEOSIDES AND NUCLEOTIDES: PHYSICAL CONSTANTS AND SPECTRAL PROPERTIES (Continued)

No.	Compound	Symbol 3-Letter	Symbol 1-Letter	Structure	Formula (Mol Wt)	Melting Point °C	$[\alpha]_D^t$	pK Basic	pK Acidic
196	7-Methylguanosine 5'-phosphate	7MeGuo-5'-P 7MeGMP	pm^7 G $-m^7$ G	(structure)	$C_{11}H_{16}N_5O_8P$ (377.25)	–	–	r	7.1
197	7-Methylguanosine 5'-diphosphate	7MeGuo-5'-P$_2$ 7MeGDP	ppm^7 G	(structure)	$C_{11}H_{17}N_5O_{11}P_2$ (457.23)	–	–	r	7.2
198	7-Methylguanosine 5'-triphosphate	7MeGuo-5'-P$_3$ 7MeGTP	$pppm^7$ G	(structure)	$C_{11}H_{18}N_5O_{14}P_3$ (537.21)	–	–	r	7.5

Acidic Spectral Data

No.	pH	λ_{max}	ε_{max} (×10⁻³)	λ_{min}	230	240	250	270	280	290
196	2	257	12	230	–	–	–	–	–	–
197	2	257	11.0	230	–	–	–	–	–	–
198	2	257	11.7	230	–	–	–	–	–	–

Neutral Spectral Data

No.	pH	λ_{max}	ε_{max} (×10⁻³)	λ_{min}	230	240	250	270	280	290
196	7.4^q	258	10.3	236	–	–	–	–	–	–
		280	8.6	271						
197	7.4^q	258	8.9	236	–	–	–	–	–	–
		280	7.3	271						
198	7.4^q	258	9.8	236	–	–	–	–	–	–
		280	8.0	271						

Alkaline Spectral Data

No.	pH	λ_{max}	ε_{max} (×10⁻³)	λ_{min}	230	240	250	270	280	290
196	8.9^p	282	8.3	242	–	0.78	0.93	1.11	1.43	1.29
	12^{pt}	268	8.6	244	–	–	–	–	–	–
197	12^{qs}	272	7.0	242	–	–	–	–	–	–
198	12^p	281	8.55	243	–	–	–	–	–	–

REFERENCES

No.	Spectral Data	pK	$[\alpha]_D^t$	Origin and Synthesis	Mass Spectra	R_f
196	334^b	334	–	C: 334,125	–	125,334
197	334	334	–	C: 334	–	334
198	334	334	–	C: 334	–	334

PURINES, PYRIMIDINES, NUCLEOSIDES AND NUCLEOTIDES: PHYSICAL CONSTANTS AND SPECTRAL PROPERTIES (Continued)

No.	Compound	Symbol (3-Letter)	Symbol (1-Letter)	Structure	Formula (Mol Wt)	Melting Point °C	$[\alpha]_D^t$	pK Basic	pK Acidic
199	Inosine 3'(2')-phosphate	Ino-3'(2')-P	Ip for 3'		$C_{10}H_{13}N_4O_8P$ (348.21)	-	-	-	-
200	Inosine 5'-phosphate	IMP / Ino-5'-P	pI		$C_{10}H_{13}N_4O_8P$ (348.21)	-	-18.4^{24} (0.9, 0.2 NHCl)	-	-
201	Inosine 5'-diphosphate / Inosinic acid	IDP / Ino-5'-P$_2$	ppI		$C_{10}H_{14}N_4O_{11}P_2$ (428.19)	-	-	-	-

Acidic Spectral Data

No.	pH	λ_{max}	ε_{max} (×10⁻³)	λ_{min}	Spectral Ratios 230	240	250	270	280	290
199	-	-	-	-	-	-	-	-	-	-
200	-	-	-	-	-	-	-	-	-	-
201	-	-	-	-	-	-	-	-	-	-

Neutral Spectral Data

No.	pH	λ_{max}	ε_{max} (×10⁻³)	λ_{min}	Spectral Ratios 230	240	250	270	280	290
199	5	248	-	222	0.63	1.32	1.59	0.63	0.29	0.04
200	6	248	12.2	22.5	-	-	1.68	-	0.25	-
201	6	248.5	12.2	-	-	-	1.68	-	0.25	-

Alkaline Spectral Data

No.	pH	λ_{max}	ε_{max} (×10⁻³)	λ_{min}	Spectral Ratios 230	240	250	270	280	290
199	-	-	-	-	-	-	-	-	-	-
200	-	-	-	-	-	-	-	-	-	-
201	-	-	-	-	-	-	-	-	-	-

REFERENCES

No.	Origin and Synthesis	$[\alpha]_D^t$	pK	Spectral Data	Mass Spectra	R_f
199	R: 90	-	-	90	-	-
200	C: 368	368	-	368,411e	-	368,411
201	C: 411	-	-	411	-	411

PURINES, PYRIMIDINES, NUCLEOSIDES AND NUCLEOTIDES: PHYSICAL CONSTANTS AND SPECTRAL PROPERTIES (Continued)

No.	Compound	Symbol (3-Letter)	Symbol (1-Letter)	Structure	Formula (Mol Wt)	Melting Point °C	$[\alpha]_D^t$	pK Basic	pK Acidic
202	1-Methylinosine 3'(2')-phosphate	1MeIno-3'(2')-P	M^1Ip for 3'		$C_{11}H_{15}N_4O_8P$ (362.24)	—	—	—	—
203	Uridine 2'-phosphate	Urd-2'-P / 2'-UMP	Up		$C_9H_{13}N_2O_9P$ (324.18)	190–191° (dec) (Diammonium salt)	$+22.3^{zz}$ (2.0, H_2O)	—	—
204	Uridine 3'-phosphate	Urd-3'-P / 3'-UMP	Up / U-		$C_9H_{13}N_2O_9P$ (324.18)	192°	$+22.3^{zz}$ (2.0, H_2O)	—	9.4

Acidic Spectral Data

No.	pH	λ_{max}	ε_{max} (×10⁻³)	λ_{min}	230	240	250	270	280	290
202	—	—	—	—	—	—	—	—	—	—
203	2	$260^{*,z}$	9.9[z]	230[z]	—	—	0.8	—	0.28	0.03
204	1	262	10	230	—	—	0.76	0.82	0.32*	0.03*

Neutral Spectral Data

No.	pH	λ_{max}	ε_{max} (×10⁻³)	λ_{min}	230	240	250	270	280	290
202	4	249	—	233	0.66	1.35	1.65	0.72	0.41	0.07
203	7	$260^{*,z}$	10.0[z]	230[z]	—	—	0.78	—	0.30	0.03
204	7	262[z]	10.0[z]	230[z]	—	—	0.73	—	0.35	0.03

Alkaline Spectral Data

No.	pH	λ_{max}	ε_{max} (×10⁻³)	λ_{min}	230	240	250	270	280	290
202	9.5	249.5	—	224	0.67	1.3	1.67	0.73	0.43	0.09
203	12	261[z]	7.3[z]	242[z]	—	—	0.85	0.85	0.25	0.02
204	13	261	7.8	241	—	—	0.83	—	0.28*	0.02*

REFERENCES

No.	Origin and Synthesis	Spectral Data	Mass Spectra	$[\alpha]_D^t$	pK	R_f
202	R: 410	R: 410	—	—	—	
203	R: 178,170,216[z]	$181^{*,zb},179^{y},90^{x}$	—	216[z]	—	258
204	C: 190 R: 178,170,216[z]	$265^{*,b},181^{zbcd},179^{e}$	—	216[z]	223	258

PURINES, PYRIMIDINES, NUCLEOSIDES AND NUCLEOTIDES: PHYSICAL CONSTANTS AND SPECTRAL PROPERTIES (Continued)

No.	Compound	Symbol (3-Letter)	Symbol (1-Letter)	Structure	Formula (Mol Wt)	Melting Point °C	$[\alpha]_D$	pK (Basic)	pK (Acidic)
205	Uridine 5'-phosphate / 5'-Uridylic acid	Urd-5'-PUMP	pU / -U		$C_9H_{13}N_2O_9P$ (324.18)	190–202° (dibrucine salt)	$+3.44^{28}$ (1.02, 10% HCl)	—	9.5
206	Uridine 5'-diphosphate	Urd-5'-P$_2$ / UDP	ppU		$C_9H_{14}N_2O_{12}P_2$ (404.16)	—	—	—	9.4
207	Uridine 5'-triphosphate	Urd-5'-P$_3$ / UTP	pppU		$C_9H_{15}N_2O_{15}P_3$ (484.15)	—	—	—	9.6

Acidic Spectral Data

No.	pH	λ_{max}	ε_{max} (×10⁻³)	λ_{min}	230	240	250	270	280	290
205	2	262	10.0	230	—	—	0.73	—	0.39	0.03
206	2	262	10.0	230	—	—	0.73	—	0.39*	0.04
207	2	262	10.0	230	0.21	0.37	0.75	0.88	0.38	—

Neutral Spectral Data

No.	pH	λ_{max}	ε_{max} (×10⁻³)	λ_{min}	230	240	250	270	280	290
205	7	262	10.0	230	0.21	0.38	0.73	0.87	0.39	0.03
206	7	262	10.0	230	—	—	0.73	—	0.39	—
207	7	262	10.0	230	0.21	0.38	0.75	0.86	0.38	—

Alkaline Spectral Data

No.	pH	λ_{max}	ε_{max} (×10⁻³)	λ_{min}	230	240	250	270	280	290
205	11	261	7.8	241	0.79	0.5	0.8	—	0.31	0.02
206	11	261	7.9	241	—	—	0.8	—	0.32	—
207	11	261	8.1	239	0.79	0.65	0.81	0.78	0.31*	—

REFERENCES

No.	Origin and Synthesis	$[\alpha]_D$	pK	Spectral Data	Mass Spectra	R_f
205	C: 264,190[a],368 R: 195 N: 198	217	212	21,183[b],184[b],179[e]	—	210[b],74
206	C: 210 N: 198	—	212	212,183[b],179*[e]	—	210
207	C: 210 N: 198,204	—	204,212	212[b],204*[e],183[b]	—	210

PURINES, PYRIMIDINES, NUCLEOSIDES AND NUCLEOTIDES: PHYSICAL CONSTANTS AND SPECTRAL PROPERTIES (Continued)

No.	Compound	Symbol 3-Letter	Symbol 1-Letter	Formula (Mol Wt)	Melting Point °C	[α]$_D^t$	pK Basic	pK Acidic
208	2-Thiouridine 5'-phosphate	2SUrd-5'-P, 2Srd-5'-P, 2SUMP	ps²U, p²S	C$_9$H$_{13}$N$_2$O$_8$PS (340.25)	–	–	–	–
209	5-(Methoxycarbonylmethyl)-2-thiouridine 3'-phosphate; 5-Carboxymethyl-2-thiouridine methyl ester 3'-phosphate	5MeCm2SUrd-3'-P, 5MeCm2Srd-3'-P	mcm⁵s²Up, mcm⁵Sp	C$_{12}$H$_{17}$N$_2$O$_{10}$PS (412.31)	–	–	–	–
210	5-(Methylaminomethyl)-2-thiouridine 3'-phosphate	5(MeNHMe)2Srd-3'-P, 5(MeNHMe)2SUrd-3'-P	mnm⁵s²Up, mnm⁵Sp	C$_{11}$H$_{18}$N$_3$O$_8$PS (383.32)	–	–	–	–

Acidic Spectral Data

No.	pH	λ$_{max}$	ε$_{max}$ (×10⁻³)	λ$_{min}$	230	240	250	270	280	290
208	1	275		243						

Neutral Spectral Data

No.	pH	λ$_{max}$	ε$_{max}$ (×10⁻³)	λ$_{min}$	230	240	250	270	280	290
208	H₂O	272		243						
209	7	275		243						

Alkaline Spectral Data

No.	pH	λ$_{max}$	ε$_{max}$ (×10⁻³)	λ$_{min}$	230	240	250	270	280	290
208	12ᵇ	241		213						

REFERENCES

No.	Spectral Data	pK	[α]$_D$	Mass Spectra	R$_f$
208	344	–	–	–	344
209	306ᵇ	–	–	–	–
210	–	–	–	–	305

No.	Origin and Synthesis
208	C: 344
209	R: 306
210	R: 305

PURINES, PYRIMIDINES, NUCLEOSIDES AND NUCLEOTIDES: PHYSICAL CONSTANTS AND SPECTRAL PROPERTIES (Continued)

No.	Compound	Symbol 3-Letter	Symbol 1-Letter	Structure	Formula (Mol Wt)	Melting Point °C	$[\alpha]_D^t$	pK Basic	pK Acidic
211	3-Methyluridine 3'(2')-phosphate	3MeUrd-3'(2')-P	m³UP, m³U- for 3'		$C_{10}H_{15}N_2O_9P$ (338.21)	–	–	–	–
212	3-Methyluridine 5'-phosphate	3MeUrd-5'-P, 3MeUMP	Pm³U, -m³U		$C_{10}H_{15}N_2O_9P$ (338.21)	–	–	–	–
213	4-Thiouridine 3'(2')-phosphate	4Srd-3'(2')-P, 4SUrd-3'(2')-P	s⁴Up ⁴SP, s⁴U- for 3'		$C_9H_{13}N_2O_8PS$ (340.25)	–	–	–	–

Acidic Spectral Data

No.	pH	λ_{max}	ε_{max} (×10⁻³)	λ_{min}	230	240	250	270	280	290
211	2*	258	–	233	–	–	–	–	–	–
		245	4.0	225						
		331	20.6*	276						

Neutral Spectral Data

No.	pH	λ_{max}	ε_{max} (×10⁻³)	λ_{min}	230	240	250	270	280	290
211	H₂O	262	8.8*	232	–	–	0.77	–	0.45	–
212	H₂O	262	8.8	225	–	–	–	–	–	–
213	5.6	245	4.0							
		331	20.6	276						

Alkaline Spectral Data

No.	pH	λ_{max}	ε_{max} (×10⁻³)	λ_{min}	230	240	250	270	280	290
211	11.6	260	9.3	233	–	–	–	–	–	–
213	13	315*	18.3*	257	–	–	–	–	–	–

REFERENCES

No.	Origin and Synthesis	$[\alpha]_D^t$	pK	Spectral Data	Mass Spectra	R_f
211	C: 173,142,174	–	–	173,174c; 142*cd	–	13,142,143,173
212	C: 344	–	–	344	–	125,344
213	C: 343 R: 144	–	–	343,144*b	–	343

PURINES, PYRIMIDINES, NUCLEOSIDES AND NUCLEOTIDES: PHYSICAL CONSTANTS AND SPECTRAL PROPERTIES (Continued)

No.	Compound	Symbol (3-Letter)	Symbol (1-Letter)	Structure	Formula (Mol Wt)	Melting Point °C	$[\alpha]_D^t$	pK (Basic)	pK (Acidic)
214	4-Thiouridine 5'-phosphate	4Srd-5'-P / 4Surd-5'-P / 4SUMP	ps4U / -s4U / p4S		$C_9H_{13}N_2O_8PS$ (340.25)	—	—	—	—
215	5-Carboxymethyluridine 3'(2')-phosphate / Uridine-5-acetic acid 3'(2')-phosphate	5CmUrd-3'(2')-P / 5CxMeUrd-3'(2')-P	cm5Up for 3'		$C_{11}H_{15}N_2O_{11}P$ (382.22)	—	—	—	~4^p
216	5-Carbamoylmethyluridine 3'(2')-phosphate / Uridine-5-acetamide 3'(2')-phosphate	5NcmUrd-3'(2')-P / 5NcMeUrd-3'(2')-P	ncm5Up for 3'		$C_{11}H_{16}N_3O_{10}P$ (381.24)	—	—	—	—

Acidic Spectral Data

No.	pH	λ_{max}	ε_{max} (×10⁻³)	λ_{min}	230	240	250	270	280	290
214										
215	2	265	9.7^h	232	0.26	0.37	0.71	0.97	0.55	0.11
216	2	266	10.0^h	232	0.31	0.38	0.71	0.98	0.55	0.11

Neutral Spectral Data

No.	pH	λ_{max}	ε_{max} (×10⁻³)	λ_{min}	230	240	250	270	280	290
214	H_2O	245 / 331	– / 20.6	225 / 274						
215	7	267	9.8^h	232	0.23	0.28	0.62	1.06	0.69	0.14
216	6	266	10.2^h	232	0.30	0.39	0.68	1.02	0.62	0.16

Alkaline Spectral Data

No.	pH	λ_{max}	ε_{max} (×10⁻³)	λ_{min}	230	240	250	270	280	290
214										
215	12.3	266	7.0^h	242	1.13	0.74	0.77	0.98	0.55	0.07
216	11.5	265	6.9^h	244	1.08	0.76	0.79	0.97	0.55	0.13

REFERENCES

No.	Origin and Synthesis	$[\alpha]_D^t$	pK	Spectral Data	Mass Spectra	R_f
214	C: 344,343	—	—	344	—	343,344
215	R: 278,410	—	278	410	—	278
216	R: 398,410	—	—	410	—	—

PURINES, PYRIMIDINES, NUCLEOSIDES AND NUCLEOTIDES: PHYSICAL CONSTANTS AND SPECTRAL PROPERTIES (Continued)

No.	Compound	Symbol 3-Letter	Symbol 1-Letter	Structure	Formula (Mol Wt)	Melting Point °C	$[\alpha]_D$	pK Basic	pK Acidic
217	5-Hydroxyuridine 5′-phosphate	5HOUrd-5′-P	po5U o5U		$C_9H_{13}N_2O_{10}P$ (340.18)	–	–	–	–
218	5-Methyluridine 3′(2′)-phosphate Ribosylthymine 3′(2′)-phosphate	5MeUrd-3′(2′)-P Thd-3′(2′)-P	M5Upm5U- Tp T-for 3′		$C_{10}H_{15}N_2O_9P$ (338.21)	–	–	–	–
219	5-Methyluridine 5′-phosphate Ribosylthymine 5′-phosphate	Thd-5′-P TMP 5MeUMP	PT -T pm5U -m5U		$C_{10}H_{15}N_2O_9P$ (338.21)	–	–12.3[26] (2.0, 0.1 N HCl)	–	–

Acidic Spectral Data

No.	pH	λ_{max}	ε_{max} (×10⁻³)	λ_{min}	Spectral Ratios 230	240	250	270	280	290
217	–	–	–	–	–	–	–	–	–	–
218	1	267*	9.8	235	–	–	0.68	1.05	0.66	0.23
219	2	267	8.8	–	–	–	–	–	–	–

Neutral Spectral Data

No.	pH	λ_{max}	ε_{max} (×10⁻³)	λ_{min}	Spectral Ratios 230	240	250	270	280	290
217	6	278	–	245	–	–	–	–	–	–
218	–	–	–	–	–	–	–	–	–	–
219	–	–	–	–	–	–	–	–	–	–

Alkaline Spectral Data

No.	pH	λ_{max}	ε_{max} (×10⁻³)	λ_{min}	Spectral Ratios 230	240	250	270	280	290
217	9	236 300	–	268	–	–	–	–	–	–
218	13	268	–	247	–	–	0.79	1.04	0.69	0.23
219	–	–	–	–	–	–	–	–	–	–

REFERENCES

No.	Origin and Synthesis	Spectral Data	pK	$[\alpha]_D$	Mass Spectra	R_f
217	C: 146,74	146	–	–	–	74
218	R: 165 C: 142	265[b],165*	–	368	–	165,142
219	C: 368	368	–	368	–	142

PURINES, PYRIMIDINES, NUCLEOSIDES AND NUCLEOTIDES: PHYSICAL CONSTANTS AND SPECTRAL PROPERTIES (Continued)

No.	Compound	Structure	Symbol 3-Letter	Symbol 1-Letter	Formula (Mol Wt)	Melting Point °C	$[\alpha]_D$	pK Basic	pK Acidic
220	5-Methyluridine 5'-diphosphate; Ribosylthymine 5'-diphosphate		Thd-5'-P$_2$; TDP; 5MeUDP	ppm5U; ppT; ppT	$C_{10}H_{16}N_2O_{12}P_2$ (418.18)	–	–	–	–
221	Pseudouridine 3'(2') phosphate β-f; Pseudouridine 3'(2')-phosphate; 5-Ribosyluracil 3'(2')-phosphate		ψrd-3'(2')-P	Ψp; ψr-; For 3'	$C_9H_{13}N_2O_9P$ (324.18)	–	–	–	9.6
222	Pseudouridine 5'-phosphate β-f; Pseudouridine 5'-phosphate; 5-Ribosyluracil 5'-phosphate		ψrd-5'-P; ψMP	Pψ; -ψ	$C_9H_{13}N_2O_9P$ (324.18)	–	–	–	–

Acidic Spectral Data

No.	pH	λ_{max}	ε_{max} (×10^{-3})	λ_{min}	230	240	250	270	280	290
220	2	268	10.0	234	0.37	0.34	0.64	1.10	0.77	0.27
221	2'	263	8.4	233	0.30	0.41	0.75	0.86	0.40*	0.07*
222	–	–	–	–	–	–	–	–	–	–

Neutral Spectral Data

No.	pH	λ_{max}	ε_{max} (×10^{-3})	λ_{min}	230	240	250	270	280	290
220	–	–	–	–	–	–	–	–	–	–
221	7	263	–	233	0.28	0.39	0.74	0.85	0.40	0.07
222	–	–	–	–	–	–	–	–	–	–

Alkaline Spectral Data

No.	pH	λ_{max}	ε_{max} (×10^{-3})	λ_{min}	230	240	250	270	280	290
220	–	–	–	–	–	–	–	–	–	–
221	12	286	8.4	246	2.13	0.75	0.64*	1.54*	2.06*	2.14*
222	12	–	–	–	–	–	–	–	1.40	–

REFERENCES

No.	Origin and Synthesis	$[\alpha]_D^t$	pK	Spectral Data	Mass Spectra	R$_f$
220	C: 175	–	–	175	–	175
221	R: 157,94	–	157	157[b],94,158,265*[b]	–	165
222	C: 158,176	–	–	158	–	158

PURINES, PYRIMIDINES, NUCLEOSIDES AND NUCLEOTIDES: PHYSICAL CONSTANTS AND SPECTRAL PROPERTIES (Continued)

No.	Compound	Symbol 3-Letter	Symbol 1-Letter	Structure	Formula (Mol Wt)	Melting Point °C	$[\alpha]_D^t$	pK Basic	pK Acidic
223	Pseudouridine 5'-diphosphate β-f; Pseudouridine 5'-diphosphate;5-Ribosyluracil 5'-diphosphate	ψrd-5'-P$_2$, ψDP			$C_9H_{14}N_2O_{12}P_2$ (404.16)	–	–	–	–
224	Orotidine 5'-phosphate 6-Carboxyuridine 5'-phosphate	Ord-5'-P, OMP, 6CxUMP	pO, -O		$C_{10}H_{13}N_2O_{11}P$ (368.19)	–	–	–	–
225	5-N-Methyl formamido-6-ribosylamino *iso* cystosine 3'(2')-phosphate[f]; 2-Amino-4-hydroxy-5-N-methylformamido-6-ribosylaminopyrimidine 3'(2')-phosphate	5MeFn6(RibNH)*iso*Cyt-3'(2')-P			$C_{11}H_{18}N_5O_9P$ (395.27)	–	–	–	–

Acidic Spectral Data

No.	pH	λ_{max}	ε_{max} (×10⁻³)	λ_{min}	230	240	250	270	280	290
223	–	–	–	–	–	–	–	–	–	–
224	–	–	–	–	–	–	–	–	–	–
225	2	273	14.0[c]	247	1.00	0.50	0.47	1.81	1.41	0.31

Neutral Spectral Data

No.	pH	λ_{max}	ε_{max} (×10⁻³)	λ_{min}	230	240	250	270	280	290
223	–	–	–	–	–	–	–	–	–	–
224	7	266	–	–	–	–	–	–	0.66	–
225	–	–	–	–	–	–	–	–	–	–

Alkaline Spectral Data

No.	pH	λ_{max}	ε_{max} (×10⁻³)	λ_{min}	230	240	250	270	280	290
223	12	–	–	–	–	–	–	–	1.30	–
224	–	–	–	–	–	–	–	–	–	–
225	13	265	10.5[c]	244	0.77	0.51	0.56	1.03	0.26	0.05

REFERENCES

No.	Origin and Synthesis	$[\alpha]_D^t$	pK	Spectral Data	Mass Spectra	R_f
223	C: 158	–	–	158	–	158
224	E: 177	–	–	177	–	–
225	C: 90	–	–	90,334[b]	–	334

PURINES, PYRIMIDINES, NUCLEOSIDES AND NUCLEOTIDES: PHYSICAL CONSTANTS AND SPECTRAL PROPERTIES (Continued)

No.	Compound	Symbol (3-Letter)	Symbol (1-Letter)	Structure	Formula (Mol Wt)	Melting Point °C	$[\alpha]_D$	pK (Basic)	pK (Acidic)
				DEOXYRIBONUCLEOTIDES					
226	Deoxyadenosine 3'-phosphate	dAdo-3'P / 3'dAMP	dAp / dA-		$C_{10}H_{14}N_5O_6P$ (331.22)	—	—	—	—
227	Deoxyadenosine 5'-phosphate	dAdo-5'-P / dAMP	pdA / -dA		$C_{10}H_{14}N_5O_6P$ (331.22)	142°	-38.0^{19} (0.23, H_2O)	~4.4	—
228	Deoxyadenosine 5'-triphosphate	dado-5'-P_3 / dATP	pppdA		$C_{10}H_{16}N_5O_{12}P_3$ (491.19)	—	—	—	—

Acidic Spectral Data

No.	pH	λ_{max}	ε_{max} (×10⁻³)	λ_{min}	230	240	250	270	280	290
226	—	—	—	—	—	—	—	—	—	—
227	2	258	14.3*	230	—	—	0.82	—	0.23	0.04
228	—	—	—	—	—	—	—	—	—	—

Neutral Spectral Data

No.	pH	λ_{max}	ε_{max} (×10⁻³)	λ_{min}	230	240	250	270	280	290
226	7	—	—	—	—	—	0.79	0.68	0.14	—
227	7	—	15.3	—	—	0.42	0.8	0.66	0.14	0.01
228	7	—	—	—	—	—	0.77	—	0.14	—

Alkaline Spectral Data

No.	pH	λ_{max}	ε_{max} (×10⁻³)	λ_{min}	230	240	250	270	280	290
226	—	—	—	—	—	—	—	—	—	—
227	—	—	—	—	—	—	—	—	—	—
228	—	—	—	—	—	—	—	—	—	—

REFERENCES

No.	Origin and Synthesis	$[\alpha]_D$	pK	Spectral Data	Mass Spectra	R_f
226	D: 263 C: 203	—	—	263	—	263
227	D: 200ª,260 C: 202	260	180	186,185*ᵉ,200,223ᶜᵈ	—	263
228	E: 209	—	—	209	—	—

PURINES, PYRIMIDINES, NUCLEOSIDES AND NUCLEOTIDES: PHYSICAL CONSTANTS AND SPECTRAL PROPERTIES (Continued)

No.	Compound	Symbol 3-Letter	Symbol 1-Letter	Structure	Formula (Mol Wt)	Melting Point °C	$[\alpha]_D$	pK Basic	pK Acidic
229	N^6-Methyldeoxyadenosine 5'-phosphate	6MedAdo-5'-P 6MedAMP d6MeAdo-5'-P	Pm6dA -m6dA	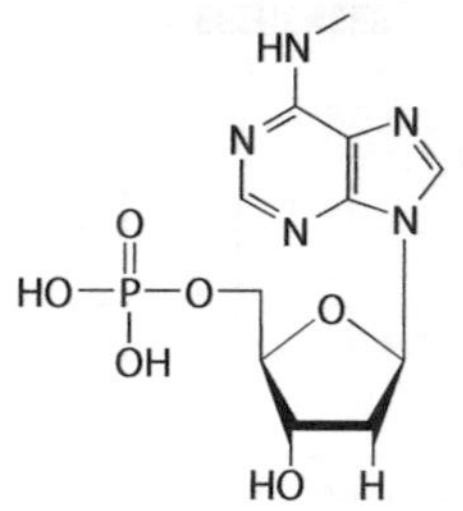	$C_{11}H_{16}N_5O_6P$ (345.25)	—	—	3.6^p	—
230	Deoxycytidine 3'-phosphate	dCyd-3'-P 3'-dCMP	dCp dC-	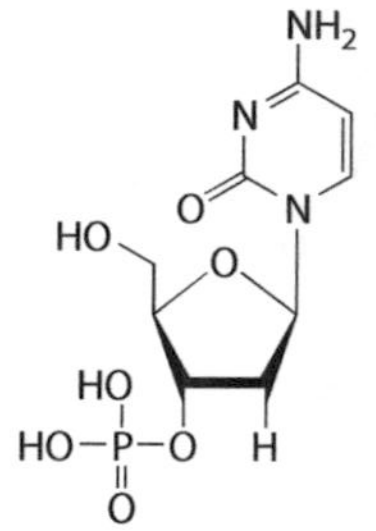	$C_9H_{14}N_3O_7P$ (307.20)	196–197° (dec)	$+57.0^{17}$ (1.35, H_2O)	—	—
231	Deoxycytidine 5'-phosphate	dCyd-5'-P dCMP	pdC -dC	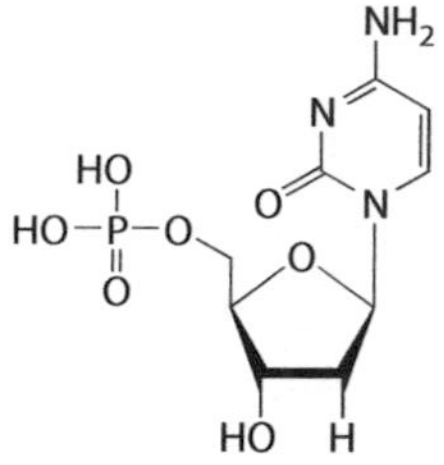	$C_9H_{14}N_3O_7P$ (307.20)	183–184° (dec)	$+35.0^{21}$ (0.2, H_2O)	4.6	—

Acidic Spectral Data

No.	pH	λ_{max}	ε_{max} (×10⁻³)	λ_{min}	230	240	250	270	280	290
229	4^a	266	—	—	0.18	0.28	0.63	1.09	0.66	0.25
230	3	—	—	—	—	—	—	—	2.0	—
231	2	280	13.5	239	—	—	0.43	—	2.12	1.55

Neutral Spectral Data

No.	pH	λ_{max}	ε_{max} (×10⁻³)	λ_{min}	230	240	250	270	280	290
229	—	—	—	—	—	—	—	—	—	—
230	7	—	—	—	—	—	0.84	1.19	0.93	—
231	7	271	9.3	249	—	0.91	0.82	1.25	0.99	0.30

Alkaline Spectral Data

No.	pH	λ_{max}	ε_{max} (×10⁻³)	λ_{min}	230	240	250	270	280	290
229	13	266	—	234	0.18	0.24	0.57	1.08	0.63	0.21
230	12	—	—	—	—	—	—	—	—	—
231	—	—	—	—	—	—	0.82	—	0.99	0.30

REFERENCES

No.	Origin and Synthesis	$[\alpha]_D^t$	pK	Spectral Data	Mass Spectra	R_f
229	D: 21	—	21	21^b	—	—
230	D: 263 C: 201,203,202	201	—	$263,201^e$	—	203,201,263
231	C: 201 D: 200	207	180	$185^b,179^e,186^e,201$	—	185,201,263,74

PURINES, PYRIMIDINES, NUCLEOSIDES AND NUCLEOTIDES: PHYSICAL CONSTANTS AND SPECTRAL PROPERTIES (Continued)

No.	Compound	Symbol 3-Letter	1-Letter	Formula (Mol Wt)	Melting Point °C	$[\alpha]_D^t$	pK Basic	pK Acidic
232	Deoxycytidine 5'-triphosphate	dCyd-5'-P₃ / dCTP	pppdC	$C_9H_{16}N_3O_{13}P_3$ (467.17)	–	–	–	–
233	5-Methyldeoxycytidine 5'-phosphate	5MedCyd-5'-P 5MedCMP / d5MeCyd-5'-P	pm⁵dC / -m⁵dC	$C_{10}H_{16}N_3O_7P$ (321.22)	–	–	4.4	–
234	5-Hydroxymethyldeoxycytidine 5'-phosphate	5HmdCyd-5'-P 5HmdCMP 5HOMedCMP	pom⁵dC / -om⁵dC / phm⁵dC* / -hm⁵dC*	$C_{10}H_{16}N_3O_8P$ (337.22)	–	–	–	–

Acidic Spectral Data

No.	pH	λmax	εmax (×10⁻³)	λmin	230	240	250	270	280	290
232	2	–	–	–	–	–	0.44	–	2.14	–
233	2	287	–	244	1.51	0.43	0.36	2.10	3.14	3.44
234	1	284	12.5	245	1.12*	0.39	0.44	1.89	2.68	2.53

Neutral Spectral Data

No.	pH	λmax	εmax (×10⁻³)	λmin	230	240	250	270	280	290
232	–	–	–	–	–	–	–	–	–	–
233	7	278	–	254	1.52	1.29	0.95	1.40	1.52	1.01
234	7	275	7.7	254	1.50	1.10	0.90	1.35	1.33	0.71

Alkaline Spectral Data

No.	pH	λmax	εmax (×10⁻³)	λmin	230	240	250	270	280	290
232	–	–	–	–	–	–	–	–	–	–
233	12	278	–	–	–	–	–	–	–	–
234	12	275	7.7	254	1.40*	1.08	0.93	1.33	1.31	0.65

REFERENCES

No.	Origin and Synthesis	$[\alpha]_D^t$	pK	Spectral Data	Mass Spectra	R_f
232	E: 209 C: 214	–	–	209	–	–
233	D: 68	–	170	68ᵇ,186	–	–
234	C: 74 E: 70 D: 171,172	–	–	74,70*bcdᵇ,171ᵈ,172*	–	74

PURINES, PYRIMIDINES, NUCLEOSIDES AND NUCLEOTIDES: PHYSICAL CONSTANTS AND SPECTRAL PROPERTIES (Continued)

No.	Compound	Symbol 3-Letter	Symbol 1-Letter	Structure	Formula (Mol Wt)	Melting Point °C	$[\alpha]_D^t$	pK Basic	pK Acidic
235	Deoxyguanosine 3'-phosphate	dGuo-3'-P / 3'-dGMP	dGp / dG-		$C_{10}H_{14}N_5O_7P$ (347.23)	–	–	–	–
236	Deoxyguanosine 5'-phosphate	dGuo-5'-P / dGMP	pdG / -dG		$C_{10}H_{14}N_5O_7P$ (347.23)	180–182°	-31^{19} (0.43, H_2O)	2.9	9.7
237	Deoxyguanosine 5'-triphosphate	dGuo-5'-P$_3$ dGTP	pppdG		$C_{10}H_{16}N_5O_{13}P_3$ (507.20)	–	–	–	–

Acidic Spectral Data

No.	pH	λ_{max}	ε_{max} (×10^{-3})	λ_{min}	230	240	250	270	280	290
235	–	–	–	–	–	–	–	–	–	–
236	1°	255	11.8	228	–	–	1.02	–	0.70	–
	2⁶	–	–	–	–	–	1.03	–	0.70	0.46
237	–	–	–	–	–	–	–	–	–	–

Neutral Spectral Data

No.	pH	λ_{max}	ε_{max} (×10^{-3})	λ_{min}	230	240	250	270	280	290
235	7	–	–	–	–	–	–	–	–	–
236	7	–	–	–	–	0.79	1.20	0.82	0.67	–
	7	–	–	–	–	–	1.13	0.81	0.67	0.27
237	7	–	–	–	–	–	1.14	–	0.66	–

Alkaline Spectral Data

No.	pH	λ_{max}	ε_{max} (×10^{-3})	λ_{min}	230	240	250	270	280	290
235	–	–	–	–	–	–	–	–	–	–
236	–	–	–	–	–	–	–	–	–	–
237	–	–	–	–	–	–	–	–	–	–

REFERENCES

No.	Origin and Synthesis	$[\alpha]_D^t$	pK	Spectral Data	Mass Spectra	R_f
235	D: 263 C: 203	–	–	263	–	263
236	D: 200,180[a],259	259	180	186,185[e],200,223[cde]	–	185,263
237	E: 209 C: 214	–	–	209	–	–

PURINES, PYRIMIDINES, NUCLEOSIDES AND NUCLEOTIDES: PHYSICAL CONSTANTS AND SPECTRAL PROPERTIES (Continued)

No.	Compound	Symbol 3-Letter	Symbol 1-Letter	Structure	Formula (Mol Wt)	Melting Point °C	$[\alpha]_D^t$	pK Basic	pK Acidic
238	7-Methyldeoxyguanosine 5′-phosphate	7MedGuo-5′-P 7MedGMP d7MeGuo-5′-P	pm⁷dG -m⁷dG		$C_{11}H_{16}N_5O_7P$ (361.24)	—	—	r	—
239	7-Methyldeoxyguanosine 5′-triphosphate	7MedGuo-5′-P₃ 7MedGTP	pppm⁷dG		$C_{11}H_{18}N_5O_{13}P_3$ (521.21)	—	—	r	7.5

Acidic Spectral Data

No.	pH	λ_{max}	ε_{max} (×10⁻³)	λ_{min}	Spectral Ratios 230	240	250	270	280	290
238	—	—	—	—	—	—	—	—	—	—
239	2	257	10.6	230						

Neutral Spectral Data

No.	pH	λ_{max}	ε_{max} (×10⁻³)	λ_{min}	Spectral Ratios 230	240	250	270	280	290
238	7ᵃ	256 283	9.8 7.8	236 271						
239	7.4ᵠ	258 280	8.9 7.25	236 271						

Alkaline Spectral Data

No.	pH	λ_{max}	ε_{max} (×10⁻³)	λ_{min}	Spectral Ratios 230	240	250	270	280	290
238										—
239	12ᵠ	281	7.9	243						

REFERENCES

No.	Origin and Synthesis	Spectral Data	pK	$[\alpha]_D^t$	Mass Spectra	R_f
238	C: 46	46	—	—	—	46
239	C: 334	334	334	—	—	334

PURINES, PYRIMIDINES, NUCLEOSIDES AND NUCLEOTIDES: PHYSICAL CONSTANTS AND SPECTRAL PROPERTIES (Continued)

No.	Compound	Symbol 3-Letter	Symbol 1-Letter	Structure	Formula (Mol Wt)	Melting Point °C	$[\alpha]_D^t$	pK Basic	pK Acidic
240	Deoxyuridine 3′-phosphate	dUrd-3′-P 3′-dUMP	dUp dU-		$C_9H_{13}N_2O_8P$ (308.18)	–	–	–	–
241	Deoxyuridine 5′-phosphate	dUrd-5P dUMP	pdU -dU		$C_8H_{13}N_2O_8P$ (308.18)	–	–	–	–
242	Deoxyuridine 5′-triphosphate	dUrd-5′-P₃ dUTP	pppdU		$C_9H_{15}N_2O_{14}P_3$ (468.15)	–	–	–	–

Acidic Spectral Data

No.	pH	λ_{max}	ε_{max} $(\times10^{-3})$	λ_{min}	230	240	250	270	280	290
240	–	–	–	–	–	–	–	–	–	–
241	2	260	9.8	231	–	–	0.72	–	–	–
242	1	262	–	–	–	–	–	–	0.45	–

Neutral Spectral Data

No.	pH	λ_{max}	ε_{max} $(\times10^{-3})$	λ_{min}	230	240	250	270	280	290
240	–	–	–	–	–	–	–	–	–	–
241	7	260	–	230	–	–	–	–	–	–
242	–	–	–	–	–	–	–	–	–	–

Alkaline Spectral Data

No.	pH	λ_{max}	ε_{max} $(\times10^{-3})$	λ_{min}	230	240	250	270	280	290
240	–	–	–	–	–	–	–	–	–	–
241	12	261	7.6ᵇ	241	–	–	–	–	–	–
242	–	–	–	–	–	–	–	–	–	–

REFERENCES

No.	Origin and Synthesis	$[\alpha]_D^t$	pK	Spectral Data	Mass Spectra	R_f
240	–	–	–	–	–	–
241	E: 229	–	–	230ᵇ	–	74
242	C: 289	–	–	289	–	–

PURINES, PYRIMIDINES, NUCLEOSIDES AND NUCLEOTIDES: PHYSICAL CONSTANTS AND SPECTRAL PROPERTIES (Continued)

No.	Compound	Symbol 3-Letter	Symbol 1-Letter	Structure	Formula (Mol Wt)	Melting Point °C	$[\alpha]_D^t$	pK Basic	pK Acidic
243	Thymidine 3'-phosphate	dThd-3'-P / 3'dTMP	dTp / dT-		$C_{10}H_{15}N_2O_8P$ (322.21)	178°q (dibrucine salt)	$+7.3^{20}$ (1.5, H_2O)	—	—
244	Thymidine 5'-phosphate	dThd-5'-P / dTMP	pdT / -dT		$C_{10}H_{15}N_2O_8P$ (322.21)	175° (dibrucine salt)	-4.4^{21} (0.4, H_2O)	—	10.0
245	Thymidine 5'-triphosphate	dThd-5'-P$_3$ / dTTP	pppdT		$C_{10}H_{17}N_2O_{14}P_3$ (482.18)	—	—	—	—

Acidic Spectral Data

No.	pH	λ_{max}	ε_{max} (×10⁻³)	λ_{min}	230	240	250	270	280	290
243	2	267	—	—	—	—	—	—	0.69	—
244	2	267	102	—	—	—	0.64	—	0.72	0.23
245	2	—	—	—	—	—	0.64	—	0.72	—

Neutral Spectral Data

No.	pH	λ_{max}	ε_{max} (×10⁻³)	λ_{min}	230	240	250	270	280	290
243	7	267	9.5	—	—	—	0.65	1.08	0.71	—
244	7	267	10.2	—	—	0.34	0.65	1.10	0.73	0.24
245	—	—	—	—	—	—	—	—	—	—

Alkaline Spectral Data

No.	pH	λ_{max}	ε_{max} (×10⁻³)	λ_{min}	230	240	250	270	280	290
243	—	—	—	—	—	—	—	—	—	—
244	12	—	—	—	—	—	0.74	—	0.67	0.17
245	—	—	—	—	—	—	—	—	—	—

REFERENCES

No.	Origin and Synthesis	$[\alpha]_D^t$	pK	Spectral Data	Mass Spectra	R_f
243	C: 262,202,187a,203 D: 263	187	—	262,187e,263e	—	187,262,263
244	C: 187,202 D: 200	207	180	185b,186e,179e,223	—	187,185,263
245	E: 209 C: 209	—	—	209	—	—

PURINES, PYRIMIDINES, NUCLEOSIDES AND NUCLEOTIDES: PHYSICAL CONSTANTS AND SPECTRAL PROPERTIES (Continued)

No.	Compound	Symbol 3-Letter	Symbol 1-Letter	Structure	Formula (Mol Wt)	Melting Point °C	$[\alpha]_D$	pK Basic	pK Acidic
246	5-Hydroxymethyldeoxyuridine 5'-phosphate	5HmdUrd-5'P 5HmdUMP 5(HOMe) dUMP	pom5 dU -om5 dU phm5 dU*		$C_{10}H_{15}N_2O_9P$ (338.21)	–	–	–	–

Acidic Spectral Data

No.	pH	λ_{max}	ε_{max} (×10⁻³)	λ_{min}	230	240	250	270	280	290
							Spectral Ratios			
246	2	264	10.2	234	0.32	0.37	0.69	0.97	0.56	0.11

Neutral Spectral Data

No.	pH	λ_{max}	ε_{max} (×10⁻³)	λ_{min}	230	240	250	270	280	290
							Spectral Ratios			
246	–	–	–	–	–	–	–	–	–	–

Alkaline Spectral Data

No.	pH	λ_{max}	ε_{max} (×10⁻³)	λ_{min}	230	240	250	270	280	290
							Spectral Ratios			
246	12	264	–	244*	1.15	0.75	0.80	0.95	0.48	0.09

REFERENCES

No.	Origin and Synthesis	$[\alpha]_D$	pK	Spectral Data	Mass Spectra	R_f
246	C: 74 D: 96,171,349	–	–	74,171* d,96	–	74

a Melting point from this reference.
b Full spectrum given.
c λ_{max} and/or λ_{min} from this reference.
d ε_{max} from this reference.
e Spectral ratios from this reference.
f pK of 2-methyl-6-methylaminoadenine. Compare the similar pK of adenine and N^6-methyladenine.[15]
g Spectral data taken on material synthesized this way then purified by paper chromatography.
h In 50% dimethylformamide (HCONMe₂).
i In 50% dimethylsulfoxide/ethanol (Me₂ SO/EtOH).
j For an explanation of this nomenclature and abbreviations, see General Remarks on Wyosine in Natural Occurrence of Modified Nucleosides.
k pK of 6-amino-5-formamidoisocytosine.
l pK of nucleotide.
m λ_{max} and ε_{max} due to adenosine.
n ε calculated from spectral data using ε_{max} acid of nucleoside.
o Decomposes at this pH.
p Determined from electrophoretic mobility.
q Values very dependent on pH (near pK).
r Basic ionization at all pH values.
s Spectral data in water and pH 11 indicate decomposition.
t Alkaline degradation product of 7-methylguanosine or nucleotide.
v Spectra in acid and neutral similar.
w ε estimated from conversion to N^6-methyladenosine 3' (2')- or 5'-phosphate using ε of 15.2 × 10³ in alkali, for the N^6-isomers.
x Based on ε of 7-methylguanosine 3'(2')-phosphate assuming quantitative conversion in alkali. For a possible error in this value see General Remarks on 7-Methylguanosine in Natural Occurrence of Modified Nucleosides.
y Cyclohexylamine salt.
z Data on mixed 2' and 3' phosphates.

The authors are indebted to a number of authors who supplied unpublished data, provided original spectra for calculations of the values or gave advice on the selection of the most reliable data. They also wish particularly to thank Mr. I. H. Flack, Mr. R. Thedford and Miss L. Csonka for their assistance in the preparation of the table.

References

1. Leonard and Deyrup, *J. Am. Chem. Soc.*, 84, 2148 (1962).
2. Shapiro and Gordon, *Biochem. Biophys. Res. Commun.*, 17, 160 (1964).
3. Chheda, Hall, Magrath, Mozejko, Schweizer, Stasiuk, and Taylor, *Biochemistry*, 8, 3278 (1969).
4. Schweizer, Chheda, Baczynskyj, and Hall, *Biochemistry*, 8, 3283 (1969).
5. Baczynskyj, Biemann, Fleysher, and Hall, *Can. J. Biochem.*, 47, 1202 (1969).
6. Hall, *Biochemistry*, 3, 769 (1964).
7. Saponara and Enger, *Nature*, 223, 1365 (1969).
8. Brookes and Lawley, *J. Chem. Soc.*, 539 (1960) and unpublished.
9. Dunn, *Biochim. Biophys. Acta*, 46, 198 (1961).
10. Jones and Robins, *J. Am. Chem. Soc.*, 85, 193 (1963) and unpublished.
11. Mandel, Srinivasan, and Borek, *Nature*, 209, 586 (1966).
12. Wacker and Ebert, *Z. Naturforsch.*, 14B, 709 (1959).
13. Lawley and Brookes, *Biochem. J.*, 89, 127 (1963).
14. Leonard, Achmatowicz, Loeppky, Carraway, Grimm, Szweykowska, Hamzi, and Skoog, *Proc. Natl. Acad. Sci. USA*, 56, 709 (1966).
15. Martin and Reese, *J. Chem. Soc.*, 1731 (1968).
16. Leonard and Fujii, *Proc. Natl. Acad. Sci. USA*, 51, 73 (1964).
17. Baddiley, Lythgoe, McNeil, and Todd, *J. Chem. Soc.*, 383 (1943).
18. Littlefield and Dunn, *Biochem. J.*, 70, 642 (1958).
19. Lynch, Robins, and Cheng, *J. Chem. Soc.*, 2973 (1958).
20. Baddiley, Lythgoe, and Todd, *J. Chem. Soc.*, 318 (1944).
21. Dunn and Smith, *Biochem. J.*, 68, 627 (1958).
22. Albert and Brown, *J. Chem. Soc.*, 2060 (1954).
23. Elion, Burgi, and Hitchings, *J. Am. Chem. Soc.*, 74, 411 (1952).
24. Broom, Townsend, Jones, and Robins, *Biochemistry*, 3, 494 (1964).
25. Adler, Weissman, and Gutman, *J. Biol. Chem.*, 230, 717 (1958).
26. Elion, *The Chemistry and Biology of Purines* CIBA Symposium, Churchill, London, 1957, 39.
27. Weissman, Bromberg, and Gutman, *J. Biol. Chem.*, 224, 407 (1957).
28. Mason, *J. Chem. Soc.*, 2071 (1954).
29. Baker, Joseph, and Schaub, *J. Org. Chem.*, 19, 631 (1954).
30. Brederick, Haas, and Martini, *Chem. Ber.*, 81, 307 (1948).
31. Hall, Robins, Stasiuk, and Thedford, *J. Am. Chem. Soc.*, 88, 2614 (1966).
32. Robins, Hall, and Thedford, *Biochemistry*, 6, 1837 (1967).
33. Elion, *J. Org. Chem.*, 27, 2478 (1962).
34. Fischer, *Chem. Ber.*, 31, 104 (1898).
35. Pal, *Biochemistry*, 1, 558 (1962).
36. Lawley and Brookes, *Biochem. J.*, 92, 19c (1964).
37. Gulland and Holiday, *J. Chem Soc.*, 765 (1936).
38. Traube and Dudley, *Chem. Ber.*, 46, 3839 (1913).
39. Pfleiderer, *Annalen*, 647, 167 (1961).
40. Smith and Dunn, *Biochem. J.*, 72, 294 (1959).
41. Haines, Reese, and Todd, *J. Chem. Soc.*, 5281 (1962).
42. Reiner and Zamenhof, *J. Biol. Chem.*, 228, 475 (1957).
43. Elion, Lange, and Hitchings, *J. Am. Chem. Soc.*, 78, 217 (1956).
44. Gerster and Robins, *J. Am. Chem. Soc.*, 87, 3752 (1965).
45. Fischer, *Chem. Ber.*, 30, 2400 (1897).
46. Lawley, *Proc. Chem. Soc.*, 290 (1957).
47. Gulland and Story, *J. Chem. Soc.*, 692 (1938).
48. Brookes and Lawley, *J. Chem. Soc.*, 3923 (1961).
49. Hall, *Biochem. Biophys. Res. Commun.*, 13, 394 (1963) and unpublished.
50. Traube and Winter, *Arch. Pharm.*, 244, 11 (1906).
51. Ogston, *J. Chem. Soc.*, 1713 (1936).
52. Cohn, unpublished.
53. Cavalieri, Fox, Stone, and Chang, *J. Am. Chem. Soc.*, 76, 1119 (1954).
54. Pfleiderer and Nübel, *Annalen*, 647, 155 (1961).
55. Ogston, *J. Chem. Soc.*, 1376 (1935).
56. Taylor, *J. Chem. Soc.*, 765 (1948).
57. Brookes and Lawley, *J. Chem. Soc.*, 1348 (1962) and unpublished.
58. Ueda and Fox, *J. Am. Chem. Soc.*, 85, 4024 (1963).
59. Szer and Shugar, *Acta Biochim. Polon.*, 13, 177 (1966).
60. Ueda and Fox, *J. Org. Chem.*, 29, 1770 (1964).
61. Brown, *J. Appl. Chem.* 5, 358 (1955).
62. Johns, *J. Biol. Chem.*, 9, 161 (1911).
63. Brown, *J. Appl Chem.*, 9, 203 (1959).
64. Hitchings, Elion, Falco, and Russell, *J. Biol. Chem.*, 177, 357 (1949).
65. Wheeler and Johnson, *Am. Chem. J.*, 31, 591 (1904).
66. Shugar and Fox, *Biochim. Biophys. Acta*, 9, 199 (1952).
67. Wyatt, *Biochem. J.*, 48, 581 (1951).
68. Cohn, *J. Am. Chem. Soc.*, 73, 1539 (1951); also Beaven, Holiday, and Johnson, in *The Nucleic Acids, I*, Chargaff and Davidson, Eds., Academic Press, New York, 1955, 520.
69. Cline, Fink, and Fink, *J. Am. Chem. Soc.*, 81, 2521 (1959).
70. Flaks and Cohen, *J. Biol. Chem.*, 234, 1501 (1959).
71. Miller, *J. Am. Chem. Soc.*, 77, 752 (1955).
72. Fissekis, Myles, and Brown, *J. Org. Chem.*, 29, 2670 (1964).
73. Wyatt and Cohen, *Biochem. J.*, 55, 774 (1953).
74. Alegria, *Biochim Biophys. Acta*, 149, 317 (1967) and unpublished.
75. Loeb and Cohen, *J. Biol. Chem.*, 234, 364 (1959).
76. Pohland, Flynn, Jones, and Shive, *J. Am. Chem. Soc.*, 73, 3247 (1951).
77. Dunn, *Biochem. J.*, 86, 14P (1963).
78. Hilbert and Johnson, *J. Am. Chem. Soc.*, 52, 2001 (1930).
79. Brown, Hoerger, and Mason, *J. Chem. Soc.*, 211 (1955).
80. Levene, Bass, and Simms, *J. Biol. Chem.*, 70, 229 (1926).
81. Scannell, Crestfield, and Allen, *Biochim. Biophys. Acta*, 32, 406 (1959).
82. Whitehead, *J. Am. Chem. Soc.*, 74, 4267 (1952).
83. Johnson and Heyl, *Am. Chem. J.*, 37, 628 (1907).
84. Wheeler and Liddle, *Am Chem. J.*, 40, 547 (1908).
85. Fox and Van Praag, *J. Am. Chem. Soc.*, 82, 486 (1960).
86. Elion, Ide, and Hitchings, *J. Am. Chem. Soc.*, 68, 2137 (1946).
87. Wang, *J. Am. Chem. Soc.*, 81, 3786 (1959).
88. Johnson and McCollum, *J. Biol. Chem.*, 1, 437 (1906).
89. Behrend and Roosen, *Annalen*, 251, 235 (1889).
90. Dunn, D. B. and Flack, I. H., unpublished.
91. Stimson, *J. Am. Chem. Soc.*, 71, 1470 (1949).
92. Johnson and Litzinger, *J. Am. Chem. Soc.*, 58, 1940 (1936).
93. Dornow and Petsch, *Annalen*, 588, 45 (1954).
94. Cohn, *J. Biol. Chem.*, 235, 1488 (1960).
95. Yu and Allen, *Biochim. Biophys. Acta*, 32, 393 (1959).
96. Kallen, Simon, and Marmur, *J. Mol. Biol.*, 5, 248 (1962).
97. Chambers and Kurkov, *Biochemistry*, 3, 326 (1964).
98. di Carlo, Schultz, and Kent, *J. Biol Chem.*, 199, 333 (1952).
99. Green and Cohen, *J. Biol. Chem.*, 225, 397 (1957).
100. Brown and Johnson, *J. Am. Chem. Soc.*, 45, 2702 (1923).
101. Fischer and Roeder, *Chem. Ber.*, 34, 3751 (1901).
102. Lengfeld and Stieglitz, *Am. Chem. J.*, 15, 504 (1893).
103. Batt, Martin, Ploeser, and Murray, *J. Am. Chem. Soc.*, 76, 3663 (1954).
104. Mitchell and Nyc, *J. Am. Chem. Soc.*, 69, 674 and 1382 (1947).
105. Bachstetz, *Chem. Ber.*, 63b, 1000 (1930).
106. Johnson and Schroeder, *J. Am. Chem. Soc.*, 54, 2941 (1932).
107. Broom and Robins, *J. Am. Chem. Soc.*, 87, 1145 (1965).
108. Khwaja and Robins, *J. Am. Chem. Soc.*, 88, 3640 (1966).
109. Hall, *Biochim. Biophys. Acta*, 68, 278 (1963) and unpublished.
110. Hall, *Biochemistry*, 4, 661 (1965) and unpublished.
111. Davoll and Lowy, *J. Am. Chem. Soc.*, 74, 1563 (1952).
112. Johnson, Thomas, and Schaeffer, *J. Am. Chem. Soc.*, 80, 699 (1958).
113. Kissman, Pidacks, and Baker, *J. Am. Chem. Soc.*, 77, 18 (1955).
114. Townsend, Robins, Loeppky, and Leonard, *J. Am. Chem. Soc.*, 86, 5320 (1964).
115. Andrews and Barber, *J. Chem. Soc.*, 2768 (1958).
116. Feldmann, Dütting, and Zachau, *Hoppe-Seyler's Z. Physiol. Chem.*, 347, 236 (1966).
117. Hall, Csonka, David, and McLennan, *Science*, 156, 69 (1967) and unpublished.
118. Hall, *Biochemistry*, 3, 876 (1964).
119. Friedrich and Bernhauer, *Chem. Ber.*, 89, 2507 (1956).
120. Montgomery and Thomas, *J. Am. Chem. Soc.*, 85, 2672 (1963).
121. Friedrich and Bernhauer, *Chem. Ber.*, 90, 465 (1957).
122. Miles, *J. Org. Chem.*, 26, 4761 (1961).
123. Brown and Weliky, *J. Biol. Chem.*, 204, 1019 (1953).

124. Furukawa, Kobayaski, Kanai, and Honjo, *Chem. Pharm. Bull. Jap.*, 13, 1273 (1965) and unpublished.
125. Haines, Reese, and Todd, *J. Chem. Soc.*, 1406 (1964).
126. Hall, *Biochem. Biophys. Res. Commun.*, 12, 361 (1963).
127. Van Montagu and Stockx, *Arch. Intern. Physiol. Biochim*, 73, 158 (1965) and unpublished.
128. Fox, van Pragg, Wempen, Doerr, Cheong, Knoll, Eidinoff, Bendich, and Brown, *J. Am. Chem. Soc.*, 81, 178 (1959).
129. Wempen, Duschinsky, Kaplan, and Fox, *J. Am. Chem. Soc.*, 83, 4755 (1961).
130. Brimacombe and Reese, *J. Chem. Soc.*, 588C (1966).
131. Nichols and Lane, *Can. J. Biochem.*, 44, 1633 (1966).
132. Dunn, *Biochim. Biophys. Acta*, 38, 176 (1960).
133. Dekker and Elmore, *J. Chem. Soc.*, 2864 (1951).
134. Cohen and Barner, *J. Biol Chem.*, 226, 631 (1957).
135. Cohen, *Cold Spring Harbor Symp. Quant. Biol.*, 18, 221 (1953).
136. Brossmer and Röhm, *Angew. Chem. Int.*, 20, 742 (1963).
137. Townsend and Robins, *J. Am. Chem. Soc.*, 85, 242 (1963).
138. Smith and Dunn, *Biochim. Biophys. Acta*, 31, 573 (1959).
139. Miles, *Biochim. Biophys. Acta*, 22, 247 (1956).
140. Visser, Barron, and Beltz, *J. Am. Chem. Soc.*, 75, 2017 (1953).
141. Levene and Tipson, *J. Biol. Chem.*, 104, 385 (1934).
142. Thedford, Fleysher, and Hall, *J. Med. Chem.*, 8, 486 (1965).
143. Brimacombe, Griffin, Haines, Haslam, and Reese, *Biochemistry*, 4, 2452 (1965).
144. Lipsett, *J. Biol Chem.*, 240, 3975 (1965).
145. Roberts and Visser, *J. Am. Chem. Soc.*, 74, 668 (1952).
146. Ueda, *Chem. Pharm. Bull. Jap.*, 8, 455 (1960).
147. Levene and La Forge, *Chem. Ber.*, 45, 608 (1912).
148. Lis and Passarge, *Arch. Biochem. Biophys.*, 114, 593 (1966).
149. Reichard, *Acta Chem. Scand.*, 9, 1275 (1955).
150. Fox, Yung, Davoll, and Brown, *J. Am. Chem. Soc.*, 78, 2117 (1956).
151. Farkas and Sorm, *Coll. Czech. Chem. Commun.*, 28, 1620 (1963).
152. Brossmer and Röhm, *Angew. Chem. Int.*, 3, 66 (1964).
153. Cohn, Kurkov, and Chambers, *Biochem. Prep.*, 10, 135 (1963).
154. Shapiro and Chambers, *J. Am. Chem. Soc.*, 83, 3920 (1961).
155. Chambers, *Progr. Nucleic Acid Res. Mol. Biol.*, 5, 349 (1966) and Shapiro, R., Reeves, R. R., and Chambers, R. W., unpublished.
156. Ofengand and Schaefer, *Biochemistry*, 4, 2832 (1965).
157. Davis and Allen, *J. Biol. Chem.*, 227, 907 (1957).
158. Chambers, Kurkov, and Shapiro, *Biochemistry*, 2, 1192 (1963).
159. Michelson and Cohn, *Biochemistry*, 1, 490 (1962).
160. Michelson, Drell, and Mitchell, *Proc. Natl. Acad. Sci. USA*, 37, 396 (1951).
161. Bergmann and Feeney, *J. Org. Chem.*, 16, 981 (1951).
162. Fox, Yung, and Bendich, *J. Am. Chem. Soc.*, 79, 2775 (1957).
163. Fox and Shugar, *Biochim. Biophys. Acta*, 9, 369 (1952).
164. Griffin and Reese, *Biochim. Biophys. Acta*, 68, 185 (1963) and unpublished.
165. Davis, Carlucci, and Roubein, *J. Biol. Chem.*, 234, 1525 (1959).
166. Ikehara, Ohtsuka, and Ishikawa, *Chem. Pharm. Bull. Jap.*, 9, 173 (1961).
167. Griffin, Haslam, and Reese, *J. Mol. Biol.*, 10, 353 (1964).
168. Ikehara, Ueda, and Ikeda, *Chem. Pharm. Bull. Jap.*, 10, 767 (1962).
169. Szer, *Biochem. Biophys. Res. Commun.*, 20, 182 (1965).
170. Cohn, *in The Nucleic Acids* I, Chargaff, Davidson, Academic Press, New York, 1955, 211.
171. Kuno and Lehman, *J. Biol. Chem.*, 237, 1266 (1962).
172. Lehman and Pratt, *J. Biol. Chem.*, 235, 3254 (1960).
173. Szer and Shugar, *Acta Biochim. Polon.*, 7, 491 (1960).
174. Letters and Michelson, *J. Chem. Soc.*, 71 (1962).
175. Griffin, Todd, and Rich, *Proc. Natl. Acad. Sci. USA*, 44, 1123 (1958) and unpublished.
176. Goldberg and Rabinowitz, *Biochim. Biophys. Acta*, 54, 202 (1961).
177. Lieberman, Kornberg, and Simms, *J. Am. Chem. Soc.*, 76, 2844 (1954).
178. Cohn, *J. Am. Chem. Soc.*, 72, 2811 (1950).
179. Cohn, in *The Nucleic Acids* I, Chargaff, Davidson, Eds., Academic Press, New York, 1955, 513.
180. Hurst, Marko, and Butler, *J. Biol. Chem.*, 204, 847 (1953).
181. Ploeser and Loring, *J. Biol. Chem.*, 178, 431 (1949).
182. Cohn, *J. Cell Comp. Physiol.*, 38, supp, 1, 21 (1951).
183. Anon., Pabst Laboratories, Circular OR-10 (1956).
184. Steiner and Beers Jr., in *Polynucleotides. Elsevier*, New York, 1961, 155.
185. Shapiro and Chargaff, *Biochim. Biophys. Acta*, 26, 596 (1957).
186. Sinsheimer, *J. Biol. Chem.*, 208, 445 (1954).
187. Michelson and Todd, *J. Chem. Soc.*, 951 (1953).
188. Clark, Kirby, and Todd, *J. Chem. Soc.*, 1497 (1957).
189. Chambers, Moffatt, and Khorana, *J. Am. Chem. Soc.*, 79, 3747 (1957).
190. Michelson and Todd, *J. Chem. Soc.*, 2476 (1949).
191. Brown, Fasman, Magrath, and Todd, *J. Chem. Soc.*, 1448 (1954).
192. Loring, Bortner, Levy, and Hammell, *J. Biol. Chem.*, 196, 807 (1952).
193. Barker, *J. Chem. Soc.*, 3396 (1954).
194. Jones and Perkins, *J. Biol. Chem.*, 62, 557 (1925).
195. Cohn and Volkin, *Arch. Biochem. Biophys.*, 35, 465 (1952).
196. Chambers, Shapiro, and Kurkov, *J. Am. Chem. Soc.*, 82, 970 (1960).
197. Brown, Haynes, and Todd, *J. Chem. Soc.*, 3299 (1950).
198. Schmitz, Hurlbert, and Potter, *J. Biol. Chem.*, 209, 41 (1954).
199. Chambers, Moffatt, and Khorana, *J. Am. Chem. Soc.*, 77, 3416 (1955).
200. Volkin, Khym, and Cohn, *J. Am. Chem. Soc.*, 73, 1533 (1951).
201. Michelson and Todd, *J. Chem. Soc.*, 34 (1954).
202. Tener, *J. Am. Chem. Soc.*, 83, 159 (1961).
203. Schaller, Weimann, Lerch, and Khorana, *J. Am. Chem. Soc.*, 85, 3821 (1963).
204. Lipton, Morell, Frieden, and Bock, *J. Am. Chem. Soc.*, 75, 5449 (1953).
205. Volkin and Cohn in *Methods of Biochemical Analysis*, I, Glick, Ed., Interscience, New York, 1954. 287.
206. Morell and Bock, Am. Chem. Soc. 126th Meeting, New York, Div. of Biol., *Abstracts*, 1954, 44C.
207. Klein and Thannhauser, *Z. Physiol. Chem.*, 231, 96 (1935).
208. Lipsett, *Cold Spring Harbor Symp. Quant. Biol.*, 31, 449 (1966).
209. Lehman, Bessman, Simms, and Kornberg, *J. Biol. Chem.*, 233, 163 (1958).
210. Hall and Khorana, *J. Am. Chem. Soc.*, 76, 5056 (1954).
211. Khorana, *J. Am. Chem. Soc.*, 76, 3517 (1954).
212. Bock, Nan-Sing Ling, Morell, and Lipton, *Arch. Biochem. Biophys.*, 62, 253 (1956).
213. Chambers and Khorana, *J. Am. Chem. Soc.*, 79, 3752 (1957).
214. Smith and Khorana, *J. Am. Chem. Soc*, 80, 1141 (1958).
215. Loring and Luthy, *J. Am. Chem. Soc.*, 73, 4215 (1951).
216. Loring, Roll, and Pierce, *J. Biol. Chem.*, 174, 729 (1948).
217. Levene and Tipson, *J. Biol. Chem.*, 106, 113 (1934).
218. Cavalieri, *J. Am. Chem. Soc.*, 75, 5268 (1953).
219. Brown and Todd, *J. Chem. Soc.*, 44 (1952).
220. Alberty, Smith, and Bock, *J. Biol. Chem.*, 193, 425 (1951).
221. Reichard, Takenaka, and Loring, *J. Biol. Chem.*, 198, 599 (1952).
222. Levene, *J. Biol. Chem.*, 41, 483 (1920).
223. California Corporation for Biochemical Research, *Properties of Nucleic Acids Derivatives*, 4th Revision, 1961.
224. Levene and Jacobs, *Chem. Ber.*, 43, 3150 (1911).
225. Chambers, Moffatt, and Khorana, *J. Am. Chem. Soc.*, 79, 4240 (1957).
226. Le Page, *Biochem. Preps.*, 1, 1, (1949).
227. Shaw, Smallwood, and Wilson, *J. Chem. Soc.*, 921C (1969).
228. Carrington, Shaw, and Wilson, *J. Chem. Soc.*, 6864 (1965).
229. Scarano, *Boll. Soc. Ital. Biol. Sper.*, 34, 728 (1958).
230. Scarano, *Boll. Soc. Ital. Biol. Sper.*, 34, 727 (1958).
231. Levene and Bass, *in The Nucleic Acids*. Chemical Catalog Co, New York, 1931.
232. Beaven, Holiday, Johnson, (1955) in *The Nucleic Acids* I, Chargaff, Davidson, Eds., Academic Press, New York, 1955, 493.
233. Hilbert, Jansen, and Hendricks, *J. Am. Chem. Soc.*, 57, 552 (1935).
234. Traube, *Chem. Ber.*, 33, 1371 (1900).
235. Davoll, Lythgoe, and Todd, *J. Chem. Soc.*, 967 (1948).
236. Elmore, *J. Chem. Soc.*, 2084 (1950).
237. Davoll and Lowy, *J. Am. Chem. Soc.*, 73, 1650 (1951).
238. Andersen, Dekker, and Todd, *J. Chem. Soc.*, 2721 (1952).

239. Klein, *Z. Physiol. Chem.*, 224, 244 (1934).
240. Deutsch, unpublished data.
241. Schindler, *Helv. Chim. Acta*, 32, 979 (1949).
242. Hotchkiss, *J. Biol. Chem.*, 175, 315 (1948).
243. Dekker and Todd, *Nature*, 166, 557 (1950).
244. Watanabe and Fox, *Angew. Chem.*, 78, 589 (1966).
245. Mizuno, Itoh, and Tagawa, *Chem. Ind.*, 1498 (1965).
246. Anon., Schwarz Bioresearch, data (1966).
247. Hoffer, Duschinsky, Fox, and Yung, *J. Am. Chem. Soc.*, 81, 4112 (1959).
248. Wood, *J. Chem. Soc.*, 89, 1839 (1906).
249. Ness and Fletcher, *J. Am. Chem. Soc.*, 82, 3434 (1960).
250. Albert, *Biochem. J.*, 54, 646 (1953).
251. Fox, Yung, Wempen, and Doerr, *J. Am. Chem. Soc.*, 79, 5060 (1957).
252. Howard, Lythgoe, and Todd, *J. Chem. Soc.*, 1052 (1947).
253. Bergmann and Dikstein, *J. Am. Chem. Soc.*, 77, 691 (1955).
254. Johnson and Mackenzie, *Am. Chem. J.*, 42, 353 (1909).
255. Levene, Simms, and Bass, *J. Biol. Chem.*, 70, 243 (1926).
256. Baddiley, Lythgoe, and Todd, *J. Chem. Soc.*, 386 (1943).
257. Robins, Dille, Willits, and Christensen, *J. Am. Chem. Soc.*, 75, 263 (1953).
258. Carter, *J. Am. Chem. Soc.*, 72, 1466 (1950).
259. Klein and Thannhauser, *Z. Physiol. Chem.*, 218, 173 (1933).
260. Klein and Thannhauser, *Z. Physiol. Chem.*, 224, 252 (1934).
261. Embden and Schmidt, *Z. Physiol. Chem.*, 181, 130 (1929).
262. Turner and Khorana, *J. Am. Chem. Soc.*, 81, 4651 (1959).
263. Cunningham, *J. Am. Chem. Soc*, 80, 2546 (1958).
264. Hall and Khorana, *J. Am. Chem. Soc.*, 77, 1871 (1955).
265. Venkstern and Baev, in *Absorption Spectra of Minor Components and Some Oligonucleotides of Ribonucleic Acid*, Science Publishing House, Moscow, 1967; English transl., *Absorption Spectra of Minor Bases, Their Nucleosides, Nucleotides and Selected Oligoribonucleotides*, Plenum Press Data Division, New York, 1965.
266. Hanze, *J. Am. Chem. Soc.*, 89, 6720, (1967).
267. Venner, *Chem. Ber.*, 93, 140 (1960).
268. Falconer, Gulland, and Story, *J. Chem. Soc.*, 1784 (1939).
269. Davoll, *J. Am. Chem. Soc.*, 73, 3174 (1951).
270. Carbon, David, and Studier, *Science*, 161, 1146 (1968) and unpublished.
271. Ueda, Iida, Ikeda, and Mizuno, *Chem. Pharm. Bull Jap.*, 16, 1788 (1968) and unpublished.
272. Ueda and Nishino, *J. Am. Chem. Soc.*, 90, 1678 (1968).
273. Ueda, Iida, Ikeda, and Mizuno, *Chem. Pharm. Bull. Jap.*, 14, 666 (1966).
274. Burrows, Armstrong, Skoog, Hecht, Boyle, Leonard, and Occolowitz, *Science,* 161, 691 (1968) and unpublished.
275. Baczynskyj, Biemann, and Hall, *Science*, 159, 1481 (1968).
276. Shaw, Warrener, Maguire, and Ralph, *J. Chem. Soc.*, 2294 (1958).
277. Strominger and Friedkin, *J. Biol. Chem.*, 208, 663 (1954).
278. Gray and Lane, *Biochemistry*, 7, 3441 (1968).
279. Johnson and Speh, *Am. Chem. J.*, 38, 602 (1907).
280. Codington, Fecher, Maguire, Thomson, and Brown, *J. Am. Chem. Soc.*, 80, 5164 (1958).
281. Brown, Todd, and Varadarajan, *J. Chem. Soc.*, 2384 (1956).
282. Bendich, Tinker, and Brown, *J. Am. Chem. Soc.*, 70, 3109 (1948).
283. Cavalieri, Bendich, Tinker, and Brown, *J. Am. Chem. Soc.*, 70, 3875 (1948).
284. Wyngaarden and Dunn, *Arch. Biochem. Biophys.*, 70, 150 (1957).
285. Lee and Wigler, *Biochemistry*, 7, 1427 (1968).
286. Lis and Passarge, *Physiol. Chem. Phys.*, 1, 68 (1969).
287. Fujii and Leonard in *Synthetic Procedures in Nucleic Acid Chemistry.*, 1, Zorbach, Tipson, Eds., Interscience, New York, 1968, 13.
288. Nishimura, Yamada, and Ishikura, *Biochim. Biophys. Acta*, 179, 517 (1969).
289. Bessman, Lehman, Adler, Zimmerman, Simms, and Kornberg, *Proc. Natl. Acad. Sci. USA*, 44, 633 (1958).
290. Chheda, *Life Sci.*, 8, 979 (1969) and unpublished.
291. Saneyoshi, Ohashi, Harada, and Nishimura, *Biochim. Biophys. Acta*, 262, 1 (1972).

292. Saneyoshi, Harada, and Nishimura, *Biochim. Biophys. Acta*, 190, 264 (1969).
293. Burrows, Armstrong, Skoog, Hecht, Boyle, Leonard, and Occolowitz, *Biochemistry*, 8, 3071 (1969).
294. Hecht, Leonard, Burrows, Armstrong, Skoog, and Occolowitz, *Science*, 166, 1272 (1969).
295. Schweizer, McGrath, and Baczynskyj, *Biochem. Biophys. Res. Commun.*, 40, 1046 (1970).
296. Ishikura, Yamada, Murao, Saneyoshi, and Nishimura, *Biochem. Biophys. Res. Commun.*, 37, 990 (1969).
297. Kimura-Harada, von Minden, McCloskey, and Nishimura, *Biochemistry*, 11, 3910 (1972).
298. Ohashi, Murao, Yahagi, von Minden, McCloskey, and Nishimura, *Biochim. Biophys. Acta*, 262, 209 (1972).
299. Harada, Gross, Kimura, Chang, Nishimura, and RajBhandary, *Biochem. Biophys. Res. Commun.*, 33, 299 (1968).
300. Ohashi, Maeda, McCloskey, and Nishimura, *Biochemistry*, 13, 2620 (1974).
301. Vorbrüggen and Strehlke, *Chem. Ber.*, 106, 3039 (1973).
302. Fissekis and Sweet, *Biochemistry*, 9, 3136 (1970).
303. Kwong and Lane, *Biochim. Biophys. Acta*, 224, 405 (1970).
304. Tumaitis and Lane, *Biochim. Biophys. Acta*, 224, 391 (1970).
305. Ohashi, Saneyoshi, Harada, Hara, and Nishimura, *Biochem. Biophys. Res. Commun.*, 40, 866 (1970).
306. Yoshida, Takeishi, and Ukita, *Biochim. Biophys. Acta*, 228, 153 (1971).
307. Kimura-Harada, Saneyoshi, and Nishimura, *FEBS Lett.*, 13, 335 (1971).
308. Murao, Saneyoski, Harada, and Nishimura, *Biochem. Biophys. Res. Commun.*, 38, 657 (1970).
309. Ishikura, Yamada, and Nishimura, *Biochim. Biophys. Acta*, 228, 471 (1971).
310. Nakanishi, Furutachi, Funamizu, Grunberger, and Weinstein, *J. Am. Chem. Soc.*, 92, 7617 (1970).
311. Thiebe, Zachau, Baczynskyj, Biemann, and Sonnenbichler, *Biochim. Biophys. Acta*, 240, 163 (1971).
312. Kasai, Goto, Takemura, Goto, and Matsuura, *Tetrahedron Lett.*, 29, 2725 (1971).
313. Nishimura, *Progr. Nucl. Res. Mol. Biol.*, 12, 49 (1972).
314. Hecht, Gupta, and Leonard, *Anal. Biochem.*, 30, 249 (1969).
315. Howlett, Johnson, Trim, Eagles, and Self, *Anal. Biochem.*, 39, 429 (1971).
316. Thiebe and Zachau, *Eur. J. Biochem.*, 5, 546 (1968).
317. Hall, *The Modified Nucleosides in Nucleic Acids.*, Columbia University Press, New York, 1971, 27.
318. Macon and Wolfenden, *Biochemistry*, 7, 3453 (1968).
319. Grimm and Leonard, *Biochemistry*, 6, 3625 (1967).
320. Funamizu, Terahara, Feinberg, and Nakanishi, *J. Am. Chem. Soc.*, 93, 6706 (1971).
321. Blobstein, Grunberger, Weinstein, and Nakanishi, *Biochemistry*, 12, 188 (1973).
322. Ivanovics, Rousseau, and Robins, *Physiol. Chem. Phys.*, 3, 489 (1971).
323. Gross, Simsek, Raba, Limburg, Heckman, and RajBhandary, *Nucl. Acid Res.*, 1, 35 (1974).
324. Yoshikami and Keller, *Biochemistry*, 10, 2969 (1971).
325. Brandon, Gallop, Marmur, Hayashi, and Nakanishi, *Nature New Biol.*, 239, 70 (1972).
326. Hayashi, Nakanishi, Brandon, and Marmur, *J. Am. Chem. Soc.*, 95, 8749 (1973).
327. Feinberg, Nakanishi, Barciszewski, Rafalski, Augustyniak, and WiewiÓrowski, *J. Am. Chem. Soc.*, 96, 7797 (1974).
328. Sasaki and Mizuno, *Chem. Pharm. Bull. Jap.*, 15, 894 (1967).
329. Yamada, Saneyoshi, Nishimura, and Ishikura, *FEBS Lett.*, 7, 207 (1970).
330. Dutta, Hong, Murphy, Mittleman, Chheda, *Biochemistry*, 14, 3144 (1975) and unpublished
331. Miller, Robin, and Astwood, *J. Am. Chem. Soc.*, 67, 2201 (1945).
332. Burrows, Armstrong, Kaminek, Skoog, Bock, Hecht, Damman, Leonard, and Occolowitz, *Biochemistry*, 9, 1867 (1970).
333. Jacobson and Bonner, *Biochem. Biophys. Res. Commun.*, 33, 716 (1968).

334. Hendler, Fürer, and Srinivasan, *Biochemistry*, 4141 (1970).
335. Yamada, Nishimura, and Ishikura, *Biochim. Biophys. Acta*, 247, 170 (1971).
336. Harkins and Freiser, *J. Am. Chem. Soc.*, 80, 1132 (1958).
337. Richter, Loeffler, and Taylor, *J. Am. Chem. Soc.*, 82, 3144 (1960).
338. Breshears, Wang, Bechtolt, and Christensen, *J. Am. Chem. Soc.*, 81, 3789 (1959).
339. Zemlicka and Sorm, *Coll. Czech. Chem. Commun.*, 30, 1880 (1965).
340. Taylor, Vogl, and Cheng, *J. Am. Chem. Soc.*, 81, 2442 (1959).
341. Biemann and McCloskey, *J. Am. Chem. Soc.*, 84, 2005 (1962).
342. Yamazaki, Kumashiro, and Takenishi, *J. Org. Chem.*, 33, 2583 (1968).
343. Saneyoshi and Sawada, *Chem. Pharm. Bull Jap.*, 17, 181 (1969).
344. Kochetkov, Budowsky, Shebaev, Yeliseeva, Grachev, and Demushkin, *Tetrahedron*, 19, 1207 (1963).
345. Saponara and Enger, *Biochim. Biophys. Acta*, 349, 61 (1974).
346. RajBhandary, Faulkner, and Stuart, *J. Biol. Chem.*, 243, 575 (1968).
347. Fink, Lanks, Goto, and Weinstein, *J. Biol. Chem.*, 10, 1873 (1971).
348. Guyot and Mentzer, *Compt. Rend.*, 246, 436 (1958).
349. Roscoe and Tucker, *Virology*, 29, 157 (1966).
350. Kissman and Weiss, *J. Org. Chem.*, 21, 1053 (1956).
351. Furukawa and Honjo, *Chem. Pharm. Bull. Jap.*, 16, 1076 (1968).
352. Wempen, Brown, Ueda, and Fox, *Biochemistry*, 4, 54 (1965).
353. Ziff and Fresco, *Biochemistry*, 8, 3242 (1969).
354. Yamazaki, Kumashiro, and Takenishi, *J. Org. Chem.*, 32, 1825 (1967).
355. Shapiro, Cohen, Shiuey, and Maurer, *Biochemistry*, 8, 238 (1969).
356. Ulbricht, *Tetrahedron*, 6,225 (1959).
357. Ichikawa, Kato, and Takenishi, *J. Het. Chem.*, 2, 253 (1965).
358. Shaw, *J. Biol. Chem.*, 185, 439 (1950).
359. Taylor and Cheng, *Tetrahedron Lett.*, 12, 9 (1959).
360. Townsend and Robins, *J. Org. Chem.*, 27, 990 (1962).
361. Scherp, *J. Am. Chem. Soc.*, 68, 912 (1946).
362. Shaw and Warrener, *J. Chem. Soc.*, 157 (1958).
363. Fox, Wempen, Hampton, and Doerr, *J. Am. Chem. Soc.*, 80, 1669 (1958).
364. Davidson and Baudisch, *J. Am. Chem. Soc.*, 48, 2379 (1926).
365. Armstrong, Evans, Burrows, Skoog, Petit, Dahl, Steward, Strominger, Leonard, Hecht, and Occolowitz, *J. Biol. Chem.*, 245, 2922 (1970).
366. Babcock and Morris, *Biochemistry*, 9, 3701 (1970).
367. Shaw, Desiderio, Tsuboyama, and McCloskey, *J. Am. Chem. Soc.*, 92, 2510 (1970).
368. Shimizu, Asai, and Nishimura, *Chem. Pharm. Bull. Jap.*, 15, 1847 (1967).
369. Martin, Reese, and Stephenson, *Biochemistry*, 7, 1406 (1968).
370. Gin and Dekker, *Biochemistry*, 7, 1413 (1968).
371. Izatt, Hansen, Rytting, and Christensen, *J. Am. Chem. Soc.*, 87, 2760 (1965).
372. Yamazaki, Kumashiro, and Takenishi, *J. Org. Chem.*, 32, 3032 (1967).
373. Davoll, Lythgoe, and Todd, *J. Chem. Soc.*, 1685 (1948).
374. McCloskey, Lawson, Tsuboyama, Krueger, and Stillwell, *J. Am. Chem. Soc.*, 90, 4182 (1968).
375. Randerath, Yu, and Randerath, *Anal. Biochem.*, 48, 172 (1972).
376. Reddy, Ro-Choi, Henning, Shibata, Choi, and Busch, *J. Biol. Chem.*, 247, 7245 (1972).
377. Yamazaki, Kumashiro, and Takenishi, *J. Org. Chem.*, 32, 3258 (1967).
378. Baddiley, Buchanan, Hardy, and Stewart, *J. Chem. Soc.*, 2893 (1959).
379. Nishimura, Shimizu, and Iwai, *Chem. Pharm. Bull. (Jap.)*, 12, 1471 (1964).
380. Wempen and Fox, *Methods Enzymol*, 12A, 59 (1967).
381. Gerster and Robins, *J. Org. Chem.*, 31, 3258 (1966).
382. Visser, in *Synthetic Procedures in Nucleic Acid Chemistry vol. 1*, Zorbach, Tipson, Eds., Interscience John Wiley & Sons, New York, 1968. 428
383. Janion and Shugar, *Acta Biochim. Polon.*, 7, 309 (1960).
384. Cerutti, Kondo, Landis, and Witkop, *J. Am. Chem. Soc.*, 90, 771 (1968).
385. Prystaš and Šorm, *Coll. Czech. Chem. Commun.*, 31, 1053 (1966).
386. Prystaš and Šorm, *Coll. Czech. Chem. Commun.*, 31, 1035 (1966).
387. Brown, Burdon, and Slatcher, *J. Chem. Soc.*, 1051 (1968).
388. Cohn, *Methods Enzymol.*, 12A, 101 (1967).
389. Anderson, Goodman, and Baker, *J. Am. Chem. Soc.*, 81, 3967 (1959).
390. Pedersen and Fletcher, *J. Am. Chem. Soc.*, 82, 5210 (1960).
391. Wempen and Fox, *Methods Enzymol.*, 12A, 76 (1967).
392. Brown, Todd, and Varadarajan, *J. Chem. Soc.*, 2388 (1956).
393. Bergmann and Burk, *J. Org. Chem.*, 20, 1501 (1955).
394. Fox, Miller, and Wempen, *J. Med. Chem.*, 9, 101 (1966).
395. Wheeler and Merriam, *Am. Chem. J.*, 29, 478 (1903).
396. Wheeler and Johnson, *Am. Chem. J.*, 29, 492 (1903).
397. Chesterfield, McOmie, and Tute, *J. Chem. Soc.*, 4590 (1960).
398. Dunn and Trigg, *John Innes Institute Report*, 1972, 142 and unpublished.
399. Schaeffer and Thomas, *J. Am. Chem. Soc.*, 80, 3738 (1958).
400. Broude, Budowsky, and Kochekov, *Mol. Biol.*, 1, 214 (1967).
401. Marmur, Brandon, Neubort, Ehrlich, Mandel, and Konvicka, *Nature New Biol.*, 1, 239, 68 (1972).
402. Kropinski, Bose, and Warren, *Biochemistry*, 12, 151 (1973).
403. Takemura, Kasai, and Goto, *J. Biochem.*, *(Japan)*, 75, 1169 (1974).
404. Hecht and McDonald, *Anal. Biochem.*, 47, 157 (1972).
405. McCloskey, Futrell, Elwood, Schram, Panzica, and Townsend, *J. Am. Chem. Soc.*, 95, 5762 (1973).
406. Hecht, *Anal. Biochem.*, 44, 262 (1971).
407. Cunningham and Gray, *Biochemistry*, 13, 543 (1974).
408. Chheda and Hong, *J. Med. Chem.*, 14, 748 (1971) and unpublished.
409. Dyson, Hall, Hong, Dutta, and Chheda, *Can. J. Biochem.*, 50, 237 (1972).
410. Dunn and Trigg, *Biochem. Soc. Trans.*, 3, 656 (1975) and unpublished.
411. P. L. Biochemicals, Biochemical reference guide & price list, (1973).
412. Cushley, Watanabe, and Fox, *J. Am. Chem. Soc.*, 89, 394 (1967).
413. Dunn and Flack, *John Innes Institute Report*, 1970, 76 and unpublished.
414. Kuntzel, Weissenbach, Wolff, Tumaitis-Kennedy, Lane, and Dirheimer, *Biochimie*, 57, 61 (1975).
415. Gray, *Biochemistry*, 13, 5453 (1974).

CHEMICAL MODIFICATION OF NUCLEIC ACIDS

Roger L. Lundblad

The chemical modification of nucleic acids is not as complex as that of proteins since there are fewer monomer units and, for all practical purposes, only nitrogen as a nucleophilic reactive group; the nitrogen is reactive as a primary and secondary amine. Reaction at the primary amine groups of, for example, adenine, is referred to an exocyclic modification whereas reaction at the imine nitrogens of pyrimidines and purine rings is referred to as an endocyclic modification. There are also ring-opening reactions and cross-linking reactions.

TABLE 1: Chemical Modification of Nucleic Acids

Reagent	Base Modified	Product	Reference
Aldehydes[a]	Most data on pyrimidines with less on purines	Various adducts	1–10
Alkylation	Purine and pyrimidines	Various product resulting from environmental agents such as ethylene oxides and nitrogen mustards	11–20
Diethylpyrocarbonate	Purine and pyrimidines	Carboxethylation of the N-7 site on the purine ring followed by ring opening; pyrimidines react at primary amino groups to yield carboethoxy derivatives[b]	21–28
Dimethyl Sulfate (Methylation)	Purines and Pyrimidines	N^7-Methylguanidine with minor reaction at the N^1 and N^3-positions; reaction also occurs at N^3 in adenine and at N^3-position in cytidine; reactivity is controlled by polynucleotide structure[c,d]	29–41
Hydrazine	Pyrimidines	Ring cleavage yielding pyrazole derivatives[e] and the ribosyl backbone; reaction used sequence analaysis and footprinting	42–47
Hydroxylamine	Purines and pyrimidines	Hydroxamate formation at "exocyclic" nitrogen; conversion of guanine to isoxazolone.	48–55
Nitrous Acid (HNO_2)	Purines and pyrimidines	Deamination; crosslinking at guanine, cytosine bases	56–64
Potassium Permanganate	Purines and Pyrmidines	Oxidation at double bonds; preferential reaction with thymidine	65–75
Sodium Bisulfate	Cytosine	Uracil (5-methylcytosine is converted to thymine)[f]	76–84

[a] e.g. formaldehyde, acetaldehyde, acrolein, crotonaldehyde; 4-hydroxy-2-nonenal (4-HNE)

[b] Diethylpyrocarbonate modification is used for DNA footprinting (Fox, K.R., Webster, R., Phelps, R.J., *et al.*, Sequence selective binding of bis-daunorubicin WP631 to DNA, *Eur.J.Biochem.* 271, 3556-3566, 2004)

[c] The N^7-position of guanine is always reactive for methylation (the N^7-position of guanine is the most reactive site in nucleic acids); methylation of guanine also occurs at the N^1-position of guanine at high concentrations of methylating agents. Methylation of the N^3-position of cytidine occurs in single-stranded DNA but is blocked in double-stranded DNA. Methylation (alkylation) also occurs at the N^1 and N^3 position of adenine but methylation is restricted in at the N^1 position in double-stranded DNA. *In vivo* methylation of DNA occurs at cytidine residues largely in CpG islands (Ehrlich, M. and Wang, R.Y., 5-Methylcytosine in eukaryotic DNA, *Science* 212, 1350-1357, 1981; Lewis, J. and Bird, A., DNA methylation and chromatin structure, *FEBS Lett.* 285, 155-159, 1991; Cheng, X., Structure and function of DNA methyltransferases, *Annu.Rev.Biophys.Biomol.Struct.* 24, 293-318, 1995; Scheule, R.K., The role of CpG motifs in immunostimulation and gene therapy, *Adv.Drug Deliv.Rev.* 44, 119-134, 2000).

[d] Base treatment of N^7-methylguanine results in opening of the imidazolium ring while N^3-methylcytidine undergoes base-catalyzed deamination to give N^3-methyluridine. Methylation of cytidine blocks conversion to thymidine by sodium bisulfite

[e] 4-methyl-5-pyrazolone with thymidylic acid; 3(5)-aminopyrazole with deoxycytidine

[f] Conversion to uracil does not occur with 5-methylcytosine; 5-methylcytosine is converted to thymine. The rate of reaction of 5-methylcytosine with sodium bisulfite is much slower than reaction of cytosine.

References for Table 1

1. Alegria, A.H., Hydroxymethylation of pyrimidine mononucleotides with formaldehyde, *Biochim.Biophys.Acta* 149, 317–324, 1967.
2. Feldman, M.Y., Reactions of nucleic acids and nucleoproteins with formaldehyde, *Prog.Nucleic Acid Res.Mol.Biol.* 13, 1–49, 1973.
3. McGhee, J.D. and von Hippel, P.H., Formaldehyde as a probe of DNA structure. I. Reaction with exocyclic amine groups of DNA bases, *Biochemistry* 25, 1281–1296, 1975.
4. McGhee, J.D. and von Hippel, P.H., Formaldehyde as a probe of DNA structure. II. Reaction with endocyclic imine groups of DNA bases, *Biochemistry* 25, 1297–1303, 1975.
5. Yamazaki, Y. and Suzuki, H., A new method of chemical modification of N^6-amino group in adenine nucleotides with formaldehyde and a thiol and its application to preparing immobilized ADP and ATP, *Eur.J.Biochem.* 92, 197–207, 1978.
6. Chung, F.L., Young, R., and Hecht, S.S., Formation of cyclic 1, N^2-propanodeoxyguanosine adducts in DNA upon reaction with acrolein or crotonaldehyde, *Cancer Res.* 44, 990–995, 1984.

7. Winter, C.K., Segall, H.J., and Haddon, W.F., Formation of cyclic adducts of deoxyguanosine with the aldehydes *trans*-4-hydroxy-2-hexenal and *trans*-4-hydroxynonenal *in vitro*, *Cancer Res.* 46, 5682–5686, 1986.

8. Kennedy, G., Slaich, P.K., Golding, B.T., and Watson, W.P., Structure and mechanism of formation of a new adduct from formaldehyde and guanosine, *Chem.Biol.Interact.* 102, 93–100, 1996.

9. Hecht, S.S., McIntee, E.J., and Wang, M., New DNA adducts of crotonaldehyde and acetaldehyde, *Toxicology* 166, 31–36, 2001.

10. Kurtz, A.J. 1, N^2-deoxyguanosine adducts of acrolein, crotonaldehyde, and *trans*-4-hydroxynonenal cross-link to peptides via Schiff base linkage, *J.Biol.Chem.* 278, 5970–5976, 2003.

11. Singer, B., The chemical effects of nucleic acid alkylation and their relation to mutagenesis and carcinogenesis, *Prog.Nucleic Res.Mol. Biol.* 15, 219–284, 1975.

12. Lawley, P.D., DNA as a target of alkylating carcinogenesis, *Br.Med. Bull.* 36, 19–24, 1980.

13. Coles, B., Effects of modifying structure on electrophilic reactions with biological nucleophiles, *Drug Metab.Rev.* 15, 1307–1334, 1984–1985.

14. Wild, C.P., Antibodies to DNA alklylation adducts as analytical tools its chemical carcinogenesis, *Mutat.Res.* 233, 219–233, 1990.

15. Lawley, P.D., Alkylation of DNA and its aftermath, *Bioessays* 17, 561–568, 1995.

16. Bolt, H.M., Quantification of endogenous carcinogens. The ethylene oxide paradox, *Biochem.Pharmacol.* 52, 1–5, 1996.

17. Rios-Blanco, M.N., Plna, K., Faller, T., *et al.*, Propylene oxide: mutatgenesis, carcinogenesis and molecular dose, *Mutat.Res.* 380, 179–197, 1997.

18. Wilson, D.S. and Szostak, J.W., In vitro selection of functional nucleic acids, *Annu.Rev.Biochem.* 68, 611–647, 1999.

19. Denny, W.A., DNA minor groove alkylating agents, *Curr.Med. Chem.* 8, 533–544, 2001.

20. Mishina, Y. and He, C., Oxidative dealkylation DNA repair mediated by the mononuclear non-heme iron AlkB proteins, *J.Inorg. Biochem.* 100, 670–678, 2006.

21. Leonard, N.J., McDonald, J.J., Henderson, R.E.I., and Reichmann, M.E., Reaction of diethyl pyrocarbonate with nucleic acid components. Adenosine. *Biochemistry* 10, 335–3342, 1971.

22. Solymosy, F., Hüvös, P., Gulyás, A., *et al.*, Diethyl pyrocarbonate, a new tool in the chemical modification of nucleic acids, *Biochim. Biophys.Acta* 238, 406–426, 1971.

23. Vincze, A., Henderson, R.E.I., McDonald, J.J., and Leonard, N.J., Reaction of diethyl pyrocarbonate with nucleic acid components. Bases and nucleosides derived from guanine, cytosine, and uracil, *J.Amer.Chem.Soc.* 95, 2677–2683, 1973.

24. Ehrenfeld, E., Interaction of Diethylpyrocarbonate with poliovirus double-stranded RNA, *Biochem.Biophys.Res.Commun.* 56, 214–219, 1974.

25. Herr, W., Diethyl pyrocarbonate: A chemical probe for secondary structure in negatively supercoiled DNA, *Proc.Nat.Acad.Sci.USA* 82, 8009–8013, 1985.

26. Johnston, B.H. and Rich, A., Chemical probes of DNA conformation: Detection of Z-DNA at nucleotide resolution, *Cell* 42, 713–724, 1985.

27. Runkel, L. and Nordheim, A., Chemical footprinting of the interaction between left-handed Z-DNA and anti-Z-DNA antibodies by Diethylpyrocarbonate carboethoxylation, *J.Mol.Biol.* 189, 487–501, 1986.

28. Buckle, M. and Buc, H., Fine mapping of DNA single-stranded regions using base-specific chemical probes: Study of an open complex formed between RNA polymerase and the *lac* UV5 promoter, *Biochemistry* 28, 4388–4396, 1989.

29. Jordan, D.O., The physical properties of nucleic acids, in *The Nucleic Acids. Chemistry and Biology*, Vol. 1, ed. E. Chargaff and J.N. Davidson., Academic Press, New York, NY, USA, Chapter 13, pps. 447–492, 1955.

30. Kanduc, D., tRNA chemical modification In vitro and in vivo formation of 1,7-dimethylguanosine at high concentrations of methylating agents, *Biochem.Biophys.Acta* 653, 9–17, 1981.

31. Singer, B., The chemical effects of nucleic acid alkylation and their relation to mutagenesis and carcinogenesis, *Prog.Nucl.Acids Res. Mol.Biol.* 15, 219–284, 1975.

32. Behmoaras, T., Toulme, J.-J., and Relene, C., Specific recognition of apurinic sites in DNA by a tryptophan-containing peptide, *Proc. Nat.Acad.Sci.USA* 78, 926–930, 1981.

33. Mhaskar, D.N., Chang, M.J.W., Hart, R.W., and D'Ambrosio, S.M., Analysis of alkylated sites at *N*-3 and *N*-7 positions of purines as an indicator for chemical carcinogens, *Cancer Res.* 41, 223–229, 1981.

34. Kirkegaard, K., Buc, H., Spassky, A., and Wang, J.C., Mapping of single-stranded regions in duplex DNA at the sequence level: Single-strand-specific cytosine Methylation in RNA polymerase-promoter complexes, *Proc.Nat.Acad.Sci.USA* 80, 2544–2548, 1983.

35. Potaman, V.N. and Sinden, R., Stabilization of triple-helical nucleic acids by basic oligopeptides, *Biochemistry* 34, 14885–14892, 1995.

36. Lawley, P.D., Effects of some chemical mitogens and carcinogens on nucleic acids, *Prog.Nucl.Acid Res.Mol.Biol.* 5, 89–131, 1996.

37. Dobner, T., Buchner, D., Zeller, T., *et al.*, Specific nucleoprotein complexes within adenovirus capsids, *Biol.Chem.* 382, 1373–1377, 2001.

38. Hock, T.D. Nick, H.S., and Agarwal, A. Upstream stimulatory factors, USF1 and USF2, bind to the human haem oxygenase-1 proximal promoter *in vivo* and regulates its transcription, *Biochem.J.* 383, 209–218, 2004.

39. Lagor, W.R., de Groh, E.D., and Ness, G.C., Diabetes alters the occupancy of the hepatic 5-hydroxy-3-methylglutaryl-CoA reductase promoter, *J.Biol.Chem.* 280, 36601–36608, 2005.

40. Haugen, S.P., Berkmen, M.B., Ross, W., *et al.*, tRNA promoter regulates by nonoptimal binding of sigma region 1.2: an additional recognition element for RNA polymerase, *Cell* 125, 1069–1082, 2006.

41. Temperli, A., Türler, H., Rüst, P. *et al.*, Studies on the nucleotide arrangement in deoxyribonucleic acids. IX. Selective degradation of pyrimidines deoxyribonucleotides, *Biochim.Biophys.Acta* 91, 462–476, 1964.

42. Cashmore, A.R. and Peterson, G.B., The degradation of DNA by hydrazine: a critical study of the suitability of the reaction for the quantitative determination of purine nucleotide sequences, *Biochim.Biophys.Acta* 174, 591–603, 1969.

43. Türler, H. and Chargaff, E., Studies on the nucleotide arrangement in deoxyribonucleic acids. XII. Apyrimidinic acid from calf-thymus deoxyribonucleic acid: preparation and properties, *Biochim. Biophys.Acta* 195, 446–455, 1969.

44. Maxam, A.M. and Gilbert, W., A new method for sequencing DNA, *Proc.Nat.Acad.Sci.USA* 74, 560–564, 1977.

45. Cashmore, A.R. and Petersen, G.B., The degradation of DNA by hydrazine: identification of 3-ureidopyrazole as a product of the hydrazinolysis of deoxycytidylic acid residues, *Nucleic Acids Res.* 5, 2485–2891, 1978.

46. Peattie, D.A., Direct chemical method for sequencing RNA, *Proc. Nat.Acad.Sci.USA* 76, 1760–1764, 1979.

47. Tolson, D.A. and Nicholson, N.H., Sequencing RNA by a combination of exonuclease digestion and uridine-specific chemical cleavage using MALDI-TOF, *Nucleic Acids Res.* 26, 446–451, 1998.

48. Small, G.D. and Gordon, M.P., Reaction of hydroxylamine and methoxyamine with the ultraviolet-induced hydrate of cytidine, *J.Mol.Biol.* 14, 281–291, 1968.

49. Brown, D.M. and Osborne, M.R., The reaction of adenosine with hydroxylamine, *Biochim.Biophys.Acta* 247, 514–518, 1971.

50. Fraenkel-Conrat, H., and Singer, B., The chemical basis for the mutagenicity of hydroxylamine and methoxyamine, *Biochim. Biophys.Acta* 262, 264–268, 1972.

51. Iida, S., Chung, K.C., and Hayatsu, H., The reaction of hydroxylamine with 4-thiouridine, *Biochim.Biophys.Acta* 308, 198–204, 1973.

52. Kasai, H. and Nishimura, S., Hydroxylation of deoxyguanosine at the C-8 position by ascorbic acid and other reducing agents, *Nucleic Acids Res.* 12, 2137–2145, 1984.

53. Johnston, B.H., Hydroxylamine and methoxyamine as probes of DNA structure, *Methods Enzymol.* 212, 180–194, 1992.

54. Simandan, T., Sun, J., and Dix, T.A., Oxidation of DNA bases, deoxyribonucleosides and homopolymers by peroxyl radicals, *Biochem.J.* 335, 233–240, 1998.

55. Tessman, I., Poddar, R.K., and Kumar, S., Identification of the altered bases in mutated single-stranded DNA. I. In vitro mutagenesis by hydroxylamine, ethyl methanesulfonate and nitrous acid, *J.Mol.Biol.* 93, 352–363, 1964.

56. Stuy, J.H., Inactivation of transforming deoxyribonucleic acid by nitrous acid, *Biochem.Biophys.Res.Commun.* 6, 328–333, 1961.

57. Horn, E.E. and Herriott, R.M., The mutagenic action of nitrous acid on "single-stranded" (denatured) Hemophilus transforming DNA, *Proc.Nat.Acad.Sci.USA* 48, 1409–1416, 1962.

58. Kotaka, T. and Baldwin, R.L., Effects of nitrous acid on the DAT copolymer as a template for DNA polymerase, *J.Mol.Biol.* 93, 323–329, 1964.

59. Carbon, J. and Curry, J.B., A change in the specificity of transfer RNA after partial deamination with nitrous acid, *Proc.Nat.Acad. Sci.USA* 59, 467–474, 1968.

60. Shapiro, R. and Yamaguchi, H., Nucleic acid reactivity and conformation I. Deamination of cytosine by nitrous acid, *Biochim. Biophys.Acta.* 281, 501–506, 1972.

61. Verly, W.G. and Lacroix, M. DNA and nitrous acid, *Biochim. Biophys.Acta* 414, 185–192, 1975.

62. Dubelman, S. and Shapiro, R., A method for the isolation of cross-linked nucleosides from DNA: application to cross-links induced by nitrous acid, *Nucleic Acids Res.* 4, 1815–1827, 1977.

63. Shapiro, R. Dubelman, S., Feinberg, A.M., et al., Isolation and identification of cross-linked nucleosides from nitrous acid treated deoxyribonucleic acid, *J.Amer.Chem.Soc.* 99, 302–303, 1977.

64. Edfeldt, N.B., Harwood, E.A., Sigurdsson, S.T. et al., Solution structure of a nitrous acid induced DNA interstrand cross-link, *Nuc.Acids Res.* 32, 2785–2794, 2004.

65. Darby, C.K., Jones, A.S., Tittensor, J.R., and Walker, R.T., Chemical degradation of DNA oxidized by permanganate, *Nature* 216, 793–794, 1967.

66. Hayatsu, H. and Ukita, T., The selective degradation of pyrimidines in nucleic acids by permanganate oxidation, *Biochem.Biophys.Res. Commun.* 29, 556–561. 1967.

67. Rubin, C.M. and Schmid, C.W., Pyrimidine-specific chemical reactions useful for DNA sequencing, *Nucleic Acids Res.* 8, 4613–4619, 1980.

68. Fritzsche, E., Hayatsu, H., Igloi, G.L., et al., The use of permanganate as a sequencing reagent for identification of 5-methylcytosine residues in DNA, *Nucleic Acisd Res.* 15, 5517–5528, 1987.

69. Sasse-Dwight, S. and Gralla, J.D., KMnO4 as a probe for *lac* promoter DNA melting and mechanism *in vivo*, *J.Biol.Chem.* 264, 8074–8081, 1989.

70. Klysik, J., Rippe, K., and Jovin, T.M., Reactivity of parallel-stranded DNA to chemical modification reagents, *Biochemistry* 29, 9831–9839, 1990.

71. Jiang, H., Zacharias, W., and Amirhaeri, S., Potassium permanganate as an *in situ* probe for B-Z and Z-Z junctions, *Nucleic Acids Res.* 19, 6943–6948, 1991.

72. Nawamura, T., Negishi, K., and Hayatsu, H., 8-Hydroxyguanine is not produced by permanganate oxidation of DNA, *Arch.Biochem. Biophys.* 311, 523–524, 1994.

73. Bailly, C. and Waring, M.J., Comparison of different footprinting methodologies for detecting binding sites for a small ligand on DNA, *J.Biomol.Struct.Dyn.* 12, 869–898, 1995.

74. Kahl, B.F. and Paule, M.R., The use of Diethylpyrocarbonate and potassium permanganate as probes for strand separation and structural distortions in DNA, *Methods Mol.Biol.* 148, 63–75, 2001.

75. Spicuglia, S., Kumar, S., Chasson, L., Potassium permanganate as a probe to map DNA-protein interactions *in vivo*, *J.Biochem. Biophys.Methods* 59, 189–194, 2004.

76. Hayatsu, H., Wataya, Y., Kai, K., and Iida, S., Reaction of sodium bisulfite with uracil, cytosine, and their derivatives, *Biochemistry* 9, 2858–2865, 1970.

77. Shapiro, R., Braverma, B., Louis, J.B., and Servis, R.E., Nucleic-acid reactivity and conformation 2. Reaction of cytosine and uracil with sodium bisulfite, *J.Biol.Chem.* 248, 4060–4064, 1973.

78. Wang, R.Y.-H., Gehrke, C.W., and Ehrlich, M., Comparison of bisulfite of 5-methyldeoxycytidine and deoxycytidine residues, *Nucleic Acids Res.* 8, 4777–4790, 1980.

79. Frommer, M., McDonald, L.E., Millar, D.S., et al., A genomic sequencing protocol that yields a positive display of 5-methylcytosine residues in individual DNA strands, *Proc.Nat.Acad.Sci.USA* 89, 1827–1831, 1992.

80. Chen, H. and Shaw, B.R., Kinetics of bisulfite-induced cytosine deamination in single-stranded DNA, *Biochemistry* 32, 3535–3539, 1993.

81. Herman, J.G., Graff, J.R., Myöhänen, S., et al., Methylation-specific PCR: A novel PCR assay for methylation status of CpG islands, *Proc.Nat.Acad.Sci.USA* 93, 9821–9826, 1996.

82. Hong, K.-M., Yang, S.-H., Guo, M., et al., Semiautomatic detection of DNA methylation at CpG islands, *BioTechniques* 38, 354–358, 2005.

83. Ordway, J.M., Bedell, J.A., Citek, R.W. et al., MethylMapper: a method for high-throughput, multilocus bisulfite sequence analysis and reporting, *BioTechniques* 39, 464–470, 2005.

84. Zhou, D., Qiao, W., Yang, L., and Lu, Z., Bisulfite-modified target DNA array for aberrant methylation analysis, *Anal.Biochem.* 351, 26–35, 2006.

There are modifications of ribose moiety in ribonucleotides such as periodate oxidation which was used in early structural analysis. Oxidation of the ribose ring has also been used to couple RNA to protein amino groups and to amino-containing matrices for affinity chromatography.

TABLE 2: Reaction of Periodate with Nucleic Acids

Reaction	Conditions	Reference
Coupling of periodate-oxidized RNA to hydrazide-agarose	140 µL 0.2 M NaIO$_4$ added to 500 – 3000 µg RNA in a volume of 1 mL 0.1 M sodium acetate, pH 5.0 for one hours at 23°C in the dark; reaction terminated with 80 µL ethylene glycol; after removal of reactants, the modified RNA was coupled to hydrazide matrix in the same solvent	1
Coupling of double-stranded RNA to agarose	12 µL 0.1 M NaIO$_4$ (sodium meta-periodate) /10 A$_{260}$ units of RNA(40 A$_{260}$ units/mL) in 0.1 M sodium acetate, pH 5.0, and incubated for 1 hr at 23°C. The reaction is terminated by precipitation of the RNA with ethanol. Coupling to agarose was accomplished in 0.1 M sodium acetate, pH 5.0	2

References for Table 2

1. Robberson, D.L. and Davidson, N., Covalent coupling of ribonucleic acid to agarose, *Biochemistry* 11, 533–537, 1972.

2. Langland, J.O., Pettiford, S.M., and Jacobs, B.L., Nucleic acid affinity chromatography: Preparation and characterization of double-stranded RNA agarose, *Protein Exp.Purif.* 6, 25–32, 1995.

1   The reaction of formaldehyde with adenine in ribonucleic acid. (Adapted from *Nucleic Acids in Chemistry and Biology*, ed. G.M. Blackburn and M.J. Galt, Oxford University Press, Oxford, UK, 1996.)

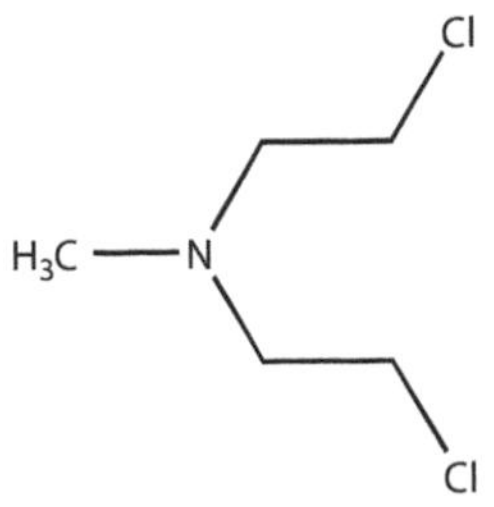

Chlormethine

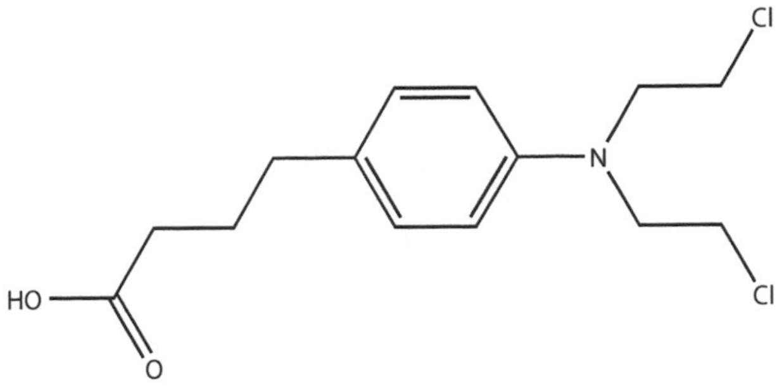

Chlorambucil

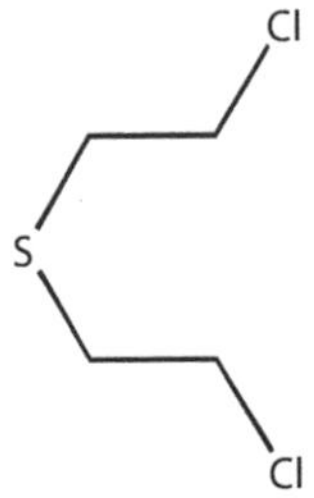

bis(2-chloroethyl) sulfide
Mustard Gas; Sulfur Mustard

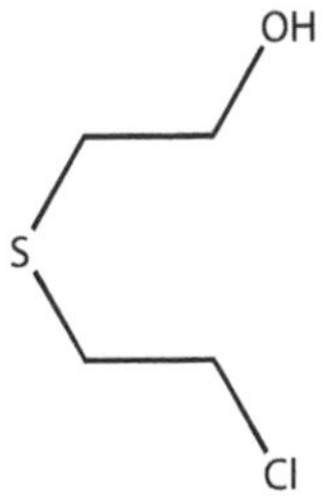

2-chloroethyl-2-hydroxyethyl sulfide
Hemisulfur Mustard

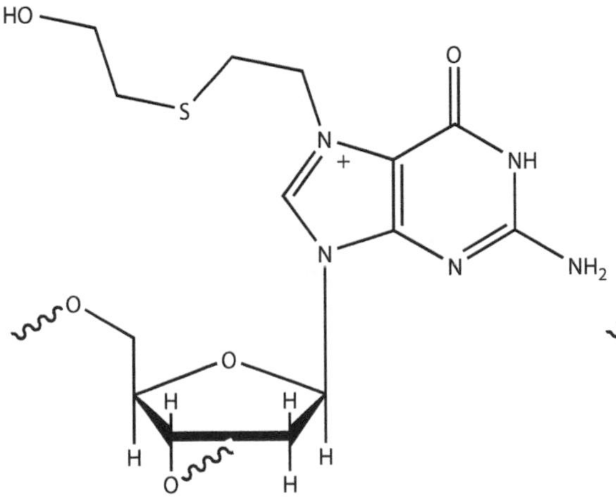

Deoxyguanyl;

Monosubstitution product with
bis(2-chloroethyl) sulfide or product
with hemisulfur mustard

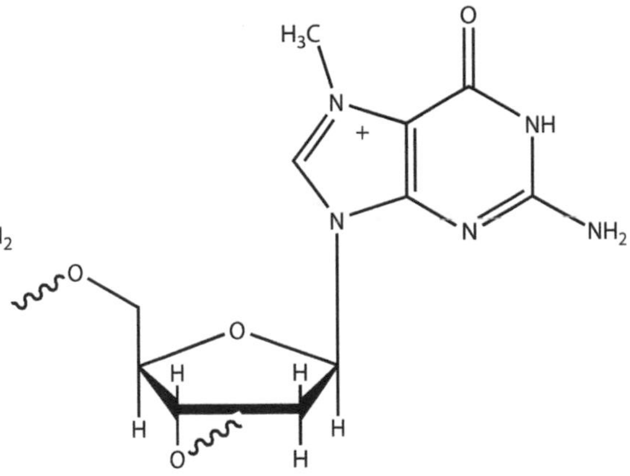

Reaction product of
deoxyguanyl residue with methyl iodide

2 Some alkylating agents for the modification of DNA. Nitrogen mustards are described as a group of bis(2-chloroalkylamines). The original mustards were chloroalkyl disulfides. Also shown is the methylation of purine with methyl iodide. The N7-position on the guanine ring is the most susceptible site for alkylation. See *Nucleic Acids in Chemistry and Biology*, ed. G.M. Blackburn and M.J. Galt, Oxford University Press, Oxford, UK, 1996; Denny, W.A., DNA minor groove alkylating agents, *Curr.Med.Chem.* 8, 533–544, 2001.

3 The reaction of diethylpyrocarbonate with adenyl and guanyl residues in ribonucleic acid.

4 The modification of purines and pyrimidines with dimethyl sulfate.

5   The degradation of cytidine with hydrazine. (Adapted from Cashmore, A.R. and Petersen, G.B., The degradation of DNA by hydrazine: identification of 3-ureidopyrazole as a product of the hydrazinolysis of deoxycytidylic acid residues, *Nucleic Acids Res.* 5, 2485–2491, 1978.)

6 The reaction of hydroxylamine with cytosine. (Adapted from Blackburn, G.M., Jarvis, S., Ryder, M.C., *et al.*, Kinetics and mechanism of reaction of hydroxylamine with cytosine and its derivatives, *J.Chem.Soc.Perkins Trans* 1, 370–375, 1975 and *Nucleic Acids in Chemistry and Biology*, ed. G.M. Blackburn and M.J. Galt, Oxford University Press, Oxford, UK, 1996.)

7 The reaction of purines and pyrimidines with nitrous acid resulting in deamination. The riboside derivative of hypoxanthine is inosine.

8 The oxidation of thymidine with potassium permanganate. Adapted from Bui, C.T., Rees, K., and Cotton, R.G.H., Permanganate oxidation reactions of DNA: Perspective in biological studies, *Nucleosides, Nucleotides, and Nucleic Acids* 22, 1835–1855, 2003.

9 The modification of cytosine with sodium bisulfite results in the formation of uracil.

10 The covalent coupling of RNA to an agarose matrix. The RNA is oxidized with periodate and then coupled to an alkyl hydrazide derivative of agarose.

General References for the Chemical Modification of Nucleic Acids

Jordan, D.O., The reaction of nucleic acids with mustard gas, *Biochem.J.* 42, 308–316, 1948.

Jordan, D.O., Nucleic acids, purines, and pyrimidines, *Annu.Rev.Biochem.* 21, 209–244, 1952.

Jordan, D.O., The physical properties of nucleic acids, in *The Nucleic Acids. Chemistry and Biology*, Vol. 1., ed. E.Chargaff and J.N. Davidson., Academic Press, New York, Chapter 13, pps. 447–492, 1955.

Lawley, P.D., Effects of some chemical mutagens and carcinogens on nucleic acids, *Prog.Nucl.Acid.Res.Mol.Biol.* 5, 89–131, 1966.

Lawley, P.D., Effects of some chemical mutagens and carcinogens on nucleic acids, *Prog.Nucleic Acid Res.Mol.Biol.* 5, 89–131, 1966.

Singer, B. and Fraenkel-Conrat, H., The role of conformation in chemical modification, *Prog.Nucl.Acid Res.Mol.Biol.* 9, 1–29. 1969.

Kochetkov, N.K. and Budowsky, E.T., The chemical modification of nucleic acids, *Prog.Nucl.Acid Res.Mol.Biol.* 9, 403–438, 1969.

Steinschneider, A., Effect of methylamine on periodate-oxidized adenosine 5'-phosphate, *Biochemistry* 10, 173–178, 1971.

Solymosy, S., Hüvös, P., Gulyás, A., *et al.*, Diethyl pyrocarbonate, a new tool in the chemical modification of nucleic acids, *Biochim. Biophys.Acta.* 238, 406–416, 1971.

Lawley, P.D., Orr, D.J., and Shah, S.A., Reaction of alkylating mutagens and carcinogens with nucleic acids: *N*-3 of guanine as a site of alkylation by *N*-methyl-*N*-nitrosourea and dimethyl sulphate, *Chem.Biol.Interact.* 4, 431–434, 1972.

Uziel, M., Periodate oxidation and amine-catalyzed elimination of the terminal nucleoside from adenylate or ribonucleic acid. Products of overoxidation, *Biochemistry* 12, 938–942, 1973.

Singer, B., The chemical effects of nucleic acid alkylation and their relation to mutagenesis and carcinogenesis, *Prog.Nucl.Acid Res.Mol. Biol.* 15, 219–284, 1975.

Maxam, A.M. and Gilbert, W., A new method for sequencing DNA, *Proc. Nat.Acad.Sci.USA* 74, 560–564, 1977.

Swenson, D.H. and Lawley, P.D., Alkylation of deoxyribonucleic acid by carcinogens dimethyl sulphate, ethylmethanesulphonate, *N-ethyl-N*-nitrosourea and *N*-methyl-*N*-nitrosourea. Relative reactivity of the phosphodiester site thymidylyl(3'-5')thymidine, *Biochem.J.* 171, 575–587, 1978.

Erhesamann, C., Baudin, F., Mougel, M., *et al.*, Probing the structure of DNA in solution, *Nucleic Acids Res.* 15, 9109–9128.

Chemistry of Nucleosides and Nucleotides, Volume 1, ed. L.B. Townsend., Plenum Press, New York, 1988.

Chemistry of Nucleosides and Nucleotides, Volume 2, ed. L.B. Townsend., Plenum Press, New York, 1991.

Oakley, E.J., DNA methylation analysis: A review of current methodologies, *Pharmacol.Therapeut.* 84, 389–400, 1991.

Glennon, R.A. and Tejon-Butl, S., Mesoionic nucleosides and heterobases, in *Chemistry of Nucleosides and Nucleotides*, Volume 2, ed. L.B. Townsend., Plenum Press, New York, Chapter 1, pps. 1–21, 1991.

Adams, R.L.P., Knowler, J.T. and Leader, D.P., *The Biochemistry of the Nucleic Acids*, 11th Edn., Chapman & Hall, London, 1992.

Brown, D.J. Evans, R.E., Cowder, W.B., and Fenn, M.D., *The Pyrimidines*, Interscience/John Wiley, New York, 1994.

Chemistry of Nucleosides and Nucleotides, Vol. 3, ed. L.B. Townsend, Plenum Press, New York, 1994.

Shaw, G., The synthesis and chemistry of imidazole and benzimidazole nucleosides and nucleotides, in *Chemistry of Nucleosides and Nucleotides*, Vol. 3, ed. L.B. Townsend., Plenum Press, New York, Chapter 4, pps. 263–420, 1994.

Nucleic Acids in Chemistry and Biology, 2nd Edn., ed. G.M. Blackburn and M.J. Gait., Oxford University Press, Oxford, UK, 1996.

Oakeley, E.J., DNA methylation analysis: a review of current methodologies, *Pharmacol. Therapeut.* 84, 389–400, 1999.

Ordway, J.M., Bedell, J.A., Citek, R.W., *et al.*, MethylMapper: A method for high-throughput, multilocus bisulfite sequence analysis and reporting, *BioTechniques* 39, 464–470, 2005.

Chen, X., Dudgeon, N., Shen, L., and Wang, J.H., Chemical modification of gene silencing oligonucleotides for drug discovery and development, *Drug Discov.Today* 10, 587–593, 2005.

Zhang, W.-Y., Du, Q., Wahlestedt, C., and Liang, Z., RNA interference with chemically modified siRNA, *Curr.Top.Med.Chem.* 6, 893–900, 2006.

POLYMERASE CHAIN REACTION

Roger L. Lundblad

The polymerase chain reaction (PCR)[1] was developed by Kerry Mullis in 1983 and is a mainstay of molecular biology. The history of the development of the PCR has been described[2] as well as its importance for biotechnology.[3,4] PCR is a method used for amplification of DNA or RNA for analysis or use in recombinant DNA technology.[5-8] There are a number of version of the PCR which are shown in Table PCR 1. Some variations of the PCR such as the panhandle PCR[9,10] and vectorette PCR[11-13] which are used for genomic sequencing are not shown in the table. Although the bulk of PCR is used for genomic diagnostics and recombinant DNA work, there is use of PCR for the amplification of barcodes in DNA chemical libraries.[14,15] Primed *in situ* labeling (PRINS) is a technical approach related to PCR where a DNA probe is used to bind to denatured cellular DNA and serve as a primer for a PCR where the product can be visualized with a label such as biotin or digoxigenin (both as dUTP derivatives).[16,17]

References

1. Mullis, K.B., and Faloona, F.A., Specific synthesis of DNA in vitro via a polymerase-catalyzed chain reaction, *Methods Enzymol.* 155, 335–350, 1987.
2. Mullis, K.B., The unusual origin of the polymerase chain reaction, *Sci. Am.* 262, 56–61, 1990.
3. Robinson, P., *Making PCR: A Story of Biotechnology,* University of Chicago Press, Chicago, IL, 1996.
4. McPherson, M., and Møller, S., *PCR,* 2nd edn., Garland Science/ Taylor & Francis, New York, 2006.
5. Dorek, M.J., ed. *Real-Time PCR,* Taylor & Francis, Abingdon, England, 2006.
6. Nolan, T., and Bustin, S.A., ed. *PCR Technology: Current Innovations,* 3rd edn., CRC Press, Boca Raton, FL, 2013.
7. Biasoni, R., and Rosi, A., ed. *Quantitative Real-Time PCR Methods and Protocols,* Humana/Springer, Clifton, NJ, 2014.
8. Basu, C., ed. *PCR Primer Design,* Humana/Springer, Clifton, NJ, 2015.
9. Jones, D.H., and Winistorfer, S.C., Sequence specific generation of a DNA panhandle permits PCR amplification of unknown flanking DNA, *Nucleic Acids Res.* 20, 595–600, 1992.
10. Megonigal, M.D., Rappaport, E.F., Wilson, R.B., et al., Panhandle PCR for cDNA: A rapid method for isolation of *MLL* fusion transcripts involving unknown partner genes, *Proc. Natl. Acad. Sci. U. S. A.,* 97, 9597–9602, 2000.
11. Arnold, C., and Hodgson, I.J., Vectorette PCR: A novel approach to genomic walking, *Genome Res.* 1, 39–42, 1991.
12. Proffitt, J., Fenton, J., Pratt, G., Yates, Z., and Morgan, G., Isolation and characterization of recombinant events involving immunoglobulin heavy chain switch regions in multiple myeloma using long distance vectorette PCR (LDV-PCR), *Leukemia* 13, 1100–1107, 1999.
13. Hilario, E., Fraser, L.G., and McNeilage, M., Trinucleotide repeats as bait for vectorette PCR: A tool for developing genetic mapping markers, *Mol. Biotechnol.* 42, 320–326, 2009.
14. Franzini, R.M., and Randolph, C., Chemical space of DNA-encoded libraries, *J. Med. Chem.* 59, 6629–6644, 2016.
15. Zimmermann, G., and Neri, D., DNA-encoded chemical libraries: Foundations and applications in lead discovery, *Drug Discov. Today* 21(11), 1828–1834, 2016.
16. Koch, J., Primed *in situ* labeling as a fast and sensitive method for the detection of specific DNA sequences in chromosomes and nuclei, *Methods* 9, 122–128, 1996.
17. Speel, E.J., Ramaekers, F.C., and Hopman, A.H., Primed *in situ* nucleic acid labeling combined with immunocytochemistry to simultaneously localize DNA and proteins in cells and chromosomes, *Methods Mol. Biol.* 226, 453–464, 2003.

DESCRIPTION OF VARIOUS TECHNOLOGIES FOR NUCLEIC ACID AMPLIFICATION BASED ON THE POLYMERASE CHAIN REACTION

PCR Technique	Description	References
PCR	The original technique uses a DNA polymerase to extend two opposed primers flanking a segment of DNA designated as the target region. Early work designated the target region as the amplicon[1,2] and this terminology is still used.[3] The fundamental process involves the initial separation of double-stranded DNA sample by heat denaturation. After cooling, primer, enzyme, Mg^{2+}, and the mixture of deoxynucleotide triphosphates in buffer (e.g., Tris) are added. This process is repeated and the original amplicon continues to be copied at a linear rate; the transcripts are transcribed at an exponential rate.[4,5] The original technique used a Klenow fragment of DNA polymerase[6] which lacked the intrinsic exonuclease activity seen with DNA polymerases. The thermal lability of the Klenow fragment required the addition of fresh enzyme after each thermal denaturation cycle.[7,8] The use of a thermostable DNA polymerase such as Taq polymerase[9] allowed the reaction to proceed without the addition of fresh enzyme at each cycle. Given the exponential nature of the PCR, it is possible to obtain a ten million-fold amplification of an amplicon.[4,7,a] This process is shown in Figure 1	1–9
Nested PCR	Nested PCR is a variation of PCR where a second set of primers internal on the amplicon relative to the original primers is used to focus on a shorter DNA sequence (Figure 1). Nested PCR is used to increase the sensitivity and fidelity of the PCR.[10-12]	10–12
Inverse PCR	Inverse PCR is a technique that permits the determination of DNA sequence flanking the target region.[13-16] This approach is dependent on the presence of one restriction site inside the target region and a different restriction site in the flanking regions. A segment of DNA containing the target sequence and flanking regions is obtained by one restriction enzyme or by reverse transcriptase. A second strand of DNA is obtained to yield a double-stranded DNA which is then circularized by DNA ligase (Figure 2). A linear DNA is obtained by restriction enzyme cleavage in the target region and a PCR product is obtained by primers directed "out" from opposing ends of the target region. Inverse PCR has been proved useful for chromosome walking.[17]	13–17
RT-PCR	RT-PCR is a PCR technique in which RNA is used as the source of amplicon. A polydT primer is frequently used for the preparation of the first cDNA copy reflecting the presence of a polyA tail on mRNA. A single primer is then used to make the second DNA chain which is then amplified with normal PCR process.[18] RT-PCR is used for the measurement of gene expression in tissues[19,20] and single cells.[20-22]	18–22

DESCRIPTION OF VARIOUS TECHNOLOGIES FOR NUCLEIC ACID AMPLIFICATION BASED ON THE POLYMERASE CHAIN REACTION (Continued)

PCR Technique	Description	References
Real-time PCR	Real-time PCR uses a fluorescent signal to measure the progress of strand duplication. This is accomplished by the use of oligonucleotide probes containing a fluorophore[23,24] which hybridizes with the PCR product or with the use of a dye such as ethidium bromide or cyanine dyes[25] which intercalate into double-stranded DNA sequence with a change in spectral characteristics.[23,26] The use of fluorescent probes to measure PCR product has permitted the development of instrumentation to measure the progress of PCR in "real-time"[27] rather than by electrophoretic analysis following amplification. Real-time RT-PCR is a method used to measure the mRNA levels.[28] In this context, the technique is referred to as quantitative real-time RT-PCR.[29]	23–29
qPCR	Current qPCR uses the measurement technologies of real-time PCR to measure the concentration of a specific DNA species.[30] Real-time PCR coupled with RT-PCR permits the accurate quantitative determination of messenger RNA concenrations.[31] There are many considerations in the application of this technique to the measurement of mRNA levels[31–34]	30–33
dPCR	dPCR is a variation of PCR where a complex DNA sample is diluted to an extent that a single drop contains a single DNA species.[35–38] This is intended to improve the specificity of the PCR with complex mixtures such as those present in the preparation of DNA libraries.[39–41] This technique is also described as digital droplet PCR.[42] dPCR has been adapted for use with microfluidic systems,[43] permitting the analysis of single cells.[44]	35–44b
Emulsion PCR	Emulsion PCR is an extension of dPCR where the components of a PCR are separated into oil droplet.[45–48] Solid-phase reaction technology with beads has been used in emulsion PCR.[49,50] Emulsion PCR has been used for amplification of single DNA molecules.[46,51]	45–51
Multiplex PCR	A process where multiple primers are used to obtain products from multiple target sequences in genomic DNA.[52] Multiplex PCR was originally used to define genomic deletions in Duchenne muscular dystrophy.[53] Multiplex PCR continues to be used for diagnosis of genomic rearrangements[54] and identification of pathogens.[55]	52–55
Anchored PCR		
Ligation PCR		

PCR, polymerase chain reaction; RT-PCR, reverse transcriptase-PCR; qPCR, quantitative PCR; dPCR, digital PCR.

[a] For example, 25 cycles with 70% amplification efficiency would produce 1 µg of PCR product from 1 pg of target sequence (From Table 1.1 in Newton, C.R., and G.A. Graham, *PCR*, 2nd edn., Bios Science, Oxford, England, 1997).

References

1. Baran, N., Lapidot, A., and Manor, H., Unusual sequence element found at the end of an amplicon, *Mol. Cell. Biol.* 7, 2636–2640, 1987.
2. Chang, F., and Li, M.M., Clinical application of amplicon-based next-generation sequencing in cancer, *Cancer Genet.* 206, 413–419, 2013.
3. Pabinger, S., Ernst, K., Pulverer, W.S., et al., Analysis and visualization tool for targeted amplicon bisulfite sequencing on Ion torrent sequencers, *PLoS One* 11(7), e0160227, 2016.
4. Newton, C.R., and Graham, A., *PCR, Introduction to Biotechniques* 2nd edn., Bios, Oxford, England, 1997.
5. McPherson, M.J., and Møller, S.G., *PCR*, Bios, Oxford, England, 2000.
6. Mullis, K.B., and Faloona, F.A., Specific synthesis of DNA *in vitro* via polymerase-catalyzed chain reaction, *Methods Enzymol.* 155, 335–350, 1987.
7. Salik, R.K., Gelfand, D.H., Stoffel, S., et al., Primer-directed enzymatic amplification of DNA with a thermostable DNA polymerase, *Science* 239, 487–491, 1988.
8. Syvänen, A.C., Bengtatröm, M., Tenhunen, J., and Söderlund, H., Quantification of polymerase chain reaction products by affinity-based hybrid collection, *Nucleic Acids Res.* 16, 11327–11338, 1988.
9. Liu, C.C., and LiCata, V.J., The stability of Taq DNA polymerase results from a reduced entropic folding penalty; identification of other thermophilic proteins with similar folding thermodynamics, *Proteins* 82, 785–793, 2014.
10. Porter-Jordan, K., Rosenberg, E.I., Keiser, J.F., et al., Nested polymerase chain reaction assay for the detection of cytomegalovirus overcomes false positives caused by contamination with fragmented DNA, *J. Med. Virol.* 30, 85–91, 1990.
11. Borchers, K., and Slater, J., A nested PCR for the detection and differentiation of EHV-1 and EHV-4, *J. Virol. Methods* 45, 331–336, 1993.
12. Mijatovic-Rustempasic, S., Esona, M.D., Williams, A.L., and Bowen, M.D., Sensitive and specific nested PCR assay for detection of rotovirus A in samples with a low viral load, *J. Virol. Methods* 236, 41–46, 2016.
13. Ochman, H., Gerber, A.S., and Hard, D.L., Genetic applications of an inverse polymerase reaction, *Genetics* 120, 621–623, 1988.
14. Zilberberg, N., and Gurevitz, M., Rapid isolation of full length cDNA clones by "inverse PCR": Purification of a scorpion cDNA family encoding α-neurotoxins, *Analyt. Biochem.* 209, 203–205, 1993.
15. Huang, S-H., Inverse polymerase chain reaction: An efficient approach to cloning cDNA ends, *Mol. Biotechnol.* 2, 15–22, 1994.
16. Pavlopoulos, A., Identification of DNA sequences that flank a known region by inverse PCR, *Methods Mol. Biol. (Molecular Methods for Evolutionary Genetics)* 772, 267–275, 2011.
17. Trinh, Q., Zhu, P., Shi, H., et al., A-T linker adapter polymerase chain reaction for determining flanking sequences by rescuing inverse PCR or thermal asymmetric interlaced PCR products, *Anal. Biochem.* 466, 24–26, 2014.
18. Ohan, N.W., and Jeikkila, J.J., Reverse transcription-polymerase chain reaction: An overview of the technique and its applications, *Biotechnol. Adv.* 11, 13–29, 1993.
19. Salonga, D.S., Danenburg, K.D., Grem, J., et al., Relative gene expression in normal and tumor tissue by quantitative RT-PCR, *Methods Mol. Biol.* 191, 83–98, 2002.
20. Hashimoto, A., Matsui, T., Tanaka, S., et al., Laser-mediated microdissection for analysis of gene expression in synovial tissue, *Modern Rheumatol.* 17, 185–190, 2007.
21. Dixon, A.K., Richardson, P.J., Pinnock, R.D., and Lee, K., Gene expression analysis at the single-cell level, *Trends Pharm. Sci.* 21, 65–70, 2000.
22. Phiilips, J.K., and Lipski, J., Single-cell RT-PCR as a tool to study gene expression in central and peripheral autonomic neurons, *Auton. Neurosci.* 86, 1–13, 2000.
23. Chminggi, M., Monereau, S., Pernet, P., et al., Specific real-time PCR vs. fluorescent dyes for serum free DNA quantification, *Clin. Chem. Lab. Med.* 45, 993–995, 2007.
24. Faltin, B., Zengele, R., and von Stetten, F., Current methods for fluorescence-based universal sequence-dependent detection of nucleic acids in homogeneous assay and clinical applications, *Clin. Chem.* 59, 1567–1582, 2013.

25. Bruijns, B.B., Tiggelaar, R.M., and Gardeniers, J.G., Fluorescent cyanine dyes for the quantification of low amounts of dsDNA, *Anal. Biochem.* 511, 74–79, 2016.

26. McCarthy, M.T., and O'Callaghan, C.A., Solid-phase-reader quantification of specific PCR products by measurement of band-specific ethidium bromide fluorescence, *Anal. Biochem.* 447, 30–32, 2014.

27. Oste, C.C., PCR Instrumentation: Where do we stand?, in *The Polymerase Chain Reaction*, ed. K.B. Mullis, F. Ferré, and R.A. Gibbs, pp. 165–173, Birkhäuser, Boston, MA, 1994.

28. Blashke, V., Reich, K., Blaschke, S., Zipprich, S., and Neumann, C., Rapid quantitation of proinflammatory and chemoattractant cytokine expression in small tissue samples and monocyte-derived dendritic cells: Validation of a new real-time RT-PCR technology, *J. Immunol. Methods* 246, 79–90, 2000.

29. Winer, J., Jung, C.K.S., Shackel, I., and Williams, W.P., Development and validation of real-time quantitative reverse transcriptase-polymerase chain reaction for monitoring gene expression in cardiac monocytes in vitro, *Anal. Biochem.* 270, 41–49, 1999.

30. Dymond, J.S., Explanatory chapter: Quantitative PCR, *Methods Enzymol.* 529, 279–289, 2013.

31. Bustin, S.A., Benes, V., Garson, J.A., et al., The MIQE guidelines: Minimum information for publication of quantitative real-time PCR experiments, *Clin. Chem.* 55, 611–622, 2009.

32. Bustin, S.A., Why the need for qPCR publication guidelines?—The case for MIQE, *Methods* 50, 217–226, 2010.

33. Lanoix, D., Lacasse, A.A., St-Pierre, J., et al., Quantitative PCR pitfalls: The case of the human placenta, *Mol. Biotechnol.* 52, 234–243, 2012.

34. Sanders, R., Mason, D.J, Foy, C.A., and Hugget, J.F., Considerations for accurate gene expression measurements by reverse transcription quantitative PCR when analyzing clinical samples, *Anal. Bioanal. Chem.* 406, 6471–6483, 2014.

35. Sykes, P.J., Neoh, S.H., Brisco, M.J., et al., Quantitation of targets for PCR by use of limiting dilution, *Biotechniques* 13, 444–449, 1992.

36. Vogelstein, B., and Kinzler, K.W., Digital PCR, *Proc. Natl. Acad. Sci. U. S. A.*, 96, 9236–9241, 1999.

37. Bizouarn, F., Introduction to Digital PCR, *Methods Mol. Biol. (Quantitative Real-Time PCR. Method and Protocols)* 1160, 27–40, 2014.

38. Huggett, J.F., Cowen, S., and Foy, C.A., Considerations for digital PCR as an accurate molecular diagnostic tool, *Clin. Chem.* 61, 79–88, 2015.

39. Persson, M.A., Combinatorial libraries, *Int. Rev. Immunol.* 10, 53–63, 1993.

40. Pollock, S., Thomas, D.Y., and Jansen, G., PCR-based unidirectional deletion method for creation of comprehensive cDNA libraries, *Biochim. Biophys. Acta* 1723, 265–269, 2005.

41. Aigrain, L., Gu, Y., and Quail, M.A., Quantification of next generation sequencing library preparation protocol efficiencies using droplet digital PCR assays—A systematic comparison of DNA library preparation kits for Illumina sequencing, *BMC Genomics* 17, 458, 2016.

42. Zonta, E., Garlan, F., Pécuchet, N., et al., Multiplex detection of rare mutations by picoliter droplet based digital PCR: Sensitivity and specificity, *PLoS One* 11(7), e0159094, 2016.

43. Zhang, Y., and Jiang, H-R., A review on continuous-flow microfluidic PCR in droplets: Advances, challenges and future, *Anal. Chim. Acta* 914, 7–16, 2016.

44. Ma, S., Loufakis, D.N., Cao, Z., et al., Diffusion-based microfluidic PCR for "one-pot" analysis of cells, *Lab Chip*, 124, 2905–2909, 2014.

45. Tawfik, D.S., and Griffiths, A.D., Man-made cell-like compartments for molecular evolution, *Nat. Biotechnol.* 16, 652–656, 1998.

46. Nakano, M., Komatsu, J., Matsuura, S-I., et al., Single-molecule PCR using water-in-oil emulsion, *J. Biotechnol.* 102, 117–124, 2003.

47. Williams, R., Peisajovich, S.G., Miller, O.J., et al., Amplification of complex gene libraries by emulsion PCR, *Nat. Methods* 3, 545–550, 2006.

48. Schültze, T., Rubelt, F., Repkow, J., et al., A streamlined protocol for emulsion polymerase chain reaction and subsequent purification, *Anal. Biochem.* 410, 155–157, 2011.

49. Takaaki, K., Takei, Y., Ohtsuka, M., et al., PCR amplification from single DNA molecules on magnetic beads in emulsion: Application for high-throughput screening for transcription factor targets, *Nucleic Acids Res.* 33, e150/1–e150/9, 2005.

50. Hueninger, T., Wessels, H., Fischer, C., Paschke-Kratzin, A., and Fischer, M., Just in time selection: A rapid semiautomated SELEX of DNA aptamers using magnetic separation and beads, emulsion, amplification, and magnetics, *Anal. Chem.* 86, 10940–10947, 2014.

51. Orkunoglu-Suer, F., Harralson, A.F., Frankfurter, D., Gindoff, P., and O'Brien, T.J., Targeted single molecule sequencing methodology for ovarian hyperstimulation syndrome, *BMC Genomics*, 16, 264, 2015.

52. Edwards, M.C., and Gibbs, R.A., Multiplex PCR: Advantages, development, and applications, *Genomic Res.* 3(4), S65–S75, 1994.

53. Chamberlain, J.S., Gibbs, R.A., Ranier, J.E., Nguyen, P.N., and Caskey, C.T., Deletion screening of the Duchenne muscular dystrophy locus via multiplex DNA amplification, *Nucleic Acids Res.* 16, 11141–11156, 1988.

54. De Lellis, L., Curia, M.C., Veschi, S., et al., Methods for routine diagnosis of genomic rearrangements: Multiplex PCR-based methods and future perspectives, *Exp. Rev. Mol. Diagn.* 8, 41–52, 2008.

55. Chang, S.S., Hseih, W.H., Liu, T.S., et al., Multiplex PCR system for rapid detection of pathogens in patients with presumed sepsis—A systemic review and meta-analysis, *PLoS One*, 8(5), e62323, 2013.

GENE EDITING

Roger L. Lundblad

Gene Editing and Designer Nucleases-Some Definitions

A *designer nuclease* is a nuclease engineered to cleave a very specific phosphodiester sequence in a duplex DNA (double-strand DNA cleavage). Current designer nucleases include meganucleases, zinc finger nucleases (ZFNs), transcription activator-like effector nucleases (TALENs), and clustered regulatory interspaced short palindromic repeat (CRISPR)-associated protein 9 (CRISPR/Cas9). TALENs and ZFNs contain a restriction nuclease, Fokl. Meganucleases and CRISPR/Cas9 contains an intrinsic nuclease function.

Gene editing is a process by which a coding DNA sequence may be edited (altered) by the process of homologous recombination. This process is controlled by a DNA cleaving enzyme referred to as a designer nuclease that causes a double-strand breakage in a very specific DNA sequence. This cleavage is "repaired" by the insertion of a specific DNA sequence showing extensive homology to the cleaved region. Gene editing can be used to add one or more nucleotides to or delete one or more nucleotides from a DNA sequence. For gene editing to be successful, "off-target" DNA cleavage must be avoided as such strand breaks would be repaired by non-homologous end-to-end joining (NHEJ) which could disrupt the integrity of message (Maggio, I., and Goncalves, A.F.V., Genome editing at the crossroads of delivery, specificity, and fidelity, *Trends Biotechnol.* 33, 280–291, 2015).

Gene targeting is a method which uses homologous recombination to delete genetic information (*knockout*) or add genetic information (*knockin*). The classic approach used homologous recombination in a mouse embryonic stem cell. The engineered embryonic stem cell is injected into a mouse blastocyst which is then implanted in a foster parent, and offspring are selected for chimeras, usually on the basis of coat color. Gene editing can be considered as a more efficient method of gene targeting for the generation of knockout gene modification (Hendriks, W.T., Warren, C.R., and Cowan, C.A., Genome editing in human pluripotent stem cells: Approaches, pitfalls, and solutions, *Cell Stem Cell* 18, 53–65, 2016) or knockin gene modification (Zhu, Z., Verma, N., González, F., Shi, Z.D., and Huangfu, D., A CRISPR/Cas-mediated selection-free knockin strategy in human embryonic stem cells, *Stem Cell Reports* 4, 1103–1111, 2015). It should be mentioned that a *knockdown* uses a different mechanism based on RNA interference (Fellmann, C., and Lowe, S.W., Stable RNA interference rules for silencing, *Nat. Cell Biol.* 16, 10–18, 2014).

Homologous recombination is a mechanism in the cell where a DNA sequence is exchanged between two similar or identical DNA molecules which serve as templates. This process is greatly facilitated by double-strand DNA cleavage (Rovet, P., Smith, F., and Jasin, M., Expression of a site-specific nuclease stimulates homologous recombination in mammalian cells, *Proc. Natl. Acad. Sci. U. S. A.* 91, 6064–6068, 1994).

Non-homologous end-to-end joining is a DNA repair process where strand breakage is repaired by ligation of DNA termini without the use of a template. This is a normal repair process but can result in translocation. It can be a complex process with the involvement of phosphodiesterases, nucleases, and polymerases (Barlett, E.J., Brissett, N.C., Plocinski, P., Carlberg, T., and Doherty, A.J., Molecular basis for DNA strand displacement by NHEJ repair polymerases, *Nucleic Acids Res.* 44, 2173–2186, 2016; Menon, V., and Povrik, L.F., End-processing nucleases and phosphodiesterases: An elite supporting cast for the non-homologous end joining pathway of DNA double-strand break repair, *DNA Repair* 43, 57–68, 2016).

Restriction nucleases (restriction endonucleases) are a group of bacterial enzymes characterized by their ability to specifically cleave palindromic sequences in double-stranded DNA. Cleavage can result in blunt ends or strands with either 3'- or 5'-overhangs. The name of a specific restriction endonuclease is derived from the first letter of the genus and the first two letters of the species; other letters can be added to further describe the source. Thus, the name for the widely used type II restriction endonuclease from *Escherichia coli* is *EcoR1*.

Designer Nucleases

The term *designer nuclease* currently refers to nucleases which can be programmed to execute double-strand DNA cleavages at a specific phosphodiester bond between two deoxyribonucleotides. The term *designer nuclease* was first used to describe a protein derivative consisting of the *trans*-activation response (TAR) RNA-binding domain of *trans*-activator of transcription protein (Tat) fused to the ribonuclease H domain of HIV-1 reverse transcriptase.[1] The resulting fusion protein specifically cleaved the HIV-1 TAR RNA. The use of the designer nucleases in the manipulation of genomic information has been referred to as gene editing.[2]

At the time of this writing (September, 2016), there are four distinct enzymes which are considered designer nucleases; the fusion of meganuclease with the TAL domain provides a derivative of the parent meganuclease, megaTALs[3] with increased specificity for double-strand DNA cleavage that provides a fifth type of designer nuclease. This is achieved by attaching a DNA recognition sequence from transcription activator-like effector (TALE) protein[4] to an meganuclease.[3] In the cited work, a fusion protein was prepared between a truncated transcription activator-like effector (TALE; TAL effector) and a meganuclease (I-AniI). The DNA recognition sequence of TALE will direct the meganuclease to the desired genomic site. There are several excellent general reviews of the use of designer nucleases in gene editing.[5–7]

Homing Endonuclease/Meganuclease

A *homing endonuclease* describes several families of double-strand DNA cleaving enzymes which are encoded primarily by mobile introns but can also be encoded by inteins.[8,9] The term *homing* is derived from genetics which describes a site-specific gene conversion event where a mobile intervening sequence is copied and transferred to a cognate allele which lack that element.[9,10] The terms *meganuclease* and *homing endonuclease* are both used in the literature with meganuclease being used more in reference to gene editing.

The most significant of the several families (Table 1) contains a signature sequence, LeuAlaGlyLeuIle-GluAlaGluGly (LAGLI-DADG),[11] which is suggested to have both a structural role and a functional role.[12] The LAGLI-DADG family can be further separated into single-motif and double-motif groups and those coded by introns (such as ICreI) or inteins (such as Pi-SceI).[12] A meganuclease was first described as an intron-encoded specific double-strand endonuclease activity in *Escherichia coli* in 1986.[13] The utility of meganuclease I-*Sce* I in enabling homologous recombination was established by Thierry and Dujon in 1992[14] and was extended for use in mammalian cells for site-specific homologous recombination by Choulika and coworkers.[15] The specificity for double-strand cleavage by meganucleases is in protein sequence, and the catalytic mechanism involves the participation of metal ions.[16] There is great interest in engineering meganucleases to improve specificity[17] and in using the engineered enzymes in agricultural applications.[18]

TALENs (Transcription Activator-Like Effector Nucleases)

TALENs are designer nucleases composed of DNA recognition domains derived from the transcription activator-like effectors (TALEs)[19–23] and the catalytic domain of FokI.[24] TALEs are proteins produced by certain bacterial plant pathogens, most notably members of the *Xanthomonas* AvrBs3 family, which support virulence.[25] TALEs possess a central domain containing tandem repeats consisting of 34 amino acids which bind to a specific DNA sequence. Specificity of binding is provided by a pair of amino acids at positions 12 and 13 in each tandem repeat referred to as the hypervariable di-residue (RVD).[19,23] The sequence of these two amino acids in the RVD determines the base bound in the DNA sequence. The Golden Gate cloning method[26] has been used to engineer TALE domains[27] for the preparation of TALENs.[28] The Platinum Gate method is a modification of the Golden Gate method and is said to produce TALENs with higher efficiencies.[29,30]

Zinc Finger Nuclease

Zinc finger nucleases (ZFNs) are conceptually similar to TALENs in that there are protein domains which recognize specific DNA sequences connected to the catalytic domain of FokI nuclease allowed for specific cleavage of DNA.[31,32] Zinc fingers are protein domains in transcription factors which bind zinc and specifically interact with DNA.[33] Since zinc fingers bind to specific bases in DNA, there has been interest in the development of engineered zinc finger proteins in biopharmaceuticals.[34] Each zinc finger binds to a specific 3 base pair sequence in a DNA molecule. Thus, for example, the use of three zinc finger domains would permit the recognition of a nine-nucleotide sequence on either side of the double-strand break catalyzed by a FokI dimer.[35] The FokI-catalyzed cleavage of the double-stranded DNA requires the formation of a dimer.[36]

CRISPR/Cas9 (Clustered Regulatory Interspaced Short Palindromic Repeat-Associated Protein 9)

CRISPR/Cas9 is a nuclease that catalyzes specific DNA double-strand breaks. CRIPR/Cas 9 was first described as an immune mechanism in prokaryotes to provide protection against bacteriophage and viruses in bacteria and archaea.[37–39] The specificity for DNA cleavage is provided by a "guide RNA"(gRNA) consisting of a trans-activating RNA (tracRNA) and a CRISPR RNA (crRNA)[40] that is associated with the enzyme. Additional specificity for cleavage is provided by obligatory binding of the Cas9 protein to PAM (protospacer adjacent motif) which is the G-rich region of the tracRNA.[41] Cas (CRISPR associated) proteins are a family of proteins with enzymatic activity directed against nucleic acids.[42–44]

The CRISPR/Cas9 protein can be engineered to bind to a specific DNA sequence without cleavage of a phosphodiester bond but blocking the binding of a protein such as transcription factor or a RNA polymerase[45] in a process called *CRISPR interference*.[45,46]

References

1. Melekhovets, Y.F., and Joshi, S., Fusion with an RNA binding domain to confer target RNA specificity to an RNase: Design and engineering of Tat-RNase H that specifically recognizes and cleaves HIV-1 RNA *in vitro*, *Nucleic. Acids Res.* 24, 1908–1912, 1996.
2. Mani, M., Kandavelou, K., Dy, F.J., Durai, S., and Chandrasegaran, S., Design, engineering, and characterization of zinc finger nucleases, *Biochem. Biophys. Res. Commun.* 335, 447–457, 2005.
3. Boissael, S., Jarjour, J., Astrakhan, A., et al., megaTALs: A rare-cleaving nuclease architecture for therapeutic genome engineering, *Nucleic Acids Res.* 42, 2591–2601, 2014.
4. Miller, J.C., Tan, S., Qiao, G., et al., A TALE nuclease architecture for efficient genome editing, *Nat. Biotechnol.* 29, 143–148, 2011.
5. Weeks, D.P., Spalding, M.H., and Yang, B., Use of designer nucleases for targeted gene and genome editing in plants, *Plant Biotechnol. J.* 14, 483–495, 2016.
6. Merkert, S., and Martin, U., Targeted genome engineering using designer nucleases: State of the art and practical guidance for application in human pluripotent stem cells, *Stem Cell Res.* 16, 377–380, 2016.
7. Maggio, I., and Goncalves, M.A.F.V., Genome editing at the crossroads of delivery, specificity, and fidelity, *Trends Biotechnol.* 33, 280–291, 2015.
8. Doolittle, R.F., The comings and goings of homing endonucleases and mobile introns, *Proc. Natl. Acad. Sci. U. S. A.* 90, 5379–5381, 1993.
9. Jurica, M.S., and Stoddard, B.L., Homing endonucleases: Structure, function and evolution, *Cell. Mol. Life Sci.* 55, 1304–1326, 1999.
10. Dujon, B., Colleaux, L., Hacquier, A., Michel, F., and Monteiulhet, C., Mitochondrial introns as mobile genetic elements: The role of intron-encoded proteins, *Basic Life Sci.* 40, 5–27, 1986.
11. Waring, R.B., Davies, R.W., Scazzocchio, C., and Brown, T.A., Internal structure of a mitochondrial intron of *Aspergillus nidulans Proc. Natl. Acad. Sci. U. S. A.* 79, 6332–6336, 1982.
12. Pingoud, A., Silva, G.H., and Wende, W., Precision genome surgery with meganucleases: A promising biopharmaceutical for gene therapy, in *Modern Biopharmaceuticals: Recent Success Stories*, ed. J. Knäblein, pp. 165–181, Wiley-Blackwell, Weinheim, Germany, 2013.

13. Colleaux, L., d'Auriol, L., Belemier, M., et al., Universal code equivalent of a yeast mitochondrial intron reading frame is expressed in *E. coli* as a specific double strand endonuclease, *Cell* 44, 521–533, 1986.

14. Thierry, A., and Dujon, B., Nested chromosomal fragmentation in yeast using the meganuclease I-*Sec* I: A new method for physical mapping of eukaryotic genomes, *Nucl. Acids Res.* 20, 5625–5631, 1992.

15. Choulika, A., Perrin, A., Dujon, B., and Nicolas, J.F., The yeast I-Sce I meganuclease induces site-directed chromosomal recombination in mammalian cells, *C. R. Acad. Sci. III* 317, 1013–1019, 1994.

16. Galburt, E.A., and Stoddard, B.L., Catalytic mechanisms of restriction and homing endonucleases, *Biochemistry* 41, 13851–13860, 2000.

17. Arnould, S., Delenda, C., Grizot, S., et al., The I-CreI meganuclease and its engineered derivatives: Application from cell modification to gene therapy, *Protein Eng. Des. Sel.* 24, 27–31, 2011.

18. D'Halluin, K., Vanderstraeten, C., Van Hulle, J., et al., Targeted molecular trait stacking in cotton through targeted double-strand break induction, *Plant Biotechnol. J.* 11, 933–941, 2013.

19. Moscou, M.J., and Bogdanova, A.J., A simple cipher governs DNA recognition by TAL effectors, *Science* 326, 1501, 2009.

20. Boch, J., Scholze, H., Schornack, S., et al., Breaking the code of DNA binding specificity of TAL-type III effectors, *Science* 326, 1509–1512, 2009.

21. Sugisaki, H., and Kanazawa, S., New restriction endonuclease from *Flovobacterium okeanokoites* (FokI) and *Micrococcus luteus* (M1uI), *Gene* 16, 73–78, 1981.

22. Boch, J., and Bonas, U., *Xanthomonas* AvrBs3 family-type effectors: Discovery and function, *Annu. Rev. Phytopathol.* 48, 419–436, 2010.

23. Meckler, J.F., Bhakta, M.S., Kim, M.-S., et al., Quantitative analysis of TALE-DNA interactions suggests polarity effects, *Nucleic Acids Res.* 41, 4118–4128, 2013.

24. Deng, D., Yan, C., Wu, J., Pan, X., and Yan, N., Revisiting the TALE repeat, *Protein Cell* 5, 297–306, 2014.

25. Miller, J.C., Zhang, L., Xia, D.F., et al., Improved specificity of TALE-based genome editing using an expanded RVD repertoire, *Nat. Methods* 12, 465–470, 2015.

26. Engler, C., Kandzia, R., and Marillonnet, S., A one pot, one step, precision cloning method with high throughput capability, *PLoS One*, 3(11), e3647, 2008.

27. Weber, E., Gruetzner, R., Werner, S., Engler, C., and Marillonnet, S., Assembly of designer TAL effectors by Golden Gate cloning, *PLoS One*, 6(5), e19722, 2011.

28. Cermak, T., Starker, C.G., and Voytas, D.F., Efficient design and assembly of custom TALENS using the Golden Gate platform, *Methods Mol. Biol.* 1239, 133–159, 2015.

29. Sakuma, T., Oschiai, H., Kaneko, T., et al., Repeating patterns of non-RVD variations in DNA-binding modules enhances TALEN activity, *Sci. Reports*, 3, 3379, 2013.

30. Sakuma, T., and Yamamoto, T., Engineering customized TALENs using the Platinum Gate TALEN kit, *Methods Mol. Biol.* 1338, 61–70, 2016.

31. Porteus, M.H., and Carroll, D., Gene targeting using zinc finger nucleases, *Nat. Biotechnol.* 23, 967–973, 2005.

32. Porteus, M.H., Mammalian gene targeting with designed zinc finger nucleases, *Mol. Ther.* 13, 438–446, 2006.

33. Berg, J., Zinc finger domains hypotheses and current knowledge, *Annu. Rev. Biophys. Biophys. Chem.* 18, 405–421, 1990.

34. Klug, A., Towards therapeutic applications of engineered zinc finger proteins, *FEBS Lett.* 579, 892–894, 2005.

35. Granja, S., Marchiq, I., Baltazar, F., and Pouysségur, J., Gene disruption using zinc finger nuclease technology, *Methods Mol. Biol.* 1165, 253–260, 2014.

36. Mani, M., Smith, J., Kandavelou, K., Berg, J.M., and Chardrasegaran, S., Binding of two zinc finger nuclease monomers to two specific sites is required for effective double-strand DNA cleavage, *Biochem. Biophys. Res. Commun.* 334, 1191–1197, 2005.

37. Barrangou, R., Fremaux, C., Deveau, H., et al., CRISPR provides acquired resistance against viruses in prokaryotes, *Science* 315, 1709–1712, 2007.

38. Sapranauskas, R., Gasiunas, G., Fremaux, C., et al., The *Streptococcus thermophilus* CRISPR/Cas systems provides immunity in *Escherichia coli*, *Nucl. Acids Res.* 39, 9275–9282, 2011.

39. Bhaya, D., Davison, M., and Barragou, R., CRISPR-Cas systems in bacterial and archaea: Versatile small RNAs, *Annu. Rev. Genet.* 45, 273–297, 2011.

40. Anders, C., and Jinek, M., *In vitro* enzymology of Cas9, *Methods Enzymol.* 546, 1–20, 2014.

41. Kleinstiver, B.P., Prew, M.A., Tsai, S.G., et al., Broadening the targeting range of *Staphylococcus aureus* CRISPR-Cas9 by modifying Pam recognition, *Nat. Biotechnol.* 33, 1293–1298, 2015.

42. Maranova, K.S., Aravind, L., Wolf, Y.I., and Koonin, E.V., Unification of Cas protein families and a simple scenario for the origin and evolution of CRISPR-Cas systems, *Biol. Direct*, 6, 38, 2011.

43. van der Oost, J., Westra, E.R., Jackson, R.N., and Wiedenheft, B., Unravelling the structural and mechanistic basis of CRISPR-Cas systems, *Nat. Rev. Microbiol.* 12, 479–492, 2014.

44. Hille, F., and Charpentier, E., CRISPR-Cas: Biology, mechanisms, and relevance, *Phil. Trans. R. Soc. B.* 371, 20150496, 2016.

45. Qi, L.S., Larson, M.H., Gilbert, L.A., et al., Repurposing CRISPR as an RNA-guided platform for sequence-specific control of gene expression, *Cell* 152, 1173–1183, 2013.

46. Cleto, S., Jensen, J.V., Wendisch, V.F., and Lu, T.K., *Corynebacterium glutamicum* metabolic engineering with CRISPR interference (CRISPRi), *ACS Synth. Biol.* 5, 375–385, 2016.

TABLE 1: Homing endonucleases[a,b]

Family[c]	Description	Cleavage[d]	References
LAGLIDADG	This family of homing endonucleases is characterized by the presence of highly conserved DNA sequence coding for a decapeptide, LAGLIDADG, or a close homolog. This sequence was first observed in the mitochondrial intron of *Aspergillus nidulans*.[1] The presence of this sequence or closely related homolog in site-specific endonuclease encoded by introns containing open reading frames suggested the existence of a protein family.[2,3] It is thought that the LAGLIDADG domain contributes to both DNA binding and double-strand DNA cleavage.[4] Many LAGLIDADG enzymes are homodimeric such as I-CreI.[5] There are monomeric forms containing two copies of the LAGLIDADG domain such as I-SecI[6] (I—designated intron-coded protein[7] and I-OmiI and I-OmiII) which can function as a monomer. The LAGLIDADG domain is important for DNA binding but does not have a direct role in catalysis.	4 nts 3'	1–7
GIY-YIG	This family of homing endonucleases is characterized by the presence of GIY separated from YIG by 10 or 11 amino acids.[8,9] The best known of GIY-YIG enzyme, I-TevI binds DNA as a monomer that catalyzes a double-strand break resulting in a 2-nucleotide 3' overhang[10] in a process that involves sequential nicking of the double-strand DNA.[11] The GIY-YIG domain does not bind tightly to DNA but is important for the catalysis of phosphoryl bond cleavage.	2 nts 3'	8–11
H–N–H	The H–N–H family of homing endonuclease is encoded by group I and group II introns.[12,13] The H–N–H domain is suggested to be involved in the binding to DNA and in the catalytic process with the participation of metal ions.[12,14] The H–N–H motif is important in the nuclease activity of colicin E9.[15]	Nicking	12–15
His-Cys Box	The His-Cys box family contains a conserved region of sequence which contains several histidine and cysteine residues[16] which have been shown to be important for endonuclease function.[17,18]	4 nts 3'	16–18
PD-(D/E)-XK	There are several homing endonucleases with I-Ssp6803I.[19,20] The PD-(D/E)-XK homing endonucleases are members of the PD-(D/E)-XK phosphodiesterase superfamily.[21]	2 nts 5'	19-21
EDxHD	One member identified in this family is I-Bth0305I.[22]	2 nts 5'	22

nts, nucleotides in overhang.

[a] The term *homing endonuclease* and *meganuclease* are both used in the literature.

[b] A nomenclature for the homing endonucleases has been developed (Belfort, M., and Roberts, R.J., Homing endonucleases: Keeping the house in order, *Nucl. Acids Res.* 25, 3379–3388, 1997; Roberts, R.J., Belfort, M., and Bestor, T., A nomenclature for restriction enzymes, DNA methyltransferases, homing endonucleases and their genes, *Nucl. Acids Res.* 31, 1805–1812, 2003; Hafez, M., and Hausner, G., Homing endonucleases: DNA scissors on a mission, *Genome* 55, 553–569, 2012).

[c] The homing endonuclease families are based on the presence of a conserved primary structure motif (McManus, H.A., Lewis, L.A., Fučíková, K., and Haugen, P., Invasion of protein coding genes by green algal ribosomal group I introns, *Molec. Phylogenet. Evolution*, 62, 109–116, 2012).

[d] All cleavages are double-stranded DNA except for H-N-H which a single-strand(nicking) but sequential action can result in double-strand cleavage (Hafez, M., and Hausner, G., Homing endonucleases: DNA scissors on a mission, *Genome* 55, 553–569, 2012).

References

1. Waring, R.B., Davies, H.W., Scazzocchio, C., and Brown, T.A., Internal structure of a mitochondrial intron of *Aspergillus nidulans*, *Proc. Natl. Acad. Sci. U. S. A.* 79, 6332–6336, 1982.

2. Shub, D.A., and Goodrich-Blair, H., Protein introns: A new home for endonucleases, *Cell* 71, 183–186, 1992.

3. Dalgaard, J.Z., Garrett, R.A., and Belfort, M., A site-specific endonuclease encoded by a typical archaeal intron, *Proc. Natl. Acad. Sci. U. S. A.* 90, 5414–5417, 1993.

4. Gristin, A., Fonfora, I., Alexeeski, A., et al., Identification of conserved features of LAGLIDADG homing endonucleases, *J. Bioinformatics Computational Biol.* 8, 453–469, 2010.

5. Heath, P.J., Stephens, K.M., Monnet, R.J., Jr., and Stoddard, B.L., The structure of I CreI, a group I intron-encoded homing endonuclease, *Nat. Struct. Biol.* 4, 468–476, 1997.

6. Beylot, B., and Spassky, A., Chemical probing shows that the intron-encoded endonuclease I-*SecI* distorts DNA through binding in monomeric form to its homing site, *J. Biol. Chem.* 276, 25243–25353, 2001.

7. Hafez, M., Guha, T.K., and Hausner, G., I-OmiI and I-OmiII: Two intron-encoded homing endonucleases within the *Opohiostoma minus rns* gene, *Fungal Biol.* 118, 721–731, 2014.

8. Michel, F., and Dujon, B., Genetic exchanges between bacteriophage T4 and filamentous fungi, *Cell* 46, 323, 1986.

9. Kowalski, J.C., Belfort, M., Stapleton, M.A., et al., Configuration of the catalytic GIY-YIG domain on intron endonuclease I-*TevI*: Coincidence of computational and molecular findings, *Nucleic Acids Res.* 27, 2115–2125, 1999.

10. Kleinstiver, B.P., Wolfs, J.M., Kolaczyk, T., et al., Monomeric site-specific nucleases for genome editing, *Proc. Natl. Acad. Sci. U. S. A.* 109, 8061–8066, 2012.

11. Kleinstiver, B.P., Wolfs, J.M., and Edgell, D.R., The monomeric GIY-YIG homing endonuclease I-MolI uses a molecular anchor and a flexible tether to sequentially nick DNA, *Nucleic Acids Res.* 41, 5413–5427, 2013.

12. Shub, D.A., Goodrich-Blair, H., and Eddy, S.R., Amino acid sequence motif of group I intron endonucleases is conserved in open reading frames of group II introns, *TIBS* 19, 402–404, 1994.

13. Gorbalenya, A.E., Self-splicing group I and group II introns encode homologous (putative) DNA endonucleases of a new family, *Protein Sci.* 3, 1117–1120, 1994.

14. Corina, L.E., Qiu, W., Desai, A., and Herrin, D.L., Biochemical and mutagenic analysis of I-CreII reveals distinct but important roles of both H-N-H and GIY-YIG motifs, *Nucleic Acids Res.* 37, 5810–5821, 2009.

15. Walker, D.C., Georgioui, T., Pommer, A.J., et al., Mutagenic scan of the H-N-H motif of colicin E9: Implications for the mechanistic enzymology of colicins, homing enzymes, and apoptotic endonucleases, *Nucleic Acids Res.* 30, 3225–3234, 2002.

16. Johansen, S., Embley, T.M., and Willassen, N.P., A family of nuclear homing endonucleases, *Nucleic Acids Res.* 21, 4405, 1993.

17. Flick, K.E., Jurica, M.S., Mnnat, R.J., Jr., and Stoddard, B.L., DNA binding and cleavage by the nuclear intron-encoded homing endonuclease I-Ppol, *Nature* 394, 96–1010, 1998.

18. Galburt, E.A., and Jurica, M.S., His-Cys box homing endonucleases, in *Homing Endonucleases and Inteins*, ed. M. Belfort, D.M. Wood, B.L. Stoddard, and V. Derbyshire, pp. 85–102, Springer, New York, 2005.

19. Orlowski, J., Boniecki, M., and Bjnicki, J.M., I-Ssp6803I: The first homing endonuclease from the PD-(D/E)XK superfamily exhibits an unusual mode of DNA recognition, *Bioinformatics* 23, 527–530, 2007.

20. Zhao, L., Bonocora, R.P., Shub, D.A., and Stoddard, B.L., The restriction fold turns to the dark side: A bacterial homing endonuclease with a PD-(D/E)-XK motif, *EMBO J.* 26, 2432–2443, 2007.

21. Steczkiewicz, K., Muszewska, A., Knizewski, L., Rychlewski, L., and Ginalski, K., Sequence, structure and functional diversity of PD-(D/E)XK phosphodiesterase superfamily, *Nucleic Acids Res.* 40, 7016–7045, 2012.

22. Taylor, G.K., Heiter, D.F., Pietrokovski, S., and Stoddard, B.L., Activity, specificity and structure of I-Bth0305I: A representative of a new homing endonuclease family, *Nucleic Acids Res.* 39, 9705–9719, 2011.

Section VI
Glycoscience

NOMENCLATURE OF CARBOHYDRATES

Carbohydrate nomenclature has an impact on stereochemistry and on the nomenclature of certain other compounds (e.g. hydroxylactones), which are often named as modified carbohydrates in *Chemical Abstracts* (CAS) and elsewhere.

For IUPAC guidelines on carbohydrate nomenclature, see:

Pure Appl. Chem., 1996, **68**, 1919–2008.
Nomenclature of Organic Chemistry (IUPAC Recommendations and Preferred IUPAC Names 2013), ed. H. A. Favre and W. H. Powell, Royal Society of Chemistry, Cambridge, 2014 and the IUPAC website.

Dictionary of Carbohydrates, ed. P. M. Collins, Taylor and Francis, Boca Raton, 2006, is recommended for an overview of all the fundamental types of carbohydrates (323 listed) and can often resolve uncertainties of nomenclature.

Fundamental Aldoses

The fundamental carbohydrates are polyhydroxyaldehydes (aldoses) and -ketones (ketoses). Of these, the most important for nomenclature are the aldoses. An aldose, $HOCH_2(CHOH)_{n-2}CHO$, has $(n-2)$ chiral centres. The stereochemical designation of a fundamental aldose is arrived at by assigning it to the D- or L-series, depending on the absolute configuration of the *highest-numbered chiral centre (penultimate carbon atom)* of the chain, together with the aldose name that defines the relative configuration of all the chiral centres, thus D-glucose. This system of

stereo-description is used extensively in organic chemistry to specify the absolute configurations of compounds that can be related to carbohydrates. When applied in this general sense, the descriptors are italicised, for example, L-*erythro*-, D-*gluco*-.

Carbohydrates may be represented as *Fischer, Haworth* or *Planar (Mills)* diagrams, as well as zigzag diagrams as used for non-carbohydrates. Figure 1 shows how these representations are related and how to go from one to another.

In a *Fischer projection* of an open-chain carbohydrate, the chain is written vertically with carbon number 1 at the top. The OH group on the highest-numbered chiral carbon atom is depicted on the right in monosaccharides of the D-series and on the left in the L-series. To go from a Fischer projection to the correct absolute configuration, the groups attached to the *horizontal* bonds are pulled *above* the plane of the paper. Rotation of a Fischer diagram by 180° in the plane of the paper is an allowed operation, which leaves the configuration unchanged. *Caution:* Rotating a Fischer projection by 90° inverts the stereochemistry. Occasionally Fischer diagrams are drawn horizontally to save space. This should never be done!

The configuration of a group of consecutive asymmetric carbon atoms (such as >CHOH) containing one to four centres of chirality is designated by one of the following configurational prefixes (shown in Table 1).

Each prefix is preceded by D- or L- depending on the configuration of the highest-numbered chiral carbon atom in the Fischer projection of the prefix.

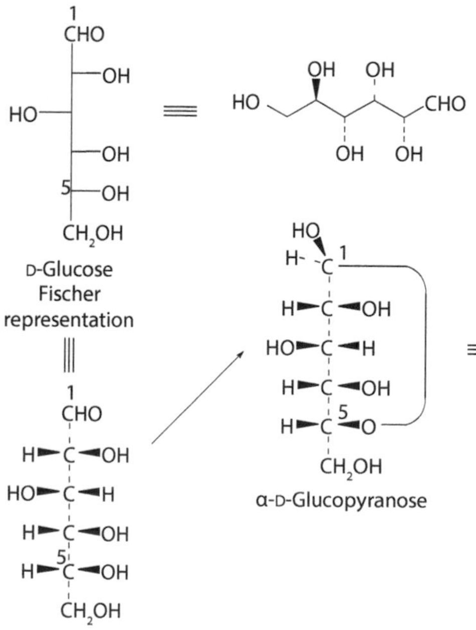

FIGURE 1 Fischer, Haworth and Mills representations of D-Glucose.

TABLE 1: Configurational Prefixes

No. of Carbon Atoms	Prefixes
1	glycero-
2	erythro-, threo-
3	arabino-, lyxo-, ribo-, xylo-
4	allo-, altro-, galacto-, gluco-, gulo-, ido-, manno-, talo-

The names of the aldoses and their formulae are:

D-Glycerose   D-Erythrose   D-Threose

D-Ribose   D-Arabinose   D-Xylose   D-Lyxose

D-Allose   D-Altrose   D-Glucose   D-Mannose

D-Gulose   D-Idose   D-Galactose   D-Talose

Strictly, carbohydrates containing one chiral centre should have their configuration specified as D- or L-*glycero*-. In practice this is often omitted, and such compounds can often be named equally well as aliphatics.

2,3-Dideoxy-D-
glycero-pentose

(S)-4,5-Dihydroxypentanal
(note different numbering)

2,3-Dideoxy-D-*glycero*-pentofuranose
= Tetrahydro-5-(hydroxymethyl)-2-furanol
(note different numbering)
or Tetrahydro-5-hydroxy-2-furanmethanol
(note different numbering)

The consecutive asymmetric carbon atoms need not be contiguous. Thus, the following four arrangements are all L-*erythro*- (X is attached to the lowest-numbered carbon atoms).

L-*erythro*-

Fundamental Ketoses

The most important ketoses are the hexos-2-uloses $HOCH_2(CH_2)_3COCH_2OH$ such as fructose. They have one less chiral centre than the aldoses of the same chain length – that is, there are only four diastereomerically different hexos-2-uloses.

The trivial names for the 2-hexuloses and their formulae are:

D-Psicose   D-Fructose   D-Sorbose   D-Tagatose

TABLE 2: Suffixes Used in Carbohydrate Nomenclature

-ose	aldose	X = CHO, Y = CH_2OH	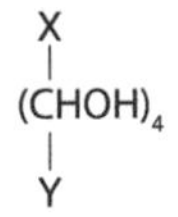
-odialdose	dialdose	X = Y = CHO	X
-onic acid	aldonic acid	X = COOH, Y = CH_2OH	$(CHOH)_4$ (Hexose series)
-uronic acid	uronic acid	X = CHO, Y = COOH	Y
-aric acid	aldaric acid	X = Y = COOH	
-itol	alditol	X = Y = CH_2OH	
-ulose	ketose	X = Y = CH_2OH	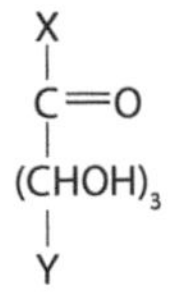 X
-osulose	ketoaldose	X = CHO, Y = CH_2OH	$C{=}O$
-ulosonic acid	ulosonic acid	X = COOH, Y = CH_2OH	$(CHOH)_3$ (2-Hexulose series)
-ulosuronic acid	ulosuronic acid	X = CHO, Y = COOH	Y
-ulosaric acid	ulosaric acid	X = Y = COOH	
-odiulose	diketose		

Modified Aldoses and Ketoses

Suffixes are employed to denote modification of functional groups in an aldose or ketose, for example, by oxidation of an OH group (Table 2).

Higher Sugars

Sugars having more than six carbon atoms are named using two prefixes, one defining the configuration at C-2 to C-5 as in a hexose and the other, which appears first in the name, defining the configuration at the remaining chiral centres.

Examples of the use of configurational prefixes are:

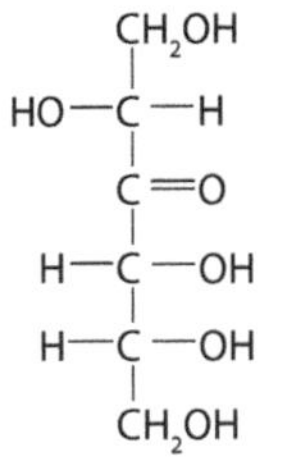

D-*arabino*-3-Hexulose 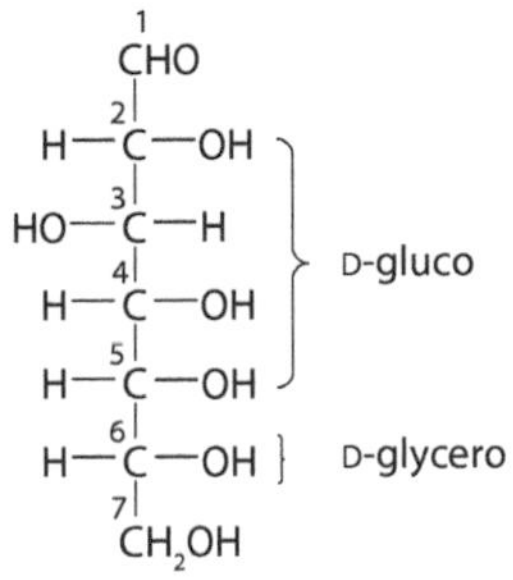   D-*glycero*-D-*gluco*-Heptose

Cyclic Forms: Anomers

When a monosaccharide exists in the heterocyclic intramolecular hemiacetal form, the size of the ring is indicated by the suffixes -*furanose*, -*pyranose* and -*septanose* for five-, six- and seven-membered rings, respectively.

Two configurations, known as anomers, may result from the formation of the ring. These are distinguished by the anomeric prefixes α- and β-, which relate the configuration of the anomeric carbon atom to the configuration at a reference chiral carbon atom (normally the highest-numbered chiral carbon atom). For example, consider the glucopyranoses:

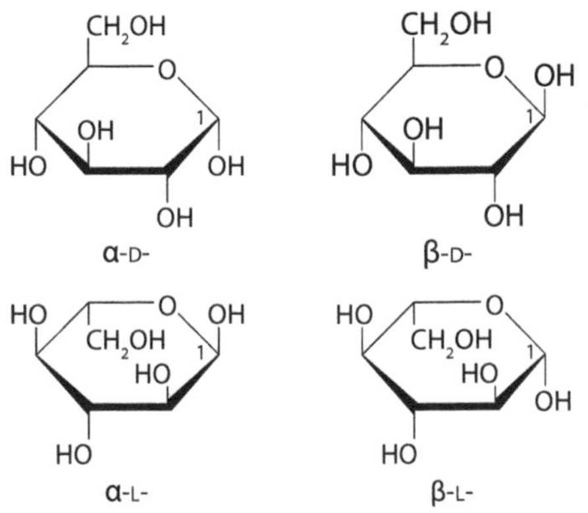

α-D-   β-D-

α-L-   β-L-

- In the D-series, the CH_2OH is projected above the ring.
- In the L-series, the CH_2OH is projected below the ring.
- In the α-series, the anomeric OH (at position 1) is on the opposite side of the ring to the CH_2OH group.
- In the β-series, the anomeric OH (at position 1) is on the same side of the ring as the CH_2OH group.

It is sometimes necessary to draw Haworth formulae with the ring in unconventional orientations (see Figure 2) if bulky substituents are to be represented or linkages in oligo- or polysaccharides denoted. Note that if the ring is inverted (diagrams g to l in Figure 2) the numbering runs anticlockwise.

Suffixes used in carbohydrate nomenclature to indicate cyclic forms are as follows:

-ose (acyclic form) → -ofuranose (five-membered ring), -opyranose (six-membered ring), -heptanose (seven-membered ring).

Similar suffixes can be constructed for dicarbonyl sugars and other modifications, for example:

-ulose	-ulopyranose
-osulose	-opyranosulose or -osulopyranose
-odialdose	-odialdopyranose

The suffixes for the acids can be modified to indicate the corresponding amide, nitriles, acid halides and so on – for example, -uronamide, -ononitrile, -ulosonyl chloride.

Glycosides

These are mixed acetals resulting from the replacement of the hydrogen atom on the anomeric (glycosidic) OH of the cyclic form of a sugar by a radical R derived from an alcohol or phenol (ROH). They are named by changing the terminal -*e* of the name of the corresponding cyclic form of the saccharide into -*ide*; the name of the R radical is put at the front of the name followed by a space.

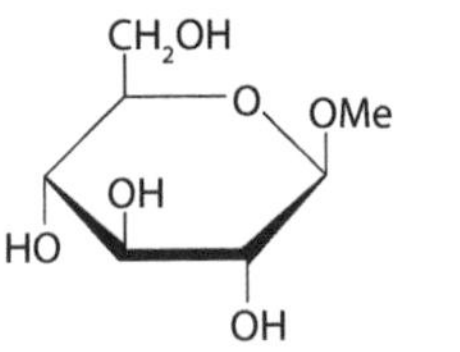

Methyl β-D-glucopyranoside

Disaccharides and Oligosaccharides

These are sugars produced where the alcohol forming the glycoside of a sugar is another sugar. Where the resulting sugar has a

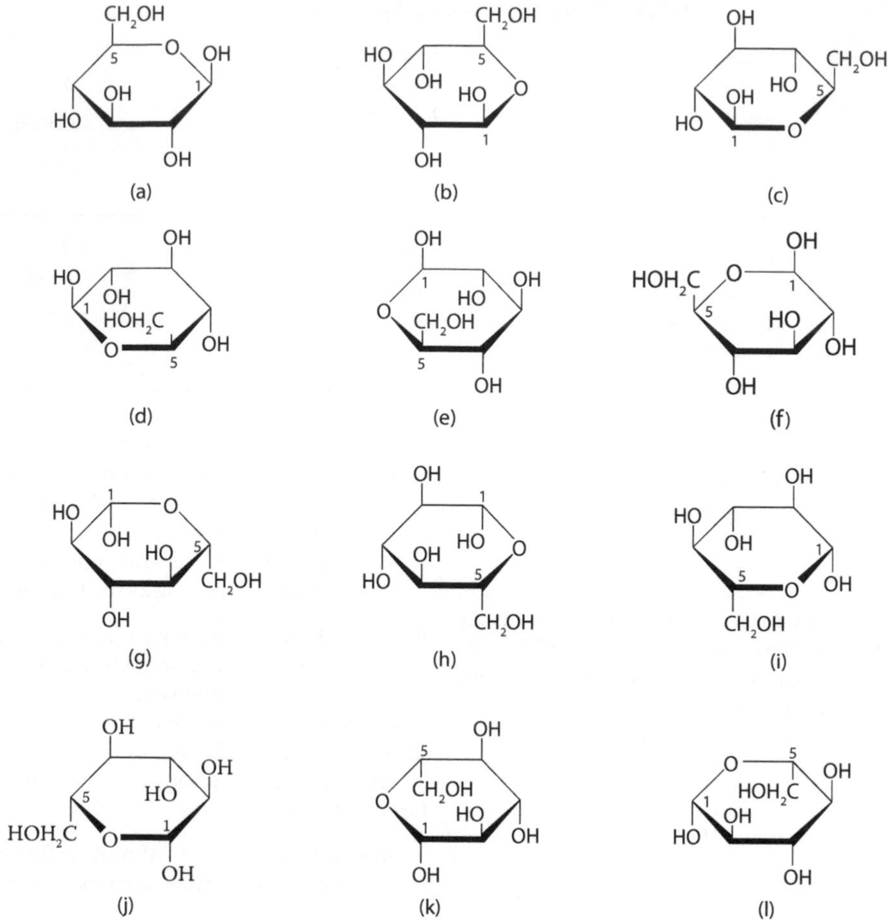

FIGURE 2   β-D-**Glucopyranose in unconventional orientations.**

(potentially) free aldehyde function, it is called a reducing disaccharide, and where both aldehyde functions are involved in the linkage (1→1) glycoside, it is a non-reducing disaccharide.

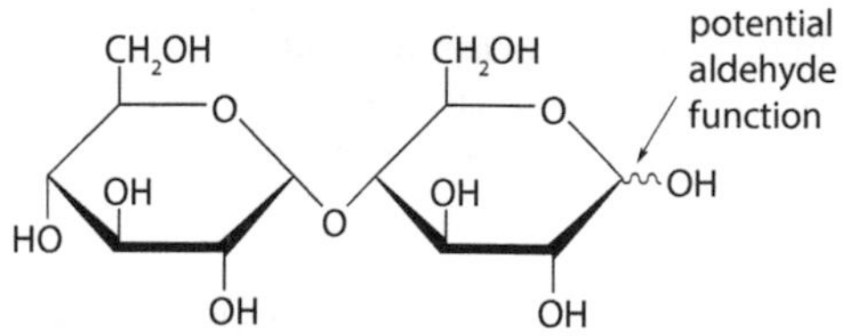

Maltose (4-*O*-α-D-Glucopyranosyl-D-glucose),
a reducing disaccharide

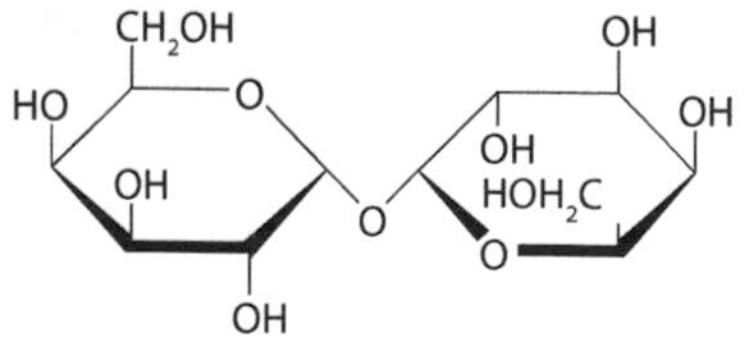

α-D-Galactopyranosyl α-D-galactopyranoside,
a non-reducing disaccharide

Chain branching is shown by nesting brackets, for example, β-D-Glucopyranosyl-(1→2)-[β-D-glucopyranosyl-(1→4)]-D-glucose.

Abbreviations for use in representing oligosaccharides are shown in Table 3.

TABLE 3: Abbreviations for Use in Representing Oligosaccharides

Hexoses	All	allose
	Alt	altrose
	Gal	galactose
	Glc	glucose
	Gul	gulose
	Ido	idose
	Man	mannose
	Tal	talose
Pentoses	Ara	arabinose
	Lyx	lyxose
	Rib	ribose
	Xyl	xylose
Other	Rha	rhamnose
	Fuc	fucose
	Fru	fructose
Suffixes	*f*	furanose
	p	pyranose
	A	uronic acid
	N	2-deoxy-2-amino sugar
Prefixes	D-	configurational descriptor
	L-	configurational descriptor
	An	anhydro

Examples are:

Ara*f*	arabinofuranose
Glc*p*	glucopyranose
Gal*p*A	galactopyranuronic acid
D-Glc*p*N	2-amino-2-deoxy-D-glucopyranose
3,6-AnGal	3,6-anhydrogalactose

See *Pure Appl. Chem.*, 1982, **54**, 1517–1522.

Trivially Named Sugars

A number of names for modified sugars, which occur frequently in natural glycosides, are in common use.

Allomethylose	6-Deoxyallose
Cymarose	2,6-Dideoxy-3-*O*-methyl-*ribo*-hexose
Diginose	2,6-Dideoxy-3-*O*-methyl-*lyxo*-hexose
Digitoxose	2,6-Dideoxy-*ribo*-hexose
Quinovose	6-Deoxyglucose
Fucose	6-Deoxygalactose
Rhamnose	6-Deoxymannose
Oleandrose	2,6-Dideoxy-3-*O*-methyl-*arabino*-hexose
Thevetose	6-Deoxy-3-*O*-methylglucose

Note that if the absolute configuration of a sugar is not clear from the literature, CAS makes certain assumptions – for example, rhamnose is assumed to be L-.

Alditols and Cyclitols

Alditols

Reduction of the carbonyl group of an aldose (or of the oxo group in a ketose) gives the series of alditols (called *tetritols*, *pentitols*, *hexitols* etc., with 4, 5, 6 carbon atoms and so on).

Because of their higher symmetry compared to the aldoses, the number of possible isomers is lower and some isomers are *meso* forms or, in the C_7 series, some isomers show pseudoasymmetry (further described in Chapter 5). Examples are shown in Figure 3.

Some isomers can therefore be named in more than one way. A choice is made according to a special carbohydrate rule, which says that allocation to the D- series takes precedence over alphabetical assignment to the parent carbohydrate diastereoisomer.

Cyclitols

The most important cyclitols are the inositols (1,2,3,4,5,6-cyclohexanehexols). The relative arrangement of the six hydroxyl groups below or above the plane of the cyclohexane ring is denoted by an italicised configurational prefix in the eight inositol stereoparents (the numerical locants indicate OH groups that are on the same side of the ring):

cis-Inositol	(1,2,3,4,5,6)
epi-Inositol	(1,2,3,4,5)
allo-Inositol	(1,2,3,4)
myo-Inositol	(1,2,3,5)
muco-Inositol	(1,2,4,5)
neo-Inositol	(1,2,3)
chiro-Inositol	(1,2,4)
scyllo-Inositol	(1,3,5)

Inositols adopt the chair conformation; the *scyllo*-isomer has no axial hydroxyl groups; the *myo*-isomer has one; *epi*-, *chiro*- and *neo*-isomers have two; and the *allo*-, *cis*- and *muco*-isomers each have three axial hydroxyl groups. In unsubstituted inositols, six isomers (*scyllo*-, *myo*-, *epi*-, *neo*-, *cis*- and *muco*-inositol) have one or more planes of symmetry and are achiral and *meso*compounds; *chiro*-inositol lacks a plane of symmetry and exists as the D- and L-forms. In *myo*-inositol, the plane of symmetry is C-2/C-5; unsymmetrically substituted derivatives on C-1, C-3, C-4, C-6

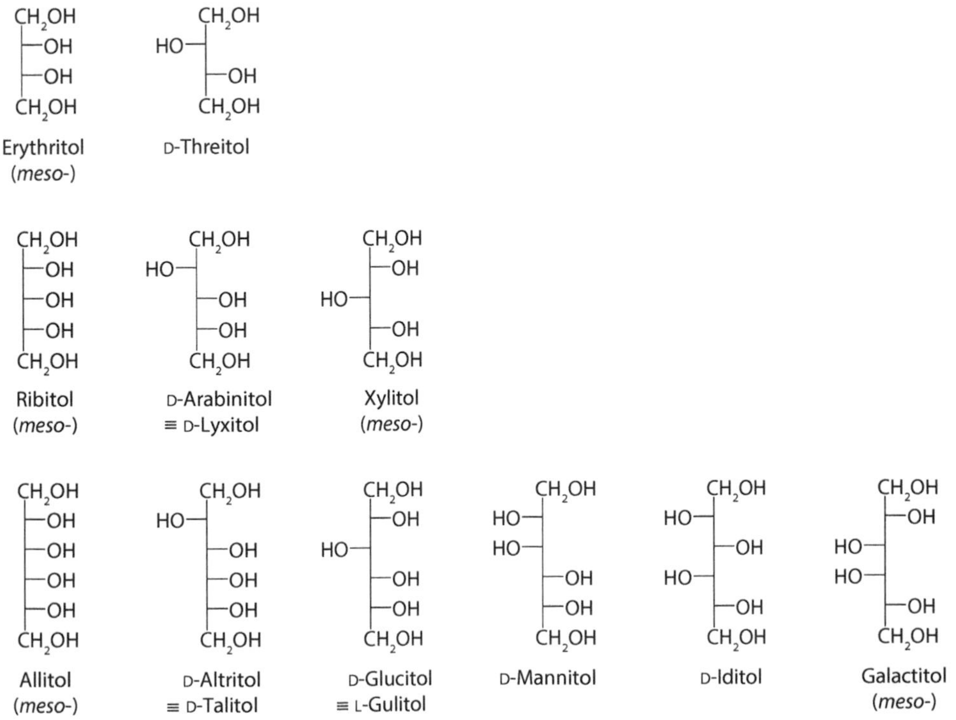

FIGURE 3 The alditols derived from the C4, C5 and C6 monosaccharides in the D-series. Degenerate symmetry means that there are only three pentitols and six hexitols.

are chiral. Substitution at C-2 and/or C-5 gives a *meso*-product. The apparent plane of symmetry in the Haworth projection of *allo*-inositol is misleading. Conformational inversion produces a non-superimposable mirror image, and at room temperature *allo*-inositol is racemic with the enantiomeric conformers in rapid equilibrium.

Assignment of Locants for Inositols

(From the IUPAC-IUB 1973 Recommendations for the Nomenclature of Cyclitols; *Biochem. J.*, 1976, **153**, 23–31; based upon proposals first issued in 1968; *Biochem. J.*, 1969, **112**, 17–28)

- The lowest locants are assigned to the set (above or below the plane) that has the most OH groups.
- For *meso*-inositols only, the C-1 locant is assigned to the lowest-numbered (prochiral) carbon atom that leads to an L rather than a D designation (see Section "Absolute Configuration").

Absolute Configuration

Using a horizontal projection of the inositol ring, if the substituent on the lowest-numbered asymmetric carbon is above the plane of the ring and the numbering is anticlockwise, the configuration is assigned D, and if clockwise, the configuration is L (illustrated in Figure 4 for *myo*-inositol 1-phosphate enantiomers; hydroxyl groups are omitted).

OPO₃H₂

1D-*myo*-Inositol 1-(dihydrogen phosphate)

H₂O₃PO

1L-*myo*-Inositol 1-(dihydrogen phosphate)

FIGURE 4   *myo*-Inositol 1-phosphate enantiomers.

Note that 1D-*myo*-inositol 1-phosphate is the same as 1L-*myo*-inositol 3-phosphate (and 1L-*myo*-inositol 1-phosphate is the same as 1D-*myo*-inositol 3-phosphate), but the lower locant has precedence over the stereochemical prefix (D or L) in naming the derivative. A consequence of applying the 1973 IUPAC-IUB rules to *myo*-inositol is that the numbering of C-2 and C-5 remains invariant, and C-2 is the axial-hydroxyl group.

Before 1968, the nomenclature for inositols assigned the symbols D- and L- to the *highest*-numbered chiral centre, C-6. This convention was based on the rules for naming carbohydrates. For substituted *myo*-inositols, in particular where C-1 and C-6 hydroxyl groups are *trans*, compounds identified in the literature before 1968 as D- are now assigned 1L-.

Locants for unsubstituted inositols other than *myo*-inositol are shown for Haworth projections in Figure 5 (hydroxyl groups are omitted).

In order to clarify the metabolic pathways for substituted *myo*-inositols (in practice, *myo*-inositol phosphates), the lowest-locant rule, which gives priority to a 1L-locant, has been relaxed and numbering based on the 1D-series is now allowed (*Biochem. J.*, 1989, **258**, 1–2). This is to allow substances related by simple chemical or biochemical transformations to carry the same labels. Thus, 1L-*myo*-inositol 1-phosphate may now be called 1D-*myo*-inositol 3-phosphate.

In a further simplification, the symbol *Ins* may be used to denote *myo*-inositol, with the numbering of the 1D-configuration implied (unless the prefix L- is explicitly added).

Further Reading

Recent advances in inositol syntheses, biochemistry and pharmacology, are reviewed by M. P. Thomas et al., *Angew. Chem. Int. Ed.*, 2016, **55**, 1614–1650.

The Supporting Information for this review (available as a downloadable pdf) is a comprehensive account of the stereochemical names, structures and ring numbering of inositol isomers and their phosphate derivatives and may be regarded as the definitive account of this topic.

Posternak, T., *The Cyclitols*, Holden-Day, San Francisco, 1965.

Hudlicky, T. and Cebulak, M., *Cyclitols and Their Derivatives: A Handbook of Physical, Spectral and Synthetic Data*, VCH, New York, 1993.

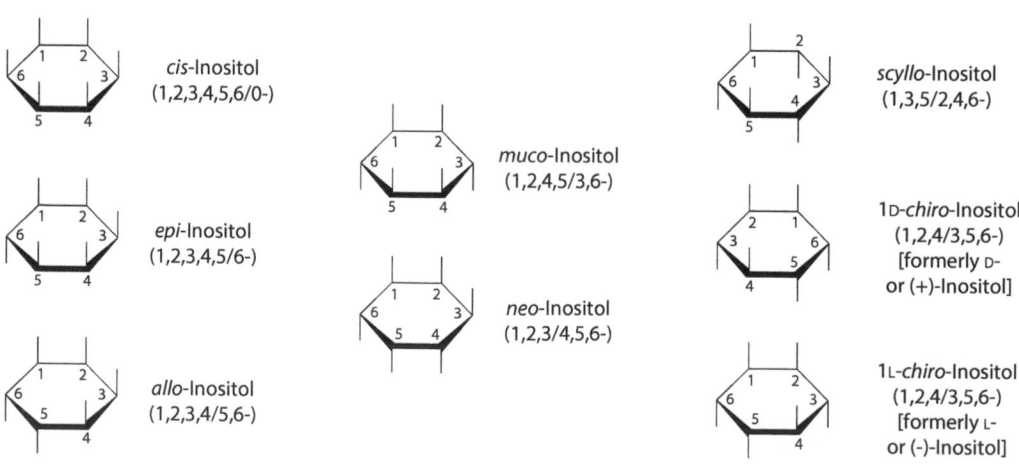

FIGURE 5   Seven inositol stereoparents. The fractional notation below the name of each isomer indicates the hydroxyl groups above/below the plane of the cyclohexane ring. Ring numbering is for the L-configuration (apart from 1D-*chiro*-inositol).

CHEMICAL MODIFICATION OF CARBOHYDRATES

Roger L. Lundblad

General References

Cumpstey, I., Chemical modification of polysaccharides, *ISRN Org. Chem.*, 2013, 417672, 2014.

Hoover, R., and Sosulski, F.W., Composition, structure, functionality, and chemical modification of legume starches: A review, *Can. J. Physiol. Pharmacol.*, 69, 79–92, 1991.

Jayakumuar, R., Nwe, N., Tokura, S., et al., Sulfated chitin and chitosan as novel biomaterials, *Int. J. Biol. Macromol.*, 40, 175–181, 2007.

Kellam, B., De Bank, P.A., and Shakesheff, K.M., Chemical modification of mammalian cell surfaces, *Chem. Soc. Rev.*, 32, 327–337k, 2003.

Lin, C.H., and Lin, C.C., Enzymatic and chemical approaches for the synthesis of sialyl glycoconjugates, *Adv. Exp. Med. Biol.*, 491, 215–230, 2001.

Stevens, C.V., Meriggi, A., and Booten, K., Chemical modification of inulin, a valuable renewable resource, and its industrial applications, *Biomacromolecules*, 2, 1–16, 2001.

Tomasik, P., and Schilling, C.H., Chemical modification of starch, *Adv. Carbohydr. Chem. Biochem.*, 59, 175–403, 2004.

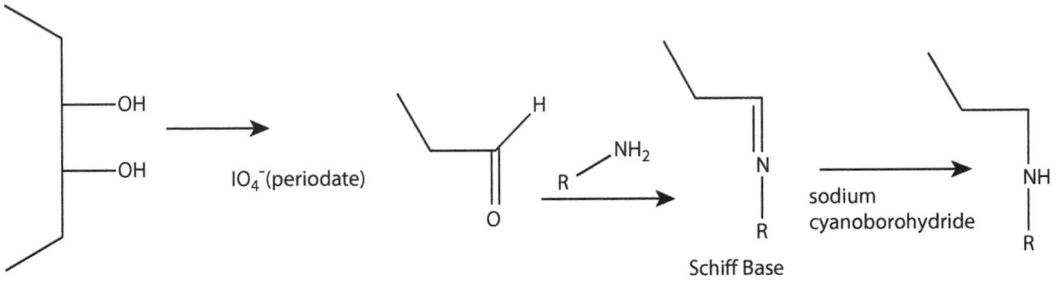

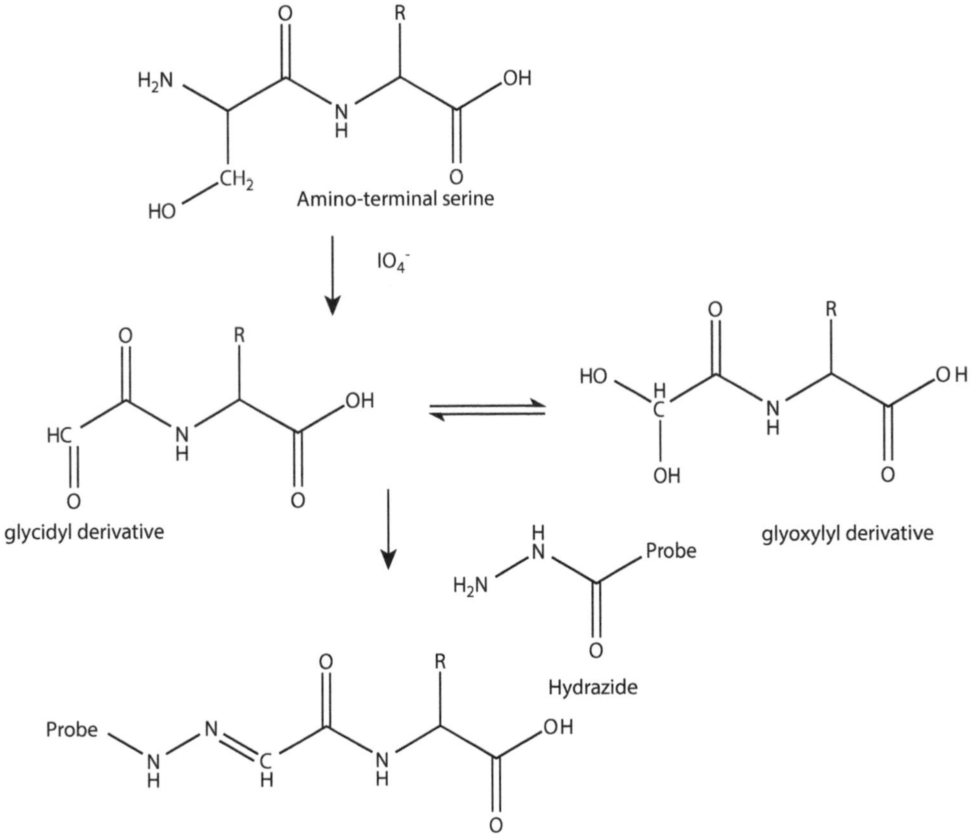

Schiff Base

Amino-terminal serine

glycidyl derivative

glyoxylyl derivative

Hydrazide

Probe

Glycol cleavage: The glycol cleavage of carbohydrates is the oxidative cleavage of a carbon–carbon bond between vicinal hydroxyl groups resulting in the formation of aldehydes which can, for example, be coupled to amino groups. Amino-terminal serine or threonine is also subjected to glycol cleavage (From Chai, W., Stoll, M.S., Cashmore, G.C., and Lawson, A.M., Specificity of mild periodate oxidation of oligosaccharide-alditols: Relevance to the analysis of the core-branching pattern of O-linked glycoprotein oligosaccharides, *Carbohydr. Res.*, 239, 107–115, 1993; Zhong, Y.L., and Shing, T.K., Efficient and facile glycol cleavage oxidation using improved silica gel-supported sodium metaperiodate, *J. Org. Chem.*, 62, 2622–2624, 1997; Balakrishnan, B., Lesieur, S., Labarre, D., and Jayakrishnan, A., Periodate oxidation of sodium alginate in water and in ethanol-water mixture: A comparative study, *Carbohydr. Res.*, 340, 1425–1429, 2005; Liu, B., Burdine, L., and Kodadek, T., Chemistry of periodate-mediated cross-linking of 3,4-dihydroxyphenylalanine-containing molecules to proteins,

J. Am. Chem. Soc., 128, 15228–15235, 2006; Chelius, D., and Shaler, T.A., Capture of peptides with N-terminal serine and threonine: A sequence-specific chemical method for peptide mixture simplification, *Bioconjug. Chem.*, 14, 205–211, 2003).

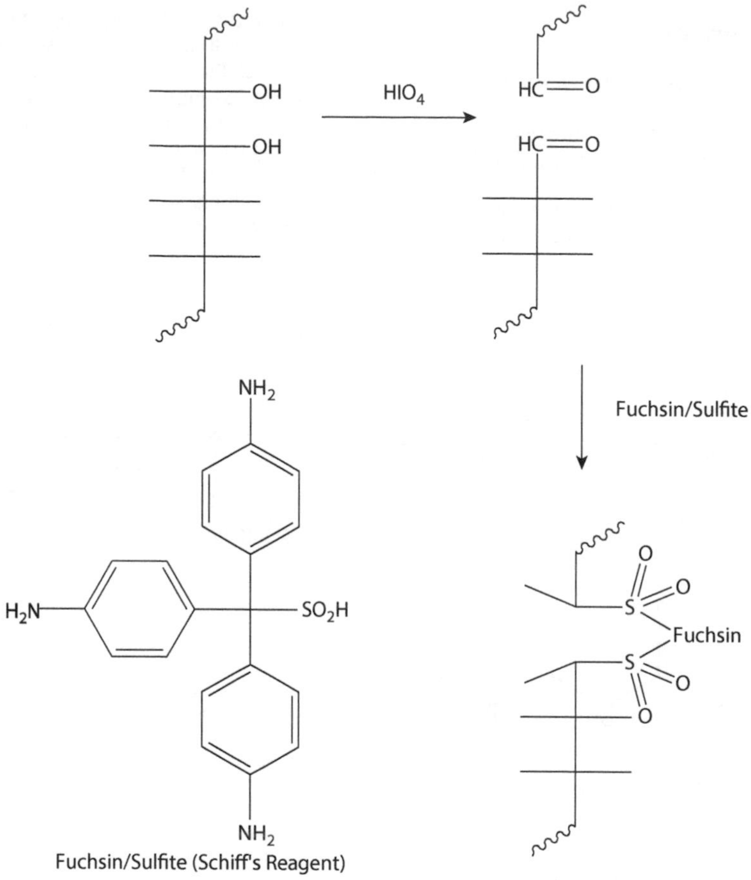

Fuchsin/Sulfite (Schiff's Reagent)

The periodic acid–Schiff (PAS) reaction for carbohydrate. This figure shows the oxidation of a vicinal diol in a monosaccharide yielding dialdehyde which then reacts with Schiff's reagent (fuchsin-sulfite). Schiff's reagent is prepared by dissolving 4-rosanilin (*p*-rosanilin) in sulfurous acid (sulfur dioxide in water). (For further information, see Jackson, E.L., and Hudson, C.S., The structure of the products of the periodic acid oxidation of starch and cellulose, *J. Am. Chem. Soc.*, 60, 988–991, 1938; Hotchkiss, R.D., A microchemical reaction resulting in the staining of polysaccharide structures in fixed tissue preparations, *Arch. Biochem.*, 16, 131–141, 1948; McManus, J.F.A., and Cason, J.E., Carbohydrate histochemistry studied by acetylation techniques, *J. Exptl. Med.*, 91, 651–654, 1950.)

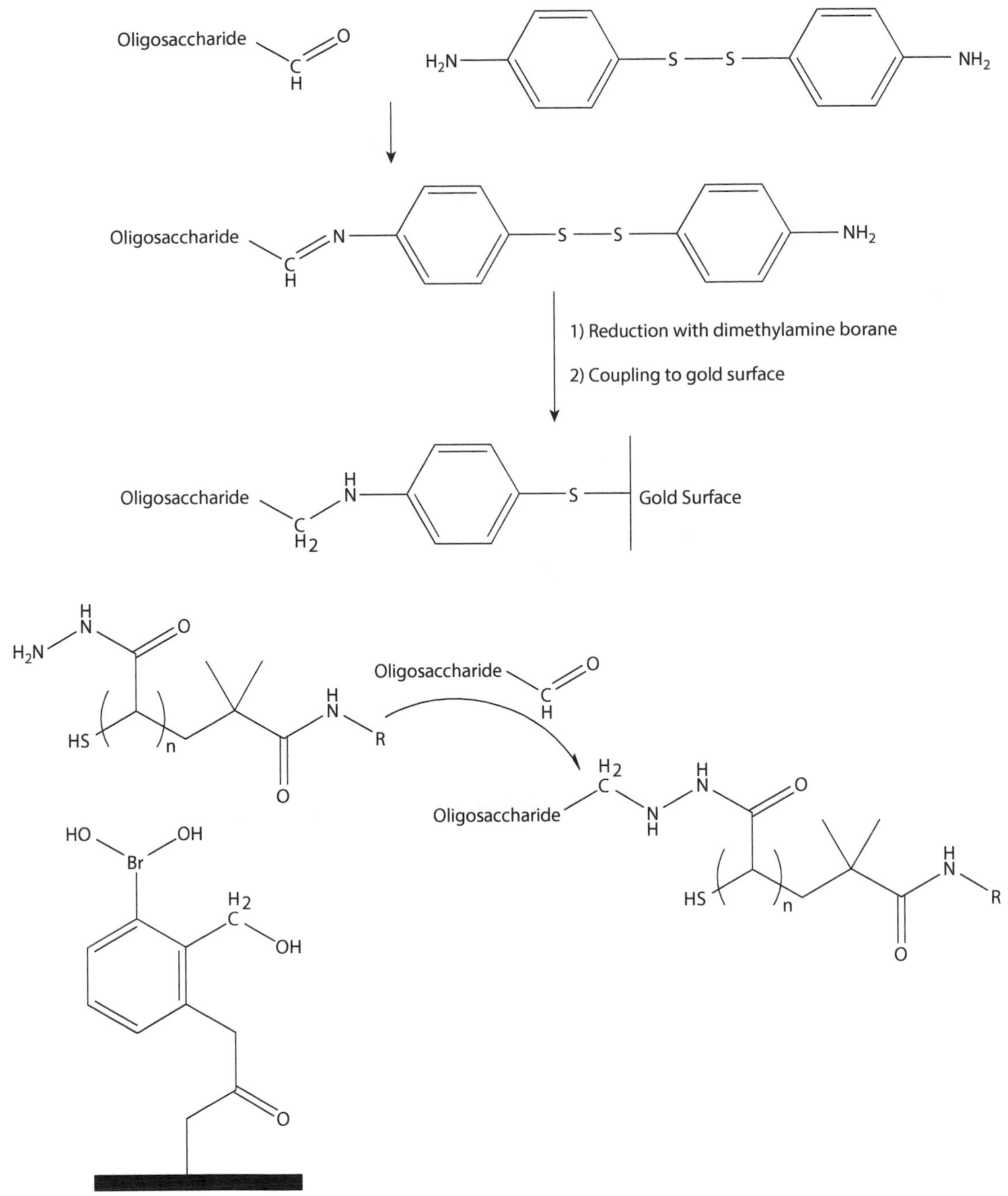

The reaction of terminal reducing sugars of oligosaccharides. This figure shows the immobilization of an oligosaccharide to a gold surface via coupling via the terminal reducing sugars. The oligosaccharide is coupled to the 4-aminodisulfide via the aldehyde function and then reduced; although disulfide is used for coupling, the interaction with the gold surface occurs via the sulfhydryl groups (From Seo, J.H., Adachi, K., and Lee, B.K., Facile and rapid direct gold surface immobilization with controlled orientation for carbohydrates, *Bioconjug. Chem.*, 18, 2197–2201, 2007). The figure shown below is the coupling of oligosaccharide to a hydrazide scaffold (From Godula, K., and Bertozzi, C.R., Synthesis of glycopolymers for microarray applications via ligation of reducing sugars to a poly(acryloyl hydrazide) scaffold, *J. Am. Chem. Soc.*, 132, 9963–9965, 2010). Also shown is the 5-amino-2-hydroxyphenyl boronic acid coupled to a matrix for use as a carbohydrate microarray (From Hsiao, H.-Y., Chen, M.-L., Wu, H.-T., et al., Fabrication of carbohydrate microarrays through boronate formation, *Chem. Commun.*, 47(4), 1187–1189, 2011).

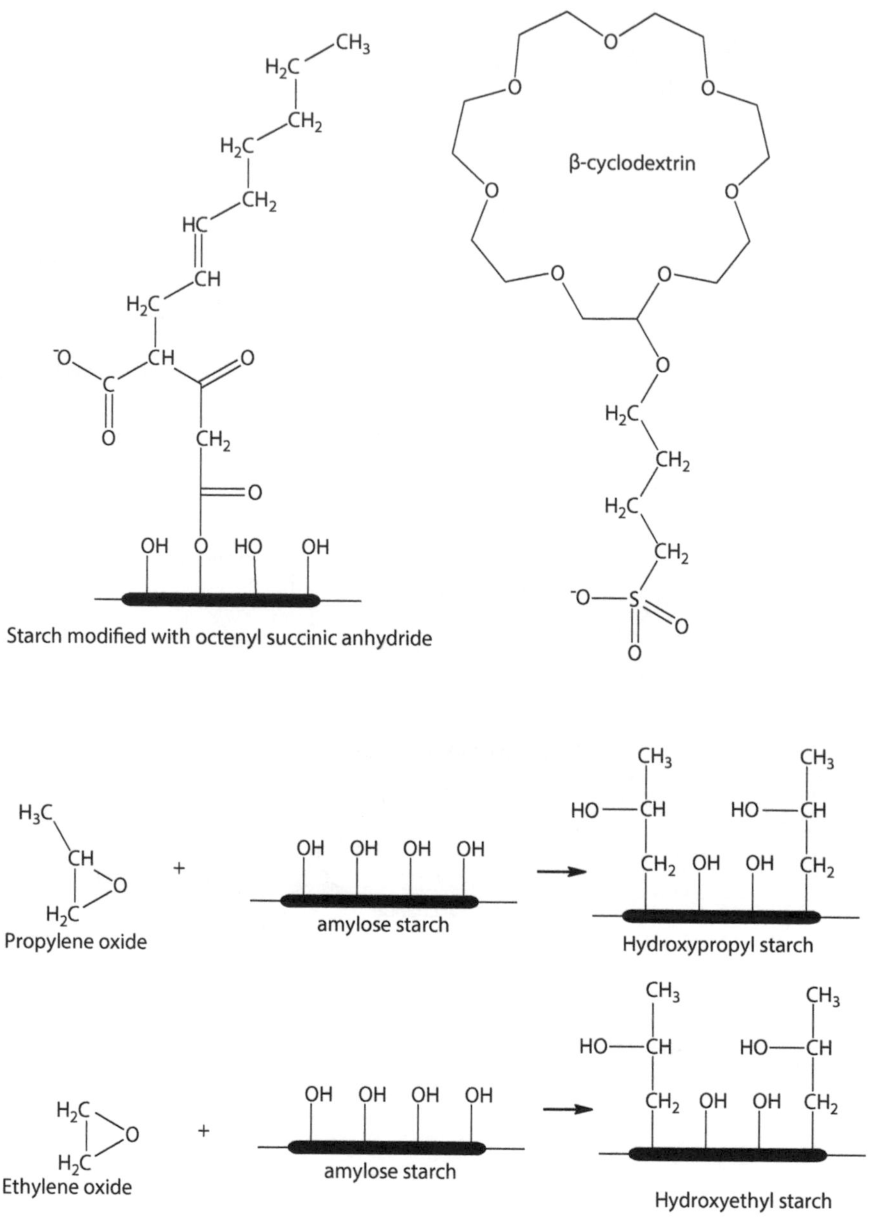

Starch modified with octenyl succinic anhydride

β-cyclodextrin

Propylene oxide + amylose starch → Hydroxypropyl starch

Ethylene oxide + amylose starch → Hydroxyethyl starch

The chemical modification of starch. This figure shows the product of the reaction of octenyl succinic anhydride with amylose starch (From Wang, J., Su, L., and Wang, S., Physicochemical properties of octenyl succinic anhydride-modified potato starch with different degrees of substitution, *J. Sci. Food Agric.*, 90, 424–429, 2010) and a schematic representation of sulfobutylether-β-cyclodextrin (From Zin, V., Rajewski, R.A., and Stella, V.J., Effect of cyclodextrin charge on complexation of neutral and charged substrates: Comparison of (SBE)$_{7M}$-β-CD to HP-β-CD, *Pharm. Res.*, 18, 667–673, 2001). Also shown is the reaction of propylene oxide with starch to form hydroxypropyl starch (From Pal, J., Singhai, P.R., and Kulkarni, P.R., A comparative account of conditions of synthesis of hydroxypropyl derivative from corn and amaranth starch, *Carbohydrate Polymers*, 43, 55–103, 2000) and with ethylene oxide to form hydroxyethyl starch.

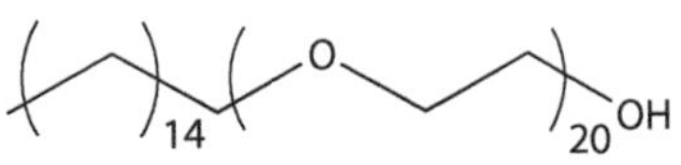

Brij 58P

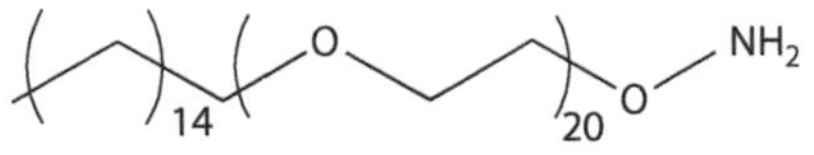

Hydroxylamine derivative

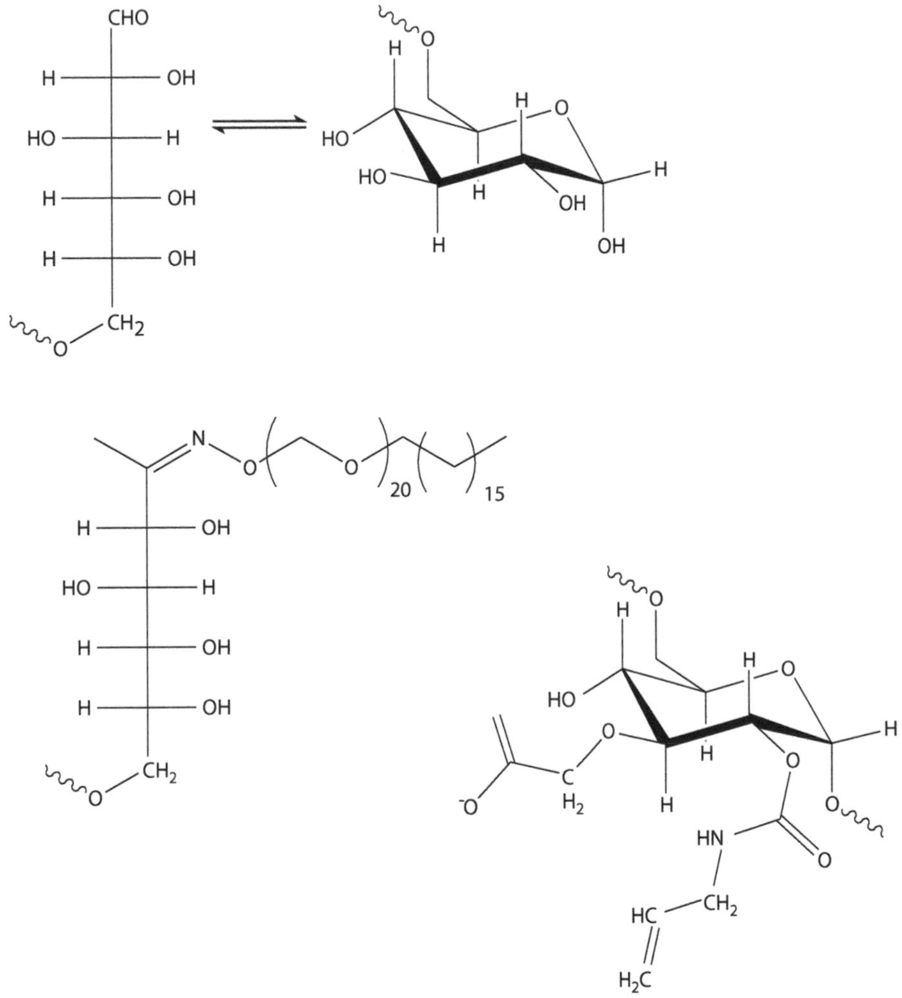

Example of the chemical modification of dextran. This figure shows the modification of dextran via the terminal reducing sugar (From Richard, A., Barras, A., Younes, A.B., et al., Minimal chemical modification of reductive end of dextran to produce an amphiphilic polysaccharide able to incorporate onto lipid nanocapsules, *Bioconjug. Chem.*, 19, 1491–1495, 2008). Also shown is a dextran derivative which can be crosslinked by UV irradiation (From Sun, G., Shen, Y.-I., Ho, C.C., et al., Functional groups affect physical and biological properties of dextran-based hydrogels, *J. Biomed. Mater. Res.*, 93A, 1080–1090, 2009).

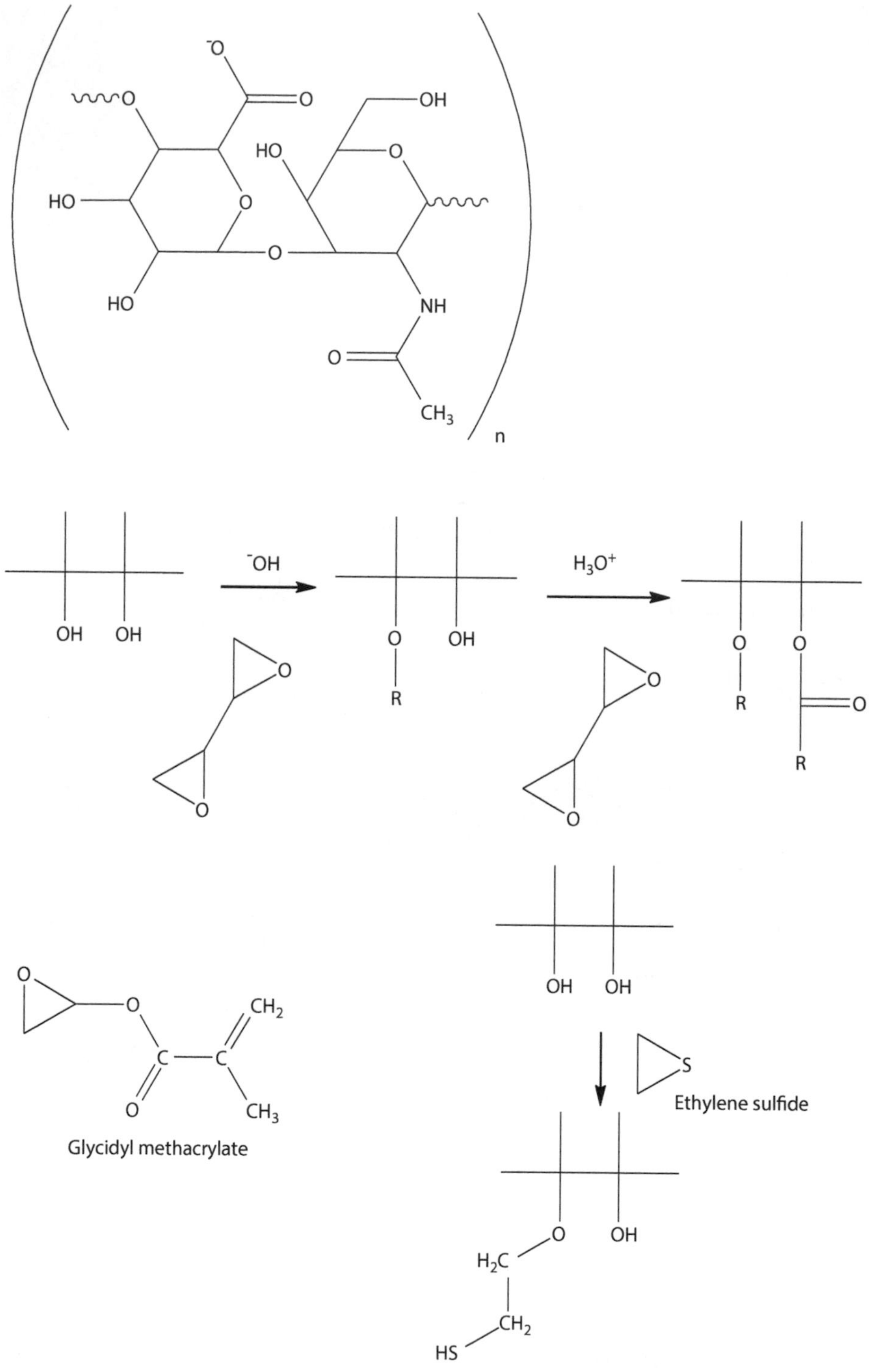

Chemical modification of hyaluronan. This figure shows a schematic structure of the repeated glucosamine-glucuronic acid disaccharide of hyaluronan and a two-step crosslinking process which uses pH as the control for differentiating between ether formation and ester formation (Zhao, X.B., Fraser, J.E., Alexander, C., et al., Synthesis and characterization of a novel double crosslinked hyaluronan hydrogel, *J. Mater. Sci. Mater. Med.*, 13, 11–16, 2002). Also shown is glycidyl methacrylate which was used for photocrosslinking of hyaluronan (Jha, A.K., Malik, M.S., Farach-Carson, M.C., et al., Hierarchically structured hyaluronic acid-based hydrogel matrices via the covalent integration of microgels into macroscopic networks, *Soft Matter*, 6, 5045–5055, 2010) and the reaction of ethylene sulfide with hyaluronan to yield a thioethyl ether derivative (Serban, M.A., Yang, G., and Prestwich, G.D., Synthesis, characterization and chondroprotective properties of a hyaluronan thioethyl ether derivative, *Biomaterials*, 29, 1388–1399, 2008).

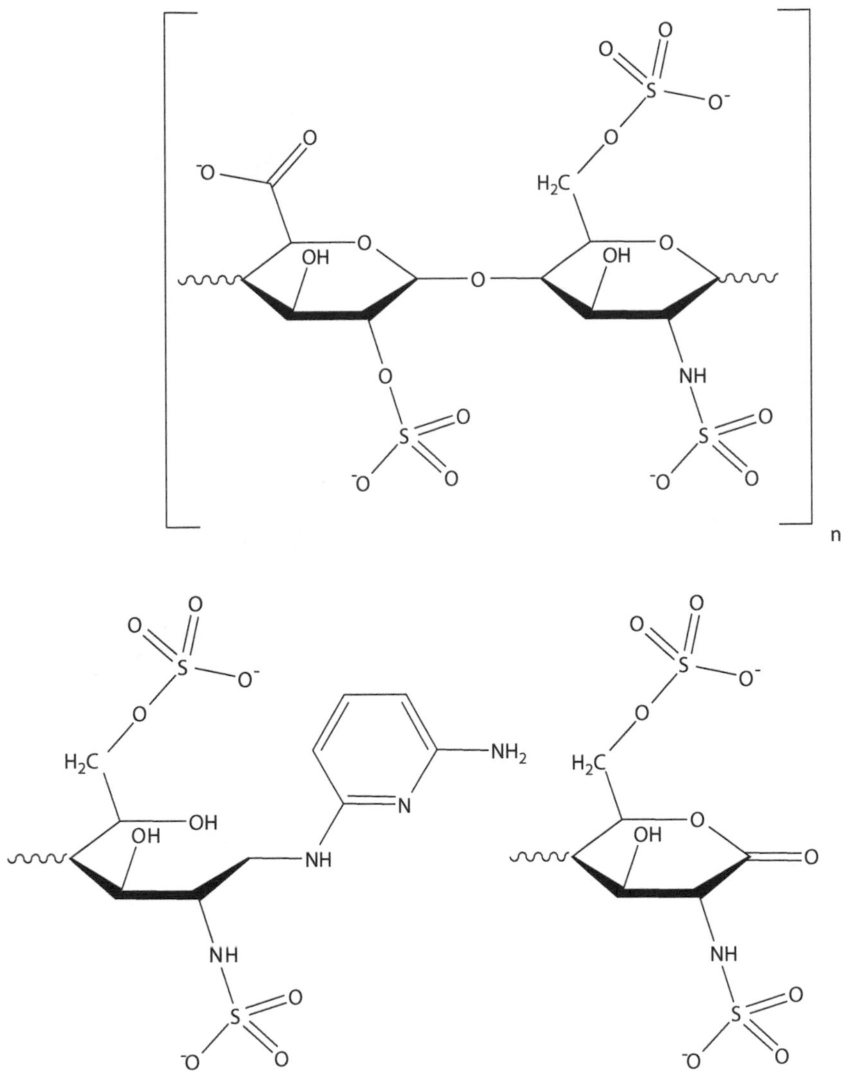

2,4-diaminopyridinyl heparin   heparin lactone

This figure shows the representation of the functional disaccharide unit with carboxyl group, O-sulfation, and N-sulfation (see Petitou, M., Casu, B., and Lindahl, U., 1976–1983, A critical period in the history of heparin: the discovery of the antithrombin binding site, *Biochimie*, 85, 83–89, 2003, for more accurate structural information). It is important to emphasize that the N-sulfated derivative is presented; the amino group may also be acetylated. Also shown are derivatives of the reducing end unit permitting orientation on a support (Nadkarni, V.D., Pervin, A., and Linhardt, R.J., Directional immobilization of heparin onto beaded supports, *Analyt. Biochem.*, 222, 59–67, 1994).

Structure and reactions of chitin and chitosan. This monomer unit of chitin is *N*-acetylglucosamine (left) which can be converted to chitosan where the monomer unit is glucosamine. Chitosan can be modified by trichloroacetic anhydride to yield the *N*-trichloroacetyl derivative which can be subjected to heterogeneous copolymerization with methyl acrylate (Jenkins, J.W., and Hudson, S.M., Heterogeneous graft copolymerization of chitosan powder with methyl acrylate using trichloroacetyl-manganese carbonyl co-initiation, *Macromolecules*, 33, 3413–3419, 2002). Also shown is the formation of a graft copolymer of carboxymethyl chitosan and methyl acrylate (El-Sherbiny, I.M., Abdel-Bary, E.M., and Harding, D.R.K., Preparation and *in vitro* evaluation of new pH-sensitive hydrogel beads for oral delivery of protein drugs, *J. Appl. Polym. Sci.*, 115, 2828–2837, 2010).

Galactose oxidase: Galactose oxidase can be used as sensors for the detection of galactose.

Leskovac, V., Trivic, S., Wohlfahrt, G., et al., Glucose oxidase from *Aspergillus niger*: The mechanism of action of oxygen, quinines, and one-electron acceptors, *Int. J. Biochem. Cell. Biol.*, 37, 731–750, 2005.

Willner, I., Baron, R., and Willner, B., Integrated nanoparticle-biomolecule systems for biosensing and bioelectronics, *Biosens. Bioelectron.*, 22, 1841–1852, 2007.

Galactose oxidase: Galactose oxidase can be used as sensors for the detection of galactose. The ability of galactose oxidase to convert the C-6 hydroxyl to an aldehyde provides a mechanism for coupling with amines via Schiff base formation.

Osuga, D.T., Feather, M.S., Shah, M.J, and Feeney, R.E., Modification of galactose and N-acetylgalactose amine residues by oxidation of C-6 hydroxyls followed by reductive amination: Model systems and antifreeze glycoproteins, *J. Prot. Chem.*, 8, 519–528, 1989.

Whittacker, J.W., The radical chemistry of galactose oxidase, *Arch. Biochem. Biophys.*, 433, 227–239, 2005.

Kondakova, L., Yanishpolskii, V., Tertykh, V., and Bulglova, T., Galactose oxidase immobilized on silica in an analytical determination of galactose-containing carbohydrates, *Analyt. Sci.*, 23, 97–101, 2007.

Alberton, D., de Olivera, L.S., Peralta, R.M. et al., Production, purification, and characterization of a novel galactose oxidase from *Fusarium acumindatum*, *J. Basic Microbiol.*, 47, 203–212, 2007.

Henderson, G.E., Isett, K.D., and Gerngross, T.U., Site-specific modification of recombinant proteins: A novel platform for modifying glycoproteins expressed in *E.coli*, *Bioconjug. Chem.*, 22, 903–912, 2011.

Dalkiran, B., Erden, P.E., and Kilic, E., Electrochemical biosensing of galactose based on carbon materials: Graphene versus multi-walled carbon nanotubes, *Anal. Bioanal. Chem.*, 408, 4329–4339, 2016.

SOME PROPERTIES OF GLYCOSAMINOGLYCANS

Roger L. Lundblad

Some Properties of Glycosaminoglycans (GAG) and Their Chemical Modification

Glycosaminoglycans are a group of large polysaccharide polymers which may contain modifications such as sulfation or N-acetylation. Glycosaminoglycans were previously described as mucopolysaccharides; the term *mucopolysaccharides* is still used.

Hyaluronan

Hyaluronan is a linear polysaccharide consisting of a repeating disaccharide with one residue possessing an acetamido group and the other a carboxylic acid (uronic acid).[1] Hyaluronan can be quite large (6000–8000 kDa). The large size and linear nature combined with the high negative charge are responsible for the viscosity of hyaluronan solution which is critical for its function as a lubricating agent.[2-5] Most of the chemical modification of hyaluronan (Figure 1) focuses on hydrogel development.[6-9] Zhao and coworkers[6] prepared a "double-crosslinked" hyaluronan hydrogel in a two-step process using the same crosslinking reagents but different reaction conditions. The first step is performed under strong alkaline conditions yielding a hyaluronan derivative crosslinked by ether bonds between hydroxyl groups (Figure 1). The second step is performed at acid pH yielding an ester derivative between carboxyl groups. Segura and coworkers[7] modified carboxyl groups with a diamine using carbodiimide chemistry as a method to attach biotin to hyaluronan. These investigators also used a poly(ethylene glycol) diepoxide to crosslink hyaluronan via hydroxyl group on the pyranose ring. Richer and coworkers[8] modified hyaluronan with 4-vinylaniline using carbodiimide technology. The modified hyaluronan was photopolymerized to the polylactic acid membrane. Jha and coworkers[9] have modified hyaluronan with glycidyl methacrylate (Figure Glyco G1) and then used photo-crosslinking to prepare hydrogels. Serban and coworkers[10] prepared a thioethyl ether derivative of hyaluronan (Figure 1) which had unique therapeutic potential. Mlcochová and coworkers[11] used cyanogen bromide coupling to prepare carbamate-linked alkyl derivatives of hyaluronan. Prestwich and Kuo[12] have a recent review of the development and use of chemically modified hyaluronan derivatives.

Heparin

Heparin is a sulfated glycosaminoglycan/proteoglycan derived from biological tissue[13,14] and is used primarily as an acute anticoagulant drug which also has an effect on lipid metabolism.[15] Heparin, with its various modifications (Figure 2) including the variable content of protein remaining from the manufacturing processes, is a heterogeneous protein with multiple sites available for modification. Iverius[16] suggested that the cyanogen bromide-coupling of heparin to agarose beads occurs via a serine or peptide residue at the reducing end of the polysaccharide. Gentry and Alexander[17] also used cyanogen bromide to prepare heparin bound to agarose. Danishefsky and coworkers[18] compared cyanogen bromide coupling of heparin to agarose with heparin coupled to aminohexyl-agarose using carbodiimide technology. Some differences were observed in the performance of the two matrices. Nadkarni and coworkers[19] modified the reducing end of heparin producing several derivatives (Figure 2). Fry and coworkers[20] used iminothiolane (Traut's reagent) to modify heparin with a terminal amino group to obtain a derivative with a free sulfhydryl available for coupling to a matrix. Other chemical modification studies on heparin have focused on inclusion in to hydrogels via crosslinking through the carboxyl or the amino group (after deacetylation).[21] Tae and workers[22] converted the carboxyl groups into thiol functions by carbodiimide-mediated reaction with cystamine. Kim and coworkers[23] also used thiolated heparin to form a hydrogel with acrylated poly(ethylene glycol) for encapsulating cells.

Chitin and Chitin Derivatives

Chitin is another long-chain glucose-based polymer (Figure 3); the monomer unit is N-acetylglucosamine.[24] Chitin is a major component of the exoskeletons of insects, crabs, lobsters, and other related organisms. Chitosan is a heterogeneous copolymer of *N-acetylglucosamine* (20%) and *N*-glucosamine (80%)[25,26] derived from chitin by alkaline hydrolysis.[27] Chitin is the second most abundant naturally occurring polysaccharide and has a role in the mineralization of the exoskeleton of arthropods (*phylum arthropoda*).[25,26] Chitin is also suggested for clinical application for hard tissue problems.[28-30] Chitin is similar to cellulose in composition (chitin is essentially a homopolymer of N-acetylglucosamine, whereas cellulose is a homopolymer of glucose), functional properties, and importance of insolubility for function with the note that chitin is more insoluble and more inert. Selective protection/deprotection can permit regioselective modification (regioselective in this sense refers to driving modification toward one of the several hydroxyl group on the pyranose ring).[31] The observation[32] that β-chitin obtained from squid is more reactive than α-chitin obtained from shrimp has proved useful in subsequent studies where trimethylsialylation was used to modify hydroxyl groups.[33] The modification of chitin can use chitin whiskers.[34,35] Chitin whiskers are microfibrils that contain protein in addition to the polysaccharide. Chitin whiskers can be incorporated into natural rubber by chemical modification to form nanocomposites.[36] Cunha and Gandini[37] have recently reviewed the progress on using chemical and/or physical modification to convert chitin and chitosan to more hydrophobic derivatives. The most useful chemical modification of chitin is the conversion to chitosan by alkaline hydrolysis.[38] The use of chitin deacetylase[39] is attracting attention as the chitosan product is more homogeneous than the product derived from alkaline hydrolysis; however, the physical characteristics of chitin present issues with respect to process efficiency.[40] The presence of a free amino group provides more opportunities for the chemical modification both in somewhat improved solubility and a reasonable nucleophile for modification.

There is considerable interest in chitosan for drug delivery including gene therapy vectors.[41-46] In addition to gene therapy applications,[47-49] Alatorre-Meda[49] has evaluated the effect of chitosan size and charge density on transfection ability. The term *valence* is used together with charge density and pH as attributes: DNA binding and transfection efficiency. The term *valence* is described by Maurstad and coworkers[50] to describe the total charge per chitosan molecule. This is different from the common

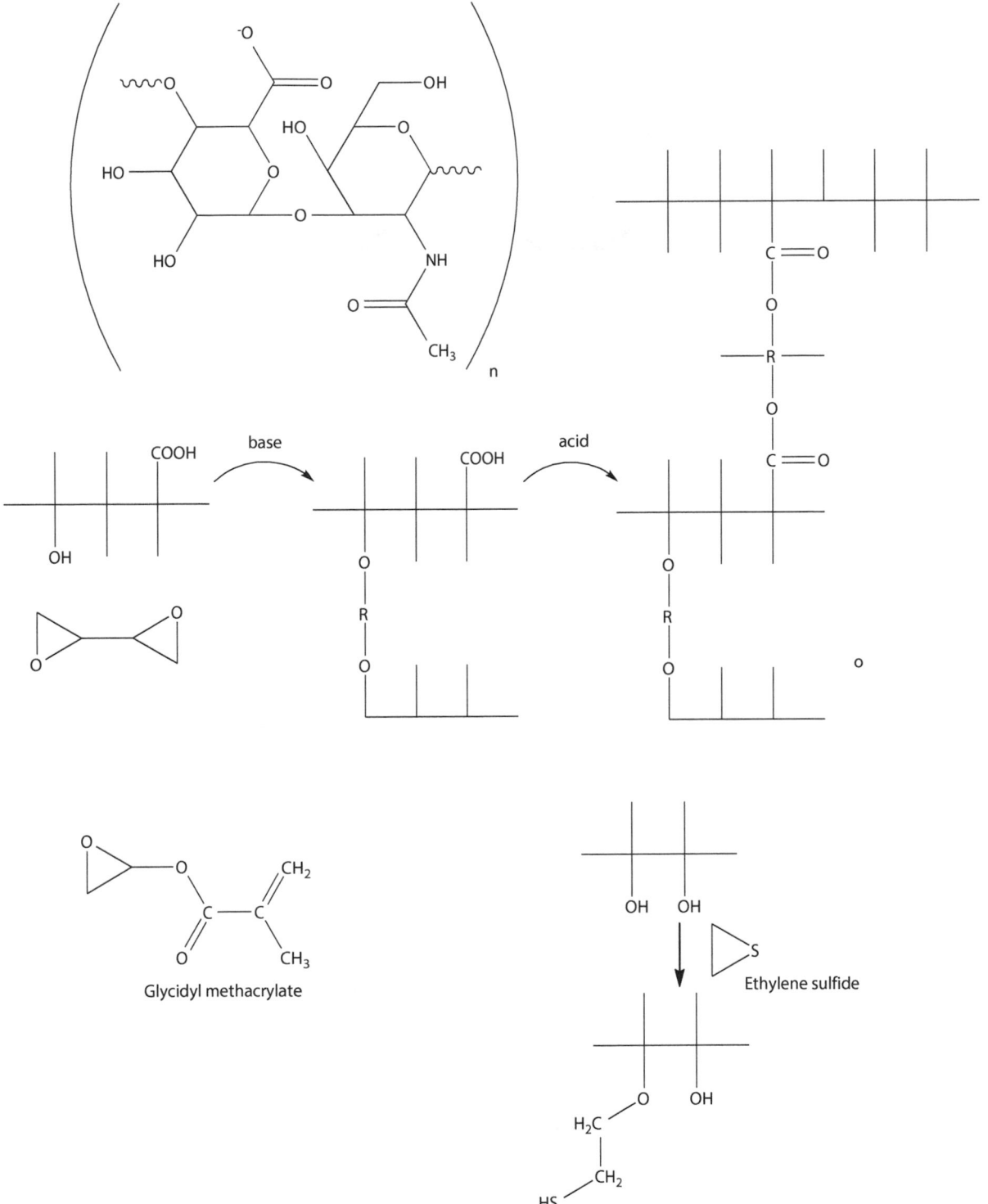

FIGURE 1 Chemical modification of hyaluronan. The figure shows a schematic structure of the repeated glucosamine-glucuronic acid disaccharide of hyaluronan. Also shown below is a process for producing hyaluronan hydrogels via a two-step crosslinking process which uses pH as the control for differentiating between ether formation and ester formation (Zhao, X.B., Fraser, J.E., Alexander, C., et al., Synthesis and characterization of a novel double crosslinked hyaluronan hydrogel, *J. Mater. Sci. Mater. Med.*, 13, 11–16, 2002). Also shown is glycidyl methacrylate which was used for photocrosslinking of hyaluronan (Jha, A.K., Malik, M.S., Farach-Carson, M.C., et al., Hierarchically structured hyaluronic acid-based hydrogel matrices via the covalent integration of microgels into macroscopic networks, *Soft Matter*, 6, 5045–5055, 2010) and the reaction of ethylene sulfide with hyaluronan to yield a thioethyl ether derivative (Serban, M.A., Yang, G., and Prestwich, G.D., Synthesis, characterization and chondroprotective properties of a hyaluronan thioethyl ether derivative, *Biomaterials*, 29, 1388–1399, 2008).

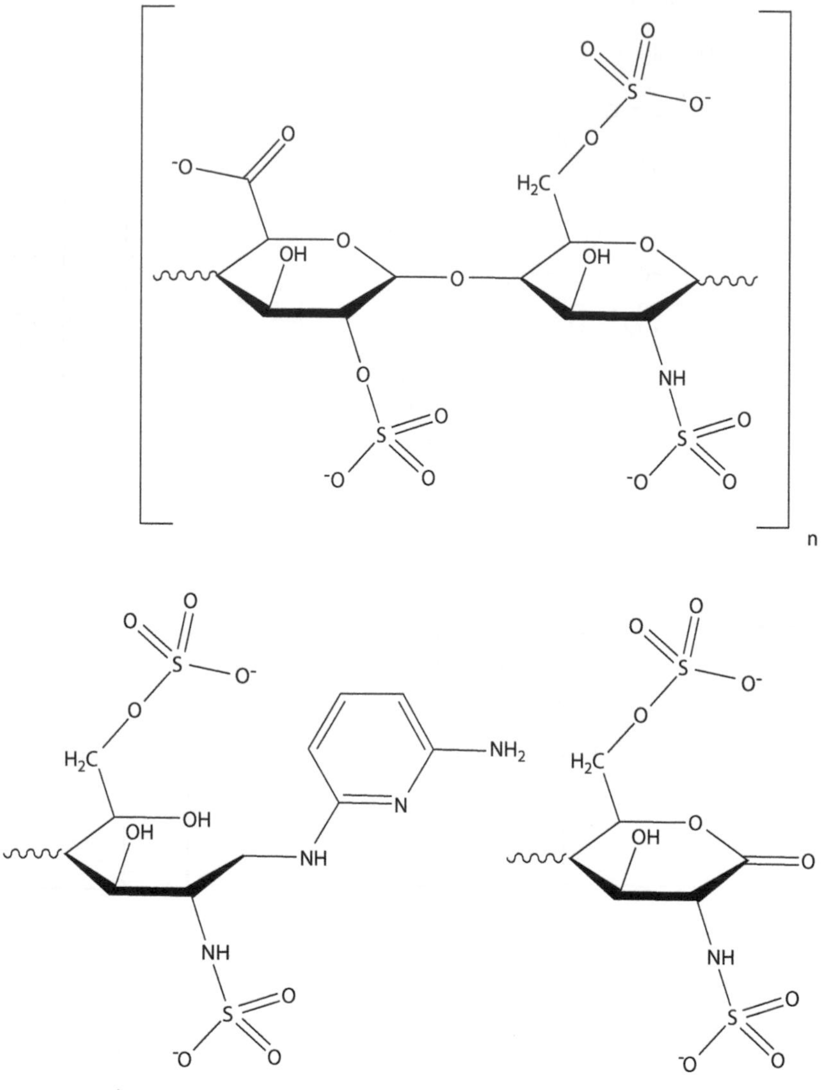

2,4-diaminopyridinyl heparin   heparin lactone

FIGURE 2 Heparin structure and chemical modification. The figure shows the representation of the functional disaccharide unit with carboxyl group, *O*-sulfation, and *N*-sulfation (see Petitou, M., Casu, B., and Lindahl, U., 1976–1983, A critical period in the history of heparin: The discovery of the antithrombin binding site, *Biochimie*, 85, 83–89, 2003, for more accurate structural information). It is important to emphasize that the *N*-sulfated derivative is presented; the amino group may also be acetylated. Also shown are derivatives of the reducing end unit permitting orientation on a support (Nadkarni, V.D., Pervin, A., and LInhardt, R.J., Directional immobilization of heparin onto beaded supports, *Analyt. Biochem.*, 222, 59–67, 1994).

understanding of valence in chemistry which refers to the number of bonding electrons in an atom. The term *valence* is also used to describe the number of antigen binding sites on an antibody or vice versa. A quick check of PubMed shows that the term *valence* is also used in psychology but the *Oxford English Dictionary*[51] is mute on this point but does define valency as strength. Chitosan is of value for colon drug delivery.[52–56]

Chitosan can be subjected to chemical modification using techniques as described above for other polysaccharides to improve characteristics for therapeutic applications.[27] This is useful time to emphasize that the various biological polymers which have been described in the current work are, in fact, chemical polymers such as polyurethane, polystyrene, or polyacrylate but differ from these polymers in the variety and complexity of the monomer units. Polysaccharides, such as chitosan, can be combined

via graft polymerization with classical polymer monomers such as methyl acrylate or acrylonitrile.[57–59] Jenkins and Hudson[57] prepared a graft polymer of chitosan and methyl acrylate using heterogeneous graft copolymerization (Figure Glyco G3). Chitosan was trifluoroacetylated and methyl acrylate polymer "built" from the trichloromethyl group upon reaction with manganese carbonyl using photoactivation. For the non-polymer chemist, the term *heterogeneous graft polymerization* describes a reaction that occurs in two phases.[60] El-Sherbiny and workers[61] address the issue of chitosan solubility by preparing the carboxymethyl derivative (Figure 3) using reaction with chloroacetic acid. This derivative was then graft copolymerized with methacrylic acid (Figure 3) and combined with alginate as biodegradable hydrogel for oral drug delivery. Graft polymerization of carboxymethyl chitosan with acrylic acid has also been reported.[62]

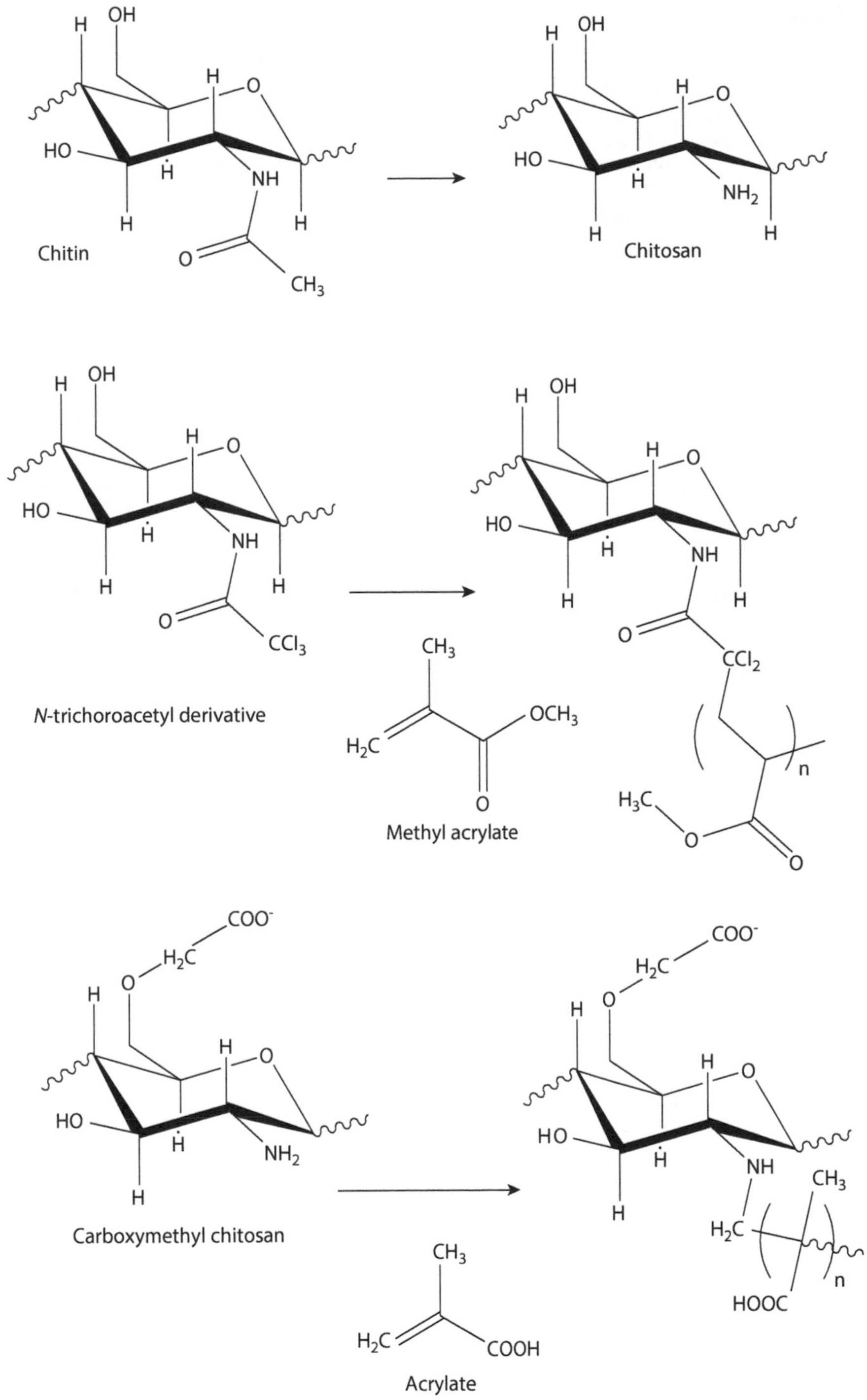

FIGURE 3 Structure and reactions of chitin and chitosan. The monomer unit of chitin is *N*-acetylglucosamine (left) which can be converted to chitosan where the monomer unit is glucosamine. Chitosan can be modified by trichloroacetic anhydride to yield the *N*-trichloroacetyl derivative which can be subjected to heterogeneous copolymerization with methyl acrylate (Jenkins, J.W., and Hudson, S.M., Heterogeneous graft copolymerization of chitosan powder with methyl acrylate using trichloroacetyl-manganese carbonyl co-initiation, *Macromolecules*, 33, 3413–3419, 2002). Also shown is the formation of a graft copolymer of carboxymethyl chitosan and methyl acrylate (El-Sherbiny, I.M., Abdel-Bary, E.M., and Harding, D.R.K., Preparation and *in vitro* evaluation of new pH-sensitive hydrogel beads for oral delivery of protein drugs, *J. Appl. Polym. Sci.*, 115, 2828–2837, 2010).

References

1. Cowman, M.K., and Matsuoka, S., Experimental approaches to hyaluronan structure, *Carbohydrate Res.* 340, 791–809, 2005.
2. Fam, H., Kontopoulou, M., and Bryant, J.T., Effect of concentration and molecular weight on the rheology of hyaluronic acid/bovine calf serum solutions, *Biorheology* 46, 31–43, 2009.
3. Guillaumie, F., Furrer, P., Felt-Baeyens, O., et al., Comparative studies of various hyaluronic acids produced by microbial fermentation for potential topical ophthalmic applications, *J. Biomed. Mater. Res. A* 92, 1421–1430, 2010.
4. Nyström, B., Kjøniksen, A.L., Beheshti, N., et al., Characterization of polyelectrolyte features in polysaccharide systems and mucin, *Adv.Colloid Interface Sci.* 158, 108–118, 2010.
5. James, D.F., Rick, G.M., and Baines, W.D., A mechanism to explain physiological lubrication, *J. Biomech. Eng.* 132, 071002, 2010.
6. Zhao, X.B., Fraser, J.E., Alexander, C., et al., Synthesis and characterization of a novel double crosslinked hyaluronan hydrogel, *J. Mater. Sci. Mater. Med.* 13, 11–16, 2002.
7. Segura, T., Anderson, B.C., Chung, P.H., et al., Crosslinked hyaluronic acid hydrogels: A strategy to functionalize and pattern, *Biomaterials* 26, 359–371, 2005.
8. Richter, C., Reinhardt, M., Giselbrecht, S., et al., Spatially controlled cell adhesion on three-dimensional substrates, *Biomed. Microdevices* 12, 787–795, 2010.
9. Jha, A.K., Malik, M.S., Farach-Carson, M.C., et al., Hierarchically structured, hyaluronic acid-based hydrogel matrices via the covalent integration of microgels into macroscopic networks, *Soft. Matter.* 6, 5045–5055, 2010.
10. Serban, M.A., Yang,G., and Prestwich, G.D., Synthesis, characterization and chondroprotective properties of a hyaluronan thioethyl ether derivative, *Biomaterials* 29, 1388–1399, 2008.
11. Mlcochová, P., Bystrický, S., Steiner, B., et al., Synthesis and characterization of new biodegradable hyaluronan alkyl derivatives, *Biopolymers* 82, 74–79, 2006.
12. Prestwich, G.D. and Kuo, J.W., Chemically-modified HA for therapy and regenerative medicine, *Curr. Pharm. Biotechnol.* 9, 242–245, 2008.
13. Lindahl, U., Structure of the heparin-protein linkage region, *Arkiv. Kemi.* 26, 101–110, 1966.
14. Seethanathan, P., and Ehrlich, K., Anticoagulant and antilipemic activities of heparin proteoglycan from bovine intestinal mucosa, *Thromb. Res.* 19, 95–102, 1980.
15. Lundblad, R.L., Brown, W.V., Mann, K.G., and Roberts, H.R., ed. *Chemistry and Biology of Heparin*, Elsevier/North Holland, New York, 1981.
16. Iverius, P.-H., Coupling of glycosaminoglycans to agarose beads (Sepharose 4B), *Biochem. J.* 124, 677–683, 1971.
17. Gentry, P.W., and Alexander, B., Specific coagulation adsorption to insoluble heparin, *Biochem. Biophys. Res. Commun.* 50, 500–509, 1973.
18. Danishefsky, I., Tzeng, F., Ahrens, M., and Klein, S., Synthesis of heparin-sepharoses and their binding with thrombin and antithrombin-heparin cofactor, *Thromb. Res.* 8, 131–140, 1976.
19. Nadkarni, V.D., Pervin, A., and Linhardt, R.J., Directional immobilization of heparin onto beaded supports, *Analyt. Biochem.* 222, 59–67, 1994.
20. Fry, A.K., Schilke, K.F.,McGuire, J., and Bird, K.E., Synthesis and anticoagulant activity of heparin immobilized "end-on" to polystyrene microspheres coated with end-group activated polyethylene oxide, *J. Biomed. Mater. Res. B.* 94, 187–198, 2010.
21. Kiick, K.L., Peptide- and protein-mediated assembly of heparinized hydrogels, *Soft Matter* 4, 29–37, 2008.
22. Tae, G., Kim, Y.J., Choi, W.I., et al., Formation of a novel heparin-based hydrogel in the presence of heparin-binding biomolecules, *Biomacromolecules* 8, 1979–1986, 2007.
23. Kim, M., Lee, J.Y., Jones, C.N., et al., Heparin-based hydrogel as a matrix for encapsulation and cultivation of primary hepatocytes, *Biomaterials* 31, 3596–3603, 2010.
24. Morgulis, S., The chemical constitution of chitin, *Science* 44, 866–867, 1916.
25. Tharanthan, R.N. and Kittur, F.S., Chitin—The undisputed biomolecule of great potential, *Crit. Rev. Food Sci. Nutr.* 43, 61–87, 2003.
26. Muzzarelli, R.A.A., *Chitin*, Pergamon Press, New York, 1977.
27. Alves, N.M., and Mann, J.F., Chitosan derivatives obtained by chemical modification for biomedical and environmental applications, *Int. J. Biol. Macromolecules* 43, 401–414, 2008.
28. Li, X., Liu, X., Dong, W., et al., In vitro evaluation of porous poly (L-lactic acid) scaffold reinforced by chitin fibers, *J. Biomed. Mater. Res. B.* 90, 503–509, 2009.
29. Ge, H., Zhao, B., Lai, Y., et al., From crabshell to chitosan-hydroxyapatite composite material via a biomorphic mineralization synthesis method, *J. Mater. Sci. Mater. Med.* 21, 1781–1787, 2010.
30. Swetha, M., Sahithi, K., Moothi, A., et al., Biocomposites containing natural polymers and hydroxyapatite for bone tissue engineering, *Int. J. Biol. Macromol.* 47, 1–4, 2010.
31. Kurita, K., Yoshida, Y., and Umemura, T., Finely selective protection and deprotection of multifunctional chitin and chitosan to synthesize key intermediates for regioselective chemical modifications, *Carbohydrate Polymers* 81, 434–440, 2010.
32. Kurita, K., Ishii, S., Tomita, K., et al., Reactivity characteristics of squid β-chitin as compared to those of shrimp chitin: High potentials of squid chitin as a starting material for facile chemical modifications, *J. Polymer Sci. A* 32, 1027–1032, 1994.
33. Kurita, K., Sugita, K., Kodaira, N., et al., Preparation and evaluation of trimethylsilylated chitin as a versatile precursor for facile chemical modifications, *Biomacromolecules* 6, 1414–1418, 2005.
34. Gopalan Nair, K., Dufresne, A., Gandni, A., and Gelgacem, M.N., Crab shell chitin whiskers reinforced natural rubber nanocomposites. 1. Processing and swelling behavior, *Biomacromolecules* 4, 657–665, 2003.
35. Lertwattanaseri, T., Ichikawa, N., Mizoguchi, T., et al., Microwave technique for efficient deacetylation of chitin nanowhiskers to a chitosan nanoscaffold, *Carbohydr. Res.* 344, 331–335, 2009.
36. Gopalan Nair, K., Dufresne, A., Gandni, A., and Gelgacem, M.N., Crab shell chitin whiskers reinforced natural rubber nanocomposites. 3. Effects of chemical modification of chitin whiskers, *Biomacromolecules* 4, 1835–1842, 2003.
37. Cunha, A.G., and Gandini, A., Turning polysaccharides into hydrophobic materials: A critical review. Part 2. Hemicelluloses, chitin/chitosan, starch, pectin and alginates, *Cellulose* 17, 1945–1065, 2010.
38. Hirano, S., and Usutani, A., Hydrogels of *N*-acylchitosans and their cellulose composites generated from the aqueous alkaline solutions, *Int. J. Biol. Macromol.* 20, 245–249, 1997.
39. Tsigos, I., Martinou, A., Kafetzopoulos, D., et al., Chitin deacetylases: New, versatile tools in biotechnology, *Trends Biotechnol.* 18, 305–312, 2000.
40. WIn, N.N., and Stevens, W.F., Shrimp chitin as substrate for fungal chitin deacetylase, *Appl. Microbiol. Biotechnol.* 57, 334–341, 2001.
41. Zhang, J., Xia, W., Liu, P., et al., Chitosan modification and pharmaceutical/biomedical applications, *Mar. Drugs* 8, 1962–1987, 2010.
42. Prabaharan, M., and Mano, J.F., Chitosan-based particles as controlled drug delivery systems, *Drug. Deliv.* 12, 41–57, 2005.
43. Park, J.H., Saravanakumar, G., Kim, K., and Kwon, I.C., Targeted delivery of low molecular drugs using chitosan and its derivatives, *Adv. Drug. Deliv. Rev.* 62, 28–41, 2010.
44. Tong, H., Qin, S., Fernandex, J.C., et al., Progress and prospects of chitosan and its derivatives as non-viral gene vectors in gene therapy, *Curr. Gene Ther.* 9, 495–502, 2009.
45. Xu, Q., Wang, C.H., and Pack, D.W., Polymeric carriers for gene delivery: Chitosan and poly(amidoamine) dendrimers, *Curr. Pharm. Des.* 16, 2350–2368, 2010.
46. Rudzinski, W.E., and Aminabhavi, T.M., Chitosan as a carrier for targeted delivery of small interfering RNA, *Int. J. Pharm.* 399, 1–11, 2010.
47. Raviña, M., Cubillo, E., Olmeda, D., et al., Hyaluronic acid/chitosan-g-poly(ethylene glycol) nanoparticles for gene therapy: An application for pDNA and siRNA delivery, *Pharm. Res.* 27, 2544–2555, 2010.

49. Alatorre-Meda, M., Taboada, P., Hartl, F., et al., The influence of chitosan valence on the complexation and transfection of DNA: The weaker the DNA-chitosan binding the higher the transfection efficiency, *Colloids Surf. B. Biointerfaces* 82, 54–62, 2011.

50. Maurstad, G., Danielsen, S., and Stokke, B.T., The influence of charge density of chitosan in the compaction of the polyanions DNA and xanthan, *Biomacromolecules* 8, 1124–1130, 2007.

51. XXX *Oxford English Dictionary*, Oxford University Press, Oxford, United Kingdom, 2010.

52. Hejazi, R., and Amiji, M., Chitosan-based gastrointestinal delivery systems, *J. Control. Release* 89, 151–165, 2003.

53. Chourasia, M.K., and Jain, S.K., Polysaccharides for colon targeted drug delivery, *Drug Deliv.* 11, 129–148, 2004.

54. Kosaraju, S.L., Colon targeted delivery systems: Review of polysaccharides for encapsulation and delivery, *Crit. Rev. Food Sci. Nutr.* 45, 251–258, 2005.

55. Saboktakin, M.R., Tabatabaie, R.M., Maharramov, A., and Ramazanov, M.A., Synthesis and characterization of chitosan hydrogels containing 5-aminosalicylic acid nanopendents for colon: Specific drug delivery, *J. Pharm. Sci.* 99, 4955–4961, 2010.

56. Kadiyala, I., Loo,Y., Roy, K., et al., Transport of chitosan-DNA nanoparticles in human intestinal M-cell model versus normal intestinal enterocytes, *Eur. J. Pharm. Sci.* 39, 103–109, 2010.

57. Jenkins, D.W., and Hudson, S.M., Heterogeneous graft copolymerization of chitosan power with methyl acrylate using trichloroacetyl-manganese carbonyl co-initiation, *Macromolecules* 35, 3413–3419, 2002.

58. Prashanth, K.V.H., and Tharanathan, R.N., Studies on graft polymerization of chitosan with synthetic monomers, *Carbohydrate Polymers* 54, 343–351, 2003.

59. Ulbricht, M., and Riedel, M., Ultrafiltration membrane surfaces with grafted polymer "tentacles": Preparation, characterization and application for covalent protein binding, *Biomaterials* 19, 1229–1237, 1998.

60. El-Sherbiny, J.M., Aldel-Bary, E.M., and Harding, D.R.K., Preparation and *In Vitro* evaluation of new, pH-sensitive hydrogel beads for oral delivery of protein drugs, *J. Appl. Polym. Sci.* 114, 2828–2837, 2010.

61. El-Sherbiny, E.M., and Elmahdy, M.M., Preparation, characterization, structure, and dynamics of carboxymethyl chitosan grafted with acrylic acid sodium salt, *J. Appl. Polym. Sci.* 118, 2134–2143, 2010.

62. Lv, P., Bin, Y., Yongqiang, C., et al., Studies on graft copolymerization of chitosan with acrylonitrile by the redox system, *Polymer* 50, 5675–5680, 2009.

SUGAR MIMETICS

Roger L. Lundblad

Glycomimetics

Glycomimetics, also referred to as sugar mimetics, are analogs of carbohydrates. They range from compounds where a nitrogen (iminosugars) or a sulfur molecule is substituted for oxygen to more complex structures that include "tags" for "click chemistry."

Bewley, C.A., ed. *Protein-Carbohydrate Interactions in Infectious Disease*, Royal Society of Chemistry, Cambridge, United Kingdom, 2006.

Cipolla, L., and Peri, F., Carbohydrate-based bioactive compounds for medicinal chemistry applications, *Mini Rev. Med. Chem.* 11, 39–54, 2011.

Chapleur, Y., ed. *Carbohydrate Mimics: Concepts and Methods*, Wiley-VCH, New York, 1998.

Compain, P., and Martin, O.R., Carbohydrate mimetics-based glycosyltransferase inhibitors, *Bioorg. Med. Chem.* 9, 3077–3092, 2001.

Jiménez-Barbera, J., Cañada, F.J., and Martin-Santamaria, S., ed. *Carbohydrates in Drug Design and Discovery*, Royal Society of Chemistry, Cambridge, United Kingdom, 2015.

Moran, A.P., and Holst, O., ed. *Microbial Glycobiology: Structure, Relevance, and Applications*, Academic Press/Elsevier, London, United Kingdom, 2009.

Roy, R., ed. *Glycomimetics: Modern Synthetic Methodology*, American Chemical Society, Washington, DC, 2005.

Saliba, R.C., and Pohl, N.L.B., Designing sugar mimetics: Non-natural pyranosides as innovative chemical tools, *Curr. Opin. Chem. Biol.* 34, 127–134, 2010.

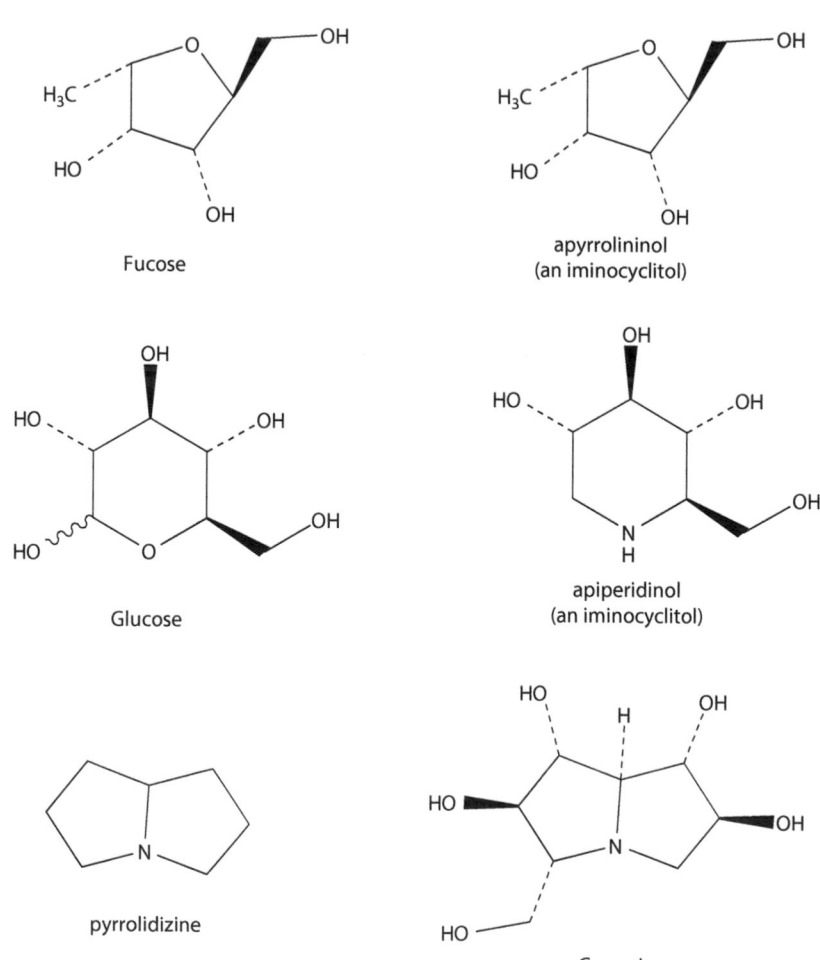

FIGURE 1 The structural basis of some glycomimetics. Ribose and hexose rings provide the structural basis for iminocyclitols which function as glycomimetics. Pyrrolidizines provide the structural basis for glycomimetics such as casuarina (Nash, R.J., Thomas, P.I., Waigh, R.D., et al., Casuarine: A very highly oxygenated pyrrolizidine alkaloid, *Tetrahedron Lett.*, 35, 7849–7852, 1994; Denmark, S.E., and Hurd, A.R., Synthesis of (+)-casuarine, *Org. Lett.*, 1, 1311–1314, 1999).

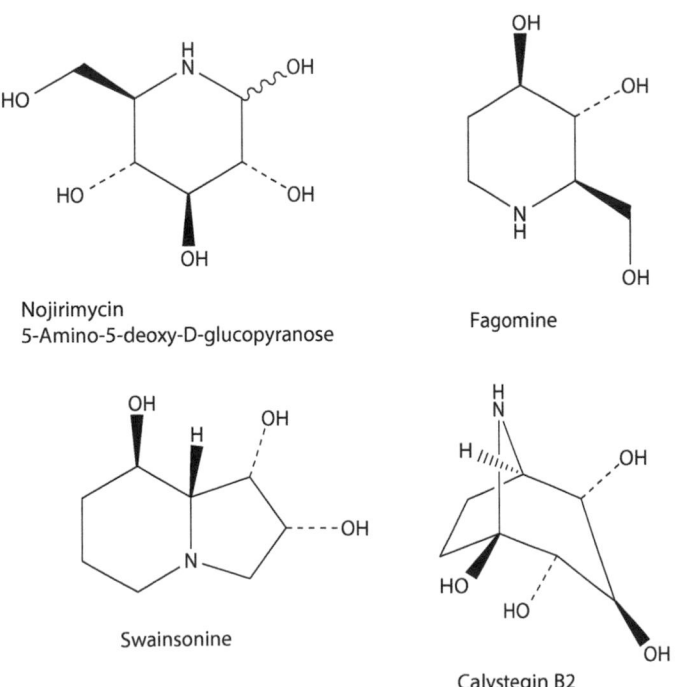

Kifor β-galactosidase 3.3 x 10⁻⁶
Kifor α-mannosidase 1.7 x 10⁻³

Pseudodisaccharide

Kifor β-galactosidase 3.3 x 10⁻⁶
Kifor α-mannosidase 1.7 x 10⁻³

Pyrrolidine derivative in equilibrium
between galactose mimic and mannose mimic

FIGURE 2 Two pyrrolidine glycomimetics with different activities reflecting equilibrium between a galactose mimic and a mannose mimic. The figure shows a pseudodisaccharide derivative with a higher activity against a β-galactosidase and a lower activity against an α-mannosidase, and also shows a less complex pyrrolidine derivative with a higher activity against an α-mannosidase than a β-galactosidase (Saotome, C., Kanie, Y., Kanie, O., and Wong, C-H., Synthesis and enzymatic evaluation of five-membered iminocyclitols and a pseudodisaccharide, *Bioorg. Med. Chem.*, 8, 2249–2261, 2000).

Nojirimycin
5-Amino-5-deoxy-D-glucopyranose

Fagomine

Swainsonine

Calystegin B2

FIGURE 3 Some naturally occurring glycomimetics (Adapted from Cipolla, L., and Peri, F., Carbohydrate-based bioactive compounds for medicinal chemistry applications, *Mini Rev. Med. Chem.*, 11, 39–54, 2011; Harit, V.K., and Ramesh, N.G., Amino-functionalized iminocyclitols: Synthetic glycomimetics of medicinal interest, *RSC Adv.*, 6, 109528–109607, 2016).

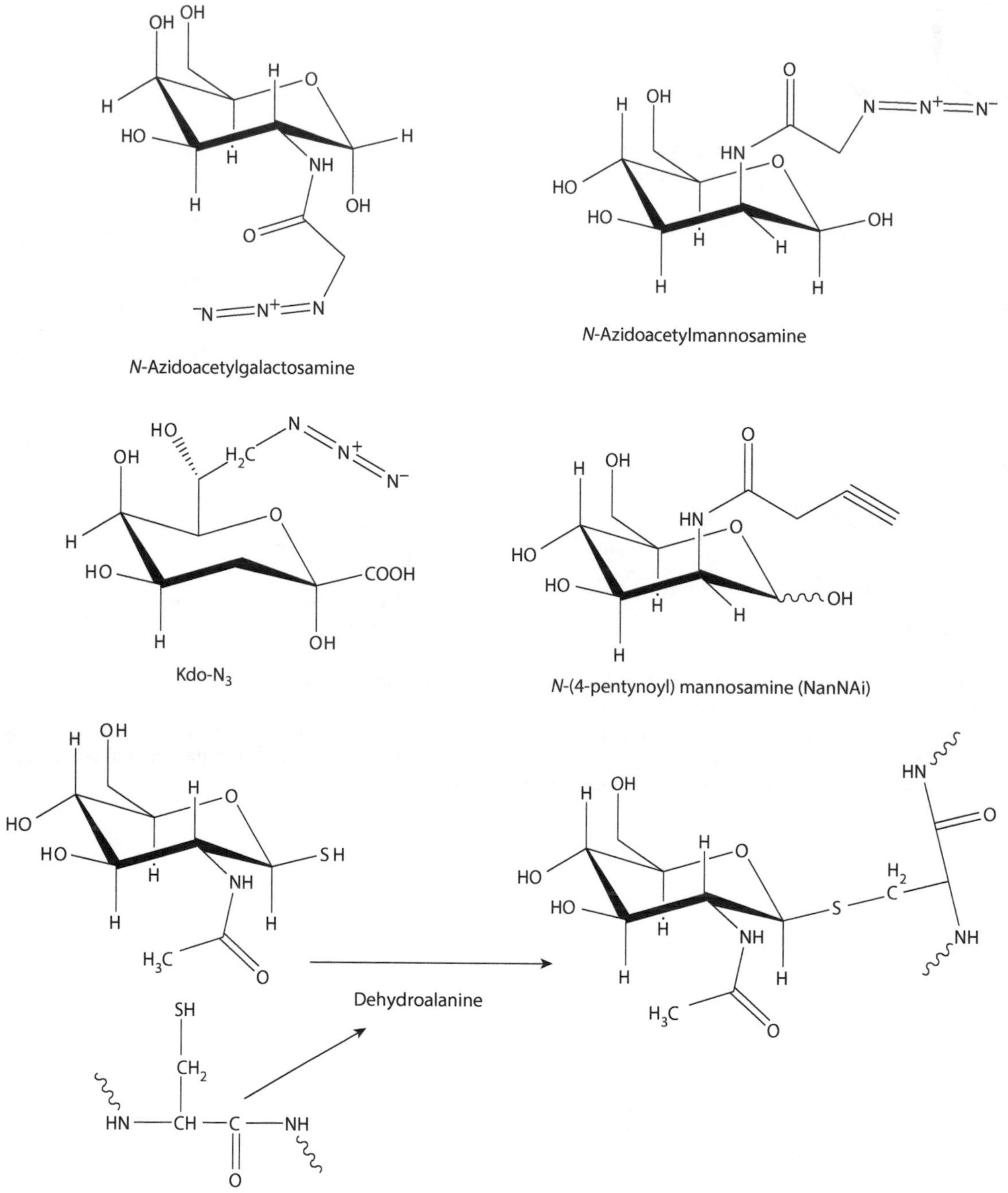

FIGURE 4 Some glycomimetic probes for chemical biology. *N*-Azidoacetylgalactosamine (Neves, A.A., Stöckmann, H., Wainman, Y.A., et al., Imaging cell surface glycosylation in vivo using "double click" chemistry, *Bioconjug. Chem.*, 24, 934–941, 2013) and *N*-azidoacetylmannosamine (Neves, A.A., Stöckmann, H., Harmston, R.R., et al., Imaging sialylated tumor cell glycans *in vivo*, *FASEB J.*, 8, 2528–2537, 2017) have been used to label glycans *in vivo*. The two derivatives are presented as peracetylated derivatives. Plant cell wall has been imaged using Kdo-N₃ (8-azido 8-deoxy 3-deoxy-D-*manno*-oct-2-ulosonic acid) (Dumont, M., Lehner, A., Vauzeilles, B., et al., Plant cell wall imaging by metabolic click-mediated labelling of rhammogalacturonan II using azido 3-deoxy-D-*manno*-oct-2-ulosonic acid, *Plant J.*, 85, 437–447, 2016). *N*-(4-Pentynol)mannosamine (NAnNAi) is taken into the cell, incorporated into a glycan, and subsequently labeled with an azide-labeled fluorescent probe (Gilomini, P.A., Lion, C., Vicogne, D., et al., A sequential bioorthogonal dual strategy: ManNAI and SiaNAI as distinct tools to unravel sialic acid metabolic pathways, *Chem. Comm.*, 52, 2318–2321, 2016). A thiol derivative of glucose is used to couple to dehydroalanine to yield an analogue for the posttranslational modification of proteins with *N*-acetylglucosamine (Lercher, L., Raj, R., Patel, N.A., et al., Generation of a synthetic GlcNAcylated nucleosome reveals regulation of stability by H2A-Thr101 GlnNAcylation, *Nat. Commun.*, 6, 7978, 2015. doi: 10.1038/ncomms8978). 8-Azido-8-deoxy-3-deoxy-D-*manno*-oct-2-ulosonic acid (8-azido 8 deoxy Kdo, Kdo-N₃) can be incorporated into a cell wall pectin and then reacted with an alkyne derivative of a fluorescent probe using click chemistry (Dumont, M., Lehner, A., Vauszeilles, B., et al., Plant cell wall imaging by metabolic click-mediated labeling of rhamnogalacturonan II using azido 3-deoxy-D-*manno*-oct-2-ulosonic acid, *Plant J.*, 85, 437–447, 2016).

INTRINSIC VISCOSITY OF POLYSACCHARIDES

Roger L. Lundblad

The intrinsic viscosity of a polymer can be considered as a measure of asymmetry and is independent of concentration (see Kyte, J., *Structure in Protein Chemistry*, 2nd edn., p. 278, Garland Science/Taylor & Francis, New York, 2007).

General References for the Study of the Viscosity of Polysaccharides

Harding, S.E., Abdelhameed, A.S., and Morris, G.A., Molecular weight distribution evaluation of polysaccharides and glycoconjugates using analytical ultracentrifugation, *Macromol. Biosci.* 10, 714–720, 2010.

Harding, S.E., The intrinsic viscosity of biological macromolecules. Progress in measurement, interpretation and application to structure in dilute solution, *Prog. Biophys. Mol. Biol.* 68, 207–262, 1997.

Carraher, C.E., Jr., *Introduction to Polymer Chemistry*, 3rd edn., CRC Press/Taylor and Francis, Boca Raton, FL, 2013.

Intrinsic Viscosity of Glycogen

Glycogen Type[a,b]	$[\eta]$ mL g^{-1}	Comment	Reference
Rabbit liver	6.1 ± 0.2[c] 5.7 ± 0.3 (RCAM)	0.1 M NaCl, 20°C RCAM modified with 2-mercapto-ethanol/iodoacetamide	1
Glycogen (commercial)	7.1	0.5 M NaOH, 30°C	2
Type VII from Mussel	6.6 (H_2O) 6.9 (0.5 M NaOH)	20°C	3,4
Rabbit liver Type III	6.8 ± 0.2	pH 7.4, phosphate-buffered saline, 20°C	5
Oyster Type II	6.5 ± 0.7	pH 7.4, phosphate-buffered saline, 20°C	5
Bovine Type IX (fast)	8.5 ± 0.4	pH 7.4, phosphate-buffered saline, 20°C	5
Mussel Type VII	8.3 ± 0.5	pH 7.4, phosphate-buffered saline, 20°C	5

[a] Unfractionated glycogen.

[b] The intrinsic viscosity of glycogen is independent of molecular mass.

[c] Viscosity of unmodified glycogen (prior to reduction with 2-mercaptoethanol).

References

1. Geddes, R., Harvey, J.D., and Wills, P.P., Hydrodynamic properties of 2-mercaptoethanol-modified glycogen, *Eur. J. Biochem.* 81, 465–477, 1977.
2. Weaver, L., Yu, L.P., and Rollings, J.E., Weighted intrinsic viscosity relationships of polysaccharides mixtures in dilute aqueous solution, *J. Appl. Polymer Sci.* 35, 1631–1637, 1988.
3. Ioan, C.E., Aberle, T., and Burchard, W., Solution properties of glycogen. 1. Dilute solutions, *Macromolecules* 32, 7444–7453, 1999.
4. Ioan, C.E., Aberle, T., and Burchard, W., Solution properties of glycogen. 2. Semidilute solutions, *Macromolecules* 32, 8655–8662, 1999.
5. Morris, G.A., Ang, S., Hill, S.E., et al., Molar mass and solution conformation of branched α(1-4), α(1-6) glucans. Part 1. Glycogens in water, *Carbohydr. Polymer.* 71, 101–108, 2008.

Intrinsic Viscosity of Hyaluronan

Hyaluronan M_w	$[\eta]$ (mL g^{-1})	Comment	Reference
91,000 Da	250.1	0.15 M NaCl, 37°C	1
236,000 Da	526.1	0.15 M NaCl, 37°C	1
660,000 Da	1173.2	0.15 M NaCl, 37°C	1
1,400,000 Da	1962.0	0.15 M NaCl, 37°C	1
3,500,000 Da	3402.2	0.15 M NaCl, 37°C	1
1,400,000 Da[a]	2500[b]	Phosphate-buffered saline, 37°C	2
1,585,000[a]	2298[b,c]	Phosphate-buffered saline, 23°C	3
150,000[a]	480[b]	Na+ salt, 0.1 mol/L ionic strength[e]	4
150,000[a]	299[b]	Na+ salt, infinite ionic strength[e]	4
150,000[a]	372[b]	TBA salt[d], 0.1 mol/L ionic strength	4
150,000[a]	295[b]	TBA salt[d], infinite ionic strength	4
Not provided[f]	1150	0.1 M NaCl, pH 2.6	5
Not provided[f]	920	10% EtOH in 0.1 M NaCl, pH 2.6	5
1,600,000	2600[b,e]	0.15 ionic strength, pH 7.0	6
1,600,000	3900[b,e]	0.015 ionic strength, pH 7.0	6
1,600,000	590[b,g]	0.15 ionic strength, pH 13.2	6
4,000,000	5900[b]	0.15 ionic strength, pH 7.0	6
4,000,000	3400[b,g]	0.15 ionic strength, pH 2.6	6
861,000	1434[b]	0.1 M NaCl/25°C	7[h]
1,435,000	2375[b]	0.1 M NaCl/25°C	7
1,150,000	1934[b]	0.1 M NaCl/25°C	7
1,600,000	2545[b]	0.1 M NaCl/25°C	7
1,400,000	2395[b]	0.1 M NaCl/25°C	7

[a] Weight average molecular weight.

[b] Reported as dL gm^{-1}; converted to mL gm^{-1} by x100.

[c] Determined by size-exclusion chromatography.

[d] Tetramethylammonium salt.

[e] The solution properties of hyaluronic acid are very sensitive to ionic strength.

[f] An early therapeutic preparation from Biotrics, Boston, Massachusetts.

[g] The solution properties of hyaluronic acid are sensitive to pH (Mathews, M.B., and Decker, L., Conformation of hyaluronan in neutral and alkaline solutions, *Biochim. Biophys. Acta*, 498, 259–263, 1977).

[h] This study also evaluated the mixtures of hyaluronan.

References

1. Mendichi, R., Soltés, L., and Schieroni, A.G., Evaluation of radius of gyration and intrinsic viscosity molar mass dependence on stiffness of hyaluronan, *Biomacromolecules* 4, 1805–1810, 2003.
2. la Gatta, A. de Rosa, M., Marzaioli, I., Bosico, T., and Schiraldi, C., A complete hyaluronan characterization using a size exclusion chromatography-triple detection array system during in vitro enzymatic degradation, *Arch. Biochem. Biophys.* 404, 21–29, 2010.
3. Harmon, P.S., Mazierz, E.P., and Liu, X.M., Detailed characterization of hyaluronan using aqueous size exclusion chromatography with triple detection and multiangle light-scattering detection, *J. Biomed. Mat. Res. B.* 1008, 1955–1960, 2012.
4. Geciova, R., Flaibani, A., Delben, F., et al., Physico-chemical properties of hyaluronan and its hydrophobic derivatives: A calorimetric and viscometric study, *Macromol. Chem. Phys.* 196, 2891–2903, 1995.
5. Park, J.W., and Chakrabarti, B., Solvent induced changes in conformation of hyaluronic acid, *Biopolymers* 16, 2807–2809, 1977.
6. Morris, E.R., Rees, D.A., and Welsh, E.J., Conformation and dynamic interactions in hyaluronate solutions, *J. Mol. Biol.* 138, 383–400, 1980.
7. Berriaud, N., Milas, M., and Rinaudo, M., Rheological study on mixtures of different molecular weight hyaluronates, *Int. J. Biol. Macromol.* 16, 137–142, 1994.

Intrinsic Viscosity of Dextran

Dextran type	[η] mL g⁻¹	Comment	Reference
Dextran T500[a]	49.1	H_2O/20°C	1
Dextran T500[a]	96.4	Ethanolamine/20°C	1
Dextran T500[a]	79.2	Dimethylsulfoxide/20°C	1
Dextran T500[a]	66.9	Formamide/20°C	1
Dextran T500[a]	58.0	Ethylene glycol/20°C[b]	1
Dextran T500[a]	45.7	H_2O/40°C	1
Dextran T500[a]	85.4	Ethanolamine/40°C	1
Dextran T500[a]	74.3	Dimethylsulfoxide/40°C	1
Dextran T500[a]	59.1	Formamide/40°C	1
Dextran T500[a]	34.7[b]	Ethylene Glycol/40°C	1
Dextran T70[c]	23	H_2O/25°C	2
Dextran T70[c]	22	1 M urea/25°C	2
Dextran T70[c]	21	1 M thiourea/25°C	2
Dextran T70[c]	20	1 M guanidine sulfate/25°C	2
20% oxidized Dextran T70[d]	20	H_2O/25°C	2
20% oxidized Dextran T70[d]	20	1 M urea/25°C	2
20% oxidized Dextran T70[d]	18	1 M thiourea/25°C	2
20% oxidized Dextran T70[d]	16	1 M guanidine sulfate/25°C	2
Dextran T40[e]	20.6	H_2O/25°C	3
Dextran T110[f]	31.1	H_2O/25°C	3
Dextran T500[g]	54.1	H_2O/25°C	3
Dextran T2000[h]	69.1	H_2O/25°C	3
Dextran T10 (9,300[i])	8.01[j]	H2O[k]	4
Dextran T20 (20,000[i])	12.08[j]	H_2O[k]	4
Dextran T40 (42,000[i])	18.63[j]	H_2O[k]	4
Dextran T70 (66,000[i])	22.91[j]	H_2O[k]	4
Dextran T110 (101,000[i])	28.36[j]	H_2O[k]	4
Dextran T150 (151,000[i])	33.18[j]	H_2O[k]	4
Dextran T250 (239,500[i])	38.24[j]	H_2O[k]	4
Dextran T550 (546,000[i])	47.20[j]	H_2O[k]	4

[a] DextranT500 from GE Healthcare, originally a Pharmacia Product. Weight average molecular weight (M_w), 500,000; number average molecular weight (M_n), 191,500. The weight average molecular weight is the average of the molecular weight of the various species in a sample, while the number average molecular weight is the total weight of the sample divided by the number of molecules in the sample. The polydispersity index (M_w/M_r) is a measure of the size homogeneity of a polymer sample.
[b] Value obtained by extrapolation of data at 25°C to 40°C.
[c] Dextran T70 with a stated molecular weight of 70,000 from Pharmacia (now GE Healthcare).
[d] Dextran T70 oxidized with periodate to form the dialdehyde derivative.
[e] Dextran T40, M_w, 40,000; M_n, 30,000 (Pharmacia data sheet)
[f] Dextran T110, M_w, 110,000; M_n, 76,000 (Pharmacia data sheet).
[g] Dextran T500, M_w, 500,000; M_n, 350,000 (Pharmacia data sheet).
[h] Dextran T2000, M_w, 200,000; M_n, 143,000 (Pharmacia Data sheet).
[i] Molecular weights determined by gel permeation chromatography (GPC) in H_2O at 30°C with Porosil®.
[j] The average intrinsic viscosity determined from the analysis of individual eluent fractions from the GPC column using a capillary viscometer.
[k] Temperature not provided for measurement of viscosity.

References

1. Antoniou, E., Buitrago, C.F., Tsianou, M., and Alexandridis, P., Solvent effects on polysaccharide conformation, *Carbohydr. Polymer.* 79, 380–390, 2010.
2. Uraz, I., and Günen, A., Comparison of molecular association of dextran and periodate-oxidized dextran in aqueous solution, *Carbohydr. Polymer.* 34, 127–130, 1997.
3. Kawaizumi, F., Nishio, N., Nomura, H., and Miyahara, Y., Calorimetric and compressibility study of aqueous solutions of dextrans with special reference to hydration and structural change of water, *Polymer J.* 13, 209–213, 1981.
4. Soeteman, A.A., Roels, J.P.M., Van Dijk, J.A.P.P., and Smit, J.A.M., Separation of dextrans by gel permeation, chromatography *J. Polymer Sci. Polymer Physics Edn.* 16, 2147–2155, 1978.

Intrinsic Viscosity of Various Polysaccharides

Sample	[η] mL g⁻¹	Comment	Reference
Xanthan[a]	15557	H_2O/20°C	1
Xanthan[a]	9290	2 mM NaCl/20°C	1
Xanthan[a]	7320	40 mM NaCl/20°C	1
Deacetylated xanthan[b]	16300	H_2O/20°C	1
Deacetylated xanthan[b]	9060	2 mM NaCl/20°C	1
Deacetylated xanthan[b]	5670	40 mM NaCl/20°C	1
Guar[c]	1200	H_2O/20°C	1
Guar[c]	1190	2 mM NaCl/20°C	1
Guar[c]	1170	40 mM NaCl/20°C	1
Amylose[d]	95.00	0.5 M NaOH	2
Amylose tris(phenylcarbamate)[e]	126	Methyl acetate/25°C	3
Amylose tris(phenylcarbamate)[e]	156	Ethyl acetate/33°C	3
Amylose tris(phenylcarbamate)[e]	226	4-methyl-2-pentanone	3
Amylose[f]	310–460	1.0 M KOH/25°C	4
Amylose[g]	74.9	H_2O/25°C	5
I₂-Amylose[h]	52.5	H_2O/25°C	5
Amylose[i]	158	H_2O/22.5°C	6
Amylose[i]	158	0.33 M KCl/22.5°C	6
Amylose[i]	500	0.2 M KOH/22.5°C	7
Amylose[i]	62	0.33 M KCl/22.5°C	7
Amylose[i]	150	0.2 M KOH	7
Amylopectin[k]	184	0.5 M NaOH	2
Amylopectin[l]	210–250	1.0 M KOH	4
Inulin[m]	4.49	H_2O/29.85°C	8
Inulin[m]	3.65	0.5 M NH₄SCN/29.85°C	8
Inulin[m]	4.30	0.5 M NaCl/29.85°C	8
Inulin[m]	4.25	0.5 M Na₂SO₄	8
Inulin[m]	15.21	Dimethylsulfoxide/29.85°C	8

[a] Xanthan, M_w 2.65 x 10⁶, 3.51% acetate, 0.9% pyruvate from Sigma Chemical Company. Xanthan contains mannose residue which contain covalently bound acetate and pyruvate.
[b] Deacylated xanthan was prepared by reaction of xanthan with 25 mM KOH in 0.1 M KCl under nitrogen at ambient temperature for 2.5 hours followed by neutralization with HCl to pH 6.5 and dialysis into deionized H_2O. Deacylated xanthan had a molecular weight of 2.36 x 10⁶, 0.32% acetate, 0.9% pyruvate.
[c] Guar (Guaran, guar gum) is a high molecular weight polysaccharide (a galactomannan) with considerable application in the food industry. Guar gum has been reported to have an M_w greater than 2 x 10⁶(Barth, H.G., and Smith, D.A., High-performance size-exclusion chromatography of guar gum, *J. Chromatog.*, 206, 410–415, 1981) but lower molecular weights have been reported (Mudgil, D., Barak, S., and Khatkar, B.S., X-ray diffraction, IR spectroscopy and thermal characterization of partially hydrolyzed guar gum, *Int. J. Biol. Macromolecules* 50, 1035–1039, 2012). The guar gum used in this study is reported to have a M_w of 1.45 x 10⁶.
[d] Amylose obtained from Serva, Germany; molecular weight not provided. Amylose is an unbranched polymer of glucose, generally of high molecular weight (Hizukuri, S., and Takagi, T., Estimation of the distribution of molecular weight for amylose by the low-angle laser-light-scattering technique combined with high-performance gel chromatography, *Carbohydrate Res.*, 134, 1–10, 1984).
[e] Molecular weight 491,000; prepared by the reaction of phenylisocyanate with amylose, polydispersity index 1.05–1.11.
[f] Purified from sago starch, M_w 1.41–22.26 x 10⁶.
[g] Potato amylose, M_w 80,000.
[h] Potato amylose, M_w 80,000, substitution with I_2, 0.13 gm I_2/g amylose.
[i] Purified from potato and crystallized from H_2O/n-butanol, molecular weight 1,700,000.
[j] Purified from potato and crystallized from H_2O/n-butanol, molecular weight 350,000.
[k] Amylopectin (From Sigma Chemical Company, molecular weight not defined).
[l] Purified from sago starch, M_w 6.7–9.73 x 10⁶.
[m] Inulin Aggregation in DMSO.

References

1. Khouryieh, H.A., Herald, T.J., Aramouni, F., and Alavi, S., Intrinsic viscosity and viscoelastic properties of xanthan/guar mixtures in dilute solutions: Effect of salt concentration on the polymer interactions, *Food Res. Intn.* 40, 883–893, 2007.
2. Weaver, L., Yu, L.P., and Rollings, J.E., Weighted intrinsic viscosity relationships for polysaccharide mixtures in dilutes aqueous solutions, *J. Appld. Polymer Sci.* 35, 1631–1637, 1988.

3. Fujii, T., Terao, K., Tsuda, M., Kitamuro, S., and Norisuye, T., Solvent dependent conformation of amylose tris(phenylcarbamate) as deduced from scattering and viscosity data, *Biopolymers* 91, 729–736, 2009.

4. Ahman, F.B., Williams, P.A., Doublier, J.L., Durand, S., and Buleon, A., Physico-chemical characterization of sago starch, *Carbohydr. Polymer.* 38, 361–370, 1999.

5. Senior, M.B., and Hamori, E., Investigation of the effect of amylose/iodine complexation on the conformation of amylose in aqueous solution, *Biopolymers* 12, 65–78, 1973.

6. Banks, W., and Greenword, C.T., Hydrodynamic properties and dimensions of linear potato amylose molecules in dilute aqueous solution, *Makromolek. Chem.* 67, 49–63, 1963.

7. Banks, W., and Greenwood, C.T., Viscosity and sedimentation studies on amylase in aqueous solution-further evidence for non-helical characteri, *Eur. Polymer J.* 5, 649–658, 1969.

8. Dan, A., Ghosh, S., and Moulik, S.P., Physicochemical studies on the biopolymer inulin: A critical evaluation of its self-aggregation, aggregate morphology, interaction with water, and thermal stability, *Biopolymers* 91, 687–699, 2009.

References

1. Vaikousi, H., Biliaderis, C.G., and Izyderczyk, M.S., Solution flow behavior and gelling properties of water-soluble barley (1-3),(1-4)-β-glucans varying in molecular size, *J. Cereal Sci.* 39, 119–137, 2004.

2. Lazaridou, A., Biliadevis, C.G., Micha-Screttas, M., and Steele, B.R., A comparative study on structure-function relationships of mixed-linkage (1→3),(1→4) linear β-D-glucans, *Food Hydrocolloids* 18, 837–855, 2004.

3. Lazaridou, A., Billadevis, C.G., and Izyderczyk, M.S., Molecular size effects on rheological properties of oat β-glucans in solutions and gels, *Food Hydrocolloids* 17, 693–712, 2003.

4. Agbenorhevi, J.K., Kontogiorgos, V., Kirby, A.R., Morris, V.J., and Tosh, S.M., Rheological and microstructural investigation of oat β-glucan isolates varying in molecular weight, *Int. J. Biol. Macromol.* 49, 369–377, 2011.

5. Tomasi, I., Marconi, O., Sileoni, V., and Perretti, G., Validation of a high-performance size-exclusion chromatography method to determine and characterize β-glucans in beer wort using a triple-detector array, *Food Chem.* 214, 176–182, 2017.

Intrinsic Viscosity of β-Glucans[a]

β-Glucan M_w	$[\eta]$ (mL g^{-1})	Comment	Reference
BLG[b] 40,000	63	H_2O/20°C	1
BLG[b] 70,000	111	H_2O/20°C	1
BLG[b] 110,000	186	H_2O/20°C	1
BLG[b] 140,00	219	H_2O/20°C	1
BLG[b] 180,000	233	H_2O/20°C	1
BLG[b] 210,000	291	H_2O/20°C	1
BLG[b] 250,000	301	H_2O/20°C	1
Oat[c] 105,000	177	H_2O/20°C	2
Oat[c] 203,000	301	H_2O/20°C	2
Bar[d] 107.000	186	H_2O/20°C	2
Bar[d] e213,000	311	H_2O/20°C	2
Whe[e] 209,000	298	H_2O/20°C	2
Lic100[f] 106,000	156	H_2O/20°C	2
OGL[g] 35,000	67	H_2O/20°C	3
OGL[g] 65,000	91	H_2O/20°C	3
OGL[g] 110,000	185	H_2O/20°C	3
OGL[g] 140,000	241	H_2O/20°C	3
OGL[g] 250,000	383	H_2O/20°C	3
OBG[c] 2,800,00	720	H_2O/20°C	4
H05[h] 252,000	230	H_2O/20°C	4
H10[h] 172,000	180	H_2O/20°C	4
H15[h] 142,000	170	H_2O/20°C	4
Beer Wort[i] 88,802	62	0.1 M $NaNO_3$ with 500 mg L^{-1} NaN_3/35°	5

[a] β-Glucans are linear polymers composed of β-D-glucose residues derived from various grains including barley and oats. β-Glucans are thought to be nutraceuticals with a broad range of effects from immunostimulation and promotion of cardiovascular health (Ulbricht, C., An evidence-based systematic review of beta-glucan by the natural standard research collaboration, *J. Diet Suppl.*, 11, 361–475, 2014; Nwachukwu, I.D., Devassy, J.G., Aluko, R.E., and Jones, J.P., Cholesterol-lowering properties of oat β-glucan and the promotion of cardiovascular health: Did Health Canada make the right call?, *Appl. Physiol. Nutr. Metab.*, 40, 535–542, 2015; Barton, C., Vigor, K., Scott, R., et al., Beta-contamination of pharmaceutical products: How much should we accept?, *Cancer Immunol. Immunother.*, 65, 1289–1301, 2016).

[b] BLG40 (M_w 40,000) was obtained from CEBA Foods AB(Now Oatly AB) (Lund, Sweden). The other (1-3),(1-4)-β-glucan fractions were obtained by acid hydrolysis (80°C, pH 2.0, 5 N H_3PO_4) of β-glucan purified from barley flour.

[c] Oat β-glucan.

[d] Barley β-glucan.

[e] Wheat β-glucan.

[f] Moss β-glucan

[g] Various oat β-glucan fractions. The 140,000 M_w and 250,000 M_w fractions were obtained from whole flours from Greek cultivars. The other β-glucans were obtained from CEBA Foods AB(Now Oatly AB) (Lund, Sweden).

[h] Various fractions obtained by the acid hydrolysis (80°C/pH 1, 0.5 h, 1.0 h, 1.5 h).

[i] β-Glucans were extracted from beer wort (wort is the liquid obtained from crushed barley which is soaked in hot water during the mashing process). The presence of β-glucans in the wort can have a negative effect on the downstream brewing process. Wort is also obtained in the process of making whiskey. Wort contains sugars used in the fermentation process).

Intrinsic Viscosity of Mixtures of Polysaccharides

Sample	$[\eta]$ mL g^{-1}	Comment	Reference
DextranT500[a]	50.7	0.5 M NaOH/30°C	1
DextranT500:DextranT70 (4:1)	47.0	0.5 M NaOH/30°C	1
DextranT500:DextranT70 (3:2)	42.0	0.5 M NaOH/30°C	1
DextranT500:DextranT70 (2:3)	34.9	0.5 M NaOH/30°C	1
DextranT500:DextranT70 (3:7)	30.7	0.5 M NaOH/30°C	1
DextranT500:DextranT70 (1:9)	25.2	0.5 M NaOH/30°C	1
DextranT70	24.7	0.5 M NaOH/30°C	1
Amylose[b]	95.0	0.5 M NaOH/30°C	1
Amylose:DextranT500 (4:1)	86.0	0.5 M NaOH/30°C	1
Amylose:DextranT500 (3:2)	73.8	0.5 M NaOH/30°C	1
Amylose:DextranT500 (2:3)	67.7	0.5 M NaOH/30°C	1
Amylose:DextranT500 (3:7)	61.8	0.5 M NaOH/30°C	1
Amylose:DextranT500 (1:4)	53.4	0.5 M NaOH/30°C	1
Amylose:DextranT500 (1:9)	52.0	0.5 M NaOH/30°C	1
Amylose:Glycogen[c] (4:1)	85.1	0.5 M NaOH/30°C	1
Amylose:Glycogen[c] (3:2)	63.5	0.5 M NaOH/30°C	1
Amylose:Glycogen[c] (2:3)	46.8	0.5 M NaOH/30°C	1
Amylose:Glycogen[c] (1:4)	32.8	0.5 M NaOH/30°C	1
Glycogen[c]	7.1	0.5 M NaOH/30°C	1
Amylose:Amylopectin[d] (4:!)	112.0	0.5 M NaOH/30°C	1
Amylose:Amylopectin[d] (3:2)	118.2	0.5 M NaOH/30°C	1
Amylose:Amylopectin[d] (2:3))	153.5	0.5 M NaOH/30°C	1
Amylose:Amylopectin[d] (1:4)	166	0.5 M NaOH/30°C	1
Amylopectin[d]	184	0.5 M NaOH/30°C	1
Xanthan[e]	15570	H$_2$O/20°C	2
Xanthan:Guar[f] (80:20)	8220	H$_2$O/20°C	2
Xanthan:Guar[f] (60:40)	6330	H$_2$O/20°C	2
Xanthan:Guar[f] (40:60)	5690	H$_2$O/20°C	2
Xanthan:Guar[f] (20:80)	3280	H$_2$O/20°C	2
Guar[f]	1200	H$_2$O/20°C	2

[a] See Table p. 523 entitled Intrinsic Viscosity of Dextran for dextran polymer information.

[b] Amylose obtained from Serva, Germany; molecular weight not provided. Amylose is a unbranched polymer of glucose, generally of high molecular weight (Hizukuri, S., and Takagi, T., Estimation of the distribution of molecular weight for amylose by the low-angle laser-light-scattering technique combined with high-performance gel chromatography, *Carbohydrate Res.* 134, 1–10, 1984).

[c] Glycogen (From Sigma Chemical Company, molecular weight not defined).

[d] Amylopectin (From Sigma Chemical Company, molecular weight not defined).

[e] Xanthan (xathan gum) is high molecular heterogeneous linear polysaccharide secreted by a number of bacterial species. Xanthan (obtained from *Xanthomanas campestris*) has been reported to have a molecular weight (M_w) of 15,000,000 with a polydispersity of 2.8 (Holzwarth, G., Molecular weight of xanthan polysaccharide, *Carbohydrate Res.* 66, 173–186, 1978).

[f] Guar (guaran, guar gum) is a high molecular weight polysaccharide (a galactomannan) with considerable application in the food industry. Guar gum has been reported to have a M_w greater than 2 x 10^6 (Barth, H.G., and Smith, D.A., High-performance size-exclusion chromatography of guar gum, *J. Chromatog.* 206, 410–415, 1981) but lower molecular weights have been reported (Mudgil, D., Barak, S., and Khatkar, B.S., X-ray diffraction, IR spectroscopy and thermal characterization of partially hydrolyzed guar gum, *Int. J. Biol. Macromolecules* 50, 1035–1039, 2012). The guar gum used in this study is reported to have a M_w of 1.45 x 10^6). The reader is directed to another study on the interaction of galactomannans with xanthan (Grisel, M., Agurni, Y., Renou, F., and Malhiac, C., Impact of fine structure of galactomannans on their interactions with xanthan: Two co-existing mechanisms to explain the synergy, *Food Hydrocolloids* 51, 449–458, 2015).

References

1. Weaver, L., Yu, L.P., and Rollings, J.E., Weighted intrinsic viscosity relationships for polysaccharide mixtures in dilutes aqueous solutions, *J. Appl. Polymer Sci.* 35, 1631–1637, 1988.
2. Khouryieh, H.A., Herald, T.J., Aramouni, F., and Alavi, S., Intrinsic viscosity and viscoelastic properties of xanthan/guar mixtures in dilute solutions: Effect of salt concentration on the polymer interactions, *Food Res. Int.* 40, 883–893, 2007.

Section VII
Chemical Biology and Drug Design

UNNATURAL AMINO ACIDS FOR INCORPORATION INTO PROTEINS

Roger L. Lundblad

Amino acids can be divided into two groups. Proteinogenic amino acids are defined as amino acids which can be incorporated into proteins.[1–4] Proteogenic amino acids are differentiated from amino acids which are subject to post translational modification[5,6] such as the γ-carboxylation of glutamic acid. Non proteinogenic (non protein) amino acids[7] such as cyclopentenylglycine[8] and l-*p*-hydroxyphenylglycine[9] are involved in metabolism and in peptide antibiotics. There has been considerable interest in the development of unnatural amino acids. While the broad definition of an unnatural amino acid is any synthetic organic carboxylic acid which contains an amino or imino function, the definition for this section is that an unnatural amino acid must be capable of incorporation into a protein in a specific manner using a biological system.[10–17]

References

1. Hardy, P.M., The protein amino acids, in *Chemistry and Biochemistry of the Amino Acids*, ed. G.C. Barrett, Chapman & Hall, London, UK, Chapter 2, pps. 6–24, 1985.
2. Szyperski, T., Biosynthetically directed fractional ¹³C-labeling of proteinogenic amino acid. No efficient analytical tool to investigate intermediary metabolism, *Eur.J.Biochem.* 232, 433–448, 1995.
3. Seebach, D., Beck, A.M., and Bierbaum, D.J., The world of β- and γ-peptides comprised of homologated proteinogenic amino acids and other components, *Chem.Biodivers.* 1, 1111–1239, 2004.
4. Chan, W.C., Higton, A., and Davis, J.J., Amino acids, in *Amino Acids, Peptides, and Proteins*, Vol. 35, ed. J.S. Davies, RSC Publishing, Cambridge, UK, pps. 1–73, 2006.
5. Walsh, C.T., Garneau-Tsodikova, S., and Gatto, G.J., Jr., Protein posttranslational modification: the chemistry of proteome diversification, *Angew.Chem.Int.Ed.Engl.* 44, 7342–7373, 2005.
6. Walsh, G. and Jeffries, R., Post-translational modifications in the context of therapeutic proteins, *Nat.Biotechnol.* 24, 1241–1252, 2006.
7. Hunt, S., The non-protein amino acids, in *Chemistry and Biochemistry of the Amino Acids*, ed. G.C. Barrett, Chapman & Hall, London, UK, Chapter 5, pps. 55–138, 1985.
8. Cramer, U. and Spener, F. Biosynthesis of cyclopentenyl fatty acids. Cyclopentenylglycine, a non-proteinogenic amino acids as precursor of cyclic fatty acids in *Flacourtiaceae*, *Eur.J.Biochem.* 94, 495–500, 1977.
9. Hubbard, B.K., Thomas, M.G., and Walsh, C.T., Biosynthesis of L-*p*-hydroxyphenylglycine, a non-proteinogenic amino acid constituent of peptide antibiotics, *Chem.Biol.* 7, 931–942, 2000.
10. Brookes, P., Studies on the incorporation of an unnatural amino acid, *p*-di-(2-hydroxy[¹⁴C₂]ethyl)amino-L-phenylalanine into proteins, *Brit. J.Cancer* 13, 313–317, 1959.
11. Anthony-Cahill, S.J., Griffith, M.C., Noren, C.J., *et al.*, Site-specific mutagenesis with unnatural amino acids, *Trends Biochem.Sci.* 14, 400–403, 1989.
12. Bain, J.D., Switzer, C., Chamberlin, A.R., and Benner, S.A., Ribosome-mediated incorporation of a non-standard amino acid into a peptide through expansion of the genetic code, *Nature* 356, 537–539, 1992.
13. Noren, C.J., Anthony-Cahill, S.J., Suich, D.J., *et al.*, In vitro expression of an amber mutation by a chemically aminoacylated transfer RNA prepared by runoff transcription, *Nucleic Acids Res.* 18, 83–88, 1990.
14. Ibba, M. and Hennecke, H., Relaxing the substrate specificity of an aminoacyl-tRNA synthetase allows *in vitro* and *in vivo* synthesis of proteins containing unnatural amino acids, *FEBS Lett.* 364, 272–275, 1995.
15. Bacher, J.M. and Ellington, A.D., The directed evolution of organismal chemistry: Unnatural amino acids and incorporation, in *Translation Mechanisms*, ed. J.Lapointe and L. Brackier-Gingras, Landes Bioscience/Kluwer Academic, New York, NY, USA, Chapter 5, pps. 80–94, 2003.
16. Magliery, T.J., Pastrnak, M., Anderson, J.C., In vitro tools and in vivo engineering: Incorporation of unnatural amino acids into proteins, in *Translation Mechanisms*, ed. J.Lapointe and L. Brackier-Gingras, Landes Bioscience/Kluwer Academic, New York, NY, USA, Chapter 6, pps. 95–114, 2003.
17. Liu, W., Brock, A., Chen, S., *et al.*, Genetic incorporation of unnatural amino acids into proteins in mammalian cells, *Nat.Methods* 4, 239–244, 2007.

	Unnatural Amino Acid	Structure	References
1	*p*-Propargyloxyphenylalanine		1–3
2	*p*-Azidophenylalanine		1,4,5
3	4-Fluorotryptophan		6–11
4	Azaleucine		12
5	*p*-Fluorophenylalanine		13–21

6	O-Methyltyrosine		22–24
7	p-Acetylphenylalanine or m-acetylphenylalanine		25–28
8	p-Iodophenylalanine		29
9	p-Benzoylphenylalanine		30–31

References for Table

1. Dieters, A., Cropp, A., Mukherji, M., et al., Adding amino acids with novel reactivity to the genetic code of *Saccharomyces cerevisiae*, *J.Amer.Chem.Soc.* 125, 11782–11783, 2003.

2. Dieters, A. and Schultz, P.G., In vivo incorporation of an alkyne into proteins in *Escherichia coli*, *Bioorg.Med.Chem.Lett.* 15, 1521–1524, 2005.

3. Iida, S., Asakura, N., Tabata, K. et al., Incorporation of unnatural amino acids into cytochrome c3 and specific viologen binding to the unnatural amino acid, *Chembiochem* 7, 1853–1855, 2006.

4. Dieters, A., Cropps, T.A., Summerer, D., et al., Site-specific PEGylation of proteins containing unnatural amino acids, *Bioorg. Med.Chem.Lett.* 14, 5743–5745, 2004.

5. Carrico, I.S., Mackarinec, S.A., Heilshorn, S.C., Lithographic patterning of photoreactive cell-adhesive proteins, *J.Am.Chem.Soc.*, in press, 2007.

6. Pratt, E.A. and Ho, C., Incorporation of fluorotryptophans into proteins of *Escherichia coli*, *Biochemistry* 14, 3035–3040, 1975.

7. Browne, D.T. and Otvos, J.D., 4-Fluorotryptophan alkaline phosphatase from *E.coli*: preparation, properties, and ¹⁹F NMR spectrum, *Biochem.Biophys.Res.Commun.* 68, 907–913, 1976.

8. Wong, C.Y. and Eftink, M.R., Incorporation of tryptophan analogues into staphylococcal nuclease: stability toward thermal and guanidine-HCl induced unfolding, *Biochemistry* 37, 8947–8953, 1998.

9. Zhang, Q.S., Shen, L., Wang, E.D., and Wang, Y.L., Biosynthesis and characterization of 4-fluorotryptophan-labeled *Escherichia coli* arginyl tRNA synthetase, *J.Protein Chem.* 18, 187–192, 1999.

10. Mohammed, F., Prentice, G.A., and Merrill, A.R., Protein-protein interaction using tryptophan analogues: novel spectroscopic probes for toxin-elongation factor-2 interactions, *Biochemistry* 40, 10273–10283, 2001.

11. Bacher, J.D. and Ellington, A.D., Selection and characterization of *Escherichia coli* variants capable of growth on an otherwise toxic tryptophan analogue, *J.Bacteriol.* 183, 5414–5425, 2001.

12. Lemeigan, B. Sonigo, P. and Marliere, P. Phenotypic suppression by incorporation of an alien amino acid, *J.Mol.Biol.* 231, 161–166, 1993.

13. Dunn, T.F. and Leach, F.R., Incorporation of p-fluorophenylalanine into protein by a cell-free system, *J.Biol.Chem.* 242, 2693–2699, 1967.

14. Rels, P.J. and Gillespie, J.M., Effects of phenylalanine and analogues of methionine and phenylalanine on the composition of wool and mouse hair, *Aust.J.Biol.Sci.* 38, 151–163, 1985.

15. Kast, P. and Hennecke, H., Amino acid substrate specificity of *Escherichia coli* phenylalanyl-tRNA synthetase altered by distinct mutations, *J.Mol.Biol.* 222, 99–124, 1991.

16. Lian, C., Le, H., Montez, B., et al., Fluorine-19 nuclear magnetic resonance spectroscopic study of fluorophenylalanine and fluorotryptophan-labeled avian egg white lysozymes, *Biochemistry* 33, 5238–5245, 1994.

17. Danielson, M.A., Biemann, M.P., Koshland, D.E.,Jr., and Falke, J.J., Attractant- and disulfide-induced conformational changes in the ligand binding domain of the chemotaxis aspartate receptor: a ¹⁹F NMR study, *Biochemistry* 33, 6100–6109, 1994.

18. Furter, R., Expansion of the genetic code: site-directed p-fluorophenylalanine incorporation in *Escherichia coli*, *Protein Sci.* 7, 419–426, 1998.

19. Minka, C., Nuber, R., Moroder, L., and Budisa, N., Noninvasive tracing of recombinant proteins with "fluorophenylalanine-fingers", *Anal.Biochem.* 284, 29-34, 2000.

20. Bann, J.G. and Frieden, C., Folding and domain-domain interactions of the chaperone PapD measured by ¹⁹F NMR, *Biochemistry* 43, 13775–13786, 2004.

21. Jackson, J.C., Hammill, J.T. , and Mehl, R.A., Site-specific incorporation of a ¹⁹F-amino acid into proteins as an NMR probe for characterizing protein structure and reactivity, *J.Am.Chem.Soc.* 129, 1160–1166, 2007.

22. Wang, L., Brock, A., and Schultz, P.G., Adding L-3-(2-naphthalyl) alanine to the genetic code of *E.coli*, *J.Amer.Chem.Soc.* 124, 1836–1837, 2002.

23. Zhang, D., Valdehi, N., Goddard, W.A., Jr., et al., Structure-based design of mutant *Methanococcus jannaschii* tyrosyl-tRNA synthetase for incorporation of O-methyl-L-tyrosine, *Proc.Natl.Acad. Sci.USA* 99, 6579–6584, 2002.

24. Zhang, Y, Wang, L., Schultz, P.G., and Wilson, I.A., Crystal structures of apo wild-type *M. jannashchii* tyrosyl-tRNA synthetase (TyrRS) and an engineered TyrRS specific for O-methyl-L-tyrosine, *Protein Sci.* 14, 1340–1349, 2005.

25. Wang, L., Zhang, Z., Brock, A., and Schultz, P.G., Addition of the keto functional group to the genetic code of *Escherichia coli*, *Proc. Natl.Acad.Sci.USA* 100, 56–61, 2003.

26. Zhang, Z., Smith, B.A., Wang, L., et al., A new strategy for the site-specific modifications of proteins in vivo, *Biochemistry* 42, 6735–6746, 2003.

27. Wu, N., Dieters, A., Cropp, T.A., et al., A genetically encoded photocaged amino acid, *J.Am.Chem.Soc.* 126, 14306–14307, 2004.

28. Taki, M. and Sisido, M., Leucyl/phenylalanyl (L/F)-tRNA-protein transferase-mediated aminoacyl transfer of a nonnatural amino acid to the N-terminal of peptides and proteins and subsequent functionalization by bioorthogonal reactions, *Biopolymers* 88, 263–271, 2007.

29. Black, K.M., Clark-Lewis, I., and Wallace, C.J., Conserved tryptophan in cytochrome c: importance of the unique side-chain features of the indole moiety, *Biochem.J.* 359, 715–720, 2001.

30. Chin, J.W., Cropp, T.A., Anderson, J.C., et al., An expanded eukaryotic genetic code, *Science* 301, 964–967, 2003.

31. Farrell, I.S., Tornoney, R., Hazen, J.L., et al., Photo-crosslinking interacting proteins with a genetically encoded benzophenone, *Nat.Methods* 2, 377–384, 2005.

STRUCTURES AND SYMBOLS FOR SYNTHETIC AMINO ACIDS INCORPORATED INTO SYNTHETIC POLYPEPTIDES

M. C. Khosla and W. E. Cohn

The amino acids included in this list are those that have been incorporated into biologically active peptides, e.g., angiotensin II,[a] to study structure-activity relationships. Most of these amino acids are synthetic and are either available commercially or have been synthesized by various investigators as structural variants of naturally occurring amino acids. However, a few of these are also naturally occurring.[b] The selection here is of those most widely used and whose representation by symbols in peptide sequences has caused problems for authors and editors. The symbols listed are those considered most in keeping with the system originated by the IUPAC-IUB Commission on Biochemical Nomenclature[c,d]

and have been chosen with an eye to internal consistency, ability to evoke the proper name, and suitability for use in sequences. Only one new one has been invented: ▲ for -yn- (triple bond), by analogy with Δ for -en- (double bond).

The list may also be useful in selecting suitable isosteres of natural amino acids. The bibliography may be helpful in synthesis, resolution, or studies of the effects of these substances on the biological activity of various peptides.

The following trivial names are listed under other names (given by the number of the entry): N-amidinoglycine (67), 6-aminocaproic acid (18), 2-aminoethanesulfonic acid (112), β,β-bis(trifluoromethyl)alanine (70), carbamoylglycine (73), 2-(2-carboxyhydrazino)propane (83), cycloleucine (15), diethylalanine (17), dihydrophenylalanine (46), dopa (57), glycocyamine (67), isolysine (52), β-lysine (52), mercaptovaline (60), α-methylalanine (21), penicillamine (60), 5-pyrrolidone-2-carboxylic acid (109), surinamine (94), tetrahydrophenylalanine (47), trimethylammoniocaproic acid (116).

---

[a] for a review of structure-activity relationships and a listing of various analogs in which a number of these amino acids have been incorporated in angiotensin molecule, see Khosla, Smeby, and Bumpus.[26]

[b] IUPAC Commission on the Nomenclature of α-Amino Acids (Recommendations 1974), *Biochemistry*, 14, 449 (1975).

[c] IUPAC-IUB Commission on Biochemical Nomenclature, Symbols for Amino-Acid Derivatives and Peptides (Recommendations 1971), *Biochemistry*, 11, 1726 (1972). See Nomenclature section.

[d] IUPAC Commission on Biochemical Nomenclature, Abbreviations and symbols for Nucleic Acids, Polynucleotides, and Their Constituents (Recommendations 1970), *J. Biol. Chem.*, 245, 5171 (1970). See Nomenclature Section.

STRUCTURE AND SYMBOLS FOR SYNTHETIC AMINO ACIDS INCORPORATED INTO SYNTHETIC POLYPEPTIDES (Continued)

No.	Structure	Name/Reference	Symbol
1	$H_2C=C(NHCOCH_3)COOH$	2-Acetamidoacrylic acid	AcAacr
2		N^α-Acetyl-2-fluorophenylalanine	AcPhe(2F)
3	$H_2N(CH_2)_4CH(NHCOCH_3)CONHCH_3$	N^α-Acetyllysine-N-methylamide	Ac-Lys-NHMe
4	$H_2NCH_2CH_2COOH$	β-Alanine[b]	βAla[c]
5	$CH_3CH_2CH(CH_3)CH(NH_2)COOH$	Alloisoleucine[b]	aIle[c]
6	$HOOC(CH_3)_3CH(NH_2)COOH$	2-Aminoadipic acid	Aad[c]
7	$HOOCCH_2CH_2CH(NH_2)CH_2COOH$	3-Aminoadipic acid	βAad[c]
8	$H_2NCH_2CH(CH_2C_6H_5)COOH$	3-Amino-2-benzylpropionic acid	βApr(αBzl)
9	$H_2NCH(CH_2C_6H_5)CH_2COOH$	3-Amino-3-benzylpropionic acid	βApr(βBzl)
10	$CH_3CH_2CH(NH_2)COOH$	2-Aminobutyric acid	Abu[c]
11	$CH_3CH(NH_2)CH_2COOH$	3-Aminobutyric acid	βAbu[c]
12	$H_2N(CH_2)_3COOH$	4-Aminobutyric acid	γAbu
13	$CH_3CH=C(NH_2)COOH$	2-Aminocrotonic acid	ACrt
14		1-Aminocyclohexane-1-carboxylic acid (cyclonorleucine)	cHxA(αCx); cNle[b]
15		1-Aminocyclopentane-1-carboxylic acid (cycloleucine)	cPeA(αCx); cLeu[c]
16	$(CH_3)_2NCH_2C≡CCH_2CH(NH_2)COOH$	2-Amino-6-dimethylamino-4-hexynoic acid (1)	αε A₂ hx(▲γ, $N^\varepsilon Me_2$)
17	$CH_3CH_2CH(CH_2CH_3)CH(NH_2)COOH$	2-Amino-3-ethylvaleric acid (diethylalanine)	Ala(βEt₂)
18	$H_2N(CH_2)_5COOH$	6-Aminohexanoic acid (6-aminocaproic acid)	εAhx[c]
19	$(CH_3)_2CHCH_2CH(NH_2)CH(OH)CH_2COOH$	4-Amino-3-hydroxy-6-methylheptanoic acid (2,3)	γAhp(βOH, εMe)
20		2-Amino-3-(2-imidazolyl)propionic acid	Apr(βIm-2)
21	$(CH_3)_2C(NH_2)COOH$	2-Aminoisobutyric acid (α-methylalanine)	Ala(αMe)
22	$H_2NCH_2SO_3H$	Aminomethanesulfonic acid	Ams
23		4-Aminomethylbenzoic acid	Bz(4Ame); Bz(4CH₂ NH₂)
24	$CH_3CH_2CH(CH_3)CH_2CH_2CH(NH_2)COOH$	2-Amino-4-methyl-hexanoic acid (4)	Ahx(γMe)
25	$CH_3CH=C(CH_3)CH_2CH_2CH(NH_2)COOH$	2-Amino-4-methyl-4-hexenoic acid (4)	Ahx(Δγ, γMe)
26	$CH_2=C(CH_3)CH_2CH_2CH_2CH(NH_2)COOH$	2-Amino-5-methyl-5-hexenoic acid (4)	Ahx(Δδ, δMe)
27	$H_2N(CH_2)_7COOH$	8-Aminooctanoic acid	ωAoc

STRUCTURE AND SYMBOLS FOR SYNTHETIC AMINO ACIDS INCORPORATED INTO SYNTHETIC POLYPEPTIDES (Continued)

No.	Structure	Name/Reference	Symbol
28		(4-Amino)phenylalanine (5)	Phe(4NH$_2$)
29		3-Amino-4-phenylbutyric acid	βAbu(γPh)
30	HOOCCH(NH$_2$)(CH$_2$)$_4$COOH	2-Aminopimelic acid	αApm
31		2-Amino-3-(2-pyridyl)propionic acid	Apr(βPrd-2)
32		2-Amino-3-(2-pyrimidyl)propionic acid	Apr(βPyr-2)^{c,d}
33	(CH$_3$)$_3$$^+$N(CH$_2$)$_4$CH(NH$_2$)COOH	2-Amino-6-(trimethylammonio)hexanoic acid	α,εA$_2$hx(N^{ε}Me$_3$)
34		3-Aminotyrosine	Tyr(3NH2)
35	HOOCCH$_2$CH(NH$_2$)CONHCH$_3$	Aspartic α-methylamide	Asp-NHMe
36	CH$_3$NHCOCH$_2$CH(NH$_2$)COOH	Aspartic β-methylamide	Asn(Me); Asp(NHMe)
37		Azetidine-2-carboxylic acid	Azt
38		Aziridinecarboxylic acid	Azr
39		Aziridinonecarboxylic acid (6)	Azro
40	(PhCH$_2$)$_2$C(NH$_2$)COOH	(α-Benzyl)phenylalanine (7)	Phe(αBzl)
41		3-Benzyltyrosine (8)	Tyr(3Bzl)
42		(4-Chloro)phenylalanine (5)	Phe(4Cl)
43	H$_2$NCONH(CH$_2$)$_3$CH(NH$_2$)COOH	Citrulline^b	Ctr
44	NCCH$_2$CH(NH$_2$)COOH	β-Cyanoalanine	Ala(βCN)
45	NCCH$_2$CH$_2$NHCH$_2$COOH	N-(2-Cyanoethyl)glycine	(CNEt)Gly; CNEt-Gly

STRUCTURE AND SYMBOLS FOR SYNTHETIC AMINO ACIDS INCORPORATED INTO SYNTHETIC POLYPEPTIDES (Continued)

No.	Structure	Name/Reference	Symbol
46		β-(1,4-Cyclohexadienyl)alanine (9) (dihydrophenylalanine)	Ala(βcHxΔ¹Δ⁵); Phe(H₂)
47		β-(Cyclohexyl)alanine (10, 20) (hexahydrophenylalanine)	Ala(βcHx); Phe(H₆)
48		α-(Cyclohexyl)glycine	Gly(cHx)
49		β-(Cyclopentyl)alanine	Ala(βcPe)
50		α-(Cyclopentyl)glycine	Gly(cPe)
51	$H_2NCH_2CH_2CH(NH_2)COOH$	2,4-Diaminobutyric acid	A_2 bu [c]
52	$H_2N(CH_2)_3CH(NH_2)CH_2COOH$	3,6-Diaminohexanoic acid (isolysine;[b] β-lysine[b])	βε A_2 hx; βLys
53	$H_2NCH_2C \equiv CCH_2CH(NH_2)COOH$	2,6-Diamino-4-hexynoic acid (11)	αεA₂ hx(▲γ)
54	$HOOCCH(NH_2)(CH_2)_3CH(NH_2)COOH$	2,2'-Diaminopimelic acid	A_2 pm [c]
55	$H_2NCH_2CH(NH_2)COOH$	2,3-Diaminopropionic acid	A_2 pr [c]
56		3,4-Dihydroxy-(α-methyl)phenylalanine [β-(3,4-Dihydroxyphenyl)-α-methylalanine]	Dopa(αMe)
57		3,4-Dihydroxyphenylalanine[b]	Dopa [b]
58		(3,4-Dihydroxyphenyl)serine	Dopa(βHO)
59	$HOOCCH_2CH(Me_2\,N \rightarrow O)COOH$	N,N-Dimethylaspartic N-oxide (12)	(O,Me₂)Asp; Me₂ (O)Asp
60	$(CH_3)_2C(SH)CH(NH_2)COOH$	β,β-Dimethylcysteine (β-mercaptovaline; penicillamine[b])	Val(βSH); Cys(βMe₂)
61	$(CH_3)_2CHCH(CH_3)CH(NHCH_3)COOH$	threo-N, β-Dimethylleucine (13)	MeLeu(βMe)
62		α,3-Dimethyltyrosine	Tyr(α,3-Me₂)

STRUCTURE AND SYMBOLS FOR SYNTHETIC AMINO ACIDS INCORPORATED INTO SYNTHETIC POLYPEPTIDES (Continued)

No.	Structure	Name/Reference	Symbol
63	$(C_6H_5)_2C(NH_2)COOH$	α,α-Diphenylglycine	Gly(Ph$_2$)
64	$CH_3CH_2SCH_2CH_2CH(NH_2)COOH$	Ethionine[b]	Eth
65	$CH_3CH_2NHCH_2COOH$	N-Ethylglycine	EtGly
66	*(imidazole structure with COOH, NH$_2$, N-ethyl)*	tele-ethylhistidine[b,c] "1-Ethylhistidine" (14) (cf. 88, 89)	His(τEt)[b,c]
67	$H_2NC(=NH)NHCH_2CO—$	Guanidinoacetyl(N-amidinoglycyl; glycocyamine)	GdnAc-: AmdGly-
68	$H_2NC(=NH)NHCH_2CH(NH_2)COOH$	β-Guanidinoalanine	Ala(βGdn)
69	$H_2NC(=NH)NH(CH_2)_3COOH$	5-Guanidinovaleric acid	Vlr(δ Gdn)
70	$(CF_3)_2CHCH(NH_2)COOH$	γ$_6$-Hexafluorovaline[β,β-bis(trifluoromethyl)alanine]	Val(γF$_6$)
71	$H_2NC(=HN)NH(CH_2)_4CH(NH_2)COOH$	Homoarginine[b]	Har[c]
72	$H_2N(CH_2)_5CH(NH_2)COOH$	Homolysine[b] (15)	Hly[c]
73	$H_2NCONHCH_2COOH$	Hydantoic acid; (carbamoylglycine)	CbmGly
74	*(hydantoin structure)*	5-Hydantoinacetyl	HydAc-
75	$CH_3CH(OH)CH_2CH_2CH(NH_2)COOH$	ε-Hydroxynorleucine (16)	Nle(ε OH)
76	*(piperidine ring structure, COOH, N–OH)*	1-Hydroxypipecolic acid (17)	Pip(1HO)
77	*(pyrrolidine ring structure, COOH, N–OH)*	1-Hydroxyproline (17)	Pro(1HO)[c]
78	*(pyrrolidine ring structure, OH, COOH)*	3-Hydroxyproline	Pro(3HO)[c]
79	*(pyrrolidine ring structure, HO, COOH)*	4-Hydroxyproline	Pro(4HO)[c]
80	$CH_3N(OH)CH_2COOH$	N-Hydroxysarcosine (17)	Sar(N-HO)
81	$HOOCCH_2CH(NH_2)CONH_2$	Isoasparagine[b]	Asp-NH$_2$[c]
82	$HOOCCH_2CH_2CH(NH_2)CONH_2$	Isoglutamine[b]	Glu-NH$_2$[c]
83	$H_2NN(CHMe_2)COOH$	2-Isopropylcarbazic acid [2-(1-carboxyhydrazino)propane]	Hdz(iPr)
84	$(CH_3)_2CHNH(CH_2)_3CH(NH_2)COOH$	N^δ-Isopropylornithine	Orn(δiPr)
85	$CH_3C(SH)(NH_2)COOH$	α-Mercaptoalanine (18)	Ala(αSH)
86	$CH_3CH(NHCH_3)COOH$	N-Methylalanine (19)	MeAla
87	$CH_3CH_2CH(CH_3)CH(NHCH_3)COOH$	N-Methylalloisoleucine (20)	(Me)alle

STRUCTURE AND SYMBOLS FOR SYNTHETIC AMINO ACIDS INCORPORATED INTO SYNTHETIC POLYPEPTIDES (Continued)

No.	Structure	Name/Reference	Symbol
88		*tele*Methylhistidine;[b,c] "1-Methylhistidine" (14, 21) (cf. 89)	His(τMe)[b,c]
89		*pros*Methylhistidine;[b,c] "3-Methylhistidine" (21) (cf. 88)	His(πMe)[b,c]
90	HOOCCH$_2$CH(NHCH$_3$)CONH$_2$	N-Methylisoasparagine (22)	MeAsp-NH$_2$
91		(N-Methyl)phenylalanine (23)	MePhe
92	CH$_3$OCH$_2$CH(NH$_2$)COOH	O-Methylserine	Ser(Me)[c]
93	CH$_3$CH(OCH$_3$)CH(NH$_2$)COOH	O-Methylthreonine	Thr(Me)[c]
94		N-Methyltyrosine (22) (surinamine)[b]	MeTyr
95		α-Methyltyrosine	Tyr(αMe)
96		O-Methyltyrosine	Tyr(OMe);Phe(4-OMe)
97		β-(1-Naphthyl)alanine	Ala(βNap-1)
98		β-(2-Naphthyl)alanine	Ala(βNap-2)
99	O$_2$NHNC(=NH)NHCH$_2$CO—	Nitroguanidinoacetyl	NGdnAc-
100	CH$_3$(CH$_2$)$_3$CH(NH$_2$)COOH	Norleucine[b] (2-aminohexanoic acid)	Nle[c]
101	CH$_3$CH$_2$CH$_2$CH(NH$_2$)COOH	Norvaline (2-aminovaleric acid)	Nva[c]
102		(Pentafluorophenyl)alanine	Ala(βPhF$_5$)
103		Phenylglycine	Gly(Ph)

STRUCTURE AND SYMBOLS FOR SYNTHETIC AMINO ACIDS INCORPORATED INTO SYNTHETIC POLYPEPTIDES (Continued)

No.	Structure	Name/Reference	Symbol
104		Pipecolic acid (piperidine-2-carboxylic acid)	Pip
105		β-(1-Pyrazolyl)alanine	Ala(βPz1)
106		β-(3-Pyrazolyl)alanine (24, 25)	Ala (βPz3)
107		β-(4-Pyrazolyl)alanine (25)	Ala(βPz4)
108		Pyro-2-aminoadipic acid	pAad; < Aad
109		Pyroglutamic acid[b] 5-pyrrolidone-2-carboxylic acid	pGlu; <Glu[c]
110	CH_3HNCH_2COOH	Sarcosine[a,] (N-methylglycine)	Sar[c]; MeGly
111	$HOOCCH_2CH_2CONH_2$	Succinamic acid	Suc-NH_2
112	$H_2NCH_2CH_2SO_3H$	Taurine (2-aminoethanesulfonic acid)	Tau
113		Thiazolidine-4-carboxylic acid	Tzl
114		β-(2-Thienyl)alanine	Ala(βThi2)
115		β-(2-Thienyl)serine	Ser(βThi2)
116	$(CH_3)_3N^+(CH_2)_5COOH$	ε-(Trimethylammonio)hexanoic acid[(ε-trimethylammonio)caproic acid]	εAhx(N[e]Me₃)
117		o-Tyrosine	Phe(2HO)
118		m-Tyrosine[b]	Phe(3HO)

Compiled by M. C. Khosla and W. E. Cohn.

References

1. Jansen, weustink, kerling, and havinga, *Rec. Trav. Chim. Pays-Bas,* 88, 819 (1969).
2. Umezawa, Aoyagi, Morishima, Matsuzaki, Hamada, and Takeuchi, *J. Antiobiot.* (Tokyo), 23, 259 (1970).
3. Morishima, Takita, and Umezawa, *J. Antibiot. (Tokyo),* 26, 115 (1973).
4. Edelson, Skinner, Ravel, and Shive, *J. Am. Chem. Soc.,* 81, 5150 (1959).
5. Houghten and Rapoport, *J. Med. Chem.,* 17, 556 (1974).
6. Miyoshi, *Bull. Chem. Soc. Jap.,* 46, 1489 (1973).
7. Rydon, *J. Chem. Soc. Perkin Trans.* 1, 2634 (1972).
8. Erickson and Merrifield, *J. Am. Chem. Soc.,* 95, 3750 (1973).
9. Nagarajan, Diamond, and Ressler, *J. Org. Chem.,* 38, 621 (1973).
10. Khosla, Leese, Maloy, Ferreira, Smeby, an Bumpus, *J. Med. Chem.,* 15, 792 (1972).
11. Jansen, Kerling, and Havinga, *Rec. Trav. Chim. Pays-Bas,* 89, 861 (1970).
12. Ikutani, *Bull. Chem. Soc. Jap.,* 43, 3602 (1970).
13. Sheehan and Ledis, *J. Am. Chem. Soc.,* 95, 875 (1973).
14. Beyerman, Maat, and Van Zon, *Rec. Trav. Chim. Pays-Bas,* 91, 246 (1972).
15. Bodanszky and Lindeberg, *J. Med. Chem.,* 14, 1197 (1971).
16. Dreyfuss, *J. Med. Chem.,* 17, 252 (1974).
17. Nagasawa, Kohlhoff, Fraser, and Mikhail, *J. Med. Chem.,* 15, 483 (1972).
18. Patel, Currie, Jr., and Olsen, *J. Org. Chem.,* 38, 126 (1973).
19. Khosla, Hall, Smeby, and Bumpus, *J. Med. Chem.,* 17, 431 (1974).
20. Khosla, Hall, Smeby, and Bumpus, *J. Med. Chem.,* 17, 1156 (1974).
21. Needleman, Marshall, and Rivier, *J. Med. Chem.,* 16, 968 (1973).
22. Khosla, Smeby, and Bumpus, Abstr. *169th Natl. Meet. Am. Chem. Soc.* Philadelphia, April 1975, MEDI 57.
23. Khosla, Smeby, and Bumpus, *J. Am. Chem. Soc.,* 94, 4721 (1972).
24. Hofmann and Bowers, *J. Med. Chem.,* 13, 1099 (1970).
25. Seeman, McGandy, and Rosenstein, *J. am. Chem. Soc.,* 94, 1717 (1972).
26. Khosla, Smeby, and Bumpus, in *Handbook of Experimental Pharmacology,* Vol. 37, Page and Bumpus, Eds., Springer-Verlag, Heidelberg, 1974, 126.

PROPERTIES OF THE α-KETO ACID ANALOGS OF AMINO ACIDS

α-Keto Acid	α-Amino Acid Analog	2,4-Dinitrophenylhydrazone Crystallization M.p. (°C)	Solvent[a]	Amino Acids After Hydrogenation (14)	Reduction by Lactic Dehydrogenase[b,g]	Decarboxylation by Yeast Decarboxylase[c]
Pyruvic	Alanine	216	h	Alanine	26,800	1,200
α-Ketoadipamic	α-Aminoadipamic acid (homoglutamine)					
α-Ketoadipic	α-Aminoadipic acid	208	h	α-Aminoadipic acid		
α-Ketobutyric	α-Aminobutyric acid	198	h	α-Aminobutyric acid	21,000	
α-Ketoheptylic	α-Aminoheptylic acid	130	e, l	α-Aminoheptylic acid	483	
α-Keto-ε-hydroxycaproic	α-Amino-ε-hydroxy-caproic acid	183	h	α-Amino-ε-hydroxy-caproic acid	181	25
Mesoxalic	α-Aminomalonic acid	205	hc	α-Aminomalonic acid, glycine		
α-Ketophenylacetic	α-Aminophenylacetic acid	193	h	α-Aminophenylacetic acid, cyclohexylglycine	2.6	0
DL-Oxalosuccinic	α-Aminotricarballylic acid					
α-Keto-δ-guanidinovaleric	Arginine	216, 267 (1)		Arginine	9.0	0
α-Ketosuccinamic	Asparagine	183		Asparagine, aspartic acid	8,930	
Oxalacetic	Aspartic acid	218	h	Aspartic acid, alanine, β-alanine	12.8	
α-Keto-δ-carbamidovaleric	Citrulline	190	h	Citrulline	4.3	0
β-Cyclohexylpyruvic	β-Cyclohexylalanine	189	h	β-Cyclohexylalanine	14.6	0
β-Sulfopyruvic	Cysteic acid	210	a	Cysteic acid, alanine	89.6	
β-Mercaptopyruvic	Cysteine	195–200 (2) 161–162 (3)		Alanine	27,000	750
α-Keto-γ-ethiolbutyric	Ethionine	131	h	Ethionine	1,650	121
α-Ketoglutaric	Glutamic acid	220	h	Glutamic acid	9.2	0
α-Ketoglutaric γ-ethyl ester	Glutamic acid γ-ethyl ester				49.0	721
α-Ketoglutaramic	Glutamine			Glutamine, glutamic acid		
Glyoxylic	Glycine	203	h	Glycine	21,100	0
β-Imidazolylpyruvic	Histidine	190–192, 240 (1)	hc, e, l	Histidine		
α-Keto-γ-hydroxybutyric	Homoserine					
DL-α-Keto-β-methylvaleric	DL-Isoleucine (or DL-alloisoleucine)	169	h	Isoleucine		
L-α-Keto-β-methylvaleric	L-Isoleucine (or D-alloisoleucine)	176	h	Isoleucine	5.0	1,000
D-α-Keto-β-methylvaleric	D-Isoleucine (or L-alloisoleucine)	176	h	Isoleucine	1.9	280
α-Ketoisocaproic	Leucine	162	h	Leucine	3.2	306
Trimethylpyruvic	tert-Leucine	180	h	tert-Leucine		
α-Keto-ε-aminocaproic	Lysine	212	h	Lysine, pipecolic acid		
α-Keto-γ-methiolbutyric	Methionine	150	h	Methionine	1,550	125
α-Keto-γ-methylsulfonylbutyric	Methionine sulfone	175	h	Methione sulfone		
α-Keto-δ-nitroguanidinovaleric	Nitroarginine	225	ac	Nitroarginine, arginine	42.6	0
α-Ketocaproic	Norleucine	153	h	Norleucine	560	
α-Ketovaleric	Norvaline	167	h	Norvaline	1,470	
α-Keto-δ-aminovaleric	Ornithine, proline	232–242 (4) 219 (5) 211–212 (6)		Ornithine, proline, pentahomoserine[d]		
Phenylpyruvic	Phenylalanine	162–164. 192–194 (7)		Phenylalanine	755	0
S-Benzyl-β-mercaptopyruvic	S-Benzylcysteine	150	a			
β-Hydroxypyruvic	Serine	162	e	Serine, alanine	26,000	0[h]
N-Succinyl-α-amino-ε-ketopimelic (15)	N-Succinyl-α,ε-diaminopimelic acid	137–143	h	N-Succinyl-α,ε-diaminopimelic acid		
DL-α-Keto-β-hydroxybutyric	DL-Threonine (or DL-allothreonine)	157–158 (8)		Threonine, α-aminobutyric acid	20,000	
β-[3,5-Diiodo-4-(3′,5′-diiodo 4′-hydroxyphenoxy)phenyl]	Thyroxine					
β-Indolylpyruvic	Tryptophan	169 (1)		Tryptophan	670	0
p-Hydroxyphenylpyruvic	Tyrosine	178	h	Tyrosine	345	0
α-Ketoisovaleric	Valine	196	h	Valine	103	922

[a] h = water; e = ethyl acetate; l = ligroin; hc = hydrochloric acid; ac = glacial acetic acid; a = ethanol.
[b] Mole × 10^{-8} of DPNH oxidized per mg of enzyme per minute at 26° (9, 10).
[c] μL. CO_2 per hour (10).
[d] α-Amino-δ-hydroxy-n-valeric acid.
[e] Originally designated d (11). Originally designated l (11).
[g] Additional data have been published on the reduction of α-keto acids by lactic dehydrogenase (12).
[h] This keto acid has been reported to be decarboxylated by yeast preparations; the reaction is much more rapid at pH 6.3 than at 5 (13).

From Meister, *Biochemistry of the Amino Acids*, 2nd ed., Academic Press, New York, 1965, 162–164. With permission.

References

1. Stumpf and Green, *J. Biol. Chem.*, 153, 387 (1944).
2. Schneider and Reinefeld, *Biochem. Z.*, 318, 507 (1948).
3. Meister, Fraser, and Tice, *J. Biol. Chem.*, 206, 561 (1954).
4. Krebs, *Enzymologia*, 7, 53 (1939).
5. Blanchard, Green, Nocito, and Ratner, *J. Biol Chem.*, 155, 421 (1944).
6. Meister, *J. Biol. Chem.*, 206, 579 (1954).
7. Fones, *J. Org. Chem.*, 17, 1534 (1952).
8. Sprinson and Chargaff, *J. Biol. Chem.*, 164, 417 (1947).
9. Meister, *J. Biol. Chem.*, 197, 309 (1953).
10. Meister, *J. Biol. Chem.*, 184, 117 (1950).
11. Meister, *J. Biol. Chem.*, 190,269 (1951).
12. Czok and Büchler, *Advanc. Protein. Chem.*, 15, 315 (1960).
13. Dickens and Williamson, *Nature*, 178, 1349 (1956).
14. Meister and Abendschein, *Anal. Chem.*, 28, 171 (1956).
15. Gilvarg, *J. Biol. Chem.*, 236, 1429 (1961).

α,β-UNSATURATED AMINO ACIDS

α,β-Unsaturated amino acids with free α-amino groups are not stable; N-acylated α,β-unsaturated amino acids are stable compounds. The α,β-unsaturated amino acids listed in this table are present in natural products in which they are stabilized by peptide bond formation. The addition of mercaptans to α,β-unsaturated amino acids and the reversible conversion to keto acids and amides are of biological significance.[1,2,11]

No.	Amino Acid/Synonym	Source	Structure	Formula (Mol Wt)	References Chemistry	References Spectral Data
1	Dehydroalanine	Nisin Subtilin	$H_2C=C(NH_2)COOH$	$C_3H_5NO_2$ 87.08	1, 2 2	1, 2 2
2	β-Methyldehydroalanine	Nisin, Subtilin Stendomycin	$H_3CCH=C(NH_2)COOH$	$C_4H_7NO_2$ 101.10	1, 2 3	1, 2 3
3	Dehydroserine	Viomycin Capreomycin	$HOHC=C(NH_2)COOH$	$C_3H_5NO_3$ 103.08	4 4	4 4
4	Dehydroleucine	Albonoursin	$(H_3C)_2CHCH=C(NH_2)COOH$	$C_6H_{11}NO_2$ 129.16	5	
5	Dehydrophenylalanine	Albonoursin	$PhCH=C(NH_2)COOH$	$C_9H_9NO_2$ 163.17	5	
6	Dehydrotryptophan	Telomycin	(indole structure)	$C_{11}H_{10}N_2O_2$ 202.21	6	6
7	Dehydroarginine	Viomycin Capreomycin	$H_2NC(=NH)$ $NHCH_2CH_2CH=C(NH_2)COOH$	$C_6H_{12}N_4O_2$ 172.19	4	4
8	Dehydroproline	Ostreogrycin A	(pyrroline structure)	$C_5H_7NO_2$ 113.11	4 7	4 7
9	Dehydrovaline	Penicillin	$(H_3C)_2C=C(NH_2)COOH$	$C_5H_9NO_2$ 115.13	8	
10	Dehydrocysteine	Micrococcin Thiostrepton	$HSCH=C(NH_2)COOH$	$C_3H_5NO_2S$	9, 10	10

Compiled by Erhard Gross.

References

1. Gross and Morell, *J. Am. Chem. Soc.*, 89, 2791 (1967).
2. Gross and Morell, *Fed. Eur. Biochem. Soc. Lett.*, 2, 61 (1968).
3. Bodanszky, Izdebski, and Muramatsu, *J. Am. Chem. Soc.*, 91, 2351 (1969).
4. Bycroft, Cameron, Croft, Hassanali-Walji, Johnson, and Webb, *Tetrahedron Lett.*, p. 5901 (1968).
5. Khokhlov and Lokshin, *Tetrahedron Lett.*, p.1881 (1963).
6. Sheehan, Mani, Nakamura, Stock, and Maeda, *J. Am. Chem. Soc.*, 90, 462 (1968).
7. Delpierre, Eastwood, Gream, Kingston, Sarin, Todd, and Williams, *J. Chem. Soc.*, p. 1653 (1966).
8. Abraham and Newton, in *Antibiotics*, Gottlieb and Shawn, Eds., Springer-Verlag, New York, 1967.
9. Brookes, Clarke, Majhofer, Mijovic, and Walker, *J. Chem. Soc.*, p. 925 (1960).
10. Bodanszky, Sheehan, Fried, Williams, and Birkhimer, *J. Am. Chem. Soc.*, 82, 4747 (1960).
11. Gross, Morell, and Craig, *Proc. Natl. Acad. Sci. U.S.A.*, 62, 953 (1969).

AMINO ACID ANTAGONISTS

Amino Acid	Analog	System	Reference
α-Alanine	α-Aminoethanesulfonic acid	Bacteria	1
		Mouse tumor	2
	Glycine	Bacteria	3
	α-Aminoisobutyric acid	Bacteria	4
	Serine	Bacteria	3
D-Alanine	D-Cycloserine	Bacterial cell wall	5–10
	O-Carbamyl-D-serine	Bacterial cell wall	11
	D-α-Aminobutyric acid	Bacterial cell wall	12
β-Alanine	β-Aminobutyric acid	Yeast	13
	Propionic acid	Bacteria	14
	Asparagine	Yeast	15
	D-Serine	Bacteria	16
Arginine	Canavanine	Yeast, *Neurospora*, bacteria	17, 18–22
		Carcinosarcoma	23
		Animals	24, 25
		Plants	26, 27
		Tissue culture	28, 29
	Lysine	Arginase	30
	Ornithine	Arginase	31
	Homoarginine	Bacteria	22, 32
Aspartic acid	Cysteic acid	Bacteria	1, 33, 34
		Bacteria	35
	β-Hydroxyaspartic acid	Bacteria	34, 36, 37
	Diaminosuccinic acid	Bacteria	36
	Aspartophenone	Bacteria, yeast	4
	α-Aminolevulinic acid	Bacteria, yeast	4
	α-Methylaspartic acid	Bacteria	38
	β-Aspartic acid hydrazide	Bacteria	38
	S-Methylcysteine sulfoxide	Bacteria	39
	β-Methylaspartic acid	Bacteria	40
	Hadacidin	Purine biosynthesis	41
Asparagine	2-Amino-2-carboxyethanesulfonamide	*Neurospora*	42
Cysteine	Allylglycine	Bacteria, yeast	43
α,ε-Diaminopimelic acid	α,α-Diaminosuberic acid	Bacteria	44
	α,α-Diaminosebacic acid	Bacteria	44
	β-Hydroxy-α,ε-diaminopimelic acid	*Escherichia coli*	45
	γ-Methyl-α,ε-diaminopimelic acid	*E. coli*	46
	Cystine	*E. coli*	47
Glutamic acid	Methionine sulfoxide	Bacteria	48, 49
		Glutamine synthesis	50
	γ-Glutamylethylamide	Bacteria	51
	β-Hydroxyglutamic acid	Bacteria	52, 53
	Methionine sulfoximine	Bacteria	54, 55
	α-Methylglutamic acid	Enzymes	56, 57
	γ-Phosphonoglutamic acid	Glutamine synthesis	58
	P-Ethyl-γ-phosphonoglutamic acid	Glutamine synthesis	58
	γ-Fluoroglutamic acid[a]	Glutamine synthesis	59
Glutamine	S-Carbamylcysteine	Bacteria	60
		Ascites cells	61
	O-Carbamylserine	Bacteria	62
	O-Carbazylserine	Bacteria	63
	3-Amino-3-carboxypropanesulfonamide	*E. coli*	64
	N-Benzylglutamine	*Streptococcus lactis*	65
	Azaserine	Enzymes	66
	6-Diazo-5-oxonorleucine	Enzymes	66
	γ-Glutamylhydrazide	*S. faecalis*	67
Glycine	α-Aminomethanesulfonic acid	Bacteriophage	68

AMINO ACID ANTAGONISTS (Continued)

Amino Acid	Analog	System	Reference
		Vaccinia virus	69
		Bacteria	1
		E. coli	4
Histidine	D-Histidine	Histidase	70
	Imidazole		70
	2-Thiazolealanine	E. coli	71
	1,2,4-Triazolealanine	E. coli	71, 72
		Salmonella	73
Isoleucine	Leucine	Bacteria	74
		Rats	75
	Methallylglycine	Bacteria, yeast	4, 43
	ω-Dehydroisoleucine	Bacteria	76
	3-Cyclopentene-1-glycine	Bacteria	77
	Cyclopentene glycine	Bacteria	78
	2-Cyclopentene-1-glycine	Bacteria	79
	O-Methylthreonine	Tumor cells	80
	β-Hydroxyleucine	Bacteria	37
Leucine	D-Leucine	Bacteria	81
	α-Aminoisoamylsulfonic acid	Bacteria	1, 33
		Mouse tumor	2
	Norvaline	Bacteria	4
	Norleucine	Bacteria	1, 4, 82
	Methallylglycine	Yeast, bacteria	4
	α-Amino-β-chlorobutyric acid	Yeast, bacteria	4
	Valine	Bacteria	83
	δ-Chloroleucine	Neurospora	84
	Isoleucine	Bacteria	85
	β-Hydroxynorleucine	Bacteria	86
	β-Hydroxyleucine	Bacteria	86
	Cyclopentene alanine	Bacteria	87
	3-Cyclopentene-1-alanine	Bacteria	88
	2-Amino-4-methylhexenoic acid	Bacteria	89
	5,′5,′5′-Trifluoroleucine	E. coli	90
	4-Azaleucine	E. coli	91
Lysine	α-Amino-ε-hydroxycaproic acid	Rat	92
	Arginine	Neurospora	93
	2,6-Diaminoheptanoic acid	Bacteria	94
	Oxalysine	Bacteria	95
	3-Aminomethylcyclohexane glycine	Bacteria	96
	3-Aminocyclohexane alanine	Bacteria	97
	trans-4-Dehydrolysine	Bacteria	98
	S-(β-Aminoethyl)cysteine	Bacteria	99
	4-Azalysine	Bacteria	
Methionine	2-Amino-5-heptenoic acid (crotylalanine)	E. coli	100
	2-Amino-4-hexenoic acid (crotylglycine)	E. coli	101
	Methoxinine	Bacteria	102
		Vaccinia virus	69
		Rats	103
	Norleucine	Bacteria	82, 104, 105
		Animal tissues	106
		Casein	107
	Ethionine	Bacteria, animals	28, 102, 105, 108–120
		Amylase	121, 122
		Yeast	123
		Tumors	124
		Pancreatic proteins	125
	Methionine sulfoximine	Bacteria	126
	Threonine	Neurospora	127
	Selenomethionine	Chlorella	128

AMINO ACID ANTAGONISTS (Continued)

Amino Acid	Analog	System	Reference
		E. coli, yeast	129–132
Ornithine	α-Amino-δ-hydroxyvaleric acid	Bacteria	21
	Canaline	Bacteria	21
Phenylalanine	α-Amino-β-phenylethanesulfonic acid	Mouse tumor	2
	Tyrosine	Bacteria	133
	β-Phenylserine	Bacteria	134–136
	Cyclohexylalanine	Rats	137
	o-Aminophenylalanine	E. coli	138
	p-Aminophenylalanine	Bacteria	139, 140
	Fluorophenylalanines	Fungi, bacteria	140–148
		Lysozyme, albumin	149
		Muscle enzymes	150
		Amylase	151
		Hemoglobin	152
		Rats	153
Phenylalanine	Chlorophenylalanines	Fungi	147
	Bromophenylalanines	Fungi	147
	β-2-Thienylalanine	Rat, bacteria, yeast	136, 154–164
		β-Galactosidase	165
	β-3-Thienylalanine	Bacteria, yeast	166
	β-2-Furylalanine	Bacteria, yeast	4
	β-3-Furylalanine	Bacteria, yeast	4
	β-2-Pyrrolealanine	Bacteria, yeast	167
	1-Cyclopentene-1-alanine	Bacteria	87
	1-Cyclohexene-1-alanine	Bacteria	87
	2-Amino-4-methyl-4-hexenoic acid	Bacteria	89
	S-(1,2-Dichlorovinyl)cysteine	E. coli	168
	β-4-Pyridylalanine	Bacteria	169
	Tryptophan	Bacteria	170
	β-2-Pyridylalanine	Bacteria	171
	β-4-Pyrazolealanine	Bacteria	171
	β-4-Thiazolealanine	Bacteria	171
	p-Nitrophenylalanine	Bacteria	140
Proline	Hydroxyproline	Fungi	172
	3,4-Dehydroproline	Bacteria, beans	173, 174
	Azetidine-2-carboxylic acid	Bacteria, beans	175, 176
		Actinomycin	177, 178
Serine	α-Methylserine	Bacteria	4
	Homoserine	Bacteria	4
	Threonine	Bacteria	179, 180
	Isoserine	Enzymes	181
Threonine	Serine	Bacteria	179, 180, 182
	β-Hydroxynorvaline	Bacteria	86, 183
	β-Hydroxynorleucine	Bacteria	86, 183
Thyroxine	Ethers of 3,5-diiodotyrosine	Tadpoles	184
Tryptophan	Methyltryptophans	Bacteria	141, 185–188
		Bacteriophage	189
	Naphthylalanines	Bacteria	190, 191
		Rat	4
	Indoleacrylic acid	Bacteria	192
	Naphthylacrylic acid	Bacteria	193
	β-(2-Benzothienyl)alanine	Bacteria	194
	Styrylacetic acid	Bacteria	193
	Indole	Bacteriophage	195
	α-Amino-β-3(indazole)propionic acid (Tryptazan)	Yeast	196
		Enzyme	197
		E. coli	198
	5-Fluorotryptophan	Enzyme	199, 200
	6-Fluorotryptophan	Enzyme	201

AMINO ACID ANTAGONISTS (Continued)

Amino Acid	Analog	System	Reference
	7-Azatryptophan	E. coli	202–205
Tyrosine	Fluorotyrosines	Fungi	147, 206
		Rat	206
	p-Aminophenylalanine	Fungi	139
	m-Nitrotyrosine	Bacteria	140
	β-(5-Hydroxy-2-pyridyl)alanine	Bacteria	207
Valine	α-Aminoisobutanesulfonic acid	Bacteria	1, 2, 33
		Vaccinia	69
	α-Aminobutyric acid	Bacteria	4, 182
	Norvaline	Bacteria	4
	Leucine, isoleucine	Bacteria	83, 182
	Methallylglycine	Bacteria, yeast	4
	β-Hydroxyvaline	Bacteria	86, 183
	ω-Dehydroalloisoleucine	Bacteria	76

ᵃ Some of the observed inhibition may be due to fluoride ion present in the amino acid preparation or formed during incubation.[208]

Courtesy of Herbert M. Kagan, Boston University School of Medicine (from Meister, A., Ed., *Biochemistry of the Amino Acids*, 2nd ed., Vol. 1, 1965, 233–238).

References

1. McIlwain, *Brit. J. Exp. Pathol.* 22, 148 (1941).
2. Greenberg and Schulman, *Science* 106, 271 (1947).
3. Snell and Guirard, *Proc. Nat. Acad. Sci. (US)* 29, 66 (1943).
4. Dittmer, *Ann. N.Y. Acad. Sci.* 52, 1274 (1950).
5. Bondi, Kornblum and Forte, *Proc. Soc. Exp. Biol. Med.* 96, 270 (1957).
6. Zygmunt, *J. Bacteriol.* 84, 154 (1962); 85, 1217 (1963).
7. Strominger, Threnn and Scott, *J. Amer. Chem. Soc.* 81, 3803 (1959).
8. Strominger, Ito and Threnn, *J. Amer. Chem. Soc.* 82, 998 (1960).
9. Neuhaus and Lynch, *Biochem. Biophys. Res. Commun.* 8, 377 (1962).
10. Moulder, Novosel and Officer, *J. Bacteriol.* 85, 707 (1963).
11. Tanaka, *Biochem. Biophys. Res. Commun.* 12, 68 (1963).
12. Snell, Radin and Ikawa, *J. Biol. Chem.* 217, 803 (1955).
13. Nielsen, *Naturwissenschaften* 31, 146 (1943).
14. Wright and Skeggs, *Arch. Biochem.* 10, 383 (1946).
15. Sarett and Cheldelin, *J. Bacteriol.* 49, 31 (1945).
16. Durham and Milligan, *Biochem. Biophys. Res. Commun.* 7, 342 (1962).
17. Richmond, *Biochem. J.* 73, 261 (1959).
18. Horowitz and Srb, *J. Biol. Chem.* 174, 371 (1948).
19. Teas, *J. Biol. Chem.* 190, 369 (1951).
20. Miller and Harrison, *Nature* 166, 1035 (1950).
21. Volcani and Snell, *J. Biol. Chem.* 174, 893 (1948).
22. Walker, *J. Biol. Chem.* 212, 207. 617 (1955).
23. Kruse, White, Carter and McCoy, *Cancer Res.* 19, 122 (1959).
24. Owaga, *J. Agr. Chem. Soc. Jap.* 10, 225 (1934); *Chem. Abstr.* 28, 4458 (1934).
25. Owaga, *J. Agr. Chem. Soc. Jap.* 11, 559 (1935); *Chem. Abstr.* 29, 740, 3379 (1935).
26. Steward, Pollard, Patchett and Witkop, *Biochim. Biophys. Acta.* 28, 308 (1958).
27. Bonner, *Amer. J. Bot.* 36, 323, 429 (1949).
28. Gros and Gros-Doulcet, *Exp. Cell. Res.* 14, 104 (1958).
29. Morgan, Morton and Pasieka, *J. Biol. Chem.* 233, 664 (1958).
30. Hunter and Downs, *J. Biol. Chem.* 157, 427 (1945).
31. Gross Z, *Physiol. Chem.* 112, 236 (1921).
32. Walker, *J. Biol. Chem.* 212, 617 (1955).
33. McIlwain, *J. Chem. Soc.* p 75 (1941).
34. Ifland and Shive, *J. Biol. Chem.* 223, 949 (1956).
35. Shive, Ackerman and Ravel, *Chem. Soc.* 69, 2567 (1947).
36. Shive and Macow, *J. Biol. Chem.* 162, 452 (1946).
37. Otani, *Arch. Biochem. Biophys.* 101, 131 (1963).
38. Roberts and Hunter, *Proc. Soc. Exp. Biol. Med.* 83, 720 (1953).
39. Arnold, Morris and Thompson, *Nature* 186, 1051 (1960).
40. Woolley *J. Biol. Chem.* 235, 3238 (1960).
41. Shigeura and Gordon, *J. Biol. Chem.* 237, 1932, 1937 (1962).
42. Heymann, Ginsberg, Gulick, Konopka and Mayer, *J. Amer. Chem. Soc.* 81, 5125 (1959).
43. Dittmer, Goering, Goodman and Cristol, *J. Amer. Chem. Soc.* 70, 2499 (1948).
44. Simmonds, *Biochem. J.* 58, 520 (1954).
45. Rhuland, *J. Bacteriol.* 73, 778 (1957).
46. Rhuland and Hamilton, *Biochim. Biophys. Acta.* 51, 525 (1961).
47. Meadow, Hoare and Work, *Biochem. J.* 66, 270 (1957).
48. Borek, Miller, Sheiness and Waelsch, *J. Biol. Chem.* 163, 347 (1946).
49. Borek and Waelsch, *Arch. Biochem.* 14, 143 (1947).
50. Elliot and Gale, *Nature* 161, 129 (1948).
51. Lichtenstein and Grossowicz, *J. Biol. Chem.* 171, 387 (1947).
52. Borek and Waelsch, *J. Biol. Chem.* 177, 135 (1949).
53. Ayengar and Roberts, *Proc. Soc. Exp. Biol. Med.* 79, 476 (1952).
54. Pace and McDermott, *Nature* 169, 415 (1952).
55. Heathcote and Pace, *Nature* 166, 353 (1950).
56. Roberts, *J. Biol. Chem.* 202, 359 (1953).
57. Lichtenstein, Ross and Cohen, *Nature* 171, 45 (1953); *J Biol. Chem.* 201, 117 (1953).
58. Mastalerz, *Arch. Immunol. Terap. Dos.* 7, 201 (1959).
59. Provided by Pattison [Buchanan, Dean and Pattison Can. J. Chem. 40, 1571 (1962)], and studied in the author's laboratory.
60. Ravel, McCord, Skinner and Shive, *J. Biol. Chem.* 232, 159 (1958).
61. Rabinovitz and Fisher, *J. Nat. Cancer Inst.* 28, 1165 (1962).
62. Skinner, McCord, Ravel and Shive, *J. Amer. Chem. Soc.* 78, 2412 (1956).
63. McCord, Ravel, Skinner and Shive, *J. Amer. Chem. Soc.* 80, 3762 (1958).
64. Reisner *J. Amer. Chem. Soc.* 78, 5102 (1956).
65. Edelson, Skinner and Shive, *J. Med. Pharm. Chem.* 1, 165 (1959).
66. Meister (1962) in *The Enzymes*, Boyer, Lardy and Myrback, Eds. Academic, New York, VI, p 247.
67. McIlwain, Roper and Hughes, *Biochem. J.* 42, 492 (1948).
68. Spizizen, *J. Infect. Dis.* 73, 212 (1943).
69. Thompson, *J. Immunol.* 55, 345 (1947).
70. Edlbacher, Baur and Becker, *Z. Physiol. Chem.* 265, 61 (1940).
71. Moyed *J. Biol. Chem.* 236, 2261 (1961).
72. Jones and Ainsworth, *J. Amer. Chem. Soc.* 77, 1538 (1955).
73. Levin and Hartman, *J. Bacteriol.* 86, 820 (1963).
74. Doudoroff, *Proc. Soc. Exp. Biol. Med.* 53, 73 (1943).
75. Harper, Benton, Winje and Elvehjem, *Arch. Biochem. Biophys.* 51, 523 (1954).
76. Parker, Skinner and Shive, *J. Biol. Chem.* 236, 3267 (1961).
77. Edelson, Fissekis, Skinner and Shive, *J. Amer. Chem. Soc.* 80, 2698 (1958).
78. Harding and Shive, *J. Biol. Chem.* 206, 401 (1954).

79. Dennis, Plant, Skinner, Sutherland and Shive, *J. Amer. Chem. Soc.* 77, 2362 (1955).
80. Rabinovitz, Olson and Greenberg, *J. Amer. Chem. Soc.* 77, 3109 (1955).
81. Fox, Fling and Bollenback, *J. Biol. Chem.* 155, 465 (1944).
82. Harding and Shive *J. Biol. Chem.* 174, 743 (1948).
83. Brickson, Henderson, Solhjell and Elvehjem, *J. Biol. Chem.* 176, 517 (1948).
84. Ryan, *Arch. Biochem. Biophys.* 36, 487 (1952).
85. Hirsh and Cohen, *Biochem. J.* 53, 25 (1953).
86. Buston and Bishop, *J. Biol. Chem.* 215, 217 (1955).
87. Pal, Skinner, Dennis and Shive, *J. Amer. Chem. Soc.* 78, 5116 (1956).
88. Edelson, Skinner, Ravel and Shive, *Arch. Biochem. Biophys.* 80, 416 (1959).
89. Edelson, Skinner, Ravel and Shive, *J. Amer. Chem. Soc.* 81, 5150 (1959).
90. Rennert and Anker, *Biochemistry* 2, 471 (1963).
91. Smith, Bayliss and McCord, *J. Arch. Biochem. Biophys.* 102, 313 (1963).
92. Page, Gaudry and Gringras, *J. Biol. Chem.* 171, 831 (1948).
93. Daermann, *Arch. Biochem.* 5, 373 (1944).
94. McLaren and Knight, *J. Amer. Chem. Soc.* 73, 4478 (1951).
95. McCord, Ravel, Skinner and Shive, *J. Amer. Chem. Soc.* 79, 5693 (1957).
96. Davis, Skinner and Shive, *Arch. Biochem. Biophys.* 87, 88 (1960).
97. Davis, Ravel, Skinner and Shive, *Arch. Biochem. Biophys.* 76, 139 (1958).
98. Davis, Skinner and Shive, *J. Amer. Chem. Soc.* 83, 2279 (1961).
99. Shiota, Folk and Tietze, *Arch. Biochem. Biophys.* 77, 372 (1958).
100. Goering, Cristol and Dittmer, *J. Amer. Chem. Soc.* 70, 3314 (1948).
101. Skinner, Edelson and Shive, *J. Amer. Chem. Soc.* 83, 2281 (1961).
102. Roblin, Lampen, English, Cole and Vaughan, *J. Amer. Chem. Soc.* 67, 290 (1945).
103. Shaffer and Critchfield, *J. Biol. Chem.* 174, 489 (1948).
104. Reisner, *J. Amer. Chem. Soc.* 78, 2132 (1956).
105. Porter and Meyers, *Arch. Biochem.* 8, 169 (1945).
106. Rabinovitz, Olson and Greenberg, *J. Biol. Chem.* 210, 837 (1954).
107. Black and Kleiber, *J. Amer. Chem. Soc.* 77, 6082 (1955).
108. Dyer *J. Biol. Chem.* 124, 519 (1938).
109. Harris and Kohn, *J, Pharmacol. Exp. Therap.* 73, 383 (1941).
110. Halvorson and Spiegelman, *J. Bacteriol.* 64, 207 (1952).
111. Simpson, Farber and Tarver, *J. Biol. Chem.* 182, 81 (1950).
112. Simmonds, Keller, Chandler and du Vigneaud, *J. Biol. Chem.* 183, 191 (1950).
113. Stekol and Weiss, *J. Biol. Chem.* 179, 1049 (1949).
114. Stekol and Weiss, *J. Biol. Chem.* 185, 577, 585 (1950).
115. Farber, Simpson and Tarver, *J. Biol. Chem.* 182, 91 (1950).
116. Keston and Wortis, *Proc. Soc. Exp. Biol. Med.* 61, 439 (1946).
117. Levine and Tarver, *J. Biol. Chem.* 192, 835 (1951).
118. Tarver (1954) in *The Proteins*, Neurath and Bailey, Eds., Academic, New York IIB, p 1199.
119. Swendseid, Swanson and Bethell, *J. Biol. Chem.* 201, 803 (1953).
120. Levy, Montanez, Murphy and Dunn, *Cancer Res.* 13, 507 (1953).
121. Yoshida, *Biochim. Biophys. Acta.* 29, 213 (1958).
122. Yoshida and Yamasaki, *Biochim. Biophys. Acta.* 34, 158 (1959).
123. Parks, *J. Biol. Chem.* 232, 169 (1958).
124. Rabinovitz, Olson and Greenberg, *J. Biol. Chem.* 227, 217 (1957).
125. Hansson and Garzo, *Biochim. Biophys. Acta.* 61, 121 (1962).
126. Heathcote, *Lancet* 257, 1130 (1949).
127. Doudney and Wagner, *Proc. Nat. Acad. Sci. U.S.* 38, 196 (1952); 39, 1043 (1953).
128. Shrift, *Amer. J. Bot.* 41, 345 (l954).
129. Cowie and Cohen, *Biochim. Biophys. Acta.* 26, 252 (1957).
130. Cohen and Cowie, *Compt. Rend. Acad. Sci.* 244, 680 (1957).
131. Blau, *Biochim. Biophys. Acta.* 49, 389 (1961).
132. Tuve and Williams, *J. Amer. Chem. Soc.* 79, 5830 (1957).
133. Beerstecher and Shive, *J. Biol. Chem.* 167, 527 (1947).
134. Beerstecher and Shive, *J. Biol. Chem.* 164, 53 (1946).
135. Fox and Warner, *J. Biol. Chem.* 210, 119 (1954).
136. Miller and Simmonds, *Science* 126, 445 (1957).
137. Baltes, Elliott, Doisy and Doisy, *J. Biol. Chem.* 194, 627 (1952).
138. Davis, Lloyd, Fletcher, Bayliss and McCord, *Arch. Biochem. Biophys.* 102, 48 (1963).
139. Burckhalter and Stephens, *J. Amer. Chem. Soc.* 73. 56 (1951).
140. Bergmann, Sicher and Volcani, *Biochem. J.* 54, 1 (1953).
141. Munier and Cohen, *Biochim. Biophys. Acta.* 21, 592 (1956).
142. Munier and Cohen, *Biochim. Biophys. Acta.* 31, 378 (1959).
143. Cohen and Munier *Biochim. Biophys. Acta.* 31, 347 (1959).
144. Cowie, Cohen, Bolton and De Robichon-Szulmajster, *Biochim. Biophys. Acta.* 34, 39 (1959).
145. Cohen, Halvorson and Spiegelman (1958) *Microsomal Particles Protein Syn. Papers. Symp. Biophys. Soc. 1st*, Cambridge, Mass, Pergamon, New York, p 100.
146. Baker, Johnson and Fox, *Biochim. Biophys. Acta.* 28, 318 (1958).
147. Mitchell and Niemann, *J. Amer. Chem. Soc.* 69, 1232 (1947).
148. Atkinson, Melvin and Fox, *Arch. Biochem. Biophys.* 31, 205 (1951).
149. Vaughan and Steinberg, *Biochim. Biophys. Acta.* 40, 230 (1960).
150. Boyer and Westhead, *Abstr. Meeting. Amer. Chem. Soc.* Washington, DC. p 2C (1958).
151. Yoshida, *Biochim. Biophys. Acta.* 41, 98 (1960).
152. Kruh and Rose, *Biochim. Biophys. Acta.* 34, 561 (1959).
153. Armstrong and Lewis, *J. Biol. Chem.* 188, 91 (1951).
154. du Vigneaud. McKennis, Simmonds, Dittmer and Brown, *J. Biol. Chem.* 159, 385 (1945).
155. Dittmer, Ellis, McKennis and du Vigneaud, *J. Biol. Chem.* 164, 761 (1946).
156. Dittmer, Hertz and Chambers, *J. Biol. Chem.* 166, 541 (1946).
157. Garst, Campaigne and Day, *J. Biol. Chem.* 180, 1013 (1949).
158. Ferger and du Vigneaud, *J. Biol. Chem.* 179, 61 (1949).
159. Drea, *J. Bacteriol.* 56, 257 (1948).
160. Dunn and Dittmer, *J. Biol. Chem.* 188, 263 (1951).
161. Kihara and Snell, *J. Biol. Chem.* 212, 83 (1955).
162. Ferger and du Vigneaud, *J. Biol. Chem.* 174, 241 (1948).
163. Dunn, *J. Biol. Chem.* 233, 411 (1958).
164. Dunn, Ravel and Shive, *J. Biol. Chem.* 219, 809 (1956).
165. Janeček and Rickenberg, *Biochim. Biophys. Acta.* 81, 108 (1964).
166. Dittmer, *J. Amer. Chem. Soc.* 71, 1205 (1949).
167. Herz, Dittmer and Cristol, *J. Amer. Chem. Soc.* 70, 504 (1948).
168. Dickie and Schultz, *Arch. Biochem. Biophys.* 100, 279, 285 (1963).
169. Elliott, Fuller and Harington *J. Chem. Soc.* p. 85 (1948).
170. Beerstecher and Shive *J. Amer. Chem. Soc.* 69, 461 (1947).
171. Lansford and Shive, *Arch. Biochem. Biophys.* 38, 347 (1952).
172. Robbins and McVeigh, *Amer. J. Bot.* 33, 638 (1946).
173. Fowden, Neale and Tristram, *Nature* 199, 35 (1963).
174. Smith, Ravel, Skinner and Shive, *Arch. Biochem. Biophys.* 99, 60 (1962).
175. Fowden and Richmond, *Biochim. Biophys. Acta.* 71, 459 (1963).
176. Fowden, *J. Exp. Bot.* 14, 387 (1963).
177. Katz and Goss, *Biochem. J.* 73, 458 (1959).
178. Katz, *Ann. N.Y. Acad. Sci.* 89, 304 (1960).
179. Meinke and Holland, *J. Biol. Chem.* 173, 535 (1948).
180. Holland and Meinke, *J. Biol. Chem.* 178, 7 (1949).
181. Leibman and Fellner, *J. Biol. Chem.* 237, 2213 (1962).
182. Gladstone, *Brit. J. Exp. Pathol.* 20, 189 (1939).
183. Buston, Churchman and Bishop, *J. Biol. Chem.* 204, 665 (1953).
184. Woolley, *J. Biol. Chem.* 164, 11 (1946).
185. Trudinger and Cohen, *Biochem. J.* 62, 488 (1956).
186. Anderson, *Science* 101, 565 (1945).
187. Fildes and Rydon, *Brit. J. Exp. Pathol.* 28, 211 (1947).
188. Marshall and Woods, *Biochem. J.* 51, ii (1952).
189. Cohen and Anderson *J. Exp. Med.* 84, 525 (1946).
190. Erlenmeyer and Grubemann, *Helv. Chim. Acta.* 30, 297 (1947).
191. Dittmer, Herz and Cristol, *J. Biol. Chem.* 173, 323 (1948).
192. Fildes, *Brit. J. Exp. Pathol.* 22, 293 (1941).
193. Block and Erlenmeyer, *Helo. Chim. Acta.* 25, 694, 1063 (1942).
194. Avakian, Mars and Martin, *J. Amer. Chem. Soc.* 70, 3075 (1948).
195. Delbrück *J. Bacteriol.* 56, 1 (1948).
196. Halvorson, Spiegelman and Hinman, *Arch. Biochem. Biophys.* 55, 512 (1956).
197. Durham and Martin, *Biochim. Biophys. Acta.* 71, 481 (1963).
198. Brawerman and Yüeas, *Arch. Biochem. Biophys.* 68, 112 (1957).
199. Moyed, *J. Biol. Chem.* 235, 1098 (1960).

200. Bergmann, Eschinazi, Sicher and Volcani, *Bull. Res. Soc. Israel* 2, 308 (1952).
201. Moyed and Friedmann, *Science* 129, 968 (1959).
202. Robison and Robison, *J. Amer. Chem. Soc.* 77, 457 (1955).
203. Pardee, Shore and Prestidge, *Biochim. Biophys. Acta.* 21, 406 (1956).
204. Pardee and Prestidge, *Biochim. Biophys. Acta.* 27, 330 (1958) .
205. Kidder and Dewey *Biochim. Biophys. Acta.* 17, 288 (1955).
206. Niemann and Rapport, *J. Amer. Chem. Soc.* 68, 1671 (1946).
207. Norton, Skinner and Shive, *J. Org. Chem.* 26, 1495 (1961).
208. Kagan, H., *unpublished studies.*

Particle Diameter

PARTICLE DIAMETER

This figure originally appeared in Sober, Ed., *Handbook of Biochemistry and Selected Data for Molecular Biology*, 2nd ed., Chemical Rubber Co., Cleveland, 1970.

WEIGHTS OF CELLS AND CELL CONSTITUENTS

Norman G. Anderson

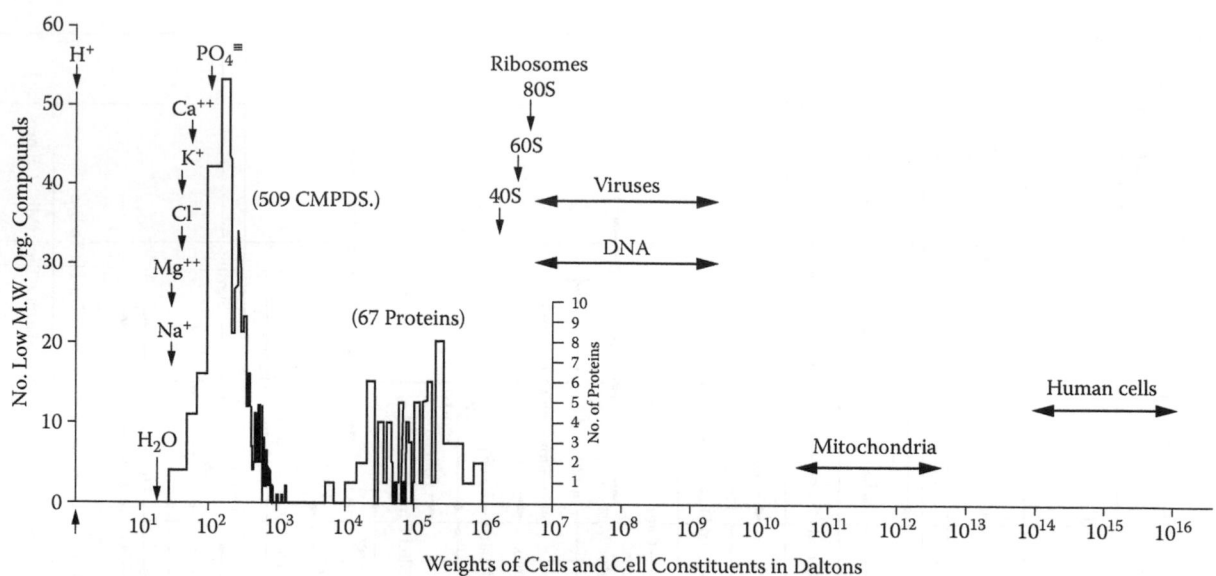

This figure originally appeared in Sober, Ed., *Handbook of Biochemistry and Selected Data for Molecular Biology,* 2nd ed., Chemical Rubber Co., Cleveland, 1970.

CLICK CHEMISTRY

Roger L. Lundblad

Click chemistry is a concept developed by Professor Barry Sharpless and his colleagues at Scripps Research Institute. The concept is based on modular components, wide in scope of application, providing high yields with benign side products.[1] There are several reactions (Figures 1 and 2) which have been referred to as click chemistry.[2]

In addition, there is thiol-ene click chemistry which has been used in polymer chemistry[3,4] as well as in maleimide-thiol click chemistry.[5] Some rate constants for various click chemistry reactions are shown in Table 1. These rate constants can be dependent on the solvent.[5–7]

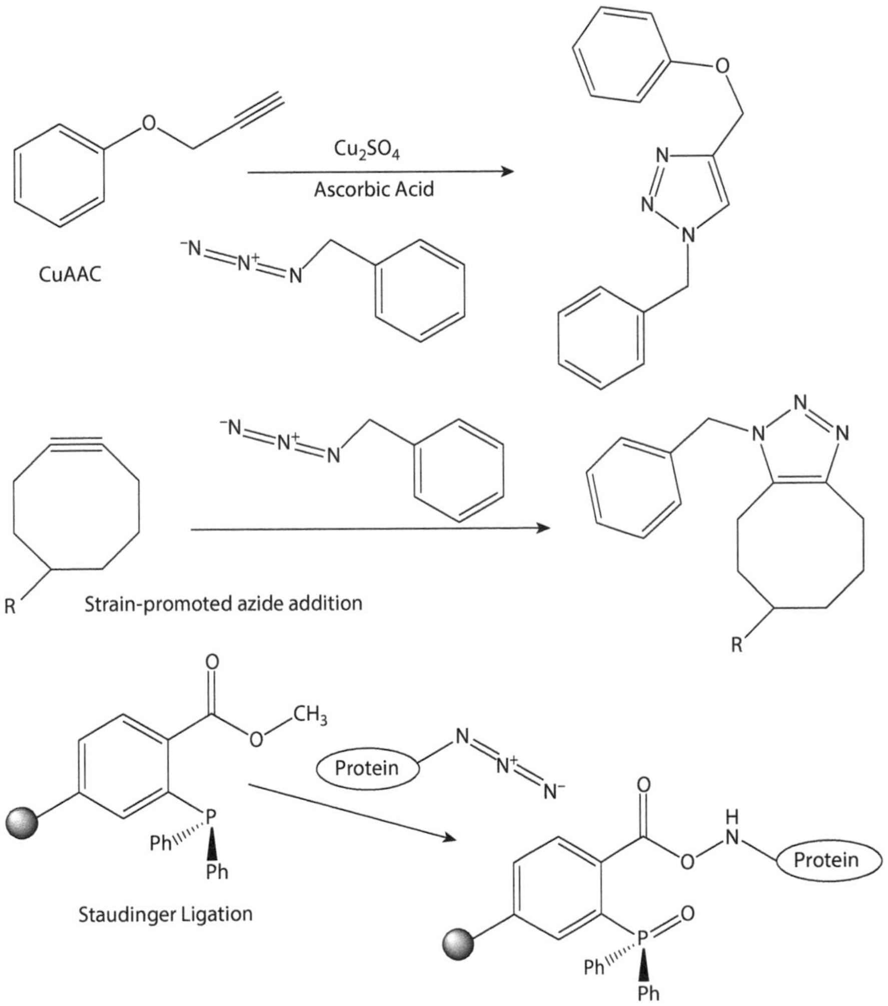

FIGURE 1 Some examples of click chemistry. CuAAC (copper catalyzed azide alkyne cycloaddition) is a cuprous ion catalyzed Huisgen cycloaddition reaction (Rostovtsev, V.V., Green, L.G., Fokin, V.V., and Sharpless, K.B., A stepwise Huisgen cycloaddition process: Copper(I)-catalyzed regioselective "ligation" of azides and terminal alkynes, *Angew. Chem., Int. Ed.* 114, 2708–2711, 2002). Strain-promoted azide addition (Leunissen, E.H., Meuleners, M.N., Verkade, J.M., et al., Copper-free click reactions with polar bicyclononyne derivatives for modulation of cellular imaging, *Chembiochem.*, 15, 1446–1451, 2014). Staudinger ligation (Hang, H.C., Yu, C., Kato, D.L., and Bertozzi, C.R., A metabolic labeling approach toward proteomic analysis of mucin-type O-linked glycosylation, *Proc. Natl. Acad. Sci. U.S.A.*, 100, 14846–14851, 2003).

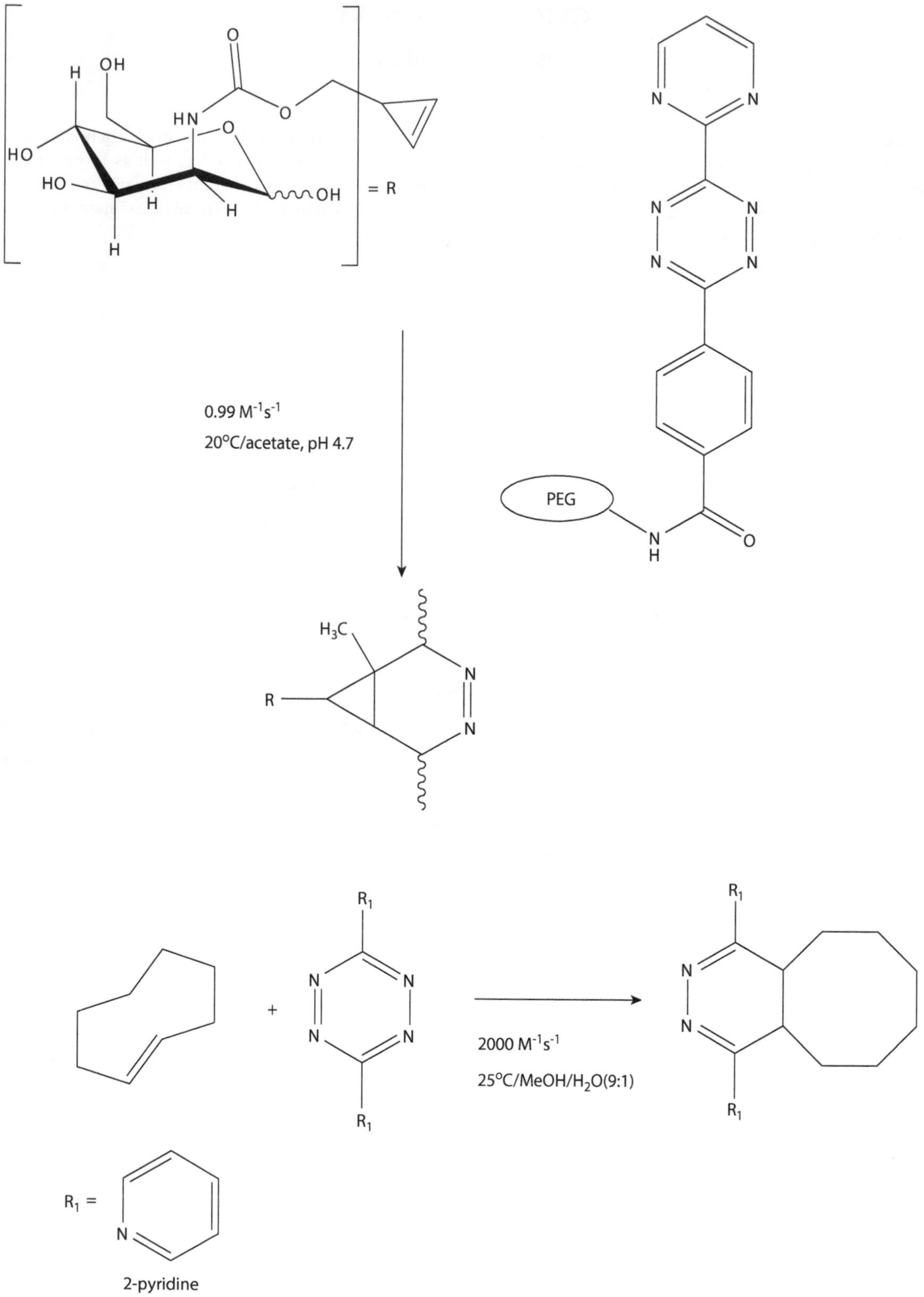

FIGURE 2 Examples of click chemistry based on inverse-electron-demand Diel-Alder reaction. At the top is shown the reaction of a cyclopropane derivative of manosamine with a tetrazine derivative containing a poly(ethylene glycol) chain. A biotin moiety may be attached to the end of the PEG chain (Späte, A.-K., Buszkmap, H., Niederwieser, A., et al., Rapid labeling of a metabolically engineered cell-surface glycoconjugates with a carbamate-linked cyclopropane reporter, *Bioconjugate Chem.*, 25, 147–154, 2014). The bottom reaction shows the reaction of *trans*-cyclooctene with a tetrazine derivative. The reaction was demonstrated to occur with at least 80% yields in cell lysate and media (Blackman, M.L., Royzen, M., and Fox, J.M., Tetrazine ligation: Fast conjugation based on inverse-electron-demand Diels-Alder reactivity, *J. Am. Chem. Soc.*, 130, 13518–13519, 2008).

References

1. Kolb, H.C., Finn, M.G., and Sharpless, K.B., Click chemistry: Diverse chemical function from a few good reactions, *Angew. Chem. Int. Ed.* 40, 2004–2021, 2004.
2. Meyer, J.-P., Adumeau, P., Lewis, J.S., and Zeglis, B.M., Click chemistry and radiochemistry: The first 10 years, *Bioconjugate Chem.* 27, 2791–2807, 2016.
3. Hoyle, C.E., and Bowman, C.N., Thiol-ene click chemistry. *Angew. Chem. Int. Ed. Engl.* 49, 1540–1573, 2010.
5. Northrop, B.H., Frayne, S.H., and Choudhary, U., Thiol-maleimide "click" chemistry: Evaluating the influence of solvent, initiator, and thiol on the reaction mechanism, kinetics, and selectivity, *Polymer Chem.* 6, 3415–3430, 2015.
4. Grim, J.C., Marozas, I.A., and Anseth, K.S., Thiol-ene photocleavage chemistry for controlled presentation of biomolecules in hydrogels, *J. Contrl. Release* 219, 95–106, 2015.
6. Blackman, M.L., Royzen, M., and Fox, J.M., Tetrazine ligation: Fast bioconjugation based on inverse-electron-demand Diels-Alder reactivity, *J. Am. Chem. Soc.* 130, 13518–13519, 2008.
7. Paredes, E., and Das, S.R., Optimization of acetonitrile co-solvent and copper stoichiometry for pseudo-ligandless click chemistry with nucleic acids, *Bioorg. Med. Chem. Lett.* 22, 5313–5316, 2012.

Reviews of Application of Click Chemistry in Biochemistry 2014–2017

1. Martell, J., and Weerapana, E., Applications of copper-catalyzed click chemistry in activity-based protein profiling, *Molecules* 19, 1378–1393, 2014.

2. Horisawa, K., Specific and quantitative labeling of biomolecules using click chemistry, *Front. Physiol.* 4, 457, 2014.
3. Musumeci, F., Schenone, S., Desogus, A., et al., Click chemistry, a potent tool in medicinal sciences, *Curr. Med. Chem.* 22, 2022–2050, 2015.
4. Patterson, D.M., and Prescher, J.A., Orthogonal bioorthogonal chemistries, *Curr. Opin. Chem. Biol.*, 28, 141–149, 2015.
5. Wang, X. Huang, B. Liu, X., and Zhan, P., Discovery of bioactive molecules from CuAAC click chemistry-based combinatorial libraries, *Drug Discovery Today* 21, 118–132, 2016.
6. Castrp. V., Rodríguez, H., and Albericio, F., An efficient click chemistry reaction on solid phase, *ACS Comb. Sci.* 18, 1–14, 2016.
7. He, X.P., Zeng, Y.L., Zang, Y., et al., Carbohydrate CuAAC click chemistry for therapy and diagnosis, *Carbohydr. Res.* 429, 1–22, 2016.
8. Tiwari, V.K., Mishra, B.B., Mishra, K.B., et al., Cu-catalyzed click reaction in carbohydrate chemistry, *Chem. Rev.* 116, 3086–3240, 2016.
9. Chen, X., and Wu, Y.-W., Selective chemical labeling of proteins, *Org. Biomol. Chem.* 14, 5417–5439, 2016.
10. Chandrasekaran, S., and Ramapanicker, R., Click chemistry route to the synthesis of unusual amino acids, peptides, triazole-fused heterocycles and pseudodisaccharides, *Chem. Rec.* 17, 63–70, 2017.

TABLE 1: Rate constants for some click chemistry reactions[a]

Reaction	K (M^{-1} s^{-1})	Reference
Aldehyde-ketone condensation[b]	0.001, 0.26	1, 2
Staudinger ligation	0.003	1, 3
Cyanobenzothiazole condensation	9–19	1, 4
Copper-catalyzed alkyne-azide cycloaddition	0.1–200	1, 5, 6
Strain-promoted azide-alkyne cycloaddition (SPAAC)	0.0012–0.96	1, 7
Substituted cyclopropene with a tetrazole in photoclick reaction	4.6; 58[c]	8
Acrylamide with a tetrazole in a photoclick reaction	9.2; 46[c]	8
Norbornene with a tetrazole in a photoclick reaction	5.8;32[c]	8
1,3-dipolar cycloadditions: diazo with unstrained dipolarophile	0.1 13.5	1, 9
Other 1,3-dipolar cycloadditions	0.13–106,00	1
Cycloaddition of fluorosydnones with alkynes	≤ 10^{4,d}	1, 10
Inverse-electron-demand Diels-Alder[e]: *trans*-cyclooctene and aliphatic azides	2.0	1, 11
Inverse-electron-demand Diels-Alder: trans-cyclooctenes with tetrazines	2000	1, 12
Cyclooctadiene with azide forming a triazoline derivative (3 + 2)[f]	0.019	13
Inverse-electron-demand Diels-Alder: triazoline derivative with subsequent reaction with a tetrazine derivative thus linking an azide to a tetrazine	297[g]	13
Inverse-electron-demand Diels-Alder: substitute cyclopropene with a tetrazine	0.0319; 2.778	14
Inverse-electron-demand Diels-Alder: carbamate-linked cyclopropene derivatives with tetrazines	0.99	15
Isonitrile (isocyano) with tetrazine (4 + 1) addition	0.052;0.077[h] 0.124;0.575[i]	16
Tris(2-carboxyethyl)phosphine reaction with acrylamide[j]	0.07	17

Compiled by Roger L Lundblad

[a] The rate constants should be considered to be approximate values. The reader is directed to the cited references for specific reaction conditions and specificity of modification.
[b] Pictet-Spengler is the best-known example (Spears, R.J., and Fascione, M.A., Site-selective incorporation and ligation protein aldehydes, *Org. Biomol. Chem.*, 14, 7622–7638, 2016).
[c] Rate constants dependent on photoactivation wavelength and tetrazole compound.
[d] Rate of reaction with cycloalkynes suggested to approach 10^4 M^{-1} s^{-1}.
[e] For a discussion of the inverse-electron-demand Diels-Alder reaction, see Wu, H., and Devaraj, N.K., Inverse electron-demand Diels-Alder bioorthogonal reactions, *Top. Curr. Chem.*, 374, 3, 2016.
[f] Reaction of the initial triazoline product with benzyl azide (second [3 + 2] cycloaddition is 0.000 M^{-1}s^{-1}).
[g] Reaction of the initial triazoline product with a tetrazine.
[h] MeOH.
[i] THF:H$_2$O (1:1).
[j] Dansyl phosphine was used to label N$^\varepsilon$-acryloyl-lysine in proteins.

References

1. Cited in Patterson, D.M., Nazarova, L.A., and Prescher, J.A., Finding the right (bioorthogonal) chemistry, *ACS Chem. Biol.* 9, 592–605, 2014.

2. Agarwal, P., van der Weijden, J., Sletten, E.M., Rabuka, D., and Bertozzi, C.R., A Pictet-Spengler ligation for protein chemical modification, *Proc. Natl. Acad. Sci. U.S.A.* 110, 46–51, 2013.

3. Lin, F.L., Hoyt, H.M., van Halbeek, H., Bergman, R.G., and Bertozzi, C.R., Mechanistic investigation of the Staudinger ligation, *J. Am. Chem. Soc.* 127, 2686–2695, 2005.

4. Nguyen, D.P., Elliott, T., Holt, M., Muir, T.W., and Chin, J.W., Genetically encoded 1,2-aminothiols facilitate rapid and site-specific protein labeling via a bio-orthogonal cyanobenzothiazole condensation, *J. Am. Chem. Soc.* 133, 11418–11421, 2011.

5. Rodionov, V.O., Presolski, S.I., Diaz, D.D., Folkin, V.V., and Finn, M.G., Ligand-accelerated Cu-catalyzed azide-alkyne cycloaddition: A mechanistic report, *J. Am. Chem. Soc.* 129, 12705–12712, 2007.

6. Machida, T., and Winssinger, N., One-step derivatization of reducing oligosaccharides for rapid and live-cell-compatible chelation-assisted CuAAC conjugation, *Chembiochem* 17, 811–815, 2016.

7. Debets, M.F., Prins, J.S., Merkx, D., et al., Synthesis of DIBAC analogues with excellent SPAAC rate constants, *Org. Biomol. Chem.* 12, 5031–5037, 2014.

8. Yu, Z., Pan, Y., Wang, Z., Wang, J., and Lin, Q., Genetically encoded cyclopropene directs rapid, photoclick-chemistry-mediated protein labeling in mammalian cells, *Angew. Chem.* 51, 10600–10604, 2012.

9. Aronoff, M.R., Gold, B., and Raines, R.T., Rapid cycloaddition of a diazo group with an unstrained dipolarophile, *Tetrahedron Lett.* 57, 2347–2350, 2016.

10. Dommerholt, J., van Rooijen, O., Borrmann, A., et al., Highly accelerated inverse electron-demand cycloaddition of electron-deficient azides with aliphatic cyclooctynes, *Nat. Comm.* 5, 5378, 2014.

11. Blackman, M.L., Royzen, M., and Fox, J.M., Tetrazine ligation: Fast bioconjugation based on inverse-demand-electron-demand Diels-Alder reactivity, *J. Am. Chem. Soc.* 130, 13518–13519, 2008.

12. Liu, H., Audisio, D., Plougastel, L., et al., Ultrafast click chemistry with fluorosydnones, *Angew. Chem. Int. Edn.* 55, 12073–12077, 2016.

13. Stöckmann, H., Neves, A.A., Day, H.A., et al., (*E,E*)-1,5-cyclooctadiene: A small and fast click-chemistry multitalent, *Chem. Commun.* 47, 7203–7205, 2011.

14. Kamber, D.N., Nazarova, L.A., Liang, Y., et al., Isomeric cyclopropenes exhibit unique bioorthogonal reactivities, *J. Am. Chem. Soc.* 135, 13680–13683, 2013.

15. Späte, A.K., Buszkamp, H., Niederwieser, A. et al., Rapid labeling of metabolically engineered cells-metabolically engineered cell-surface glycoconjugates with a carbamate-linked cyclopropene reporter, *Bioconjugate Chem.* 25, 147–154, 2014.

16. Stöckmann, H., Neves, A.A., Stairs, S., Brindle, K.M., and Leeper, F.J., Exploring isonitrile-based click chemistry for ligation with biomolecules, *Org. Biomol. Chem.* 9, 7303–7305, 2011.

17. Lee, Y.-J., Kurra, Y., and Liu, W.R., Phospha-Michael addition as a new click reaction for protein functionalization, *Chembiochem* 17, 456–461, 2016.

A LISTING OF LOG P VALUES, WATER SOLUBILITY, AND MOLECULAR WEIGHT FOR SOME SELECTED CHEMICALS[a]

Roger L. Lundblad

Compound	M.W.	Log P[b]	Water Solubility(gm/L)[c]
Acetamide	59.07	−1.26	2.25×10^3
Acetic acid	60.05	−0.17	10×10^3
Acetic anhydride	102.09	−0.58	1.2×10^2
Acetoacetic acid	102.1	−0.98	1×10^3
Acetoin	88.11	−0.36	1×10^3
Acetone	58.08	−0.24	1×10^3
Acetophenone	120.15	1.58	6.13
N-Acetylcysteinamide	162.21	−0.29	5.8
N-Acetylcysteine		−0.64	
N-Aceylmethionine		−0.49	
Acetylsalicylic acid	180.16	1.19	4.6
Acridine	179.22	3.40	0.03
Acrolein	56.06	−0.01	2.13×10^2
Acrylamide	71.08	−0.67	6.4×10^2
Adenine	135.13	−0.09	1.0
Adenosine	267.25	−1.05	8.2
Alanine	89.09	−2.96	1.7×10^2
Aldosterone		1.08	
9-Aminoacridine	194.23	2.74	0.02
4-Aminobenzoic acid (p-aminobenzoic acid; PABA)	151.17	1.03	9.89
4-Aminobutyric acid (γ-aminobutyric acid; GABA)	103.12	−3.17	1.3×10^3
6-Aminohexanoic acid (ε-aminocaproic acid)	131.18	−2.95	5.05×10^2
Ammonium picrate	246.14	−1.40	1.6×10^2
Aniline		0.9	
Anisole		2.11	
ANS (1-amino-2-naphthalenesulfonic acid)	222.25	−0.97	2.23
Anthracene		4.45	
Arabinose	150.13	−3.02	1×10^3
Arginine	174.20	−4.20	1.82×10^2
Ascorbic acid	176.13	−1.64	1×10^3
Asparagine	132.12	−3.82	29.4
Aspartic acid	133.10	−3.89	5.0
Barbital (5,5-diethylbarbituric acid)	184.20	0.65	7
Barbituric acid	128.1	−1.47	
Benzamide	121.14	0.64	13.5
Benzamidine	120.16	0.65	27.9
Benzene	78.11	2.13	0.002
Benzoic acid	122.12	1.87	3.4
Betaine	117.15	−4.93	6.11×10^2
Biuret (imidodicarbonic acid)	103.08		1.5
Bromoacetic acid	138.95	0.41	93
2-Bromopropionic acid	152.98	0.92`	29.9
2,3-Butanediol	90.12	−0.36	7.6×10^2
2,3-Butanedione	86.09	−1.34	2×10^2
Butyl urea	116.16	0.41	46.3
3-Butyl hydroxy urea	132.16	0.32	23.5
Cacodylic acid	138.00	0.36	2×10^3
Carbon tetrachloride	153.82	2.83	0.8
Cholesterol	386.67	8.74	0.9
Chloroacetamide	93.51	−0.53	90
Chloroacetic anhydride	170.98	−0.07	68
Chloroacetyl chloride	112.94	−0.22	1.6×10^2
Chloroform	119.38	1.97	8
6-Chloroindole	151.60	3.25	0.1
p-Chloromercuribenzoic acid	357.16	1.48	0.3
Chlorosuccinic acid	152.54	−0.57	1.8×10^2
Cholic acid	405.58	2.02	0.2
Citric acid	192.13	−1.72	5.92×10^2
Congo red	696.68	2.63	1.2×10^2

A LISTING OF LOG P VALUES, WATER SOLUBILITY, AND MOLECULAR WEIGHT FOR SOME SELECTED CHEMICALS[a] (Continued)

Compound	M.W.	Log P[b]	Water Solubility(gm/L)[c]
Corticosterone		1.94	
Cortisone		2.88	
Creatine	132.14	−3.72	13.3
Creatinine	113.12	−1.76	80
Crotonaldehyde (2-butenal)	70.09	0.60	1.8×10^2
Cyanoacetic acid	85.06	−0.76	7.7×10^2
Cyanogen	52.04	0.07	1.2×10^2
Cyanuric acid	129.08	0.61	2
Cyclohexanone		0.81	
Cysteine	121.16	−2.49	1.1×10^2
Cystine	240.30	−5.08	0.2
Cytidine	243.22	−2.51	1.8×10^2
Cytosine	111.10	−1.73	8
Deoxycholic acid	392.58	3.50	0.04
Deoxycorticosterone		2.88	
Dexamethasone		2.01	
Diazomethane	42.04	2.00	2
Dichloromethane		1.2	
Dicumarol	336.30	2.07	0.1
Diethyl ether (ethyl ether; ether)	74.1	0.9	
Diethylsuberate	230.31	3.35	0.7
Diethylsulfone	122.19	−0.59	1.4×10^2
N,N-Diethyl urea	116.2	0.1	4
Dihydroxyacetone	88.11	−0.49	16.2
Diketene	84.08	−0.39	5.3×10^2
Dimethylformamide		−1.04	
Dimethylguanidine	87.13	−0.95	1.6
Dimethylsulfoxide	78.13	−1.35	1×10^3
Dimethylphthalate		1.56	
1,4-Dinitrobenzene		1.47	
2,4-Dinitrophenol		1.55	
EDTA	292.25	−3.86	1
EDTA, sodium salt	360.17	−13.17	1×10^3
Ethanol (ethyl alcohol)	46.07	−0.31	$1 \times 10^{+3}$
N-Hydroxy-1-ethylurea	104.11	−0.10	7
N-Ethylnicotinamide	150.18	0.31	41.2
N-Hydroxyurea	104.11	−0.76	
Estradiol		2.69	
N-Ethylthiourea	104.17	−0.21	24
Ethylurea	88.11	−0.74	26.4
Ethylene glycol	2.07	−1.36	1×10^3
Ethylene oxide	44.05	−0.30	1×10^3
Fluorescein	333.32	3.35	0.05
Fluoroacetone	76.07	−0.39	286
Folic acid	441.41	−2.00	0.002
Formaldehyde	30.03	0.35	400
Formic acid	48.03	−0.54	1×10^3
Galactose	180.16	−2.43	683
Glucose	180.16	−1.88	1.2×10^3
Glutamic acid	147.10	−3.69	8.6
Glutamine	146.15	−3.64	41
Glycerol	92.10	−1.76	1×10^3
Glycine	75.10	−3.21	2.5×10^2
Glyoxal	58.04	−1.66	1×10^3
Glyoxylic acid	74.04	−1.40	1×10^3
Guanidine	59.07	−1.63	1.8
Guanine	151.13	−0.91	2.1
Guanosine	283.25	−1.90	0.7
Hexanal	100.16	1.78	6
Hydroxyproline	131.13	−3.17	395
Hydroxyurea	76.06	−1.80	224

A LISTING OF LOG P VALUES, WATER SOLUBILITY, AND MOLECULAR WEIGHT FOR SOME SELECTED CHEMICALS[a] (Continued)

Compound	M.W.	Log P[b]	Water Solubility(gm/L)[c]
Imidazole	68.08	−0.08	160
Indole	117.15	2.14	4
Inositol	180.16	−2.08	143
Iodoacetamide	184.96	−0.19	76
Isoleucine	131.18	−1.70	34
Isopropanol	60.10	0.05	1×10^3
Lactic acid	90.08	−0.72	1×10^3
Lactose	342.30	−5.43	195
Leucine	131.18	−1.52	22
Linoleic acid	280.45	7.05	0.00004
Lysine	146.19	−3.05	1×10^3
Maleic anhydride	98.06	1.62	5
Maltose	342.30	−5.43	780
Mannitol	182.17	−3.10	216
Mercaptoacetic acid	92.12	0.09	1×10^3
2-Mercaptobenzoic acid	154.19	2.39	0.7
Methane	16.04	1.09	0.002
Methanol	32.04	−0.77	1×10^3
Methionine	149.21	−1.87	57
Methotrexate	454.45	−1.85	2.6
Methylene blue	319.86	5.85	44
N-Methyl glycine	89.09	−2.78	300
5-Methylindole	131.18	2.68	0.5
Methyl isocyanate	57.05	0.79	29
Methylmalonic acid	118.09	−0.83	680
Methyl methacrylate	86.09	0.80	49
Methylmethane sulfonate	110.13	−0.66	1×10^3
Methyl thiocyanate	73.12	0.73	32
N-Methyl thiourea	119.21	−0.69	240
Methyl urea	74.08	−1.40	100
Naphthalene	128.17	3.29	220
Nicotinic acid	123.11	0.36	18
Ornithine	132.16	−4.22	1×10^3
Orotic acid	156.10	−0.83	2
Oxalic acid	90.06	−2.22	
Oxindole	133.15	1.16	9
Palmitic acid	256.43	7.17	0.0008
Paraldehyde	132.16	0.67	112
Pentobarbital	226.28	2.10	0.7
Phenol	94.11	1.46	83
Phenylalanine	165.19	−1.52	22
Phosgene	98.02	−0.71	475
Proline	115.13	−2.54	131
Prostaglandin E2	352.48	2.82	0.006
Propylamine	59.11	0.48	1×10^3
Propylene oxide	58.08	0.03	595
Pyridine	79.10	0.65	1×10^3
Pyridoxal	203.63	−3.32	500
Pyridoxal-5-phosphate	247.15	0.37	20
Pyridoxine	169.18	−0.77	282
Pyruvic acid	88.06	−1.24	1×10^3
Ribose	150.13	−2.32	
Sarin	140.10	0.72	1×10^3
Serine	105.09	−3.07	425
Sorbic acid	112.13	1.33	2
Sorbitol	182.17	−2.20	3×10^3
Stearic acid	284.49	8.23	0.03
Succinic anhydride	100.07	0.81	24
Succinimide	99.09	−0.85	196
Sucrose	342.30	−3.70	2.12×10^3
Testosterone	288.43	3.32	0.03

A LISTING OF LOG P VALUES, WATER SOLUBILITY, AND MOLECULAR WEIGHT FOR SOME SELECTED CHEMICALS[a] (Continued)

Compound	M.W.	Log P[b]	Water Solubility(gm/L)[c]
Tetrahydrofuran	72.11	0.46	1×10^3
Threonine	119.12	−2.94	97
Toluene	92.14	2.73	0.5
2,4,6-Trinitrobenzene	257.12	0.23	21
Tryptophan	204.23	−1.06	12
Urea	60.06	−2.11	545
Valine	117.15	−2.26	60

Compiled by Roger L Lundblad.

[a] Adapted from *Handbook of Physical Properties of Organic Chemicals*, ed. P.H. Howard and W.M. Meylan, CRC Press, Boca Raton, FL, 1997.

[b] $\text{Log } P = \log \dfrac{[\text{Concentration in 1 − octanol}]}{[\text{concentration in water}]}$

See above Howard and Meylan and following for discussion of log P (log of partitioning coefficient for a substance between 1-octanol and water.

[c] Solubility values taken from various literature sources and in some cases are approximations.

General References

Chuman, H., Mori, A., Tanaka, H., Prediction of the 1-octanol/H2O partition coefficient, Log *P*, by *Ab Initio* calculations: hydrogen-bonding effect of organic solutes on Log *P*, *Analyt.Sci.* 18, 1015–1020, 2002.

Hansch, C. and Leo, A., *Exploring QSAR. Fundamentals and Applications in Chemistry and Biology*, American Chemical Society, Washington, DC, 1995.

Uttamsingh, V., Keller, D.A., and Anders, M.W., Acylase I-catalyzed deacetylation of N-acetyl-L-cysteine and S-Alkyl-N-acetyl-L-cysteines, *Chem.Res.Toxicol.* 11, 800–809, 1998

Yalkowsky, S.H. and He, Y., *Handbook of Aqueous Solubility Data*, CRC Press, Boca Raton, Florida, 2003.

Halling, P.J., Thermodynamic predictions for biocatalysis in nonconventional media: theory, tests, and recommendations for experimental design and analysis, *Enzyme Microb.Technol.* 16, 178–206, 1994.

Abrahams, M.H., Du, C.M., and Platts, J.A., Lipophilicity of the nitrophenols, *J.Org.Chem.* 65, 7114–7718, 2000.

Lipinski, C.A., Lombardo, F., Dominy, B.W., and Feeney, P.J., Experimental and computational approaches to estimate solubility and permeability in drug discovery and development settings, *Adv.Drug.Deliv. Rev.* 46, 3–26, 2001.

Valko, K., Du, C.M., Bevan, C., Reynolds, D.P., and Abraham, M.H., Rapid method for the estimation of octanol/water partition coefficient (Log Poct) from gradient RP-HPLC retention and a hydrogen bond acidity term ($\Sigma \alpha_2 H$), *Curr.Medicin.Chem.* 8, 1137–1146, 2001.

Avdeef, A., Physicochemical profiling (solubility, permeability and charge state), *Curr.Top.Med.Chem.* 1, 277–351, 2001.

Section VIII
Physical and Chemical Data

IUBMB-IUPAC JOINT COMMISSION ON BIOCHEMICAL NOMENCLATURE (JCBN) RECOMMENDATIONS FOR NOMENCLATURE AND TABLES IN BIOCHEMICAL THERMODYNAMICS

(IUPAC Recommendations 1994)

http://www.chem.qmul.ac.uk/iubmb/thermod/

Robert A. Alberty

Department of Chemistry, Massachusetts Institute of Technology, Cambridge, Massachusetts 02139, USA

*Membership of the Panel on Biochemical Thermodynamics during the preparation of this report (1991–1993) was as follows:

Convener: R. A. Alberty (USA); A. Cornish-Bowden (France); Q. H. Gibson (USA); R. N. Goldberg (USA); G. G. Hammes (USA); W. Jencks (USA); K. F. Tipton (Ireland); R. Veech (USA); H. V. Westerhoff (Netherlands); E. C. Webb (Australia).

†Membership of the IUBMB–IUPAC Joint Commission on Biochemical Nomenclature (JCBN):

Chairman: J. F. G Vliegenthart (Netherlands); *Secretary*: A. J. Barrett (UK); A. Chester (Sweden); D. Coucouvanis (USA); C Liébecq (Belgium); K. Tipton (Ireland); P. Venetianer (Hungary); *Associate Members*: H. B. F. Dixon (UK); J. C. Rigg (Netherlands).

Chemical equations are written in terms of specific ionic and elemental species and balance elements and charge, whereas biochemical equations are written in terms of reactants that often consist of species in equilibrium with each other and do not balance elements that are assumed fixed, such as hydrogen at constant pH. Both kinds of reaction equations are needed in biochemistry. When the pH and the free concentrations of certain metal ions are specified, the apparent equilibrium constant K' for a biochemical reaction is written in terms of sums of species and can be used to calculate a standard transformed Gibbs energy of reaction $\Delta_r G'^\circ$. Transformed thermodynamic properties can be calculated directly from conventional thermodynamic properties of species. Calorimetry or the dependence of K' on temperature can be used to obtain the standard transformed enthalpy of reaction $\Delta_r H'^\circ$. Standard transformed Gibbs energies of formation $\Delta_f G'^\circ(i)$ and standard transformed enthalpies of formation $\Delta_f H'^\circ(i)$ for reactants (sums of species) can be calculated at various T, pH, pMg, and ionic strength (I) if sufficient information about the chemical reactions involved is available. These quantities can also/be calculated from measurement of K' for a number of reactions under the desired conditions. Tables can be used to calculate $\Delta_r G'^\circ$ and $\Delta_r H'^\circ$ for many more reactions.

Contents

1. Preamble

In 1976 an Interunion Commission on Biothermodynamics (IUPAC, IUB, IUPAB) published *Recommendations for Measurement and Presentation of Biochemical Equilibrium Data* (ref. 1). This report recommended symbols, units, and terminology for biochemical equilibrium data and standard conditions for equilibrium measurements. These recommendations have served biochemistry well, but subsequent developments indicate that new recommendations and an expanded nomenclature are needed. In 1985 the Interunion Commission on Biothermodynamics published *Recommendations for the Presentation of Thermodynamic and Related Data in Biology (1985)* (ref. 2).

Before discussing the new recommendations, some of the basic recommendations of 1976 are reviewed and the recommended changes in these basic matters are given.

Reproduced from:
Pure & Appl. Chem., Vol. 66, No.8, pp. 1641–1666, 1994.
© 1994 IUPAC

2. Basic 1976 Recommendations on Symbols and Nomenclature

In the 1976 *Recommendations* (ref. 1), the overall reaction for the hydrolysis of ATP to ADP was written as

$$\text{total ATP} + \text{H}_2\text{O} = \text{total ADP} + \text{total P}_i \tag{1}$$

and the expressions for the apparent equilibrium constant K' and the apparent standard Gibbs energy change $\Delta G^{\circ\prime}$ were written as[*]

$$K' = \frac{[\text{total ADP}][\text{total P}_i]}{[\text{total ATP}]} \tag{2}$$

$$\Delta G^{0\prime} = -RT \ln \frac{[\text{total ADP}][\text{total P}_i]}{[\text{total ATP}]} \tag{3}$$

where these are equilibrium concentrations, recommended to be molar concentrations. The 1976 Recommendations further recommended that information about the experimental conditions could be indicated by writing $K_c'(\text{pH} = x, \text{etc.})$ and $\Delta G_c^{\circ\prime}(\text{pH} = x,$ etc.), where the subscript c indicates that molar concentrations are used. The 1976 Recommendations pointed out that the hydrolysis of ATP can also be formulated in terms of particular species of reactants and products. For example, at high pH and in the absence of magnesium ion

$$\text{ATP}^{4-} + \text{H}_2\text{O} = \text{ADP}^{3-} + \text{P}_i^{2-} + \text{H}^+ \tag{4}$$

leads to the equilibrium constant expression

$$K_{\text{ATP}^{4-}} = \frac{[\text{ADP}^3][\text{P}_i^2][\text{H}^+]}{[\text{ATP}^{4-}]} \tag{5}$$

where the equilibrium constant $K_{\text{ATP}}4-$ is independent of pH. The 1976 *Recommendations* went on to show how K' is related to $K_{\text{ATP}}4-$.

3. Corresponding New Recommendations

The new recommendation is that reaction 1 be should be written as

$$\text{ATP} + \text{H}_2\text{O} = \text{ADP} + \text{P}_i \tag{6}$$

where ATP refers to an equilibrium mixture of ATP^{4-}, HATP^{3-}, $\text{H}_2\text{ATP}^{2-}$, MgATP^{2-}, MgHATP^-, and Mg_2ATP at the specified pH and pMg. This is referred to as a *biochemical equation* to emphasize that it describes the reaction that occurs at specified pH and pMg. The apparent equilibrium constant K' is made up of the equilibrium concentrations of the reactants relative to the standard state concentration c°, which is 1 M; note that M is an abbreviation for mol L^{-1}.

$$K' = \frac{([\text{ADP}]/c^\circ)[\text{P}_i]/c^\circ)}{([\text{ATP}]/c^\circ} = \frac{[\text{ADP}][\text{P}_i]}{[\text{ATP}]c^\circ} \tag{7}$$

The term c° arises in the derivation of this equilibrium constant expression from the fundamental equation of thermodynamics and makes the equilibrium constant dimensionless. The logarithm of K' can only be taken if it is dimensionless (ref. 3). The standard state concentration used is an absolutely essential piece of information for the interpretation of the numerical value of an equilibrium constant. The apparent equilibrium constant K' is a function

of T, P, pH, pMg, and I (ionic strength). Various metal ions may be involved, but Mg^{2+} is used as an example. As described below,

$$\Delta_r G^{\prime\circ} = -RT \ln K' \tag{8}$$

where $\Delta_r G^{\prime\circ}$ is the standard transformed Gibbs energy of reaction. The important point is that when the pH, and sometimes the free concentrations of certain metal ions, are specified, the criterion of equilibrium is the transformed Gibbs energy G' (ref. 4, 5). The reason for this name is discussed later in the section on transformed thermodynamic properties. Since the apparent equilibrium constant K' yields the standard value (the change from the initial state with the separated reactants at c° to the final state with separated products at c°) of the change in the transformed Gibbs energy G', the superscript $\circ$ comes after the prime in $\Delta_r G^{\prime\circ}$. The subscript r (recommended in ref. 3) refers to a reaction and is not necessary, but it is useful in distinguishing the standard transformed Gibbs energy of reaction from the standard transformed Gibbs energy of formation $\Delta_f G^{\prime\circ}(i)$ of reactant i, which is discussed below.

The hydrolysis of ATP can also be described by means of a *chemical equation* such as

$$\text{ATP}^{4-} + \text{H}_2\text{O} = \text{ADP}^{3-} + \text{HPO}_4^{2-} + \text{H}^+ \tag{9}$$

A *chemical equation* balances atoms and charge, but a *biochemical equation* does not balance H if the pH is specified or Mg if pMg is specified, and therefore does not balance charge. Equation 9 differs from equation 4 in one way that is significant but not of major importance. Writing HPO_4^{2-}, rather than P_i^{2-} is a move in the direction of showing that atoms and charge balance in equation 9. Strictly speaking ATP^{4-} ought to be written $\text{C}_{10}\text{H}_{12}\text{O}_{13}\text{N}_5\text{P}_3^{4-}$. That is not necessary or advocated here, but we will see later that the atomic composition of a biochemical species is used in calculating standard transformed thermodynamic properties. Chemical equation 9 leads to the following equilibrium constant expression

$$K = \frac{[\text{ADP}^{3-}][\text{HPO}_4^{2-}][\text{H}^4]}{[\text{ATP}^{4-}](c^\circ)^2} \tag{10}$$

where $c^\circ = 1$ M. The equilibrium constant K is a function of T, P, and I. This equilibrium constant expression does not completely describe the equilibrium that is reached except at high pH and in the absence of Mg^{2+}. Chemical equations like equation 4 are useful in analyzing biochemical reactions and are often referred to as reference equations; thus, the corresponding equilibrium constants may be represented by K_{ref}. The effect of Mg^{2+} is discussed here, but this should be taken as only an example because the effects of other metal ions can be handled in the same manner.

4. Additional New Recommendations

4.1 Recommendations Concerning Chemical Reactions

The thermodynamics of reactions of species in aqueous solution is discussed in every textbook on physical chemistry, but this section is included to contrast the nomenclature with that of the next section and to respond to the special needs of biochemistry. As mentioned in section 3, equilibrium constants of chemical reactions that are used in biochemistry are taken to be functions of T, P, and I. Therefore, the standard thermodynamic properties are also functions of T, P, and I. The standard Gibbs energy of reaction $\Delta_r G^\circ$ for reaction 9 is calculated using

$$\Delta_r G^\circ = -RT \ln K \tag{11}$$

and there are corresponding values of $\Delta_r H^\circ$ and $\Delta_r S^\circ$ that are related by

$$\Delta_r G^\circ = \Delta_r H^\circ - T\Delta_r S^\circ \tag{12}$$

---

[*] *Note* Abbreviations used in this document are: AMP, adenosine 5'-monophosphate; ADP, adenosine 5'-diphosphate; ATP, adenosine 5'-triphosphate; Glc, glucose; Glc-6-P, glucose 6-phosphate; P$_i$, orthophosphate. The designator (aq) is understood as being appended to all species that exist in aqueous solution.

The standard enthalpy of reaction is given by

$$\Delta_r H° = RT\left[\frac{\partial \ln K}{\partial T}\right]_{P,I} \quad (13)$$

If $\Delta_r H°$ is independent of temperature in the range considered, it can be calculated using

$$\Delta_r H° = [RT_1T_2/(T_2 - T_1)] \ln (K_2/K_1) \quad (14)$$

If the standard molar heat capacity change $\Delta_r CP°$ is not equal to zero and is independent of temperature, the standard molar enthalpy of reaction varies with temperature according to

$$\Delta_r H°(T) = \Delta_r H°(T^*) + \Delta_r C_p°(T - T^*) \quad (15)$$

The reference temperature T^* is usually taken as 298.15 K. In this case, $\Delta_r G°$ and K vary with temperature according to (ref. 6)

$$\Delta_r G°(T) = - RT \ln K(T)$$
$$= \Delta_r H°(T^*) + \Delta_r C_p°(T - T^*) + T\{\Delta_r G°(T^*) \quad (16)$$
$$- \Delta_r H°(T^*)\}/T^* - T \Delta_r C_p° \ln (T/T^*)$$

Additional terms containing $(\partial\Delta_r C_P°/\partial T)_P$ and higher order derivatives may be needed for extremely accurate data or for a very wide temperature range.

Equations 13 and 14 are exact only when the equilibrium constants are based on a molality standard state. If the equilibrium constants were determined with a standard state based on molarity, these equilibrium constants should be converted to a molality basis prior to using equation 13. For dilute aqueous solutions, $m_i = c_i/\rho$ where m_i and c_i are, respectively, the molality and the molarity of substance i and ρ is the mass density of water in kg L^{-1}. If this conversion is not made, there is an error of $RT^2(\partial \ln\rho/\partial T)_{P,I}$ for each unsymmetrical term in the equilibrium constant. This quantity is equal to 0.187 kJ mol^{-1} for dilute aqueous solutions at 298.15 K. Similar statements pertain to equations 27 and 28, which are given later in this document.

Since the standard thermodynamic properties $\Delta_r G°$ and $\Delta_r H°$ apply to the change from the initial state with the separated reactants at $c°$ to the final state with separated products at $c°$, it is of interest to calculate the changes in the thermodynamic properties under conditions where the reactants and products have specified concentrations other than $c°$. The change in Gibbs energy $\Delta_r G$ in an isothermal reaction in which the reactants and products are not all in their standard states, that is, not all at 1 M, is given by

$$\Delta_r G = \Delta_r G° + RT\ln Q \quad (17)$$

where Q is the reaction quotient of specified concentrations of species. The reaction quotient has the same form as the equilibrium constant expression, but the concentrations are arbitrary, rather than being equilibrium concentrations. Ideal solutions are assumed. The change in Gibbs energy $\Delta_r G$ in an isothermal reaction is related to the change in enthalpy $\Delta_r H$ and change in entropy $\Delta_r S$ by

$$\Delta_r G = \Delta_r H - T\Delta_r S \quad (18)$$

The corresponding changes in entropy and enthalpy are given by

$$\Delta_r S = \Delta_r S° - R\ln Q \quad (19)$$

$$\Delta_r H = \Delta_r H° \quad (20)$$

The standard reaction entropy can be calculated from the standard molar entropies of the reacting species: $\Delta_r S° = \Sigma v_i°(i)$, where v_i is the stoichiometric number (positive for products and negative for reactants) of species i.

The electromotive force E of an electrochemical cell is proportional to the $\Delta_r G$ for the cell reaction.

$$\Delta_r G = - |v_e|FE \quad (21)$$

where $|v_e|$ is the number of electrons transferred in the cell reaction and F is the Faraday constant (96 485.31 C mol^{-1}). Substituting equation 17 yields

$$E = E° - \frac{RT}{|v_e|F}\ln Q \quad (22)$$

where $E° = - \Delta_r G°/|v_e|F$ is the standard electromotive force, that is the electromotive force when all of the species are in their standard states, but at the ionic strength specified for $\Delta_r G°$. The electromotive force for a cell is equal to the difference in the electromotive forces of the half cells.

The standard Gibbs energy and enthalpy of reaction can be calculated from the formation properties of the species.

$$\Delta_r G° = \Sigma v_i\Delta_f G°(i) \quad (23)$$

$$\Delta_r H° = \Sigma v_i\Delta_f H°(i) \quad (24)$$

where the v_i is the stoichiometric numbers of species i. The standard entropy of formation of species i can be calculated using

$$\Delta_f S°(i) = [\Delta_f H°(i) - \Delta_f G°(i)]/T \quad (25)$$

Two special needs of biochemistry are illustrated by considering the seven species in Table 1. The first part of Table 1 gives the standard thermodynamic properties as they are found in the standard thermodynamic tables (see Appendix). The standard thermodynamic tables give the standard formation properties for the standard state, which is the state in a hypothetical ideal solution with a concentration of 1 M but the properties of an infinitely dilute solution and the activity of the solvent equal to unity. This means that the tabulated thermodynamic properties apply at $I = 0$. Since many biochemical reactions are studied at about $I = 0.25$ M, the tabulated values of $\Delta_f G°(i)$ and $\Delta_f H°(i)$ in *The NBS Tables of Chemical Thermodynamic Properties* and the *CODATA Key Values for Thermodynamics* have to be corrected to ionic strength 0.25 M, as described in Section 5.3. The values at $I = 0.25$ M are given in the second part of Table 1. No adjustments are made for H_2O, $MgHPO_4$, and glucose because the ionic strength adjustment is negligible for neutral species. We will see in Section 5.1 that the transformed Gibbs energy G' is the criterion of equilibrium at specified pH and pMg. In Section 5.4 we will see that the calculation of transformed thermodynamic properties involves the adjustment of the standard formation properties of species to the desired pH and pMg by use of formation reactions involving H^+ and Mg^{2+}. The standard transformed formation properties of species can be calculated at any given pH and pMg in the range for which the acid dissociation constants and magnesium complex dissociation constants are known. However, for the purpose of making tables, it is necessary to choose a pH and pMg that is of general interest. For the tables given here, pH = 7 and pMg = 3 are used because they are close to the values in many living cells. Table II shows the result of these calculations for the species in Table I. The ions H^+ and Mg^{2+} do not appear in this table because it applies at pH = 7 and pMg = 3. These methods have been applied to calculate the transformed formation properties of P_i (ref. 4); glucose 6-phosphate (ref. 5); adenosine, AMP, ADP, and ATP (ref. 7).

Tables 1 and 2 can be extended by use of measured equilibrium constants and enthalpies of reaction for enzyme-catalyzed reactions. For example, the species of glucose 6-phosphate can be added to these two tables because the equilibrium constant for the hydrolysis of glucose 6-phosphate has been measured

TABLE 1: Standard Formation Properties of Aqueous Species at 298.15 K.

	$\Delta_f H°$/kJ mol^{-1}	$\Delta_f G°$/kJ mol^{-1}
	I = 0 M	
H_2O	−285.83	−237.19
H^+	0.00	0.00
Mg^{2+}	−467.00	−455.30
HPO_4^{2-}	−1299.00	−1096.10
$H_2PO_4^-$	−1302.60	−1137.30
$MgHPO_4$	−1753.80	−1566.87
Glucose	−1262.19	−915.90
	I = 0.25 M	
H_2O	−285.83	−237.19
H^+	0.41	-0.81
Mg^{2+}	−465.36	−458.54
HPO_4^{2-}	−1297.36	−1099.34
$H_2PO_4^-$	−1302.19	−1138.11
$MgHPO_4$	−1753.80	−1566.87
Glucose	−1262.19	−915.90

TABLE 2: Standard Transformed Formation Properties of Species at 298.15 K, pH = 7, pMg = 3, and I = 0.25 M.

	$\Delta_f H'°$/kJ mol^{-1}	$\Delta_f G'°$/kJ mol^{-1}
H_2O	−286.65	−155.66
HPO_4^{2-}	−1297.77	−1058.57
$H_2PO_4^-$	−1303.01	−1056.58
$MgHPO_4$	−1288.85	−1050.44
Glucose	−1267.11	−426.70

at several temperatures, and because the acid dissociation constant and magnesium complex dissociation constant for glucose 6-phosphate are known at more than one temperature. However, as the standard thermodynamic properties are not known for any species of adenosine, AMP, ADP, or ATP, it is necessary to adopt the convention that $\Delta_f G° = \Delta_f H° = 0$ for adenosine in dilute aqueous solution at each temperature. This convention was introduced for H^+ a long time ago. This method has been used to calculate the standard enthalpies and standard Gibbs energies of formation of adenosine phosphate species relative to H_2ADP^- at 298.15 K (ref. 8). When this convention is used, it is not possible to calculate the enthalpy of combustion of adenosine, but it is possible to calculate $\Delta_f G°$ and $\Delta_f H°$ for reactions of adenosine that do not reduce it to CO_2, H_2O, and N_2. If the standard thermodynamic properties of all of the species of a reactant are known, $\Delta_f G'°$ and $\Delta_f H'°$ can be calculated at any specified pH and pMg, as described in the next section. When $\Delta_f G°$ and $\Delta_f H°$ are eventually determined for adenosine in dilute aqueous solution, the values of $\Delta_f G°$ and $\Delta_f H°$ of the other species in the ATP series can be calculated, but this will not alter the equilibrium constants and enthalpies of reaction that can be calculated using the tables calculated using the assumption that $\Delta_f G° = \Delta_f H° = 0$ for adenosine.

In making these calculations, the pH has been defined by $pH = - \log_{10}([H^+]/c°)$, rather than in terms of the activity, as it is in more precise measurements. The reason for doing this is that approximations are involved in the interpretation of equilibrium experiments on biochemical reactions at the electrolyte concentrations of living cells. Even Na^+ and K^+ ions are bound weakly by highly charged species of biochemical reactants, like ATP. As an approximation the acid dissociation constants and magnesium complex dissociation constants are taken to be functions of the ionic strength and the different effects of Na^+ and K^+ are ignored. These approximations can be avoided in more precise work, but only at the cost of a large increase in the number of parameters and the amount of experimental work required.

4.2 Recommendations Concerning Biochemical Reactions

When pH and pMg are specified, a whole new set of transformed thermodynamic properties come into play (ref. 4, 5). These properties are different from the usual Gibbs energy G, enthalpy H, entropy S, and heat capacity at constant pressure C_P, and they are referred to as the transformed Gibbs energy G', transformed enthalpy H', transformed entropy S', and transformed heat capacity at constant pressure Cp'. The standard transformed Gibbs energy of reaction $\Delta_r G'°$ is made up of contributions from the standard transformed enthalpy of reaction $\Delta_r H'°$ and the standard transformed entropy of reaction $\Delta_r S'°$.

$$\Delta_r G'° = \Delta_r H'° - T\Delta_r S'° \tag{26}$$

The standard transformed enthalpy of reaction is given by

$$\Delta_r H'° = RT^2 \left(\frac{\partial \ln K'}{\partial T} \right)_{P,pH,pMg,I} \tag{27}$$

If $\Delta_r H'°$ is independent of temperature in the range considered, it can be calculated using

$$\Delta_r H'° = [RT_1 T_2/(T_2 - T_1)] \ln (K_2'/K_1') \tag{28}$$

where K_2' and K_1' are measured at the same P, pH, pMg, and I. If $\Delta_r H'°$ is dependent on temperature, a more complicated equation involving an additional parameter $\Delta_r C_P'°$, the standard transformed heat capacity of reaction at constant pressure, can be used with the assumption that

$$\Delta_r H'°(T) = \Delta_r H'°(298.15 \text{ K}) + (T - 298.15 \text{ K})\Delta_r C_P'° \tag{29}$$

This more complicated equation is analogous to equation 16. The standard transformed reaction entropy can be calculated from the standard transformed molar entropies of the reacting species: $\Delta_1 S° = \sum_i \nu \frac{i}{-} \bar{S}°(i)$, where the ν_i' are the apparent stoichiometric numbers (positive for products and negative for reactants) of the reactants i in a biochemical reaction written in terms of reactants (sums of species) (for example, reaction 6).

The standard transformed enthalpy of reaction $\Delta_r H'°$ can also be calculated from calorimetric measurements. When that is done it is necessary to make corrections for the enthalpies of reaction caused by the change $\Delta_r N(H^+)$ in the binding of H^+ and in the change $\Delta_r N (Mg^{2+})$ in the binding of Mg^{2+} in the reaction (see equation 38 below). The change in binding of an ion in a biochemical reaction is equal to the number of ions bound by the products at the specified pH and pMg minus the number of the ions bound by the reactants. Note that $\Delta_r N (H^+)$ and $\Delta_r N(Mg^{2+})$ are dimensionless.

The change in binding of H^+ and Mg^{2+} in a biochemical reaction can be calculated if the acid dissociation constants and magnesium complex dissociation constants for the reactants are known; the equilibrium constant for the biochemical reaction itself does not have to be known for this calculation. Earlier calculations of the production of H^+ and Mg^{2+} used a different sign convention (ref. 9). The changes in binding $\Delta_r N(H^+)$ and $\Delta_r N(Mg^{2+})$ are given by

$$\Delta_r N(H^+) = \sum \nu_i' \bar{N}_H(i) \tag{30}$$

$$\Delta_r N(Mg^{2+}) = \sum \nu_i' \bar{N}_{Mg}(i) \tag{31}$$

where the ν_i' are the apparent stoichiometric numbers of the reactants i in a biochemical reaction. $\bar{N}_H(i)$ is the number of H bound by an average molecule of reactant i at T, P, pH, pMg, and I. $\bar{N}_H(i)$ is calculated from $\sum r_i N_H(i)$ where r_i is the mole fraction of species i in the equilibrium mixture of the species of the reactant at the specified pH and pMg. $N_H(i)$ is the number of hydrogen atoms in species i. The average numbers $\bar{N}_H(i)$ and $\bar{N}_{Mg}(i)$ can be included in tables of transformed thermodynamic properties at specified pH and pMg so that $\Delta_r N(H^+)$ and $\Delta_r N(Mg^{2+})$ can be readily calculated for biochemical reactions. The sign and magnitude of $\Delta_r N(H^+)$ and $\Delta_r N(Mg^{2+})$ are important because they determine the effect of pH and pMg on the apparent equilibrium constant K'. It can be shown (ref. 9, 10) that

$$\Delta_r N(H^+) = -\left(\frac{\partial \log_{10} K'}{\partial pH}\right)_{T,P,pMg,I} \qquad (32)$$

$$\Delta_r N(Mg^{2+}) = -\left(\frac{\partial \log_{10} K'}{\partial pMg}\right)_{T,P,pH,I} \qquad (33)$$

where the logarithms are $\log_{10}$. A pHstat can be used to measure $\Delta_r N(H^+)$ directly.

Since the standard transformed thermodynamic properties $\Delta_r G'^\circ$ and $\Delta_r H'^\circ$ apply to the change from the initial state with the separated reactants at c° to the final state with separated products at c°, it is of interest to calculate the changes in the transformed thermodynamic properties under conditions where the reactants and products have the concentrations they do in a living cell. The change in transformed Gibbs energy $\Delta_r G'$ in an isothermal reaction in which the reactants and products are not all in their standard states, that is, not all at 1 M, is given by

$$\Delta_r G' = \Delta_r G'^\circ + RT \ln Q' \qquad (34)$$

where Q' is the apparent reaction quotient of specified concentrations of reactants (sums of species). The change in transformed Gibbs energy $\Delta_r G'$ in an isothermal reaction at specified pH and pMg is related to the change in transformed enthalpy $\Delta_r H'$ and change in transformed entropy $\Delta_r S'$ by

$$\Delta_r G' = \Delta_r H' - T\Delta_r S' \qquad (35)$$

The corresponding changes in transformed entropy and transformed enthalpy are given by

$$\Delta_r S' = \Delta_r S'^\circ - R \ln Q' \qquad (36)$$

$$\Delta_r H' = \Delta_r H'^\circ \qquad (37)$$

The calorimetrically determined enthalpy of reaction $\Delta_r H(cal)$ includes the enthalpies of reaction of H^+ and Mg^{2+} (consumed or produced) with the buffer at the specified T, P, pH, pMg, and I. The standard transformed enthalpy of reaction $\Delta_r H'^\circ$ can be calculated using (ref. 11)

$$\Delta_r H'^\circ = \Delta_r H(cal) - \Delta_r N(H^+)\Delta_r H^\circ(HBuff)$$
$$- \Delta_r N(Mg^{2+})\Delta_r H^\circ(MgBuff) \qquad (38)$$

$\Delta_r H^\circ(HBuff)$ is the standard enthalpy for the acid dissociation of the buffer, and $\Delta_r H^\circ(MgBuff)$ is the standard enthalpy for the dissociation of the magnesium complex formed with the buffer. The values of $\Delta_r N(H^+)$ and $\Delta_r N(Mg^{2+})$ can be determined experimentally using equations 32 and 33, or they can be calculated if sufficient data on acid and magnesium complex dissociation constants are available.

When the pH is specified, the electromotive force of an electrochemical cell can be discussed in terms of the concentrations of reactants (sums of species) rather than species. When this is done the electromotive force of the cell or of a half cell is referred to as the apparent electromotive force E'. When this is done equation 34 becomes

$$E' = E'^\circ - \frac{RT}{|v_e|F} \ln Q' \qquad (39)$$

where $E'^\circ = -\Delta_r G'^\circ / |v_e|F$ is the standard apparent electromotive force at that pH. The symbol E'° is also used for the standard apparent reduction potential for an electrode reaction.

Biochemists have not had the advantage of having tables of standard formation properties of reactants at some standard set of conditions involving pH and pMg. Currently, information on biochemical reactions is tabulated as standard transformed Gibbs energies of reaction $\Delta_r G'^\circ$ and, in some cases, standard transformed enthalpies of reaction $\Delta_r H'^\circ$ at specified, T, P, pH, pMg, and I. Standard transformed formation properties have not been calculated because of lack of thermodynamic information to connect reactants in aqueous solution with the elements in their standard states and because of lack of knowlege as to how to calculate standard thermodynamic properties for a reactant like ATP that is made up of an equilibrium mixture of species at a given pH and pMg. The solution to the first problem is to assign zeros to a minimum number of species. This is what is done with $H^+(aq)$ a long time ago. The solution to the second problem is that when pH and pMg are specified, the various species ATP^{4-}, $HATP^{3-}$, $MgATP^{2-}$, etc. of ATP become pseudoisomers. That is, the relative concentrations of the various species are then a function of temperature only. At a given T, P, pH, pMg, and I, the relative concentrations can be calculated, and the standard transformed thermodynamic properties of ATP (sum of species) can be calculated. The equations for doing this are given in Section 5.2. Thus, ATP at a given pH and pMg can be treated like a single species with the properties $\Delta_f G'^\circ$, $\Delta_f H'^\circ$, and $\Delta_f S'^\circ$.

When pH and pMg are specified, the transformed formation properties (indicated by a subscript f) of reactants are defined by (ref. 4)

$$\Delta_r G'^\circ = \Sigma \, v_i' \Delta_f G'^\circ(i) \qquad (40)$$

$$\Delta_r H'^\circ = \Sigma \, v_i' \Delta_f H'^\circ(i) \qquad (41)$$

where the v_i' are the apparent stoichiometric numbers of the reactants i in a biochemical reaction written in terms of reactants. These formation properties apply to reactants like ATP (that is, sums of species) at a specified T, P, pH, pMg, and I. The corresponding standard transformed entropy of formation of a reactant like ATP can be calculated using

$$\Delta_f G'^\circ(i) = \Delta_f H'^\circ(i) - T \Delta_f S'^\circ(i) \qquad (42)$$

Table 3 gives standard transformed enthalpies of formation and standard transformed Gibbs energies of formation that have been calculated at 298.15 K, pH = 7, pMg = 3, and I = 0.25 M (ref. 7). The values for creatine phosphate are based on the recent work of Teague and Dobson (ref. 12). The adjustment of standard formation properties of species to standard transformed formation

TABLE 3: Standard Transformed Formation Properties of Reactants (sums of species) at 298.15 K, pH = 7, pMg = 3, and I = 0.25 M. This Table Uses the Convention that $D_fG^\circ = D_fH^\circ = 0$ for Adenosine in Dilute Aqueous Solution

	$\Delta_f H'^\circ$/kJ mol^{-1}	$\Delta_f G'^\circ$/kJ mol^{-1}
ATP	−2981.79	−2102.88
ADP	−2000.19	−1231.48
AMP	−1016.59	−360.38
A (adenosine)	−5.34	529.96
Glc-6-P	−2279.09	−1318.99
Glc (glucose)	−1267.11	−426.70
CrP	−1509.75	−750.37
Cr (creatine)	−540.08	107.69
P$_i$	−1299.13	−1059.55
H$_2$O(l)	−286.65	−155.66

properties at the desired pH and pMg has been mentioned in connection with Table 2. When a reactant exists as a single species at pH = 7 and pMg = 3, the transformed formation properties of the species in Table 2 go directly into Table 3. Water has to be included in this table because its formation properties must be used in equations 40 and 41, even though it does not appear in the expression for the apparent equilibrium constant. When a reactant exists at pH = 7 and pMg = 3 as an equilibrium mixture of species, isomer group thermodynamics (see Section 5.2) has to be used to calculate standard transformed formation properties (Table 3) for that reactant.

The large number of significant figures in Table 1 might appear to indicate that these thermodynamic properties are known very accurately, but this is misleading. The values in such a table are used only by subtracting them from other values in the table, and so the only things that are important are differences between values. The values have to be given in the table with enough significant figures so that thermodynamic information in the differences is not lost. The following examples illustrate uses of this table.

This kind of table will make it easier to make thermodynamic calculations on systems of enzymatic reactions, like glycolysis. Currently, to calculate $\Delta_r G'^{\circ}$ for the net reaction of glycolysis, 10 reactions must be added and $\Delta_r G'^{\circ}$ must be multiplied by 2 for some of them.

Example 1. Calculate $\Delta_r G'^{\circ}$, $\Delta_r H'^{\circ}$, $\Delta_r S'^{\circ}$, and K' for the glucokinase reaction (EC 2.7.1.2) (ref. 13) at 298.15 K, pH = 7, pMg = 3, and $I = 0.25$ M.

ATP + Glc = ADP + Glc-6-P
$\Delta_r G'^{\circ} = (-1231.48 - 1318.99 + 2102.88 + 426.70)$ kJ mol^{-1}
$= -20.89$ kJ mol^{-1}
$\Delta_r H'^{\circ} = (-2000.19 - 2279.09 + 2981.79 + 1267.11)$ kJ mol^{-1}
$= -30.38$ kJ mol^{-1}
$\Delta_r S'^{\circ} = (-30.38 + 20.89) \times 10^3$ J mol^{-1}/298.15 K $= -31.83$ J K^{-1} mol^{-1}

$$K' = \exp\left(\frac{20\,890 \text{ Jmol}^{-1}}{8.3145 \text{ JK}^{-1} \times 298.15\text{K}}\right) = 4.57 \times 10^3$$

Example 2. Calculate $\Delta_r G'$, $\Delta_r H'$, and $\Delta_r S'$ for the glucokinase reaction at 298.15 K, pH = 7, pMg = 3, and $I = 0.25$ M when the reactant concentrations are [ATP] = 10^{-5} M, [ADP] = 10^{-3} M, [Glc] = 10^{-4} M, and [Glc-6-P] = 10^{-2} M.

$Q' = (10^{-3})(10^{-2})/(10^{-5})(10^{-4}) = 10^4$
$\Delta_r G' = \Delta_r G'^{\circ} + RT\ln Q' = -20.89 + (8.3145 \times 10^{-3})(298.15)\ln 10^4 = 1.94$ kJ mol^{-1}

Since $\Delta_r G'$ is positive, the glucokinase reaction cannot occur in the forward direction under these conditions.

$\Delta_r H' = \Delta_r H'^{\circ} = -30.38$ kJ mol^{-1}
$\Delta_r S' = \Delta_r S'^{\circ} - R\ln Q' = -108.41$ J K^{-1} mol^{-1}

Note that

$\Delta_r G' = \Delta_r H' - T\Delta_r S' = -30.38 - (298.15)(-0.10841) = 1.94$ kJ mol^{-1}

4.3 The Importance of Distinguishing Between Chemical Equations and Biochemical Equations

Both types of equations are needed in biochemistry. Chemical equations are needed when it is important to keep track of all of the atoms and charges in a reaction, as in discussing the mechanism of chemical change. Biochemical reactions are needed to answer the question as to whether a reaction goes in the forward or backward direction at specified T, P, pH, pMg, and I, or for calculating the equilibrium extent of such a reaction. Therefore,

it is essential to be able to distinguish between these two types of equations on sight. The reaction equations in *Enzyme Nomenclature* [ref. 13] are almost exclusively biochemical equations. In the case of the hydrolysis of adenosine triphosphate to adenosine diphosphate and inorganic phosphate, it is clear that equation 9 is a chemical equation and equation 6 is a biochemical equation. Equation 6 does not indicate that hydrogen ions or magnesium ions are conserved, but it is meant to indicate that C, O, N, and P are conserved. Equation 6 indicates the form of the expression for the apparent equilibrium constant K' at specified T, P, pH, pMg, and I. Equation 9 indicates that electric charge is conserved, and the abbreviations ATP^{4-} and ADP^{3-} can be replaced by the atomic compositions of these ions to show that C, H, O, N, and P are conserved. Equation 9 indicates the form of the expression for the equilibrium constant K at specified T, P, and I. Currently, the hydrolysis of ATP is often represented by ATP + H_2O = ADP + Pi + H$^+$ in textbooks and research papers, but this is a hybrid of a chemical equation and a biochemical equation and does not have an equilibrium constant. Furthermore, this "equation" does not give the correct stoichiometry. The correct stoichiometry with respect to H$^+$ is obtained by use of equation 32 and is $\Delta_r N(H^+) = 0.62$ at 298.15 K, 1 bar, pH = 7, pMg = 3, and $I = 0.25$ M. The convention is that H_2O is omitted in the equilibrium expression for K or K' when reactions in dilute aqueous solutions are considered.

In writing biochemical equations, words are often used to avoid the implication that hydrogen atoms and charge are being balanced, but it is important to understand that all other atoms are balanced. For example,

$$\text{pyruvate + carbonate + ATP = oxaloacetate + ADP + P}_i \quad (43)$$

is a biochemical equation and

$$C_3H_3O_3^- + HCO_3^- + ATP^{4-} = C_4H_2O_5^{2-} + ADP^{3-} + HPO_4^{2-} + H^+. \quad (44)$$

is a chemical reaction. There is no unique way to write a chemical reaction; for example, this equation could be written with $H_2PO_4^-$ and no H$^+$ on the right hand side. It can also be written with CO_2 on the left-hand side, but then it is necessary to be clear about whether this CO_2 is in the solution or gas phase. In equation 43 the word carbonate refers to the sum of the species CO_2, H_2CO_3, HCO_3^-, and CO_3^{2-} in aqueous solutions.

It is important to realize that $K' = K$ for reactions where the reactants are nonelectrolytes (ref. 14). An example is the hydrolysis of sucrose to glucose and fructose. Of course sugars do have ionizable groups, but we are usually not interested in the dissociations that occur above pH = 12. For racemases, $K' = K$. There are other reactions for which K' is approximately equal to K because a product has very nearly the same acid dissociation constant as a reactant.

The need to clearly distinguish between biochemical equations and chemical equations raises problems with some abbreviations that are widely used. For example, the use of NAD$^+$ in a biochemical equation makes it look like this charge should be balanced. NAD$^+$ is also not a suitable abbreviation for use in a chemical equation because it is actually a negative ion.

Chemical equations and biochemical equations should not be added or subtracted from each other because their sum or difference does not lead to an equation that has an equilibrium constant. On the other hand, chemical equations can be added to chemical equations, and biochemical equations can be added to biochemical equations.

The net equation for a system of biochemical reactions can also be written as a chemical equation or a biochemical equation, but the equilibrium constants are, of course, in general different.

Net equations in the form of biochemical equations are especially useful for determining whether the system of reactions goes in the forward or backward direction at specified T, P, pH, pMg, and I.

These recommendations apply also to reactions catalyzed by RNA enzymes (ref. 15), catalytic antibodies (ref. 16), and synthetic enzymes (ref. 17) (sometimes called ribozymes, abzymes, and synzymes, respectively). The reactions catalyzed have apparent equilibrium constants K' that are functions of pH and free concentratioins of certain metal ions. Both biochemical equations and chemical equations can be written for these reactions if the reactants are weak acids or bind metal ions.

4.4 Experimental Matters

In reporting results on equilibrium measurements on biochemical reactions it is extremely important to give enough information to specify T, P, pH, pMg (or free concentration of any other cation that is bound by reactants), and I at equilibrium. The most difficult of these variables are pMg and I. The calculation of pMg in principle requires information on the composition of the solution in terms of species, and this requires information on the dissociation constants of all of the weak acids and magnesium complex ions. However, if the metal ion binding constants of the buffer are known and the reactants are at low concentrations compared with the buffer, the concentrations of free metal ions can be calculated approximately. It is important to specify the composition of the solution and calculate the ionic strength, even if it can only be done approximately. Other important issues are the purities of materials, the methods of analysis, the question as to whether the same value of apparent equilibrium constant was obtained from both directions, and assignment of uncertainties. For calorimetric measurements, it is important to measure the extent of reaction. An important part of any thermodynamic investigation is the clear specification of the substances used and the reaction(s) studied. It is very helpful to readers to give *Enzyme Nomenclature* (ref. 13) identification numbers of enzymes and Chemical Abstracts Services registry numbers for reactants. IUPAC has published a "Guide to the Procedures for the Publication of Thermodynamic Data" (ref. 18), and CODATA has published a "Guide for the Presentation in the Primary Literature of Numerical Data Derived from Experiments" (ref. 19).

It is recommended that equilibrium and calorimetric measurements on biochemical reactions be carried out over as wide a range of temperature, pH, pMg, and I as is practical. For the study of biochemical reactions under "near physiological conditions," the following set of conditions is recommended: T = 310.15 K, pH = 7.0, pMg = 3.0, and I = 0.25 M. It is also recognized that there is no unique set of physiological conditions and that for many purposes it will be necessary and desirable to study biochemical reactions under different sets of conditions.

For the purpose of relating results obtained on biochemical reactions to the main body of thermodynamic data (NBS Tables and other tables listed in the Appendix) the results of experiments should be treated so as to yield results for a chemical (reference) reaction at T = 298.15 K and I = 0. If this calculation is done, the method of data reduction and all auxiliary data used should be reported. It is also recognized that while a standard state based upon the concentration scale has been widely used in biochemistry, the molality scale has significant advantages for many purposes and can also be used for the study of biochemical reactions and for the calculation of thermodynamic properties.

5. Thermodynamic Background

5.1 Transformed Thermodynamic Properties

The definition of a transformed Gibbs energy is a continuation of a process that starts with the first and second laws of thermodynamics, but is not always discussed in terms of Legendre transforms. The combined first and second law for a closed system involving only pressure-volume work is

$$dU = TdS - PdV \qquad (45)$$

where U is the internal energy and S is the entropy. The criterion for spontaneous change at specified S and V is $(dU)_{S,V} \leq 0$. That is, if S and V are held constant, U can only decrease and is at a minimum at equilibrium. To obtain a criterion at specified S and P, the enthalpy was defined by the Legendre transform $H = U + PV$ so that $(dH)_{S,P} \leq 0$. To obtain a criterion at specifed T and V, the Helmholtz energy was defined by the Legendre transform $A = U - TS$ so that $(dA)_{T,V} \leq 0$. To obtain a criterion at specified T and P, the Gibbs energy was defined by the Legendre transform $G = H - TS$ so that $(dG)_{T,P} \leq 0$. The Gibbs energy is especially useful because it provides the criterion for equilibrium at specified T and P. Two Legendre transforms can be combined. For example, the internal energy can be transformed directly to G by use of $G = U + PV - TS$. Alberty and Oppenheim (ref. 20, 21) used a Legendre transform to develop a criterion for equilibrium for the alkylation of benzene by ethylene at a specified partial pressure of ethylene. Wyman and Gill (ref. 22) have described the use of transformed Gibbs energies in describing macromolecular components in solution.

In 1992, Alberty (refs. 4, 5) used the Legendre transform

$$G' = G - n'(H^+)\mu(H^+) - n'(Mg^{2+})\mu(Mg^{2+}) \qquad (46)$$

to define a transformed Gibbs energy G' in terms of the Gibbs energy G. Here $n'(H^+)$ is the total amount of H^+ in the system (bound and unbound) and $\mu(H^+)$ is the specified chemical potential for H^+, which is given for an ideal solution by

$$\mu(H^+) = \mu(H^+)^\circ + RT \ln ([H^+]/c^\circ) \qquad (47)$$

where $\mu(H^+)^\circ$ is the chemical potential of H^+ at 1 M in an ideal solution at specified T, P, and I. The transformed Gibbs energy G' is defined in order to obtain a criterion of spontaneous change at T, P, pH, and pMg. It can be shown that $(dG')_{T,P,pH,pMg} \leq 0$, so that G' is at a minimum when T, P, pH, and pMg are held constant. This is the fundamental justification for the use of G' in biochemistry. Under the appropriate circumstances, the magnesium term can be left out or be replaced by a term in another metal ion. The reaction is generally an enzyme-catalyzed reaction, but these concepts apply to any reaction involving a weak acid or metal ion complex when the pH and concentration of free metal ion at equilibrium are specified.

A consequence of equation 46 is that the chemical potential μ_i of each species in the system is replaced by the transformed chemical potential μ_i' given by

$$\mu_i' = \mu_i - N_H(i)\mu(H^+) - N_{Mg}(i)\mu(Mg^{2+}) \qquad (48)$$

where $N_H(i)$ is the number of hydrogen atoms in species i and $N_{Mg}(i)$ is the number of magnesium atoms in species i.

Although thermodynamic derivations are carried out using the chemical potential, in actual calculations, the chemical potential μ_i of species i is replaced by the Gibbs energy of formation $\Delta_f G_i$

and the transformed chemical potential μ_i' of species i is replaced by the transformed Gibbs energy of formation $\Delta_f G_i'$, where

$$\Delta_f G_i = \Delta_f G_i^\circ + RT \ln ([i]/c^\circ) \tag{49}$$

$$\Delta_f G_i' = \Delta_f G_i'^\circ + RT \ln ([i]/c^\circ) \tag{50}$$

for ideal solutions. The calculation of $\Delta_f G_i'^\circ$ for a species is discussed in Section 5.4 and the calculation of $\Delta_f G_i'^\circ$ for a reactant is discussed in Section 5.5.

Once the $\Delta_f G_i'^\circ$ for the species ($H_2PO_4^-$, HPO_4^{2-}, $MgHPO_4$) of P_i, for example, have been calculated, the next question is how can these values be combined to obtain the value of $\Delta_f G_i'^\circ$ for P_i? The equations for this calculation are given in the next section.

5.2 Isomer Group Thermodynamics

A problem that has to be faced in biochemical thermodynamics at specified pH and pMg is that a reactant may consist of various species in equilibrium at the specified pH and pMg. Fortunately, a group of isomers (or pseudoisomers) in equilibrium with each other have thermodynamic properties just like a species does, but we refer to the properties of a pseudoisomer group as transformed properties. The problem of calculating a standard transformed Gibbs energy of formation of a reactant like ATP also arises when a reactant exists in isomeric forms (or hydrated and unhydrated forms), even if it is not a weak acid and does not complex with metal ions, so first we discuss a simple isomerization. The thing that characterizes an isomer group in ideal solutions is that the distribution within the isomer group is a function of temperature only. For such solutions, the standard Gibbs energy of formation of an isomer group $\Delta_f G^\circ(\text{iso})$ can be calculated from the standard Gibbs energies of formation $\Delta_f G_i^\circ$ of the various isomers using (ref. 23)

$$\Delta_f G^\circ(\text{iso}) = -RT \ln \sum_{i=1}^{N_I} \exp\left(-\Delta_f G_i^\circ / RT\right) \tag{51}$$

where N_I is the number of isomers in the isomer group. The standard enthalpy of formation $\Delta_f H^\circ(\text{iso})$ of the isomer group can be calculated using (ref. 24)

$$\Delta_f H^\circ(\text{iso}) = \sum_{i=1}^{N_I} r_i \Delta_f H_i^\circ \tag{52}$$

where r_i is the equilibrium mole fraction of the ith species within the isomer group that is given by

$$r_i = \exp\{[\Delta_f G^\circ(\text{iso}) - \Delta_f G_i^\circ]/RT\} \tag{53}$$

The standard entropy of formation of the isomer group $\Delta_f S^\circ(\text{iso})$ is given by

$$\Delta_f S^\circ(\text{iso}) = \sum_{i=1}^{N_I} r_i \Delta_f S_i^\circ - R \sum_{i=1}^{N_I} r_2 \ln r_i \tag{54}$$

These equations can be used for pseudoisomer groups (for example, the species of ATP at specified pH and pMg) by using the transformed thermodynamic properties of the species.

For pseudoisomer groups, equations 51, 52, and 53 become

$$\Delta_f G'^\circ(\text{reactant}) = -RT \ln \sum_{i=1}^{N_I} \exp(-\Delta_f G_i'^\circ/RT) \tag{55}$$

$$\Delta_f H'^\circ(\text{reactant}) = \sum_{i=1}^{N_I} r_i \Delta_f H_i'^\circ \tag{56}$$

$$r_i = \exp\{[\Delta_f G'^\circ(\text{reactant}) - \Delta_f G_i'^\circ]/RT\} \tag{57}$$

where i refers to a species at specified pH and specified free concentrations of metal ions that are bound.

5.3 Adjustment for Ionic Strength

The ionic strength has a significant effect on the thermodynamic properties of ions, and the extended Debye-Huckel theory can be used to adjust the standard Gibbs energy of formation and the standard enthalpy of formation of ion i to the desired ionic strength (ref. 25–28). At 298.15 K these adjustments can be approximated by

$$\Delta_f G_i^\circ(I) = \Delta_f G_i^\circ(I = 0) - 2.91482 z_i^2 I^{1/2}/(1 + BI^{1/2}) \tag{58}$$

$$\Delta_f H_i^\circ(I) = \Delta_f H_i^\circ(I = 0) + 1.4775 z_i^2 I^{1/2}/(1 + BI^{1/2}) \tag{59}$$

where kJ mol^{-1} are used, z_i is the charge on ion i, and $B = 1.6$ L$^{1/2}$ mol$^{-1/2}$. Since for H$^+$, $\Delta_f G^\circ = 0$ and $\Delta_f H^\circ = 0$ at each temperature at $I = 0$, $\Delta_f G^\circ(\text{H}^+, 298.15 \text{ K}, I = 0.25 \text{ M}) = -0.81$ kJ mol^{-1} and $\Delta_f H^\circ(\text{H}^+, 298.15 \text{ K}, I = 0.25 \text{ M}) = 0.41$ kJ mol^{-1}. For the purpose of these recommendations, pH $= -\log_{10}([\text{H}^+]/c^\circ)$ and pMg $= -\log_{10}([\text{Mg}^{2+}]/c^\circ)$, as discussed above Section 4.1.

The adjustment of thermodynamic quantities from one solution composition to another using ionic strength effects alone is an approximation that works well at low ionic strengths (< 0.1 M) but it can fail at higher ionic strengths. Rigorous treatments require the use of interaction parameters (ref. 29) and a knowledge of the composition of the solution. While a substantial body of information on these parameters exists for aqueous inorganic solutions, there is very little of this type of data available for biochemical substances. Therefore, it is important that complete information on the compositions of the solutions used in equilibrium and calorimetric measurements be reported so that when values of these interaction parameters eventually become available, the results can be treated in a more rigorous manner. Specific ion effects are especially important when nucleic acids, proteins, and other polyelectrolytes are involved (refs. 30, 31).

5.4 Adjustment of Standard Thermodynamic Properties of Species to the Desired pH and pMg

When pH and pMg are specified, the various species of ATP, for example, become pseudoisomers; that is their relative concentrations are a function of temperature only. The procedure for calculating the transformed chemical potential μ_i' of a species has been indicated in equation 48. For actual calculations the chemical potentials μ_i of species are replaced with $\Delta_f G_i$ (see equation 49), and the transformed chemical potentials μ_i' of species are replaced with $\Delta_f G_i'$ (see equation 50). Thus equation 48 for a species can be written

$$\Delta_f G_i'^\circ = \Delta_f G_i^\circ - N_H(i)[\Delta_f G^\circ(\text{H}^+) + RT\ln([\text{H}^+]/c^\circ)] - N_{Mg}(i)[\Delta_f G^\circ(\text{Mg}^{2+}) + RT\ln([\text{Mg}^{2+}]/c^\circ)] \tag{60}$$

where $N_H(i)$ is the number of hydrogen atoms in species i. The corresponding equation for the standard transformed enthalpy of formation of species i is

$$\Delta_f H_i'^\circ = \Delta_f H_i^\circ - NH(i)\Delta_f H^\circ(\text{H}^+) - NMg(i)\Delta_f H^\circ(\text{Mg}^{2+}) \tag{61}$$

since the enthalpy of an ion in an ideal solution is independent of its concentration.

In adjusting standard Gibbs energies of formation to a specified pH, there is the question as to whether to count all of the hydrogens or only those involved in the reaction under consideration. However, the recommendation here is to adjust for all of the hydrogens in a species because all of them may be ultimately removed in biochemical reactions. This has been done in Tables 2 and 3.

There is a simple way to look at the standard transformed Gibbs energy of formation $\Delta_f G_i'^\circ$ and the standard transformed enthalpy of formation $\Delta_f H_i'^\circ$ of species i, and that is that they are the changes in formation reactions of the species with H^+ at the specified pH and Mg^{2+} at the specified pMg on the left-hand side of the formation reaction (ref. 32). For $H_2PO_4^-$,

$$P(s) + 2O_2(g) + 2H^+(pH = 7) + 3e^- = H_2PO_4^- \qquad (62)$$

$$\Delta_f G'^\circ(H_2PO_4^-) = \Delta_f G^\circ(H_2PO_4^-) - 2\{\Delta_f G^\circ(H^+) + RT \ln 10^{-pH}\} \qquad (63)$$

$$\Delta_f H'^\circ(H_2PO_4^-) = \Delta_f H^\circ(H_2PO_4^-) - 2\Delta_f H^\circ(H^+) \qquad (64)$$

The quantities $\Delta_f G^\circ(H^+)$ and $\Delta_f H^\circ(H^+)$ are included because they are equal to zero only at zero ionic strength. The electrons required to balance the formation reaction are assigned $\Delta_f G^\circ(e^-) = \Delta_f H^\circ(e^-) = 0$. This calculation can be made with either the standard thermodynamic properties at $I = 0$ or at some specified ionic strength.

The calculation of $\Delta_f G'^\circ$ and $\Delta_f H'^\circ$ for HPO_4^{2-} and $MgHPO_4$ follow this same pattern, with $Mg^{2+}(pMg = 3)$ also on the left-hand side of the formation reaction of $MgHPO_4$.

For a pseudoisomer group in which $\Delta_f G^\circ$ and $\Delta_f H^\circ$ are not known for any species, zero values have to be assigned to one of the species, as described in Section 4.1.

5.5 Calculation of the Standard Formation Properties of a Pseudoisomer Group at Specified ph and pmg

$H_2PO_4^-$, HPO_4^{2-} and $MgHPO_4$ form a pseudoisomer group when pH and pMg are specified. Therefore, equations 55–57 can be used to calculate $\Delta_f G'^\circ(P_i)$ and $\Delta_f H'^\circ(P_i)$ for inorganic phosphate at the desired pH and pMg. These calculations have been made for inorganic phosphate and glucose 6-phosphate at pH = 7 and pMg = 3 by Alberty (ref. 4), and for adenosine, AMP, ADP, and ATP by Alberty and Goldberg (ref. 7) using the convention that $\Delta_f G^\circ = \Delta_f H^\circ = 0$ for neutral adenosine.

For less common and more complicated reactants, the acid dissociation constants and magnesium complex dissociation constants may not be known. The $\Delta_f G_i'^\circ$ values of the reactants at pH = 7 and pMg = 3 can, however, be calculated if K' has been measured at pH = 7 and pMg = 3 for a reaction in which $\Delta_f G_i'^\circ$ is known for the other reactants. For example, this approach can be used to calculate $\Delta_f G_i'^\circ$ for the reactants in glycolysis.

5.6 The Actual Experiment and Thought Experiments

In the laboratory, a biochemical equilibrium experiment is actually carried out at specified T and P, and the pH is measured at equilibrium. Buffers are used to hold the pH constant, but there may be a change in the pH if the catalyzed reaction produces or consumes acid. pMg at equilibrium has to be calculated, and this can be done accurately only if the acid dissociation constants and magnesium complex dissociation constants are known for all of the reactants and buffer

components (ref. 12, 33). In the absence of this information pMg can be calculated approximately if the buffer binds H^+ and Mg^{2+}, these dissociation constants are known, and the concentrations of the reactants are much smaller than the concentration of the buffer components that are primarily responsible for the binding of Mg^{2+}. We can hope that some day there will be a pMg electrode as convenient as the pH electrode.

When we interpret the thermodynamics of a biochemical equilibrium experiment, we use an idealized thought experiment that is equivalent to the laboratory experiment. In the laboratory experiment, the buffer determines the approximate pH, but the pH will drift if H^+ is produced or consumed. The pH should be measured at equilibrium because the composition and $\Delta_r G'^\circ$ and $\Delta_r H'^\circ$ depend on this pH. Since the experimental results depend on the final pH, we can imagine that the experiment was carried out in a reaction vessel with a semipermeable membrane (permeable to H^+ and an anion, and impermeable to other reactants) with a pH reservoir on the other side. If the binding of H^+ by the products is greater than that of the reactants, H^+ will diffuse in from the pH reservoir as the reaction proceeds. If the binding of H^+ by the reactants is greater, H^+ will diffuse out of the reaction vessel as the reaction proceeds. Thus hydrogen ion is not conserved in the reaction vessel in this idealized thought experiment. Similar statements can be made about Mg^{2+}. In calorimetric experiments, corrections have to be made for the enthalpies of reaction due to the production of H^+ and Mg^{2+} to obtain $\Delta_r H'^\circ$, as mentioned earlier.

The thermodynamic interpretation of the apparent equilibrium constant K' uses $\Delta_f G'^\circ$ and $\Delta_r H'^\circ$. These quantities correspond with another thought experiment in which the separated reactants, each at 1 M at the specified T, P, final pH, final pMg, and I react to form the separated products, each at 1 M at the specified T, P, final pH, final pMg, and I.

5.7 Linear Algebra

It is generally understood that chemical equations conserve atoms and charge, but it is not generally known how the conservation equations for a chemical reaction system can be calculated from a set of chemical equations or how an independent set of chemical equations can be calculated from the conservation equations for the system. Nor is it well known that conservation equations in addition to atom and charge balances may arise from the mechanism of reaction. The quantitative treatment of conservation equations and chemical reactions requires the use of matrices and matrix operations (ref. 10, 23). When the equilibrium concentrations of species such as H^+ and Mg^{2+} are specified, these species and electric charge are not conserved, and so a biochemical equation should not indicate that they are conserved. The current practice of using words like acetate and symbols like ATP and P_i is satisfactory provided that people understand the reason for using these words and symbols. It should be possible to distinguish between chemical equations and biochemical equations on sight, and this means that different symbols should be used for the reactants in these two types of equations.

A set of simple chemical equations has been discussed from the viewpoint of linear algebra (ref. 34). The hydrolysis of ATP to ADP and P_i at specified pH has also been discussed from the viewpoint of linear algebra which shows why the 4 chemical equations reduce down to a single biochemical equation (ref. 35).

The conservation matrix for a biochemical reaction is especially useful for the identification of the constraints in addition to element balances (ref. 36).

6. Recommendations on Thermodynamic Tables

The papers by Alberty (ref. 5) and Alberty and Goldberg (ref. 7) show four types of tables of thermodynamic properties of biochemical reactants: (1) $\Delta_f G^\circ$ and $\Delta_f H^\circ$ for species at 298.15 K, 1 bar (0.1 MPa), $I = 0$. (2) $\Delta_f G^\circ$ and $\Delta_f H^\circ$ for species at 298.15 K, 1 bar, $I = 0.25$ M. (3) $\Delta_f G'^\circ$ and $\Delta_f H'^\circ$ for species at 298.15 K, 1 bar, pH = 7, pMg = 3, and $I = 0.25$ M. (4) $\Delta_f G'^\circ$ and $\Delta_f H'^\circ$ for reactants (sum of species) at 298.15 K, 1 bar, pH = 7, pMg = 3, and $I = 0.25$ M. Table 1 contains the most basic information for calculating $\Delta_f G^\circ$ and $\Delta_f H^\circ$ for reference reactions at $I = 0$ and corresponds with the NBS and CODATA Tables. Table 4 is the most convenient for calculating $\Delta_r G'^\circ$ and $\Delta_r H'^\circ$ under normal experimental conditions of 298.15 K, 1 bar, pH = 7, pMg = 3, and $I = 0.25$ M. Currently, thermodynamic information in biochemistry is stored as K' and $\Delta_r H'^\circ$ when pH and pMg are specified and as K and $\Delta_r H^\circ$ for reactions in terms of species. In order to calculate K' and $\Delta_r H'^\circ$ or K and $\Delta_r H^\circ$ for a reaction that has not been studied, it is currently necessary to add and subtract known reactions. It would be more convenient to be able to look up reactants in a table and add and subtract their formation properties to calculate K' and $\Delta_r H'^\circ$ or K and $\Delta_r H^\circ$, as is usually done for chemical reactions. One reactant can be involved in hundreds of reactions, and so it is more economical to focus on the reactants. The usefulness of such a table increases rapidly with its length. As mentioned in Section 4.3 columns for $N_H(i)$ and $N_{Mg}(i)$ can be included so that the change in binding of H and Mg at specified T, P, pH, pMg, and I can be readily calculated by use of equations 30 and 31.

The choice of 298.15 K, 1 bar, pH = 7, pMg = 3, and $I = 0.25$ M is arbitrary, but these conditions are often used. Tables can be constructed for other conditions (T, pH, pMg, and I) if sufficient information is available. H_2O has to be included in this table because its $\Delta_f G'^\circ(H_2O)$ and $\Delta_f H'^\circ(H_2O)$ have to be included in the summations in equations 40 and 41 when it is a reactant, even though H_2O is omitted in the expression for the apparent equilibrium constant.

The most basic principle is that thermodynamic tables on biochemical reactants at pH = 7 and pMg = 3 should be consistent with the usual thermodynamic tables to as great an extent as possible. A great deal is already known about the thermodynamics of reactions in aqueous solution, and this is all of potential value in biochemistry. The standard transformed formation properties of inorganic phosphate and glucose 6-phosphate at pH = 7 and pMg = 3 can be calculated since the standard formation properties of inorganic phosphate and glucose are well known and the properties of glucose 6-phosphate can be calculated from $\Delta_r G'^\circ$ and $\Delta_r H'^\circ$ for the glucose 6-phosphatase reaction. This is true for many other biochemical reactants. Sometimes it is necessary to use the convention that $\Delta_f G^\circ = \Delta_f H^\circ = 0$ for a reference species, as described in the discussion of the ATP series. It is difficult and expensive to obtain these missing data because biochemical reactants are often rather large molecules and contain a large number of elements. The methods described here make it possible to calculate $\Delta_f G'^\circ$ and $\Delta_f H'^\circ$ for P_i, glucose 6-phosphate, adenosine, AMP, ADP, and ATP at temperatures in the approximate range 273–320 K, pH in the approximate range 3–10, pMg in the range above about 2, and ionic strengths in the approximate range 0–0.35 M. Since the choice of reference species is arbitrary to a certain extent, it is desirable to have international agreement on these choices. This agreement is required so that thermodynamic properties in different tables of this type can be used together.

For many biochemical reactants, the acid and magnesium complex dissociation constants have not been measured, but this does not mean that these reactants cannot be included in a table of $\Delta_f G'^\circ$ and $\Delta_f H'^\circ$ at 298.15 K, pH = 7, pMg = 3, and $I = 0.25$ M. What is required is that the apparent equilibrium constant K' for a reaction involving this reactant (or pair of reactants) with reactants with known properties has been determined at pH = 7, pMg = 3, and $I = 0.25$ M at more than one temperature. If the pKs of a reactant are unknown, there is a problem in calculating the equilibrium pMg, but this uncertainty may not be large if the concentration of Mg^{2+} is controlled by a buffer with known binding properties and the equilibrium concentration of the reactants is low.

The fact that biochemical reactions are often organized in series will facilitate the construction of thermodynamic tables. When a series starts or ends with a reactant with known formation properties, knowlege of the apparent equilibrium constants in the series makes it possible to calculate $\Delta_f G'^\circ$ for reactants in the series at pH = 7. For example, consider glycolysis for which the apparent equilibrium constants for the 10 reactions have been known for some time. Since the standard transformed thermodynamic properties of glucose in aqueous solution are known, the $\Delta_f G'^\circ$ values for the 17 reactants at pH = 7, including pyruvate, can be calculated with just one problem. Since $\Delta_f G^\circ$ is not known for NAD or NADH, one of the species has to be assigned $\Delta_f G^\circ = \Delta_f H^\circ = 0$. Since the thermodynamic properties of pyruvate are known, this provides a check on the calculation of $\Delta_f G_i'^\circ$ of the reactants in glycolysis.

The following conventions are recommended:

1. When a reactant exists only in an electrically neutral form at pH = 7 and pMg = 3 and $\Delta_f G^\circ$ and $\Delta_f H^\circ$ for that form in dilute aqueous solution are known, the values of $\Delta_f G'^\circ$ and $\Delta_f H'^\circ$ are calculated by adjusting for the content of H. An example is glucose.

2. When a reactant exists in a single ionized form in the neighborhood of pH = 7 and pMg = 3, the values of $\Delta_f G^\circ$ and $\Delta_f H^\circ$ for that form in the usual tables (which apply at $I = 0$) have to be adjusted to $I = 0.25$ M with the extended Debye-Hückel theory and adjusted for H to obtain the entry to the table of $\Delta_f G'^\circ$ and $\Delta_f H'^\circ$ values. Obviously, thermodynamic properties of H^+ and Mg^{2+} will not be found in the table of $\Delta_f G'^\circ$ values. Also, ions like Ca^{2+} which bind significantly with multiply charged negative species of biochemical reactants cannot be put in the table because they require treatment like Mg^{2+}. Values of $\Delta_f G^\circ$ and $\Delta_f H^\circ$ for Krebs cycle intermediates that exist at pH = 7 and pMg = 3 in a single ionic form calculated by Miller and Smith-Magowan (Appendix, ref. 8) can be adjusted for H and Mg and used in the proposed table after the values have been corrected to $I = 0.25$ M. An example is succinate.

3. When a reactant exists in several ionized or complexed forms that are at equilibrium at pH = 7 and pMg = 3 and the standard thermodynamic properties of all of the ionized and complexed forms are known, the values of $\Delta_f G'^\circ$ and $\Delta_f H'^\circ$ of reactants at pH = 7, pMg = 3, $I = 0.25$ M can be calculated using isomer group thermodynamics. Examples are inorganic phosphate (P_i), pyrophosphate, carbonate, citrate, and glucose 6-phosphate.

4. When a reactant exists in several ionized or complexed forms with known dissociation constants and $\Delta_f G^\circ$ and $\Delta_f H^\circ$ are not known for any species of the reactant, $\Delta_f G'^\circ$ and $\Delta_f H'^\circ$ for the species can only be calculated by assigning one of them $\Delta_f G^\circ = \Delta_f H^\circ = 0$ in dilute aqueous solution. The $\Delta_f G^\circ$ and $\Delta_f H^\circ$ values of the various species have to

be adjusted to an ionic strength of 0.25 M and adjusted for H and Mg, so that $\Delta_f G'^\circ$ and $\Delta_f H'^\circ$ can be calculated for the reactant (sum of species) by use of isomer group thermodynamics, as illustrated here for the ATP series. NAD and NADH also provide an example, which is a little different because the acid and magnesium complex dissociation constants are believed to be identical.

5. If acid dissociation and magnesium dissociation constants are not known for a reactant, it can still be put into a table at pH = 7 and pMg = 3 if apparent equilibrium constants have been measured under these conditions for a reaction involving this reactant with other reactants whose transformed thermodynamic properties are known. Examples are the many reactants in glycolysis other than glucose, ATP, ADP, Pi, NAD, NADH, and H_2O.

6. It is not necessary to have columns in tables for $\Delta_f S'^\circ$ and $\Delta_f S^\circ$ because these can be treated as dependent properties and can be calculated from equations 25 and 42.

7. Nomenclature

Symbol	Name	Unit
A	extensive Helmholtz energy of a system	kJ
B	parameter in the extended Debye-Hückel theory	$L^{-1/2}\,mol^{-1/2}$
ci	concentration of species i	$mol\,L^{-1}$
c°	standard state concentration (1 M)	$mol\,L^{-1}$
$\Delta_r C_P{}^\circ$	standard heat capacity at constant pressure of reaction at T, P, and I	$J\,K^{-1}\,mol^{-1}$
$\Delta_r C_P{}'^\circ$	standard transformed heat capacity of reaction at constant T, P, pH, pMg, and I	$J\,K^{-1}\,mol^{-1}$
E	electromotive force	V
E°	standard electromotive force of a cell or half cell	V
E'	apparent electromotive force at specified pH	V
E'°	standard apparent electromotive force of a cell or half cell at specified pH	V
F	Faraday constant (96 485.31 C mol⁻¹)	$C\,mol^{-1}$
G	extensive Gibbs energy of a system	kJ
G'	extensive transformed Gibbs energy of a system	kJ
$\Delta_r G$	reaction Gibbs energy for specified concentrations of species at specified T, P, and I	$kJ\,mol^{-1}$
$\Delta_r G^\circ$	standard reaction Gibbs energy of a specified reaction in terms of species at specified T, P, and I	$kJ\,mol^{-1}$
$\Delta_r G'$	transformed reaction Gibbs energy in terms of reactants (sums of species) for specified concentrations of reactants and products at specified T, P, pH, pMg, and I	$kJ\,mol^{-1}$
$\Delta_r G'^\circ$	standard transformed reaction Gibbs energy of a specified reaction in terms of reactants (sums of species) at specified T, P, pH, pMg and I	$kJ\,mol^{-1}$
$\Delta_f G(i)$	Gibbs energy of formation of species i at a specified concentration of i and specified T, P, and I	$kJ\,mol^{-1}$
$\Delta_f G^\circ(i)$	standard Gibbs energy of formation of species i at specified T, P, and I	$kJ\,mol^{-1}$
$\Delta_f G'(i)$	transformed Gibbs energy of formation of species i or reactant i (sum of species) at specified concentration and specified T, P, pH, pMg, and I	$kJ\,mol^{-1}$
$\Delta_f G'^\circ(i)$	standard transformed Gibbs energy of formation of species i or reactant i (sum of species) at specified T, P, pH, pMg, and I	$kJ\,mol^{-1}$
H	extensive enthalpy of a system	kJ
H'	extensive transformed enthalpy of a system	kJ
$\Delta_r H(cal)$	calorimetrically determined enthalpy of reaction that includes the enthalpies of reaction of H⁺ and Mg²⁺ (consumed or produced) with any buffer in solution	$kJ\,mol^{-1}$
$\Delta_r H$	enthalpy of reaction of a specified reaction in terms of species at specified T, P, and I	$kJ\,mol^{-1}$
$\Delta_r H^\circ$	standard enthalpy of reaction of a specified reaction in terms of species at specified T, P, and I	$kJ\,mol^{-1}$
$\Delta_r H'$	transformed enthalpy of reaction of a specified reaction in terms of reactants (sums of species) for specified concentrations of reactants and products at specified T, P, pH, pMg, and I	$kJ\,mol^{-1}$
$\Delta_r H'^\circ$	standard transformed enthalpy of a specified reaction in terms of reactants (sums of species) at specified T, P, pH, pMg and I	$kJ\,mol^{-1}$
$\Delta_f H(i)$	enthalpy of formation of species i at specified T, P, and I	$kJ\,mol^{-1}$
$\Delta_f H^\circ(i)$	standard enthalpy of formation of species i at specified T, P, and I	$kJ\,mol^{-1}$
$\Delta_f H'(i)$	transformed enthalpy of formation of species i or reactant i (sum of species) at specified T, P, pH, pMg, and I	$kJ\,mol^{-1}$
$\Delta_f H'^\circ(i)$	standard transformed enthalpy of formation of species i or reactant i (sum of species) at specified T, P, pH, pMg, and I	$kJ\,mol^{-1}$
I	ionic strength	$mol\,L^{-1}$
K	equilibrium constant for a specified reaction written in terms of concentrations of species at specified T, P, and I (omitting H_2O when it is a reactant)	dimensionless
K'	apparent equilibrium constant for a specified reaction written in terms of concentrations of reactants (sums of species) at specified T, P, pH, pMg, and I (omitting H_2O when it is a reactant)	dimensionless
m_i	molality of i	$mol\,kg^{-1}$
n_i or $n(i)$	amount of species i	mol
$n'(i)$	amount of species (bound and unbound) or amount of reactant i (that is, sum of species)	mol
$N_H(i)$	number of H atoms in species i	dimensionless
$N_{Mg}(i)$	number of Mg atoms in species i	dimensionless
$\bar{N}_H(i)$	average number of H atoms in reactant i at specified T, P, pH, pMg, and I	dimensionless
$\Delta_r N(H^+)$	change in binding of H⁺ in a biochemical reaction at specified T, P, pH, pMg, and I	dimensionless
$\Delta_r N(Mg^{2+})$	change in binding of Mg⁺² in a biochemical reaction at specified T, P, pH, pMg, and I	dimensionless
N_i	number of isomers in an isomer group	dimensionless
pH	$-\log_{10}([H^+]/c^\circ)$	dimensionless
pMg	$-\log_{10}([Mg^{2+}]/c^\circ)$	dimensionless
pX	$-\log_{10}([X]/c^\circ)$	dimensionless
P	pressure	bar
Q	reaction quotient of specified concentrations of species in the same form as the equilibrium constant expression	dimensionless
Q'	apparent reaction quotient of specified concentrations of reactants and products (sum of species) in the same form as the apparent equilibrium constant expression	dimensionless
R	gas constant (8.31451 J K⁻¹ mol⁻¹)	$J\,K^{-1}\,mol^{-1}$
r_i or $r(i)$	equilibrium mole fraction of i within a specified class of molecules	dimensionless
S	extensive entropy of a system	$J\,K^{-1}$
S'	extensive transformed entropy of a system	$J\,K^{-1}$
$S'^\circ(i)$	standard molar entropy of species i at specified T, P, and I	$J\,K^{-1}\,mol^{-1}$
$S'^\circ(i)$	standard molar transformed entropy of species i or reactant i at specified T, P, pH, pMg, and I	$J\,K^{-1}\,mol^{-1}$
$\Delta_r S$	entropy of reaction of a specified reaction in terms of species at specified T, P, and I	$J\,K^{-1}\,mol^{-1}$
$\Delta_r S^\circ$	standard entropy of reaction of a specified reaction in terms of ionic species at specified T, P, and I	$J\,K^{-1}\,mol^{-1}$
$\Delta_r S'$	transformed entropy of reaction of a specified reaction in terms of reactants (sums of species) for specified concentrations of reactants and products at specified T, P, pH, pMg, and I	$J\,K^{-1}\,mol^{-1}$
$\Delta_r S'^\circ$	standard transformed entropy of a specified reaction in terms of sums of species at specified T, P, pH, pMg and I	$J\,K^{-1}\,mol^{-1}$
$\Delta_f S^\circ(i)$	standard entropy of formation of species i at specified T, P, and I	$J\,K^{-1}\,mol^{-1}$
$\Delta_f S'^\circ(i)$	standard transformed entropy of formation of species i or reactant i (sum of species) at specified T, P, pH, pMg, and I	$J\,K^{-1}\,mol^{-1}$
T	temperature	K
U	extensive internal energy of a system	kJ
V	volume	L
z_i	charge of ion i with sign	dimensionless
ρ	density	$kg\,m^{-3}$
$\mu(i)$	chemical potential of species i at specified T, P, and I	$kJ\,mol^{-1}$
$\mu'(i)$	transformed chemical potential of species i or reactant (sum of species) at specified T, P, pH, pMg, and I [can be replaced by $\Delta_f G'(i)$]i	$kJ\,mol^{-1}$
$\mu^\circ(i)$	standard chemical potential of species i at specified T, P, and I [can be replaced by $\Delta_f G^\circ(i)$]	$kJ\,mol^{-1}$
ν_e	number of electrons in a cell reaction	dimensionless
ν_i or $\nu(i)$	stoichiometric number of species i in a specified chemical reaction	dimensionless
$\nu'(i)$	apparent stoichiometric number of reactant i in a specified biochemical reaction	dimensionless

8. References

1. Wadsö, I., Gutfreund, H., Privlov, P., Edsall, J. T., Jencks, W. P., Strong, G. T., and Biltonen, R. L. (1976) Recommendations for Measurement and Presentation of Biochemical Equilibrium Data, *J. Biol. Chem.* 251, 6879-6885; (1976) *Q. Rev. Biophys.* 9, 439–456.
2. Wadsö, I., and Biltonen, R. L.(1985) Recommendations for the Presentation of Thermodynamic Data and Related Data in Biology, *Eur. J. Biochem.* 153, 429–434.
3. Mills, I., Cvitas, T., Homann, K., Kallay, N., and Kuchitsu, K. (1988 and 1993) *Quantities, Units and Symbols in Physical Chemistry*, Blackwell Scientific Publications, Oxford.
4. Alberty, R. A. (1992) *Biophys. Chem.* 42, 117–131.
5. Alberty, R. A. (1992) *Biophys. Chem.* 43, 239–254.
6. Clarke, E. C. W., and D. N. Glew, D. N. (1966) *Trans. Faraday Soc.* 62, 539–547.
7. Alberty, R. A., and Goldberg, R. N. (1992) *Biochemistry 31*, 10610–10615.
8. Wilhoit, R. C. (1969) *Thermodynamic Properties of Biochemical Substances, in Biochemical Microcalorimetry*, H. D. Brown, ed., Academic Press, New York.
9. Alberty, R. A. (1969) *J. Biol. Chem.* 244, 3290–3302.
10. Alberty, R. A. (1992) *J. Phys. Chem.* 96, 9614–9621.
11. Alberty, R. A., and Goldberg, R. N. (1993) *Biophys. Chem.* 47, 213–223.
12. Teague, W. E., and Dobson, G. P. (1992) *J. Biol. Chem.* 267, 14084–14093.
13. Webb, E. C. (1992) *Enzyme Nomenclature*, Academic Press, San Diego.
14. Alberty, R. A., and Cornish-Bowden, A. (1993) *Trends Biochem. Sci. 18*, 288–291.
15. Cech, T. R., Herschlag, D., Piccirilli, J. A., and Pyle, J. A. (1992) *J. Biol. Chem.* 256, 17479–82.
16. Blackburn, G. M., Kang, A. S., Kingsbury, G. A., and Burton, D. R. (1989) *Biochem. J.* 262, 381–391.
17. Pike, V. W. (1987) in *Biotechnology* (H.-J. Rehm and G. Reed, eds.), vol. 7a, 466–485, Verlag-Chemie.
18. "A Guide to the Procedures for the Publication of Thermodynamic Data", (1972) *PureAppl. Chem.* 289, 399–408. (Prepared by the IUPAC Commission on Thermodynamics and Thermochemistry.)
19. "Guide for the Presentation in the Primary Literature of Numerical Data Derived from Experiments". (February 1974) Prepared by a CODATA Task Group. Published in *National Standard Reference Data System News.*
20. Alberty, R. A., and Oppenheim, I. (1988) *J. Chem. Phys.* 89, 3689–3693.
21. Alberty, R. A., and Oppenheim, I. (1992) *J. Chem. Phys.* 96, 9050–9054.
22. Wyman, J., and Gill, S. J. (1990) *Binding and Linkage*, University Science Books, Mill Valley, CA.
23. Smith, W. R., and Missen, R. W. (1982) *Chemical Reaction Equilibrium Analysis: Theory and Algorithms*, Wiley-Interscience, New York.
24. Alberty, R. A. (1983) *I & EC Fund. 22*, 318–321.
25. Goldberg, R. N., and Tewari, Y. B. (1989) *J. Phys. Chem. Ref. Data 18*, 809–880.
26. Larson, J. W., Tewari, Y. B., and Goldberg, R. N. (1993) *J. Chem. Thermodyn. 25*, 73–90.
27. Goldberg, R. N., and Tewari, Y. B. (1991) *Biophys. Chem. 40*, 241–261.
28. Clarke, E. C. W., and Glew, D. N. (1980) *J. Chem. Soc., Faraday Trans. 1 76*, 1911–1916.
29. Pitzer, K. S. (1991) Ion Interaction Approach: Theory and Data Correlation, in *Activity Coefficients in Electrolyte Solutions*, 2nd Edition, K. S. Pitzer, editor, CRC Press, Boca Raton, Fla.
30. Record, M. T., Anderson, C. F., and Lohman, T. M. (1978) *Q. Rev. Biophys. 11*, 2.
31. Anderson, C. F., and Record, M. T. (1993) *J. Phys. Chem. 97*, 7116–7126.
32. Alberty, R. A. (1993) *Pure Appl. Chem. 65*, 883–888.
33. Guynn, R. W., and Veech, R. L. (1973) *J. Biol. Chem. 248*, 6966–6972.
34. Alberty, R. A. (1991) *J. Chem. Educ. 68*, 984.
35. Alberty, R. A. (1992) *J. Chem. Educ. 69*, 493.
36. Alberty, R. A. (1994) *Biophys. Chem. 49*, 251–261.

9. Appendix: Survey of Current Biochemical Thermodynamic Tables

(The reader is cautioned on distinguishing chemical reactions from biochemical reactions.)

1. Burton, K., Appendix in Krebs, H. A., and Kornberg, H. L. (1957) *Energy Transformations in Living Matter*, Springer-Verlag, Berlin.
2. Atkinson, M. R., and R. K. Morton, R. K. (1960) in *Comparative Biochemistry*, Volume II, *Free Energy and Biological Function*, Florkin, M., and Mason, H. (eds.), Academic Press, New York.
3. Wilhoit, R. C. (1969) *Thermodynamic Properties of Biochemical Substances, in Biochemical Microcalorimetry*, H. D. Brown (ed.), Academic Press, New York. This article gives standard thermodynamic properties of a large number of species at zero ionic strength. In a separate table standard enthalpies and standard Gibbs energies of formation of adenosine phosphate species are given relative to H_2ADP- at 298.15 K.
4. Thauer, R. K., Jungermann, K., and Decker, K. (1977) *Bacteriological Reviews 41*, 100–179. Standard Gibbs energies of formation of many species of biochemical interest at 298.15 K. Table of standard Gibbs energies of reaction corrected to pH 7 by adding $m\Delta f G$ °(H+), where m is the net number of protons in the reaction.
5. Goldberg, R. N. (1984) *Compiled thermodynamic data sources for aqueous and biochemical systems: An annotated bibliography (1930-1983)*, National Bureau of Standards Special Publication 685, U. S. Government Printing Office, Washington, D. C. A general and relatively complete guide to compilations of thermodynamic data on biochemical and aqueous systems.
6. Rekharsky, M. V., Galchenko, G. L., Egorov, A. M., and Berezin, I. V. (1986) Thermodynamics of Enzymatic Reactions, in *Thermodynamic Data for Biochemistry and Biotechnology*, H.-J. Hinz (ed.), Springer-Verlag, Berlin. Tables of $\Delta_r H°$, $\Delta_r G°$, and $\Delta r S°$ at pH 7 and 298.15 K, but the reactions are written in terms of ionic species so that there is a question about the interpretation of the parameters.
7. Goldberg, R. N., and Tewari, Y. B. (1989) Thermodynamic and Transport Properties of Carbohydrates and their Monophosphates: The Pentoses and Hexoses, *J. Phys. Chem. Ref. Data 18*, 809-880. Values on a very large number of reactions at 298.15 K carefully extrapolated to zero ionic strength. $\Delta_f H°$ and $\Delta_f G°$ for a large number of sugars and their phosphate esters.
8. Miller, S. L., and Smith-Magowan, D. (1990) The Thermodynamics of the Krebs Cycle and Related Compounds, *J. Phys. Chem. Ref. Data 19*, 1049–1073. A critical evaluation for a large number of reactions and properties of substances at 298.15 K.
9. Goldberg, R. N., and Tewari, Y. B. (1991) Thermodynamics of the Disproportionation of adenosine 5′-diphosphate to adenosine 5′-triphosphate and Adenosine 5′-monophosphate, *Biophys. Chem. 40*, 241–261. Very complete survey of data on this reaction and on the acid dissociation and magnesium complex dissociations involved.
10. Goldberg, R. N., Tewari, Y. B., Bell, D., Fazio, K., and Anderson, E. (1993) Thermodynamics of Enzyme-Catalyzed Reactions; Part 1. Oxidoreductases, *J. Phys. Chem. Ref. Data* 515–582. This review contains tables of apparent equilibrium constants and standard transformed molar enthalpies for the biochemical reactions catalyzed by the oxidoreductases.
11. Goldberg, R. N., and Tewari, Y. B. (1994) Thermodynamics of Enzyme-Catalyzed Reactions: Part 2. Transferases, *J. Phys. Chem. Ref. Data 23*, 547–617.

Standard Thermodynamic Tables

1. Wagman, D. D., Evans, W. H., Parker, V. B., Schumm, R. H., Halow, I., Bailey, S. M., Churney, K. L., and Nutall, R. L. (1982) *The NBS Tables of Chemical Thermodynamic Properties, J. Phys. Chem. Ref. Data* 11, Suppl. 2.
2. Cox, J. D., Wagman, D. D., and Medvedev, M. V. (1989) *CODATA Key Values for Thermodynamics*, Hemisphere, Washington, D. C.

STANDARD TRANSFORMED GIBBS ENERGIES OF FORMATION FOR BIOCHEMICAL REACTANTS

Robert N. Goldberg and Robert A. Alberty

This table contains values of the standard transformed Gibbs energies of formation $\Delta_f G'^{\circ}$ for 130 biochemical reactants. Values of $\Delta_f G'^{\circ}$ are given at pH 7.0, the temperature 298.15 K, and the pressure 100 kPa for three ionic strengths: $I = 0$, $I = 0.1$ mol/L and $I = 0.25$ mol/L. The table can be used for calculating apparent equilibrium constants K' and standard apparent reduction potentials E'° for biochemical reactions. Such a listing is more compact than tabulating the actual apparent equilibrium constants or standard apparent reduction potentials, which would require a very large number of reactant–product combinations. In the table, all reactants are in aqueous solution unless indicated otherwise.

A biochemical reactant is a sum of species. For example, ATP consists of an equilibrium mixture of the aqueous species ATP^{4-}, $HATP^{3-}$, H_2ATP^{2-}, $MgATP^{2-}$, etc. Similarly, phosphate refers to the equilibrium mixture of the aqueous species PO_4^{3-}, HPO_4^{2-}, $H_2PO_4^{-}$, H_3PO_4, $MgHPO_4$, etc. Biochemical reactions are written using biochemical reactants in terms of an apparent equilibrium constant K', which is distinct from the standard equilibrium constant K. This subject is discussed in an IUPAC report (see Reference 1 below).

The apparent equilibrium constant K' and the standard transformed Gibbs energy change $\Delta_r G'^{\circ}$ for a biochemical reaction can be calculated from the $\Delta_f G'^{\circ}$ values by using the relationship

$$-RT \ln K' = \Delta_r G'^{\circ} = \Sigma v'_i \Delta_f G'^{\circ},$$

where the summation is over all of the biochemical reactants. The quantity v'_i is the stoichiometric number of reactant i (v'_i is positive for reactants on the right side of the equation and negative for reactants on the left side); R is the gas constant. As an example, the hydrolysis reaction of ATP is

$$ATP + H_2O(l) = ADP + phosphate.$$

At pH 7.00 and $I = 0.25$ M, $\Delta_r G'^{\circ}$ and K' are calculated as follows:

$$\Delta_r G'^{\circ} = \{-1424.70 - 1059.49 - (-2292.50 - 155.66)\} \cdot (kJ\ mol^{-1})$$
$$= -36.03\ kJ\ mol^{-1}$$

$$K' = \exp[-(-36030\ J\ mol^{-1})/\{(8.3145\ J\ mol^{-2}\ K^{-1}) \cdot (298.15K)\}]$$
$$= 2.05 \cdot 10^{6}$$

An example involving a biochemical half-cell reaction is

$$acetaldehyde(aq) + 2\ e^{-} = ethanol(aq).$$

At 298.15 K, pH 7.00, and $I = 0$, the standard apparent reduction potential E'° can be calculated as follows

$$E'^{\circ} = -(1/nF) \cdot \{\Delta_f G'^{\circ}\ (ethanol) - \Delta_f G'^{\circ}\ (acetaldehyde)\},$$

where n is the number of electrons in the half-cell reaction and F is the Faraday constant. Then,

$$E'^{\circ} = [-1/2 \cdot 9.6485 \cdot 10^4\ C\ mol^{-1})] \cdot (58.10 \cdot 10^3\ J\ mol^{-1}$$
$$- 20.83 \cdot 10^3\ J\ mol^{-1}) = -0.193\ V$$

References

1. Alberty, R.A., Cornish-Bowden, A., Gibson, Q.H., Goldberg, R.N., Hammes, G., Jencks, W., Tipton, K.F, Veech, R., Westerhoff, H.V., and Webb, E.C. *Pure Appl. Chem.* 66, 1641–1666, 1994.
2. Alberty, R.A., *Arch. Biochem. Biophys.*, 353, 116-130, 1998; 358, 25–39, 1998.
3. Alberty, R.A., *Thermodynamics of Biochemical Reactions,* Wiley-Interscience, New York, 2003.
4. Alberty, R.A., *BasicBiochemData2: Data and Programs for Biochemical Thermodynamics,* <http://library.wolfram.com/infocenter/MathSource/797>.

Reactant	$\Delta_f G'^{\circ}$(I = 0) kJ mol⁻¹	$\Delta_f G'^{\circ}$(I = 0.1 M) kJ mol⁻¹	$\Delta_f G'^{\circ}$(I = 0.25 M) kJ mol⁻¹
Acetaldehyde	20.83	23.27	24.06
Acetate	−249.46	−248.23	−247.83
Acetone	80.04	83.71	84.90
Acetyl Coenzyme A	−60.49	−58.65	−58.06
Acetylphosphate	−1109.34	−1107.57	−1107.02
cis-Aconitate	−797.26	−800.93	−802.12
Adenine	510.45	513.51	514.50
Adenosine	324.93	332.89	335.46
Adenosine 5′-diphosphate (ADP)	−1428.93	−1425.55	−1424.70
Adenosine 5′-monophosphate (AMP)	−562.04	−556.53	−554.83
Adenosine 5′-triphosphate (ATP)	−2292.61	−2292.16	−2292.50
D-Alanine	−91.31	−87.02	−85.64
Ammonia	80.50	82.34	82.93
D-Arabinose	−342.67	−336.55	−334.57
L-Asparagine	−206.28	−201.38	−199.80
L-Aspartate	−456.14	−453.08	−452.09

STANDARD TRANSFORMED GIBBS ENERGIES OF FORMATION FOR BIOCHEMICAL REACTANTS (Continued)

Reactant	$\Delta_f G'^\circ (I = 0)$ kJ mol^{-1}	$\Delta_f G'^\circ (I = 0.1$ M$)$ kJ mol^{-1}	$\Delta_f G'^\circ (I = 0.25$ M$)$ kJ mol^{-1}
1,3-Biphosphoglycerate	−2202.06	−2205.69	−2207.30
Butanoate	−72.94	−69.26	−68.08
1-Butanol	227.72	233.84	235.82
Citrate	−963.46	−965.49	−966.23
Isocitrate	−956.82	−958.84	−959.58
Coenzyme A (CoA)	−7.98	−7.43	−7.26
CO(aq)	−119.90	−119.90	−119.90
CO(g)	−137.17	−137.17	−137.17
CO_2(aq)[total]	−547.33	−547.15	−547.10
CO_2(g)	−394.36	−394.36	−394.36
Creatine	100.41	105.92	107.69
Creatinine	256.55	260.84	262.22
L-Cysteine	−59.23	−55.01	−53.65
L-Cystine	−187.03	−179.69	−177.32
Cytochrome c [oxidized]	0.00	−5.51	−7.29
Cytochrome c [reduced]	−24.51	−26.96	−27.75
Dihydroxyacetone phosphate	−1096.60	−1095.91	−1095.70
Ethanol	58.10	61.77	62.96
Ethyl acetate	−18.00	−13.10	−11.52
Ferredoxin [oxidized]	0.00	−0.61	−0.81
Ferredoxin [reduced]	38.07	38.07	38.07
Flavine adenine dinucleotide (FAD) [oxidized]	1238.65	1255.17	1260.51
Flavine adenine dinucleotide (FAD) [reduced]	1279.68	1297.43	1303.16
Flavin adenine dinucleotide-enzyme (FADenz) [oxidized]	1238.65	1255.17	1260.51
Flavin adenine dinucleotide-enzyme (FADenz) [reduced]	1229.96	1247.71	1253.44
Flavin mononucleotide (FMN) [oxidized]	759.17	768.35	771.32
Flavin mononucleotide (FMN) [reduced]	800.20	810.61	813.97
Formate	−311.04	−311.04	−311.04
D-Fructose	−436.03	−428.69	−426.32
D-Fructose 1,6-diphosphate	−2202.84	−2205.66	−2206.78
D-Fructose 6-phosphate	−1321.71	−1317.16	−1315.74
Fumarate	−521.97	−523.19	−523.58
D-Galactose	−429.45	−422.11	−419.74
α-D-Galactose 1-phosphate	−1317.50	−1313.01	−1311.60
D-Glucose	−436.42	−429.08	−426.71
α-D-Glucose 1-phosphate	−1318.03	−1313.34	−1311.89
D-Glucose 6-phosphate	−1325.00	−1320.37	−1318.92
Glutamate	−377.82	−373.54	−372.16
D-Glutamine	−128.46	−122.34	−120.36
Glutathione [oxidized]	1198.69	1214.60	1219.74
Glutathione [reduced]	625.75	634.76	637.62
Glutathione-coenzyme A	563.49	572.06	574.83
D-Glyceraldehyde 3-phosphate	−1088.94	−1088.25	−1088.04
Glycerol	−177.83	−172.93	−171.35
sn-Glycerol 3-phosphate	−1080.22	−1077.83	−1077.13
Glycine	−180.13	−177.07	−176.08
Glycolate	−411.08	−409.86	−409.46
Glycylglycine	−200.55	−195.65	−194.07
Glyoxylate	−428.64	−428.64	−428.64
H_2(aq)	97.51	98.74	99.13
H_2(g)	79.91	81.14	81.53
H_2O(l)	−157.28	−156.05	−155.66
H_2O_2(aq)	−54.12	−52.89	−52.50
3-Hydroxypropanoate	−318.62	−316.17	−315.38
Hypoxanthine	249.33	251.77	252.56
Indole	503.49	507.78	509.16
Lactate	−316.94	−314.49	−313.70
Lactose	−688.29	−674.83	−670.48
L-Leucine	167.18	175.14	177.71

STANDARD TRANSFORMED GIBBS ENERGIES OF FORMATION FOR BIOCHEMICAL REACTANTS (Continued)

Reactant	$\Delta_f G'^\circ (I = 0)$ kJ mol^{-1}	$\Delta_f G'^\circ (I = 0.1$ M$)$ kJ mol^{-1}	$\Delta_f G'^\circ (I = 0.25$ M$)$ kJ mol^{-1}
L-Isoleucine	175.53	183.49	186.06
D-Lyxose	−349.58	−343.46	−341.48
Malate	−682.88	−682.85	−682.85
Maltose	−695.65	−682.19	−677.84
D-Mannitol	−383.22	−374.65	−371.89
Mannose	−430.52	−423.18	−420.81
Methane(aq)	125.50	127.94	128.73
Methane(g)	109.11	111.55	112.34
Methanol	−15.48	−13.04	−12.25
L-Methionine	−63.40	−56.67	−54.49
N_2(aq)	18.70	18.70	18.70
N_2(g)	0.00	0.00	0.00
Nicotinamide Adenine Dinucleotide (NAD) [oxidized]	1038.86	1054.17	1059.11
Nicotinamide Adenine Dinucleotide (NAD) [reduced]	1101.47	1115.55	1120.09
Nicotinamide Adenine Dinucleotide Phosphate (NADP) [oxidized]	163.73	173.52	176.68
Nicotinamide Adenine Dinucleotide Phosphate (NADP) [reduced]	229.67	235.79	237.77
O_2(aq)	16.40	16.40	16.40
O_2(g)	0.00	0.00	0.00
Oxalate	−673.90	−676.35	−677.14
Oxaloacetate	−713.38	−714.60	−715.00
Oxalosuccinate	−979.05	−979.05	−979.05
2-Oxoglutarate	−633.58	−633.58	−633.58
Palmitate	979.25	997.61	1003.54
L-Phenylalanine	232.42	239.15	241.33
Phosphate	−1058.56	−1059.17	−1059.49
2-Phospho-D-glycerate	−1340.72	−1341.32	−1341.79
3-Phospho-D-glycerate	−1346.38	−1347.19	−1347.73
Phosphoenolpyruvate	−1185.46	−1188.53	−1189.73
1-Propanol	143.84	148.74	150.32
2-Propanol	134.42	139.32	140.90
Pyrophosphate	−1934.95	−1939.13	−1940.66
Pyruvate	−352.40	−351.18	−350.78
Retinal	1118.78	1135.91	1141.45
Retinol	1170.78	1189.14	1195.07
Ribose	−339.23	−333.11	−331.13
Ribose 1-phosphate	−1215.87	−1212.24	−1211.14
Ribose 5-phosphate	−1223.95	−1220.32	−1219.22
Ribulose	−336.38	−330.26	−328.28
L-Serine	−231.18	−226.89	−225.51
Sorbose	−432.47	−425.13	−422.76
Succinate	−530.72	−530.65	−530.64
Succinyl Coenzyme A	−349.90	−348.06	−347.47
Sucrose	−685.66	−672.20	−667.85
Thioredoxin [oxidized]	0.00	0.00	0.00
Thioredoxin [reduced]	54.32	55.41	55.74
L-Tryptophan	364.78	372.12	374.49
L-Tyrosine	68.82	75.55	77.73
Ubiquinone [oxidized]	3596.07	3651.15	3668.94
Ubiquinone [reduced]	3586.06	3642.37	3660.55
Urate	−206.03	−204.81	−204.41
Urea	−42.97	−40.53	−39.74
Uric acid	−197.07	−194.63	−193.84
L-Valine	80.87	87.60	89.78
D-Xylose	−350.93	−344.81	−342.83
D-Xylulose	−346.59	−340.47	−338.49

ENTHALPY, ENTROPY, AND FREE ENERGY VALUES FOR BIOCHEMICAL REDOX REACTIONS

(Data are reported for pH 7.0 and 298 K)

Oxidation Half Reaction	$E^{\circ\prime}$ –Volts	ΔG kJ Mole^{-1}	ΔH kJ Mole^{-1}	ΔS J Mole^{-1} Deg^{-1}	References (Enthalpy Data)
Non protein reactions					
2 Cys $\rightleftharpoons$ (Cys)$_2$ + 2H$^+$ + 2e$^-$	0.32	−61.5	40.2	341	1, 2
2GSH $\rightleftharpoons$ (GS)$_2$ + 2H$^+$ + 2e$^-$	0.23	−44.4	25.1	233	1, 2
2HOC$_2$H$_4$SH $\rightleftharpoons$ (HOC$_2$H$_4$S)$_2$ + 2H$^+$ + 2e$^-$	—	—	38.1	—	1, 2
L(+)Lactate $\rightleftharpoons$ pyruvate + 2H$^+$ + 2e$^-$	0.18	−34.7	78.2	379	1, 2
H$_4$Folate $\rightleftharpoons$ H$_2$ folate + 2H$^+$ + 2e$^-$	0.18	−34.7	211.7	828	3
Ascorbate $\rightleftharpoons$ dehydroascorbate+2H$^+$ + 2e$^-$	−0.06	11.7	77.8	222	—
FMNH$_2$ $\rightleftharpoons$ FMN + 2H$^+$ + 2e$^-$	−0.22	42.3	56.1	46.0	4
Hydroquinone $\rightleftharpoons$ benzoquinone + 2H$^+$ + 2e$^-$	−0.29	55.6	177.4	408	1, 2
NADH $\rightleftharpoons$ NAD$^+$ + H$^+$ + 2e$^-$	−0.32	61.6	29.2	−108	2, 5, 6
NADPH $\rightleftharpoons$ NADP$^+$ + H$^+$ + 2e$^-$	−0.324	62.4	25.3	−124	2, 5, 7
Fe(CN)$_6$ $\rightleftharpoons$ Fe(CN)$_6^{-3}$ + e$^-$	−0.36	69.4	111.7	142	8[a]
Protein reactions					
Fe(II)hemerythrin $\rightleftharpoons$ Fe(III)hemerythrin + e$^-$	—	—	102.5	—	9
Ferrocytochrome c $\rightleftharpoons$ Ferrocytochrome c + e$^-$ (mammalian)	−0.26	25	59	114	1
Ferrocytochrome c $\rightleftharpoons$ Ferrocytochrome c + e$^-$ (bacterial)	—	—	79.5	—	1

Compiled by Neal Langerman.

[a] This reaction is the commonly used reference reaction.

References

1. Watt and Sturtevant, personal communication.
2. Schott and Sturtevant, personal communication.
3. Rothman, Kisliuk, and Langerman, *J. Biol. Chem.*, 248, 7845 (1973).
4. Beaudette and Langerman, *Arch. Biochem. Biophys.*, 161, 125 (1974).
5. Burton, *Biochem. J.*, 143, 365 (1974).
6. Poe, Gutfreund, and Estabrook, *Arch. Biochem. Biophys.*, 122, 204 (1967).
7. Engel and Dalziel, *Biochem. J.*, 105, 691 (1967).
8. Hanania, Irvine, Eaton, and George, *J. Phys. Chem.*, 71, 2022 (1967).
9. Langerman and Sturtevant, *Biochemistry*, 10, 2809 (1971).

OXIDATION-REDUCTION POTENTIALS, ABSORBANCE BANDS, AND MOLAR ABSORBANCE OF COMPOUNDS USED IN BIOCHEMICAL STUDIES

Paul A. Loach

In addition to the references[1-5,7,8] in the table, other generally used sources of oxidation-reduction data are: *Biochemist's Handbook*, D. Van Nostrand Co., Princeton, N.J. (1961); *The Encyclopedia of Electrochemistry*, C. A. Hampel, Ed., Reinhold Publishing Corp. New York (1964); *Oxidation-Reduction Potentials in Bacteriology and Biochemistry*, sixth ed., L. F. Hewitt, McCorquodale and Co. Ltd., London, (1950); *Biochemisches Taschenbuch* part II, Springer-Verlag, New York, (1964).

The oxidation-reduction couples are listed according to decreasing values of $E°$ or $E°'$. When both values are available, the order is according to $E°'$. Unless otherwise indicated, $E°'$ is the mid-point potential for a particular couple at pH7. Temperatures are not listed; most of the data are relevant to room temperature (20°C to 30°C). When more exact conditions are desired (ionic strength, concentration, temperature, nature of data used to derive $E°$ or $E°'$) the reader should consult the reference listed.

	System	$E°$	$E°'$	λ_{max}	E_{mM}	Reference
1.	$F_2(gas)/F^-$	2.87	—	—	—	1
2.	$H_2N_2O_2/N_2$ (gas)	2.65	—	—	—	1
3.	$S_2O_8^{2-}/SO_4^{2-}$	2.0	—	—	—	1
4.	H_2O_2/H_2O	1.77	—	—	—	1
5.	MnO_4^-/MnO_2	1.69	—	—	—	1
6.	$HClO_2/HClO$	1.64	—	—	—	1
7.	H_5IO_6/IO_3^-	1.6	—	—	—	1
8.	MnO_4^-/Mn^{2+}	1.51	—	—	—	1
9.	Mn^{3+}/Mn^{2+}	1.4	—	—	—	2
10.	$Cl_2(gas)/Cl^-$	1.359	—	—	—	1
11.	$ClO_2(gas)/HClO_2$	1.27	—	—	—	1
12.	MnO_2/Mn^{2+}	1.23	—	—	—	1
13.	$[Mn^{3+}(PO_4)_2]^{3-}/[Mn^{2+}(PO_4)_2]^{4-}$	1.22	—	—	—	2
14.	Pt^{2+}/Pt	1.2	—	—	—	1
15.	IO_3^-/I_2	1.19	—	—	—	1
16.	ClO_4^-/ClO_3^-	1.19	—	—	—	1
17.	$ClO_3^-/ClO_2(gas)$	1.15	—	—	—	1
18.	$[Cu^{3+}(IO_6)_2]^{7-}/[Cu^{2+}(IO_6)_2]^{8-}$, pH 8	—	1.1	—	—	2
	pH 12		0.7			
19.	Br_2/Br^-	1.087	—	—	—	1
20.	$N_2O_4(gas)/HNO_2$	1.07	—	—	—	1
21.	Fe^{3+}/Fe^{2+} O-phenanthroline	1.06	—	—	—	3
22.	$[IrCl_6]^{2-}/[IrCl_6]^{3-}$	1.05	—	—	—	1
23.	VO_3^-/VO^{2+}	1.0	—	—	—	2
24.	IO_4^-/IO_3^-	1.375	0.96	—	—	2
25.	$HNO_2/NO(gas)$	0.99	—	—	—	1
26.	*p*-Toluenesulfochloramide, Na salt (Chloramine-T)	1.52	0.90	—	—	2
27.	Nitrosoguanidine/Nitroguanidine	0.85	—	—	—	4
28.	O_2/H_2O	1.229	0.816	—	—	1
29.	NO_3^-/N_2O_4 (gas)	0.80	—	—	—	1
30.	Ag^+/Ag	0.7994	—	—	—	1
31.	1,2-Benzoquinone	0.792	—	—	—	5
32.	Hg_2^{2+}/Hg	0.792	—	—	—	1
33.	Zn Octaethylporphyrin (methanol)	—	0.78	—	—	71
34.	Fe^{3+}/Fe^{2+}	0.771	—	—	—	1
35.	$[Mo^{3+}(CN)_6]^{3-}/[Mo^{2+}(CN)_6]^{4-}$	0.73	—	—	—	5
36.	Porphyrexide	—	0.725	—	—	5
37.	Pyrogallol	0.713	—	—	—	5
38.	$NO(gas)/H_2N_2O_2$	0.71	—	—	—	1
39.	Hg^{2+}/Hg_2^{2+}	0.91	—	—	—	1
40.	1,2-Naphthoquinone-4-sulfonate	0.628	—	—	—	5
41.	Mn^{4+}/Mn^{3+} Hematoporphyrin IX, pH 9.9	—	0.626	400(ox)	70	6
42.	MnO_4^-/MnO_4^{2-}	0.6	—	—	—	1
43.	$S_2O_6^{2-}/H_2SO_3$	0.6	—	—	—	1
44.	$[W(CN)_8]^{3-}/[W(CN)_8]^{4-}$	0.57	—	—	—	5
45.	Porphyrindin	—	0.565	—	—	5
46.	NH_2OH/NH_4	—	0.562	—	—	7
47.	$H_3AsO_4/HAsO_2$	0.56	—	—	—	1

OXIDATION-REDUCTION POTENTIALS, ABSORBANCE BANDS AND MOLAR ABSORBANCE
OF COMPOUNDS USED IN BIOCHEMICAL STUDIES (Continued)

	System	$E°$	$E°'$	λ_{max}	E_{mM}	Reference
48.	o-Tolidine	—	0.55	—	—	5
49.	Cu^{2+}/Cu^+ Hemocyanin	—	0.540	350	—	8, 9
				600		
50.	I_2/I^-	0.536	—	—	—	1
51.	Cu^+/Cu	0.521	—	—	—	1
52.	Bacteriochlorophyll a (methanol)	—	0.52	—	—	71
53.	$S_2O_3^{2-}/S$	0.5	—	—	—	1
54.	$S_2O_4^{2-}/S_2O_3^{2-}$	1.03	0.484	—	—	1,7
55.	MoO_2^{2+}/MoO^{3+}	0.48	—	—	—	1
56.	Phenylhydrazine sulfonate	0.437	—	—	—	5
57.	2-Methyl-1,4-naphthoquinone (Menadione-Vitamin K_3)	0.422	—	—	—	5
58.	P_{700}	—	0.43	—	—	10
59.	$P_{890}(P_{0.44})$	—	0.44	—	—	11, 12 13, 14
60.	NO_3^-/NO_2^-	0.94	0.421	—	—	1, 7
61.	$H_2SO_3/S_2O_3^{2-}$	0.40	—	—	—	1
62.	2,5-Dihydroxy-1,4-benzoquinone	—	0.38	—	—	5
63.	Adrenalin	0.809	0.380	—	—	4, 5
64.	p-Aminodimethylaniline	—	0.38	—	—	5
65.	Fe^{3+}/Fe^{2+} Cytochrome f	—	0.365	413(ox)	—	66
				423(red)		
				525(red)		
				555(red)		
66.	$[Fe(CN)_6]^{3-}/[Fe(CN)_6]^{4-}$	—	0.36	—	—	5
				420(ox)	1.000	15
67.	o-Quinone/Diphenol		0.35	—	—	5
68.	Fe^{3+}/Fe^{2+} Cytochrome c_{550} (R. rubrum)	—	0.338	409(ox)	—	16
				416(red)		
				521(red)		
				550(red)		
69.	Cu^{2+}/Cu	0.337	—	—	—	1
70.	Fe^{3+}/Fe^{2+} Acetate, pH 5	—	0.34	—	—	5
71.	Fe^{3+}/Fe^{2+} Cytochrome c_5 (Azotobacter)	—	0.32	420(red)	—	17
				526(red)		
				555(red)		
72.	$As5^+/As^{3+}$	—	0.316	—	—	2
73.	p-Aminophenol	0.779	0.314	—	—	5
74.	$O_2(gas)/H_2O_2$	0.69	0.295	—	—	7
75.	Fe^{3+}/Fe^{2+} Cyt. c_4 (Azotobacter)	—	0.30	411(ox)	115.8	17
				416(red)	157.2	
				522(red)	17.6	
				551(red)	23.8	
76.	Fe^{3+}/Fe^{2+} Cyt c_{552} (Pseudomonas)	—	0.300	409(ox)	—	36
				416(red)		
				520(red)		
				552(red)		
77.	1,4-Benzoquinone	0.699	0.293	—	—	5
78.	Fe^{3+}/Fe^{2+} Cyt a	—	0.29	—	—	18
79.	p-Quinone/Hydroquinone	—	0.28	—	—	5
80.	2,6-Dibromo-2'-SO_3H indophenol	—	0.273	—	—	5
81.	Fe^{3+}/Fe^{2+} Malonate, pH 4	—	0.26	—	—	5
82.	2,5-Dihydroxyphenylacetic acid (Homogentisic acid)	0.687	0.260	—	—	5
83.	Fe^{3+}/Fe^{2+} Salicylate, pH 4	—	0.26	—	—	5
84.	Fe^{3+}/Fe^{2+} Cyt c	—	0.254	407(ox)	—	19, 20
				415(red)	125	
				521(red)	15.9	
				550(red)	27.7	
85.	2,6,2'-Trichloroindophenol	—	0.254	—	—	5
86.	Fe^{3+}/Fe^{2+} Chlorocruorin(pyridine)$_2$	—	0.246	434(red)		29
				544(red)		
				562(red)		
87.	Indophenol	—	0.228	—	—	5
88.	o-Toluidine Blue	0.677	0.224	—	—	5
89.	Phenol Blue	—	0.224	—	—	5

OXIDATION-REDUCTION POTENTIALS, ABSORBANCE BANDS AND MOLAR ABSORBANCE
OF COMPOUNDS USED IN BIOCHEMICAL STUDIES (Continued)

	System	$E°$	$E°'$	λ_{max}	E_{mM}	Reference
90.	Fe^{3+}/Fe^{2+} Cyt c_1	—	0.22	410(ox)		37
				418(red)	116	
				524(red)	11.6	
				554(red)	24.1	
91.	Fe^{3+}/Fe^{2+} Mesoporphyrin poly D, L-(lysine-phenylalanine), pH 4	—	0.22		—	21
92.	Fe^{3+}/Fe^{2+} Cyt b_2 (yeast)	—	0.219	—	—	22
93.	2,6-Dichlorophenolindophenol (DCPIP)	—	0.217	600	20.6	5, 23
94.	2,6-Dibromoindophenol	—	0.216	—	—	5
95.	Janus Green	—	0.21	—	—	5
96.	3-Aminothiazine	—	0.208	—	—	5
97.	Butyryl-Co A dehydrogenase $FAD^+/FADH_2$ (Cu present)	—	0.187	—	—	24
98.	Fe^{3+}/Fe^{2+} Hemoglobin (H 6.0),	—	0.17	500(ox)	9.0	25, 26
				630(ox)	4.0	27
	pH 7.0	—	0.144	—	—	26, 28
99.	SO_4^{2-}/H_2SO_3	0.17	—	—	—	1
100.	2,6-Dibromo-2'-methoxyindophenol	—	0.161	—	—	5
101.	Sn^{4+}/Sn^{2+}	—	0.15	—	—	2
102.	Adrenodoxin	—	0.15	414(ox)	5.7	9
103.	2,6-Dimethylindophenol	—	0.148	—	—	5
104.	1,2-Naphthoquinone	0.547	0.143	—	—	4
105.	Fe^{3+}/Fe^{2+} PPIX(pyridine)$_2$,	—	0.137	419(red)	192	29
				525(red)	17.5	30
				557(red)	34.4	
	pH9	—	0.09	—	—	5
106.	I-Naphthol-2-sulfonate indophenol	—	0.123	—	—	5
107.	Fe^{3+}/Fe^{2+} Cyt$_{553}$ (R. spheroides)	—	0.120	412(ox)	—	31
				418(red)		
				523(red)		
				553(red)		
108.	Toluylene Blue	—	0.115	—	—	5
109.	Fe^{3+}/Fe^{2+} Cyt$_{552}$ (Chromatium)	—	0.100	410(ox)	—	16
				417(red)		
				525(red)		
				552(red)		
110.	Ubiquinone/Ubihydroquinone (in 95% ethanol)	0.542	0.10	275	15	32
111.	TiO^{2+}/Ti^{3+}	—	0.10	—	—	3
112.	$S_4O_6^{2-}/S_2O_3^{2-}$	0.08	—	—	—	1
113.	Dehydroascorbic acid/ascorbic acid,	—	0.058	—	—	5
	pH 4	—	0.166	—	—	7
	pH 8.7	—	−0.012	—	—	2
114.	N-Methylphenazinium methosulfate (PMS)	—	0.08	387(ox)	23.8	33
				388(semi-		5
				450 (quinone)		
115.	Fe^{3+}/Fe^{2+} Cyt b (mitochondrial)	—	0.077	—	—	34
			0.050	429	114	
				532		
				561	21	
			−0.040			18
116.	$[W^{5+}(OH^-)_4(CN^-)_4]^{3-}/[W^{4+}/OH^-)_4(CN^-)_4]^{4-}$	—	0.07	—	—	35
117.	Thionine	0.563	0.064	—	—	5
118.	Thioindigo-tetrasulfonate	0.409	0.063	—	—	5
119.	Phenazine ethosulfate	—	0.055	—	—	5
120.	Cresyl Blue	0.583	0.047	632	—	5
121.	Fe^{3+}/Fe^{2+} Myoglobin	—	0.046	500(ox)	9.1	28, 27
				630(ox)	3.5	
122.	Fe^{3+}/Fe^{2+} Cyt b_3 (plants)	—	0.040	560(red)	—	39
				529(red)	—	
123.	1,4-Naphthoquinone	0.470	0.036	—	—	5
124.	Toluidine Blue	0.534	0.034	—	—	5
125.	Fumaric/Succinate	—	0.031	—	—	7
126.	$[Ni(C_{10}H_{10})]^+/Ni(C_{10}H_{10})$	—	0.03	—	—	40
127.	Thiazine Blue	—	0.027	—	—	5
128.	Gallocyanine	—	0.021	—	—	5

OXIDATION-REDUCTION POTENTIALS, ABSORBANCE BANDS AND MOLAR ABSORBANCE
OF COMPOUNDS USED IN BIOCHEMICAL STUDIES (Continued)

	System	$E°$	$E°'$	λ_{max}	E_{mM}	Reference
129.	Fe^{3+}/Fe^{2+} Cyt b_5 (microsomal)	—	0.02	413(ox)	117	41
				423(red)	170	
				526(red)	13	
				555(red)	26	
130.	Thioindigo disulfonate	0.347	0.014	—	—	5
131.	Methylene Blue	0.532	0.011	688(ox)	—	5
132.	Fe^{3+}/Fe^{2+} Methylated heme undecapeptide of Cyt c (pyridine)	—	0.008	—	—	68
133.	Fe^{3+}/Fe^{2+} Hematoporphyrin (pyridine)$_2$	—	+0.004	519(red)	—	8, 29
				545(red)		
134.	Fe^{3+}/Fe^{2+} Oxalate	—	0.002	—	—	5
135.	3-Methyl-9-phenyl isoalloxazine	—	−0.002	—	—	5
136.	Fe^{3+}/Fe^{2+} Cytochromoid c (*Chromatium*)	—	−0.040	406(ox)	—	42
				418(red)		
				525(red)		
				552(red)		
137.	Fe^{3+}/Fe^{2+} Cytochromoid c (*R. rubrum*)	—	−0.008	390(ox)	—	70
				424(red)		
				568(red)		
138.	Crotonyl-CoA/Butyryl-CoA	—	−0.015	—	—	38
139.	Pyocyanine	0.235	−0.034	690(ox)	4.5	33
			−0.038	370		5
140.	Indigo-tetrasulfonate	0.365	−0.046	—	—	5
141.	2-Methyl-3-phytyl-1,4-naphthoquinone (Vitamin K_1/ Dihydro-Vitamin K_1)	0.363	−0.05	—	—	5
142.	Luciferin	—	−0.05	—	—	4
				490(ox)	8.85	
				380(ox)	10.8	
143.	Fe^{3+}/Fe^{2+} Rubredoxin		−0.057	333(ox)	6.3	69
				311(red)	10.8	
144.	Fe^{3+}/Fe^{2+} Cyt b_6 (Chloroplasts)	—	−0.06	563(red)	—	43
145.	Methyl Capri Blue	0.477	−0.061	—	—	5
146.	Fe^{3+}/Fe^{2+} Mesoporphyrin (pyridine)$_2$	—	−0.063	—	—	8
147.	$H_2O_3/HS_2O_4^-$	−0.08	—	—	—	1
148.	Fe^{3+}/Fe^{2+} Mesoporphyrin poly-D, L-(glu- phe), pH 9	—	−0.07	—	—	21
149.	Xanthine oxidase	—	−0.08	—	—	5
150.	Indigo-trisulfonate	0.332	−0.081	—	—	5
151.	Fe^{3+}/Fe^{2+}1, 3, 5, 8-Tetramethyl porphyrin-6,7-dipropionic acid methyl ester-2,4-disulfonic acid	—	−0.09	—	—	44
152.	Thiohistidine	—	−0.09	—	—	4
153.	$[V(C_{10}H_{10})]^{2+}/[V(C_{10}H_{10})]^+$	—	−0.08	—	—	40
154.	Glyoxylate/Glycollate	—	−0.090	—	—	7
155.	Fe^{3+}/Fe^{2+} Heme undecapeptide from Cyt c (pyridine)	—	−0.092	403(ox)	117	68
				413(red)	155	
				521(red)		
				551(red)		
156.	6,8,9-Trimethyl isoalloxazine	—	−0.109	—	—	5
157.	Chloraphine	0.274	−0.115	—	—	5
158.	CO_2(gas)/CO(gas)	−0.12	—	—	—	1
159.	Yellow enzyme FMN/FMNH$_2$	—	−0.122	—	—	45
160.	Indigo-disulfonate	0.291	−0.125	—	—	5
161.	9-Phenyl isoalloxazine	—	−0.126	—	—	4
162.	Vitamin K reductase	—	−0.127	—	—	46
163.	Fe^{3+}/Fe^{2+} PPIX (histidine)$_2$, pH9.5	—	−0.138	—	—	5
164.	2-OH-1,4-Naphthoquinone	—	−0.139	—	—	5
165.	Thioglycolic acid	—	−0.14	—	—	4
166.	Fe^{3+}/Fe^{2+} (Pyrophosphate)	—	−0.14	—	—	5
167.	2-Amino-*N*-methyl phenazine methosulfate	—	−0.145	—	—	5
168.	Indigo-monosulfonate	0.262	−0.157	—	—	5
169.	Hydroxypyruvate/Glycerate	—	−0.158	—	—	7
170.	Oxaloacetate/Malate	—	−0.166	—	—	47
171.	Brilliant Alizarin Blue	—	−0.173	—	—	5
172.	Alloxazine	—	−0.170	—	—	5
173.	Mn^{3+}/Mn^{2+} Methyl pheophorbide a	—	−0.180	370(ox)	39	48
				425(ox)	31	
				475(ox)	13	

OXIDATION-REDUCTION POTENTIALS, ABSORBANCE BANDS AND MOLAR ABSORBANCE
OF COMPOUNDS USED IN BIOCHEMICAL STUDIES (Continued)

	System	$E°$	$E°'$	λ_{max}	E_{mM}	Reference
				665(ox)	17	
				418(red)	120	
				647(red)	24	
174.	2-Methyl-3-hydroxy-1,4-naphthoquinone (Phthiocol)	—	−0.180	—	—	5
		—	—	—	—	4
175.	9-Methylisoalloxazine	—	−0.183	—	—	
176.	Fe^{3+}/Fe^{2+} PPIX (CN⁻)₂, pH9.9	—	−0.183	—	—	5
177.	Anthraquinone-2,6-disulfonate	0.228	−0.184	—	—	5
178.	Pyruvate/Lactate	—	−0.185	—	—	4
			−0.190			7
179.	Fe^{3+}/Fe^{2+} Protoporphyrin IX (borate buffer), pH 8.2	—	−0.188	—	—	4, 49
180.	Neutral Blue	0.17	−0.19	—	—	5
181.	Dihydroxy acetone-P/	—	−0.19	—	—	4
	α-Glycero-P		−0.192	—	—	7
182.	Acetaldehyde/Ethanol	—	−0.197	—	—	4, 7
183.	$[Ti(C_{10}H_{10})]^{2+}/[Ti(C_{10}H_{10})]^{+}$	—	−0.20	—	—	40
184.	$SO_4^{2-}/S_2O_6^{2-}$	−0.2	—	—	—	1
185.	Fe^{3+}/Fe^{2+} Heme undecapeptide, Cyt c (imidazole)	—	−0.201	—	—	68
186.	Riboflavin	—	−0.208	260	27.7	4
				375(ox)	10.6	
				450(ox)	12.2	50
187.	Fe^{3+}/Fe^{2+} Cyt c₃ (*Desulforibro desulfuricans*)	—	−0.205	410(ox)	—	51
				419(red)		
				525(red)		
				553(red)	4.2	
188.	Fe^{3+}/Fe^{2+} Heme octapeptide from Cyt c	—	−0.205	397(ox)	140	52
				414(red)	128	
				520(red)	6	
				550(red)	10	
189.	$[Ru(NH_3)_6]^{3+}/[Ru(NH_3)_6]^{2+}$	—	−0.214	—	—	53
190.	Fe^{3+}/Fe^{2+} Heme octapeptide from Cyt c (imidazole)	—	−0.217	405(ox)	122	68
				416(red)	162	
				520(red)		
				550(red)		
191.	Anthraquinone-1-sulfonate	0.195	−0.218	—	—	5
192.	FMN/FMNH₂, pH 7.09	—	−0.219	260	27.1	54
			−0.211	375(ox)	10.4	50
				450(ox)	12.2	
193.	FAD/FADH₂	—	−0.219	260	37	54
				375(ox)	9.3	
				450(ox)	11.3	
194.	6,7,9-Trimethyl-isoalloxazine (Lumiflavin)	—	−0.223	—	—	54
195.	Janus Green B	—	−0.225	—	—	5
196.	Fe^{3+}/Fe^{2+} Protoporphyrin IX (phosphate buffer), pH 8.2	—	−0.226	395(ox)	55	4
				495(ox)	7	30
				620(ox)	6	
197.	Glutathione	—	−0.23	—	—	7, 5
			−0.34			
198.	Acetoacetyl CoA/B-OH-Butyryl CoA	—	−0.238	—	—	7
199.	S(rhombic)/H₂S	0.14	−0.243	—	—	1, 7
200.	Acetylmethyl carbinol/butane-2,3-diol	—	−0.244	—	—	7
201.	Fe^{3+}/Fe^{2+} Copoporphyrin (CN⁻)₂, pH 9.6	—	−0.247	—	—	5
202.	3-Acetylpyridine-NAD	—	−0.248	—	—	55
203.	Phenosafranine	0.280	−0.252	—	—	5
204.	V^{3+}/V^{2+}	−0.255	—	—	—	5
205.	Co^{3+}/Co^{2+} Mesoporphyrin (pyridine)₂	—	−0.265	—	—	5
206.	Mn^{3+}/Mn^{2+}Hematoporphyrin IX dimethyl ester	—	−0.268	—	—	6
207.	Fe^{3+}/Fe^{2+} Peroxidase (horseradish)	—	−0.271	415(ox)	60	56, 27, 57
				500(ox)	10.0	
				640(ox)	3.0	
208.	Fruotose-sorbitol	—	−0.272	—	—	5
209.	H₃PO₄/H₃PO₃	−0.276	—	—	—	1
210.	Rosindulin 2G	0.139	−0.281	—	—	5
211.	Thionicotinamide-NAD	—	−0.285	400(red)	—	58

OXIDATION-REDUCTION POTENTIALS, ABSORBANCE BANDS AND MOLAR ABSORBANCE
OF COMPOUNDS USED IN BIOCHEMICAL STUDIES (Continued)

	System	E°	E°′	λ_{max}	E_{mM}	Reference
212.	Acetone/Isopropanol	—	−0.281	—	—	5
			−0.286			
213.	Safranine T	0.235	−0.289	—	—	5
214	Lipoic acid	—	−0.29	—	—	5
215.	Indulin Scarlet	0.047	−0.299	—	—	5
216.	Thiophenol	—	−0.30	—	—	4
217.	4-Aminoacridine	—	−0.301	—	—	59
218.	Acridine	—	−0.313	—	—	59
219.	NAD$^+$/NADH	−0.105	−0.320	259(ox)	18	7, 50
				259(red)	15	
				339(red)	6.2	
220.	NADP$^+$/NADPH	—	−0.324	259(ox)	18	7, 50
				259(red)	15	
				339(red)	6.2	
221.	Neutral Red	0.240	−0.325	—	—	5
222.	Cystine/Cysteine	—	−0.340	240(ox) (shoulder)	0.050	7
223.	Lipoyl dehydrogenase	—	−0.34	—	—	60
224.	NAD$^+$/α-NADH	—	−0.341	259(ox)	17	61
				346(red)		
225.	Mn^{3+}/Mn^{2+} Hematoporphyrin IX	—	−0.342	370(ox)	79	6
				460(ox)	50	
				545(ox)	12	
				770(ox)	1.3	
				416(red)	175	
				545(red)	18	
226.	Acetoacetate/β-hydroxybutyrate	—	−0.346	—	—	7
227.	Uric acid/Xanthine	—	−0.36	—	—	7
228.	Benzyl viologen	—	−0.36	—	—	5
229.	Gluconolactone/Glucose	—	−0.364	—	—	7
230.	3-Aminoacridine	—	−0.369	—	—	59
231.	Xanthine/Hypoxanthine	—	−0.371	248.5(ox)	10.2	7, 50
				278(ox)	8.9	
232.	Mn^{3+}/Mn^{2+} Mesoporphyrin (pyridine)$_2$	—	−0.387	—	—	5
233.	1-Aminoacridine	—	−0.394	—	—	59
234.	Cr^{3+}/Cr^{2+}	−0.40	—	—	—	1, 2
235.	N-Methyl nicotinamide	—	−0.419	—	—	5
236.	CO$_2$/Formate	−0.20	−0.42	—	—	1
237.	Fe^{3+}/Fe^{2+} Ferredoxin (Clostridium)	—	−0.413	300(ox)		65
				390(ox)	6	
238.	H$^+$/H$_2$	0.000	−0.421	—	—	5
239.	Fe^{3+}/Fe^{2+} Ferredoxin (spinach)	—	−0.432	325	—	65
				420(ox)		
				463(ox)		
240.	Methyl violgoen	—	−0.44	—	—	5
241.	Xanthine oxidase	—	−0.45	—	—	63
242.	SO$_4^{2-}$/SO$_3^{2-}$	—	−0.454	—	—	7
243.	Gluconate/Glucose	—	−0.44	—	—	62
			−0.47			7
244.	2-Aminoacridine	—	−0.486		—	59
245.	Oxalate/Glyoxalate	—	−0.50		—	7
246.	H$_3$PO$_3$/H$_3$PO$_2$	−0.50	—	—	—	1
247.	SO$_3^{2-}$/S$_2$O$_4^{2-}$	—	−0.527	—	—	7
			−0.471			
248.	Acetate/acetaldehyde	—	−0.581	—	—	7
			−0.589			
249.	2,8-Diaminoacridine	—	−0.731	—	—	59
250.	SiO$_2$/Si	−0.86	—	—	—	1
251.	5-Aminoacridine	—	−0.916	—	—	59
252.	N$_2$(gas)/H$_3$NOH$^+$	−1.87	—	—	—	1
253.	Formamidine sulfinic acid	—	−1.5	—	—	64

Compiled by Paul A. Loach.

References

1. Latimer, in *The Oxidation States of the Elements and Their Potentials in Aqueous Solution*, 2nd ed., Prentice-Hall, New York, 1952.
2. Berka, Vulterin, and Zyka, in *Newer Redox Titrants*, Pergamon Press, New York, 1965.
3. Koltoff, Belcher, Stenger, and Matsuyama, in *Volumetric Analysis*, Vol. III. Interscience, New York, 1957.
4. Lardy, in *Respiratory Enzymes*, Burgess, Minneapolis, 1949.
5. Clark, in *Oxidation-Reduction Potentials of Organic Systems*, Williams & Wilkins, Baltimore, 1960.
6. Loach and Calvin, *Biochemistry*, 2, 361 (1963).
7. Burton, *Ergeb. Physiol.*, 49, 275 (1957).
8. Martell and Calvin, in *Chemistry of Metal Chelate Complexes*, Prentice-Hall, New York, 1958.
9. Klotz and Klotz, *Science*, 121, 477 (1955).
10. Kok, *Biochim. Biophys. Acta*, 48, 527 (1961).
11. Goodheer, *Biochim. Biophys. Acta*, 38, 389 (1960).
12. Clayton, *Photochem. Photobiol.*, 1, 201 (1962).
13. Loach, Androes, Maksim, and Calvin, *Photochem. Photobiol*, 2, 443 (1963).
14. Kuntz, Loach, and Calvin, *Biophys. J.*, 4, 277 (1964).
15. Minakami, Ringler, and Singer, *J. Biol. Chem.*, 237, 569 (1962).
16. Kamen and Vernon, *Biochim. Biophys. Acta*, 17, 10 (1955).
17. Tissieres, *Biochem. J.*, 64, 582 (1956).
18. Ball, *Biochem. Z.*, 295, 262 (1938).
19. Rodkey and Ball, *J. Biol. Chem.*, 182, 17 (1950).
20. Theorell and Åkeson, *J. Am. Chem. Soc.*, 63, 1804 (1941).
21. Lautsch, Brouer, and Becker, *Z. Electrochem.*, 61, 174 (1957).
22. Cutolo, *Arzneimittelforsch*, 8, 581 (1958).
23. Armstrong, *Biochim. Biophys. Acta*, 86, 194 (1964).
24. Green, Mii, Mahler, and Bock, *J. Biol. Chem.*, 206, 1 (1954).
25. Havemann, *Biochem. Z.*, 314, 118 (1943).
26. Taylor and Hastings, *J. Biol. Chem.*, 131, 649 (1939).
27. George, Beetleston, and Griffith, in *Symposia on Hematin Enzymes*, Canberra, 1959.
28. Taylor and Morgan, *J. Biol. Chem.*, 144, 15 (1942).
29. Falk, in *Porphyrins and Metalloporphyrins*, Elsevier, New York, 1964.
30. Shack and Clark, *J. Biol. Chem.*, 171, 143 (1947).
31. Orlando, *Biochim. Biophys. Acta*, 57, 373 (1962).
32. Morton, Gloor, Schindler, Wilson, Chopard-dit-Jean, Hemming, Isler, Leat, Pennock, Ruegg, Schwieter, and Wiss, *Helv. Chim. Acta*, 41, 2343 (1958).
33. Jagendorf and Marguiliea, *Arch. Biochem. Biophys.*, 90, 184 (1960).
34. Holton and Colpa-Boonstra, *Biochem. J.*, 76, 179 (1960).
35. Mikhalevich and Litvinchuk, *Zh. Neorgan. Khim.*, 9, 2391 (1964).
36. Kamen and Lakeda, *Biochim. Biophys. Acta*, 21, 518 (1956).
37. Green, Jarnefelt, and Tisdale, *Biochim. Biophys. Acta*, 31, 34 (1959).
38. Hauge, *J. Am. Chem. Soc.*, 78, 5266 (1956).
39. Hartree, *Advanc. Enzymol.*, 18, 1 (1957).
40. Pauson, *Quart. Rev.*, 9, 391 (1955).
41. Velick and Strittmatter, *J. Biol. Chem.*, 221, 265 (1956).
42. Newton and Kamen, *Biochim. Biophys. Acta*, 21, 71 (1956).
43. Hill, *Nature*, 174, 501 (1954).
44. Walter, *J. Biol. Chem.*, 196, 151 (1952).
45. Vestling, *Acta Chem. Scand.*, 9, 1600 (1955).
46. Martius and Marki, *Biochem. Z.*, 333, 111 (1960).
47. Burton and Wilson, *Biochem. J.*, 54, 86 (1953).
48. Loach and Calvin, *Nature*, 22, 343 (1964).
49. Cowgill and Clark, *J. Biol. Chem.*, 198, 33 (1952).
50. Weber, in *Biochemist's Handbook*, Long, Ed., Spon, London, 1961., 81.
51. Postgate, *Biochim. Biophys. Acta*, 18, 427 (1955).
52. Harbury and Loach, *J. Biol. Chem.*, 235, 3640 (1960).
53. Endicott, and Taube, *Inorg. Chem.*, 4, 437 (1965).
54. Lowe and Clark, *J. Biol. Chem.*, 221, 983 (1956).
55. Rodkey, *J. Biol. Chem.*, 234, 188 (1959).
56. Harbury, *J. Biol. Chem.*, 225, 1009 (1957).
57. Theotell, *Enzymologia*, 10, 3 (1942).
58. Anderson and Kaplan, *J. Biol. Chem.*, 234, 1226 (1959).
59. Breyer, Buchanan, and Duewell, *J. Chem. Soc.*, 360, 000 (1944).
60. Searls and Sanadi, *Proc. Natl. Acad. Sci. (USA)*, 45, 697 (1957).
61. Kaplan, in *The Enzymes*, 2nd, ed., Vol. 3, Boyer, Lardy, and Myrbäck, Eds., Academic Press, New York, 1960, 105.
62. Strecker and Korkes, *J. Biol. Chem.*, 196, 769 (1952).
63. Mackler, Mahler, and Green, *J. Biol. Chem.*, 210, 149 (1954).
64. Shashova, *Biochemistry*, 3, 1719 (1964).
65. Tagawa and Arnon, *Nature*, 195, 537 (1962).
66. Davenport and Hill, *Proc. R. Soc. B (England)*, 139, 327 (1952).
67. Wateri and Kimura, *Biochem. Biophys. Res. Commun.*, 24, 106 (1966).
68. Harbury and Loach, *J. Biol. Chem.*, 235, 3646 (1960).
69. Lovenberg and Sobel, *Proc. Natl. Acad. Sci. (USA)*, 54, 193 (1965).
70. Bartsch and Kamen, *J. Biol. Chem.*, 230, 41 (1958).
71. Fuhrhop and Mauzerall, *J. Am. Chem. Soc.*, 91, 4174 (1969).

CALORIMETRIC ΔH VALUES ACCOMPANYING CONFORMATIONAL CHANGES OF MACROMOLECULES IN SOLUTION

Macromolecule	Mol	$S_{20,w}$	Solvent	pH[a]	Concentration[a]	Temperature[b] °C	Type of Transition	Type of Measurement	ΔH° kcal/mol	Ref.
Pepsin	3.5×10^5	—	0.05 M phosphate and about 0.15 M KCl	7.16	0.2–0.5%	15	Denaturation	Heat of mixing	22[c]	1, 2
				6.41		35			69[c]	
Trypsin	2.0×10^4	—	0.1 M NaCl	1.4–2.5	0.2–0.5%	25	Denaturation	Heat of mixing	8.0	3
Fibrin	3.3×10^5	—	1.0 M NaBr-acetate, phosphate	6.08	2.91%	25	Polymerization	Heat of mixing	–19	4
				6.88			Clotting		–44.5	
Fibrinogen	3.3×10^5	—	Phosphate	6–8.5	5 g/l	25	Clotting	Heat of mixing	–44	5
Mercaptalbumin	6.7×10^4	—	0.1 M NaCl	2.8–4.7	2–3.5%	25	Denaturation	Heat of mixing	1.5–3.4[d]	3, 6
						15			1.5[d]	6
Ferrihemoglobin	6.8×10^4	—	0.02 M sodium formate	3.2–3.8	0.76%	25	Denaturation	Heat of mixing	10 ± 0.3	7
Horse serum albumin	6.9×10^4	—			0.61, 1.17%	15			–76 ± 1.6	
			0.1 M glycine	7.0	2%	55	Denaturation	Heat capacity	90 ± 15	8
						68			75 ± 10	
						76			55 ± 7	
Myoglobin sperm whale	1.78×10^4	—	0.15 M KCl	4.5	3 g/l	30	Denaturation	Heat of mixing	40	9
	1.76×10^4		0.1 M glycine	9.5	3.0 g/l	85		Heat capacity	200	41, 42
				10.6		78			178	
				11.0		72			134	
				11.5		63			100	
				12.25		50			73	
Ribonuclease A	1.37×10^4	—	0.15 M KCl	2.8	1.385 and 2.69%	43	Denaturation	Heat capacity	70 ± 1	10
			0.1 M KCl	2.2	0.5–1.0 g/l	45		Heat of mixing	109 ± 5	11
			0.15 M KCl	2.8	1.5%	44		Heat capacity	86.5 ± 4.4	12
			Water	7.80	3.41–7.22%	60			99 ± 8	75
			1.5 M urea		7.14%	55			87 ± 4	76
			2 M urea		4.86–7.43%	53.5			83 ± 5	75
			2.5 M urea		7.26%	52			81 ± 13	76
			3 M urea		5.73%	48.5			71 ± 4	75
			4 M urea		7.02%	46			68 ± 6	76
			1 M guanidine HCl		4.61%	50			79 ± 1	76
			2 M guanidine HCl		4.31%	37.5			55 ± 3	75
			1 M hexa-methylene-tetramine		9.5	61			99 ± 2	75
			2 M hexamethylenetetramine		4.7–14.4%	60			105 ± 10	
			15 mM cacodylate	9.24	5.16–6.63%	61			99 ± 2	75
			0.1 M glycine, acetate	2.4	0.1–1.0%	36			52	65
				3.3		47			66	
				3.7		50			73	
				4.44		54			77	
				6.0		59			89	

CALORIMETRIC ΔH VALUES ACCOMPANYING CONFORMATIONAL CHANGES OF MACROMOLECULES IN SOLUTION (Continued)

Macromolecule	Mol	$S_{20,w}$	Solvent	pH^a	Concentration^a	Temperature^b °C	Type of Transition	Type of Measurement	ΔH^c kcal/mol	Ref.
Ribonuclease—bovine pancreatic	1.37×10^4	—	0.04 M glycine	5.5	2.0 g/l	69.0	Denaturation	Heat capacity	115.0	43, 44
				4.0		57.0			108.0	
				3.3		49.0			97.0	
				2.75		42.0			91.5	
			HCl	0.36	0.5%	31.5			61	64
				1.05		29.9			59	
			0.2 M glycine	2.02		31.2			66	
				2.80	0.1–2.7%	40.6			88	
				3.28	0.5%	45.8			105	
			0.2 M acetate	4.04		52.3			126	
				5.00		57.8			151	
				6.23		60.8			155	
			0.2 M NaCl	7.00		61.3			168	
				7.80		61.2			178	
Ribonuclease S'	—	—	15 mM cacodylate	7.0	5.16–6.63%	47.1	Denaturation	Heat capacity	111	75
Ribonuclease S protein	—	—	15 mM cacodylate	7.0	5.16–6.63%	37.6	Denaturation	Heat capacity	55	75
Ribonuclease S	—	—	15 mM cacodylate	7.0	5.16–6.63%	47.7	Denaturation	Heat capacity	107	75
			0.3 M NaCl		75 µM S-protein	5	S-protein+S-peptide=RNase S'	Heat of mixing	–23.6	55
						10			–25.2	
						15			–28.4	
						20			–33.3	
						25			–39.8	
						30			–47.9	
						35			–57.5	
						40			–68.8	
						0	S-protein+Met (O$_2$)-S-13-Peptide=Met (O$_2$)-13-RNase S'		–18.9	
						5			–19.8	
						10			–21.9	
						15			–25.0	
						20			–29.2	
						25			–34.4	
						30			–40.6	
						35			–47.8	
						40			–56.0	
Tropocollagen Rat skin	3.6×10^5	—	Acetic acid, no salt	3.5	0.1–0.4 g/l	40.8	Denaturation	Heat capacity	1.53 residue	39, 40
Pike skin	3.6×10^5	—	Acetic acid, no salt	3.5	0.1–0.4 g/l	30.6	Denaturation	Heat capacity	1.24 residue	39, 40
Merlang skin	3.6×10^5	—	Acetic acid, no salt	3.5	0.1–0.4 g/l	21.5	Denaturation	Heat capacity	0.88 residue	39, 40
Cod skin	3.6×10^5	—	Acetic acid, no salt	3.5	0.1–0.4 g/l	20.0	Denaturation	Heat capacity	0.75 residue	39, 40
Lysozyme — egg white^h	1.45×10^4	—	0.1 M phosphate	5.37	5.34–6.16%	76.5	Denaturation	Heat capacity	138 ± 7	62
			4 M urea		5.23–9.67%	65.5			103 ± 7	
			7 M urea		5.92%	55.0			80 ± 3	

CALORIMETRIC ΔH VALUES ACCOMPANYING CONFORMATIONAL CHANGES OF MACROMOLECULES IN SOLUTION (Continued)

Macromolecule	Mol	$S_{20,w}$	Solvent	pH^a	Concentration^a	Temperature^b °C	Type of Transition	Type of Measurement	ΔH^e kcal/mol	Ref.
Lysozyme — egg white^h (Continued)	1.43×10^4		1 M guanidine HCl		4.40%	67.5			103 ± 6	44
			2 M guanidine HCl		5.22%	58			85 ± 4	
			1 M hexa-methylene-tetramine		4.72–5.53%	—			121 ± 9	
			2 M hexa-methylene-tetramine		5.72%				121 ± 6	
			0.04 M glycine	4.5	10–5.0 g/l	78.5			141	
				4.0		77.0			134	
				3.0		74.5			133	
				2.6		69.0			125	
				2.5		66.0			119	
				2.0		56.0			106	
				1.5		48.0			91	
Ovalbumin	4.5×10^4	—	Water-HCl	1.0	2.5%	46		Heat of mixing	56 ± 8	13
			3 M guanidine HCl	1.25	4.47–22.4 g/l	25		Heat capacity	30 ± 3	61
			0.1 M glycine	10.0	~2%	77.5	Denaturation		210 ± 13	60
				9		73			172 ± 13	
				5		68			119 ± 13	
				4.5		62			95 ± 13	
				4		57			84 ± 13	
				3		52			45 ± 13	
Chymotrypsin	—	—	0.01 M KCl	2.0 ± 0.08	2.0–10.0 g/l	25	Denaturation	Heat of mixing	50 ± 10	50
						40			110	
Chymotrypsinogen	2.57×10^4	—	0.01 M KCl	2.0 ± 0.08	2.0–10.0 g/l	50	Denaturation	Heat of mixing	123	50
			Water HCl	1.95	0.21–0.26%	40.6	Denaturation	Heat of mixing	103	51
				2.03		42.0			102	
				2.08		42.0			99	
			0.05 M glycine HCl	2.59		48.0			126	
				2.99		53.9			145	
				3.02		54.2			135	
Me₂ SO-chymotrypsin	—	—	0.01 M KCl	2.0 ± 0.08	2.0–10.0 g/l	25	Denaturation	Heat of mixing	32	50
						40			73	
Chymotrypsin-bovine	2.52×10^4	—	0.04 M glycine	4.0	1.0–5.0 g/l	56.4	Denaturation	Heat capacity	162	44, 46
				3.4		55.4			155	
				3.1		52.0			149	
				2.8		48.6			142	
				2.6		44.8			132	
				2.2		38.2			108	
Chymotrypsinogen A	—	—	0.1 M NaCl, 0.1 M hydro-cinnamate	7.4	0.4 mM	25	Activation to π chymotrypsin	Heat of mixing	0 ± 0.5	66
	2.51×10^4		HCl	3	5.92%	56	Denaturation	Heat capacity	154 ± 8	76
				2	6.77%	42.5			112 ± 3	
π Chymotrypsin	—	—	Various NaCl, CaCl₂, and buffers	7.4	0.06–0.7 mM	25	Conversion to δ-chymotrypsin	Heat of mixing	−2 ± 1	66
α-Chymotrypsinogen	2.45×10^4	—	0.01 M glycine acetate	2.3	0.1–1.0%	43	Denaturation	Heat capacity	78	41

CALORIMETRIC ΔH VALUES ACCOMPANYING CONFORMATIONAL CHANGES OF MACROMOLECULES IN SOLUTION (Continued)

Macromolecule	Mol	$S_{20,w}$	Solvent	pH[a]	Concentration[a]	Temperature[b] °C	Type of Transition	Type of Measurement	ΔH[c] kcal/mol	Ref.
α-Chymotrypsinogen (Continued)				2.6					102	
				2.8					110	
				3.4					130	
				4.0					140	
				5.0					148	
α-Chymotrypsin	—	—	0.05 M phosphate, 0.2 M KCl	7.8	0.1–0.4 mM	25	Dimerization	Heat of mixing	−17.1 ± 1.2	67
Cytochrome c bovine heart	1.24×10^4	—	0.04 M Glycine	4.8	1.0–5.0 g/l	78.0	Denaturation	Heat capacity	107	44, 47
				4.5		77.0			103	
				3.9		72.0			96	
				3.7		70.0			93	
				3.4		66.0			84	
				3.2		62.0			77	
				3.0		59.0			70	
				2.8		52.5			60	
Poly (β-benzyl-l-aspartate)	—	—	5.2 mol % $CHCl_2CO_2H$, 94.8 mol % $CHCl_2CHCl_2$	—	0–1%	−0.8	Coil-helix	Heat of mixing	0.358 residue	13
			5.7 mol % $CHCl_2CO_2H$, 94.3 mol % $CHCl_2CHCl_2$			7.4			0.334 residue	
			6.0 mol % $CHCl_2CO_2H$, 94.0 mol % $CHCl_2CHCl_2$			17.8			0.298 residue	
			6.4 mol % $CHCl_2CO_2H$, 93.6 mol % $CHCl_2CHCl_2$			28.8			0.229 residue	
			93.3 mol % $CHCl_2CO_2H$, 6.7 mol % $CHCl_2CHCl_2$			38.0			0.169 residue	
Poly (γ-benzyl-l-glutamate)	5×10^5	—	47 mol % $CHCl_2CO_2H$, 53 mol % $CHCl_3$	—	2–3 wt/vol%	0	Coil-helix	Heat capacity	0.75 residue	73
			51 mol % $CHCl_2CO_2H$, 49 mol % $CHCl_3$			2			0.71 residue	
			56 mol % $CHCl_2CO_2H$, 44 mol % $CHCl_3$			9			0.68 residue	
			62 mol % $CHCl_2CO_2H$, 38 mol % $CHCl_3$			15			0.61 residue	
			78 mol % $CHCl_2CO_2H$, 22 mol % $CHCl_3$			41			0.40 residue	
			46 mol % $CHCl_2CO_2H$, 54 mol % $CHCl_2CHCl_2$			−21			0.84 residue	
			52 mol % $CHCl_2CO_2H$, 48 mol % $CHCl_2CHCl_2$			−15			0.80 residue	
			65 mol % $CHCl_2CO_2H$, 35 mol % $CHCl_2CHCl_2$			3			0.72 residue	
			74 mol % $CHCl_2CO_2H$, 26 mol % $CHCl_2CHCl_2$			14			0.57 residue	
			79 mol % $CHCl_2CO_2H$, 21 mol % $CHCl_2CHCl_2$			21			0.84 residue	
			81 mol % $CHCl_2CO_2H$, 19 mol % $CHCl_2CHCl_2$			39			0.30 residue	
			37 mol % $CHCl_2CO_2H$, 63 mol % CH_2ClCH_2Cl			−24			0.86 residue	

CALORIMETRIC ΔH VALUES ACCOMPANYING CONFORMATIONAL CHANGES OF MACROMOLECULES IN SOLUTION (Continued)

Macromolecule	Mol	$S_{20,w}$	Solvent	pH[a]	Concentration[a]	Temperature[b] °C	Type of Transition	Type of Measurement	ΔH[c] kcal/mol	Ref.
Poly (γ-benzyl-l-glutamate) (Continued)			47 mol % $CHCl_2CO_2H$, 53 mol % CH_2ClCH_2Cl			−10			0.81 residue	
			56 mol % $CHCl_2CO_2H$, 44 mol % CH_2ClCH_2Cl			2			0.73 residue	
			63 mol % $CHCl_2CO_2H$, 37 mol % CH_2ClCH_2Cl			13			0.66 residue	
			69 mol % $CHCl_2CO_2H$, 31 mol % CH_2ClCH_2Cl			23			0.56 residue	
			74 mol % $CHCl_2CO_2H$, 26 mol % CH_2ClCH_2Cl			31			0.49 residue	
			77 mol % $CHCl_2CO_2H$, 23 mol % CH_2ClCH_2Cl			40			0.36 residue	14, 15
	2.35×10^5		19 wt % CH_2ClCH_2Cl, 81 wt % $CHCl_2CO_2H$		0.257 m residue	32			0.43 residue	
					0.132 m residue				0.68 residue	
					0.068 m residue				0.81 residue	
					C → 0				0.95 ± 0.03 residue	
	2.7×10^5		25 vol % CH_2ClCH_2Cl, 75 vol % $CHCl_2CO_2H$		0.097 m residue	26		Heat of solution	0.525 ± 0.08 residue	16
	1.6×10^5		($CHCl_2CO_2H$–CH_2ClCH_2Cl) →100% $CHCl_2CO_2H$		7 mM residue	30		Heat of solution	0.70 ± 0.05 residue	17
	3.5×10^5		CH_2ClCH_2Cl–$CHCl_2CO_2H$ 82 wt % $CHCl_2CO_2H$		0.25 m residue	37		Heat capacity	0.38 residue	18
			83 wt % $CHCl_2CO_2H$		0.07 m residue	43			0.79 residue	
					0.25 m residue	40			0.32 residue	
					0.13 m residue	44			0.62 residue	
					0.07 m residue	46			0.78 residue	
			85 wt % $CHCl_2CO_2H$		0.25 m residue	46			0.29 residue	
					0.13 m residue	50			0.58 residue	
					0.07 m residue	53			0.76 residue	
			88 wt % $CHCl_2CO_2H$		0.25 m residue	—			0.26 residue	
					0.13 m residue				0.55 residue	
					0.07 m residue				0.74 residue	
	2.9×10^5		25 vol % $CHCl_3$, 75 vol % $CHCl_2CO_2H$		0.139–0.082 m residue	25		Heat of mixing	1.0 ± 0.1 residue	31
	1.6×10^5		20 vol % CH_2ClCH_2Cl, 80 vol % $CHCl_2CO_2H$		2 g/l	30		Heat of solution	0.65 ± 0.3 residue	32
			25 vol % $CHCl_3$, 75 vol % $CHCl_2CO_2H$						0.65 ± 0.3 residue	
	2.0×10^5		25 vol % CH_2ClCH_2Cl, 75 vol % $CHCl_2CO_2H$		0.123–0.7 m residue	25		Heat of mixing	0.75 ± 0.2 residue	33
	3.5×10^4		75 vol % $CHCl_2CO_2H$, 25 vol % CH_2ClCH_2Cl		3%	—		Heat capacity	0.3 ± 0.8 residue	58
	4.5×10^4								0.38 ± 0.8 residue	
	9.9×10^4								0.49 ± 0.5 residue	
	29.0×10^4								0.615 ± 0.8 residue	
	33.5×10^4								0.59 ± 0.8 residue	

CALORIMETRIC ΔH VALUES ACCOMPANYING CONFORMATIONAL CHANGES OF MACROMOLECULES IN SOLUTION (Continued)

Macromolecule	Mol	$S_{20,w}$	Solvent	pH[a]	Concentration[a]	Temperature[b] °C	Type of Transition	Type of Measurement	ΔH* kcal/mol	Ref.
Poly (γ-benzyl-l-glutamate) (Continued)	43.5×10^4								0.60 ± 0.5 residue	
	55.0×10^4								0.515 ± 0.6 residue	19
Poly-γ-benzyl-l-glutamate (deuterated)	2.7×10^5		34 vol % CH_2ClCH_2Cl, 66 vol % $CHCl_2CO_2H$	—	3%	8.5	Coil-helix	Heat capacity	0.67 ± 0.05 residue	
			18 vol % CH_2ClCH_2Cl, 82 vol % $CHCl_2CO_2H$			40			0.38 ± 0.05 residue	
Poly (N-γ-car-bobenzoxy-l-α-γ-diaminobutric acid)	—		CH_2ClCH_2Cl/ $CHCl_2CO_2H$	—	~2 g/l	30	Solvation	Heat of solution	-0.6 residue	68
Poly (N-δ-carbobenzoxy-l-ornithine)	—		CH_2ClCH_2Cl/ $CHCl_2CO_2H$	—	~2 g/l	30	Order-disorder	Heat of solution	0.255 ± .025 residue	
							Order-disorder		-0.65 residue	
Poly(l-lysine)	1.1×10^5		0.1 M KCl	6.0	0.25%	15, 25	Coil-helix	Heat of mixing	1.2 residue	63
							α-β		0 residue	
Poly (ε-carbobenzoxy-l-lysine)	7.5×10^5		CH_2ClCH_2Cl/ $CHCl_2CO_2H$	—	0.1%	15, 25	Coil-helix	Heat of mixing	0.62 ± 0.04 residue	59
	1.5×10^5									
	2.75×10^5		37 vol % $CHCl_2CO_2H$, 63 vol % $CHCl_3$	—	3%	26	Coil-helix	Heat capacity	0.21 ± 0.06 residue	20
Poly (l-glutamic acid)	$0.4-1.0 \times 10^5$		0.1 M KCl	4.5-5.5	0.5 g/l	30	Coil-helix	Heat of mixing	-1.1 ± 0.2 residue	21
Poly (γ-ethyl-l-glutamate)	1.3×10^5		40 vol % CH_2ClCH_2Cl, 60 vol % $CHCl_2CO_2H$	—	2 g/l	30	Coil-helix	Heat of solution	0.65 ± 0.3 residue	32
	4.0×10^5		35 vol % CH_2ClCH_2Cl, 65 vol % $CHCl_2CO_2H$						0.65 ± 0.3 base pair	
Salmon DNA	—	21.7	0.1 M NaCl	6.0	0.15-0.6 g/l	25	Acid denaturation	Heat of mixing	8.31 base pair	23, 24
Herring spermatozoa DNA	—	—	0.015 M NaCl, 1.5 mM citrate	—	1%	75	Thermal denaturation	Heat capacity	5 base pair	15
Ps. fluorescens DNA	—	20.1	0.1 M NaCl	6.0	0.15-0.6 g/l	25	Acid denaturation	Heat of mixing	7.83 base pair	24
S. marcessens DNA	—	17.4	0.1 M NaCl	6.0	0.15-0.6 g/l	25	Acid denaturation	Heat of mixing	7.83 base pair	24
Sea urchin DNA	—	23.3	0.1 M NaCl	6.0	0.15-0.6 g/l	25	Acid denaturation	Heat of mixing	8.03 base pair	24
Calf thymus DNA	$>10^6$	—	0.015 M NaCl, 1.5 mM citrate	6.0	10 g/l	72	Thermal denaturation	Heat capacity	7.0 ± 0.5 base pair	25
			0.15 M Phosphate	11.3	~4 mM base pair	34	Denaturation		8.3 ± 0.5 base pair	52
				11.15		44.2			9.5 ± 0.5 base pair	
				11.00		47.2			9.5 ± 0.5 base pair	
				10.90		50.6			9.3 ± 0.5 base pair	
				10.70		56.6			10.0 ± 0.7 base pair	
				10.60		58.8			9.1 ± 0.5 base pair	
				10.45		63.5			9.2 ± 0.7 base pair	
				10.30		68.8			10.4 ± 0.7 base pair	
			1 mM phosphate, 1.5 mM Na^+	7.0		58.05			6.4 ± 0.3 base pair	
			1 mM phosphate, 6.5 mM Na^+			64.5			6.8 ± 0.3 base pair	
			1 mM phosphate, 11.2 mM Na^+			68.8			6.9 ± 0.3 base pair	
			1 mM phosphate, 51 mM Na^+			77.0			7.2 ± 0.3 base pair	
Cl. perfrigens DNA	—		1.0 mM KCl, 1.5 mM sodium citrate	7.0	5-6 g/l	55	Denaturation	Heat capacity	7.73 base pair	53
M. lysodeikticus DNA	—		1.0 mM KCl, 1.5 mM sodium citrate	7.0	5-6 g/l	79	Denaturation	Heat capacity	8.52 base pair	53
T2 phage DNA	—		3 mM phosphate, 0.2 M NaCl	7.0	0.5 g/l	84.8	Denaturation	Heat capacity	9.65 base pair	37

CALORIMETRIC ΔH VALUES ACCOMPANYING CONFORMATIONAL CHANGES OF MACROMOLECULES IN SOLUTION (Continued)

Macromolecule	Mol	$S_{20,w}$	Solvent	pH^a	Concentration[a]	Temperature[b] °C	Type of Transition	Type of Measurement	ΔH^c kcal/mol	Ref.
T$_2$ phage DNA (Continued)			3 mM phosphate, 0.115 M NaCl			81.2			9.42 base pair	
			3 mM phosphate, 0.057 M NaCl			75.0			9.28 base pair	
			3 mM phosphate, 0.036 M NaCl			71.5			9.14 base pair	
			3 mM phosphate, 0.014 M NaCl			66.0			9.15 base pair	
			3 mM phosphate, 0.009 M NaCl			69.0			8.90 base pair	
			3 mM phosphate, 0.2 M NaCl	8.5		82.5			8.94 base pair	
			3 mM phosphate, glycine	8.9		76.5			8.03 base pair	
			3 mM glycine, 0.2 M NaCl	9.3		71.8			7.78 base pair	
				9.6		66.3			7.14 base pair	
			3 mM citrate, phosphate, 0.20 M NaCl	5.4		84.0			9.40 base pair	37, 38
			3 mM citrate, 0.20 M NaCl	4.8		82.3			8.57 base pair	
				4.3		76.0			6.60 base pair	
				4.0		71.5			5.43 base pair	
				3.8		68.0			5.00 base pair	
				3.5		64.0			4.70 base pair	
				3.2		55.0			7.00 base pair	
Salmon sperm DNA	—	—	1.0 mM HCl, 1.5 mM sodium citrate	7.0	5–6 g/l	60.6	Denaturation	Heat capacity	7.84 base pair	53
M$_4$ coliphage DNA	4 × 10^7	—	0.015 M HCl, 0.1 M KCl, 2.2 M urea, citrate	3.25	0.045–0.066 g/l	27	Denaturation	Heat of mixing	9.5 ± 1.5 base pair	69
tRNA^{Phe}-yeast	—	—	0.01 M tris, 50 μM Mg^{2+}	7.0	~0.12%	66.5	Unfolding	Heat capacity	140	48
			0.01 M tris, 0.1 mM Mg^{2+}			70			156	
			0.01 M tris, 0.25 mM Mg^{2+}			73			216	
			0.01 M tris, 5 mM Mg^{2+}			80.5			248	
			5 mM phosphate, 0.1 M NaCl, 0.2 mM Mg^{2+}			68			175	
			5 mM NaCl, 1 mM MgCl$_2$	7.2	~10 μM	57		Heat of mixing	123 ± 25	49
			5 mM citrate, 1 mM MgSO$_4$	6.5	0.06–0.08 mM	49		Heat capacity	200 ± 30	71
			5 mM citrate, 5 mM MgSO$_4$			70			250 ± 20	
			5 mM citrate, 0.08 M MgSO$_4$, 0.5 M NaCl			76.5			240 ± 20	
			5 mM citrate, 8 mM MgSO$_4$, 0.1 M NaCl			76.5			240 ± 20	
			5 mM citrate, 0.08 M MgSO$_4$, 0.5 M NaCl			76.5			240 ± 20	
						76.5			220 ± 20	
			5 mM citrate, 0.02 M MgSO$_4$			79			230 ± 20	
			5 mM citrate 10 mM MgSO$_4$	6.5	1.25–2.5 g/l	60		Heat of mixing	310	71
Poly(A-U)	—	4.5–10.0 Poly(U), 8.0–12.0 Poly(A)	0.1 M KCl, 0.01 M cacodylate	6.6	20 mM—50 μM nucleotide	25	Poly (A)+ Poly (U)=Poly(A-U)	Heat of mixing	−5.9 ± 0.2 base pair	26
			0.5 M KCl, 0.01 M cacodylate						−5.9 ± 0.2 base pair	
			1.0 M KCl, 0.01 M cacodylate						−4.75 ± 0.3 base pair	

CALORIMETRIC ΔH VALUES ACCOMPANYING CONFORMATIONAL CHANGES OF MACROMOLECULES IN SOLUTION (Continued)

Macromolecule	Mol	$S_{20,w}$	Solvent	pH[a]	Concentration[a]	Temperature[b] °C	Type of Transition	Type of Measurement	ΔH[e] kcal/mol	Ref.
Poly(A·U) (Continued)		2.1–12.2 Poly(A)	0.1 M KCl, 0.01 M cacodylate						−5.95 ± 0.1 base pair	2
		6.1 Poly(A), 7.2 Poly(U)	0.1 M KCl, 0.01 M cacodylate	7.0	35 mM nucleotide	10			−6.29 ± 0.19 base pair[f]	
						25			−6.97 ± 0.17 base pair[f]	
						40			−7.72 ± 0.29 base pair[f]	
			0.1 M NaCl, 0.01 M cacodylate	6.8	80 mM nucleotide	24			−5.95 ± 0.1 base pair	
						37			−6.50 ± 0.1 base pair	
			0.5 M NaCl, 0.01 M cacodylate			37			−6.69 ± 0.1 base pair	
	~10⁵		0.01 M citrate, 0.057 M NaCl		8.5 mM base pair	49		Heat capacity	−6.7 base pair	29
			0.01 M citrate, 0.10 M NaCl			54.8			−7.2 base pair	
			0.01 M citrate, 15 M NaCl			58.4			−7.7 base pair	
	—	—				85–90		Extrapolated	−8.5 ± 0.5 base pair	34
		9.53 Poly(A), 6.15 Poly(U)	0.018 M NaCl, 5 mM cacodylate	6.9–7.0	5.0 mM nucleotide	44.5		Heat capacity	−7.38 ± 0.08 base pair	
			0.043 M NaCl, 5 mM cacodylate			51.3			−7.95 ± 0.07 base pair	
			0.103 M NaCl, 0.01 M cacodylate		6.04 mM nucleotide	58.3			−8.20 ± 0.2 base pair	
			0.104 M NaCl, 0.01 M cacodylate		5.0 mM nucleotide	58.2			−8.20 ± 0.24 base pair	
		7.56 Poly(A), 5.62 Poly(U)	0.011 M KCl, 5 mM cacodylate			35.9			−6.44 ± 0.22 base pair	3
			0.012 M KCl, 5 mM cacodylate			36.2			−6.44 ± 0.22 base pair	
			0.040 M KCl, 5 mM cacodylate		2.28 mM nucleotide	47			−6.83 ± 0.33 base pair	
			0.054 M KCl, 5 mM cacodylate		5.0 mM nucleotide	48.7			−6.85 ± 0.11 base pair	
			0.055 M KCl, 5 mM cacodylate			48.8			−6.85 ± 0.11 base pair	
	~10⁵		0.06 M cations, 3.3 mM citrate	6.5	3.76 mM base pair	49.4			6.8 ± 0.4 base pair	3
			0.063 M cations, 3.3 mM citrate		1.88 mM base pair	51.2			−6.9 ± 0.4 base pair	
			0.06 M cations, 3.3 mM citrate		0.984 mM base pair	51			−6.9 ± 0.4 base pair	
			0.46 M cations, 0.01 M citrate	6.8	Not given	56.1			−8.2 base pair	36
						70.0			−8.8 base pair	
			0.50 M cations, 0.01 M citrate			54.1			−8.1 base pair	
						71.6			−8.7 base pair	
			0.57 M cations, 0.01 M citrate			53.5			−8.0 base pair	
						74.5			−8.9 base pair	
						95		Extrapolated	−9.5 ± 0.5 base pair	
			5 mM NaCl		8.5 mM nucleotide	45.8	Poly(A) + Poly(U)= Poly(A·U)	Heat capacity	−6.6 base pair	70
			5 mM NaCl, D₂O			47.7			−6.6 base pair	
			0.1 M NaCl, 0.01 M cacodylate			24	Poly(A·U)+Poly(U)= Poly(A·2U)	Heat of mixing	−3.82 ± 0.1 (A·2U) residue	28
						37			−3.5 ± 0.5 (A·2U) residue	

CALORIMETRIC ΔH VALUES ACCOMPANYING CONFORMATIONAL CHANGES OF MACROMOLECULES IN SOLUTION (Continued)

Macromolecule	Mol	$S_{20,w}$	Solvent	pH[a]	Concentration[a]	Temperature[b] °C	Type of Transition	Type of Measurement	ΔH[e] kcal/mol	Ref.
	—	7.56 Poly(A), 5.62 Poly(U)	0.5 M NaCl, 0.01 M cacodylate			24			−3.80 ± 01 (A·2U) residue	
						37			−4.09 ± 0.1 (A·2U) residue	36
			0.015 M KCl, 5 mM cacodylate		7.72 mM nucleotide	28.4		Heat capacity	−1.24 ± 0.1 (A·2U) residue	
	—	9.53 Poly(A), 6.15 Poly(U)	0.018 M NaCl, 5 mM cacodylate	6.9–7.0	7.50 mM nucleotide	28.6			−1.24 ± 0.15 (A·2U) residue	34
			0.019 M NaCl, 5 mM cacodylate		5.0 mM nucleotide	32.6		Heat capacity	−1.29 ± 0.16 (A·2U) residue	
						31.5			−1.29 ± 0.16 (A·2U) residue	
	~10⁵	—	0.46 M cations, 0.01 M citrate	6.8	Not given	56.1			−4.1 ± 2 (A·2U) residue	
			0.50 M cacodylate 0.01 M citrate			54.1			−4.3 ± 2 (A·2U) residue	
			0.57 M cations, 0.01 M cacodylate			53.1			−4.2 ± 2 (A·2U) residue	
	~10⁵		0.01 M citrate, 0.5 M NaCl			54.3	2 Poly(A·U)=Poly(A·2U)+Poly(A)		3.2 (A·2U) residue	29
						85–90		Extrapolated	4.5 ± 0.5 (A·2U) residue	
	—	9.53 Poly(A), 6.15 Poly(U)	0.263 M NaCl, 0.01 M cacodylate	6.9–7.0	5.0 mM nucleotide	57.5		Heat capacity	2.76 ± 0.1 (A·2U) residue	34
			0.46 M cations, .01 M citrate	6.8	Not given	56.1			4.1 (A·2U) residue	
			0.50 M cations, .0 M citrate			54.1			3.8 (A·2U) residue	36
			0.57 M cations, .01 M citrate			53.5			3.8 (A·2U) residue	
						95		Extrapolated	5.1 ± 0.5 (A·2U) residue	
			0.01 M citrate, 0.50 M cations			72.1	Poly(A·2U)=Poly(A)+ 2 Poly(U)		11.9 (A·2U) residue	
						85–90			12.5 ± 0.5 (A·2U) residue	
	—	7.56 Poly A, 5.62 Poly U	268 M NaCl, 0.01 M cacodylate	6.9–7.0	7.0 mM nucleotide	67.9		Heat capacity	12.7 ± 0.13 (A·2U) residue	34
			5.5 mM KCl, 5mM cacodylate		6.0 mM nucleotide	49.1			10.0 ± 0.25 (A·2U) residue	
			5.6 mM KCl, 5mM cacodylate		5.6 mM nucleotide	49.3			10.0 ± 0.25 (A·2U) residue	
	~10⁵	—	0.46 M cations, 0.01 M citrate	6.8	Not given	70.0			12.9 (A·2U) residue	36
			0.50 M cations, 0.01 M cacodylate			71.6			13.0 (A·2U) residue	
			0.57 M cations, 0.01 M cacodylate			74.5			13.1 (A·2U) residue	
						95	Poly(A)+2 Poly(U)=Poly(A·U) +Poly(U)	Extrapolated	13.5 ± 0.5 (A·2U) residue	
	—	9.53 Poly(A), 6.15 Poly(U)	1.8 mM NaCl, 5 mM cacodylate	6.9–7.0	7.5 mM nucleotide	45.5		Heat capacity	−8.38 ± 0.14 (A·U) residue	34
			1.9 mM NaCl, 5 mM cacodylate			45.0			−8.38 ± 0.14 (A·U) residue	
	—	7.56 Poly(A), 5.62 Poly(U)	1.5 mM KCl, 5 mM cacodylate		7.72 mM nucleotide	38.8			−7.49 ± 0.23 (A·U) residue	
					7.50 mM nucleotide	38.6			−7.49 ± 0.23 (A·U) residue	
Poly A	~10⁵	4.23	0.1 M NaCl, 0.01 M tris	7.30	C → 0 from 0.37–1.34 g/l	35	Helix-coil	Heat capacity	9.4 residue	3
		—	Various salt concentrations	6.8	7.8 mM base pair	90–95		Extrapolated	4.5 ± 2 residue	
			0.20 M citrate, 0.15 M NaCl, HCl	5.50	0.0132 m nucleotide	31.5	Double helix-coil	Heat capacity	3.36 base pair	2

CALORIMETRIC ΔH VALUES ACCOMPANYING CONFORMATIONAL CHANGES OF MACROMOLECULES IN SOLUTION (Continued)

Macromolecule	Mol	$S_{20,w}$	Solvent	pH[a]	Concentration[a]	Temperature[b] °C	Type of Transition	Type of Measurement	ΔH[e] kcal/mol	Ref.
Poly A (Continued)				5.30		39.2			4.09 base pair	
				5.06		47.1			4.67 base pair	
				4.89		56.6			5.13 base pair	
				4.70		65.5			5.57 base pair	
				4.20		85.5			5.90 base pair	
	—	6.1	0.1 M KC1, 0.01 M cacodylate	4.0		10		Heat of mixing	1.80 ± 0.25[g] residue	27
						25			2.74 ± 0.20[g] residue	
Poly(dA·dT)	—	—	5 mM NaCl, 1 mM cacodylate, 1 mM citrate	7.0	5.9–11.6 mM base pair	40	Helix-coil	Heat capacity	7.9 ± 0.14 base pair	56
Poly(I·C)	5 × 10⁵	—	.01 M citrate, .063 m Na⁺	6.9 ± 0.1	1.8 mm base pair	54.1	Poly(I)+Poly(C)= Poly(I·C)	Heat capacity	-6.5 ± 0.4 base pair	54
			.01 M citrate, 0.104 m Na⁺		1.78 mm base pair	60.8			6.8 ± 0.4 base pair	
			.01 M citrate, 0.303 m Na⁺			67.6			-7.6 ± 0.4 base pair	
			.01 M citrate, 0.503 m Na⁺			70.7			-7.9 ± 0.4 base pair	
			.01 M citrate, 1.003 m Na⁺			73.9			-8.0 ± 0.4 base pair	
	—		0.02–0.2 M NaCl	8.0	70 mM base pair	20		Heat of mixing	-5.59 ± 0.02 base pair	57
			0.1–0.4 M NaCl			37			-5.59 ± 0.01 base pair	
Poly(I)	—	—	0.1 M citrate, 1.0 m Na⁺	6.9 ± 0.1	1.79 mM base pair	43.6	Triple helix-coil	Heat capacity	-1.9 ± 0.4 residue	54
PolyC	—	—	1 mM acetate, 0.01 M Na⁺	3.68	~2.8 g/l	40	Double helix-coil	Heat capacity	4.06 base pair	72
				4.33		63			5.20 base pair	
				4.48		75			5.25 base pair	
				4.55		74			5.27 base pair	
				4.85		72			5.12 base pair	
				5.20		61			4.95 base pair	
				5.50		54			4.34 base pair	
				5.76		47			3.62 base pair	

Compiled by Gordon C. Kresheck.

a Final value in mixing experiments; *m* is used for molal concentration; M for molar.
b Transition temperature for heat capacity experiments.
c These values depend upon the choice of expressing pepsin.
d Value depended upon commercial source of protein.
e The manner of treating ionization changes and baseline shifts varies from worker to worker and may introduce differences between the results reported by different laboratories. The latter is discussed in some detail in Reference 48 for heat capacity measurements.
f Heat change corrected for unfolding poly A before reaction.
g These calorimetric data were recalculated by Stevens and Felsenfeld[77] to yield values of 6.5 and 8.5 kcal mol nucleotide for the single helix-coil transition.
h Data are also found in Reference 74 for this protein, although complete experimental conditions were not given.

References

1. Buzzell and Sturtevant, *J. Am. Chem. Soc.*, 74, 1983 (1952).
2. Sturtevant, *J. Phys. Chem.*, 58, 97 (1954).
3. Gutfreund and Sturtevant, *J. Am. Chem. Soc.*, 75, 5447 (1953).
4. Sturtevant, Laskowski, Donnelly, and Scheraga, *J. Am. Chem. Soc.*, 77, 6163 (1955).
5. Laki and Kitzinger, *Nature (Lond.)*, 178, 985 (1956).
6. Bro and Sturtevant, *J. Am. Chem. Soc.*, 80, 1789 (1958).
7. Forrest and Sturtevant, *J. Am. Chem. Soc.*, 82, 585 (1960).
8. Privalov and Monaselidze, *Biofizika*, 8, 420 (1963).
9. Hermans and Rialdi, *Biochemistry*, 4, 1277 (1965).
10. Beck, Gill, and Downing, *J. Am. Chem. Soc.*, 87, 901 (1965).
11. Kresheck and Scheraga, *J. Am. Chem. Soc.*, 88, 4588 (1966).
12. Danforth, Krakauer, and Sturtevant, *Rev. Sci. Instrum.*, 38, 484 (1967).
13. McKnight, Ph.D. thesis, University of Massachusetts, 1974.
14. Ackermann and Ruterjans, *Z. Phys. Chem.*, 41, 116 (1964).
15. Ackermann and Ruterjans, *Ber Bunsenges Phys. Chem.*, 68, 850 (1964).
16. Karasz, O'Reilly, and Bair, *Nature (Lond.)*, 202, 693 (1964).
17. Giacometti and Turolla, *Z. Phys. Chem.*, 51, 108 (1966).
18. Ackermann and Neumann, *Biopolymers*, 5, 649 (1967).
19. Karasz and O'Reilly, *Biopolymers*, 4, 1015 (1966).
20. Karasz, O'Reilly, and Bair, *Biopolymers*, 3, 241 (1965).
21. Rialdi and Hermans, *J. Am. Chem. Soc.*, 88, 5719 (1966).
22. Klump, Neumann, and Ackermann, *Biopolymers*, 7, 423 (1969).
23. Sturtevant and Geiduschek, *J. Am. Chem. Soc.*, 80, 2911 (1958).
24. Bunville, Geiduschek, Rawitscher, and Sturtevant, *Biopolymers*, 3, 213 (1965).
25. Ruterjans, thesis, University of Munster, Germany, 1965.
26. Steiner and Kitzinger, *Nature (Lond.)*, 194, 1172 (1962).
27. Rawitscher, Ross, and Sturtevant, *J. Am. Chem. Soc.*, 85, 1915 (1963).
28. Ross and Scruggs, *Biopolymers*, 3, 491 (1965).
29. Neumann and Ackermann, *J. Phys. Chem.*, 71, 2377 (1967).
30. Epand and Scheraga, *J. Am. Chem. Soc.*, 89, 3888 (1967).
31. Kagemoto and Fugishiro, *Makromol. Chem.*, 114, 139 (1968).
32. Giacometti, Turolla, and Boni, *Biopolymers*, 6, 441 (1968).
33. Kagemoto and Jujishiro, *Biopolymers*, 6, 1753 (1968).
34. Krakauer and Sturtevant, *Biopolymers*, 6, 491 (1968).
35. Hinz, Schmitz, and Ackermann, *Biopolymers*, 7, 611 (1969).
36. Neumann and Ackermann, *J. Phys. Chem.*, 73, 2170 (1969).
37. Privalov, *Mol. Biol.* (Mosc.), 3, 690 (1969).
38. Privalov, Ptitsyn, and Birstein, *Biopolymers*, 8, 559 (1969).
39. Privalov, *Biofizika*, 13, 955 (1968).
40. Privalov and Tiktopulo, *Biopolymers*, 9, 127 (1970).
41. Privalov, Khechinashvili, and Atanasov, *Biopolymers*, 10, 1865 (1971).
42. Atanasov, Khechinashvili, and Privalov, *Mol. Biol.* (Mosc.), 6, 33 (1972).
43. Privalov, Tiktopulo, and Khechinashvili, *Int. J. Protein Peptide Res.*, 5, 229 (1973).
44. Privalov and Khechinashvili, *J. Mol. Biol.*, 86, 665 (1974).
45. Khechinashvili, Privalov, and Tiktopulo, *FEBS Lett.*, 30, 57 (1973).
46. Tischenko, Tiltopulo, and Privalov, *Biofizika*, 19, 400 (1974).
47. Khechinashvili and Privalov, *Biofizika*, 19, 14 (1974).
48. Brandts, Jackson, and Ting, *Biochemistry*, 13, 3595 (1974).
49. Levy, Rialdi, and Biltonen, *Biochemistry*, 11, 4138 (1972).
50. Biltonen, Schwartz, and Wadsö, *Biochemistry*, 10, 3417 (1971).
51. Jackson and Brandts, *Biochemistry*, 9, 2294 (1970).
52. Shiao and Sturtevant, *Biopolymers*, 12, 1829 (1973).
53. Klump and Ackermann, *Biopolymers*, 10, 513 (1971).
54. Hinz, Haar, and Ackermann, *Biopolymers*, 9, 923 (1970).
55. Hearn, Richards, Sturtevant, and Watt, *Biochemistry*, 10, 806 (1971).
56. Scheffler and Sturtevant, *J. Mol. Biol.*, 42, 577 (1969).
57. Ross and Scruggs, *J. Mol. Biol.*, 45, 567 (1969).
58. Kagemoto and Karasz, *Analytical Calorimetry*. Vol. 2, Plenum Press, New York, 1970, 147.
59. Giacometti, Turolla, and Boni, *Biopolymers*, 9, 979 (1970).
60. Privalov, *Biofizika*, 3, 308 (1963).
61. Atha and Ackers, *J. Biol. Chem.*, 246, 5845 (1971).
62. Delben and Crescenzi, *Biochim. Biophys. Acta*, 194, 615 (1969).
63. Chou and Scheraga, *Biopolymers*, 10, 657 (1971).
64. Tsong, Hearn, Warthall, and Sturtevant, *Biochemistry*, 9, 2666 (1970).
65. Gerassimov and Mikhailov, *Soobshch. Akad. Nauk Gruz. SSSR*, 64, 185 (1971).
66. Sturtevant and Beres, *Biochemistry*, 10, 2120 (1971).
67. Shiao and Sturtevant, *Biochemistry*, 8, 4910 (1969).
68. Giacometti, Turolla, and Verdini, *J. Am. Chem. Soc.*, 93, 3092 (1971).
69. Rialdi and Profumo, *Biopolymers*, 6, 899 (1968).
70. Klump, *Biopolymers*, 11, 2331 (1972).
71. Bode, Schernau, and Ackermann, *Biophys. Chem.*, 1, 214 (1974).
72. Klump, in press.
73. Simon and Karasz, *Thermochim. Acta*, 8, 97 (1974).
74. McKnight and Karasz, *Thermochim. Acta*, 5, 339 (1973).
75. Delben, Crescenzi, and Quadrifoglio, *Int. J. Protein Peptide Res.*, 3, 57 (1971).
76. Crescenzi and Delben, *Int. J. Protein Peptide Res.*, 3, 57 (1971).
77. Stevens and Felsenfeld, *Biopolymers*, 2, 293 (1964).

FREE ENERGIES OF HYDROLYSIS AND DECARBOXYLATION

William P. Jencks

One of the reasons that there has been so much confusion and disagreement regarding the free energies of hydrolysis of "energy-rich" compounds of biochemical interest is that it is uncommon for any two workers to express their results according to the same nomenclature and conventions. The following summary may be helpful in making use of these tables of free energies of hydrolysis and decarboxylation.

The equilibrium constant, K_I, for the hydrolysis of an ester may be expressed according to the Equation 1 and the free energy of hydrolysis according to Equation 2, using the convention that the concentration of water is expressed in the same units as the other reactants and pure water is 55.5 M. For glycine ethyl ester the values of K_I = 0.43 and $\Delta G°$ = +500 cal/mol at 39° reflect

$$K_1 = \frac{[RCOOH][HOR']}{[RCOOR'][HOH]} \tag{1}$$

$$\Delta G_I° = -RT \ln K_I \tag{2}$$

the fact that –OH and $-OC_2H_5$ have approximately the same affinity for the carbonyl group.

For biochemical reactions, which usually take place in dilute aqueous solution, it is generally more convenient to take the activity of pure water as 1.0, and this convention will be adopted here. For glycine ethyl ester the values of K_I = 24 and $\Delta G°_1$ = –1,970 cal/mol according to this convention reflect the fact that the driving force toward hydrolysis which results from the high concentration of water compared to the other reactants is hidden in the equilibrium expression by the convention that the activity of liquid water is 1.0. This extra driving force amounts to –RT in 55.5 $\cong$ –2,400 cal/mol and is one reason that free energies of hydrolysis expressed according to this convention are unlikely to be equal to heats of hydrolysis. The standard states of the other reactants according to this convention are ideal 1 M solutions of the non-ionized species. This commonly leads to difficulty for a compound such as glycine which does not exist in a non-ionized form in appreciable concentration and the standard state is commonly modified, as in the case of the values for glycine ethyl ester given here, to refer to a species in which the *reacting* groups are non-ionized; i.e., to H^+_3 NCH_2COOH. instead of H_2 NCH_2 COOH. This convention, which we shall call convention I, gives a single value of $\Delta G°$ which is true regardless of the pH. Its use requires that only the actual concentrations (or activities) of the *particular ionic species* which are given in the equilibrium expression be included in calculations. For example, in order to calculate the free energy of hydrolysis of glycine ethyl ester from the results of an experiment carried out at pH 3.0, it is necessary to insert the concentration of H^+_3 NCH_2 COOH which is present at equilibrium at this pH, not the stoichiometric concentration of total glycine.

It is often convenient, especially when the ionization constants of the reactants are not accurately known, to use convention II in which the concentrations (or activities) of the reactants are given in terms of some convenient ionic species that is present under the conditions of the experiments and any hydrogen ions present in the equilibrium expression are included. For glycine ethyl ester this is shown in Equations 3 and 4 and the value of $\Delta G_{II}°$ is + 1,440

cal/mol. As in the case of convention I, this convention refers only to the concentrations of the particular

$$K_{II} = \frac{[RCOO^-][H^+][HOR']}{[RCOOR'][HOH]} \tag{3}$$

$$\Delta G_{II}° = -RT \ln K_{II} \tag{4}$$

ionic species given in the equilibrium expression which may be present in a given solution. The $G_{II}°$ value of $\Delta G_{II}°$ is independent of pH.

To interconvert these pH-independent free energies with free energies which hold for stoichiometric concentrations of reactants and products at a given pH, which would be found experimentally, it is only necessary to substitute in Equation 5 the actual concentrations present at the desired pH of the particular ionic species of the reactants which are present at that pH,

$$\Delta G' = \Delta G° + RT \ln \frac{[products]}{[reactants]} \tag{5}$$

including any hydrogen ions given off or taken up in the reaction. Equation 5 is the basic equation which relates concentrations (or activities) to free energies. When a reaction is at equilibrium $\Delta G'$ = 0 and the standard free energy is then a logarithmic function of the *equilibrium* concentrations of the reactants and products (Equation 6). When the reactants and products are all in the standard state of activity 1.0 the concentration term drops out and the free energy of the system is equal to the standard free energy of the reaction (Equation 7).

$$\Delta G° = -RT \ln \frac{[C]_{eq}[D]_{eq}}{[A]_{eq}[B]_{eq}} = -RT \ln K \tag{6}$$

$$\Delta G' = \Delta G° + RT \ln \frac{1 \times 1}{1 \times 1} = \Delta G° \tag{7}$$

Thus, the standard free energy is the difference in free energy between a system in which all the reactants and products are in the standard states ($\Delta G'$ = $\Delta G°$) and the same system at equilibrium ($\Delta G°$ = 0).

A useful special case of Equation 5 is the situation in which the total concentrations of all reactants and products, except hydrogen ion, are 1.0 M at a given pH. This gives a value of $\Delta G°'$ which refers to 1.0 M *total concentrations of all the ionic species* of the reactants and products and is *true only at the specified pH*. This convention III is the convention which refers most directly to experimental results and is most useful in making comparisons of free energies of hydrolysis under physiological conditions. $\Delta G°'$ is also sometimes referred to as $\Delta G'$, $\Delta G°_{anal}$ $\Delta G°_{exp}$ and (unfortunately) as $\Delta G°$.

For example, the value of $\Delta G°'$ for glycine ethyl ester is calculated from the $\Delta G°$ of convention I by inserting the fraction of the 1 M total glycine that is present as the free acid at pH 7.0, as shown in Equation 8.

$$\Delta G^{\circ\prime} = \Delta G_I^{\circ} + RT \ln \frac{[RCOOH][HOR']}{[RCOOR'][HOH]}$$

$$= +500 + 1{,}420 \log \frac{(1\times10^{-4,-6})(1)}{(0.85)(1)} \qquad (8)$$

$$= -8{,}400 \text{ cal/mol}$$

The fact that glycine ethyl ester is only 85% in the protonated form at pH 7.0 introduces a further small correction. The same value of $\Delta G^{\circ\prime}$ may be calculated from the ΔG° of convention II by inserting the hydrogen ion activity at pH 7.0 into the equilibrium expression (Equation 9), because at pH 7 glycine is entirely in the form of the carboxylate anion, which is the form which is used in the equilibrium expression according to this convention.

$$\Delta G^{\circ\prime} = \Delta G_{II}^{\circ} + RT \ln \frac{[RCOO^-][H^+][HOR']}{[RCOOR'][HOH]}$$

$$= 1{,}440 + 1{,}420 \log \frac{(1)(10^{-7})(1)}{(0.85)(1)} \qquad (9)$$

$$= -8400 \text{ cal/mol}$$

These interconversions between pH-independent and pH-dependent free energies may generally be carried out without difficulty if the following two simple rules are followed:

1. The equilibrium expression for the pH-independent equilibrium constant and free energy of hydrolysis may include any desired ionic species of the reactants, but must be based on a *balanced equation* for the reaction which includes any *hydrogen ions* which are given off or taken up.
2. The actual concentrations (or activities) of the *particular ionic species* given in this expression and which are present at a given pH value must be substituted in the expression for the pH-independent equilibrium constant or free energy.

A final convention gives the molar free energy of hydrolysis under conditions in which the reactants are at concentrations other than 1.0 M. For glycine ethyl ester at pH 7.0 under conditions in which the reactants and products, except for water and hydrogen ion, are present at a concentration of 10^{-3} M, the free energy of hydrolysis is –12,660 cal/mol, as shown in Equation 10. The importance of specifying and understanding the particular convention that is being used is illustrated by the range of values from +1,440 to –12,660 calories/mole for the free energy of hydrolysis of glycine ethyl ester according to the different conventions. At pH 7 and under physiological conditions, glycine ethyl ester has a free energy of hydrolysis which clearly places it in the category of "high-energy" or "energy-rich" compounds. All of these conventions are correct and are useful for different purposes.

$$\Delta G' = \Delta G_{pH7}^{\circ\prime} + RT \ln \frac{[gly]_{tot}[HOEt]_{tot}}{[glyOEt]_{tot}[HOH]}$$

$$= -8{,}400 + 1{,}420 \log \frac{(10^{-3})(10^{-3})}{(10^{-3})(1)} \qquad (10)$$

$$= 12{,}660 \text{ cal/mol}$$

Complexation of the compounds which are involved in an equilibrium with other compounds which may be present in the solution is a common cause of difficulty in the determination of equilibria and free energies of hydrolysis. The most important example of this in biochemical reactions is the binding of magnesium and other ions to phosphate and polyphosphates. This problem may be dealt with in several ways:

1. The reaction may be carried out under conditions in which the complexing ions are present in negligible concentrations compared to the compounds involved in the equilibrium under study.
2. The concentrations of the free and complexed species of the reactants and ions may be calculated from equilibrium constants for complex formation, which must be determined in separate experiments or be obtained from the literature. There is still some disagreement in the literature as to the correct values for these complexing constants for many compounds and ions of biochemical importance.
3. The reaction may be carried out in the presence of an excess of ions under conditions in which most of the reactants exist in the form of the complex. The equilibrium constant and free energy are then obtained for this particular set of experimental conditions or may be expressed in terms of reactions of the complexed species. For example, the affinity of Mg^{2+} toward ATP^{4-} and toward ATP^{3-} is much larger than that toward HPO_4^{2-}, so that the equilibrium in the presence of excess Mg^{2+} may be expressed according to Equation 11. Most of the free energies of hydrolysis of polyphosphate compounds which are given in these tables refer to conditions in which Mg^{2+} is present in excess and most or all of the polyphosphates exist as the magnesium complexes. There is still no general agreement regarding these values.

$$K = \frac{[Mg \cdot ADP^-][HPO_4^=][H^+]}{[Mg \cdot ATP^=][H_2O]} \qquad (11)$$

The free energies in these tables generally refer to concentrations rather than activities of the reactants. Thermodynamic values extrapolated to zero ionic strength are of theoretical interest, but have not often been obtained for reactions of biochemical importance.

It is worth noting that these equilibria refer only to aqueous solutions, and that a large fraction of a cell or cell particle is not aqueous. The perturbation of equilibria that may occur in nonaqueous systems is illustrated by the fact that esters of long chain fatty acids can be formed at equilibrium in a nonaqueous phase which is in contact with neutral buffer, although the equilibrium in the buffer solution is far toward hydrolysis.

It cannot be pointed out too often that thermodynamic measurements and conventions say nothing about the *pathway* by which a reaction takes place; i.e., the equilibrium state of a system under a given set of experimental conditions is the same regardless of the pathway by which equilibrium is attained. Thus, the common practice of calling a particular ionic species the "reactive" species from an observed change in the stoichiometric equilibrium position of a reaction with changing pH is incorrect. It is this independence of reaction pathway that makes it equally legitimate to specify the equilibrium constant of a reaction according to any of a number of equations which contain different ionic species of reactants and products; the only requirement is that the equations balance. Different equilibrium constants will be obtained, of course, from the different equations.

Further information regarding the methods for dealing with free energies of hydrolysis may be found in References 1–4. Carpenter[5] has prepared a useful summary of the dependence on pH of $\Delta G^{\circ\prime}$ for several classes of compounds of biochemical interest.

FREE ENERGIES OF HYDROLYSIS OF THIOL ESTERS[a]

Compound	$-\Delta G^{\circ a}$	$-G^{\circ\prime}{}_{PH7}{}^b$	Reference
N,S-Diacetyl-β-mercaptoethylamine	4,460	7,520	4
S-Acetylmercaptoacetate	4,140	7,200	4
S-Acetyhnercaptopropanol	4,400	7,460	9
2-Diethylaminoethane thioacetate	—	7,470[c]	8
S-Acetylthiophenol	—	7,450[c]	8
2-Di*iso*propylaminoethane thioacetate	—	6,720[c]	8
S-Acetylglutathione	—	7,500[c]	8
	—	7,830[d]	7
Acetyl coenzyme A,	—[c]	7,520[e]	4
pH 7.2	—	7,100[f]	15
	—	7,370[g]	7, 16

Compiled by William P. Jencks.

[a] Standard free energy of hydrolysis based on a standard state of 1 M concentrations of the *uncharged* reactants and products and an activity of pure water of 1.0 (convention I).

[b] Standard free energy of hydrolysis at pH 7.0 based on a standard state of 1 M total stoichiometric concentration of reactants and products, except hydrogen ion, and on an activity of pure water of 1.0 (convention III). Values for derivatives of acetic acid are based on a thermodynamic pK_a of 4.76 for acetic acid and a ΔG for ionization of acetic acid at pH 7.0 of 3,060 cal/mol. Values for $\Delta G^{\circ\prime}{}_{PH7}{}^b$ for acetate derivatives based on a pK'_a of 4.63 ± 0.02 at ionic strength 0.2 to 1.0[12] are 180 cal/mol more negative.

[c] Based on Reference 8 and 4-pyridinealdoxime acetate (see previous table).

[d] Based on Reference 7 and acetylimidazole (see following table).

[e] Based on N,S-diacetyl-β-mercaptoethylamine.

[f] Based on the equilibria for the condensation of acetate and acetyl coenzyme A with oxaloacetate to give citrate with the correction for citrate ionization recalculated as described in the text above.

[g] Based on equilibria with acetyl phosphate and acetylimidazol.[7,16]

FREE ENERGIES OF HYDROLYSIS OF ESTERS OF ACETIC ACID AND RELATED COMPOUNDS AT 25°

Compound	$-\Delta G^{\circ a}$	$-G^{\circ\prime}{}_{PH7}{}^b$	Reference
Acetic anhydride	15,700	21,800	6
p-Nitrophenyl acetate	9,430	13,010	3
m-Nitrophenyl acetate	8,550	11,610	3
p-Chlorophenyl acetate	7,590	10,650	3
Phenyl acetate	7,390	10,450	3
p-Methylphenyl acetate	6,890	9,950	3
p-Methoxyphenyl acetate	6,590	9,650	3
Acetyl hypochlorite	ca. 5,950	ca. 9,214	13, 14[f]
Acetyl phosphate	6,690[c]	10,300	7, 3
N,O-Diacetyl-N- methylhydroxylamine[d]	6,190	9,250	3
4-Pyridinealdoxime acetate[c] (37°)	5,670	8,730	8
Glycine ethyl ester (39°)	1,970	8,400	9
Valyl RNA (30°)	2,000[g]	8,400[g]	10
Trifluoroethyl acetate	4,970	8,030	4
Acetylcarnitine (35°)	4,150	7,210	4, 11
Acetylcholine	2,940	6,000	4
Chloroethyl acetate	2,840	5,900	4
Methoxyethyl acetate	2,180	5,240	4
Ethyl acetate	1,660	4,720	4

Compiled by William P. Jencks.

[a] Standard free energy of hydrolysis based on a standard state of 1 M concentrations of the *uncharged* reactants and products and an activity of pure water of 1.0 (convention I).

[b] Standard free energy of hydrolysis at pH 7.0 based on a standard state of 1 M total stoichiometric concentration of reactants and products, except hydrogen ion, and on an activity of pure water of 1.0 (convention III). Values for derivatives of acetic acid are based on a thermodynamic pK_a of 4.76 for acetic acid and a ΔG for ionization of acetic acid at pH 7.0 of 3,060 cal/mol. Values for $\Delta G^{\circ\prime}{}_{PH7}$ for acetate derivatives based on a pK'_a of 4.63 ± 0.02 at ionic strength 0.2 to 1.0[12] are 180 cal/mol more negative.

[c] For the dianions of acetyl phosphate and phosphate.

[d] For hydrolysis of the ester.

[e] Based on (closely similar) equilibrium constants with several thiol esters and the ΔG° for N,S-dicetyl-β-mercaptoethylamine.

[f] From the data of De la Mare in acetic acid containing traces of water[13] and an ionization constant of 4.1×10^{-8} for hypochlorous acid.[14]

[g] Based on Reference 10. $\Delta G^{\circ\prime}{}_{pH7.0} = -7,700$ for ATP (→ PP and AMP), and pK_a valine = 2.32.

FREE ENERGIES OF HYDROLYSIS OF AMIDES

Compound	$-\Delta G^{\circ\prime}{}_{PH7}{}^a$	Reference
Acetylimidazole	12,970	3
10-Formyltetrahydrofolic acid (pH 7.7, 37°)	5,830[b]	17
Asparagine	3,600	18
Glutamine	3,400	18
N-Dimethylpropionamide	2,100[c]	19
Propionamide	2,100[c]	19
Hippurylanilide (pH 5.0, 39°)	1,470	20
Benzoyltyrosyl-glycylanilide (pH 6.5, 23°)	1,360	21
Benzoyltyrosyl-glycinamide	420[d]	22
N-Acetyltyrosine hydroxamic acid	1,870	23
Acetohydroxamic acid	−200	23
N-Methylpropionamide	−300[c]	19

Compiled by William P. Jencks.

[a] Standard free energy of hydrolysis at pH 7.0 based on a standard state of 1 M total stoichiometric concentration of reactants and products, except hydrogen ion, and on an activity of pure water of 1.0 (convention III).

[b] Based on Reference 17 and $\Delta G^{\circ\prime}{}_{PH7}$ 7.7 = −8,030 cal/mol for ATP.

[c] Data for other simple amides at elevated temperatures are given in Reference 19.

[d] For cleavage of the peptide bond, to fully ionized products.

FREE ENERGIES OF HYDROLYSIS OF PHOSPHATES[a]

Compound	$-\Delta G^{\circ\prime b}$	Reference
Phosphoenolpyruvate, pH 7.0	14,800	24
pH 7.4–8.4	12,800[b]	2
β-Aspartyl phosphate, pH 8.0, 15°	13,000[c]	25
Carbamyl phosphate, pH 9.5	ca. 12,300[d]	26
3-Phosphoglyceroyl phosphate, pH 6.9	11,800	2
Acetyl phosphate, pH 7.0	10,300	7, 3
Creatine phosphate, pH 7.0, 7.5, 37°	10,300	27
Phosphoarginine, pH 8.0, excess Mg++	7,700[e]	28
Uridine diphosphate glucose (glycoside cleavage), pH 7.6	7,300	29
Adenosine triphosphate ($\rightarrow$ AMP, PP), pH 7.0, excess Mg++	7,700[f]	4, 9
pH 7.5, excess Mg++	10,300[g]	30
Adenosine triphosphate ($\rightarrow$ ADP, Pi), 37°, pH 7.0, excess Mg++	7,300	31–33
25°, pH 7.4, $10^{-3}M$ Mg++	8,800	44
25°, pH 7.4, 0 Mg++	9,600	44
Pyrophosphate, pH 7.0	8,000	24
pH 7.0, 0.005 M Mg++	4,500	24
Cytidine-2′-3′-phosphate (cyclic)$\rightarrow$ 3′-phosphate, pH 7.0	5,000	34
Glucose-1-phosphate, 25°, pH 7.0	5,000	35
N-Acetylethanolamine phosphate, pH 7.0	2,900	36
Glucose-6-phosphate, 25°, pH 7.0	3,300	35
α-Glycerophosphate, 38°, pH 8.5	2,200	37
pH 5.8	2,600	3
Hexose-6-phosphates, 38°, pH 8.5	2,800 ± 200	37
pH 5.8	3,200 ± 200	37

Compiled by William P. Jencks.

[a] For a more detailed compilation, see Reference 2.
[b] Standard free energy of hydrolysis based on a standard state of 1 M total stoichiometric concentration of reactants and products, except hydrogen ion, and on an activity of pure water of 1.0 (convention III).
[c] Based on Reference 25 and $-\Delta G^{\circ\prime}_{PH\,8.0}$ = –8,400 cal/mol for ATP.
[d] Based on Reference 26 and $\Delta G^{\circ\prime}_{pH\,9.5}$ = –10,440 cal/mol for ATP.
[e] Based on Reference 28 and $\Delta G^{\circ\prime}_{pH\,8\cdot0}$ = –8,400 cal/mol for ATP.
[f] Based on acetyl coenzyme A and the ATP-activated synthesis of acetyl coenzyme A.
[g] Based on a series of equilibria and the assumption of the similarity of the terminal phosphates of ATP and ADP. This value is not consistent with the preceding estimate.

FREE ENERGIES OF HYDROLYSIS OF GLYCOSIDES

Compound	$-\Delta G^{\circ\prime}_{PH7}$[a]	Reference
Uridine diphosphoglucose (pH 7.6)	7,300[b,c,d]	29
Sucrose	7,000[b]	38
Levan (fructofuranoside 2-6-fructose)	5,000[b]	39
Glucose-1-phosphate	5,000	35
Maltose	4,000	39
Glycogen	4,000	39
Amylose (α(l-4)glucosidic)	3,400	39

Compiled by William P. Jencks.

[a] Standard free energy of hydrolysis at pH 7.0 based on a standard state of 1 M total stoichiometric concentration of reactants and products, except hydrogen ion, and on an activity of pure water of 1.0 (convention III).
[b] Based on a corrected value for sucrose hydrolysis in Reference 38.
[c] Recalculated from K = 1.6, $\Delta G^{\circ\prime}$ = –300 from the data of Reference 29.
[d] The values for thymidine diphosphoglucose and adenosine diphosphoglucose are very similar.[4,5,46]

References

1. Johnson, in *The Enzymes*, Vol. 3, 2nd ed., Boyer, Lardy, Myrbäck, Eds., Academic, New York, 1960, chap, 21, 407.
2. Atkinson and Morton, in *Comparative Biochemistry*, Vol. 2,. Florkin and Mason, Eds., Academic, New York, 1960, chap. 1, 1.
3. Gerstein and Jeacks, *J. Am. Chem. Soc.*, 86, 4655 (1964).

FREE ENERGIES OF DECARBOXYLATION

Compound	$-\Delta G^{\circ a}$	Reference
Oxaloacetate$^-$ $\leftrightarrows$ Pyruvate$^-$ + HCO_3^-	6,200	24
Methylmalonyl-CoA $\leftrightarrows$ Propionyl- CoA + HCO_3^-		
30°	6,200[b]	24,40
28°	7,510[c]	41
Enzyme-biotin-CO_2 $\leftrightarrows$ Enzyrne-biotin + HCO_3^-(pH 7.0, 0°)	4,700	43

Compiled by William P. Jencks.

[a] Based on the indicated ionic species of reactants and products. Units are cal/mole.
[b] Based on oxaloacetate decarboxylation and K for carbon dioxide transfer; K = [pyruvate] [D-methyl-malonyl-CoA] / [propionyl-CoA] =1.0.[47]
[c] Based on ATP-coupled carboxylation and $-\Delta G^{\circ\prime}_{PH8.1}$ = –8.540 for ATP hydrolysis. The corresponding value at 37° from the data of Reference 42 is –11.500 cal/mol.[42]

4. Jencks and Gilchrist, *J. Am. Chem. Soc.*, 86, 4651 (1964).
5. Carpenter, *J. Am. Chem. Soc.*, 82, 1111 (1960).
6. Jencks, Barley, Barnett, and Gilchrist, *J. Am. Chem. Soc.*, 88, 4464 (1966).
7. Stadtman, in *The Mechanism of Enzyme Action*, McElroy and Glass, Eds., Johns Hopkins, Baltimore, 1954, 581
8. O'Neill, Kohl, and Epstein, *Biochem. Pharm.*, 8, 399 (1961).
9. Jencks, Cordes, and Carriuolo, *J. Biol. Chem.*, 235, 3608 (1960).
10. Berg, Bergmann, Ofengand, and Dieckmann, *J. Biol. Chem.*, 236, 1726 (1961).
11. Fritz, Schultz, and Srere, *J. Biol. Chem.*, 238, 2509 (1963).
12. Bjerrum, Schwarzenbach, and Sillén, Stability Constants. Chemical Society, London, 1957.
13. De la Mare, Hilton, and Vernon, *J. Chem. Soc.*, 4039 (1960).
14. Mauger and Soper, *J. Chem. Soc.*, p. 71 (1946).
15. Tate and Datta, *Biochem. J.*, 94, 470 (1965).
16. Sly and Stadtman, *J. Biol. Chem.*, 238, 2639 (1963).
17. Himes and Rabinowitz, *J. Biol. Chem.*, 237, 2903 (1962).
18. Benzinger, Kitzinger, Hems, and Burton, *Biochem. J.*, 71, 400 (1959).
19. Morawetz and Otaki, *J. Am. Chem. Soc.*, 85, 463 (1963).
20. Carty and Kirschenbaum, *Biochim. Biophys. Acta*, 110, 399 (1965).
21. Gawron, Glaid, Boyle, and Odstrchel, *Arch. Biochem. Biophys.*, 95, 203 (1961).
22. Dobry, Fruton, and Sturtevant, *J. Biol. Chem.*, 195, 149 (1952).
23. Jencks, Caplow, Gilchrist, and Kallen, *Biochemistry*, 1313 (1963).
24. Wood, Davis, and Lochmüller, *J. Biol. Chem.*, 241, 5692 (1966).
25. Black and Wright, *J. Biol. Chem.*, 213, 27 (1955).
26. Jones and Lipmann, *Proc. Natl. Acad. Sci. U.S.A.*, 46, 1194 (1960).
27. Kuby and Noltmann in *The Enzymes* Vol. 4, 2nd. ed., Boyer, Lardy and Myrbäck, Eds., Academic, New York,1962, chap 31, 515
28. Uhr, Marcus, and Morrison, *J. Biol. Chem.*, 241, 5428 (1966).
29. Avigad, *J. Biol. Chem.*, 239, 3613 (1964).
30. Schuegraf, Ratner, and Warner, *J. Biol. Chem.*, 235, 3597 (1960).
31. Atkinson, Johnson, and Morton, *Nature*, 184, 1925 (1959).
32. Robbins and Boyer, *J. Biol. Chem.*, 224, 121 (1957).
33. Benzinger, Kitzinger, Hems, and Burton, *Biochem. J.*, 71, 400 (1959).
34. Bahr, Cathou, and Hammes, *J. Biol. Chem.*, 240, 3372 (1965).
35. Atkinson, Johnson, and Morton, *Biochem. J.*, 79, 12 (1961).
36. Dayan and Wilson, *Biochim. Biophys. Acta*, 77, 446 (1963).
37. Meyerhof and Green, *J. Biol. Chem.*, 178, 655 (1949).
38. Neufeld and Hassid, *Adv Carbohyd. Chem.*, 18, 309 (1963) (footnote 166, p.329).
39. Dedonder, *Ann. Rev. Biochem.*, 30, 347 (1961).
40. Wood and Stjernholm, *Proc. Natl. Acad. Sci. U.S.A.*, 47, 289 (1961).
41. Kaziro, Grossman, and Ochoa, *J. Biol. Chem.*, 240, 64 (1965).
42. Halenz, Feng, Hegre, and Lane, *J. Biol. Chem.*, 237, 2140 (1962).
43. Wood, Lochmüller, Riepertinger, and Lynen, *Biochem. Z.*, 337, 247 (1963).
44. Alberty, R. A., personal communication.
45. Avigad and Milnetr, *Meth. Enzymol.*, 8, 341 (1966).
46. Murata, Sugiyama, Minimikawa, and Akazawa, *Arch. Biochem. Biophys.*, 113, 34 (1966).
47. Wood, H., *personal communication.*

DECI-NORMAL SOLUTIONS OF OXIDATION AND REDUCTION REAGENTS

Atomic and molecular weights in the following table are based upon the 1965 atomic weight scale and the isotope C-12. The weight in grams of the compound in 1 cc of the following deci-normal solutions is found by dividing the H equivalent in the last column by 1,000.

Name	Formula	Atomic or Molecular Weight	Hydrogen Equivalent	0.1 Hydrogen Equivalent in g
Antimony	Sb	121.75	$\frac{1}{2}$ Sb	6.0875
Arsenic	As	74.9216	$\frac{1}{2}$ As	3.7461
Arsenic trisulfide	As_2S_3	246.0352	$\frac{1}{2}$ As_2S_3	6.1509
Arsenous oxide	As_2O_3	197.8414	$\frac{1}{4}$ As_2O_3	4.9460
Barium peroxide	BaO_2	169.3388	$\frac{1}{2}$ BaO_2	8.4669
Barium peroxide hydrate	$BaO_2 \cdot 8H_2O$	313.4615	$\frac{1}{2}$ BaO_2 $8H_2O$	15.6730
Calcium	Ca	40.08	$\frac{1}{2}$ Ca	2.004
Calcium carbonate	$CaCO_3$	100.0894	$\frac{1}{2}$ $CaCO_3$	5.0045
Calcium hypochlorite	$Ca(OCl)_2$	142.9848	$\frac{1}{4}$ $Ca(OCl)_2$	3.5746
Calcium oxide	CaO	56.0794	$\frac{1}{2}$ CaO	2.8040
Chlorine	Cl	35.453	Cl	3.5453
Chromium trioxide	CrO_3	99.9942	$\frac{1}{3}$ CrO_3	3.3331
Ferrous ammonium sulfate	$FeSO_4(NH_4)SO_4 \cdot 6H_2O$	392.0764	$FeSO_4(NH_4)_2SO_4 \cdot 6H_2O$	39.2076
Hydroferrocyanic acid	$H_4Fe(CN)_6$	215.9860	$H_4Fe(CN)_6$	21.5986
Hydrogen peroxide	H_2O_2	34.0147	$\frac{1}{2}$ H_2O_2	1.7007
Hydrogen sulfide	H_2S	34.0799	$\frac{1}{2}$ H_2S	1.7040
Iodine	I	126.9044	I	12.6904
Iron	Fe	55.847	Fe	5.5847
Iron oxide (ferrous)	FeO	71.8464	FeO	7.1846
Iron oxide (ferric)	Fe_2O_3	159.6922	$\frac{1}{2}$ Fe_2O_3	7.9846
Lead peroxide	PbO_2	239.1888	$\frac{1}{2}$ PbO_2	11.9594
Manganese dioxide	MnO_2	86.9368	$\frac{1}{2}$ MnO_2	4.3468
Nitric acid	HNO_3	63.0129	$\frac{1}{3}$ HNO_3	2.1004
Nitrogen trioxide	N_2O_3	76.0116	$\frac{1}{4}$ N_2O_3	1.9002
Nitrogen pentoxide	N_2O_5	108.0104	$\frac{1}{5}$ N_2O_5	1.8001
Oxalic acid	$C_2H_2O_4$	90.0358	$\frac{1}{2}$ $C_2H_2O_4$	4.5018
Oxalic acid hydrate	$C_2H_2O_4 \cdot 2H_2O$	126.0665	$\frac{1}{2}$ $C_2H_2O_4 \cdot 2H_2O$	6.3033
Oxygen	O	15.9994	$\frac{1}{2}$ O	0.8000
Potassium dichromate	$K_2Cr_2O_7$	294.1918	$\frac{1}{6}$ $K_2Cr_2O_7$	4.9032
Potassium chlorate	$KClO_3$	122.5532	$\frac{1}{6}$ $KClO_3$	2.0425
Potassium chromate	K_2CrO_4	194.1076	$\frac{1}{3}$ K_2CrO_4	6.4733
Potassium ferrocyanide	$K_4Fe(CN)_6$	368.3621	$K_4Fe(CN)_6$	36.8362
Potassium ferrocyanide	$K_4Fe(CN)_6 \cdot 3H_2O$	422.4081	$K_4Fe(CN)_6 \cdot 3H_2O$	42.2408
Potassium iodide	KI	166.0064	KI	16.6006
Potassium nitrate	KNO_3	101.1069	$\frac{1}{3}$ KNO_3	3.3702
Potassium perchlorate	$KClO_4$	138.5526	$\frac{1}{8}$ $KC1O_4$	1.7319
Potassium permanganate	$KMnO_4$	158.0376	$\frac{1}{5}$ $KMnO_4$	3.1608
Sodium chlorate	$NaClO_3$	106.4410	$\frac{1}{6}$ $NaClO_3$	1.7740
Sodium nitrate	$NaNO_3$	84.9947	$\frac{1}{3}$ $NaNO_3$	2.8332
Sodium thiosulfate	$Na_2S_2O_3 \cdot 5H_2O$	248.1825	$Na_2S_2O_3 \cdot 5H_2O$	24.8183
Stannous chloride	$SnCl_2$	189.5960	$\frac{1}{2}$ $SnCl_2$	9.4798
Stannous oxide	SnO	134.6894	$\frac{1}{2}$ SnO	6.7345
Sulfur dioxide	SO_2	64.0628	$\frac{1}{2}$ SO_2	3.2031
Tin	Sn	118.69	$\frac{1}{2}$ Sn	5.935

This table originally appeared in Sober, Ed., *Handbook of Biochemistry and Selected Data for Molecular Biology*, 2nd ed., Chemical Rubber Co., Cleveland, 1970.

GUIDELINES FOR POTENTIOMETRIC MEASUREMENTS IN SUSPENSIONS PART A—THE SUSPENSION EFFECT[1]

(IUPAC Technical Report)

Srecko F.Oman[1], M. Filomena Camões[2], Kipton J. Powell[3], Raj Rajagopalan[4], and Petra Spitzer[5]

[1]Faculty of Chemistry and Chemical Technology, University of Ljubljana, Aškerčeva 5,1000 Ljubljana, Slovenia
[2]Departamento de Química e Bioquímica, University of Lisbon (CECUL/DQB), Faculdade de Sciências da Universidade de Lisboa, Edificio C8, Pt-1749-016, Lisboa, Portugal
[3]Department of Chemistry, University of Canterbury, Christchurch, New Zealand
[4]Department of Chemical and Biomolecular Engineering, National University of Singapore, 117576, The Republic of Singapore
[5]Physikalisch-Technische Bundesanstalt (PTB), Postfach 3345, D-38023, Braunschweig, Germany

*Membership of the Analytical Chemistry Division during the final preparation of this report:

President: R. Lobinski (France); *Titular Members:* K. J. Powell (New Zealand); A. Fajgelj (Slovenia); R. M. Smith (UK); M. Bonardi (Italy); P. De Bièvre (Belgium); B. Hibbert (Australia); J.-Å. Jönsson (Sweden); J. Labuda (Slovakia); W. Lund (Norway); *Associate Members:* Z. Chai (China); H. Gamsjäger (Austria); U. Karst (Germany); D. W. Kutner (Poland); P. Minkkinen (Finland); K. Murray (USA); *National Representatives:* C. Balarew (Bulgaria); E. Dominguez (Spain); S. Kocaoba (Turkey); Z. Mester (Canada); B. Spivakov (Russia); W. Wang (China); E. Zagatto (Brazil); *Provisional Member:* N. Torto (Botswana).

Abstract: An explanation of the origin and interpretation of the suspension effect (SE) is presented in accordance with "pH Measurement: IUPAC Recommendations 2002" [*Pure Appl. Chem.* **74**, 2169 (2002)]. It is based on an analysis of detailed schemes of suspension potentiometric cells and confirmed with experimental results. Historically, the term "suspension effect" evolved during attempts to determine electrochemically the thermodynamically defined activity of H^+ (aq) in suspensions. The experimental SE arises also in determining other pIon values, analogous to pH values.

The SE relates to the observation that for the potential generated when a pair of electrodes (e.g., reference electrode, RE, and glass electrode) is placed in a suspension, the measured cell voltage is different from that measured when they are both placed in the separate equilibrium solution (eqs). The SE is defined here as the sum of: (1) the difference between the mixed potential of the indicator electrode (IE) in a suspension and the IE potential placed in the separated eqs; and (2) the anomalous liquid junction potential of the RE placed in the suspension. It is not the consequence of a boundary potential between the sediment and its eqs in the suspension potentiometric cells as is stated in the current definition of the SE.

Keywords: operational definition of suspension effect; suspension effect; pH; suspension potentiometric cell; IUPAC Analytical Chemistry Division; pIon; boundary potential; mixed potential; soil pH; anomalous liquid junction potential

1. The Suspension Effect Explained on the Basis of Analysis of Potentiometric Cells

1.1 Introduction

Potentiometry is an electroanalytical technique based on the measurement of the potential of an electrochemical cell, composed of a measuring and a reference electrode (RE), both immersed in the measuring solution to be measured.

In homogeneous solutions, direct potentiometry is used for the estimation of ion activities (e.g., pH) and potentiometric titrations for determination of the amount concentration of ionic species. These measuring techniques are also applied to suspensions or sols of different materials (containing positively or negatively charged particles) in aqueous dispersion media. Although pH measurement in soil suspensions is highly relevant to this work, ion exchanger suspensions were chosen preferentially as models due to their simplicity.

The most frequently applied direct potentiometric method is the measurement of pH. Therefore, the determination of pH is selected to explain the essential procedures and experimental set-up for the potentiometric techniques applied to suspensions or sols.

The most recent definitions, procedures, and terminology relating to pH measurements in dilute aqueous solutions in the temperature range 5–50 °C are given in the IUPAC Recommendations 2002 [1]. In this reference, the glass electrode cell V is proposed for practical pH measurements [1, p. 2187]:

reference electrode | KCl ($c \geq 3.5$ mol dm^{-3})

solution pH(X) | glass electrode (cell V)

Typically, the galvanic cells used for practical pH measurements conform to the characteristics of cell V; therefore, the results obtained in these practical pH measurements approximate results obtained by cell V.

Although "the quantity pH is intended to be a measure of the activity of hydrogen ions in [homogeneous] solutions" [1], and measurements using cell V include an unknown liquid junction potential, cell V is also used for practical measurement of pH in suspensions with the electrodes usually positioned in different phases.

When pH is measured in (i) a suspension (or its sediment) or (ii) in its equilibrium solution (eqs), the measured pH value

[1] Reproduced from:
Pure & Appl. Chem., Vol. 79, No.1, pp. 67–79, 2007.
doi: 10.1351/pac200779010067
© 2007 IUPAC

in each of these constituent parts is different, even though the total system is in equilibrium. None of these pH values represents the (thermodynamically) true H$^+$ activity in a suspension. This observation has caused serious problems for the theory and practice of pH measurements, problems which remain unresolved.

1.2 Consideration of the "Glass Electrode Cell" Containing a Suspension

The term "suspension" should mean a *uniform equilibrated multiphase system*. It can be separated into the eqs and the sediment. If, when separated, the eqs and the sediment remain in physical and electrical contact, they represent a *combined suspension system*. The separated supernatant, obtained by sedimentation, centrifugation, or filtration, does not necessarily give absolutely equivalent solutions, yet they can be considered eqs, because the differences between them can be neglected with respect to the characteristics of the measured values.

In this work, the term "suspension" means the dispersion of electrically charged solid particles in water or in an aqueous solution. The origin of the charges can be adsorption or ionization, or as a property of the ion exchanger beads. The positively or negatively charged particles of different sizes found in soils provide another example. However, for this document (and in the literature that it relies upon) ion exchanger particles (which, depending on solution pH lower than 7 will be mostly in the H$^+$ form) were chosen as a representative example for the study of pH measurements in suspension. These particles reduce the experimental effort and make a simple approach possible. Experiments showed essentially the same results when particles of other types were used [2].

The bulk liquid (of any electrolyte concentration) in the suspension will be identical to the supernatant of this suspension, when it is separated in whatever manner into two parts. It is different from that in the diffusion layers of individual particles, which are responsible for the mixed electrode potential when they are in contact with the glass electrode part of the pH electrode (Section 1.4). The diffusion layer of individual particles contributes to the anomalous liquid junction potential observed in pH measurements in suspensions.

The two separated parts are (i) the *sediment*, which can be considered the most concentrated suspension possible, and (ii) the clear (homogeneous, non-turbid) solution above it. This solution is called the eqs, if the suspension is equilibrated before separation. It is proposed to call the combination of an eqs and sediment, which are in physical and electrical contact, a *combined suspension system*.

For pH measurement in a combined suspension system, the following specific positions for the glass and REs are possible:

1. both electrodes are positioned in the eqs;
2. both electrodes are in the sediment;
3. the glass electrode is in the sediment and the RE is in the eqs; or
4. the electrodes are in the reverse position from that in 3.

   In addition, it is possible to measure the pH in each *separated suspension component*, which means that:
5. both electrodes are in the separated "eqs" or
6. both electrodes are in the separated sediment.

   The pH measurement is possible also with
7. both electrodes in the original, (nonseparated) equilibrated suspension, the concentration of which should (ideally) be practically constant during the measurement.

In a suspension in equilibrium, the electrochemical potential $\tilde{\mu}_{H^+}$ is equal throughout the system, therefore, the different electrode arrangements 1 to 7 could be expected to give the same pH values. Nevertheless, the electrode combinations 1 and 2 and the analogous pair 5 and 6 show large (and nearly equal) pH differences, as do the combinations 3 and 4. These pH differences were named the *suspension effect* (SE) for the first time in 1930 [5,6]. Subsequently, the nature of this effect has been studied intensively by many authors; a list of references may be found in reviews, e.g., [4,7–9]. However, there has been no consensus on the origin of, or explanation for, the SE.

An acceptable explanation of this phenomenon follows from a detailed analysis of the suspension cells (combinations 1 and 2, or 5 and 6) and from their cell potential differences, ΔE, from which the corresponding pH differences can be calculated; this explanation is supported by recent experimental observations [3].

1.3 Detailed Schemes for Potentiometric Cells Used in Suspensions

Scheme 1 shows both electrodes in the eqs (combined with sediment, system 1, or separated, system 5).

$$[A]\ Ag\,|\,AgCl\,|\,KCl\,\|\!|\,\|\,KCl\,\|\ eqs\,(H^+)\ \|\,HCl\,|\,AgCl\,|\,Ag\qquad E_A$$
$$E_{ref1}\qquad E_j(S_A)\quad E_j(A)\qquad\qquad E_g(A)\qquad E_{ref2}\quad (\equiv E_{soln})$$

Scheme 1

Here, S indicates the separator (membrane) of the salt bridge and G the glass membrane of the glass electrode. The symbol $\|\|$ represents the region of the KCl solution in the separator and that in the contact range of eqs with KCl solution diffused from the RE. (The extent of the KCl layer in eqs is exaggerated in the scheme.) E_{ref} is the potential of the RE, E_g is the potential of the glass electrode. $E_j(S_A)$ and $E_j(A)$ are the liquid junction potentials; these are of negligible magnitude due to the approximately equal transport numbers of K$^+$ and Cl$^-$, as established by potentiometric measurements [3,13].

This scheme is equivalent to that for cell V (above), but considers the interphases in detail.

Scheme 2 shows both electrodes in the sediment (combined with eqs, or separated, systems 2 and 6, respectively).

$$[B]\ Ag\,|\,AgCl\,|\,KCl\,\|\!|\,\|\,KCl,HX\,\|\!|\,\|\ eqs\,(H^+),\,HX\,\|\!\|\,HCl\,|\,AgCl\,|\,Ag\qquad E_B$$
$$E_{ref1}\qquad E_j(S_B)\qquad E_{j\ anomal}(B)\qquad\qquad E_{g\ mix}(B)\qquad E_{ref}\quad (\equiv E_{susp})$$

Scheme 2

Again, S, G, and $\|\|$ have the same meaning as in scheme [A]. The symbol $\|$ represents the ion exchanger X (sediment of X in H$^+$ form) bathed in KCl solution which diffuses from the RE, and the symbol $\|\|$ means the ion exchanger X (in H$^+$ form) dispersed in eqs. The sign $\|\!\|$ represents the glass electrode in intimate contact with the suspension particles (HX) and entrained eqs; this evokes the mixed electrode potential. $E_{j,anomal}$ is the anomalous liquid junction potential and $E_{g,mix}$ is the mixed potential of the glass electrode. $E_j(S_B)$ is negligible [3], and E_{ref} is defined as in [A].

When comparing cells [A] and [B], the first component of the potential difference arises from junction potentials, viz. $E_j(A) + E_j(S_A) - E_{j,anomal}(B) - E_j(S_B)$, which can be approximated to $E_j(A) - E_{j,anomal}(B)$, as $E_j(S_A)$ and $E_j(S_B)$ are negligible [3]. This difference occurs because in cell [B] the filling solution, which diffuses from the salt bridge into the suspension, exchanges K^+ for the H^+ counter-ions of the particles, which changes the ion arrangement in the suspension and most importantly affects the approximate equality of ion transport numbers in the KCl diffusion front. This effect is termed an anomalous liquid junction potential and represents the *suspension effect of the second kind*, SE 2, as defined in [2,3,10]. The second component of the potential difference is $E_{g',mix}(B) - E_g(A)$; this results from the small suspension particles making intimate contact with the electrode surface, and is called the *suspension effect of the first kind*, SE 1 [3,11]. This arises because the electrode is in contact with the (true) eqs and at the same time in intimate contact with charged particles. In the latter contact regions, an overlapping of the double layers of the particles and the electrode occurs and causes a different H^+ activity in comparison with the activity existing in contacts of eqs with the electrode. This gives rise to a mixed potential [2,3,12], as discussed in Section 1.4.

It is evident that the cell potentials E_A and E_B will differ in two component potentials: (1) $E_j(A)$ and $E_{j,anomal}(B)$ and (2) $E_g(A)$ and $E_{g',mix}(B)$. As both electrodes are in the same phase there can be no boundary potential component $E_{boundary}$, either in E_A or in E_B.

Scheme 3, System 3, shows the glass electrode in the sediment and RE in the eqs of a "combined suspension system" in equilibrium.

$$\begin{array}{cccccc} & S & & & G & \\ [C]\ Ag\mid AgCl\mid KCl\ \vdots\!\vdots\ KCl\ \vdots\ eqs\ \vdots\ eqs,\ HX\ \vdots\!\!\vdots\ HCl\mid AgCl\mid Ag & & & & & E_C \\ E_{ref1} & E_j(S_C)\quad E_j(C)\quad E_b & & & E_{g\,mix}(C) & E_{ref2} \end{array}$$

Scheme 3

The boundary potential is represented by E_b (= $E_{boundary}$); all other symbols have the analogous meanings as above. The cell potential E_C differs from the potential E_A (Scheme 1) only in the potential of the glass electrode because, as discussed below, E_b is negligible [3]. In [A] the potential of the glass electrode $E_g(A)$ is a single potential, because the electrode is in contact with a homogeneous solution. However, in [C] it is a multiple or mixed electrode potential, as in [B].

The potential E_b (also known as a Donnan potential) at the eqs/sediment boundary is often considered, without foundation, as arising from an effective semipermeable membrane. It has been established experimentally [2,3] that when, for example, the movable electrode penetrates the sediment phase ("perforates" the "fictitious membrane") no measurable step-change of the electrode potential occurs. Thus, $E_b = 0$ and can be neglected. However, the electrode potential changes proportionately with progressive immersion of the electrode in the sediment. This is in accordance with the above interpretation that a mixed potential forms.

A Donnan potential exists at the solid–solution interface around individual particles (because the fixed ions inside the particles cannot cross the interfaces), but it does not exist where the bulk eqs is constricted in the interstitial eqs channels between the particles.

1.4 Analysis of the Schemes and Findings
Potential at the Eqs/Sediment Boundary

Analysis of the above cell schemes shows that the effect of suspended sediment material on two electrochemical processes is responsible for the SE. The SE is not a result of a hypothetical membrane and the corresponding potential, which might be ascribed to the boundary between the eqs and the sediment. It

has been established experimentally that $E_b \approx 0$ [2,3] both in control experiments, which included an appropriate agitation of the RE in the suspension, and in experiments in which a restrained flow of the solution filling the salt bridge was used or the direction of the flow was reversed.

Liquid Junction Potential

The liquid junction potential formed at the contact of the RE salt bridge with the sediment can show a much greater value than when in contact with the eqs.

The experiments carried out using a "movable electrode" to establish the existence of the "hypothetical membrane" between eqs and the sediment [10] showed that the *cause* of this change in liquid junction potential is, in fact, ion exchange between the sediment particles and the electrolyte solution flowing from the salt bridge [10]. This change in cell potential begins even before the tip of the salt bridge of the movable RE penetrates the interface [10]. This explanation is also accepted in Galster's monograph on pH measurement [13].

The ions of the diffused filling solution may exchange with counterions (e.g., H^+) in the (colloid) particle double layers and change the solution composition in the particle environment, which will affect *the approximately equal ion transport numbers of the diffusing electrolyte solution*. This is the fundamental reason for the development and maintenance of the *anomalous liquid junction potential*, which can be regarded as the *nature* of the changed potential. This potential can be considered as a systematic error of measurement and can be eliminated (as described in Section 2.6). The magnitude of this potential is usually of the order of some tens of mV, but it can attain more than 100 mV [2,3,7,8].

Indicator Electrode (IE) Potential and its Duration

The change of the IE potential when the electrode comes into intimate contact with the charged particles can also be followed by means of the above-mentioned movable electrode. Experiments confirm the interpretation that the overlapping of the electrode double layer with the double layers of particles is the *cause* of the potential change of the IE when introduced into a suspension [3,4,11,12]. If in the combined suspension system, a movable IE perforates the fictitious membrane, where a phase boundary potential difference between supernatant and the slurry phase should exist, an instantaneous electrode potential change would occur, but it does not! By a step-by-step movement of the electrode into the bulk of the suspension, a progressive increase of the electrode surface in contact with particles occurs and the electrode potential changes in parallel. This leads to the interpretation that the electrode potential change in the suspension depends on surface processes at the electrode and not on effects associated with a membrane. With further penetration of the electrode into the suspension, the contact regions on the electrode surface increase and with this the influence on the value of the mixed potential.

After the introduction of the electrode into the suspension and establishment of contacts with the particles, the electrode potential becomes an *irreversible mixed potential* [12], because two electrochemical reactions proceed simultaneously on the same electrode surface. This potential remains essentially constant for a period of time which exceeds the time required for a potentiometric measurement. This mixed potential can be regarded as the *nature* of the changed IE potential in suspensions, which cannot be eliminated from any measurement. The mixed potential in cells [B] or [C] depends on the species, smoothness of the electrode and the particles, the ionic strength of the solution, and the particle charge and size [11,12]. Its value is usually not greater than some tens of mV.

The potentiometric cell, represented schematically by cell [C], is generally adopted as the most suitable for soil pH measurements. The analysis of its scheme shows that $E_j(B)$ (required in cell [B]) is replaced by $E_j(C)$ (which is ≈ 0) and E_b (which is $= 0$). The cell potential E_C changes measurably only when the mixed potential of the IE $E_g(C_{mix})$ changes. The systematic RE error is eliminated from the cell potential because the filling solution of the RE does not flow into the suspension. From the steady-state potential E_C, a useful approximation of the pH of a suspension can be calculated, because E_C depends on the contribution to the H$^+$ activity from both the particles and the eqs. If the eqs is not completely free from colloidal particles, this may represent (at most) a small uncertainty which must be taken into account.

The interpretation of the experimental results obtained in the study of hydrogen ion activity in suspensions [12] is applicable in general to a potentiometric estimation of ion activities in suspensions measured with different ion-selective electrodes (ISEs) in combination with the RE. For the latter measurements, the symbol pH used in this work should be replaced by the symbol pIon.

1.5 Conclusions

In the publication "Measurement of pH: IUPAC Recommendations 2002" [1], cell V is recommended for practical pH measurement *in solutions*. Because this cell is identical to the pH cells most frequently used in laboratory measurements in the past, the results from both are equivalent and in accordance with the recommendations. Cell V and some other cells are used also for pH measurements *in suspensions*, with the electrodes positioned usually separately, the glass electrode in the sediment, and the RE in its eqs. The pH values measured separately in the suspension (or in its sediment) or in the eqs are different, even though the suspension and solution are in equilibrium. This pH difference, which can be expressed in terms of the corresponding differences in the cell potentials, ΔE, is called the "suspension effect".

An analysis of the detailed schemes for the potentiometric cells used in such suspension measurements provides an acceptable explanation of the SE. The SE is the sum of two galvanic potential changes, which occur when the electrodes are transferred from the eqs to the suspension (or sediment):

1. The change in potential of the IE, which changes to *an irreversible mixed potential probe* (a consequence of the overlapping of the diffuse double layers of the electrode with the double layers of particles, when the electrode makes intimate contact with them).
2. The change in the liquid junction potential that exists between the salt-bridge solution of the RE and either the eqs or the suspension. In the latter case, contact of the flowing electrolyte from the salt bridge with the suspension particles gives rise to *an anomalous junction potential*.

Each of these phenomena has been confirmed with experiments [2–4,10–12].

Measurements on the suspension potentiometric cell [B] shows no evidence for a potential boundary (as is also the case in cell [A]), characterized as a "semipermeable membrane". Experiments have established that there is *no measurable boundary potential* existing between the eqs and the sediment. Therefore, the SE does not include a measurable boundary potential; the SE cannot be interpreted as a boundary or Donnan potential.

2. Guidelines for Practical pH Measurements in Soil Suspensions

2.1 Introduction

The revised view of potentiometric measurements in suspensions (Section 1), which takes into account the currently presented definition of the SE and its interpretation in "Guidelines for potentiometric measurements in suspensions: Part B. Guidelines for practical pH measurements in soil suspensions (IUPAC Recommendations 2007)" [*Pure Appl. Chem.* **79**, 81 (2007)], provides an explanation for the results obtained by different potentiometric measurement techniques when applied to suspensions. This is important especially in the determination of soil pH.

Each of the different methods used provides a soil pH value, which is often neither clearly defined nor understood. The results can involve a large uncertainty and may only approximate the actual pH value. Only one experimental method is considered to provide a pH value with acceptable uncertainty in regard to the influence of soil solution components on a plant. However, a comparison of results obtained by several potentiometric methods can give a meaningful insight to the true H$^+$ activity in the suspensions.

The SE that contributes to the measurement value should not be considered a very significant characteristic of a suspension, but rather it is a troublesome difference between two cell potentials, both of which affect the determination of the *actual pH value of the suspension*. The thermodynamically defined H$^+$ ion activity in a suspension cannot be equated with any potentiometrically determined pH value.

The methods for pH measurement in dilute aqueous solutions, as in IUPAC Recommendations 2002 [6], are taken as the basis for pH measurements of suspensions. From the definition and interpretation of the SE presented here, a revised view of pH measurements in suspensions becomes possible. The effects, which occur in the measurement system due to the suspension characteristics, are analyzed below for five different measurement protocols applied to cells which contain the eqs or the suspension. These effects influence the potential difference measured in suspension potentiometric cells. Each of these measurement protocols is applicable to soil pH measurements. Advice is given on the reasonable choice and use of electrodes in suspension measurements.

To codify the different expressions of the suspension pH (soil pH), measured by cell [C] or cell V, some expressions can be proposed that specify the technique used.

The term "direct suspension pH" is used when the original sample is measured directly by cell V [1], with both electrodes in the original suspension (or soil), analogous to the pH measurement in solutions (noted as, e.g., "direct soil pH"). The term "modified direct pH" is used when the suspension is modified in any way before measurement (e.g., with water or electrolyte solution added to the original sample); this must be explicitly noted (e.g., "modified direct soil pH (1:2 w)") and the notation explained.

The term "effective suspension pH" can be used in the case where the original suspension is separated into two parts (combined suspension system) and the pH is measured with the IE in the sediment and the RE in the eqs of the cell [C], either without any prior modification of the suspension ("effective soil pH") or with a modification of the suspension ("modified effective" suspension pH). In this case, any water or solution added to the original sample must be noted explicitly (e.g., "modified effective soil pH (1:5 KCl)"). Each of these measurements is considered to give an approximation to the true pH in soil solution, that is the pH to which an object immersed in this suspension (e.g., a root) could be exposed.

The *true* pH means the pH value measured in the clear eqs separated from the equilibrated original suspension (e.g., "true soil pH"). Analogous to the above, the term "modified true" is used when the sample was modified before measurements (e.g., "modified true soil pH (1:2 CaCl₂))". These values, in combination with the direct pH values, are used for determination of the SE.

For routine work, the corresponding abbreviations are proposed:

D soil pH, MD soil pH (1:2 w)
E soil pH, ME soil pH (2:5 KCl)
T soil pH, MT soil pH (1:5 CaCl₂), etc.

The values should be valid for measurements at 20 °C; "w" means distilled water, "KCl" 1 mol kg⁻¹ solution and "CaCl₂" 0.01 mol kg⁻¹ solution of salts, if not indicated otherwise.

2.2 Nature of Suspensions and Their Relation to the pH Electrode Potential

In this report, the aqueous suspensions considered are defined as *charged solid particles* of not strictly determined sizes, which are dispersed in an aqueous *dispersing medium* (water or aqueous solution). This medium surrounds the particles permanently, even when they are settled and form a suspension *sediment*. In a suspension of, for example, ion exchanger beads (declared to be in H⁺-form), which are in equilibrium with the surrounding eqs, the particles together with their double layers may contain a larger or smaller concentration of H⁺ than that existing in the bulk solution. These charged particles could be regarded as reservoirs of ions that are blocked from the eqs by an equilibrium Donnan potential. Thus, a suspension contains at least two phases of either similar or different activity of H⁺.

The electrochemical potential λ_{H^+} is the same throughout the whole equilibrated suspension system. Therefore, *the pH of the eqs* can be considered to be the true pH value of the whole interstitial solution in a suspension or sediment (which is not disturbed by the measurement). The pH of the eqs can be measured practically by means of cell V, defined in IUPAC Recommendations 2002 [1]. In the case of an equilibrated soil suspension, it could be considered as the true soil pH value.

When the pH electrode is placed into the suspension, the particles do not influence its electrode potential during the measurement [7,10] until the reservoirs come into intimate contact with the electrode, resulting in an overlapping of the double layers of both. As a consequence of contact regions, the number depending on the particle size, the IE potential changes [12]. The change is proportional to the ratio of contact surfaces to the total electrode surface and to the double-layer thicknesses.

Whereas the potential of the pH glass electrode positioned in the eqs follows the Nernst equation, it changes to an *irreversible mixed (or corrosion) potential* when the electrode is transferred to the *corresponding suspension or sediment*, as described in Section 1.4. Different electrodes may show different mixed potentials in the same suspension, and the same electrode may show different mixed potentials when it contacts particles of different sizes in the same suspension.

The contents of reservoirs can be estimated approximately by selected methods given in Section 2.5.

2.3 Nature of Suspensions and Their Relation to the Reference Electrode Potential

The *heterogeneous character of suspensions* also influences the potential of the reference part of the potentiometric cell (represented by the RE connected with the salt bridge), which is immersed in the suspension. The liquid junction potential

between the RE and its salt bridge remains unchanged during the cell potential measurement. The liquid junction potential between the filling solution of the salt bridge (containing cations and anions of approximately equal transport numbers) and the eqs can practically be neglected. In contrast, the liquid junction potential between the diffused filling solution of the salt bridge and the suspension particles can be significant. It is called the *anomalous liquid junction potential*. In regard to the measurement technique, it represents a systematic error of measurement, and can be eliminated only by avoiding the salt-bridge filling solution from coming in contact with the suspension particles.

2.4 Relationship between the Suspension–Equilibrium Solution–Sediment and the Positioning of the Electrodes

Because the origin and cause of the SEs have not been clarified since the beginning of their study (in 1930), different modified techniques were introduced into routine determination of soil pH which give different and not clearly explained, nevertheless useful, results.

With regard to the electrode positioning in a uniform or in a combined system, the following classification of potentiometric techniques is possible: both electrodes placed (1) in the original suspension system, (2) in the eqs of the suspension, (3) in the suspension sediment, or (4) the IE in the sediment and RE in the eqs of the suspension, and (5) in the reverse mode to (4).

In these methods, the above-mentioned relations between the electrodes and the measured medium must be considered, and for 4 and 5 also the possible influence of the boundary between the sediment and the eqs on the measured cell potential. As described in Section 1.5 no measurable (Donnan) boundary potential exists at this interface; thus, it is not a "virtual continuous semipermeable membrane", as has been shown in control experiments [3,12]. Nevertheless, in spite of this fact, in some recent publications it is erroneously assumed that a boundary potential between the eqs and the sediment is the main contributor to the SE [16–18].

2.5 Discussion of Modified Methods of pH Measurements in Soil Suspensions

This part provides guidelines for pH measurement. With the aid of the proposed definition and interpretation of the SE in "Guidelines for potentiometric measurements in suspensions: Part B. Guidelines for practical pH measurements in soil suspensions (IUPAC Recommendations 2007)" [*Pure Appl. Chem.* **79**, 81 (2007)], processes and techniques are discussed and the significance of the results obtained is explained.

The in situ *"soil pH"* can be measured only in wet soil if it contains enough water so that the *water activity a* ≈ 1. If this is not the case, deionized or rain water is added to the soil to obtain a homogenized wet *soil paste*, similar to the original wet soil. In these cases, the suspension is not separated into the eqs and the sediment. Measurements of pH with both electrodes in nearly dry soils are meaningless from a sheer physicochemical point of view.

In *routine pH measurements*, a greater amount of water is added to the soil to form a diluted aqueous suspension. This must *be equilibrated and separated into sediment and the corresponding eqs*. In laboratory measurements, a complete separation is performed by centrifugation, otherwise the separation is obtained by sedimentation, in which case the imperfect separation must be taken into account in assessing the uncertainty of the result. For better-defined results, the air-dried pulverized soil is sieved, mixed with deionized water in known proportions by mass, and the pH is measured in the eqs after separation. The result for a 1:2 soil/water system can be given as "soil pH (1:2 w)". Different soil/water proportions show different pH values, which need a suitable interpretation to give useful information. Protocols for the sampling of soil populations are described in "Terminology in soil sampling (IUPAC Recommendations 2005)" [19].

Method 1 (Cell Potential E₁)

The *direct pH measurement of the original suspension* by means of cell V (analogous to IUPAC Recommendations 2002, which is recommended for measurement in homogeneous solutions), with *both electrodes placed in the soil suspension*, gives a result which is different from those obtained with other methods. This pH_1 value has *no reasonable pH meaning*, because it is calculated from a cell potential E_1, which contains the unknown mixed potential of the IE and the anomalous liquid junction potential, the latter representing a systematic error of the measurement (Scheme 2 in Section 1.3). These two potentials are responsible for the SE. Nevertheless, pH_1 can be used in comparison with other pH_n values as a repeatable suspension characteristic. Also, the *pH of a soil paste* can be considered as a result of Method 1 with the same significance.

Method 2 (Cell Potential E₂)

In this method, a known amount of water or of salt solution is added to the soil sample and the equilibrated suspension separated into the eqs and the sediment. For pH measurement, *both electrodes are positioned in the eqs*, which may, or may not, be in contact with the sediment. The cell potential E_2 is equivalent to the difference of the electrode potentials E_A of the cell [A] in Section 1.3. The value pH_2 calculated from E_2 is not influenced by the diffuse layer of the suspended particles. This pH value can be adopted as the pH of the whole suspension system if the suspension is not disturbed by the measurement.

The amount of water added to the original suspension must be reported with the results. The air-dried soil-to-liquid mass ratio of the suspension should be reproducible with acceptable precision as it determines the measured cell potential. The ratio should be expressed explicitly; e.g., for the ratio 1:2 as $E_2(1:2\ w)$ for water, or $E_2(1:2\ KCl)$ for KCl solution and $E_2(1:2\ CaCl_2)$ for $CaCl_2$ solution, whichever is used as the dispersing medium. The comparison of E_2 values, obtained in water-eqs and solution-eqs, respectively, allows an estimation of the amount of H^+ set free from particles for different soil-to-liquid ratios after these were exchanged by K^+ or Ca^{2+} [7]. In routine work, the measured E_2 values are expressed as corresponding pH_2 values. These can be regarded as the best defined, "true pH" value measured for a suspension.

Method 3 (Cell Potential E₃)

The measurement is performed with *both electrodes in the separated sediment* of a suspension and is *equivalent to that in Method 1*, except for the fact that the particle concentration is the maximum possible. The sediment may, or may not, be in contact with the separated part of eqs. The cell scheme is given in Section 1.3, Scheme 2. Both E_j and E_g contribute to pH_3, and it cannot be used for pH evaluation of a suspension, but it is used for the determination of the total SE as described in the definition of the SE.

Method 4 (Cell Potential E₄)

4(a) The electrode position in Method 4 is obtained by transferring *the IE* from the eqs, as it is positioned in Method 2, *into the sediment, while the RE remains in eqs*. As can be seen from the cell [C] (Scheme 3 in Section 1.3), the IE potential changes to a mixed potential, the value of which depends on the pH of the eqs and on the H^+ activity of the diffuse layer of the contacting suspension particles. Because the RE potential and the diffusion potential remain unchanged, the measured cell potential E_4 differs from E_2 by the potential difference ΔE known as SE 1 (Section 1.3). For an equilibrated suspension soil/water ratio of ½, this is given by $\Delta E_{4-2}(1:2\ w) = E_4 - E_2$. The pH_4 values obtained with the same IE in different (soil) suspensions allow an *approximate comparison* of the H^+ activity to which a (charged) surface similar to that of the IE (e.g., of a root in the measured soil) could be exposed, when coming in contact with the particles of these soils. Any change in pH_4 indicates a change of the electrode mixed potential, which depends on the particle contacts with the electrode surface.

Except for a method only applicable to the laboratory, where the filling solution of the salt bridge is exposed to a negative pressure [2], three other variations of Method 4 are used in routine practice, 4(b), (c), and (d). In these, the amount of the separated eqs is minimal and contact of the salt-bridge filling solution with the particles is avoided.

4(b) In this method, only a small amount of the eqs is needed for a measurement. It employs an RE connected with the suspension by two salt bridges in series (double salt bridge), of which the second one is filled with eqs.

4(c) In this modification, a strip of filter paper wetted with eqs is used for the electrolytic connection between the suspension and the salt bridge. When brought into contact with the suspension [9], a minimal amount of the clear eqs diffuses along the strip to the salt bridge.

4(d) In this method, a special combination electrode is used which, during the measurement, has only the pH sensing element in contact with the suspension. The eqs "climbs up" the specially prepared surface of the electrode stem to form the contact with the salt-bridge solution. In this case, the combination electrode does not *measure pH without the SE*, as it is often declared, because the presence of the SE 1 is unavoidable.

Method 4 is used very frequently in routine work, because the measured pH_4 values, though not absolutely repeatable, depend on the sum of H^+ activities contributed from the eqs and from the particles.

Method 5 (Cell Potential E₅)

In this method, the IE is placed in the eqs and the RE in the sediment. It is used solely when the anomalous liquid junction potential (i.e., the systematic error of measurement), equal to the cell potential difference $\Delta E_{5-2} = E_5 - E_2$, is to be determined. The derived pH_5 value is not very relevant in routine work. From the methods discussed above, the most appropriate one can be used to obtain the information of interest. An illustration of the above methods applied to soil pH measurement is presented in [7]. It is seen that different soils show different pH_2 values (and pH differences), which can be used for the characterization of these soils in agronomy. The treatise relating to soil pH measurement can be applied—*cum grano salis*—to the general potentiometric pIon measurement in soils and in other suspensions. It should be emphasized once more that, by measurement of the voltage of any suspension galvanic cell no thermodynamically defined quantity can be obtained.

2.6 Devices and Their Application in Practical "Soil pH" Measurements

Because these guidelines are based on the IUPAC Recommendations 2002 [1], the definitions given in that Glossary for pH measurement in real solutions, are also valid when applied to pH measurement in suspensions. Nevertheless, some additional points should be noted.

The *electrodes* used may be "single" or "combination", but combination ones are suitable only in some cases.

Single IEs used in suspensions should be glass or other solid-state ISE, having smooth surfaces and providing fast responses and reproducible results. Electrodes of the second kind (e.g., Ag/AgCl, Sb/Sb$_2$O$_3$) do not have smooth surfaces, and for this and other reasons they show a greater or unexpected contribution to the SE [12].

The *single RE* may be constructed with one salt bridge which is filled with the same filling solution as the electrode ("half bridge"). Two salt bridges in series (a double salt bridge) are also feasible. The term "double salt bridge" in this case is more appropriate than the term "double junction" electrode. Both kinds of salt bridge are sealed with a separator (capillary, porous ceramic plug, frit, ground glass sleeve, or other). From the separator of the single salt bridge, which is in contact with the measured medium, its filling solution (e.g., saturated KCl solution of the RE half-cell) always flows or diffuses, even if the filling solution is gel- stabilized [10,14,15]. This can give rise to an anomalous liquid junction potential when it contacts the suspension particles. This can be minimized if the final half of the double salt bridge and the separator are filled with, for example, the eqs of the measured suspension for both the test solution measurements and the electrode calibration. It must be emphasized that the filling solution which flows from the separator to the sediment boundary can cause large systematic errors, even if the separator is placed in eqs near this boundary [10]. This can be minimized with a shielding tube, which is pulled onto the salt bridge and perforated by a small side-aperture (about 1.5 cm above the bottom of the tube), providing liquid and electrical contact between the two sides [11].

Combination electrodes are often used for measurements in suspensions. They are not suitable for measurements in *combined suspension systems*, except if the electrode is placed so that its indicator half-cell is connected with the sediment and the reference half-cell with the eqs so that SE 2 is minimized. The cell voltages measured with combination electrodes, the IE of which is immersed in a suspension, always include SE 1, notwithstanding that the electrodes are often declared to "measure soil pH without suspension effect", as found in advertisements. Only some combination electrodes of special construction could possibly eliminate SE 2. *ISFET (combined) electrodes* also cannot avoid the SE in suspension measurements as the experiments showed; the results are therefore equivalent to those obtained with method 1.

For measurements in suspensions, the electrodes must be *placed* in the suspension in such a way that any differentiation in particle sizes around the sensing element of the electrode is avoided and a stable position of the electrodes is assured.

The instruments for voltage measurement should have a high input resistance (as pH meters generally have). The potential differences of the suspension potentiometric cells, which have relatively small ohmic inner resistances (e.g., cells with the metal or solid membrane used as a halogenide IE), can be measured with voltmeters of smaller input resistance, but the readings are not stable and are difficult to interpret.

References

1. R. P. Buck, S. Rondinini, A. K. Covington, F. G. K. Baucke, C. M. A. Brett, M. F. Camoes, M. J. T. Milton, T. Mussini, R. Naumann, K. W. Pratt, R Spitzer G. S. Wilson. *Pure Appl. Chem.* **74**, 2169 (2002).
2. S. F. Oman, I. Lipar. *Electrochim. Acta* **42**, 15 (1997).
3. S. Oman. *Talanta* **51**, 21 (2000).
4. J. Th. G. Overbeek. *J. Colloid Sci.* **8**, 593 (1953).
5. H. Pallmann. *Kolloid Beih.* **30**, 334 (1930).
6. G. Wiegner. *Kolloid-Z.* **51**, 49 (1930).
7. S. F. Oman. *Acta Chim. Slov.* **47**, 519 (2000).
8. Yu. M. Chernoberezhskii. "The Suspension Effect" in *Surface and Colloid Science.* 2nd ed., Vol. 12, E. Matijevic (Ed.), pp. 359–453, Plenum Press, New York (1982).
9. T. R. Yu. *Ion-Selective Electrode Rev.* **7**, 165 (1985).
10. Lehrwerk Chemie, Vol. 5, G. Ackermann et al. *Elektrolytgleichgewichte und Elektrochemie*, 4th ed., p. 70, VEB Deutscher Verlag, Leipzig (1985).
11. S. Oman, A. Godec. *Electrochim. Acta* **36**, 59 (1991).
12. S. F. Oman. *Acta Chim. Slov.* **51**, 189 (2004).
13. H. Galster. *pH Measurement*, Chaps. 3.2, 3.4, 6.2, VCH, Weinheim (1991).
14. A. K. Covington. *Ion-Selective Electrode Methodology*, Vol. I, p. 60, CRC Press, Boca Raton (1980).
15. R. E. Dohner, D. Wegmann, W. E. Morf, W. Simon. *Anal. Chem.* **58**, 2585 (1986).
16. R. P. Buck, E. Lindner. *Pure Appl. Chem.* **66**, 2533 (1994).
17. D. H. Everett, L. K. Koopal. *Chem. Int.* **25**, 18 (2003) and refs. therein.
18. R. J. Hunter. *Colloid Science*, 2nd ed., p. 354, Oxford University Press, New York (2001).
19. P. de Zorzi, S. Barbizzi, M. Belli, G. Ciceri, A. Fajgelj, D. Moore, U. Sansone, M. Van der Perk. *Pure Appl. Chem.* **77**, 827 (2005).

IONIZATION CONSTANTS OF ACIDS AND BASES

W. P. Jencks and J. Regenstein

These pK'_a values were taken from the original literature and from several extensive compilations of such data, of which the most important are

> Albert, *Ionization Constants of Acids and Bases*, Methuen, London, 1962.
>
> Bell, *The Proton in Chemistry*, 2nd ed., Cornell, Ithaca, New York, 1973.
>
> Brown, McDaniel, and Häfliger, in Braude and Nachod, *Determination of Organic Structures by Physical Methods*, Academic Press, New York, 1955.
>
> Kortum, Vogel, and Andrussow, *Dissociation Constants of Organic Acids in Aqueous Solution*, Butterworths, London, 1961.
>
> Perrin, *Dissociation Constants of Organic Bases in Aqueous Solution*, Butterworths, London, 1965.
>
> Yukawa, Ed., *Handbook of Organic Structural Analysis*, Benjamin, New York, 1965.

A particularly valuable source of dissociation constants obtained under a variety of experimental conditions is provided by Sillen, L. G. and Martell, A. E., Eds., *Stability Constants*, Special Publications No. 17 and 25, Chemical Society, London, 1964 and 1971. This compilation also lists association constants of metals for a variety of inorganic and organic ligands.

The compounds selected were those which were thought most likely to be useful to biochemists and chemists and these compilations should be consulted for information on compounds which are not included here.

All values are reported as $pK'_a = -\log K'_a = 14 - pK'_b$. K'_a is the ionization constant

$$\frac{[H^+][A^-]}{[HA]} \text{ or } \frac{[H^+][B]}{[HB^+]} \text{ or } \frac{[A^{n-1}][H^+]}{[HA^n]}$$

Temperatures are not indicated because variations of pK'_a with temperature are generally smaller than the variations of the data from different sources for other reasons, but most of the data were obtained at or near 25°. Ionization constants which are reported as thermodynamic values at 25° are indicated with an asterisk, *, but some of these may only represent values measured at low ionic strength.

These pK'_a values and a measured pH should not be used to obtain an *exact* measure of the ratio of acid to base in a given solution. Ionic strength and specific salt effects, as well as possible errors in the reported pK'_a values, are likely to make such estimates inaccurate. It should be kept in mind that the effect of increasing ionic strength is generally to decrease the apparent pK'_a of neutral and anionic acids and to increase the pK_a of cationic acids. These effects are particularly large for polyanions, such as phosphates.

There is some intentional redundancy in the tables to facilitate the location of listings for compounds that might be listed in several sections. The pK'_a values for amines refer to the ionization of the conjugate acids of the amines except for a few nitrogen acids, which undergo an acidic ionization.

The pH of a solution at a given ionic strength and temperature is given by

$$pH = pK'_a + \log \frac{(base)}{(acid)}$$

in which the pK'_a is measured under the same experimental conditions. The following relationships are useful to have readily available to estimate the ratio of acid to base at a given pH or to estimate the buffer ration of acid required to give a given pH; the compiler keeps a copy of these numbers on his desk.

For graphical plots of a large number of substituted phosphorus compounds see Ref. (83). For complex chelating agents of aliphatic amines, see also Reference 77.

Fraction Base or Acid	pH
5% or 95%	$pK'_a \pm 1.25$
10% or 90%	$pK'_a \pm 0.95$
15% or 85%	$pK'_a \pm 0.75$
20% or 80%	$pK'_a \pm 0.60$
25% or 75%	$pK'_a \pm 0.48$
30% or 70%	$pK'_a \pm 0.37$
35% or 65%	$pK'_a \pm 0.27$
40% or 60%	$pK'_a \pm 0.18$
45% or 55%	$pK'_a \pm 0.09$
50% or 50%	$pK'_a \pm 0$

INORGANIC ACIDS

Compound	pK'_a	Reference	Compound	pK'_a	Reference
AgOH	3.96	4	$H_3P_2O_7^-$	2.36*	77
$Al(OH)_3$	11.2	28	$H_2P_2O_7^{2-}$	6.60*	77
$As(OH)_3$	9.22	28	$HP_2O_7^{3-}$	9.25*	77
H_3AsO_4	2.22, 7.0, 13.0	28	$HReO_4$	−1.25	30
$H_2AsO_4^-$	6.98*	77	HSCN	0.85	77
$HAsO_4^{2-}$	11.53*	77	H_3SiO_3	10.0	34
H_3AsO_3	9.22*	—	H_2S	7.00*	77
H_3AuO_3	13.3, 16.0	78	HS^-	12.92*	77
H_3BO_3	9.23	28	H_2SO_3	1.9, 7.0, 1.76*	28, 77
$H_2B_4O_7$	4.00	34	H_2SO_4	1.9	28
$HB_4O_7^-$	9.00	34	HSO_3^-	7.21*	77
$Be(OH)_2$	3.7	4	HSO_4^-	1.99*	77
HBr	−9.00	31	$H_2S_2O_3$	0.60,* 1.72*	77
HOBr	8.7	28	$H_2S_2O_4$	1.9	29
HOCl	7.53, 7.46	28, 33	H_2Se	3.89*	77
$HClO_2$	2.0	28	HSe^-	11.00*	77
$HClO_3$	−1.00	28	H_2SeO_3	2.6, 8.3; 2.62*	28
HCN	9.40	34	$HSeO_3^-$	8.32	77
H_2CO_3	6.37, 6.35,* 3.77*	34, 23	H_2SeO_4	Strong, 2.0	28
HCO_3^-	10.33*	—	$HSeO_4^-$	2.00	34
H_2CrO_4	−0.98, 0.74	30, 77	$HSbO_2$	11.0	34
$HCrO_4^-$	6.50*	2, 30	HTe	5.00	34
HOCN	3.92	34	H_2Te	2.64, 11.0	34, 78
HF	3.17*	77	H_2TeO_3	2.7, 8.0	28
H_3GaO_3	10.32, 11.7	78	$Te(OH)_6$	6.2, 8.8	28
H_2GeO_3	8.59, 12.72	34, 78	H_2VO_4	8.95	30
$Ge(OH)_4$	8.68, 12.7	28	HVO_4^{2-}	14.4	30
HI	−10.0	31	$H_4V_6O_{17}$	1.96	78
HOI	11.0	28	Cacodylic acid	1.57,* 6.27*	99
HIO_3	0.8	28	$(CH_3)_2As(O)OH$		
$H_4IO_6^-$	6.00	34			
H_5IO_6	1.64, 1.55, 8.27	34, 28, 78			
	3.29, 6.70, 15.0	—		**SUBSTITUTED AsO_3H_2**	
$HMnO_4$	−2.25	30	CH_3-	3.61,* 8.18*	97
NH_3OH^+	5.98*	12	CH_3CH_2-	3.89,* 8.35*	—
NH_4^+	9.24*	77	$CH_3(CH_2)_4-$	4.14,* 10.07*	—
HN_3	4.72*	77	$CH_3(CH_2)_5-$	4.16,* 9.19*	—
H_3N	33	153	$COOH(CH_2)-$	2.94,* 4.67,* 7.68*	—
HNCS	~−2.0	143	$COOH(CH_2)_4-$	2.00,* 4.89,* 7.74*	—
HNO_2	3.29	28	$o-CH_3C_6H_4-$	3.82,* 8.85*	—
HNO_3	−1.3	28	$m-CH_3C_6H_4-$	3.82,* 8.60*	—
$N_2H_5^+$	7.99*	77	$p-CH_3C_6H_4-$	3.70,* 8.68*	—
$H_2N_2O_2$	7.05	34	$o-NH_2C_6H_4-$	3.77,* 8.66*	—
$H_2N_2O_2^-$	11.0	34	$m-NH_2C_6H_4-$	4.05,* 8.62*	—
H_2NSO_3H	1.0	80	$p-NH_2C_6H_4-$	4.05,* 8.92*	—
H_2OsO_5	12.1	34			
H_2O	15.7	—		**HYDRATED METAL IONS**	
H_3O^+	−1.7	—	Ti^{3+}	1.15	98
$Pb(OH)_2$	6.48 (10.92)	4, 78	Bi^{+3}	1.58	—
PH_3	27	156	Fe^{+3}	2.80	—
H_3PO_2	2.0, 2.23,* 1.07	28, 77	Hg^{+2}	2.60, 3.70	—
H_3PO_4	2.12*	77	Sn^{+2}	4.00	—
$H_2PO_4^-$	7.21*	77	Cr^{+3}	3.80	—
HPO_4^{2-}	12.32*	77	Al^{+3}	4.96	—
H_3PO_5	1.12, 5.51, 12.80	102	Sc^{+3}	4.96	—
H_3PO_3	2.0, 1.07	28, 77	Fe^{+2}	8.30	—
$H_2PO_3^-$	6.58*	77	Cu^{+2}	8.30	—
$H_4P_2O_7$	1.52*	77	Ni^{+2}	9.30	—
			Zn^{+2}	9.60, 10.84	—

* Thermodynamic value.

PHOSPHATES AND PHOSPHONATES

Compound	pK'_a	Reference	Compound	pK'_a	Reference
PHOSPHATES			*PHOSPHONATES (Continued)*		
Phosphate	2.12,* 7.21,* 12.32*	77	($^-$OOCCH$_2$)$_2$NH$^+$-(CH$_2$)$_2$-	6.54	57
Glyceric acid 2-phosphate	3.6, 7.1	53	CH$_2$I-	1.30, 6.72	57
Enolpyruvic acid	3.5, 6.4	53		2.45, 7.00	57
Methyl-	1.54, 6.31	55	C$_6$H$_5$CH=CH-	2.00, 7.1	57
Ethyl-	1.60, 6.62	55	HOCH$_2$-	1.91, 7.15	57
n-Propyl-	1.88, 6.67	55		2.1	57
n-Butyl-	1.80, 6.84	55	C$_6$H$_5$NH(CH$_2$)$_3$-	7.17	57
Dimethyl-	1.29	55	Br(CH$_2$)$_2$-	2.25, 7.3	57
Diethyl-	1.39	55	CH$_3$(CH$_2$)$_5$CH(COO$^-$)-	7.5	57
Di-*n*-propyl-	1.59	55	C$_6$H$_5$CH$_2$-	2.3, 7.55	57
Di-*n*-butyl-	1.72	55	NH$_3$$^+$(CH$_2$)$_4$-	2.55, 7.55	57
Glucose-3-	0.84, 5.67	56	NH$_3$$^+$(CH$_2$)$_5$-	2.6, 7.6	57
Glucose-4-	0.84, 5.67	56	NH$_3$$^+$(CH$_2$)$_{10}$-	8.00	57
α-Glycero-	1.40, 6.44	54	$^-$OOC(CH$_2$)$_{10}$-	8.25	57
β-Glycero-	1.37, 6.34	54	(CH$_3$)$_3$SiCH$_2$-	3.22, 8.70	57
3-Phosphoglyceric acid	1.42, 3.42	54	C$_6$H$_5$CH$_2$-	3.3[†], 8.4[†]	57
2-Phosphoglyceric acid	1.42, 3.55, 7.1	—	(C$_6$H$_5$)$_3$C-	3.85[†], 9.00[†]	57
Peroxymonophosphoric acid	4.85	69			
Diphosphoglyceric acid	7.40, 7.99	54	*ARYLPHOSPHONIC ACIDS*		
Glyceraldehyde-	2.10, 6.75	54	2X-RC$_6$H$_3$PO$_3$H$_2$	—	57
Dioxyacetone-	1.77, 6.45	54	X R		—
Hexose di-	1.52, 6.31	54	Cl 4-O$_2$N	1.12, 6.14	—
Fructose-6-	0.97, 6.11	54	Br 5-O$_2$N	6.14	—
Glucose-6-	0.94, 6.11	54	Cl 5-Cl	6.63	—
Glucose-1-	1.10, 6.13	54	Cl H	1.63, 6.98	—
Pyrophosphoric acid	0.9, 2.0, 6.6, 9.4	54	Br H	1.64, 7.00	—
Phosphopyruvic acid	3.5, 6.38	54	Br 5-CH$_3$	1.81, 7.15	—
DL-Phosphoserine	6.19	145	Cl 4-NH$_2$	7.33	—
Creatine phosphate	2.7, 4.5	54	CH$_3$O 4-O$_2$N	1.53, 6.96	—
Arginine phosphate	2.8, 4.5, 9.6, 11.2	54	CH$_3$O H	2.16, 7.77	—
Amino phosphate	(−0.9), 2.8, 8.2	54	CH$_3$O 4-NH$_2$	8.22	—
Trimetaphosphate	2.05	77	HO 4-O$_2$N	1.22, 5.39	—
Trimethyl phosphine	8.80*	99	O$_2$N H	1.45, 6.74	—
Triphosphate	8.90, 6.26, 2.30	77	F H	1.64, 6.80	—
Tetrametaphosphate	2.74	77	I H	1.74, 7.06	—
Fluorophosphate	0.55, 4.8	56	NH$_2$ H	7.29	—
See also under *Nucleic Acid Derivatives*			CH$_3$ H	2.10, 7.68	—
			C$_6$H$_5$ H	8.13	—
PHOSPHONATES			HOOC H	1.71, 9.17	—
H$_2$O$_3$P(CH$_2$)$_4$PO$_3$H$_2$	< 2, 2.75, 7.54, 8.38	57			
H$_2$O$_3$P(CH$_2$)$_3$PO$_3$H$_2$	< 2, 2.65, 7.34, 8.35	57	*SUBSTITUTED-PO$_2$H$_2$*		
H$_2$O$_3$PCH$_2$CH(CH$_3$)-PO$_3$H$_2$	< 2, 2.6, 7.00, 9.27	57	CH$_3$-	3.08*	97
H$_2$O$_3$PCH$_2$PO$_3$H$_2$	< 2, 2.57, 6.87, 10.33	57	CH$_3$CH$_2$-	3.29*	97
Methyl-	2.35, 7.1*	57, 97	CH$_3$(CH$_2$)$_2$-	3.46*	97
Ethyl-	2.43, 7.85*	57, 97	(CH$_3$)$_2$CH-	3.56*	97
n-Propyl-	2.45, 8.18*	57, 97	CH$_3$(CH$_2$)$_3$-	3.41*	97
Isopropyl-	2.55, 7.75	57	(CH$_3$)$_3$C-	4.24*	97
n-Butyl-	2.59, 8.19	57	C$_6$H$_5$-	2.1*	97
Isobutyl-	2.70, 8.43	57	*p*-BrC$_6$H$_4$-	2.1*	97
s-Butyl-	2.74, 8.48	57	*p*-CH$_3$OC$_6$H$_4$-	2.35*	97
t-Butyl-	2.79, 8.88	57	*p*-(CH$_3$)$_2$N-	2.1*, 4.1*	97
Neopentyl-	2.84, 8.65	57			
1,1-Dimethylpropyl-	2.88, 8.96	57			
n-Hexyl-	2.6, 7.9	57			
n-Dodecyl-	8.25	57			
CH$_3$(CH$_2$)$_5$CH(COOH)-	1	57			
CF$_3$-	1.16, 3.93	57			
CCl$_3$-	1.63, 4.81	57			
NH$_3$$^+CH_2$-	2.35, 5.9	57			
($^-$OOCCH$_2$)$_2$NH$^+$CH$_2$-	5.57	57			
CHCl$_2$-	1.14, 5.61	57			
CH$_2$Cl-	1.40, 6.30	57			
CH$_2$Br-	1.14, 6.52	57			

	pK'_a				
X=	−H		−NH$_3$$^+$		Ref. 2
X(CH$_2$)PO$_3$H$_2$	2.35	7.1	1.85	5.35	—
X(CH$_2$)$_2$PO$_3$H$_2$	2.45	7.85	2.45	7.00	—
X(CH$_2$)$_4$PO$_3$H$_2$	—	—	2.55	7.55	—
X(CH$_2$)$_5$PO$_3$H$_2$	—	—	2.6	7.65	—
X(CH$_2$)$_6$PO$_3$H$_2$	2.6	7.9	—	—	—
X(CH$_2$)$_{10}$PO$_3$H$_2$	—	—	—	8.00	—

* Thermodynamic value.

[†] These values were obtained in 50 per cent ethanol.

For graphical plots of a large number of substituted phosphorus compounds see Ref. 83.

CARBOXYLIC ACIDS

Compound	pK_a	Reference
	ALIPHATIC	
Acetic Acids, Substituted		
H-	4.76*	2
O$_2$N-	1.68*	2
(CH$_3$)$_3$N$^+$-	1.83*	2
(CH$_3$)$_2$NH$^+$-	1.95	2
CH$_3$NH$_2^+$-	2.16*	2
NH$_3^+$-	2.31*	2
CH$_3$SO$_2$-	2.36*	2
NC-	2.43*	2
C$_6$H$_5$SO$_2$-	2.44	2
HO$_2$C-	2.83*	2
C$_6$H$_5$SO-	2.66	2
F-	2.66	2
Cl-	2.86*	2
Br-	2.86	2
Cl$_2$-	1.29	2
F$_2$-	1.24	2
Br$_2$	1.48	142
Br$_3$-	0.66	2
Cl$_3$-	0.65	2
F$_3$-	0.23, (−0.26)	2
HON-	3.01	2
F$_3$C-	3.07*	2
ClF$_2$	0.46	159
N$_3$-	3.03	2
I-	3.12	2
C$_6$H$_5$O-	3.12	2
C$_2$H$_5$O$_2$C-	3.35	2
C$_6$H$_5$S-	3.52*	2
CH$_3$O-	3.53	2
NCS-	3.58	2
CH$_3$CO-	3.58*	2
C$_2$H$_5$O-	3.60	2
n-C$_3$H$_7$O-	3.65	2
n-C$_4$H$_9$O-	3.66	2
Sec. -C$_4$H$_9$O-	3.67	2
HS-	3.67*	2
i-C$_3$H$_7$O-	3.69*	2
CH$_3$S-	3.72*	2
i-C$_3$H$_7$S-	3.72*	2
C$_6$H$_5$CH$_2$S-	3.73*	2
C$_2$H$_5$S-	3.74*	2
n-C$_3$H$_7$S-	3.77*	2
n-C$_4$H$_9$S-	3.81*	2
HO-	3.83*	2
−O$_3$S-	4.05	2
(C$_6$H$_5$)$_3$CS-	4.30*	2
C$_6$H$_5$-	4.31*	2
CH$_2$=CH-	4.35*	2
CH$_3$-	4.88*	2
−O$_2$Se-	5.43	2
−O$_2$C-	5.69*	2
(CH$_3$)$_2$-	4.86	2
(C$_6$H$_5$CH$_2$)$_2$-	4.57	2
(C$_6$H$_5$)$_2$	3.96	2
(CH$_3$)$_3$-	5.01	2
CH$_3$CHOH-	3.9	2
(CH$_3$CH$_2$)$_2$-	4.74	
(CH$_3$)$_2$ (CN)-	2.43	
(CH$_3$)$_2$ C(CN)-	2.40	
HC≡C-	1.84	142
CH$_3$C≡C-	2.60	142
C$_6$H$_5$C≡C-	2.23	142
CH$_3$CH=CH-	4.69	142
C$_6$H$_5$CH=CH-	4.44	142
3,5-Di-NO$_2$C$_6$H$_5$-	2.82	142
OHC-	3.32	142
C$_6$H$_5$CO-	1.32	142

* Thermodynamic value.

Substituent	Propionic		Butyric			Valeric	
	α	β	α	β	γ	α	δ
	STRAIGHT-CHAIN, SUBSTITUTED						
H-	4.88	—	4.82*	—	—	4.86*	—
O$_2$N-	—	3.81	—	—	—	—	—
(CH$_3$)$_3$N$^+$-	—	—	—	—	—	—	—
H$_3$N$^+$-	2.34	3.60	—	—	4.23	—	4.27*
NC-	2.43	3.99*	—	—	4.44*	—	—
HO$_2$C-	—	4.19*	—	—	4.34*	—	4.42*
Cl-	2.80	4.08	2.84	4.06	4.52	—	4.70
Br-	2.98	4.02	2.99	—	4.58	—	4.72
HON=	3.32	4.01	3.15	—	—	3.19	4.64
F$_3$C-	—	4.18*	—	—	4.49	—	—
I–	3.12	4.06	—	—	4.64	—	4.77
C$_6$H$_5$O-	3.11	4.27	3.17	—	—	—	—
C$_2$H$_5$O$_2$C-	—	4.52	—	—	—	—	4.60
CH$_3$O-	3.52	4.46	—	—	4.68	—	4.72
CH$_3$CO-	—	4.60	—	—	4.67	—	4.72
C$_2$H$_5$O-	3.61	4.50	—	—	4.70	—	—
HS-	3.70*	4.34*	—	—	—	—	—
HO-	3.86*	4.51	4.22	4.52	4.72	3.89	—
-O$_3$S-	4.22	—	—	—	—	—	—
C$_6$H$_5$-	4.31	4.66*	—	—	4.76*	—	—
H$_2$CCH-	—	4.68*	—	—	4.72*	—	—
CH$_3$-	4.86*	4.82*	4.78	4.78*	4.86*	—	4.88*
-O$_2$Se-	5.48	6.00	5.48	—	—	5.48	—
-O$_2$C-	—	5.48*	—	—	5.42*	—	5.41*

Compound	pK_a	Reference
	GENERAL ALIPHATIC	
Acetoacetic	3.58	6
Acetopyruvic	2.61, 7.85 (enol)	6
Aconitic, trans-	2.80, 4.46	6
Adipamic	4.37	101
Aminomalonic	3.32, 9.83	77
Betaine	1.84	6
α-Bromobutyric	2.97	77
N-Butylaminoacetic	2.29, 10.07	77
Caproic	4.88	101
Caprylic	4.89	101
N-(Carbamoylmethyl)- iminodiacetic	2.30, 6.60	77
β-Carboxymethylamino- propionic	3.61, 9.46	77
2-Carboxyethyliminodiacetic	2.06, 3.69, 9.66	77
Citric	3.09, 4.75, 5.41	6
Crotonic	4.69	6
Cyanomethyliminodiacetic	3.06, 4.34	77
Cyclohexane carboxylic	4.90	153
Cyclopentane carboxylic	4.99	153
Cyclopropane carboxylic	4.83	153
α-Diaminobutyric	1.85, 8.24, 10.44	77
α,β-Diaminopropionic	1.23, 6.69	77
Di-(carboxymethyl)- aminomethylphosphonic	2.25, 5.57, 10.76	77
Diethylaminoacetic	2.04, 10.47	77
Dihydroxyfumaric	1.14	6
α,β-Dimercaptosuccinic	2.40, 3.46, 9.44, 11.82	77
Dimethylaminoacetic	2.08, 9.80	77
2,2-Dimethylbutanoic	4.93	131
2,2-Dimethylpropionic	5.03	131
2-Ethylbutanoic	4.75	131
α-Ethylbutyric	4.74	130
Ethyl hydrogen adipate	4.60	101
Ethyl hydrogen diethyl-malonate	3.64	101
Ethyl hydrogen dimethyl-malonate	3.52	101
Ethyl hydrogen ethyl-malonate	3.40	101
Ethyl hydrogen malonate	3.35	101

CARBOXYLIC ACIDS (Continued)

Compound	pK_a	Reference
GENERAL ALIPHATIC (Continued)		
Ethyl hydrogen methyl-malonate	3.41	101
Ethyl hydrogen sebacate	4.84	101
Ethyl hydrogen suberate	4.84	101
Ethyl hydrogen succinate	4.52	101
N-Ethylaminoacetic	2.30, 10.10	77
Ethylenediaminetetraacetic	2.00, 2.67, 0.26, 6.16, 10.26, 0.96	6, 94
Ethylenediamine-N,N-diacetic	5.58, 11.05	77
Formic	3.77*	2
Fumaric	3.03, 4.54	6
Gluconic	3.86*	77
Glutaramic	4.40	101
Glyceric	3.55	6
Glycolic	3.82	6
Glyoxylic	3.32	6
Heptanoic	4.89	131
Hexanoic	4.86	129
Homogentisic	4.40	6
α-Hydroxybutyric	3.65	77
β-Hydroxybutyric	4.39	77
N-2-Hydroxyethyliminodiacetic	2.2, 8.73	77
β-Hydroxypropionic	3.73	77
3-Hydroxypropyliminodiacetic	2.06, 9.24	77
Iminodiacetic	2.98*, 9.89*	77
Iminodipropionic	4.11, 9.61	77
β-Iodopropionic	4.04*	77
Isobutyric	4.86*	77
Isocaproic	4.85	130
Isohexanoic	4.85	129
Isovaleric	4.78	129
N-Isopropylaminoacetic	2.36, 10.06	77
α-Keto-β-methyl valeric	2.3	6
Lactic	3.86	6
Maleic	1.93, 6.58	6
Malic	3.40, 5.2	6
Malonamic	3.64	101
Mandelic	3.41	77
α-Mercaptobutyric	3.53	77
2-Mercaptoethyliminodiacetic	−2.14, 8.17, 10.79	77
2-Methoxyethyliminodiacetic	2.2, 8.96	77
N-Methylaminoacetic	2.24, 10.01	77
Methyl hydrogen succinate	4.49	101
Methyliminodiacetic	2.81, 10.18	77
2-Methylthioethyliminodiacetic	2.1, 8.91	77
Nitrilotriacetic	3.03, 3.07, 10.70	77
Octanoic	4.90	131
Oenanthylic	4.89	77
Oxalic	1.25, 4.14	77
Oxalacetic (*trans*-enol)	2.56, 4.37	6, 97
(*cis*-enol)	2.15, 4.06	6
Pelargonic	4.95	101
Pentanoic	4.84	131
2-Methyl-	4.78	131
3-Methyl-	4.77	131
4-Methyl-	4.85	131
2,2-Dimethyl-	4.97	131
2-Phosphonoethyliminodiacetic	1.95, 2.45, 6.54, 10.46	77
Pivalic	5.05	153
N-n-Propylaminoacetic	2.25, 10.03	77
Protocatechuic	4.48	6
Pyruvic	2.50	6
Succinamic	4.54	101
N-2-Sulfoethyliminodiacetic	1.92, 2.28, 8.16	77
Tartaric D or L	2.89, 4.16	6
meso-	3.22, 4.85	6
Thiophene-2-carboxylic	3.53	129
Vinylacetic	4.42	6

Compound	pK_a	Reference
GENERAL ALIPHATIC (Continued)		
$CH_3CH_2OCH_2COOH$	3.65*	97
$o\text{-}CH_3C_6H_4OCH_2COOH$	3.23*	97
$m\text{-}CH_3C_6H_4OCH_2COOH$	3.20*	97
$p\text{-}CH_3C_6H_4OCH_2COOH$	3.22*	97
$2,6\text{-}(CH_3)_2C_6H_3OCH_2\text{-}COOH$	3.36*	97
$o\text{-}CH_3OC_6H_4OCH_2COOH$	3.23*	97
$m\text{-}CH_3OC_6H_4OCH_2\text{-}COOH$	3.14*	97
$p\text{-}CH_3OC_6H_4OCH_2COOH$	3.21	97
$CH_3COCH_2COCOOH$	2.58*, 8.50*	97
$CH_3CH(OH)COOCH\text{-}(CH_3)COOH$	2.95*	97
$CH_2ClCH(OH)COOH$	3.12*	97
$CH_3CH(OH)CHClCOOH$	2.59*	97
$CH_3CHClCH(OH)COOH$	3.08*	97
$CH_2ClC(CH_3)(OH)COOH$	3.20*	97
$COOHCHClCH(OH)\text{-}COOH$	2.32*	97
$CH_3COOC(CH_2COOH)_2\text{-}COOH$	2.49*	97

SULFUR CONTAINING CARBOXYLIC ACIDS

Compound	pK_a	Reference
$HOOCH_2SCH_2COOH$	3.30*, 4.50*	97
$HOOCCH_2SCH_2SCH_2\text{-}COOH$	3.31*, 4.34*	97
$HOOCCH_2S(CH_2)_5SCH_2\text{-}COOH$	3.49*, 4.41*	97
$CH_3SCH(CH_3)SCH_2\text{-}COOH$	3.77*	97
$(CH_3)_2CHSCH(CH_3)\text{-}COOH$	3.78*	97

Compound	pK_a	Reference
$CH_3\text{-}CH\text{-}COOH$ $\quad\vert$ $\quad S$ $\quad\vert$ $HOOC\text{-}CH\text{-}CH_3$	4.62*	97
$CH_3\text{-}CH\text{-}COOH$ $\quad\vert$ $\quad S$ $\quad\vert$ $CH_3\text{-}CH\text{-}COOH$	4.57*	97
$CH_3\text{-}CH\text{-}COOH$ $\quad\vert$ $\quad S\text{-}S$ $\quad\vert$ $CH_3\text{-}CH\text{-}COOH$	3.14*	97
$CH_3\text{-}CH\text{-}COOH$ $\quad\vert$ $\quad S\text{-}S$ $\quad\vert$ $COOH\text{-}CH\text{-}CH_3$	3.15*	97
$HOOC(CH_2)_9S(CH_2)_2\text{-}NH_2$	4.00*, 8.30*	97
$HOOC(CH_2)_{10}S(CH_2)_2\text{-}NH_2$	2.6*, 9.6*	97
$CH_3SO_2CH(CH_3)COOH$	2.44*	97

UNSATURATED ACIDS, CIS AND TRANS

$$R_1CH=CR_2COOH$$

R_1	R_2	*cis*-Acid	*trans*-Acid	Reference
H-	H-	4.25*	4.25*	2
CH_3-	H-	4.44*	4.69*	2
Cl-	H-	3.32	3.65	2
C_6H_5-	H-	3.88*	4.44*	2
$o\text{-}ClC_6H_4$-	H-	3.91	4.41	2
$o\text{-}BrC_6H_4$-	H-	4.02	4.41	2
CH_3-	CH_3-	4.30	5.02	2
C_6H_5-	H-	5.26†	5.58†	2
$2,4,6\text{-}(CH_3)_3\text{-}C_6H_2$-	H-	6.12†	5.70†	2
C_6H_5-	CH_3-	4.98†	5.98†	2

* Thermodynamic value.

CARBOXYLIC ACIDS (Continued)

Compound	pK_a	Reference
UNSATURATED DICARBOXYLIC ACIDS*		
Acetylenediacrboxylic	1.73, 4.40	2
Bromofumaric	1.46, 3.57	2
Bromomaleic	1.45, 4.62	2
Chlorofumaric	1.78, 3.81	2
Chloromaleic	1.72, 3.86	2
Citraconic (Dimethylmaleic acid)	2.29, 6.15	2
Fumaric	3.02, 4.38	2
Itaconic (I-Propene-2,3-dicarboxylic acid)	3.85, 5.45	2
Maleic	1.92, 6.23	2
Mesaconic (Dimethylfumaric acid)	3.09, 4.75	2
Phthalic	2.95, 5.41	2
Δ^1-Tetrahydrophthalic	3.01, 5.34	2
ALICYCLIC DICARBOXYLIC ACIDS		
cis-Caronic (1,1-dimethylcyclopropane-2,3-dicarboxylic acid)	2.34*, 8.31*	2
trans-Caronic	3.83*, 5.32*	2
1,2-(trans-Cyclopropanedicarboxylic	3.65*, 5.13*	2
1,2-cis-Cyclopropanedicarboxylic	3.33*, 6.47*	2
trans-Ethyleneoxide-dicarboxylic	1.93, 3.25	2
1,2-trans-Cyclobutanedicarboxylic	3.94, 5.55	132
1,3-trans-Cyclobutanedicarboxylic	3.81, 5.28	2
1,2-trans-Cyclopentanedicarboxylic	3.89, 5.91	2
1,3-trans-Cyclopentanedicarboxylic	4.40, 5.45	2
1,2-trans-Cyclohexanedicarboxylic	4.18, 5.93	2
1,3-trans-Cyclohexanedicarboxylic	4.31, 5.73	2
1,4-trans-Cyclohexanedicarboxylic	4.18, 5.42	2
cis-Ethyleneoxidedicarboxylic	1.94, 3.92	2
1,2-cis-Cyclobutanedicarboxylic	4.16, 6.23	132
1,3-cis-Cyclobutanedicarboxylic	4.03, 5.31	2
1,2-cis-Cyclopentanedicarboxylic	4.37, 6.51	2
1,3-cis-Cyclopentanedicarboxylic	4.23, 5.53	2
1,2-cis-Cyclohexanedicarboxylic	4.34, 6.76	2
1,3-cis-Cyclohexanedicarboxylic	4.10, 5.46	2
1,4-cis-Cyclohexanedicarboxylic	4.44, 5.79	2
HYDROXYCYCLOHEXANECARBOXYLIC ACIDS		
Cyclohexanecarboxylic	4.90	2
cis-1,2-	4.80	2
cis-1,3-	4.60	2
cis-1,4-	4.84	2
trans-1,2-	4.68	2
trans-1,3-	4.82	2
trans-1,4-	4.68	2
BICYCLO(2.2.2)OCTANE-1-CARBOXYLIC ACIDS, 4-SUBSTITUTED		
H-	6.75	2
$C_2H_5O_2C$-	6.31	2
NC-	5.90	2
HO-	6.33	2
Br-	6.08	2
DICARBOXYLIC ACIDS AND DERIVATIVES*		
Oxalic	1.23, 4.19	2
Malonic	2.83, 5.69	2
Methyl-	3.05, 5.76	2
Ethyl-	2.99, 5.83	2
Ethylisoamyl-	2.50, 7.31	129
n-Propyl-	3.00, 5.84	2
i-Propyl-	2.94, 5.88	2
Dimethyl-	3.17, 6.06	2
Methylethyl-	2.86, 6.41	2
Diethyl-	2.21, 7.29	2

Compound	pK_a	Reference
DICARBOXYLIC ACIDS AND DERIVATIVES* (Continued)		
Diisopropyl-	2.12, 8.85	136
Ethyl-n-propyl-	2.15, 7.43	2
Di-n-propyl-	2.07, 7.51	2
Glutaric	4.34, 5.42	2
β-Methyl-	4.25, 6.22	2
β-Ethyl-	4.29, 6.33	2
β-Isopropyl-	4.30, 5.51	129
β-n-Propyl-	4.31. 6.39	2
β,β-Dimethyl-	3.70, 6.29	2
β,β -Methylethyl-	3.62, 6.70	2
β,β-Diethyl-	3.62, 7.12	2
β,β-Di-n-propyl-	3.69, 7.31	2
β,β-Pentamethylene-	3.49, 6.96	129
Succinic	4.19, 5.48	2
Methyl-	4.07, 5.64	101
Ethyl-	4.07, 5.89	101
Tetramethyl-	3.50, 7.28	2
DL-1:2-Dichloro-	1.68, 3.18	20
meso-1:2-Dichloro-	1.74, 3.24	20
DL-1:2-Dibromo-	1.48	20
meso-1:2-Dibromo-	1.42, 2.97	20
DL-1:2-Dimethyl-	3.93, 6.00	20
meso-1:2-Dimethyl-	3.77, 5.36	20
D-Tartaric	3.03, 4.45	20
meso-Tartaric	3.29, 4.92	20
Adipic	4.42, 5.41	2
Pimelic	4.48, 5.42	2
Suberic	4.52, 5.40	2
Azelaic	4.55, 5.41	2
LYSERGIC ACID AND DERIVATIVES		
Ergometrine	6.8	2
Ergometrinine	7.3	2
Dihydroergometrine	7.4	2
α-Dihydrolysergol	8.3	2
β-Dihydrolysergol	8.2	2
6-Methylergoline	8.85	2
Lysergic acid	7.8, 3.3	2
Isolysergic acid	8.4, 3.4	2
α-Dihydrolysergic	8.3, 3.6	2
γ-Dihydrolysergic	8.6, 3.6	2
For complex chelating agents, see also Ref. (84).		
AROMATIC		
Anthracene-1-COOH	3.69	2
Anthracene-9-COOH	3.65	2
2-Furan-COOH	3.16	153
3-Furan-COOH	3.95	153
Naphthalene-2-COOH	4.17	2
Naphthalene-1-COOH	3.69	2
Naphthol-1-COOH	9.85	153
Naphthol-2-COOH	9.63	153
1-Phenyl-5-methyl-1,2,3-triazole-4-COOH	3.73	126
1-Phenyl-1,2,3-triazole-4-COOH	2.88	126
1-Phenyl-1,2,3-triazole-4,5-(COOH)$_2$	2.13, 4.93	126
2-Pyrrole-COOH	4.45	153
2-Thiophen-COOH	3.53	153
3-Thiophen-COOH	4.10	153
1,2,3-Triazole-4-COOH	3.22, 8.73	126
1,2,3-Triazole-4,5-(COOH)$_2$	1.86, 5.90, 9.30	126

* Thermodynamic value.

CARBOXYLIC ACIDS (Continued)

Benzoic Acid	ortho	meta	para	Reference	Compound	pK_a	Reference
		AROMATIC (Continued)				*ORTHO-SUBSTITUTED BENZOIC ACIDS*	
Substituted Benzoic Acids				2, 97, 100, 101	2-CH$_3$-	3.91*	2
					2-t-C$_4$H$_9$-	3.46	2
					2,6-(CH$_3$)$_2$-	3.21	2
H-	4.20*	—	—	—	2,3,4,6-(CH$_3$)$_4$-	4.00	2
O$_2$N-	2.17*	3.45*	3.44	—	2,3,5,6-(CH$_3$)$_4$-	3.52	2
CH$_3$CO-	4.14	3.83	3.70	—	2-C$_2$H$_5$-	3.77	2
CH$_3$SO$_2$-	—	3.64*	3.52*	—	2-C$_6$H$_5$-	3.46*	2
CH$_3$S-	—	5.53	5.74	—	2,4,6-(CH$_3$)$_3$-	3.43	2
HS-	5.02	5.42	5.56	—	2,3,4,5-(CH$_3$)$_4$-	4.22	2
Br-	2.85*	3.81*	4.00*	—	2,4-OH-	3.22*	97
F-	3.27*	3.87*	4.14*	—	2,6-OH-	1.22*	97
CH$_3$O-	4.09*	4.09*	4.47*	—			
n-C$_3$H$_7$O-	4.24*	4.20*	4.46*	—			
n-C$_4$H$_9$O-	—	4.25*	4.53*	—			
C$_6$H$_5$O-	3.53*	3.95*	4.52*	—			
CH$_3$-	3.91*	4.24*	4.34*	—			
(CH$_3$)$_2$CH-	—	—	4.35*	—			
(CH$_3$)$_3$N+-	1.37	3.45	3.43	—			
NC-	3.14*	3.60*	3.55*	—			
HO$_2$C-	2.95*	3.54	3.51	—			
F$_3$C-	—	3.79	—	—			
HO-	2.98*	4.08*	4.58*	—			
I-	2.86*	3.86*	3.93	—			
Cl-	2.94*	3.83*	3.99*	—			
(CH$_3$)$_3$Si-	—	4.24*	4.27*	—			
C$_2$H$_5$O-	4.21*	4.17*	4.45*	—			
i-C$_3$H$_7$O-	4.24*	4.15*	4.68*	—			
n-C$_5$H$_{11}$O-	—	—	4.55*	—			
C$_6$H$_5$-	3.46*	—	—	—			
CH$_3$CH$_2$-	3.77	—	4.35*	—			
(CH$_3$)$_3$C-	3.46	4.28	4.40*	—			
NH$_2$-	2.05*	3.07*	2.38*	—			
	4.95*	4.73*	4.89*	—			
SO$_2$NH$_2$-	—	3.54	3.47	—			
CH$_3$CO$_2$-	3.48	4.00	4.38	—			
CH$_3$CONH-	3.63	4.07	4.28	—			
-HO$_3$P-	3.78	4.03	3.95	—			
-O$_3$S-	—	4.15	4.11	—			
(CH$_3$)$_2$N-	8.42	5.10	5.03	—			
-HO$_3$As-	—	—	4.22	—			
-O$_2$C-	5.41	4.60	4.82	—			
CH$_3$NH-	5.33	5.10	5.04	—			

Acid	Position of Carboxyl	pK^I	pK^{II}	pK^{III}	pK^{IV}	pK^V	pK^{VI}
			BENZENE POLYCARBOXYLIC ACIDS (2)				
Benzoic	1	4.17*	—	—	—	—	—
Phthalic	1, 2	2.98*	5.28*	—	—	—	—
Isophthalic	1, 3	3.46*	4.46*	—	—	—	—
Terephthalic	1, 4	3.51*	4.82*	—	—	—	—
Hemimellitic	1, 2, 3	2.80*	4.20*	5.87*	—	—	—
Trimellitic	1, 2, 4	2.52*	3.84*	5.20*	—	—	—
Trimesic	1, 3, 5	3.12*	3.89*	4.70*	—	—	—
Mellophanic	1, 2, 3, 4	2.06*	3.25*	4.73*	6.21*	—	—
Prehnitic	1, 2, 3, 5	2.38*	3.51*	4.44*	5.81*	—	—
Pyromellitic	1, 2, 4, 5	1.92*	2.87*	4.49*	5.63*	—	—
Benzenepentacarboxylic	1, 2, 3, 4, 5	1.80*	2.73*	3.97*	5.25*	6.46*	—
Mellitic	1, 2, 3, 4, 5, 6	1.40*	2.19*	3.31*	4.78*	5.89*	6.96*

* Thermodynamic value.

PHENOLS

Phenol	ortho	meta	para	Reference
H-	9.95*	—	—	52, 97, 100, 153
(CH$_3$)$_3$N$^+$-	7.42	8	8	—
CH$_3$SO$_2$-	—	8.40	7.83	—
CH$_3$CO-	—	9.19	8.05	—
C$_2$H$_5$O$_2$C-	—	—	8.50*	—
C$_3$H$_5$CH$_2$O$_2$C-	—	—	8.41*	—
Br-	8.42*	9.11*	9.34	—
F-	8.81*	9.28*	9.95*	—
HO-	9.48	9.44	9.96	—
CH$_3$-	10.28*	10.08	10.19*	—
CH$_3$O-	9.93	9.65	10.20	—
-O$_2$C-	13.82	9.94*	9.39*	153
—O$_3$P-	—	10.2	9.9	—
C$_6$H$_5$-	9.93	9.59	9.51	—
O$_2$N-	7.23*	8.35*	7.14*	—
OCH-	6.79	8.00	7.66	—
NC-	—	8.61	7.95	—
CH$_3$O$_2$C-	—	—	8.47*	—
n-C$_4$H$_9$O$_2$C-	—	—	8.47*	—
I-	8.51	9.17*	9.31	—
Cl-	8.48*	9.02*	9.38*	—
CH$_3$S-	—	9.53	9.53	—
HOCH$_2$-	9.92*	9.83*	9.82*	—
C$_2$H$_5$-	10.2	9.9	10.0	—
H$_2$N-	9.71	9.87	10.30	—
-O$_3$S-	—	9.29	9.03	—
—O$_3$As-	—	—	8.37	—
NO-	—	—	6.35	—
H$_2$NCO-	8.37*	—	—	—

Name	pK$_a$	Reference
POLYSUBSTITUTED PHENOLS		
2,3-Dimethyl-	10.54	101
2,4-Dimethyl-	10.60	101
2,5-Dimethyl-	10.41	101
2,6-Dimethyl-	10.63	101
2,4,5-Trimethyl-	10.88	101
2,3,5-Trimethyl-	10.69	101

Name	pK$_a$	Reference
POLYSUBSTITUTED PHENOLS (Continued)		
3,4-Dimethyl-	10.36	101
3,5-Dimethyl-	10.19	101
2,4-Dichloro-	7.85	101
3-Chloro-2-nitro-	6.75	101
3-Chloro-4-nitro-	6.80	101
3-Bromo-2-nitro-	6.78	101
3-Bromo-4-nitro-	6.84	101
3-Iodo-2-nitro-	6.89	101
3-Iodo-4-nitro-	6.94	101
2,4-Dinitro-	4.11	101
2,5-Dinitro-	5.22	101
2,6-Dinitro-	5.23	101
3,4-Dinitro-	5.42	101
2,4,6-Trinitro-	0.96	101
2-Chloro-4-nitro-	5.45	79
2-Nitro-4-chloro-	6.46	79
2-OCH$_3$-4-CH$_2$CH=CH$_2$-	10.00*	97
2-OCH$_3$-4-OHC-	7.40*	97
2-OCH$_3$-6-OHC-	7.91*	97
2-OCH$_3$-5-OHC-	8.89*	97
Chromotropic acid	5.36, 15.6	6
2-Amino-4,5-dimethylphenol hydrochloride	10.4, 5.28	51
4,5-Dihydroxybenzene-1,3-disulfonic acid	7.66, 12.6	77
Kojic acid	9.40	77
Resorcinol	9.15 (30°)	50
3-Hydroxyanthranilic acid	10.09, 5.20	51
2-Aminophenol hydrochloride	9.99, 4.86	51
SUBSTITUTED CATECHOLS		
3-Nitro-	6.66	101
4-Nitro-	6.89	101
3,4-Dinitro-	4.39	101
4-Formyl-	7.36	101
4-Hydroxyiminomethyl-	8.68	101
3-Methyl-	9.28	101
3-Methoxy-	9.28	101
4-Benzoyl-	7.74	101
4-Cyano-	7.72	101

* Thermodynamic value.

ALCOHOLS AND OTHER OXYGEN ACIDS

ALCOHOLS, SIMPLE

Compound	pK_a	Reference
Choline	13.9	6
CF_3CH_2OH	12.43	63
$CF_3CH(OH)CH_3$	11.8	63
$C_3F_7CH_2OH$	11.4†	63
$(C_3F_7)_2CHOH$	10.6†	63
$CH{\equiv}CCH_2OH$	13.55	64
$C(CH_2OH)_4$	14.1	64
$CH_2OHCHOHCH_2OH$	14.4	64
CH_2OHCH_2OH	14.77	64
$CH_3OCH_2CH_2OH$	14.82	64
CH_3OH	15.54	64
$CH_2{=}CHCH_2OH$	~15.52	64
H_2O	15.74	64
CH_3CH_2OH	16	64
CCl_3CH_2OH	12.24	64
$CHF_2CH_2CH_2OH$	12.74	64
$CHCl_2CH_2OH$	12.89	64
CH_2ClCH_2OH	14.31	64
$CF_3C(CH_3)_2OH$	11.6	64
$HOCH_2CF_2CF_2CH_2OH$	11	64
$C_3F_7CH(C_2F_5)OH$	10.48	65
$(C_3F_7)_2CHOH$	10.52	65
$(CF_3)_2CHOH$	9.3	108
$(CF_3)_3COH$	5.4	108
$(CF_3)C(OH)CF_2NO$	3.9	108
$(CF_3)_2C(CH_3)OH$	9.6	122
$(CF_3)_2CHOH$	9.3	122
$(CF_3)_2C(CClF_2)OH$	5.3	122
$(CF_3)_2C(CCl_3)OH$	5.1	122
F_2CHCH_2OH	13.11	142
FCH_2CH_2OH	14.20	142
Br_3CCH_2OH	12.70	142
Br_2CHCH_2OH	13.29	142
$BrCH_2CH_2OH$	14.38	142
ICH_2CH_2OH	14.56	142
$NCCH_2CH_2OH$	14.03	142
$C_2H_5OCH_2CH_2OH$	14.98	142
$C_6H_5OCH_2CH_2OH$	14.60	142
$C_6H_5CH_2CH_2OH$	15.48	142
$HOCH_2CH_2OH$	15.11	142
$C_2H_5CH_2OH$	15.92	142
$C_3H_7CH_2OH$	15.87	142
$i\text{-}C_3H_7CH_2OH$	15.91	142
$(CH_3)_3CCH_2OH$	16.04	142
$CH_3C{\equiv}CCH_2OH$	14.16	142
$C_6H_5C{\equiv}CCH_2OH$	13.87	142
$CH_2{=}CHCH_2OH$	15.48	142
$CH_3CH{=}CHCH_2OH$	15.80	142
$C_6H_5CH{=}CHCH_2OH$	15.62	142
$C_6H_5CH_2OH$	15.44	142
$3,5\text{-}Di\text{-}NO_2C_6H_3CH_2OH$	14.43	142
$OHCCH_2OH$	14.80	142
CH_3COCH_2OH	14.19	142
$C_6H_5COCH_2OH$	13.33	142

HYDROXAMIC ACIDS

Compound	pK_a	Reference
Aceto-	9.40	68
o-Aminobenzo-	9.17	93
p-Aminobenzo-	9.32	93
Benzo-	8.88	68
n-Butyro-	9.48	68
Chloroaceto-	8.40	93
p-Chlorobenzo-	9.59	68
p-Chlorophenoxyaceto-	8.75	93
Cyclohexano-	9.75	93
Formo-	8.65	93
Furo-	8.45	72
Glycine-	7.40	72
Hexano-	9.75	93
Hippuro-	8.80	72
p-Hydroxybenzo-	8.93	93
N-Hydroxyphthalimide	7.00, 6.10	71, 72
Indole-3-aceto-	9.58	93
L-Lacto-	9.35	93
D-Lysine-	7.93	93
L-Lysine-	7.93	93
p-Methylbenzo-	8.90	72
p-Methoxybenzo-	9.00	68
α-Naphtho-	~7.7	68
Nicotin-	8.30	72
isoNicotin-	7.85	72
Nicotin-methiodide	6.46	72
m-Nitrobenzo-	8.07	72
p-Nitrobenzo-	8.01	93
Phenylaceto	9.19	68
N-Phenylbenzo-	9.15	93
N-Phenylnicotino-	8.00	93
Phthalo-	9.48	93
Picolin-	8.50	72
Propiono-	9.46	68
Pyrimidine-2-carbox-	7.88	72
Salicyl-	7.43	72
Tropo-	9.09	72
L-Tyrosine	9.20	93

OXIMES

Compound	pK_a	Reference
Acet-	12.42	18
Acetophenone	11.48	18
Benzophenone	11.3	18
Benzoquinoline mon-	6.25	93
1,2,3-Cyclohexanetrionetri-	8.0	76
Diethyl ket-	12.6	18
Isonitrosoacetone (INA)	8.3	76
Isonitrosoacetylacetone (INAA)	7.4	76
5-Methyl-1,2,3-cyclohexanetrione-1,3-di-	8.3	76
5-Methyl-1,2,3-cyclohexanetrionetri-	8.0	76
Phenylglyoxald-	8.30	93
Pyridine-2-ald-	3.56*, 10.17*	99
Pyridine-3-ald-	3.94*, 10.32*	99
Pyridine-4-ald-	4.58*, 9.91*	99
Pyridine-4-aldoxime dodeciodide	8.50	93
Pyridine-2-aldoxime heptiodide	8.00	93
Pyridine-2-aldoxime methiodide	8.00	93
Pyridine-3-aldoxime methiodide	9.20	93
Pyridine-4-aldoxime methiodide	8.50	93
Pyridine-4-aldoxime pentiodide	8.50	93
3-Pyridine-1,2-ethanedione-2-oxime methiodide	7.20	93
4-Pyridine-1,2-ethanedione-2-oxime methiodide	7.10	93

Substituted Triphenylmethanols in

CARBONIUM IONS

Substituted Triphenylmethanols	H_2SO_4	$HClO_4$	HNO_3	Ref. 66
4,4′,4″-Trimethoxy-	0.82	0.82	0.80	
4,4′-Dimethoxy-	−1.24	−1.14	−1.11	
4-Methoxy-	−3.40	−3.56	−3.41	
4-Methyl-	−5.41	−5.67	—	
4-Trideuteriomethyl-	−5.43	−5.67	—	
3,3′,3″-Trimethyl-	−6.35	−5.95	—	
Unsubstituted triphenylmethanol	−6.63	−6.89	−6.60	
4,4′,4″-Trichloro-	−7.74	−8.01	—	
4-Nitro-	−9.15	−9.76	—	

* Thermodynamic value.
† 50% aqueous methanol.

ALCOHOLS AND OTHER OXYGEN ACIDS (Continued)

PEROXIDES, ROOH

R=	H	CH_3	C_2H_5	iso-C_3H_7	$tert$-C_4H_9	iso-C_4H_9	Reference
	11.6	11.5	11.8	12.1	12.8	12.8	70

Compound	pK'_a	Reference
	PEROXY ACIDS	
Acetic	8.2	70
n-Butyric	8.2	70
Formic	7.1	70
Peroxydiphosphoric	5.18, 7.68	85
Peroxymonophosphoric	4.85	90
Peroxymonosulfuric	9.4	69
Propionic	8.1	70

X	2—	3—	4—
	PYRIDINE 1-OXIDES AND DERIVATIVES (Ref. 99, 47, 67)		
H-	0.79	—	—
CH_3CONH-	−0.42*	0.99*	1.59*
H_2N-	2.67*	1.47*	3.59*
$C_6H_5CH_2S$-	−0.23*	—	2.09*
HOOC-	—	0.09	−0.48
	—	2.73*	2.86*
$(CH_3)_2N$-	2.27*	—	3.88*
HO-	5.97*	—	5.76*
CH_3O-	1.23*	—	2.05*
CH_3NH-	2.61*	—	3.85*
C_6H_5-	0.77*	0.74*	0.83*
CH_3-	2.61*	1.08*	1.29*
C_2H_5O-	1.18*	—	—
$C_6H_5CH_2O$-	—	—	1.99
NO_2-	—	—	−1.7
$COOC_4H_9$-	—	0.03	—

PYRIDINE 1-OXIDES AND DERIVATIVES

2-Amino-1-methoxypyridinium perchlorate	12.4	67
4-Amino-1-methoxypyridinium perchlorate	>11	67
1-Benzyloxypyrid-2-one	−1.7	67
1-Benzyloxypyrid-4-one	2.58	67
4-Dimethylamino-1-methoxypyridinium perchlorate	>11	67
2-Methylamino-1-methoxypyridinium toluene-p-sulfonate	>11	67
1-Methoxypyrid-2-one	−1.3	67
1-Methoxypyrid-4-one	2.57	67
3-R-Pyrazine-1-Oxides		
R=CN—	−1.12	121
Cl—	−1.05	121
CH_3O—	−0.45	121

* Thermodynamic value.

Compound	pK'_a	Reference
PYRIDINE 1-OXIDES AND DERIVATIVES (Continued)		
NH_2—	−1.92, 1.50	121
H—	0.05	121
CH_3—	0.46	121
$(CH_3)_2N$—	−1.77, 1.34	121
N (ring)	−1.80, 1.34	121
SULFINIC ACIDS		
Benzene-	1.84, 2.16	73
p-Bromobenzene-	1.89	73
p-Chlorobenzene-	1.81	73
m-Nitrobenzene-	1.88	73
p-Nitrobenzene-	1.86	73
p-Toluene-	1.99	73
OTHER OXYGEN ACIDS		
CF_3CH_2NHOH	11.3	108
$(CF_3)_2CHNHOH$	8.5	108
$(CF_3)_3CNHOH$	5.9	108
CF_3CHNOH	8.9	108
$(CF_3)_2CNOH$	6.0	108
Glutaconic dialdehyde	5.75	153
Hydroxylamine	13.7	133
Mannitol	13.5	100
Sucrose	12.7	100
Phenylboric acid	8.86	100
Pyridine-4-aldehyde	12.20	153
β-Phenylethylboric acid	10	100
Lyxose	12.11	25
Ribose	12.11	25
2-Deoxyribose	12.61	25
Xylose	12.15	25
Arabinose	12.34	25
Fructose	12.03	25
2-Deoxyglucose	12.52	25
Galactose	12.35	25
$(CF_3)_2C(OH)_2$	6.58	108
$(CF_2Cl)_2C(OH)_2$	6.67	108
$(CF_2H)_2C(OH)_2$	8.79	108
$CF_2ClCF_2HC(OH)_2$	7.90	108
Trimethylamine-N-oxide	4.6	18
Triethylamine-N-oxide	5.13*	99
Acetaldehyde hydrate	13.48	91
Formaldehyde hydrate	13.29	91
Glucose	12.43*	97
Mannose	13.50*	97
Sorbose	13.57	97
Acetamide-H+	−0.025	149, 150
Chloroacetamide-H+	−0.26	149, 150
Dichloroacetamide-H	−0.26	149, 150
N-Methylacetamide-H+	0.26	149, 150
N,N-Dimethylacetamide-H+	0.62	149, 150
Biotin-H+	−1.13	149, 150
Desthiobiotin-H+	−0.97	149, 150
Dimethylurea-H+	−0.20	149, 150
Formamide-H+	0.12	149, 150
N,N-Diethylformamide-H+	0.36	149, 150
N,N-Dimethylformamide-H+	0.18	149, 150
N-Methylformamide-H+	0.52	149, 150
Imidazolidone-H+	−1.05	149, 150
$(CH_3)_2CHCH(OH)_2$	13.77	160
$CH_3CH(OH)_2$	13.57	160
$CH_2(OH)_2$	13.27	160
$CF_3CH(OH)_2$	10.20	160
$CCl_3CH(OH)_2$	10.04	160
$C_6H_5C(OH)_2CF_3$	10.00	160

AMINO ACIDS

Compound	pK_a	Reference	Compound	pK_a	Reference
Alanine	2.34, 9.69	6	**4-Aminophenylacetic acid**	3.60, 5.26	99
N-Acetyl-	3.72	97	**2-Aminophenylarsonic acid**	3.77, 8.66	99
Amide	8.02*	99	**2-Aminophenylboric acid**	4.53, 9.31	99
3-(2-Aminoethyldithio)-	8.28, 9.30	99	**β-Aminopropionic acid**	3.55*, 10.23*	97
Carbamyl-	3.89	99	**4-Aminosalicylic acid**	1.78, 3.63	99
N-Ethyl-	2.22, 10.22	99	α-Aminotricarballylic acid	2.10, 3.60, 4.60, 9.82	99
N-Methyl-	2.22, 10.19	99	α-Aminovaleric acid	4.20	130
N-n-Propyl-	2.21, 10.19	99	2-Anilinoethylsulfonic acid	3.80	99
β-(2-Pyridyl)-	1.37, 4.02, 9.22	99	**Arginine**	12.48, 2.17, 9.04	6
β-(3-Pyridyl)-	1.77, 4.64, 9.10	99	**Argininosuccinic acid**	>12, 1.62, 9.58, 2.70, 4.26	—
β-(4-Pyridyl)-	4.85	99	**Asparagine**	2.02, 8.8	6
β-Alanine	3.60, 10.19	6	α-Hydroxy-	2.28, 7.20	99
N-Acetyl-	4.44	129	β-Hydroxy-	2.09, 8.29	99
Carbamyl-	4.49	129	**Aspartic acid**	2.09, 3.86, 9.82	99
Allothreonine	2.11, 9.01	99	Diamide	7.00	99
O-Methyl-	1.92, 8.90	99	Hydroxy-	1.91, 3.51, 9.11	99
γ-Aminoacetoacetic acid	2.9, 8.3	99	**Azaserine**	8.55	101
α-Aminoadipic acid	2.14, 4.21	101	m-Benzbetaine	3.22	99
2-Aminobenzoic acid	2.19, 4.95	99	f-Benzbetaine	3.25	99
N,N-Dimethyl-	1.4, 8.49	99	Betaine	1.84	99
3-Hydroxy-	5.19, 10.12	99	**γ-Butyrobetaine**	3.94	99
N-Methyl-	1.97, 5.34	99	**Canaline**	2.40-, 3.70, 9.20	99
3-Aminobenzoic acid	3.29, 5.10	99	**Canavanine**	2.50, 6.60, 9.25	99
4-Aminobenzoic acid	2.50, 4.87	99	L-**Citrulline**	2.43, 9.41	99
4-Aminobutylphosphonic acid	2.55, 7.55, 10.9	99	**Creatine**	2.67, 11.02	6
4-Aminobutylsulphonic acid	10.65	99	**Creatinine**	4.84, 9.2	6
α-Aminobutyric acid	2.55, 9.60	6	**Cycloserine**	4.4, 7.4	101
Carbamoyl-α-amino-n-butyric	3.89	129	**Cysteine**	10.78, 1.71, 8.33	6
γ-Aminobutyric acid	4.23, 10.43	6	Ethyl ester	6.69, 9.17	99
Carbamyl-	4.68	129	Methyl ester	6.56, 8.99	99
2-Aminobutyric acid	2.27, 9.68	99	S-Ethyl-	1.94, 8.69	99
α-Amino-n-caproic acid	2.33	129	S-Methyl-	8.75	99
ε-Aminocaproic acid	4.37	129	**Cystine**	1.65, 7.85	6
10-Aminodecylphosphonic acid	8.0, 11.25	99	L-**Cystine diamide**	5.93, 6.90	99
10-Aminodecylsulphonic acid	11.35	99	**2,4-Diaminobutyric acid**	1.85, 8.28, 10.50	99
10-Amino-n-dodecanoic acid	4.648	99	**2,3-Diaminopropionic acid**	1.23, 6.73, 9.56	99
Aminoethylphosphoric acid	2.45, 7.0, 10.8	99	**2,7-Diaminosuberic acid**	1.84, 2.64, 9.23, 9.89	99
2-Aminoethylsulphoric acid	8.95	99	**3-Dimethylaminopropionic acid**	9.85	99
ω-Aminoheptanoic acid	4.50	136	**Formamidinoglutaric acid**	2.7, 4.4, 11.3	99
6-Aminohexanoic acid	4.37, 10.81	99	**Formamidinoacetic acid**	2.6, 11.5	99
α-Aminoisobutyric acid	2.36, 10.21	6	**Glutamic acid**	2.19, 4.25, 9.67	6
Carbamyl-	4.46	129	Diethyl ester	7.04	99
α-Aminoisocaproic acid	2.33	129	γ-Monobenzyl ester	2.17, 9.00	99
α-Aminoisovaleric acid	2.29	129	α-Monoethyl ester	3.85, 7.84	99
δ-Aminolaevulinic acid	4.05, 8.90	99	γ-Monoethyl ester	2.15, 9.19	99
Aminomethylphosphonic acid	2.35, 5.9	99	**Glutamine**	2.17, 9.13	6
Aminomethylsulfonic acid	5.75	99	**Glycine**	2.34, 9.6	6
α-Amino-β-methyl-n-valeric acid	2.32	129	N-Acetyl-	3.67	99
1-Aminonaphthalene-2-sulfonic acid	1.71	99	N,N-Bis(2-hydroxyethyl)-	2.50, 8.11	99
2-Aminonaphthalene-1-sulfonic acid	2.35	99	N-n-Butyl-	2.35, 10.25	99
3-Amino-1-naphthoic acid	2.61, 4.39	99	Carbamyl-	3.88*	97
4-Aminopentanoic acid	3.97, 10.46	99	Chloroacetyl-	3.38*	97
5-Aminopentylsulfonic acid	10.95	99			

* Thermodynamic value.

AMINO ACIDS (Continued)

Compound	pK_a	Reference	Compound	pK_a	Reference
N,N-Diethyl-	2.04, 10.47	99	*o*-Fluoro-	2.12*, 9.01*	97
Dihydroxyethyl-	8.08*	97	*m*-Fluoro-	2.10*, 8.98*	97
N,N-Dimethyl-	2.08–, 9.80	99	*p*-Fluoro-	2.13*, 9.05*	97
N-Ethyl-	2.34*, 10.23	99	*p*-HOSO$_2$NH-	1.99*, 8.64*, 10.26*	97
Ethyl ester	7.83	99	α-Methyl-	9.57	99
Formyl-	3.43*	97	Methyl ester	7.00	99
N-Isobutyl-	2.35, 10.12	99	**Phenylglycine**	1.83, 4.39	99
Methyl ester	7.73	99	*m*-Chloro-	1.05, 3.93	99
Histamine	5.0, 9.7	6	*p*-Chloro-	1.46, 4.04	99
Histidine	6.0, 1.82, 9.17	6	*m*-Cyano-	0.28, 3.78	99
Amide	5.78, 7.64	99	*m*-Methyl-	1.89, 4.60	99
2-Mercapto-	1.84, 8.47, 11.4	99	*p*-Methyl-	1.97, 4.85	99
1-Methyl-	6.58, 8.60	99	**Proline**	1.99, 10.60	6
2-Methyl-	1.7, 7.2, 9.5	99	**2-Pyrrolidone-5-carboxylic acid**	3.32	6
Methyl ester	7.33, 5.38	99	(glutamic acid)		
Homocysteine	2.22, 8.87	101	**Sarcosine**	2.23, 10.01	6
β-Hydroxyglutamate	2.27, 4.29, 9.66	99	Amide	8.31*	99
N-Hydroxyethylethylenediamine- triacetic acid			*N*-Dimethylamide	8.82*	99
			N-Methylamide	8.24*	99
Hydroxylysine	2.13, 8.62, 9.67	6	**Serine**	2.21, 9.15	6
Hydroxyproline	1.92, 9.73	6	Amide	7.30	99
Imidazolelactic acid	2.96, 7.35	99	Methyl ester	7.10	99
Isoasparagine	2.97, 8.02	99	**Taurine**	1.5, 8.74	6
N-Acetyl-	3.99	151	**Thiolhistidine**	<1.5, 11.4, 1.84, 8.47	6
N-Carbobenzoxy-	4.05	151	**Threonine**	2.63, 10.43	6
Isocreatine	2.84	99	*O*-Methyl-	2.02, 9.00	101
Isoglutamine	3.81, 7.88	99	**5,5,5-Trifluoroleucine**	2.05, 8.92	111
N-Acetyl-	4.34	151	**6,6,6-Trifluoronorleucine**	2.164, 9.46	111
N-Carbobenzoxy-	4.39	151	**4,4,4-Trifluorothreonine**	1.55, 7.82	111
Isoleucine	2.36, 9.68	6	**4,4,4-Trifluorovaline**	1.54, 8.10	111
Isoserine	2.72, 9.33	99	**Tryptophan**	2.38, 9.39	6
Leucine	2.36, 9.60	6	Amide	7.5	99
Amide	7.80	99	**Tyrosine**	10.07, 2.20, 9.11	6
Ethyl ester	7.57	99	Amide	7.48, 9.89	99
Lombricine	8.9	99	3,5-Dibromo-	2.17, 6.45, 7.60	99
Lysine	2.18, 8.95	6	3,5-Dichloro-	2.22, 6.47, 7.62	99
Hydroxy-	2.13, 8.62, 9.67	99	Diiodo-	6.48, 2.12, 7.82	6
Methionine	2.28, 9.21	6	Ethyl ester	7.33, 9.80	22
Amide	7.53	99	*O*-Methyl-	9.27	21
N-Methylaminodiacetic acid	2.15	129	*O*-Methyl, ethyl ester	7.31	22
Nitrilotriacetic acid	1.88, 2.48, 4.28	129	*N*-Trimethyl-	9.75	21
Norleucine	2.39, 9.76	6	**Urocanic acid**	5.8, 3.5	—
Norvaline	2.30, 9.78	99	**Valine**	2.32, 9.62	6
Octopine	1.40, 2.30, 8.72, 11.34	99	Amide	8.00	99
Ornithine	1.71, 8.69	6	Hydroxy-	2.55, 9.77	99
Phenylalanine	1.83, 9.13	6	β-Mercapto-	2.0, 8.0, 10.5	99
Amide	7.22	99	CH$_3$CH$_2$OCONHCH$_2$COOH	3.66*	97
o-Chloro-	2.23, 8.94	99	CH$_3$CONH(CH$_2$)$_2$COOH	4.45	97
m-Chloro-	2.17, 8.91	99	NH$_2$CONH(CH$_2$)$_2$COOH	4.49	97
p-Chloro-	2.08, 8.96	99	DL-CH$_3$CH$_2$CH(NH$_2$)COOH	2.29, 9.83	97
3,4-Dihydroxy-	2.32*, 8.68*, 9.88*	97	CH$_3$CONHCH(CH$_2$CH$_3$)COOH	3.72	97
2,4-Diiodo-3-hydroxy-	2.12*, 6.48*, 7.82*	97	NH$_2$CONHCH(CH$_2$CH$_3$)COOH	3.89	97
			NH$_2$CONH(CH$_2$)$_3$COOH	4.68	97
			(CH$_3$)$_2$C(NH$_2$)COOH	2.36*, 10.205*	97
			NH$_2$CONHCH(CH$_3$)$_2$COOH	4.46	97
			DL-CH$_3$(CH$_2$)$_2$CH(NH$_2$)COOH	4.36*, 9.72*	97
			CH$_3$CH$_2$CH(NH$_2$)CH$_2$COOH	4.02*, 10.40*	97

* Thermodynamic value.

AMINO ACIDS (Continued)

Compound	pK'_a	Reference	Compound	pK_a	Reference
$NH_2(CH_2)_4COOH$	4.20*, 10.69*	97	$(COOHCH_2CH_2)_2N(CH_2)_2N(CH_2CH_2COOH)$	3.00*, 3.43*, 6.77*, 9.60*	97
DL-$(CH_3)_2CHCH(NH_2)COOH$	2.29, 9.74	97	NH_2COCH_2COOH	3.64*	97
$NH_2(CH_2)_5COOH$	4.43*, 10.75*	97	$NH_2CO(CH_2)_2COOH$	4.54*	97
$NH_2(CH_2)_{11}COOH$	4.65*	97	$NH_2CO(CH_2)_3COOH$	4.60*	97
$NH_2(CH_2)_3CH(NH_2)COOH$	1.94*, 8.65*, 10.76*	97	$NH_2CO(CH_2)_4COOH$	4.63*	97
$NH_2CONH(CH_2)_3CH(NH_2)COOH$	2.43*, 9.41*	97			
$COOH(CH_2)_2CH(NH_2)COOCH_2CH_3$	3.85*, 7.84*	97	Oxyproline	1.92*, 9.73*	97
$CH_3CH_2OCO(CH_2)_2CH(NH_2)COOH$	2.15*, 9.19*	97			
$COOHCH_2NHCH_2COOH$	2.54*, 9.12*	97			
$COOHCH_2N(CH_3)CH_2COOH$	2.15*, 10.09*	97	$COOHCH_2CH(OH)CH(NH_2)COOH$	2.32*, 4.23*, 9.56*	97
$N(CH_2COOH)_3$	2.96*, 10.23	97	$CH_3CH_2SCH_2CH(NH_2)COOH$	2.03*, 8.60*	97
$COOH(CH_2)_2NHCH_2COOH$	3.61*, 9.46*	97	$CF_3(CH_2)_3CH(NH_2)COOH$	2.16*, 9.46*	97
$COOH(CH_2)_2NH(CH_2)_2COOH$	4.11*, 9.61*	97	$CF_3CH(CH_3)CH_2CH(NH_2)COOH$	2.05*, 8.94*	97
$COOHCH_2NH(CH_2)_2NHCH_2COOH$	6.42*, 9.46*	97	$CF_3(CH_2)_2CH(NH_2)COOH$	2.04*, 8.92*	97
$(CH_3)_2N(CH_2)_2N(CH_2COOH)_2$	6.05*, 10.07*	97	$CF_3CH(CH_3)CH(NH_2)COOH$	1.54*, 8.10*	97
$(COOHCH_2)_2N(CH_2)_2N(CH_2COOH)_2$	6.27*, 10.95*	97	$CF_3CH_2CH(NH_2)COOH$	1.60*, 8.17*	97
$COOH(CH_2)_2N(CH_2COOH)$ $(CH_2)_2N(CH_2COOH(CH_2)_2COOH$	3.00*, 3.79*, 5.98*, 9.83*	97	$CF_3CH(OH)CH(NH_2)COOH$	1.55*, 7.82*	97
			$CF_3CH(NH_2)CH_2COOH$	2.76*, 5.82*	97
$COOH(CH_2)_2NH(CH_2)_2NH(CH_2)_2\ COOH$	6.87*, 9.60*	97			

* Thermodynamic value.

PEPTIDES

Compound	pK'$_a$	Reference	Compound	pK'$_a$	Reference
Ala-Ala-(LD)	3.12, 8.30	27	Gly-Ala-Ala-Gly	3.30, 7.93	99
Ala-Ala-(LL)	3.30, 8.14	27	Gly-Asp	2.81, 4.45, 8.60	99
Ala-Ala-Ala-(3D)	3.39, 8.06	27	Gly-asparagine	2.82, 7.20	99
Ala-Ala-Ala-(DLL)	3.37, 8.06	27	Gly-Gly	3.06, 8.13	6
Ala-Ala-Ala-Ala-(DLLL)	3.42, 7.99	27	Gly-Gly-cystine	2.71, 7.94	99
Ala-Ala-Ala-(3L)	3.39, 8.03	27	Gly-Gly-Gly	3.26, 7.91	23
Ala-Ala-Ala-Ala-(4L)	3.42, 7.94	27	Gly-His	6.79, 8.20	99
Ala-Ala-Ala-(LDL)	3.31, 8.13	27	Gly-Leu	3.10, 8.41	99
Ala-Ala-Ala-Ala-(LDLL)	3.22, 7.99	27	Gly-Pro	2.81, 8.65	99
Ala-Ala-Ala-(LLD)	3.37, 8.05	27	Gly-sarcosine	2.98, 8.57	99
Ala-Ala-Ala-Ala-(LLDL)	3.24, 7.93	27	Gly-Ser	2.92, 8.10	99
Ala-Gly	3.16, 8.24	27	Gly-Ser-Gly	3.23, 7.99	99
Ala-Gly-Gly	3.19, 8.15	99	Gly-Trp	8.06	99
Ala-Lys-Ala-(3L)	3.15, 7.65, 10.30	27	Gly-Tyr	2.93, 8.45, 10.49	99
Ala-Lys-Ala-(LDL)	3.33, 7.97, 10.36	27	Gly-Val	3.15, 8.18	99
Ala-Lys-Ala-(LDLL)	3.32, 8.01, 10.37	27	His-Gly	2.36, 6.27, 8.57	99
Ala-Lys-Ala-(LLD)	3.29, 7.84, 10.49	27	His-His	5.54, 6.80, 7.82	99
Ala-Lys-Ala-Ala-(4L)	3.58, 8.01, 10.58	27	Leu-asparagine	2.83, 8.23	99
Ala-Lys-Ala-Ala-Ala-(5L)	3.53, 7.75, 10.35	27	Leu-Tyr	2.87, 8.36, 10.28	99
Ala-Lys-Ala-Ala-Ala-(LDLLL)	3.30, 7.85, 10.29	27	Lys-Ala-(LD)	3.00, 7.74, 10.63	27
β-Ala-1-methylhistidine	2.64, 7.04, 9.49	99	Lys-Ala-(LL)	3.22, 7.62, 10.70	27
Ala-Pro	3.04, 8.38	99	Lys-Glu	2.98, 4.47, 8.45, 11.30	99
β-Ala-Bis	2.73, 6.87, 9.73	99	Lys-Lys-(LD)	2.85, 7.53, 9.92, 10.98	27
Anserine	7.0, 2.65, 9.5	6	Lys-Lys-(LL)	3.01, 7.53, 10.05, 11.01	27
Asparaginyl-Gly	2.90, 7.25	99	Lys-Lys-Lys-(3L)	3.08, 7.34, 9.80, 10.54, 11.32	27
Asp-Asp	2.70, 3.40, 4.70, 8.26	99	Lys-Lys-Lys-(LDD)	2.94, 7.14, 9.60, 10.38, 11.09	27
α-Aspartyl-histidine	2.45, 3.02, 6.82, 7.98	99	Lys-Lys-Lys-(LDL)	2.91, 7.29, 9.79, 10.54, 11.42	27
β-Aspartyl-histidine	1.93, 2.95, 6.93, 8.72	99	Met-Met	2.22, 9.27	99
Asp-Gly	2.10, 4.53, 9.07	99	Methyl-Leu-Gly	3.29, 7.82	99
Asp-Tyr	2.13, 3.57, 8.92, 10.23	99	Phe-Ala-Arg	2.60, 7.54, 12.43	99
Carnosine	6.83, 9.51	6	Phe-Gly	3.13, 7.62	99
Cys-Cys	2.65, 7.27, 9.35, 10.85	99	Phenylalanylglycine amide	6.72	99
Cys-Gly-Gly	3.13, 6.36, 6.95	99	Pro-Gly	3.19, 8.97	99
Cys-Gly-Gly-Gly-Gly	3.21, 6.01, 6.87	99	Sarcosyl-Gly	3.14, 8.66	99
L-Cystinylcystine	1.87, 2.94, 6.53, 7.66	99	Sarcosyl-Leu	3.15, 8.67	99
N,N-Dimethylglycyl-glycine	3.11, 8.09	99	Sarcosylsarcosine	2.89, 9.18	99
N,N-Dimethyl-leucyl-glycine	7.78	99	Ser-Gly	3.10, 7.33	99
Glutaminyl-glutamic acid	3.14, 4.38, 7.62	99	Ser-Leu	3.08, 7.45	99
Glutaminyl-glycine	3.15, 7.52	99	Tyr-Tyr	3.52, 7.68, 9.80, 10.26	99
Glutathione	3.59, 8.75, 9.65	77	Val-Gly	3.23, 8.00	99
Glutathione, oxidized	3.15, 4.03, 8.57, 9.54	77			
Gly-Ala (L), (D)	3.17, 8.23	27			
Gly-Ala-Ala (LD)	3.30, 8.17	27			
Gly-Ala-Ala (LL)	3.38, 8.10	27			

NITROGEN COMPOUNDS

X	XNH_3^+	$XCH_2NH_3^+$	$X(CH_2)_2NH_3^+$	$X(CH_2)_3NH_3^+$	$X(CH_2)_4NH_3^+$	$X(CH_2)_5NH_3^+$	Reference
			ALIPHATIC AMINES, SIMPLE				
Primary Amines							
H–	9.25*	10.64*	10.67*	10.58*	10.61*	10.63	2
HF_2C–	—	7.52	—	—	—	—	—
RO_2C–	—	7.75	9.13	9.71	10.15*	10.37	2
HO–	5.96*	—	9.50*	—	—	—	—
C_6H_5–	4.58*	9.37*	9.83*	10.20*	10.39*	10.49*	2
H_2N–	8.12*	—	9.98	10.65*	10.84*	11.05*	2
$H_2C=CH$–	—	9.69	—	—	—	—	—
CH_3–	10.64*	10.67*	10.58*	10.61*	10.63*	10.64*	2

X	Me_2N	–H	$–NH_3^+$	$–CO_2^-$	$–SO_3^-$	$–PO_3^-$	Reference
$X-NH_3^+$		9.25*	-0.88	—	1	10.25	2
$X(CH_2)NH_3^+$		10.64	—	9.77	5.75	10.8	2
$X(CH_2)_2NH_3^+$	5.98, 9.30	10.67	—	10.19	9.20	10.8	2, 118
$X(CH_2)_3NH_3^+$	9.91, 7.67	10.58	8.59	10.43	10.05	—	2, 118
$X(CH_2)_4NH_3^+$	8.44, 10.17	10.61	9.31	10.77	10.65	10.9	2, 118
$X(CH_2)_5NH_3^+$	9.07, 10.44	10.63	9.74	10.75	10.95	11.0	2, 118
$X(CH_2)_8NH_3^+$		10.65	10.10	—	—	—	2
$X(C_2)_{10}NH_3^+$		10.64	—	—	11.35	11.25	2

For complex chelating agents of aliphatic amines, see also Ref. 7.

Compound	pK'_a	Reference	Compound	pK'_a	Reference
PRIMARY AMINES			*PRIMARY AMINES (Continued)*		
1-Acetamido-2-aminoethane	9.05*	99	2-Amino-3-hydroxyindan	8.13*	99
1-Acetoxy-2-aminoethane	9.1	99	1-Amino-2-hydroxy-2-methylpropane	9.25*	99
Acetylhydrazine	3.24*	99	2-Amino-1-hydroxy-2-methylpropane	9.71*	99
β-Alanine ester	9.13	1	1-Amino-5-hydroxypentane	10.46*	99
Allylamine	9.49	1	1-Amino-3-hydroxypropane	9.96*	99
1-Amino-2-benzamidoethane	9.13*	99	2-Amino-1-hydroxypropane	9.43*	99
1-Amino-2-benzylaminoethane	6.48*, 9.41*	99	1-Amino-2-(2-hydroxypropyl)aminoethane	6.94*, 9.86*	99
1-Amino-2-bromoethane	8.49*	99	1-Amino-2-(3-hydroxypropyl)aminoethane	6.78*, 9.67*	99
1-Amino-3-bromopropane	8.93*	99	2-Aminoindan	9.57*	99
1-Amino-2-butylaminoethane	7.53*, 10.30*	99	5-Aminoindan	5.31*	99
(3-Amino)butylbenzene	9.79*	99	1-Amino-2-isopropylaminoethane	7.70*, 10.62*	99
(4-Amino)butylbenzene	10.36*	99	Aminomalonic acid	3.32, 9.83	77
γ-Amino-n-butyric acid ester	9.71	1	1-Amino-2-mercaptoethane	8.27*, 10.53*	99
1-Amino-2-diethylaminoethane	7.07*, 10.02*	99	1-Amino-2-methylbutane	10.64	99
1-Amino-2-dimethylaminoethane	6.63*, 9.53*	99	1-Amino-3-methylbutane	10.60*	99
1-Amino-2,2-dimethylpropane	10.24*	99	2-Amino-2-methylbutane	10.72*	99
1-Amino-2-ethylaminoethane	7.63*, 10.56*	99	1-Amino-3-methylcyclohexane	10.56* cis, 10.61* trans	99
1-(2-Aminoethyl)piperidine	6.38*, 9.89*	99	1-Amino-2-methylpropane	10.72*	99
2-Aminoethylsulfonic acid	9.08	77	2-Amino-2-methylpropane	10.68*	99
(2-Aminoethyl)trimethylammonium chloride	7.1	99	1-Amino-2-methylaminoethane	6.86*, 10.15*	99
1-Aminofluorene	3.87*	99	1-Amino-2-methylthioethane	9.49*	99
2-Aminofluorene	4.64*	99	1-Aminononane	10.64*	99
3-Aminofluorene	4.82*	99	1-Aminooctane	10.65*	99
4-Aminofluorene	3.39*	99	2-Aminooctane	10.49*	99
1-Amino-2-furfurylaminoethane	6.20*, 9.72*	99	1-Aminopentane	10.63*	99
1-Aminoheptane	10.66*	99	3-Aminopentane	10.42*	99
2-Aminoheptane	10.67*	99	1-Amino-2-propylaminoethane	8.24*, 11.04*	99
1-Aminohexane	10.56*	99	1-Aminoprop-2-ene	9.49*	99
1-Amino-4-hydroxybutane	10.35*	99	1-Aminoprop-2-yne	8.15*	99
2-Amino-1-hydroxybutane	9.52*	99	1-Aminotetradecane	10.62*	99
1-Amino-2-hydroxycycloheptane	9.25*	99	1-Amino-3.3,3-trichloropropane	9.65*	99
1-Amino-2-hydroxycyclopentane	9.70* cis, 9.28 trans	99	Benzamide	-1.85	99
2-Amino-2'-hydroxydiethyl sulfide	9.04, 9.41	77, 99	Benzoylhydrazine	2.97	114
1-Amino-2-(2-hydroxyethyl)aminoethane	6.83*, 9.82*	99			

* Thermodynamic value.

NITROGEN COMPOUNDS (Continued)

Compound	pK_a	Reference	Compound	pK_a	Reference
PRIMARY AMINES (Continued)			*PRIMARY AMINES (Continued)*		
Benzyl-	9.34	1	Methyl benzimidate	5.8*	99
bis(2-aminoethyl)disulfide	8.82*, 9.16*	99	*N*-Methylethylenedi-	7.56, 10.40	77
1,2-bis(2-aminoethyl)thioethane	8.69*, 9.62*	99	2-Methylthioethyl-	9.18	77
1,2-bisglycylamidoethane	7.63*, 8.35*	99	Octyl-	10.65	153
n-Butyl-	10.59	1	*neo*-Pentyl-	10.21	1
t-Butyl-	10.55	1	Phenylamyl-	10.49	2
N-*n*-Butylethylenedi-	7.53, 10.30	77	(δ-Phenylbutyl-	10.40	2
Carbamylmethyl-	7.93	153	β-Phenylethyl-	9.83	1
N-(Carbamoylmethyl)iminodiacetic acid	2.30, 6.60	77	Phenylmethyl-	9.34	153
Cyanoethyl-	7.7	153	γ-Phenylpropyl-	10.20	1
Cyanomethyl-	5.34	153	Propionamide	−0.49*	99
Ethoxycarbonylethyl-	9.13	153	*n*-Propyl-	10.53	1
Cyclohexyl-	10.64	1	*N*-*n*-Propylethylenedi-	7.54, 10.34	77
Cyclohexylmethyl	10.49	1	*sec*-Butyl-	10.56	1
1,4-Diaminobutane-	9.24, 10.72	146	Semicarbazide	3.65*	99
2,3-Diaminobutane, *meso*	6.92, 9.97	77	1,2,3-Triaminopropane	3.72, 7.95, 9.59	77
2,3-Diaminobutane, *racemic*	6.91, 10.00	77	Triaminotriethyl-	8.56, 9.59, 10.29	77
2,2′-Diaminodiethyl-	3.58, 8.86, 9.65	77	β,β′,β″-Triaminotriethyl-	8.42, 9.44, 10.13	87
2,2′-Diaminodiethyl sulfide	8.84, 9.64	77	2,2,2-Trichloroethyl-	5.47*	99
2,3-Diamino-2,3-dimethylbutane	6.56, 10.13	77	2-Trienylmethyl-	8.92	77
1,3-Diamino-2,2-dimethylpropane	8.18, 10.22	77	Triethylenedi-	8.8*	—
3,3′-Diamino-*n*-propyl-	8.02, 9.70, 10.70	77	Trifluoroethyl-	5.7	10
N,N-Di-(2-aminoethyl)ethylenedi-	3.32, 6.67, 9.20, 9.92	77	Trimethylsilylmethyl-	10.96	1
1,2-Di-(2-aminoethylthio)ethane	8.42, 9.32	77	Thioacetamide	−1.76*	99
1,3-Diamino-2-hydroxypropane	7.93*, 9.69*	99	Tris-(hydroxymethyl)aminomethane	8.10	77
1,2-Diamino-2-methylpropane	6.79, 10.00	77	Undecyl-	10.63	153
1,3-Diaminopropan-2-ol	8.23, 9.68	77	Vinylmethyl-	9.69	153
1,2-Diaminopropane	7.13*, 10.00*	99	CF₃SO₂−	5.8	128
1,3-Diaminopropane	8.64*, 10.62*	99			
β-Difluoroethyl-	7.52	1	*SECONDARY AMINES*		
N,N-Diglycylethylenedi-	7.63, 8.35	77	*N*-(2-Acetamido)-2-aminoethane-sulfonic acid	6.9	108
2,3-Dimethoxybenzyl-	9.41*	99	Acetamidoglycine	7.7	108
3,4-Dimethoxybenzyl-	9.39*	99	Acetanilide	0.61	4
N,N-Diethylethylenedi-	7.07, 10.02	77	1-Acetylpiperazine	7.94*	99
N,N-Dimethylethylenedi-	6.63, 9.53	77	Allylmethyl-	10.11	1
4-4′-Diaminostilbene	3.9*, 5.2*	99	*N*-2-Aminoethylpiperazine	8.51*, 9.63*	99
1-Dimethylamino-3-hydrazinobutane	5.90*, 9.23*	99	Aminomethylcyclohexane	10.59*	99
Ethanol-	9.50	1	1-4-Benzoquinoneimine	3.9*	99
Ethyl-	10.63	1	*N*-Benzoylpiperazine	7.78	1
Ethylenedi-	9.98, 7.52	1, 77	Benzylethyl-	9.68	1
Ethylenediamine-*N,N*-diacetic acid	7.63, 8.35	77	Benzylmethyl-	9.58	1
N-Ethylethylenedi-	7.63, 10.56	77	α-Benzylpyrrolidine	10.36	2
Furfuryl-	8.89	77	α-Benzylpyrroline-	7.08	2
D-Glucos-	7.75*	99	1,2-Bisethylaminoethane	7.70*, 10.46*	99
Glycine ester	7.75	1	1,2-Bisfurfurylaminoethane	5.74*, 8.61*	99
Hexadecyl-	10.61	153	1,2-Bisisopropylaminoethane	7.59*, 10.40*	99
Hydrazine	8.10	1	1,2-Bismethylaminoethane	7.40*, 10.16*	99
N-(2-Hydroxyethyl)ethylenedi-	6.83, 9.82	77	1,2-Bispropylaminoethane	7.53*, 10.27*	99
Hydroxyl-	5.97	1	*N*-Butylaminoacetic acid	2.29, 10.07	77
2-Hydroxy-3-methoxybenzylamine	8.70, 11.06*	99	*t*-Butylcyclohexyl-	11.23	1
3-Hydroxy-2-methoxybenzylamine	8.89*, 10.54*	99	*N*-Carbethoxypiperazine	8.28	1
4-Hydroxy-3-methoxybenzylamine	8.94*, 10.52*	99	β-Carboxymethylaminopropionic acid	3.61, 9.46	77
2-(2-Hydroxypropylamino)ethyl-	6.94, 9.86	77	*cis*-2,6-Dimethylpiperidine	10.92	3
2-(3-Hydroxypropylamino)ethyl-	6.78, 9.76	77	α-Cyclohexylpyrrolidine	10.80	2
N-Isopropylethylenedi-	7.70, 10.62	77	α-Cyclohexylpyrroline	7.95	2
Isopropyl-	10.63	1	Diallyl-	9.29	1
Mercaptoethyl-	8.27, 10.53	77	Di-*n*-butyl-	11.25	1
Methoxy-	4.60*	12	Diethyl-	10.98	1
Methoxycarbonylmethyl-	7.66	153	*N,N*-Diethylethylenedi-	7.70, 10.46	77
2-Methoxyethyl-	9.20	77	Di-(trimethylsilylmethyl)-	11.40	1
Methyl-	10.62	1	Di-(hydroxyethyl)amine	8.88*	99
N-Methylaminoacetic acid	2.24, 10.01	77	Diisobutyl-	10.50	1
Methyl-α-amino-β-mercaptopropionate	6.56, 8.99	77	Diisopropyl-	11.05	1
			Dimethyl-	10.64	1

* Thermodynamic value.

NITROGEN COMPOUNDS (Continued)

Compound	pK_a	Reference
SECONDARY AMINES (Continued)		
N,N'-Dimethylethylenedi-	7.40, 10.16	77
N,O-Dimethylhydroxyl-	4.75*	12
1-Diphenylmethoxy-2-methylaminoethane	9.12*	99
Di-*n*-propyl-	11.00	1
N,N'-Di-*n*-propylethylenedi-	8.14, 10.97	77
Di-*sec*-butyl-	11.01	1
N-Ethylaminoacetic acid	2.30, 10.10	77
Ethylenediamine- *N,N'*-diacetic acid	6.42, 9.46	77
α-Ethylpyrrolidine	10.43	2
α-Ethylpyrroline	7.43	2
Iminodiacetic acid	2.98, 9.89	77
Iminodipropionic acid	4.11, 9.61	77
N-Isopropylaminoacetic acid	2.36, 10.06	77
Methylaminocyclopentane	10.85*	99
1-Methylaminoprop-2-ene	10.11*	99
N-Methylglucamine	9.62*	99
N-Methylhydroxyl-	5.96*	12
N-Methylmethoxy-	4.75	1
2-Methylpiperidine	11.08*	99
3-Methylpiperidine	11.07*	99
Methyltrifluorethyl-	6.05	10
Morpholine	8.36	1
Piperazine	5.68, 9.82	77
Piperidine	11.22	1
N-n-Propylaminoacetic acid	2.28, 10.03	77
1-Propylaminopropane	11.00	11
Pyrrolidine	11.27	1
α-(*p*-Tolyl)-pyrrolidine	10.01	2
α-(*p*-Tolyl)pyrroline	7.59	2
1-Tosylpiperazine	7.39	3
Trimethyleneimine	11.29	1
N-Tris(hydroxymethyl)methylglycine	8.15	108
TERTIARY AMINES		
N-(2-Acetamido)iminodiacetic acid	6.6	99
1-Acetyl-2-diethylaminoethane	9.04*	99
Allyldimethyl-	8.73	1
N-Allylmorpholine	7.05	1
N-Allylpiperidine	9.68	1
4-(2-Aminoethyl)morpholine	4.84, 9.45	77
1-Benzoyl-4-methylpiperazine	6.78*	99
1-Benzylcarbonyl-2-diethylaminoethane	9.40*	99
1-Acetyl-2-dimethylaminoethane	8.37*	99
1-Benzylcarbonyl-2-dimethylaminoethane	8.30*	99
Benzyldiethyl-	9.48	1
Benzyldimethyl-	8.93	1
Bis(2-chloroethyl)aminoethane	6.55*	99
1-Bis(2-chloroethyl)amino-2-methoxyethane	5.45*	99
1,2-Bisdimethylaminopropane	5.40*, 9.49*	99
1,3-Bisdimethylaminopropane	7.7*, 9.8*	99
N,N-Bis(2-hydroxyethyl)-2-aminoethanesulfonic acid	7.15	99
N,N-Bis(2-hydroxyethyl)glycine	8.35	99
1-*n*-Butylpiperidine	10.47*	99
1-*n*-Butyl-2-methyl-Δ²-pyrroline	11.90	2
1-Chloro-2-diethylaminoethane	8.80*	99
N-Chloro-*N*-ethylaminoethane	1.02*	99
N-Chloro-*N*-methylaminomethane	0.46*	99
1-Cyanomethylpiperidine	4.55*	99
Diallylmethyl-	8.79	1
Diethylaminoacetic acid	2.04, 10.47	77

Compound	pK_a	Reference
TERTIARY AMINES (Continued)		
1-Diethylaminobutan-(4)-	10.1	5
1-Diethylaminohexan-(6)-	10.1	5
1-Diethylaminohexanethiol-(6)-	10.1	5
1-Diethylaminopropan-(3)-	8.0, 10.5	5
N-Diethylcysteamine	7.8, 10.75	5
Di-(2-hydroxyethyl)aminoacetic acid	8.08	77
Dimethylaminoacetic acid	2.08, 9.80	77
1-Dimethylamino-2-hydroxyethane	9.31*	99
1-Dimethylaminoprop-2-ene	8.64*	99
1-Dimethylaminoprop-2-yne	6.97*	99
Dimethyl-*n*-butyl-	10.02	1
Dimethyl-*t*-butyl-	10.52	1
N-Dimethylcysteamine	7.95, 10.7	5
Dimethylethyl-	9.99	1
N-Dimethylhydroxylamine	5.20*	12
Dimethylisobutyl-	9.91	1
Dimethylisopropyl-	10.30	1
N,N-Dimethylmethoxy-	3.65	1
1,2-Dimethylpiperidine	10.26	2
Dimethyl-*n*-propyl-	9.99	1
1,2-Dimethylpyrrolidine	10.26	2
1,2-Dimethyl-Δ²-pyrroline	11.94	2
Dimethyl-*sec*-butyl-	10.40	1
1,2-Dimethyl-Δ²-tetrahydropyridine	11.57	2
Dimethyltrifluoroethyl-	4.75	10
l-Dipropylaminopropane	10.26*	99
N-Dipropylcysteamine	8.00, 10.8	5
1-Ethoxycarbonyl-4-methylpiperazine	7.31*	99
N-Ethyl-*cis*-2,3-iminobutane	8.56	7
N-Ethyl-1,2-iminobutane	8.18	7
1-Ethyl-2-methylpiperidine	10.70	2
l-Ethyl-2-methyl-Δ²-pyrroline	11.92	2
1-Ethyl-2-methylpyrrolidine	10.64	2
1-Ethyl-2-methyl-Δ²-tetrahydropyridine	11.57	2
N-Ethylmorpholine	7.70	1
N-Ethylpiperidine	10.40	1
N-Ethyl-*trans*-2,3-iminobutane	9.47	7
Hexamethylenetetra-	5.13	77
N-2-Hydroxyethyliminodiacetic acid	2.2, 8.73	77
N-2-Hydroxyethylpiperazine-*N'*-2-ethanesulfonic acid	7.55	99
1-Hydroxy-2-(2-hydroxyethylmethyl)aminoethane	8.52*	99
1,2-Iminoethane	7.93	7
1-Methyl-2-*n*-butylpyrrolidine	10.24	2
1-Methyl-2-*n*-butyl-Δ²-pyrroline	11.90	2
N-β-Mercaptoethylmorpholine	6.65, 9.8	5
N-β-Mercaptoetnylpiperidine	7.95, 11.05	5
Methyl-β-diethylaminoethylsulfide	9.8	5
Methyldiethyl-	10.29	1
Methyliminodiacetic acid	2.81, 10.18	77
1-Methyl-4-nitrosopiperazine	5.93*	99
N-Methylmorpholine	7.41	1
N-Methylpiperidine	10.08	1
N-Methylpyrrolidine	10.46	1
N-Methyltrimethyleneimine	10.40	1
2-(*N*-Morpholino)ethanesulfonic acid	6.15	99
Piperazine-*N,N'*-bis(2-ethanesulfonic acid	6.8	99
Propargyldimethyl-	7.05	1
Propargylethyldimethyl-	8.88	1
Propargylmethyldimethyl-	8.33	1
1-*n*-Propylpiperidine	10.48	2
Triallyl-	8.31	1
Tri-*n*-butyl-	10.89	1

* Thermodynamic value.

NITROGEN COMPOUNDS (Continued)

Compound	pK'$_a$	Reference
TERTIARY AMINES (Continued)		
Triethanol-	7.77	1
Triethyl-	10.65	1
Triethylenedi-	4.18, 8.19,	77
Trimethyl-	9.76	1
	2.97, 8.82	116
Trimethylhydroxylamine	3.65	12
Tri-*n*-propyl-	10.65	1
N-Tris(hydroxymethyl)-methyl-2-aminoethanesulfonic acid	7.5	99
$(CH_3)_2NCH_3$	9.76	119
$(CH_3CH_2)_2NCH_3$	10.29	119
$(CH_2)_2\ NCH_3$ *N*-Methylaziridine	7.86	119
$(CH_2)_3\ NCH_3$ *N*-Methylazetidine	10.40	119
$(CH_2)_4\ NCH_3$ *N*-Methylpyrrolidine	10.46	119
$(CH_2)_5\ NCH_3$ *N*-Methylpiperidine	10.08	119

BENZYLAMINES, MONOSUBSTITUTED

	2	3	4	99
Chloro-	5.20*	—	—	—
Methoxy-	9.70*	9.15*	9.47*	—
Methyl-	9.19*	9.33*	9.36*	—
Sulfamoyl-	8.53*	8.55*	8.52*	—
	10.11*	10.14*	10.08*	—

Compound	pK'$_a$	Reference
CYANOAMINES		
N-Piperidine-CH$_2$CN		8
Et$_2$NCN	−2.0	8
Et$_2$N(CH$_2$)$_2$CN	7.65	8
Et$_2$N(CH$_2$)$_4$CN	10.08	8
Et$_2$NC(CH$_3$)$_2$CN	9.13	8
EtN(CH$_2$CN)$_2$	−0.6	8
EtN(CH$_2$CH$_2$CN)$_2$	4.55	8
H$_2$NCH$_2$CN	5.34	8
N-Amphetamine-(CH$_2$)$_2$-CN	7.23	8
N-Norcodeine-(CH$_2$)$_2$CN	5.68	8
Dimethylcyanimide	1.2	9
Diethylcyanimide	1.2	9
Aminoacetonitrile	5.3	9
Diethylaminoacetonitrile	4.5	9
2-Amino-2-cyanopropane	5.3	9
β-Isopropylaminopropionitrile	8.0	9
β-Diethylaminopropionitrile	7.6	9
1-Amino-2-cyanoethane	7.7*	99
Et$_2$NCH$_2$CN	4.55	8
Et$_2$N(CH$_2$)$_3$CN	9.29	8
Et$_2$N(CH$_2$)$_5$CN	10.46	8
HN(CH$_2$CN)$_2$	0.2	8
HN(CH$_2$CH$_2$CN)$_2$	5.26	8
N(CH$_2$CH$_2$CN)$_3$	1.1	8
N-Piperidine-C(CH$_3$)$_2$CN	9.22	8
N-Methamphetamine-(CH$_2$)$_2$CN	6.95	8
Methyl cyanamide	1.2	9
Ethyl cyanamide	1.2	9
Cyanamide	1.1	9
Dimethylaminoacetonitrile	4.2	9

* Thermodynamic value.

Compound	pK'$_a$	Reference
CYANOAMINES (Continued)		
β-Aminopropionitrile	7.7	9
β-Dimethylaminopropionitrile	7.0	9
β,β"-Dicyanodiethylamine	5.2	9
CYCLIC AMINES		
1,2-Iminoethane	7.98	7
cis-2,3-Iminobutane	8.72	7
1,2-Imino-2-methylpropane	8.61	7
1,2-Iminobutane	8.29	7
trans-2,3-Iminobutane	8.69	7
In 80 percent methyl cellosolve:		
Pentamethylene-	9.99	2
Hexamethylene-	10.00	2
Heptamethylene-	9.77	2
Octamethylene	9.39	2
Nonamethylene-	9.14	2
Decamethylene-	9.04	2
Undecamethylene-	9.31	2
Dodecamethylene-	9.31	2
Tridecamethylene-	9.35	2
Tetradecamethylene-	9.35	2
Hexadecamethylene-	9.29	2
Heptadecamethylene-	9.27	2
Cyclohexyl-	9.82	2
Cycloheptyl-	9.99	2
Cycloöctyl-	10.01	2
Cyclononyl-	9.95	2
Cyclodecyl-	9.85	2
Cycloundecyl-	9.71	2
Cyclododecyl-	9.62	2
Cyclotridecyl-	9.63	2
Cyclotetradecyl-	9.54	2
Cyclopentadecyl-	9.54	2
Cycloheptadecyl-	9.57	2
Cyclooctadecyl-	9.54	2
PHENYLETHYLAMINES		
2-Phenylethylamine	9.78	11
N-Methyl-2-(3,4-dihydroxyphenyl)-ethylamine	8.78	11
N-Methyl-2-phenyl-	10.31	11
Epinephrine	8.55	11
Arterenol	8.55	11
		11

R$_1$	R$_2$	R$_3$	R$_4$	pK'$_a$
H	H	H	H	9.78
H	H	OH	H	8.90
H	OH	OH	H	8.81
OH	H	OH	H	8.67
H	OH	H	H	9.22
OH	OH	H	H	8.93
OH	OH	OH	H	8.58
H	H	H	CH$_3$	10.31
H	H	OH	CH$_3$	9.31
H	OH	OH	CH$_3$	8.62
OH	H	OH	CH$_3$	8.89
H	OH	H	CH$_3$	9.36
OH	OH	H	CH$_3$	8.78
OH	OH	OH	CH$_3$	8.55

NITROGEN COMPOUNDS (Continued)

Compound	pK'_a	Reference	Compound	pK'_a	Reference
ALKALOIDS AND DERIVATIVES			*ALKALOIDS AND DERIVATIVES (Continued)*		
Acetylscopolamine	7.35*	99	10-Hydroxycodeine	7.12*	99
Aconitine	8.35*	99	Hyoscyamine	9.68*	99
Alypine	3.8*, 9.5*	99	Isolysergic acid	3.33*, 8.46*	99
Anhydroplatynecine	9.40*	99	Isopilocarpine	7.18*	99
Apomorphine	7.20*, 8.92*	99	Isoretronecanol	10.83*	99
Aposcopolamine	7.72*	99	Lysergic acid	3.32*, 7.82*	99
Arecaidine	9.07*	99	N-Methyl-1-benzoylecgonine	8.65*	99
Arecaidine methyl ester	7.64*	99	6-Methyl ergoline	8.87*	99
Arecoline	7.41*	99	Morphine	8.07*, 9.85*	99
Aspidospermine	7.63*	99	Myosmine	5.26*	99
Atropine	9.85*	99	Narceine	3.5*, 9.3*	99
Benzoylecgonine	11.80*	99	Narcotine	5.86*	99
Benzoylecgonine methyl ester	8.74*	99	Nicotine	3.13*, 8.02*	99
N-Benzyltriacanthine	5.94*	99	Nicotine dimethohydroxide	7.88*, 10.23*	99
Berberine	11.73*	99	Nicotine isomethohydroxide	5.35*, 11.72*	99
Brucine	2.50*, 8.16*	99	Nicotine methohydroxide	8.54*, 12.04*	99
N-Butylveratramine	7.20*	99	Nicotine monomethobromide	3.09*	99
Cevadine	9.05*	99	Nicotine oxide	5.00*	99
Cinchonidine	4.17*, 8.40*	99	Nicotyrine	4.76*	99
Cinchonine	4.28*, 8.35*	99	Norcodeine	5.68*	99
Cocaine	8.39*	99	Norcurarine	8.5*	99
Codeine	8.21*	99	Norhyoscyamine	10.28*	99
Colchicine	1.85*	99	Nornicotyrine	4.35*	99
Cupreine	7.63*	99	Optochine	4.05*, 8.5*	99
Cytisine	1.20*, 8.12*	99	Papaverine	6.40*	99
Deacetylaspidospermine	2.70*, 8.45*	99	Pelletierine	9.45*	99
Desoxyretronecine	9.51*	99	N-Pentylveratramine	7.28*	99
Dicodide	7.95*	99	Perlolidine	4.01*, 11.39*	99
Dihydroarecaidine	9.70*	99	Perloline	8.54*	99
Dihydroarecaidine, methyl ester	8.39*	99	Physostigmine	1.96*, 8.08*	99
Dihydrocodeine	8.75	99	Pilocarpate	7.47*	99
α-Dihydrolysergic acid	3.57*, 8.45*	99	Pilocarpine	1.63*, 7.05*	99
γ-Dihydrolysergic acid	3.60*, 8.71*	99	Piperine	1.98*	99
Dihydromorphine	9.35*	99	Platynecine	10.20*	99
Dihydroergonovine	7.38*	99	N-Propylveratramine	7.20*	
α-Dihydrolysergol	8.30*	99	Pseudoecgonine	9.70*	99
β-Dihydrolysergol	8.23*	99	Pseudoecgonine methyl ester	8.15*	99
Dihydronicotyrine	7.07*	99	Pseudotropine	9.86*	99
Dilaudide	7.8*	99	Quinidine	4.2*, 8.77*	99
Ecgonine	10.91	99	Quinine	4.32*, 8.4*	99
Ecgonine methyl ester	9.16*	99	Retronecanol	10.88*	99
Emetine	7.56*, 8.43*	99	Retronecine	8.88*	99
Ergobasine	6.79*	99	Scopolamine	7.55*	99
Ergobasinine	7.43*	99	Scopoline	8.20*	99
Ergometrinine	7.32*	99	Sempervirine	10.6*	99
Ergonovine	6.73*	99	Solanine	7.54*	99
Ethylmorphine	8.08*	99	Sparteine	4.80*, 11.96*	99
N-Ethylveratramine	7.40*	99	Stovaine	7.9*	99
β-Eucaine	9.35*	99	Strychnine	8.26*	99
Eucodal	8.6*	99	Tetradehydroyohimbine	10.69*	99
Gelsemine	9.79*	99	Tetrahydro-α-morphimethine	8.65*	99
Harmine	7.61*	99	Tetrahydroserpentine	10.55*	99
Harmol	7.86*, 9.51*	99	Thebaine	8.15*	99
Heliotridane	11.40*	99	Theobromine	10.00*	99
Heliotridene	10.55*	99	Theophylline	8.6*	99
Heroin	7.6*	99	Triacanthine	6.0*	99
Homatropine	9.7*	99	Tropacocaine	9.88*	99
Hydrastine	6.63*	99	Tropine	10.33*	99
Hydrastinine	11.58*	99	Veratramine	7.49*	99
Hydroquinine	8.87*	99	Yohimbine	3*, 7.45*	99

* Thermodynamic value.

NITROGEN COMPOUNDS (Continued)

ANILINES (2,99)

Monosubstituted

Substituent	ortho	meta	para
H-	4.62*	4.64*	4.58*
(CH₃)₃N⁺-	—	2.26	2.51
CH₃O₂C-	2.16	3.56	2.30
CH₃SO₂-	—	2.68*	1.48
CH₃S-	—	4.05	4.40
Br-	2.60*	3.51*	3.91*
F-	2.96*	3.38*	4.52*
CH₃O-	4.49*	4.20*	5.29*
C₆H₅-	3.78*	4.18	4.27*
(CH₃)₃C-	3.78	—	—
-O₃S-	—	3.80	3.32
H₃N⁺-	1.3	2.65	3.29
O₂N-	−0.28*	2.45*	0.98*,1.11*
HO₂C-	2.04	3.05	2.32
C₂H₅O₂C-	2.10	—	2.38
F₃C-	—	3.49*	2.57*
HO-	4.72	4.17	5.50
Cl-	2.62*	3.32*	3.81*
(CH₃)₃Si-	—	4.64*	4.36*
C₂H₅O-	4.47*	4.17*	5.25*
CH₃-	4.38*	4.67*	5.07*
-HO₃As-	3.77	4.05	4.05
H₂N-	4.47	4.88	6.08
CH₃CO-	2.22*	3.59*	2.19*
CN-	0.95*	2.75	1.74
C₂H₅-	4.37*	4.70*	—
C₆H₅CO-	—	—	2.17*
n-Butyl	4.26*	—	—
t-Butyl	5.03*	4.66*	4.95*
HCO-	—	—	1.76*
I-	2.60*	3.61*	3.78*
Isopropyl-	4.42*	4.67*	—
HS-	3.00*	—	—
	6.59*	—	—
Sulfamoyl	1.0*	2.90*	2.02*

Compound	pK′ₐ	Reference
3-Amino-2,6-dihydroxyaniline	2.9*, 5.6*, 9.3*, 11.5*	99
3-Amino-4,6-dihydroxyaniline	3.8*, 6.0*, 9.8*, 12.0*	99
3-Amino-2-hydroxyaniline	2.7*, 5.5*, 10.5*	99

Compound	pK′ₐ	Reference
3-Amino-4-hydroxyaniline	3.1*, 5.7*, 10.5*	99
4-Bromo-2,6-dimethylaniline	3.54*	99
3-Bromo-4-methylaniline	3.98*	99
4-Bromo-2-methylaniline	3.58*	99
3,5-di-t-Butylaniline	4.97	88
3-Chloro-5-methoxyaniline	3.10	88
3-Chloro-4-methylaniline	4.05*	88
2,4-Diaminoaniline	3.7*, 6.1*	99
2,4-Dibromoaniline	2.3*	99
2,6-Dibromoaniline	0.38*	99
3,5-Dibromoaniline	2.34*	99
2,4-Dichloroaniline	2.05*	99
2,5-Dichloroaniline	1.57*	99
3,5-Dichloroaniline	2.37	138
2,4-Dihydroxyaniline	5.7*, 9.3*, 11.3*	99
2,6-Dihydroxyaniline	5.1*, 9.3*, 11.6*	99
3,5-Diiodoaniline	2.37	138
3,5-Dimethoxyaniline	3.82	88
3-Methoxy-5-nitroaniline	2.11	88
2,3-Dimethylaniline	4.70*	99
2,4-Dimethylaniline	4.84*	99
2,5-Dimethylaniline	4.57*	99
2,6-Dimethylaniline	3.89*	99
3,4-Dimethylaniline	5.17*	99
3,5-Dimethylaniline	4.91*	99
2,4-Dinitroaniline	−4.27	120
3,5-Dinitroaniline	0.23	138
2,3,5,6-Tetramethylaniline	4.30*	99
2,4,6-Trimethylaniline	4.38*	99
3,4,5-Trimethylaniline	5.12*	99

	pK₁	pK₂	Ref.
3-Amino-5-nitrobenzoic acid	1.55	3.55	147
methyl ester	1.47	—	147
ethyl ester	1.52	—	147
Ethyl N-(m-carboxyphenyl)glycinate	1.15	4.30	147
Ethyl N-(m-methoxycarbonylphenyl)glycinate	1.06	—	147
Ethyl N-(m-ethoxycarbonylphenyl)glycinate	1.11	—	147
Ethyl N-phenylglycinate	2.08	—	147
Methyl N-phenylglycinate	2.07	—	147
Ethyl N-(p-carboxyphenyl)glycinate	—	4.88	147

N-SUBSTITUTED ANILINES

R	C₆H₅NHR	C₆H₅N(CH₃)R	C₆H₅NR₂	2-CH₃C₆H₄NHR (2)	2-CH₃C₆H₄NR₂
H-	4.58	4.85	4.58	4.39	4.39
CH₃-	4.85	5.06	5.06	4.59	5.86
C₂H₅-	5.11	5.98	6.56	4.92	7.18
n-C₃H₇-	5.02	—	5.59	—	—
n-C₄H₉-	4.95	—	~5.7	—	—
i-C₄H₉-	—	5.20	—	—	—
sec-C₄H₉-	—	6.03	—	—	—
t-C₆H₁₂-	6.30	—	—	—	—
Cyclopentyl-	5.30	6.71	—	5.07	—
Cyclohexyl-	5.60	6.35	—	5.34	—
t-C₄H₉	6.95	7.52	—	6.49	—

* Thermodynamic value.

NITROGEN COMPOUNDS (Continued)

N-SUBSTITUTED ANILINES[119]

R=	4-$NO_2C_6H_4R$	4-$HOOCC_6H_4R$	C_6H_5R
$(CH_3)_2N-$	0.65	1.40	4.22 4.39
CH_3CH_2N-	1.75	2.45	5.71 5.85
$(CH_2)_3$ -N- Azetidine	0.34		5.59 4.08
$(CH_2)_4$ -N- Pyrrolidine	−0.42	0.39	3.71 3.45 3.24
$(CH_2)_5$ -N- Piperidine	2.46	2.67	4.60 5.22 4.93
$(CH_2)_6$ -N- Hexahydroazepine	−0.15		

Compound	pK_a	Reference
N,N-DIETHYL-		
2,4-Dinitro-	0.18*	99
2-Methyl-	7.23*	99
3-Methyl-	7.12*	99
4-Methyl-	7.13*	99
4-Nitroso-	4.11*	99
N,N-DIMETHYL-		
H–	5.07	52
m-NO_2-	2.63	52
m-CN-	2.97	52
p-NO_2	0.61	52
p-CN-	1.78	52
p-NO-	4.54	52
N-DIMETHYL-, IN 50% ETHANOL		
H-	4.21, 4.09	2
m-CH_3-	4.66	2
p-C_2H_5-	4.69	2
o-$(CH_3)_2$CH-	5.05	2
p-$CH_3CH_2CH_2CH_2$-	4.62	2
o-$(CH_3)_3$C-	4.26	2
p-I-	3.43, 2.73	2
p-Br-	3.52, 2.82	2
p-Cl-	3.33	2
m-$(CH_3)_3$Si-	4.41	2
o-CH_3O-	5.49	2
o-CH_3-	5.15, 5.07	2
p-CH_3-	4.94	2
p-$CH_3CH_2CH_2$-	4.43	2
p-$(CH_3)_2$CH-	4.77	2
p-$(CH_3)_2$CHCH$_2$-	4.19	2
p-$(CH_3)_3$C-	4.65	2
m-Br-	3.08	2
m-Cl-	3.09	2
p-F-	4.01	2
p-$(CH_3)_3$Si-	3.99	2
p-CH_3O-	5.14, 5.16	2
N-Methyl		
4-Chloro-	3.9*	99
4-Chloro, 2-nitro-	−1.49*	99
2-Methyl-	4.62*	99
3-Methyl-	5.00*	99
4-Methyl-	5.36*	99
2-Methoxycarbonyl-	3.53*	99
4-Methoxycarbonyl-	2.32*	99

Compound	pK_a	Reference
ORTHO-SUBSTITUTED, IN 50% ETHANOL		
H-	4.25	2
2-CH_3-	3.98, 4.09	2
2,3-$(CH_3)_2$-	4.42	2
2,4-$(CH_3)_2$-	4.61	2
2,5-$(CH_3)_2$-	4.17, 4.23	2
2,6-$(CH_3)_2$-	3.42, 3.49	2
3,5-$(CH_3)_2$-	4.48	2
2-CH_3-	4.09	2
2-$(CH_3)_2$CH-	4.06	2
2-$(CH_3)_3$C-	3.38	2
2,6-$(CH_3)_2$-4-$(CH_3)_3$C-	3.88	2
2,4-$(CH_3)_2$-6-$(CH_3)_3$C-	3.43	2
2-CH_3-4,6-$(CH_3)_3$C-	3.31	2
2,4,6-$[(CH_3)_3C]_3$-	< 2	2
2-NITROANILINE		
R=H-	−0.29	120
4-CH_3O-	0.77	120
4-CH_3-	0.43	120
4-F-	−0.44	120
4-Cl-	−1.03	120
4-Br-	−1.05	120
4-CF_3-	−2.25	120
4-CH_3OCO	−2.61	120
4-NO_2-	−4.27	120
4-CH_3CO-	−2.85	120
4-HO-	1.20	120
3-CH_3-	−0.09	120
3-CH_3O-	−0.72	120
3-Cl-	−1.48	120
3-Br-	−1.48	120
3-NO_2-	−2.49	120
3-HO-	−0.55	120
6-NITROANILINE		
R=2-Cl-	−2.41	120
2-NO_2-	−5.56	120
2,4-Cl_2-	−3.16	120
4-CH_3-2-NO_2-	−4.45	120
2-4-$(NO_2)_2$-	−10.23	120
OTHER ANILINE DERIVATIVES, IN 50% ETHANOL		
Unhindered aniline	4.19	40
p-Aminodiphenyl	3.81	40
2-Naphthylamine	3.77	40

* Thermodynamic value.

NITROGEN COMPOUNDS (Continued)

Compound		pK_a	Reference	Compound		pK_a	Reference
3-Phenanthrylamine		3.59	40				
Hindered-*o*-aminodiphenyl		3.03	40		SUBSTITUTED NAPHTHYLAMINES		
peri					OH	3.30	88
1-Naphthylamine		3.40	40		CH_3	3.96	88
9-Phenanthrylamine		3.19	40		Cl	2.71	88
3-Aminopyrene		2.91	40	2-NH_2,5-X	NO_2	3.01	88
meso					OH	4.07	88
9-Anthrylamine		2.7	40	1-NH_2,5-X	NO_2	2.73	88
m-Aminodiphenyl		3.82	40		OH	3.96	88
2-Aminofluorene		4.21	40		Cl	3.34	88
2-Phenanthrylamine		3.60	40		NH_2	4.21	88
2-Anthrylamine		3.40	40	1-NH_2,7-X	NO_2	2.55	88
1-Phenanthrylamine		3.23	40		Cl	3.48	88
1-Anthrylamine		3.22	40		OCH_3	4.07	88
					OH	4.20	88
O-AMINOPHENOLS				1-NH_2,2-X	NO_2	−1.74	88
3-Hydroxyanthranilic acid		10.09, 5.20	51	1-X,2-NH_2	NO_2	−0.85	88
2-Aminophenol hydrochloride		9.99, 4.86	51	1-NH_2,8-X	NO_2	2.79	88
2-Amino-4,5-dimethyl- phenolhydrochloride		10.40, 5.28	51	2-NH_2,4-X	NO_2	2.43	88
					CN	2.66	88
INDICATORS					Cl	3.38	88
p-Aminoazobenzene		2.82, 2.76			Br	3.40	88
4-Chloro-2-nitroaniline		−1.02, −1.03	60		I	3.41	88
4,6 Dichloro-2-nitroaniline		−3.61, −3.32	60		$COOCH_3$	3.38	88
6-Bromo-2,4-dinitroaniline		−6.64, −6.71	60		OCH_3	4.05	88
N,N-Dimethyl-2,4- dinitroaniline		−1.00	60	1-NH_2,6-X	NO_2	2.89	88
p-Nitrodiphenylamine		−2.4 to −2.9, −2.50	60	X	Cl	3.48	88
4-Methyl-2,6-dinitroaniline		−3.96, −4.44	60		OCH_3	3.90	88
					OH	3.97	88
SUBSTITUTED NAPHTHYLAMINES				2-NH_2, 7-X	NO_2	3.10	88
1-NH_2-		3.92*	2		Cl	3.71	88
1-NH_2-2-NO_2-		−1.6	2		OCH_3	4.19	88
1-NH_2-3-NO_2-		2.22	2		OH	4.25	88
1-NH_2-4-NO_2-		0.54	2		NH_2	4.66	88
1-NH_2-5-NO_2-		2.80	2	2-NH_2,6-X	NO_2	2.62	88
1-NH_2-6-NO_2-		3.15	2		OCH_3	4.64	88
1-NH_2-7-NO_2-		2.83	2	2-NH_2,8-X	NO_2	2.73	88
1-NH_2-8-NO_2-		2.79	2	1-NH_2,4-X	NO_2	0.54	88
1-NH_2-2- SO_3-		1.71	2		Br	3.21	88
1-NH_2-3- SO_3-		3.20*	2	2-NH_2,3-X	NO_2	1.48	88
1-NH_2-4- SO_3-		2.81*	2				
1-NH_2-5- SO_3-		3.69*	2				
1-NH_2-6- SO_3-		3.80*	2	HETEROCYCLIC COMPOUNDS			
1-NH_2-7- SO_3-		3.66*	2	Adenine		4.15, 9.80	6
1-NH_2-8- SO_3-		5.03*	2	Adenine deoxyriboside-5′-phosphoric acid		4.4, 6.4	99
2-NH_2-		4.11*	2	Adenosine		3.63, 12.5	6, 99
2-NH_2-1-NO_2-		−1.0	2	1-Oxide		2.25, 12.86	99
2-NH_2-3- NO_2-		2.93	2	ADP		3.95, 6.3, (7.20*)	36, 113
2-NH_2-4- NO_2-		2.63	2	5-Amino-1(β-D-ribosyluronic acid)uracil		3.06	99
2-NH_2-5- NO_2-		3.16	2	2′-AMP		3.81, 6.17	6
2-NH_2-6- NO_2-		2.75	2	3′-AMP		3.74, 5.92	6
2-NH_2-7- NO_2-		3.13	2	5′-AMP		3.74, 6.2–6.4	6
2-NH_2-8- NO_2-		2.86	2	5-Aminouridine		3.11	99
2-NH_2-1-SO_3-		2.35	2	1-D-Arabinosyl-5-methylcytosine		4.1	99
2-NH_2-4-SO_3-		3.70	2	ATP		4.00 (4.1), 6.5 (7.68*)	36, 113
2-NH_2-5-SO_3-		3.96*	2	Barbital		7.85, 12.7	37
2-NH_2-6-SO_3-		3.74*	2	Barbituric acid		3.9, 12.5	37
2-NH_2-7-SO_3-		3.95*	2	*N-n*-Butyl-5-fluoro-2′-deoxycytidine		2.21	99
2-NH_2-8-SO_3-		3.89*	2	CDP		4.44, (7.18*)	6, 113
2-Naphthylamine	X	4.16	88	CDP (deoxy)		4.8, 6.6	6
1-NH_2,3-X	NO_2	2.07	88	2′-CMP		4.3–4.4, 6.19*	6
	CN	2.26	88	3′-CMP		4.16–4.31, 6.04	6
	Cl	2.66	88	5′-CMP		4.5, 6.3	6
	Br	2.67	88	CTP		4.6, 6.4, (7.65*)	6, 113
	I	2.82	88	Cytidine		4.22, 12.5	35
	$COOCH_3$	3.12	88	Cytosine		4.45, 12.2	6
	OCH_3	3.26	88				

* Thermodynamic value.

NITROGEN COMPOUNDS (Continued)

Compound	pK′$_a$	Reference	Compound	pK′$_a$	Reference
NUCLEOSIDES, NUCLEOTIDES, AND RELATED COMPOUNDS (Continued)			**NUCLEOSIDES, NUCLEOTIDES, AND RELATED COMPOUNDS (Continued)**		
Cytosine (deoxy)	4.25, ~13	6, 101	5-Methylcytidine	4.21	99
Deoxycytidine-5′-phosphoric acid	4.6, 6.6	99	5-Methylcytidylic acid	4.4	99
2,6-Diaminopurine	5.09, 10.77	6	5-Methyicytosine	4.6, 12.4	6
N,N-Dimethylcytidine	3.58	99	5-Methylcytosine deoxyriboside	4.5, 13.0	6
N,N-Dimethyl-2′-deoxycytidine	3.75	99	5-Methylcytosine deoxyriboside 5-phosphate	4.4, 13	6, 100
N-Ethyl-5-fluoro-2′-deoxycytidine	2.21	99	N-Methyl-2′-deoxycytidine	3.97	99
5-Fluorocytidine	2.22	99	5-Methyl-2′-deoxycytidine	4.33	99
5-Fluoro-2′-deoxycytidine	2.39	99	1-Methyluracil	9.95	37
5-Fluoro-N,N-dimethyl-2′-deoxycytidine	1.89	99	3-Methyluracil	9.75	37
5-Fluoro-N-methyl-2′-deoxycytidine	2.14	99	1-Methylxanthine	7.7, 12.05	38
GDP	2.9, 9.6, 6.3, (7.19*)	6, 113	3-Methylxanthine	8.5, (8.1), 11.3	38
1-D-Glucopyranosylcytosine	3.78	99	7-Methylxanthine	8.5, (8.3)	38
GMP (2′+3′)	2.3, 9.36, 0.7, 5.9	6	9-Methylxanthine	6.3	38
5′-GMP	2.4, 9.4, 6.1	6	Orotic acid	2.8, 9.45, 13	6
5′-GMP (deoxy)	2.9, 9.7, 6.4	6	Purine	2.52, 8.90	37
GTP	3.3, 9.3, 6.5, (7.65*)	6, 113	Pyrimidine	1.30	37
Guanine	3.3, 9.2, 12.3	6	Thymidine	9.8	6
Guanine deoxyriboside-3′-phosphoric acid	2.9, 6.4, 9.7	99	Thymine	0, 9.9, >13.0	6
Guanosine	1.6, 9.16, 12.5	35	5′-TMP	10.0, 1.6, 6.5	6
Guanosine-3′-phosphoric acid	0.7, 2.3, 5.92, 9.38	99	UDP	9.4, 6.5, (7.16*)	6, 113
Guanosine (deoxy)	1.6–2.2, 9.16–9.5	6	UMP(2′+3′)	9.43, 1.02, 5.88	6
Hypoxanthine	1.98, 8.94, 12.10	6	5′-UMP	9.5, 6.4	6
5′-IMP	8.9, 1.54, 6.04	6	Uracil	0.5, 9.5, 13.0	6
Inosine	1.2, 8.75, 12.5	6, 35	Uracil deoxyriboside	9.3, >13	6, 101
ITP	7.68*	113	Uric acid	5.4, 10.3	6
IDP	7.18*	113	Uridine	9.17, 12.5	35
N-Methylcytidine	3.88	99	UTP	9.5, 6.6, (7.58*)	6, 113
1-Methylcytidine	8.7	99	Xanthine	0.8, 7.44, 11.12	6
			Xanthosine	0, 5.5, 13.0	6

HETEROCYCLIC BASES

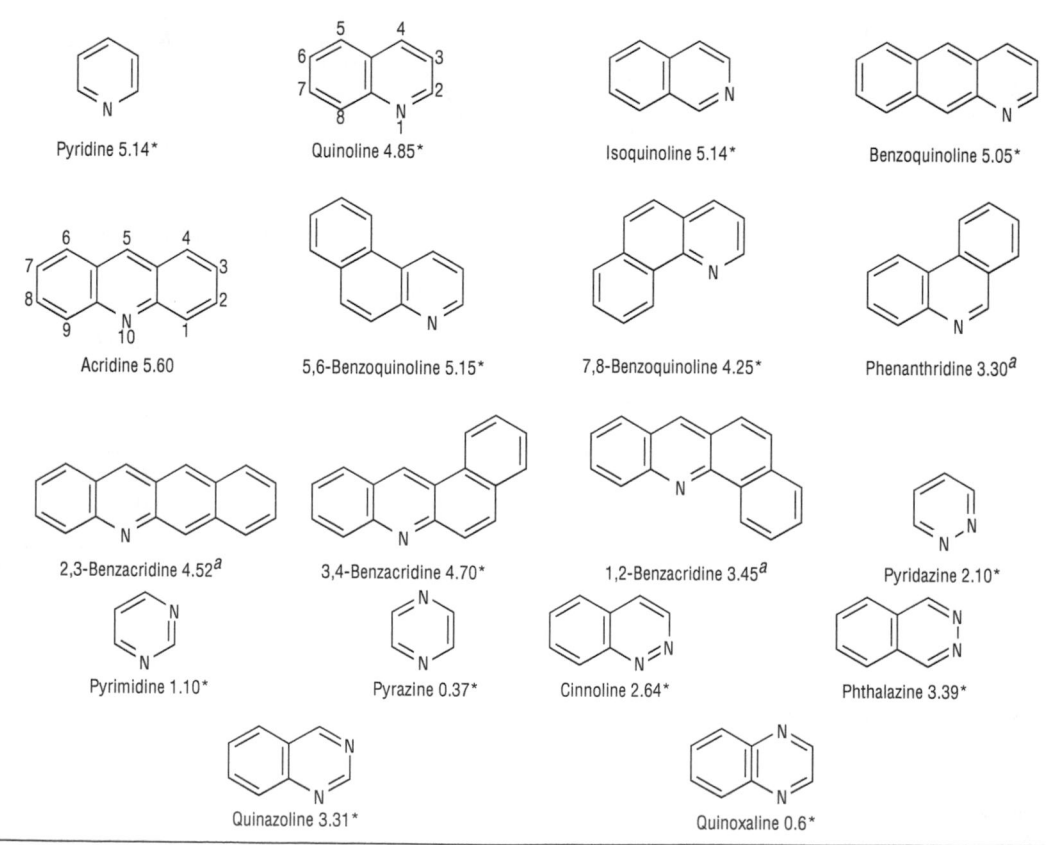

Pyridine 5.14*   Quinoline 4.85*   Isoquinoline 5.14*   Benzoquinoline 5.05*

Acridine 5.60   5,6-Benzoquinoline 5.15*   7,8-Benzoquinoline 4.25*   Phenanthridine 3.30[a]

2,3-Benzacridine 4.52[a]   3,4-Benzacridine 4.70*   1,2-Benzacridine 3.45[a]   Pyridazine 2.10*

Pyrimidine 1.10*   Pyrazine 0.37*   Cinnoline 2.64*   Phthalazine 3.39*

Quinazoline 3.31*   Quinoxaline 0.6*

* Thermodynamic value.
[a] In 50% EtOH

NITROGEN COMPOUNDS (Continued)

Acridine	1-	2-	3-	4-	5-	9-
H-	5.60*	4.11[a]	—	—	—	—
H_2N-	4.40*	8.04*	5.88*	6.04*	9.99*	9.95*
	3.59[a]	7.61[a]	5.03[a]	5.50[a]	9.45[a]	—
HO-	4.18[a]	4.86[a]	5.52	4.45[a]	−0.32	—
	10.7[a]	9.9[a]	8.81	9.4[a]	>12	—
CH_3-	3.95[a]	—	4.60[a]	—	4.70[a]	—
H_2N-(1-CH_3–)-	—	—	—	4.79[a]	9.73[a]	3.22[a]
I,9-$(CH_3)_2$-	2.88[a]	—	—	—	—	—
COOH-	—	5.26*	—	7.76*	—	5.0*

Reference 3, 39, 99

Compound	pK'_a	Reference
HETEROCYCLICS (Continued)		
Acridine	5.62	39
3-Amino-7-carboxy-	2.3*, 9.0*	99
3-Amino-6-chloro-	7.22*	99
3-Amino-7-chloro-	6.91*	99
9-Amino-1-hydroxy-	5.57*	99
9-Amino-2-hydroxy-	7.67*	99
9-Amino-3-hydroxy-	6.59*	99
9-Amino-4-hydroxy-	7.01*	99
3-Amino-7-sulfo-	7.6*	99
2,7-Diamino-	6.14*	99
3,6-Diamino-	9.65*	99
3,7-Diamino-	8.11	99
3,9-Diamino-	8.11	99
5-Methoxy-	7	39
9-Methoxy-	−0.32*	99
2-Sulpho-	4.78*	99
Aureomycin	3.30, 7.44, 9.27	77
Azacycloundecane 1-Methyl-6-hydroxy-7-oxo-	9.1*	99
Azaindole		
4-	6.9	154
5-	8.3	154
6-	8.0	154
7-	4.6	154
3,4-Di-	4.0, 11.1	154
3,5-Di-	6.1, 10.9	154
2,5, 7-Tri-	2.8, 9.5	154
4-Amino-2, 5, 7-tri-	4.6, 10.8	154
Azepine Hexahydro-	11.07*	99
Azetidine	11.29*	99
Aziridine	8.01*	99
1:2-Benzacridine	3.45[a]	19
5-Amino-	8.13[a]	19
7-Amino-	4.05[a]	19
8-Amino-	6.72, 5.97[a]	19
4′,5-Diamino-	8.44[a]	19
2:3-Benzacridine	4.52[a]	19
5-Acetamido-	4.56[a]	19
5-Amino-	9.72[a]	19
7-Amino-	5.38[a]	19
5-Amino-6, 7, 8, 9-tetrahydro-	9.66[a]	19
3:4-Benzacridine	4.70, 4.16[a]	19
8-Acetamido-	4.48[a]	19
5-Amino-	8.4|[a]	19
7-Amino-	5.03[a]	19
8-Amino-	7.42, (651)[a]	19
8-Dimethylamino-	7.31, 6.99	19

* Thermodynamic value.
[a] In 50% alcohol

Compound	pK'_a	Reference
HETEROCYCLICS (Continued)		
Benzimidazole	5.4, 12.78	43, 86, 99, 107
2-Amino-	7.51*	—
5-Amino-	3.04*, 6.07*	—
6-Amino-	3.0, 6.0	—
2-Aminomethyl-	7.69*, 3.46*	—
1-α-D-Arabopyranosyl-	4.19*	—
1-α-L-Arabopyranosyl-	4.06*	—
1-α-L-Arabopyranosyl-5,6-dimethyl-	4.56*	—
1-α-L-Arabopyranosyl-5-methyl-	4.30	—
1-Ethyl-	5.59*	—
2-Ethyl-	6.18*	—
1-β-D-Glucopyranosyl-	3.97*	—
1-β-D-Glucopyranosyl-5, 6-dimethyl-	4.60*	—
1-β-D-Glucopyranosyl-5-methyl-	4.29*	—
4-Hydroxy-	5.3, 9.5	—
4-Hydroxy-6-amino-	5.9	—
1-Hydroxymethyl-	5.41*	—
2-Hydroxymethyl-	5.40*, 11.55*	—
4-Hydroxy-6-nitro-	3.05	—
4-Methoxy-	5.1	—
1-Methyl-	5.54*	—
2-Methyl-	5.58	—
4-Methyl-	5.65*	—
5-Methyl-	5.78*	—
2-Methyl-4-hydroxy-6-amino-	6.65	—
1-Methyl-2-hydroxymethyl-	5.55, 11.45	—
2-Methyl-4-hydroxy-6-nitro-	3.9	—
4-Nitro-	3.33*	—
5-Nitro-	3.48*	—
6-Nitro-	3.05, 10.6	—
5-F-	1.67*, 4.92*	123, 124
5-Br-	1.98*, 4.66*	123, 124
5-CF_3-	2.28*, 4.22*	123, 124
5-Cl-	1.94*, 4.70*	123, 124
Benzo[c]cinnoline	2.20*	99
6,7-Benzoquinazoline	5.2*	99
5,6-Benzoquinoline	5.15, 3.90[a]	19
4-Amino-	7.99[a]	19
2-Amino-4-methyl-	7.14, 6.51[a]	19
4-Amino-2-methyl-	8.45[a]	19
1′-Amino-	5.03	19
3′-Amino-	4.02[a]	19
4′-Amino-	5.20, 4.10[a]	19
2′,4′-Diamino-	4.91[a]	19
2-Methyl-	4.44[a]	19
6,7-Benzoquinoline	5.05, 3.84[a]	19
3-Amino-	4.78, 3.73[a]	19
4-Amino-	8.75[a]	19
4-Amino-2-methyl-	9.45[a]	19
4-Amino-2-methyl-8-chloro-	5.95[a]	19
8-Chloro-	2.5[a]	19
3,4-Diamino-	8.15[a]	19
7,8-Benzoquinoline	4.25, 3.15[a]	19
4-Amino-	7.68[a]	19
2-Amino-4-methyl-	6.74, 6.02[a]	19
4-Amino-2-methyl-	7.96[a]	19
6-Amino-2-methyl-	5.23[a]	19
1′-Amino-2-methyl-	4.75[a]	19
Benzoxazole	(decomp.)	19
2-Amino-	3.73	19
Benzthiazole	1.2, 0.1[a]	19
2-Amino-	4.51	19
Benztriazole	1.6, 8.64*	19
Bispidine	10.25*	99

NITROGEN COMPOUNDS (Continued)

Compound	pK'_a	Reference	Compound	pK'_a	Reference
HETEROCYCLICS (Continued)			*HETEROCYCLICS (Continued)*		
Caffeine	0.61	4	3-Methyl-5,5-pentamethylene-2-thio-	11.23	42
Cinchonine	7.2	4	5:5-Pentamethylene-2-thio-	8.79	42
Cinnoline	2.70, 2.29	19, 39	3:5:5-Trimethyl-2-thio-	10.80	42
4-Amino-	6.84	19	Imidazoles	7.05, 14.52	107
3-Hydroxy-	8.64, 0.21	39	4-(2-Acetoxyethyl)-	6.97*	99
4-Hydroxy-	9.27, 0.35	39	N-Acetyl-	3.6	99
5-Hydroxy-	7.40, 1.92	39	N-Acetylhistidine	7.05	43
6-Hydroxy-	7.52, 3.65	39	4-Aminomethyl-	9.37*, 4.71*	99
7-Hydroxy-	7.56, 3.31	39	5-Amino-4-(N-methylcarboxamidino)-	9.5*	99
8-Hydroxy-	8.20, 2.74	39	4-Bromo-	3.7	43
4-Methoxy-	3.21	39	4-Carbamoyl-	3.7*, 11.8*	99
4-Methylthio-	3.09*	99	4-(3-Carbamoylpropyl)-	6.52*	99
5,6,7,8-Tetrahydro-	4.30*	99	Carbobenzoxy-l-histidyl-l-tyrosine ethyl ester	6.25	43
α,α'-Dipyridyl	4.43	6	4-(2′,4′-Dihydroxyphenyl)-	6.45	43
4.5-Diazaindan	4.12*	99	4-Chloro-1-methyl-	6.23*	99
1,4-Diazaindene	6.92*	99	2,4-Dimethyl-	8.36*	99
1,5-Diazaindene	8.24*	99	2,4-Dinitro-	2.85	106
1,6-Diazaindene	7.93*	99	2,5-Dinitro-	2.85	106
1,7-Diazaindene	4.57*	99	2,4-Diphenyl-	5.64*, 12.53*	99
Flavone	−1.2	154	2,5-Diphenyl-	5.64, 12.53	107
Δ²-Dihydro-2-methyl-	11.1	154	4,5-Diphenyl-	5.90*, 12.80*	99
Furan, 2-(2-aminoethylaminomethyl)-	6.54*, 9.87*	99	1-Ethyl-	7.30*	99
Furan, 3-(2-aminoethylaminomethyl)-	6.70*, 9.86*	99	2-Ethyl-	8.00	99
Furan, 2-aminomethyl-	8.89	99	1H-Imidazo[4,5-b]pyridine	3.92*, 11.11*	99
Gramine	16.00	152	1H-Imidazo[4, 5-c]pyridine	6.10*, 10.88*	99
5-Benzyloxy-	16.90	152	Imidazolidines		
Histamine	6.0	43	2-Imino-1-methyl-4-oxo-	4.80*	99
Histidine methyl ester	5.2, 7.1	43	2-Imino-4-oxo-	4.76*	99
4-Hydroxymethyl-	6.39	99	n-Nitrimino-	−1.36*	99
2-(2-Imidazolyl)-	4.53*	99	2-Imidazoline		
4-(3-Methoxycarbonylpropyl)-	7.3	99	2-(N-Benzylanilinomethyl)-	2.45*, 10.13*	99
1-Methyl-	6.95*	99	2-(3-Diethylamino-1-phenyl)propyl-	8.41*, 10.09*	99
2-Methyl-	7.85	99	2-(3-Dimethylamino-1-phenyl)propyl-	7.98*, 9.99*	99
4-Methyl-	7.51	99	2-Diphenylmethyl-	9.78*	99
1-Methyl-4-chloro-	3.10	106	Imidazoline		
1-Methyl-5-chloro-	4.75	106	2-(3-(2-Hydroxynaphthyl))-	7.01*, 10.85*	99
1-Methyl-4-nitro-	−0.53*	99	2-(2-Hydroxyphenyl)-	6.63*, 12.58*	99
1-Methyl-5-nitro-	2.13*	99	4-Methyl-5-carboxylic acid-	2.49, 7.02	144
1-Methyl-4-phenyl-	5.78*	99	1-Methyl-2-carboxylic acid-	1.26, 7.25	144
2-Nitro-	7.15	106	1H-Indazole	1.22*, 14*	99
4-Nitro-	−0.05*	99	3-Amino-	3.12*	99
5-Nitro-	9.20	106	4-Amino-	3.26*	99
4-Nitro-5-chloro-	5.85	106	5-Amino-	5.12*	99
5-Nitro-4-chloro-	5.85	106	6-Amino-	3.99*	99
2-Phenyl-	6.48*, 13.32*	99	7-Amino-	3.02*	99
4-Phenyl-	6.10*, 13.42*	99	Indole	−2.4*	99
5-Phenyl-	6.10, 13.42	107	Indole	−3.6, 16.97	154, 152
4-(2-Pyridyl)-	5.42*	99	2-Amino-	8.15*	99
2,4,5-Trimethyl-	8.92*	99	2-Amino-1-methyl-	9.60*	99
Hydantoin	9.16	42	1,2-Dimethyl-	0.34*	99
5:5-Dimethyl-2-thio-	8.71	42	2,3-Dimethyl-	−1.10*	99
5:5-Diphenyl-2-thio-	7.69	42	1-Methyl-	−1.80	99
5-Isopropyl-2-thio-	8.70	42	2-Methyl-	−0.10*	99
1-Methyl-5,5-pentamethylene-2-thio-	9.25	42	3-Methyl-	−3.35*	99
			3-Formyl-	12.36	152
			3-Acetyl-	12.99	152
			5-Nitro-	14.75	152
			5-Cyano-	15.24	152
			5-Bromo-	16.13	152
			5-Fluoro-	16.30	152
			4-Fluoro-	16.30	152

* Thermodynamic value.

NITROGEN COMPOUNDS (Continued)

Compound	pK'a	Reference	Compound	pK'a	Reference
HETEROCYCLICS (Continued)			*HETEROCYCLICS (Continued)*		
2-Carboxylate-	17.13	152	5-NO$_2$-2-Carboxylate	14.91	152
3-Carboxylate-	15.59	152	5-Br-2-Carboxylate	16.10	152
5-Carboxylate-	16.92	152	5-MeO-2-Carboxylate	17.03	152
3-Acetic acid-	16.90	152	Isoalloxazine, 7,8 dichloro-		
3-Carbinol-	16.50	152	10-(3-Dibutylaminopropyl)-	8.0*	99
L-Tryptophanol	16.91	152	10-(4-Diethylaminobutyl)-	9.7*	99
L-Tryptophan	16.82	152	10-(2-Diethylaminoethyl)-	7.7*	99
4-Methyltryptophan	16.90	152	10-(5-Diethylaminopropyl)-	9.1*	99
5-Hydroxytryptophan	19.20	152	10-(3-Piperidinopropyl)-	9.0*	99
6-Methoxytryptophan	16.70	152	Isoxazole	1.3*	27
Tryptamine	16.60	152	3,5-Dimethyl-	–2*	27
Serotonin	19.50	152	4,5-Dimethyl-	0*	27
Gramine	16.00	152	3-Methyl-	–1*	27
5-Benzyloxydramine	16.90	152	5-Methyl-	2.3*	27
Skatole	16.60	152	3,4,5-Trimethyl-	–1*	27

	1	3	4	5	6	7	8	Reference
Isoquinoline	5.46	5.14	—	—	—	—	—	19, 44, 99
OH-	–1.2	2.18*	4.78*	5.40	5.85	5.68*	5.66	—
	—	9.62*	8.70*	8.45	9.15	8.90*	8.40	—
NH$_2$-	7.59*	5.05	6.26*	5.59	7.16*	6.20*	6.04*	—
CH$_3$-	—	5.64*	—	—	—	—	—	—
Br-	—	—	3.31*	—	—	—	—	—
SH-	–1.9*	0.39*	—	—	—	—	—	—
	10.86*	8.62*	—	—	—	—	—	—
CH$_3$O-	3.01*	—	—	—	—	—	—	—
CH$_3$S-	3.89*	3.37*	—	—	—	—	—	—
NO$_2$-	—	—	1.35*	3.49*	3.43*	3.57*	3.55*	—

Compound	pK'a	Reference	Compound	pK'a	Reference
HETEROCYCLICS (Continued)			*HETEROCYCLICS (Continued)*		
Isoquinoline			2-Ethyl-	6.13*, 12.9*	99
1,2,3,4-Tetrahydro-	9.4	154	2-Hydroxy-	11.66*	99
Isoquinoline-*N*-oxide	1.01	47	2-Methyl-	6.10*, 12.9*	99
Morpholine	8.39*	99	1,5-Naphthyridine	2.84*	99
N-(3-Acetyl-3,3-diphenyl)propyl-	6.83*	99	1,6-Naphthyridine	3.76*	99
N-(2-Acetyl-2-phenyl)ethyl-	6.23*	99	1,7-Naphthyridine	3.61*	99
N-Allyl-	7.02*	99	1,8-Naphthyridine	3.36*	99
N-(2-Amino)ethyl-	4.84*, 9.45*	99	8-Hydroxy-6-methyl-1,6-naphthyridinium chloride	4.34	44
N-(2-Benzylcarbonyl-2-phenyl)ethyl-	6.17*	99	8-Hydroxy-1,6-naphthyridine	4.08	44
N-(2-Bis-2-hydroxypropyl)aminoethyl-	7.9*	99	Oxazoline		
N-(3-Cyano-3,3-diphenyl)propyl-	6.04*	99	4-Carbamoyl-2-phenyl-	2.9	96
N-(3-Cyano-1-methyl-3,3-diphenyl)propyl-	5.5*, 8.4*	99	2-Methyl-Δ^2-	5.5	96
N-(2-Diphenylmethyl-carbonyl)ethyl-	6.39*	99	2-Phenyl-Δ^2-	4.4	96
N-(3,3-Diphenyl)propyl-	7.20*	99	4-Methyl-	1.07	144
N-(3,3-Diphenyl-3-propyl-carbonyl)propyl-	7.17*	99	Ethyl-4-Methyl-5-carboxylate-	0.83	144
N-Ethyl-	7.67*	99	4-Methyl-5-carboxylic acid-	0.95, 2.88	144
N-(3-Ethylcarbonyl-3,3-diphenyl)propyl-	6.95*	99	Perimidine	6.35*	99
N-(3-Ethylcarbonyl-1-methyl-3,3-diphenyl)propyl	6.68*	99	3,4-Pentamethylene-5,6,7,8-tetrahydrocinnoline	6.03*	99
N-(3-Ethylcarbonyl-2-methyl-3,3-diphenyl)propyl-	7.12*	99	1,5-Phenanthroline	0.75*, 4.10	99
N-(2-Hydroxy-3-morpholino)propyl-	5.00*, 6.98*	99	1,7-Phenanthroline	1,4	99
N-Methyl-	7.38*	99	1,10-Phenanthroline	4.84*	99
N-(1-Methyl-3,3-diphenyl)propyl-	6.85*	99	4-Bromo-	4.01*	99
N-(2-Morpholino)ethyl-	3.63*, 6.65*	99	3-Chloro-	3.97*	99
N-(3-Morpholino)propyl-	6.25*, 7.25*	99	4-Chloro-	4.30*	99
1(3)*H*-Naphth[l,2-d]imidazole	5.27*	99	5-Chloro-	4.24*	99
1*H*-Naphth[2,3-d]imidazole	5.21*. 12.58*	99	4-Cyano-	3.56*	99
2-Amino-	6.99*	99	3-Ethyl-	4.96*	99
2-Carboxymethylthio-	1.9*, 4.72*	99			

* Thermodynamic value.

NITROGEN COMPOUNDS (Continued)

Compound	pK'_a	Reference	Compound	pK'_a	Reference
HETEROCYCLICS (Continued)			*HETEROCYCLICS (Continued)*		
4-Ethyl-	5.42*	99	2,4-di-OH-	< 1.0, 7.91	101
4-Hydroxy-	2.17*	99	2,6-di-OH-	6.7, 11.6	101
2-Methyl-	4.98*	99	2,7-di-OH-	5.83, 10.07	101
3-Methyl-	4.98*	99	4,6-di-OH-	6.08, 9.73	101
5-Methyl-	5.26*	99	4,7-di-OH-	6.82, 10.02	101
5-Nitro-	3.55*	99	6,7-di-OH-	6.87, 10.0	101
2-Phenyl-	4.88*	99	2,4,6-tri-OH-	5.73, 9.41	101
3-Phenyl-	4.80*	99	3,4,7-tri-OH-	3.61	101
4-Phenyl-	4.88*	99	4-OH-6-Me-	8.19	101
5-Phenyl-	4.70*	99	4-OH-7-Me-	8.09	101
o-Phenanthroline	4.27[a], 5.2	19	6-OH-5-Me-	3.73, 10.6	101
p-Phenanthroline	3.12[a]	19	7-OH-8-Me-	1.1	101
1:10-Diamino-3,8-dimethyl-	8.76[a], 6.31[a]	19	2-OH-1-Me-	<1, 11.43	101
6-*m*-Phenanthroline	3.11[a]	19	2-OH-3-Me-	1, 11.01	101
1-Amino-	ca. 7.3, 7.29[a]	19	2-OH-3,6,7-tri-Me-	< 2 , 11.36	101
Phenazine	1.23	39	2-OH-6,7,8-tri-Me-	< 2, 10.26	101
1-Amino-	2.6[a]	19	4-OH-1-Me-	1.25	101
2-Amino-	4.75, 3.46[a]	19	4-OH-3-Me-	−0.47	101
1,3-Diamino-	5.64[a]		4-OH-6,7-di-Me-	8.39	101
2,3-Diamino-	4.74	19	4-OH-6,7,8-tri-Me-	4.70, 9.46	101
2:7-Diamino-	4.63, 3.9[a]	19	7,8-Dihydro-6-OH-	4.78, 10.54	101
1-Hydroxy-	1.61*, 8.33*		5,6-Dihydro-7-OH-	3.36, 9.94	101
2-Hydroxy-	7.5, 2.6	99	5,6-Dihydro-6,7-di-OH-5-Me-	2.91, 9.33	101
Phenanthridine	4.65	39	5,6-Dihydro-4,7-di-OH-6-Me-	8.43, 11.40	101
2-Amino-9-methyl-	5.66[a]	44	4,7-di-OH-6-CHO-	5.93, 9.31	101
6-Amino-	6.88	19	4,7-di-OH-6-COOH-	ca. 3, 6.69, 10.15	101
7-Amino-9-methyl-	5.23[a]	40	2-MeO-	2.13	101
9-Amino-	7.31, 6.75[a]	19	4-MeO-	1.04	101
2:7-Diamino-9-methyl-	6.26[a]	19	6-MeO-	3.60	101
2-Hydroxy-	8.79, 4.82	19	7-MeO-	1.64	101
6-Hydroxy-	8.43, 5.35	44	2-NH$_2$-	4.29	101
7-Hydroxy-	4.38, 8.68	44	4-NH$_2$-	3.51	101
9-Hydroxy (phenanthridone)	<−1.5	44	6-NH$_2$-	4.15	101
9-Methoxy-	2.38	44	7-NH$_2$-	2.96	101
2,7,9-Triamino-	8.06[a]	44	2,4-di-NH$_2$-	5.32	101
Phenothiazine		19	4,6-di-NH$_2$-	4.37	101
10-(2-Diethylaminoethyl)-	9.06*	99	4,7-di-NH$_2$-	4.97	101
10-(2-Dimethylaminobutyl)-	9.02*	99	2,4,7-tri-NH$_2$-	6.03	101
10-(2-Dimethylaminoethyl)-	8.66*	99	4,6,7-tri-NH$_2$-	5.57	101
3,7-Diamino-	5.3, 4.4	154	2,4,6,7-tetra-NH$_2$-	6.86	101
Phthalazine	3.47	19	2-MeNH-	3.64	101
1-Amino-	6.60	19	4-MeNH-	4.33	101
1-Hydroxy-	11.99, −2	39	2-Me$_2$N-	3.03	101
1-Mercapto-	−3.43*, 9.99*	99	4-Me$_2$N-	4.33	101
1-Methoxy-	3.73*	99	6-Me$_2$N-	4.31	101
1-Methyl-	4.37*	99	7-Me$_2$N-	2.56	101
1-Methylthio-	3.44*	99	2-NH$_2$-7-OH-	1.5*, 7.50*	99
1-Phenyl-	3.51*	99	2-NH$_2$-4-CH$_3$O-	3.44*	99
Picolinic acid	5.52	4	2-NH$_2$-4-CH$_3$-	2.81*	99
Trimethyl(2,6-di-tert-butyl-4-picolyl)ammonium	3.51	125	2-NH$_2$-6-CH$_3$-	4.03*	99
Pteridines	4.12	101	2-NH$_2$-7-CH$_3$-	3.73*	99
6-Cl-	3.68*	99	4-NH$_2$-2-CH$_3$-	4.28*	99
2-Me-	4.87	101	2-NH$_2$-4-OH-	2.31, 7.92	101
4-Me-	2.94	101	4-NH$_2$-2-OH-	3.21, 9.97	101
7-Me-	3.49	101	2-NH$_2$-4,6-di-OH-	1.6, 6.3, 9.23	101
6,7-di-Me-	2.93	101	2-MeCONH-	2.67	101
2,6,7-tri-Me-	3.76	101	4-MeCONH-	1.21	101
2-OH-	< 2, 11.13	101	4-H$_2$NNH-	4.00	101
4-OH-	< 1.5, 7.98	101	2-SH-	9.98	101
6-OH-	3.67, 6.7	101	4-SH-	6.81	101
7-OH-	1.2, 6.41	101	7-SH-	5.5	101
			2-MeS-	2.2	101
			4-MeS-	2.59	101

NITROGEN COMPOUNDS (Continued)

Compound	pK'_a	Reference	Compound	pK'_a	Reference
HETEROCYCLICS (Continued)			*HETEROCYCLICS (Continued)*		
7-MeS-	2.49	101	2,6,8-tri-NH$_2$-	2.41, 6.23, 10.96	101
4-MeS-7-Me-	< 2	101	6-MeNH-	1, 4.18, 9.99	101
4-SH-7-Me-	7.02	101	8-MeNH-	4.78, 9.56	101
3,4-Dihydro-2-OH-	0*, 12.6*	99	2-Me$_2$N-	4.02, 10.22	101
3,4-Dihydro-4-OH-	4.75*, 11.25*	99	6-Me$_2$N-	<1, 3.84, 10.5	101
5,6-Dihydro-4-OH-	2.94*, 10.24*	99	8-Me$_2$N-	1, 4.80, 9.73	101
7,8-Dihydro-2-OH-	3.46*	99	2-C$_6$H$_5$NH-	4.2, 10.1	101
7,8-Dihydro-4-OH-	0.32*, 12.13*	99	2-Me-6-MeNH-	5.08	101
6-OH-2-CH$_3$-	4.65*, 6.33*	99	2-NH$_2$-6-OH-(Guanine)	3.3, 9.2, 12.3	101
6-OH-4-CH$_3$-	4.08*, 6.41*	99	6-NH$_2$-2-OH-	4.51, 8.99	101
6-OH-7-CH$_3$-	3.69*, 7.20*		2-NH$_2$-6-SH-	8.2, 11.6	101
7,8-Dihydro-4,6-dimethyl-	6.0	154	6-CHO-	2.4, 8.8	101
5,6,7,8-Tetrahydro-	6.6	154	6-HONH-	3.88, 9.88, >12	101
5,6,7,8-Tetrahydro-5-formyl-	5.0	154	6-NH$_2$CONH-	2.35, 9.95	101
5,6,7,8-Tetrahydro-4-methyl-	6.7	154	6-CN-	ca. 0.3, 6.88	101
5,6,7,8-Tetrahydro-4-hydroxy-	3.9, 10.1	154	6-CF$_3$-	0, 7.35	101
Pteridines			8-CF$_3$-	1.0, 5.12	101
7-OH-2-CH$_3$-	1.68*, 6.70*	99	6-Me-	2.6, 9.02	101
3-Methyl-4-pteridone	−0.47	44	8-Me-	2.85, 9.37	101
1-Methyl-4-pteridone	1.25	44	9-Me-	2.36	101
Pteroylglutamic acid	8.26	77	8-Ph-	2.68, 8.09	101
Purine	2.39, 8.93	101	2-OH-	8.43, 11.90	101
2-Amino-6,8-bistrifluoro-methyl-	0.3*, 5.02*	99	6-OH- (Hypoxanthine)	8.94, 12.10	101
6-Amino-9-cyclohexyl-amino-	4.19*	99	8-OH-	8.24, >12	101
2-Amino-8-phenyl-	3.97*, 9.21*	99	2,8-di-OH-	7.65, 9.7	101
2-Amino-6-trifluoromethyl-	1.85*, 8.87*	99	2,6-di-OH- (Xanthine)	7.44, 11.12	101
8-Carboxy-	0*, 2.93*, 9.41*	99	1-Me-2,6-di-OH-	7.7, 12.5	101
6-Chloro-	7.85*	99	3-Me-2,6-di-OH-	8.33, 11.9	101
6-Cyclohexylamino-	4.2*, 10.2*	99	7-Me-2,6-di-OH-	8.7, 10.7	191
9-Cyclohexyl-6-cyclohexyl-amino-	4.4*	99	1,3-di-Me-2,6-di-OH-	8.81	101
2,6-Diamino-8-trifluoro-methyl-	3.68*, 7.55*	99	1,7-di Me-2,6-di-OH-	8.71	101
1,6-Dihydro-1,7-dimethyl-6-oxo-	2.13*	99	3,7-di Me-2,6-di-OH-	9.97	101
7,8-Dihydro-7,9-dimethyl-8-oxo-	2.8*	99	2,6,8-tri-OH- (Uric acid)	5.75, 10.3	101
1,2-Dihydro-8-hydroxy-1-methyl-2-oxo-	−0.5*, 7.0*, 13.0*	99	2,6,8-tri-OH-3-Me-	5.75, >12	101
1,6-Dihydro-8-hydroxy-1-methyl-6-oxo-	8.54*, 11.87*	99	2,6,8-tri-OH-1-Me-	5.75, 10.6	101
2,3-Dihydro-8-hydroxy-3-methyl-2-oxo-	1.25*, 8.0*, 13.0*	99	2,6,8-tri-OH-1,3-di-Me-	5.75	101
1,6-Dihydro-6-imino-1-methyl-	11.0*, 7.0*	99	2,6,8-tri-OH-3,7-di-Me-	5.5, 12	101
1,2-Dihydro-1-methyl-2-oxo-	1.8*, 8.80*	99	2,6,8-tri-OH-1,3,7-tri-Me-	6.0	101
1,2-Dihydro-2-oxo-1-β-d-ribofuranosyl-	1.5*, 8.55*	99	2,6,8-tri-OH-3,7,9-tri-Me-	8.35	101
6-Dimethylcarbamoyl-	0*, 7.9*	99	6-OH-9-Me-	1.86, 9.32	101
6-(Ethoxycarbonyl)amino-	2.4*, 9.63*, 12.2*	99	8-OH-7-Me-	2.69, 8.20	101
6-Ethylamino-2-methyl-	5.01*	99	8-OH-9-Me-	2.80, 9.05	101
6-Hydrazonomethyl-	2.8*, 9.2*	99	2-MeO-	2.44, 9.2	101
8-Hydroxymethyl-	2.58*, 8.83*	99	6-MeO-	1.98, 8.94	101
6-Hydroxy-2-trifluoro-methyl-	1.1*, 5.1*, 11.2*	99	8-MeO-	3.14, 7.73	101
7-Methyl-	2.25*	99	Xanthine	7.53, 11.63	101
8-Methylthio-	2.92*, 7.70*	99	1-Me-	7.7, 12.05	101
Purine 1-oxide, 6-amino-	2.69*, 8.845*, 15.4*	99	3-Me-	8.10, 11.3	101
2-SH-	7.15*, 10.4	101	7-Me-	8.30	101
6-SH-	7.77, 10.84	101	9-Me-	6.25	101
8-SH-	6.64, 11.64	101	Hypoxanthine	8.8, 12.0	101
2-MeS-	8.91	101	Uric acid	5.78, 5.85	101
6-MeS-	8.74	101	Pyrazine	1.1 (0.6)	49, 39
2-NH$_2$-	−0.28, 3.80, 9.93	101	3-Acetyl-2-aminomethylene-amino-	5.49*	99
6-NH$_2$- (adenine)	<1, 4.22, 9.8	101	2-Amidino-3-methylamino-	8.96*	99
8-NH$_2$-	4.68, 9.36	101	2-Amino-	3.14	19
2,6-di-NH$_2$-	<1, 5.09, 10.7	101	2-Amino-3-carboxy-	3.70*	99
			2-Carbomoyl-	−0.5*	99
			2-Carbamoyl-3-methyl-amino-	2.09*	99
			2,3-Dicarboxy-	0.9*, 3.57*	99
			2,5-Dimethyl-	2.1	49
			2,6-Dimethyl-	2.5*	99

* Thermodynamic value.

NITROGEN COMPOUNDS (Continued)

HETEROCYCLICS (Continued)

Compound	pK'_a	Reference
2-Dimethylamino-	3.24*	99
2-Hydroxy-	−0.1*, 8.25*	99
2-Mercapto	−0.73*, 6.34*	99
2-Methoxy-	0.75	39
2-Methyl-	−5.25*, 1.45*	99
1-Methyl-2-pyrazone	−0.04	39
2-Methylamino-	3.39*	99
2-Methylthio-	0.48*	99
2-Sulphanilamido-	6.04*	99
2,3,5,6-Tetramethyl-	2.8	49
Trimethyl-	−0.35*, 2.8*	99
Pyrazole	2.48	99
3-(2-Aminoethyl)-	2.02*, 9.61*	99
1,3-Dimethyl-	3.11*	99
3,5-Dimethyl-	4.38*	99
1-Methyl-	2.04*	99
3-Methyl-	3.56*	99
Pyrazolo[4,5-4,5]pyrimidine 6-Amino-	4.96*, 10.19*	99
Pyrazolo[5',4'-4,5]pyrimidine	2.80*, 9.58*	99
6-Amino-	4.55*, 10.88*	99
6-Amino-1'-melhyl-	4.28*	99
6-Amino-2'-methyl-	5.37*, 11.34*	99
6-Amino-3'-methyl-	4.57*, 11.15*	99
6-Anilino-	3.88*	99
6-Benzylamino-	4.12*, 10.97*	99
2,6-Diamino-	4.63*, 11.25*	99
6-Diethylamino-	4.67*	99
6-Dimethylamino-	4.49*, 11	99
6-Ethylamino-	4.56*, 10.94*	99
6-Furfurylamino-	3.97*	99
6-Isopropylamino-	4.58*, 11.03*	99
6-Methylamino-	4.49*, 10.59*	99
1-Methyl-	2.46*	99
6-Methylthio-	1.0*, 9.69*	99
6-Phenethylamino-	4.34*	99
Pyridazine	2.33	19
3-Amino-	5.19	19
4-Amino-	6.65*	99
3-Amino-6-methyl-	5.29*	99
3-n-Butyl-	3.49*	99
3-Carbamoyl-	1.0*	99
4-Carbamoyl-	1.0*	99
3,5-Dihydroxy-	−2.2*	99
3,6-Dihydroxy-	5.67, −2.2, 13	39
3,6-Dimethoxy-	1.61	39
3,4-Dimethyl-	4.10*	99
3,5-Dimethyl-	4.11*	99
3,6-Dimethyl-	3.99*	99
4,5-Dimethyl-	4.13*	99
3-Hydroxy-	10.46, −1.8	39
4-Hydroxy-	8.68, 1.07	39
4-Hydroxy-2-methylpyridazinium chloride	1.74	44
3-Mercapto-	−2.68*. 8.32*	99
4-Mercapto-	−0.75*, 6.55*	99
3-Methoxy-	2.52	39
4-Methoxy-	3.70	39
3-Methyl-	3.46*	99
4-Methyl-	3.53*	99
3-Methylthio-	2.26*	99
4-Methylthio-	3.24*	99
3-Sulfanilamido-	7.06*	99

HETEROCYCLICS (Continued)

Compound	2-	3-	4-
Pyridine (2, 46–48, 88, 99, 105, 117,140)			
H-	5.17*	—	—
Cl-	0.72*	2.84*	3.88
I-	1.82*	3.25*	4.02*
CH3CH2-	5.97*	5.70*	6.02*
(CH3)3C-	5.76*	5.82*	5.99*
HO-	0.75	4.86	3.27
	11.62	8.72	11.09
NO2-	−2.06	0.81	1.23
SO3-	—	2.9	—
CH3O-	3.28	4.88	6.62
C2H5O-	—	—	6.67
F-	−0.44*	2.97*	—
Br-	0.90*	2.84*	3.82
CH3-	5.97*	5.68*	6.02*
(CH3)2CH-	5.83*	5.72*	6.02*
CH3CO-	—	3.18*	—
CONH2-	2.10	3.40	3.61
NC-	−0.26*	1.45	1.90*
CH3CONH-	4.09*	4.46	5.87
EtOOC-	—	3.35	3.45
NH2-	6.71*	6.03*	9.11
	−7.6	−1.5	−6.3
C6H5CONH-	3.33*	3.80*	5.32*
COOH-	0.99*	2.00*	1.77*
	5.39*	4.83*	4.84*
HCO-	3.80*	3.80*	4.77*
	12.80*	13.10*	12.20*
H2NNHCO-	—	1.86*	1.82*
	3.86*	3.29*	3.52*
	12.27*	11.47*	10.79*
HS-	−1.07*	2.26*	1.43*
	10.00*	7.03*	8.86*
CH3OCO-	2.21*	3.13*	3.26*
CH3NH-	—	—	9.66
CH3S-	3.59*	4.42*	5.94*
C6H5-	4.48*	4.80*	5.55*
CH2=CH-	4.98*	—	5.62*
Benzyl-	5.13*	—	—
Benzylthio-	3.23*	—	5.41*
t-Butyl-	5.76*	5.82*	5.99*
Dimethylaminoethyl-	3.46*	4.30*	4.66*
	8.75*	8.86*	8.70*
Dimethylaminomethyl-	2.58*	3.17*	3.39*
	8.12*	8.00*	7.66*
Hexyl-	5.95*	—	—
Methanesulfonamido-	1.10*	3.43*	3.64*
	8.02*	7.02*	9.07*
N-Methylacetamido-	2.01*	3.52*	4.62*
N-Methylbenzamido-	1.44*	3.66*	4.68*
N-Methylmethanesulfonamido-	1.73*	3.94*	5.14*
Piperidineoethyl-	3.59*	4.25*	4.68*
	9.29*	8.81*	9.06*
Piperidinomethyl-	2.61*	3.16*	3.90*
	8.51*	8.30*	7.88*
2-Pyridyl-	4.44*	—	—
3-Pyridyl-	4.42*	4.60*	—
	1.52*	3.0*	—
4-Pyridyl-	4.77*	4.85*	4.82*
	1.19*	3.0*	

* Thermodynamic value.

NITROGEN COMPOUNDS (Continued)

HETEROCYCLICS (Continued)

Compound	pK_a	Reference	Compound	pK_a	Reference
Pyridine-N-oxides: see oxygen acids			4,5-Diamino-2-chloro-	4.79, 0.08	105
Pyridines			2,3-Diamino-6-chloro-	3.02, −0.91	105
2,3-Me₂-	6.60	48	2,4-Dichloro-5-amino-	0.73	105
2,4-Me₂-	6.72	48	2:4-Dihydroxy-	13, 1.37, 6.50	39
2,5-Me₂-	6.47	48	4-Ethoxy-3-nitro-	2.67	105
2,6-Me₂-	6.77	48	2-Hydroxy-3-nitro-	−4.00, 8.52	105
3,4-Me₂-	6.52	48	4-Hydroxy-3-nitro-	−0.70, 7.65	105
3,5-Me₂-	6.14	48	1-Methyl-2-pyridone	0.32	39
2,4,6-Me₃-	7.48	48	1-Methyl-4-pyridone	3.33	39
2-Me,5-Et-	6.51	48	4-Methylamino-3-nitro-	5.19	105
2-Amino-3-nitro-	2.38	105	1-Methylpyrid-2-one acetylimine	7.12	46
2-Amino-3-nitro-	2.42, −12.4	141	1-Methylpyrid-4-one acetylimine	11.03	46
2-Amino-5-nitro-	2.80, −12.1	141	1-Methylpyrid-4-one benzylimine	9.89	46
3-Amino-2-nitro-	0.02, −9.07	141	2,4,6-Trihydroxy-	4.6, 9.0, 13.00	39
4-Amino-3-nitro-	5.04	105	Trimethyl(2,6-di-tert-butyl-4-pyridyl) ammonium ion	1.65	125
3-Amino-4-methylamino-	0.38, 9.57	105	Trimethyl(2-tert-butyl-6-pyridyl)ammonium ion	<−1	125
4-Amino-3-methylamino-	0.12, 9.37	105	Dimethyl(2,6-di-tert-butyl-4-pyridyl) ammonium ion	1.6	125
2-Amyl-	6.00*	45	Δ′-Tetrahydro-2-methyl-	9.6	154
2-Benzamido-	3.33	46	Δ′-Tetrahydro-1,2-dimethyl-	11.4	154
2-Benzyl-	5.13	45	1,4-Dihydro-1,4,4-trimethyl-	7.4	154
2-Chloro-3-nitro-	−2.6	105	Pyrimidines		
2,3-Diamino-	7.00, −0.01	105			
3,4-Diamino-	9.14, 0.49	105			

	pK_a	3,4-(NH₂)₂	3-NH₂	4-NH₂	5-NH₂	6-NH₂	2-NH₂
2-OH[140,141]		−0.87	2.78	−5.14	−0.61	−6.12	
		4.16		2.65	3.77	2.32	
		13.43		13.54	11.65	11.38	
2-OMe		5.68, 1.06	3.35	−5.86			
				7.05	4.28	4.64	
1-Me-2=O	0.32		2.94		0.05	2.09	
1-Me-4=O	3.33		3.88				
4-OH			0.04				−6.58
			3.84				5.04
			11.38				10.69
4-OMe			7.30				
2-NH₂			−12.1		−10.7	−3.73	
			0.38		1.97	6.00	7.62
			6.73		6.46		
3-NH₂				−10.7			
				0.80			
				9.19			

Monosubstituted(99)	2	4	5	Compound	pK_a	Reference
Amino-	3.45*	5.69*	2.51*	Cytidine	4.08, 12.5	134
n-Butylamino-	4.14*	—	—	Cytosine	4.60, 12.16	101
Carboxy-	−1.13*	—	—	5-Me-cytosine	4.6, 12.4	101
	2.85*	—	—	Isocytosine	4.01, 9.42	101
Dimethylamino-	3.93*	6.32*	—	Thymine	9.90	134
Ethylamino-	3.89*	—	—	Thymidine	9.79	134
Hydroxy-	2.15*	1.66*	1.85*	Uracil	9.45	101
	9.20*	8.63*	6.80*	Uridine	9.30, 12.59	134
Mercapto-	1.35*	0.68*	—	1-Me-	9.99	101
	7.10*	6.94*	—	3-Me-	9.71	101
Methoxy-	<1	2.5*	—	5-Me-	9.94	101
Methyl-	—	1.91*	—	1,3-di-Me-	None	101
Methylamino-	3.79*	6.09*	—	Orotic acid	2.40, 9.45	101
Methylthio-	0.59*	—	—			
Sulfanilamido-	6.34*	6.17*	6.22*			
	2.0*	—	—			

* Thermodynamic value.

NITROGEN COMPOUNDS (Continued)

Compound	pK_a	Reference	Compound	pK_a	Reference
HETEROCYCLICS (Continued)			*HETEROCYCLICS (Continued)*		
Pyrimidines, substituted			4-Amino-	7.23*	—
4,6-Bisdimethylamino-	6.34*	99	5-Amino-	0.99*, 3.93*	99
4,5-Bismethylamino-	6.77*	99	4-Amino-6-chloro-	3.55*	99
4,6-Bismethylamino-	6.32*	99	5-Amino-4,6-dihydroxy-	3.6*, 8.9*	99
5-Bromo-2,4-dihydroxy-	−7.25*, 7.83*	99	6-Amino-5-formylamino-4-hydroxy-	2.5*, 9.9*	99
5-Bromo-2-methylamino-	2.09*	99	4-Amino-6-hydroxy-	3.30*, 10.81*	99
4-Butylamino-2-hydroxy-	4.67*	99	4-Amino-6-hydroxy-5-methyl-	3.58*, 11.10*	99
4-Butylamino-2-mercapto-	3.2*, 11.15*	99	4-Amino-6-methyl-	7.7*	99
4-Carboxy-6-hydroxy-	2.8*, 8.4*	99	5-Amino-6-methylthio-	5.44*	99
2-Chloro-4-methylamino-	2.90*	99	4,5-Diamino-	2.50*, 7.60*	99
4-Chloro-2-methylamino-	2.59*	99	4,6-Diamino-	6.81*	99
4-Chloro-6-dimethylamino-	2.42*	99	Pyrimidines, 4-amino substituted		
4-Chloro-6-methylamino-	2.24*	99	5-Aminomethyl-2-methyl-	4.0*, 7.1*	99
1,2-Dihydro-2-imino-1-methyl-	10.71*	99	5-Carboxymethylamino-	2.99*, 6.70*	99
1,4-Dihydro-4-imino-1-methyl-	12.18	99	6-Chloro-	2.10*	—
l,2-Dihydro-1-methyl-2-oxo-	2.45*	99	6-Chloro-2-methylamino-	3.79*	99
1,4-Dihydro-1-methyl-4-oxo-	2.02*	99	1,2-Dihydro-1,5-dimethyl-2-oxo	4.69*	99
1,6-Dihydro-1-methyl-6-oxo-	1.79*	99	1,6-Dihydro-6-imino-1-methyl-	11.94*	99
1,2-Dihydro-1-methyl-2-thio-	1.66*	99	1,2-Dihydro-1-methyl-2-oxo-	4.57*	99
1,4-Dihydro-1-methyl-6-thio-	0.56*	99	1,6-Dihydro-1-methyl-6-oxo-	0.98*	99
2,4-Dihydroxy-	−3.38*, 9.45*	99	2,3-Dihydro-3-methyl-2-oxo-	7.4*	99
2,4-Dihydroxy-5-amino-	3.20, 8.52	140	5-Fluoro-2-hydroxy-	2.90*	99
2,6-Dihydroxy-4-amino-	0.00, 8.69, 15.32	140	2-Hydroxy-	4.60*, 12.16*	99
2,6-Dihydroxy-4,5-diamino-	4.56	140	6-Hydroxy-	1.36*, 10.08*	99
2,6-(=0)-1,3-Methyl-4,5-diamino-	4.44	140	2-Hydroxy-5-methyl-	4.6*, 12.4*	99
4,5-Dihydroxy-	1.99*, 7.52*, 11.69*	99	6-Hydroxy-2-methylamino-	3.20*, 11.06*	99
4,6-Dihydroxy-	5.4	39	2-Hydroxy-5-nitro-	7.40*	99
4,6-Dimethyl-	2.7*	99	2-Mercapto-	3.29*, 10.66*	99
4-Dimethylamino-2-hydroxy-	4.21*	99	2-Methoxy-	5.3*	99
4-Dimethylamino-6-hydroxy-	1.22*, 10.49*	99	6-Methoxy-	4.00*	99
4,6-Dimethyl-2-methyl-amino-	5.23*	99	6-Methyl-	6.16*	99
4-Dimethylamino-2-methoxy-	6.13*	99	2-Methylamino-	7.53*	99
4-Dimethylamino-6-methoxy-	4.27*	99	6-Methylamino-	6.30*	99
4-Ethoxy-2-hydroxy-	1.00*, 10.7*	99	6-Methylamino-5-nitro-	2.73*	99
4-Ethylamino-2-mercapto-	3.08*, 11.15*	99	5-Trifluoroacetamido-	3.91*	99
4-Ethylamino-2-hydroxy-	4.56*	99	5-Amino-	6.00*	99
5-Ethyl-2-methylamino-	4.29*	99	6-Amino-	5.99*	99
4-Hydroxy-5-methoxy-	1.75*, 8.64*	99	6-Amino-5-bromo-	4.20*	99
2-Hydroxy-4-methyl-	3.06*, 9.9*	99	5-Amino-2-chloro-	2.63*	99
4-Hydroxy-6-methyl-	2.06*, 9.1*	99	5-Amino-2-chloro-6-ethoxycarbonyl-	1.27*	99
2-Mercapto-4-methyl-	2.1*, 8.1*	99	5-Amino-6-dimethylamino-6-ethoxycarbonyl-	−2.03*, 6.47*	99
4-Mercapto-6-methyl-	1.8*, 7.3*	99	5-Amino-6-ethoxycarbonyl-2-hydroxy-	−3.21*, 3.22*	99
2-Mercapto-4-methyl-amino-	3.07*, 11.12*	99	5-Amino-6-ethoxycarbonyl-2-mercapto-	2.11*	99
4-Methyl-2-methylthio-	1.86*	99	5-Amino-6-hydroxy-	1.28*, 3.54*, 9.89*	99
4-Methyl-6-methylthio-	3.16*	99	5-Amino-2-hydroxy-	4.34*, 11.48*	99
4-Methyl-2-sulphanilamido-	7.06*	99	6-Amino-2-hydroxy-	6.47*, 11.98*	99
1,4,5,6-Tetrahydro-	13.0	99	5-Amino-2-mercapto-	2.93*, 10.42*	99
1,4,5,6-Tetrahydro-2-amino-	14.1	154	5-Amino-2-methylthio-	5.03*	99
2,4,6-Trihydroxy- (Barbituric acid)	3.9, 12.5	39	5,6-Diamino-	1.41*, 5.75*	99
2,4,5-Trihydroxy- (Bobarbituric acid)	8.11, 11.48	39	Pyrimidines, 5-amino substituted		
Pyrimidines, 2-amino substituted			4-Carboxy-6-carboxy-methylamino-2-chloro-	3.05*, 4.48*	99
5-Bromo-	1.95*	99	4-Carboxy-6-carboxy-methylamino-2-dimethylamino-	9.85*	99
4-Chloro-1,6-dihydro-6-imino-1-methyl-	9.87*	99	4-(1-Carboxyethylidene)imino-	3.04*, 7.10*	99
4-Diethylaminoethylamino-5,6-dimethyl-	7.9*, 9.7*	99	4-Carboxymethylamino-	2.9*, 6.59*	99
4-Diethylaminoethylamino-6-methyl-	7.5*, 9.55*	99	2-Ethoxy-4-ethoxycarbonyl-6-ethoxycarbonylmethyl-amino-	4.58*	99
1,4-Dihydro-4-imino-1-methyl-	12.9*	99			
4,5-Dimethyl-	5.0*	99	4-Methyl-	3.06*	99
4,6-Dimethyl-	4.85	39	1-Methyl-2-pyrimidone	2.50	39
4-Dimethylamino-	7.94*	99	1-Methyl-4-pyrimidone	1.8	39
4,6-Diphenyl-	3.74*	99	3-Methyl-4-pyrimidone	1.84	39
4-Hydroxy-	3.91*, 9.54*	99			
4-Methyl-	4.11*	99			
5-Nitro-	0.35	99			
1,4,5,6-Tetrahydro-	14.11*	99			

* Thermodynamic value.

NITROGEN COMPOUNDS (Continued)

Compound	pK_a	Reference	Compound	pK_a	Reference
4-Pyrone	0.1	154	2-Benzyl-	10.31*	99
2,6-Dimethyl-	0.4	154	1-n-Butyl-2-methyl-	10.61*	99
3-Hydroxy-	7.9	154	2-n-Butyl-1-methyl-	10.20*	99
Pyrrole	17.51	152	2-Carbamoyl-	8.82*	99
2,4-Dimethyl-	2.55*	99	1-Cyanomethyl-	4.8*	99
2,5-Dimethyl-	−0.71*	99	2-Cyclohexyl-	10.76*	99
3,4-Dimethyl-	0.66*	99	1,2-Dimethyl-	10.20*	99
3-Ethyl-2,4-dimethyl-	3.54*	99	1-Ethyl-2-methyl-	10.56*	99
1-Methyl-	−2.90*	99	1-Methyl-	10.32*	99
2-Methyl-	−0.21	99	2-(p-Tolyl)-	9.95	99
3-Methyl-	−1.00	99	2-Pyrrolines		
2,3,4,5-Tetramethyl-	3.77	99	2-Benzyl-	7.06*	99
2,3,4-Trimethyl-	3.94	99	2-n-Butyl-1-methyl-	11.84*	99
2,3,5-Trimethyl-	2.00	99	2-Cyclohexyl-	7.91*	99
Δ'-Dihydro-l,2-dimethyl-	11.9	154	1,2-Dimethyl-	11.90*	99
Δ'-Dihydro-2-ethyl-	7.9	154	1-Ethyl-2-methyl-	11.84*	99
Δ³-Dihydro-1-methyl-	9.9	154	2-Phenyl-	6.7	99
Pyrrolidine	11.27*	99			
3-Amino-2,5-dioxo-	5.9*, 9.0*	99			
1-(2-Aminoethyl)-	6.56*. 9.74*	99			

Quinazoline(19,39,99)	2	4	5	6	7	8
NH₂-	4.43	5.73	3.56*	3.2ᵃ	4.59*	2.4ᵃ
OH-	1.30	2.12	3.62*	3.12	3.20*	3.41
CH₃O-	1.31	3.13	3.39*	2.83*	2.87*	3.49*
Cl-	−1.6	—	3.73*	3.53*	3.25*	3.28*
SH-	0.26*	1.51*	—	—	—	—
	8.18*	8.47*	—	—	—	—
CH₃-	4.50*	2.44*	3.61*	3.39*	3.15*	3.18*
CH₃S-	1.60*	2.97*	—	—	—	—
NO₂-	—	—	3.73*	4.16*	4.03*	3.98*

Compound	pK_a	Reference
3,4-Dihydro-	1.47, 9.2	99, 154
3,4-Dihydro-2-methyl-	10.2	154
3,4-Dihydro-3-methyl-	9.2	154
3,4-Dihydro-3-methyl-4-hydroxy	7.6	154
2:4-Dihydroxy-	9.78, 2.5	39
2,4-Dimethyl-	3.58*	99
3-Methiodide	7.26	39
3-Oxide	1.47*	99
1,2,3,4-Tetrahydro-	10.2	154

Quinoline(2,44,99)		3	4	5	6	7	8
H−	4.85*	4.80	4.69*	—	—	—	—
H₂N-	7.25*	4.86*	9.08*	5.37*	5.54*	6.56*	3.90*
HO-	−0.36	4.30	2.27	5.20	5.17	5.48	5.13
	11.74	8.06	11.25	8.54	8.88	8.85	9.89
CH₃	5.42	5.14	5.20	4.62	4.92	5.08	4.60
	5.8	—	5.6	—	—	—	—
F−	—	2.36*	—	3.68*	4.00*	4.04*	3.08*
HO₂C-	4.96*	4.62*	4.53*	4.81*	4.98*	4.97*	7.20*
Br-	1.05*	2.75*	—	3.62*	3.91*	3.87*	3.33*
Cl-	—	2.63*	3.72*	3.65*	3.99*	3.85*	3.12*
HS-	1.44*	2.29*	0.77*	—	—	—	—
	10.25*	6.17*	8.87*	—	—	—	—
CH₃O-	3.16*	—	6.45*	—	5.03*	—	—
CH₃S-	3.67*	3.84*	5.85*	4.46*	4.71*	—	3.46*
O₂N-	—	1.03	—	2.69*	2.72*	2.40*	2.55*

* Thermodynamic value.
ᵃ In 50% ethanol on methanol

NITROGEN COMPOUNDS (Continued)

Compound	pK_a	Reference	Compound	pK_a	Reference
HETEROCYCLICS (Continued)			*HETEROCYCLICS (Continued)*		
Quinoline			4-COO-	10.55	158
4-Amino-7-chloro-	8.23*	99	4-COOCH₃-	9.46	158
4-Amino-8-hydroxy-	6.91*, 10.71*	99	4-COOC₂H₅-	9.44	158
5-Amino-8-hydroxy-	5.67*, 11.24*	99	4-CO CH₃-	9.45	158
4-Amino-6-methoxy-	8.93*	99	4CONH₂ -	9.38	158
8-Amino-6-methoxy-	3.38*	99	4-CN-	8.07	158
6-Bromo-4-chloro-	2.83*	99	4-OH-	9.44	158
4-Chloro-6-ethoxy-	3.82*	99	4-OCH₃-	9.31	158
4-Chloro-6-fluoro-	2.95*	99	4-OCOCH₃-	8.99	158
4-Chloro-6-methoxy-	3.93	99	4-Cl-	8.62	158
4-Chloro-6-methyl-	3.96	99	4-Br-	8.49	158
4,6-Dichloro-	2.81	99	4-I-	8.70	158
2:4-Diamino-	9.45	19	4-NH₂-	10.10	158
1,4-Dihydro-4-imino-1-methyl-	12.4*	99	4-NHCH₃-	10.28	158
1,2-Dihydro-1-methyl-2-oxo-	−0.71*	99	4-N(CH₃)₂-	10.11	158
1,2-Dihydro-1-methyl-2-thio-	−1.6	99	4-NHCOCH₃-	9.54	158
2:4-Dihydroxy-	5.86, 0.76	39	4-NHCOOC₂H₅-	9.57	158
2,3-Dimethyl-	4.94*	99	4-NO₂-	7.65	158
2,4-Dimethyl-	5.12*	99	Riboflavin	9.93	77
2,6-Dimethyl-	6.1*	99	Serotonine	19.50	152
2,7-Dimethyl-	5.02*	99	Sulfadiazine	6.48	6
2,8-Dimethyl-	4.11*	99	Sulfapyridine	8.43	6
1-Methyl-2-quinolone	−0.71	39	Sulfaguanidine	11.25	6
1-Methyl-4-quinolone	2.46	39	Sulfathiazole	7.12	6
1,2,3,4-Tetrahydro-	5.0	154	Terramycin	3.10, 7.26, 9.11	77
Quinoxaline	0.8, 0.56	19, 39	1,4,5,8-Tetraazanaphthalene	2.47*	99
2-Amino-	3.96	19	Tetramethylenediamine1,2,4,5-Tetrazine	10.7	4
5-Amino-	2.62	19	3,6-Diethyl-1,4-dihydro-	4.23*	99
6-Amino-	2.95	19	1,4-Dihydro-	2.25*	99
2-Carbamoyl-	−0.4*	99	Tetrazole	4.9	51
2:3-Diamino-	4.70	19	5-Chloro-	2.1	51
2:3-Dihydroxy-	9.52	39	5-Amino-	1.8,6.0	51
2-Hydroxy-	9.08, −1.37	39	1,2,4-Thiadiazole		
4-Hydroxy-	10.01, 2.85	39	3-Amino-5-phenyl-	0.1*	99
5-Hydroxy-	8.65, 0.9	39	5-Amino-3-phenyl-	1.4*	99
6-Hydroxy-	7.92, 1.40	39	1,3,4-Thiadiazole		
5-Hydroxy-1-methyl-quinoxaliniumchloride	5.74	44	2-Amino-5-phenyl-	2.9*	99
1,2,3,4-Tetrahydro-	2.1, 4.8	154	2-Benzylamino-5-phenyl-	2.5*	99
2-Mercapto-	−1.24*, 7.20*	99	2-Ethylamino-5-phenyl-	3.05*	99
1-Methiodide-	5.74	39	2-Methylamino-5-phenyl-	2.8*	99
2-Methoxy-	0.28*	99	Thiazine		
2-Methyl-	0.95*	99	Δ²-Dihydro-2-methyl-	7.6	154
2-Methylamino-	4.07*	99	1,4-Thiazine		
2-Methylthio-	0.29*	99	Tetrahydro-	8.40*	99
1,5-Naphthyridine	2.91	39	Thiazole	2.44*	99
Quinuclidine	10.95*	99	2-Amino-	5.36, 5.39	99, 41
3-Carbamoyl-	9.67*	99	5-Carbamoyl-	0.6*	99
3-Cyano-	7.81*	99	4-Methyl-5-carboxylic acid-	3.51	144
3-Phenyl-	10.23*	99	4-Methyl-2-carboxylic acid-	1.20, 3.18	144
4-CH₃-	10.88	158	Δ²-Dihydro-2-methyl-	5.2	154
4-CH₂CH₂-	10.95	158	1,3,4-Thiazole 2-Nitramino-	−2.5*	99
4-CH(CH₂)₃-	11.02	158	Thiazolidine	6.22*, 6.31	99, 95
4-C(CH₂)₂-	11.07	158	4-Carboxy-	1.42*, 6.30*	99
4-CH=CH₂-	10.60	158	4-Carboxylate methyl ester	4.00	95
4-C₆H₆-	10.20	158	4-Methoxycarbonyl-	3.91*	99
4-CH₂OH-	10.45	158	Thiazolo[5,4-*d*]pyrimidine		
4-CH₂ OCH₃-	10.50	158	7-Amino-	2.74*	99
4-CH₂OCOCH₃-	10.27	158	7-Methylamino-	2.81*	99
4-CH₂OTs-	9.87	158	Thiophene		
4-CH₂Cl-	10.19	158	2-(2-Aminoethylaminomethyl)-	6.29*, 9.77	99
4-CH₂Br-	10.13	158	2-Aminomethyl-	8.92	99
4-CH₂I-	10.12	158	1,2,4-Triazanaphthalene	−0.82*	99
4-CH(OH)₂-	9.90	158	1,3,5-Triazanaphthalene		
			4-Hydroxy-	8.98*	99

* Thermodynamic value.

NITROGEN COMPOUNDS (Continued)

Compound	pK_a	Reference	Compound	pK_a	Reference
HETEROCYCLICS (Continued)			*HETEROCYCLICS (Continued)*		
1,3,8-Triazanaphthalene			4,5 Dibromo-	5.37	126
2-Hydroxy-	1.81*, 10.06	99	1-Phenyl-5-methyl-4-carboxylic acid-	3.73	126
1,4,5-Triazanaphthalene	1.20	39	1-Phenyl-4-carboxylic acid-	2.88	126
8-Hydroxy-	8.76, 0.60	39	1-Phenyl-4,5-dicarboxylic acid-	2.13, 4.93	126
1,4,6-Triazanaphthalene	3.05*	99	4-Carboxylic acid-	3.22, 8.73	126
5-Hydroxy-	11.05, 0.78	39	4,5-Dicarboxylic acid-	1.86 5.90, 9.30	126
1,2,4-Triazine			1,2,3-Triazole	1.17*, 9.51*	99
3-Amino-	3.09*	99	1-Methyl-	1.25*	99
1,3,5-Triazine			1,2,4-Triazole	10.3, 2.3	154
2-Amino-4,6-bisethylamino-	6.18*	99	3,5-Dimethyl-	3.8	154
2-Amino-4,6-dimethyl-	3.56*	99	3,5-Diamino-	12.1, 4.4	154
2,4-Diamino-	5.88*	99	3-Methyl-	10.7, 3.3	154
2,4-Diamino-6-guanidino-	9.4*	99	3-Amino-	11.1, 4.0	154
2:4-Dihydroxy-	6.5	39	3-Chloro-	8.1	154
2,4,6-Triamino-	5.1*	99	3,5-Dichloro-	5.2	154
2,4,6-Trisdi(2-hydroxy)ethylamino-	4.70*	99	l,2,3-Triazolo(5′,4′-4,5)pyrimidine	2.03*, 4.96*	99
2,4,6-Trisguanidino-	4.6*, 7.6*, 10.3*	99	Tryptamine	16.60	152
2,4,6-Trishydroxymethylamino-	4.0*	99	Tryptophan	16.82	152
Triazole			4-Methyl-	16.90	152
Benzo-	8.38	126	5-Hydroxy-	19.20	152

* Thermodynamic value.

SPECIAL NITROGEN COMPOUNDS

Compound	pK_a	Reference	Compound	pK_a	Reference
AMIDINES AND GUANIDINES			*C-SUBSTITUTED-N-PHENYLAMIDINIUM IONS*		
Acetamidine	12.52	19	EtO-	7.71	114
			H_2N-	10.77	114
C-SUBSTITUTED AMIDINIUM IONS			MeO-	7.41	114
BuO-	10.15	114	MeS-	7.14	114
CH_2CHCH_2O-	9.70	114	PhNH-	10.42	144
EtO-	10.02	114			
Me-	12.41	114	*AMIDOXIMES*		
Me_2N-	13.4	114	Benz-	4.99	17
MeO-	9.72	114	Malon-	~4.77	17
MeS-	9.83	114	Ox-	3.02	17
NH_2-	13.86	114	α-Phenylacet-	5.24	17
Ph-	11.6	114	Succin-	3.11, 5.97	17
PrO-	10.16	114	o-Tolu-	4.03	17
1-Chloro-4-*N*′- methylguanidino benzene	12.6*	99	p-Tolu-	5.14	17
1-Chloro-4-*N*²-methylguanidino benzene	10.85*				
Diguanide	3.07, 13.25	99	*HYDRAZINES (30°)*		
Ethyl-	3.08, 11.47	99	Hydrazine	8.07	13
Ethylene-	11.34, 1.74, 2.88, 11.76	77	Acet-	3.24	15
Methyl-	3.00, 11.42	99	*N,N*-Diethyl-	7.71	13
Phenyl-	2.16, 10.71	77	*N,N*′-Diethyl-	7.78	13
Guanidine	13.6	99	*N,N*-Dimethyl-	7.21	13
Acetyl-	8.26	99	*N,N*′-Dimethyl-	7.52	13
2-Anthryl-	11.0	99	Ethyl-	7.99	13
Carbamoyl-	3.76	99	Glycylhydrazide	2.38, 7.69	15
N,N′-Dimethyl-	13.4	99	Isonicotinhydrazide	1.85, 3.54, 10.77	77
N,N′-Dimethyl-	13.6	99	Methyl-	7.87	13
N,N′-Diphenyl-	10.12	99	Phenyl-	5.21 (15°)	14
N-Methyl-	13.4	99	Tetramethyl-	6.30	13
N-Methyl-*N*′-nitro-	12.40	99	Trimethyl-	6.56	13
2-Naphthyl-	10.7	99	$HOCH_2CH_2$-	7.12	148
Nitro-	−0.55, 12.20	99	C_6H_5-CH_2-	6.83	148
Nitroamino-	−1, 10.60	99	C_6H_5-$O(CH_2)_2$-	6.80	148
Nitroso-	2.13, 11.70	99	C_2H_5OOC-CH_2-	5.97	148
Pentamethyl-	13.8	99	NC-$(CH_2)_2$-	5.91	148
N-Phenyl-	10.77	99	CHF_2-CF_2-$CH(CH_3)$-	5.59	148
N,N,N′-Trimethyl-	13.6	99	$HC≡C$-CH_2-	5.46	148
N,N′,*N*′-Trimethyl-	13.9	99	CF_3-CH_2-	5.38	148
Triphenyl-	9.10	99	$CHF_2(CF_2)_3$ -CH_2-	5.34	148
			C_6H_5-$CH(CF_3)$-	4.88	148
1-SUBSTITUTED GUANIDINIUM IONS					
CN-	−0.4	114	*HYDRAZONES OF*		
H_2NCO-	7.85	114	Benzophenone	3.85	
MeO-	7.46	114	p-Chloro-	3.53	16
$^-O_2CCH_2O$-	7.51	114	p, p′-Dimethoxy-	4.38	16
O-Methylisourea	9.80	20	p,p′-Dichloro-	3.13	16
N-Phenyl-	7.3	20	p-Methoxyacetophenone	4.94	16
S-Methylisothiourea	9.83	20	Phenyl-2-thienyl ketone	3.80	16
N-Phenyl-	7.14	20			
			SEMICARBAZONES OF		
1-Substituted 3-Nitroguanidines			Acetone	1.33	14
Bz-	8.10	114	Acetaldehyde	1.10	14
EtO_2CCH_2-	11.20	114	Benzaldehyde	0.96	14
H_2NCO-	7.50	114	Furfural	1.44	14
$NCCH_2$-	9.30	114	Pyruvic acid	0.59	14
NH_2-	10.60	114	Semicarbazide	3.66	14
Ph-	10.50	114			
			NITROGEN ACIDS		
* Thermodynamic value.			Dimedone	5.23	18
			Diphenylthiocarbazone	4.5	6
			Nitrourea	4.57	18
			Nitrourethane	3.28	18
			Phthalimide	8.30	18

SPECIAL NITROGEN COMPOUNDS (Continued)

Compound	pK'_a	Reference	Compound	pK'_a	Reference
			Diphenylthiocarbazone	4.5	6
	OTHER		Thiourea	−0.96	4
Acetamide	−0.51	4	Urea	0.18	4,99
Azobenzene	−2.48*	99	*O*-Allyl-	9.70	99
4-Amino-3′-methyl-	−2.88*	99	*O*-*n*-Butyl-	10.15	99
4-Amino-4′-methyl-	3.04	99	*O*-Cyclohexyl-	10.19	99
4-Dimethylamino-	−1.3*, 3.226*	99	*O*-Isobutyl-	10.30	99
4-Hydroxy-	−0.93*, 8.2	99	*O*-Isopentyl-	10.11	99
Benzamide			*O*-Methyl	0.9	99
3,5-Dinitro-4-methyl-	−2.77	110	*O*-Methyl-	9.72	99
4-Methoxy-	−1.46	110	*O*-Phenethyl-	10.03	99
3-Nitro-	−2.25	110	Phenyl-	−0.3	99
2,3,6-Trichloro-	−3.10	110	*N*-Phenyl-*O*-methyl-	7.3	20
3,4,5-Trimethoxy-	−1.86	110	*N*-Propyl-	10.16	99

* Thermodynamic value.

THIOLS

Compound	pK_a	Reference	Compound	pK_a	Reference
N-Acetylcysteine	9.52	112	o-Mercaptophenylacetic acid	4.28, 7.67	59
N-Acetyl-β-mercaptoisoleucine	10.30	112	2-Mercaptopropionic acid	4.32, 10.30	153
N-Acetylpenicillamine	9.90	112	Methyl cysteine	6.5, (7.5)	81
O-Aminothiophenol	6.59	81	Methyl [β-diethylaminoethyl] sulfide	9.8	5
p-Chlorothiophenol	7.50	81	Methyl thioglycolate	7.8	23
Cysteine	1.8, 8.3, 10.8	23	p-Nitrobenzenethiol	5.1	58
Cysteine ethyl ester	6.53, 9.05	112	Penicillamine	7.90, 10.42	112
Cysteinylcysteine	2.65, 7.27, 9.35, 10.85	23	Thiocyanic acid	−1.84	104
1-Diethylaminobutane-(4)	10.1	5	Thioglycolic acid	3.67, 10.31	23
1-Diethylaminohexane-(6)	10.1	5	Thiophenol	7.8, 6.52	59, 81, 82
1-Diethylaminopropane-(3)	8.0, 10.5	5	Pentafluoro-	2.68	155
N-Diethylcysteamine	7.8, 10.75	5	p-Me-	6.82	157
N-Dimethylcysteamine	7.95, 10.7	5	p-OMe-	6.77	157
N-Dipropylcysteamine	8.00, 10.8	5	m-Me-	6.66	157
Ethyl mercaptan	10.50	81	m-OMe-	6.38	157
Glutathione	2.12, 3.59, 8.75, 9.65	23	p-Cl-	6.13	157
DL-Homocysteine	8.70, 10.46	112	p-Br-	6.02	157
2-Mercaptoethanesulfonate	7.53 (9.1)	81	m-Cl-	5.78	157
Mercaptoethanol	9.5	23	p-COMe-	5.33	157
Mercaptoethylamine	8.6, 10.75	23	m-NO₂-	5.24	157
N-β-Mercaptoethylmorpholine	6.65, 9.8	5	p-NO₂	4.71, 4.50	157
N-β-Mercaptoethylpiperidine	7.95, 11.05	5	l-Thio-D-sorbitol	9.35	81
β-Mercaptoisoleucine	8.10, 10.6	112	N-Trimethyl cysteine	8.6	23

X=	−H	−S−	−SH	X=	−H	−S−	−SH
X(CH₂)₂SH	12.0	13.96	10.75	X(CH₂)₃SH	—	13.24	11.14
X(CH₂)₄SH	12.4	13.25	11.50	X(CH₂)₅SH	—	13.27	11.82

Compound	pK_a	Reference	Compound	pK_a	Reference
Mercaptans, RSH			n-C₃H₇-	10.65	82
R			t-C₄H₉-	11.05	82
C₆H₅CH₂-	9.43	82	(CH₃)₂CH-	10.86*	103
HOCH₂CH(OH)CH₂-	9.51	82	(CH₃)₃C-	11.22*	103
CH₂=CHCH₂-	9.96	82	HOCH₂CH₂-	9.72	103
n-C₄H₉-	10.66	82	CH₃CONHCH₂CH₂-	9.92	103
t-C₅H₁₁-	11.21	82	−OCOCH₂-	10.68*	103
C₂H₅OCOCH₂-	7.95	82	⁻OCOCH₂CH₂-	10.84*	103
C₂H₅OCH₂CH₂-	9.38	82	o-⁻OCOC₆H₄-	8.88*	103
HOCH₂CH(OH)CH₂-	9.66	82	p-⁻OCOC₆H₄-	5.80*	103
			CH₃CO-	3.62*	103

* Thermodynamic value.

CARBON ACIDS

Compound	pK_a	Reference	Compound	pK_a	Reference
Acetone	c. 20	24	$CH_3COCH_2COCH_3$	9	74
Acetonitrile	c. 25	24	$CH_3COCHBrCOCH_3$	7	74
Acetylacetone	8.95	24	$CH_3COCH_2COCF_3$	4.7	74
Benzoylacetone (enol)	8.23	24	$C_6H_5COCH_2NC_5H_5$	10.51	74
Diacetylacetone	7.42	153	$CH(COCH_3)_3$	5.85	74
Dihydroresorcinol	5.26	153	$CH_3SO_2CH_3$	c. 23	74
Ethyl acetoacetate	10.68	153	$CH(SO_2CH_3)_3$	Strong	74
Dimethylsulfone	14	24	$C_2H_5O_2CCH_2CN$	9	74
Hydrocyanic acid	9.21	25	$CH_3CO_2C_2H_5$	c. 24.5	74
Nitroethane	8.44	153	$CHC_2H_5(CO_2C_2H_5)_2$	15	74
Nitromethane	10.21	153	CH_3CONH_2	c. 25	74
2-Nitropropane	7.74	18	$CH_2(CO_2C_2H_5)_2$	13.3	74
Saccharin	1.6	18	CH_3CO_2H	c. 24	74
Triacetylmethane	5.81	153	(2-thienyl)$COCH_2CCF_3$	6.10	74
CH_4	40	127			
$CH(NO_2)_3$	0	127	2-(ethoxycarbonyl)cyclohexanone ($CO_2C_2H_5$)	10.96	74
CH_3CN	25	127			
$CH_2(CN)_3$	12	127	2-acetylcyclopentanone ($COCH_3$)	7.82	74
$CH(CN)_3$	0	127			
$CH_3CHClNO_2$	7	74	2-(ethoxycarbonyl)cyclopentanone ($CO_2C_2H_5$)	10.5	74
$CH_3COCH_2NO_2$	5.1	74			
$CH(NO_2)_3$	Strong	74	2-acetylcyclohexanone (CCH_3)	10.1	74
$CH_3COCHCl_2$	15	74			
$CH_3COCHC_2H_5CO_2C_2H_5$	12.7	74	$CH_2(CHO)_2$	5	74
$CH_3COCHCH_3COCH_3$	11	74			
$CH_3COCH_2COC_6H_5$	9.4	74			
$C_6H_5COCH_2COCF_3$	6.82	74			
CH_3COCH_2CHO	5.92	74			
$CH_3COCH_2CO_2CH_3$	10	74			
$CH_3SO_2CH_2SO_2CH_3$	14	74			
$CH_3SO_2CH(COCH_3)_2$	4.3	74			
$C_2H_5O_2CCH_2NO_2$	5.82	74			
$CH_2(NO_2)_2$	3.57	74			
CH_3COCH_2Cl	c. 16.5	74			
$CH_3COCH_2CO_2C_2H_5$	10.68	74			

$RC(NO_2)_2H$ R=	pK_a	References
CH_3-	5.13	127
CH_3CH_2-	5.49	127
$CH_3CH_2CH_2-$	5.35	127
$(CH_3)_2CHCH_2-$	5.36	127
$CH_3(CH_2)_2CH_2-$	5.34	127
$CH_3(CH_2)_3CH_2-$	5.37	127
$CH_3(CH_2)_4CH_2-$	5.46	127
$CH_3(CH_2)_5CH_2-$	5.46	127
$CH_3(CH_2)_6CH_2-$	5.46	127
$CH_3(CH_2)_7CH_2-$	5.45	127
$CH_2=CHCH_2-$	4.95	127
$HOCH_2CH_2-$	4.44	127
$H-$	3.57	127
C_6H_5-	3.71	127
$CH(NO_2)_2CH_2-$	1.09	127
$CH_3C(NO_2)_2CH_2-$	1.35	127
$CH_3OOCCH_2CH_2-$	4.34	127
CH_3OCH_2-	3.48	127
$N{\equiv}CCH_2CH_2-$	3.45	127
$O_2NCH_2CH_2$	3.24	127
CH_3OOCCH_2-	3.08	127
$(CH_3)_3NCH_2-$	-1.87	127
$N{\equiv}CCH_2-$	2.27	127
$(CH_3)_2CH-$	6.71	127

MISCELLANEOUS

Compound	pK_a	Reference	Compound	pK_a	Reference
ANTIBIOTICS AND VITAMINS			*INDICATORS AND DYES (Continued)*		
Chlorotetracycline	3.30, 7.44, 9.27	99	Neutral red	7.4	28
5-Desoxypyridoxal	4.17, 8.14	99	Nile blue A	2.4	99
Dimethyloxytetracycline	7.5, 9.4	99	Phenol blue	−6.5, 4.8	99
Isochlorotetracycline	3.1, 6.7, 8.3	99	Phenolindophenol	−5.3, 0.95, 8.1	99
O-Methylpyridoxal	4.75	99	Phenol red	8.03	97
Oxytetracycline	3.27, 7.32, 9.11	99	Pinachrom (M)	7.31	99
Pyridoxal	4.20, 8.66, 13	99	N-Propylanilinesulfonephthalein	1.57, 13.11	99
Pyridoxal 5-phosphate	4.14, 6.20 8.69	99	Propylhelianthin	3.95	99
Pyridoxamine	3.31, 7.90, 10.4	99	Pyronine B	7.7	99
Pyridoxamine 5-phosphate	2.5, 3.69, 5.76, 8.61, 10.92	99	Quinaldine red	2.63	99
Pyridoxine	5.00, 8.96	99	Rhodamine B	3.2	99
Riboflavin	10.02	99	Safranin O	6.4	99
Tetracycline	3.30, 7.68, 9.69	99	Thioflavine T	2.7	99
			Thionine	6.9	99
INDICATORS AND DYES			Thymol blue (1)	1.65	28
Acridine red	3.1	99	Thymol blue (2)	9.2	28
Anilinesulfonephthalein	1.59, 12.26	99	Toluidine blue 0	7.5	99
N-Benzylanilinesulfonephthalein	0.30, 12.76	99	Tropeoline 00	2.0	28
Bindschedler's green	−2.5	99			
Bismarck brown Y	5.0	99	*PORPHYRINS, BILE PIGMENTS AND STEROIDS*		
Brilliant cresyl blue	3.2	99	Biliverdin	3	99
Bromocresol green	4.9	28	Chlorin e_6	1.9	99
Bromocresol purple	6.46	97	Chlorin p_6 trimethyl ester	1.4	99
Bromophenol blue	4.1	28	Coproporphyrin I	7.13, 4.2	99
Bromothymol blue	7.3	28	Deuteroporphyrin IX dimethyl ester disulfonic acid	0.3, 4.7	99
Butylhelianthin	4.01	99	Dipyrrylmethene	8.50	99
Chlorophenol blue	4.43	97	Mesobiliviolin	4.0	99
Chlorophenol red	7.96	97	N-Methyl coproporphyrin I	0.7, 11.3	99
Chrysoidin Y	5.3	99	N-Methyl coproporphyrin I methyl esterl	0.7, 8.3	99
Congo red	4.19	97	Methylphaeophorbid a	0.2	99
m-Cresol purple	1.70	97	Methylphaeophorbid b	−0.1, 1.9	99
Cyanine	8.62	99	Phaeopurpurin 18 methyl ester	−0.2, 2.1	99
N-Ethylanilinesulfonephthalein	1.73, 13.20	99	Phyllochlorin	2.1, 4.6	99
Ethylhelianthin	4.34	99	Phylloporphyrin	2.5, 5	99
Hexylhelianthin	3.71	99	Pyrrochlorin	2.0, 4.5	99
Iodophenol blue	2.19	97	Pyrroporphyrin	2.0, 4.5	99
N-Methylanilinesulfonephthalein	1.36, 12.94	99	Rhodin g_7	1.6	99
Methylene blue	3.8	99	Rhodochlorin dimethyl ester	0.9	99
Methylene green	3.2	99	b-Rhodochlorin dimethyl ester	0.2, 2.8	99
Methylhelianthin	3.76	99	Rhodoporphyrin	1.2, 3.7	99
Methyl orange	3.45	28	Stercobilin	7.60	99
Methyl red (1)	2.3	28	d-Urobilin	7.20	99
Methyl red (2)	5.0	28	i-Urobilin	7.40	99
Methyl yellow	3.25	28			

References

1. Hall, *J. Am. Chem. Soc.*, 79, 5441 (1957).
2. Brown, McDaniel, Häfliger, in *Determination of Organic Structures by Physical Methods.*, Braude, Nachod, Eds., Academic Press, New York, 1955, P. 567.
3. Hall, *J. Am. Chem. Soc.*, 79, 5439 (1957).
4. Hodgman, Ed., *Handbook of Chemistry and Physics,* The Chemical Rubber Co., Cleveland, 1951. p.1636
5. Franzen, *Chem. Ber.*, 90, 623 (1957).
6. Dawson, Elliott, Elliott, and Jones, *Data for Biochemical Research,* Clarendon, Oxford, 1959.
7. Buist and Lucas, *J. Am. Chem. Soc.*, 79, 6157 (1957).
8. Stevenson and Williamson, *J. Am. Chem. Soc.*, 80, 5943 (1958).
9. Soloway and Lipschitz, *J. Org. Chem.*, 23, 613 (1958).
10. Bissell and Finger, *J. Org. Chem.*, 24, 1256 (1959).
11. Tuckerman, Mayer, and Nachod, *J. Am. Chem. Soc.*, 81, 92 (1959).
12. Bissot, Parry, and Campbell, *J. Am. Chem. Soc.*, 79, 796 (1957).
13. Hinman, *J. Org. Chem.*, 23, 1587 (1958).
14. Conant and Bartlett, *J. Am. Chem. Soc.*, 54, 2881 (1932).
15. Lindegreen and Niemann, *J. Am. Chem. Soc.*, 71, 1504 (1949).
16. Harnsberger, Cochran, and Szmant, *J. Am. Chem. Soc.*, 77, 5048 (1955).
17. Pearse and Pflaum, *J. Am. Chem. Soc.*, 81, 6505 (1959).
18. Bell and Higginson, *Proc. Roy. Soc.*, 197A, 141 (1949).
19. Albert, Goldacre, and Phillips, *J. Chem. Soc.*, 2240 (1948).
20. Dippy, Hughes, and Rozanski, *J. Chem. Soc.*, 2492 (1959).
21. Edsall, Martin, Bruce, and Hollingworth, *Proc. Natl. Acad. Sci. U.S.*, 44, 505 (1958).
22. Martin, Edsall, Wetlaufer, and Hollingworth, *J. Biol. Chem.*, 233, 1429 (1958).
23. Edsall and Wyman, *Biophysical Chemistry,* Academic Press, New York, 1958.
24. Pearson and Dillon, *J. Am. Chem. Soc.*, 75, 2439 (1953).
25. Ang, *J. Chem. Soc.*, 3822 (1959).
26. Martin and Fernelius, *J. Am. Chem. Soc.*, 81, 1509 (1959).
27. Ellenbogen, *J. Am. Chem. Soc.*, 74, 5198 (1952).

28. Kolthoff and Elving, *Treatise on Analytical Chemistry.*, Interscience Encyclopedia, New York, 1959,1.

29. Edwards, *J. Am. Chem. Soc.*, 76, 1540 (1954).

30. Bailey, Carrington, Lott, and Symons, *J. Chem. Soc.*, 290 (1960).

31. Brownstein and Stillman, *J. Phys. Chem.*, 63, 2061 (1959).

32. Meier and Schwarzenbach, *Helv. Chim. Acta*, 40, 907 (1957).

33. Ingham and Morrison, *J. Chem. Soc.*, 1200 (1933).

34. Hildebrand, *Principles of Chemistry*, Macmillan, New York, 1940.

35. Baddiley, in *The Nucleic Acids*, Chargaff and Davidson, Eds., Academic Press, New York, I, 1955, 137.

36. Circular OR-18, *Pabst Laboratories*, Milwaukee, Wisc, April 1961.

37. Bendich, in *The Nucleic Acids*, Chargaff and Davidson, Eds., Academic Press, New York, I, 1955, 81.

38. Jordan, *in The Nucleic Acids*, Chargaff and Davidson, Eds., Academic Press, New York, I, 1955, 447.

39. Albert and Phillips, *J. Chem. Soc.*, 1294 (1956).

40. Elliott and Mason, *J. Chem. Soc.*, 2352 (1959).

41. Angyal and Angyal, *J. Chem. Soc.*, 1461 (1952).

42. Edward and Nielsen, *J. Chem. Soc.*, 5075 (1957).

43. Bruice and Schmir, *J. Am. Chem. Soc.*, 80, 148 (1958).

44. Mason, *J. Chem. Soc.*, 674 (1958).

45. Linnell, *J. Org. Chem.*, 25, 290 (1960).

46. Jones and Katrizky, *J. Chem. Soc.*, 1317 (1959).

47. Jaffee and Doak, *J. Am. Chem. Soc.*, 77, 4441 (1955).

48. Clarke and Rothwell, *J. Chem. Soc.*, 1885 (1960).

49. Keyworth, *J. Org. Chem.*, 24, 1355 (1959).

50. Gawron, Duggan, and Grelecki, *Anal. Chem.*, 24, 969 (1952).

51. Sims, *J. Chem. Soc.*, 3648 (1959).

52. Fickling, Fischer, Mann, Packer, and Vaughan, *J. Am. Chem. Soc.*, 81, 4226 (1959).

53. Wold and Ballou, *J. Biol. Chem.*, 227, 301 (1957).

54. McElroy and Glass, *Phosphorus Metabolism.* Johns Hopkins, Baltimore, I, 1951.

55. Kumler and Eiler, *J. Am. Chem. Soc.*, 65, 2355 (1943).

56. Van Wazer, *Phosphorus and its Compounds*, Inter-Science, New York, I, 1958.

57. Freedman and Doak, *Chem. Rev.*, 57, 479 (1957).

58. Ellman, *Arch. Biochem. Biophys.*, 74, 443 (1958).

59. Pascal and Tarbell, *J. Am. Chem. Soc.*, 79, 6015 (1957).

60. Bascombe and Bell, *J. Chem. Soc.*, 1096 (1959).

61. Gawron and Draus, *J. Am. Chem. Soc.*, 80, 5392 (1958).

62. Mukherjee and Grunwald, *J. Phys. Chem.*, 62, 1311 (1958).

63. Ballinger and Long, *J. Am. Chem. Soc.*, 81, 1050 (1959).

64. Ballinger and Long, *J. Am. Chem. Soc.*, 82, 795 (1960).

65. Haszeldine, *J. Chem. Soc.*, 1757 (1953).

66. Deno, Berkheimer, Evans, and Peterson, *J. Am. Chem. Soc.*, 81, 2344 (1959).

67. Gardner and Katritzky, *J. Chem. Soc.*, 4375 (1957).

68. Wise and Brandt, *J. Am. Chem. Soc.*, 77, 1058 (1955).

69. Fortnum, Battaglia, Cohen, and Edwards, *J. Am. Chem. Soc.*, 82, 778 (1960).

70. Everett and Minkoff, *Trans. Faraday. Soc.*, 49, 410 (1953).

71. Bauer and Miarka, *J. Am. Chem. Soc.*, 79, 1983 (1957).

72. Green, Sainsbury, Saville, and Stansfield, *J. Chem. Soc.*, 1583 (1958).

73. Burkhard, Sellers, DeCou, and Lambert, *J. Org. Chem.*, 24, 767 (1959).

74. Bell, *The Proton in Chemistry*, Cornell, Ithaca, 1959.

75. Stewart and Maeser, *J. Am. Chem. Soc.*, 46, 2583 (1924).

76. Jencks and Carriuolo, *J. Am. Chem. Soc.*, 82, 1778 (1960).

77. Bjerrum, Schwarzenbach, and Sillen, *Stability Constants of Metal-Ion Complexes, Part I, IInorganic Ligands*, Chemical Society, London, 1957.

78. Parsons, *Handbook of Electrochemical Constants*, Butterworths, London, 1959.

79. Bower and Robinson, *J. Phys. Chem.*, 64, 1078 (1960).

80. Candlin and Wilkins, *J. Chem. Soc.*, 4236 (1960).

81. Danehy and Noel, *J. Am. Chem. Soc.*, 82, 2511 (1960).

82. Kreevoy, Harper, Duvall, Wilgus, and Ditsch, *J. Am. Chem. Soc.*, 82, 4899 (1960).

83. Kabachnik, Mastrukova, Shipov, and Melentyeva, *Tetrahedron.*, 9, 10 (1960).

84. Bjerrum, Schwarzenbach, and Sillen, *Stability Constants of Metal-Ion Complexes, Part I, Organic Ligands,* Chemical Society, London, 1957.

85. Crutchfield and Edwards, *J. Am. Chem. Soc.*, 82, 3533 (1960).

86. Lane and Quinlan, *J. Am. Chem. Soc.*, 82, 2994, 2997 (1960).

87. Moeller and Ferrús, *J. Phys. Chem.*, 64, 1083 (1960).

88. Bryson, *J. Am. Chem. Soc.*, 82, 4858, 4862, 4871 (1960).

89. Henderson and Streuli, *J. Am. Chem. Soc.*, 82, 5791 (1960).

90. Fortnum, Battaglia, Cohen, and Edwards, *J. Am. Chem. Soc.*, 82, 778 (1960).

91. Bell and McTigue, *J. Chem. Soc.*, 2983 (1960).

92. Li, Miller, Solony, and Gillis, *J. Am. Chem. Soc.*, 82, 3737 (1960).

93. Cohen and Erlanger, *J. Am. Chem. Soc.*, 82, 3928 (1960).

94. Olson and Margerum, *J. Am. Chem. Soc.*, 82, 5602 (1960).

95. Ratner and Clarke, *J. Am. Chem. Soc.*, 59, 200 (1937).

96. Porter, Rydon, and Schofield, *Nature*, 182, 927 (1958).

97. Kortum, Vogel, and Andrussow, *Dissociation Constants of Organic Acids and Aqueous Solution,* Butterworths, London, 1961.

98. King, *Qualitative Analysis and Electrolytic Solutions,* Harcourt Brace, New York, 1959.

99. Perrin, *Dissociation Constants of Organic Bases in Aqueous Solution,* Butterworths, London, 1965.

100. Albert and Serjeant, *Ionization Constants of Acids and Bases.*, John Wiley & Sons, New York, 1962.

101. Yukawa, Eds., *Handbook of Organic Structural Analysis.* Benjamin, New York, 1965, 584.

102. Battaglia and Edwards, *Inorg. Chem.*, 4, 552 (1965).

103. Irving, Nelander, and Wadsö, *Acta Chem. Scand.*, 18, 769 (1964).

104. Morgan, Stedman, and Whincup, *J. Chem. Soc.*, 4813 (1965).

105. Barlin, *J. Chem. Soc.*, 2150 (1964).

106. Gallo, Pasqualucci, Radaell, and Lancini, *J. Org. Chem.*, 29, 862 (1964).

107. Walba and Isensee, *J. Org. Chem.*, 26, 2789 (1961).

108. DYatkin, Mochalina, and Knunyants, *Tetrahedron.*, 21, 2991 (1965).

109. Bell and McTigue, *J. Chem. Soc.*, 2985 (1960).

110. Yates and Riordan, *Can. J. Chem.*, 43, 2328 (1965).

111. *Tables for Identification of Organic Compounds*, Chemical Rubber Co., 3rd ed., 1967.

112. Friedman, Cavins, and Wall, *J. Am. Chem. Soc.*, 87, 3672 (1965).

113. Phillips, Eisenberg, George, and Rutman, *J. Biol. Chem.*, 240, 4393 (1965).

114. Charton, *J. Org. Chem.*, 30, 969 (1965).

115. Good, Winget, Winter, Connolly, Izawa, and Singh, *Biochemistry*, 5, 467 (1966).

116. Paelotti, Stern, and Vacca, *J. Phys. Chem.*, 69, 3759 (1965).

117. Spinner, *J. Chem. Soc.*, 3855 (1963).

118. Hine, Via, and Jensen, *J. Org. Chem.*, 36, 2926 (1971).

119. Eastes, Aldridge, Minesinger, and Kamlet, *J. Org. Chem.*, 36, 3847 (1971).

120. Kamlet and Minesinger, *J. Org. Chem.*, 36, 610 (1971).

121. Paulder and Humphrey, *J. Org. Chem.*, 35, 3467 (1970).

122. Filler and Schure, *J. Org. Chem.*, 32, 1217 (1967).

123. Walba, Stiggall, and Coutts, *J. Org. Chem.*, 32, 1954 (1967).

124. Walba and Ruiz-Velasco, *J. Org. Chem.*, 34, 3315 (1969).

125. Deutsch and Cheung, *J. Org. Chem.*, 38, 1124 (1973).

126. Hansen, West, Baca, and Blank, *J. Am. Chem. Soc.*, 90, 6588 (1971).

127. Sitzman, Adolph, and Kamlet, *J. Am. Chem. Soc.*, 90, 2815 (1968).

128. Hendrickson, Bergeron, Giga, and Sternbach, *J. Am. Chem. Soc.*, 95, 3412 (1973).

129. Christensen, Izatt, and Hansen, *J. Am. Chem. Soc.*, 89, 213 (1967).

130. Christensen, Oscarson, and Izatt, *J. Am. Chem. Soc.*, 90, 5949 (1968).

131. Christensen, Slade, Smith, Izatt, and Tsang, *J. Am. Chem. Soc.*, 92, 4164 (1970).

132. Bloomfield and Fuchs, *J. Chem. Soc. B.*, 363 (1970).

133. Hughes, Nicklin, and Shrimanker, *J. Chem. Soc.*, B, 3485 (1971).

134. Christensen, Rytting, and Izatt, *J. Chem. Soc.*, B, 1643 (1970).

135. Christensen, Rytting, and Izatt, *J. Chem. Soc.*, B, 1646 (1970).

136. Ives and Prasad, *J. Chem. Soc.*, B, 1652 (1970).

137. Ives and Mosely, *J. Chem. Soc.*, B, 1655 (1970).

138. Bolton and Hall, *J. Chem. Soc., B*, 1247 (1970).
139. Chuchani and Frohlich, *J Chem. Soc., B*, 1417 (1970).
140. Barlin and Pfleinderer, *J. Chem. Soc., B*, 1425 (1971).
141. Bellobono and Favini, *J. Chem. Soc., B*, 2034 (1971).
142. Takahashi, Cohen, Miller, and Peake, *J. Org. Chem.*, 36, 1205 (1971).
143. Crowell and Hankins, *J. Phys. Chem.*, 73, 1380 (1969).
144. Haake and Bausher, *J. Phys. Chem.*, 72, 2213 (1968).
145. Mäkitie and Mirttinen, *Suomen Kemistilehti, B*, 44, 155 (1971).
146. Koskinen and Nikkilä, *Suomen Kemistilehti, B*, 45, 89 (1971).
147. Serjeant, *Aust. J. Chem.*, 22, 1189 (1969).
148. Pollet and VandenEynde, *Bull. Soc. Chim. Belges*, 77, 341 (1968).
149. Wada and Takenaka, *Bull. Chem. Soc. Jap.*, 44, 2877 (1971).

150. Caplow, *Biochemistry*, 8, 2656 (1969).
151. Nozaki and Tanford, *J. Biol. Chem.*, 242, 4731 (1967).
152. Yagil, *Tetrahedron*, 23, 2855 (1967).
153. Albert, *Ionization Constants of Acids and Bases*, Methuen and Co. Ltd, London, 1962.
154. Albert, *Heterocyclic Chemistry*, Athalone Press, London, 1968.
155. Jencks and Salvesen, *J. Am. Chem. Soc.*, 93, 4433 (1971).
156. Bell, *The Proton in Chemistry*, 2nd ed., Cornell, Ithaca, N.Y., 1973.
157. DeMaria, Fini, and Hall, *J. Chem. Soc. Perkin II*, 1969 (1973).
158. Ceppi, Eckhardt, and Grob, *Tetrahedron Lett.*, 37, 3627 (1973).
159. Kurz and Farrar, *J. Am. Chem. Soc.*, 91, 6057 (1969).
160. Hine and Koser, *J. Org. Chem.*, 36, 1348 (1971).

GUIDELINES FOR NMR MEASUREMENTS FOR DETERMINATION OF HIGH AND LOW pK_a VALUES

(IUPAC Technical Report)

Konstantin Popov[1,2], Hannu Rönkkömäki[3], and Lauri H. J. Lajunen[4]

[1]*Institute of Reagents and High Purity Substances (IREA), Bogorodsky val-3, 107258, Moscow, Russia;* [2]*Moscow State University of Food Production, Volokolamskoye Sh. 11, 125080 Moscow, Russia;* [3]*Finnish Institute of Occupational Health, Oulu Regional Institute of Occupational Health, Laboratory of Chemistry, Aapistie 1 FIN-90220 Oulu, Finland;* [4]*Department of Chemistry, University of Oulu, P.O. Box 3000, FIN-90014 Oulu, Finland*

Abstract: Factors affecting the NMR titration procedures for the determination of pK_a values in strongly basic and strongly acidic aqueous solutions ($2 \geq \mathrm{pH} \geq 0$ and $14 \geq \mathrm{pH} \geq 12$) are analyzed. Guidelines for experimental procedure and publication protocols are formulated. These include: calculation of the equilibrium H^+ concentration in a sample; avoidance of measurement with glass electrode in highly acidic (basic) solutions; exclusion of D_2O as a solvent; use of an individual sample isolated from air for each pH value; use of external reference and lock compounds; use of a medium of constant ionic strength with clear indication of the supporting electrolyte and of the way the contribution of any ligand to the ionic strength of the medium is accounted for; use of the NMR technique in a way that eliminates sample heating to facilitate better sample temperature control (e.g., ^1H-coupled NMR for nuclei other than protons, GD-mode, CPD-mode, etc.); use of Me_4NCl/Me_4NOH or KCl/KOH as a supporting electrolyte in basic solution rather than sodium salts in order to eliminate errors arising from NaOH association; verification of the independence of the NMR chemical shift from background electrolyte composition and concentration; use of extrapolation procedures.

Keywords: NMR titration; dissociation constants; acidity constants; chemical shift dependence on medium; high and low pK measurement; IUPAC Analytical Chemistry Division.

Introduction

Numerical data for acid–base equilibria (lg K_a values) have contributed significantly to the theoretical foundation of modern organic and inorganic chemistry [1,2]. In particular, the ligand acid dissociation constants (pK_a) correlate strongly with complex stability for many classes of ligands [3]. The related linear Gibbs energy relationships may be used for prediction of metal complex stability constants K_{ML} in cases where their direct experimental measurement is difficult or impossible [2,4,5].

Many important acid–base equilibria take place in highly basic or highly acidic aqueous solutions. For strongly acidic aquametal ions (e.g., Tl^{III}, Bi^{III}, Ti^{IV}, Th^{IV}, Be^{II}, Pd^{II}), the measurement of stability constants frequently requires solutions of low pH (pH $\geq$ 2) [6], while complex formation frequently involves ligands with very small pK_a values. By contrast, many technologies and complexation reactions require pH $\geq$ 12 [7] and ligands that are strongly basic (e.g., phosphonates, anionic forms of sugars, hydroxybenzoates, polyamines). In both cases, the application of glass electrode-based potentiometry does not give reliable results [8].

In recent years, a variety of new techniques have been developed as alternatives to the classical potentiometric titration procedure.

Among these is nuclear magnetic resonance (NMR), which has a unique application for microscopic acid dissociation constant measurements [9] as well as for work in highly basic and highly acidic media [1,6–8]. Although early reports on the use of the NMR technique were not promising [1], later work revealed good concurrence with potentiometric results for compounds with pK_a values in the range $11 \geq pK_a \geq 3$ [10–11]. Recently, fully automated pH-NMR titration equipment for protonation studies has been reported [10a,10c,12–14]. However, the pK_a values estimated from NMR measurements in strongly basic (acidic) solutions often differ significantly from those obtained by potentiometry. The higher reliability of equilibrium data based on NMR measurements in the ranges $2 \geq \mathrm{pH}$ and $\mathrm{pH} \geq 12$ is widely recognized [7,8b,8c,8d,12,13].

At the same time, diverse experimental conditions have been used for protonation and stability constant measurements by NMR. This affects the reliability and the comparison of the resulting equilibrium constants. Further, many authors have not used a standard approach to the chemical shift reference application, preparation of samples, pD/pH corrections, ionic strength control, etc. [11,14–17]. This in turn has resulted in a considerable disparity among the calculated constants. The present report is therefore focused on general recommendations for the application of NMR spectroscopy to the determination of protonation (dissociation) constants in aqueous solution, with an emphasis on titration procedures in highly acidic or highly basic media ($2 \geq \mathrm{pH} \geq 0$ and $14 \geq \mathrm{pH} \geq 12$). At the same time, it provides some guidelines for the critical treatment of the NMR-based pK_a values published earlier.

Reproduced From:
Pure Appl. Chem., Vol. 78, N0.3, pp. 663–675, 2006.
doi:10.1351/pac200678030663
© 2006 IUPAC

Factors Affecting the Accuracy of NMR Titrations

Acid dissociation constants can be expressed in terms of activity (thermodynamic constants) or concentrations (concentration, conditional constants). In the former case, the activity constant $K_a = a_H a_L/a_{HL}a°$, or a mixed activity-concentration constant $K_a = a_H[L]/[HL]c°$ are considered, where $c° = 1$ mol dm^{-3} is the standard amount concentration; $a°$ is the corresponding activity; a_H, a_L, a_{HL} represent activities; and [H], [L], [HL] amount concentrations of H$^+$, L$^-$, and HL species, respectively. IUPAC recommends for solution equilibrium studies the determination of concentration-based constants $K_a = [H] [L]/[HL]c°$ [18,19]. In the present paper, the term pK_a always indicates the concentration constant valid for a particular ionic strength I and temperature, while pH corresponds to the concentration p[H] scale (p[H$^+$]); i.e., we define p[H] $= -$lg $\{[H^+]/c°\}$ unless otherwise is stated. In a similar way, p[D] should correspond to $-$lg $\{[D^+]/c°\}$. This requires either calibration of a pH meter by solutions with known [D$^+$] at a particular I, or the direct calculation of [D$^+$] in strongly basic (acidic) solutions when the concentration of L can be neglected. However, this ideal condition is seldom if ever fulfilled, and the common practice is based on the "pH meter readings" in D$_2$O solutions after the pH meter was calibrated in H$_2$O buffer solution [8a] (see eqs. 5–7 and further discussion). Obviously, this approach gives some value of pD as unclear function of activity a_D and cannot be recommended for work in concentrated (>0.1 mol dm^{-3}) solutions of bases (acids).

For the dissociation equilibrium of the protonated ligand HL (charge numbers are neglected):

$$HL \rightleftharpoons L + H \tag{1}$$

the acidity constant K_a is defined at a particular ionic strength I as $K_a = [L][H]/[HL]c°$. Then p$K_a = -$lg $K_a = $ p[H] + lg ([HL]/[L]) and at half-neutralization p[H] becomes a reasonable estimate of pK_a as [HL] = [L] and lg ([HL]/[L]) = 0.

However, many research groups use the NMR technique for D$_2$O solutions and therefore operate with measurements of pD in terms of activity as indicated earlier. The corresponding mixed activity-concentration constant is denoted here as K_a(D$_2$O) $= a_D[L]/[DL]c°$. Then the K_a(D$_2$O) values are recalculated by means

of some empirical and very arbitrary equations (see further discussion) into some equilibrium activity-concentration constant K_a(H$_2$O), which is supposed to indicate $K_a = a_H[L]/[HL]c°$ for H$_2$O solutions, although there is no rigorous background for that supposition.

From the p[H] dependence of the chemical shift, the pK_a can be determined, using ^{1}H, ^{13}C, ^{14}N, ^{15}N, ^{31}P, ^{19}F, or any other NMR-active nucleus in a ligand [9a]. Since proton dissociation from HL changes the electron density, species HL and L reveal different chemical shifts, denoted as δ_{HL} and δ_L. Most acids in aqueous solutions are characterized by rapid proton-transfer reactions on the NMR time-scale. Thus, the observed chemical shift of any one nucleus represents the single concentration-weighted average δ_{obs} of the chemical shifts for the nucleus of each chemical species in the equilibrium:

$$\delta_{obs} = x_{HL}\delta_{HL} + x_L\delta_L \tag{2}$$

where x_{HL} and x_L denote the mole fractions of equilibrium species HL and L. The dynamically averaged chemical shift δ_{obs} provides a good measure for the degree of ionization (proton dissociation):

$$x_L = (\delta_{obs} - \delta_{HL})/(\delta_L - \delta_{HL}) \tag{3}$$

The mole fractions can be expressed in terms of p[H] and pK_a [1,13]:

$$pK_a = p[H] + lg[(\delta_L - \delta_{obs})/(\delta_{obs} - \delta_{HL})] \tag{4}$$

It is easy to demonstrate from eq. 4 that: (a) for an acid HL, a plot of δ_{obs} vs. p[H] has the shape of a titration curve lying between the asymptotes δ_L and δ_{HL}, with a point of inflection at p[H] = pK_a, $\delta_{obs} = (\delta_1 + \delta_{HL})/2$; (b) the titration curve is symmetrical about the inflection point (Fig. 1), which gives a possible simple method of estimating pK_a, δ_L, and δ_{HL}.

The normal procedure for a NMR titration is based on the dependence of the chemical shift δ_{obs} on p[H], with subsequent treatment of experimental data via routine software. Therefore, three constants are to be found from the δ_{obs} vs. p[H] data by computer analysis of this nonlinear equation, and preliminary values can often be found directly from the plot. A significant advantage of the NMR technique is associated with the possibility of titrating a mixture of ligands, including impurities, if the

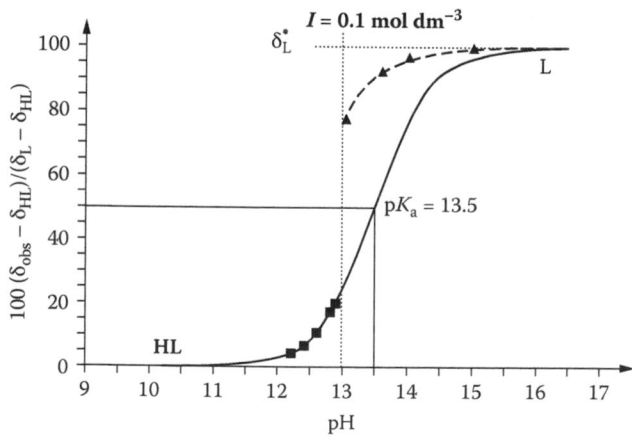

FIGURE 1 Simulated NMR titration curve for the hypothetical 0.001 mol dm^{-3} acid HL with pK_a = 13.5 at I = 0.1 mol dm^{-3} (solid line), plotted by SPECIES [35]. Squares refer to hypothetical experimental NMR-titration points at I = 0.1 mol dm^{-3}. Their range is limited by the ionic strength I (high pH limit) and by the requirement [OH$^-$] $\gg$ [HL] (low pH limit). Dashed line and triangles refer to a simulated NMR titration of the same acid at I = 1.0 mol dm^{-3}, which provides the value δ_L^* directly or via extrapolation.

total concentration of the ligands (and therefore of impurities associated with the ligands) is much less then the base (acid) concentration.

It is important to stress that for classical potentiometry with a glass electrode the inflection point can be observed only if pK_a is close to $(pK_w)^{1/2}$ [1]. For a NMR titration, the situation is completely different. As far as only mole fractions, instead of the total acid concentration, are involved in the data evaluation, NMR facilitates pK_a measurement outside the range of potentiometry if high or low p[H] are determined by means other than glass electrode readings [13]. Thus, the main sources of errors in NMR-based pK_a determinations are the accuracy and precision of δ_{obs} and p[H] values.

Chemical Shifts

General conventions for chemical shifts are comprehensively considered in recent IUPAC recommendations [20]. In the present paper, we will focus only on specific problems associated with NMR-based pK_a determinations, bearing in mind that many research groups involved in solution chemistry equilibria still do not have modern NMR equipment and have to work with routine spectrometers. It is essential that the chemical shift measurement being made for each datum point is reliable. Another important requirement is to obtain from the set of chemical shifts such a pK_a value that can pass comparison with other equilibrium constants.

As described in ref. [20], there are three types of referencing method that could reasonably be applied in titrations: *internal referencing, substitution method,* and *external referencing.* These methods all have various advantages and disadvantages in relevance to NMR titration.

Internal referencing may lead to intermolecular interactions between ligand, solvent, and reference compound. Further, in many spectrometers the sample must normally include a deuterium-containing molecule for magnetic field stabilization ("lock"). For many purposes, all these interactions can be safely ignored, but for NMR-based titrations at high and low p[H] a considerable caution is needed. The use of D_2O (as the "lock") instead of H_2O as a solvent, and the addition of uncontrolled "small" amounts of a reference compound like sodium 3-(trimethylsilyl) propane-1-sulfonate (DSS), dimethyl sulfoxide (DMSO), *tert*-butylalcohol or 1, 4-dioxane inside a sample (internally), became common practice for ^1H and ^{13}C NMR [12,15,16]. In some cases (^{13}C NMR), the added reference compound is itself deuterated (e.g., $(^2H_6)$DMSO or DSS, deuterated at the CH_2 positions), thus providing the lock signal as well. Modern NMR techniques give the possibility to work with very low concentrations of DSS. Therefore, it gives a negligible contribution to ionic strength and to solution properties. It is demonstrated to be effective at p[H] 0–1 [12]. At the same time, little is known about the properties of internal references at elevated p[H]. Nevertheless, any internal substance can potentially participate in association processes either with the cation under complex formation study or with the background electrolyte and is therefore generally undesirable from the point of view of equilibrium studies.

For ^1H NMR titrations, the use of D_2O as a solvent instead of H_2O is a common procedure. This is usually done to eliminate masking of a substrate peak by the H_2O resonance [15–17]. The use of D_2O internally raises the problems of how to effect pD measurement with a standard glass electrode, as well as the relationship between p$K_a(H_2O)$ and p$K_a(D_2O)$. The proposed simple empirical eq. 5 derived for ionic strength $I = 0.001–0.01$ mol dm^{-3} and 25°C [21] to obtain values on the conventional pD scale from glass electrode readings is widely accepted, although it is frequently used far outside of the originally intended ionic strength and temperature limits:

$$pD = pH\text{-meter reading}^* +0.40 \qquad (5)$$

Some authors, however, use eqs. 6 or 7 [22,23]:

$$pD = pH\text{-meter reading} + 0.44 \ (22°C, I = 0.01 \text{mol dm}^{-3}) \qquad (6)$$

$$pD = pH\text{-meter reading} + 0.50 \ (22°C, I = 0.1 \text{mol dm}^{-3}) \qquad (7)$$

Although the difference between pD values calculated by different equations is not large, it is a substantial contribution to systematic error, even for low ionic strength and room temperature, but particularly for high ionic strengths and high temperatures.

There is an even greater diversity of relationships between p$K_a(H_2O)$ and p$K_a(D_2O)$. Both quantities are ionic strength-dependent. The proposed empirical equations yield significantly different results and seem very arbitrary: relationships depend on the nature and number of compounds studied [24–26]. It is observed that the activity coefficient products undergo significant changes when one goes from light to heavy water [27]. It is obvious that at present a correct extrapolation of p$K_a(D_2O)$ to an aqueous phase p$K_a(H_2O)$ is not possible, and that the systematic errors for calculated values are outside the accepted uncertainty for p$K_a(H_2O)$ values derived directly from NMR measurements with external D_2O. Besides, p$K_a(D_2O)$ values can hardly pass comparison with other equilibrium constants measured in H_2O, and their use for complex formation equilibria in H_2O is very doubtful. Assuming the above difficulties, the use of internal D_2O is not recommended.

For ^{31}P NMR, the use of internal referencing at high and low p[H] is difficult, and external reference application is widely used and recommended [7c,7d,8b,8c,11a,11b,16,17a,17b].

Substitution method uses measurement of sample and reference spectra in two separate experiments. It became feasible due to implementation of stable, internally locked spectrometers. In this procedure, the sample and reference materials are not mixed. This benefits the equilibrium study. If locking is not used, the magnet should not be reshimmed between running the sample and reference solution, since this changes the applied magnetic field [20]. This can become a disadvantage for time-consuming ^{13}C NMR-based equilibrium experiments because the ligand concentrations have to be small.

External referencing involves sample and reference contained separately in coaxial cylindrical tubes. A single spectrum is recorded, which includes signals from both the sample and the reference. It is also an ideal situation for equilibrium study as far as both reference and "lock" substances are separated from the ligand solution. The external reference procedure generally requires corrections arising from differences in bulk magnetic susceptibility between sample and reference [20]. This is important for precise chemical shift measurements, but for the relative change of δ_{obs} between δ_L and δ_{HL} for a series of nearly identical aqueous solutions in a narrow pH range (either p[H] 0–2 or 12–14) with constant ionic strength and a constant sample volume it is insignificant. Numerous measurements of ^{31}P NMR-based pK_a values revealed no influence from this factor [7c,7d,8b, 8c,11a,11b,16,17a,11b]. Alternatively, magic-angle spinning could be used. Therefore, such a technique seems to be the preferable choice.

---

* pH-meter reading for solutions in D_2O when the pH electrodes are calibrated with standard aqueous buffers.

p[H] Values and Titration Procedure

An important source of error in NMR-based pK_a determinations is the accuracy and precision of the p[H] values. Determining extreme values of p[H] requires special attention, since glass electrodes cannot be used reliably [8a,8c,12,13]. Therefore, the traditional single-sample NMR titration is recommended [8c,13,27,29,30]. A set of individual samples with constant monoprotic acid HL (or ligand L) concentration (e.g., 0.01 mol dm^{-3}), constant ionic strength (e.g., 1 mol dm^{-3}) and varying p[H] value are prepared one-by-one ("constant volume titration") in such a way that a strong acid or a strong base added for desired p[H] adjustment is taken in a significant excess over HL or L (e.g., 0.1–1.0 mol dm^{-3}). This permits the equilibrium p[H] value to be calculated reliably as it is equated to the total amount of a strong acid (strong base) added to the sample [27]. Since each sample is prepared individually from stock solutions, the ionic strength can be very precisely controlled [12]. The use of "lock" and reference substances externally excludes their undesirable influence on the equilibrium system. Alternatively, in an approach developed by Hägele [13], the glass electrode can be completely avoided by adding an indicator molecule to the sample for in situ p[H] monitoring. However, this method is primarily based on the procedure stated above.

The proposed method is equally valid for both strongly acidic (pH < 2) and strongly basic (pH > 12) solutions, although some peculiarities do exist in the latter. For the acidic medium, p[H] is directly derived from the total strong acid concentration. In the case of highly basic solutions, the initially calculated p[OH$^-$] values have to be converted to the p[H] scale, using appropriate pK_w values to allow calculation of the corresponding pK_a values. Some important issues that restrict the application of the above method and influence the data quality should also be considered.

Titration Procedure and Titration Curve Treatment

A full-scale NMR titration for a single proton equilibrium 1 will provide values of δ_{HL}, δ_L, and some intermediate chemical shift values applicable to a particular pH at a constant I. Ideally, a titration spans over 4 pH units with the half-neutralization point in the middle of this pH range. For extremely high or low pK_a, this condition is not achievable: for $pK_a = 13.5$, the value for δ_L has to be measured at pH 15.5, while for $pK_a = 0.5$ a direct observation of δ_{HL} requires pH = –1.5.

If the ionic strength is 1.0 mol dm^{-3} (NaCl/NaOH), then the highest pH attainable at 25°C (pH$_{max}$) is less than 13.72 (pK_w for 1 mol dm^{-3} NaOH[*]), while for $I = 0.1$ mol dm^{-3} NaCl/NaOH pH$_{max}$ < 12.78 (limitation due to pK_w and I). Thus for $pK_a = 13.5$ at $I = 1.0$ mol dm^{-3} (NaCl/NaOH) only about 80 % of the titration curve is accessible, providing a value for δ_{HL} and a half-neutralization point, but not for δ_L. In the case of $I = 0.1$ mol dm^{-3} (NaCl/NaOH[*]), about 30 % of the full curve can be obtained experimentally, but excluding the half-neutralization point and δ_L, Fig. 1 (square points). Although comprehensive software (SigmaPlot, WinEQNMR) permits calculation of pK_a and δ_L values for very weak acids on the basis of data at different pH values below that for the half-neutralization point, the corresponding constants have a large error. But in some cases, the programs fail

to produce results and experimental measurement of high pK_a at low ionic strength becomes impossible. This can be illustrated by the last dissociation step of nitrilotris (methylenephosphonic acid) (NTPH, H_6ntph) and ethylenediaminetetra (methylenephosphonic acid) (EDTPH, H_8edtph)[†], Table 1.

On the other hand, if the initial δ_{HL} experimental value and the subsequent 30–40 % of a complete titration curve are supported by at least one final high pH titration point to provide δ_L, then the precision of the pK_a calculation becomes sufficiently high and the measurement becomes feasible.

For those nuclei with chemical shift poorly dependent on the ionic strength and nature of the supporting electrolyte (the case of ^{31}P and ^{13}C), δ_L can be obtained by titration of the same system at a higher or even uncontrolled ionic strength until the "plateau" is reached (triangle points, Fig. 1). The resultant δ_L^* is very close to δ_L, e.g., δ_L ($I = 0.1$ mol dm^{-3}) ~ δ_L^* ($I = 1.0$ mol dm^{-3}). Then the following two-step procedure is recommended. The first step involves the titration of a ligand at a sufficiently high ionic strength, e.g., 1.0 mol dm^{-3} NaCl (triangles in Fig. 1) or 1.5 mol dm^{-3} NaCl, etc., rather than in 0.1 mol dm^{-3} NaCl. This gives two advantages. The first is that the pH$_{max}$ is shifted from 12.78 to ca. 14. The second derives from the fact that sodium ion forms weak complexes with L (e.g., phosphonic acids). Therefore, the whole titration curve is shifted to a lower pH range as the total sodium concentration is increased. Both of these factors facilitated the direct observation of a "plateau" corresponding to δ_L^* ($I = 1$ mol dm^{-3}).

Due to the fact that δ_L (0.1 mol dm^{-3} NaCl) is practically equal to δ_L^* (1 mol dm^{-3} NaCl), then the δ_L^*-value could be used instead of δ_L along with experimental points obtained for $I = 0.1$ mol dm^{-3} (square points, Fig. 1). Therefore, within the second step, δ_L^* is assigned to a conventional pH = 16 or pH = 17, where the titration curve definitely has a plateau. A titration is repeated for 0.1 mol dm^{-3} NaCl solutions, a δ_L^* point is added to the experimental data set, and a pK_a^* value is calculated. The subsequent treatment of the united data reveals a significant increase in the accuracy of pK_a. This can be seen from Table 1, where both constants pK_a (calculated without δ_L^*) and pK_a^* (calculated with a δ_L^* point) are represented. If δ_L is significantly dependent on ionic strength, then the extrapolation procedure proposed by Popov, Lajunen, and Rönkkömäki [28,29] could be applied.

Ligand Concentration

Calculation of p[H] from the acid stoichiometry requires a low ligand concentration: for a monoprotic acid $C_{HL} < 0.01 I$. Recent developments of the NMR technique make it possible to now work with very dilute solutions. In case of the organophosphonates, concentrations C_L ~ 0.001 mol dm^{-3} are quite suitable for ^{31}P NMR titrations [28,29].

By contrast, for ^{13}C NMR titrations, the ligand concentration has to be rather high (about 0.1 mol dm^{-3}) in order to perform the titration in a reasonable time. Therefore, the equilibrium [OH$^-$] cannot be equal to the total [OH$^-$] added to the system. For this case (e.g., 0.1 mol dm^{-3} HL), another two-step procedure reported for sucrose dissociation constant measurements [31] is recommended. In the first step, the equilibrium [OH$^-$] is taken as equal to the total [OH$^-$] added, and the full titration curve is plotted, mathematically treated, and the pK_a, δ_L, and δ_{HL} values are calculated. The difference between δ_L and δ_{HL} chemical shifts defines the linear scale of OH$^-$ consumption by the ligand: 0 mol dm^{-3}

---

[*] Reliable values for pK_w are measured only for some common supporting electrolytes, e.g., NaCl, NaClO$_4$, KNO$_3$, etc. For 1 mol dm^{-3} NaOH, the pK_w value found for 1 mol dm^{-3} NaCl is valid as far as the difference in corresponding activity coefficients is negligible. The same situation is observed for the 0.1 mol dm^{-3} NaCl/NaOH system. However, it is not the case for a complete substitution of 1 mol dm^{-3} NO$_3^-$ for OH$^-$ or of 1 mol dm^{-3} K$^+$ (Na$^+$) for H$^+$ (acidic solutions).

[†] The PINs (preferred IUPAC names) for NTPH and EDTPH are: [nitrilo-tris(methylene)]tris(phosphonic acid) and ethane-1, 2-diyldinitrilotetra-kis(methylene)tetrakis(phosphonic acid).

TABLE 1: Dissociation Constants pK_a for Hedtph^{-7} and Hntph^{-5} Derived from ^{31}P NMR Measurements by SigmaPlot Data Treatment[a]

Ligand	I/(mol dm^{-3})	t/°C	pK_a	pK_a*	Reference
Hedtph^{-7}	0.1 (KNO$_3$)	25	Calculation failed	13.29 ± 0.07	[28]
	0.15 (NaCl)	37	13 ± 1	12.86 ± 0.07	[28]
Hntph^{-5}	0.1 (KNO$_3$)	25	12.2 ± 0.3	12.9 ± 0.1	[29]

[a] pK_a and pK_a* represent constants calculated without δ$_L$* and with δ$_L$* values, respectively; see text for other explanations.

TABLE 2: Dissociation Constant of 0.1 mol dm^{-3} Sucrose (HL) from ^{13}C NMR Titration at 60°C in 1 mol dm^{-3} NaCl/NaOH [31]

Procedure	δ$_L$/ppm	δ$_{HL}$/ppm	pK_a	R
One-step data treatment	103.00	101.98	12.40 ± 0.05	0.999
Two-step data treatment	102.96	101.98	12.30 ± 0.05	0.999

(δ$_{HL}$) and 0.1 mol dm^{-3} (δ$_L$) for a 0.1 mol dm^{-3} solution of L. Within the second step, all the experimental values δ$_{obs}$ are treated again with redefined values of p[OH], and an improved value of pK_a is calculated. As indicated in Table 2, the correction due to the second step reveals a systematic error of 0.1 in pK_a.

Background Electrolyte and Ionic Strength

To date, the background electrolyte effect on chemical shifts has been inadequately studied. Equilibrium concentration products are ionic strength-dependent, yet numerous NMR titration experiments have been performed without ionic strength control [14c,16c], and have produced pK_a values in reasonable agreement with potentiometric results. In part, this arises from the fact that the chemical shifts depend on concentrations, rather than the activities of various species in solution [32]. The best agreement has been demonstrated for systems studied by ^{13}C and ^{31}P NMR [28,29,33]. For the ^{13}C and ^{31}P NMR resonances in alkylcarboxylic and alkylphosphonic acids, the chemical shifts correlate linearly with the background electrolyte concentration. However, this effect is normally negligible in comparison with that associated with a ligand dissociation or complex formation. This fact offers a unique possibility to use ^{13}C and ^{31}P NMR chemical shifts, δ$_L$, of a ligand, measured at high pH and high ionic strength, for calculations of pK_a at low ionic strength [28,29]. General observation reveals that the chemical shift depends on both the nature of the nucleus and its position in the ligand. The ^{31}P nuclei in phosphonic ($-PO_3H_2$, $-PO_3H^-$, $-PO_3^{2-}$) as well as ^{13}C nuclei in carboxylate or methylenic groups ($-CO_2^-$, $-CH_2^-$, $-CH_3$) are relatively isolated from solution by oxygen or hydrogen atoms. Thus, their chemical shifts are mostly sensitive to the substrate intramolecular processes (deprotonation/protonation, complex formation), while the solvent changes give

the least contribution. On the other hand, the nuclei that contact the solvent directly, e.g., ^{133}Cs$^+$, ^{35}Cl$^-$, are more affected by medium effects. Therefore, a NMR titration under variable ionic strength is not desirable, unless the independence of chemical shift δ on ionic strength I is demonstrated.

Among the supporting electrolytes for 14 ≥ pH ≥ 12, the use of 1.0 mol dm^{-3} Me$_4$NCl/Me$_4$NOH is recommended as there is no reported evidence for Me$_4$NOH self-association. In the case of KOH and NaOH, corrections for base self-association could be needed. The uncertainty is associated with imprecise knowledge of the MOH stability constants. Table 3 represents the estimation of errors if the MOH stability constants recommended by Baes and Mesmer [34] are used. Table 3 also demonstrates that for NaOH solutions the pH scale has to be corrected, while for KOH no correction is needed. However, it should be mentioned that Martell [35] gives significantly higher stability constants for MOH ion pairing. Thus, the corresponding corrections could be larger.

Another important issue for NMR titration is the need for a clear indication as to whether the contribution of the ligand to the total ionic strength is considered or not. For monobasic acids, this contribution could be negligible, but it is not the case for polyprotic substrates such as EDTPH. In basic 0.01 mol dm^{-3} solutions of EDTPH, the ligand contribution to the total ionic strength constitutes 0.25 mol dm^{-3} for Hedtph^{-7} and 0.33 for edtph^{-8}.

Special care should be taken over supporting electrolyte purity. Indeed, in 1 mol dm^{-3} Me$_4$NCl/Me$_4$NOH medium, the concentration of Ca^{2+} impurities in the supporting electrolyte can be comparable with the ligand content in the system [8c].

Another important peculiarity of the titration procedure at high and low pH arises from a complete substitution of either cation or anion. Indeed, within the constant background electrolyte concentration, e.g., 1 mol dm^{-3} at 25°C, the ionic strength can change significantly. For example, the complete substitution of 1 mol dm^{-3} KNO$_3$ for 1 mol dm^{-3} KOH induces the change of mean activity coefficient from 0.444 to 0.733. In the same way, a substitution of 1 mol dm^{-3} KNO$_3$ for 1 mol dm^{-3} HNO$_3$ results in a change of activity coefficient from 0.444 to 0.730. At the same time for 1 mol dm^{-3} NaCl/NaOH system, the corresponding

TABLE 3: Calculated −lg {[H$^+$]/mol dm^{-3}} for MOH Solutions in 0.1 and 1.0 mol dm^{-3} MCl/MOH[a]

MOH	Total [OH$^-$], mol dm^{-3}	Free[a] [OH$^-$], mol dm^{-3}	pH Calculated without correction for MOH Association	pH Corrected for MOH Association[a]	ΔpH
NaOH	0.1000	0.0947	12.75	12.73	0.02
	1.00	0.69	13.75	13.54	0.21
KOH	0.1000	0.0998	13.15	13.15	0.00
	1.00	0.91	14.15	14.11	0.04

[a] Free [OH−] is calculated with the SPECIES software [36] using MOH stability constants lg K_1 from [34] (for ionic strength 1.0 mol dm^{-3} lg K_1 = −0.5 for NaOH and −0.8 for KOH), [H$^+$] is calculated from [OH$^-$] using pK_w = 13.75 for 1 mol dm^{-3} NaCl and 14.16 for 1 mol dm^{-3} KCl [37].

change is negligible (0.657 and 0.674)[*]. Therefore, a proper choice of supporting electrolyte, or clear indication of corresponding corrections, is needed.

Temperature

Dissociation constants, as well as pK_w, are temperature-dependent [35]. A temperature variation of 20–30°C can result in a change of 0.2–0.3 in pK_a (or more). Especially critical are the high pK_a – values. For example, for Hntph^{-5} dissociation $\Delta H = -38.8$ kJ mol^{-1} for $I = 0.1$ mol dm^{-3} and 25°C ([36], Mini Database). Therefore, $pK_a = 13.30$ at 25°C and 12.98 at 40°C. The difference in 0.1 pK_a unit per 5°C is significant for dissociation constant. The temperature dependence of pK_w additionally affects all the measurements in basic solutions. For example, in 0.51 mol dm^{-3} NaCl solutions, pK_w changes from 13.71 (25°C) to 12.96 (50°C). In this respect, the noise associated with ^{1}H-decoupling widely used in early NMR measurements might have led to some errors in pK_a values due to significant energy dissipation and therefore to a sample heating. Although modern multipulse decoupling methods (GD-mode, CPD-mode) dissipate less energy, some caution is needed to control the process. In some cases, ^{1}H-coupled spectra are the better choice.

Guidelines

Recommendations for NMR titrations in solutions of high and low pH ($2 \geq$ pH ≥ 0 and $14 \geq$ pH ≥ 12) are intended to be a supplement to the IUPAC guidelines for the determination of stability constants [19] and to a standard format for the publication of stability constant measurements [38] considering the peculiarities of NMR spectroscopy mentioned above. Some of these requirements are also valid for the range $12 \geq$ pH ≥ 2.

1. Within the NMR titration procedure at high and low pH solutions ($2 \geq$ pH ≥ 0 and $14 \geq$ pH ≥ 12), the equilibrium H$^+$ concentration should be calculated from solution stoichiometry, not measured with a glass electrode. For this reason, the ligand concentration has to be ≤ 0.001 mol dm^{-3}. For higher ligand concentrations, the titration is possible, but corrections for strong base (strong acid) consumption by a ligand are necessary.
2. Arrangement of a titration procedure. Sets of samples should be prepared in such a way that the concentration of the ligand and the total ionic strength remain constant, while the supporting electrolyte composition is varied from sample to sample to provide different concentrations of OH$^-$ or H$^+$. For highly basic solutions, the total concentration of added base should be much greater than the ligand concentration ([OH$^-$] >> [L]). For highly acidic media, the same requirement applies to [H$^+$] ([H$^+$] >> [L]). Thus, the total concentration of added base (acid) can be treated as the equilibrium concentration (i.e., the OH$^-$ or H$^+$ consumption by the substrate can be neglected). This circumvents the problems associated with pH measurements with the glass electrode. An additional advantage of such an approach is that the protonation constants are derived in terms of concentration, not activity.
3. A medium of constant ionic strength should be used, with clear indication of the supporting electrolyte and of the

way the contribution of the deprotonated ligand and of the change in a background electrolyte composition (e.g., change of [Cl$^-$] for [OH$^-$] or [Cl$^-$] for [H$^+$]) to medium ionic strength is taken into account.
4. The supporting electrolytes Me$_4$NCl/Me$_4$NOH or KCl/KOH should be used in basic solution rather than NaCl/NaOH of LiCl/LiOH in order to eliminate errors arising from NaOH and LiOH association. A clear indication of the pK_w used is necessary.
5. External reference and "lock" compounds should be used to eliminate any possible interactions with the ligand and additional changes of the medium.
6. Water should be used as a solvent rather then D$_2$O or H$_2$O/D$_2$O mixtures. This eliminates the need for pD/pH corrections and makes the pK_a values obtained comparable and compatible with values derived from potentiometric measurements performed in H$_2$O.
7. An NMR procedure should be selected, and described clearly, that will minimize possible sample heating (e.g., ^{1}H-coupled NMR, GD-technique, etc.) and provide confidence in temperature control.
8. The calculation of pK_a requires the chemical shift value for the free ligand L (δ_L) and for the protonated species HL (δ_{HL}) along with a number of intermediate experimental values. This is seldom possible for high (low) pH range. In those cases where the δ_{HL} or δ_L value is not available due to ionic strength (and pH) limitations, it should be derived either directly from higher ionic strength measurements (for ionic strength-independent resonance) or by an extrapolation of high ionic strength values to the lower I used in the experiment (for ionic strength-dependent resonance).

Acknowledgments

The authors are grateful to the IUPAC Analytical Chemistry Division for support within the Grant 2001-038-2-500 as well as to the Finnish Academy of Science, which supported preparation of the present paper in part. We are also thankful to K. J. Powell, P. M. May, E. D. Becker, and R. K. Harris for valuable comments and suggestions.

References

1. R. F. Cookson. *Chem. Rev.* **74**, 5 (1974).
2. H. Irving, H. S. Rossotti. *Acta Chem. Scand.* **10**, 72 (1956).
3. (a) H. H. Jensen, L. Lyngbye, M. Bols. *Angew. Chem.* **40** (2001); (b) C. M. Chang, M. K. Wung. *TheoChem.* **417**, 237 (1997); (c) G. Thirot. *Bull. Soc. Chim. Fr.* 3559 (1967).
4. (a) T. Shi, L. I. Elding. *Inorg. Chem.* **36**, 528 (1997); (b) G. Anderegg. *Inorg. Chim. Acta* **180**, 69 (1991); (c) P. R. Wells. *Linear Free Energy Relationships*, Academic Press, London (1968).
5. R. M. Smith, A. E. Martell, R. J. Motekaitis. *Inorg. Chim. Acta* **99**, 207 (1985).
6. (a) S. Nakamura, K. Yamashita. *Phosphorus Res. Bull.* **11**, 1 (2000); (b) P. Coupe, D. Williams, H. Lyn. *J. Chem. Soc., Perkin Trans.* 2 1595 (2001); (c) V. B. Fainerman, D. Vollhardt, R. Johann. *Langmiur* **16**, 7731 (2000); (d) A. S. Goldstein. U.S. Pat. 5929008 (1999); (e) S. R. Chen, M. G. F. Thomas. Eur. Pat. EP 564232 (1993) and Eur. Pat. EP 564248; (f) P. G. Yohannes, K. Bowman-James. *Inorg. Chim. Acta* **209**, 115 (1993); (j) K. M. Thompson, W. P. Griffith, M. Spiro. *J. Chem. Soc., Faraday Trans.* **89**, 1203 (1993); (h) E. Okutsu, Y. Kudo, S. Hori, K. Hasanuma. Japan Pat. JP 67073147 (1986); (i) R. R. Dague, J. N. Veenstra, T. W. McKim. *J. Water Pollut. Control Fed.* **52**, 2204 (1980).

---

[*] Mean activity coefficients are taken from *CRC Handbook of Chemistry and Physics*, 82nd ed., R. Lide (Ed.), CRC Press, Boca Raton, FL (2001–2003).

7. (a) E. Matczak-Jon, B. Kurzak, W. Sawka-Dobrowolska, P. Kafarski, B. Lejczak. *J. Chem. Soc., Dalton Trans.* 3455 (1996); (b) L. Alderighi, A. Bianchi, L. Biondi, L. Calabi, M. De Miranda, P. Gans, S. Ghelli, R Losi, L. Paleari, A. Sabatini, A. Vacca. *J. Chem. Soc., Perkin Trans. 2* 2741 (1999); (c) J. Rohovec, M. Kyvala, P. Vojtisek, P. Hermann. I. Lukes. *Eur. J. Inorg. Chem. Soc.* 195 (2000); (d) I. Lukes, L. Blaha, F. Kesner, J. Rohovec, R. Hermann. *J. Chem. Soc., Dalton Trans.* 2629 (1997).

8. (a) R. G. Bates. *Determination of pH: Theory and Practice*, 2nd ed., John Wiley, New York (1973); (b) I. Lukes, K. Bazakas, R. Hermann, R. Vojtisek. *J. Chem. Soc., Dalton Trans.* 939 (1992); (c) K. Popov, E. Niskanen, H. Rönkkömäki, L. H. J. Lajunen. *New J. Chem.* **23** (1999).

9. (a) D. L. Rabenstein, S. P. Hari, A. Kaerner. *Anal. Chem.* **69**, 4310 (1997); (b) D. L. Rabenstein, T. L. Soyer. *Anal. Chem.* **48**, 1141 (1976).

10. (a) J. Glaser, U. Henriksson, T. Klason. *Acta Chem. Scand.* **A40**, 344 (1986); (b) D. T. Major, A. Laxer, B. Fisher. *J. Org. Chem.* **67**, 790 (2002); (c) F. Reneiro, C. Guillou, C. Frassinetti, S. Ghelli. *Anal. Biochem.* **319**, 179 (2003); (d) C. Frassineti, S. Ghelli, P. Gans, A. Sabatini, M. S. Moruzzi, A. Vacca. *Anal. Biochem.* **231**, 374 (1995).

11. (a) H. Rönkkömäki, J. Jokisaari, L. H. J. Lajunen. *Acta Chem. Scand.* **47**, 331 (1993); (b) K. Sawada, T. Miyagawa, T. Sakaguchi, K. Doi. *J. Chem. Soc., Dalton Trans.* 3777 (1993).

12. Z. Szakacs, G. Hägele. *Talanta* **62**, 819 (2004).

13. Z. Szakacs, G. Hägele, R. Tyka. *Anal. Chim. Acta* **522**, 247 (2004).

14. (a) M. Peters, L. Siegfried, T. A. Kaden. *J. Chem. Soc., Dalton Trans.* 1603 (1999); (b) J. Ollig, G. Haegele. *Comput. Chem.* **19**, 287 (1995); (c) H.-Z. Cai, T. A. Kaden. *Helv. Chim. Acta* **77**, 383 (1994).

15. R. Delgado, L. C. Siegfried, T. Kaden. *Helv. Chim. Acta* **73**, 140 (1990).

16. (a) T. G. Appleton, J. R. Hall, A. D. Harris, H. A. Kimlin, I. J. McMahon. *Austr. J. Chem.* **37**, 1833 (1984); (b) T. G. Appleton, J. R. Hall, I. J. McMahon. *Inorg. Chem.* **25**, 726 (1986); (c) T. G. Appleton, J. R. Hall, S. F. Ralph, C. S. M. Thompson. *Inorg. Chem.* **28**, 1989 (1989).

17. (a) I. N. Marov, L. V. Ruzaikina, V. A. Ryabukhin, P. A. Korovaikov, N. M. Dyatlova. *Koord. Khim. (Russ. J. Coord. Chem.)* **3**, 1334 (1977); (b) I. N. Marov, L. V. Ruzaikina, V. A. Ryabukhin, R. A. Korovaikov, A. V. Sokolov. *Koord. Khim. (Russ. J. Coord. Chem.)* **6**, 375 (1980); (c) B. Song, J. Reuber, C. Ochs, F. E. Hahn, T. Luegger, C. Orvig. *Inorg. Chem.* **40**, 1527 (2001).

18. A. Braibanti, G. Ostacoli, P. Paoletti, L. D. Pettit, S. Sammartano. *Pure Appl. Chem.* **59**, 1721 (1987).

19. G. H. Nancollas, M. B. Tomson. *Pure Appl. Chem.* **54**, 2675 (1982).

20. R. K. Harris, E. D. Becker, S. M. Cabral de Menezes, R. Goodfellow, P. Granger. *Pure Appl. Chem.* **73**, 1795 (2001).

21. R K. Glasoe, F. A. Long. *J. Phys. Chem.* **64**, 188 (1960).

22. K. Mikkelsen, S. O. Nielsen. *J. Phys. Chem.* **64**, 632 (1960).

23. C. F. G. C. Geraldes, A. M. Urbano, M. C. Apoim, A. D. Sherry, K.-T. Kuan, R. Rajagopalan, F. Maton, R. N. Muller. *Magn. Reson. Imaging* **13**, 401 (1995).

24. S. R Dagnall, D. N. Hague, M. E. McAdam, A. D. Moreton. *J. Chem. Soc., Faraday Trans. 1* **81**, 1483 (1985).

25. R. Delgado, J. J. R. Frausto Da Silva, M. T. S. Amorim, M. F. Cabral, S. Chaves, J. Costa. *Anal. Chim. Acta* **245**, 271 (1991).

26. C. A. Blindauer, A. Holy, H. Dvorakova, H. Sigel. *J. Chem. Soc., Perkin Trans. 2* 2353 (1997).

27. R Salomaa, A. Vesala, S. Vesala. *Acta Chem. Scand.* **23**, 2107 (1969).

28. K. Popov, A. Popov, H. Rönkkömäki, A. Vendilo, L. H. J. Lajunen. *J. Solution Chem.* **31**, 511 (2002).

29. A. Popov, H. Rönkkömäki, L. H. J. Lajunen, A. Vendilo, K. Popov. *Inorg. Chim. Acta* **353**, 1 (2003).

30. G. Grossmann, K. A. Burkov, G. Hägele, L. A. Myund, C. Verwey, S. Hermens, S. M. Arat-ool. *Inorg. Chim. Acta* **357**, 797 (2004).

31. K. Popov, N. Sultanova, H. Rönkkömäki, M. Hannu-Kuure, L. H. J. Lajunen, I. F. Bugaenko, V. I. Tuzhilkin. *Food Chem.* **96**, 248 (2006).

32. C. A. Eckert, M. M. McNiel, B. A. Scott, L. A. Halas. *AIChE J.* **32**, 820 (1986).

33. K. Popov, N. Sultanova, H. Rönkkömäki, M. Hannu-Kuure, L. H. J. Lajunen. Unpublished data on acetate ion ^{13}C chemical shift dependence on background electrolyte concentration.

34. C. F. Baes Jr., R. E. Mesmer. *The Hydrolysis of Cations*, John Wiley, New York (1976).

35. NIST Standard Reference Database 46. NIST Critically Selected Stability Constants of Metal Complexes, Version 4.0, compiled by A. E. Martell, R. M. Smith, R. J. Motekaitis, Texas A&M University (1997).

36. IUPAC Stability Constants Database (for Windows 95/98), Version 4.06, compiled by L. D. Pettit, K. J. Powell, Academic Software and K. J. Powell, Sourby Old Farm, Timble, UK (1999); available from <www.acadsoft.co.uk>.

37. I. Kron, S. L. Marshall, P. M. May, G. T. Hefter, E. Königsberger. *Monatsh. Chem.* **126**, 819 (1995).

38. D. Tuck. *Pure. Appl. Chem.* **61**, 1161 (1989).

MEASUREMENT AND INTERPRETATION OF ELECTROKINETIC PHENOMENA

(IUPAC Technical Report)

A. V Delgado[1], F. González-Caballero[1], R. J. Hunter[2], L. K. Koopal[3], and J. Lyklema[3]

[1]*University of Granada, Granada, Spain;* [2]*University of Sydney, Sydney, Australia;*
[3]*Wageningen University, Wageningen, The Netherlands*

With contributions from (in alphabetical order): S. Alkafeef, College of Technological Studies, Hadyia, Kuwait; E. Chibowski, Maria Curie Sklodowska University, Lublin, Poland; C. Grosse, Universidad Nacional de Tucumán, Tucumán, Argentina; A. S. Dukhin, Dispersion Technology, Inc., New York, USA; S. S. Dukhin, Institute of Water Chemistry, National Academy of Science, Kiev, Ukraine; K. Furusawa, University of Tsukuba, Tsukuba, Japan; R. Jack, Malvern Instruments, Ltd., Worcestershire, UK; N. Kallay, University of Zagreb, Zagreb, Croatia; M. Kaszuba, Malvern Instruments, Ltd., Worcestershire, UK; M. Kosmulski, Technical University of Lublin, Lublin, Poland; R. Nöremberg, BASF AG, Ludwigshafen, Germany; R. W. O'Brien, Colloidal Dynamics, Inc., Sydney, Australia; V. Ribitsch, University of Graz, Graz, Austria; V. N. Shilov, Institute of Biocolloid Chemistry, National Academy of Science, Kiev, Ukraine; F. Simon, Institut für Polymerforschung, Dresden, Germany; C. Werner; Institut für Polymerforschung, Dresden, Germany; A. Zhukov, University of St. Petersburg, Russia; R. Zimmermann, Institut für Polymerforschung, Dresden, Germany

*Membership of the Division Committee during preparation of this report (2004–2005) was as follows:

President: R. D. Weir (Canada); *Vice President:* C. M. A. Brett (Portugal); *Secretary:* M. J. Rossi (Switzerland); *Titular Members:* G. H. Atkinson (USA); W. Baumeister (Germany); R. Fernández-Prini (Argentina); J. G. Frey (UK); R. M. Lynden-Bell (UK); J. Maier (Germany); Z.-Q. Tian (China); *Associate Members:* S. Califano (Italy); S. Cabral de Menezes (Brazil); A. J. McQuillan (New Zealand); D. Platikanov (Bulgaria); C. A. Royer (France); *National Representatives:* J. Ralston (Australia); M. Oivanen (Finland); J. W. Park (Korea); S. Aldoshin (Russia); G. Vesnaver (Slovenia); E. L. J. Breet (South Africa).

Abstract: In this report, the status quo and recent progress in electrokinetics are reviewed. Practical rules are recommended for performing electrokinetic measurements and interpreting their results in terms of well-defined quantities, the most familiar being the ζ-potential or electrokinetic potential. This potential is a property of charged interfaces, and it should be independent of the technique used for its determination. However, often the ζ-potential is not the only property electrokinetically characterizing the electrical state of the interfacial region; the excess conductivity of the stagnant layer is an additional parameter. The requirement to obtain the ζ-potential is that electrokinetic theories be correctly used and applied within their range of validity. Basic theories and their application ranges are discussed. A thorough description of the main electrokinetic methods is given; special attention is paid to their ranges of applicability as well as to the validity of the underlying theoretical models. Electrokinetic consistency tests are proposed in order to assess the validity of the ζ-potentials obtained. The recommendations given in the report apply mainly to smooth and homogeneous solid particles and plugs in aqueous systems; some attention is paid to nonaqueous media and less ideal surfaces.

Keywords: Electrokinetics; zeta potential; conductivity; aqueous systems; surface conductivity; IUPAC Physical and Biophysical Chemistry Division.

Contents

Reproduced From:
Pure Appl. Chem., Vol. 77, No. 10, pp. 1753–1805, 2005.
DOI:10.1351/pac200577101753
© 2005 IUPAC

1. Introduction

1.1 Electrokinetic Phenomena

Electrokinetic phenomena (EKP) can be loosely defined as all those phenomena involving tangential fluid motion adjacent to a charged surface. They are manifestations of the electrical properties of interfaces under steady-state and isothermal conditions. In practice, they are often the only source of information available on those properties. For this reason, their study constitutes one of the classical branches of colloid science, *electrokinetics*, which has been developed in close connection with the theories of the electrical double layer (EDL) and of electrostatic surface forces [1–4].

From the point of view of nonequilibrium thermodynamics, EKP are typically cross-phenomena, because thermodynamic forces of a certain kind create fluxes of another type. For instance, in *electro-osmosis* and *electrophoresis*, an electric force leads to a mechanical motion, and in *streaming current* (*potential*), an applied mechanical force produces an electric current (potential). First-order phenomena may also provide valuable information about the electrical state of the interface: for instance, an external electric field causes the appearance of a *surface current*, which flows along the interfacial region and is controlled by the *surface conductivity* of the latter. If the applied field is alternating, the *electric permittivity* of the system as a function of frequency will display one or more relaxations. The characteristic frequency and amplitude of these relaxations may yield additional information about the electrical state of the interface. We consider these first-order phenomena as *closely related* to EKP.

1.2 Definitions

Here follows a brief description of the main and related EKP [1–9].

- *Electrophoresis* is the movement of charged colloidal particles or polyelectrolytes, immersed in a liquid, under the influence of an external electric field. The *electrophoretic velocity, v_e* (m s^{-1}), is the velocity during electrophoresis. The *electrophoretic mobility, u_e* (m^2 V^{-1} s^{-1}), is the magnitude of the velocity divided by the magnitude of the electric field strength. The mobility is counted positive if the particles move toward lower potential (negative electrode) and negative in the opposite case.

- *Electro-osmosis* is the motion of a liquid through an immobilized set of particles, a porous plug, a capillary, or a membrane, in response to an applied electric field. It is the result of the force exerted by the field on the counter-charge in the liquid inside the charged capillaries, pores, etc. The moving ions drag the liquid in which they are embedded along. The *electro-osmotic velocity, v_{eo}* (m s^{-1}), is the uniform velocity of the liquid far from the charged interface. Usually, the measured quantity is the volume flow rate of liquid (m^3 s^{-1}) through the capillary, plug, or membrane, divided by the electric field strength, $Q_{to\ eo}$ (m^4 V^{-1} s^{-1}), or divided by the electric current, $Q_{to\ eo}$ (m^3 C^{-1}). A related concept is the *electro-osmotic counter-pressure, Δp_{eo}* (Pa), the pressure difference that must be applied across the system to stop the electro-osmotic volume flow. The value Δp_{eo} is considered to be positive if the high pressure is on the higher electric potential side.

- *Streaming potential (difference), U_{str}* (V), is the potential difference at zero electric current, caused by the flow of liquid under a pressure gradient through a capillary, plug, diaphragm, or membrane. The difference is measured across the plug or between the ends of the capillary. Streaming potentials are created by charge accumulation caused by the flow of counter-charges inside capillaries or pores.

- *Streaming current, I_{str}* (A), is the current through the plug when the two electrodes are relaxed and short-circuited. The *streaming current density, j_{str}* (A m^{-2}), is the streaming current per area.

- *Dielectric dispersion* is the change of the electric permittivity of a suspension of colloidal particles with the frequency of an applied alternating current (ac) field. For low and middle frequencies, this change is connected with the polarization of the ionic atmosphere. Often, only the low-frequency dielectric dispersion (LFDD) is investigated.

- *Sedimentation potential, U_{sed}* (V), is the potential difference sensed by two identical electrodes placed some vertical distance L apart in a suspension in which particles are sedimenting under the effect of gravity. The electric field generated, U_{sed}/L, is known as the *sedimentation field, E_{sed}* (V m^{-1}). When the sedimentation is produced by a centrifugal field, the phenomenon is called *centrifugation potential*.

- *Colloid vibration potential, U_{CV}* (V), measures the ac potential difference generated between two identical relaxed electrodes, placed in the dispersion, if the latter is subjected to an (ultra)sonic field. When a sound wave travels through a colloidal suspension of particles whose density differs from that of the surrounding medium, inertial forces induced by the vibration of the suspension give rise to a motion of the charged particles relative to the liquid, causing an alternating electromotive force. The manifestations of this electromotive force may be measured, depending on the relation between the impedance of the suspension and that of the measuring instrument, either as U_{CV} or as *colloid vibration current, I_{CV}* (A).

- *Electrokinetic sonic amplitude* (ESA) method provides the *amplitude, A_{ESA}* (Pa), of the (ultra)sonic field created by an ac electric field in a dispersion; it is the counterpart of the colloid vibration potential method.

- *Surface conduction* is the excess electrical conduction tangential to a charged surface. It will be represented by the *surface conductivity, K^σ* (S), and its magnitude with respect to the bulk conductivity is frequently accounted for by the *Dukhin number, Du* (see eq. 12 below).

1.3 Model of Charges and Potentials in the Vicinity of a Surface

1.3.1 Charges

The electrical state of a charged surface is determined by the spatial distribution of ions around it. Such a distribution of charges has traditionally been called EDL, although it is often more complex than just two layers, and some authors have proposed the term "electrical interfacial layer". We propose here to keep the traditional terminology, which is used widely in the field. The simplest picture of the EDL is a physical model in which one layer of the EDL is envisaged as a fixed charge, the surface or titratable charge, firmly bound to the particle or solid surface, while the other layer is distributed more or less diffusely within the solution in contact with the surface. This layer contains an excess of counterions (ions opposite in sign to the fixed charge), and has a deficit of co-ions (ions of the same sign as the fixed charge).

For most purposes, a more elaborate model is necessary [3,10]: the uncharged region between the surface and the locus of hydrated counterions is called the *Stern layer*, whereas ions beyond it form the *diffuse layer* or *Gouy layer* (also, Gouy–Chapman layer). In some cases, the separation of the EDL into a charge-free Stern layer and a diffuse layer is not sufficient to interpret experiments. The Stern layer is then subdivided into an *inner Helmholtz layer* (IHL), bounded by the surface and the *inner Helmholtz plane* (IHP) and an *outer Helmholtz layer* (OHL), located between the IHP and the *outer Helmholtz plane* (OHP). This situation is shown in Fig. 1 for a simple case. The necessity of this subdivision may occur when some ion types (possessing a chemical affinity for the surface in addition to purely Coulombic interactions), are specifically adsorbed on the surface, whereas other ion types interact with the surface charge only through electrostatic forces. The IHP is the locus of the former ions, and the OHP determines the beginning of the diffuse layer, which is the generic part of the EDL (i.e., the part governed by purely electrostatic forces). The fixed surface-charge density is denoted σ^0, the charge density at the IHP σ^i, and that in the diffuse layer σ^d. As the system is electroneutral,

$$\sigma^0 + \sigma^i + \sigma^d = 0 \qquad (1)$$

1.3.2 Potentials

As isolated particles cannot be linked directly to an external circuit, it is not possible to change their *surface potential* at will by applying an external field. Contrary to mercury and other electrodes, the surface potential, ψ^0, of a solid is therefore not capable of operational definition, meaning that it cannot be unambiguously measured without making model assumptions. As a consequence, for disperse systems it is the surface charge that is the primary parameter, rather than the surface potential. The potential at the OHP, at distance d from the surface, is called the *diffuse-layer potential, ψ^d* (sometimes also known as

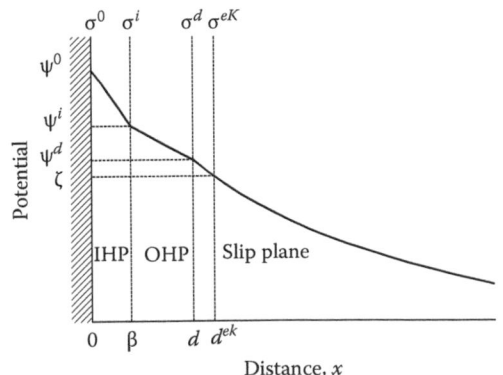

FIGURE 1 Schematic representation of the charges and potentials at a positively charged interface. The region between the surface (electric potential ψ^0; charge density σ^0) and the IHP (distance β from the surface) is free of charge. The IHP (electric potential ψ^i; charge density σ^i) is the locus of specifically adsorbed ions. The diffuse layer starts at $x = d$ (OHP), with potential ψ^d and charge density σ^d. The slip plane or shear plane is located at $x = d^{ek}$. The potential at the slip plane is the *electrokinetic* or *zeta-potential*, ζ; the *electrokinetic charge density* is σ^{ek}.

Stern potential): it is the potential at the beginning of the diffuse part of the double layer. The potential at the IHP, located at distance β ($0 \leq \beta \leq d$) from the surface, the *IHP potential*, is given the symbol ψ^i. All potentials are defined with respect to the potential in bulk solution.

Concerning the ions in the EDL, some further comments can be of interest. Usually, a distinction is made between *indifferent* and *specifically adsorbing* ions. Indifferent ions adsorb through Coulomb forces only; hence, they are repelled by surfaces of like sign, attracted by surfaces of opposite sign, and do not preferentially adsorb on an uncharged surface. Specifically adsorbing ions possess a chemical or specific affinity for the surface in addition to the Coulomb interaction, where chemical or specific is a collective adjective, embracing all interactions other than those purely Coulombic. It was recommended in [10], and is now commonly in use to restrict the notion of *surface ions* to those that are constituents of the solid, and hence are present on the surface, and to proton and hydroxyl ions. The former are covalently adsorbed. The latter are included because they are always present in aqueous solutions, their adsorption can be measured (e.g., by potentiometric titration) and they have, for many surfaces, a particularly high affinity. The term *specifically adsorbed* then applies to the sorption of all other ions having a specific affinity to the surface in addition to the generic Coulombic contribution. Specifically adsorbed charges are located within the Stern layer.

1.4 Plane of Shear, Electrokinetic Potential, and Electrokinetic Charge Density

Tangential liquid flow along a charged solid surface can be caused by an external electric field (*electrophoresis, electroosmosis*) or by an applied mechanical force (*streaming potential, current*). Experience and recent molecular dynamic simulations [11] have shown that in such tangential motion usually a very thin layer of fluid adheres to the surface: it is called the *hydrodynamically stagnant layer*, which extends from the surface to some specified distance, d^{ek}, where a so-called hydrodynamic slip plane is assumed to exist. For distances to the wall, $x < d^{ek}$, one has the *stagnant layer* in which no hydrodynamic flows can develop. Thus, we can speak of a distance-dependent viscosity with

roughly a step-function dependence [12]. The space charge for $x > d^{ek}$ is hydrodynamically mobile and electro-kinetically active, and a particle (if spherical) behaves hydrodynamically as if it had a radius $a + d^{ek}$. The space charge for $x < d^{ek}$ is hydrodynamically immobile, but can still be electrically conducting. The potential at the plane where slip with respect to bulk solution is postulated to occur is identified as the *electrokinetic* or *zeta-potential*, ζ. The diffuse charge at the solution side of the slip plane equals the negative of the *electrokinetic (particle) charge*, σ^{ek}.

General experience indicates that the plane of shear is located very close to the OHP. Both planes are abstractions of reality. The OHP is interpreted as a sharp boundary between the diffuse and the non diffuse parts of the EDL, but it is very difficult to locate it exactly. Likewise, the slip plane is interpreted as a sharp boundary between the hydrodynamically mobile and immobile fluid. In reality, none of these transitions is sharp. However, liquid motion may be hindered in the region where ions experience strong interactions with the surface. Therefore, it is feasible that the immobilization of the fluid extends further out of the surface than the beginning of the diffuse part of the EDL. This means that, in practice, the ζ-potential is equal to or lower in magnitude than the diffuse-layer potential, ψ^d. In the latter case, the difference between ψ^d and ζ is a function of the ionic strength: at low ionic strength, the decay of the potential as a function of distance is small and $\zeta = \psi^d$; at high ionic strength, the decay is steeper and $|\zeta| \leq |\psi^d|$. A similar reasoning applies to the electrokinetic charge, as compared to the diffuse charge.

1.5 Basic Problem: Evaluation of ζ-Potentials

The notion of slip plane is generally accepted in spite of the fact that there is no unambiguous way of locating it. It is also accepted that ζ is fully defined by the nature of the surface, its charge (often determined by pH), the electrolyte concentration in the solution, and the nature of the electrolyte and of the solvent. It can be said that for any interface with all these parameters fixed, ζ is a well-defined property.

Experience demonstrates that different researchers often find different ζ-potentials for supposedly identical interfaces. Sometimes, the surfaces are not in fact identical: the high specific surface area and surface reactivity of colloidal systems make ζ very sensitive to even minor amounts of impurities in solution. This can partly explain variations in electrokinetic determinations from one laboratory to another. Alternatively, since ζ is not a directly measurable property, it may be that an inappropriate model has been used to convert the electrokinetic signal into a ζ-potential. The level of sophistication required (for the model) depends on the situation and on the particular phenomena investigated. The choice of measuring technique and of the theory used depends to a large extent on the purpose of the electrokinetic investigation.

There are instances in which the use of simple models can be justified, even if they do not yield the correct ζ-potential. For example, if electrokinetic measurements are used as a sort of quality-control tool, one is interested in rapidly (online) detecting modifications in the electrical state of the interface rather than in obtaining accurate ζ-potentials. On the other hand, when the purpose is to compare the calculated values of ζ of a system under given conditions using different electrokinetic techniques, it may be essential to find a true ζ-potential. The same applies to those cases in which ζ will be used to perform calculations of other physical quantities, such as the Gibbs interaction energy between particles. Furthermore, there may be situations in which the use of simple theories may be misleading even for simple quality control. For example, there are ranges of ζ-potential and double-layer thickness for which the electrophoretic mobility does not depend linearly on ζ, as assumed in the simple models. Two samples might have the same true ζ-potential and quite different mobilities because of their different sizes. The simple theory would lead us to believe that their electrical surface characteristics are different when they are not.

An important complicating factor in the reliable estimation of ζ is the possibility that charges behind the plane of shear may contribute to the excess conductivity of the double layer (*stagnant-layer* or *inner-layer* conductivity.) If it is assumed that charges located between the surface and the plane of shear are electrokinetically inactive, then the ζ-potential will be the only interfacial quantity explaining the observed electrokinetic signal.

Otherwise, a correct quantitative explanation of EKP will require the additional estimation of the stagnant-layer conductivity (SLC). This requires more elaborate treatments [2,3,13–17] than standard or classical theories, in which only conduction at the solution side of the plane of shear is considered.

It should be noted that there are a number of situations where electrokinetic measurements, without further interpretation, provide extremely useful and unequivocal information, of great value for technological purposes. The most important of these situations are

- Identification of the isoelectric point (or point of zero z-potential) in titrations with a potential determining ion (e.g., pH titration).
- Identification of the isoelectric point in titrations with other ionic reagents such as surfactants or polyelectrolytes.
- Identification of a plateau in the adsorption of an ionic species indicating optimum dosage for a dispersing agent.

In these cases, the complications and digressions, which are discussed below, are essentially irrelevant. The electrokinetic property (or the estimated ζ-potential) is then zero or constant and that fact alone is of value.

1.6 Purpose of the Document

The present document is intended to deal mainly with the following issues, related to the role of the different EKP as tools for surface chemistry research. Specifically, its aims are:

- Describe and codify the main and related EKP and the quantities involved in their definitions.
- Give a general overview of the main experimental techniques that are available for electrokinetic characterization.
- Discuss the models for the conversion of the experimental signal into ζ-potential and, where appropriate, other double-layer characteristics.
- Identify the validity range of such models, and the way in which they should be applied to any particular experimental situation.

The report first discusses the most widely used EKP and techniques, such as electrophoresis, streaming-potential, streaming current, or electro-osmosis. Attention is also paid to the rapidly growing techniques based on dielectric dispersion and electro-acoustics.

2. Elementary Theory of Electrokinetic Phenomena

All electrokinetic effects originate from two generic phenomena, namely, the *electro-osmotic flow* and the *convective electric surface current* within the EDL. For nonconducting solids, Smoluchowski [18] derived equations for these generic

phenomena, which allowed an extension of the theory to all other specific EKP. Smoluchowski's theory is valid for any shape of a particle or pores inside a solid, provided the (local) curvature radius a largely exceeds the Debye length κ^{-1}:

$$\kappa a \gg 1 \qquad (2)$$

where κ is defined as

$$\kappa = \left\{ \frac{\sum_{i=1}^{N} e^2 z_i^2 n_i}{\varepsilon_{rs}\varepsilon_0 kT} \right\}^{1/2} \qquad (3)$$

with e the elementary charge, z_i, n_i the charge number and number concentration of ion i (the solution contains N ionic species), ε_{rs} the relative permittivity of the electrolyte solution, ε_0 the electric permittivity of vacuum, k the Boltzmann constant, and T the thermodynamic temperature. Note that under condition (2), a curved surface can be considered as flat for any small section of the double layer. This condition is traditionally called the "thin double-layer approximation", but we do not recommend this language, and we rather refer to this as the "large κa limit". Many aqueous dispersions satisfy this condition, but not those for very small particles in low ionic strength media.

Electro-osmotic flow is the liquid flow along any section of the double layer under the action of the tangential component E_t of an external field E. In Smoluchowski's theory, this field is considered to be independent of the presence of the double layer, i.e., the distortion of the latter is ignored'. Also, because the EDL is assumed to be very thin compared to the particle radius, the hydrodynamic and electric field lines are parallel for large κa. Under these conditions, it can be shown [3] that at a large distance from the surface the liquid velocity (electro-osmotic velocity), v_{eo}, is given by

$$v_{eo} = -\frac{\varepsilon_{rs}\varepsilon_0 \zeta}{\eta} E \qquad (4)$$

where η is the dynamic viscosity of the liquid. This is the *Smoluchowski equation for the electro-osmotic slip velocity*. From this, the electro-osmotic flow rate of liquid per current, $Q_{eo,I}$ ($m^3\ s^{-1}\ A^{-1}$), can be derived

$$Q_{eo,I} = \frac{Q_{eo}}{I} = -\frac{\varepsilon_{rs}\varepsilon_0 \zeta}{\eta K_L} \qquad (5)$$

K_L being the bulk liquid conductivity ($S\ m^{-1}$) and I the electric current (A).

It is impossible to quantify the distribution of the electric field and the velocity in pores with unknown or complex geometry. However, this fundamental difficulty is avoided for $\kappa\alpha \gg 1$, when eqs. 4 and 5 are valid [3].

Electrophoresis is the counterpart of *electro-osmosis*. In the latter, the liquid moves with respect to a solid body when an electric field is applied, whereas during electrophoresis the liquid as a whole is at rest, while the particle moves with respect to the liquid under the influence of the electric field. In both phenomena, such influence on the double layer controls the relative motions of the liquid and the solid body. Hence, the results obtained in considering electro-osmosis can be readily applied for obtaining the corresponding formula for electrophoresis. The expression for the electrophoretic velocity, that is, the velocity of the particle

---

' The approximation that the structure of the double layer is not affected by the applied field is one of the most restrictive assumptions of the elementary theory of EKP.

with respect to a medium at rest, becomes, after changing the sign in eq. 4

$$v_e = \frac{\varepsilon_{rs}\varepsilon_0 \zeta}{\eta} E \qquad (6)$$

and the electrophoretic mobility, u_e

$$u_e = \frac{\varepsilon_{rs}\varepsilon_0 \zeta}{\eta} \qquad (7)$$

This equation is known as the *Helmholtz–Smoluchowski* (HS) equation for electrophoresis.

Let us consider a capillary with circular cross-section of radius a and length L with charged walls. A pressure difference between the two ends of the capillary, Δp, is produced externally to drive the liquid through the capillary. Since the fluid near the interface carries an excess of charge equal to σ^{ek}, its motion will produce an electric current known as *streaming current, I_{str}*:

$$I_{str} = -\frac{\varepsilon_{rs}\varepsilon_0\, a^2}{\eta} \frac{\Delta p}{L} \zeta \qquad (8)$$

The observation of this current is only possible if the extremes of the capillary are connected through a low-resistance external circuit (short-circuit conditions). If this resistance is high (open circuit), transport of ions by this current leads to the accumulation of charges of opposite signs between the two ends of the capillary and, consequently, to the appearance of a potential difference across the length of the capillary, the *streaming-potential, U_{str}*. This gives rise to a *conduction current, I_c*:

$$I_c = K_L\, a^2 \frac{U_{str}}{L} \qquad (9)$$

The value of the *streaming-potential* is obtained by the condition of equality of the conduction and streaming currents (the net current vanishes)

$$\frac{U_{str}}{\Delta p} = \frac{\varepsilon_{rs}\varepsilon_0 \zeta}{\eta K_L} \qquad (10)$$

For large κa, eq. 10 is also valid for porous bodies.

As described, the theory is incomplete in mainly three aspects: (i) it does not include the treatment of strongly curved surfaces (i.e., surfaces for which the condition $\kappa a \gg 1$ does not apply); (ii) it neglects the effect of *surface conduction* both in the diffuse and the inner part of the EDL; and (iii) it neglects EDL polarization. Concerning the first point, the theoretical analysis described above is based on the assumption that the interface is flat or that its radius of curvature at any point is much larger than the double-layer thickness. When this condition is not fulfilled, the Smoluchowski theory ceases to be valid, no matter the existence or not of surface conduction of any kind. However, theoretical treatments have been devised to deal with these surface curvature effects. Roughly, in order to check if such corrections are needed, one should simply calculate the product κa, where a is a characteristic radius of curvature (e.g., particle radius, pore or capillary radius). When describing the methods below, we will give details about analytical or numerical procedures that can be used to account for this effect.

With respect to surface conductivity, a detailed account is given in Section 3 and mention will be made to it where necessary in the description of the methods. Here, it may suffice to say that it may be important when the ζ-potential is moderately large (>50 mV, say.)

Finally, the *polarization* of the double layer implies accumulation of excess charge on one side of the colloidal particle and depletion on the other. The resulting induced dipole is the source of an electric field distribution that is superimposed on the applied field and affects the relative solid/liquid motion. The extent of polarization depends on surface conductivity, and its role in electrokinetics will be discussed together with the methodologies.

3. Surface Conductivity and Electrokinetic Phenomena

Surface conduction is the name given to the excess electric conduction that takes place in dispersed systems owing to the presence of the electric double layers. Excess charges in them may move under the influence of electric fields applied tangentially to the surface. The phenomenon is quantified in terms of the *surface conductivity, K^σ*, which is the surface equivalent to the bulk conductivity, K_L. K^σ is a surface excess quantity just as the surface concentration Γ_i of a certain species i. Whatever the charge distribution, K^σ can always be defined through the two-dimensional analog of Ohm's law

$$j^\sigma = K^\sigma E \qquad (11)$$

where j^σ is the (excess) *surface current density* (A m^{-1}).

A measure of the relative importance of surface conductivity is given by the dimensionless Dukhin number, Du, relating surface (K^σ) and bulk (K_L) conductivities

$$Du = \frac{K^\sigma}{K_L a} \qquad (12)$$

where a is the local curvature radius of the surface. For a colloidal system, the total conductivity, K, can be expressed as the sum of a solution contribution and a surface contribution. For instance, for a cylindrical capillary, the following expression results:

$$K = \left(K_L + 2K^\sigma/a\right) = K_L(1 + 2Du) \qquad (13)$$

The factor 2 in eq. 13 applies for cylindrical geometry. For other geometries, its value may be different.

As mentioned, HS theory does not consider surface conduction, and only the solution conductivity, K_L, is taken into account to derive the tangential electric field within the double layer. Thus, in addition to eq. 2, the applicability of the HS theory requires

$$Du \ll 1 \qquad (14)$$

The surface conductivity can have contributions owing to the diffuse-layer charge outside the plane of shear, $K^{\sigma d}$, and to the stagnant layer $K^{\sigma i}$:

$$K^\sigma = K^{\sigma d} + K^{\sigma i} \qquad (15)$$

Accordingly, Du can be written as

$$Du = \frac{K^{\sigma d}}{K_L a} + \frac{K^{\sigma i}}{K_L a} = Du^d + Du^i \qquad (16)$$

The $K^{\sigma d}$ contribution is called the *Bikerman surface conductivity* after Bikerman, who found a simple equation for $K^{\sigma d}$ (Eq. 17). The SLC may include a contribution due to the specifically adsorbed charge and another one due to the part of the diffuse-layer charge that may reside behind the plane of shear. The charge on the solid surface is generally assumed to be immobile; it does not contribute to K^σ.

The conductivity in the diffuse double layer outside the plane of shear, $K^{\sigma d}$, consists of two parts: a migration contribution, caused by the movement of charges with respect to the liquid; and a convective contribution, due to the electro-osmotic liquid flow beyond the shear plane, which gives rise to an additional mobility of the charges and hence leads to an extra contribution to $K^{\sigma d}$. For the calculation of $K^{\sigma d}$, the Bikerman equation (eq. 17, see below) can be used. This equation expresses $K^{\sigma d}$ as a function of the electrolyte and double-layer parameters. For a symmetrical z-z electrolyte, a convenient expression is

$$K^{\sigma d} = \frac{2e^2 N_A z^2 c}{kT\kappa}\left[D_+(e^{-ze\zeta/2kT}-1)\left(1+\frac{3m_+}{z^2}\right) + D_-(e^{ze\zeta/2kT}-1)\left[1+\frac{3m_-}{z^2}\right]\right]$$ (17)

where c is the electrolyte amount concentration (mol m^{-3}), N_A is the Avogadro constant (mol^{-1}), and m_+ (m_-) is the dimensionless mobility of the cations (anions)

$$m_\pm = \frac{2}{3}\left(\frac{kT}{e}\right)^2\frac{\varepsilon_{rs}\varepsilon_0}{\eta D_\pm}$$ (18)

where $D_\pm$ (m^2 s^{-1}) are the ionic diffusion coefficients. The parameters $m_\pm$ indicate the relative contribution of electro-osmosis to the surface conductivity.

The extent to which K^σ influences the electrokinetic behavior of the systems depends on the value of Du. For the Bikerman part of the conductivity, Du^d can be written explicitly. For a symmetrical z-z electrolyte and identical cation and anion diffusion coefficients so that $m_+ = m_- = m$:

$$Du^d \equiv \frac{K^{\sigma d}}{K_L a} = \frac{2}{\kappa a}\left(1+\frac{3m}{z^2}\right)\left[\cosh\left(\frac{ze\zeta}{2kT}\right)-1\right]$$ (19)

From this equation, it follows that Du^d is small if $\kappa a \gg 1$, and ζ is small. Substitution of this expression for Du^d in eq. 16 yields

$$Du = \frac{2}{\kappa a}\left(1+\frac{3m}{z^2}\right)\left[\cosh\left(\frac{ze\zeta}{2kT}\right)-1\right]\left(1+\frac{K^{\sigma i}}{K^{\sigma d}}\right)$$ (20)

This equation shows that, in general, Du is dependent on the ζ-potential, the ion mobility in bulk solution, and $K^{\sigma i}/K^{\sigma d}$. Now, the condition $Du \ll 1$ required for application of the HS theory is achieved for $\kappa a \gg 1$, rather low values of ζ, and $K^{\sigma i}/K^{\sigma d} < 1$.

4. Methods

4.1 Electrophoresis
4.1.1 Operational Definitions; Recommended Symbols and Terminology; Relationship Between the Measured Quantity and ζ-Potential
Electrophoresis is the translation of a colloidal particle or polyelectrolyte, immersed in a liquid, under the action of an externally applied field, E, constant in time and position-independent. For uniform and not very strong electric fields, a linear relationship exists between the steady-state *electrophoretic velocity*, v_e (attained by the particle roughly a few milliseconds after application of the field) and the applied field

$$v_e = u_e E$$ (21)

where u_e is the quantity of interest, the *electrophoretic mobility*.

4.1.2 How and Under Which Conditions the Electrophoretic Mobility can Be Converted into ζ-Potential
As discussed above, it is not always possible to rigorously obtain the ζ-potential from measurements of electrophoretic mobility only. We give here some guidelines to check whether the system under study can be described with the standard electrokinetic models:

a. Calculate κa for the suspension.
b. If $\kappa a \gg 1$ ($\kappa a > 20$, say), we are in the large κa regime, and simple analytical models are available.
   b.1 Obtain the mobility u_e for a range of indifferent electrolyte concentrations. If u_e decreases with increasing electrolyte concentration, use the HS formula, eq. 7, to obtain ζ.
      b.1.1 If the ζ value obtained is low ($\zeta \le 50$ mV, say), concentration polarization is negligible, and one can trust the value of ζ.
      b.1.2 If ζ is rather high ($\zeta > 50$ mV, say), then HS theory is not applicable. One has to use more elaborate models. The possibilities are: (i) the numerical calculations of O'Brien and White [22]; (ii) the equation derived by Dukhin and Semenikhin [5] for symmetrical z-z electrolytes

$$\frac{3}{2}\frac{\eta e}{\varepsilon_{rs}\varepsilon_0 kT}u_e = \frac{3y^{ek}}{2}-6$$
$$\times\left(\frac{y^{ek}(1+3m/z^2)\sinh^2(zy^{ek}/4)+[2z^{-1}\sinh(zy^{ek}/2)-3my^{ek}]\ln\cosh(zy^{ek}/4)}{\kappa a+8(1+3m/z^2)\sinh^2(zy^{ek}/4)-(24m/z^2)\ln\cosh(zy^{ek}/4)}\right)$$ (22)

where m was defined in eq. 18 and

$$y^{ek} = \frac{e\zeta}{kT}$$ (23)

is the dimensionless ζ-potential. For aqueous solutions, m is about 0.15. O'Brien [4] found that eq. 22 can be simplified by neglecting terms of order $(\kappa a)^{-1}$ as follows:

$$\frac{3}{2}\frac{\eta e}{\varepsilon_{rs}\varepsilon_0 kT}u_e$$
$$= \frac{3}{2}y^{ek} - \frac{6\left[\frac{y^{ek}}{2}-\frac{\ln 2}{z}\{1-\exp(-zy^{ek})\}\right]}{2+\frac{\kappa a}{1+3m/z^2}\exp\left(-\frac{zy^{ek}}{2}\right)}$$ (24)

Note that both the numerical calculations and eqs. 22 and 24 automatically account for diffuse-layer conductivity.

b.2 If a maximum in u_e (or in the apparent ζ-potential deduced from the HS formula) vs. electrolyte concentration is found, the effect of stagnant-layer conduction is likely significant. For low ζ-potentials, when concentration polarization is negligible, the following expression can be used [23]:

$$u_e = \frac{\varepsilon_{rs}\varepsilon_0}{\eta}\zeta\left[1+\frac{Du}{1+Du}\left(\frac{kT}{e|\zeta|}\frac{2\ln 2}{z}-1\right)\right]$$ (25)

with Du including both the stagnant- and diffuse-layer conductivities. This requires additional information about the value of $K^{\sigma i}$ (see Section 3).

c. If κa is low, the O'Brien and White [22] numerical calculations remain valid, but there are also several analytical approximations. For $\kappa a < 1$, the *Hückel–Onsager* (HO) equation applies [4]:

$$u_e = \frac{2}{3}\frac{\varepsilon_{rs}\varepsilon_0}{\eta}\zeta \qquad (26)$$

d. For the transition range between low and high κa, Henry's formula can be applied if ζ is presumed to be low (<50 mV; in such conditions, surface conductivity and concentration polarization are negligible). For a nonconducting sphere, Henry derived the following expression:

$$u_e = \frac{2}{3}\frac{\varepsilon_{rs}\varepsilon_0}{\eta}\zeta\, f_1(\kappa a) \qquad (27)$$

where the function f_1 varies smoothly from 1.0, for low values of κa, to 1.5 as κa approaches infinity. Henry [24] gave two series expansions for the function f_1 one for small κa and one for large κa. Ohshima [25] has provided an approximate analytical expression which duplicates the Henry expansion almost exactly. Ohshima's relation is

$$f_1(\kappa a) = 1 + \frac{1}{2}\left[1 + \left(\frac{2.5}{\kappa a[1 + 2\exp(-\kappa a)]}\right)\right]^{-3} \qquad (28)$$

Equation 27 can be used in the calculation of the electrophoretic mobility of particles with nonzero bulk conductivity, K_p. With that aim, it can be modified to read [2]

$$u_e = \frac{2}{3}\frac{\varepsilon_{rs}\varepsilon_0}{\eta}\zeta \times F_1(\kappa a, K_p) \qquad (29)$$

$$F_1(\kappa a, K_p) = 1 + \frac{2 - 2K_{rel}}{1 + K_{rel}}[f_1(\kappa a) - 1] \qquad (30)$$

with

$$K_{rel} = \frac{K_p}{K_L} \qquad (31)$$

e. If SLC is likely for a system with low κa, then as discussed before, ζ ceases to be the only parameter needed for a full characterization of the EDL, and additional information on K^σ is required (see Section 3). Numerical calculations like those of Zukoski and Saville [9] or Mangelsdorf and White [10–12] can be used.

Figure 2a allows a comparison to be established between the predictions of the different models mentioned, for the case of spheres. For the κa chosen, the curvature is enough for the HS theory to be in error, the more so the higher $|\zeta|$. According to Henry's treatment, the electrophoretic mobility is lower than predicted by the simpler HS equation. Note also that Henry's theory fails for low-to-moderate ζ-potentials; this is a consequence of its neglecting concentration polarization. The full O'Brien and White theory demonstrates that as ζ increases, the mobility is lower than predicted by either Henry's or HS calculations. The existence of surface conduction can account for this. In addition, for sufficiently high ζ-potential, the effect of concentration polarization is a further reduction of the mobility, which goes through a maximum and eventually decreases with the increase of ζ-potential.

The effect of κa on the $u_e(\zeta)$ relationship is depicted in Fig. 2b. Note that the maximum is more pronounced with the larger κa,

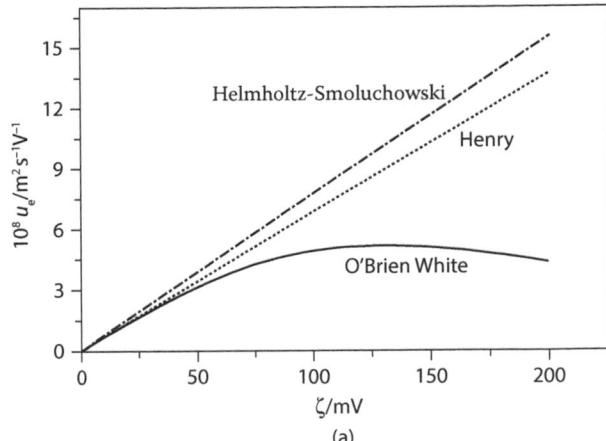

(a)

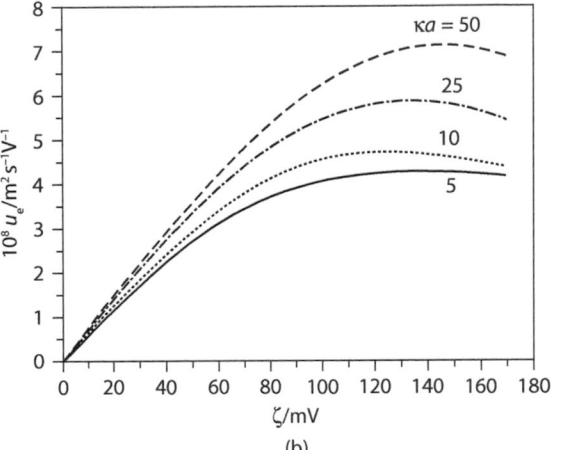

(b)

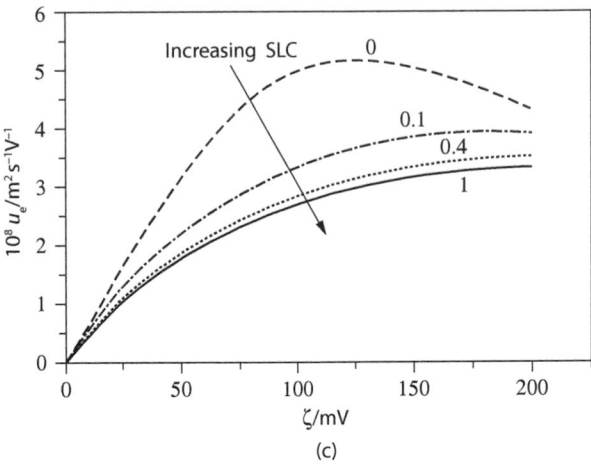

(c)

FIGURE 2 (a) Electrophoretic mobility u_e plotted as a function of the ζ-potential according to different theoretical treatments, all neglecting SLC: HS, O'Brien–White (full theory), Henry (no surface conductance), for $\kappa a = 15$. (b) Role of κa on the mobility-ζ relationship (O'Brien–White theory). (c) Effect of SLC on the electrophoretic mobility-ζ-potential relationship for the same suspensions as in part (a). The ratios between the diffusion coefficients of counterions in the stagnant layer and in the bulk electrolyte are indicated (the upper curve corresponds to zero SLC).

and that the electrophoretic mobility increases (in the range of κa shown) with the former. Finally, Fig. 2c demonstrates the drastic change that can occur in the mobility-ζ-potential trends if SLC is present. This quantity always tends to decrease u_e, as the total surface conductivity is increased, as compared to the case of diffuse-layer conductivity alone.

4.1.3 Experimental Techniques Available: Samples

i. Earlier techniques, at present seldom used in colloid science:

- *Moving boundary* [26]. In this method, a boundary is mechanically produced between the suspension and its equilibrium serum. When the electric field is applied, the migration of the solid particles provokes a displacement of the solid/liquid separation whose velocity is in fact proportional to v_e. The traditional moving-boundary method contributed to a great extent to the knowledge of proteins and polyelectrolytes as well as of colloids. It inspired gel electrophoresis, presently essential in such important fields as genetic analysis.

- *Mass transport* electrophoresis [27]. The mass transport method is based on the fact the application of a known potential difference to the suspension causes the particles to migrate from a reservoir to a detachable collection chamber. The electrophoretic mobility is deduced from data on the amount of particles moved after a certain time, which can be determined by simply weighing the collection chamber or otherwise analyzing its contents.

ii. Microscopic (visual) microelectrophoresis
Probably the most widespread method until the 1980s, microscopic (visual) microelectrophoresis is based on the direct observation, with a suitable magnifying optics, of individual particles in their electrophoretic motion. In fact, it is not the particle that is seen, but a bright dot on a dark background, due to the Tyndall effect, that is the strong lateral light scattering of colloidal particles.

Size range of samples
The ultramicroscope is necessary for particles smaller than 0.1 μm. Particles about 0.5 μm can be directly observed using a travelling microscope illuminated with a strong (cold) light source.

Advantages and prerequisites of the technique
- The particles are directly observed in their medium.
- The suspensions to be studied should be stable and dilute; if they are not, individual particles cannot be identified under the microscope. However, in dilute systems; the aggregation times are very long, even in the worst conditions, so that velocities can likely be measured.

Problems involved in the technique and proposed actions to solve them
- Its main limitations are the bias and subjectivity of the observer, who can easily select only a narrow range of velocities, which might be little representative of the true average value of the suspension. Furthermore, measurements usually take a fairly long time, and this can bring about additional problems such as Joule heating, pH changes, and so on. Hence, some manufacturers of commercial apparatus have modified their designs to include automatic tracking by digital image processing.

- Recall that electrophoresis is the movement of the particles with respect to the fluid, which is assumed to be at rest. However, the observed velocity is in fact relative to the instrument, and this is a source of error, as an electro-osmotic flow of liquid is also induced by the external field if the cell walls are charged, which is often the case. If the cell is open, the velocity over its section would be constant and equal to its value at the outer double-layer boundary. However, in almost all experimental set-ups, the measuring cell is closed, and the electro-osmotic counter-pressure provokes a liquid flow of Poiseuille type. The resulting velocity profile for the case of a cylindrical channel is given by [4]

$$v_L = v_{eo}\left(2\frac{r^2}{a^2}-1\right) \tag{32}$$

where v_{eo} is the electro-osmotic liquid velocity in the channel, a is the capillary radius, and r is the radial distance from the cylinder axis. From eq. 32, it is clear that $v_L = 0$ if $r = a/\sqrt{2}$, so that the true electrophoretic velocity will be displayed only by particles moving in a cylindrical shell placed at 0.292 a from the channel wall. It is easy to estimate the uncertainties associated with errors in the measuring position: if $a \sim 2$ mm and the microscope has a focus depth of ~50 μm, then an error of 2% in the velocity will be always present. A more accurate, although time-consuming method, consists in measuring the whole parabolic velocity profile to check for absence of systematic errors. These arguments also apply to electrophoresis cells with rectangular or square cross-sections.

Some authors (see, e.g., [28]) have suggested that a procedure to avoid this problem would be to cover the cell walls, whatever their geometry, with a layer of uncharged chemical species, for instance, polyacrylamide. However, it is possible that after some usage, the layer gets detached from the walls, and this would mask the electrophoretic velocity measured at an arbitrary depth, with an electro-osmotic contribution, the absence of which can only be ascertained by measuring u_e of standard, stable particles, which in turn remains an open problem in electrokinetics.

A more recent suggestion [29] is to perform the electrophoresis measurements in an alternating field with frequency much larger than the reciprocal of the characteristic time τ for steady electro-osmosis (τ ~ 1 s), but smaller than that of steady electrophoresis (τ ~ 10^{-4} s). Under such conditions, no electro-osmotic flow can develop and hence the velocity of the particle is independent of the position in the cell.

Another way of overcoming the electro-osmosis problem is to place both electrodes providing the external field inside the cell, completely surrounded by the suspension; since no net external field acts on the charged layer close to the cell walls, the associated electro-osmotic flow will not exist [30].

iii. Electrophoretic light scattering (ELS)
These are automated methods based on the analysis of the (laser) light scattered by moving particles [31–34]. They have different principles of operation [35]. The most frequently used method, known as laser Doppler velocimetry, is based on the analysis of the intensity autocorrelation function of the scattered light. The method of phase analysis light scattering (PALS) [36–38] has the adavantage of being suited for particles moving very slowly, for instance, close to their isoelectric point. The method is capable of detecting electrophoretic

mobilities as low as 10^{-12} m^2 V^{-1} s^{-1}, that is, 10^{-4} µm s^{-1}/V cm^{-1} in practical mobility units (note that mobilities typically measurable with standard techniques must be above $\sim10^{-9}$ m^2 V^{-1} s^{-1}). These techniques are rapid, and measurements can be made in a few seconds. The results obtained are very reproducible, with typical standard deviations less than 2 %. A small amount of sample is required for analysis, often a few millilitres of a suitable dispersion. However, dilution of the sample may be required, and therefore the sample preparation technique becomes very important.

Samples that can be studied

a. **Sample composition**

Measurements can be made of any colloidal dispersion where the continuous phase is a transparent liquid and the dispersed phase has a refractive index which differs from that of the continuous phase.

b. **Size range of samples**

The lower size limit is dependent upon the sample concentration, the refractive index difference between disperse and continuous phase, and the quality of the optics and performance of the instrument. Particle sizes down to 5 nm can be measured under optimum conditions.

The upper size limit is dependent upon the rate of sedimentation of particles (which is related to particle size and density). ELS methods are inherently directional in their measurement plane. Hence, for a horizontal field, samples can be measured while they are sedimenting. Measurement is possible so long as there are particles present in the detection volume. Typically, measurements are possible for particles with diameters below 30 µm.

c. **Sample conductivity**

The conductivity of samples that can be measured ranges from that of particles dispersed in deionized water up to media containing greater than physiological saline. In high salt concentration, the Joule heating of the sample will affect the particle mobility, and thermostating of the cell is not at all easy. Reduction of the applied voltage decreases this effect, but will also reduce the resolution obtainable from the measurement.

The presence of some ions in the medium is recommended (e.g., 10^{-4} mol/L NaCl) as this will stabilize the field in the cell and will improve the repeatability of measurements. Furthermore, some salt is always needed anyway because otherwise the double layer becomes ill-defined.

d. **Sample viscosity**

There is no particular limit as to the viscosity range of samples that can be measured. But it must be emphasized that increasing the viscosity of the medium will reduce the mobility of the particles and may require longer observation times, with the subsequent increased risk of Joule heating.

e. **Permittivity**

Measurements in a large variety of solvents are possible, depending on the instrument configuration.

f. **Fluorescence**

Sample fluorescence results in a reduction in the signal-to-noise ratio of the measurement. In severe cases, this may completely inhibit measurements.

Sample preparation

Many samples will be too concentrated for direct measurement and will require dilution. How this dilution is carried out is critical. The aim of sample preparation is to preserve the existing state of the particle surface during the process of dilution. One way to ensure this is by filtering or gently centrifuging some clear liquid from the original sample and using this to dilute the original concentrated sample. In this way, the equilibrium between surface and liquid is perfectly maintained. If extraction of a supernatant is not possible, then just letting a sample naturally sediment and using the fine particles left in the supernatant is a good alternative method. The possibility also exists of dialyzing the concentrate against a solution of the desired ionic composition. Another method is to imitate the original medium as closely as possible. This should be done with regard to pH, concentration of each ionic species in the medium, and concentration of any other additive that might be present.

However, attention must be paid to the possible modification of the surface compositon upon dilution, particularly when polymers or polyelectrolytes are in solution [39]. Also, if the particles are positively charged, care must be taken to avoid long storage in glass containers, as dissolution of glass can lead to adsorption of negatively charged species on the particles. For emulsion systems, dilution is always problematic, because changing the phase volume ratio may alter the surface properties due to differential solubility effects.

Ranges of electrolyte and particle concentration that can be investigated

Microelectrophoresis is a technique where samples must be dilute enough for particles not to interfere with each other. For any system under investigation, it is recommended that an experiment should be done to check the effect of concentration on the mobility. The concentration range which can be studied will depend upon the suitability of the sample (e.g., size, refractive index) and the optics of the instrument. By way of example, a 200-nm polystyrene latex standard (particle refractive index 1.59, particle absorbance 0.001) dispersed in water (refractive index 1.33) can be measured at a solids concentration ranging from 2×10^{-3} to 1×10^{-6} g/cm^3.

Standard samples for checking correct instrument operation

Microelectrophoresis ELS instruments are constructed from basic physical principles and as such need not be calibrated. The correctness of their operation can only be verified by measuring a sample of which the ζ-potential is known. A pioneering study in this direction was performed in 1970 by a group of Japanese surface and colloid chemists, forming a committee under the Division of Surface Chemistry in the Japan Oil Chemists Society [6,39]. This group measured and compared ζ-potentials of samples of titanium dioxide, silver iodide, silica, microcapsules, and some polymer latexes. The study involved different devices in nine laboratories, and concluded that the negatively charged PSSNa (polystyrene-sodium *p*-vinylbenzenesulfonate copolymer) particles prepared as described in [40] could be a very useful standard, providing reliable and reproducible mobility data. Currently, there is no negative ζ-potential standard available from the U.S. National Institute of Standards and Technology (NIST).

A positively charged sample available from NIST is Standard Reference Material (SRM) 1980. It contains a 500 mg/L goethite (α–FeOOH) suspension saturated with 100 µmol/g phosphate in a 5×10^{-2} mol/L sodium perchlorate electrolyte solution at a pH of 2.5. When prepared according to the procedure supplied by NIST, the certified value and uncertainty for the positive electrophoretic mobility of SRM1980 is 2.53 ± 0.12 µm s^{-1}/V cm^{-1}. This will give a ζ-potential of +32.0 ± 1.5 mV if the HS equation (eq. 7) is used.

4.2 Streaming Current and Streaming Potential

4.2.1 Operational Definitions; Recommended Symbols and Terminology; Conversion of the Measured Quantities into ζ-Potential

The phenomena of streaming current and streaming potential occur in capillaries and plugs and are caused by the charge displacement in the EDL as a result of an applied pressure inducing the liquid phase to move tangentially to the solid. The *streaming current* can be detected directly by measuring the electric current between two positions, one upstream and the other downstream. This can be carried out via nonpolarizable electrodes, connected to an electrometer of sufficiently low internal resistance.

4.2.1.1 Streaming Current

The first quantity of interest is the *streaming current per pressure drop*, $I_{str}/\Delta p$ (SI units: A Pa^{-1}), where I_{str} is the measured current, and Δp the pressure drop. The relation between $I_{str}/\Delta p$ and ζ-potential has been found for a number of cases:

a. If $\kappa a \gg 1$ (a is the capillary radius), the HS formula can be used

$$\frac{I_{str}}{\Delta p} = -\frac{\varepsilon_{rs}\varepsilon_0\zeta}{\eta}\frac{A_c}{L} \tag{33}$$

where A_c is the capillary cross-section, and L its length. If instead of a single capillary, the experimental system is a porous plug or a membrane, eq. 33 remains approximately valid, provided that $\kappa a \gg 1$ everywhere in the pore walls. In the case of porous plugs, attention has to be paid to the fact that a plug is not a system of straight parallel capillaries, but a random distribution of particles with a resulting porosity and tortuosity, for which an equivalent capillary length and cross-section is just a simplified model. In addition, the use of eq. 33 requires that the conduction current in the system is determined solely by the bulk conductivity of the supporting solution. It often happens that surface conductivity is important, and, besides that, the ions in the plug behave with a lower mobility than in solution.

A_c/L can be estimated experimentally as follows [40,41]. Measure the resistance, R_∞, of the plug or capillary wetted by a highly concentrated (above 10^{-2} mol/L, say) electrolyte solution, with conductivity K_L^∞. Since for such a high ionic strength the double-layer contribution to the overall conductivity is negligible, we may write

$$\frac{A_c}{L} = \frac{1}{K_L^\infty R_\infty} \tag{34}$$

In addition, theoretical or semi-empirical models exist that relate the apparent values of A_c and L (external dimensions of the plug) to the volume fraction, ϕ, of solids in the plug. For instance, according to [42]

$$\frac{A_c}{L} = \frac{A_c^{ap}}{L^{ap}}\exp(B\phi) \tag{35}$$

where B is an empirical constant that can be experimentally determined by measuring the electro-osmotic volume flow for different plug porosities. In eq. 35, L^{ap} and A_c^{ap} are the apparent (externally measured) length and cross-sectional area of the plug, respectively. An alternative expression was proposed in [43]:

$$\frac{A_c}{L} = \frac{A_c^{ap}}{L^{ap}}\phi_L^{-5/2} \tag{36}$$

where ϕ_L is the volume fraction of liquid in the plug (or void volume fraction). Other estimates of A_c/L can be found in [44–46].

For the case of a close packing of spheres, theoretical treatments are available involving the calculation of streaming current using cell models. No simple expressions can be given in this case; see [3,47–52] for details.

b. If κa is intermediate ($\kappa a \approx 1$–10, say), the HS equation is not valid. For low ζ, curvature effects can be corrected by means of the Burgen and Nakache theory [4,49]:

$$\frac{I_{str}}{\Delta p} = \frac{\varepsilon_{rs}\varepsilon_0\zeta}{\eta}\frac{A_c}{L}[1-G(\kappa a)] \tag{37}$$

where

$$G(\kappa a) = \frac{\tanh(\kappa a)}{\kappa a} \tag{38}$$

for slit-shaped capillaries ($2a$ corresponds in this case to the separation of the parallel solid walls). In the case of cylindrical capillaries of radius a, the calculattion was first carried out by Rice and Whitehead [50]. They found that the function $G(\kappa a)$ in eq. 37 reads

$$G(\kappa a) = \frac{2I_1(\kappa a)}{\kappa a I_0(\kappa a)} \tag{39}$$

where I_0 and I_1 are the zeroth- and first-order modified Bessel functions of the first kind, respectively. Fig. 3 illustrates the importance of this curvature correction.

c. If the ζ-potential is not low and κa is small, no simple expression for I_{str} can be given, and only numerical procedures are available [52].

4.2.1.2 Streaming Potential

The *streaming potential difference* (briefly, streaming potential) U_{str} can be measured between two electrodes, upstream and downstream in the liquid flow, connected via a high-input impedance voltmeter. The quantity of interest is, in this case, the ratio between the streaming potential and the pressure drop, $U_{str}/\Delta p$ (V Pa^{-1}). The conversion into ζ-potentials can be realized in a number of cases.

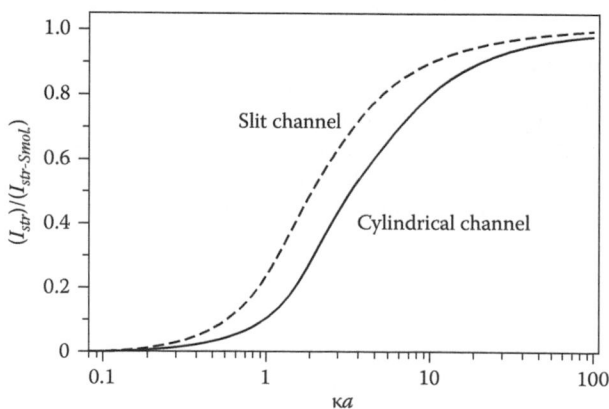

FIGURE 3 Streaming current divided by the applied pressure difference, eqs. 37 and 39, relative to the Smoluchowski formula, eq. 33, plotted as a function of the product κa (a: capillary radius, or slit half-width) for slit- and cylindrical-shaped capillaries.

a. If $\kappa a \gg 1$ and surface conduction can be neglected, the HS formula can be used:

$$\frac{U_{str}}{\Delta p} = \frac{\varepsilon_{rs}\varepsilon_0\zeta}{\eta}\frac{1}{K_L} \tag{40}$$

b. The most frequent case (except for high ionic strengths, or high K_L) is that surface conductance, K^σ, is significant. Then the following equation should be used:

$$\frac{U_{str}}{\Delta p} = \frac{\varepsilon_{rs}\varepsilon_0\zeta}{\eta}\frac{1}{K_L(1+2Du)} \tag{41}$$

where Du is given by eqs. 12 and 20.

An empirical way of taking into account the existence of surface conductivity is to measure the resistance R^∞ of the plug or capillary in a highly concentrated electrolyte solution of conductivity K_L^∞. As for such a solution, Du is negligible, one can write

$$K_L^\infty R_\infty = \left(K_L + \frac{2K^\sigma}{a}\right)R_s \tag{42}$$

where R_s is the resistance of the plug in the solution under study, of conductivity K_L. Now, eq. 41 can be approximated by

$$\frac{U_{str}}{\Delta p} = \frac{\varepsilon_{rs}\varepsilon_0\zeta}{\eta}\frac{R_S}{K_L^\infty R_\infty} \tag{43}$$

c. If κa is intermediate ($\kappa a \sim 1...10$) and the ζ-potential is low, Rice and Whitehead's corrections are needed [50]. For a cylindrical capillary, the result is

$$\frac{U_{str}}{\Delta p} = \frac{\varepsilon_{rs}\varepsilon_0\zeta}{\eta}\frac{R_S}{K_L^\infty R_\infty}\frac{1 - \dfrac{2I_1(\kappa a)}{\kappa a I_0(\kappa a)}}{1 - \beta\left[1 - \dfrac{2I_1(\kappa a)}{\kappa a I_0(\kappa a)}\dfrac{I_1^2(\kappa a)}{I_0^2(\kappa a)}\right]} \tag{44}$$

where

$$\beta = \frac{(\varepsilon_{rs}\varepsilon_0\kappa\zeta)^2}{\eta}\frac{R_S}{K_L^\infty R_\infty} \tag{45}$$

Figure 4 illustrates some results that can be obtained by using eq. 44.

d. As in the case of streaming current, for high ζ-potentials, only numerical methods are available (see, e.g., [53] for details).

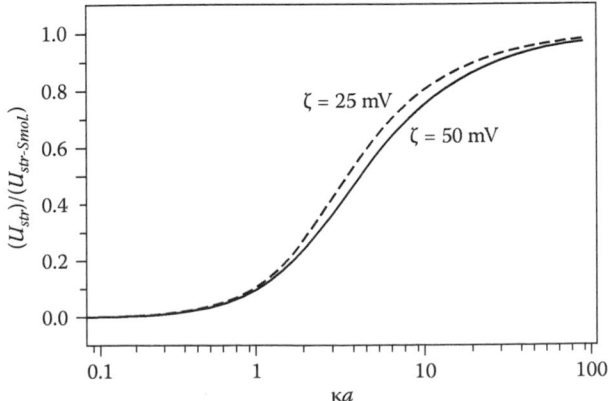

FIGURE 4 Streaming potential divided by the applied pressure difference, eq. 44, relative to its Smoluchowski value, eq. 40, as a function of the product κa (a: capillary radius), for the ζ-potentials indicated. Surface conductance is neglected.

In practice, instead of potential or current measurements for just one driving pressure, the streaming potential and streaming current are mostly measured at various pressure differences applied in both directions across the capillary system, and the slopes of the functions $U_{str} = U_{str}(\Delta p)$ and $I_{str} = I_{str}(\Delta p)$ are used to calculate the ζ-potential. This makes it possible to detect electrode asymmetry effects and correct for them. It is also advisable to verify that the Δp dependencies are linear and pass through the origin.

4.2.2 Samples that can Be Studied

Streaming potential/current measurements can be applied to study macroscopic interfaces of materials of different shape. Single capillaries made of flat sample surfaces (rectangular capillaries) and cylindrical capillaries can be used to produce micro-channels for streaming potential/current measurements. Further, parallel capillaries and irregular capillary systems such as fiber bundles, membranes, and particle plugs can also be studied. Recall, however, the precautions already mentioned in connection with the interpretation of results in the case of plugs of particles. Other effects, including temperature gradients, Donnan potentials, or membrane potential can contribute to the observed streaming potential or electro-osmotic flow. An additional condition is the constancy of the capillary geometry during the course of the experiment. Reversibility of the signal upon variations in the sign and magnitude of Δp is a criterion for such constancy.

Most of the materials studied so far by streaming potential/current measurements, including synthetic polymers and inorganic non-metals, are insulating. Either bulk materials or thin films on top of carriers can be characterized. In addition, in some cases, semiconductors [54] and even bulk metals [55] have been studied, proving the general feasibility of the experiment.

Note that streaming potential/current measurements on samples of different geometries (flat plates, particle plugs, fiber bundles, cylindrical capillaries,...) each require their own set-up.

4.2.3 Sample Preparation

The samples to be studied by streaming potential/current measurements have to be mechanically and chemically stable in the aqueous solutions used for the experiment. First, the geometry of the plug must be consolidated in the measuring cell. This can be checked by rinsing with the equilibrium liquid through repeatedly applying Δp in both directions until finding a constant signal. Another issue to consider is the necessity that the solid has reached chemical equilibrium with the permeating liquid; this may require making the plug from a suspension of the correct composition, followed by rinsing. Checking that the experimental signal does not change during the course of measurement may be a good practice. The presence or formation of air bubbles in the capillary system has to be avoided.

4.2.3.1 Standard Samples

No standard samples have been developed specifically so far for streaming potential/current measurements, although several materials have been frequently analyzed and may, therefore, serve as potential reference samples [56,57].

4.2.3.2 Range of Electrolyte Concentrations

From the operational standpoint, there is no lower limit to the ionic strength of the systems to be investigated by these methods, although in the case of narrow channels, very low ionic strengths require effective electrical insulation of the set-up in order to prevent short-circuiting. However, such low ionic strength values can only be attained if the solid sample is extremely pure and insoluble. The upper value of electrolyte concentration depends on the sensitivity of the electrometer and on the applied pressure difference; usually, solutions above 10^{-1} mol/L of 1-1 charge-type electrolyte are difficult to measure by the present techniques.

4.3 Electro-Osmosis

4.3.1 Operational Definitions; Recommended Symbols and Terminology; Conversion of the Measured Quantities into ζ-Potential

In electro-osmosis, a flow of liquid is produced when an electric field E is applied to a charged capillary or porous plug immersed in an electrolyte solution. If $\kappa a \gg 1$ everywhere at the solid/liquid interface, far from that interface the liquid will attain a constant (i.e., independent of the position in the channel) velocity (the electro-osmotic velocity) v_{eo}, given by eq. 4. If such a velocity cannot be measured, the convenient physical quantity becomes the *eoelectro-osmotic flow rate*, Q_{eo} ($m^3\ s^{-1}$), given by

$$Q_{eo} = \iint_{A_c} v_{eo} \cdot ds \qquad (46)$$

where dS is the elementary surface vector at the location in the channel where the fluid velocity is v_{eo}. The counterparts of Q_{eo} are $Q_{eo,E}$ (flow rate divided by electric field) and $Q_{eo,I}$ (flow rate divided by current). These are the quantities that can be related to the ζ-potential. As before, several cases can be distinguished:

a. If $\kappa a \gg 1$ and there is no surface conduction:

$$Q_{eo,E} \equiv \frac{Q_{eo}}{E} = -\frac{\varepsilon_{rs}\varepsilon_0 \zeta}{\eta} A_c$$

$$Q_{eo,I} \equiv \frac{Q_{eo}}{I} = -\frac{\varepsilon_{rs}\varepsilon_0 \zeta}{\eta} \frac{1}{K_L} \qquad (47)$$

b. With surface conduction, the expression for $Q_{eo,E}$ is as in eq. 47, and that for $Q_{eo,I}$ is

$$Q_{eo,I} = -\frac{\varepsilon_{rs}\varepsilon_0 \zeta}{\eta} \frac{1}{K_L(1+2Du)} \qquad (48)$$

In eq. 48, the empirical approach for the estimation of Du can be followed:

$$Q_{eo,I} = -\frac{\varepsilon_{rs}\varepsilon_0 \zeta}{\eta} \frac{R_S}{K_L^\infty R_\infty} \qquad (49)$$

c. Low ζ-potential, finite surface conduction, and arbitrary capillary radius [46]:

$$Q_{eo,E} = -\frac{\varepsilon_{rs}\varepsilon_0 \zeta}{\eta} A_c[1 - G(\kappa a)]$$

$$Q_{eo,I} = -\frac{\varepsilon_{rs}\varepsilon_0 \zeta}{\eta} \frac{[1 - G(\kappa a)]}{K_L(1+2Du)} \qquad (50)$$

$$\cong -\frac{\varepsilon_{rs}\varepsilon_0 \zeta}{\eta} \frac{R_S[1 - G(\kappa a)]}{K_L^\infty R_\infty}$$

where the function $G(\kappa a)$ is given by eq. 38.

d. When ζ is high and the condition $\kappa a \gg 1$ is not fulfilled, no simple expression can be given for Q_{eo}.

As in the case of streaming potential and current, the procedures described can be also applied to either plugs or membranes. If the electric field E is the independent variable (see eq. 47), then A_c must be estimated. In that situation, the recommendations suggested in Section 4.2.1 can be used, since eq. 47 can be written as

$$\frac{Q_{eo,E}}{\Delta V_{ext}} = -\frac{\varepsilon_{rs}\varepsilon_0 \zeta}{\eta} \frac{A_c}{L} \qquad (51)$$

where ΔV_{ext} is the applied potential difference.

4.3.2 Samples that can Be Studied

The same samples as with streaming current/potential, see Section 4.2.2.

4.3.3 Sample Preparation and Standard Samples

See Section 4.2.3 referring to streaming potential/current determination.

4.4 Experimental Determination of Surface Conductivity

Surface conductivities are excess quantities and cannot be directly measured. There are, in principle, three methods to estimate them.

i. In the case of plugs, measure the plug conductivity K_{plug} as a function of K_L. The latter can be changed by adjusting the electrolyte concentration. The plot of K_{plug} vs. K_L has a large linear range which can be extrapolated to $K_L = 0$ where the intercept represents K^σ. This method requires a plug and seems relatively straightforward.

ii. For capillaries, deduce K^σ from the radius dependence of the streaming potential, using eq. 41 and the definition of Du (eq. 12). This method is rather direct, but requires a range of capillaries with different radii, but identical surface properties [58,59].

iii. Utilize the observation that, when surface conductivity is not properly accounted for, different electrokinetic techniques may give different values for the ζ-potential of the same material under the same solution conditions. Correct the theories by inclusion of the appropriate surface conductivity, and find in this way the value of K^σ that harmonizes the ζ-potential. This method requires insight into the theoretical backgrounds [60,61], and it works best if the two electrokinetic techniques have a rather different sensitivity for surface conduction (such as electrophoresis and LFDD).

In many cases, it is found that the surface conductivity obtained in one of these ways exceeds $K^{\sigma d}$, sometimes by orders of magnitude. This means that $K^{\sigma i}$ is substantial. The procedure for obtaining $K^{\sigma i}$ consists of subtracting $K^{\sigma d}$ from K^σ. For $K^{\sigma d}$, Bikerman's equation (eq. 17) can be used. The method is not direct because this evaluation requires the ζ-potential, which is one of the unknowns; hence, iteration is required.

4.5 Dielectric Dispersion

4.5.1 Operational Definitions; Recommended Symbols and Terminology; Conversion of the Measured Quantities into ζ-potential

The phenomenon of dielectric dispersion in colloidal suspensions involves the study of the dependence on the frequency of the applied electric field of the electric permittivity and/or the electric conductivity of disperse systems. When dealing with such heterogeneous systems as colloidal dispersions, these quantities are defined as the electric permittivity and conductivity of a sample of homogeneous material, that when placed between the electrodes of the measuring cell, would have the same resistance and capacitance as the suspension. The dielectric investigation of dispersed systems involves determinations of their *complex permittivity*, $\varepsilon^*(\omega)$ (F m^{-1}) and *complex conductivity* $K^*(\omega)$ (S m^{-1}) as a function of the frequency ω (rad s^{-1}) of the applied ac field. These quantities are related to the volume, surface, and geometrical characteristics of the dispersed particles, the nature of the dispersion medium, and also to the concentration of particles, expressed either in terms of volume fraction, ϕ (dimensionless) or number concentration N (m^{-3}).

It is common to use the relative permittivity $\varepsilon_r^*(\omega)$ (dimensionless), instead of the permittivity

$$\varepsilon^*(\omega) = \varepsilon_r^*(\omega)\varepsilon_0 \tag{52}$$

ε_0 being the permittivity of vacuum. $K^*(\omega)$ and $\varepsilon^*(\omega)$ are not independent quantities:

$$K^*(\omega) = K_{DC} - i\omega\varepsilon^*(\omega) = K_{DC} - i\omega\varepsilon_0\varepsilon_r^*(\omega) \tag{53}$$

or, equivalently,

$$\mathrm{Re}[K(\omega)] = K_{DC} + \omega\varepsilon_0\,\mathrm{Im}[\varepsilon_r^*(\omega)]$$
$$\mathrm{Im}[K^*(\omega)] = -\omega\varepsilon_0\,\mathrm{Re}[\varepsilon_r^*(\omega)] \tag{54}$$

where K_{DC} is the direct-current (zero frequency) conductivity of the system.

The complex conductivity K^* of the suspension can be expressed as

$$K^*(\omega) = K_L + \delta K^*(\omega) \tag{55}$$

where $\delta K^*(\omega)$ is usually called *conductivity increment* of the suspension. Similarly, the complex dielectric constant of the suspension can be written in terms of a *relative permittivity increment* or, briefly, *dielectric increment* $\delta\varepsilon_r^*(\omega)$:

$$\varepsilon_r^*(\omega) = \varepsilon_{rs} + \delta\varepsilon_r^*(\omega) \tag{56}$$

As in homogeneous materials, the electric permittivity is the macroscopic manifestation of the electrical polarizability of the suspension components. Mostly, more than one relaxation frequency is observed, each associated with one of the various mechanisms contributing to the system's polarization. Hence, the investigation of the frequency dependence of the electric permittivity or conductivity allows us to obtain information about the characteristics of the disperse system that are responsible for the polarization of the particles.

The frequency range over which the dielectric dispersion of suspensions in electrolyte solutions is usually measured extends between 0.1 kHz and several hundred MHz. In order to define in this frame the *low-frequency* and *high-frequency* ranges, it is convenient to introduce an important concept dealing with a point in the frequency scale. This frequency corresponds to the *reciprocal of the Maxwell–Wagner–O'Konski relaxation time* τ_{MWO}

$$\omega_{MWO} \equiv \frac{1}{\tau_{MWO}} \equiv \frac{(1-\phi)K_p + (2+\phi)K_L}{\varepsilon_0\left[(1-\phi)\varepsilon_{rp} + (2+\phi)\varepsilon_{rs}\right]\varepsilon_{rs}} \tag{57}$$

and it is called the Maxwell–Wagner–O'Konski relaxation frequency. In eq. 57, ε_{rp} is the relative permittivity of the dispersed particles. For low volume fractions and low permittivity of the particles ($\varepsilon_{rp} \ll \varepsilon_{rs}$), this expression reduces to

$$\tau_{MWO} \approx \frac{\varepsilon_{rs}\varepsilon_0}{K_L} \approx \frac{1}{2D\kappa^2} \tag{58}$$

where D is the mean diffusion coefficient of ions in solution. The last term in eq. 58 suggests that τ_{MWO} roughly corresponds in this case to the time needed for ions to diffuse a distance of the order of one Debye length. In fact, in such conditions τ_{MWO} equals τ_{el}, the so-called *relaxation time of the electrolyte solution*. It is a measure of the time required for charges in the electrolyte solution to recover their equilibrium distribution after ceasing an external perturbation. Its role in the time domain is similar to the role of κ^{-1} in assessing the double-layer thickness.

The low-frequency range can be defined by the inequality

$$\omega < \omega_{MWO} \tag{59}$$

For these frequencies, the characteristic value of the *conduction current density* in the electrolyte solution significantly exceeds the *displacement current density*, and the spatial distribution of the local electric fields in the disperse system is mainly determined by the distribution of ionic currents. The frequency dependence shown by the permittivity of colloidal systems in this frequency range is known as low-frequency dielectric dispersion or LFDD.

In the high-frequency range, determined by the inequality

$$\omega > \omega_{MWO} \tag{60}$$

the characteristic value of the displacement current density exceeds that of conduction currents, and the space distribution of the local electric fields is determined by polarization of the molecular dipoles, rather than by the distribution of ions.

4.6 Dielectric Dispersion and ζ-Potential: Models

a. **Middle-frequency range:** Maxwell–Wagner–O'Konski relaxation

There are various mechanisms for the polarization of a heterogeneous material, each of which is always associated with some property that differs between the solid, the liquid, and their interface. The most widely known mechanism of dielectric dispersion, the *Maxwell–Wagner dispersion*, occurs when the two contacting phases have different conductivities and electric permittivities. If the ratio ε_{rp}/K_p is different from that of the dispersion medium, i.e., if

$$\frac{\varepsilon_{rp}}{K_p} \neq \frac{\varepsilon_{rs}}{K_L} \tag{61}$$

the conditions of continuity of the normal components of the current density and the electrostatic induction on both sides of the surface are inconsistent with each other. This results in the formation of free ionic charges near the surface. The finite time needed for the formation of such a free charge is in fact responsible for the Maxwell–Wagner dielectric dispersion.

In the Maxwell–Wagner model, no specific properties are assumed for the surface, which is simply considered as a geometrical boundary between homogeneous phases. The Maxwell–Wagner model was generalized by O'Konski [61], who first took the surface conductivity K^σ explicitly into account. In his treatment, the conductivity of the particle is modified to include the contributions of both the solid material and the excess surface conductivity. This effective conductivity will be called K_{pef}:

$$K_{pef} = K_p + \frac{2K^\sigma}{a} \tag{62}$$

Both the conductivity and the dielectric constant can be considered as parts of a complex electric permittivity of any of the system's components. Thus, for the dispersion medium

$$\varepsilon_{rs}^{*} = \varepsilon_{rs} - i\frac{K_{L}}{\omega\varepsilon_{0}} \qquad (63)$$

and for the particle

$$\varepsilon_{rp}^{*} = \varepsilon_{rp} - i\frac{K_{pef}}{\omega\varepsilon_{0}} \qquad (64)$$

In terms of these quantities, the Maxwell–Wagner–O'Konski theory gives the following expression for the complex dielectric constant of the suspension:

$$\varepsilon_{r}^{*} = \varepsilon_{rs}^{*}\frac{\varepsilon_{rp}^{*} + 2\varepsilon_{rs}^{*} + 2\phi(\varepsilon_{rp}^{*} - \varepsilon_{rs}^{*})}{\varepsilon_{rp}^{*} + 2\varepsilon_{rs}^{*} - \phi(\varepsilon_{rp}^{*} - \varepsilon_{rs}^{*})} \qquad (65)$$

b. **Low-frequency range:** dilute suspensions of nonconducting spherical particles with $\kappa a \gg 1$, and negligible $K^{\sigma i}$

At moderate or high ζ-potentials, mobile counterions are more abundant than coions in the EDL. Therefore, the contribution of the counterions and the coions to surface currents in the EDL differs from their contribution to currents in the bulk solution. Such difference gives rise to the existence of a field-induced perturbation of the electrolyte concentration, $\delta c(r)$, in the vicinity of the polarized particle. The ionic diffusion caused by $\delta c(r)$ provokes a low-frequency dependence of the particle's dipole coefficient, C_{0}^{*} (see below). This is the origin of the LFDD (α-dispersion) displayed by colloidal suspensions. Recall that the dipole coefficient relates the dipole moment d^{*} to the applied field E. For the case of a spherical particle of radius a, the dipole coefficient is defined through the relation

$$d^{*} = 4\pi\varepsilon_{rs}\varepsilon_{0}a^{3}C_{0}^{*}E \qquad (66)$$

The calculation of this quantity proves to be essential for evaluation of the dielectric dispersion of the suspension [63–65]. A model for the calculation of the low-frequency conductivity increment $\delta K^{*}(\omega)$ and relative permittivity increment $\delta\varepsilon_{r}^{*}(\omega)$ from the dipole coefficient C_{0}^{*} when $\kappa a \gg 1$ is described in Appendix I. There it is shown that, in the absence of SLC, the only parameter of the solid/liquid interface that is needed to account for LFDD is the ζ-potential.

The overall behavior is illustrated in Fig. 5 for a dilute dispersion of spherical nonconducting particles ($a = 100$ nm, $\varepsilon_{rp} = 2$) in a 10^{-3} mol/L KCl solution ($\varepsilon_{rs} = 78.5$), and with negligible ionic conduction in the stagnant layer. In this figure, we plot the variation of the real and imaginary parts of $\delta\varepsilon_{r}^{*}$ with frequency. Note the very significant effect of the double-layer polarization on the low-frequency dielectric constant of a suspension. The variation with frequency is also noticeable, and both the α- (around 10^{5} s⁻¹) and Maxwell–Wagner ($\sim 2 \times 10^{7}$ s⁻¹) relaxations are observed, the amplitude of the latter being much smaller than that of the former for the conditions chosen. No other electrokinetic technique can provide such a clear account of the double-layer relaxation processes. The effect of ζ-potential on the frequency dependence of the dielectric constant is plotted in Fig. 6: the dielectric increment always increases

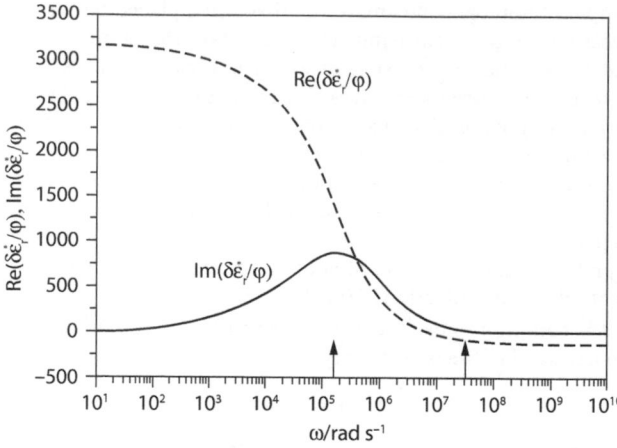

FIGURE 5 Real and imaginary parts of the dielectric increment $\delta\varepsilon_{r}^{*}$ (divided by the volume fraction ϕ) for dilute suspensions of 100-nm particles in KCl solution, as a function of the frequency of the applied field for $\kappa a = 10$ and $\zeta = 100$ mV. The arrows indicate the approximate location of the α (low frequency) and Maxwell–Wagner–O'Konski relaxations.

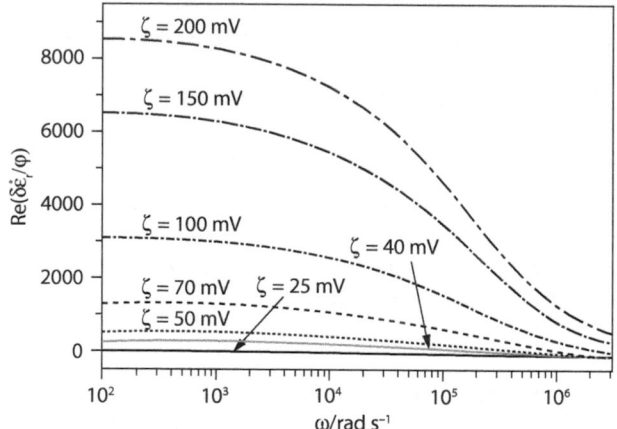

FIGURE 6 Real part of the dielectric increment $\delta\varepsilon_{r}^{*}$ (per volume fraction) as a function of the frequency of the applied field for dilute suspensions of 100-nm particles in KCl solution. The ζ-potentials are indicated, and in all cases, $\kappa a = 10$.

with ζ, as a consequence of the larger concentration of counterions in the EDL: all processes responsible for LFDD are amplified for this reason.

The procedure for obtaining ζ from LFDD measurements is somewhat involved. It is advisable to determine experimentally the dielectric constant (or, equivalently, the conductivity) of the suspension over a wide frequency range, and use eqs. I.2 and I.3 (see Appendix I) to estimate the LFDD curve that best fits the data. A simpler routine is to measure only the low-frequency values, and deduce ζ using the same equations, but substituting $\omega = 0$. However, the main experimental problems occur at low frequencies (see Section 4.5.3).

c. Dilute suspensions of nonconducting spherical particles with arbitrary κa, and negligible $K^{\sigma i}$

In this situation, there are no analytical expressions relating LFDD measurements to ζ. Instead, numerical calculations based on DeLacey and White's treatment [66] are recommended. As before, the computing routine should be constructed to perform the calculations a number of times with different ζ-potentials as inputs, until agreement between theory and experiment is obtained over a wide frequency range (or, at least, at low frequencies).

d. Dilute suspensions of nonconducting spherical particles with κa ≫ 1 and SLC

The problem of generalizing the theory by taking into account surface conduction caused by ions situated in the hydrodynamically stagnant layer has been dealt with in [60,61,64]. In theoretical treatments, SLC is equated to conduction within the Stern layer.

According to these models, the dielectric dispersion is determined by both ζ and $K^{\sigma i}$. This means that, as discussed before, additional information on $K^{\sigma i}$ (see the methods described in Section 4.4) must accompany the dielectric dispersion measurements. Using dielectric dispersion data alone can only yield information about the total surface conductivity [66].

e. Dilute suspensions of nonconducting spherical particles with arbitrary κa and SLC.

Only numerical methods are available if this is the physical nature of the system under study. The reader is referred to [13–16,61,62,67–69]. Figure 7 illustrates how important the effect of SLC on $\text{Re}[\delta\varepsilon_r^*(\omega)]$ can be for the same conditions as in Fig. 5. Roughly, the possibility of increased ionic mobilities in the stagnant layer brings about a systematically larger dielectric increment of the suspension: surface currents are larger for a conducting stagnant layer, and hence the electrolyte concentration gradients, ultimately responsible for the dielectric dispersion, will also be increased.

f. Nondilute suspensions of nonconducting spherical particles with large κa and negligible $K^{\sigma i}$

Considering that many suspensions of technological interest are rather concentrated, the possibilities of LFDD in the characterization of moderately concentrated suspensions have also received attention. This requires establishing a theoretical basis relating the dielectric or conductivity increments of such systems to the concentration of particles [70–72]. Here, we focus on a simplified model [73] that allows the calculation of the volume-fraction dependence

of both the low-frequency value of the real part of $\delta\varepsilon_r^*$, and of the characteristic time τ_α of the α-relaxation. The starting point is the assumption that L_D, the length scale over which ionic diffusion takes place around the particle, can be averaged in the following way between the values of a very dilute ($L_D \approx a$) and a very concentrated ($L_D \approx b - a$; b is half the average distance between the centers of neighboring particles) dispersion:

$$L_D = \left(\frac{1}{a^2} + \frac{1}{(b-a)^2} \right)^{-1/2} \qquad (67)$$

or, in terms of the particle volume fraction

$$L_D = a\left(1 + \frac{1}{(\phi^{-1/3}-1)^2} \right)^{-1/2} \qquad (68)$$

From these expressions, the simplified model allows us to obtain the dielectric increment at low frequency as follows. Let us call

$$\Delta\varepsilon(0) \equiv \frac{\text{Re}[\delta\varepsilon_r^*(0)]}{\phi} \qquad (69)$$

the *specific* (i.e., per unit volume fraction) *dielectric increment* (for ω → 0). In the case of dilute suspensions, this quantity is a constant (independent of φ), that we denote $\Delta\varepsilon_d(0)$:

$$\Delta\varepsilon(0) \equiv \frac{\text{Re}[\delta\varepsilon_r^*(0)]}{\phi}\bigg|_{\phi\to 0} \qquad (70)$$

The model allows us to relate eq. 69 with eq. 70 through the volume-fraction dependence of L_D:

$$\Delta\varepsilon(0) = \Delta\varepsilon_d(0)\left(1 + \frac{1}{(\phi^{-1/3}-1)^2} \right)^{-3/2} \qquad (71)$$

A similar relationship can be established between dilute and concentrated suspensions in the case of the relaxation frequency $\omega_\alpha = 1/\tau_\alpha$:

$$\omega_\alpha = \omega_{\alpha d}\left(1 + \frac{1}{(\phi^{-1/3}-1)^2} \right) \qquad (72)$$

where $\omega_{\alpha d}$ is the reciprocal of the relaxation time for a dilute suspension. Using this model, the dielectric increment and characteristic frequency of a concentrated suspension can be related to those corresponding to the dilute case which, in turn, can be related, as discussed above, to the ζ-potential and other double-layer parameters. A general treatment of the problem, valid for arbitrary values of κa and ζ can be found in [74].

Summing up, we can say that the dielectric dispersion of suspensions is an interesting physical phenomenon, extremely sensitive to the characteristics of the particles, the solution, and their interface. It can provide invaluable information on the dynamics of the EDL and the processes through which it is altered by the application of an external field. Because of the experimental difficulties involved in its determination, it is unlikely that dielectric dispersion measurements alone can be useful as a tool to obtain the ζ-potential of the dispersed particles.

4.6.1 Experimental Techniques Available

One of the most usual techniques for measuring the dielectric permittivity and/or the conductivity of suspensions as a

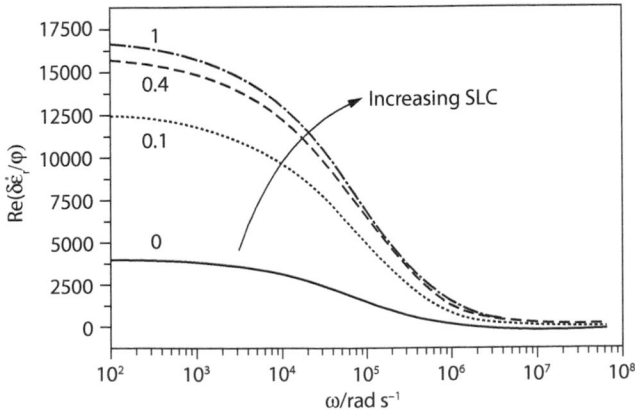

FIGURE 7 Real part of the dielectric increment (per volume fraction) of dilute suspensions as in Fig. 5. The curves correspond to increasing importance of SLC; the ratios between the diffusion coefficients of counterions in the stagnant layer and in the bulk electrolyte are indicated (the lower curve corresponds to zero SLC).

function of the frequency of the applied field, is based on the use of a conductivity cell connected to an impedance analyzer. This technique has been widely employed since it was first proposed by Fricke and Curtis [75]. In most modern set-ups, the distance between electrodes can be changed (see, e.g., [69,76–79]). The need for variable electrode separation stems from the problem of electrode polarization at low frequencies, since at sufficiently low frequencies the electrode impedance dominates over that of the sample. The method makes use of the assumption that electrode polarization does not depend on their distance. A so-called *quadrupole method* has been recently introduced [80] in which the correction for electrode polarization is optimally carried out by proper calibration. Furthermore, the method based on the evaluation of the logarithmic derivative of the imaginary part of raw $\varepsilon^*(\omega)$ data also seems to be promising [81].

These are not, however, the only possible procedures. A four-electrode method has also been employed with success [60,61,68] in this case, since the sensing and current-supplying electrodes are different, polarization is not the main problem, but the electronics of the experimental set-up is rather complicated.

4.6.2 Samples for LFDD Measurements

There are no particular restrictions to the kind of colloidal particles that can be studied with the LFDD technique. The obvious precautions involve avoiding sedimentation of the particles during measurement, and control of the stability of the suspensions. LFDD quantities are most sensitive to particle size, particle concentration, and temperature. Hence, the constancy of the latter is essential. Another important concern deals with the effect of electrode polarization. Particularly at low frequencies, electrode polarization can be substantial and completely invalidate the data. This fact imposes severe limitations on the electrolyte concentrations that can be studied; it is very hard to obtain data for ionic strengths in excess of 1 to 5 mmol L^{-1}.

4.7 Electroacoustics

4.7.1 Operational Definitions; Recommended Symbols and Terminology; Experimentally Available Quantities

Terminology

The term "electroacoustics" refers to two kinds of closely related phenomena:

- *Colloid vibration current* (I_{CV}) and *colloid vibration potential* (U_{CV}) are two phenomena in which a sound wave is passed through a colloidal dispersion and, as a result, electrical currents and fields arise in the suspension. When the wave travels through a dispersion of particles whose density differs from that of the surrounding medium, inertial forces induced by the vibration of the suspension give rise to a motion of the charged particles relative to the liquid, causing an alternating electromotive force. The manifestations of this electromotive force may be measured in a way depending on the relation between the impedance of the suspension and the properties of the measuring instrument, either as I_{CV} (for small impedance of the meter) or as U_{CV} (for large one).
- The reciprocal effect of the above two phenomena is the electrokinetic sonic amplitude (ESA), in which an alternating electric field is applied to a suspension and a sound wave arises as a result of the motion of the particles caused by their ac electrophoresis.

Colloid vibration potential/current may be considered as the ac analog of sedimentation potential/current. Similarly, ESA may be considered as the ac analog of classical electrophoresis. The relationships between electroacoustics and classical EKP may be used for testing modern electroacoustic theories, which should at least provide the correct limiting transitions to the well-known and well-established results of the classical electrokinetic theory. A very important advantage of the electroacoustic techniques is the possibility they offer to be applied to concentrated dispersions.

4.7.1.1 Experimentally Available Quantities

4.7.1.1.1 Colloid vibration potential (U_{CV}) If a standing sound wave is established in a suspension, a voltage difference can be measured between two different points in the standing wave. If measured at zero current flow, it is referred to as *colloid vibration* potential. The measured voltage is due to the motion of the particles: it alternates at the frequency of the sound wave and is proportional to another measured value, ΔP, which is the pressure difference between the two points of the wave. The kinetic coefficient, equal to the ratio

$$\frac{U_{CV}}{\Delta p} = \frac{U_{CV}}{\Delta p}\left(\omega, \phi, \Delta\rho/\rho, K^{\sigma i}, \zeta, \eta, a\right) \qquad (73)$$

characterizes the suspension. In eq. 73, $\Delta\rho$ is the difference in density between the particles and the suspending fluid, of density ρ.

4.7.1.1.2 Colloid vibration current (I_{CV}) If the measurements of the electric signal caused by the sound wave in the suspension, are carried out under zero U_{CV} conditions (short-circuited), an ac I_{CV} can be measured. Its value, measured between two different points in the standing wave, is also proportional to the pressure difference between those two points, and the kinetic coefficient $I_{CV}/\Delta p$ characterizes the suspension and is closely related to $U_{CV}/\Delta p$:

$$\frac{I_{CV}}{\Delta p} = \frac{I_{CV}}{\Delta p}\left(\omega, \phi, \Delta\rho/\rho, K^{\sigma i}, \zeta, \eta, a\right) = K^* \frac{U_{CV}}{\Delta p} \qquad (74)$$

4.7.1.1.3 Electrokinetic sonic amplitude (ESA) This refers to the measurement of the sound wave amplitude, which is caused by the application of an alternating electric field to a suspension of particles of which the density is different from that of the suspending medium. The ESA signal (i.e., the amplitude A_{ESA} of the sound pressure wave generated by the applied electric field) is proportional to the field strength E, and the kinetic coefficient A_{ESA}/E can be expressed as a function of the characteristics of the suspension

$$\frac{A_{ESA}}{E} = \frac{A_{ESA}}{E}(\omega, \phi, \Delta\rho/\rho, K^{\sigma i}, \zeta) \qquad (75)$$

Measurement of I_{CV} or A_{ESA} rather than U_{CV} has the operational advantage that it enables measurement of the kinetic characteristics, $I_{CV}/\Delta p$ and A_{ESA}/E, which are independent of the complex conductivity K^* of the suspension, and thus knowledge of K^* is not a prerequisite for the extraction of the ζ-potential from the interpretation of the electroacoustic measurements. Note, however, that if SLC is significant, as with the other EKP, additional measurements will be needed, as both ζ and $K^{\sigma i}$ are required to fully characterize the interface.

4.7.2 Estimation of the ζ-Potential from U_{CV}, I_{CV} or A_{ESA}

There are two recent methods for the theoretical interpretation of the data of electroacoustic measurements and extracting from them a value for the ζ-potential. One is based on the symmetry relation proposed in [82,83] to express both kinds of electroacoustic phenomena (colloid vibration potential/current and ESA) in terms of the same quantity, namely the *dynamic electrophoretic mobility*, u_d^*, which is the complex, frequency-dependent analog of the normal direct current (dc) electrophoretic mobility. The second method is based on the direct evaluation of I_{CV} without using the symmetry relations, and hence it is not necessarily based on the concept of dynamic electrophoretic mobility. Both methods for ζ-potential determination from electroacoustic measurements are briefly described below.

Using the dynamic mobility method has some advantages: (i) the zero frequency limiting value of u_d^* is the normal electrophoretic mobility, and (ii) the frequency dependence of u_d^* can be used to estimate not only the ζ-potential, but also (for particle radius > −40 nm) the particle size distribution. Since the calculation of the ζ-potential in the general case requires a knowledge of κa it is helpful to have available the most appropriate estimate of the average particle size (most colloidal dispersions are polydisperse, and there are many possible "average" sizes which might be chosen). Although the calculation of the ζ-potential from the experimental measurements would be a rather laborious procedure, the necessary software for effecting the conversion is provided as an integral part of the available measuring systems, for both dilute and moderately concentrated sols. The effects of SLC can also be eliminated in some cases, without access to alternative measuring devices, simply by undertaking a titration with an indifferent electrolyte.

In the case of methods based on the direct evaluation of I_{CV}, the use of different frequencies, if available, or of acoustic attenuation measurements, allows the determination of particle size distributions.

4.8 Method Based on the Concept of Dynamic Electrophoretic Mobility

The symmetry relations lead to the following expressions, relating the different electroacoustic phenomena to the dynamic electrophoretic mobility, u_d^* [82,83]:

$$\frac{U_{CV}}{\Delta p} \propto \phi \frac{\Delta \rho}{\rho} \frac{u_d^*}{K^*} \tag{76}$$

$$\frac{I_{CV}}{\Delta p} \propto \phi \frac{\Delta \rho}{\rho} u_d^* \tag{77}$$

$$\frac{A_{ESA}}{E} \propto \phi \frac{\Delta \rho}{\rho} u_d^* \tag{78}$$

Although the kinetic coefficients on the right-hand side of these relations (both magnitude and phase) can be readily measured at any particle concentration, there is some difficulty (see below) in the conversion of u_d^* to a ζ-potential, except for the simplest case of spherical particles in fairly dilute suspensions (up to a few vol %). In this respect, the situation is similar to that for the more conventional electrophoretic procedures. There are, though, some offsetting advantages. In particular, the ability to operate on concentrated systems obviates the problems of contamination which beset some other procedures. It also makes possible meaningful measurements on real systems without the need for extensive dilution, which can compromise the estimation of ζ-potential, especially in emulsions systems.

4.9 Dilute Systems (up to ~4 vol %)

1. For a dilute suspension of spherical particles with $\kappa a \gg 1$ and arbitrary ζ-potential, the following equation can be used [84], which relates the dynamic mobility with the ζ-potential and other particle properties:

$$u_d^* = \left(\frac{2\varepsilon_{rs}\varepsilon_0\zeta}{3\eta}\right)(1+f)G(\alpha) \tag{79}$$

The restriction concerning double-layer thickness requires in practice that $\kappa a > \sim 20$ for reliable results, although the error is usually tolerable down to about $\kappa a = 13$.

The function f is a measure of the tangential electric field around the particle surface. It is a complex quantity, given by

$$f = \frac{1+i\omega'-[2Du+i\omega'(\varepsilon_{rp}/\varepsilon_{rs})]}{2(1+i\omega')+[2Du+i\omega'(\varepsilon_{rp}/\varepsilon_{rs})]} \tag{80}$$

where $\omega' \equiv \omega\varepsilon_{rs}\varepsilon0/K_L$ is the ratio of the measurement frequency, ε, to the Maxwell–Wagner relaxation frequency of the electrolyte. If it can be assumed that the tangential current around the particle is carried essentially by ions outside the shear surface, then Du is given by the Du^d (eqs. 16–19); see also [85]*.

The function $G(\alpha)$ is also complex and given by

$$G(\alpha) = \frac{1+(1+i)\sqrt{\alpha/2}}{1+(1+i)\sqrt{\alpha/2}+i\frac{\alpha}{9}(3+2\Delta\rho/\rho)} \tag{81}$$

It is a direct measure of the inertia effect. The dimensionless parameter α is defined as

$$\alpha = \frac{\omega a^2 \rho}{\eta} \tag{82}$$

so G is strongly dependent on the particle size. G varies monotonically from a value of unity, with zero phase angle, when a is small (less than 0.1 μm typically) to a minimum of zero and a phase lag of $\pi/4$ when a is large (say, $a > 10$ μm).

Equations 80–82 are, as mentioned above, applicable to systems of arbitrary ζ-potential, even when conduction occurs in the stagnant layer, in which case Du in eq. 80 must be properly evaluated. They have been amply confirmed by measurements on model suspensions [86], and have proved to be of particular value in the estimation of high ζ-potentials [87]. The maximum that appears in the plot of dc mobility against ζ-potential ([22], see also Fig. 2) gives rise to an ambiguity in the assignment of the ζ-potential, which does not occur when the full dynamic mobility spectrum is available.

2. For double layers with $\kappa a < \sim 20$, there are approximate analytical expressions [88,89] for dilute suspensions of spheres, but they are valid only for low ζ-potentials. They have been checked against the numerical solutions for general κa and ζ [90,91], and those numerical calculations have been subjected to an experimental check in [92].

3. The effect of particle shape has been studied in [93,94], again in the limit of dilute systems with thin double layers. This analysis has been extended in [95] to derive formulae for cylindrical particles with zero permittivity and low ζ-potentials, but for arbitrary κa. The results are consistent with those of [93,94].

---

* If this assumption breaks down, Du must be estimated by reference to a suitable surface conductance model or, preferably, by direct measurement of the conductivity over the frequency range involved in the measurement (normally from about 1 to 40 MHz) [86]. Another procedure involved the analysis of the results of a salt titration (see previous subsection).

4.10 Concentrated Systems

The problem of considering the effect on the electroacoustic signal of hydrodynamic or electrostatic interactions between particles in concentrated suspensions was first theoretically tackled [96] by using the cell model of Levine and Neale [97,98] to provide a solution that was claimed to be valid for U_{CV} measurements on concentrated systems (see [87] for a discussion on the validity of such approach in the high-frequency range).

It is possible to deal with concentrated systems at high frequency without using cell models in the case of near neutrally buoyant systems (where the relative density compared to water is in the range 0.9–1.5) using a procedure developed by O'Brien [99, 100]. In that case, the interparticle interactions can be treated as pairwise additive and only nearest-neighbor interactions need to be taken into account. An alternative approach is to estimate the effects of particle concentration considering in detail the behavior of a pair of particles in all possible orientations [101,102]. Empirical relations have been developed that appear to represent the interaction effects for more concentrated suspensions up to volume fractions of 30% at least. In [103], an example can be found where the dynamic mobility was analyzed assuming the system to be dilute. The resulting value of the ζ-potential (ζ_{app}) was then corrected for concentration using the semi-empirical relation:

$$\zeta_{corr} = \zeta_{app} \exp\{2\phi[1+s(\phi)]\}, \quad \text{with } s(\phi) = \frac{1}{1+(0.1/\phi)^4} \quad (83)$$

Finally, O'Brien et al. [104] have recently developed an effective analytical solution to the concentration problem for the dynamic mobility.

4.11 Method Based on the Direct Evaluation of the I_{CV}

This approach [105] applies a "coupled phase model" [106–109] for describing the speed of the particle relative to the liquid. The Kuwabara cell model [110] yields the required hydrodynamic parameters, such as the drag coefficient, whereas the Shilov–Zharkikh cell model [111] was used for the generalization of the Kuwabara cell model to the electrokinetic part of the problem.

The method allows the study of polydisperse systems without using any superposition assumption. It is important in concentrated systems, where superposition does not work because of the interactions between particles.

An independent exact expression for I_{CV} in the quasi-stationary case of low frequency, using Onsager's relationship and the HS equation, and neglecting the surface conductivity effect ($Du \ll 1$), is [105]

$$I_{CV}\big|_{\omega \to 0} = \frac{\varepsilon_{rs}\varepsilon_0 \zeta K_{DC}\phi}{\eta K_L} \frac{(\rho_p - \rho_S)}{\rho_S} \frac{dp}{dx} \quad (84)$$

where x is the coordinate in the direction of propagation of the pressure wave, ρ_S is the density of the suspension (not of the dispersion medium: this is essential for concentrated suspensions, see [112]). Equation 84 is the analog of the HS equation for stationary electrophoretic mobility. It has been claimed to be valid over the same wide range of real dispersions, with particles of any shape and size, and any concentration.

4.11.1 Experimental Procedures

In the basic experimental procedures, an ac voltage is applied to a transducer that produces a sound wave which travels down a delay line and passes into the suspension. This acoustic excitation causes a very small periodic displacement of the fluid. Although the particles tend to stay at rest because of their inertia, the ionic cloud surrounding them tends to move with the fluid to create a

small oscillating dipole moment. The dipole moment from each particle adds up to create an electric field that can be sensed by the receiving transducer. The voltage difference that then appears between the electrodes (measured at zero current flow) is proportional to U_{CV}. The current, measured under short-circuit conditions, is a measure of I_{CV}. Alternatively, an ac electric field can be applied across the electrodes. A sound wave is thereby generated near the electrodes in the suspension, and this wave travels along the delay line to the transducer. The transducer output is then a measure of the ESA effect. For both techniques, measurements can be performed for just one frequency or for a set of frequencies ranging between 1 and 100 MHz, depending on the instrument.

Recently, the term *electroacoustic spectrometry* has been coined to refer to the measurement of the dynamic mobility as a function of frequency (see Fig. 8 for some examples of the kind of spectra that can be obtained). The plot of magnitude and phase of u_d^* over a range of (MHz) frequencies may yield information about the particle size as well as the ζ-potential [86,113], provided the particles are in a suitable size range (roughly 0.05 μm < a < 5 μm). For smaller particles, the signal provides a measure of the ζ-potential, but an independent estimate of size is needed for quantitative results. That can be provided by, for instance, ultrasonic attenuation measurements with the same device.

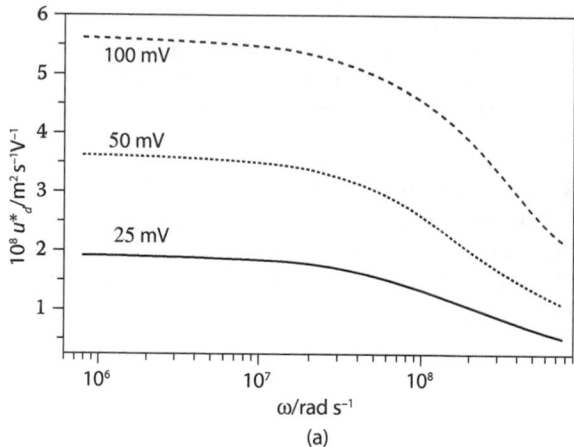

(a)

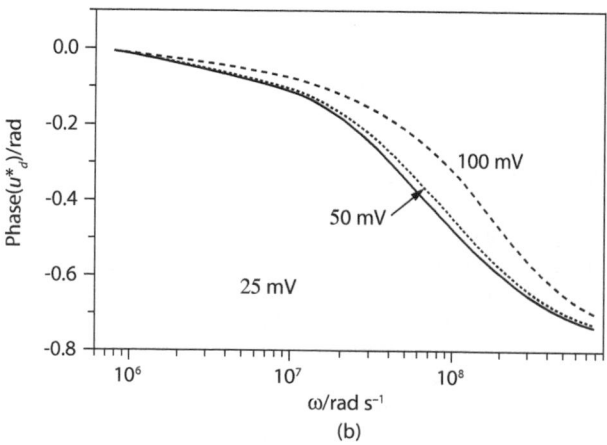

(b)

FIGURE 8 Modulus (a) and phase angle (b) of the dynamic mobility of spherical particles in a KCl solution with $\kappa a = 20$ as a function of frequency for different ζ-potentials; cf., eqs. 80–82. Parameters: particle radius 100 nm; dielectric constant of the particles (dispersion medium): 2 (78.54); density of the particles (dispersion medium): 5×10^3 (1×10^3) kg m^{-3}.

4.11.2 Samples for Calibration

The original validation of the ESA technique was achieved by comparing the theoretical dynamic mobility spectrum, as given by eqs. 80–82, with the experimentally measured values. That comparison has been done for a number of silica, alumina, titania, and goethite samples, and some pharmaceutical emulsion samples [86]. Presently, the calibration standard is a salt solution (potassium dodecatungstosilicate). This salt has a significant ESA signal that can be calculated from its known transport and equilibrium thermodynamic properties (namely, the transport numbers and partial molar volumes of the ions) [85]. Once calibrated, the instrument allows a direct measure of both the size and ζ-potential of the particles. When applied to monodisperse suspensions of spherical particles, the instrument gives results that agree, for both size and ζ-potential, with more conventional methods.

In I_{CV} measurements, calibration is often carried out using a colloid with known ζ-potential, such as Ludox™ (commercially available colloidal silica), which is diluted to a mass concentration of 0.1 g/cm³ with 10^{-2} mol L^{-1} KCl.

5. Electrokinetics in Nonaqueous Systems

5.1 Difference with Aqueous Systems: Permittivity

The majority of the investigations of EKP are devoted to aqueous systems, for which the main charging mechanisms of solid/water interfaces have been established and the EDL properties are fairly well known. All general theories of EKP assume that the equations relating them to the ζ-potential are applicable to any liquid medium characterized by two bulk properties: *electric permittivity* $\varepsilon_{rs}\varepsilon_0$ and *viscosity* η. The value of ε_{rs} is an important parameter of the liquid phase, because it determines the dissociation of the electrolytes embedded in it. Most nonaqueous solvents are less polar than water, and hence ε_{rs} is lower. All liquids can be classified roughly as nonpolar ($\varepsilon_{rs} \leq 5$), weakly polar ($5 < \varepsilon_{rs} \leq 12$), moderately polar ($12 < \varepsilon_{rs} \leq 40$), and polar ($\varepsilon_{rs} > 40$).

For $\varepsilon_{rs} > 40$, dissociation of most dissolved electrolytes is complete, and all equations concerning EDL or EKP remain unmodified, except that a lower value for ε_{rs} has to be used. For moderately polar solvents, the electrolyte dissociation is incomplete, which means that the concentration of charged species (i.e., the species that play a role in EDL or EKP) may be lower than the corresponding electrolyte concentration. Moreover, the charge number of the charge carriers can become lower. For instance, in solutions of $Ba(NO_3)_2$, we may find not (only) Ba^{2+} and NO_3^- ions, but (also) $Ba(NO_3)^+$ complexes. The category of weakly polar solvents is a transition to the class of nonpolar liquids, for which the relative permittivity (at infinite frequency) equals the square of the index of refraction. Such liquids exhibit no self-dissociation, and the notion of electrolytes almost completely dissociated loses its meaning. However, even in such media, special types of molecules may dissociate to some extent and give rise to the formation of EDL and EKP. It is this group that we shall now emphasize.

Unlike in aqueous media, dissociation in these solvents occurs only for potential electrolytes that contain ions of widely different sizes. Once dissociation occurs, the tendency for re-dissociation is relatively small because the charge on the larger ion is distributed over a large area. However, the concentration of ions (c_+, c_-) is very small. An indication of the magnitude of c_+ and c_- can be obtained from conductivity measurements.

Particles embedded in such a liquid can become charged when one type of ion can be preferentially adsorbed. Typically, the resulting surface charges, σ^0, are orders of magnitude lower than

in aqueous systems. However, because of the very low EDL capacitance, the resulting surface potentials, ψ^0, are of the same order of magnitude as in aqueous systems.

The very slow decay of the potential with distance has two consequences. First, as the decay between surface and slip plane is negligible, $\psi^0 \approx \zeta$. This simplifies the analysis. Second, the slow decay implies that colloid particles "feel" each other's presence at long range. So, even dilute sols may behave physically as "concentrated" and formation of small clusters of coagulated particles is typical.

Interestingly, electrophoresis can help in making a distinction between concentrated and dilute systems by studying the dependence of the electrophoretic mobility on the concentration of dispersed particles. If there is no dependence, the behavior is that of a dilute system. In this case, equations devised for dilute systems can be used. Otherwise, the behavior is effectively that of a concentrated system, and ESA or U_{CV} measurements are more appropriate [86].

5.2 Experimental Requirements of Electrokinetic Techniques

The methods described are also applicable to electrokinetic measurements in nonaqueous systems, but some precautions need to be taken. Microelectrophoresis cells are often designed for aqueous and water-like media whose conductivity is high relative to that of the material from which the cell is made. A homogeneous electric field between the electrodes of such cells filled with well- or moderately conducting liquids is readily achieved. However, when the cell is filled with a low-conductivity liquid, the homogeneity of the electric field can be disturbed by the more conducting cell walls and/or by the surface conduction due to adsorption of traces of water dissolved from the solvents of low polarity on the more hydrophilic cell walls. Special precautions (coating the walls with hydrophobic layers) are necessary to improve the field characteristics. The electric field in cells of regular geometrical shape is calculated from the measured current density and the conductivity of the nonaqueous liquid. Because of the low ionic strength of the latter, electrode polarization may occur and it can sometimes be observed as bubble formation. Hence, an additional pair of electrodes is often used for the measurements of the voltage gradient across the cell.

For the correct measurement of the *streaming potential* in nonaqueous systems, attention must be paid to ensure that the resistance of the capillary, plug, or diaphragm filled with liquid is at least 100 times less than the input impedance of the electrical measuring device. The usual practice is to use millivoltmeter-electrometers with input resistance higher than 10^{14} Ω and platinum gauze electrodes placed in contact with the ends of the capillary or plug for both resistance and streaming potential measurements. The resistance is usually measured with an ac bridge in the case of polar solvents (typical frequencies used are around a few kHz) and by dc methods in the case of nonpolar or weakly polar liquids. The use of data recording on the electrometer output is common practice to check the rate of attainment of equilibrium and possible polarization effects.

5.3 Conversion of Electrokinetic Data into ζ-Potentials

The first step in interpreting the electrokinetic behavior of nonaqueous systems must be to check whether the system behaves as a dilute or as a concentrated system (see Section 5.2). In the dilute regime, all theories described for aqueous systems can be used, provided one can find the right values of the essential parameters κa, K_p, and K^σ.

The calculation of κ requires knowledge of the ionic strength of the solution; this, in turn, can be estimated from the measurement of the dialysate conductivity, K_L, and knowledge of the mobilities and valences of the ionic species.

The effective conductivity of the solid particle, K_{pef}, including its surface conductivity* can be calculated from the experimental values of conductivities of the liquid K_L and of a dilute suspension of particles, K, with volume fraction ϕ using either Street's equation

$$\frac{K_{pef}}{K^L} = 1 + \frac{2}{3}\frac{\frac{K}{K_L}-1}{\phi} \tag{85}$$

or Dukhin's equation

$$\frac{K_{pef}}{K^L} = 2\frac{(1-\phi)-\frac{K}{K_L}(1+\phi/2)}{(1-\phi)\frac{K}{K_L}-(1+2\phi)} \tag{86}$$

which accounts for interfacial polarization.

For the estimation of the ζ-potential in the case of electrophoresis, considering that low κa values are not rare, it is suggested to use Henry's theory, after substitution of K_{pef} estimated as described above, for the particle conductivity. In formulas, it is suggested to employ eqs. 29 and 30.

Concerning streaming potential/current or electro-osmotic flow measurements, all the above-mentioned features of nonaqueous systems must be taken into account to obtain correct values of ζ-potential from this sort of data in either single capillaries, porous plugs, or diaphragms. In view of the low κa values normally attained by nonaqueous systems, the Rice and Whitehead curvature corrections are recommended [50]; see eqs. 37–39, 44, and 50.

Finally, electroacoustic characterization of ζ-potential in nonaqueous suspensions requires subtraction of the background arising from the equilibrium dispersion medium. This is imperative because the electroacoustic signal generated by particles in low- or nonpolar media is very weak. It is recommended to make measurements at several volume fractions in order to ensure that the signal comes, in fact, from the particles.

Note that there is one more issue that complicates the formulation of a rigorous electrokinetic theory in concentrated nonaqueous systems, namely, the conductivity of a dispersion of particles in such media becomes position-dependent, as the double layers of the particles may occupy most of the volume of the suspension. This is a significant theoretical obstacle in the elaboration of the theory. In the case of EKP based on the application of nonstationary fields (dielectric dispersion, electroacoustics), this problem can be overcome. This is possible because one of the peculiarities of low- and nonpolar liquids compared to aqueous systems is the very low value of the Maxwell–Wagner–O'Konski frequency, eqs. 57 and 58. This means that in the modern electroacoustic methods based on the application of electric or ultrasound fields in the MHz frequency region, all effects related to conductivity

can be neglected, because that frequency range is well above the Maxwell–Wagner characteristic frequency of the liquid. This makes electroacoustic techniques most suitable for the electrokinetic characterization of suspensions in nonaqueous media.

6. Remarks on Non-Ideal Surfaces

6.1 General Comments

The general theory of EKP described so far strictly applies to *ideal, nonporous,* and *rigid* surfaces or particles. By *ideal*, we mean smooth (down to the scale of molecular diameters) and chemically homogeneous, and we use *rigid* to describe those particles and surfaces that do not deform under shear. We will briefly indicate interfaces that are nonporous and rigid as *hard interfaces.* For hard particles and surfaces, there is a sharp change of density in the transition between the particle or surface and the surrounding medium. Hard particles effectively lead to stacking of water (solvent, in general) molecules; that is, only for hard surfaces the notion of a stagnant layer close to the real surface is conceptually simple. Not many surfaces fulfill these conditions. For instance, polystyrenesulfonate latex colloid has, in fact, a heterogeneous interface: the hydrophilic sulfate end-groups of its polymer chains occupy some 10 % of the total surface of the particles, the remainder being hydrophobic styrene. Moreover, the sulfate groups will protrude somewhat into the solution. Generally speaking, many interfaces are far from molecularly smooth, as they may contain pores or can be somewhat deformable. Such interfaces can briefly be indicated as *soft interfaces.* For soft interfaces, such as, for instance, rigid particles with "soft" or "hairy" polymer layers, gel-type penetrable particles and water–air or water–oil interfaces, the molecular densities vary gradually across the phase boundary. A main problem in such cases is the description of the hydrodynamics, and in some cases it is even questionable if a discrete slip plane can be defined operationally.

The difficulties encountered when interpreting experimental results obtained for non-ideal interfaces depend on the type and magnitude of the non-idealities and on the aim of the measurements. In practice, one can always measure some quantity (like u_e), apply some equation (like HS) to compute what we can call an "effective" ζ-potential, but the physical interpretation of such a ζ-potential is ambiguous. We must keep in mind that the obtained value has only a relative meaning and should not be confused with an actual electrostatic potential close to the surface. Nevertheless, such an "effective ζ" can help us in practice, because it may give some feeling for the sign and magnitude of the part of the double-layer charge that controls the interaction between particles. When the purpose of the measurement is to obtain a realistic value of the ζ-potential, there is no general recipe. It may be appropriate to use more than one electrokinetic method and to take into account the specific details of the non-ideality as well as possible in each model for the calculation of the ζ-potential. If the ζ-potentials resulting from both methods are similar, physical meaning can be assigned to this value.

Below, we will discuss different forms of non-ideality in somewhat more detail. We will mainly point out what the difficulties are, how these can be dealt with and where relevant literature can be found.

6.2 Hard Surfaces

Some typical examples of non-ideal particles that still can be considered as hard are discussed below. Attention is paid to size and shape effects, surface roughness, and surface heterogeneity. For hard non-ideal surfaces, both the stagnant-layer concept

---

* The low conductivity of nonaqueous media with respect to aqueous solutions is the main reason why often the finite bulk conductivity of the dielectric solids cannot be neglected. In contrast, if one can assume that no water is adsorbed at the interface, any SLC effect can be neglected. Furthermore, the joint adsorption of the ionic species of both signs or (and) the adsorption of such polar species as water at the solid/liquid interface can produce an abnormally high surface conduction. This is not due to the excess of free charges in the EDL, commonly taken into account in the parameter K^σ of the generalized theories of EKP. Rather, it is conditioned by the presence of thin, highly conducting adsorption layers. Therefore, the ratio K_{pef}/K_L is an important parameter that has to be estimated for nonaqueous systems.

and the ζ-potential remain locally defined and experimental data provide some average electrokinetic quantity that will lead to an average ζ-potential. The kind of averaging may depend on the electrokinetic method used, therefore, different methods may give different average ζ-potentials.

6.2.1 Size Effects

For rigid particles that are spherical with a homogeneous charge density, but differ in size, a rigorous value of the ζ-potential can be found if the electrokinetic quantity measured is independent of the particle radius, a. In general, this will be the case for $\kappa a \gg 1$ (HS limit). In the case of electrophoresis, the mobility is also independent of a for $\kappa a < 1$ (HO limit). For other cases, the particle size will come into play and most of the time an average radius has to be used to calculate an average ζ-potential [3,114]. The type of average radius used will, in principle, affect the average ζ-potential. Furthermore, different EKP may require different averages. For instance, in [115] it was found that a simple number average is suitable for analysis of electrophoresis in polydisperse systems; a volume average, on the other hand, was found to be the best choice when discussing dielectric dispersion. In principle, the best solution would be found if the full size distribution is measured, but even in such a case the signal-processing procedure must be taken into account. For instance, in ELS methods, the scattering of light by particles of different sizes is determinant for the average u_e value found by the instrument. In this context, measuring the dynamic mobility spectrum may be useful in providing information on both the size and the ζ-potential from the same signal.

6.2.2 Shape Effects

For nonspherical particles (cylinders, discs, rods, etc.) of homogeneous ζ-potential, the induced dipole moment is different for different orientations with respect to the applied field (i.e., it acquires a tensorial character). Only when the systems are sufficiently simple (cylinders, rods) is it sufficient to distinguish between a parallel and a normal orientation of the dipoles to the applied field [116]. In spite of these additional difficulties, some approximate approaches to either the electrophoresis [117–120] or the permittivity [121,122] of suspensions of nonspherical particles are available.

A more complicated situation arises if the particles are polydisperse in shape and size. Except if $\kappa a \gg 1$ (HS equation valid) or if $\kappa a \ll 1$ (HO limit), the only (approximate) approach is to define an "equivalent spherical particle" (for instance, one having the same volume as the particle under study) and use theories developed for spheres. In that case, the "average" ζ-potential that is obtained depends on the type(s) of polydispersity of the sample and the definition used for the "equivalent sphere".

6.2.3 Surface Roughness

Most theories described so far assume that the interface is smooth down to a molecular scale. However, even the surfaces prepared with the strictest precautions show some degree of roughness, which will be characterized by R, the typical dimension of the mountains or valleys present on the surface. However, surface roughness (with R as a measure of the roughness size) affects the position of the plane of shear except in conditions where $\kappa R \gg 1$ (HS limit) or $\kappa R \ll 1$ (roughness not seen). If it is assumed that the outer parts of the asperities determine the position of the slip plane, there will be diffusely bound or even free ions in the valleys. This will inevitably lead to large surface conductivities behind the apparent slip plane, and to an additional mechanism of stagnancy [6,116,123]. Due care must be taken to measure this conductivity and to take it into account in evaluating the ζ-potentials. Experiments with surfaces of well-defined roughness are required to gain further insight in the complications.

We will not proceed with a more thorough description of these highly specialized—and mostly unsolved—topics. As a rule of thumb, we recommned that the reader deal with an interface of known, high roughness to use a simple approach based on the calculation of an effective ζ-potential obtained under the assumption that the interface is smooth, but to refrain from using this effective ζ for further calculations. This is particularly true if the estimation of interaction energies between the particles is sought, as it has been shown [124] that asperities have a considerable effect on both electrostatic and van der Waals forces between colloid particles.

6.2.4 Chemical Surface Heterogeneity

In general, chemical surface heterogeneity will also lead to surface charge heterogeneity. When the charges do not protrude into the solution, the position of the slip plane is unaffected. With charge heterogeneity, often two extreme cases are considered: (1) a *random* or *regular* heterogeneity that is assumed to lead to one (smeared-out) surface charge density and also one (averaged) electrokinetic potential and electrokinetic charge density at given solution conditions; and (2) a *patchwise* heterogeneity with large patches. The patches will lead to an inhomogenous charge distribution. In this case, it is usually assumed that each patch has its own smeared-out charge density at given solution conditions. The characteristic size of the patches should be at least of the order of the Debye length, otherwise the surface may be considered as regularly heterogeneous with one smeared-out charge density over the entire surface. Particles with random heterogeneity can be treated in the same way as particles with a homogeneous charge density, so it does not present additional problems.

The patchwise heterogeneity case applies, for instance, to surfaces with different crystal faces. The electrokinetic theory for this type of surface has been considered by several authors [118,119, 125,126]. Anderson et al. [127–129] have also performed experimental checks on the validity of some theoretical predictions. In the case of spherical particles, it has been demonstrated [130] that their motion depends on the first, second, and third moments of the ζ-potential distribution along the surface of the particle. It is important to note that the second moment (dipole moment) brings about a rotational motion superimposed on the translational (when present) electrophoretic motion. Clay particles [126, 131], with anionic charges at the plate surfaces and pH-dependent charges at the edges, are typical examples of systems with patchwise heterogeneous surfaces.

A rather specific situation may appear in the case of sparse polyelectrolyte adsorption onto oppositely charged surfaces. This may lead to a mosaic-type charge distribution [132,133]. Not only the very concepts of slip plane and hence ζ-potential are doubtful here, but also electrokinetic data alone can lead us to erroneous conclusions. For instance, one can find a high $|u_e|$ value for particles with attached polyelectrolytes and from this predict a high colloidal stability. This might not be found, since the patchwise nature of the charges might induce flocculation even in systems that have considerable average ζ-potential. Such instability will be due to attraction between oppositely charged patches (corresponding to regions with and without adsorbed polyelectrolyte).

6.3 Soft Particles

Some familiar examples in which the interface must be considered as soft are discussed below. The examples refer to two different groups. The first consists of hard particles with hairy, grafted, or adsorbed layers and of particles that are (partially) penetrable. The hydrodynamic permeability and the conductivity in the permeable layer make the interpretation of the data complicated. The second group are the water–oil or water–air interfaces. Droplets and bubbles comprise a specific class of "soft" particles, for which the definition of the slip plane is an academic question. When and how this issue can be solved depends on the surface active components present at the interface.

6.3.1 Charged Particles With a Soft Uncharged Layer

For a good understanding of charged hard particles covered by nonionic surfactants or uncharged polymers, the position of the slip plane and conduction behind the slip plane must be considered. It is very useful to also investigate the bare particles. Neutral adsorbed layers reduce the tangential fluid flow and the tangential electric current near a particle surface, but to a different extent [134]. Both reductions have to be considered for a correct interpretation of the electrokinetic results. By doing this, the comparison of the results between bare and covered particles may give information about the net particle potential and effective particle charge, the surface charge adjustment, and the adsorbed-layer thickness [135]. Let us mention that electro-acoustic studies of the dynamic mobility spectrum of particles coated with adsorbed neutral polymer can give information on the thickness of the adsorbed layer and the shift of the slip plane due to the polymer [136].

6.3.2 Uncharged Particles With a Soft Charged Layer

The surface of many latex particles can be considered as being itself uncharged, but with charged groups at the end of oligomeric or polymeric "hairs" that protrude into the solution. The extension of the "hairs" from the surface into the liquid determines the position of the apparent slip plane. Due to the ion penetrability of the stagnant layer, the ionic strength will affect the distance between the surface and this (apparent) slip plane, and the electric conduction in the stagnant layer and this will lead to a more complex ionic strength dependence of the ζ-potential than with rigid particles. Some studies account for these effects through the introduction of a "softness factor" [137,138] as a fitting parameter. Stein [139] discusses the electrokinetics of polystyrene latex particles in more detail. Hidalgo-Álvarez et al. [140] discuss the anomalous electrokinetic behavior of polymer colloids in general.

6.3.3 Charged Particles With a Soft Charged Layer

Charged particles with adsorbed or grafted polyelectrolyte or ionic surfactant layers fall in this class. The complications arising with these systems are similar to those mentioned for the uncharged surfaces with charged layers. Adsorbed layers impede tangential fluid flow; therefore, in the presence of the bound layer the hydrodynamic particle radius increases and the apparent slip plane is moved outwards. This affects the tangential electric current. In most cases, the particle surface and the bound layers will have opposite charges, and, therefore, the electrostatic potential profile is rather complicated. The EKP will be dominated by conduction within the slip plane and the potential at the hydrodynamic boundary relatively far away from the surface [114,141,142]. To unravel the situation, a systematic investigation is required that considers the electrokinetic behavior of both uncovered and covered particles, the shift of the apparent slip plane and the conduction behind the slip plane. When qualitative information is required with respect to the net charge of the particle plus adsorbed layer, the sign of the ζ-potential is important, as it will indicate whether the particle charge is overcompensated or not (within the plane of shear).

6.3.4 Ion-Penetrable or Partially Penetrable Particles

Some proteins, many biological cells, and other natural particles are penetrable for water and ions. The most important complications for the description of the electrokinetic behavior of such particles are associated with the conductivity, the dielectric constant, and the liquid transport inside the particles. An additional complication occurs when the particles are able to swell depending on the solution conditions.

When the particles are only partially penetrable, we may consider them as hard with a gel-like corona. This situation is very similar to hard particles coated with a polyelectrolyte layer. In the limit of a very small particle with a very thick corona, the penetrable particle limit results. The simplest models assume that the electrical potential inside the gel layer is the Donnan potential, whereas the hindered motion of liquid in it is represented by a friction parameter incorporated in the Navier–Stokes equation [143–146]. Ohshima's theory of electrophoresis of soft spheres basically ranges from hard particles to penetrable particles. References to his work can be found in his review on EKP [140].

Systems with biological or medical relevance that have received some systematic attention are protein-coated latex particles [147], electrophoresis of biological cells [148], liposomes [149], and bacteria [150].

6.3.5 Liquid Droplets and Gas Bubbles in a Liquid

The electrophoresis of uncontaminated liquid droplets and gas bubbles in a liquid show quite different behavior from that of rigid particles. The main reason is that flow may also occur within the droplets or bubbles because there is momentum transfer across the interface. The classical notion of a slip plane loses its meaning. Due to the flow inside the droplet or bubble, the tangential velocity of the liquid surrounding the droplet does not have to become zero at the surface of the particle. As a result, the electrophoretic mobility is higher than for a corresponding rigid body. However, to model this situation and to arrive at a conversion of the mobility to a ζ-potential is not a trivial task. As there is no slip plane, even the HS model cannot be applied.

In general, however, droplets or bubbles are not stable without an adsorbed layer of a surface active component (surfactant, polymer, poly electrolyte, protein). Most layers will make the surface inextensible (rigid) if (nearly) completely covered. In this case, the surface behaves as rigid, and it is possible to use the treatments for rigid particles [3]. Even the presence of the double layer itself, through the primary electroviscous effect, makes momentum transfer to the liquid drop very slight [151].

For partially covered bubbles (as in flotation), the situation is more complex; surface inhomogeneities may occur under the influence of shear, and Marangoni effects become important. Problems arise with regard to the definition of the slip plane, its location, and the charge inhomogeneity [152].

7. Discussion and Recommendations

From the analyses given above, it will be clear that the computation of the ζ-potential from experimental data is not always a trivial task. For each method, the fundamental requirement for the conversion of experimental data is that models should be correctly used within their range of applicability. The bottom line is that the ζ-potential does exist as a characteristic of a charged surface under fixed conditions. This is fortunate, because otherwise, how could two authors compare their results with the same material using two electrokinetic techniques, or even two different versions of the same technique?

This means that we must focus on the correct use of the existing theories, and in their improvement, if necessary. The sometimes-asked question: "Is the computed ζ-potential independent of the technique used?" must be answered with *yes*, because ζ-potentials are unique characteristics for the charge state of interfaces under given conditions. Whether by different techniques identical ζ-potentials are indeed observed depends on the quality of both the technique and the interpretation. Measuring different electrokinetic properties for a given material in a given liquid medium, and checking the equality of ζ-potentials using appropriate models, is what Lyklema calls an *electrokinetic consistency test* [3], and what Dukhin and Derjaguin called *integrated electrosurface investigation* [5].

Another related question that could be asked is "Is the ζ-potential the only property characterizing the electrical equilibrium state of the interfacial region?" The answer is *most often it is not*. Most recent models and experimental results demonstrate that in the majority of cases the conductivity behind the slip plane must also be taken into account. This implies that for a correct evaluation, the Du number should also be measured. Using Du only to characterize the interface has, in general, no practical interest either. One experimental electrokinetic technique suffices only if $K^{\sigma i}/K^{\sigma d}$ is small because then $Du(\zeta,K^{\sigma i}) \approx Du(\zeta)$. The problem now is how does one know that $K^{\sigma i}$ is in fact that small? We have some possibilities:

- If we have also access to the value of the potentiometrically measured surface charge, $\sigma 0$, the values of σek (calculated from the value of the z-potential obtained by neglecting conductance behind the slip plane) and d can be compared. This comparison allows us to reach a first estimate of σi. From σi Ksi could be estimated assuming—as appears to be the case, at least for monovalent counterions—that the mobilities of ions in the inner layer are comparable to those in the bulk. When $Du(z,Ksi) \approx Du(z,0) = Du(z)$, the calculated value of z is correct, otherwise, it has to be recalculated taking the inner-layer conduction into account.

- In the case of capillaries or plugs, the total conductivity and the streaming potential can be measured. An initial value of Ksd can be obtained from z using Bikerman's equation, and Ksi can be calculated. The improved value of z can now be obtained using a suitable model including inner-layer conduction, and again Kσd and Ksi can be obtained. If the difference between z computed without and with finite Ksi is high, we should go back to the calculation of z and iterate till the difference between two steps is small.

If these approaches are not possible, there is no other way but employing different electrokinetic techniques on the same sample and performing the consistency test. In this respect, the best procedure would be using one technique in which neglecting $K^{\sigma i}$ underestimates ζ (electrophoresis, streaming potential, e.g.), and another in which ζ is overestimated (dc conductivity, dielectric dispersion) [3].

For practical reasons—not every worker has available the numerical routines required for nonanalytical theories—another question emerges: "When can we use with confidence HS equations for the different types of electrokinetic data?"

Although most published data on ζ-potentials are based on the various versions of the HS equation for EKP, let us stress that this approach is correct only if (eq. 2) $\kappa a \gg 1$, where a is a characteristic dimension of the system (curvature radius of the solid particle, capillary radius, equivalent pore radius of the plug,...), and furthermore, the surface conductance of any kind must be low,

i.e., $Du(\zeta,K^{\sigma i}) \ll 1$. Thus, in the absence of independent information about $K^{\sigma i}$, additional electrokinetic determinations can only be avoided for sufficiently large particles and high electrolyte concentrations.

Another caveat can be given, even if the previously mentioned conditions on dimensions and Dukhin number are met. For concentrated systems, the possibility of the overlap of the double layers of neighboring particles cannot be neglected if the concentration of the dispersed solids in a suspension or a plug is high. In such cases, the validity of the HS equation is also doubtful and cell models for either electrophoresis, streaming potential, or electroosmosis are required. Use of the latter two kinds of experiments or of electroacoustic or LFDD measurements is recommended. In all cases, a proper model accounting for interparticle interaction must be available.

8. Appendix I. Calculation of the Low-Frequency Dielectric Dispersion of Suspensions

Neglecting SLC, the complex conductivity increment is related to the dipole coefficient as follows [62–64]:

$$\delta K^*(\omega) = \frac{3\phi}{a^3} K_L C_0^* = \delta K^*\big|_{\omega\to 0} + 9\phi K_L \frac{(R^+ - R^-)H}{2AS} \frac{i\omega\tau_\alpha}{1+\sqrt{S}\sqrt{i\omega\tau_\alpha}+i\omega\tau_\alpha} \quad (I.1)$$

Its low-frequency value is a real quantity:

$$\delta K^*\big|_{\omega\to 0} = 3\phi K_L\left(\frac{2Du(\zeta)-1}{2Du(\zeta)+2} - \frac{3(R^+ - R^-)H}{2B}\right) \quad (I.2)$$

The dielectric increment of the suspension can be calculated from $\delta K^*\big|_{\omega\to 0}$ as follows:

$$\delta\varepsilon_r^*(\omega) = -\frac{1}{\omega\varepsilon_0}\left(\delta K^* - \delta K^*\big|_{\omega=0}\right)$$
$$= \frac{9}{2}\phi\varepsilon_{rs}' \frac{\tau_\alpha}{\tau_{el}} \frac{(R^+ - R^-)H}{AS} \frac{1}{1+\sqrt{S}\sqrt{i\omega\tau_\alpha}+i\omega\tau_\alpha} \quad (I.3)$$

Here:

$$R^\pm = 4\frac{\exp(\mp\frac{zy^{ek}}{2})-1}{\kappa a} + 6m^\pm\left[\frac{\exp(\mp\frac{zy^{ek}}{2})-1}{\kappa a} \pm z\frac{zy^{ek}}{\kappa a}\right] \quad (I.4)$$

and

$$\tau_\alpha = \frac{a^2}{2D_{ef}}\frac{1}{S} \quad (I.5)$$

is the value of the relaxation time of the low-frequency dispersion. It is assumed that the dispersion medium is an aqueous solution of an electrolyte of *z-z* charge type. The definitions of the other quantities appearing in eqs. I.1–5 and the ζ-potential are as follows:

$$D_{ef} = \frac{2D^+D^-}{D^+ + D^-} \quad (I.6)$$

$$A = 4Du(\zeta)+4 \quad (I.7)$$

$$B = (R^+ + 2)(R^- + 2) - U^+ - U^- - (U^+ R^- + U^- R^+)/2 \quad (I.8)$$

$$S = \frac{B}{A} \quad (I.9)$$

$$H = \frac{(R^+ - R^-)(1 - z^2 \Delta^2) - U^+ + U^- + z\Delta(U^+ + U^-)}{A} \quad (I.10)$$

$$U^{\pm} = \frac{48 m^{\pm}}{\kappa a} \ln\left[\cosh \frac{z y_\zeta}{4}\right] \quad (I.11)$$

$$\Delta = \frac{D^- - D^+}{z\left(D^- + D^+\right)} \quad (I.12)$$

The factor $1/S$ is of the order of unity, and comparison of eqs. 58 and I.5 leads to the important conclusion that

$$\frac{\tau_\alpha}{\tau_{MWO}} \approx (\kappa a)^2 \quad (I.13)$$

This means that for the case of $\kappa a \gg 1$, the characteristic frequency for the α-dispersion is $(\kappa a)^2$ times lower than that of the Maxwell–Wagner dispersion.

9. Acknowledgments

Financial assistance from IUPAC is gratefully acknowledged. The Coordinators of the MIEP working party wish to thank all members for their effort in preparing their contributions, suggestions, and remarks.

10. References

1. S. S. Dukhin. *Adv. Colloid Interface Sci.* **61**, 17 (1995).
2. R. J. Hunter. *Foundations of Colloid Science*, Chap. 8, Oxford University Press, Oxford (2001).
3. J. Lyklema. *Fundamentals of Interfaces and Colloid Science*, Vol. II, Chaps. 3, 4, Academic Press, New York (1995).
4. R. J. Hunter. *Zeta Potential in Colloid Science*, Academic Press, New York (1981).
5. S. S. Dukhin and B. V. Derjaguin. "Electrokinetic phenomena", in *Surface and Colloid Science*, Vol. 7, Chap. 2, E. Matijević (Ed.), John Wiley, New York (1974).
6. A. V. Delgado (Ed.). *Interfacial Electrokinetics and Electrophoresis*, Marcel Dekker, New York (2001).
7. Manual of symbols and terminology for physicochemical uantities and units, Appendix II: Definitions, terminology and symbols in colloid and surface chemistry. Part I. *Pure Appl. Chem.* **31**, 577 (1972).
8. I. Mills, T. Cvitaš, K. Homann, N. Kallay, K. Kuchitsu. *Quantities, Units and Symbols in Physical Chemistry*, 2nd ed., Sect. 2.14, International Union of Pure and Applied Chemistry, Blackwell Science, Oxford (1993).
9. A. D. McNaught and A. Wilkinson. *Compendium of Chemical Terminology. IUPAC Recommendations*, 2nd ed., International Union of Pure and Applied Chemistry, Blackwell Science, Oxford (1997).
10. J. Lyklema. *Pure Appl. Chem.* **63**, 885 (1995).
11. J. Lyklema, S. Rovillard, J. de Coninck. *Langmuir* **14**, 5659 (1998).
12. J. W. Lorimer. *J. Membr. Sci.* **14**, 275 (1983).
13. C. F. Zukoski and D. A. Saville. *J. Colloid Interface Sci.* **114**, 32 (1986).
14. C. S. Mangelsdorf and L. R. White. *J. Chem. Soc., Faraday Trans.* **86**, 2859 (1990).
15. C. S. Mangelsdorf and L. R. White. *J. Chem. Soc., Faraday Trans.* **94**, 2441 (1998).
16. C. S. Mangelsdorf and L. R. White. *J. Chem. Soc., Faraday Trans.* **94**, 2583 (1998).
17. J. Lyklema and M. Minor. *Colloids Surf., A* **140**, 33 (1998).
18. M. von Smoluchowski. In *Handbuch der Electrizität und des Magnetismus (Graetz)*, Vol. II, p. 366, Barth, Leipzig (1921).
19. J. J. Bikerman. *Z. Physik. Chem.* **A163**, 378 (1933).
20. J. J. Bikerman. *Kolloid Z.* **72**, 100 (1935).
21. J. J. Bikerman. *Trans. Faraday Soc.* **36**, 154 (1940).
22. R. W. O'Brien and L. R. White. *J. Chem. Soc., Faraday Trans. II* **74**, 1607 (1978).
23. R. W. O'Brien and R. J. Hunter. *Can. J. Chem.* **59**, 1878 (1981).
24. D. C. Henry. *Proc. R. Soc. London* **A133**, 106 (1931).
25. H. Ohshima. *J. Colloid Interface Sci.* **168**, 269 (1994).
26. R. P. Tison. *J. Colloid Interface Sci.* **60**, 519 (1977).
27. A. Homola and A. A. Robertson. *J. Colloid Interface Sci.* **51**, 202 (1975).
28. K. Furusawa, Y. Kimura, T. Tagawa. In *Polymer Adsorption and Dispersion Stability*, E. D. Goddard and B. Vincent (Eds.), ACS Symposium Series Vol. 240, p. 131, American Chemical Society, Washington, DC (1984).
29. M. Minor, A. J. van der Linde, H. P. van Leeuwen, J. Lyklema. *J. Colloid Interface Sci.* **189**, 370 (1997).
30. E. E. Uzgiris. *Rev. Sci. Instrum.* **45**, 74 (1974).
31. R. Ware and W. H. Flygare. *J. Colloid Interface Sci.* **39**, 670 (1972).
32. E. E. Uzgiris. *Optics Comm.* **6**, 55 (1972).
33. E. Malher, D. Martin, C. Duvivier. *Studia Biophys.* **90**, 33 (1982).
34. E. Malher, D. Martin, C. Duvivier, B. Volochine, J. F. Stolz. *Biorheology* **19**, 647 (1982).
35. K. Oka and K. Furusawa. In *Electrical Phenomena at Interfaces*, H. Ohshima and K. Furusawa (Eds.), Chap. 8, Marcel Dekker, New York (1998).
36. J. F. Miller, K. Schätzel, B. Vincent. *J. Colloid Interface Sci.* **143**, 532 (1991).
37. F. Manerwatson, W. Tscharnuter, J. Miller. *Colloids Surfaces A* **140**, 53 (1988).
38. J. F. Miller, O. Velev, S. C. C. Wu, H. J. Ploehn. *J. Colloid Interface Sci.* **174**, 490 (1995).
39. Japanese Surface and Colloid Chemical Group (Japan Oil Chemists Soc.). *Yukagaku* **25**, 239 (1975).
40. F. Fairbrother and H. Mastin. *J. Chem. Soc.* 2319 (1924).
41. D. R. Briggs. *J. Phys. Chem.* **32**, 641 (1928).
42. M. Chang and A. A. Robertson. *Can. J. Chem. Eng.* **45**, 66 (1967).
43. G. J. Biefer and S. G. Mason. *Trans. Faraday Soc.* **55**, 1234 (1959).
44. J. Happel and P. A. Ast. *Chem. Eng. Sci.* **11**, 286 (1960).
45. J. Schurz and G. Erk. *Progr. Colloid Polym. Sci.* **71**, 44 (1985).
46. S. Levine, G. Neale, N. Epstein. *J. Colloid Interface Sci.* **57**, 424 (1976).
47. J. L. Anderson and W. H. Koh. *J. Colloid Interface Sci.* **59**, 149 (1977).
48. S. Levine, J. R. Marriot, G. Neale, N. Epstein. *J. Colloid Interface Sci.* **52**, 136 (1975).
49. D. Burgreen and F. R. Nakache. *J. Phys. Chem.* **68**, 1084 (1964).
50. C. L. Rice and P. Whitehead. *J. Phys. Chem.* **69**, 4017 (1965).
51. R. W. O'Brien and W. T. Perrins. *J. Colloid Interface Sci.* **99**, 20 (1984).
52. D. Erickson and D. Li. *J. Colloid Interface Sci.* **237**, 283 (2001).
53. A. Szymczyk, B. Aoubiza, R Fievet, J. Pagetti. *J. Colloid Interface Sci.* **192**, 105 (2001).
54. N. Spanos and P. G. Koutsoukos. *J. Colloid Interface Sci.* **214**, 85 (1999).
55. J. M. Gierbers, J. M. Kleijn, M. A. Cohen-Stuart. *J. Colloid Interface Sci.* **248**, 88 (2002).
56. O. El-Gholabzouri, M. A. Cabrerizo, R. Hidalgo-Álvarez. *J. Colloid Interface Sci.* **261**, 386 (2003).
57. A. Pettersson and J. B. Rosenholm. *Langmuir* **18**, 8447 (2002).
58. J. Th. G. Overbeek. In *Colloid Science*, Vol. I, H. R. Kruyt (Ed.), Chap. V, Elsevier, Amsterdam (1952).
59. C. Werner, R. Zimmermann, T. Kratzmüller. *Colloids Surf., A* **192**, 205 (2001).
60. J. Kijlstra, H. P. van Leeuwen, J. Lyklema. *Langmuir* **9**, 1625 (1993).
61. J. Kijlstra, H. P. van Leeuwen, J. Lyklema. *J. Chem. Soc., Faraday Trans.* **88**, 3441 (1992).
62. C. T. O'Konski. *J. Phys. Chem.* **64**, 605 (1960).
63. S. S. Dukhin and V. N. Shilov. *Dielectric Phenomena and the Double Layer in Disperse Systems and Poly electrolytes*, John Wiley, Jerusalem (1974).

64. C. Grosse and V. N. Shilov. *J. Phys. Chem.* **100**, 1771 (1996).
65. B. Nettleblad and G. A. Niklasson. *J. Colloid Interface Sci.* **181**, 165 (1996).
66. E. H. B. DeLacey and L. R. White. *J. Chem. Soc. Faraday Trans. II* **77**, 2007 (1981).
67. V. N. Shilov, A. V. Delgado, F. González-Caballero, C. Grosse. *Colloids Surf., A* **192**, 253 (2001).
68. L. A. Rosen, J. C. Baygents, D. A. Saville. *J. Chem. Phys.* **98**, 4183 (1993).
69. F. J. Arroyo, F. Carrique, T. Bellini, A. V. Delgado. *J. Colloid Interface Sci.* **210**, 194 (1999).
70. E. Vogel and H. Pauli. *J. Chem. Phys.* **89**, 3830 (1988).
71. Yu. B. Borkovskaja and V. N. Shilov. *Colloid J.* **54**, 173 (1992).
72. V. N. Shilov and Yu. B. Borkovskaja. *Colloid J.* **56**, 647 (1994).
73. A. V. Delgado, F. J. Arroyo, F. Gonzalez-Caballero, V. N. Shilov, Y. Borkovskaja. *Colloids Surf., A* **140**, 139 (1998).
74. F. Carrique, F. J. Arroyo, M. L. Jiménez, A. V. Delgado. *J. Chem. Phys.* **118**, 1945 (2003).
75. H. Fricke and H. J. Curtis. *J. Phys. Chem.* **41**, 729 (1937).
76. F. J. Arroyo, F. Carrique, A. V. Delgado. *J. Colloid Interface Sci.* **217**, 411 (1999).
77. M. M. Springer, A. Korteweg, J. Lyklema. *J. Electroanal. Chem.* **153**, 55 (1983).
78. K. Lim and E. I. Frances. *J. Colloid Interface Sci.* **110**, 201 (1986).
79. C. Grosse, A. J. Hill, K. R. Foster. *J. Colloid Interface Sci.* **127**, 167 (1989).
80. C. Grosse and M. C. Tirado. *Mater. Res. Soc. Symp. Proc.* **430**, 287 (1996).
81. M. L. Jiménez, F. J. Arroyo, J. van Turnhout, A. V. Delgado. *J. Colloid Interface Sci.* **249**, 327 (2002).
82. R. W. O'Brien. *J. Fluid Mech.* **212**, 81 (1990).
83. R. W. O'Brien, B. R. Midmore, A. Lamb, R. J. Hunter. *Faraday Discuss. Chem Soc.* **90**, 301 (1990).
84. R. W. O'Brien. *J. Fluid Mech.* **190**, 71 (1988).
85. R. W. O'Brien, D. Cannon, W. N. Rowlands. *J. Colloid Interface Sci.* **173**, 406 (1995).
86. R. J. Hunter. *Colloids Surf., A* **141**, 37 (1998).
87. R. J. Hunter and R. W. O'Brien. *Colloids Surf., A* **126**, 123 (1997).
88. R. W. O'Brien. U.S. Patent 5,059,909 (1991).
89. R. P. Sawatsky and A. J. Babchin. *J. Fluid Mech.* **246**, 321 (1993).
90. C. S. Mangelsdorf and L. R. White. *J. Colloid Interface Sci.* **160**, 275 (1993).
91. C. S. Mangelsdorf and L. R. White. *J. Chem. Soc., Faraday Trans.* **88**, 3567 (1992).
92. S. E. Gibb and R. J. Hunter. *J. Colloid Interface Sci.* **224**, 99 (2000).
93. M. Loewenberg and R. W. O'Brien. *J. Colloid Interface Sci.* **150**, 158 (1992).
94. M. Loewenberg. *J. Fluid Mech.* **278**, 149 (1994).
95. H. Ohshima. *J. Colloid Interface Sci.* **185**, 131 (1997).
96. B. J. Marlow, D. Fairhurst, H. P. Pendse. *Langmuir* **4**, 611 (1988).
97. S. Levine and G. Neale. *J. Colloid Interface Sci.* **47**, 520 (1974).
98. S. Levine and G. Neale. *J. Colloid Interface Sci.* **49**, (1974).
99. R. W. O'Brien, W. N. Rowlands, R. J. Hunter. In *Electro-acoustics for Characterization of Particulates and Suspensions*, S. B. Malghan (Ed.), NIST Special Publication 856, pp. 1–22, National Institute of Standards and Technology, Washington, DC (1993).
100. R. J. Hunter. "Electrokinetic characterization of emulsions", in *Encyclopaedic Handbook of Emulsion Technology*, J. Sjoblom (Ed.), Chap. 7, Marcel Dekker, New York (2001).
101. P. Rider and R. W. O'Brien. *J. Fluid Mech.* **257**, 607 (1993).
102. J. Ennis, A. A. Shugai, S. L. Carnie. *J. Colloid Interface Sci.* **223**, 21 (2000).
103. S. B. Johnson, A. S. Russell, P. J. Scales. *Colloids Surf, A* **141**, 119 (1998).
104. R. W. O'Brien, A. Jones, W. N. Rowlands. *Colloids Surf, A* **218**, 89 (2003).
105. A. S. Dukhin, V. N. Shilov, H. Ohshima, P. J. Goetz. *Langmuir* **15**, 6692 (1999).
106. A. H. Harker and J. A. G. Temple. *J. Phys. D.: Appl. Phys.* **21**, 1576 (1988).
107. R. L. Gibson and M. N. Toksoz. *J. Acoust. Soc. Amer.* **85**, 1925 (1989).
108. A. S. Dukhin and P. J. Goetz. *Langmuir* **12**, 4987 (1996).
109. A. S. Ahuja. *J. Appl. Phys.* **44**, 4863 (1973).
110. S. Kuwabara. *J. Phys. Soc. Jpn.* **14**, 527 (1959).
111. V. N. Shilov, N. I. Zharkikh, Y. B. Borkovskaya. *Colloid J.* **43**, 434 (1981).
112. A. S. Dukhin, V. N. Shilov, H. Ohshima, P. J. Goetz. In *Interfacial Electrokinetics and Electrophoresis*, A. V. Delgado (Ed.), Chap. 17, Marcel Dekker, New York (2001).
113. R. J. Hunter and R. W. O'Brien. In *Encyclopedia of Colloid and Surface Science*, A. Hubbard (Ed.), p. 1722, Marcel Dekker, New York (2002).
114. H. Ohshima. In *Electrical Phenomena at Interfaces. Fundamentals, Measurements and Applications*, H. Ohshima and K. Furusawa (Eds.), Chap. 2, Marcel Dekker, New York (2002).
115. F. Carrique, F. J. Arroyo, A. V. Delgado. *J. Colloid Interface Sci.* **206**, 206 (1998).
116. S. S. Dukhin. *Adv. Colloid Interface Sci.* **44**, 1 (1993).
117. R. W. O'Brien and D. N. Ward. *J. Colloid Interface Sci.* **121**, 402 (1988).
118. M. C. Fair and J. L. Anderson. *J. Colloid Interface Sci.* **127**, 388 (1989).
119. D. Velegol, J. L. Anderson, Y. Solomentsev. In *Interfacial Electrokinetics and Electrophoresis*, A. V. Delgado (Ed.), Chap. 6, Marcel Dekker, New York (2002).
120. J. Y. Kim and B. J. Yoon. In *Interfacial Electrokinetics and Electrophoresis*, A. V. Delgado (Ed.), Chap. 7, Marcel Dekker, New York (2002).
121. C. Grosse and V. N. Shilov. *J. Colloid Interface Sci.* **193**, 178 (1997).
122. C. Grosse, S. Pedrosa, V. N. Shilov. *J. Colloid Interface Sci.* **220**, 31 (1999).
123. S. S. Dukhin, R. Zimmermann, C. Werner. *Colloids Surf., A* **195**, 103 (2001).
124. J. Y. Walz. *Adv. Colloid Interface Sci.* **74**, 119 (1998).
125. S. A. Allison. *Macromolecules* **29**, 7391 (1996).
126. M. Teubner. *J. Chem. Phys.* **76**, 5564 (1982).
127. M. C. Fair and J. L. Anderson. *Langmuir* **8**, 2850 (1992).
128. D. Velegol, J. L. Anderson, S. Garoff. *Langmuir* **12**, 675 (1996).
129. J. L. Anderson, D. Velegol, S. Garoff. *Langmuir* **16**, 3372 (2000).
130. J. L. Anderson. *J. Colloid Interface Sci.* **105**, 45 (1985).
131. H. van Olphen. *An Introduction to Clay Colloid Chemistry*, John Wiley, New York (1977).
132. S. Akari, W. Schrepp, D. Horn. *Langmuir* **12**, 857 (1996).
133. K. E. Bremmell, G. J. Jameson, S. Biggs. *Colloids Surf., A* **139**, 199 (1998).
134. M. A. Cohen-Stuart, F. H. W. Waajen, S. S. Dukhin. *Colloid Polym. Sci.* **262**, 423 (1984).
135. L. K. Koopal, V. Hlady, J. Lyklema. *J. Colloid Interface Sci.* **121**, 49 (1988).
136. L. Kong, J. K. Beattie, R. J. Hunter. *Phys. Chem. Chem. Phys.* **3**, 87 (2001).
137. H. Ohshima. *J. Colloid Interface Sci.* **163**, 474 (1995).
138. H. Ohshima and K. Makino. *Colloids Surf., A* **109**, 71 (1996).
139. H. N. Stein. In *Interfacial Electrokinetics and Electrophoresis*, A. V. Delgado (Ed.), Chap. 21, Marcel Dekker, New York (2002).
140. R. Hidalgo-Álvarez, A. Martín, A. Fernández, D. Bastos, F. Martínez, F. J. de las Nieves. *Adv. Colloid Interface Sci.* **67**, 1 (1996).
141. H. Ohshima. In *Interfacial Electrokinetics and Electrophoresis*, A. V. Delgado, (Ed.), Chap. 5, Marcel Dekker, New York (2002).
142. H. J. Keh. In *Interfacial Electrokinetics and Electrophoresis*, A. V. Delgado (Ed.), Chap. 15, Marcel Dekker, New York (2002).
143. C. Tanford and J. A. Reynolds. *Biochim. Biophys. Acta* **457**, 133 (1976).
144. D. Stigter. *Cell Biophys.* **11**, 139 (1987).
145. D. Stigter. *J. Phys. Chem. B* **104**, 3402 (2000).
146. R. J. Hill, D. A. Saville, W. B. Russel. *J. Colloid Interface Sci.* **258**, 56 (2003).
147. A. Martín-Rodríguez, J. L. Ortega-Vinuesa, R. Hidalgo-Álvarez. In *Interfacial Electrokinetics and Electrophoresis*, A. V. Delgado (Ed.), Chap. 22, Marcel Dekker, New York (2002).
148. E. Lee, F. Y. Yen, J. P. Hsu. In *Interfacial Electrokinetics and Electrophoresis*, A. V. Delgado (Ed.), Chap. 23, Marcel Dekker, New York (2002).
149. R. Barchini, H. P. van Leewen, J. Lyklema. *Langmuir* **16**, 8238 (2000).
150. A. Van der Wal, M. Minor, W. Norde, A. J. B. Zehnder, J. Lyklema. *Langmuir* **13**, 165 (1997).
151. S. A. Nespolo, M. A. Bevan, D. Y. C. Chan, F. Grieser, G. W. Stevens. *Langmuir* **17**, 7210 (2001).
152. C. Yang, T. Dabros, D. Li, J. Czarnecki, J. H. Masliyah. *J. Colloid Interface Sci.* **243**, 128 (2001).

11. List of Symbols

Note: SI base (or derived) units are given in parentheses for all quantities, except dimensionless ones.

a (m)	particle radius, local curvature radius, capillary radius		N_A (mol^{-1})	Avogadro constant
A_c (m^2)	capillary cross-section		n_i (m^{-3})	number concentration of type i ions
A_c^{ap} (m^2)	apparent (externally measured) capillary cross-section		Q_{eo} (m^3 s^{-1})	electro-osmotic flow rate
			$Q_{eo,E}$ (m^4 s^{-1} V^{-1})	electro-osmotic flow rate per electric field
A_{ESA} (Pa)	electrokinetic sonic amplitude		$Q_{eo,I}$ (m^3 C^{-1})	electro-osmotic flow rate per current
b (m)	half distance between neighboring particles		r (m)	spherical or cylindrical radial coordinate
c (mol m^{-3})	electrolyte concentration		R (m)	roughness of a surface
$c_+(c_-)$ (mol m^{-3})	concentration of cations (anions)		R_s (Ω)	electrical resistance of a capillary or porous plug in an arbitrary solution
C_0^*	dipole coefficient of particles		R_∞ (Ω)	electrical resistance of a capillary or porous plug in a concentrated ionic solution
d (m)	distance between the surface and the outer Helmholtz plane			
d^* (C m)	complex dipole moment		T (K)	thermodynamic temperature
d^{ek} (m)	distance between the surface and the slip plane		u_d^* (m^2 s^{-1} V^{-1})	dynamic electrophoretic mobility
D (m^2 s^{-1})	diffusion coefficient of counterions (or average diffusion coefficient of ions)		U_{CV} (V)	colloid vibration potential
$D+$ ($D-$) (m^2 s^{-1})	diffusion coefficient of cations (anions)		v_e (m^2 s^{-1} V^{-1})	electrophoretic mobility
			U_{sed} (V)	sedimentation potential
Du	Dukhin number		U_{str} (V)	streaming potential
Du^d	Dukhin number associated with diffuse-layer conductivity		v_e (m s^{-1})	electrophoretic velocity
			v_{eo} (m s^{-1})	electro-osmotic velocity
Du^i	Dukhin number associated with stagnant-layer conductivity		v_L (m s^{-1})	liquid velocity in electrophoresis cell
			y^{ek}	dimensionless ζ-potential
e (C)	elementary charge		z	common charge number of ions in a symmetrical electrolyte
E (V m^{-1})	applied electric field			
E_{sed} (V m^{-1})	sedimentation field		z_i	charge number of type i ions
E_t (V m^{-1})	tangential component of external field		α	relaxation of double-layer polarization, degree of electrolyte dissociation, dimensionless parameter used in electroacoustics
F (C mol^{-1})	Faraday constant			
$f_1(\kappa a)$, $F_1(\kappa a, Kp)$	Henry's functions			
I (A)	electric current intensity		β (m)	distance between the solid surface and the inner Hemholtz plane (see also eq. 45 for another use of this symbol)
$I_0 I_1$	zeroth- (first-) order modified Bessel functions of the first kind			
			Γ_i (m^{-2})	surface concentration of type i ions
I_c (A)	conduction current		δ_c (mol m^{-3})	field-induced perturbation of electrolyte amount concentration
I_{CV} (A)	colloid vibration current			
I_{str} (A)	streaming current		δK^* (S m^{-1})	conductivity increment of a suspension
j^σ (Am^{-1})	surface current density		$\delta_{\varepsilon r}$	relative dielectric increment of a suspension
j_{str} (A m^{-2})	streaming current density		Δ_p (Pa)	applied pressure difference
k (J K^{-1})	Boltzmann constant		Δ_{peo} (Pa)	electro-osmotic counter-pressure
K (S m^{-1})	total conductivity of a colloidal system		$\Delta Vext$ (V)	applied potential difference
K_{DC} (S m^{-1})	direct current conductivity of a suspension		$\Delta_\varepsilon(0)$	low-frequency dielectric increment per volume fraction
K_L (S m^{-1})	conductivity of dispersion medium			
K_L^∞ (Sm^{-1})	conductivity of a highly concentrated ionic solution		$\Delta_{\varepsilon d}(0)$	value of $\Delta\varepsilon(0)$ for suspensions with low volume fractions
K_p (S m^{-1})	conductivity of particles		$\Delta\rho$ (kg m^{-3})	density difference between particles and dispersion medium
K_{plug} (S m^{-1})	conductivity of a plug of particles			
K_{pef} (S m^{-1})	effective conductivity of particles		ε^* (F m^{-1})	complex electric permittivity of a suspension
K_{rel}	ratio between particle and liquid conductivities		ε_r^*	complex relative permittivity of a suspension
K^* (S m^{-1})	complex conductivity of a suspension			
K^σ (S)	surface conductivity		ε_{rp}	relative permittivity of the particle
$K^{\sigma d}$ (S)	diffuse-layer surface conductivity		ε_{rp}^*	complex relative permittivity of a particle
$K^{\sigma i}$ (S)	stagnant-layer surface conductivity		ε_{rs}	relative permittivity of the dispersion medium
L (m)	capillary length, characteristic dimension		ε_{rs}^*	complex relative permittivity of the dispersion medium
L^{ap} (m)	apparent (externally measured) capillary cross-section			
L_D (m)	ionic diffusion length		ε_0 (F m^{-1})	electric permittivity of vacuum
m	dimensionless ionic mobility of counterions		ζ (V)	electrokinetic or ζ-potential
$m+$ ($m-$)	dimensionless ionic mobility of cations (anions)		ζ_{app} (V)	electrokinetic or ζ-potential not corrected for the effect of particle concentration
n (m^{-3})	number concentration of particles			
			η (Pa s)	dynamic viscosity

κ (m^{-1})	reciprocal Debye length	ϕ	volume fraction of solids
ρ (kg m^{-3})	density of dispersion medium	ϕ_L	volume fraction of liquid in a plug
ρ_p (kg m^{-3})	density of particles	ψ^d (V)	diffuse-layer potential
ρ_s (kg m^{-3})	density of a suspension	ψ^i (V)	inner Helmholtz plane potential
σ^d (C m^{-2})	diffuse charge density	ψ^0 (V)	surface potential
σ^{ek} (C m^{-2})	electrokinetic charge density	ω (s^{-1})	angular frequency of an ac electric field
σ^i (C m^{-2})	surface charge density at the inner Helmholtz plane	ω_{MWO} (s^{-1})	Maxwell–Wagner–O'Konski characteristic frequency
σ^0 (C m^{-2})	titratable surface charge density		
τ_{MWO} (s)	characteristic time of the Maxwell–Wagner–O'Konski relaxation	ω_α (s^{-1})	characteristic frequency of the α-relaxation
$\tau\alpha$ (s)	relaxation time of the low-frequency dispersion	$\omega_{\alpha d}$ (s^{-1})	characteristic frequency of the α-relaxation for a dilute suspension

MEASUREMENT OF pH DEFINITION, STANDARDS, AND PROCEDURES

(IUPAC Recommendations 2002)

Working Party on pH

R. P. Buck (Chairman)[1], S. Rondinini (Secretary)[2,‡], A. K. Covington (Editor)[3], F. G. K. Baucke[4], C. M. A. Brett[5], M. F. Camões[6], M. J. T. Milton[7], T. Mussini[8], R. Naumann[9], K. W. Pratt[10], P. Spitzer[11], and G. S. Wilson[12]

[1]101 Creekview Circle, Carrboro, NC 27510, USA; [2]Dipartimento di Chimica Fisica ed Elettrochimica, Università di Milano, Via Golgi 19, I-20133 Milano, Italy; [3]Department of Chemistry, The University, Bedson Building, Newcastle Upon Tyne, NE1 7RU, UK; [4]Schott Glasswerke, P.O. Box 2480, D-55014 Mainz, Germany; [5]Departamento de Química, Universidade de Coimbra, P-3004-535 Coimbra, Portugal; [6]Departamento de Química e Bioquimica, University of Lisbon (SPQ/DQBFCUL), Faculdade de Ciencias, Edificio CI-5 Piso, P-1700 Lisboa, Portugal; [7]National Physical Laboratory, Centre for Optical and Environmental Metrology, Queen's Road, Teddington, Middlesex TW11 0LW, UK; [8]Dipartimento di Chimica Fisica ed Elettrochimica, Università di Milano, Via Golgi 19, I-20133 Milano, Italy; [9]MPI for Polymer Research, Ackermannweg 10, D-55128 Mainz, Germany; [10]Chemistry B324, Stop 8393, National Institute of Standards and Technology, 100 Bureau Drive, ACSL, Room A349, Gaithersburg, MD 20899-8393, USA; [11]Physikalisch-Technische Bundesanstalt (PTB), Postfach 33 45, D-38023 Braunschweig, Germany; [12]Department of Chemistry, University of Kansas, Lawrence, KS 66045, USA

Abstract: The definition of a "primary method of measurement" [1] has permitted a full consideration of the definition of primary standards for pH, determined by a primary method (cell without transference, Harned cell), of the definition of secondary standards by secondary methods, and of the question whether pH, as a conventional quantity, can be incorporated within the internationally accepted system of measurement, the International System of Units (SI, Système International d'Unités). This approach has enabled resolution of the previous compromise IUPAC 1985 Recommendations [2]. Furthermore, incorporation of the uncertainties for the primary method, and for all subsequent measurements, permits the uncertainties for all procedures to be linked to the primary standards by an unbroken chain of comparisons. Thus, a rational choice can be made by the analyst of the appropriate procedure to achieve the target uncertainty of sample pH. Accordingly, this document explains IUPAC recommended definitions, procedures, and terminology relating to pH measurements in dilute aqueous solutions in the temperature range 5–50 °C. Details are given of the primary and secondary methods for measuring pH and the rationale for the assignment of pH values with appropriate uncertainties to selected primary and secondary substances.

Contents

Reproduced from:
Pure Appl. Chem., Vol. 74, No. 11, pp. 2169–2200, 2002.
© 2002 IUPAC
‡ Corresponding author

Abbreviations Used

BIPM	Bureau International des Poids et Mesures, France
CRMs	certified reference materials
EUROMET	European Collaboration in Metrology (Measurement Standards)
NBS	National Bureau of Standards, USA, now NIST
NIST	National Institute of Science and Technology, USA
NMIs	national metrological institutes
PS	primary standard
LJP	liquid junction potential
RLJP	residual liquid junction potential
SS	secondary standard

1. Introduction and Scope

1.1 pH, a Single Ion Quantity

The concept of pH is unique among the commonly encountered physicochemical quantities listed in the IUPAC Green Book [3] in that, in terms of its definition [4],

$$pH = -\lg a_H$$

it involves a single ion quantity, the activity of the hydrogen ion, which is immeasurable by any thermodynamically valid method and requires a convention for its evaluation.

1.2 Cells without Transference, Harned Cells

As will be shown in Section 4, primary pH standard values can be determined from electrochemical data from the cell without transference using the hydrogen gas electrode, known as the Harned cell. These primary standards have *good* reproducibility and *low* uncertainty. Cells involving glass electrodes and liquid junctions have considerably *higher* uncertainties, as will be discussed later (Sections 5.1, 10.1). Using evaluated uncertainties, it is possible to rank reference materials as primary or secondary in terms of the methods used for assigning pH values to them. This ranking of primary (PS) or secondary (SS) standards is consistent with the metrological requirement that measurements are traceable with stated uncertainties to national, or international, standards by an unbroken chain of comparisons each with its own stated uncertainty. The accepted definition of traceability is given in Section 12.4. If the uncertainty of such measurements is calculated to include the hydrogen ion activity convention (Section 4.6), then the result can also be traceable to the internationally accepted SI system of units.

1.3 Primary pH Standards

In Section 4 of this document, the procedure used to assign primary standard [pH(PS)] values to primary standards is described. The only method that meets the stringent criteria of a primary method of measurement for measuring pH is based on the Harned cell (Cell I). This method, extensively developed by R. G. Bates [5] and collaborators at NBS (later NIST), is now adopted in national metrological institutes (NMIs) worldwide, and the procedure is approved in this document with slight modifications (Section 3.2) to comply with the requirements of a primary method.

1.4 Secondary Standards Derived From Measurements on the Harned Cell (Cell I)

Values assigned by Harned cell measurements to substances that do not entirely fulfill the criteria for primary standard status are secondary standards (SS), with pH(SS) values, and are discussed in Section 8.1.

1.5 Secondary Standards Derived From Primary Standards by Measuring Differences in pH

Methods that can be used to obtain the difference in pH between buffer solutions are discussed in Sections 8.2–8.5 of these Recommendations. These methods involve cells that are practically more convenient than the Harned cell, but have greater uncertainties associated with the results. They enable the pH of other buffers to be compared with primary standard buffers that have been measured with a Harned cell. It is recommended that these are secondary methods, and buffers measured in this way are secondary standards (SS), with pH(SS) values.

1.6 Traceability

This hierarchical approach to primary and secondary measurements facilitates the availability of traceable buffers for laboratory calibrations. Recommended procedures for carrying out these calibrations to achieve specified uncertainties are given in Section 11.

1.7 Scope

The recommendations in this Report relate to analytical laboratory determinations of pH of dilute aqueous solutions (≤ 0.1 mol kg^{-1}). Systems including partially aqueous mixed solvents, biological measurements, heavy water solvent, natural waters, and high-temperature measurements are excluded from this Report.

1.8 Uncertainty Estimates

The Annex (Section 13) includes typical uncertainty estimates for the use of the cells and measurements described.

2. Activity and the Definition of pH

2.1 Hydrogen Ion Activity

pH was originally defined by Sørensen in 1909 [6] in terms of the concentration of hydrogen ions (in modern nomenclature) as pH = $-\lg(c_H/c°)$ where c_H is the hydrogen ion concentration in mol dm^{-3}, and $c° = 1$ mol dm^{-3} is the standard amount concentration. Subsequently [4], it has been accepted that it is more satisfactory to define pH in terms of the relative activity of hydrogen ions in solution

$$pH = -\lg a_H = -\lg(m_H \gamma_H/m°) \tag{1}$$

where a_H is the relative (molality basis) activity and γ_H is the molal activity coefficient of the hydrogen ion H$^+$ at the molality m_H, and $m°$ is the standard molality. The quantity pH is intended to be a measure of the activity of hydrogen ions in solution. However, since it is defined in terms of a quantity that cannot be measured by a thermodynamically valid method, eq. 1 can be only a *notional definition* of pH.

3. Traceability and Primary Methods of Measurement

3.1 Relation to SI

Since pH, a single ion quantity, is not determinable in terms of a fundamental (or base) unit of any measurement system, there was some difficulty previously in providing a proper basis for the traceability of pH measurements. A satisfactory approach is now available in that pH determinations can be incorporated into the SI if they can be traced to measurements made using a method that fulfills the definition of a "Primary method of measurement" [1].

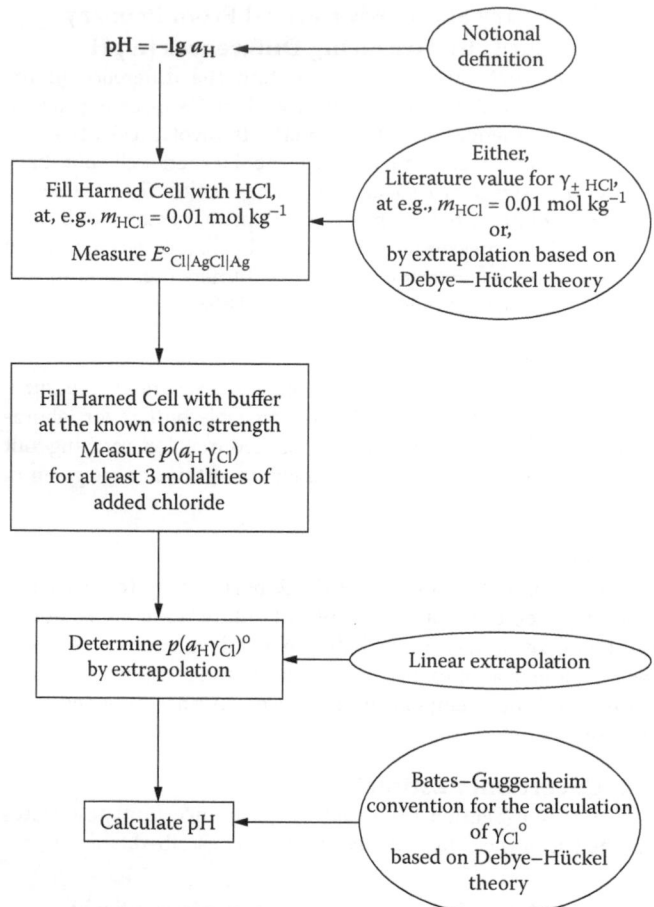

FIGURE 1 Operation of the Harned cell as a primary method for the measurement of absolute pH.

3.2 Primary Method of Measurement

The accepted definition of a primary method of measurement is given in Section 12.1. The essential feature of such a method is that it must operate according to a well-defined measurement equation in which all of the variables can be determined experimentally in terms of SI units. Any limitation in the determination of the experimental variables, or in the theory, must be included within the estimated uncertainty of the method if traceability to the SI is to be established. If a convention is used without an estimate of its uncertainty, true traceability to the SI would not be established. In the following section, it is shown that the Harned cell fulfills the definition of a primary method for the measurement of the acidity function, $p(a_H\gamma_{Cl})$, and subsequently of the pH of buffer solutions.

4. Harned Cell as a Primary Method for the Absolute Measurement of pH

4.1 Harned Cell

The cell without transference defined by

$$Pt \mid H_2 \mid buffer\ S,\ Cl^- \mid AgCl \mid Ag \qquad Cell\ I$$

known as the Harned cell [7], and containing standard buffer, S, and chloride ions, in the form of potassium or sodium chloride, which are added in order to use the silver–silver chloride electrode. The application of the Nernst equation to the spontaneous cell reaction:

$$^{1/2}H_2 + AgCl \rightarrow Ag(s) + H^+ + Cl^-$$

yields the potential difference E_I of the cell [corrected to 1 atm (101.325 kPa), the partial pressure of hydrogen gas used in electrochemistry in preference to 100 kPa] as

$$E_I = E^\circ - [(RT/F)\ln 10]\ lg[(m_H\gamma_H/m^\circ)(m_{Cl}\gamma_{Cl}/m^\circ)] \qquad (2)$$

which can be rearranged, since $a_H = m_H\gamma_H/m^\circ$, to give the acidity function

$$p(a_H\gamma_{Cl}) = -lg(a_H\gamma_{Cl}) = (E_I - E^\circ)/[(RT/F)\ln 10] + lg(m_{Cl}/m^\circ) \qquad (2')$$

where E° is the standard potential difference of the cell, and hence of the silver–silver chloride electrode, and γ_{Cl} is the activity coefficient of the chloride ion.

Note 1: The sign of the standard electrode potential of an electrochemical reaction is that displayed on a high-impedance voltmeter when the lead attached to standard hydrogen electrode is connected to the minus pole of the voltmeter.

The steps in the use of the cell are summarized in Figure. 1 and described in the following paragraphs.

The standard potential difference of the silver–silver chloride electrode, E°, is determined from a Harned cell in which only HCl is present at a fixed molality (e.g., $m = 0.01$ mol kg^{-1}). The application of the Nernst equation to the HCl cell

$$Pt \mid H2 \mid HCl(m) \mid AgCl \mid Ag \qquad Cell\ Ia$$

gives

$$E_{Ia} = E^\circ - [(2RT/F)\ln 10]\ lg[(m_{HCl}/m^\circ)(\gamma_{\pm HCl})] \qquad (3)$$

where E_{Ia} has been corrected to 1 atmosphere partial pressure of hydrogen gas (101.325 kPa) and $\gamma_{\pm HCl}$ is the mean ionic activity coefficient of HCl.

4.2 Activity Coefficient of HCl

The values of the activity coefficient ($\gamma_{\pm HCl}$) at molality 0.01 mol kg^{-1} and various temperatures are given by Bates and Robinson [8]. The standard potential difference depends in some not entirely understood way on the method of preparation of the electrodes, but individual determinations of the activity coefficient of HCl at 0.01 mol kg^{-1} are more uniform than values of E°. Hence, the practical determination of the potential difference of the cell with HCl at 0.01 mol kg^{-1} is recommended at 298.15 K at which the mean ionic activity coefficient is 0.904. Dickson [9] concluded that it is not necessary to repeat the measurement of E° at other temperatures, but that it is satisfactory to correct published smoothed values by the observed difference in E° at 298.15 K.

4.3 Acidity Function

In NMIs, measurements of Cells I and Ia are often done simultaneously in a thermostat bath. Subtracting eq. 3 from eq. 2 gives

$$\Delta E = E_I - E_{Ia} = -[(RT/F)\ln 10]\{lg[(m_H\gamma_H/m^\circ)(m_{Cl}\gamma_{Cl}/m^\circ)] - lg[(m_{HCl}/m^\circ)^2\gamma^2_{\pm HCl}]\} \qquad (4)$$

which is independent of the standard potential difference. Therefore, the subsequently calculated pH does not depend on the standard potential difference and hence does not depend on the assumption that the standard potential of the hydrogen electrode, $E^\circ(H^+|H_2) = 0$ at all temperatures. Therefore, the Harned cell can give an exact comparison between hydrogen ion activities at two different temperatures (in contrast to statements found elsewhere, see, for example, ref. [5]).

The quantity $p(a_H\gamma_{Cl}) = -lg(a_H\gamma_{Cl})$, on the left-hand side of eq. 2', is called the acidity function [5]. To obtain the quantity pH (according to eq. 1), from the acidity function, it is necessary to evaluate $\lg \gamma_{Cl}$ by independent means. This is done in two steps: (i) the value of $\lg(a_H \gamma_{Cl})$ at zero chloride molality, $\lg(a_H \gamma_{Cl})^\circ$, is evaluated and (ii) a value for the activity of the chloride ion γ°_{Cl}, at zero chloride molality (sometimes referred to as the limiting or "trace" activity coefficient [9]) is calculated using the Bates–Guggenheim convention [10]. These two steps are described in the following paragraphs.

4.4 Extrapolation of Acidity Function to Zero Chloride Molality

The value of $\lg(a_H \gamma_{Cl})^\circ$ corresponding to zero chloride molality is determined by linear extrapolation of measurements using Harned cells with at least three added molalities of sodium or potassium chloride ($I < 0.1$ mol kg^{-1}, see Sections 4.5 and 12.6)

$$-\lg(a_H \gamma_{Cl}) = -\lg(a_H \gamma_{Cl})^\circ + Sm_{Cl} \qquad (5)$$

where S is an empirical, temperature-dependent constant. The extrapolation is linear, which is expected from Brønsted's observations [11] that specific ion interactions between oppositely charged ions are dominant in mixed strong electrolyte systems at constant molality or ionic strength. However, these acidity function measurements are made on mixtures of weak and strong electrolytes at constant buffer molality, but not constant total molality. It can be shown [12] that provided the change in ionic strength on addition of chloride is less than 20 %, the extrapolation will be linear without detectable curvature. If the latter, less-convenient method of preparation of constant total molality solutions is used, Bates [5] has reported that, for equimolal phosphate buffer, the two methods extrapolate to the same intercept. In an alternative procedure, often useful for partially aqueous mixed solvents where the above extrapolation appears to be curved, multiple application of the Bates–Guggenheim convention to each solution composition gives identical results within the estimated uncertainty of the two intercepts.

4.5 Bates–Guggenheim Convention

The activity coefficient of chloride (like the activity coefficient of the hydrogen ion) is an immeasurable quantity. However, in solutions of low ionic strength ($I < 0.1$ mol kg^{-1}), it is possible to calculate the activity coefficient of chloride ion using the Debye–Hückel theory. This is done by adopting the Bates–Guggenheim convention, which assumes the trace activity coefficient of the chloride ion γ°_{Cl} is given by the expression [10]

$$\lg \gamma^\circ_{Cl} = -AI^{1/2}/(1 + Ba\, I^{1/2}) \qquad (6)$$

where A is the Debye–Hückel temperature-dependent constant (limiting slope), a is the *mean* distance of closest approach of the ions (ion size parameter), Ba is set equal to 1.5 (mol kg^{-1})$^{-1/2}$ at all temperatures in the range 5–50 °C, and I is the ionic strength of the buffer (which, for its evaluation requires knowledge of appropriate acid dissociation constants). Values of A as a function of temperature can be found in Table 14 and of B, which is effectively unaffected by revision of dielectric constant data, in Bates [5]. When the numerical value of $Ba = 1.5$ (i.e., without units) is introduced into eq. 6 it should be written as

$$\lg \gamma^\circ_{Cl} = -AI^{1/2}/[1 + 1.5\,(I/m^\circ)^{1/2}] \qquad (6')$$

The various stages in the assignment of primary standard pH values are combined in eq. 7, which is derived from eqs. 2', 5, 6',

$$pH(PS) = \lim m_{Cl} \to 0\ \{(E_I - E^\circ)/[(RT/F)\ln 10] + \lg(m_{Cl}/m^\circ)\} \\ - AI^{1/2}/[1 + 1.5\,(I/m^\circ)^{1/2}], \qquad (7)$$

and the steps are summarized schematically in Figure. 1.

5. Sources of Uncertainty in the Use of the Harned Cell

5.1 Potential Primary Method and Uncertainty Evaluation

The presentation of the procedure in Section 4 highlights the fact that assumptions based on electrolyte theories [7] are used at three points in the method:

i. The Debye–Hückel theory is the basis of the extrapolation procedure to calculate the value for the standard potential of the silver–silver chloride electrode, even though it is a published value of $\gamma_{\pm HCl}$ at, e.g., $m = 0.01$ mol kg^{-1}, that is recommended (Section 4.2) to facilitate E° determination.

iii. Specific ion interaction theory is the basis for using a linear extrapolation to zero chloride (but the change in ionic strength produced by addition of chloride should be restricted to no more than 20 %).

iii. The Debye–Hückel theory is the basis for the Bates–Guggenheim convention used for the calculation of the trace activity coefficient, γ°_{Cl}.

In the first two cases, the inadequacies of electrolyte theories are sources of uncertainty that limit the extent to which the measured pH is a true representation of $\lg a_H$. In the third case, the use of eq. 6 or 7 is a convention, since the value for Ba is not directly determinable experimentally. Previous recommendations have not included the uncertainty in Ba explicitly within the calculation of the uncertainty of the measurement.

Since eq. 2 is derived from the Nernst equation applied to the thermodynamically well-behaved platinum–hydrogen and silver–silver chloride electrodes, it is recommended that, when used to measure $-\lg(a_H \gamma_{Cl})$ in aqueous solutions, the Harned cell *potentially* meets the agreed definition of a primary method for the measurement. The word "potentially" has been included to emphasize that the method can only achieve primary status if it is operated with the highest metrological qualities (see Sections 6.1–6.2). Additionally, if the Bates–Guggenheim convention is used for the calculation of $\lg \gamma^\circ_{Cl}$, the Harned cell *potentially* meets the agreed definition of a primary method for the measurement of pH, subject to this convention if a realistic estimate of its uncertainty is included. The uncertainty budget for the primary method of measurement by the Harned cell (Cell I) is given in the Annex, Section 13.

Note 2: The experimental uncertainty for a typical primary pH(PS) measurement is of the order of 0.004 (see Table 4).

5.2 Evaluation of Uncertainty of the Bates–Guggenheim Convention

In order for a measurement of pH made with a Harned cell to be traceable to the SI system, an estimate of the uncertainty of each step must be included in the result. Hence, it is recommended that an estimate of the uncertainty of 0.01 (95% confidence interval) in pH associated with the Bates–Guggenheim convention is used. The extent to which the Bates–Guggenheim convention represents the "true" (but immeasurable) activity coefficient of the chloride ion can be calculated by varying the coefficient Ba between 1.0 and 2.0 (mol kg^{-1})$^{1/2}$. This corresponds to varying the ion-size parameter between 0.3 and 0.6 nm, yielding a range of ±0.012 (at $I = 0.1$ mol kg^{-1}) and ±0.007 (at $I = 0.05$ mol kg^{-1}) for γ°_{Cl} calculated using equation [7]. Hence, an uncertainty of 0.01 should cover the full extent of variation. This must be included in the uncertainty of pH values that are to be regarded as traceable to the SI. pH values stated without this contribution to their uncertainty cannot be considered to be traceable to the SI.

5.2 Hydrogen Ion Concentration

It is rarely required to calculate hydrogen ion concentration from measured pH. Should such a calculation be required, the only consistent, logical way of doing it is to assume $\gamma_H = \gamma_{Cl}$ and set the latter to the appropriate Bates–Guggenheim conventional value. The uncertainties are then those derived from the Bates–Guggenheim convention.

5.3 Possible Future Approaches

Any model of electrolyte solutions that takes into account both electrostatic and specific interactions for individual solutions would be an improvement over use of the Bates–Guggenheim convention. It is hardly reasonable that a fixed value of the ion-size parameter should be appropriate for a diversity of selected buffer solutions. It is hoped that the Pitzer model of electrolytes [13], which uses a virial equation approach, will provide such an improvement, but data in the literature are insufficiently extensive to make these calculations at the present time. From limited work at 25 °C done on phosphate and carbonate buffers, it seems that changes to Bates–Guggenheim recommended values will be small [14]. It is possible that some anomalies attributed to liquid junction potentials (LJPs) may be resolved.

6. Primary Buffer Solutions and their Required Properties

6.1 Requisites for Highest Metrological Quality

In the previous sections, it has been shown that the Harned cell provides a primary method for the determination of pH. In order for a particular buffer solution to be considered a primary buffer solution, it must be of the "highest metrological" quality [15] in accordance with the definition of a primary standard. It is recommended that it have the following attributes [5: p. 95;16,17]:

- High buffer value in the range 0.016–0.07 (mol OH⁻)/pH
- Small dilution value at half concentration (change in pH with change in buffer concentration) in the range 0.01–0.20
- Small dependence of pH on temperature less than ±0.01 K⁻¹
- Low residual LJP <0.01 in pH (see Section 7)
- Ionic strength ≤0.1 mol kg⁻¹ to permit applicability of the Bates–Guggenheim convention
- NMI certificate for specific batch
- Reproducible purity of preparation (lot-to-lot differences of |ΔpH(PS)| < 0.003)
- Long-term stability of stored solid material

Values for the above and other important parameters for the selected primary buffer materials (see Section 6.2) are given in Table 1.

Note 3: The long-term stability of the solid compounds (>5 years) is a requirement not met by borax [16]. There are also doubts about the extent of polyborate formation in 0.05 mol kg⁻¹ borax solutions, and hence this solution is not accorded primary status.

6.2 Primary Standard Buffers

Since there can be significant variations in the purity of samples of a buffer of the same nominal chemical composition, it is essential that the primary buffer material used has been certified with values that have been measured with Cell I. The Harned cell has been used by many NMIs for accurate measurements of pH of buffer solutions. Comparisons of such measurements have been carried out under EUROMET collaboration [18], which have

demonstrated the high comparability of measurements (0.005 in pH) in different laboratories of samples from the same batch of buffer material. Typical values of the pH(PS) of the seven solutions from the six accepted primary standard reference buffers, which meet the conditions stated in Section 6.1, are listed in Table 2. These listed pH(PS) values have been derived from certificates issued by NBS/NIST over the past 35 years. Batch-to-batch variations in purity can result in changes in the pH value of samples of at most 0.003. The typical values in Table 2 should not be used in place of the certified value (from a Harned cell measurement) for a specific batch of buffer material.

The required attributes listed in Section 6.1 effectively limit the range of primary buffers available to between pH 3 and 10 (at 25 °C). Calcium hydroxide and potassium tetroxalate have been excluded because the contribution of hydroxide or hydrogen ions to the ionic strength is significant. Also excluded are the nitrogen bases of the type BH⁺ [such as tris(hydroxymethyl)aminomethane and piperazine phosphate] and the zwitterionic buffers (e.g., HEPES and MOPS [19]). These do not comply because either the Bates–Guggenheim convention is not applicable, or the LJPs are high. This means the choice of primary standards is restricted to buffers derived from oxy-carbon, -phosphorus, -boron, and mono-, di-, and tri-protic carboxylic acids. In the future, other buffer systems may fulfill the requirements listed in Section 6.1.

7. Consistency of Primary Buffer Solutions

7.1 Consistency and the Liquid Junction Potential

Primary methods of measurement are made with cells without transference as described in Sections 1–6. Less-complex, secondary methods use cells with transference, which contain liquid junctions. A single LJP is immeasurable, but differences in LJP can be estimated. LJPs vary with the composition of the solutions forming the junction and the geometry of the junction.

Equation 7 for Cell I applied successively to two primary standard buffers, PS_1, PS_2, gives

$$\Delta pH_I = pH_I(PS_2) - pH_I(PS_1) = \lim m_{Cl\to 0}\{E_I(PS_2)/k - E_I(PS_1)/k\}$$
$$- A\{I_{(2)}^{1/2}/[1 + 1.5\,(I_{(2)}/m°)^{1/2}] - I_{(1)}^{1/2}/[1 + 1.5\,(I_{(1)}/m°)^{1/2}]\} \quad (8)$$

where $k = (RT/F)\ln 10$ and the last term is the ratio of trace chloride activity coefficients $\lg[\gamma°_{Cl(2)}/\gamma°_{Cl(1)}]$, conventionally evaluated via B-G eq. 6′.

Note 4: Since the convention may unevenly affect the $\gamma°_{Cl(2)}$ and $\gamma°_{Cl(1)}$ estimations, ΔpH_I differs from the true value by the unknown contribution: $\lg[\gamma°_{Cl(2)}/\gamma°_{Cl(1)}] - A\{I_{(1)}^{1/2}/[1 + 1.5(I_{(1)}/m°)^{1/2}] - I_{(2)}^{1/2}/[1 + 1.5(I_{(2)}/m°)^{1/2}]\}$.

A second method of comparison is by measurement of Cell II in which there is a salt bridge with two free-diffusion liquid junctions

$$\text{Pt} \mid H_2 \mid PS_2 \; \vdots \; KCl \; (\geq 3.5 \text{ mol dm}^{-3}) \; \vdots \; PS_1 \mid H_2 \mid \text{Pt} \quad \text{Cell II}$$

for which the spontaneous cell reaction is a dilution,

$$H^+(PS_1) \to H^+(PS_2)$$

which gives the pH difference from Cell II as

$$\Delta pH_{II} = pH_{II}(PS_2) - pH_{II}(PS_1) = E_{II}/k - [(E_{j2} - E_{j1})/k] \quad (9)$$

where the subscript II is used to indicate that the pH difference between the same two buffer solutions is now obtained from

TABLE 1: Summary of Useful Properties of Some Primary and Secondary Standard Buffer Substances and Solutions [5]

Salt or Solid Substance	Molecular Formula	Molality/mol kg^{-1}	MolarMass/g mol^{-1}	Density/ g dm^{-3}	Amount Conc. at 20 °C/ mol dm^{-3}	Mass/g to Make 1 dm^3	Dilution Value $\Delta pH_{1/2}$	Buffer Value (β)/ mol $OH^-\ dm^{-3}$	pH Temperature Coefficient/ K^{-1}
Potassium tetroxalate dihydrate	$KH_3C_4O_8 \cdot 2H_2O$	0.1	254.191	1.0091	0.09875	25.101			
Potassium tetroxalate dihydrate	$KH_3C_4O_8 \cdot 2H_2O$	0.05	254.191	1.0032	0.04965	12.620	0.186	0.070	0.001
Potassium hydrogen tartrate (sat. at 25 °C)	$KHC_4H_4O_6$	0.0341	188.18	1.0036	0.034	6.4	0.049	0.027	-0.0014
Potassium dihydrogen citrate	$KH_2C_6H_5O_7$	0.05	230.22	1.0029	0.04958	11.41	0.024	0.034	-0.022
Potassium hydrogen phthalate	$KHC_8H_4O_4$	0.05	204.44	1.0017	0.04958	10.12	0.052	0.016	0.00012
Disodium hydrogen orthophosphate +	Na_2HPO_4	0.025	141.958	1.0038	0.02492	3.5379	0.080	0.029	-0.0028
potassium dihydrogen orthophosphate	KH_2PO_4	0.025	136.085			3.3912			
Disodium hydrogen orthophosphate +	Na_2HPO_4	0.03043	141.959	1.0020	0.03032	4.302	0.07	0.016	-0.0028
potassium dihydrogen orthophosphate	KH_2PO_4	0.00869	136.085		0.008665	1.179			
Disodium tetraborate decahydrate	$Na_2B_4O_7 \cdot 10H_2O$	0.05	381.367	1.0075	0.04985	19.012			
Disodium tetraborate decahydrate	$Na_2B_4O_7 \cdot 10H_2O$	0.01	381.367	1.0001	0.00998	3.806	0.01	0.020	-0.0082
Sodium hydrogen carbonate +	$NaHCO_3$	0.025	84.01	1.0013	0.02492	2.092	0.079	0.029	-0.0096
sodium carbonate	Na_2CO_3	0.025	105.99			2.640			
Calcium hydroxide (sat. at 25°C)	$Ca(OH)_2$	0.0203	74.09	0.9991	0.02025	1.5	-0.28	0.09	-0.033

TABLE 2: Typical Values of pH(PS) for Primary Standards at 0–50 °C (see Section 6.2)

Primary Standards (PS)	Temp./°C										
	0	5	10	15	20	25	30	35	37	40	50
Sat. potassium hydrogen tartrate (at 25 °C)						3.557	3.552	3.549	3.548	3.547	3.549
0.05 mol kg⁻¹ potassium dihydrogen citrate	3.863	3.840	3.820	3.802	3.788	3.776	3.766	3.759	3.756	3.754	3.749
0.05 mol kg⁻¹ potassium hydrogen phthalate	4.000	3.998	3.997	3.998	4.000	4.005	4.011	4.018	4.022	4.027	4.050
0.025 mol kg⁻¹ disodium hydrogen phosphate + 0.025 mol kg⁻¹ potassium dihydrogen phosphate	6.984	6.951	6.923	6.900	6.881	6.865	6.853	6.844	6.841	6.838	6.833
0.03043 mol kg⁻¹ disodium hydrogen phosphate + 0.008695 mol kg⁻¹ potassium dihydrogen phosphate	7.534	7.500	7.472	7.448	7.429	7.413	7.400	7.389	7.386	7.380	7.367
0.01 mol kg⁻¹ disodium tetraborate	9.464	9.395	9.332	9.276	9.225	9.180	9.139	9.102	9.088	9.068	9.011
0.025 mol kg⁻¹ sodium hydrogen carbonate + 0.025 mol kg⁻¹ sodium carbonate	10.317	10.245	10.179	10.118	10.062	10.012	9.966	9.926	9.910	9.889	9.828

Cell II. ΔpH_{II} differs from ΔpH_I (and both differ from the true value ΔpH_t) since it depends on unknown quantity, the residual LJP, RLJP = $(E_{j2} - E_{j1})$, whose exact value could be determined if the true ΔpH were known.

Note 5: The subject of liquid junction effects in ion-selective electrode potentiometry has been comprehensively reviewed [20]. Harper [21] and Bagg [22] have made computer calculations of LJPs for simple three-ion junctions (such as HCl + KCl), the only ones for which mobility and activity coefficient data are available. Breer, Ratkje, and Olsen [23] have thoroughly examined the possible errors arising from the commonly made approximations in calculating LJPs for three-ion junctions. They concluded that the assumption of linear concentration profiles has less-severe consequences (~0.1–1.0 mV) than the other two assumptions of the Henderson treatment, namely constant mobilities and neglect of activity coefficients, which can lead to errors in the order of 10 mV. Breer et al. concluded that their calculations supported an earlier statement [24] that in ion-selective electrode potentiometry, the theoretical Nernst slope, even for dilute sample solutions, could never be attained because of liquid junction effects.

Note 6: According to IUPAC recommendations on nomenclature and symbols [3], a single vertical bar (|) is used to represent a phase boundary, a dashed vertical bar (¦) represents a liquid–liquid junction between two electrolyte solutions (across which a potential difference will occur), and a double dashed vertical bar (¦¦) represents a similar liquid junction, in which the LJP is assumed to be effectively zero (~1 % of cell potential difference). Hence, terms such as that in square brackets on the right-hand side of eq. 9 are usually ignored, and the liquid junction is represented by ¦¦. However, in the Annex, the symbol ¦ is used because the error associated with the liquid junction is included in the analysis. For ease of comparison, numbers of related equations in the main text and in the Annex are indicated.

Note 7: The polarity of Cell II will be negative on the left, i.e., − | +, when pH(PS₂) > pH(PS₁). The LJP E_j of a single liquid junction is defined as the difference in (Galvani) potential contributions to the total cell potential difference arising at the interface from the buffer solution less that from the KCl solution. For instance, in Cell II, $E_{j1} = E(S_1) − E(KCl)$ and $E_{j2} = E(S_2) − E(KCl)$. It is negative when the buffer solution of interest is acidic and positive when it is alkaline, provided that E_j is principally caused by the hydrogen, or hydroxide, ion content of the solution of interest

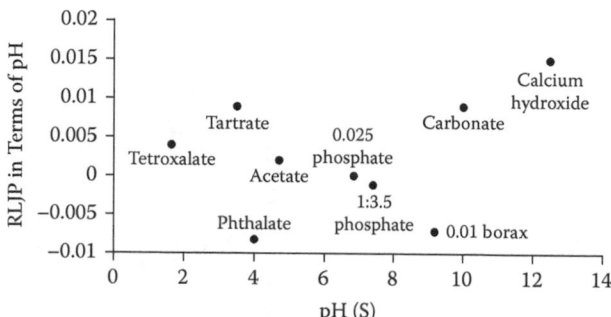

FIGURE 2 Some values of residual LJPs in terms of pH with reference to the value for 0.025 mol kg⁻¹ Na₂HPO₄ + 0.025 mol kg⁻¹ KH₂PO₄ (0.025 phosphate buffer) taken as zero [25].

(and only to a smaller degree by its alkali ions or anions). The residual liquid junction potential (RLJP), the difference E_j(right) − E_j(left), depends on the relative magnitudes of the individual E_j values and has the opposite polarity to the potential difference E of the cell. Hence, in Cell II the RLJP, $E_{j1}(PS_1) − E_{j2}(PS_2)$, has a polarity + | − when pH(S₂) > pH(S₁).

Notwithstanding the foregoing, comparison of pH_{II} values from the Cell II with two liquid junctions (eq. 9) with the assigned pH_I(PS) values for the same two primary buffers measured with Cell I (eq. 8) makes an estimation of RLJPs possible [5]:

$$[pH_I(PS_2) − pH_{II}(PS_2)] − [pH_I(PS_1) − pH_{II}(PS_1)]$$
$$= (E_{j2} − E_{j1})/k = RLJP \qquad (10)$$

With the value of RLJP set equal to zero for equimolal phosphate buffer (taken as PS₁) then $[pH_I(PS_2) − pH_{II}(PS_2)]$ is plotted against pH(PS). Results for free-diffusion liquid junctions formed in a capillary tube with cylindrical symmetry at 25 °C are shown in Figure 2 [25, and refs. cited therein].

Note 8: For 0.05 mol kg⁻¹ tetroxalate, the published values [26] for Cell II with free-diffusion junctions are wrong [27,28].

Values such as those shown in Figure 2 give an indication of the extent of possible systematic uncertainties for primary standard buffers arising from three sources:

i. Experimental uncertainties, including any variations in the chemical purity of primary buffer materials (or variations in the preparation of the solutions) if measurements of Cells I and II were not made in the same laboratory at the same occasion.

ii. Variation in RLJPs between primary buffers.
iii. Inconsistencies resulting from the application of the Bates–Guggenheim convention to chemically different buffer solutions of ionic strengths less than 0.1 mol kg^{-1}.

It may be concluded from examination of the results in Figure 2, that a consistency no better than 0.01 can be ascribed to the primary pH standard solutions of Table 2 in the pH range 3–10. This value will be greater for less reproducibly formed liquid junctions than the free-diffusion type with cylindrical symmetry.

Note 9: Considering the conventional nature of eq. 10, and that the irreproducibility of formation of geometry-dependent devices exceeds possible bias between carefully formed junctions of known geometry, the RLJP contribution, which is included in the difference between measured potential differences of cells with transference, is treated as a statistical, and not a systematic error.

Note 10: Values of RLJP depend on the Bates–Guggenheim convention through the last term in eq. 8 and would be different if another convention were chosen. This interdependence of the single ion activity coefficient and the LJP may be emphasized by noting that it would be possible *arbitrarily* to reduce RLJP values to zero for each buffer by adjusting the ion-size parameter in eq. 6.

7.2 Computational Approach to Consistency

The consistency between conventionally assigned pH values can also be assessed by a computational approach. The pH values of standard buffer solutions have been calculated from literature values of acid dissociation constants by an iterative process. The arbitrary extension of the Batcs–Guggenheim convention for chloride ion, to all ions, leads to the calculation of ionic activity coefficients of all ionic species, ionic strength, buffer capacity, and calculated pH values. The consistency of these values with primary pH values obtained using Cell I was 0.01 or lower between 10 and 40 °C [29,30].

8. Secondary Standards and Secondary Methods of Measurement

8.1 Secondary Standards Derived From Harned Cell Measurements

Substances that do not fulfill all the criteria for primary standards but to which pH values can be assigned using Cell I are considered to be secondary standards. Reasons for their exclusion as primary standards include, inter alia:

i. Difficulties in achieving consistent, suitable chemical quality (e.g., acetic acid is a liquid).
ii. High LJP, or inappropriateness of the Bates–Guggenheim convention (e.g., other charge-type buffers).

Therefore, they do not comply with the stringent criterion for a primary measurement of being of the highest metrological quality. Nevertheless, their pH(SS) values can be determined. Their consistency with the primary standards should be checked with the method described in Section 7. The primary and secondary standard materials should be accompanied by certificates from NMIs in order for them to be described as certified reference materials (CRMs). Some illustrative pH(SS) values for secondary standard materials [5,17,25,31,32] are given in Table 3.

8.2 Secondary Standards Derived From Primary Standards

In most applications, the use of a high-accuracy primary standard for pH measurements is not justified, if a traceable secondary standard of sufficient accuracy is available. Several designs of cells are available for comparing the pH values of two buffer solutions. However, there is no primary method for measuring the *difference* in pH between two buffer solutions for reasons given in Section 8.6. Such measurements could involve either using a cell successively with two buffers, or a single measurement with a cell containing two buffer solutions separated by one or two liquid junctions.

8.3 Secondary Standards Derived from Primary Standards of the Same Nominal Composition Using Cells without Salt Bridge

The most direct way of comparing pH(PS) and pH(SS) is by means of the single-junction Cell III [33].

$$Pt \mid H_2 \mid buffer\ S_2 \mathbin{\vdots} buffer\ S_1 \mid H_2 \mid Pt \qquad Cell\ III$$

The cell reaction for the spontaneous dilution reaction is the same as for Cell II, and the pH difference is given, see Note 6, by

$$pH(S_2) - pH(S_1) = E_{III}/k \qquad (11)\ cf.\ (A\text{-}7)$$

The buffer solutions containing identical Pt $\mid$ H$_2$ electrodes with an identical hydrogen pressure are in direct contact via a vertical sintered glass disk of a suitable porosity (40 μm). The LJP formed between the two standards of nominally the same composition will be particularly small and is estimated to be in the μV range. It will, therefore, be less than 10 % of the potential difference

TABLE 3: Values of pH(SS) of Some Secondary Standards from Harned Cell I Measurements

Secondary Standards	Temp./°C									
	0	5	10	15	20	25	30	37	40	50
0.05 mol kg^{-1} potassium tetroxalate[a] [5,17]		1.67	1.67	1.67	1.68	1.68	1.68	1.69	1.69	1.71
0.05 mol kg^{-1} sodium hydrogen diglycolate[b] [31]		3.47	3.47	3.48	3.48	3.49	3.50	3.52	3.53	3.56
0.1 mol dm^{-3} acetic acid + 0.1 mol dm^{-3} sodium acetate [25]	4.68	4.67	4.67	4.66	4.66	4.65	4.65	4.66	4.66	4.68
0.1 mol dm^{-3} acetic acid + 0.1 mol dm^{-3} sodium acetate [25]	4.74	4.73	4.73	4.72	4.72	4.72	4.72	4.73	4.73	4.75
0.02 mol kg^{-1} piperazine phosphate[c] [32]	6.58	6.51	6.45	6.39	6.34	6.29	6.24	6.16	6.14	6.06
0.05 mol kg^{-1} tris hydrochloride + 0.01667 mol kg^{-1} tris[c] [5]	8.47	8.30	8.14	7.99	7.84	7.70	7.56	7.38	7.31	7.07
0.05 mol kg^{-1} disodium tetraborate	9.51	9.43	9.36	9.30	9.25	9.19	9.15	9.09	9.07	9.01
Saturated (at 25°C) calcium hydroxide [5]	13.42	13.21	13.00	12.81	12.63	12.45	12.29	12.07	11.98	11.71

[a] potassium trihydrogen dioxalate (KH$_3$C$_4$O$_8$).
[b] sodium hydrogen 2,2'-oxydiacetate.
[c] 2-amino-2-(hydroxymethyl)-1,3 propanediol or tris(hydroxymethyl)aminomethane.

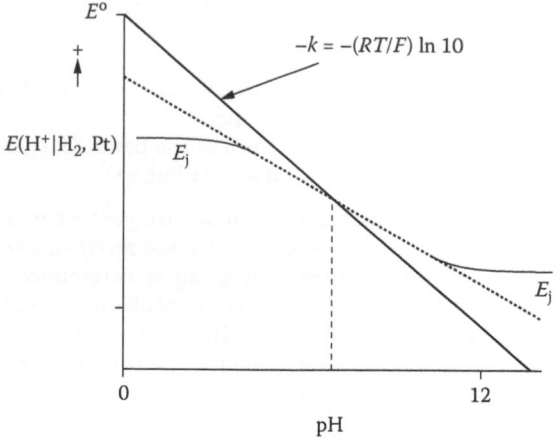

FIGURE 3 Schematic plot of the variation of potential difference (————) for the cell‑$Ag|AgCl|KCl$ H^+ (buffer)$|H2|Pt^+$ with pH and illustrating the choice of sign convention. The effect of LJP is indicated (————) with its variation of pH as given by the Henderson equation (see, e.g., ref. [5]). The approximate linearity (————) in the middle pH region should be noted. Both lines have been grossly exaggerated in their deviation from the Nernst line since otherwise they would be indistinguishable from each other and the Nernst line. For the calomel electrode $Hg|Hg_2Cl_2|KCl$ and the thallium amalgam$|$thallium(I) chloride electrode $Hg|Tl(Hg)|TlCl|KCl$, or any other constant potential reference electrode, the diagram is the same.

measured if the pH(S) values of the standard solutions are in the range $3 \leq$ pH(S) ≤ 11 and the difference in their pH(S) values is not larger than 0.02. Under these conditions, the LJP is not dominated by the hydrogen and hydroxyl ions but by the other ions (anions, alkali metal ions). The proper functioning of the cell can be checked by measuring the potential difference when both sides of the cell contain the same solution.

8.4 Secondary Standards Derived from Primary Standards Using Cells with Salt Bridge

The cell that includes a hydrogen electrode [corrected to 1 atm (101.325 kPa) partial pressure of hydrogen] and a reference electrode, the filling solution of which is a saturated or high concentration of the almost equitransferent electrolyte, potassium chloride, hence minimizing the LJP, is, see Note 6:

$$Ag|AgC|KCl\ (\geq 3.5\ \text{mol dm}^{-3})\ \vdots\ \text{buffer S} \mid H_2 \mid Pt \qquad \text{Cell IV}$$

Note 11: Other electrolytes, e.g., rubidium or cesium chloride, are more equitransferent [34].

Note 12: Cell IV is written in the direction: *reference| indicator*

i. for conformity of treatment of all hydrogen ion-responsive electrodes and ion-selective electrodes with various choices of reference electrode, and partly,

ii. for the practical reason that pH meters usually have one low impedance socket for the reference electrode, assumed negative, and a high-impedance terminal with a different plug, usually for a glass electrode.

With this convention, whatever the form of hydrogen ion-responsive electrode used (e.g., glass or quinhydrone), or whatever the reference electrode, the potential of the hydrogen-ion

responsive electrode always decreases (becomes more negative) with increasing pH (see Figure 3).

This convention was used in the 1985 document [2] and is also consistent with the treatment of ion-selective electrodes [35]. In effect, it focuses attention on the indicator electrode, for which the potential is then given by the Nernst equation for the single-electrode potential, written as a reduction process, in accord with the Stockholm convention [36]:

$$\text{For Ox} + ne^- \rightarrow \text{Red}, E = E° - (k/n)\ \lg(a_{\text{red}}/a_{\text{ox}})$$

(where a is activity), or, for the hydrogen gas electrode at 1 atm partial pressure of hydrogen gas:

$$H^+ + e^- \rightarrow {}^{1/2}H_2\ \ E = E° + k\lg a_{H^+} = E° - k\text{pH}$$

The equation for Cell IV is, therefore:

$$\text{pH(S)} = -[E_{\text{IV}}(S) - E_{\text{IV}}°']/k \qquad (12)$$

in which $E_{\text{IV}}°'$ is the standard potential, which includes the term $\lg a_{\text{Cl}}/m°$, and E_j is the LJP.

Note 13: Mercury–mercury(I) chloride (calomel) and thallium amalgam–thallium (I) chloride reference electrodes are alternative choices to the silver–silver chloride electrode in Cell IV.

The consecutive use of two such cells containing buffers S_1 and S_2 gives the pH difference of the solutions

$$\text{pH(S}_2) - \text{pH(S}_1) = -[E_{\text{IV}}(S_2) - E_{\text{IV}}(S_1)]/k \qquad (13)\ cf.\ (A\text{-}8)$$

Note 14: Experimentally, a three-limb electrode vessel allowing simultaneous measurement of two Cell IIs may be used [25] with the advantage that the stability with time of the electrodes and of the liquid junctions can be checked. The measurement of cells of type II, which has a salt bridge with two liquid junctions, has been discussed in Section 7.

Cells II and IV may also be used to measure the value of secondary buffer standards that are not compatible with the silver–silver chloride electrode used in Cell I. Since the LJPs in Cells II and IV are minimized by the use of an equitransferent salt, these cells are suitable for use with secondary buffers that have a different concentration and/or an ionic strength greater than the limit ($I \leq 0.1$ mol kg^{-1}) imposed by the Bates–Guggenheim convention. They may, however, also be used for comparing solutions of the same nominal composition.

8.5 Secondary Standards From Glass Electrode Cells

Measurements cannot be made with a hydrogen electrode in Cell IV, for example, if the buffer is reduced by hydrogen gas at the platinum (or palladium-coated platinum) electrode. Cell V involving a glass electrode and silver–silver chloride reference electrode may be used instead in consecutive measurements, with two buffers S_1, S_2 (see Section 11 for details).

8.6 Secondary Methods

The equations given for Cells II to V show that these cannot be considered primary (ratio) methods for measuring pH difference [1], (see also Section 12.1) because the cell reactions involve transference, or the irreversible inter-diffusion of ions, and hence an LJP contribution to the measured potential difference. The value of this potential difference depends on the ionic constituents, their concentrations and the geometry of the liquid junction between the solutions. Hence, the measurement equations contain terms that, although small, are not quantifiable, and the methods are secondary not primary.

9. Consistency of Secondary Standard Buffer Solutions Established with Respect to Primary Standards

9.1 Summary of Procedures for Establishing Secondary Standards

The following procedures may be distinguished for establishing secondary standards (SS) with respect to primary standards:

i. For SS of the same nominal composition as PS, use Cells III or II.
ii. For SS of different composition, use Cells IV or II.
iii. For SS not compatible with platinum hydrogen electrode, use Cell V (see Section 11.1).

Although any of Cells II to V could be used for certification of secondary standards with stated uncertainty, employing different procedures would lead to inconsistencies. It would be difficult to define specific terminology to distinguish each of these procedures or to define any rigorous hierarchy for them. Hence, the methods should include estimates of the typical uncertainty for each. The choice between methods should be made according to the uncertainty required for the application (see Section 10 and Table 4).

9.2 Secondary Standard Evaluation from Primary Standards of the Same Composition

It is strongly recommended that the preferred method for assigning secondary standards should be a procedure in which measurements are made with respect to the primary buffer of nominally the same chemical composition. All secondary standards should be accompanied by a certificate relating to that particular batch of reference material as significant batch-to-batch variations are likely to occur. Some secondary standards are disseminated in solution form. The uncertainty of the pH values of such solutions may be larger than those for material disseminated in solid form.

9.3 Secondary Standard Evaluation When There is no Primary Standard of the Same Composition

It may sometimes be necessary to set up a secondary standard when there is no primary standard of the same chemical composition available. It will, therefore, be necessary to use either Cells II, IV, or V, and a primary or secondary standard buffer of different chemical composition. Buffers measured in this way will have a different status from those measured with respect to primary standards because they are not directly traceable to a primary standard of the same chemical composition. This different status should be reflected in the, usually larger, uncertainty quoted for such a buffer. Since this situation will only occur for buffers when a primary standard is not available, no special nomenclature is recommended to distinguish the different routes to secondary standards. Secondary buffers of a composition different from those of primary standards can also be derived from measurements on Cell I, provided the buffer is compatible with Cell I. However, the uncertainty of such standards should reflect the limitations of the secondary standard (see Table 4).

10. Target Uncertainties for the Measurement of Secondary Buffer Solutions

10.1 Uncertainties of Secondary Standards Derived from Primary Standards

Cells II to IV (and occasionally Cell V) are used to measure secondary standards with respect to primary standards. In each case, the limitations associated with the measurement method will result in a greater uncertainty for the secondary standard than the primary standard from which it was derived.

Target uncertainties are listed in Table 4. However, these uncertainties do not take into account the uncertainty contribution arising from the adoption of the Bates–Guggenheim convention to achieve traceability to SI units.

10.2 Uncertainty Evaluation [37]

Summaries of typical uncertainty calculations for Cells I–V are given in the Annex (Section 13).

11. Calibration of pH Meter-Electrode Assemblies and Target Uncertainties for Unknowns

11.1 Glass Electrode Cells

Practical pH measurements are carried out by means of Cell V reference electrode | KCl ($c \geq 3.5$ mol dm^{-3}) ¦¦ solution[pH(S) or pH(X)] | glass electrode Cell V and pH(X) is obtained, see Note 6, from eq. 14

TABLE 4: Summary of Recommended Target Uncertainties

	U(pH) (For coverage factor 2)	Comments
PRIMARY STANDARDS		
Uncertainty of PS measured (by an NMI) with Harned Cell I	0.004	
Repeatability of PS measured (by an NMI) with Harned Cell I	0.0015	
Reproducibility of measurements in comparisons with Harned Cell I	0.003	EUROMET comparisons
Typical variations between batches of PS buffers	0.003	
SECONDARY STANDARDS		
Value of SS compared with same PS material with Cell III	0.004	increase in uncertainty is negligible relative to PS used e.g., biological buffers
Value of SS measured in Harned Cell I	0.01	
Value of SS labeled against different PS with Cell II or IV	0.015	
Value of SS (not compatible with Pt | H$_2$) measured with Cell V	0.02	example based on phthalate
ELECTRODE CALIBRATION		
Multipoint (5-point) calibration	0.01–0.03	
Calibration (2-point) by bracketing	0.02–0.03	
Calibration (1-point), ΔpH = 3 and assumed slope	0.3	

Note: None of the above includes the uncertainty associated with the Bates–Guggenheim convention so the results cannot be considered to be traceable to SI (see Section 5.2).

$$pH(X) = pH(S) - [E_V(X) - E_V(S)] \qquad (14)$$

This is a one-point calibration (see Section 11.3).

These cells often use glass electrodes in the form of single probes or combination electrodes (glass and reference electrodes fashioned into a single probe, a so-called "combination electrode").

The potential difference of Cell V is made up of contributions arising from the potentials of the glass and reference electrodes and the liquid junction (see Section 7.1).

Various random and systematic effects must be noted when using these cells for pH measurements:

i. Glass electrodes may exhibit a slope of the E vs. pH function smaller than the theoretical value [$k = (RT/F)\ln 10$], often called a sub-Nernstian response or practical slope k', which is experimentally determinable. A theoretical explanation for the sub-Nernstian response of pH glass electrodes in terms of the dissociation of functional groups at the glass surface has been given [38].

ii. The response of the glass electrode may vary with time, history of use, and memory effects. It is recommended that the response time and the drift of the electrodes be taken into account [39].

iii. The potential of the glass electrode is strongly temperature-dependent, as to a lesser extent are the other two terms. Calibrations and measurements should, therefore, be carried out under temperature-controlled conditions.

iv. The LJP varies with the composition of the solutions forming the junction, e.g., with pH (see Figure 2). Hence, it will change if one solution [pH(S) or pH(X)] in Cell V is replaced by another. It is also affected by the geometry of the liquid junction device. Hence, it may be different if a free-diffusion type junction, such as that used to measure the RLJP (see Section 7.1), is replaced by another type, such as a sleeve, ceramic diaphragm, fiber, or platinum junction [39,40].

v. Liquid junction devices, particularly some commercial designs, may suffer from memory and clogging effects.

vi. The LJP may be subject to hydrodynamic effects, e.g., stirring.

Since these effects introduce errors of unknown magnitude, the measurement of an unknown sample requires a suitable calibration procedure. Three procedures are in common use based on calibrations at one point (one-point calibration), two points (two-point calibration or bracketing), and a series of points (multipoint calibration).

11.2 Target Uncertainties for Unknowns

Uncertainties in pH(X) are obtained, as shown below, by several procedures involving different numbers of experiments. Numerical values of these uncertainties obtained from the different calibration procedures are, therefore, not directly comparable. It is, therefore, not possible at the present time to make a universal recommendation of the best procedure to adopt for all applications. Hence, the target uncertainty for the unknown is given, which the operator of a pH meter electrode assembly may reasonably seek to achieve. Values are given for each of the three techniques (see Table 4), but the uncertainties attainable experimentally are critically dependent on the factors listed in Section 11.1 above, on the quality of the electrodes, and on the experimental technique for changing solutions.

In order to obtain the overall uncertainty of the measurement, uncertainties of the respective pH(PS) or pH(SS) values must be taken into account (see Table 4). Target uncertainties given below, and in Table 4, refer to calibrations performed by the use of standard buffer solutions with an uncertainty U[pH(PS)] or U[pH(SS)] d 0.01. The overall uncertainty becomes higher if standards with higher uncertainties are used.

11.3 One-Point Calibration

A single-point calibration is insufficient to determine both slope and one-point parameters. The theoretical value for the slope can be assumed, but the practical slope may be up to 5% lower. Alternatively, a value for the practical slope can be assumed from the manufacturer's prior calibration. The one-point calibration, therefore, yields only an estimate of pH(X). Since both parameters may change with age of the electrodes, this is not a reliable procedure. Based on a measurement for which ΔpH = |pH(X) − pH(S)| = 5, the expanded uncertainty would be U = 0.5 in pH(X) for k' = 0.95k, but assumed theoretical, or U = 0.3 in pH(X) for ΔpH = |pH(X) − pH(S)| = 3 (see Table 4). This approach could be satisfactory for certain applications. The uncertainty will decrease with decreasing difference pH(X) − pH(S) and be smaller if k' is known from prior calibration.

11.4 Two-Point Calibration {Target Uncertainty, U[pH(X)] = 0.02–0.03 at 25 °C}

In the majority of practical applications, glass electrodes cells (Cell V) are calibrated by two-point calibration, or bracketing, procedure using two standard buffer solutions, with pH values pH(S_1) and pH(S_2), bracketing the unknown pH(X). Bracketing is often taken to mean that the pH(S_1) and pH(S_2) buffers selected should be those that are immediately above and below pH(X). This may not be appropriate in all situations and choice of a wider range may be better.

If the respective potential differences measured are $E_V(S_1)$, $E_V(S_2)$, and $E_V(X)$, the pH value of the unknown, pH(X), is obtained from eq. 15

$$pH(X) = pH(S_1) - [E_V(X) - E_V(S_1)]/k' \quad (15) \text{ cf. (A-10)}$$

where the practical slope factor (k') is given by

$$k' = [EV(S_1) - E_V(S_2)]/[pH(S_2) - pH(S_1)] \qquad (16)$$

An example is given in the Annex, Section 13.

11.5 Multipoint Calibration {Target Uncertainty: U[pH(X)] = 0.01–0.03 at 25 °C}

Multipoint calibration is carried out using up to five standard buffers [39,40]. The use of more than five points does not yield any significant improvement in the statistical information obtainable.

The calibration function of Cell V is given by eq. 17

$$E_V(S) = E_V^\circ - k'pH(S) \qquad (17) \text{ cf. (A-11)}$$

where $E_V(S)$ is the measured potential difference when the solution of pH(S) in Cell V is a primary or secondary standard buffer. The intercept, or "standard potential", E_V° and k', the practical slope are determined by linear regression of eq. 17 [39–41].

pH(X) of an unknown solution is then obtained from the potential difference, $E_V(X)$, by

$$pH(X) = [E_V^\circ - E_V(X)]/k' \qquad (18) \text{ cf. (A-12)}$$

Additional quantities obtainable from the regression procedure applied to eq. 17 are the uncertainties $u(k')$ and $u(E_V{}^\circ)$ [40]. Multipoint calibration is recommended when minimum uncertainty and maximum consistency are required over a wide range of pH(X) values. This applies, however, only to that range of pH values in which the calibration function is truly linear. In nonlinear regions of the calibration function, the two-point method has clear advantages provided that pH(S₁) and pH(S₂) are selected to be as close to pH(X) as possible.

Details of the uncertainty computations for the multipoint calibration have been given [40], and an example is given in the Annex. The uncertainties are recommended as a means of checking the performance characteristics of pH meter-electrode assemblies [40]. By careful selection of electrodes for multipoint calibration, uncertainties of the unknown pH(X) can be kept as low as $U[\text{pH(X)}] = 0.01$.

In modern microprocessor pH meters, potential differences are often transformed automatically into pH values. Details of the calculations involved in such transformations, including the uncertainties, are available [41].

12. Glossary [2,15,44]

12.1 Primary Method of Measurement

A primary method of measurement is a method having the highest metrological qualities, whose operation can be completely described and understood, for which a complete uncertainty statement can be written down in terms of SI units.

A primary direct method measures the value of an unknown without reference to a standard of the same quantity.

A primary ratio method measures the value of a ratio of an unknown to a standard of the same quantity; its operation must be completely described by a measurement equation.

12.2 Primary Standard

Standard that is designated or widely acknowledged as having the highest metrological qualities and whose value is accepted without reference to other standards of the same quantity.

12.3 Secondary Standard

Standard whose value is assigned by comparison with a primary standard of the same quantity.

12.4 Traceability

Property of the result of a measurement or the value of a standard whereby it can be related to stated references, usually national or international standards, through an unbroken chain of comparisons all having stated uncertainties. The concept is often expressed by the adjective traceable. The unbroken chain of comparisons is called a traceability chain.

12.5 Primary pH Standards

Aqueous solutions of selected reference buffer solutions to which pH(PS) values have been assigned over the temperature range 0–50 °C from measurements on cells without transference, called Harned cells, by use of the Bates–Guggenheim convention.

12.6 Bates–Guggenheim Convention

A convention based on a form of the Debye–Hückel equation that approximates the logarithm of the single ion activity coefficient of chloride and uses a fixed value of 1.5 for the product Ba in the denominator at all temperatures in the range 0–50 °C (see eqs. 4, 5) and ionic strength of the buffer < 0.1 mol kg⁻¹.

12.7 Secondary pH Standards

Values that may be assigned to secondary standard pH(SS) solutions at each temperature:

    i. with reference to [pH(PS)] values of a primary standard of the same nominal composition by Cell III,
    ii. with reference to [pH(PS)] values of a primary standard of different composition by Cells II, IV or V, or
    iii. by use of Cell I.

Note 15: This is an exception to the usual definition, see Section 12.3.

12.8 pH Glass Electrode

Hydrogen-ion responsive electrode usually consisting of a bulb, or other suitable form, of special glass attached to a stem of high-resistance glass complete with internal reference electrode and internal filling solution system. Other geometrical forms may be appropriate for special applications, e.g., capillary electrode for measurement of blood pH.

12.9 Glass Electrode Error

Deviation of a glass electrode from the hydrogen-ion response function. An example often encountered is the error due to sodium ions at alkaline pH values, which by convention is regarded as positive.

12.10 Hydrogen Gas Electrode

A thin foil of platinum electrolytically coated with a finely divided deposit of platinum or (in the case of a reducible substance) palladium metal, which catalyzes the electrode reaction: $H^+ + e \rightarrow \frac{1}{2} H_2$ in solutions saturated with hydrogen gas. It is customary to correct measured values to standard 1 atm (101.325 kPa) partial pressure of hydrogen gas.

12.11 Reference Electrode

External electrode system that comprises an inner element, usually silver–silver chloride, mercury–mercury(I) chloride (calomel), or thallium amalgam–thallium(I) chloride, a chamber containing the appropriate filling solution (see 12.14), and a device for forming a liquid junction (e.g., capillary) ceramic plug, frit, or ground glass sleeve.

12.12 Liquid Junction

Any junction between two electrolyte solutions of different composition. Across such a junction there arises a potential difference, called the liquid junction potential. In Cells II, IV, and V, the junction is between the pH standard or unknown solution and the filling solution, or the bridge solution (q.v.), of the reference electrode.

12.13 Residual Liquid Junction Potential Error

Error arising from breakdown in the assumption that the LJPs cancel in Cell II when solution X is substituted for solution S in Cell V.

12.14 Filling Solution (of a Reference Electrode)

Solution containing the anion to which the reference electrode of Cells IV and V is reversible, e.g., chloride for silver–silver chloride electrode. In the absence of a bridge solution (q.v.), a high concentration of filling solution comprising almost equitransferent cations and anions is employed as a means of maintaining the LJP small and approximately constant on substitution of unknown solution for standard solution(s).

12.15 Bridge (or Salt Bridge) Solution (of a Double Junction Reference Electrode)

Solution of high concentration of inert salt, preferably comprising cations and anions of equal mobility, optionally interposed between the reference electrode filling and both the unknown and standard solution, when the test solution and filling solution are chemically incompatible. This procedure introduces into the cell a second liquid junction formed, usually, in a similar way to the first.

12.16 Calibration

Set of operations that establish, under specified conditions, the relationship between values of quantities indicated by a measuring instrument, or measuring system, or values represented by a material measure or a reference material, and the corresponding values realized by standards.

12.17 Uncertainty (of a Measurement)

Parameter, associated with the result of a measurement, which characterizes the dispersion of the values that could reasonably be attributed to the measurand.

12.18 Standard Uncertainty, u_x

Uncertainty of the result of a measurement expressed as a standard deviation.

12.19 Combined Standard Uncertainty, $u_c(y)$

Standard uncertainty of the result of a measurement when that result is obtained from the values of a number of other quantities, equal to the positive square root of a sum of terms, the terms being the variances, or covariances of these other quantities, weighted according to how the measurement result varies with changes in these quantities.

12.20 Expanded uncertainty, U

Quantity defining an interval about the result of a measurement that may be expected to encompass a large fraction of the distribution of values that could reasonably be attributed to the measurand.

Note 16: The fraction may be viewed as the coverage probability or level of confidence of the interval.

Note 17: To associate a specific level of confidence with the interval defined by the expanded uncertainty requires explicit or implicit assumptions regarding the probability distribution characterized by the measurement result and its combined standard uncertainty. The level of confidence that may be attributed to this interval can be known only to the extent to which such assumptions may be justified.

Note 18: Expanded uncertainty is sometimes termed overall uncertainty.

12.21 Coverage Factor

Numerical factor used as a multiplier of the combined standard uncertainty in order to obtain an expanded uncertainty

Note 19: A coverage factor is typically in the range 2 to 3. The value 2 is used throughout in the Annex.

13. Annex: Measurement Uncertainty

Examples are given of uncertainty budgets for pH measurements at the primary, secondary, and working level. The calculations are done in accordance with published procedures [15,37].

When a measurement (y) results from the values of a number of other quantities, $y = f(x_1, x_2, \ldots x_i)$, the combined standard uncertainty of the measurement is obtained from the square root of the expression

$$u_c^2(y) = \sum_{i=1}^{n} \left(\frac{\partial f}{\partial x_i} \right) \cdot u^2(x_i)$$

where $\frac{\partial f}{\partial x_i}$ is called the sensitivity coefficient (c_i). This equation holds for uncorrelated quantities. The ∂x_i equation for correlated quantities is more complex.

The uncertainty stated is the expanded uncertainty, U, obtained by multiplying the standard uncertainty, $u_c(y)$, by an appropriate coverage factor. When the result has a large number of degrees of freedom, the use of a value of 2 leads to approximately 95% confidence that the true value lies in the range $\pm U$. The value of 2 will be used throughout this Annex.

The following sections give illustrative examples of the uncertainty calculations for Cells I–V.

After the assessment of uncertainties, there should be a reappraisal of experimental design factors and statistical treatment of the data, with due regard for economic factors before the adoption of more elaborate procedures.

A.1 Uncertainty Budget for the Primary Method of Measurement Using Cell I

Experimental details have been published [42–45].

A.1.1 Measurement Equations

The primary method for the determination of pH(PS) values consists of the following steps (Section 4.1):

1. Determination of the standard potential of the Ag | AgCl electrode from the acid-filled cell (Cell Ia)

$$E^\circ = E_a + 2k \lg(m_{HCl}/m^\circ) + 2k \lg \gamma_{HCl} - (k/2) \lg(p^\circ/p_{H_2})$$

$$\text{(A-2) cf. (3)}$$

where $E_{Ia} = E_a - (k/2) \lg(p^\circ/p_{H_2})$, $k = (RT/F)\ln 10$, p_{H_2} is the partial pressure of hydrogen in Cell Ia, and p° is the standard pressure.

TABLE 6: Calculation of Standard Uncertainty of the Standard Potential of the Silver–Silver Chloride Electrode (E°) from Measurements in $m_{HCl} = 0.01$ mol kg^{-1}

Quantity	Estimate x_i	Standard Uncertainty $u(x_i)$	Sensitivity Coefficient $|c_i|$	Uncertainty Contribution $u_i(y)$
E/V	0.464	2×10^{-5}	1	2×10^{-5}
T/K	298.15	8×10^{-3}	8.1×10^{-4}	6.7×10^{-6}
m_{HCl}/mol kg^{-1}	0.01	1×10^{-5}	5.14	5.1×10^{-5}
p_{H_2}/kPa	101.000	0.003	1.3×10^{-7}	4.2×10^{-7}
$\Delta E(\text{Ag/AgCl})$/V Bias potential	3.5×10^{-5}	3.5×10^{-5}	1	3.5×10^{-5}
$\gamma_\pm$	0.9042	9.3×10^{-4}	0.0568	5.2×10^{-6}

$u_c(E^\circ) = 6.5 \times 10^{-5}$ V

Note 20: The uncertainty of method used for the determination of hydrochloric acid concentration is critical. The uncertainty quoted here is for potentiometric silver chloride titration. The uncertainty for coulometry is about 10 times lower.

TABLE 7: Calculation of the Standard Uncertainty of the Acidity Function $\lg(a_H\gamma_{Cl})$ for $m_{Cl} = 0.005$ mol kg^{-1}

Quantity	Estimate x_i	Standard Uncertainty $u(x_i)$	Sensitivity Coefficient $|c_i|$	Uncertainty Contribution $u_i(y)$
E/V	0.770	2×10^{-5}	16.9	3.4×10^{-4}
$E°/V$	0.222	6.5×10^{-5}	16.9	1.1×10^{-3}
T/K	298.15	8×10^{-3}	0.031	2.5×10^{-4}
$m_{Cl}/$mol kg^{-1}	0.005	2.2×10^{-6}	86.86	1.9×10^{-4}
$p_{H_2}/$kPa	101.000	0.003	2.2×10^{-6}	7×10^{-6}
$\Delta E(\text{Ag/AgCl})/V$	3.5×10^{-5}	3.5×10^{-5}	16.9	5.9×10^{-4}

$u_c[\lg(a_H\gamma_{Cl})] = 0.0013$

Note 21: If, as is usual practice in some NMIs [42–44], acid and buffer cells are measured at the same time, then the pressure measuring instrument uncertainty quoted above (0.003 kPa) cancels, but there remains the possibility of a much smaller bubbler depth variation between cells.

TABLE 8: S_1 = Primary Buffer, pH(PS) = 4.005, u(pH) = 0.003; S_2 = Secondary Buffer, pH(SS) = 6.86. Free-Diffusion Junctions with Cylindrical Symmetry Formed in Vertical Tubes Were Used [25]

Quantity	Estimate x_i	Standard Uncertainty $u(x_i)$	Sensitivity Coefficient $|c_i|$	Uncertainty Contribution $u_i(y)$
pH(S_1)	4.005	0.003	1	0.003
E_{II}/V	0.2	1×10^{-5}	16.9	1.7×10^{-4}
$(E_{j2} - E_{j1})/V$	3.5×10^{-4}	3.5×10^{-4}	16.9	6×10^{-3}
T/K	298.15	0.1	1.2×10^{-5}	1.2×10^{-6}

$u_c[\text{pH}(S_2)] = 0.007$

Note 22: The error in E_{II} is estimated as the scatter from 3 measurements. The RLJP contribution is estimated from Figure 2 as 0.006 in pH; it is the principal contribution to the uncertainty.

2. Determination of the acidity function, $p(a_H\gamma_{Cl})$, in the buffer-filled cell (Cell I)

$$-\lg(a_H\gamma_{Cl}) = (E_b - E°)/k + \lg(m_{Cl}/m°)$$
$$-(1/2)\lg(p°/p_{H_2}), \qquad \text{(A-3) cf. (2)}$$

where $E_I = E_b - (k/2)\lg(p°/p_{H_2})$, p_{H_2} is the partial pressure of hydrogen in Cell I, and $p°$ the standard pressure.

3. Extrapolation of the acidity function to zero chloride concentration

$$-\lg(a_H\gamma_{Cl}) = -\lg(a_H\gamma_{Cl})° + Sm_{Cl} \qquad \text{(A-4) cf. (5)}$$

4. pH Determination

$$\text{pH(PS)} = -\lg(a_H\gamma_{Cl})° + \lg\gamma°_{Cl} \qquad \text{(A-5)}$$

where $\lg\gamma°_{Cl}$ is calculated from the Bates–Guggenheim convention (see eq. 6). Values of the Debye–Hückel limiting law slope for 0 to 50 °C are given in Table 14 [46].

A.1.2 Uncertainty Budget

Example: PS = 0.025 mol kg^{-1} disodium hydrogen phosphate + 0.025 mol kg^{-1} potassium dihydrogen phosphate.

The standard uncertainty due to the extrapolation to zero added chloride concentration (Section 4.4) depends in detail on the number of data points available and the concentration range. Consequently, it is not discussed in detail here. This calculation may increase the expanded uncertainty (of the acidity function at zero concentration) to $U = 0.004$.

As discussed in Section 5.2, the uncertainty due to the use of the Bates–Guggenheim convention includes two components:

i. The uncertainty of the convention itself, and this is estimated to be approximately 0.01. This contribution to the uncertainty is required if the result is to be traceable to SI, but will not be included in the uncertainty of "conventional" pH values.

ii. The contribution to the uncertainty from the value of the ionic strength should be calculated for each individual case.

The typical uncertainty for Cell I is between $U = 0.003$ and $U = 0.004$.

A.2 Uncertainty Budget for Secondary pH Buffer using Cell II

$$\text{Pt} | H_2 | S_2 \,\vdots\, \text{KCl} (\geq 3.5 \text{ mol dm}^{-3}) \,\vdots\, S_1 | H_2 | \text{Pt} \qquad \text{Cell II}$$

where S_1 and S_2 are different buffers.

A.2.1 Measurement Equations
1. Determination of pH(S_2) pH$_{II}$(S_2)

$$-\text{pH}_{II}(S_1) = E_{II}/k - (E_{j2} - E_{j1})/k \qquad \text{(A-6) cf. (9)}$$

2. Theoretical slope, $k = (RT/F)\ln 10$

A.2.2 Uncertainty Budget
Therefore, $U[\text{pH}(S_2)] = 0.014$.

A.3 Uncertainty Budget for Secondary pH Buffer using Cell III

$$\text{Pt} | H_2 | \text{Buffer } S_2 \,\vdots\, \text{Buffer } S_1 | H_2 | \text{Pt} \qquad \text{Cell III}$$

A.3.1 Measurement Equations
1. $\text{pH}(S_2) - \text{pH}(S_1) = (E_{III} + E_j)/k \qquad \text{(A-7) cf. (11)}$
2. $k = (RT/F)\ln 10$

For experimental details, see refs. [16,33,38].

Therefore, U[pH(S_2)] = 0.004. The uncertainty is no more than that of the primary standard PS_1.

A.4 Uncertainty Budget for Secondary pH Buffer using Cell IV

$$Ag \mid AgCl \mid KCl \ (\geq 3.5 \ mol \ dm^{-3}) \mid buffer$$
$$S_1 \ or \ S_2 \mid H_2 \mid Pt \qquad Cell \ IV$$

A.4.1 Measurement Equations
1. Determination of pH(S_2)

$$pH_{IV}(S_2) - pH_{IV}(S_1) = -[E_{IV}(S_2) - E_{IV}(S_1)]/k$$
$$- (E_{j2} - E_{j1})/k \qquad (A-8) \ cf. \ (13)$$

2. Theoretical slope, $k = (RT/F)\ln 10$

A.4.2 Uncertainty Budget
Therefore, U[pH(S_2)] = 0.016.

A.5 Uncertainty Budget for Unknown pH(X) Buffer Determination using Cell V

$$Ag \mid AgCl \mid KCl \ (\geq 3.5 \ mol \ dm^{-3}) \mid Buffer \ pH(S) \ or$$
$$pH(X) \mid glass \ electrode \qquad Cell \ V$$

A.5.1 Measurement Equations: 2-Point Calibration (Bracketing)
1. Determination of the practical slope (k')

$$k' = [(E_V(S_2) - E_V(S_1)]/[pH(S_2) - pH(S_1)] \quad (A-9) \ cf. \ (16)$$

2. Measurement of unknown solution (X)

$$(X) \ pH(X) = pH(S_1)$$

$$-[E_V(X) - E_V(S_1)]/k' - (E_{j2} - E_{j1})/k' \quad (A-10) \ cf. \ (15)$$

A.5.2 Uncertainty Budget
Example of two-point calibration (bracketing) with a pH combination electrode [47].

TABLE 9: pH (S_2) Determination. S_1 = Primary Standard (PS) and S_2 = Secondary Standard (SS) are of the Same Nominal Composition. Example: 0.025 mol kg⁻¹ Disodium Hydrogen Phosphate + 0.025 mol kg⁻¹ Potassium Dihydrogen Phosphate, PS_1 = 6.865, u(pH) = 0.002

Quantity	Estimate x_i	Standard Uncertainty $u(x_i)$	Sensitivity Coefficient $\|c_i\|$	Uncertainty Contribution $u_i(y)$
pH(PS_1)	6.865	2×10^{-3}	1	2×10^{-3}
$[E(S_2) - E(S_1)]$/V	1×10^{-4}	1×10^{-6}	16.9	16.9×10^{-6}
$[E_{id}(S_2) - E_{id}(S_1)]$/V	1×10^{-6}	1×10^{-6}	16.9	1.7×10^{-5}
Ej/V	1×10^{-5}	1×10^{-5}	16.9	16.9×10^{-5}
T/K	298.15	2×10^{-3}	5×10^{-6}	1×10^{-8}

u_c[pH(S_2)] = 0.002

Note 23: $[E_{id}(S_2) - E_{id}(S_1)]$ is the difference in cell potential when both compartments are filled with solution made up from the same sample of buffer material. The estimate of E_j comes from the observations made of the result of perturbing the pH of samples by small additions of strong acid or alkali, and supported by Henderson equation considerations, that E_j contributes about 10 % to the total cell potential difference [33].

TABLE 10: Example from the Work of Paabo and Bates [5] Supplemented by Private Communication from Bates to Covington. S_1 = 0.05 mol kg⁻¹ Equimolal Phosphate; S_2 = 0.05 mol kg⁻¹ Potassium Hydrogen Phthalate. KCl = 3.5 mol dm⁻³. S_1 = Primary Buffer PS_1, pH = 6.86, u(pH) = 0.003, S_2 = Secondary Buffer SS_2, pH = 4.01

Quantity	Estimate x_i	Standard Uncertainty $u(x_i)$	Sensitivity Coefficient $\|c_i\|$	Uncertainty Contribution $u_i(y)$
pH(S_1)	6.86	0.003	1	0.003
ΔE_{IV}/V	0.2	2.5×10^{-4}	16.9	4×10^{-3}
$(E_{j2} - E_{j1})$/V	3.5×10^{-4}	3.5×10^{-4}	16.9	6×10^{-3}
T/K	298.15	0.1	1.78×10^{-3}	1.78×10^{-4}

u_c[pH(S_2)] = 0.008

Note 24: The estimate of the error in ΔE_{IV} comes from an investigation of several 3.5 mol dm⁻³ KCl calomel electrodes in phosphate solutions. The RLJP contribution for free-diffusion junctions is estimated from Figure 2 as 0.006 in pH.

TABLE 11: Primary Buffers PS_1, pH = 7.4, u(pH) = 0.003; PS_2, pH = 4.01, u(pH) = 0.003. Practical Slope (k') Determination

Quantity	Estimate x_i	Standard Uncertainty $u(x_i)$	Sensitivity Coefficient $\|c_i\|$	Uncertainty Contribution $u_i(y)$
ΔE/V	0.2	5×10^{-4}	2.95×10^{-1}	1.5×10^{-4}
T/K	298.15	0.1	1.98×10^{-4}	1.98×10^{-5}
$(E_{j2} - E_{j1})$/V	6×10^{-4}	6×10^{-4}	2.95×10^{-1}	1.8×10^{-4}
ΔpH	3.39	4.24×10^{-3}	1.75×10^{-2}	7.40×10^{-5}

$u_c(k')$ = 2.3×10^{-4}

TABLE 12: pH(X) Determination

Quantity	Estimate x_i	Standard Uncertainty $u(x_i)$	Sensitivity Coefficient $|c_i|$	Uncertainty Contribution $u_i(y)$
pH(S$_1$)	7.4	0.003	1	0.003
ΔE/V	0.03	1.40×10^{-5}	16.95	2.37×10^{-4}
$(E_{j2} - E_{j1})$/V	6.00×10^{-4}	6.00×10^{-4}	16.95	1.01×10^{-2}
k'/V	0.059	2.3×10^{-4}	9.01	2.1×10^{-3}

$u_c[\text{pH(X)}] = 1.6 \times 10^{-2}$
Note 25: The estimated error in ΔE comes from replicates. The RLJP is estimated as 0.6 mV. Therefore, $U[\text{pH(X)}] = 0.021$.

TABLE 13:

Quantity	Estimate x_i	Standard Uncertainty $u(x_i)$	Sensitivity Coefficient $|c_i|$	Uncertainty Contribution $u_i(y)$
$E°$/V	−0.427	5×10^{-4}	16.96	0.0085
T/K	298.15	0.058	1.98×10^{-4}	1.15×10^{-5}
$E(X)$/V	0.016	2×10^{-4}	16.9	0.0034
k'/V	0.059	0.076×10^{-3}	67.6	0.0051

$u_c[\text{pH(X)}] = 0.005$
Note 26: There is no explicit RLJP error assessment as it is assessed statistically by regression analysis.

TABLE 14: Values of the Relative Permittivity of Water [46] and the Debye–Hückel limiting Law Slope for Activity Coefficients as lg γ in eq. 6. Values are for 100.000 kPa, but the Difference from 101.325 kPa (1 atm) is Negligible

$t/°C$	Relative Permittivity	A/mol$^{-\frac{1}{2}}$ kg$^{\frac{1}{2}}$
0	87.90	0.4904
5	85.90	0.4941
10	83.96	0.4978
15	82.06	0.5017
20	80.20	0.5058
25	78.38	0.5100
30	76.60	0.5145
35	74.86	0.5192
40	73.17	0.5241
45	71.50	0.5292
50	69.88	0.5345

A.5.3 Measurement Equations for Multipoint Calibration

$$E_V(S) = E_V° - k'\text{pH(S)} \qquad \text{(A-11) cf. (17)}$$

$$\text{pH(X)} = [E_V° - E_V(X)]/k' \qquad \text{(A-12) cf. (18)}$$

Uncertainty budget:

Example: Standard buffers pH(S$_1$) = 3.557, pH(S$_2$) = 4.008, pH(S$_3$) = 6.865, pH(S$_4$) = 7.416, pH(S$_5$) = 9.182; pH(X) was a "ready-to-use" buffer solution with a nominal pH of 7.

A combination electrode with capillary liquid junction was used. For experimental details, see ref. [41]; and for details of the calculations, see ref. [45].

The uncertainty will be different arising from the RLJPs if an alternative selection of the five standard buffers was used. The uncertainty attained will be dependent on the design and quality of the commercial electrodes selected.

Therefore, $U[\text{pH(X)}] = 0.01$.

14. Summary of Recommendations

- IUPAC recommended definitions, procedures, and terminology are described relating to pH measurements in dilute aqueous solutions in the temperature range 0–50 °C.

- The recent definition of *primary method of measurement* permits the definition of primary standards for pH, determined by a primary method (cell without transference, called the Harned cell) and of secondary standards for pH.

- pH is a conventional quantity and values are based on the Bates–Guggenheim convention. The assigned uncertainty of the Bates–Guggenheim convention is 0.01 in pH. By accepting this value, pH becomes traceable to the internationally accepted SI system of measurement.

- The required attributes (listed in Section 6.1) for primary standard materials effectively limit the number of primary substances to six, from which seven primary standards are defined in the pH range 3–10 (at 25 °C). Values of pH(PS) from 0–50 °C are given in Table 2.

- Methods that can be used to obtain the difference in pH between buffer solutions are discussed in Section 8. These methods include the use of cells with transference that are practically more convenient to use than the Harned cell, but have greater uncertainties associated with the results.

- Incorporation of the uncertainties for the primary method, and for all subsequent measurements, permits the uncertainties for all procedures to be linked to the primary standards by an unbroken chain of comparisons. Despite its conventional basis, the definition of pH, the establishment of pH standards, and the procedures for pH determination are self-consistent within the confidence limits determined by the uncertainty budgets.

- Comparison of values from the cell with liquid junction with the assigned pH(PS) values of the same primary buffers measured with Cell I makes the estimation of values of the RLJPs possible (Section 7), and the consistency of the seven primary standards can be estimated.

- The Annex (Section 13) to this document includes typical uncertainty estimates for the five cells and measurements described, which are summarized in Table 4.

- The hierarchical approach to primary and secondary measurements facilitates the availability of recommended procedures for carrying out laboratory calibrations with traceable buffers grouped to achieve specified target uncertainties of unknowns (Section 11). The three calibration procedures in common use, one-point, two-point (bracketing), and multipoint, are described in terms of target uncertainties.

15. References

1. BIPM. *Com. Cons. Quantité de Matière* **4** (1998). See also: M. J. T. Milton and T. J. Quinn. *Metrologia* **38**, 289 (2001).
2. A. K. Covington, R. G. Bates, R. A. Durst. *Pure Appl. Chem.* **57**, 531 (1985).
3. IUPAC. *Quantities, Units and Symbols in Physical Chemistry*, 2nd ed., Blackwell Scientific, Oxford (1993).
4. S. P. L. Sørensen and K. L. Linderstrøm-Lang. *C. R. Trav. Lab. Carlsberg* **15**, 6 (1924).
5. R. G. Bates. *Determination of pH*, Wiley, New York (1973).
6. S. P. L. Sørensen. *C. R. Trav. Lab. Carlsberg* **8**, 1 (1909).
7. H. S. Harned and B. B. Owen. *The Physical Chemistry of Electrolytic Solutions*, Chap. 14, Reinhold, New York (1958).
8. R. G. Bates and R. A. Robinson. *J. Solution Chem.* **9**, 455 (1980).
9. A. G. Dickson. *J. Chem. Thermodyn.* **19**, 993 (1987).
10. R. G. Bates and E. A. Guggenheim. *Pure Appl. Chem.* **1**, 163 (1960).
11. J. N. Brønsted. *J. Am. Chem. Soc.* **42**, 761 (1920); **44**, 877, 938 (1922); **45**, 2898 (1923).
12. A. K. Covington. Unpublished.
13. K. S. Pitzer. In K. S. Pitzer (Ed.), *Activity Coefficients in Electrolyte Solutions*, 2nd ed., p. 91, CRC Press, Boca Raton, FL (1991).
14. A. K. Covington and M. I. A. Ferra. *J. Solution Chem.* **23**, 1 (1994).
15. *International Vocabulary of Basic and General Terms in Metrology* (VIM), 2nd ed., Beuth Verlag, Berlin (1994).
16. R. Naumann, Ch. Alexander-Weber, F. G. K. Baucke. *Fresenius' J. Anal. Chem.* **349**, 603 (1994).
17. R. G. Bates. *J. Res. Natl. Bur. Stand., Phys. Chem.* **66A** (2), 179 (1962).
18. P. Spitzer. *Metrologia* **33**, 95 (1996); **34**, 375 (1997).
19. N. E. Good, G. D. Wright, W. Winter, T. N. Connolly, S. Isawa, K. M. M. Singh. *Biochem. J.* **5**, 467 (1966).
20. A. K. Covington and M. J. F. Rebelo. *Ion-Sel. Electrode Rev.* **5**, 93 (1983).
21. H. W. Harper. *J. Phys. Chem.* **89**, 1659 (1985).
22. J. Bagg. *Electrochim. Acta* **35**, 361, 367 (1990); **37**, 719 (1992).
23. J. Breer, S. K. Ratkje, G.-F. Olsen. *Z. Phys. Chem.* **174**, 179 (1991).
24. A. K. Covington. *Anal. Chim. Acta* **127**, 1 (1981).
25. A. K. Covington and M. J. F. Rebelo. *Anal. Chim. Acta* **200**, 245 (1987).
26. D. J. Alner, J. J. Greczek, A. G. Smeeth. *J. Chem. Soc. A* 1205 (1967).
27. F. G. K. Baucke. *Electrochim. Acta* **24**, 95 (1979).
28. A. K. Clark and A. K. Covington. Unpublished.
29. M. J. G. H. M. Lito, M. F. G. F. C. Camoes, M. I. A. Ferra, A. K. Covington. *Anal. Chim. Acta* **239**, 129 (1990).
30. M. F. G. F. C. Camoes, M. J. G. H. M. Lito, M. I. A. Ferra, A. K. Covington. *Pure Appl. Chem.* **69**, 1325 (1997).
31. A. K. Covington and J. Cairns. *J. Solution Chem.* **9**, 517 (1980).
32. H. B. Hetzer, R. A. Robinson, R. G. Bates. *Anal. Chem.* **40**, 634 (1968).
33. F. G. K. Baucke. *Electroanal. Chem.* **368**, 67 (1994).
34. P. R. Mussini, A. Galli, S. Rondinini. *J. Appl. Electrochem.* **20**, 651 (1990); C. Buizza, P. R. Mussini, T. Mussini, S. Rondinini. *J. Appl. Electrochem.* **26**, 337 (1996).
35. R. P. Buck and E. Lindner. *Pure Appl. Chem.* **66**, 2527 (1994).
36. J. Christensen. *J. Am. Chem. Soc.* **82**, 5517 (1960).
37. *Guide to the Expression of Uncertainty* (GUM), BIPM, IEC, IFCC, ISO, IUPAC, IUPAP, OIML (1993).
38. F. G. K. Baucke. *Anal. Chem.* **66**, 4519 (1994).
39. F. G. K. Baucke, R. Naumann, C. Alexander-Weber. *Anal. Chem.* **65**, 3244 (1993).
40. R. Naumann, F. G. K. Baucke, P. Spitzer. In *PTB-Report W-68*, P. Spitzer (Ed.), pp. 38–51, Physikalisch-Technische Bundesanstalt, Braunschweig (1997).
41. S. Ebel. In *PTB-Report W-68*, P. Spitzer (Ed.), pp. 57–73, Physikalisch-Technische Bundesanstalt, Braunschweig (1997).
42. H. B. Kristensen, A. Salomon, G. Kokholm. *Anal. Chem.* **63**, 885 (1991).
43. P. Spitzer, R. Eberhadt, I. Schmidt, U. Sudmeier. *Fresenius' J. Anal. Chem.* **356**, 178 (1996).
44. Y. Ch. Wu, W. F. Koch, R. A. Durst. *NBS Special Publication*, 260, p. 53, Washington, DC (1988).
45. BSI/ISO 11095 *Linear calibration using reference materials* (1996).
46. D. A. Archer and P. Wang. *J. Phys. Chem. Ref. Data* **19**, 371 (1990). See also D. J. Bradley and K. S. Pitzer. *J. Phys. Chem.* **83**, 1599 and errata 3799 (1979); D. P. Fernandez, A. R. H. Goodwin, E. W. Lemmon, J. M. H. Levelt Sengers, R. C. Williams. *J. Phys. Chem. Ref. Data* **26**, 1125 (1997).
47. A. K. Covington, R. Kataky, R. A. Lampitt. Unpublished.

GENERAL COMMENTS ON BUFFERS

Roger L. Lundblad

The major factor in biological pH control in eukaryotic cells is the carbon dioxide-bicarbonate-carbonate buffer (Scheme I) system.[1-4] There other biological buffers such as bulk protein and phosphate anions which can provide some buffering effect, metabolites such as lactic acid which can lower pH and tris(hydroxymethylaminomethyl) methane, (THAM®) has been used to treat acid base disorders.[5-7] pH control in prokaryotic cells is mediated by membrane transport of various ions including hydrogen, potassium and sodium.[8-10]

Scheme I

$CO_2 + H_2O = H_2CO_3$; $H_2CO_3 + H_2O = HCO_3^{-1} + H_3O^+$
× (pKa 6.15); $HCO_3^{-1} + H_2O = CO_3^{-2-}$ (pKa 10.3)
See Jungas, R.L., Best literature values for the pK of carbonic and phosphoric acid under physiological conditions, *Anal. Biochem.* 349, 1–15, 2006.

In the laboratory, the bicarbonate/carbonate buffer system can only be used in the far alkaline range (pH 9-11) and unless "fixed" by a suitable cation such as sodium, can be volatile. A variety of buffers, most notably the "Good" buffers which were developed by Norman Good and colleagues,[10a] have been developed over the years to provide pH control in *in vitro* experiments. While effective in controlling pH, the numerous non-buffer effects that buffer salts have on experimental systems are somewhat less appreciated. Some effects, such as observed with phosphate buffers, are based on biologically significant interactions with proteins and, as such, demonstrate specificity. Other effects, such as metal ion chelation, can be considered general. There are some effects where the stability of a reagent is dependent on both pH and buffer species. One example is provided by the stability of phenylmethylsulfonyl fluoride (PMSF).[11] PMSF was less stable in Tris buffer than in either HEPES or phosphate buffer; PMSF is less stable in HEPES than in phosphate buffer. Activity was measured by the ability of PMSF to inhibit chymotrypsin; all activity was lost in Tris (10 mM; pH 7.5) after one hour at 25°C while activity was fully retained in phosphate (10 mM, pH 7.5). This is likely a reflection of the nucleophilic property of Tris[12,13] which appears to be enhanced in the presence of divalent cations such as zinc.[14] The loss of activity, presumably the result of the hydrolysis of the fluoride to hydroxyl function, is more marked at more alkaline pH. Tris can also function as phosphoacceptor in assays for alkaline phosphatase but was not as effective as 2-amino-2-methyl-1,3-propanediol.[15] The various nitrogen-based buffers such as Tris, HEPES, CAP, and BICINE influence colorimetric protein assays.[16-18] Other specific examples are presented in Table 1.

References

1. Lubman, R.L. and Crandall, E.D., Regulation of intracellular pH in alveolar epithelial cells, *Amer.J.Physiol.* 262, L1–L14, 1992.
2. Lyall, V. and Biber, T.O.L., Potential-induced changes in intracellular pH, *Amer.J.Physiol.* 266, F685–F696, 1994.
3. Palmer, L.G., Intracellular pH as a regulator of Na^+ transport, *J.Membrane Biol.* 184, 305–311, 2001.
4. Vaughn-Jones, R.D. and Spitzer, K.W., Role of bicarbonate in the regulation of intracellular pH in the mammalian ventricular myocyte, *Biochem.Cell Biol.* 80, 579–596, 2002.
5. Henschler, D., Trispuffer(TAHM) als therapeuticum, *Deutsch. Med.Wochenschr.* 88, 1328–1331, 1963.
6. Nahas, G.G., Sutin, K.M., Fermon, C., et al, Guidelines for the treatment of acidaemia with THAM, *Drugs* 55, 191–224, 1998.
7. Rehm, M. and Finsterer, U., Treating intraoperative hypercholoremic acidosis with sodium bicarbonate or tris-hydroxymethyl amino methane, *Anesthes.Analg.* 96, 1201–1208, 2003.
8. Kashket, E.R. and Wong, P.T., The intracellular pH of *Escherichia coli*, *Biochim.Biophys.Acta* 193, 212–214, 1969.
9. Padan, E. and Schuldiner, S., Intracellular pH regulation in bacterial cells, *Methods Enzymol.* 125, 327–352, 1986.
10. Booth, I.R., The regulation of intracellular pH in bacteria, *Novartis Found.Symp.* 221, 19–28, 1999.
10a. Good, N.E., Winget, G.D., Winter, W., et al., Hydrogen ion buffers for biological research, *Biochemistry* 5, 467–477, 1966.
11. James, G.T., Inactivation of the protease inhibitor phenylmethylsulfonyl fluoride in buffers, *Anal.Biochem.* 86, 574–579, 1978.
12. Acharya, A.S., Roy, R.P., and Dorai, B., Aldimine to ketoamine isomerization (Amadori rearrangement) potential at the individual nonenzymic glycation sites of hemoglobin A: preferential inhibition of glycation by nucleophiles at sites of low isomerization potential, *J.Protein Chem.* 10, 345–358, 1991.
13. Mattson, A., Boutelje, J., Csoregh, I., et al., Enhanced stereoselectivity in pig liver esterase catalyzed diester hydrolysis. The role of a competitive inhibitor, *Bioorg.Med.Chem.* 2, 501–508, 1994.
14. Tomida, H. and Schwartz, M.A., Further studies on the catalysis of hydrolysis and aminolysis of benzylpenicillin by metal chelates, *J.Pharm.Sci.* 72, 331–335, 1983.
15. Stinson, R.A., Kinetic parameters for the cleaved substrate, and enzyme and substrate stability, vary with the phosphoacceptor in alkaline phosphatase catalysis, *Clin.Chem.* 39, 2293–2297, 1993.

TABLE 1: Effects of Buffers

Buffer	Observation
ACES	Competitive inhibitor of γ-aminobutyric acid receptor binding.[1]
ADA	Competitive inhibitor of γ-aminobutyric acid receptor binding;[1] chelation of calcium ions.[2]
BES	Interacts with DNA yielding distortion of DNA electrophoretograms.[3]
BICINE	Chelation of calcium ions;[2] protects liver alcohol dehydrogenase from inactivation by iodoacetic acid.[4]
Borate	Anomalous complex formation with nucleic acids;[5] complex formation with carbohydrates;[6,7] participant in the modification of arginine residues by 1,2-cyclohexanedione.[8]
Cacodylic Acid	Reaction with sulfhydryl compounds.[9]
Carbonate	Enhances rate of reaction of phenylglyoxal with arginine residues in proteins;[10] modulation of peroxynitrite reactions with proteins;[11,12] modulation of Cu^{2+} oxidation reactions.[13-15]
Citrate	Chelation of calcium ions.[2]
HEPES	Free radical generation[16,17] and complexation of copper ions;[18] reported adverse effects in tissue culture.[19,20]
MES	Complexes copper ions.[21]
MOPS	Adverse effect on smooth muscle contraction;[22] Oxidation of metal ions;[22] formation of nitric oxide donors on incubation with peroxynitrite;[24] slow reaction with hydrogen peroxide.[25]
Phosphate	Catalysis of the racemization of 5-phenylhydantoins.[26,27]
PIPES	Binding to bile salt-stimulated lipase;[28] variation in physiological response based on vendor source;[29] inhibition of a K^+-activated phosphatase.[30]
TES	Interaction with extracellular matrices;[31] inhibition of the interaction of proteoglycans with type 1 collagen.[32]
Tricine	Chelating agent;[2] tricine radicals have been reported in the presence of peroxide-forming enzymes.[33]
Tris	Nucleophile[34,35] and enzyme inhibitor.[36]

16. Kaushal, V. and Barnes, L.D., Effect of zwitterionic buffers on measurement of small masses of protein with bicinchoninic acid, *Anal. Biochem.* 157, 291–294, 1986.
17. Lleu, P.L. and Rebel, G., Interference of Good's buffers other biological buffers with protein determination, *Anal.Biochem.* 192, 215–218, 1991.
18. Sapan, C.V., Lundblad, R.L., and Price, N.C., Colorimetric protein assay techniques, *Biotechnol.Appl.Biochem.* 29, 99–108, 1999.

References to Table 1

1. Tunnicliff, G. and Smith, J.A., Competitive inhibition of gamma-aminobutyric acid receptor binding by N-hydroxyethylepiperazine-N-2-ethanesulfonic acid and related buffers, *J.Neurochem.* 36, 1122–1126, 1981.
2. Durham, A.C., A survey of readily available chelators for buffering calcium ion concentrations in physiological solutions, *Cell Calcium* 4, 33–46, 1983.
3. Stellwagen, N.C., Bossi, A., Gelfi, C. and Righetti, P.G., DNA and buffers: Are there any noninteracting neutral pH buffers?, *Anal. Biochem.* 287, 167–175, 2000.
4. Syvertsen, C. and McKinley-McKee, J.S., Affinity labelling of liver alcohol dehydrogenase. Effect of pH and buffers on affinity labelling with iodoacetic acid and (R,S)-2- bromo-3-(5-imidazolyl)propionic acid, *Eur.J.Biochem.* 117, 165–170, 1981.
5. Biyani, M. and Nishigaki, K., Sequence-specific and nonspecific mobilities of single-stranded oligonucleotides observed by changing the borate buffer concentration, *Electrophoresis* 24, 628–633, 2003.
6. Zittle, Z.A., Reaction of borate with substances of biological interest, *Adv.Enzymol.Relat.Sub.Biochem.* 12, 493–527, 1951.
7. Weitzman, S., Scott, V., and Keegstra, K., Analysis of glycoproteins as borate complexes by polyacrylamide gel electrophoresis, *Anal. Biochem.* 438–449, 1979.
8. Patthy, L. and Smith, E.L., Reversible modification of arginine residues. Application to sequence studies by restriction of tryptic hydrolysis to lysine residues, *J.Biol.Chem.* 250, 557–564, 1975.
9. Jacobson, K.B., Murphey, J.B., and Sarma, B.D., Reaction of cacodylic acid with organic thiols, *FEBS Lett.* 22, 80–82, 1972.
10. Cheung, S.T. and Fonda, M.L., Reaction of phenylglyoxal with arginine. The effect of buffers and pH, *Biochem.Biophys.Res.Commun.* 90, 940–947, 1979.
11. Uppu, R.M., Squadrito, G.L., and Pryor, W.A., Acceleration of peroxynitrite oxidations by carbon dioxide, *Arch.Biochem.Biophys.* 327, 335–343, 1996.
12. Denicola, A., Freeman, B.A., Trujillo, M., and Radi, R., Peroxynitrite reaction with carbon dioxide/bicarbonate: kinetics and influence on peroxynitrite-mediated oxidations, *Arch.Biochem.Biophys.* 333, 49–58, 1996.
13. Munday, R., Munday, C.M. and Winterbourn, C.C., Inhibition of copper-catalyzed cysteine oxidation by nanomolar concentrations of iron salts, *Free Rad.Biol.Med.* 36, 757–764, 2004.
14. Jansson, P.J., Del Castillo, U., Lindqvist, C., and Nordstrom, T., Effects of iron on vitamin C/copper-induced hydroxyl radical generation in bicarbonate-rich water, *Free Rad.Res.* 39, 565–570, 2005.
15. Ramirez, D.C., Mejiba, S.E. and Mason, R.P., Copper-catalyzed protein oxidation and its modulation by carbon dioxide: enhancement of protein radicals in cells, *J.Biol.Chem.* 280, 27402–27411, 2005.
16. Tadolini, B., Iron autoxidation in Mops and Hepes buffers, *Free Radic.Res.Commun.* 4, 149–160, 1987.
17. Simpson, J.A., Cheeseman, K.H., Smith, S.E., and Dean, R.T., Free-radical generation by copper ions and hydrogen peroxide. Stimulation by Hepes buffer, *Biochem.J.* 254, 519–523, 1988.
18. Sokolowska, M. and Bal, W., Cu(II) complexation by "non-coordinating" N-2-hydroxyethylpiperazine-N'-ethanesulfonic acid (HEPES buffer), *J.Inorg.Biochem.* 99, 1653–1660, 2005.
19. Bowman, C.M., Berger, E.M., Butler, E.N. *et al.*, HEPES may stimulate cultured endothelial-cells to make growth-retarding oxygen metabolites, *In Vitro Cell.Devel.Biol.* 21, 140–142, 1985.
20. Magonet, E., Briffeuil, E., Polimay, Y., and Ronveaux, M.F., Adverse-effects of HEPES on human-endothelial cells in culture, *Anticancer Res.* 7, 901, 1987.
21. Mash, H.E., Chin, Y.P., Sigg, L., *et al.*, Complexation of copper by zwitterionic aminosulfonic (Good) buffers, *Anal.Chem.* 75, 671–677, 2003.
22. Altura, B.M., Carella, A., and Altura, B.T., Adverse effects of Tris, HEPES, and MOPS buffers on contractile responses of arterial and venous smooth muscle induced by prostaglandins, *Prostaglandins Med.* 5, 123–130, 1980.
23. Tadolini, B., and Sechi, A.M., Iron oxidation in Mops and Hepes buffers, *Free Radic.Res.Commun.* 4, 149–160, 1987.
24. Schmidt, K., Pfeiffer, S., and Meyer, B., Reaction of peroxynitrite with HEPES or MOPS results in the formation of nitric oxide donors, *Free Radic.Biol.Med.* 24, 859–862, 1998.
25. Zhao, G. and Chasteen, J.D., Oxidation of Good's buffers by hydrogen peroxide, *Anal.Biochem.* 349, 262–267, 2006.
26. Dudley, K.H. and Bius, D.L., Buffer catalysis of the racemization reaction of some 5-phenylhydantoins and its relation to in vivo metabolism of ethotoin, *Drug.Metab.Dispos.* 4, 340–348, 1976.
27. Lazarus, R.A., Chemical racemization of 5-benzylhydantoin, *J.Org. Chem.* 55, 4755–4757, 1990.
28. Moore, S.A., Kingston, R.L., Loomes, K.M., *et al.*, The structure of truncated recombinant human bile salt-stimulated lipase reveals bile salt-independent conformational flexibility at the active-site loop and provides insight into heparin binding, *J.Mol.Biol.* 312, 511–523, 2001.
29. Schmidt, J., Mangold, C., and Deitmer, J., Membrane responses evoked by organic buffers in identified leech neurones, *J.Exp.Biol.* 199, 327–335, 1996.
30. Robinson, J.D. and Davis, R.L., Buffer, pH, and ionic strength effects on the (Na$^+$ + K$^+$)-ATPase, *Biochim.Biophys.Acta* 912, 343–347, 1987.
31. Poole, C.A., Reilly, H.C., and Flint, M.H., The adverse effects of HEPES, TES, and BES zwitterionic buffers on the ultrastructure of cultured chick embryo epiphyseal chondrocytes, *In Vitro* 18, 755–765, 1982.
32. Pogány, G., Hernandez, D.J., and Vogel, K.G., The in Vitro interaction of proteoglycans with type I collagen is modulated by phosphate, *Archs.Biochem.Biophys.* 313, 102–111, 1994.
33. Grande, H.J. and Van der Ploeg, K.R., Tricine radicals as formed in the presence of peroxide producing enzymes, *FEBS Lett.* 95, 352–356, 1978.
34. Oliver, R.W. and Viswanatha, T., Reaction of tris(hydroxymethyl) aminomethane with cinnamoyl imidazole and cinnamoyltrypsin, *Biochim.Biophys.Acta* 156, 422–425, 1968.
35. Ray, T., Mills, A., and Dyson, P., Tris-dependent oxidative DNA strand scission during electrophoresis, *Electrophoresis* 16, 888–894, 1995.
36. Qi, Z., Li, X., Sun, D., *et al.*, Effect of Tris on catalytic activity of MP-11, *Bioelectrochemistry* 68, 40–47, 2006.

LIST OF BUFFERS

Common Name	Chemical Name	M.W	Properties and Comment
ACES	2-[2-amino-2-oxoethyl)amino] ethanesulfonic acid	182.20	One of the several "Good" buffers

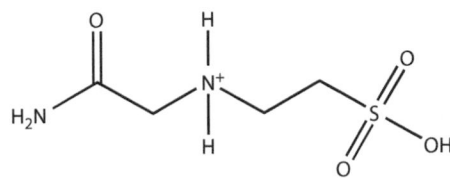

Good, N.E., Winget, G.D., Winter, W., *et al.*, Hydrogen ion buffers for biological research, *Biochemistry* 5, 467–477, 1966; Tunnicliff, G. and Smith, J.A., Competitive inhibition of gamma-aminobutyric acid receptor binding by N-hydroxyethylpiperazine-N'-2-ethanesulfonic acid and related buffers, *J.Neurochem.* 36, 1122–1126, 1981; Chappel, D.J., N-[(carbamoylmethyl)amino] ethanesulfonic acid improves phenotyping of α-1-antitrypsin by isoelectric focusing on agarose gel, *Clin.Chem.* 31, 1384–1386, 1985; Liu, Q., Li, X., and Sommer, S.S., pk-Matched running buffers for gel electrophoresis, *Anal.Biochem.* 270, 112–122, 1999; Taha, M., Buffers for the physiological pH range: acidic dissociation constants of zwitterionic compounds in various hydroorganic media, *Ann.Chim.* 95, 105–109, 2005.

| Acetic Acid/Sodium Acetate | acetic acid (usually with sodium hydroxide to provide sodium acetate | 60.0/82.0 | Frequently used in chromatography with cation exchange matrices below pH 6.0; therapeutic use for acid-base disorders; buffer for peritoneal dialysis. It is an organic acid and a natural product (as is the case with citrate and phosphate) |

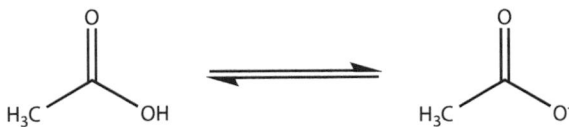

Chohan, I.S., Vermylen, J., Singh, I. *et al.*, Sodium acetate buffer: a diluent of choice in the clot lysis time technique, *Thromb.Diath.Haemorrh.* 33, 226–229, 1975; Lim, C.K. and Peters, T.J., Ammonium acetate: a general purpose buffer for clinical applications of high-performance liquid chromatography, *J.Chromatog.* 3126, 397–406, 1984; Kodama, C., Kodama, T., and Yosizawa, Z., Methods for analysis of urinary glycosaminoglycans, *J.Chromatog.* 429, 293–313, 1988; Stegmann, S., Norgren, R.B., Jr., and Lehman, M.N., Citric acid-ammonium acetate buffer, *Biotech.Histochem.* 1, 27–28,1991; Cuvelier, A., Bourguignon, J., Muir, J.F., *et al.*, Substitution of carbonate by acetate buffer for IgG coating in sandwich ELISA, *J.Immunoassay* 17, 371–382, 1996; Urbansky, E.T., Cooper, B.T., and Margerum, D.W., Disproportionation kinetics of hypoiodous acid as catalyzed and suppressed by acetic acid-acetate buffer, *Inorg.Chem.* 36, 1338–1344, 1997; Watanabe, N., Shirakami, Y., Tomiyoshi, K., *et al.*, Direct labeling of macroaggregated albumin with indium-111-chloride using acetate buffer, *J.Nucl.Med.* 38, 1590–1592, 1997; Righetti, P.G. and Gelfi, C., Capillary electrophoresis of DNA in the 20-500 bp range: recent developments, *J.Biochem.Biophys.Methods* 41, 75–90, 1999; Sen Gupta, K.K., Pal, B., and Begum, B.A., Reactivity of some sugars and sugar phosphates toward gold (III) in sodium acetate-acetic acid buffer medium, *Carbohydr.Res.* 330, 115–123, 2001. Citations for clinical use: Man, N.K., Itakura, Y., Chauveau, P., and Yamauchi, T., Acetate-free biofiltration: state of the art, *Contrib.Nephrol.* 108, 87–93, 1994; Maiorca, R., Cancarini, G.C., Zubani, R., *et al.*, Differing dialysis treatment strategies and outcome, *Nephrol.Dial.Transplant.* 11(Suppl 2), 134–139, 1996; Naka, T. and Bellomo, R., Bench-to-bedside review: Treating acid-base abnormalities in the intensive care unit – the role of renal replacement therapy, *Crit.Care* 8, 108–114, 2004; Khanna, A. and Kurtzman, N.A., Metabolic alkalosis, *J.Nephrol.* 19(Suppl 9), S86–S96, 2006.

| ADA | N-(2-amino-2-oxoethyl)-N-(carboxymethyl)glycineN-(2-acetamido)iminodiacetic acid | 190.2 | A "Good" buffer |

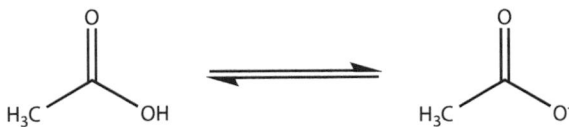

LIST OF BUFFERS (Continued)

Common Name	Chemical Name	M.W	Properties and Comment

Good, N.E., Winget, G.D., Winter, W., *et al.*, Hydrogen ion buffers for biological research, *Biochemistry* 5, 467–477, 1966; Tunnicliff, G. and Smith, J.A., Competitive inhibition of gamma-aminobutyric acid receptor binding by *N*-2-hydroxyethylpiperazine-*N'*-2-*e*-ethanesulfonic acid and related buffers, *J.Neurochem.* 36, 1122–1126, 1981; Durham, A.C., A survey of readily available chelators for buffering calcium ion concentrations in physiological solutions, *Cell Calcium* 4, 33–46, 1983; Kaushal, V. and Barnes, L.D., Effect of zwitterionic buffers on measurement of small masses of protein with bicinchoninic acid, *Anal.Biochem.* 157, 291–294, 1986; Robinson, J.D. and Davis, R.L., Buffer, pH, and ionic strength effects on the (Na$^+$, + K$^+$)-ATPase, *Biochim.Biophys.Acta* 912, 343–347, 1987; Pietrzkowski, E and Korohoda, W., Extracellular ATP and ADA-buffer enable chick embryo fibroblasts to grow in secondary culture in protein-free, hormone-free, extracellular growth factor-free media, *Folia Histochem.Cytobiol.* 26, 143–152, 1988; Righetti, P.G., Chiari, M., and Gelfi, C., Immobilized pH gradients: effect of salts, added carrier ampholytes and voltage gradients on protein patterns, *Electrophoresis* 9, 65–73, 1988; Bers, D.M., Hryshko, L.V., Harrison, S.M., and Dawson, D.D., Citrate decreases contraction and Ca current in cardiac muscle independent of its buffering action, *Am.J.Physiol.* 260, C900–C909, 1991; Delaney, J.P., Kimm, G.E., and Bonsack, M.E., The influence of luminal pH on the severity of acute radiation enteritis, *Int.J.Radiat.Biol.* 61, 381–386, 1992; Taha, M., Buffers for the physiological pH range: acidic dissociation constants of zwitterionic compounds in various hydroorganic media, *Ann.Chim.* 95, 105–109, 2005.

BES — *N,N*-bis(2-hydroxyethyl)-2-aminoethanesulfonic acid; *N,N*-bis(2-hydroxyethyl)taurine — 213.3 — A "Good" buffer, not frequently used, similar to MES, HEPES

Good, N.E., Winget, G.D., Winter, W., *et al.*, Hydrogen ion buffers for biological research, *Biochemistry* 5, 467–477, 1966; Kaushal, V. and Barnes, L.D., Effect of zwitterionic buffers on the measurement of small masses of protein with bicinchoninic acid, *Anal.Biochem.* 157, 291–294, 1986; MacKerrow, S.D., Merry, J.M., and Hoeprich, P.D., Effects of buffers on testing of Candida species susceptibility to flucytosine, *J.Clin.Microbiol.* 25, 885–888, 1987; Tuli, R.K. and Holtz, W., The effect of zwitterionic buffers on the feasibility of Boer goat semen, *Theriogenology* 37, 947–951, 1992; Stellwagen, N.C., Bossi, A., Gelfi, C., and Righetti, P.G., DNA and buffers: are there any noninteracting, neutral pH buffers, *Anal.Biochem.* 287, 167–175, 2000; Hosse, M. and Wilkinson, K.J., Determination of electrophoretic mobilities and hydrodynamic radii of three humic substances as a function of pH and ionic strength, *Environ.Sci.Technol.* 35, 4301–4306, 2002; Taha, M., Buffers for the physiological pH range: acidic dissociation contstants of zwitterionic compounds in various hydroorganic media, *Ann.Chim.* 95, 105–109, 2005.

Bicine — *N,N*-bis-(2-hydroxyethyl)glycine; *N,N*-bis(2-hydroxyethyl)amino-acetic acid — 163.2

Kanfer, J.N., Base exchange reactions of the phospholipids in rat brain particles, *J.Lipid Res.* 13, 468–476, 1972; Williams-Smith, D.L., Bray, R.C., Barber, M.J., *et al.*, Changes in apparent pH on freezing aqueous buffer solutions and their relevance to biochemical electron-paramagnetic-resonance spectroscopy, *Biochem.J.* 167, 593–600, 1977; Syvertsen, C. and McKinley-McKee, J.S., Affinity labeling of liver alcohol dehydrogenase. Effects of pH and buffers on affinity labeling with iodoacetic acid and (R, S)-2-bromo-3-(5-imidazoyl)propionic acid, *Eur.J.Biochem.* 117, 165–170, 1981; Ito, S., Takaoka, T., Mori, H., and Teruo, A., A sensitive new method for measurement of guanase with 8-azaguanine in bicine bis-hydroxy ethyl glycine buffer as substrate, *Clin.Chim.Acta* 115, 135–144, 1981; Nakon, R., Krishnamoorthy, C.R., Free-metal ion depletion by "Good's" buffers, *Science* 221, 749–750, 1983; Ito, S., Xu,Y., Keyser, A.J., and Peters, R.L., Histochemical demonstration of guanase in human liver with guanine in bicine buffer as substrate, *Histochem.J.* 16, 489–499, 1984; Roy, R.N., Gibbons, J.J, Baker, G., and Bates, R.G., Standard electromotive force of the H$_2$-AgCL:Ag cell in 30, 40, and 50 mass% dimethyl sulfoxide/water from -20 to 25°; pK$_2$ and pH values for a standard "Bicine" buffer solution at subzero temperatures, *Cryobiology* 21, 672–681, 1984; Vaidya, N.R., Gothoskar, B.P., and Banerji, A.P., Column isoelectric focusing in nature pH gradients generated by biological buffers, *Electrophoresis* 11, 156–161, 1990; Wiltfang, J., Arold, N., and Neuhoff, V., A new multiphasic buffer system for sodium sulfate-polyacrylamide gel electrophoresis of proteins and peptides with molecular masses 100,000-1000, and their detection with picomolar sensitivity, *Electrophoresis* 12, 352–366, 1991; Rabilloud, T., Vuillard, L., Gilly, C., and Lawrence, J.J., Silver-staining of proteins in polyacrylamide gels: a general overview, *Cell.Mol. Biol.* 40, 57–75, 1994; Gordon-Weeks, R., Koren'kov, V.D., Steele, S.H., and Leigh, R.A., Tris is a competitive inhibitor of K+ activation of the vacuolar H+-pumping pyrophosphatase, *Plant Physiol.* 114, 901–905, 1997; Luo, Q., Andrade, J.D., and Caldwell, K.D., Thin-layer ion-exchange chromatography of proteins, *J.Chromatog. A* 816, 97–105, 1998; Churchill, T.A. and Kneteman, N.M., Investigation of a primary requirement of organ preservation solutions: supplemental buffering agents improve hepatic energy production during cold storage, *Transplanation* 65, 551–559, 1998; Taha, M., Thermodynamic study of the second-stage dissociation of *N,N*-bis-(2-hydroxyethyl)glycine (bicine) in water at different ionic strength and different solvent mixtures, *Ann.Chim.* 94, 971–978, 2004; Taha, M., Buffers for the physiological pH range: acidic dissociation constants of zwitterionic compounds in various hydroorganic media, *Ann.Chim.* 95, 105–109, 2005; Williams, T.I., Combs, J.C., Thakur, A.P., *et al.*, A novel Bicine running buffer system for doubled sodium dodecyl sulfate – polyacrylamide gel electrophoresis of membrane proteins, *Electrophoresis* 27, 2984–2995, 2006.

LIST OF BUFFERS (Continued)

Common Name	Chemical Name	M.W	Properties and Comment
Borate: Sodium Borate (sodium tetraborate/Boric Acid	$Na_2B_4O_7/H_3BO_3$Sodium borate decahydrate is borax)	61.8/201.2	Borate buffers have long history of use; borate well-known for interaction with carbohydrates; participates in the reversible modification of arginine residues by 1,2-cyclohexanedione

$$B(OH)_3 + 2H_2O \rightleftharpoons B(OH)_4^- + H_3O^+$$

Adjutantis, G., Electrophoretic separation of filter paper of the soluble liver-cell proteins of the rat using borate buffer, *Nature* 173, 539-540, 1954; Consden, R. and Powell, M.N., The use of borate buffer in paper electrophoresis of serum, *J.Clin.Pathol.* 8, 150–152, 1955; Cooper, D.R., Effect of borate buffer on the electrophoresis of serum, *Nature* 181, 713–714, 1958; Cooper, D.R., Effect of borate buffer on the electrophoresis of serum, *Nature* 181, 713–714, 1958; Poduslo, J.F., Glycoprotein molecular-weight estimation using sodium dodecyl sulfate-pore gradient electrophoresis: Comparison of Tris-glycine and Tris-borate-EDTA buffer systems, *Anal.Biochem.* 114, 131–139, 1981; Shukun, S.A. and Zav'yalov, V.P., Peculiar features of application of pH gradients formed in borate buffer with a polyhydroxy compound for separation of proteins in a free-flow electrophoretic apparatus, *J.Chromatog.* 496, 121–128, 1989; Patton, W.F., Chung-Welch, N., Lopez, M.F., *et al.*, Tris-tricine and Tris-borate buffer systems provide better estimates of huma mesothelial cell intermediate filament protein molecular weights than the standard Tris-glycine system, *Anal.Biochem.* 197, 25–33, 1991; Roden, L., Yu, H., Jin, J., and Greenshields, J., Separation of *N*-acetylglucosamine and *N*-acetylmannosamine by chromatography on Sephadex in borate buffer, *Anal. Biochem.* 209, 188–191, 1993; Yokota, H., van den Engh, G., Mostert, M., and Trask, B.J., Treatment of cells with alkaline borate buffer extends the capability of interphase FISH mapping, *Genomics* 25, 485–491, 1995; Biyani, M. and Nishigaki, K., Sequence-specific and nonspecific mobilities of single-stranded oliogonucleotides observed by changing the borate buffer concentration, *Electrophoresis* 24, 628–633, 2003; Zhao, Y., Yang, X., Jiang, R. *et al.*, Chiral separation of synthetic vicinal diol compounds by capillary zone electrophoresis with borate buffer and β-cyclodextrin as buffer additives, *Anal.Sci.* 22, 747–751, 2006. Articles focusing on the interaction of borate with carbohydrates and other polyols include: Zittle, C.A., Reaction of borate with substances of biological interest, *Adv.Enzymol.Relat.Sub.Biochem.* 12, 493–527, 1951; Larsson, U.B. and Samuelson, O. Anion exchange separation of organic acids in borate medium: influence of the temperature, *J.Chromatog.* 19, 404–411, 1965; Lin, F.M. and Pomeranz, Y., Effect of borate on colorimetric determinations of carbohydrates by the phenol-sulfuric acid method, *Anal.Biochem.* 24, 128–131, 1968; Haug, A., The influence of borate and calcium on the gel formation of a sulfated polysaccharide from *Ulva lactuca*, *Acta Chem.Scand. B.* 30, 562–566, 1976; Weitzman, S., Scott, V., and Keegstra, K., Analysis of glycoproteins as borate complexes by polyacrylamide gel electrophoresis, *Anal.Biochem.* 97, 438–449, 1979; Honda, S., Takahashi, M., Kakehi, K. and Ganno, S., Rapid, automated analysis of monosaccharides by high-performance anion-exchange chromatograpy of borate complexes with fluorometric detection using 2-cyanoacetamide, *Anal.Biochem.* 113, 130–138, 1981; Rothman, R.J. and Warren, L., Analysis of IgG glycopeptides by alkaline borate gel filtration chromatography, *Biochim.Biophys.Acta* 955, 143–153, 1988; Todd, P. and Elsasser, W., Nonamphometric isoelectric focusing: II. Stablity of borate-glycerol pH gradients in recycling isoelectric focusing, *Electrophoresis* 11, 947–952, 1990. Selected studies on the effect of borate on the modification of arginine with 1,2-cyclohexanedione include: Patthy, L. and Smith, E.L., Reversible modification of arginine residues. Application to sequence studies by restriction of tryptic hydrolysis to lysine residues, *J.Biol.Chem.* 250, 557–564, 1975; Patthy, L. and Smith, E.L., Identification of functional arginine residues in ribonuclease A and lysozyme, *J.Biol.Chem.* 250, 565–569,1975; Menegatti, E., Ferroni, R., Benassi, C.A., and Rocchi, R., Arginine modification in Kunitz bovine trypsin inhibitor through 1,2-cyclohexanedione, *Int.J.Pept.Protein Res.* 10, 146–152, 1977; Kozik, A., Guevara, I. and Zak, Z., 1,2-Cyclohexanedione modification of arginine residues in egg-white riboflavin-binding protein, *Int.J.Biochem.* 20, 707–711, 1988.

Cacodylic Acid	Dimethylarsinic Acid	138.10	Buffer salt in neutral pH range; largely replaced because of toxicity.

McAlpine, J.C., Histochemical demonstration of the activation of rat acetylcholinesterase by sodium cacodylate and cacodylic acid using the thioacetic acid method, *J.R.Microsc.Soc.* 82, 95–106, 1963; Jacobson, K.B., Murphy, J.B., and Das Sarma, B., Reaction of cacodylic acid with organic thiols, *FEBS Lett.* 22, 80–82, 1972; Travers, F., Douzou, P., Pederson, T., and Gunsalus. I.C., Ternary solvents to investigate proteins at sub-zero temperature, *Biochimie* 57, 43–48, 1975; Young, C.W., Dessources, C., Hodas, S., and Bittar, E.S., Use of cationic disc electrophoresis near neutral pH in the evaluation of trace proteins in human plasma, *Cancer Res.* 35, 1991–1995, 1975; Chirpich, T.P., The effect of different buffers on terminal deoxynucleotidyl transferase activity, *Biochim.Biophys.Acta* 518, 535–538, 1978; Nunes, J.F., Aguas, A.P., and Soares, J.O., Growth of fungi in cacodylate buffer, *Stain Technol.* 55, 191–192, 1980; Caswell, A.H. and Bruschwig, J.P., Identification and extraction of proteins that compose the triad junction of skeletal muscle, *J.Cell Biol.* 99, 929–939, 1984; Parks, J.C. and Cohen, G.M., Glutaraldehyde fixatives for preserving the chick's inner ear, *Acta Otolaryngol.* 98, 72–80, 1984; Song, A.H. and Asher, S.A., Internal intensity standards for heme protein UV resonance Raman studies: Excitation profiles of cacodylic acid and sodium selenate, *Biochemistry* 30, 1199–1205, 1991; Henney, P.J., Johnson, E.L., and Cothran, E.G., A new buffer system for acid PAGE typing of equine protease inhibitor, *Anim.Genet.* 25, 363–364, 1994; Jezewska, M.J., Rajendran, S., and Bujalowski, W., Interactions of the 8-kDa domain of rat DNA polymerase beta with DNA, *Biochemistry* 40, 3295–3307, 2001; Kenyon, E.M. and Hughes, M.F., A concise review of the toxicity and carcinogenicity of dimethylarsinic acid, *Toxicology* 160, 227–236, 2001; Cohen, S.M., Arnold, L.L., Eldan, M., *et al.*, Methylated arsenicals: the implications of metabolism and carcinogenicity studies in rodents to human risk management, *Crit.Rev.Toxicol.* 99–133, 2006.

LIST OF BUFFERS (Continued)

Common Name	Chemical Name	M.W	Properties and Comment
CAPS	3-(cyclohexylamino)-1-propanesulfonic acid	221.3	A zwitterionic buffer similar to a "Good" buffer

Lad, P.J. and Leffert, H.L., Rat liver alcohol dehydrogenase. I. Purification and characterization, *Anal.Biochem.* 133, 350–361, 1983; Kaushal, V. and Barnes, L.D., Effect of zwitterionic buffers on measurement of small masses of protein with bicinchoninic acid, *Anal.Biochem.* 157, 291–294, 1986; Himmel, H.M. and Heller, W., Studies on the interference of selected substances with two modifications of the Lowry protein determination, *J.Clin.Chem. Clin.Biochem.* 25, 909–913, 1987; Nguyen, A.L., Luong, J.H., and Masson, C., Determination of nucleotides in fish tissues using capillary electrophoresis, *Anal.Chem.* 62, 2490–2493, 1990; Jin, Y. and Cerletti, N., Western blotting of transforming growth factor β2. Optimization of the electrophoretic transfer, *Appl.Theor.Electrophor.* 3, 85–90, 1992; Ng, L.T., Selwyn, M.J., and Choo, H.L., Effect of buffers and osmolality on anion uniport across the mitochondrial inner membrane, *Biochim.Biophys.Acta* 1143, 29–37, 1993; Venosa, R.A., Kotsias, B.A., and Horowicz, P., Frog striated muscle is permeable to hydroxide and buffer anions, *J.Membr.Biol.* 139, 57–74, 1994; Righetti, P.G., Bossi, A. and Gelfi, C., Capillary isoelectric focusing and isoelectric buffers: an evolving scenario, *J.Capillary Electrophor.* 4, 47–59, 1997; Bienvenut, W.V., Deon, C., Sanchez, J.C., and Hochstrasser, D.F., *Anal.Biochem.* 307, 297–303, 2002; Zaitseva, J., Holland, I.B., and Schmitt, L., The role of CAPS buffer in expanding the crystallization space of the nucleotide-binding domain of the ABC transporter haemolysin B from *Escherichia coli*, *Acta Crystallogr.D.Biol.Crystallogr.* 60, 1076–1084, 2004; Kannamkumarath, S.S., Wuilloud, R.G., and Caruso, J.A., Studies of various elements of nutritional and toxicological interest associated with different molecular weight fractions in Brazil nuts, *J.Agric.Food Chem.* 52, 5773–5780, 2004; Hautala, J.T., Wiedmer, S.K., and Riekkola, M.L., Influence of pH on formation and stability of phosphatidylcholine/phosphatidylserine coatings in fused-silica capillaries, *Electrophoresis* 26, 176–186, 2005; Taha, M., Buffers for the physiological pH range: acidic dissociation constants of zwitterionic compounds in various hydroorganic media, *Ann.Chim.* 95, 105–109, 2005; Tu, J., Halsall, H.B., Seliskar, C.J. *et al.*, Estimation of logP(ow) values for neutral and basic compounds by microchip microemulsion electrokinetic chromatography with indirect fluorometric detection (muMEEKC-IFD), *J.Pharm.Biomed.Anal.* 38, 1–7, 2005.

CAPSO	3-(Cyclohexylamino)-2-hydroxy-1-propanesulfonic acid	237.3	A zwitterionic buffer similar to a "Good" buffer

Delaney, J.P., Kimm, G.E., and Bonsack, M.E., The influence of lumenal pH on the severity of acute radiation enteritis, *Int.J.Radiat.Biol.* 61, 381–386, 1992; McGregor, D.P., Forster, S., Steven, J. *et al.*, Simultaneous detection of microorganisms in soil suspension based on PCR amplification of bacterial 16S rRNA fragments, *BioTechniques* 21, 463–466, 1996; Liu, Q. Li, X., and Somer, S.S. pK-Matched running buffers for gel electrophoresis, *Anal.Biochem.* 270, 112–122, 1999; Quiros, M., Parker, M.C., and Turner, N.J., Tuning lipase enantioselectivity in organic media using solid-state buffers, *J.Org.Chem.* 66, 5074–5079, 2001; Okuda, M., Iwahori, K., Yamashita, I., and Yoshimura, H., Fabrication of nickel and chromium nanoparticles using the protein cage of apoferritin, *Biotechnol.Bioeng.* 84, 187–194, 2003; Vespalec, R., Vlckova, M., and Horakova, H., Aggregation and other intermolecular interactions of biological buffers observed by capillary electrophoresis and UV photometry, *J.Chromatog.A* 1051, 75–84, 2004; Taha, M., Buffers for the physiological pH range: acidic dissociation constants of zwitterionic compounds in various hydroorganic media, *Ann.Chim.* 95, 105–109, 2005.

Carbonate	Sodium bicarbonate Sodium Carbonate Ammonium bicarbonate ammonium carbonate;		The ammonium salt system is a volatile buffer. The carbonate buffer is considered to be a physiological buffer. Bicarbonate buffers are used in renal dialysis.

Nagasawa, K. and Uchiyama, H., Preparation and properties of biologically active fluorescent heparins, *Biochim.Biophys.Acta* 544, 430–440, 1978; Horejsi, V. and Hilgert, I., Simple polyacrylamide gel electrophoresis in continuous carbonate buffer system suitable for the analysis of ascites fluids of hybridoma bearing mice, *J.Immunol.Methods* 86, 103–105, 1986; Chang, G.G. and Shiao, S.L., Possible kinetic mechanism of human placental alkaline phosphatase in vivo as implemented in reverse micelles, *Eur.J. Biochem.* 220, 861–870, 1994; Steinitz, M. and Tamir, S., An improved method to create nitrocellulose particles suitable for the immobilization of antigen and antibody, *J.Immunol.Methods* 187, 171–177, 1995; Wang, Z., Gurel, O., Baatz, J.E. and Notter, R.H., Acylation of pulmonary surfactant protein-C is required for its optimal surface active interactions with phospholipids, *J.Biol.Chem.* 271, 19104–19109, 1996; Petersen, A. and Steckhan, E., Continuous indirect electrochemical regeneration of galactose oxidase, *Bioorg.Med.Chem.* 7, 2203–2208, 1999; Medda, R., Padiglia, A., Messana, T., *et al.*, Separation of diadenosine polyphosphates by capillary electrophoresis, *Electrophoresis* 21, 2412–2416, 2000; Bartzatt, R., Fluorescent labeling of drugs and simple organic compounds containing amine functional groups, utilizing dansyl chloride in Na$_2$CO$_3$ buffer, *J.Pharmacol.Toxicol.Methods* 45, 247–253, 2001; Bruno, F., Curini, R., Di Corcia, A., *et al.*, Determination of surfactants and some of their metabolites in untreated and anaerobically digested sewage sludge by subcritical water extraction followed by liquid chromatography-mass spectrometry, *Environ.Sci. Technol.* 36, 4156–4161, 2002; Chen, X.L., Sun, C.Y., Zhang, Y.Z., and Gao, P.J., Effects of different buffers on the thermostability and autolysis of a cold-adapted proteases MCP-01, *J.Protein Chem.* 21,523–527, 2002; Duman, M., Saber, R., and Piskin, E., A new approach for immobilization of

List of Buffers

LIST OF BUFFERS (Continued)

Common Name	Chemical Name	M.W	Properties and Comment

oligonucleotides onto piezoelectric quartz crystal for preparation of a nucleic acid sensor following hybridization, *Biosens.Bioelectron.* 18, 1355–1363, 2003; Talu, G.F. and Diyamandoglu, V., Formate ion decomposition in water under UV irradiation at 253.7 nm, *Environ.Sci.Technol.* 38, 3984–3993, 2004; Dwight, S.J., Gaylord, B.S., Hong, J.W., and Bazan, G.C., Perturbation of fluorescence by nonspecific interactions between anionic poly(phenylenevinylene)s and proteins. Implications for biosensors, *J.Am.Chem.Soc.* 126, 16850–16859, 2004; Willems, A.V., Deforce, D.L., Van Peteghem, C.H., and Van Bocxlaer, J.F., Development of a quality control method for the characterization of oligonucleotides by capillary zone electrophoresis-electrospray ionization-quadrupole time of flight-mass spectrometry, *Electrophoresis* 26, 1412–1423, 2005; Asberg, P.,Bjork, P., Hook, F., and Inganas, O., Hydrogels from a water-soluble zwitterionic polythiophene: dynamics under pH change and biomolecular interactions observed using quartz crystal microbalance with dissipation monitoring, *Langmuir* 21, 7292–7298, 2005; Shah, M., Meija, J., Cabovska, B., and Caruso, J.A., Determination of phosphoric acid triesters in human plasma using solid-phase microextraction and gas chromatography coupled to inductively coupled plasma mass spectrometry, *J.Chromatog.A.* 1103, 329–336, 2006; Di Pasqua, A.J., Goodisman, J., Kerwood, D.J. *et al.*, Activation of carboplatin by carbonate, *Chem Res.Toxicol.* 18, 139–149, 2006; Ormond, D.R. and Kral, T.A., Washing methogenic cells with the liquid fraction from a Mars soil stimulant and water mixture, *J.Microbiol. Methods* 67, 603–605, 2006; Binter, A., Goodisman, J., and Dabrowiak, J.C., Formation of monofunctional cisplatinin-DNA adducts in carbonate buffer, *J.Inorg.Biochem.* 100, 1219–1224, 2006. Alkaline carbonate buffers have been used as the medium for proteins for application to microplates for immunoassays such as ELISA assays (Rote, N.S., Taylor, N.L. Shigeoka, A.O., *et al.*, Enzyme-linked immunosorbent assay for group B streptococcal antibodies, *Infect. Immun.* 27, 118–123, 1980; Hubschle, O.J., Lorenz, R.J., and Matheka, H.D., Enzyme-linked immunosorbent assay for detection of bluetongue virus antibodies, *Am.J.Vet.Res.* 42, 61–65, 1981; Solling, H., and Dinesen, B., The development of a rapid ELISA for IgE utilizing commercially available reagents, *Clin.Chim.Acta* 130, 71–83, 1983; Mowat, W.P. and Dawson, S., Detection and identification of plant viruses by ELISA using crude sap extracts and unfractionated antisera, *J.Virol.Methods* 15, 233–247, 1987; Ferris, N.P., Powell, H., and Donaldson, A.I., Use of pre-coated immunoplates and freeze-dried reagents for the diagnosis of foot-and-mouth disease and swine vesicular disease by enzyme-linked immunosorbent assay [ELISA], *J.Virol. Methods* 19,197–206, 1988; Cutler, S.J. and Wright, D.J., Comparison of immunofluorescence and enzyme linked immunosorbent assays for diagnosing Lyme disease, *J.Clin.Pathol.* 42, 869–871, 1989; Oshima, M. and Atassi, M.Z., Comparison of peptide-coating conditions in solid phase assays for detection of anti-peptide antibodies, *Immunol.Invest.* 18, 841–851, 1989; Martin, R.R., Relationships among luteoviruses based on nucleic acid hybridization and serological studies, *Intervirology* 31,23–30, 1990; Houen, G. and Koch, C., A non-denaturing enzyme linked immunosorbent assay with protein preadsorbed onto aluminum hydroxide, *J.Immunol.Methods* 200, 99–105, 1997; Shrivastav, T.G., Basu, A., and Kariya, K.P., Substitution of carbonate buffer by water for IgG immobilization in enzyme linked immunosorbent assay, *J.Immunoassay Immunochem.* 24, 191–203, 2003). Bicarbonate buffers also have an effect on the reaction of phenylglyoxal with proteins (Cheung, S.T. and Fonda, M.L., Reaction of phenylglyoxal with arginine. The effect of buffers and pH, *Biochem.Biophys.Res.Commun.* 90, 940–947, 1979). Bicarbonate also enhances the binding of iron to transferrin(Matinaho, S., Karhumäki, P., and Parkkinen, J., Bicarbonate inhibits the growth of *Staphylococcus epidermidis* in platelet concentrates by lowering the level of non-transferrin-bound iron, *Transfusion* 45, 1768–173, 2005.

| Cholamine | (2-aminoethyl) trimethyl-ammonium chloride hydrochloride | | |

Blasie, C.A. and Berg, J.M., Structure-based thermodynamic analysis of a coupled metal binding-protein folding reaction involving a zinc finger peptide, *Biochemistry* 41, 15068–15073, 2002; Zwiorek, K., Kloeckner, J., Wagner, E., and Coester, C., Gelatin nanoparticles as a new and simple gene delivery system, *J.Pharm.Pharm.Sci.* 7, 22–28, 2005.

| Citric Acid | 2-hydroxy-1,2,3-propanetricarboxylic acid | 192.1 | Compounds found in a variety of biological tissues and cells; involved in energy metabolism (citric acid cycle; Krebs cycle; Krebs, H.A., The citric acid cycle and the Szent-Gyorgyi cycle in pigeon breast muscle, *Biochem.J.* 34, 775–779, 1940). Also used as biological buffer. |

Citric acid has three carboxylic acid functions which permits buffering capacity from pH 2.0 to pH 12. Citric acid also chelate divalent cations and is used an anticoagulant for the collection of blood based its ability to chelate calcium ions. Chelation of metal ions is responsible for the observed inhibition of many enzymes. For early observations, see Smith, E.G., Dipeptidases, *Methods Enzymol.* 2, 93–114, 1955; McDonald, M.R., Deoxyribonucleases, *Methods Enzymol.* 2, 437–447, 1955; Kornberg, A., Adenosine phosphokinase, *Methods Enzymol.* 2, 497–500, 1955; Koshland, D.E., Jr., Preparation and properties of acetyl phosphatase, *Methods Enzymol.* 2, 556–556, 1955. The ability to chelate calcium serves as the basis for use as a decalcification agent. The polyvalent nature of citrate provide some unique characteristics such as the differentiation of muscle fiber types for histochemistry (Matoba, H., and Gollnick, P.D., Influence of ionic composition, buffering agent, and pH on the histochemical demonstration of myofibrillar actomyosin ATPase, *Histochemistry* 80, 609–614, 1984) and the activation of "prothrombin"(Seegers, W.H., McClaughery, R.I., and Fahey, J.L., Some properties of purified prothrombin and its activation with sodium citrate, *Blood* 5, 421–433, 1950; Lanchantin, G.F., Friedman, J.A., and Hart, D.W., The conversion of human prothrombin to thrombin by sodium citrate. Analysis of the reaction mixture, *J.Biol.Chem.* 240, 3276–3282.

LIST OF BUFFERS (Continued)

Common Name	Chemical Name	M.W	Properties and Comment

1965; Aronson, D.L. and Mustafa, A.J., The activation of human factor X in sodium citrate: the role of factor VII, *Thromb.Haemostas.* 36, 104–114, 1976). Citrate is a polyvalent anion and like other polyvalent anions such as phosphate and sulfate, citrate can cause a "salting-out" phenomena (Hegardt, F.G. and Pie, A., Sodium citrate salting-out of the human blood serum proteins, *Rev.Esp.Fisiol.* 24, 161–168, 1968; Carrea, G., Pasta, P., and Vecchio, G., Effect of the lyotropic series of anions on denaturation and renaturation of 20-β-hydroxysteroid dehydrogenase, *Biochim.Biophys.Acta* 784, 16–23, 1984; Nakano, T., Yuasa, H., and Kanaya, Y., Suppression of agglomeration in fluidized bed coating. III. Hofmeister series in suppression of particle agglomeration, *Pharm.Res.* 16, 1616–1620, 1999; Nakano, T. and Yuasa, H., Suppression of agglomeration in fluidized bed coating. IV. Effects of sodium citrate concentration on the suppression of particle agglomeration and the physical properties of HPMC film, *Int.J.Pharm.* 215, 3–12, 2001; Mani, N. and Jun, H.W., Microencapsulation of a hydrophilic drug into a hydrophobic matrix using a salting-out procedure. I: Development and optimization of the process using factorial design, *J.Microencapsulation* 21, 125–135, 2004). Citrate also has an effect on partitioning in aqueous two-phase systems (Andrews, B.A., Schmidt, A.S., and Asenjo, J.A., Correlation for the partition behavior of proteins in aqueous two-phase systems: effect of surface hydrophobicity and charge, *Biotechnol.Bioeng.* 90, 380–390, 2005). Citrate has proved useful in the solubilization of proteins, usually, but not always, from mineralized/calcified matrices (Faludi, E. and Harsanyi, V., The effect of Na₃-citrate on the solubility of cryoprecipitate [citrate effect of cryoprecipitate], *Haematologia* 14, 207–214, 1981; Myllyla, R., Preparation of antibodies to chick-embryo galactosylhydroxylysyl glucosyltransferase and their use for an immunological characterization of the enzyme of collagen synthesis, *Biochim.Biophys.Acta* 658, 299–307, 1981; Guy, O., Robles-Diaz, G., Adrich, Z., *et al.*, Protein content of precipitates present in pancreatic juice of alcoholic subjects and patients with chronic calcifying pancreatitis, *Gastroenterology* 84, 102–107, 1983; Collingwood, T.N., Shanmugam, M., Daniel, R.M., and Langdon, A.G., M[III]-facilitated recovery and concentration of enzymes from mesophilic and thermophilic organisms, *J.Biochem. Biophys.Methods* 19, 281–286, 1989). Citrate is useful for dissociating protein complexes in some situations by binding to specific anion binding sites; the ability of citrate to function as a buffering at low pH is an advantage [Kuo, T.T., Chow, T.Y., Lin, X.T., *et al.*, Specific dissociation of phage Xp12 by sodium citrate, *J.Gen.Virol.* 10,199–202, 1971(in this case, the dissociation is reflection of metal ion binding; the dissociation is associated with the loss of biological activity – see Lark, K.G. and Adams, M.H., The stability of phage as a function of the ionic environment, *Cold Spring Harbor Symposium on Quantitative Biology*, 18, 171–183, 1953); Sheffery, M. and Newton, A., Reconstitution and purification of flagellar filaments from *Caulobacter crescentus*, *J.Bacteriol.* 132, 1027–1030, 1977; Brooks, S.P. and Nicholls, P., Anion and ionic strength effects upon the oxidation of cytochrome c by cytochrome c oxidase, *Biochim.Biophys.Acta* 680, 33–43, 1982; Berliner, L.J., Sugawara, Y., and Fenton, J.W., 2nd, Human alpha-thrombin binding to nonpolymerized fibrin-Sepharose: evidence for an anionic binding region, *Biochemistry* 24, 7005–7009, 1985; Kella, N.K. and Kinsella, J.E., Structural stability of beta-lactoglobulin in the presence of kosmotropic salts. A kinetic and thermodynamic study, *Int.J.Pept.Protein Res.* 32, 396–405, 1988; Oe, H., Takahashi, N., Doi. E., and Hirose, M., Effects of anion binding on the conformations of the two domains of ovotransferrin, *J.Biochem.* 106, 858–863, 1989; Polakova, K., Karpatova, M., and Russ, G., Dissociation of β-2-microglobulin is responsible for selective reduction of HLA class I antigenicity following acid treatment of cells, *Mol.Immunol.* 30, 1223–1230, 1993; Lecker, D.N. and Khan, A., Model for inactivation of α-amylase in the presence of salts: theoretical and experimental studies, *Biotechnol.Prog.* 14, 621–625, 1998; Rabiller-Baudry, M. and Chaufer, B., Small molecular ion adsorption on proteins and DNAs revealed by separation techniques, *J.Chromatog.B.Analyt.Technol.Biomed.Life.Sci.* 797, 331–345, 2003; Raibekas, A.A., Bures, E.J., Siska, C.C., *et al.*, Anion binding and controlled aggregation of human interleukin-1 receptor antagonist, *Biochemistry* 44, 9871–9879, 2005). A special application of citrate dissociation of protein complexes is the isolation and dissociation of antigen-antibody complexes (Woodroffe, A.J. and Wilson, C.B., An evaluation of elution techniques in the study of immune complex glomerulonephritis, *J.Immunol.* 118, 1788–1794, 1977; Ehrlich, R. and Witz, I.P., The elution of antibodies from viable murine tumor cells, *J.Immunol.Methods* 26, 345–353, 1979; McIntosh, R.M., Garcia, R., Rubio, L., *et al.*, Evidence of an autologous immune complex pathogenic mechanism in acute poststreptococcal glomerulonephritis, *Kidney Int.* 14, 501–510, 1978; Theofilopoulos, A.N., Eisenberg, R.A., and Dixon, F.J., Isolation of circulating immune complexes using Raji cells. Separation of antigens from immune complexes and production of antiserum, *J.Clin.Invest.* 61, 1570–1581, 1978; Tomino, Y., Sakai, H., Endoh, M., *et al.*, Cross-reactivity of eluted antibodies from renal tissues of patients with Henoch-Schonlein purpura nephritis and IgA nephropathy, *Am.J.Nephrol.* 3, 315–318, 1983). A more complex and poorly understood application of citrate buffers is in epitope retrieval (Shi, S.R., Chaiwun, B., Young, L., *et al.*, Antigen retrieval techniques utilizing citrate buffer or urea solution for immunohistochemical demonstration of androgen receptor in formalin-fixed paraffin sections, *J.Histochem.Cytochem.* 41, 1599–1604, 1993; Langlois, N.E., King, G., Herriot, R., and Thompson, W.D., Non-enzymatic retrieval of antigen permits staining of follicle centre cells by the rabbit polyclonal antibody to protein gene product 9.5, *J.Pathol.* 173, 249–253, 1994; Leong, A.S., Microwaves in diagnostic immunohistochemistry, *Eur.J.Morphol.* 34, 381–383, 1996; Lucas, D.R., al-Abbadi, M., Teabaczka, P., *et al.*, c-Kit expression in desmoid fibroblastosis. Comparative immunohistochemical evaluation of two commercial antibodies, *Am.J.Clin.Pathol.* 119, 339–345, 2003). Additional work has indicated that citrate is useful but not unique for epitope retrieval (Imam, S.A., Young, L., Chaiwun, B., and Taylor, C.B., Comparison of two microwave based antigen-retrieval solutions in unmasking epitopes in formalin-fixed tissues for immunostaining, *Anticancer Res.* 15, 1153–1158, 1995; Pileri, S.A., Roncador, G., Ceccarelli, C., *et al.*, Antigen retrieval techniques in immunohistochemistry: comparison of different methods, *J.Pathol.* 183, 116–123, 1997; Rocken, C. and Roessner, A., An evaluation of antigen retrieval procedures for immunoelectron microscopic classification of amyloid deposits, *J.Histochem.Cytochem.* 47, 1385–1394, 1999). Citrate buffer has been useful in affinity chromatography (Ishikawa, K. and Iwai, K., Affinity chromatography of cysteine-containing histone, *J.Biochem.* 77, 391–398, 1975; Chadha, K.C., Grob, P.M., Mikulski, A.J., *et al.*, Copper chelate affinity chromatography of human fibroblast and leucocyte interferons, *J.Gen.Virol.* 43, 701-706, 1979; Tanaka, H., Sasaki, I., Yamashita, K. *et al.*, Affinity chromatography of porcine pancreas deoxyribonuclease I on DNA-binding Sepharose under non-digestive conditions, using its substrate-binding site, *J.Biochem.* 88, 797–806, 1980 Smith, R.L. and Griffin, C.A., Separation of plasma fibronectin from associated hemagglutinating activity by elution from gelatin-agarose at pH 5.5, *Thromb.Res.* 37, 91–101, 1985). Citrate is also used for immunoaffinity chromatography including chromatography on Protein A (Martin, L.N., Separation of guinea pig IgG subclasses by affinity chromatography on protein A-Sepharose, *J.Immunol.Methods* 52, 205–212, 1982; Compton, B.J., Lewis, M.A., Whigham, F., *et al.*, Analtyical potential of protein A for affinity chromatography of polyclonal and monoclonal antibodies, *Anal.Chem.* 61, 1314–1317, 1989; Giraudi, G. and Baggiani, C. Strategy for fractionating high-affinity antibodies to steroid hormones by affinity chromatography, *Analyst* 121, 939–944, 1996; Arakawa, T., Philo, J.S., Tsumoto, K., *et al.*, Elution of antibodies from a Protein-A column by aqueous arginine solutions, *Protein Expr.Purif.* 36, 244–248, 2004; Ghose, S., McNerney, T., and Hubbard, B., Protein A affinity chromatography for capture and purification of monoclonal antibody and Fc-fusion protein: Practical considerations for process development, in *Process Scale Bioseparations for the Biopharmaceutical Industry*, ed. A.A. Shukla, M.R. Etzel, and S. Gadam, , ed. A.A. Shukla, M.R. Etzel, and S. Gadam, CRC/Taylor & Francis, Boca Raton, FL., Chapter 16, pps. 462–489, 2007).

LIST OF BUFFERS (Continued)

Common Name	Chemical Name	M.W	Properties and Comment
HEPES	4-(2-hydroxyethyl)-1-piperizineethanesulfonic acid	238.3	a "Good" buffer; reagent purity has been an issue; metal ion binding must be considered; there are buffer-specific effects which are poorly understood; component of tissue fixing technique

Good, N.E., Winget, G.D., Winter, W., *et al.*, Hydrogen ion buffers for biological research, *Biochemistry* 5, 467–477, 1966; Turner, L.V. and Manchester, K.L., Interference of HEPES with the Lowry method, *Science* 170, 649, 1970; Chirpich, T.P., The effect of different buffers on terminal deoxynucleotidyl transferase activity, *Biochim.Biophys.Acta* 518, 535–538, 1978; Tadolini, B., Iron autoxidation in Mops and Hepes buffers, *Free Radic.Res. Commun.* 4, 149–160, 1987; Simpson, J.A., Cheeseman, K.H., Smith, S.E., and Dean, R.T., Free-radical generation by copper ions and hydrogen peroxide. Stimulation by Hepes buffer, *Biochem.J.* 254, 519–523, 1988; Abas, L. and Guppy M., Acetate: a contaminant in Hepes buffer, *Anal.Biochem.* 229, 131–140, 1995; Schmidt, K., Pfeiffer, S., and Mayer, B., Reaction of peroxynitrite with HEPES or MOPS results in the formation of nitric oxide donors, *Free Radic. Biol.Med.* 24, 859–862, 1998; Wiedorn, K.H., Olert, J., Stacy, R.A., *et al.*, HOPE – a new fixing technique enables preservation and extraction of high molecular weight DNA and RNA of >20 kb from paraffin-embedded tissues. Hepes-glutamic acid buffer mediated Organic solvent Protection Effect, *Pathol.Res.Pract.* 198, 735–740, 2002; Fulop, L., Szigeti, G., Magyar, J., *et al.*, Differences in electrophysiological and contractile properties of mammalian cardiac tissues bathed in bicarbonate – and HEPES-buffered solutions, *Acta Physiol.Scand.*178, 11–18, 2003; Mash, H.E., Chin, Y.P., Sigg, L., *et al.*, Complexation of copper by zwitterionic aminosulfonic (good) buffers, *Anal.Chem.* 75, 671–677, 2003 Sokolowska, M., and Bal, W., Cu(II) complexation by "non-coordinating" N-2-hydroxyethylpiperazine-N'-ethanesulfonic acid (HEPES buffer), *J.Inorg.Biochem.* 99, 1653–1660, 2005; ; Zhao, G. and Chasteen, N.D., Oxidation of Good's buffers by hydrogen peroxide, *Anal.Biochem.* 349, 262–267, 2006; Hartman, R.F. and Rose, S.D., Kinetics and mechanism of the addition of nucleophiles to alpha,beta-unsaturated thiol esters, *J.Org.Chem.* 71, 6342–6350, 2006.

MES	1-morpholineethanesulfonic acid; 2-(4-morpholino)ethanesulfonate	198.2	A "Good" buffer

Good, N.E., Winget, G.D., Winter, W., *et al.*, Hydrogen ion buffers for biological research, *Biochemistry* 5, 467–477, 1966; Bugbee, B.G. and Salisbury, F.B., An evaluation of MES (2(N-morpholino)ethanesulfonic acid) and Amberlite 1RC-50 as pH buffers for nutrient growth studies, *J.Plant Nutr.* 8, 567–583, 1985; Kaushal, V. and Barnes, L.D., Effect of zwitterionic buffers on measurement of small masses of proiten with bicinchoninic acid, *Anal.Biochem.* 157, 291–294, 1986; Grady, J.K., Chasteen, N.D., and Harris, D.C., Radicals from "Good's buffers, *Anal.Biochem.* 173, 111–115, 1988; Le Hir, M., Impurity in buffer substances mimics the effect of ATP on soluble 5'-nucleotidase, *Enzyme* 45, 194–199, 1991; Pedrotti, B., Soffientini, A., and Islam, K., Sulphonate buffers affect the recovery of microtubule-associated proteins MAP1 and MAP2: evidence that MAP1A promotes microtubule assembly, *Cell Motil. Cytoskeleton* 25, 234–242, 1993; Vasseur, M., Frangne, R., and Alvarado, F., Buffer-dependent pH sensitivity of the fluorescent chloride-indicator dye SPQ, *Am.J.Physiol.* 264, C27–C31, 1993; Frick, J. and Mitchell, C.A., Stabilization of pH in solid-matrix hydroponic systems, *HortScience* 28, 981–984, 1993; Yu, Q., Kandegedara, A., Xu, Y., and Rorabacher, D.B., Avoiding interferences from Good's buffers: A continguous series of noncomplexing tertiary amine buffers covering the entire range of pH 3-11, *Anal.Biochem.* 253, 50–56, 1997; Gelfi, C., Vigano, A., Curcio, M., *et al.*, Single-strand conformation polymorphism analysis by capillary zone electrophoresis in neutral pH buffer, *Electrophoresis* 21, 785–791, 2000; Walsh, M.K., Wang, X., and Weimer, B.C., Optimizing the immobilization of single-stranded DNA onto glass beads, *J.Biochem.Biophys.Methods* 47, 221–231, 2001; Hosse, M. and Wilkinson, K.J., Determination of electrophoretic mobilities and hydrodynamic radii of three humic substances as a function of pH and ionic strength, *Environ.Sci.Technol.* 35, 4301–4306, 2001; Mash, H.E., Chin, Y.P., Sigg, L., *et al.*, Complexation of copper by zwitterionic aminosulfonic (good) buffers, *Anal.Chem.* 75, 671–677, 2003; Ozkara, S., Akgol, S., Canak, Y., and Denizli, A., A novel magnetic adsorbent for immunoglobulin-g purification in a magnetically stabilized fluidized bed, *Biotechnol.Prog.* 20, 1169–1175, 2004; Hachmann, J.P. and Amshey, J.W., Models of protein modification in Tris-glycine and neutral pH Bis-Tris gels during electrophoresis: effect of pH, *Anal.Biochem.* 342, 237–345, 2005; Krajewska, B. and Ciurli, S., Jack bean (*Canavalia ensiformis*) urease. Probing acid-base groups of the active site by pH variation, *Plant Physiol.Biochem.* 43, 651–658, 2005; Zhao, G. and Chasteen, N.D., Oxidation of Good's buffers by hydrogen peroxide, *Anal.Biochem.* 349, 262–267, 2006.

LIST OF BUFFERS (Continued)

Common Name	Chemical Name	M.W	Properties and Comment
MOPS	3-(*N*-morpholino)propanesulfonic acid;4-morpholinepropanesulfonic acid	209.3	A "Good" buffer

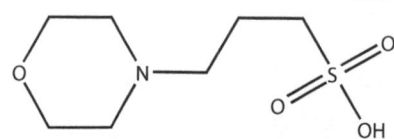

Good, N.E., Winget, G.D., Winter, W., *et al.*, Hydrogen ion buffers for biological research, *Biochemistry* 5, 467-477, 1966; Altura, B.M., Altura, B.M., Carella, A. and Altura, B.T., Adverse effects of Tris, HEPES and MOPS buffers on contractile responses of arterial and venous smooth muscle induced by prostaglandins, *Prostaglandins Med.* 5, 123-130, 1980; Tadolini, B., Iron autoxidation in Mops and Hepes buffers, *Free Radic.Res.Commun.* 4, 149-160, 1987;Tadolini, B. and Sechi, A.M., Iron oxidation in Mops buffer. Effect of phosphorus containing compounds, *Free Radic.Res.Commun.* 4, 161-172, 1987; Tadolini, B., Iron oxidation in Mops buffer. Effect of EDTA,. hydrogen peroxide and FeCl$_3$, *Free Radic.Res.Commun.* 4, 172-182, 1987; Ishihara, H. and Welsh, M.J., Block by MOPS reveals a conformation change in the CFTR pore produced by ATP hydrolysis, *Am.J.Physiol.* 273, C1278-C1289, 1997; Schmidt, K., Pfeiffer, S., and Meyer, B., Reaction of peroxynitrite with HEPES or MOPS results in the formation of nitric oxide donors, *Free Radic.Biol. Med.* 24, 859-862, 1998; Hodges, G.R. and Ingold, K.U., Superoxide, amine buffers and tetranitromethane: a novel free radical chain reaction, *Free Radic. Res.* 33, 547-550, 2000; Corona-Izquierdo, F.P. and Membrillo-Hernandez, J., Biofilm formation in *Escherichia coli* is affected by 3-(*N*-morpholino)propane sulfonate (MOPS), *Res.Microbiol.* 153, 181-185, 2002; Mash, H.E., Chin, Y.P., Sigg, L., *et al.*, Complexation of copper by zwitterionic aminosulfonic (good) buffers, *Anal.Chem.* 75, 671-677, 2003; Denizli, A., Alkan, M., Garipcan, B., *et al.*, Novel metal-chelate affinity adsorbent for purification of immunoglobulin-G from human plasma, *J.Chromatog.B.Analyt.Technol.Biomed.Life.Sci.* 795, 93-103, 2003; Emir, S., Say, R., Yavuz, H., and Denizli, A., A new metal chelate affinity adsorbent for cytochrome C, *Biotechnol.Prog.* 20, 223-228, 2004; Cvetkovic, A., Zomerdijk, M., Straathof, A.J., *et al.*, Adsorption of fluorescein by protein crystals, *Biotechnol.Bioeng.* 87, 658-668, 2004; Zhao, G. and Chasteen, J.D., Oxidation of Good's buffers by hydrogen peroxide, *Anal.Biochem.* 349, 2620267, 2006; Vrakas, D., Giaginis, C. and Tsantili-Kakoulidou, A., Different retention behavior of structurally diverse basic and neutral drugs in immobilized artificial membrane and reversed-phase high performance liquid chromatography: comparison with octanol-water partitioning, *J.Chromatog.A.* 1116, 158-164, 2006; de Carmen Candia-Plata, M., Garcia, J., Guzman, R., *et al.*, Isolation of human serum immunoglobulins with a new salt-promoted adsorbent, *J.Chromatog.A.* 1118, 211-217, 2006.

Phosphate

Phosphate buffers are among the most common buffers used for biological studies. It is noted that the use of phosphate solutions in early transfusion medicine lead to the discovery of the importance of calcium ions in blood coagulation (Hutchin, P., History of blood transfusion: A tercentennial look, *Surgery* 64, 685–700, 1968). Phosphate-buffer saline (PBS; generally 0.01 M sodium phosphate – 0.14 M NaCl, pH 7.2 – Note, an incredible variation in PBS exists so it is necessary to verify composition – the only common factor that this writer finds is 0.01 M (10 mM) phosphate) is extensively used. Sodium phosphate buffers are the most common but there is extensive use of potassium phosphate buffers and mixtures of sodium and potassium. Unfortunately many investigators simply refer to phosphate buffer without respect to counter ion. Also, investigators will prepare a stock solution of sodium phosphate[usually sodium dihydrogen phosphate (sodium phosphate, monobasic) or disodium hydrogen phosphate (sodium phosphate, dibasic) and adjust pH as required with (usually) hydrochloric acid and/or sodium hydrogen. This is not preferable and, if used, must be described in the text to permit other investigators to repeat the experiment. pH changes in phosphate buffers during freezing can be dramatic due to precipitation of phosphate buffer salts (van den Berg, L. and Rose, D., Effect of freezing on the pH and composition of sodium and potassium phosphate solutions: The reciprocal system KH$_2$PO$_4$-Na$_2$PO$_4$-H$_2$O, *Arch.Biochem.Biophys.* 81, 319–329, 1959; Murase, N. and Franks, F., Salt precipitation during the freeze-concentration of phosphate buffer solutions, *Biophys.Chem.* 34, 393–300, 1989; Pikal-Cleland, K.A. and Carpenter, J.F., Lyophilization-induced protein denaturation in phosphate buffer systems: monomeric and tetrameric beta-galactosidase, *J.Pharm.Sci.* 90, 1255–1268, 2001; Gomez, G., Pikal, M., and Rodriguez-Hornedo, N., Effect of initial buffer composition on pH changes during far-from-equilibrium freezing of sodium phosphate buffer solutions, *Pharm.Res.* 18, 90–97, 2001; Pikal-Cleland, K.A., Cleland, J.L., Anchorodoquy, T.J. and Carpenter, J.F., Effect of glycine on pH changes and protein stability during freeze-thawing in phosphate buffer systems, *J.Pharm .Sci.* 91, 1969–1979, 2002). Phosphate bind divalent cations in solutions

LIST OF BUFFERS (Continued)

Common Name	Chemical Name	M.W	Properties and Comment

and can form insoluble salts. Phosphate influences biological reactions by binding cations such as calcium, platinum and iron (Staum, M.M., Incompatibility of phosphate buffer in 99^m Tc-sulfur colloid containing aluminum ion, *J.Nucl.Med.* 13, 386–387, 1972; Frank, G.B., Antagonism by phosphate buffer of the twitch ions in isolated muscle fibers produced by calcium-free solutions, *Can.J.Physiol.Pharmacol.* 56, 523–526, 1978; Hasegawa, K., Hashi, K., and Okada, R., Physicochemical stability of pharmaceutical phosphate buffer solutions. I. Complexation behavior of Ca(II) with additives in phosphate buffer solutions, *J.Parenter.Sci.Technol.* 36, 128–133, 1982; Abe, K., Kogure, K., Arai, H., and Nakano, M., Ascorbate induced lipid peroxidation results in loss of receptor binding in tris, but not in phosphate, buffer. Implications for the involvement of metal ions, *Biochem.Int.* 11, 341–348, 1985; Pedersen, H.B., Josephsen, J., and Keerszan, G., Phosphate buffer and salt medium concentrations affect the inactivation of T4 phage by platinum(II) complexes, *Chem.Biol.Interact.* 54, 1–8, 1985; Kuzuya, M., Yamada, K., Hayashi, T., *et al.*, Oxidation of low-density lipoprotein by copper and iron in phosphate buffer, *Biochim.Biophys.Acta* 1084, 198–201, 1991. Also see Wolf, W.J., and Sly, D.A., Effects of buffer cations on chromatography of proteins on hydroxylapatite, *J.Chromatog.* 15, 247–250, 1964; Taborsky, G., Oxidative modification of proteins in the presence of ferrous ion and air. Effect of ionic constituents of the reaction medium on the nature of the oxidation products, *Biochemistry* 12, 1341–1348, 1973; Millsap, K.W., Reid, G., van der Mei, H.C., and Busscher, H.J., Adhesion of *Lactobacillus* species in urine and phosphate buffer to silicone rubber and glass under flow, *Biomaterials* 18, 87–91, 1997; Gebauer, P. and Bocek, P., New aspects of buffering with multivalent weak acids in capillary zone electrophoresis: pros and cons of the phosphate buffer, *Electrophoresis* 21, 2809–2813, 2000; Gebauer, P., Pantuikova, P. and Bocek, P., Capillary zone electrophoresis in phosphate buffer – known or unknown?, *J.Chromatog.A* 894, 89–93, 2000; Buchanan, D.D., Jameson, E.E., Perlette, J., *et al.*, Effect of buffer, electric field, and separation time on detection of aptamers-ligand complexes for affinity probe capillary electrophoresis, *Electrophoresis* 24, 1375–1382, 2003; Ahmad, I., Fasihullah, Z. and Vaid, F.H., Effect of phosphate buffer on photodegradation reactions of riboflavin in aqueous solution, *J.Photochem.Photobiol.B* 78, 229–234, 2005.

| PIPES | piperazine-*N*,*N*'-bis(2-ethanesulfonic acid)1,4-piperazinediethane sulfonic acid | 302.4 | A "Good" buffer |

Good, N.E., Winget, G.D., Winter, W., *et al.*, Hydrogen ion buffers for biological research, *Biochemistry* 5, 467–477, 1966; Olmsted, J.B. and Borisy, G.G., Ionic and nucleotide requirements for microtubule polymerization in vitro, *Biochemistry* 14, 2996–3005, 1975; Baur, P.S. and Stacey, T.R., The use of PIPES buffer in the fixation of mammalian and marine tissues for electron microscopy, *J.Micros.* 109, 315–327, 1977; Schiff, R.I. and Gennaro, J.F., Jr., The influence of the buffer on maintenance of tissue liquid in specimens for scanning electron microscopy, *Scan.Electron Microsc.* (3), 449–458, 1979; Altura, B.M., Altura, B.T., Carella, A., and Turlapty, P.D., Adverse effects of artificial buffers on contractile responses of arterial and venous smooth muscles, *Br.J.Pharmacol.* 69, 207–214, 1980; Syvertsen, C. and McKinley-McKee, J.S., Affinity labeling of liver alcohol dehydrogenase. Effects of pH and buffers on affinity labelling with iodoacetic acid and (*R,S*-2-bromo-3-(5-imidazolyl)propionic acid, *Eur.J.Biochem.* 117, 165–170, 1981; Roy, R.N., Gibbons, J.J., Padron, J.L., *et al.*, Revised values of the paH of monosodium 1,4-piperazinediethanesulfonate ("Pipes") in water other buffers in isotonic saline at various temperatures, *Clin.Chem.* 27, 1787–1788, 1981; Waxman, P.G., del Campo, A.A., Lowe, M.C., and Hamel, E., Induction of polymerization of purified tubulin by sulfonate buffers. Marked differences between 4-morpholineethananesulfonate (Mes) and 1,4-piperazineethanesulfonate(Pipes), *Eur.J.Biochem.* 129, 129–136, 1981; Yamamoto, K. and Ogawa, K., Effects of NaOH-PIPES buffer used in aldehyde fixative on alkaline phosphatase activity in rat hepatocytes, *Histochemistry* 77, 339–351, 1983; Haviernick, S., Lalague, E.D., Corvellec, M.R., *et al.*, The use of Hanks'—pipes buffers in the preparation of human, normal leukocytes for TEM observation, *J.Microsc.* 135, 83–88, 1984; Simpson, J.A., Cheeseman, K.H., Smith, S.E., and Dean, R.T., Free-radical generation by copper ions and hydrogen peroxide. Stimulation by Hepes buffers, *Biochem.J.* 254, 519–523, 1988; Prutz, W.A. The interaction between hydrogen peroxide and the DNA-Cu(I) complex: effects of pH and buffers, *Z.Naturforsch.* 45, 1197–1206, 1990; Le Hir, M., Impurity in buffer substances mimics the effects of ATP on soluble 5'-nucleotidase, *Enzyme* 45, 194–199, 1991; Lee, B.H. and Nowak, T., Influence of pH on the Mn^{2+} activation of and binding to yeast enolase: a functional study, *Biochemistry* 31, 2165–2171, 1992; Tedokon, M., Suzuki, K., Kayamori, Y., *et al.*, Enzymatic assay of inorganic phosphate with the use of sucrose phosphorylase and phosphoglucomutase, *Clin.Chem.* 38, 512–515, 1992; Correla, J.J., Lipscomb, L.D., Dabrowiak, J.C., *et al.*, Cleavage of tubulin by vandate ion, *Arch.Biochem.Biophys.* 309, 94–104, 1994; Schmidt, J., Mangold, C., and Deitmer, J., Membrane responses evoked by organic buffers in identified leech neurones, *J.Exp.Biol.* 199, 327–335, 1996; Yu, Q., Kandegedara, A., Xu, Y., and Rorabacher, D.B., Avoiding interferences from Good's buffers: A contiguous series of noncomplexing tertiary amine buffers covering the entire pH range of pH 3-11, *Anal.Biochem.* 253, 50–56, 1997; Rover Junior, L., Fernandes, J.C., de Oliveira Neto, G., *et al.*, Study of NADH stability using ultraviolet-visible spectrophotometric analysis and factorial design, *Anal.Biochem.* 260, 50–55, 1998; Moore, S.A., Kingston, R.L., Loomes, K.M., *et al.*, The structure of truncated recombinant human bile salt-stimulated lipase reveals bile salt-independent conformational flexibility at the active-site loop and provides insights into heparin binding, *J.Mol.Biol.* 3 12, 511–523, 2001; Sani, R.K., Peyton, B.M., and Dohnalkova, A., Toxic effects of uranium on *Desulfovibrio desulfuricans* G20, *Environ. Toxicol.Chem.* 25, 1231–1238, 2006.

LIST OF BUFFERS (Continued)

Common Name	Chemical Name	M.W	Properties and Comment
TES	N-tris(hydroxymethyl) methyl-2-aminoethane-sulfonic acid	229.3	A "Good" buffer.

Good, N.E., Winget, G.D., Winter, W., et al., Hydrogen ion buffers for biological research, *Biochemistry* 5, 467–477, 1966; Itagaki, A. and Kimura, G., Tes and HEPES buffers in mammalian cell cultures and viral studies: problem of carbon dioxide requirement, *Exp.Cell Res.* 83, 351–361, 1974; Bridges, S. and Ward, B., Effect of hydrogen ion buffers on photosynthetic oxygen evolution in the blue-green alga, *Agmenellum quadruplicatum, Microbios* 15, 49–56, 1976; Bailyes, E.M., Luzio, J.P., and Newby, A.C., The use of a zwitterionic detergent in the solubilization and purification of the intrinsic membrane protein 5'-nucleotidase, *Biochem.Soc.Trans.* 9, 140–141, 1981; Poole, C.A., Reilly, H.C., and Flint, M.H., The adverse effects of HEPES, TES, and BES zwitterionic buffers on the ultrastructure of cultured chick embryo epiphyseal chondrocytes, *In Vitro* 18, 755–765, 1982; Nakon, R. and Krishnamoorthy, C.R., Free-metal ion depletion by "Good's" buffers, *Science* 221, 749–750, 1983; del Castillo, J., Escalona de Motta, G., Eterovic, V.A., and Ferchmin, P.A., Succinyl derivatives of N-tris (hydroxylmethyl) methyl-2-aminoethane sulphonic acid: their effects on the frog neuromuscular junction, *Br.J.Pharmacol.* 84, 275–288, 1985; Kaushal, V. and Varnes, L.D., Effect of zwitterionic buffers on measurement of small masses of protein with bicinchoninic acid, *Anal.Biochem.* 157, 291–294, 1986; Bhattacharyya, A. and Yanagimachi, R., Synthetic organic pH buffers can support fertilization of guinea pig eggs, but not as efficiently as bicarbonate buffer, *Gamete Res.* 19, 123–129, 1988; Veeck, L.L., TES and Tris (TEST)-yolk buffer systems, sperm function testing, and in vitro fertilization, *Fertil.Steril.* 58, 484–486, 1992; Kragh-Hansen, U. and Vorum, H., Quantitative analyses of the interaction between calcium ions and human serum albumin, *Clin.Chem.* 39, 202–208, 1993; Jacobs, B.R., Caulfield, J., and Boldt, J., Analysis of TEST (TES and Tris) yolk buffer effects of human sperm, *Fertil.Steril.* 63, 1064–1070, 1995; Stellwagne, N.C., Bossi, A., Gelfi, C., and Righetti, P.G., DNA and buffers: are there any noninteracting, neutral pH buffers?, *Anal.Biochem.* 287, 167–175, 2000; Taylor, J., Hamilton, K.L., and Butt, A.G., HCO_3^- potentiates the cAMP-dependent secretory response of the human distal colon through a DIDS-sensitive pathway, *Pflugers Arch.* 442, 256–262, 2001; Taha, M., Buffers for the physiological pH range: acidic dissociation constants of zwitterionic compounds in various hydroorganic media, *Ann.Chim.* 95, 105–109, 2005.

| Tricine | N-[tris(hydroxymethyl) methyl] glycine; N-[2-hydroxy-1,1-bis-(hydroxymethyl)ethyl] glycine | 179.2 | A "Good" buffer which is also used as a chelating agent, useful for cupric ions. Tricine is also used to complex technetium-99(99mTc) in cancer therapy. |

Garder, R.S., The use of tricine buffer in animal tissue cultures, *J.Cell Biol.* 42, 320–321, 1969; Spendlove, R.S., Crosbie, R.B., Hayes, S.F., and Keeler, R.F., TRICINE-buffered tissue culture media for control of mycoplasma contaminants, *Proc.Soc.Exptl.Biol.Med.* 137, 258–263, 1971; Bates, R.G., Roy, R.N., and Robinson, R.A., Buffer standards of tris(hydroxymethyl)methylglycine ("tricine") for the physiological range pH 7.2 to 8.5, *Anal.Chem.* 45, 1663–1666, 1973; Roy, R.N., Robinson, R.A., and Bates, R.G., Thermodynamics of the two dissociation steps of N-tris(hydroxymethyl)methylglycine ("tricine") in water from 5 to 50 degrees, *J.Amer.Chem.Soc.* 95, 8231–8235, 1973; Grande, H.J. and van der Ploeg, K.R., Tricine radicals as formed in the presence of peroxide producing enzymes, *FEBS Lett.* 95, 352-356, 1978; Roy, R.N., Gibbons, J.J., and Baker, G.E., Acid dissociation constants and pH values for standard "bes" and "tricine" buffer solutions in 30, 40, and 50 mass% dimethyl sulfoxide/water between 25 and -25°C, *Cryobiology* 22, 589–600, 1985; Hall, M.S. and Leach, F.R., Stability of firefly luciferase in tricine buffer and in a commercial enzyme stabilizer, *J.Biolumin.Chemilumin.* 2, 41–44, 1988; Patton, W.F., Chung-Welch, N., Lopez, M.F., *et al,,* Tris-tricine and tris-borate buffer systems provide better estimates of human mesothelial cell intermediate filament protein molecular weights than the standard Tris-glycine system, *Anal.Biochem.* 197, 25–33, 1991; [99mTc]tricine: a useful precursor complex for the radiolabeling of hydrazinonicotinate protein conjugates, *Bioconjugate Chem.* 6, 635–638, 1995; Wisdom, G.B., Molecular weight determinations using polyacrylamide gel electrophoresis with tris-tricine buffers, *Methods Mol.Biol.* 73, 97–100, 1997; Barrett, J.A., Crocker, A.C., Damphousee, D.J.. Biological evaluation of thrombus imaging agents utilizing water soluble phospines and tricine as coligands when used to label a hydrazinonicotinamide-modified cyclic glycoprotein IIb/IIIa receptor antagonist with 99mTc, *Bioconjug.Chem.* 8, 155–160, 1997; Bangard, M., Behe, M., Guhlke, S., *et al.,* Detection of somatostatin receptor-positive tumours using the new 99mTc-tricine-HYNIC-D-Phe1-Tyr3-octreotide: first results in patients and comparison with 111In-D-Phe1-octreotide, *Eur.J.Nucl.Med.* 27, 628–637, 2000; Ramos silva, M., Paixao, J.A. , Matos Beja, A., and Alte da Veiga, L., Conformational flexibility of tricine as a chelating agent in catena-poly-[[(tricinato)copper(II)]-mu-chloro], *Acta Crystallogr.C.* 57, 9–11, 2001; Silva, M.R., Paixo, J.A., Beja, A., and Alte da Veiga, L., N-[Tris(hydroxymethyl)methyl]glycine(tricine), *Acta Crystallogr.C.* 57, 421–422, 2001;

LIST OF BUFFERS (Continued)

Common Name	Chemical Name	M.W	Properties and Comment

Su, Z.F., He, J., Rusckowski, M., and Hnatowich, D.J., In vitro cell studies of technetium-99m-labeled RGD-HYNIC peptide, a comparison of tricine and EDDA as co-ligands, *Nucl.Med.Biol.* 30, 141–149, 2003; Le, Q.T. and Katunuma, N., Detection of protease inhibitors by a reverse zymography method, performed in a tris(hydroxylmethyl)aminomethane-Tricine buffer system, *Anal.Biochem.* 324, 237–240, 2004.

Triethanolamine	tris(2-hydroxyethyl) amine	149.2	Buffer; transdermal transfer reagent

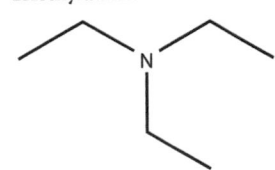

Fitzgerald, J.W., The tris-catalyzed isomerization of potassium D-glucose 6-*O*-sulfate, *Can.J.Biochem.* 53, 906–910, 1975; Buhl, S.N., Jackson, K.Y., and Graffunder, B., Optimal reaction conditions for assaying human lactate dehydrogenase pyruvate-to-lactate at 25, 30, and 37 degrees C, *Clin.Chem.* 24, 261–266, 1978; Myohanen, T.A., Bouriotas, V., and Dean, P.D. Affinity chromatography of yeast alpha-glucosidase using ligand-mediated chromatography on immobilized phenylboronic acids, *Biochem.J.* 197, 683–688, 1981; Shinomiya, Y., Kato, N., Imazawa, M., and Miyamoto, K., Enzyme immunoassay of the myelin basic protein, *J.Neurochem.* 39, 1291–1296, 1982; Arita, M., Iwamori, M., Higuchi, T., and Nagai, Y., 1,1,3,3-tetramethylurea and triethanolaminme as a new useful matrix for fast atom bombardment mass spectrometry of gangliosides and neutral glycosphingolipids, *J.Biochem.* 93, 319–322, 1983; Cao, H. and Preiss, J., Evidence for essential arginine residues at the active site of maize branching enzymes, *J.Protein Chem.* 15, 291–304, 1996; Knaak, J.B., Leung, H.W., Stott, W.T., *et al.*, Toxicology of mono-, di-, and triethanolamine, *Rev.Environ.Contim.Toxicol.* 149, 1–86, 1997; Liu, Q., Li, X., and Sommer, S.S., pK-matched running buffers for gel electrophoresis, *Anal.Biochem.* 270, 112–122, 1999; Sanger-van de Griend, C.E., Enantiomeric separation of glycyl dipeptides by capillary electrophoresis with cyclodextrins as chiral selectors, *Electrophoresis* 20, 3417–3424, 1999; Fang, L., Kobayashi, Y., Numajiri, S., *et al.*, The enhancing effect of a triethanolamine-ethanol-isopropyl myristate mixed system on the skin permeation of acidic drugs, *Biol.Pharm.Bull.* 25, 1339–1344, 2002; Musial, W. and Kubis, A., Effect of some anionic polymers of pH of triethanolamine aqueous solutions, *Polim.Med.* 34, 21–29, 2004.

Triethylamine	*N,N*-diethylethanamine	101.2	ion-pair reagent; buffer

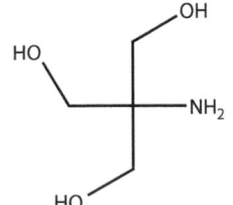

Brind, J.L., Kuo, S.W., Chervinsky, K., and Orentreich, N., A new reversed phase, paired-ion thin-layer chromatographic method for steroid sulfate separations, *Steroids* 52, 561–570, 1988; Koves, E.M., Use of high-performance liquid chromatography-diode array detection in forensic toxicology, *J.Chromatog.A* 692, 103–119, 1995; Cole, S.R. and Dorsey, J.G., Cyclohexylamine additives for enhanced peptide separations in reversed phase liquid chromatography, *Biomed.Chromatog.* 11, 167–171, 1997; Gilar, M., and Bouvier, E.S.P., Purification of crude DNA oligonucleotides by solid-phase extraction and reversed-phase high-performance liquid chromatography, *J.Chromatog.A* 890, 167–177, 2000; Loos, R. and Barcelo, D., Determination of haloacetic acids in aqueous environments by solid-phase extraction followed by ion-pair liquid chromatography-electrospray ionization mass spectrometric detection, *J.Chromatog.A.* 938, 45–55, 2001; Gilar, M., Fountain, K.J., Budman, Y., *et al.*, Ion-pair reversed phase high-performance liquid chromatography analysis of oligonucleotides: retention prediction, *J.Chromatog.A.* 958, 167–182, 2002; El-dawy, M.A., Mabrouk, M.M., and El-Barbary, F.A., Liquid chromatographic determination of fluoxetine, *J.Pharm.Biomed.Anal.* 30, 561–571, 2002; Yang, X., Zhang, X., Li, A., *et al.*, Comprehensive two-dimensional separations based on capillary high-performance liquid chromatography and microchip electrophoresis, *Electrophoresis* 24, 1451–1457, 2003; Murphey, A.T., Brown-Augsburger, P., Yu, R.Z., *et al.*, Development of an ion-pair reverse-phase liquid chromatographic/tandem mass spectrometry method for the determination of an 18-mer phosphorothioate oligonucleotide in mouse liver tissue, *Eur.J.Mass Spectrom.* 11, 209–215, 2005; Xie, G., Sueishi, Y., and Yamamoto, S., Analysis of the effects of protic, aprotic, and multi-component solvents on the fluorescence emission of naphthalene and its exciplex with triethylamine, *J.Fluoresc.* 15, 475–483, 2005.

Tris	tris(hydroxymethyl)aminomethylmethane	121.14	Buffer

LIST OF BUFFERS (Continued)

Common Name	Chemical Name	M.W	Properties and Comment

Bernhard, S.A., Ionization constants and heats of tris(hydroxymethyl)aminomethane and phosphate buffers, *J.Biol.Chem.* 218, 961–969, 1956; Rapp, R.D. and Memminger, M.M., Tris (hydroxymethyl)aminomethane as an electrophoresis buffer, *Am.J.Clin.Pathol.* 31, 400–403, 1959; Rodkey, F.L., Tris(hydroxymethyl)aminomethane as a standard for Kjeldahl nitrogen analysis, *Clin.Chem.* 10, 606–610, 1964; Oliver, R.W. and Viswanatha, T., Reaction of tris(hydroxymethyl)aminomethane with cinnamoyl imidazole and cinnamoyltrypsin, *Biochim.Biophys.Acta* 156, 422–425, 1968; Douzou, P., Enzymology at sub-zero temperatures, *Mol.Cell.Biochem.* 1, 15–27, 1973; The tris-catalyzed isomerization of potassium D-glucose 6-O-sulfate, *Can.J.Biochem.* 53, 906–910, 1975; Visconti, M.A. and Castrucci, A.M., Tris buffer effects on melanophore aggegrating responses, *Comp.Biochem. Physiol.C* 82, 501–503 1985; Stambler, B.S., Grant, A.O., Broughton, A., and Strauss, H.C., Influences of buffers on dV/dtmax recovery kinetics with lidocaine in myocardium, *Am.J.Physiol.* 249, H663–H671, 1985; Nakano, M. and Tauchi, H., Difference in activation by Tris(hydroxymethyl) aminomethane of Ca,Mg-ATPase activity between young and old rat skeletal muscles, *Mech.Aging.Dev.* 36, 287–294, 1986; Oliveira, L., Araujo-Viel, M.S., Juliano, L., and Prado, E.S., Substrate activation of porcine kallikrein N-α derivatives of arginine 4-nitroanilides, *Biochemistry* 26, 5032–5035, 1987; Ashworth, C.D. and Nelson, D.R., Antimicrobial potentiation of irrigation solutions containing tris-[hydroxymethyl] aminomethane-EDTA, *J.Am.Vet.Med. Assoc.* 197, 1513–1514, 1990; Schacker, M., Foth, H., Schluter, J., and Kahl, R., Oxidation of tris to one-carbon compounds in a radical-producing model system, in microsomes, in hepatocytes and in rats, *Free Radic.Res.Commun.* 11, 339–347, 1991; Weber, R.E., Use of ionic and zwitterionic (Tris/BisTris and HEPES) buffers in studies on hemoglobin function, *J.Appl.Physiol.* 72, 1611–1615, 1992; Veeck, L.L., TES and Tris (TEST)-yolk buffer systems, sperm function testing, and in vitro fertilization, *Fertil.Steril.* 58, 484–486, 1992; Shiraishi, H., Kataoka, M., Morita, Y., and Umemoto, J., Interaction of hydroxyl radicals with tris (hydroxymethyl) aminomethane and Good's buffers containing hydroxymethyl or hydroxyethyl residues produce formaldehyde, *Free Radic.Res.Commun.* 19, 315–321, 1993; Vasseur, M., Frangne, R., and Alvarado, F., Buffer-dependent pH sensitivity of the fluorescent chloride-indicator dye SPQ, *Am.J.Physiol.* 264, C27–C31, 1993; Niedernhofer, L.J., Riley, M., Schnez-Boutand, N., *et al.*, Temperature dependent formation of a conjugate between tris(hydroxymethyl)aminomethane buffer and the malondialdehyde-DNA adduct pyrimidopurinone, *Chem.Res.Toxicol.* 10, 556–561, 1997; Trivic, S., Leskovac, V., Zeremski, J., *et al.*, Influence of Tris(hydroxymethyl)aminomethane on kinetic mechanism of yeast alcohol dehydrogenase, *J.Enzyme Inhib.* 13, 57–68, 1998; Afifi, N.N., Using difference spectrophotometry to study the influence of different ions and buffer systems on drug protein binding, *Drug Dev.Ind.Pharm.* 25, 735–743, 1999; AbouHaider, M.G. and Ivanov, I.G., Non-enzymatic RNA hydrolysis promotedby the combined catalytic activity of buffers and magnesium ions, *Z.Naturforsch.* 54, 542–548, 1999; Shihabi, Z.K., Stacking of discontinuous buffers in capillary zone electrophoresis, *Electrophoresis* 21, 2872–2878, 2000; Stellwagen, N.C, Bossi, A., Gelfi, C., and Righetti, P.G., DNA and buffers: are theire any nointeracting, neutral pH buffers?, *Anal.Biochem.* 287, 167–175, 2000;Burcham, P.C., Fontaine, F.R., Petersen, D.R., and Pyke, S.M., Reactivity of Tris(hydroxymethyl) aminomethane confounds immunodetection of acrolein-adducted proteins, *Chem.Res.Toxicol.* 16, 1196–1201, 2003; Koval, D., Kasicka, V., and Zuskova, I., Investigation of the effect of ionic strength of Tris-acetate background electrolyte on electrophoretic mobilities of mono-, di-, and trivalent organic anions by capillary electrophoresis, *Electrophoresis* 26, 3221–3231, 2005; Kinoshita, T., Yamaguchi, A., and Tada, T., Tris(hydroxymethyl)aminomethane induced conformational change and crystal-packing contraction of porcine pancreatic elastase, *Acta Crystallograph. Sect.F .Struct. Biol. Cryst.Commun.* 62, 623–626, 2006; Qi, Z., Li, X., Sun, D., *et al,*, Effect of Tris on catalytic activity of MP-11, *Bioelectrochemistry* 68, 40–47, 2006.

BRØNSTED ACIDITIES

Roger L. Lundblad

Definition: A molecule (conjugate acid) which liberates a proton in solution; the residual molecular ion is a conjugate base

$EH_x \rightarrow EH_{x-1}$
  –Acid strength depends on the strength of the E-H bond.
  –Electronegativity of E influences the polarity of the E-H bond
  –Energy of solvation of $[EH_{x-1}]^-$ – small anions have more favorable solvation energies
pKa values of EH_x
CH_4 –58
NH_3 39
OH_2 14
SH_2 7
SeH_2 4
TeH_2 3
FH 3

Mingo, D.M.P., *Essential Trends of Inorganic Chemistry*, Oxford University Press, Oxford, United Kingdom, 1998.

Lewis Acids

Definition: A molecule which can accept electrons.

$AlCl_3 + Cl^- \rightarrow [AlCl_4]^-$

Lewis Base is an electron donor, for example PR_3—which becomes a "stronger" base as the electron donating properties of the R group increases as long as the Lewis acid is a simple electron acceptor and steric effects are not important.

References

Blackwell, J.A. and Carr, S.W., The role of Lewis Acid-Base processes in ligand-exchange chromatography of benzoic acid derivatives on zirconium oxide, *Anal.Chem.* 64, 853–862, 1992.
Hancock, R.D., Bartolotti, L.J., and Kaltsoyannis, N., Density functional theory-based prediction of some aqueous-phase chemistry of superheavy element 111. Roentgenium(I) is the 'softest' metal ion, *Inorg.Chem.* 45, 10780–10785, 2006.

BUFFER SOLUTIONS

No.	Name	Range of pH Value	Temperature (°C)	ΔpH/K
	GENERAL BUFFERS			
1	KCl/HCl (Clark and Lubs)[2]	1.0–2.2	Room	0
2	Glycine/HCl (Sørensen)[3]	1.2–3.4	Room	0
3	Na citrate/HCl (Sørensen)[3]	1.2–5.0	Room	0
4	K biphthalate/HCl (Clark and Lubs)[2]	2.4–4.0	20	+ 0.001
5	K biphthalate/NaOH (Clark and Lubs)[2]	4.2–6.2	20	
6	Na citrate/NaOH (Sørensen)[3]	5.2–6.6	20	+ 0.004
7	Phosphate (Sørensen).[3]	5.0–8.0	20	− 0.003
8	Barbital-Na/HCl (Michaelis)[4]	7.0–9.0	18	
9	Na borate/HCl (Sørensen)[3]	7.8–9.2	20	− 0.005
10	Glycine/NaOH (Sørensen)[3]	8.6–12.8	20	− 0.025
11	Na borate/NaOH (Sørensen)[3]	9.4–10.6	20	− 0.01
	UNIVERSAL BUFFERS			
12	Citric acid/phosphate (McIlvaine)[5]	2.2–7.8	21	
13	Citrate-phosphate-borate/HCl (Teorell and Stenhagen)[6]	2.0–12.0	20	
14	Britton-Robinson[7]	2.6–11.8	25	At low pH:0 At high pH: − 0.02
	BUFFERS FOR BIOLOGICAL MEDIA			
15	Acetate (Walpole)[8–10]	3.8–5.6	25	
16	Dimethylglutaric acid/NaOH[11]	3.2–7.6	21	
17	Piperazine/HCl[12,13]	4.6–6.4	20	
		8.8–10.6		
18	Tetraethylethylenediamine[a,13]	5.0–6.8	20	
		8.2–10.0		
19	Tris maleate[9,14]	5.2–8.6	23	
20	Dimethylaminoethylamine[a,13]	5.6–7.4	20	
		8.6–10.4		
21	Imidazole/HCl[15]	6.2–7.8	25	
22	Triethanolamine/HCl[16]	7.9–8.8	25	
23	N-Dimethylaminoleucylglycine/NaOH[17]	7.0–8.8	23	− 0.015
24	Tris/HCl[9]	7.2–9.0	23	− 0.02
25	2-Amino-2-methylpropane-1,3-diol/HCl[9,14]	7.8–10.0	23	
26	Carbonate (Delory and King)[9,8]	9.2–10.8	20	

[a] Can be combined with tris buffer to give a cationic universal buffer (see Semenza et al.[13]).

BUFFER SOLUTIONS (Continued)

pH	1	2	3	4	5	6	7	8	9	10	11	12	13	14	15	16a	16b	17	18	19	20	21	22	23	24	25	26
1.0	54.2	—	—	—	—	—	—	—	—	—	—	—	—	—	—	—	—	—	—	—	—	—	—	—	—	—	—
1.2	36.0	11.1	9.0	—	—	—	—	—	—	—	—	—	—	—	—	—	—	—	—	—	—	—	—	—	—	—	—
1.4	23.2	26.4	17.9	—	—	—	—	—	—	—	—	—	—	—	—	—	—	—	—	—	—	—	—	—	—	—	—
1.6	14.7	36.2	23.6	—	—	—	—	—	—	—	—	—	—	—	—	—	—	—	—	—	—	—	—	—	—	—	—
1.8	9.3	43.9	27.6	—	—	—	—	—	—	—	—	—	—	—	—	—	—	—	—	—	—	—	—	—	—	—	—
2.0	5.9	50.7	30.2	—	—	—	—	—	—	—	—	—	74.4	—	—	—	—	—	—	—	—	—	—	—	—	—	—
2.2	3.8	56.5	32.2	—	—	—	—	—	—	—	—	98.8	68.8	—	—	—	—	—	—	—	—	—	—	—	—	—	—
2.4	—	62.3	34.1	41.0	—	—	—	—	—	—	—	94.5	64.6	—	—	—	—	—	—	—	—	—	—	—	—	—	—
2.6	—	68.4	36.0	34.3	—	—	—	—	—	—	—	90.0	63.3	1.6	—	—	—	—	—	—	—	—	—	—	—	—	—
2.8	—	74.7	37.9	27.8	—	—	—	—	—	—	—	85.1	58.9	3.6	—	—	—	—	—	—	—	—	—	—	—	—	—
3.0	—	81.0	39.9	21.6	—	—	—	—	—	—	—	80.3	56.9	5.7	—	—	—	—	—	—	—	—	—	—	—	—	—
3.2	—	86.2	42.1	15.9	—	—	—	—	—	—	—	76.0	55.2	7.8	—	7.0	14.4	—	—	—	—	—	—	—	—	—	—
3.4	—	90.3	44.8	10.9	—	—	—	—	—	—	—	72.0	53.9	9.9	—	13.3	20.9	—	—	—	—	—	—	—	—	—	—
3.6	—	—	47.8	6.7	—	—	—	—	—	—	—	68.4	52.9	11.7	—	20.7	26.8	—	—	—	—	—	—	—	—	—	—
3.8	—	—	51.2	3.3	—	—	—	—	—	—	—	65.1	51.8	13.5	—	26.3	32.4	—	—	—	—	—	—	—	—	—	—
4.0	—	—	55.1	0.0	3.0	—	—	—	—	—	—	62.0	50.7	15.3	10.9	32.4	36.6	—	—	—	—	—	—	—	—	—	—
4.2	—	—	60.0	—	6.7	—	—	—	—	—	—	59.1	49.7	17.5	16.6	36.2	40.3	—	—	—	—	—	—	—	—	—	—
4.4	—	—	66.4	—	11.1	—	—	—	—	—	—	56.4	48.6	19.7	23.9	39.3	43.1	—	—	—	—	—	—	—	—	—	—
4.6	—	—	74.9	—	16.5	—	—	—	—	—	—	53.7	47.5	21.9	33.5	41.3	45.7	—	—	—	—	—	—	—	—	—	—
4.8	—	—	85.6	—	22.6	87.1	—	—	—	—	—	51.2	46.4	24.1	44.9	43.5	48.3	—	—	—	—	—	—	—	—	—	—
5.0	—	—	100.0	—	28.8	78.0	99.2	—	—	—	—	49.0	45.4	26.3	56.6	45.7	51.5	94.3	94.3	—	94.3	—	—	—	—	—	—
5.2	—	—	—	—	34.4	70.3	98.4	—	—	—	—	46.9	44.3	28.6	67.8	48.4	53.6	91.5	91.5	3.2	91.7	—	—	—	—	—	—
5.4	—	—	—	—	39.1	64.5	97.3	—	—	—	—	44.7	43.2	31.0	76.8	51.3	58.2	87.8	87.8	5.0	88.0	—	—	—	—	—	—
5.6	—	—	—	—	42.4	60.3	95.5	—	—	—	—	42.4	42.0	33.4	84.0	55.0	63.6	83.6	83.1	7.3	83.3	—	—	—	—	—	—
5.8	—	—	—	—	45.0	57.2	92.8	—	—	—	—	40.0	40.8	35.8	89.3	58.8	68.7	77.6	77.6	9.7	77.9	—	—	—	—	—	—
6.0	—	—	—	—	46.7	54.8	88.9	—	—	—	—	37.4	39.7	38.3	—	63.9	73.6	71.8	71.7	12.4	72.0	43.4	—	—	—	—	—
6.2	—	—	—	—	—	53.2	83.0	—	—	—	—	34.5	38.4	40.8	—	69.5	78.5	66.5	66.4	15.2	66.6	40.4	—	—	—	—	—
6.4	—	—	—	—	—	—	75.4	—	—	—	—	31.4	37.0	43.3	—	74.1	83.3	61.8	61.7	17.9	61.9	36.5	—	—	—	—	—
6.6	—	—	—	—	—	—	65.3	—	—	—	—	27.9	35.6	45.8	—	83.5	87.4	58.2	58.0	20.8	58.1	31.4	86.2	86.4	44.7	43.9	—
6.8	—	—	—	—	—	—	53.4	53.3	—	—	—	23.5	34.2	48.3	—	87.4	91.0	55.5	55.3	22.2	55.3	25.4	79.6	80.6	42.0	41.6	—
7.0	—	—	—	—	—	—	41.3	55.0	—	—	—	19.0	32.9	50.9	—	90.0	93.2	—	—	23.7	—	19.6	71.3	72.8	39.3	38.4	—
7.2	—	—	—	—	—	—	29.6	57.6	—	—	—	13.8	31.7	53.4	—	91.8	94.9	—	—	25.2	—	14.6	62.0	63.2	33.7	34.8	—
7.4	—	—	—	—	—	—	19.7	60.8	—	—	—	9.8	30.6	55.8	—	93.0	95.8	—	—	26.7	—	10.2	52.0	52.1	27.9	30.7	—
7.6	—	—	—	—	—	—	12.8	65.2	53.0	—	—	6.8	29.6	58.2	—	93.8	96.8	—	—	28.6	—	6.6	42.0	41.1	22.9	23.3	—
7.8	—	—	—	—	—	—	7.4	70.6	55.4	—	—	4.6	28.8	60.5	—	—	—	—	—	31.2	—	—	31.9	31.4	17.3	17.7	—
8.0	—	—	—	—	—	—	3.7	75.9	58.0	—	—	—	28.1	62.8	—	—	—	—	—	33.9	—	—	22.5	23.0	13.0	13.3	—
8.2	—	—	—	—	—	—	—	81.2	62.1	—	—	—	27.6	65.0	—	—	—	—	—	36.9	—	—	16.0	15.9	8.8	—	—
8.4	—	—	—	—	—	—	—	86.2	66.9	—	—	—	27.0	67.2	—	—	—	—	—	39.9	—	—	11.7	10.3	5.3	—	—
8.6	—	—	—	—	—	—	—	90.1	73.6	94.7	—	—	26.3	69.3	—	—	—	45.5	46.4	42.7	45.4	—	—	—	—	—	—
8.8	—	—	—	—	—	—	—	93.2	83.5	92.0	—	—	25.2	71.3	—	—	—	43.2	43.9	—	42.8	—	—	—	—	—	—
9.0	—	—	—	—	—	—	—	—	95.6	88.4	—	—	24.0	73.2	—	—	—	40.0	40.9	—	39.2	—	—	—	—	—	—
9.2	—	—	—	—	—	—	—	—	—	84.0	—	—	22.6	75.1	—	—	—	35.8	36.8	—	34.7	—	—	—	—	—	10.0
9.4	—	—	—	—	—	—	—	—	—	78.9	87.0	—	21.4	77.0	—	—	—	30.8	31.8	—	29.3	—	—	—	—	9.2	18.4
9.6	—	—	—	—	—	—	—	—	—	73.2	75.5	—	20.2	78.8	—	—	—	25.0	26.2	—	23.6	—	—	—	—	5.2	29.3
9.8	—	—	—	—	—	—	—	—	—	67.2	65.1	—	19.0	80.4	—	—	—	19.4	20.4	—	19.0	—	—	—	—	4.1	42.0
10.0	—	—	—	—	—	—	—	—	—	62.5	59.6	—	18.1	81.8	—	—	—	14.3	15.2	—	13.1	—	—	—	—	2.3	53.4
10.2	—	—	—	—	—	—	—	—	—	58.8	56.4	—	17.1	83.1	—	—	—	10.0	10.8	—	9.2	—	—	—	—	—	63.7
10.4	—	—	—	—	—	—	—	—	—	55.7	54.1	—	16.5	84.3	—	—	—	—	7.4	—	6.2	—	—	—	—	—	73.1

BUFFER SOLUTIONS (Continued)

pH	1	2	3	4	5	6	7	8	9	10	11	12	13	14	15	16a	16b	17	18	19	20	21	22	23	24	25	26	pH
10.6	—	—	—	—	—	—	—	—	—	53.6	52.3	—	16.0	85.4	—	—	—	6.9	—	—	—	—	—	—	—	—	81.2	10.6
10.8	—	—	—	—	—	—	—	—	—	52.2	—	—	15.5	86.5	—	—	—	—	—	—	—	—	—	—	—	—	87.9	10.8
11.0	—	—	—	—	—	—	—	—	—	51.2	—	—	14.7	87.8	—	—	—	—	—	—	—	—	—	—	—	—	—	11.0
11.2	—	—	—	—	—	—	—	—	—	50.4	—	—	13.5	89.3	—	—	—	—	—	—	—	—	—	—	—	—	—	11.2
11.4	—	—	—	—	—	—	—	—	—	49.5	—	—	11.7	91.3	—	—	—	—	—	—	—	—	—	—	—	—	—	11.4
11.6	—	—	—	—	—	—	—	—	—	48.7	—	—	9.1	94.5	—	—	—	—	—	—	—	—	—	—	—	—	—	11.6
11.8	—	—	—	—	—	—	—	—	—	47.6	—	—	5.5	99.0	—	—	—	—	—	—	—	—	—	—	—	—	—	11.8
12.0	—	—	—	—	—	—	—	—	—	46.0	—	—	1.3	—	—	—	—	—	—	—	—	—	—	—	—	—	—	12.0
12.2	—	—	—	—	—	—	—	—	—	43.2	—	—	—	—	—	—	—	—	—	—	—	—	—	—	—	—	—	12.2
12.4	—	—	—	—	—	—	—	—	—	39.1	—	—	—	—	—	—	—	—	—	—	—	—	—	—	—	—	—	12.4
12.6	—	—	—	—	—	—	—	—	—	31.8	—	—	—	—	—	—	—	—	—	—	—	—	—	—	—	—	—	12.6
12.8	—	—	—	—	—	—	—	—	—	21.4	—	—	—	—	—	—	—	—	—	—	—	—	—	—	—	—	—	12.8

Note: The table gives the volumes x (in ml) of the stock solutions listed that are required to make up a buffer solution of the desired pH value.

BUFFER SOLUTIONS (Continued)

Stock solutions and their amount of substance concentrations or mass and/or volume contents of the solutes

No	A	B	Composition of the Buffer
1	KCl 0.2 mol l^{-1} (14.91 g l^{-1})	HCl 0.2 mol l^{-1}	25 ml A + x ml B made up to 100 ml
2	Glycine 0.1 mol l^{-1} + NaCl 0.1 mol l^{-1} (1 l solution contains 7.507 g glycine + 5.844 g NaCl)	HCl 0.1 mol l^{-1}	x ml A + (100 − x) ml B
3	Disodium citrate 0.1 mol l^{-1} (1 l solution contains 21.01 g citric acid monohydrate + 200 ml NaOH 1 mol l^{-1})	HCl 0.1 mol l^{-1}	x ml A + (100 − x) ml B
4	Potassium biphthalate 0.1 mol l^{-1} (20.42 g l^{-1})	HCl 0.1 mol l^{-1}	50 ml A + x ml B made up to 100 ml
5	As No. 4	NaOH 0.1 mol l^{-1}	50 ml A + x ml B made up to 100 ml
6	As No. 3	NaOH 0.1 mol l^{-1}	x ml A + (100 − x) ml B
7	Potassium dihydrogen phosphate 1/15 mol l^{-1} (9.073 g l^{-1})	Disodium phosphate 1/15 mol l^{-1} (Na$_2$HPO$_4$ · 2 H$_2$O, 11.87 g l^{-1})	x ml A + (100 − x) ml B
8	Barbital-Na 0.1 mol l^{-1} (20.62 g l^{-1})	HCl 0.1 l^{-1}	x ml A + (100 − x) ml B
9	Boric acid, half-neutralized, 0.2 mol l^{-1} (corresponds to 0.05 mol l^{-1} borax solution; 1 l solution contains 12.37 g boric acid 100 ml NaOH 1 mol l^{-1})	HCl 0.1 mol l^{-1}	x ml A + (100 − x) ml B
10	As No. 2	NaOH 0.1 mol l^{-1}	x ml A + (100 − x) ml B
11	As No. 9	NaOH 0.1 mol l^{-1}	x ml A + (100 − x) ml B
12	Citric acid 0.1 mol l^{-1} (citric acid monohydrate 21.01 g l^{-1})	Disodium phosphate 0.2 mol l^{-1} (Na$_2$HPO$_4$ · 2 H$_2$O, 35.60 g l^{-1})	x ml A + (100 − x) ml B
13	To 100 ml citric acid and 100 ml phosphoric acid solution, each equivalent to 100 ml NaOH 1 mol l^{-1}, add 3.54 g boric acid and 343 ml NaOH 1 mol l^{-1}and make up to 1 l of solution	HCl 0.1 l^{-1}	20 ml A + x ml B made up to 100 l
14	Citric acid, potassium hydrogen phosphate, barbital, and boric acid, all 0.02857 mol l^{-1} (1 l solution contains 6.004 g citric acid monohydrate, 3.888 g potassium hydrogen phosphate, 5.263 g barbital, 1.767 g boric acid)	NaOH 0.2 mol l^{-1}	100 ml A + x ml B
15	Sodium acetate 0.1 mol l^{-1} (1 l solution contains 8.204 g C$_2$H$_3$O$_2$Na or 13.61 g C$_2$H$_3$O$_2$Na · 3 H$_2$O)	Acetic acid 0.1 mol l^{-1} (6.005 g l^{-1})	x ml A + (100 − x) ml B
16a	Dimethylglutaric acid 0.1 mol l^{-1} (16.02 g l^{-1})	NaOH 0.2 mol l^{-1}	(a) 100 ml A + x ml B made up to 1000 ml
16b	Dimethylglutaric acid 0.1 mol l^{-1} (16.02 g l^{-1})	NaOH 0.2 mol l^{-1}	(b) 100 ml A + x ml B + 5.844 g NaCl made up to 1000 ml NaCl – 0.1 mol l^{-1}
17	Piperazine 1 mol l^{-1} (86.14 g l^{-1})	HCl 0.1 mol l^{-1}	5 ml A + x ml B made up to 100 ml
18	Tetraethylethylenediamine 1 mol l^{-1} (172.32 g l^{-1})	HCl 0.1 mol l^{-1}	5 ml A + x ml B made up to 100 ml
19	Tris acid maleate 0.2 mol l^{-1} [1 l solution contains 24.23 g tris(hydroxymethyl)aminomethane + 23.21 g maleic acid or 19.61 g maleic annydride]	NaOH 0.2 mol l^{-1}	25 ml A + x ml B made up to 100 ml
20	Dimethylaminoethylamine 1 mol l^{-1} (88 g l^{-1})	HCl 0.1 mol l^{-1}	5 ml A + x ml B made up to 100 ml
21	Imidazole 0.2 mol l^{-1} (13.62 g l^{-1})	HCl 0.1 mol l^{-1}	25 ml A + x ml B made up to 100 ml
22	Triethanolamine 0.5 mol l^{-1} + ethylenediamine-tetraacetic acid disodium salt (1 l solution contains 74.60 g C$_6$H$_{15}$O$_3$N + 20 g C$_{10}$H$_{14}$O$_8$N$_2$ · Na$_2$ · 2 H$_2$O)	HCl 0.05 mol l^{-1}	10 ml A + x ml B made up to 100 ml
23	N-Dimethylaminoleucylglycine 0.1 mol l^{-1} + NaCl 0.2 mol l^{-1} (1 l solution contains 24.33 g C$_{10}$H$_{20}$O$_3$N$_2$ · ½ H$_2$O + 11.69 g NaCl)	NaOH 1 mol l^{-1} 100 ml made up to 1 l with solution A	x ml A + (100−x) ml B
24	Tris 0.2 mol l^{-1} [tris(hydroxymethyl)aminomethane 24.23 g l^{-1}]	HCl 0.1 mol l^{-1}	25 ml A + x ml B made up to 100 ml
25	2-Amino-2-methylpropane-1,3-diol 0.1 mol l^{-1} (10.51 g l^{-1})	HCl 0.1 mol l^{-1}	50 ml A + x ml B made up to 100 ml
26	Sodium carbonate anhydrous 0.1 mol l^{-1} (10.60g l^{-1})	Sodium bicarbonate 0.1 mol l^{-1} (8.401 g l^{-1})	x ml A + (100−x) ml B

Source: From Lenter, C, Ed., *Geigy Scientific Tables*, 8th ed., volume 3, Ciba-Geigy, Basel, 1984, pages 58–60. With permission.

Note: When not otherwise specified, both stock and buffer solutions should be made up with distilled water free of CO$_2$. Only standard reagents should be used. If there is any doubt as to the purity or water content of solutions, their amount of substance concentration must be checked by titration. The volumes x (in ml) of stock solutions required to make up a buffer solution of the desired pH value are given in the table on the next page.

AMINE BUFFERS USEFUL FOR BIOLOGICAL RESEARCH

Norman Good

All of these amines are highly polar, water-soluble substances. Their advantages and disadvantages must be determined empirically for each biological reaction system. For best buffering performance they should be used at pH's close to the pKa, preferably within ± 0.5 pH units of the pKa and never more than ± 1.0 unit from the pKa. Note that the pKa's, and therefore the pH's of buffered solutions, change with temperature in the manner indicated.

Chemical Name	Trivial Name or Acronym	Structure	pKa at 20°C	ΔpKa/°C
2-(N-Morpholino)ethanesulfonic acid	MES		6.15	− 0.011
Bis(2-hydroxyethyl)imino-tris-(hydroxymethyl)methane	Bistris	$(HOCH_2CH_2)_2=N-C\equiv(CH_2OH)_3$	6.5	—
N-(2-Acetamido)iminodiacetic acid	ADA[a]		6.6	− 0.011
Piperazine-N,N'-bis(2-ethanesulfonic acid)	PIPES		6.8	− 0.0085
1,3-Bis[tris(hydroxymethyl)methylamino] propane	Bistrispropane	$(HOCH_2)_3\equiv C-NH(CH_2)_3\ NH-C\equiv(CH_2\ OH)_3$	6.8 (9.0)	—
N-(Acetamido)-2-aminoethanesulfonic acid	ACES	$H_2NCOCH_2\ N^+H_2CH_2CH_2SO_3^-$	6.9	− 0.020
3-(N-Morpholino)propanesulfonic acid	MOPS		7.15	− 0.013
N,N'-Bis(2-hydroxyethyl)-2-amino-ethanesulfonic acid	BES	$(HOCH_2CH_2)_2=N^+HCH_2CH_2SO_3^-$	7.15	− 0.016
N-Tris(hydroxymethyl)methyl-2-aminoethanesulfonic acid	TES	$(HOCH_2)_3\equiv C-N^+H_2CH_2CH_2SO_3^-$	7.5	− 0.020
N-2-Hydroxyethylpiperazine-N'-ethanesulfonic acid	HEPES[b]		7.55	− 0.014
N-2-Hydroxyethylpiperazine-N'-propanesulfonic acid	HEPPS[b]		8.1	− 0.015
N-Tris(hydroxymethyl)methylglycine	Tricine[a]	$(HOCH_2)_3\equiv C-N^+H_2CH_2COO^-$	8.15	− 0.021
Tris(hydroxymethyl)aminomethane	Tris	$(HOCH_2)_3\equiv CNH_2$	8.3	− 0.031
N,N-Bis(2-hydroxyethyl)glycine	Bicine[a]	$(HOCH_2CH_2)_2=N^+HCH_2COO^-$	8.35	− 0.018
Glycylglycine	Glycylglycine[a]	$H_3N^+CH_2CONHCH_2COO^-$	8.4	− 0.028
N-Tris(hydroxymethyl)methyl-3-amino-propanesulfonic acid	TAPS	$(HOCH_2)_3\equiv C-N^+H_2(CH_2)_3SO_3^-$	8.55	− 0.027
1,3-Bis[tris(hydroxymethyl)-methylamino]propane	Bistrispropane	$(HOCH_2)_3\equiv C-NH(CH_2)_3NH-C\equiv(CH_2OH)_3$	9.0 (6.8)	—
Glycine	Glycine[a]	$H_3N^+CH_2COO^-$	9.9	—

Compiled by Norman Good.

[a] These substances may bind certain di- and polyvalent cations and therefore they may sometimes be useful for providing constant, low level concentrations of free heavy metal ions (heavy metal buffering).

[b] These substances interfere with and preclude the Folin protein assay.

For further information on these and other buffers, see Good and Izawa, in *Methods in Enzymology, Part B,* Vol. 24, Pietro, Ed., Academic Press, New York, 1972, 53.

PREPARATION OF BUFFERS FOR USE IN ENZYME STUDIES*

G. Gomori

The buffers described in this section are suitable for use either in enzymatic or histochemical studies. The accuracy of the tables is within ± 0.05 pH at 23°. In most cases the pH values will not be off by more than ± 0.12 pH even at 37° and at molarities slightly different from those given (usually 0.05 M).

The methods of preparation described are not necessarily identical with those of the original authors. The titration curves of the majority of the buffers recommended have been redetermined by the writer. The buffers are arranged in the order of ascending pH range. For more complete data on phosphate and acetate buffers over a wide range of concentrations, see Vol. I [10].*

*From Gomori, in *Methods in Enzymology*, Vol. 1, Colowick and Kaplan, Eds., Academic Press, New York, 1955, 138. With permission.

TABLE 1: Hydrochloric Acid-Potassium Chloride Buffer*

x	pH
97.0	1.0
78.0	1.1
64.5	1.2
51.0	1.3
41.5	1.4
33.3	1.5
26.3	1.6
20.6	1.7
16.6	1.8
13.2	1.9
10.6	2.0
8.4	2.1
6.7	2.2

* Stock solutions.

A: 0.2 M solution of KCl (14.91 g in 1,000 ml).
B: 0.2 M HCl 50 ml of A + x ml of B, diluted to a total of 200 ml.

Reference

1. Clark and Lubs, *J. Bacteriol.*, 2, 1 (1917).

TABLE 2: Glycine-HCL Buffer*

x	pH	x	pH
5.0	3.6	16.8	2.8
6.4	3.4	24.2	2.6
8.2	3.2	32.4	2.4
11.4	3.0	44.0	2.2

* Stock solutions.

A: 0.2 M solution of glycine (15.01 g in 1,000 ml).
B: 0.2 M HCl 50 ml of A + x ml of B, diluted to a total of 200 ml.

Reference

1. Sørensen, *Biochem. Z.*, 21, 131 (1909); 22, 352 (1909).

TABLE 3: Phthalate-Hydrochloric Acid Buffer*

x	pH	x	pH
46.7	2.2	14.7	3.2
39.6	2.4	9.9	3.4
33.0	2.6	6.0	3.6
26.4	2.8	2.63	3.8
20.3	3.0		

* Stock solutions.

A: 0.2 M solution of potassium acid phthalate (40.84 g in 1,000 ml).
B: 0.2 M HCl 50 ml of A + x ml of B, diluted to a total of 200 ml.

Reference

1. Clark and Lubs, *J. Bacteriol.*, 2, 1 (1917).

TABLE 4: Aconitate Buffer*

x	pH	x	pH
15.0	2.5	83.0	4.3
21.0	2.7	90.0	4.5
28.0	2.9	97.0	4.7
36.0	3.1	103.0	4.9
44.0	3.3	108.0	5.1
52.0	3.5	113.0	5.3
60.0	3.7	119.0	5.5
68.0	3.9	126.0	5.7
76.0	4.1		

* Stock solutions.

A: 0.5 M solution of aconitic acid (87.05 g in 1,000 ml).
B: 0.2 M NaOH 20 ml of A + x ml of B, diluted to a total of 200 ml.

Reference

1. Gomori, unpublished data.

TABLE 5: Citrate Buffer*

x	y	pH
46.5	3.5	3.0
43.7	6.3	3.2
40.0	10.0	3.4
37.0	13.0	3.6
35.0	15.0	3.8
33.0	17.0	4.0
31.5	18.5	4.2
28.0	22.0	4.4
25.5	24.5	4.6
23.0	27.0	4.8
20.5	29.5	5.0
18.0	32.0	5.2
16.0	34.0	5.4
13.7	36.3	5.6
11.8	38.2	5.8
9.5	41.5	6.0
7.2	42.8	6.2

* Stock solutions.

A: 0.1 M solution of citric acid (21.01 g in 1,000 ml).

B: 0.1 M solution of sodium citrate (29.41 g $C_6H_5O_7Na_3 \cdot 2H_2O$ in 1,000 ml; the use of the salt with 5½ H_2O is not recommended). x ml of A + y ml of B, diluted to a total of 100 ml.

Reference

1. Lillie, *Histopathologic Technique*, Blakiston, Philadelphia and Toronto, 1948.

TABLE 6: Acetate Buffer*

x	y	pH
46.3	3.7	3.6
44.0	6.0	3.8
41.0	9.0	4.0
36.8	13.2	4.2
30.5	19.5	4.4
25.5	24.5	4.6
20.0	30.0	4.8
14.8	35.2	5.0
10.5	39.5	5.2
8.8	41.2	5.4
4.8	45.2	5.6

* Stock solutions.

A: 0.2 M solution of acetic acid (11.55 ml in 1,000 ml).

B: 0.2 M solution of sodium acetate (16.4 g of $C_2H_3O_2Na$ or 27.2 g of $C_2H_3O_2Na \cdot 3H_2O$ in 1,000 ml) x ml of A + y ml of B, diluted to a total of 100 ml.

Reference

1. Walpole, *J. Chem. Soc.*, 105, 2501 (1914).

TABLE 7: Citrate-Phosphate Buffer*

x	y	pH
44.6	5.4	2.6
42.2	7.8	2.8
39.8	10.2	3.0
37.7	12.3	3.2
35.9	14.1	3.4
33.9	16.1	3.6
32.3	17.7	3.8
30.7	19.3	4.0
29.4	20.6	4.2
27.8	22.2	4.4
26.7	23.3	4.6
25.2	24.8	4.8
24.3	25.7	5.0
23.3	26.7	5.2
22.2	27.8	5.4
21.0	29.0	5.6
19.7	30.3	5.8
17.9	32.1	6.0
16.9	33.1	6.2
15.4	34.6	6.4
13.6	36.4	6.6
9.1	40.9	6.8
6.5	43.6	7.0

* Stock solutions.

A: 0.1 M solution of citric acid (19.21 g in 1,000 ml).

B: 0.2 M solution of dibasic sodium phosphate (53.65 g of $Na_2HPO_4 \cdot 7H_2O$ or 71.7 g of $Na_2HPO_4 \cdot 12H_2O$ in 1,000 ml) x ml of A + y ml of B, diluted to a total of 100 ml.

Reference

1. McIlvaine, *J. Biol. Chem.*, 49, 183 (1921).

TABLE 8: Succinate Buffer*

x	pH	x	pH
7.5	3.8	26.7	5.0
10.0	4.0	30.3	5.2
13.3	4.2	34.2	5.4
16.7	4.4	37.5	5.6
20.0	4.6	40.7	5.8
23.5	4.8	43.5	6.0

* Stock solutions.

A: 0.2 M solution of succinic acid (23.6 g in 1,000 ml).

B: 0.2 M NaOH 25 ml of A + x ml of B, diluted to a total of 100 ml.

Reference

1. Gomori, unpublished, data.

TABLE 9: Phthalate-Sodium Hydroxide Buffer*

x	pH	x	pH
3.7	4.2	30.0	5.2
7.5	4.4	35.5	5.4
12.2	4.6	39.8	5.6
17.7	4.8	43.0	5.8
23.9	5.0	45.5	6.0

* Stock solutions.

A: 0.2 M solution of potassium acid phthalate (40.84 g in 100 ml).

B: 0.2 M NaOH 50 ml of A + x ml of B, diluted to a total of 200 ml.

Reference

1. Clark and Lubs, *J. Bacteriol.*, 2, 1 (1917).

TABLE 10: Maleate Buffer*

x	pH	x	pH
7.2	5.2	33.0	6.2
10.5	5.4	38.0	6.4
15.3	5.6	41.6	6.6
20.8	5.8	44.4	6.8
26.9	6.0		

* Stock solutions

A: 0.2 M solution of acid sodium maleate (8 g of NaOH + 23.2 g of maleic acid or 19.6 g of maleic anhydride in 1,000 ml).

B: 0.2 M NaOH 50 ml of A + x ml of B, diluted to a total of 200 ml.

Reference

1. Temple, *J. Am. Chem. Soc.*, 51, 1754 (1929).

TABLE 11: Cacodylate Buffer*

x	pH	x	pH
2.7	7.4	29.6	6.0
4.2	7.2	34.8	5.8
6.3	7.0	39.2	5.6
9.3	6.8	43.0	5.4
13.3	6.6	45.0	5.2
18.3	6.4	47.0	5.0
23.8	6.2		

* Stock solutions.

A: 0.2 M solution of sodium cacodylate (42.8 g of $Na(CH_3)_2$ $AsO_2 \cdot 3H_2O$ in 1,000 ml).

B: 0.2 M HCl 50 ml of A + x ml of B, diluted to a total of 200 ml.

Reference

1. Plumel, *Bull. Soc. Chim. Biol.*, 30, 129 (1949).

TABLE 12: Phosphate Buffer*

x	y	pH	x	y	pH
93.5	6.5	5.7	45.0	55.0	6.9
92.0	8.0	5.8	39.0	61.0	7.0
90.0	10.0	5.9	33.0	67.0	7.1
87.7	12.3	6.0	28.0	72.0	7.2
85.0	15.0	6.1	23.0	77.0	7.3
81.5	18.5	6.2	19.0	81.0	7.4
77.5	22.5	6.3	16.0	84.0	7.5
73.5	26.5	6.4	13.0	87.0	7.6
68.5	31.5	6.5	10.5	90.5	7.7
62.5	37.5	6.6	8.5	91.5	7.8
56.5	43.5	6.7	7.0	93.0	7.9
51.0	49.0	6.8	5.3	94.7	8.0

* Stock solutions.

A: 0.2 M solution of monobasic sodium phosphate (27.8 g in 1,000 ml).

B: 0.2 M solution of dibasic sodium phosphate (53.65 g of $Na_2HPO_4 \cdot 7H_2O$ or 71.7 g of $Na_2HPO_4 \cdot 12H_2O$ in 1,000 ml) x ml of A + y ml of B, diluted to a total of 200 ml.

Reference

1. Sørensen, *Biochem. Z.*, 21, 131 (1909); 22, 352 (1909).

TABLE 13: Tris(Hydroxymethyl)Aminomethane-Maleate (Tris-Maleate) Buffer*†

x	pH	x	pH
7.0	5.2	48.0	7.0
10.8	5.4	51.0	7.2
15.5	5.6	54.0	7.4
20.5	5.8	58.0	7.6
26.0	6.0	63.5	7.8
31.5	6.2	69.0	8.0
37.0	6.4	75.0	8.2
42.5	6.6	81.0	8.4
45.0	6.8	86.5	8.6

* Stock solutions.

A: 0.2 M solution of Tris acid maleate (24.2 g. of tris(hydroxymethyl)aminomethane + 23.2 g of maleic acid or 19.6 g of maleic anhydride in 1,000 ml).

B: 0.2 M NaOH 50 ml of A + x ml of B, diluted to a total of 200 ml.

† A buffer-grade Tris can be obtained from the Sigma Chemical Co., St. Louis, MO., or From Matheson Coleman & Bell, East Rutherford, NJ.

Reference

1. Gomori, *Proc. Soc. Exp. Biol. Med.*, 68, 354 (1948).

TABLE 14: Barbital Buffer*†

x	pH
1.5	9.2
2.5	9.0
4.0	8.8
6.0	8.6
9.0	8.4
12.7	8.2
17.5	8.0
22.5	7.8
27.5	7.6
32.5	7.4
39.0	7.2
43.0	7.0
45.0	6.8

* Stock solutions.

A: 0.2 M solution of sodium barbital (veronal) (41.2 g in 1,000 ml).

B: 0.2 M HCl 50 ml of A + x ml of B, diluted to a total of 200 ml.

†Solutions more concentrated than 0.05 M may crystallize on standing, especially in the cold.

Reference

1. Michaelis, *J. Biol. Chem.*, 87, 33 (1930).

TABLE 15: Tris(Hydroxymethyl)-Aminomethane (Tris) Buffer*†

x	pH
5.0	9.0
8.1	8.8
12.2	8.6
16.5	8.4
21.9	8.2
26.8	8.0
32.5	7.8
38.4	7.6
41.4	7.4
44.2	7.2

* Stock solutions.

A: 0.2 M solution of tris(hydroxymethyl)aminomethane (24.2 g in 1,000 ml).

B: 0.2 M HCl 50 ml of A + x ml of B, diluted to a total of 200 ml.

† A buffer-grade Tris can be obtained from the Sigma Chemical Co., St. Louis, MO., or from Matheson Coleman & Bell, East Rutherford, NJ.

TABLE 16: Boric Acid-Borax Buffer*

x	pH	x	pH
2.0	7.6	22.5	8.7
3.1	7.8	30.0	8.8
4.9	8.0	42.5	8.9
7.3	8.2	59.0	9.0
11.5	8.4	83.0	9.1
17.5	8.6	115.0	9.2

* Stock solutions.

A: 0.2 M solution of boric acid (12.4 g in 1,000 ml).
B: 0.05 M solution of borax (19.05 g in 1,000 ml; 0.2 M in terms of sodium borate) 50 ml of A + x ml of B, diluted to a total of 200 ml.

Reference

1. Holmes, *Anat. Rec.*, 86, 163 (1943).

TABLE 17: 2-Amino-2-Methyl-1,3-Propanediol (Ammediol) Buffer*

x	pH	x	pH
2.0	10.0	22.0	8.8
3.7	9.8	29.5	8.6
5.7	9.6	34.0	8.4
8.5	9.4	37.7	8.2
12.5	9.2	41.0	8.0
16.7	9.0	43.5	7.8

* Stock solutions.

A: 0.2 M solution of 2-amino-2-methyl-1,3-propanediol (21.03 g in 1,000 ml).
B: 0.2 M HCl 50 ml of A + x ml of B, diluted to a total of 200 ml.

Reference

1. Gomori, *Proc. Soc. Exp. Biol. Med.*, 62, 33 (1946).

TABLE 18: Glycine-NaOH Buffer*

x	pH	x	pH
4.0	8.6	22.4	9.6
6.0	8.8	27.2	9.8
8.8	9.0	32.0	10.0
12.0	9.2	38.6	10.4
16.8	9.4	45.5	10.6

* Stock solutions

A: 0.2 M solution of glycine (15.01 g in 1,000 ml).
B: 0.2 M NaOH 50 ml of A + x ml of B, diluted to a total of 200 ml.

Reference

1. Sørensen, *Biochem. Z.*, 21, 131 (1909); 22, 352 (1909).

TABLE 19: Borax-NaOH Buffer*

x	pH
0.0	9.28
7.0	9.35
11.0	9.4
17.6	9.5
23.0	9.6
29.0	9.7
34.0	9.8
38.6	9.9
43.0	10.0
46.0	10.1

* Stock solutions.

A: 0.05 M solution of borax (19.05 g in 1,000 ml; 0.02 M in terms of sodium borate).
B: 0.2 M NaOH 50 ml of A + x ml of B, diluted to a total of 200 ml.

Reference

1. Clark and Lubs, *J. Bacteriol.*, 2, 1 (1917).

TABLE 20: Carbonate-Bicarbonate Buffer*

x	y	pH
4.0	46.0	9.2
7.5	42.5	9.3
9.5	40.5	9.4
13.0	37.0	9.5
16.0	34.0	9.6
19.5	30.5	9.7
22.0	28.0	9.8
25.0	25.0	9.9
27.5	22.5	10.0
30.0	20.0	10.1
33.0	17.0	10.2
35.5	14.5	10.3
38.5	11.5	10.4
40.5	9.5	10.5
42.5	7.5	10.6
45.0	5.0	10.7

* Stock solutions.

A: 0.2 M solution of anhydrous sodium carbonate (21.2 g in 1,000 ml).
B: 0.2 M solution of sodium bicarbonate (16.8 g in 1,000 ml) x ml of A + y ml of B, diluted to a total of 200.

Reference

1. Delory and King, *Biochem. J.*, 39, 245 (1945).

INDICATORS FOR VOLUMETRIC WORK AND PH DETERMINATIONS

Indicator	Chemical Name	Acid Color	pH Range	Basic Color	Preparation
Methyl violet 6B	Tetra and pentamethylated *p*-rosaniline hydrochloride	Y	0.1–1.5	B	pH: 0.25% water
Metacresol purple (acid range)	*m*-Cresolsulfonphthalein	R	0.5–2.5	Y	pH: 0.10 g. in 13.6 ml. 0.02 *N* NaOH, diluted to 250 ml. with water
Metanil yellow	4-Phenylamino-azobenzene-3′-sulfonic acid	R	1.2–2.3	Y	pH: 0.25% in ethanol
p-Xylenol blue (acid range)	1,4-Dimethyl-5-hydroxybenzenesulfonphthalein	R	1.2–2.8	Y	pH: 0.04% in ethanol
Thymol blue (acid range)	Thymolsulfonphthalein	R	1.2–2.8	Y	pH: 0.1 g. in 10.75 ml. 0.02 *N* NaOH, diluted to 250 ml. with water
Tropaeolin OO	Sodium *p*-diphenylamino-azobenzenesulfonate	R	1.4–2.6	Y	pH: 0.1% in water Vol.: 1% in water
Quinaldine red	2-(*p*-Dimethylaminostyryl)quinoline ethiodide	C	1.4–3.2	R	Vol.: 0.1% in ethanol
Benzopurpurine 4B	Ditolyl-diazo-bis-α-naphthyl-amine-4-sulfonic acid	B-V	1.3–4.0	R	pH, vol.: 0.1% in water
Methyl violet 6B	Tetra and pentamethylated *p*-rosaniline hydrochloride	B	1.5–3.2	V	pH, vol.: 0.25% in water
2,4-Dinitrophenol		C	2.6–4.0	Y	pH, vol.: 0.1 g. in 5 ml. ethanol, diluted to 100 ml. with water
Methyl yellow	*p*-Dimethylaminoazobenzene	R	2.9–4.0	Y	pH, vol.: 0.05% in ethanol
Bromphenol blue	Tetrabromophenolsulfonphthalein	Y	3.0–4.6	B	pH: 0.1 g. in 7.45 ml. 0.02 *N* NaOH, diluted to 250 ml. with water
Tetrabromophenol blue	Tetrabromophenol-tetrabromosulfon-phthalein	Y	3.0–4.6	B	pH: 0.1 g. in 5.00 ml. 0.02 *N* NaOH, diluted to 250 ml. with water
Direct purple	Disodium 4,4′-bis(2-amino-1-naphthylazo)-2,2′-stilbenedisulfonate	B-P	3.0–4.6	R	Vol.: 0.1 g. in 7.35 ml. 0.02 *N* NaOH, diluted to 100 ml. with water
Congo red	Diphenyl-diazo-bis-1-naphthylamine-4-sodium sulfonate	B	3.0–5.2	R	pH: 0.1% in water
Methyl orange	4′-Dimethylaminoazobenzene-4-sodium sulfonate	R	3.1–4.4	Y	Vol.: 0.1% in water
Brom-chlorphenol blue	Dibromodichlorophenolsulfonphthalein	Y	3.2–4.8	B	pH: 0.1 g. in 8.6 ml. 0.02 *N* NaOH, diluted to 250 ml. with water Vol.: 0.04% in ethanol
p-Ethoxychrysoidine	4′-Ethoxy-2,4-diaminoazobenzene	R	3.5–5.5	Y	Vol.: 0.1% in ethanol
α-Naphthyl red		R	3.7–5.0	Y	Vol.: 0.1% in ethanol
Sodium alizarinsulfonate	Dihydroxyanthraquinone sodium sulfonate	Y	3.7–5.2	V	pH, vol.: 1% in water
Bromcresol green	Tetrabromo-*m*-cresolsulfonphthalein	Y	3.8–5.4	B	pH: 0.10 g. in 7.15 ml. 0.02 *N* NaOH, diluted to 250 ml. with water
2,5-Dinitrophenol		C	4.0–5.8	Y	pH, vol.: 0.10 g. in 20 ml. Ethanol, then dilute to 100 ml. with water
Methyl red	4′-Dimethylaminoazobenzene-2-carboxylic acid	R	4.2–6.2	Y	pH: 0.10 g. in 18.6 ml. 0.02 *N* NaOH, diluted to 250 ml. with water Vol.: 0.1% in ethanol
Lacmoid		R	4.4–6.2	B	Vol.: 0.5% in ethanol
Azolitmin		R	4.5–8.3	B	Vol.: 0.5% in water
Litmus		R	4.5–8.3	B	Vol.: 0.5% in water
Cochineal	Complex hydroxyanthraquinone derivative	R	4.8–6.2	V	Vol.: Triturate 1 g. with 20 ml. Ethanol and 60 ml. water, let stand 4 days, and filter
Hematoxylin		Y	5.0–6.0	V	Vol.: 0.5% in ethanol.
Chlorphenol red	Dichlorophenolsulfonphthalein	Y	5.0–6.6	R	pH: 0.1 g. in 11.8 ml. 0.02 *N* NaOH, diluted to 250 ml. with water Vol.: 0.04% in ethanol
Bromcresol purple	Dibromo-*o*-cresolsulfonphthalein	Y	5.2–6.8	Pu	pH: 0.1 g. in 9.25 ml. 0.02 *N* NaOH, diluted to 250 ml with water Vol.: 0.02% in ethanol
Bromphenol red	Dibromophenolsulfonphthalein	Y	5.2–7.0	R	pH: 0.l g. in 9.75 ml. 0.02 *N* NaOH, diluted to 250 ml. with water Vol.: 0.04% in ethanol
Alizarin	1,2-Dihydroxyanthraquinone	Y	5.5–6.8	R	Vol.: 0.1% in ethanol
Dibromophenoltetrabromo-phenolsulfonphthalein		Y	5.6–7.2	Pu	pH: 0.1 g. in 1.21 ml. 0.1 *N* NaOH, diluted to 250 ml. with water
p-Nitrophenol		C	5.6–7.6	Y	pH, vol.: 0.25% in water
Bromothymol blue	Dibromothymolsulfonphthalein	Y	6.0–7.6	B	pH: 0.1 g. in 8 ml. 0.02 *N* NaOH, diluted to 250 ml. with water Vol.: 0.1% in 50% ethanol
Indo-oxine	5,8-Quinolinequinone-8-hydroxy-5-quinolyl-5-imide	R	6.0–8.0	B	Vol.: 0.05% in ethanol
Cucumin		Y	6.0–8.0	Br-R	Vol: saturated aq. soln.
Quinoline blue	Cyanine	C	6.6–8.6	B	Vol.: 1% in ethanol
Phenol red	Phenolsulfonphthalein	Y	6.8–8.4	R	pH: 0.1 g. in 14.20 ml. 0.02 *N* NaOH, diluted to 250 ml. with water Vol.: 0.1% in ethanol
Neutral red	2-Methyl-3-amino-6-dimethylaminophenazine	R	6.8–8.0	Y	pH, vol.: 0.1 g. in 70 ml. ethanol, diluted to 100 ml. with water
Rosolic acid aurin; corallin		Y	6.8–8.2	R	pH, vol.: 1% in 50% ethanol
Cresol red	*o*-Cresolsulfonphthalein	Y	7.2–8.8	R	pH: 0.1 g. in 13.1 ml. 0.02 *N* NaOH, diluted to 250 ml. with water Vol.: 0.1% in ethanol
α-Naphtholphthalein		P	7.3–8.7	G	pH. vol.: 0.1% in 50% ethanol
Metacresol purple (alkaline range)	*m*-Cresolsulfonphthalein	Y	7.4–9.0	P	pH: 0.1 g. in 13.1 ml. 0.02 *N* NaOH, diluted to 250 ml. with water Vol.: 0.1% in ethanol

INDICATORS FOR VOLUMETRIC WORK AND PH DETERMINATIONS (Continued)

Indicator	Chemical Name	Acid Color	pH Range	Basic Color	Preparation
Ethylbis-2,4-dinitrophenylacetate		C	7.5–9.1	B	Vol.: saturated soln. in equal volumes of acetone and ethanol
Tropaeolin OOO No. 1	Sodium α-naphtholazobenzene-sulfonate	Y	7.6–8.9	R	Vol.: 0.1% in water
Thymol blue (alkaline range)	Thymolsulfonphthalein	Y	8.0–9.6	B	pH: 0.l g. in 10.75 ml. 0.02 N NaOH, diluted to 250 ml. with water Vol.: 0.1% in ethanol
p-Xylenol blue	1,4-Dimethyl-5-hydroxybenzenesulfonphthalein	Y	8.0–9.6	B	pH, vol.: 0.04% in elhanol
o-Cresolphthalein		C	8.2–9.8	R	pH, vol.: 0.04% in ethanol
α-Naphtholbenzein		Y	8.5–9.8	G	pH, vol.: 1% in ethanol
Phenolphthalein	3,3-Bis(p-hydroxyphenyl)-phthalide	C	8.2–10	R	Vol.: 1% in ethanol
Thymolphthalein		C	9.3–10.5	B	pH, vol.: 0.1% in ethanol
Nile blue A	Aminonaphthodiethylaminophenoxazine sulfate	B	10–11	P	Vol.: 0.1% in water
Alizarin yellow GG	3-Carboxy-4-hydroxy-3′-nitroazobenzene	Y	10–12	L	pH, vol.: 0.1% in 50% ethanol
Alizarin yellow R	3-Carboxy-4-hydroxy-4′-nitroazobenzene sodium salt	Y	10.2–12.0	R	pH, vol.: 0.1% in water
Poirrer's blue C4B		B	11–13	R	pH: 0.2% in water
Tropaeolin O	p-Benzenesulfonic acid-azoresorcinol	Y	11–13	O	pH: 0.1% in water
Nitramine	Picrylnitromethylamine	C	10.8–13	Br	pH: 0.1% in 70% ethanol
1,3,5-Trinitrobenzene		C	11.5–14	O	pH: 0.1% in ethanol
Indigo carmine	Sodium indigodisulfonate	B	11.6–14	Y	pH: 0.25% in 50% ethanol

Note: The indicator colors are abbreviated as follows: B, blue; Br, brown; C, colorless; G, green; L, lilac; O, orange; P, pink; Pu, purple; R, red; V, violet; and Y, yellow.

MIXED INDICATORS

Composition	Solvent	Transition pH	Acid Color	Transition Color	Basic Color
Dimethyl yellow, 0.05% + Methylene blue, 0.05%	alc.	3.2	Blue–violet	—	Green
Methyl orange, 0.02% + Xylene cyanole FF, 0.28%	50% alc.	3.9	Red	Gray	Green
Methyl yellow, 0.08% + Methylene blue, 0.004%	alc.	3.9	Pink	Straw–pink	Yellow–green
Methyl orange, 0.1% + Indigocarmine, 0.25%	aq.	4.1	Violet	Gray	Yellow–green
Bromcresol green, 0.1% + Methyl orange, 0.02%	aq.	4.3	Orange	Light green	Dark green
Bromcresol green, 0.075% + Methyl red, 0.05%	alc.	5.1	Wine–red	—	Green
Methyl red, 0.1% + Methylene blue, 0.05%	alc.	5.4	Red–violet	Dirty blue	Green
Bromcresol green, 0.05% + Chlorphenol red, 0.05%	aq.	6.1	Yellow–green	—	Blue–violet
Bromcresol purple, 0.05% + Bromthymol blue, 0.05%	aq.	6.7	Yellow	Violet	Violet–blue
Neutral red, 0.05% + Methylene blue, 0.05%	alc.	7.0	Violet–blue	Violet–blue	Green
Bromthymol blue, 0.05% + Phenol red, 0.05%	aq.	7.5	Yellow	Violet	Dark violet
Cresol red, 0.025% + Thymol blue, 0.15%	aq.	8.3	Yellow	Rose	Violet
Phenolphthalein, 0.033% + Methyl green, 0.067%	alc.	8.9	Green	Gray–blue	Violet
Phenolphthalein, 0.075% + Thymol blue, 0.025%	50% alc.	9.0	Yellow	Green	Violet
Phenolphthalein, 0.067% + Naphtholphthalein, 0.033%	50% alc.	9.6	Pale rose	—	Violet
Phenolphthalein, 0.033% + Nile blue, 0.133%	alc.	10.0	Blue	Violet	Red
Alizarin yellow, 0.033% + Nile blue, 0.133%	alc.	10.8	Green	—	Red–brown

ACID AND BASE INDICATORS

The following is a brief list of some acid-base indicators (a more comprehensive listing is available in the *CRC Handbook of Chemistry and Physics*, CRC Press, Boca Raton, FL, USA, Section 8). There is extensive use of acid-base indicators in the measurement of intracellular pH, as indicators for enzyme-catalyzed reactions, and in the measurement of material transfer across membranes and detection of changes in solid matrices.

Some Acid-Base Indicators (pH Indicators)

Indicator Dye	Acid Color	Basic Color	pKa	pH Range
Cresol Red (I) (*o*cresolsulfonephthalein)	Red	Yellow		0.2 – 1.8
Crystal Violet	Green	Blue		0.0 – 2.0
Thymol Blue (I) (thymolsulfonephthalein)	Red	Yellow	1.6	1.2 – 2.8
Cresol Purple(metacresol purple; *m*-cresolpurple)	Red	Yellow	1.5	1.2 – 2.8
Bromophenol Blue	Yellow	Blue	4.1	3.0 – 4.6
Congo Red	Blue/Violet	Red		3.0 – 5.2
Methyl Red	Red	Yellow	5.1	4.4 – 6.3
Neutral Red	Red	Yellow	7.4	6.8 – 8.0
Phenol Red(phenolsulfonphthalein)	Yellow	Red	8.0	6.8 – 8.4
Cresol Red (II)	Yellow	Purple	8.4	7.3 – 8.8
Cresol Purple (II)	Yellow	Purple	8.3	7.4 – 9.0
Thymol Blue (II)	Yellow	Blue	9.2	8.0 – 9.6
Phenolphthalein	Colorless	Red	9.6	8.3 – 10.0
Nile Blue	Blue	Red	10.0	9.0 – 10.4
Nitramine (picrymethylnitramine)	Colorless	Orange-Brown		10.8 – 12.8

Acid-Base Indicators in Organic Solvents

Indicator	pKa		
	H$_2$0	Dimethylformamide	2-Propanol
Thymol Blue (I)	1.7		5.0
Cresol Red(I)			4.3
Bromophenol Blue	4.1		8.8
Neutral Red	7.4		7.2
Phenol Red	8.0	15.4	15.4
Cresol Purple	8.3	15.2	

References for the Use of Acid-Base Indicators

Hammett, L.P. and Deyrup, A.J., A series of simple basic indicators. I. The acidity functions of mixtures of sulfuric and perchloric acids with water, *J.Amer.Chem.Soc.* 54, 2721–2739, 1932.

Gardner, K.J., Use of acid-base indicator for quantitative paper chromatography of sugars, *Nature* 176, 929–930, 1955.

Meikle, R.W., Paper chromatography of 2-halogenated carboxylic acids: *N,N*-dimethyl-*p*-phenylazoaniline as an acid-base indicator reagent, *Nature* 196, 61, 1962.

Kolthoff, I.M., Bhowmik, S., and Chantooni, M.K., Acid-base indicator properties of sulfonephthaleins and benzeins in acetonitrile, *Proc. Nat.Acad.Sci.USA* 56, 1370–1376, 1966.

Chance, B. and Scarpa, A., Acid-base indicator for the measurement of rapid changes in hydrogen ion concentration, *Methods Enzymol.* 24, 336–342, 1972.

Benkovic, P.A., Hegazi, M., Cunningham, B.A., and Benkovic, S.J., Investigation of the pre-steady state kinetics of fructose bisphosphatase by employment of an indicator method, *Biochemistry* 18, 830–860, 1979.

Smith, M.A. and Thompson, R.A., A method for the estimation of the activity of the inhibitor of the first component of complement, *J.Clin.Pathol.* 33, 167–170, 1980.

Kogure, K., Alonso, O.F., and Martinez, E., A topographical measurement of brain pH, *Brain Res.* 195, 95–109, 1980.

Kiernan, J.A, Chromoxane cyanine R. I. Physical and chemical properties of the dye and of some its iron complexes, *J.Microsc.* 143, 13–23, 1984.

Paradiso, A.M., Tsien, R.Y., and Machen, T.E., Na$^+$-H$^+$ exchange in gastric glands as measured with a cytoplasmic-trapped, fluorescent pH indicator, *Proc.Nat.Acad.Sci.USA* 81, 7436–7440, 1984.

Mera, S.L. and Davies, J.D., Differential Congo red staining: the effects of pH, non-aqueous solvents and the substrate, *Histochem.J.* 16, 195–210, 1984.

Horie, K., Hagihara, H., Wada, A., and Fukutome, H., A highly sensitive photometric method for proton release or uptake: difference photometry, *Anal.Biochem.* 137, 80–87, 1984.

Krchnak, V., Vagner, J., and Lebl, M., Noninvasive continuous monitoring of solid-phase peptide synthesis by acid-base indicator, *Int.J.Pept. Protein Res.* 32, 415–416, 1988.

Rosenberg, R.M., Herreid, R.M., Piazza, G.J., and O'Leary, M.N., Indicator assay for amino acid decarboxylases, *Anal.Biochem.* 181, 55–65, 1989.

Weiner, I.D. and Hamm, L.L., Use of fluorescent dye BCECF to measure intracellular pH in cortical collecting tubule, *Am.J.Physiol(Renal, Fluid, Electrolyte Physiol.)*, 256, F957–F964, 1989.

Bassnett, S., Reinisch, L., and Beebe, D.C., Intracellular pH measurement using single excitation-dual emission fluorescence ratios, *Am.J.Physiol.(Cell Physiol.)* 258, C171–C178, 1990.

Anderson, R.E, Bjorkman, D. and McGreavy, J.M., Alteration of gastric surface cell pH regulation by sodium taurocholate, *J.Surg.Res.* 50, 65–71, 1991.

Tortorello, M.L., Trotter, K.M., Angelos, S.M., *et al.*, Microtiter plate assays for the measurement of phage adsorption and infection in *Lactococcus* and *Enterococcus*, *Anal.Biochem.* 192, 362–366, 1991.

Raley-Sussman, K.M., Sapolsky, R.M., and Kopito, R.R., Cl⁻ . HCO₃⁻- exchange function differs in adult and fetal rat hippocampal neurons, *Brain Res.* 614, 308–314, 1993.

Reusch, H.P., Reusch, R., Rosskopf, D., *et al.*, Na$^+$/H$^+$ exchange in human lymphocytes and platelets in chronic and subacute metabolic acidosis, *J.Clin.Invest.* 92, 858–865, 1993.

Mehta, V.D., Kulkarni, P.V., Mason, R.P., *et al.*, 6-Fluoropyridoxal: a novel probe of cellular pH using ¹⁹F NMR spectroscopy, *FEBS Lett.* 349, 234–238, 1994.

Optiz, N., Merten, E., and Acker, H., Evidence for redistribution-associated intracellular pH shifts of the pH-sensitive fluoroprobe carboxy SNARF-1, *Pflugers Arch.* 427, 332–342, 1994.

Webb, B., Frame, J., Zhao, Z., *et al.*, Molecular entrapment of small molecules within the interior of horse spleen ferritin, *Arch.Biochem. Biophys.* 309, 178–183, 1994.

Zhou, Y., Marcus, E.M., Haugland, R.P., and Opas, M., Use of a new fluorescent probe, seminaphthofluorescein-calcein, for determination of intracellular pH by simulateneous dual-emission imaging laser scanning confocal microscopy, *J.Cell Physiol.* 164, 9–16, 1995.

Scheef, C.A., Oelkrug, D., and Schmidt, P.C., Surface acidity of solid pharmaceutical excipients III. Excipients for solid dosage forms, *Eur.J.Pharm.Biopharm.* 46, 209–213, 1998.

Shao, P.G. and Bailey, L.C., Porcine insulin biodegradable polyester microspheres: stability and in vitro release characteristics, *Pharm.Dev. Technol.* 5, 1–9, 2000.

Silver, R.B., Breton, S. and Brown, D., Potassium depletion increases proton pump (H(+)-ATPase) activity in intercalated cells of cortical collecting duct, *Am.J.Physiol.Renal Physiol.* 279, F195–F202, 2000.

Chu, Y.I., Penland, R.L., and Wilhemus, K.R., Colorimetric indicators of microbial contamination in corneal preservation, *Cornea* 19, 517–520, 2000.

Jayaraman, S., Song, Y., and Verkman, A.S., Airway surface liquid pH in well-differentiated airway epithelial cell cultures and mouse trachea, *Am.J.Physiol.Cell Physiol.* 281, C1504–155, 2001.

Yu, E., Pan, J., and Zhou, H.M., A direct continuous pH-spectrophotometric assay for arginine kinase activity, *Protein Pept.Lett.* 9, 545–552, 2002.

Hur, O., Niks, D., Casino, P., and Dunn, M.F., Proton transfer in the β-reaction catalyzed by tryptophan synthase, *Biochemistry* 41, 9991–10001, 2002.

Sun, C. and Berg, J.C, A review of the different techniques for solid surface acid-base characterization, *Adv.Colloid Interface Sci.* 105, 1510175, 2003.

Li, J., Chatterjee, K., Medek, A., *et al.*, Acid-base characterization of bromophenol blue-citrate buffer systems in the amorphous state, *J.Pharm.Sci.* 93, 697–712, 2004.

Balderas-Hernandez, P, Rojas-Hernandez, A., Galvan, M., and Ramirez-Silva, M.T., Spectrophotometric study of the system Hg(II)-thymol blue-H₂O and its evidence through electrochemical means, *Spectrochimica Acta A Mol.Biomol.Spectrosc.* 60, 569–577, 2004.

Gilman, J.B. and Vaida, V., Permeability of acetic acid through organic films at the air-aqueous interface, *J.Phys.Chem.A Mol.Spectros.Kinet. Environ.Gen.Theory* 110, 7581–7587, 2006.

Sanchez-Armass, S., Sennoune, S.R., Maiti, D., *et al.*, Spectral imaging microscopy demonstrates cytoplasmic pH oscillations in glial cells, *Am.J.Physiol.Cell Physiol.* 290, C524–C538, 2006.

General Acid-Base Indicators

Widmer, M., Titrimety, in *Encyclopedia of Analytical Chemistry*, ed. R.A. Meyers, John Wiley & Sons, Ltd., Chichester, UK, pps. 13624–13636, 2002.

Encyclopedia of Analytical Sciences, ed. A. Townshend, Academic Press, London, 1995.

Butler, J.N., *Ionic Equilibrium. Solubility and pH Calculations*, John Wiley & Sons, New York, NY, USA, 1998.

Westcott, G.C., *pH Measurements*, Academic Press, New York, NY, USA, 1978.

Kotyk, A. and Slavík, J., *Intracellular pH and Its Measurement*, CRC Press, Boca Raton, FL, USA, 1989.

Britton, H.T.S., *Hydrogen Ions. Their Determination and Importance in Pure and Industrial Chemistry*, D.Van Nostrand, New York, NY, USA, 1932.

Kolthoft, I.M.(trans. Rosenblum, C.), *Acid-Base Indicators(Säure-Basen Indicatoren)*, MacMillan Company, New York, NY, USA, 1937.

Kolthoff, I.M. and Laitinen, H.A., *pH and Electro Titration. The Colorimetric and Potentiometric Determination of pH, Potentiometry, Conductometry, and Voltometry(Polarography). Outline of Electrometric Titration*, John Wiley & Sons, Inc., New York, NY, USA, 1941.

Webber, R.B., *The Book of pH*, George Newnes Ltd., London, UK, 1957.

Fritz, J.S., *Acid-Base Titrations in Nonaqueous Solvents*, G. Frederick Smith Chemical Company, Columbus, Ohio, 1952.

Clark, W.M. *The Determination of Hydrogen Ions*, 2nd edn., Williams & Wilkins, Baltimore, MD, USA, 1927.

Radhuraman, B., Gustavson, G, van Hal, R.E.G., *et al.*, Extended-range spectroscopic pH measurement using optimized mixtures of dyes, *Appl.Spectrosc.* 60, 1461–1468, 2006.

Non-Aqueous Titration

Kolade, Y.T., Adegbolagun, O.M., Idowu, O.S. *et al.*, Comparative determination of halofantrine tablets by titrimetry, spectrophotometry and liquid chromatography, *Afr.J.Med.Med.Sci.* 35, 79–84, 2006.

Mera, S.L. and Davies, J.D., Differential congo red staining: the effects of pH, non-aqueous solvents and the substrate, *Histochem.J.* 16, 195–210, 1984.

Cresol Purple

Schindler, J.F., Naranjo, P.A., Honaberger, D.A., *et al.*, Haloalkane dehalogenase: Steady-state kinetics and halide inhibition, *Biochemistry* 38, 5772–5778, 1999.

Phenolphthalein

King, B.F., Liu, M., Townsend-Nicholson, A., *et al.*, Antagonism of ATP responses at P2X receptor subtypes by the pH indicator dye, phenol red, *Br.J.Pharmacol.* 145, 313–322, 2005.

Riccio, M.L., Rossolini, G.M., Lombardi, G., *et al.*, Expression cloning of different bacterial phosphatase-encoding genes by Histochemical screening of genomic libraries onto an indicator medium containing phenolphthalein diphosphate and methyl green, *J.Appl.Microbiol.* 82, 177185, 1997.

Gerber, H., Colorimetric determination of alkaline phosphatase as indicator of mammalian feces in corn meal: collaborative study, *J.Assoc. Off.Anal.Chem.* 69, 496–498, 1986.

50a. Khalifab, R.G., The carbon dioxide hydration activity of carbonic anhydrase. I. Stop-flow kinetic studies on the native human isoenzymes B and C, *J.Biol.Chem.* 246, 2561–2573, 1971.

Cresol Red

Borucki, B., Davanthan, S., Otto, H., *et al.*, Kinetics of proton uptake and dye binding by photoactive yellow protein in wild type and the E46Q and E46A mutants, *Biochemistry* 41, 10026–10037, 2002.

Actis, L.A., Smoot, J.C., Baracin, C.E., and Findlay, R.H., Comparison of differential plating media and two chromatographic techniques for the detection of histamine production in bacteria, *J.Microbiol. Methods* 39, 79–90, 1999.

Jeronimo, P.C., Araujo, A.N., Montenegro, M.C., *et al.*, Flow-through sol-gel optical biosensor for the colorimetric determination of acetazolamide, *Analyst* 130, 1190–1197, 2005.

Nakamura, N. and Amao, Y., Optical sensor for carbon dioxide combining colorimetric change of a pH indicator and a reference luminescent dye, *Anal.Bioanal.Chem.* 376, 642–646, 2003.

Yu, Z., Pan, J., and Zhou, H.M., A direct continuous pH-spectrophotometric assay for arginine kinase activity, *Protein Pept.Lett.* 9, 545–552, 2002.

58a. Caselli, M., Mangone, A., Paoliollo, P., and Traini, A., Determination of the acid dissociation constant of bromocresol green and cresol red in water/AOT/isooctane reverse micelles by multiple linear regression and extended principal component analysis, *Ann.Chim.* 92, 501–512, 2002.

Actis, L.A., Smoot, J.C, Barancin, C.E., and Findlay, R.H., Comparison of differential plating media and two chromatographic techniques for the detection of histamine production in bacteria, *J.Microbiol. Methods* 39, 79–90, 1999.

Grabner, R., Influence of cationic amphiphilic drugs on the phosophatidylcholine hydrolysis by phospholipase A2, *Biochem.Pharmacol.* 36, 1063–1067, 1987.

Horie, K., Hagihara, H., Wada, A., and Fukutome, H., A highly sensitive photometric method for proton release or uptake: difference photometry, *Anal.Biochem.* 137, 80–87, 1984.

Velthuys, B.R., A third site of proton translocation in green plant photosynthetic electron transport, *Proc.Nat.Acad.Sci.USA* 75, 6031–6034, 1978.

Crystal Violet

Kolade, Y.T., Adegboagun, O.M. Iodwu, O.S., *et al.*, Comparative determination of halofantrine tablets by titrimetry, spectrophometry and liquid chromatography, *Afr.J.Med.Med.Sci.* 35, 79–84, 2006.

Bornscheuer, U.T., Altenbuchner, J., and Meyer, J.H., Directed evolution of an esterase for the stereoselective resolution of a key intermediate in the synthesis of epothilones, *Biotechnol.Bioeng.* 58, 554–559, 1998.

Nakayasu, H., Crystal violet as an indicator dye for nonequilibrium pH gradient.

Congo Red

Mera, S.L., and Davies, J.D., Differential Congo red staining: the effects of pH, non-aqueous solvents and the substrate, *Histochem.J.* 16, 195–210, 1984.

Schneider, R.L., Chung, E.B., Leffall, L.D., Jr., and Syphax, B., Delineation of the canine gastric antrum with pH probe and dye indicator, *J.Natl. Med.Assoc.* 63, 202–204, 1971.

Xu, S., Kramer, M., and Haag, R., pH-Responsive dendritic core-shell architectures as amphiphilic nanocarriers for polar drugs, *J.Drug Target.* 14, 367–374, 2006.

Sekine, H., Iijima, K., Koike, T., *et al.*, Regional differences in the recovery of gastric acid secretion after *Helicobacter pylori* eradication: evaluations with Congo red chromoendoscopy, *Gastrointest.Endosc.* 64, 686–690, 2006.

Parrish, N.M., Ko, C.G., Dick, J.D., *et al.*, Growth, Congo Red agar colony morphotypes and antibiotic susceptibility testing of *Mycobacterium avium* subspecies paratuberculosis, *Clin.Med.Res.* 2, 107–114, 2004.

Thymol Blue

Balderas-Hernandez, P., Rojas-Hernandez, A., Galvan, M., and Ramirez-Silva, M.T., Spectrophotometric study of the system Hg(II)-thymol blue-H$_2$O and its evidence through electrochemical means, *Spectrochim.Acta A Mol.Biomol.Spectrosc.* 60, 569–577, 2004.

Nakamura, N. and Amao, Y., Optical sensor for carbon dioxide combining colorimetric change of a pH indicator and a reference luminescent dye, *Anal.Bioanal.Chem.* 376, 642–646, 2003.

Dowding, C.E., Borda, M.J., Fey, M.V., and Sparks, D.L., A new method for gaining insight into the chemistry of drying mineral surfaces using ATR-FTIR, *J.Colloid Interface Sci.* 292, 148–151, 2005.

Saika, P.M., Bora, M., and Dutta, R.K., Acid-base equilibrium of anionic dyes partially bound to micelles of nonionic surfactants, *J.Colloid Interface Sci.* 285, 382–387, 2005.

Bromophenol Blue

Govindarajan, R., Chatterjee, K., Gatlin, L., *et al.*, Impact of freeze-drying on ionization of sulfonphthalein probe molecule in trehalose-citrate systems, *J.Pharm.Sci.* 95, 1498–1510, 2006.

Suzuki, Y., Theoretical analysis concerning the characterization of a dye-binding method for determining serum protein based on protein error of pH indicator: effect of buffer concentration of the color reagent on the color development, *Anal.Sci.* 21, 83–88, 2005.

Li, J., Chatterjee, K., Medek, A. *et al.*, Acid-base characteristics of bromophenol blue-citrate buffer system in the amorphous state, *J.Pharm. Sci.* 93, 697–712, 2004.

Shao, P.G. and Bailey, L.C., Porcine insulin biodegradable polyester microspheres: stability and in vitro release characteristics, *Pharm.Dev. Technol.* 5, 1–9, 2000.

Koren, R. and Hammes, G.G., A kinetic study of protein-protein interactions, *Biochemistry* 15, 1165–1171, 1976.

Methyl Red

Katsuda, T., Ooshima, H., Azuma, M., and Kato, J., New detection method for hydrogen gas for screening hydrogen-producing microorganisms using water-soluble Wilkinson's catalyst derivative, *J.Biosci. Bioeng.* 102, 220–226, 2006.

Benedict, J.B., Cohen, D.E., Lovell, S., *et al.*, What is syncrystallization? States of the pH indicator methyl red in crystals of phthalic acid, *J.Am.Chem.Soc.* 128, 5548–5559, 2006.

Pelechova, J., Petrova, L., Ujcova, E. and Martinkova, L., Selection of a hyper-producing strain of *Aspergillus niger* for biosynthesis of citric acid on unusual carbon substrates, *Folia Microbiol.* 35, 138–142, 1990.

Phenol Red

Govindarajan, R., Chatterjee, K., Gatlin, L., *et al.*, Impact of freeze-drying on ionization of sulfonphthalein probe molecule in trehalose-citrate systems, *J.Pharm.Sci.* 95, 1498–1510, 2006.

Chu, A., Morris, K., Greenberg, R. and Zhou, D. Stimulus induced pH changes in retinal implants, *Conf.Proc.IEEE Eng.Med.Biol.Soc.* 6, 4160–4162, 2004.

Deng, C. and Chen ,R.R., A pH-sensitive assy for galactosyltransferase, *Anal.Biochem.* 330, 219–226, 2004.

Still, K., Reading, L., and Scutt, A., Effects of phenol red on CRU-f differentiation and formation, *Calcif.Tissue Int.* 73, 173–179, 2003.

Hur, O., Nik, D., Casino, P., and Dunn, M.F., Proton transfers in the β-reaction catalyzed by tryptophan synthase, *Biochemistry* 41, 9991–10001, 2002.

Oh, K.H., Nam, S.H., and Kim, H.S., Directed evolution of N-carbamyl-D-amino acid amidohydrolase for simultaneous improvement of oxidative and thermal stability, *Biotechnol.Prog.* 18, 413–417, 2002.

Girard, P., Jordan, M., Tsao, M. and Wurm, F.M., Small-scale bioreactor system for process development and optimization, *Biochem.Eng.J.* 7, 117–119, 2001.

Jarrett, J.T, Choi, C.Y. and Matthews, R.G., Changes in protonation associated with substrate binding and Cob(I)alamin formation in cobalamin-dependent methionine synthase, *Biochemistry* 36, 15739–15748, 1997.

Ahmed, Z. and Connor, J.A., Intracellular pH changes induced by calcium influx during electrical activity in molluscan neurons, *J.Gen.Physiol.* 75, 403–426, 1980.

Connor, J.A. and Ahmed, Z., Diffusion of ions and indicator dyes in neural cytoplasm, *Cell.Mol.Neurobiol.* 4, 53–66, 1984.

Clark, A.M. and Perrin, D.D., A re-investigation of the question of activators of carbonic anhydrase, *Biochem.J.* 48, 495–502, 1951.

Nile Blue

Lie, C.-W., Shulok, J.R., Wong, Y.-K., *et al.*, Photosensitization, uptake, and retention of phenoxazine Nile Blue derivatives in human bladder carcinoma cells, *Cancer Res.* 51, 1109–1114, 1991.

SPECIFIC GRAVITY OF LIQUIDS

Specific gravity and density are not identical although the abbreviation "d" is frequently used to designate specific gravity. Specific gravity and density are numerically equal when water is the standard of reference for specific gravity and g/ml is the unit designation for density.

The numerical value for specific gravity is usually written with a superscript (indicating the temperature of the liquid) and a subscript (indicating the temperature of the liquid to which it is referred), thus d_4^{25} 1.724 or sp. gr. 1.724_4^{25}.

When these are omitted in this table, the specific gravity at 20°C referred to water at 4°C is intended. When the standard of reference is not specified, for liquids and solids, it is understood to be water.

Water is most dense at 4°C, hence the sp. gr. of a liquid with reference to water will be higher at all other temperatures than it is at 4°C. To obtain the sp. gr. with reference to water at the same temperature as the liquid, multiply the sp. gr. of $\frac{15}{4}$, $\frac{20}{4}$, or $\frac{25}{4}$ by 1.001, 1.002, or 1.003, respectively.

(Items listed in the order of increasing specific gravities)

Liquid	Specific Gravity	Liquid	Specific Gravity
n-Pentane	0.626	n-Octylamine	0.779_{20}^{20}
n-Hexane	0.660	Isoamyl ether	0.781_{15}^{15}
1-Butyne	0.668_4^0	Propionitrile	0.783
Dimethylamine	0.680_4^0	Acetonitrile	0.783_{25}^{25}
Isoprene	0.681	n-Butyl ether	0.784_4^0
n-Heptane	0.684	Isopropyl alcohol	0.785
2-Butyne	0.688^{25}	Isovaleronitrile	0.788
1,5-Hexadiene	0.688	Butyl alcohol, tertiary	0.789
Isopropylamine	0.694_4^{15}	Methanol, anhydrous	0.791
Butylamine, tertiary	0.696	Acetone	0.792
Triethylboron	0.696^{23}	Isobutyraldehyde	0.794
Ethylamine	0.706_4^0	Acrylonitrile	0.797
Diethylamine	0.711_4^{18}	Ethyl alcohol, anhydrous	$0.798_{15.56}^{15.56}$
2,4-Hexadiene	0.711	Valeronitrile	0.801
Diethyl ether	0.713	Isovaleraldehyde	0.803_4^{17}
n-Nonane	0.716	n-Propyl alcohol	0.804
Triethylamine	0.723_4^{25}	Allyl ether	0.805_0^{18}
Butylamine, secondary	0.724	Ethyl methyl ketone	0.805
Isopropyl ether	0.726	Isobutyl alcohol	0.806_4^{15}
Ethyl methyl ether	0.726_4^0	Propionaldehyde	0.807
2,4-Heptadiene	$0.733_4^{21.5}$	Butyl alcohol, secondary	0.808
Isobutylamine	0.724_4^{25}	Amyl alcohol, tertiary	0.809
Propyl ether	0.736	Methyl propyl ketone	0.809
Methyl propyl ether	0.738	n-Butyl alcohol	0.810
Dipropylamine	0.738	Cycloheptane	0.810
Ethyl n-propyl ether	0.739	Cyclohexene	0.810
n-Butylamine	0.740	Isoamyl alcohol	0.813_4^{15}
Undecane	0.741	Ethyl propyl ketone	$0.813_4^{21.8}$
N,N-Dimethylamylamine	0.743	pri-n-Amyl alcohol	0.814
Ethyl isopropyl ether	0.745_4^0	Heptyl ether	0.815_4^0
Isoamylamine	0.751	Diethyl ketone	0.816_4^{19}
Cyclopentane	0.751	Ethyl alcohol, 95 per cent	$0.816_{15.56}^{15.56}$
Butyl ethyl ether	0.752	Butyraldehyde	0.817
Isohexylamine	0.758_4^{25}	Dipropyl ketone	0.817
Isobutyl ether	0.761_4^{15}	Ethyl butyl ketone	0.818
Allylamine	0.761	n-Hexyl methyl ketone	0.819
n-Amylamine	0.761	1-Hexanol	0.819
Butyl methyl ether	0.764_4^0	3-Hexanol	0.819
Allyl ether ether	0.765	Isoamyl alcohol, secondary	0.819
n-Dodecane	0.766_4^0	Pinacolin	0.821_4^0
Dibutylamine	0.767	Amyl methyl ketone	0.822_4^{15}
n-Butyl ether	0.769_{20}^{20}	Cycloheptene	0.823
Cyclopentene	0.774	n-Octyl alcohol	0.825
n-Heptylamine	0.777	2-Undecanone	0.826
Cyclohexane	0.778	Light Liquid Petrolatum	$0.828-0.880_{25}^{25}$

SPECIFIC GRAVITY OF LIQUIDS (Continued)

Liquid	Specific Gravity	Liquid	Specific Gravity
2-Hexanol	0.829^0_4	Caraway oil	$0.900\text{--}0.910^{25}_{25}$
n-Decyl alcohol	0.829	Ethyl acetate	0.902
n-Undecylaldehyde	0.830	Linoleic acid	0.903
Butyl methyl ketone	0.830^0_4	Cubeb oil	$0.905\text{--}0.925^{25}_{25}$
1-Undecanol	0.833^{23}_4	Eucalyptus oil	$0.905\text{--}0.925^{25}_{25}$
Acrolein	0.841	Diethyl Carbitol	0.907
Orange oil	$0.842\text{--}0.846^{25}_{25}$	Styrene	0.907
Bitter orange oil	$0.845\text{--}0.851^{25}_{25}$	Undecylenic acid	0.908^{25}_4
Butyl chloride, tertiary	0.847^{15}_4	Olive oil	$0.910\text{--}0.915^{25}_{25}$
Rose oil	$0.848\text{--}0.863^{30}_{15}$	Expressed almond oil	$0.910\text{--}0.915^{25}_{25}$
Lemon oil	$0.849\text{--}0855^{25}_{25}$	Persic oil	$0.910\text{--}0.923^{25}_{25}$
Amyl ether ketone	0.850^0_4	Thyme oil	$0.910\text{--}0.935^{25}_{25}$
n-Amyl nitrite	0.853	n-Butyl nitrite	0.911^0_4
Rectified turpentine oil	$0.853\text{--}0.862^{25}_{25}$	Peanut oil	$0.912\text{--}0.920^{25}_{25}$
Dwarf pine needle oil	$0.853\text{--}0.871^{25}_{25}$	Mustard oil	$0.914\text{--}0.916^{15}_{15}$
Allyl alcohol	0.854	Corn oil	$0.914\text{--}0.921^{25}_{25}$
Mesityl oxide	0.854	Methyl propionate	0.915
Myristica oil	$0.854\text{--}0.910^{25}_{25}$	Glycerin trioleate	0.915
p-Cymene	0.857	Cottonseed oil	$0.915\text{--}0.921^{25}_{25}$
dl-Pinene	0.858	Sesame oil	$0.916\text{--}0.921^{25}_{25}$
Isopropyl chloride	0.859	Spearmint oil	$0.917\text{--}0.934^{25}_{25}$
2-Diethylaminoethanol	0.860^{25}_{25}	Cardamom oil	$0.917\text{--}0.947^{25}_{25}$
Liquid Petrolatum	$0.860\text{--}0.905^{25}_{25}$	Coconut oil	$0.918\text{--}0.923^{25}_{25}$
Piperidine	0.861	Cod liver oil	$0.918\text{--}0.927^{25}_{25}$
Cumene	0.863	Halibut liver oil	$0.920\text{--}0.930^{25}_{25}$
Coriander oil	$0.863\text{--}0.875^{25}_{25}$	Eucalyptol	$0.921\text{--}0.923^{25}_{25}$
Orange flower oil	$0.863\text{--}0.880^{25}_{25}$	Ethyl format	0.924^{25}_4
Phytol	0.864^0_4	Soya oil	$0.924\text{--}0.927^{15}_{15}$
m-Xylene	0.864	Linseed oil	$0.925\text{--}0.935^{25}_{25}$
Toluene	0.866	Pine oil	$0.927\text{--}0.940^{25}_{25}$
Ethyl benzene	0.867	Methyl acetate	0.928
m-Cymene	0.870	Cellosolve	0.930
Isoamyl acetate	0.870^{25}_4	Ionone	$0.933\text{--}0.937^{25}_{25}$
Isopropyl acetate	0.870	N,N-Diethylaniline	0.935
Isobutyl nitrite	0.870^{20}_{20}	Furan	0.937
Butyl chloride, secondary	0.871	Allyl chloride	0.938
Octyl acetate	0.873^{20}_{20}	Valeric acid	0.942
Isobutyl acetate	0.875	Castor oil	$0.945\text{--}0.965^{25}_{25}$
Isoamyl nitrite	0.875^{25}_{25}	Cyclohexanone	0.948
Bergamot oil	$0.875\text{--}0.880^{25}_{25}$	Pyrrole	0.948
Lavender oil	$0.875\text{--}0.888^{25}_{25}$	Cyclopentanone	0.948
o-Cymene	0.876	Cyclopentanol	0.949
Benzene	0.879^{15}_4	Isobutyric acid	0.949
Amyl acetate	0.879^{20}_{20}	2-Picoline	0.950^{15}
Geraniol	0.881^{16}_4	Chenopodium oil	$0.950\text{--}0.980^{25}_{25}$
n-Amyl chloride	0.883	Myrcia oil	$0.950\text{--}0.990^{25}_{25}$
Isobutyl chloride	0.883^{15}	Cycloheptanone	0.951
n-Butyl chloride	0.884	Fennel oil	$0.953\text{--}0.973^{25}_{25}$
Pine needle oil	$0.884\text{--}0.886^{15}_{15}$	Dimethylaniline	0.956
Citronella oil	$0.885\text{--}0.912^{25}_{25}$	4-Picoline	0.957^{15}_4
2-Dimethylaminoethanol	0.887	3-Picoline	0.961^{15}_4
n-Propyl acetate	0.887	Indan	0.965
1-Menthol	0.890^{15}_{15}	Methyl cellosolve	0.966
Propyl chloride	0.890^{20}_{20}	Phenetole	0.967
Isoamyl chloride	0.893	Vitamin K_1	0.967^{25}_{25}
Rosemary oil	$0.894\text{--}0.912^{25}_{25}$	Tetralin	0.970
Oleic acid	0.895^{18}_4	Carvacrol	0.976
Isodurene	0.896^0_4	Pyridine	0.978^{25}_4
Peppermint oil	$0.896\text{--}0.908^{25}_{25}$	Anise oil	$0.978\text{--}0.988^{25}_{25}$
o-Xylene	0.897	Ethyl urethan	0.981
Ethyl nitrite	0.900^{15}_{15}	Benzylamine	0.983^{19}_4
		Benzyl acetone	0.989^{17}_{23}

SPECIFIC GRAVITY OF LIQUIDS (Continued)

Liquid	Specific Gravity	Liquid	Specific Gravity
m-Toluidine	0.989	Aldol	1.103
Carbitol	0.990	Acetyl chloride	1.105
Dimethyl glyoxal	0.990_{15}^{15}	Ethyl nitrate	1.105
Isoamyl benzoate	0.993_4^{19}	Chlorobenzene	1.107
Paraldehyde	0.994	Polyethylene Glycol 400	$1.110–1.140_{25}^{25}$
Anisole	0.995	Cinnamaldehyde	1.112_4^{15}
Isoamyl nitrate	0.996_4^{22}	Benzyl benzoate	1.118_4^{25}
Morpholine	0.999	Diethylene glycol	1.118_{20}^{20}
Water	0.9970_4^{0}	Anisaldehyde	1.123
Water	0.9999_{20}^{20}	Diethyl phthalate	1.123_4^{25}
Water	$1.0000_{4.08}^{4.08}$	Triethanolamine	1.124
Isobutyl benzoate	1.002_4^{15}	Polyethylene Glycol 300	$1.124–1.130_{25}^{25}$
o-Toluidine	1.004	Furfuryl alcohol	1.130
Indene	1.006	Nitromethane	1.130
Nicotine	1.009	Formamide	1.134
Benzonitrile	1.010_{15}^{15}	Ethyl salicylate	1.136_4^{15}
Hydrazine	1.011_4^{15}	*m*-Nitrotoluene	1.157
Ethanolamine	1.018	Ethyl chloroacetate	1.159
Pimenta oil	$1.018–1.048_{25}^{25}$	Furfural	1.160
Aniline	1.022	Glycerol triacetate	1.161
Sparteine	1.023	*o*-Nitrotoluene	1.163
Phenylethyl alcohol	1.024_4^{15}	Salicylaldehyde	1.167
Dibenzylamine	1.026	Methyl salicylate	1.184_{25}^{25}
Chloroacetal	1.026_4^{16}	Dimethyl phthalate	1.189_{25}^{25}
Acetophenone	1.033_{15}^{15}	Nitrobenzene	1.205_4^{15}
1,4-Dioxane	1.034	Isoamyl bromide	1.210_4^{15}
m-Cresol	1.034	Benzoyl chloride	1.219_{15}^{15}
Glycerol tributyrate	1.035	*sym.*-Dichloroethyl ether	1.222
Propylene glycol	1.036_4^{25}	Butyl bromide, tertiary	1.222
Phlorol	1.037^{12}	Formic acid	1.226_4^{15}
Butyl nitrate, secondary	1.038_4^{0}	Methyl chloroacetate	1.238_{20}^{20}
Bitter almond oil	$1.038–1.060_{25}^{25}$	Amyl bromide	1.246_4^{0}
Clove oil	$1.038–1.060_{25}^{25}$	Lactic acid (*dl*)	1.249_4^{15}
Ethyl succinate	1.040	*.uns.*-Ethylene dichloride	1.252
Benzyl ether	1.043	Butyl bromide, secondary	1.258
Benzyl alcohol	1.045_4^{25}	Glycerol	1.260
Cinnamon oil	$1.045–1.063_{25}^{25}$	Carbon disulfide	1.263
o-Cresol	1.047	*n*-Butyl bromide	1.269_4^{25}
n-Butyl phthalate	1.047	Isobutyl bromide	1.272_4^{15}
n-Butyl nitrate	1.048_4^{0}	*sym.*-Dichloroethylene	1.291_4^{15}
Acetic acid (glacial)	1.049_{25}^{25}	*o*-Dichlorobenzene	1.307_{20}^{20}
Benzaldehyde	1.050_4^{15}	Isopropyl bromide	1.310
Ethyl benzoate	1.051_4^{15}	Ethylsulfuric acid	1.316_4^{17}
Ethyl malonate	1.055	Methylene chloride	1.335_4^{15}
Benzyl acetate	1.057_4^{16}	*n*-Propyl bromide	1.353
Allyl benzoate	1.058_{15}^{15}	*m*-Xylyl bromide	1.371_4^{23}
n-Propyl nitrate	1.058	Benzotrichloride	1.380_4^{15}
Succinaldehyde	1.064	Ethyl trichloroacetate	1.383
Thiophene	1.064	Allyl bromide	1.398
Methyl carbonate	1.065_4^{17}	Ethyl bromide	1.430
Eugenol	1.066	Benzyl bromide	1.438_0^{22}
p-Chlorotoluene	1.070	Hydrogen peroxide, anhydrous	1.465_4^{0}
m-Chlorotoluene	1.072	Trichloroethylene	1.465
Diethyl maleate	1.074_{15}^{15}	Chloroform	1.498_{15}^{15}
Benzofuran	1.078_{15}^{15}	Bromobenzene	1.499_{15}^{15}
o-Chlorotoluene	1.082	Chloral	1.512
Acetic anhydride	1.087_4^{15}	Trichloroethanol	1.550_{20}^{20}
o-Anisidine	1.092	Dichloroacetic acid	1.563
Methyl benzoate	1.094_4^{15}	Benzoyl bromide	1.570_4^{15}
Quinoline	1.095	Glycerophosphoric acid	1.590_4^{19}
m-Anisidine	1.096	Nitroglycerin	1.592_4^{25}
Diethanolamine	1.097	Carbon tetrachloride	1.595
Benzyl chloride	1.103_4^{18}		

SPECIFIC GRAVITY OF LIQUIDS (Continued)

Liquid	Specific Gravity	Liquid	Specific Gravity
Tetrachloroethane	1.600	Ethylene dibromide	2.172_{25}^{25}
Tetrachloroethylene	1.631_4^{15}	Methyl iodide	2.251
Chloropicrin	1.651	Bromal	2.300_4^{15}
Diphosgene	1.653_4^{14}	Methylene bromide	2.495
Thionyl chloride	$1.655^{10.4}$	Bromoform	2.890
Acetyl bromide	1.663_4^{16}	Tetrabromoethane	2.964
Isopropyl iodide	1.703	Methylene iodide	3.325
Ethyl iodide	1.933	Mercury	13.546
Ethylene bromide	2.170_4^{25}		

Reprinted from *The Merck Index* (1960), 7th ed., Merck and Co., Rahway, N.J., pp. 1532–1535, with permission of the copyright owner.

PROPERTIES OF SOME SOLVENTS

Roger L. Lundblad

PROPERTIES OF SOME SOLVENTS USEFUL IN BIOCHEMISTRY AND MOLECULAR BIOLOGY[a]

	Solvent	Molecular weight	Freezing point (°C)	Boiling point (°C$_{760}$)	Density (°C)[b]	Viscosity (mPa s)[c]	Log P	pKa	UV cutoff[d] (nm)
1	H$_2$O	18	0	100	1.00	0.89	–	14	190
2	MeOH	32.04	–97.8	64.7	0.79	0.54	–0.77	15.3	206
3	EtOH	46.07	–114	78.4	0.79	1.07	–0.31	15.9	205
4	nPrOH	60.10	–127	97.2	0.80	2.26	0.25	16.1	210
5	iPrOH	60.10	–87.9	82.3	0.79	2.04	0.05	17.1	205
6	nBuOH	74.12	–88.6	117.6	0.81	2.54	0.88	16.1	180
7	Acn[e]	41.05	–44	81.6	0.79	0.35	–0.34		255
8	Acetone	58.08	–94.9	56.1	0.79	0.32	–0.24		265
9	HOAc	60.05	16.7	118	1.05	1.06	0.017	4.76	255
10	EtOAc	88.10	–83.8	77.1	0.90	0.42	0.73		265
11	EG	60.07	–13	197.6	1.1	16.9	1.93[f]		
12	HCOOH	46.03	8.4	100.8	1.2	1.6	–0.54		
13	TFA	144.2	–15.4	72.4	1.5	0.93	–0.25	0.3	
14	DMSO	78.13	18.5	189	1.1	2.47	–1.35	35.1	286
15	Formamide[g]	45.05	2.5	211	1.1	3.34	–1.51		275
16	DMF	73.09	–60.3	152.8	0.94	0.80	–1.01		263
17	CHCl$_3$	119.38	–63.4	61.2	1.48	5.63	1.27		245
18	CCl$_4$	153.83	–23	76.8	1.59	2.03	2.83		233
19	CHCl$_2$	84.93	–95	40	1.33	0.44	1.25		233
20	Dioxane	88.11	11.8	101.2	1.03	1.18	–0.27		215
21	THF	72.16	–108.5	65	0.89	0.53	0.46		212
22	DMAc	87.12	–20	163	0.94	0.92	–0.77		268
23	n-heptane	100.2	–90.5	98.4	0.68	0.42	4.66		200
24	n-hexane	86.18	–95.4	68.7	0.66	0.33	3.90		200
25	Toluene	92.14	–94.9	110.6	0.86	0.56	2.73		284

DMF, dimethyl formamide; DMSO, dimethyl sulfoxide; EG, ethylene glycol (Ethane, 1,2-diol); TFA, trifluoroacetic acid; DMAc, N,N-dimethylacetamide; THF, tetrahydrofuran.

[a] This information has been obtained from a variety of sources. For general reference, the following references are recommended:

    1. PubChem. https://pubchem.ncbi.nih.gov.

    2. *CRC Handbook of Chemistry and Physics*, CRC Press/Taylor & Francis, Boca Raton, FL.

    3. *The Merck Index: An Encyclopedia of Chemicals, Drugs, and Biologicals*, ed. M.J. O'Neil, Royal Society of Chemistry, Cambridge, United Kingdom, 2013 (and previous editions published by Merck and Company, Whitehouse Station, NJ).

    4. Shugar, G.J. and Dean, J.A., *The Chemists Ready Reference Handbook*, McGraw-Hill, New York, 1990.

    5. Lide, D.R., *Basic Laboratory and Industrial Chemicals*, CRC Press, Boca Raton, FL, 1993.

    6. Bruno, T.J. and Svoronos, P.D.N., *Handbook of Basic Tables for Chemical Analysis*, CRC Press, Boca Raton, FL, 1989.

    7. Ramis-Ramos, G., García-Álvarez_Coque, M.C., Solvent selection in liquid chromatography, in *Liquid Chromatography Fundamental and Instructions*, ed. S. Fanali, P.R. Haddad, C.R. Poole, P. Schoenmakers, and D. Lloyd, pp. 225–249, Elsevier, Amsterdam, Netherlands, 2013.

    8. Seaver, C. and Sadek, P., Solvent selection. Part I. UV absorption characteristics, *LCGC* 12, 742, 1994.

[b] Normalized to water = 1.00 g/cm^3 (1 cm^3 = 1 mL).

[c] Millepascals second (mPa s); millepascals second = centipoise.

[d] UV cutoff defined as wavelength where solvent has 1 AU in 1 cm pathlength.

[e] For additional discussion on the use of acetonitrile in HPLC (see Welch, J., Brkovic, T., Schafer, W., and Gong, X., Performance to burn? Re-evaluating the choice of acetonitrile as the platform solvent for analytical HPLC, *Green Chem.* 11, 1232–1238, 2009).

[f] T-value of -1.36 has also been reported for the log P for ethylene glycol.

[g] For additional discussion of the use of formamide as a solvent for capillary zone electrophoresis (see Porras, S.P., and Kenndler, E., Formamide as solvent for capillary zone electrophoresis, *Electrophoresis* 25, 2946–2958, 2004).

EFFECT OF ORGANIC SOLVENTS ON THE pKa OF VARIOUS ACIDS[a]

Compound	^w_wpKa	^s_wpKa							
		MeOH[b]	EtOH	EG	PG	Me$_2$SO	DMF	Dioxane	THF
GlyGly (pKa1)	3.15	3.47	3.46	3.43	3.44	3.55	3.46	3.63	3.51
HOAc	4.59	4.90	4.95	4.82	4.86	4.96	4.95	5.28	5.29
Benzoic acid[c]	3.98	4.53	-	-	-	4.51	4.52	4.59	4.95
Imidazole	7.13	6.88	6.88	7.02	6.92	6.72	6.58	6.79	=
HEPES (pKa1)	2.94	2.84	2.88	3.10	2.96	2.87	2.86	2.94	2.88
HEPES (pKa2)	7.54	7.46	7.47	7.66	7.52	7.46	7.38	7.51	7.45
MES	6.14	6.07	6.04	6.30	6.18	6.04	5.97	6.08	—
Tris	8.23	8.16	8.12	8.31	8.24	8.14	8.04	8.20	-
TAPS	8.46	8.45	8.43	8.54	8.48	8.37	8.32	8.52	8.43
Boric acid	9.29	9.42	9.90	8.18[d]	7.98[d]	10.50	10.23	10.12	—
KH$_2$PO$_4$	6.91	7.39	7.40	7.24	7.25	7.64	7.44	7.49	—

GlyGly, ;HOAc, acetic acid; HEPES, N-(2-hydroxyethyl)-piperazine-N'-2-ethanesulfonic acid; MES, 2-(N-morpholino)-ethanesulfonic acid; Tris, tris(hydroxymethyl)aminomethane; TAPS, 3-[[tris(hydroxymethyl)methyl]amino]propanesulfonic acid; MeOH, methanol; EtOH, ethanol; EG, ethylene glycol; PG, propylene glycol; Me$_2$SO, dimethyl sulfoxide; DMF, dimethylformamide; THF, tetrahydrofuran.

[a] Data taken from Grace, S., and Dunaway-Mariano, D., Examination of the solvent perturbation technique as a method to identify enzyme catalytic groups, *Biochemistry* 22, 4238–4247, 1983.

[b] Solvent at 25% (V/V by preparation).

[c] For a more detailed study on the effect of organic solvents see Rubino, J.T. and Berryhill, W.S., Effects of solvent polarity on the acid dissociation-constants of benzoic acid, *J. Pharm. Sci.* 75, 182–186, 1986.

[d] The effect of ethylene glycol and propylene glycol on boric acid reflects the complexation of polyhydroxy compounds with boric acids resulting in a decrease in pH. A similar effect has been observed with monosaccharides (Shubhada, S., and Sundaram, P.V., The role of pH change caused by the addition of water-miscible organic solvents in the destabilization of an enzyme, *Enzyme Microb. Technol.* 17, 330–335, 1994).

EFFECT OF ACETONITRILE OR METHANOL ON THE pKa OF SOME ORGANIC ACIDS

Buffer	pKa						
	Water	20% Acn	40% Acn	60% Acn	20% MeOH[e]	40% MeOH[e]	60% MeOH[e]
Formic acid[a,b]	3.72	3.96 (3.99)[c]	4.40 (4.54)	4.87 (5.33)	–	–	–
Acetic acid[d]	4.74	(5.17)	(5.76)	(6.62)	5.05	5.43	5.66
Citrate (k$_1$)[d]	3.16	(3.49)	(3.90)	(4.45)	3.44	3.84	4.30
Citrate (k$_2$)[d]	4.79	(5.14)	(5.60)	(6.28)	6.40	7.39	7.96
Boric acid[a]	9.23	9.85 (9.88)	10.43 (10.57)	11.00 (11.45)			
Carbonic acid	10.35	10.82 (10.85)	11.31 (11.45)	11.62 (12.08)			
H$_3$PO$_4$	2.21	(2.62)	(3.11)	(3.75)	2.63	3.09	3.68
H$_2$PO$_4$	7.23	(7.60)	(8.08)	(8.73)	7.55	8.04	8.75
Tris	8.08	7.94 (7.97)	7.85 (7.99)	7.72 (8.18)			
NH$_4$	9.29	(9.21)	(9.19)	(9.34)	9.11	8.97	8.82

[a] Subirats, X., Bosch, E., and Rosés, M., Retention of ionizable compounds on high-performance liquid chromatography XVII pH variation in mobile phases containing formic acids, piperazine, tris, boric acid, and carbonate as buffering systems and acetonitrile as organic modified, *J. Chromatog. A*, 1216, 2491–2498, 2009.

[b] The pKa values for neutral acids increase with the addition of organic solvent with a sharp increase in pH to about 60–70% solvent, whereas cationic acids (e.g., Tris, ammonia) show a decrease in pKa values to about 80% solvent with a sharp increase in pKa values at higher concentrations (Cox, B.G., Acids, bases, and salts in mixed-aqueous solvents, *Org. Process Res. Dev.* 19, 1800–1808, 2015).

[c] Numbers in parentheses are values obtained with a solvent containing reference buffer (^s_spKa); values without parentheses are obtained with aqueous reference buffer (^s_wpKa). This is IUPAC nomenclature where the superscript indicates the media of the sample (s being solvent), while the subscript indicates the media for the reference solvent (w being water) (*IUPAC Compendium of Analytical Nomenclature. Definitive Rules 1997*, Blackwell, Oxford, England, 1998).

[d] Subirats, X., Bosch, E., and Rosés, M., Retention of ionizable compounds on high-performance liquid chromatography XV. Estimation of the pH variation of aqueous buffers with the change of the acetonitrile fraction of the mobile phase, *J. Chromatog. A* 1059, 33–42, 2004.

[e] Subirats, X., Bosch, E., and Rosés, M., Retention of ionizable compounds on high-performance liquid chromatography XVII Estimation of the pH variation of aqueous buffers with the change in methanol fraction of the mobile phase, *J. Chromatog. A* 1138, 203–214, 2007.

CHANGE IN pH ON ADDITION OF SOLVENT TO SEVERAL BUFFERS SYSTEMS[a]

Buffer	^w_wpH	^s_wpH						
		20% ACN	40% ACN	60% ACN	20% MeOH	40% MeOH	60% MeOH	80% MeOH
0.01 M Acetate	3.50	3.83	4.16	4.48	3.75	4.09	4.48	4.90
	4.00	4.45	4.90	5.36	4.30	4.71	5.17	5.68
	5.00	5.46	5,91	6.37	5.30	5.72	6.19	6.70
0.05 M Acetate	3.50	3.95	4.39	4.84	3.79	4.19	4.65	5.14
	4.00	4.46	4.91	5.37	4.30	4.71	5.17	5.68
	5.00	5.46	5.91	6.37	5.30	5.71	6.18	6.68
0.01 M Citrate	4.00	4.31	4.62	4.94	4.31	4.75	5.24	5.78
	6.00	6.40	6.79	7.19	6.38	6.89	7.49	8.13
	7.50	7.90	8.30	8.69	7.87	8.38	8.96	9.59
0.05 M Citrate	4.00	4.32	4.64	4.96	4.32	4.76	5.26	5.81
	6.00	6.38	6.75	7.13	6.37	6.87	7.44	8.07
	7.50	7.88	8.25	8.63	7.86	8.36	8.92	9.54
0.01 M Phosphate	3.50	3.77	4.04	4.30	3.82	4.27	4.77	5.32
	6.50	6.88	7.20	7.55	6.90	7.45	8.08	8.76
	8.00	8.35	8.70	9.05	8.38	8.91	9.51	10.16
0.05 M Phosphate	3.50	3.84	4.18	4.53	3.88	4.39	4.99	5.63
	6.50	6.84	7.18	7.53	6.90	7.44	8.06	8.74
	8.00	8.34	8.68	9.03	8.39	8.92	9.52	10.18
0.01 M NH$_4$	8.00	7.88	7.76	7.64	7.86	7.73	7.59	7.45
	10.00	9.88	9.76	9.64	9.87	9.73	9.60	9.47
0.05 M NH$_4$	8.00	7.88	7.76	7.64	7.86	7.73	7.59	7.45
	10.00	9.94	9.76	9.64	9.86	9.73	9.59	9.46

[a] Data are taken from Subirats, X., Rosés, M., and Bosch, E., On the effects of organic solvent composition on the pH of buffer HPLC mobile phases and the pKa of analytes—A review, *Sep. Purif. Rev.*, 36, 231–255, 2007.

POLARITY OF SOLVENTS USED IN CHROMATOGRAPHY[a]

	Solvent	Solvent polarity (P')[b]	Solvent polarity (P')[b,c]	Solvent polarity (P')[d]	Eluuotropic solvent strength (E°)[g] Al_2O_3 [e]	Solvent polarity[h] (E_T^N)[f]	Solvation ability (A)[g]	Dielectric constant (E_r)[h]
1	H_2O	10.2	1.00			1.00	2.00	80.1
2	MeOH	5.1	0.5		0.95	0.762	1.25	33
3	EtOH	4.3	0.4	4.4		0.654	1.11	25.3
4	nPrOH	3.9	0.4	4.1		0.617	1.08	20.8
5	iPrOH	3.9	0.4	3.9	0.82	0.546		20.2
6	nBuOH	3.9	0.4	4.1		0.586		17.8
7	Acn	5.8	0.6	5.6	0.79	0.460	1.22	36.6
8	Acetone					0.355	1.06	21.0
9	HOAc	6.0	0.6	6.1		0.228	1.06	6.2
10	EtOAc	4.4	0.4	4.2	0.58	0.221	0.79	6.1
11	EG	6.9	0.7			0.790	1.62	41.4
12	HCOOH				6.1	0.728		51.1
13	TFA						1.72	8.4
14	DMSO	7.2	0.7		7.3	0.444		47.2
15	Formamide	9.6	0.9			0.775	1.65	111
16	DMF	6.4	0.6	6.3		0.386	1.23	38.3
17	$CHCl_3$	4.1	0.4	4.3	0.40	0.259	1.15	4.7
18	CCl_4	1.6	0.2	1.6	0.18	0.052	0.43	2.2
19	$CHCl_2$	3.1	0.3	4.3	0.42	0.309	1.13	8.9
20	Dioxane	4.8		5.3	0.63	0.164	0.86	2.2
21	THF	4.0		4.3		0.207	0.84	7.5
22	DMAc	6.5		6.5				38.9
23	n-heptane							1.9
24	n-hexane	0.1		-0.14				1.9
25	Toluene	2.4		2.7				2.4

DMF, dimethyl formamide; DMSO, dimethyl sulfoxide; EG, ethylene glycol (Ethane, 1,2-diol); TFA, trifluoroacetic acid; DMAc, N,N-dimethylacetamide

[a] This information has been obtained from a variety of sources. For general reference, the following references are recommended:

1. PubChem (https://pubchem.ncbi.nih.gov).
2. CRC Handbook of Chemistry and Physics, CRC Press/Taylor & Francis, Boca Raton, Florida, USA.
3. The Merck Index: An encyclopedia of chemicals, drugs, and biologicals, ed. M.J. O'Neil, Royal Society of Chemistry, Cambridge, United Kingdom, 2013 (and previous editions published by Merck and Company, Whitehouse Station, New Jersey, USA).
4. Shugar, G.J. and Dean, J.A., The Chemists Ready Reference Handbook, McGraw-Hill, New York, New York, 1990.
5. Lide, D.R., Basic Laboratory and Industrial Chemicals, CRC Press, Boca Raton, Florida, USA, 1993.
6. Bruno, T.J. and Svoronos, P.D.N., Handbook of Basic Tables for Chemical Analysis, CRC Press, Boca Raton, Florida, USA, 1989.
7. Ramis-Ramos, G., García-Álvarez_Coque, M.C., Solvent selection in liquid chromatography, in Liquid Chromatography Fundamental and Instructions, ed. S. Fanali, P.R. Haddad, C.R. Poole, P. Schoenmakers, and D. Lloyd, Chapter 10, pp. 225–249, Elsevier, Amsterdam, Netherlands, 2013.
8. Seaver, C. and Sadek, P., Solvent selection. Part I. UV absorption characteristics, LCGC 12, 742, 1994.

[b] Solvent polarity (P') as defined by Snyder (Snyder, L.R., Classification of the solvent properties of common liquids, J. Chromatog. Sci., 16, 223–234, 1978). P' is a global estimation of solvent strength (polarity) including acidity, basicity, and dipolar characteristics.

[c] Normalized to water = 1; not taken to more significant figures than original data.

[d] Solvent polarity (P') slightly modified (Rutan, S.C., Carr, P.W., Cheung, W.J., et al., Re-evaluation of the solvent triangle and comparison to solvatochromic-based scales of solvent strength and selectivity, J. Chromatog. A., 463, 21–37, 1989).

[e] Eluotropic is a measure of the adsorption interaction of a solvent with a specific stationary phase. In this example, the stationary phase is a normal phase thin layer (planar) chromatography (Gocan, S., Eluotropic series of solvents for TLC, in Encyclopedia of Chromatography, 3rd edn., ed. J. Cazes, pp. 730–735, CRC Press/Taylor & Francis, Boca Raton, Florida, USA, 2010).

[f] E_T^N is $E_T^{(30)}$ normalized to water = 1. $E_T^{(30)}$ is an empirical scale of solvent polarity (Reichardt, C., Pyridinium N-phenolate betaine dyes as empirical indicators of solvent polarity: Some new findings, Pure Appl. Chem., 76, 1909–1919, 2004. Data shown are taken from Reichardt, C., Solvatochromic dyes as solvent polarity indicators, Chem. Rev., 94, 2319–2358, 1994. $E_T^{(30)}$ is the molar electronic transition energy of pyridinium N-phenolate betaine dye; E_T^N is obtained from the normalization of $E_T^{(30)}$ using water as the most polar solvent and tetramethylsilane as the most nonpolar solvent. Units of $E_T^{(30)}$ are kcal mol^{-1}, while E_T^N is dimensionless.

[g] A measure of solvation—a combination of anion-solvating ability and cation-solvating ability considered a measure of solvent polarity (Reichardt, C. and Welton, T., Solvents and Solvent Effects in Organic Chemistry, 4th edn., Wiley-VCH, Weinheim, New Jersey, 2011).

[h] Also referred to as permittivity; shown here is the relative permittivity which is the ratio of actual permittivity to permittivity in a vacuum.

CHEMICALS COMMONLY USED IN BIOCHEMISTRY AND MOLECULAR BIOLOGY AND THEIR PROPERTIES

Roger L. Lundblad

Common Name	Chemical Name	M.W.	Properties and Comment
Acetaldehyde	Acetaldehyde, Ethanal	44.05	Manufacturing intermediate; modification of amino groups; toxic chemical; first product in detoxification of ethanol.

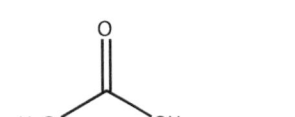

Acetaldehyde + H_2O ⇌ *gem*-diol form (approximately 60%)

Burton, R.M. and Stadtman, E.R., The oxidation of acetaldehyde to acetyl coenzyme A, *J. Biol. Chem.* 202, 873–890, 1953; Gruber, M. and Wesselius, J.C., Nature of the inhibition of yeast carboxylase by acetaldehyde, *Biochim. Biophys. Acta* 57, 171–173, 1962; Holzer, H., da Fonseca-Wollheim, F., Kohlhaw, G., and Woenckhaus, C.W., Active forms of acetaldehyde, pyruvate, and glycolic aldehyde, *Ann. N.Y. Acad. Sci.* 98, 453–465, 1962; Brooks, P.J. and Theruvathu, J.A., DNA adducts from acetaldehyde: implications for alcohol-related carcinogenesis, *Alcohol* 35, 187–193, 2005; Tyulina, O.V., Prokopieva, V.D., Boldyrev, A.A., and Johnson, P., Erthyrocyte and plasma protein modification in alcoholism: a possible role of acetaldehyde, *Biochim. Biophys. Acta* 1762, 558–563, 2006; Pluskota-Karwatka, D., Pawlowicz, A.J., and Kronberg, L., Formation of malonaldehyde-acetaldehyde conjugate adducts in calf thymus DNA, *Chem. Res. Toxicol.* 19, 921–926, 2006.

Acetic Acid	Acetic Acid, Glacial	60.05	Solvent (particular use in the extraction of collagen from tissue), buffer component (used in urea-acetic acid electrophoresis). Use in endoscopy as mucous-resolving agent.

Banfield, A.G., Age changes in the acetic acid-soluble collagen in human skin, *Arch. Pathol.* 68, 680–684, 1959; Steven, F.S. and Tristram, G.R., The denaturation of acetic acid-soluble calf-skin collagen. Changes in optical rotation, viscosity, and susceptibility towards enzymes during serial denaturation in solutions of urea, *Biochem. J.* 85, 207–210, 1962; Neumark, T. and Marot, I., The formation of acetic-acid soluble collagen under polarization and electron microscrope, *Acta Histochem.* 23, 71–79, 1966; Valfleteren, J.R., Sequential two-dimensional and acetic acid/urea/Triton X-100 gel electrophoresis of proteins, *Anal. Biochem.* 177, 388–391, 1989; Smith, B.J., Acetic acid-urea polyacrylamide gel electrophoresis of proteins, *Methods Mol. Biol.* 32, 39–47, 1994; Banfield, W.G., MacKay, C.M., and Brindley, D.C., Quantitative changes in acetic acid-extractable collagen of hamster skin related to anatomical site and age, *Gerontologia* 12, 231–236, 1996; Lian, J.B., Morris, S., Faris, B. et al., The effects of acetic acid and pepsin on the crosslinkages and ultrastructure of corneal collagen, *Biochim. Biophys. Acta.* 328, 193–204, 1973; Canto, M.I., Chromoendoscopy and magnifying endoscopy for Barrett's esophagus, *Clin.Gastroenterol.Hepatol.* 3 (7 Suppl. 1), S12–S15, 2005; Sionkowska, A., Flash photolysis and pulse radiolysis studies on collagen Type I in acetic acid solution, *J. Photochem. Photobiol. B* 84, 38–45, 2006.

CHEMICALS COMMONLY USED IN BIOCHEMISTRY AND MOLECULAR BIOLOGY AND THEIR PROPERTIES (Continued)

Common Name	Chemical Name	M.W.	Properties and Comment
Acetic Anhydride	Acetic Anhydride	102.07	Protein modification (trace labeling of amino groups); modification of amino groups and hydroxyl groups.

Jencks, W.P., Barley, F., Barnett, R., and Gilchrest, M., The free energy of hydrolysis of acetic anhydride, *J. Am. Chem. Soc.* 88, 4464–4467, 1966; Cromwell, L.D. and Stark, G.D., Determination of the carboxyl termini of proteins with ammonium thiocyanate and acetic anhydride, with direct identification of the thiohydantoins, *Biochemistry* 8, 4735–4740, 1969; Montelaro, R.C. and Rueckert, R.R., Radiolabeling of proteins and viruses *in vitro* by acetylation with radioactive acetic anhydride, *J. Biol. Chem.* 250, 1413–1421, 1975; Valente, A.J. and Walton, K.W., The binding of acetic anhydride- and citraconic anhydride-modified human low-density lipoprotein to mouse peritoneal macrophages. The evidence for separate binding sites, *Biochim. Biophys. Acta* 792, 16–24, 1984; Fojo, A.T., Reuben, P.M., Whitney, P.L., and Awad, W.M., Jr., Effect of glycerol on protein acetylation by acetic anhydride, *Arch. Biochem. Biophys.* 240, 43–50, 1985; Buechler, J.A., Vedvick, T.A., and Taylor, S.S., Differential labeling of the catalytic subunit of cAMP-dependent protein kinase with acetic anhydride: substrate-induced conformational changes, *Biochemistry* 28, 3018–3024, 1989; Baker, G.B., Coutts, R.T., and Holt, A., Derivatization with acetic anhydride: applications to the analysis of biogenic amines and psychiatric drugs by gas chromatography and mass spectrometry, *J. Pharmacol. Toxicol. Methods* 31, 141–148, 1994; Ohta, H., Ruan, F., Hakomori, S., and Igarashi, Y., Quantification of free Sphingosine in cultured cells by acetylation with radioactive acetic anhydride, *Anal. Biochem.* 222, 489–494, 1994; Yadav, S.P., Brew, K., and Puett, D., Holoprotein formation of human chorionic gonadotropin: differential trace labeling with acetic anhydride, *Mol. Endocrinol.* 8, 1547–1558, 1994; Miyazaki, K. and Tsugita, A., C-terminal sequencing method for peptides and proteins by the reaction with a vapor of perfluoric acid in acetic anhydride, *Proteomics* 4, 11–19, 2004.

Acetone	Dimethyl Ketone; 2-propanone	58.08	Solvent, protein purification (acetone powders); rare reaction with amino groups.

La Du, B., Jr. and Greenberg, D.M., The tyrosine oxidation system of liver. I. Extracts of rat liver acetone powder, *J. Biol. Chem.* 190, 245–255, 1951; Korn, E.D. and Payza, A.N., The degradation of heparin by bacterial enzymes. II. Acetone powder extracts, *J. Biol. Chem.* 223, 859–864, 1956; Ohtsuki, K., Taguchi, K., Sato, K., and Kawabata, M., Purification of ginger proteases by DEAE-Sepharose and isoelectric focusing, *Biochim. Biophys. Acta* 1243, 181–184, 1995; Selden, L.A., Kinosian, H.J., Estes, J.E., and Gershman, L.C., Crosslinked dimers with nucleating activity in actin prepared from muscle acetone powder, *Biochemistry* 39, 64–74, 2000; Abadir, W.F., Nakhla, V., and Chong, F., Removal of superglue from the external ear using acetone: case report and literature review, *J. Laryngol. Otol.* 109, 1219–1221, 1995; Jones, A.W., Elimination half-life of acetone in humans: case reports and review of the literature, *J. Anal. Toxicol.* 24, 8–10, 2000; Huang, L.P. and Guo, P., Use of acetone to attain highly active and soluble DNA packaging protein Gp16 of Phi29 for ATPase assay, *Virology* 312, 449–457, 2003; Paska, C., Bogi, K., Szilak, L. et al., Effect of formalin, acetone, and RNAlater fixatives on tissue preservation and different size amplicons by real-time PCR from paraffin-embedded tissues, *Diagn. Mol. Pathol.* 13, 234–240, 2004; Kuksis, A., Ravandi, A., and Schneider, M., Covalent binding of acetone to aminophospholipids *in vitro* and *in vivo*, *Ann. N.Y. Acad. Sci.* 1043, 417–439, 2005; Perera, A., Sokolic, F., Almasy, L. et al., On the evaluation of the Kirkwood–Buff integrals of aqueous acetone mixtures, *J. Chem. Physics* 123, 23503, 2005; Zhou, J., Tao, G., Liu, Q. et al., Equilibrium yields of mono- and di-lauroyl mannoses through lipase-catalyzed condensation in acetone in the presence of molecular sieves, *Biotechnol. Lett.* 28, 395–400, 2006.

Acetonitrile	Ethenenitrile, Methyl Cyanide	41.05	Chromatography solvent, general solvent.

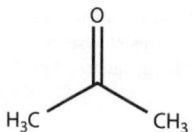

CHEMICALS COMMONLY USED IN BIOCHEMISTRY AND MOLECULAR BIOLOGY AND THEIR PROPERTIES (Continued)

Common Name	Chemical Name	M.W.	Properties and Comment

Hodgkinson, S.C. and Lowry, P.J., Hydrophobic-interaction chromatography and anion-exchange chromatography in the presence of acetonitrile. A two-step purification method for human prolactin, *Biochem. J.* 199, 619–627, 1981; Wolf-Coporda, A., Plavsic, F., and Vrhovac, B., Determination of biological equivalence of two atenolol preparations, *Int. J. Clin. Pharmacol. Ther. Toxicol.* 25, 567–571, 1987; Fischer, U., Zeitschel, U., and Jakubke, H.D., Chymotrypsin-catalyzed peptide synthesis in an acetonitrile-water-system: studies on the efficiency of nucleophiles, *Biomed. Biochim. Acta* 50, S131–S135, 1991; Haas, R. and Rosenberry, T.L., Protein denaturation by addition and removal of acetonitrile: application to tryptic digestion of acetylcholinesterase, *Anal. Biochem.* 224, 425–427, 1995; Joansson, A., Mosbach, K., and Mansson, M.O., Horse liver alcohol dehydrogenase can accept NADP+ as coenzyme in high concentrations of acetonitrile, *Eur. J. Biochem.* 227, 551–555, 1995; Barbosa, J., Sanz-Nebot, V., and Toro, I., Solvatochromic parameter values and pH in acetonitrile-water mixtures. Optimization of mobile phase for the separation of peptides by high-performance liquid chromatography, *J. Chromatog. A* 725, 249–260, 1996; Barbosa, J., Hernandez-Cassou, S., Sanz-Nebot, V., and Toro, I., Variation of acidity constants of peptides in acetonitrile-water mixtures with solvent composition: effect of preferential salvation, *J. Pept. Res.* 50, 14–24, 1997; Badock, V., Steinhusen, U., Bommert, K., and Otto, A., Prefractionation of protein samples for proteome analysis using reversed-phase high-performance liquid chromatography, *Electrophoresis* 22, 2856–2864, 2001; Yoshida, T., Peptide separation by hydrophilic-interaction chromatography: a review, *J. Biochem. Biophys. Methods* 60, 265–280, 2004: Kamau, P. and Jordan, R.B., Complex formation constants for the aqueous copper(I)-acetonitrile system by a simple general method, *Inorg. Chem.* 40, 3879–3883, 2001; Nagy, P.I. and Erhardt, P.W., Monte Carlo simulations of the solution structure of simple alcohols in water-acetonitrile mixtures, *J. Phys. Chem. B Condens. Matter Mater. Surf. Interfaces Biophys.* 109, 5855–5872, 2005; Kutt, A., Leito, I., Kaljurand, I. et al., A comprehensive self-consistent spectrophotometric acidity scale of neutral Bronstad acids in acetonitrile, *J. Org. Chem.* 71, 2829–2938, 2006.

Common Name	Chemical Name	M.W.	Properties and Comment
Acetyl Chloride	Ethanoyl Chloride	78.50	Acetylating agent.

Hallaq, Y., Becker, T.C., Manno, C.S., and Laposata, M., Use of acetyl chloride/methanol for assumed selective methylation of plasma nonesterified fatty acids results in significant methylation of esterified fatty acids, *Lipids* 28, 355–360, 1993; Shenoy, N.R., Shively, J.E., and Bailey, J.M., Studies in C-terminal sequencing: new reagents for the synthesis of peptidylthiohydantoins, *J. Protein Chem.* 12, 195–205, 1993; Bosscher, G., Meetsma, A., and van De Grampel, J.C., Novel organo-substituted cyclophosphazenes via reaction of a monohydro cyclophosphazene and acetyl chloride, *Inorg. Chem.* 35, 6646–6650, 1996; Mo, B., Li, J., and Liang, S., A method for preparation of amino acid thiohydantoins from free amino acids activated by acetyl chloride for development of protein C-terminal sequencing, *Anal. Biochem.* 249, 207–211, 1997; Studer, J., Purdie, N., and Krouse, J.A., Friedel–Crafts acylation as a quality control assay for steroids, *Appl. Spectros.* 57, 791–796, 2003.

Common Name	Chemical Name	M.W.	Properties and Comment
Acetylcysteine	N-acetyl-L-cysteine	163.2	Mild reducing agent for clinical chemistry (creatine kinase); therapeutic use for aminoacetophen intoxication; some other claimed indications.

Szasz, G., Gruber, W., and Bernt, E., Creatine kinase in serum. I. Determination of optimum reaction conditions, *Clin. Chem.* 22, 650–656, 1976; Holdiness, M.R., Clinical pharmacokinetics of N-acetylcysteine, *Clin. Pharmacokinet.* 20, 123–134, 1991; Kelley, G.S., Clinical applications of N-acetylcysteine, *Altern. Med. Rev.* 3, 114–127, 1998; Schumann, G., Bonora, R., Ceriotti, F. et al., IFCC primary reference procedures for the measurement of catalytic activity concentrations of enzymes at 37°C. Part 2. Reference procedure for the measurement of catalytic concentration of creatine kinase, *Clin. Chem. Lab. Med.* 40, 635–642, 2002; Zafarullah, M., Li, W.Q., Sylvester, J., and Ahmad, M., Molecular mechanisms of N-acetylcysteine actions, *Cell. Mol. Life Sci.* 60, 6–20, 2003; Marzullo, L., An update of N-acetylcysteine treatment for acute aminoacetophen toxicity in children, *Curr. Opin. Pediatr.* 17, 239–245, 2005; Aitio, M.L., N-acetylcysteine — passé-partout or much ado about nothing? *Br. J. Clin. Pharmacol.* 61, 5–15, 2006.

CHEMICALS COMMONLY USED IN BIOCHEMISTRY AND MOLECULAR BIOLOGY AND THEIR PROPERTIES (Continued)

Common Name	Chemical Name	M.W.	Properties and Comment
N-Acetylimidazole	1-acetyl-1*H*-imidazole	110.12	Reagent for modification of tyrosyl residues in proteins.

Lundblad, R.L., *Chemical Reagents for Protein Modification*, CRC Press, Boca Raton, FL, 2004; Gorbunoff, M.J., Exposure of tyrosine residues in proteins. 3. The reaction of cyanuric fluoride and *N*-acetylimidazole with ovalbumin, chymotrypsinogen, and trypsinogen, *Biochemistry* 44, 719–725, 1969; Houston, L.L. and Walsh, K.A., The transient inactivation of trypsin by mild acetylation with *N*-acetylimidazole, *Biochemistry* 9, 156–166, 1970; Shifrin, S. and Solis, B.G., Reaction of *N*-acetylimidazole with L-asparaginase, *Mol. Pharmacol.* 8, 561–564, 1972; Ota, Y., Nakamura, H., and Samejima, T., The change of stability and activity of thermolysin by acetylation with *N*-acetylimidazole, *J. Biochem.* 72, 521–527, 1972; Kasai, H., Takahashi, K., and Ando, T., Chemical modification of tyrosine residues in ribonuclease T1 with *N*-acetylimidazole and *p*-diazobenzenesulfonic acid, *J. Biochem.* 81, 1751–1758, 1977; Zhao, X., Gorewit, R.C., and Currie, W.B., Effects of *N*-acetylimidazole on oxytocin binding in bovine mammary tissue, *J. Recept. Res.* 10, 287–298, 1990; Wells, I. and Marnett, L.J., Acetylation of prostaglandin endoperoxide synthase by *N*-acetylimidazole: comparison to acetylation by aspirin, *Biochemistry* 31, 9520–9525, 1992; Cymes, G.D., Iglesias, M.M., and Wolfenstein-Todel, C., Chemical modification of ovine prolactin with *N*-acetylimidazole, *Int. J. Pept. Protein Res.* 42, 33–38, 1993; Zhang, F., Gao, J., Weng, J. et al., Structural and functional differences of three groups of tyrosine residues by acetylation of *N*-acetylimidazole in manganese-stabilizing protein, *Biochemistry* 44, 719–725, 2005.

Acetylsalicylic Acid	2-(acetoxy)benzoic Acid; Aspirin	180.16	Analgesic, anti-inflammatory; mild acetylating agent.

Hawkins, D., Pinckard, R.N., and Farr, R.S., Acetylation of human serum albumin by acetylsalicylic acid, *Science* 160, 780–781, 1968; Kalatzis, E., Reactions of aminoacetophen in pharmaceutical dosage forms: its proposed acetylation by acetylsalicylic acid, *J. Pharm. Sci.* 59, 193–196, 1970; Pinckard, R.N., Hawkins, D., and Farr, R.S., The inhibitory effect of salicylate on the actylation of human albumin by acetylsalicylic acid, *Arthritis Rheum.* 13, 361–368, 1970; Van Der Ouderaa, F.J., Buytenhek, M., Nugteren, D.H., and Van Dorp, D.A., Acetylation of prostaglandin endoperoxide synthetase with acetylsalicylic acid, *Eur. J. Biochem.* 109, 1–8, 1980; Rainsford, K.D., Schweitzer, A., and Brune, K., Distribution of the acetyl compared with the salicyl moiety of acetylsalicylic acid. Acetylation of macromolecules in organs wherein side effects are manifest, *Biochem. Pharmacol.* 32, 1301–1308, 1983; Liu, L.R. and Parrott, E.L., Solid-state reaction between sulfadiazine and acetylsalicyclic acid, *J. Pharm. Sci.* 80, 564–566, 1991; Minchin, R.F., Ilett, K.F., Teitel, C.H. et al., Direct *O*-acetylation of *N*-hydroxy arylamines by acetylsalicylic acid to form carcinogen-DNA adducts, *Carcinogenesis* 13, 663–667, 1992.

Acrylamide	2-propenamide	71.08	Monomer unit of polyacrylamide in gels, hydrogels, hard polymers; environmental carcinogen; fluorescence quencher.

CHEMICALS COMMONLY USED IN BIOCHEMISTRY AND MOLECULAR BIOLOGY AND THEIR PROPERTIES (Continued)

Common Name	Chemical Name	M.W.	Properties and Comment

Eftink, M.R. and Ghiron, C.A., Fluorescence quenching studies with proteins, *Anal. Biochem.* 114, 199–227, 1981; Dearfield, K.L., Abernathy, C.O., Ottley, M.S. et al., Acrylamide: its metabolism, developmental and reproductive effects, *Mutat. Res.* 195, 45–77, 1988; Williams, L.R., Staining nucleic acids and proteins in electrophoresis gels, *Biotech. Histochem.* 76, 127–132, 2001; Hamden, M., Bordini, E., Galvani, M., and Righetti, P.G., Protein alkylation by acrylamide, its *N*-substituted derivatives and crosslinkers and its relevance to proteomics: a matrix-assisted laser desorption/ionization-time of flight-mass spectrometry study, *Electrophoresis* 22, 1633–1644, 2001; Cioni, P. and Strambini, G.B., Tryptophan phosphorescence and pressure effects on protein structure, *Biochim. Biophys. Acta* 1595, 116–130, 2002; Taeymans, D., Wood, J., Ashby, P. et al., A review of acrylamide: an industry perspective on research, analysis, formation, and control, *Crit. Rev. Food Sci. Nutr.* 44, 323–347, 2004; Rice, J.M., The carcinogenicity of acrylamide, *Mutat. Res.* 580, 3–20, 2005; Besaratinia, A. and Pfeifer, G.P., DNA adduction and mutagenic properties of acrylamide, *Mutat. Res.* 580, 31–40, 2005; Hoenicke, K. and Gaterman, R., Studies on the stability of acrylamide in food during storage, *J. AOAC Int.* 88, 268–273, 2005; Castle, L. and Ericksson, S., Analytical methods used to measure acrylamide concentrations in foods, *J. AOAC Int.* 88, 274–284, 2005; Stadler, R.H., Acrylamide formation in different foods and potential strategies for reduction, *Adv. Exp. Med. Biol.* 561, 157–169, 2005; Lopachin, R.M. and Decaprio, A.P., Protein adduct formation as a molecular mechanism in neurotoxicity, *Toxicol. Sci.* 86, 214–225, 2005.

Gamma (γ)-aminobutyric Acid (GABA)	4-aminobutanoic acid	103.12	Neurotransmitter.

Mandel, P. and DeFeudis, F.V., Eds., *GABA—Biochemistry and CNS Functions*, Plenum Press, New York, 1979; Costa, E. and Di Chiara, G., *GABA and Benzodiazepine Receptors*, Raven Press, New York, 1981; Racagni, G. and Donoso, A.O., *GABA and Endocrine Function*, Raven Press, New York, 1986; Squires, R.F., *GABA and Benzodiazepine Receptors*, CRC Press, Boca Raton, FL, 1988; Martin, D.L. and Olsen, R.W., *GABA in the Nervous System: The View at Fifty Years*, Lippincott, Williams & Wilkins, Philadelphia, PA, 2000.

Amiloride	3,5-diamino-*N*-(aminoiminomethyl)-6-chloropyrazinecarboxamide	229.63	Sodium ion channel blocker.

Benos, D.J., A molecular probe of sodium transport in tissues and cells, *Am. J. Physiol.* 242, C131–C145, 1982; Garty, H., Molecular properties of epithelial, amiloride-blockable Na⁺ channels, *FASEB J.* 8, 522–528, 1994; Barbry, P. and Lazdunski, M., Structure and regulation of the amiloride-sensitive epithelial sodium channel, *Ion Channels* 4, 115–167, 1996; Kleyman, T.R., Sheng, S., Kosari, F., and Kieber-Emmons, T., Mechanism of action of amiloride: a molecular perspective, *Semin. Nephrol.* 19, 524–532, 1999; Alvarez de la Rosa, D., Canessa, C.M., Fyfe, G.K., and Zhang, P., Structure and regulation of amiloride-sensitive sodium channels, *Annu. Rev. Physiol.* 62, 573–594, 2000; Haddad, J.J., Amiloride and the regulation of NF-κ β: an unsung crosstalk and missing link between fluid dynamics and oxidative stress-related inflammation — controversy or pseudo-controversy, *Biochem. Biophys. Res. Commun.* 327, 373–381, 2005.

2-Aminopyridine	α-aminopyridine	94.12	Precursor for synthesis of pharmaceuticals and reagents; used to derivatize carbohydrates for analysis; blocker of K+ channels.

CHEMICALS COMMONLY USED IN BIOCHEMISTRY AND MOLECULAR BIOLOGY AND THEIR PROPERTIES (Continued)

Common Name	Chemical Name	M.W.	Properties and Comment

Hase, S., Hara, S., and Matsushima, Y., Tagging of sugars with a fluorescent compound, 2-aminopyridine, *J. Biochem.* 85, 217–220, 1979; Hase, S., Ibuki, T., and Ikenaka, T., Reexamination of the pyridylamination used for fluorescence labeling of oligosaccharides and its application to glycoproteins, *J. Biochem.* 95, 197–203, 1984; Chen, C. and Zheng, X., Development of the new antimalarial drug pyronaridine: a review, *Biomed. Environ. Sci.* 5, 149–160, 1992; Hase, S., Analysis of sugar chains by pyridylamination, *Methods Mol. Biol.* 14, 69–80, 1993; Oefner, P.J. and Chiesa, C., Capillary electrophoresis of carbohydrates, *Glycobiology* 4, 397–412, 1994; Dyukova, V.I., Shilova, N.V., Galanina, O.E. et al., Design of carbohydrate multiarrays, *Biochim. Biophys. Acta* 1760, 603–609, 2006; Takegawa, Y., Deguchi, K., Keira, T. et al., Separation of isomeric 2-aminopyridine derivatized *N*-glycans and *N*-glycopeptides of human serum immunoglobulin G by using a zwitterionic type of hydrophilic-interaction chromatography, *J. Chromatog. A* 1113, 177–181, 2006; Suzuki, S., Fujimori, T., and Yodoshi, M., Recovery of free oligosaccharides from derivatives labeled by reductive amination, *Anal. Biochem.* 354, 94–103, 2006; Caballero, N.A., Melendez, F.J., Munoz-Caro, C., and Nino, A., Theoretical prediction of relative and absolute pK(a) values of aminopyridine, *Biophys. Chem.*, 124, 155–160, 2006.

Ammonium Bicarbonate   Acid Ammonium Carbonate   79.06   Volatile buffer salt.

Gibbons, G.R., Page, J.D., and Chaney, S.G., Treatment of DNA with ammonium bicarbonate or thiourea can lead to underestimation of platinum-DNA monoadducts, *Cancer Chemother. Pharmacol.* 29, 112–116, 1991; Sorenson, S.B., Sorenson, T.L., and Breddam, K., Fragmentation of protein by *S. aureus* strain V8 protease. Ammonium bicarbonate strongly inhibits the enzyme but does not improve the selectivity for glutamic acid, *FEBS Lett.* 294, 195–197, 1991; Fichtinger-Schepman, A.M., van Dijk-Knijnenburg, H.C., Dijt, F.J. et al., Effects of thiourea and ammonium bicarbonate on the formation and stability of bifunctional cisplatin-DNA adducts: consequences for the accurate quantification of adducts in (cellular) DNA, *J. Inorg. Biochem.* 58, 177–191, 1995; Overcashier, D.E., Brooks, D.A., Costantino, H.R., and Hus, C.C., Preparation of excipient-free recombinant human tissue-type plasminogen activator by lyophilization from ammonium bicarbonate solution: an investigation of the two-stage sublimation process, *J. Pharm. Sci.* 86, 455–459, 1997.

ANS   1-anilino-8-naphthalenenesulfonate   299.4   Fluorescent probe for protein conformation; considered a hydrophobic probe; study of molten globules.

Ferguson, R.N., Edelhoch, H., Saroff, H.A. et al., Negative cooperativity in the binding of thyroxine to human serum prealbumin. Preparation of tritium-labeled 8-anilino-1-naphthalenesulfonic acid, *Biochemistry* 14, 282–289, 1975; Ogasahara, K., Koike, K., Hamada, M., and Hiraoka, T., Interaction of hydrophobic probes with the apoenzyme of pig heart lipoamide dehydrogenase, *J. Biochem.* 79, 967–975, 1976; De Campos Vidal, B., The use of the fluorescence probe 8-anilinonaphthalene sulfate (ANS) for collagen and elastin histochemistry, *J. Histochem. Cytochem.* 26, 196–201, 1978; Royer, C.A., Fluorescence spectroscopy, *Methods Mol. Biol.* 40, 65–89, 1995; Celej, M.S., Dassie, S.A., Freire, E. et al., Ligand-induced thermostability in proteins: thermodynamic analysis of ANS-albumin interaction, *Biochim. Biophys. Acta* 1750, 122–133, 2005; Banerjee, T. and Kishore, N., Binding of 8-anilinonaphthalene sulfonate to dimeric and tetrameric concanavalin A: energetics and its implications on saccharide binding studied by isothermal titration calorimetry and spectroscopy, *J. Phys. Chem. B Condens. Matter Mater. Surf. Interfaces Biophys.* 110, 7022–7028, 2006; Sahu, K., Mondal, S.K., Ghosh, S. et al., Temperature dependence of salvation dynamics and anisotropy decay in a protein: ANS in bovine serum albumin, *J. Chem. Phys.* 124, 124909, 2006; Wang, G., Gao, Y., and Geng, M.L., Analysis of heterogeneous fluorescence decays in proteins. Using fluorescence lifetime of 8-anilino-1-naphthalenesulfonate to probe apomyoglobin unfolding at equilibrium, *Biochim. Biophys. Acta* 1760, 1125–1137, 2006; Greene, L.H., Wijesinha-Bettoni, R., and Redfield, C., Characterization of the molten globule of human serum retinol-binding protein using NMR spectroscopy, *Biochemistry* 45, 9475–9484, 2006.

CHEMICALS COMMONLY USED IN BIOCHEMISTRY AND MOLECULAR BIOLOGY AND THEIR PROPERTIES (Continued)

Common Name	Chemical Name	M.W.	Properties and Comment
Arachidonic Acid	5,8,11,14(all *cis*)-eicosatetraenoic acid	304.5	Essential fatty acid; precursor of prostaglandins, thromboxanes, and leukotrienes.

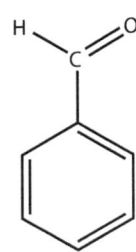

Moncada, S. and Vane, J.R., Interaction between anti-inflammatory drugs and inflammatory mediators. A reference to products of arachidonic acid metabolism, *Agents Actions Suppl.* 3, 141–149, 1977; Moncada, S. and Higgs, E.A., Metabolism of arachidonic acid, *Ann. N.Y. Acad. Sci.* 522, 454–463, 1988; Piomelli, D., Arachidonic acid in cell signaling, *Curr. Opin. Cell Biol.* 5, 274–280, 1993; Janssen-Timmen, U., Tomic, I., Specht, E. et al., The arachidonic acid cascade, eicosanoids, and signal transduction, *Ann. N.Y. Acad. Sci.* 733, 325–334, 1994; Wang, X. and Stocco, D.M., Cyclic AMP and arachidonic acid: a tale of two pathways, *Mol. Cell. Endocrinol.* 158, 7–12, 1999; Brash, A.R., Arachidonic acid as a bioactive molecule, *J. Clin. Invest.* 107, 1339–1345, 2001; Luo, M., Flamand, N., and Brock, T.G., Metabolism of arachidonic acid to eicosanoids within the nucleus, *Biochim. Biophys. Acta* 1761, 618–625, 2006; Balboa, M.A. and Balsinde, J., Oxidative stress and arachidonic acid mobilization, *Biochim. Biophys. Acta* 1761, 385–391, 2006.

Ascorbic Acid	Vitamin C; 3-oxo-L-gulofuranolactone	176.13	Nutrition, antioxidant (reducing agent); possible antimicrobial function.

Ascorbic acid   Dehydroascorbic acid

Barnes, M.J. and Kodicek, E., Biological hydroxylations and ascorbic acid with special regard to collagen metabolism, *Vitam. Horm.* 30, 1–43, 1972; Leibovitz, B. and Siegel, B.V., Ascorbic acid and the immune response, *Adv. Exp. Med. Biol.* 135, 1–25, 1981; England, S. and Seifter, S., The biochemical functions of ascorbic acid, *Annu. Rev. Nutr.* 6, 365–406, 1986; Levine, M. and Hartzell, W., Ascorbic acid: the concept of optimum requirements, *Ann. N.Y. Acad. Sci.* 498, 424–444, 1987; Padh, H., Cellular functions of ascorbic acid, *Biochem. Cell Biol.* 68, 1166–1173, 1990; Meister, A., On the antioxidant effects of ascorbic acid and glutathione, *Biochem. Pharmacol.* 44, 1905–1915, 1992; Wolf, G., Uptake of ascorbic acid by human neutrophils, *Nutr. Rev.* 51, 337–338, 1993; Kimoto, E., Terada, S., and Yamaguchi, T., Analysis of ascorbic acid, dehydroascorbic acid, and transformation products by ion-pairing high-performance liquid chromatography with multiwavelength ultraviolet and electrochemical detection, *Methods Enzymol.* 279, 3–12, 1997; May, J.M., How does ascorbic acid prevent endothelial dysfunction? *Free Rad. Biol. Med.* 28, 1421–1429, 2000; Smirnoff, N. and Wheeler, G.L., Ascorbic acid in plants: biosynthesis and function, *Crit. Rev. Biochem. Mol. Biol.* 35, 291–314, 2000; Arrigoni, O. and De Tullio, M.C., Ascorbic acid: much more than just an antioxidant, *Biochim. Biophys. Acta* 1569, 1–9, 2002; Akyon, Y., Effect of antioxidant on the immune response of *Helicobacter pyrlori, Clin. Microbiol. Infect.* 8, 438–441, 2002; Takanaga, H., MacKenzie, B., and Hediger, M.A., Sodium-dependent ascorbic acid transporter family SLC23, *Pflügers Arch.* 447, 677–682, 2004.

Benzaldehyde	Benzoic Aldehyde; Essential Oil of Almond	106.12	Intermediate in manufacture of pharmaceuticals, flavors; reacts with amino groups, semicarbidizide.

CHEMICALS COMMONLY USED IN BIOCHEMISTRY AND MOLECULAR BIOLOGY AND THEIR PROPERTIES (Continued)

Common Name	Chemical Name	M.W.	Properties and Comment

Chalmers, R.M., Keen, J.N., and Fewson, C.A., Comparison of benzyl alcohol dehydrogenases and benzaldehyde dehydrogenases from the benzyl alcohol and mandelate pathways in *Acinetobacter calcoaceticus* and the TOL-plasmid-encoded toluene pathway in *Pseudomonas putida*. *N*-terminal amino acid sequences, amino acid composition, and immunological cross-reactions, *Biochem. J.* 273, 99–107, 1991; Pettersen, E.O., Larsen, R.O., Borretzen, B. et al., Increased effect of benzaldehyde by exchanging the hydrogen in the formyl group with deuterium, *Anticancer Res.* 11, 369–373, 1991; Nierop Groot, M.N. and de Bont, J.A.M., Conversion of phenylalanine to benzaldehyde initiated by an amino-transferase in *Lactobacillus plantarum*, *Appl. Environ. Microbiol.* 64, 3009–3013, 1998; Podyminogin, M.A., Lukhtanov, E.A., and Reed, M.W., Attachment of benzaldehyde-modified oligodeoxynucleotide probes to semicarbazide-coated glass, *Nucleic Acids Res.* 29, 5090–5098, 2001; Kurchan, A.N. and Kutateladze, A.G., Amino acid-based dithiazines: synthesis and photofragmentation of their benzaldehyde adducts, *Org. Lett.* 4, 4129–4131, 2002; Kneen, M.M., Pogozheva, I.D., Kenyon, G.L., and McLeish, M.J., Exploring the active site of benzaldehyde lyase by modeling and mutagenesis, *Biochim. Biophys. Acta* 1753, 263–271, 2005; Mosbacher, T.G., Mueller, M., and Schultz, G.E., Structure and mechanism of the ThDP-dependent benzaldehyde lyase from *Pseudomonas fluorescens*, *FEBS J.* 272, 6067–6076, 2005; Sudareva, N.N. and Chubarova, E.V., Time-dependent conversion of benzyl alcohol to benzaldehyde and benzoic acid in aqueous solution, *J. Pharm. Biomed. Anal.* 41, 1380–1385, 2006.

Benzamidine HCl   156.61   Inhibitor of trypticlike serine proteases.

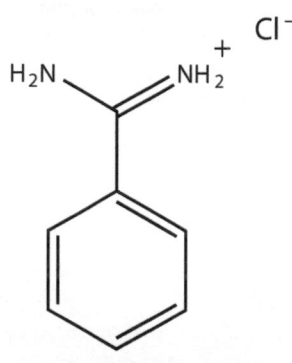

Ensinck, J.W., Shepard, C., Dudl, R.J., and Williams, R.H., Use of benzamidine as a proteolytic inhibitor in the radio-immunoassay of glucagon in plasma, *J. Clin. Endocrinol. Metab.* 35, 463–467, 1972; Bode, W. and Schwager, P., The refined crystal structure of bovine beta-trypsin at 1.8 Å resolution. II. Crystallographic refinement, calcium-binding site, benzamidine-binding site and active site at pH 7.0, *J. Mol. Biol.* 98, 693–717, 1975; Nastruzzi, C., Feriotto, G., Barbieri, R. et al., Differential effects of benzamidine derivatives on the expression of *c-myc* and HLA-DR alpha genes in a human B-lymphoid tumor cell line, *Cancer Lett.* 38, 297–305, 1988; Clement, B., Schmitt, S., and Zimmerman, M., Enzymatic reduction of benzamidoxime to benzamidine, *Arch. Pharm.* 321, 955–956, 1988; Clement, B., Immel, M., Schmitt, S., and Steinman, U., Biotransformation of benzamidine and benzamidoxime *in vivo*, *Arch. Pharm.* 326, 807–812, 1993; Renatus, M., Bode, W., Huber, R. et al., Structural and functional analysis of benzamidine-based inhibitors in complex with trypsin: implications for the inhibition of factor Xa, tPA, and urokinase, *J. Med. Chem.* 41, 5445–5456, 1998; Henriques, R.S., Fonseca, N., and Ramos, M.J., On the modeling of snake venom serine proteinase interactions with benzamidine-based thrombin inhibitors, *Protein Sci.* 13, 2355–2369, 2004; Gustavsson, J., Farenmark, J., and Johansson, B.L., Quantitative determination of the ligand content in benzamidine Sepharose® 4 Fast Flow media with ion-pair chromatography, *J. Chromatog. A* 1070, 103–109, 2005.

Benzene   Benzene   78.11   Solvent; a xenobiotic.

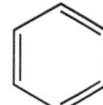

Lovley, D.R., Anaerobic benzene degradation, *Biodegradation* 11, 107–116, 2000; Snyder, R., Xenobiotic metabolism and the mechanism(s) of benzene toxicity, *Drug Metab. Rev.* 36, 531–547, 2004; Rana, S.V. and Verma, Y., Biochemical toxicity of benzene, *J. Environ. Biol.* 26, 157–168, 2005; Lin, Y.S., McKelvey, W., Waidyanatha, S., and Rappaport, S.M., Variability of albumin adducts of 1,4-benzoquinone, a toxic metabolite of benzene, in human volunteers, *Biomarkers* 11, 14–27, 2006; Baron, M. and Kowalewski, V.J., The liquid water-benzene system, *J. Phys. Chem. A Mol. Spectrosc. Kinet. Environ. Gen. Theory* 100, 7122–7129, 2006; Chambers, D.M., McElprang, D.O., Waterhouse, M.G., and Blount, B.C., An improved approach for accurate quantitation of benzene, toluene, ethylbenzene, xylene, and styrene in blood, *Anal. Chem.* 78, 5375–5383, 2006.

| **Benzidine** | *p*-benzidine; (1,1'-biphenyl)-4,4'-diamine | 184.24 | Precursor for azo dyes; mutagenic agent; forensic analysis for bloodstains based on reactivity with hemoglobin. |

CHEMICALS COMMONLY USED IN BIOCHEMISTRY AND MOLECULAR BIOLOGY AND THEIR PROPERTIES (Continued)

Common Name	Chemical Name	M.W.	Properties and Comment

Ahlquist, D.A. and Schwartz, S., Use of leuco-dyes in the quantitative colorimetric microdetermination of hemoglobin and other heme compounds, *Clin. Chem.* 21, 362–369, 1975; Josephy, P.D., Benzidine: mechanisms of oxidative activation and mutagensis, *Fed. Proc.* 45, 2465–2470, 1986; Choudhary, G., Human health perspectives on environmental exposure to benzidine: a review, *Chemosphere* 32, 267–291, 1996; Madeira, P., Nunes, M.R., Borges, C. et al., Benzidine photodegradation: a mass spectrometry and UV spectroscopy combined study, *Rapid Commun. Mass Spectrom.* 19, 2015–2020, 2005; Saitoh, T., Yoshida, S., and Ichikawa, J., Naphthalene-1,8-diylbis(diphenylmethylium) as an organic two-electron oxidant: benzidine synthesis via oxidative self-coupling of *N,N*-dialkylanilines, *J. Org. Chem.* 71, 6414–6419, 2006.

Common Name	Chemical Name	M.W.	Properties and Comment
BIG CHAP/Deoxy BIG CHAP	*N,N*-bis(3-d-gluconamido-propyl) cholamide/*N,N*-bis(3-d-gluconamido-propyl) deoxycholamide	878.1/ 862.1	Nonionic detergents; protein solubilization, adenovirus gene transfer enhancement.

Bonelli, F.S. and Jonas, A., Reaction of lecithin: cholesterol acyltransferase with a water-soluble substrate: effects of surfactants, *Biochim. Biophys. Acta* 1166, 92–98, 1993; Aigner, A., Jager, M., Pasternack, R. et al., Purification and characterization of cysteine-*S*-conjugate *N*-acetyltransferase from pig kidney, *Biochem. J.* 317, 213–218, 1996; Mechref, Y. and Eirassi, Z., Micellar electrokinetic capillary chromatography with *in-situ* charged micelles. 4. Evaluation of novel chiral micelles consisting of steroidal glycoside surfactant borate complexes, *J. Chromatog. A* 724, 285–296, 1996; Abe, S., Kunii, S., Fujita, T., and Hiraiwa, K., Detection of human seminal gamma-glutamyl transpeptidase in stains using sandwich ELISA, *Forensic Sci. Int.* 91, 19–28, 1998; Akutsu, Y., Nakajima-Kambe, T., Nomura, N., and Nakahara, T., Purification and properties of a polyester polyurethane-degrading enzyme form *Comamonas acidovorans* TB-35, *Appl. Environ. Microbiol.* 64, 62–67, 1998: Connor, R.J., Engler, H., Machemer, T. et al., Identification of polyamides that enhance adenovirus-mediated gene expression in the urothelium, *Gene Therapy* 8, 41–48, 2001; Vajdos, F.F., Ultsch, M., Schaffer, M.L. et al., Crystal structure of human insulin-like growth factor-1: detergent binding inhibits binding protein interactions, *Biochemistry* 40, 11022–11029, 2001; Kuball, J., Wen, S.F., Leissner, J. et al., Successful adenovirus-mediated wild-type p53 gene transfer in patients with bladder cancer by intravesical vector instillation, *J. Clin. Oncol.* 20, 957–965, 2002; Susasara, K.M., Xia, F., Gronke, R.S., and Cramer, S.M., Application of hydrophobic interaction displacement chromatography for an industrial protein purification, *Biotechnol. Bioeng.* 82, 330–339, 2003; Ishibashi, A. and Nakashima, N., Individual dissolution of single-walled carbon nanotubes in aqueous solutions of steroid or sugar compounds and their Raman and near-IR spectral properties, *Chemistry*, 12, 7595–7602, 2006.

CHEMICALS COMMONLY USED IN BIOCHEMISTRY AND MOLECULAR BIOLOGY AND THEIR PROPERTIES (Continued)

Common Name	Chemical Name	M.W.	Properties and Comment
Biotin	Coenzyme R	244.31	Coenzyme function in carboxylation reactions; growth factor; tight binding to avidin used for affinity interactions.

Biotin

Knappe, J., Mechanism of biotin action, *Annu. Rev. Biochem.* 39, 757–776, 1970; Dunn, M.J., Detection of proteins on blots using the avidin-biotin system, *Methods Mol. Biol.* 32, 227–232, 1994; Wisdom, G.B., Enzyme and biotin labeling of antibody, *Methods Mol. Biol.* 32, 433–440, 1994; Wilbur, D.S., Pathare, P.M, Hamlin, D.K. et al., Development of new biotin/streptavidin reagents for pretargeting, *Biomol. Eng.* 16, 113–118, 1999; Jitrapakdee, S. and Wallace, J.C., The biotin enzyme family: conserved structural motifs and domain rearrangements, *Curr. Protein Pept. Sci.* 4, 217–229, 2003; Nikolau, B.J., Ohlrogge, J.B., and Wurtels, E.S., Plant biotin-containing carboxylases, *Arch. Biochem. Biophys.* 414, 211–222, 2003; Fernandez-Mejia, C., Pharmacological effects of biotin, *J. Nutri. Biochem.* 16, 424–427, 2005; Wilchek, M., Bayer, E.A., and Livnah, O., Essentials of biorecognition: the (strept)avidin-biotin system as a model for protein–protein and protein–ligand interactions, *Immunol. Lett.* 103, 27–32, 2006; Furuyama, T. and Henikoff, S., Biotin-tag affinity purification of a centromeric nucleosome assembly complex, *Cell Cycle* 5, 1269–1274, 2006; Streaker, E.D. and Beckett, D., Nonenzymatic biotinylation of a biotin carboxyl carrier protein: unusual reactivity of the physiological target lysine, *Protein Sci.* 15, 1928–1935, 2006; Raichur, A.M., Voros, J., Textor, M., and Fery, A., Adhesion of polyelectrolyte microcapsules through biotin-streptavidin specific interaction, *Biomacromolecules* 7, 2331–2336, 2006. For biotin switch assay, see Martinez-Ruiz, A. and Lamas, S., Detection and identification of S-nitrosylated proteins in endothelial cells, *Methods Enzymol.* 396, 131–139, 2005; Huang, B. and Chen, C., An ascorbate-dependent artifact that interferes with the interpretation of the biotin switch assay, *Free Radic. Biol. Med.* 41, 562–567, 2006; Gladwin, M.T., Wang, X., and Hogg, N., Methodological vexation about thiol oxidation versus S-nitrosation — a commentary on "An ascorbate-dependent artifact that interferes with the interpretation of the biotin-switch assay," *Free Radic. Biol. Med.* 41, 557–561, 2006.

| Biuret | Imidodicarbonic Diamide | 103.08 | Prepared by heating urea, reaction with cupric ions in base yields red-purple (the biuret reaction); nonprotein nitrogen (NPN) nutritional source. |

Jensen, H.L. and Schroder, M., Urea and biuret as nitrogen sources for *Rhizobium* spp., *J. Appl. Bacteriol.* 28, 473–478, 1965; Ronca, G., Competitive inhibition of adenosine deaminase by urea, guanidine, biuret, and guanylurea, *Biochim. Biophys. Acta* 132, 214–216, 1967; Oltjen, R.R., Slyter, L.L., Kozak, A.S., and Williams, E.E., Jr., Evaluation of urea, biuret, urea phosphate, and uric acid as NPN sources for cattle, *J. Nutr.* 94, 193–202, 1968; Tsai, H.Y. and Weber, S.G., Electrochemical detection of oligopeptides through the precolumn formation of biuret complexes, *J. Chromatog.* 542, 345–350, 1991; Gawron, A.J. and Lunte, S.M., Optimization of the conditions for biuret complex formation for the determination of peptides by capillary electrophoresis with ultraviolet detection, *Clin. Chem.* 51, 1411–1419, 2000; Roth, J., O'Leary, D.J., Wade, C.G. et al., Conformational analysis of alkylated biuret and triuret: evidence for helicity and helical inversion in oligoisocyates, *Org. Lett.* 2, 3063–3066, 2000; Hortin, G.L., and Mellinger, B., Cross-reactivity of amino acids and other compounds in the biuret reaction: interference with urinary peptide measurements, *Clin. Chem.* 51, 1411–1419, 2005.

| Boric Acid | o-boric Acid | 61.83 | Buffer salt, manufacturing; complexes with carbohydrates and other polyhydroxyl compounds; therapeutic use as a topic antibacterial/antifungal agent. |

$$B(OH)_3 + 2H_2O \rightleftharpoons B(OH)_4^- + H_3O^+$$

CHEMICALS COMMONLY USED IN BIOCHEMISTRY AND MOLECULAR BIOLOGY AND THEIR PROPERTIES (Continued)

Common Name	Chemical Name	M.W.	Properties and Comment

Sciarra, J.J. and Monte Bovi, A.J., Study of the boric acid–glycerin complex. II. Formation of the complex at elevated temperature, *J. Pharm. Sci.* 51, 238–242, 1962; Walborg, E.F., Jr. and Lantz, R.S., Separation and quantitation of saccharides by ion-exchange chromatography utilizing boric acid–glycerol buffers, *Anal. Biochem.* 22, 123–133, 1968; Lerch, B. and Stegemann, H., Gel electrophoresis of proteins in borate buffer. Influence of some compounds complexing with boric acid, *Anal. Biochem.* 29, 76–83, 1969; Walborg, E.F., Jr., Ray, D.B., and Ohrberg, L.E., Ion-exchange chromatography of saccharides: an improved system utilizing boric acid/2,3-butanediol buffers, *Anal. Biochem.* 29, 433–440, 1969; Chen, F.T. and Sternberg, J.C., Characterization of proteins by capillary electrophoresis in fused-silica columns: review on serum protein anlaysis and application to immunoassays, *Electrophoresis* 15, 13–21, 1994; Allen, R.C. and Doktycz, M.J., Discontinuous electrophoresis revisited: a review of the process, *Appl. Theor. Electrophor.* 6, 1–9, 1996; Manoravi, P., Joseph, M., Sivakumar, N., and Balasubramanian, H., Determination of isotopic ratio of boron in boric acid using laser mass spectrometry, *Anal. Sci.* 21, 1453–1455, 2005; De Muynck, C., Beauprez, J., Soetaert, W., and Vandamme, E.J., Boric acid as a mobile phase additive for high-performance liquid chromatography separation of ribose, arabinose, and ribulose, *J. Chromatog. A* 1101, 115–121, 2006; Herrmannova, M., Kirvankova, L., Bartos, M., and Vytras, K., Direct simultaneous determination of eight sweeteners in foods by capillary isotachophoresis, *J. Sep. Sci.* 29, 1132–1137, 2006; Alencar de Queiroz, A.A., Abraham, G.A., Pires Camillo, M.A. et al., Physicochemical and antimicrobial properties of boron-complexed polyglycerol-chitosan dendrimers, *J. Biomater. Sci. Polym. Ed.* 17, 689–707, 2006; Ringdahl, E.N., Recurrent vulvovaginal candidiasis, *Mol. Med.* 103, 165–168, 2006.

Common Name	Chemical Name	M.W.	Properties and Comment
BNPS-Skatole	(2-[2′-nitrophenyl-sulfenyl]-3-methyl-3′-bromoindolenine	363.23	Tryptophan modification, peptide-bond cleavage; derived from skatole, which is also known as boar taint.

Boulanger, P., Lemay, P., Blair, G.E., and Russell, W.C., Characterization of adenovirus protein IX, *J. Gen. Virol.* 44, 783–800, 1979; Russell, J., Kathendler, J., Kowalski, K. et al., The single tryptophan residue of human placental lactogen. Effects of modification and cleavage on biological activity and protein conformation, *J. Biol. Chem.* 256, 304–307, 1981; Moskaitis, J.E. and Campagnoni, A.T., A comparison of the dodecyl sulfate-induced precipitation of the myelin basic protein with other water-soluble proteins, *Neurochem. Res.* 11, 299–315, 1986; Mahboub, S., Richard, C., Delacourte, A., and Han, K.K., Applications of chemical cleavage procedures to the peptide mapping of neurofilament triplet protein bands in sodium dodecyl sulfate-polyacrylamide gel electrophoresis, *Anal. Biochem.* 154, 171–182, 1986; Rahali, V. and Gueguen, J., Chemical cleavage of bovine beta-lactoglobulin by BPNS-skatole for preparative purposes: comparative study of hydrolytic procedure and peptide characterization, *J. Protein Chem.* 18, 1–12, 1999; Swamy, N., Addo, J., Vskokovic, M.R., and Ray, R., Probing the vitamin D sterol-binding pocket of human vitamin D-binding protein with bromoacetate affinity-labeling reagents containing the affinity probe at C-3, C-6, C-11, and C-19 positions of parent vitamin D sterols, *Arch. Biochem. Biophys.* 373, 471–478, 2000; Celestina, F. and Suryanarayana, T., Biochemical characterization and helix-stabilizing properties of HSNP-C′ from the thermophilic archaeon *Sulfolobus acidocaldarius*, *Biochem. Biophys. Res. Commun.* 267, 614–618, 2000; Kibbey, M.M., Jameson, M.J., Eaton, E.M., and Rosenzweig, S.A., Insulinlike growth factor binding protein-2: contributions of the C-terminal domain to insulinlike growth factor-1 binding, *Mol. Pharmacol.* 69, 833–845, 2006.

Common Name	Chemical Name	M.W.	Properties and Comment
p-**Bromophenacyl Bromide**	2-bromo-1-(4-bromophenyl)ethanone; 4-bromophenacyl bromide	277.04	Modification of various residues in proteins: reagent for identification of carboxylic acids; phospholipase A2 inhibitor.

CHEMICALS COMMONLY USED IN BIOCHEMISTRY AND MOLECULAR BIOLOGY AND THEIR PROPERTIES (Continued)

Common Name	Chemical Name	M.W.	Properties and Comment

Erlanger, B.F., Vratrsanos, S.M., Wasserman, N., and Cooper, A.G., A chemical investigation of the active center of pepsin, *Biochem. Biophys. Res. Commun.* 23, 243–245, 1966; Yang, C.C. and King, K., Chemical modification of the histidine residue in basic phospholipase A2 from the venom of *Naja nigricollis*, *Biochim. Biophys. Acta.* 614, 373–388, 1980; Darke, P.L., Jarvis, A.A., Deems, R.A., and Dennis, E.A., Further characterization and *N*-terminal sequence of cobra venom phospholipase A2, *Biochim. Biophys. Acta* 626, 154–161, 1980; Ackerman, S.K., Matter, L., and Douglas, S.D., Effects of acid proteinase inhibitors on human neutrophil chemotaxis and lysosomal enzyme release. II. Bromophenacyl bromide and 1,2-epoxy-3-(*p*-nitrophenoxy)propane, *Clin. Immunol. Immunopathol.* 26, 213–222, 1983; Carine, K. and Hudig, D., Assessment of a role for phospholipase A2 and arachidonic acid metabolism in human lymphocyte natural cytotoxicity, *Cell Immunol.* 87, 270–283, 1984; Duque, R.E., Fantone, J.C., Kramer, C. et al., Inhibition of neutrophil activation by *p*-bromophenacyl bromide and its effects on phospholipase A2, *Br. J. Pharmacol.* 88, 463–472, 1986; Zhukova, A., Gogvadze, G., and Gogvadze, V., *p*-bromophenacyl bromide prevents cumene hydroperoxide-induced mitochondrial permeability transition by inhibiting pyridine nucleotide oxidation, *Redox Rep.* 9, 117–121, 2004; Thommesen, L. and Laegreid, A., Distinct differences between TNF receptor 1- and TNR receptor 2-mediated activation of NF-κβ* *J. Biochem. Mol. Biol.* 38, 281–289, 2005; Yue, H.Y., Fujita, T., and Kumamoto, E., Phospholipase A2 activation by melittin enhances spontaneous glutamatergic excitatory transmission in rat substantia gelatinosa neurons, *Neuroscience* 135, 485–495, 2005; Costa-Junior, H.M., Hamaty, F.C., de Silva Farias, R. et al., Apoptosis-inducing factor of a cytotoxic T-cell line: involvement of a secretory phospholipase A(2), *Cell Tissue Res.* 324, 255–266, 2006; Marchi-Salvador, D.P., Fernandes, C.A., Amui, S.F. et al., Crystallization and preliminary X-ray diffraction analysis of a myotoxic Lys49-PLA2 from *Bothrops jararacussu* venom complexed with *p*-bromophenacyl bromide, *Acta Crystallograph. Sect. F Struct. Biol. Cryst. Commun.* 62, 600–603, 2006.

Common Name	Chemical Name	M.W.	Properties and Comment
Calcium Chloride	CaCl$_2$	110.98	Anhydrous form as drying agent for organic solvents, variety of manufacturing uses; meat quality enhancement; therapeutic use in electrolyte replacement and bone cements; source of calcium ions for biological assays.

Barratt, J.O., Thrombin and calcium chloride in relation to coagulation, *Biochem. J.* 9, 511–543, 1915; Van der Meer, C., Effect of calcium chloride on choline esterase, *Nature* 171, 78–79, 1952; Bhat, R. and Ahluwalia, J.C., Effect of calcium chloride on the conformation of proteins. Thermodynamic studies of some model compounds, *Int. J. Pept. Protein Res.* 30, 145–152, 1987; Furihata, C., Sudo, K., and Matsushima, T., Calcium chloride inhibits stimulation of replicative DNA synthesis by sodium chloride in the pyloric mucosa of rat stomach, *Carcinogenesis* 10, 2135–2137, 1989; Ishikawa, K., Ueyama, Y., Mano, T. et al., Self-setting barrier membrane for guided tissue regeneration method: initial evaluation of alginate membrane made with sodium alginate and calcium chloride aqueous solutions, *J. Biomed. Mater. Res.* 47, 111–115, 1999; Vujevic, M., Vidakovic-Cifrek, Z., Tkalec, M. et al., Calcium chloride and calcium bromide aqueous solutions of technical and analytical grade in Lemna bioassay, *Chemosphere* 41, 1535–1542, 2000; Miyazaki, T., Ohtsuki, C., Kyomoto, M. et al., Bioactive PMMA bone cement prepared by modification with methacryloxypropyltrimethoxysilane and calcium chloride, *J. Biomed. Mater. Res. A* 67, 1417–1423, 2003; Harris, S.E., Huff-Lonegan, E., Lonergan, S.M. et al., Antioxidant status affects color stability and tenderness of calcium chloride-injected beef, *J. Anim. Sci.* 79, 666–677, 2001; Behrends, J.M., Goodson, K.J., Koohmaraie, M. et al., Beef customer satisfaction: factors affecting consumer evaluations of calcium chloride-injected top sirloin steaks when given instructions for preparation, *J. Anim. Sci.* 83, 2869–2875, 2005.

Common Name	Chemical Name	M.W.	Properties and Comment
Cetyl Pyridinium Chloride	1-hexadecylpyridinium chloride	350.01	Cationic detergent; precipitating agent and staining agent for glycosaminoglycans; antimicrobial agent.

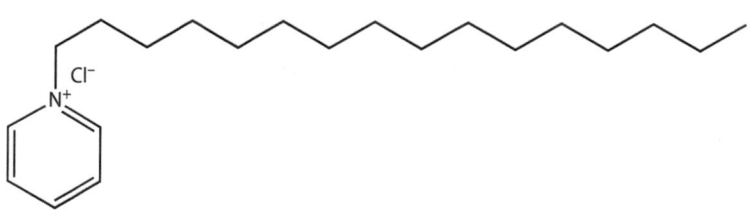

Laurent, T.C. and Scott, J.E., Molecular weight fractionation of polyanions by cetylpyridinium chloride in salt solutions, *Nature* 202, 661–662, 1964; Kiss, A., Linss, W., and Geyer, G., CPC-PTA section staining of acid glycans, *Acta Histochem.* 64, 183–186, 1979; Khan, M.Y. and Newman, S.A., An assay for heparin by decrease in color yield (DECOY) of a protein-dye-binding reaction, *Anal. Biochem.* 187, 124–128, 1990; Chardin, H., Septier, D., and Goldberg, M., Visualization of glycosaminoglycans in rat incisor predentin and dentin with cetylpyridinium chloride-glutaraldehyde as fixative, *J. Histochem. Cytochem.* 38, 885–894, 1990; Chardin, H., Gokani, J.P., Septier, D. et al., Structural variations of different oral basement membranes revealed by cationic dyes and detergent added to aldehyde fixative solution, *Histochem. J.* 24, 375–382, 1992; Agren, U.M., Tammi, R., and Tammi, M., A dot-blot assay of metabolically radiolabeled hyaluronan, *Anal. Biochem.* 217, 311–315, 1994; Maccari, F. and Volpi, N., Glycosaminoglycan blotting on nitrocellulose membranes treated with cetylpyridinium chloride afer agarose-gel electrophoretic separation, *Electrophoresis* 23, 3270–3277, 2002; Maccari, F. and Volpi, N., Direct and specific recognition of glycosaminoglycans by antibodies after their separation by agarose gel electrophoresis and blotting on cetylpyridinium chloride-treated nitrocellulose membranes, *Electrophoresis* 24, 1347–1352, 2003.

CHEMICALS COMMONLY USED IN BIOCHEMISTRY AND MOLECULAR BIOLOGY AND THEIR PROPERTIES (Continued)

Common Name	Chemical Name	M.W.	Properties and Comment
CHAPS	3-[(3-cholamidopropyl)-dimethylammonio]-1-propanesulfonate	614.89	Detergent, solubilizing agent; extensive use for the solubilization of membrane proteins.

Hjelmeland, L.M., A nondenaturing zwitterionic detergent for membrane biochemistry: design and synthesis, *Proc. Natl. Acad. Sci. USA* 77, 6368–6370, 1980; Giradot, J.M. and Johnson, B.C., A new detergent for the solubilization of the vitamin K–dependent carboxylation system from liver microsomes: comparison with triton X-100, *Anal. Biochem.* 121, 315–320, 1982; Liscia, D.S., Alhadi, T., and Vonderhaar, B.K., Solubilization of active prolactin receptors by a nondenaturing zwitterionic detergent, *J. Biol. Chem.* 257, 9401–9405, 1982; Womack, M.D., Kendall, D.A., and MacDonald, R.C., Detergent effects on enzyme activity and solubilization of lipid bilayer membranes, *Biochim. Biophys. Acta* 733, 210–215, 1983; Klaerke, D.A. and Jorgensen, P.L., Role of Ca^{2+}-activated K$^+$ channel in regulation of NaCl reabsorption in thick ascending limb of Henle's loop, *Comp. Biochem. Physiol. A* 90, 757–765, 1988; Kuriyama, K., Nakayasu, H., Mizutani, H. et al., Cerebral GABAB receptor: proposed mechanisms of action and purification procedures, *Neurochem. Res.* 18, 377–383, 1993; Koumanov, K.S., Wolf, C., and Quinn, P.J., Lipid composition of membrane domains, *Subcell. Biochem.* 37, 153–163, 2004.

Chloroform	Trichloromethane	177.38	Used for extraction of lipids, usually in combination with methanol.

Stevan, M.A. and Lyman, R.L., Investigations on extraction of rat plasma phospholipids, *Proc. Soc. Exp. Biol. Med.* 114, 16–20, 1963; Wells, M.A. and Dittmer, J.C., A microanalytical technique for the quantitative determination of twenty-four classes of brain lipids, *Biochemistry* 5, 3405–3418, 1966; Colacicco, G. and Rapaport, M.M., A simplified preparation of phosphatidyl inositol, *J. Lipid. Res.* 8, 513–515, 1967; Curtis, P.J., Solubility of mitochondrial membrane proteins in acidic organic solvents, *Biochim. Biophys. Acta* 183, 239–241, 1969; Privett, O.S., Dougherty, K.A., and Castell, J.D., Quantitative analysis of lipid classes, *Am. J. Clin. Nutr.* 24, 1265–1275, 1971; Claire, M., Jacotot, B., and Robert, L., Characterization of lipids associated with macromolecules of the intercellular matrix of human aorta, *Connect. Tissue Res.* 4, 61–71, 1976; St. John, L.C. and Bell, F.P., Extraction and fractionation of lipids from biological tissues, cells, organelles, and fluids, *Biotechniques* 7, 476–481, 1989; Dean, N.M. and Beaven, M.A., Methods for the analysis of inositol phosphates, *Anal. Biochem.* 183, 199–209, 1989; Singh, A.K. and Jiang, Y., Quantitative chromatographic analysis of inositol phospholipids and related compounds, *J. Chromatog. B Biomed. Appl.* 671, 255–280, 1995.

CHEMICALS COMMONLY USED IN BIOCHEMISTRY AND MOLECULAR BIOLOGY AND THEIR PROPERTIES (Continued)

Common Name	Chemical Name	M.W.	Properties and Comment
Cholesterol		386.66	The most common sterol in man and other higher animals. Cholesterol is essential for the synthesis of a variety of compounds including estrogens and vitamin D; also membrane component.

Cholesterol

Doree, C., The occurrence and distribution of cholesterol and allied bodies in the animal kingdom, *Biochem. J.* 4, 72–106, 1909; Heilbron, I.M., Kamm, E.D., and Morton, R.A., The absorption spectrum of cholesterol and its biological significance with reference to vitamin D. Part I: Preliminary observations, *Biochem. J.* 21, 78–85, 1927; Cook, R.P., Ed., *Cholesterol: Chemistry, Biochemistry, and Pathology*, Academic Press, New York, 1958; Vahouny, G.V. and Treadwell, C.R., Enzymatic synthesis and hydrolysis of cholesterol esters, *Methods Biochem. Anal.* 16, 219–272, 1968; Heftmann, E., *Steroid Biochemistry*, Academic Press, New York, 1970; Nestel, P.J., Cholesterol turnover in man, *Adv. Lipid Res.* 8, 1–39, 1970; Dennick, R.G., The intracellular organization of cholesterol biosynthesis. A review, *Steroids Lipids Res.* 3, 236–256, 1972; J. Polonovski, Ed., *Cholesterol Metabolism and Lipolytic Enzymes*, Masson Publications, New York, 1977; Gibbons, G.F., Mitrooulos, K.A., and Myant, N.B., *Biochemistry of Cholesterol*, Elsevier, Amsterdam, 1982; Bittman, R., *Cholesterol: Its Functions and Metabolism in Biology and Medicine*, Plenum Press, New York, 1997; Oram, J.P. and Heinecke, J.W., ATP-binding cassette transporter A1: a cell cholesterol exporter that protects against cardiovascular disease, *Physiol. Rev.* 85, 1343–1372, 2005; Holtta-Vuori, M. and Ikonen, E., Endosomal cholesterol traffic: vesicular and non-vesicular mechanisms meet, *Biochem. Soc. Trans.* 34, 392–394, 2006; Cuchel, M. and Rader, D.J., Macrophage reverse cholesterol transport: key to the regression of atherosclerosis? *Circulation* 113, 2548–2555, 2006.

Cholic Acid		408.57	Component of bile; detergent.

Schreiber, A.J. and Simon, F.R., Overview of clinical aspects of bile salt physiology, *J. Pediatr. Gastroenterol. Nutr.* 2, 337–345, 1983; Chiang, J.Y., Regulation of bile acid synthesis, *Front. Biosci.* 3, dl176–dl193, 1998; Cybulsky, M.I., Lichtman, A.H., Hajra, L., and Iiyama, K., Leukocyte adhesion molecules in atherogenesis, *Clin. Chim. Acta* 286, 207–218, 1999.

CHEMICALS COMMONLY USED IN BIOCHEMISTRY AND MOLECULAR BIOLOGY AND THEIR PROPERTIES (Continued)

Common Name	Chemical Name	M.W.	Properties and Comment
Citraconic Anhydride	Methylmaleic Anhydride	112.1	Reversible modification of amino groups.

Dixon, H.B. and Perham, R.N., Reversible blocking of amino groups with citraconic anhydride, *Biochem. J.* 109, 312–314, 1968; Gibbons, I. and Perham, R.N., The reaction of aldolase with 2-methylmaleic anhydride, *Biochem. J.* 116, 843–849, 1970; Yankeelov, J.A., Jr. and Acree, D., Methylmaleic anhydride as a reversible blocking agent during specific arginine modification, *Biochem. Biophys. Res. Commun.* 42, 886–891, 1971; Takahashi, K., Specific modification of arginine residues in proteins with ninhydrin, *J. Biochem.* 80, 1173–1176, 1976; Brinegar, A.C. and Kinsella, J.E., Reversible modification of lysine in soybean proteins, using citraconic anhydride: characterization of physical and chemical changes in soy protein isolate, the 7S globulin, and lipoxygenase, *J. Agric. Food Chem.* 28, 818–824, 1980; Shetty, J.K. and Kensella, J.F., Ready separation of proteins from nucleoprotein complexes by reversible modification of lysine residues, *Biochem. J.* 191, 269–272, 1980; Yang, H. and Frey, P.A., Dimeric cluster with a single reactive amino group, *Biochemistry* 23, 3863–3868, 1984; Bindels, J.G., Misdom, L.W., and Hoenders, H.J., The reaction of citraconic anhydride with bovine alpha-crystallin lysine residues. Surface probing and dissociation-reassociation studies, *Biochim. Biophys. Acta* 828, 255–260, 1985; Al jamal, J.A., Characterization of different reactive lysines in bovine heart mitochondrial porin, *Biol. Chem.* 383, 1967–1970, 2002; Kadlik, V., Strohalm, M., and Kodicek, M., Citraconylation — a simple method for high protein sequence coverage in MALDI-TOF mass spectrometry, *Biochem. Biophys. Res. Commun.* 305, 1091–1093, 2003.

Coomassie Brilliant Blue G-250	CI Acid Blue 90	854	Most often used for the colorimetric determination of protein.

Bradford, M.M., A rapid and sensitive method for the quantitation of microgram quantities of protein utilizing the principle of protein-dye binding *Anal. Biochem.* 72, 248–254, 1976; Saleemuddin, M., Ahmad, H., and Husain, A., A simple, rapid, and sensitive procedure for the assay of endoproteases using Coomassie Brilliant Blue G-250, *Anal. Biochem.* 105, 202–206, 1980; van Wilgenburg, M.G., Werkman, E.M., van Gorkom, W.H., and Soons, J.B., Criticism of the use of Coomassie Brilliant Blue G-250 for the quantitative determination of proteins, *J.Clin. Chem.Clin. Biochem.* 19, 301–304, 1981; Mattoo, R.L., Ishaq, M., and Saleemuddin, M., Protein assay by Coomassie Brilliant Blue G-250-binding method is unsuitable for plant tissues rich in phenols and phenolases, *Anal. Biochem.* 163, 376–384, 1987; Lott, J.A., Stephan, V.A., and Pritchard, K.A., Jr., Evaluation of the Coomassie Brilliant Blue G-250 method for urinary proteins, *Clin. Chem.* 29, 1946–1950, 1983; Fanger, B.O., Adaptation of the Bradford protein assay to membrane-bound proteins by solubilizing in glucopyranoside detergents, *Anal. Biochem.* 162, 11–17, 1987; Marshall, T. and Williams, K.M., Recovery of proteins by Coomassie Brilliant Blue precipitation prior to electrophoresis, *Electrophoresis* 13, 887–888, 1992; Sapan, C.V., Lundblad, R.L., and Price, N.C., Colorimetric protein assay techniques, *Biotechnol. Appl. Biochem.* 29, 99–108, 1999.

CHEMICALS COMMONLY USED IN BIOCHEMISTRY AND MOLECULAR BIOLOGY AND THEIR PROPERTIES (Continued)

Common Name	Chemical Name	M.W.	Properties and Comment
Coomassie Brilliant Blue R-250	CI Acid Blue 83	826	Most often used for the detection of proteins on solid matrices such as polyacrylamide gels.

Vesterberg, O., Hansen, L., and Sjosten, A., Staining of proteins after isoelectric focusing in gels by a new procedure, *Biochim. Biophys. Acta* 491, 160–166, 1977; Micko, S. and Schlaepfer, W.W., Metachromasy of peripheral nerve collagen on polyacrylamide gels stained with Coomassie Brilliant Blue R-250, *Anal. Biochem.* 88, 566–572, 1978; Osset, M., Pinol, M., Fallon, M.J. et al., Interference of the carbohydrate moiety in Coomassie Brilliant Blue R-250 protein staining, *Electrophoresis* 10, 271–273, 1989; Pryor, J.L., Xu, W., and Hamilton, D.W., Immunodetection after complete destaining of Coomassie blue-stained proteins on immobilon-PVDF, *Anal. Biochem.* 202, 100–104, 1992; Metkar, S.S., Mahajan, S.K., and Sainis, J.K., Modified procedure for nonspecific protein staining on nitrocellulose paper using Coomassie Brilliant Blue R-250, *Anal. Biochem.* 227, 389–391, 1995; Kundu, S.K., Robey, W.G., Nabors, P. et al., Purification of commercial Coomassie Brilliant Blue R-250 and characterization of the chromogenic fractions, *Anal. Biochem.* 235, 134–140, 1996; Choi, J.K., Yoon, S.H., Hong, H.Y. et al., A modified Coomassie blue staining of proteins in polyacrylamide gels with Bismark brown R, *Anal. Biochem.* 236, 82–84, 1996; Moritz, R.L., Eddes, J.S., Reid, G.E., and Simpson, R.J., *S*- pyridylethylation of intact polyacrylamide gels and *in situ* digestion of electrophoretically separated proteins: a rapid mass spectrometric method for identifying cysteine-containing peptides, *Electrophoresis* 17, 907–917, 1996; Choi, J.K. and Yoo, G.S., Fast protein staining in sodium dodecyl sulfate polyacrylamide gel using counter ion-dyes, Coomassie Brilliant Blue R-250, and neutral red, *Arch. Pharm. Res.* 25, 704–708, 2002; Bonar, E., Dubin, A., Bierczynska-Krzysik, A. et al., Identification of major cellular proteins synthesized in response to interleukin-1 and interleukin-6 in human hepatoma HepG2 cells, *Cytokine* 33, 111–117, 2006.

Cy 2		714	Fluorescent label used in proteomics and gene expression; use for internal standard.

CHEMICALS COMMONLY USED IN BIOCHEMISTRY AND MOLECULAR BIOLOGY AND THEIR PROPERTIES (Continued)

Common Name	Chemical Name	M.W.	Properties and Comment

Tonge, R., Shaw, J., Middleton, B. et al., Validation and development of fluorescence two-dimensional differential gel electrophoresis proteomics technology, *Proteomics* 1, 377–396, 2001; Chan, H.L., Gharbi, S., Gaffney, P.R. et al., Proteomic analysis of redox- and ErbB2-dependent changes in mammary luminal epithelial cells using cysteine- and lysine-labeling two-dimensional difference gel electrophoresis, *Proteomics* 5, 2908–2926, 2005; Misek, D.E., Kuick, R., Wang, H. et al., A wide range of protein isoforms in serum and plasma uncovered by a quantitative intact protein analysis system, *Proteomics* 5, 3343–3352, 2005; Doutette, P., Navet, R., Gerkens, P. et al., Steatosis-induced proteomic changes in liver mitochondria evidenced by two-dimensional differential in-gel electrophoresis, *J. Proteome Res.* 4, 2024–2031, 2005.

Cy 3		911.0	Fluorescent label used in proteomics and gene expression; in combination with Cy 5 is used for FRET-based assays.

Brismar, H. and Ulfake, B., Fluorescence lifetime measurements in confocal microscopy of neurons labeled with multiple fluorophores, *Nat. Biotechnol.* 15, 373–377, 1997; Strohmaier, A.R., Porwol, T., Acker, H., and Spiess, E., Tomography of cells by confocal laser scanning microscopy and computer-assisted three-dimensional image reconstruction: localization of cathepsin B in tumor cells penetrating collagen gels *in vitro*, *J. Histochem. Cytochem.* 45, 975–983, 1997; Alexandre, I., Hamels, S., Dufour, S. et al., Colorimetric silver detection of DNA microarrays, *Anal. Biochem.* 295, 1–8, 2001; Shaw, J., Rowlinson, R., Nickson, J. et al., Evaluation of saturation labeling two-dimensional difference gel electrophoresis fluorescent dyes, *Proteomics* 3, 1181–1195, 2003.

CHEMICALS COMMONLY USED IN BIOCHEMISTRY AND MOLECULAR BIOLOGY AND THEIR PROPERTIES (Continued)

Common Name	Chemical Name	M.W.	Properties and Comment
Cy 5		937.1	Fluorescent label used in proteomics and gene expression; also used in histochemistry.

Uchihara, T., Nakamura, A., Nagaoka, U. et al., Dual enhancement of double immunofluorescent signals by CARD: participation of ubiquitin during formation of neurofibrillary tangles, *Histochem. Cell Biol.* 114, 447–451, 2000; Duthie, R.S., Kalve, I.M., Samols, S.B. et al., Novel cyanine dye-based dideoxynucleoside triphosphates for DNA sequencing, *Bioconjug. Chem.* 13, 699–706, 2002; Graves, E.E., Yessayan., D., Turner, G. et al., Validation of *in vivo* fluorochrome concentrations measured using fluorescence molecular tomography, *J. Biomed. Opt.* 10, 44019, 2005; Lapeyre, M., Leprince, J., Massonneau, M. et al., Aryldithioethyloxycarbonyl (Ardec): a new family of amine-protecting groups removable under mild reducing conditions and their applications to peptide synthesis, *Chemistry* 12, 3655–3671, 2006; Tang, X., Morris, S.L., Langone, J.J., and Bockstahler, L.E., Simple and effective method for generating single-stranded DNA targets and probes, *Biotechniques* 40, 759–763, 2006.

α-**Cyano-4-hydroxycinnamic Acid**	4-HCCA; Cinnamate	189.2	Used as matrix substance for MALDI; transport inhibitor and enzyme inhibitor.

CHEMICALS COMMONLY USED IN BIOCHEMISTRY AND MOLECULAR BIOLOGY AND THEIR PROPERTIES (Continued)

Common Name	Chemical Name	M.W.	Properties and Comment

Gobom, J., Schuerenberg, M., Mueller, M. et al., α-cyano-4-hydroxycinnamic acid affinity sample preparation. A protocol for MALDI-MS peptide analysis in proteomics, *Anal. Chem.* 73, 434–438, 2001; Zhu, X. and Papayannopoulos, I.A., Improvement in the detection of low concentration protein digests on a MALDI TOF/TOF workstation by reducing α-cyano-4-hydroxycinnamic acid adduct ions, *J. Biomol. Tech.* 14, 298–307, 2003; Neubert, H., Halket, J.M., Fernandez Ocana, M., and Patel, R.K., MALDI post-source decay and LIFT-TOF/TOF investigation of α-cyano-4-hydroxycinnamic acid cluster interferences, *J. Am. Soc. Mass Spectrom.* 15, 336–343, 2004; Kobayashi, T., Kawai, H., Suzuki, T. et al., Improved sensitivity for insulin in matrix-assisted laser desorption/ionization time-of-flight mass spectrometry by premixing α-cyano-4-hydroxycinnamic acid with transferrin, *Rapid Commun. Mass Spectrom.* 18, 1156–1160, 2004; Pshenichnyuk, S.A. and Asfandiarov, N.L., The role of free electrons in MALDI: electron capture by molecules of α-cyano-4-hydroxycinnamic acid, *Eur. J. Mass Spectrom.* 10, 477–486, 2004; Bogan, M.J., Bakhoum, S.F., and Agnes, G.R., Promotion of α-cyano-4-hydroxycinnamic acid and peptide cocrystallization within levitated droplets with net charge, *J. Am. Soc. Mass Spectrom.* 16, 254–262, 2005. As enzyme inhibitor: Clarke, P.D., Clift, D.L., Dooledeniya, M. et al., Effects of α-cyano-4-hydroxycinnamic acid on fatigue and recovery of isolated mouse muscle, *J. Muscle Res. Cell Motil.* 16, 611–617, 1995; Del Prete, E., Lutz, T.A., and Scharrer, E., Inhibition of glucose oxidation by α-cyano-4-hydroxycinnamic acid stimulates feeding in rats, *Physiol. Behav.* 80, 489–498, 2004; Briski, K.P. and Patil, G.D., Induction of Fox immunoreactivity labeling in rat forebrain metabolic loci by caudal fourth ventricular infusion of the monocarboxylate transporter inhibitor, α-cyano-4-hydroxycinnamic acid, *Neuroendocrinology* 82, 49–57, 2005.

Cyanogen	C_2N_2; Ethanedinitrile	53.03	Protein crosslinking at salt bridges.

$$N \equiv C - C \equiv N$$

Ghenbot, G., Emge, T., and Day, R.A., Identification of the sites of modification of bovine carbonic anhydrase II (BCA II) by the salt bridge reagent cyanogen, C_2N_2, *Biochim. Biophys. Acta* 1161, 59–65, 1993; Karagozler, A.A., Ghenbot, G., and Day, R.A., Cyanogen as a selective probe for carbonic anhydrase hydrolase, *Biopolymers* 33, 687–692, 1993; Winters, M.S. and Day, R.A., Identification of amino acid residues participating in intermolecular salt bridges between self-associating proteins, *Anal. Biochem.* 309, 48–59, 2002; Winters, M.S. and Day, R.A., Detecting protein–protein interactions in the intact cell of *Bacillus subtilis* (ATCC 6633), *J. Bacteriol.* 185, 4268–4275, 2003.

Cyanogen Bromide	CNBr; Bromide Cyanide	105.9	Protein modification; cleavage of peptide bonds; coupled nucleophiles to polyhydroxyl matrices; environmental toxicon derived from monobromamine and cyanide.

$$Br - C \equiv N$$

Hofmann, T., The purification and properties of fragments of trypsinogen obtained by cyanogen bromide cleavage, *Biochemistry* 3, 356–364, 1964; Chu, R.C. and Yasunobu, K.T., The reaction of cyanogen bromide and *N*-bromosuccinimide with some cytochromes C, *Biochim. Biophys. Acta* 89, 148–149, 1964; Inglis, A.S. and Edman, P., Mechanism of cyanogen bromide reaction with methionine in peptides and proteins. I. Formation of imidate and methyl thiocyanate, *Anal. Biochem.* 37, 73–80, 1970; Kagedal, L. and Akerstrom, S., Binding of covalent proteins to polysaccharides by cyanogen bromide and organic cyanates. I. Preparation of soluble glycine-, insulin- and ampicillin-dextran, *Acta Chem. Scand.* 25, 1855–1899, 1971; Sipe, J.D. and Schaefer, F.V., Preparation of solid-phase immunosorbents by coupling human serum proteins to cyanogen bromide–activated agarose, *Appl. Microbiol.* 25, 880–884, 1973; March, S.C., Parikh, I., and Cuatrecasas, P., A simplified method for cyanogen bromide activation of agarose for affinity chromatography, *Anal. Biochem.* 60, 149–152, 1974; Boulware, D.W., Goldsworthy, P.D., Nardella, F.A., and Mannik, M., Cyanogen bromide cleaves Fc fragments of pooled human IgG at both methionine and tryptophan residues, *Mol. Immunol.* 22, 1317–1322, 1985; Jaggi, K.S. and Gangal, S.V., Monitoring of active groups of cyanogen bromide-activated paper discs used as allergosorbent, *Int. Arch. Allergy Appl. Immunol.* 89, 311–313, 1989; Villa, S., De Fazio, G., and Canosi, U., Cyanogen bromide cleavage at methionine residues of polypeptides containing disulfide bonds, *Anal. Biochem.* 177, 161–164, 1989; Luo, K.X., Hurley, T.R., and Sefton, B.M., Cyanogen bromide cleavage and proteolytic peptide mapping of proteins immobilized to membranes, *Methods Enzymol.* 201, 149–152, 1991; Jennissen, H.P., Cyanogen bromide and tresyl chloride chemistry revisited: the special reactivity of agarose as a chromatographic and biomaterial support for immobilizing novel chemical groups, *J. Mol. Recognit.* 8, 116–124, 1995; Kaiser, R. and Metzka, L., Enhancement of cyanogen bromide cleavage yields for methionyl-serine and methionyl-threonine peptide bonds, *Anal. Biochem.* 266, 1–8, 1999; Kraft, P., Mills, J., and Dratz, E., Mass spectrometric analysis of cyanogen bromide fragments of integral membrane proteins at the picomole level: application to rhodopsin, *Anal. Biochem.* 292, 76–86, 2001; Kuhn, K., Thompson, A., Prinz, T. et al., Isolation of *N*-terminal protein sequence tags from cyanogen bromide-cleaved proteins as a novel approach to investigate hydrophobic proteins, *J. Proteome Res.* 2, 598–609, 2003; Macmillan, D. and Arham, L., Cyanogen bromide cleavage generates fragments suitable for expressed protein and glycoprotein ligation, *J. Am. Chem. Soc.* 126, 9530–9531, 2004; Lei, H., Minear, R.A., and Marinas, B.J., Cyanogen bromide formation from the reactions of monobromamine and dibromamine with cyanide ions, *Environ. Sci. Technol.* 40, 2559–2564, 2006.

CHEMICALS COMMONLY USED IN BIOCHEMISTRY AND MOLECULAR BIOLOGY AND THEIR PROPERTIES (Continued)

Common Name	Chemical Name	M.W.	Properties and Comment
Cyanuric Chloride	2,4,6-trichloro-1,3,5-triazine	184.41	Coupling of carbohydrates to proteins; more recently for coupling of nucleic acid to microarray platforms.

Gray, B.M., ELISA methodology for polysaccharide antigens: protein coupling of polysaccharides for adsorption to plastic tubes, *J. Immunol. Methods* 28, 187–192, 1979: Horak, D., Rittich, B., Safar, J. et al., Properties of RNase A immobilized on magnetic poly(2-hydroxyethyl methacrylate) microspheres, *Biotechnol. Prog.* 17, 447–452, 2001; Lee, P.H., Sawan, S.P., Modrusan, Z. et al., An efficient binding chemistry for glass polynucleotide microarrays, *Bioconjug. Chem.* 13, 97–103, 2002; Steinberg, G., Stromsborg, K., Thomas, L. et al., Strategies for covalent attachment of DNA to beads, *Biopolymers* 73, 597–605, 2004; Abuknesha, R.A., Luk, C.Y., Griffith, H.H. et al., Efficient labeling of antibodies with horseradish peroxidase using cyanuric chloride, *J. Immunol. Methods* 306, 211–217, 2005.

1,2-Cyclohexylenedinitrilotetraacetic acid	CDTA		Chelating agent suggested to have specificity for manganese ions; weaker for other metal ions such as ferric.

Tandon, S.K. and Singh, J., Removal of manganese by chelating agents from brain and liver of manganese, *Toxicology* 5, 237–241, 1975; Hazell, A.S., Normandin, L., Norenberg, M.D., Kennedy, G., and Yi, J.H., Alzheimer type II astrocyte changes following sub-acute exposure to manganese, *Neurosci. Lett.*, 396, 167–171, 2006; Hassler, C.S. and Twiss, M.R., Bioavailability of iron sensed by a phytoplanktonic Fe-bioreporter, *Environ. Sci. Tech.* 40, 2544–2551, 2006.

Dansyl Chloride	5-(dimethylamino)-1-naphthalenesulfonyl chloride	269.8	Fluorescent label for proteins; amino acid analysis.

Hill, R.D. and Laing, R.R., Specific reaction of dansyl chloride with one lysine residue in rennin, *Biochim. Biophys. Acta* 132, 188–190, 1967; Chen, R.F., Fluorescent protein-dye conjugates. I. Heterogeneity of sites on serum albumin labeled by dansyl chloride, *Arch. Biochem. Biophys.* 128, 163–175, 1968; Chen, R.F., Dansyl-labeled protein modified with dansyl chloride: activity effects and fluorescence properties, *Anal. Biochem.* 25, 412–416, 1968; Brown, C.S. and Cunningham, L.W., Reaction of reactive sulfydryl groups of creatine kinase with dansyl chloride, *Biochemistry* 9, 3878–3885, 1970; Hsieh, W.T. and Matthews, K.S., Lactose repressor protein modified with dansyl chloride: activity effects and fluorescence properties, *Biochemistry* 34, 3043–3049, 1985;

CHEMICALS COMMONLY USED IN BIOCHEMISTRY AND MOLECULAR BIOLOGY AND THEIR PROPERTIES (Continued)

Common Name	Chemical Name	M.W.	Properties and Comment

Scouten, W.H., van den Tweel, W., Kranenburg, H., and Dekker, M., Colored sulfonyl chloride as an activated agent for hydroxylic matrices, *Methods Enzymol.* 135, 79–84, 1987; Martin, M.A., Lin, B., Del Castillo, B., The use of fluorescent probes in pharmaceutical analysis, *J. Pharm. Biomed. Anal.* 6, 573–583, 1988; Walker, J.M., The dansyl method for identifying *N*-terminal amino acids, *Methods Mol. Biol.* 32, 321–328, 1994; Walker, J.M., The dansyl-Edman method for peptide sequencing, *Methods Mol. Biol.* 32, 329–334, 1994; Pin, S. and Royer, C.A., High-pressure fluorescence methods for observing subunit dissociation in hemoglobin, *Methods Enzymol.* 323, 42–55, 1994; Rangarajan, B., Coons, L.S., and Scarnton, A.B., Characterization of hydrogels using luminescence spectroscopy, *Biomaterials* 17, 649–661, 1996; Kang, X., Xiao, J., Huang, X., and Gu, X., Optimization of dansyl derivatization and chromatographic conditions in the determination of neuroactive amino acids of biological samples, *Clin. Chim. Acta* 366, 352–356, 2006.

DCC *N,N* '-dicyclohexylcarbodiimide   206.33   Activates carboxyl groups to react with hydroxyl groups to form esters and with amines to form an amide bond; used to modify ion-transporting ATPases. Lack of water solubility has presented challenges.

Chau, A.S. and Terry, K., Analysis of pesticides by chemical derivatization. I. A new procedure for the formation of 2-chloroethyl esters of ten herbicidal acids, *J. Assoc. Off. Anal. Chem.* 58, 1294–1301, 1975; Patel, L. and Kaback, H.R., The role of the carbodiimide-reactive component of the adenosine-5'-triphosphatase complex in the proton permeability of *Escherichia coli* membrane vesicles, *Biochemistry* 15, 2741–2746, 1976; Esch, F.S., Bohlen, P., Otsuka, A.S. et al., Inactivation of the bovine mitochondrial F1-ATPase with dicyclohexyl[^{14}C]carbodiimide leads to the modification of a specific glutamic acid residue in the beta subunit, *J. Biol. Chem.* 256, 9084–9089, 1981; Hsu, C.M. and Rosen, B.P., Characterization of the catalytic subunit of an anion pump, *J. Biol. Chem.* 264, 17349–17354, 1989; Gurdag, S., Khandare, J., Stapels, S. et al., Activity of dendrimer-methotrexate conjugates on methotrexate-sensitive and -resistant cell lines, *Bioconjug. Chem.* 17, 275–283, 2006; Vgenopoulou, I., Gemperli, A.C., and Steuber, J., Specific modification of a Na$^+$ binding site in NADH: quinone oxidoreductase from *Klebsiella pneumoniae* with dicyclohexylcarbodiimide, *J. Bacteriol.* 188, 3264–3272, 2006; Ferguson, S.A., Keis, S., and Cook, G.M., Biochemical and molecular characterization of a Na$^+$-translocating F1Fo-ATPase from the thermophilic bacterium *Clostridium paradoxum, J. Bacteriol.* 188, 5045–5054, 2006.

Deoxycholic Acid   Desoxycholic Acid   392.57   Detergent, nanoparticles.

Akare, S. and Martinez, J.D., Bile acid-induced hydrophobicity-dependent membrane alterations, *Biochim. Biophys. Acta* 1735, 59–67, 2005; Chae, S.Y., Son, S., Lee, M. et al., Deoxycholic acid-conjugated chitosan oligosaccharide nanoparticles for efficient gene carrier, *J. Control. Release* 109, 330–344, 2005; Dall'Agnol, M., Bernstein, C., Bernstein, H. et al., Identification of *S*-nitrosylated proteins after chronic exposure of colon epithelial cells to deoxycholate, *Proteomics* 6, 1654–1662, 2006; Dotis, J., Simitsopoulou, M., Dalakiouridou, M. et al. Effects of lipid formulations of amphotericin B on activity of human monocytes against *Aspirgillus fumigatus, Antimicrob. Agents Chemother.* 128, 3490–3491, 2006; Darragh, J., Hunter, M., Pohler, E. et al., The calcium-binding domain of the stress protein SEP53 is required for survival in response to deoxycholic acid-mediated injury, *FEBS J.* 273, 1930–1947, 2006.

CHEMICALS COMMONLY USED IN BIOCHEMISTRY AND MOLECULAR BIOLOGY AND THEIR PROPERTIES (Continued)

Common Name	Chemical Name	M.W.	Properties and Comment
Deuterium Oxide D$_2$O	"Heavy Water"	20.03	Structural studies in proteins, enzyme kinetics; *in vivo* studies of metabolic flux.

Cohen, A.H., Wilkinson, R.R., and Fisher, H.F., Location of deuterium oxide solvent isotope effects in the glutamate dehydrogenase reaction, *J. Biol. Chem.* 250, 5343–5246, 1975; Rosenberry, T.L., Catalysis by acetylcholinesterase: evidence that the rate-limiting step for acylation with certain substrates precedes general acid-base catalysis, *Proc. Natl. Acad. Sci. USA* 72, 3834–3838, 1975; Viggiano, G., Ho, N.T., and Ho, C., Proton nuclear magnetic resonance and biochemical studies of oxygenation of human adult hemoglobin in deuterium oxide, *Biochemistry* 18, 5238–5247, 1979; Bonnete, F., Madern, D., and Zaccai, G., Stability against denaturation mechanisms in halophilic malate dehydrogenase "adapt" to solvent conditions, *J. Mol. Biol.* 244, 436–447, 1994; Thompson, J.F., Bush, K.J., and Nance, S.L., Pancreatic lipase activity in deuterium oxide, *Proc. Soc. Exp. Biol. Med.* 122, 502–505, 1996; Dufner, D. and Previs, S.F., Measuring *in vivo* metabolism using heavy water, *Curr. Opin. Clin. Nutr. Metab. Care* 6, 511–517, 2003; O'Donnell, A.H., Yao, X., and Byers, L.D., Solvent isotope effects on alpha-glucosidase, *Biochem. Biophys. Acta* 1703, 63–67, 2004; Hellerstein, M.K. and Murphy, E., Stable isotope-mass spectrometric measurements of molecular fluxes *in vivo*: emerging applications in drug development, *Curr. Opin. Mol. Ther.* 6, 249–264, 2004; Mazon, H., Marcillat, O., Forest, E., and Vial, C., Local dynamics measured by hydrogen/deuterium exchange and mass spectrometry of the creatine kinase digested by two proteases, *Biochimie* 87, 1101–1110, 2005; Carmieli, R., Papo, N., Zimmerman, H. et al., Utilizing ESEEM spectrscopy to locate the position of specific regions of membrane-active peptides within model membranes, *Biophys. J.* 90, 492–505, 2006.

| DFP | Diisopropylphosphorofluoridate; Isofluorophate | 184.15 | Classic cholinesterase inhibitor; inhibitor of serine proteases, some nonspecific reaction tyrosine. |

Baker, B.R., Factors in the design of active-site-directed irreversible inhibitors, *J. Pharm. Sci.* 53, 347–364, 1964; Dixon, G.H. and Schachter, H., The chemical modification of chymotrypsin, *Can. J. Biochem. Physiol.* 42, 695–714, 1964; Singer, S.J., Covalent labeling active site, *Adv. Protein Chem.* 22, 1–54, 1967; Kassell, B. and Kay, J., Zymogens of proteolytic enzymes, *Science* 180, 1022–1027, 1973; Fujino, T., Watanabe, K., Beppu, M. et al., Identification of oxidized protein hydrolase of human erythrocytes as acylpeptide hydrolase, *Biochim. Biophys. Acta* 1478, 102–112, 2000; Manco, G., Camardello, L., Febbraio, F. et al., Homology modeling and identification of serine 160 as nucleophile as the active site in a thermostable carboxylesterase from the archeon *Archaeoglobus fulgidus, Protein Eng.* 13, 197–200, 2000; Gopal, S., Rastogi, V., Ashman, W., and Mulbry, W., Mutagenesis of organophosphorous hydrolase to enhance hydrolysis of the nerve agent VX, *Biochem. Biophys. Res. Commun.* 279, 516–519, 2000; Yeung, D.T., Lenz, D.E., and Cerasoli, D.M., Analysis of active-site amino acid residues of human serum paraoxanse using competitive substrates, *FEBS J.* 272, 2225–2230, 2005; D'Souza, C.A., Wood, D.D., She, Y.M., and Moscarello, M.A., Autocatalytic cleavage of myelin basic protein: an alternative to molecular mimicry, *Biochemistry* 44, 12905–12913, 2005.

| Dichloromethane | Methylene Chloride | 84.9 | Lipid solvent; isolation of sterols, frequently used in combination with methanol. |

Bouillon, R., Kerkhove, P.V., and De Moor, P., Measurement of 25-hydroxyvitamin D3 in serum, *Clin. Chem.* 22, 364–368, 1976; Redhwi, A.A., Anderson, D.C., and Smith, G.N., A simple method for the isolation of vitamin D metabolites from plasma extracts, *Steroids* 39, 149–154, 1982; Scholtz, R., Wackett, L.P., Egli, C. et al., Dichloromethane dehalogenase with improved catalytic activity isolated form a fast-growing dichloromethane-utilizing bacterium, *J. Bacteriol.* 170, 5698–5704, 1988; Russo, M.V., Goretti, G., and Liberti, A., Direct headspace gas chromatographic determination of dichloromethane in decaffeinated green and roasted coffee, *J. Chromatog.* 465, 429–433, 1989; Shimizu, M., Kamchi, S., Nishii, Y., and Yamada, S., Synthesis of a reagent for fluorescence-labeling of vitamin D and its use in assaying vitamin D metabolites, *Anal. Biochem.* 194, 77–81, 1991; Rodriguez-Palmero, M., de la Presa-Owens, S., Castellote-Bargallo, A.I. et al., Determination of sterol content in different food samples by capillary gas chromatography, *J. Chromatog. A* 672, 267–272, 1994; Raghuvanshi, R.S., Goyal, S., Singh, O., and Panda, A.K., Stabilization of dichloromethane-induced protein denaturation during microencapsulation, *Pharm. Dev. Technol.* 3, 269–276, 1998; El Jaber-Vazdekis, N., Gutierrez-Nicolas, F., Ravelo, A.G., and Zarate, R., Studies on tropane alkaloid extraction by volatile organic solvents: dichloromethane vs. chloroform, *Phytochem. Anal.* 17, 107–113, 2006.

CHEMICALS COMMONLY USED IN BIOCHEMISTRY AND MOLECULAR BIOLOGY AND THEIR PROPERTIES (Continued)

Common Name	Chemical Name	M.W.	Properties and Comment
Diethyldithiocarbamate	Ditiocarb; Dithiocarb; DTC	171.3 (Na)	Chelating agent with particular affinity for Pb, Cu, Zn, Ni; colorimetric determination of Cu.

Matsuba, Y. and Takahashi, Y., Spectrophotometric determination of copper with *N,N,N',N'*-tetraethylthiuram disulfide and an application of this method for studies on subcellular distribution of copper in rat brains, *Anal. Biochem.* 36, 182–191, 1970, Koutensky, J., Eybl, V., Koutenska, M. et al., Influence of sodium diethyldithiocarbamate on the toxicity and distribution of copper in mice, *Eur. J. Pharmacol.* 14, 389–392, 1971; Xu, H. and Mitchell, C.L., Chelation of zinc by diethyldithiocarbamate facilitates bursting induced by mixed antidromic plus orthodromic activation of mossy fibers in hippocampal slices, *Brain Res.* 624, 162–170, 1993; Liu, J., Shigenaga, M.K., Yan, L.J. et al., Antioxidant activity of diethyldithiocarbamate, *Free Radic. Res.* 24, 461–472, 1996; Zhang, Y., Wade, K.L., Prestera, T., and Talalav, P., Quantitative determination of isothiocyanates, dithiocarbamates, carbon disulfide, and related thiocarbonyl compounds by cyclocondensation with 1,2-benzenedithiol, *Anal. Biochem.* 239, 160–167, 1996; Shoener, D.F., Olsen, M.A., Cummings, P.G., and Basic, C., Electrospray ionization of neutral metal dithiocarbamate complexes using in-source oxidation, *J. Mass Spectrom.* 34, 1069–1078, 1999; Turner, B.J., Lopes, E.C., and Cheema, S.S., Inducible superoxide dismutase 1 aggregation in transgenic amyotrophic lateral sclerosis mouse fibroblasts, *J. Cell Biochem.* 91, 1074–1084, 2004; Xu, K.Y. and Kuppusamy, P., Dual effects of copper-zinc superoxide dismutase, *Biochem. Biophys. Res. Commun.* 336, 1190–1193, 2005; Jiang, X., Sun, S., Liang, A. et al., Luminescence properties of metal(II)-diethyldithiocarbamate chelate complex particles and its analytical application, *J. Fluoresc.* 15, 859–864, 2005; Wang, J.S. and Chiu, K.H., Mass balance of metal species in supercritical fluid extraction using sodium diethyldithio-carbamate and dibuylammonium dibutyldithiocarbamate, *Anal. Sci.* 22, 363–369, 2006.

Diethylpyrocarbonate (DEPC)	Ethoxyformic Anhydride	162.1	Reagent for modification of proteins and DNA; used as a sterilizing agent; RNAse inhibitor for RNA purification; preservative for wine and fruit fluids.

Wolf, B., Lesnaw, J.A., and Reichmann, M.E., A mechanism of the irreversible inactivation of bovine pancreatic ribonuclease by diethylpyrocarbonate. A general reaction of diethylpyrocarbonate with proteins, *Eur. J. Biochem.* 13, 519–525, 1970; Splittstoesser, D.F. and Wilkison, M., Some factors affecting the activity of diethylpyrocarbonate as a sterilant, *Appl. Microbiol.* 25, 853–857, 1973; Fedorcsak, I., Ehrenberg, L., and Solymosy, F., Diethylpyrocarbonate does not degrade RNA, *Biochem. Biophys. Res. Commun.* 65, 490–496, 1975; Berger, S.L., Diethylpyrocarbonate: an examination of its properties in buffered solutions with a new assay technique, *Anal. Biochem.* 67, 428–437, 1975; Lloyd, A.G. and Drake, J.J., Problems posed by essential food preservatives, *Br. Med. Bull.* 31, 214–219, 1975; Ehrenberg, L., Fedorcsak, I., and Solymosy, F., Diethylpyrocarbonate in nucleic acid research, *Prog. Nucleic Acid Res. Mol. Biol.* 16, 189–262, 1976; Saluz, H.P. and Jost, J.P., Approaches to characterize protein–DNA interactions *in vivo*, *Crit. Rev. Eurkaryot. Gene Expr.* 3, 1–29, 1993; Bailly, C. and Waring, M.J., Diethylpyrocarbonate and osmium tetroxide as probes for drug-induced changes in DNA conformation *in vitro*, *Methods Mol. Biol.* 90, 51–59, 1997; Mabic, S. and Kano, I., Impact of purified water quality on molecular biology experiments, *Clin. Chem. Lab. Med.* 41, 486–491, 2003; Colleluori, D.M., Reczkowski, R.S., Emig, F.A. et al., Probing the role of the hyper-reactive histidine residue of argininase, *Arch. Biochem. Biophys.* 444, 15–26, 2005; Wu, S.N. and Chang, H.D., Diethylpyrocarbonate, a histidine-modifying agent, directly stimulates activity of ATP-sensitive potassium channels in pituitary GH(3) cells, *Biochem. Pharmacol.* 71, 615–623, 2006.

Dimedone	5,5-dimethyl-1,3-cyclohexanedione	140.18	Originally described as reagent for assay of aldehydes; used as a specific modifier of sulfenic acid.

CHEMICALS COMMONLY USED IN BIOCHEMISTRY AND MOLECULAR BIOLOGY AND THEIR PROPERTIES (Continued)

Common Name	Chemical Name	M.W.	Properties and Comment

Bulmer, D., Dimedone as an aldehyde-blocking reagent to facilitate the histochemical determination of glycogen, *Stain Technol.* 34, 95–98, 1959; Sawicki, E. and Carnes, R.A., Spectrophotofluorimetric determination of aldehydes with dimedone and other reagents, *Mikrochim. Acta* 1, 95–98, 1968; Benitez, L.V. and Allison, W.S., The inactivation of the acyl phosphatase activity catalyzed by the sulfenic acid form of glyceraldehyde 3-phosphate dehydrogenase by dimedone and olefins, *J. Biol. Chem.* 249, 6234–6243, 1974; Huszti, Z. and Tyihak, E., Formation of formaldehyde from *S*-adenosyl-L-[methyl-³H] methionine during enzymic transmethylation of histamine, *FEBS Lett.* 209, 362–366, 1986; Sardi, E. and Tyihak, E., Sample determination of formaldehyde in dimedone adduct form in biological samples by high-performance liquid chromatography, *Biomed. Chromatog.* 8, 313–314, 1994; Demaster, A.G., Quast, B.J., Redfern, B., and Nagasawa, H.T., Reaction of nitric oxide with the free sulfhydryl group of human serum albumin yields a sulfenic acid and nitrous oxide, *Biochemistry* 34, 14494–14949, 1995; Rozylo, T.K., Siembida, R., and Tyihak, E., Measurement of formaldehyde as dimedone adduct and potential formaldehyde precursors in hard tissues of human teeth by overpressurized layer chromatography, *Biomed. Chromatog.* 13, 513–515, 1999; Percival, M.D., Ouellet, M., Campagnolo, C. et al., Inhibition of cathepsin K by nitric oxide donors: evidence for the formation of mixed disulfides and a sulfenic acid, *Biochemistry* 38, 13574–13583, 1999; Carballal, S., Radi, R., Kirk, M.C. et al., Sulfenic acid formation in human serum albumin by hydrogen peroxide and peroxynitrite, *Biochemistry* 42, 9906–9914, 2003; Poole, L.B., Zeng, B.-B., Knaggs, S.A., Yakuba, M., and King, S.B., Synthesis of chemical probes to map sulfenic acid modifications on proteins, *Bioconjugate Chem.* 16, 1624–1628, 2005; Kaiserov, K., Srivastava, S., Hoetker, J.D. et al., Redox activation of aldose reductase in the ischemic heart, *J. Biol. Chem.* 281, 15110–15120, 2006.

Dimethylformamide (DMF)   *N,N*-dimethylformamide   73.09   Solvent.

Eliezer, N. and Silberberg, A., Structure of branched poly-alpha-amino acids in dimethylformamide. I. Light scattering, *Biopolymers* 5, 95–104, 1967; Bonner, O.D., Bednarek, J.M., and Arisman, R.K., Heat capacities of ureas and water in water and dimethylformamide, *J. Am. Chem. Soc.* 99, 2898–2902, 1977; Sasson, S. and Notides, A.C., The effects of dimethylformamide on the interaction of the estrogen receptor with estradiol, *J. Steroid Biochem.* 29, 491–495, 1988; Jeffers, R.J., Feng, R.Q., Fowlkes, J.B. et al., Dimethylformamide as an enhancer of cavitation-induced cell lysis *in vitro*, *J. Acoust. Soc. Am.* 97, 669–676, 1995; You, L. and Arnold, F.H., Directed evolution of subtilisin E in *Bacillus subtilis* to enhance total activity in aqueous dimethylformamide, *Protein Eng.* 9, 77–83, 1996; Szabo, P.T. and Kele, Z., Electrospray mass spectrometry of hydrophobic compounds using dimethyl sulfoxide and dimethylformamide, *Rapid Commun. Mass Spectrom.* 15, 2415–2419, 2001; Nishida, Y., Shingu, Y., Dohi, H., and Kobayashi, K., One-pot alpha-glycosylation method using Appel agents in *N,N*-dimethylformamide, *Org. Lett.* 5, 2377–2380, 2003; Shingu, Y., Miyachi, A., Miura, Y. et al., One-pot alpha-glycosylation pathway via the generation *in situ* of alpha-glycopyranosyl imidates I *N,N*-dimethylformamide, *Carbohydr. Res.* 340, 2236–2244, 2005; Porras, S.P. and Kenndler, E., Capillary electrophoresis in *N,N*-dimethylformamide, *Electrophoresis* 26, 3279–3291, 2005; Wei, Q., Zhang, H., Duan, C. et al., High sensitive fluorophotometric determination of nucleic acids with pyronine G sensitized by *N,N*-dimethylformamide, *Ann. Chim.* 96, 273–284, 2006.

Dimethyl Suberimidate (DMS)   Crosslinking agent.

Davies, G.E. and Stark, G.R., Use of dimethyl suberimidate, a crosslinking reagent, in studying the subunit structure of oligomeric proteins, *Proc. Natl. Acad. Sci. USA* 66, 651–656, 1970; Hassell, J. and Hand, A.R., Tissue fixation with diimidoesters as an alternative to aldehydes. I. Comparison of crosslinking and ultrastructure obtained with dimethylsuberimidate and glutaraldehyde, *J. Histochem. Cytochem.* 22, 223–229, 1974; Thomas, J.O., Chemical crosslinking of histones, *Methods Enzymol.* 170, 549–571, 1989; Roth, M.R., Avery, R.B., and Welti, R., Crosslinking of phosphatidylethanolamine neighbors with dimethylsuberimidate is sensitive to the lipid phase, *Biochim. Biophys. Acta* 986, 217–224, 1989; Redl, B., Walleczek, J., Soffler-Meilicke, M., and Stoffler, G., Immunoblotting analysis of protein–protein crosslinks within the 50S ribosomal subunit of *Escherichia coli*. A study using dimethylsuberimidate as crosslinking reagent, *Eur. J. Biochem.* 181, 351–256, 1989; Konig, S., Hubner, G., and Schellenberger, A., Crosslinking of pyruvate decarboxylase-characterization of the native and substrate-activated enzyme states, *Biomed. Biochim. Acta* 49, 465–471, 1990; Chen, J.C., von Lintig, F.C., Jones, S.B. et al., High-efficiency solid-phase capture using glass beads bonded to microcentrifuge tubes: immunoprecipitation of proteins from cell extracts and assessment of ras activation, *Anal. Biochem.* 302, 298–304, 2002; Dufes, C., Muller, J.M., Couet, W. et al., Anticancer drug delivery with transferrin-targeted polymeric chitosan vesicles, *Pharm. Res.* 21, 101–107, 2004; Levchenko, V. and Jackson, V., Histone release during transcription: NAP1 forms a complex with H2A and H2B and facilitates a topologically dependent release of H3 and H4 from the nucleosome, *Biochemistry* 43, 2358–2372, 2004; Jastrzebska, M., Barwinski, B., Mroz, I. et al., Atomic force microscopy investigation of chemically stabilized pericardium tissue, *Eur. Phys. J. E* 16, 381–388, 2005.

CHEMICALS COMMONLY USED IN BIOCHEMISTRY AND MOLECULAR BIOLOGY AND THEIR PROPERTIES (Continued)

Common Name	Chemical Name	M.W.	Properties and Comment
Dimethyl Sulfate		126.1	Methylating agent; methylation of nucleic acids; used for a process called footprinting to identify sites of protein–nucleic acid interaction.

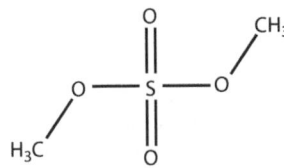

Nielsen, P.E., *In vivo* footprinting: studies of protein–DNA interactions in gene regulation, *Bioessay* 11, 152–155, 1989; Saluz, H.P. and Jost, J.P., Approaches to characterize protein–DNA interactions *in vivo*, *Crit. Rev. Eurkaryot. Gene Expr.* 3, 1–29, 1993; Saluz, H.P. and Jost, J.P., *In vivo* DNA footprinting by linear amplification, *Methods Mol. Biol.* 31, 317–329, 1994; Paul, A.L. and Ferl, R.J., *In vivo* footprinting of protein–DNA interactions, *Methods Cell Biol.* 49, 391–400, 1995; Gregory, P.D., Barbaric, S., and Horz, W., Analyzing chromatin structure and transcription factor binding in yeast, *Methods* 15, 295–302, 1998; Simpson, R.T., *In vivo* to analyze chromatin structrure, *Curr. Opin. Genet. Dev.* 9, 225–229, 1999; Nawrocki, A.R., Goldring, C.E., Kostadinova, R.M. et al., *In vivo* footprinting of the human 11β-hydroxysteroid dehydro-genase type 2 promoter: evidence for cell-specific regulation by Sp1 and Sp3, *J. Biol. Chem.* 277, 14647–14656, 2002; McGarry, K.C., Ryan, V.T., Grimwade, J.E., and Leonard, A.C., Two discriminatory binding sites in the *Escherichia coli* replication origin are required for DNA stand opening by initiator DnaA-ATP, *Proc. Natl. Acad. Sci. USA* 101, 2811–2816, 2004; Kellersberger, K.A., Yu, E., Kruppa, G.H. et al., Two-down characterization of nucleic acids modified by structural probes using high-resolution tandem mass spectrometry and automated data interpretation, *Anal. Chem.* 76, 2438–2445, 2004; Matthews, D.H., Disney, M.D., Childs, J.L. et al., Incorporating chemical modification constraints into a dynamic programming algorithm for prediction of RNA secondary structure, *Proc. Natl. Acad. Sci. USA* 101, 7287–7292, 2004; Forstemann, K. and Lingner, J., Telomerase limits the extent of base pairing between template RNA and temomeric DNA, *EMBO Rep.* 6, 361–366, 2005; Kore, A.R. and Parmar, G., An industrial process for selective synthesis of 7-methyl guanosine 5′-diphosphate: versatile synthon for synthesis of mRNA cap analogues, *Nucleosides Nucleotides Nucleic Acids* 25, 337–340, 2006.

Dioxane	1,4-diethylene Dioxide	88.1	Solvent.

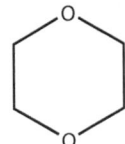

Sideri, C.N. and Osol, A., A note on the purification of dioxane for use in preparing nonaqueous titrants, *J. Am. Pharm. Am. Pharm. Assoc.* 42, 586, 1953; Martel, R.W. and Kraus, C.A., The association of ions in dioxane-water mixtures at 25 degrees, *Proc. Natl. Acad. Sci. USA* 41, 9–20, 1955; Mercier, P.L. and Kraus, C.A, The ion-pair equilibrium of electrolyte solutions in dioxane-water mixtures, *Proc. Natl. Acad. Sci. USA* 41, 1033–1041, 1995; Inagami, T., and Sturtevant, J.M., The trypsin-catalyzed hydrolysis of benzoyl-L-arginine ethyl ester. I. The kinetics in dioxane-water mixtures, *Biochim. Biophys. Acta* 38, 64–79, 1980; Zaeklj, A. and Gros, M., Electrophoresis of lipoprotein, prestained with Sudan Black B, dissolved in a mixture of dioxane and ethylene glycol, *Clin. Chim. Acta* 5, 947, 1960; Krasner, J. and McMenamy, R.H., The binding of indole compounds to bovine plasma albumin. Effects of potassium chloride, urea, dioxane, and glycine, *J. Biol. Chem.* 241, 4186–4196, 1966; Smith, R.R. and Canady, W.J., Solvation effects upon the thermodynamic substrate activity: correlation with the kinetics of enzyme-catalyzed reactions. II. More complex interactions of alpha-chymotrypsin with dioxane and acetone which are also competitive inhibitors, *Biophys. Chem.* 43, 189–195, 1992; Forti, F.L., Goissis, G., and Plepis, A.M., Modifications on collagen structures promoted by 1,4-dioxane improve thermal and biological properties of bovine pericardium as a biomaterial, *J. Biomater. Appl.* 20, 267–285, 2006.

Dithiothreitol	1,4-dithiothreitol; DTT; Cleland's Reagent; *threo*-2,3-dihydroxy-1,4-dithiolbutane	154.3	Reducing agent.

CHEMICALS COMMONLY USED IN BIOCHEMISTRY AND MOLECULAR BIOLOGY AND THEIR PROPERTIES (Continued)

Common Name	Chemical Name	M.W.	Properties and Comment

Cleland, W.W., Dithiothreitol, a new protective reagent for SH groups, *Biochemistry* 3, 480–482, 1964; Gorin, G., Fulford, R., and Deonier, R.C., Reaction of lysozyme with dithiothreitol and other mercaptans, *Experientia* 24, 26–27, 1968; Stanton, M. and Viswantha, T., Reduction of chymotryptin A by dithiothreitol, *Can. J. Biochem.* 49, 1233–1235, 1971; Warren, W.A., Activation of serum creatine kinase by dithiothreitol, *Clin. Chem.* 18, 473–475, 1972; Hase, S. and Walter, R., Symmetrical disulfide bonds as *S*-protecting groups and their cleavage by dithiothreitol: synthesis of oxytocin with high biological activity, *Int. J. Pept. Protein Res.* 5, 283–288, 1973; Fleisch, J.H., Krzan, M.C., and Titus, E., Alterations in pharmacologic receptor activity by dithiothreitol, *Am. J. Physiol.* 227, 1243–1248, 1974; Olsen, J. and Davis, L., The oxidation of dithiothreitol by peroxidases and oxygen, *Biochim. Biophys. Acta.* 445, 324–329, 1976; Chao, L.P., Spectrophotometric determination of choline acetyltransferase in the presence of dithiothreitol, *Anal. Biochem.* 85, 20–24, 1978; Fukada, H. and Takahashi, K., Calorimetric study of the oxidation of dithiothreitol, *J. Biochem.* 87, 1105–1110, 1980; Alliegro, M.C., Effects of dithiothreitol on protein activity unrelated to thiol-disulfide exchange: for consideration in the analysis of protein function with Cleland's reagent, *Anal. Biochem.* 282, 102–106, 2000; Rhee, S.S. and Burke, D.H., Tris(2-carboxyethyl)phosphine stabilization of RNA: comparison with dithiothreitol for use with nucleic acid and thiophosphoryl chemistry, *Anal. Biochem.* 325, 137–143, 2004; Pan, J.C., Cheng, Y., Hui, E.F., and Zhou, H.M., Implications of the role of reactive cysteine in arginine kinase: reactivation kinetics of 5,5'-dithiobis-(2-nitrobenzoic acid)-modified arginine kinase reactivated by dithiothreitol, *Biochem. Biophys. Res. Commun.* 317, 539–544, 2004; Thaxton, C.S., Hill, H.D., Georganopoulou, D.G. et al., A bio-barcode assay based upon dithiothreitol-induced oligonucleotide release, *Anal. Chem.* 77, 8174–8178, 2005.

DMSO	Dimethylsulfoxide	78.13	Solvent; suggested therapeutic use; effect on cellular function; cyropreservative.

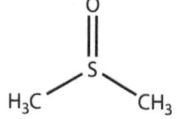

Huggins, C.E., Reversible agglomeration used to remove dimethylsulfoxide from large volumes of frozen blood, *Science* 139, 504–505, 1963; Yehle, A.V. and Doe, R.H., Stabilization of *Bacillus subtilis* phage with dimethylsulfoxide, *Can. J. Microbiol.* 11, 745–746, 1965; Fowler, A.V. and Zabin, I., Effects of dimethylsulfoxide on the lactose operon of *Escherichia coli*, *J. Bacteriol.* 92, 353–357, 1966; Williams, A.E. and Vinograd, J., The buoyant behavior of RNA and DNA in cesium sulfate solutions containing dimethylsulfoxide, *Biochim. Biophys. Acta* 228, 423–439, 1971; Levine, W.G., The effect of dimethylsulfoxide on the binding of 3-methylcholanthrene to rat liver fractions, *Res. Commun. Chem. Pathol. Pharmacol.* 4, 511–518, 1972; Fink, A.L, The trypsin-catalyzed hydrolysis of *N*-alpha-benzoyl-L-lysine *p*-nitrophenyl ester in dimethylsulfoxide at subzero temperatures, *J. Biol. Chem.* 249, 5072–5932, 1974; Hutton, J.R. and Wetmur, J.G., Activity of endonuclease S1 in denaturing solvents: dimethylsulfoxide, dimethylformamide, formamide, and formaldehyde, *Biochim. Biophys. Res. Commun.* 66, 942–948, 1975; Gal, A., De Groot, N., and Hochberg, A.A., The effect of dimethylsulfoxide on ribosomal fractions from rat liver, *FEBS Lett.* 94, 25–27, 1978; Barnett, R.E., The effects of dimethylsulfoxide and glycerol on Na+, K+-ATPase, and membrane structure, *Cryobiology* 15, 227–229, 1978; Borzini, P., Assali, G., Riva, M.R. et al., Platelet cryopreservation using dimethylsulfoxide/ polyethylene glycol/sugar mixture as cryopreserving solution, *Vox Sang.* 64, 248–249, 1993; West, R.T., Garza, L.A., II, Winchester, W.R., and Walmsley, J.A., Conformation, hydrogen bonding, and aggregate formation of guanosine 5'-monophosphate and guanosine in dimethylsulfoxide, *Nucleic Acids Res.* 22, 5128–5134, 1994; Bhattacharjya, S. and Balarma, P., Effects of organic solvents on protein structures: observation of a structured helical core in hen egg-white lysozyme in aqueous dimethylsulfoxide, *Proteins* 29, 492–507, 1997; Simala-Grant, J.L. and Weiner, J.H., Modulation of the substrate specificity of *Escherichia coli* dimethylsulfoxide reductase, *Eur. J. Biochem.* 251, 510–515, 1998; Tsuzuki, W., Ue, A., and Kitamura, Y., Effect of dimethylsulfoxide on hydrolysis of lipase, *Biosci. Biotechnol. Biochem.* 65, 2078–2082, 2001; Pedersen, N.R., Halling, P.J., Pedersen, L.H. et al., Efficient transesterification of sucrose catalyzed by the metalloprotease thermolysin in dimethylsulfoxide, *FEBS Lett.* 519, 181–184, 2002; Fan, C., Lu, J., Zhang, W., and Li, G., Enhanced electron-transfer reactivity of cytochrome b5 by dimethylsulfoxide and *N,N'*-dimethylformamide, *Anal. Sci.* 18, 1031–1033, 2002; Tait, M.A. and Hik, D.S., Is dimethylsulfoxide a reliable solvent for extracting chlorophyll under field conditions? *Photosynth. Res.* 78, 87–91, 2003; Malinin, G.I. and Malinin, T.I., Effects of dimethylsulfoxide on the ultrastructure of fixed cells, *Biotech. Histochem.* 79, 65–69, 2004; Clapisson, G., Salinas, C., Malacher, P. et al., Cryopreservation with hydroxyethylstarch (HES) + dimethylsulfoxide (DMSO) gives better results than DMSO alone, *Bull. Cancer* 91, E97–E102, 2004.

EDC	1-ethyl-(3-dimethylaminopropyl) carbodiimide; *N*-(3-dimethylaminopropyl)-*N'*-ethylcarbodiimide	191.7 (HCl)	Water-soluble carbodiimide for the modification of carboxyl groups in proteins; zero-length crosslinking proteins; activation of carboxyl groups for amidation reactions, as for the coupling of amino-nucleotides to matrices for DNA microarrays.

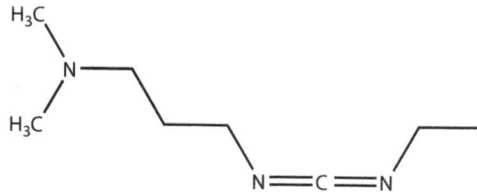

CHEMICALS COMMONLY USED IN BIOCHEMISTRY AND MOLECULAR BIOLOGY AND THEIR PROPERTIES (Continued)

Common Name	Chemical Name	M.W.	Properties and Comment

Lin, T.Y. and Koshland, D.E., Jr., Carboxyl group modification and the activity of lysozyme, *J. Biol. Chem.* 244, 505–508, 1969; Carraway, K.L., Spoerl, P., and Koshland, D.E., Jr., Carboxyl group modification in chymotrypsin and chymotrypsinogen, *J. Mol. Biol.* 42, 133–137, 1969; Yamada, H., Imoto, T., Fujita, K. et al., Selective modification of aspartic acid-101 in lysozyme by carbodiimide reaction, *Biochemistry* 20, 4836–4842, 1981; Buisson, M. and Reboud, A.M., Carbodiimide-induced protein-RNA crosslinking in mammalian subunits, *FEBS Lett.* 148, 247–250, 1982; Millett, F., Darley-Usmar, V., and Capaldi, R.A., Cytochrome c is crosslinked to subunit II of cytochrome c oxidase by a water-soluble carbodiimide, *Biochemistry* 21, 3857–3862, 1982; Chen, S.C., Fluorometric determination of carbodiimides with trans-aconitic acid, *Anal. Biochem.* 132, 272–275, 1983; Davis, L.E., Roth, S.A., and Anderson, B., Antisera specificities to 1-ethyl-3-(3-dimethylaminopropyl) carbodiimide adducts of proteins, *Immunology* 53, 435–441, 1984; Ueda, T., Yamada, H., and Imoto, T., Highly controlled carbodiimide reaction for the modification of lysozyme. Modification of Leu129 or As119, *Protein Eng.* 1, 189–193, 1987; Ghosh, M.K., Kildsig, D.O., and Mitra, A.K., Preparation and characterization of methotrexate-immunoglobulin conjugates, *Drug. Des. Deliv.* 4, 13–25, 1989; Grabarek, Z. and Gergely, J., Zero-length crosslinking procedure with the use of active esters, *Anal. Biochem.* 185, 131–135, 1990; Gilles, M.A., Hudson, A.Q., and Borders, C.L., Jr., Stability of water-soluble carbodiimides in aqueous solutions, *Anal. Biochem.* 184, 244–248, 1990; Soinila, S., Mpitsos, G.J., and Soinila, J., Immunohistochemistry of enkephalins: model studies on hapten-carrier conjugates and fixation methods, *J. Histochem. Cytochem.* 40, 231–239, 1992; Soper, S.A., Hashimoto, M., Situma, C. et al., Fabrication of DNA microarrays onto polymer substrates using UV modification protocols with integration into microfluidic platforms for the sensing of low-abundant DNA point mutations, *Methods* 37, 103–113, 2005.

Common Name	Chemical Name	M.W.	Properties and Comment
EDTA	Ethylenediaminetetraacetic acid	292.24	Chelating agent; some metal ion-EDTA complexes (i.e., Fe^{2+}-EDTA) function as chemical nucleases.

Flaschka, H.A., *EDTA Titrations: An Introduction to Theory and Practice*, Pergamon Press, Oxford, UK, 1964; West, T.S., *Complexometry with EDTA and Related Reagents*, BDH Chemicals Ltd., Poole (Dorset), UK, 1969; Pribil, R., *Analytical Applications of EDTA and Related Compounds*, Pergamon Press, Oxford, UK, 1972; Papavassiliou, A.G., Chemical nucleases as probes for studying DNA–protein interactions, *Biochem. J.* 305, 345–357, 1995; Martell, A.E., and Hancock, R.D., *Metal Complexes in Aqueous Solutions*, Plenum Press, New York, 1996; Loizos, N. and Darst, S.A, Mapping protein–ligand interactions by footprinting, a radical idea, *Structure* 6, 691–695, 1998; Franklin, S.J., Lanthanide-mediated DNA hydrolysis, *Curr. Opin. Chem. Biol.* 5, 201–208, 2001; Heyduk, T., Baichoo, N., and Henduk, E., Hydroxyl radical footprinting of proteins using metal ion complexes, *Met. Ions Biol. Syst.* 38, 255–287, 2001; Orlikowsky, T.W., Neunhoeffer, F., Goelz, R. et al., Evaluation of IL-8-concentrations in plasma and lyszed EDTA-blood in healthy neonates and those with suspected early onset bacterial infection, *Pediatr. Res.* 56, 804–809, 2004; Matt, T., Martinez-Yamout, M.A., Dyson, H.J., and Wright, P.E., The CBP/p300 TAZ1 domain in its native state is not a binding partner of MDM2, *Biochem. J.* 381, 685–691, 2004; Nyborg, J.K. and Peersen, O.B., That zincing feeling: the effects of EDTA on the behavior of zinc-binding transcriptional regulators, *Biochem. J.* 381, e3–e4, 2004; Haberz, P., Rodriguez-Castanada, F., Junker, J. et al., Two new chiral EDTA-based metal chelates for weak alignment of proteins in solution, *Org. Lett.* 8, 1275–1278, 2006.

Common Name	Chemical Name	M.W.	Properties and Comment
Ellman's Reagent	5,5′-dithiobis[2-nitro-benzoic] acid	396.35	Reagent for determination of sulfydryl groups/disulfide bonds.

CHEMICALS COMMONLY USED IN BIOCHEMISTRY AND MOLECULAR BIOLOGY AND THEIR PROPERTIES (Continued)

Common Name	Chemical Name	M.W.	Properties and Comment

Ellman, G.L., Tissue sulfhydryl groups, *Arch. Biochem. Biophys.* 82, 70–77, 1959; Boyne, A.F. and Ellman, G.L., A methodology for analysis of tissue sulfydryl components, *Anal. Biochem.* 46, 639–653, 1972; Brocklehurst, K., Kierstan, M., and Little, G., The reaction of papain with Ellman's reagent (5,5′-dithiobis-(2-nitrobenzoate), *Biochem. J.* 128, 811–816, 1972; Weitzman, P.D., A critical reexamination of the reaction of sulfite with DTNB, *Anal. Biochem.* 64, 628–630, 1975; Hull, H.H., Chang, R., and Kaplan, L.J., On the location of the sulfhydryl group in bovine plasma albumin, *Biochim. Biophys. Acta* 400, 132–136, 1975; Banas, T., Banas, B., and Wolny, M., Kinetic studies of the reactivity of the sulfhydryl groups of glyceraldehyde-3-phosphate dehydrogenase, *Eur. J. Biochem.* 68, 313–319, 1976; der Terrossian, E. and Kassab, R., Preparation and properties of *S*-cyano derivatives of creatine kinase, *Eur. J. Biochem.* 70, 623–628, 1976; Riddles, P.W., Blakeley, R.L., and Zerner, B., Ellman's reagent: 5,5′-dithiobis(2-nitrobenzoic acid) — a reexamination, *Anal. Biochem.* 94, 75–81, 1979; Luthra, N.P., Dunlap, R.B., and Odom, J.D., Characterization of a new sulfhydryl group reagent: 6, 6′- diselenobis-(3-nitrobenzoic acid), a selenium analog of Ellman's reagent, *Anal. Biochem.* 117, 94–102, 1981; Di Simplicio, P., Tiezzi, A., Moscatelli, A. et al., The SH-SS exchange reaction between the Ellman's reagent and protein-containing SH groups as a method for determining conformational states: tubulin, *Ital. J. Biochem.* 38, 83–90, 1989; Woodward, J., Tate, J., Herrmann, P.C., and Evans, B.R., Comparison of Ellman's reagent with *N*-(1-pyrenyl)maleimide for the determination of free sulfhydryl groups in reduced cellobiohydrolase I from *Trichoderma reesei, J. Biochem. Biophys. Methods* 26, 121–129, 1993; Berlich, M., Menge, S., Bruns, I. et al., Coumarins give misleading absorbance with Ellman's reagent suggestive of thiol conjugates, *Analyst* 127, 333–336, 2002; Riener, C.K., Kada, G., and Gruber, H.J., Quick measurement of protein sulfhydryls of Ellman's reagents and with 4,4′-dithiopyridine, *Anal. Bio. Anal. Chem.* 373, 266–276, 2002; Zhu, J., Dhimitruka, I., and Pei, D., 5-(2-aminoethyl)dithio-2-nitrobenzoate as a more base-stable alternative to Ellman's reagent, *Org. Lett.* 6, 3809–3812, 2004; Owusu-Apenten, R., Colorimetric analysis of protein sulfhydryl groups in milk: applications and processing effects, *Crit. Rev. Food Sci. Nutr.* 45, 1–23, 2005.

Ethanolamine	Glycinol	61.08	Buffer component; component of a phospholipid (phosphatidyl ethanolamine, PE).

Vance, D.E. and Ridgway, N.D., The methylation of phosophatidylethanolamine, *Prog. Lipid Res.* 27, 61–79, 1988; Louwagie, M., Rabilloud, T., and Garin, J., Use of ethanolamine for sample stacking in capillary electrophoresis, *Electrophoresis* 19, 2440–2444, 1998; de Nogales, V., Ruiz, R., Roses. M. et al., Background electrolytes in 50% methanol/water for the determination of acidity constants of basic drugs by capillary zone electrophoresis, *J. Chromatog. A* 1123, 113–120, 2006.

Ethidium Bromide		394.31	

Sela, I., Fluorescence of nucleic acids with ethidium bromide: an indication of the configurative state of nucleic acids, *Biochim. Biophys. Acta* 190, 216–219, 1969; Le Pecq, J.B., Use of ethidium bromide for separation and determination of nucleic acids of various conformational forms and measurement of their associated enzymes, *Methods Biochem. Anal.* 20, 41–86, 1971; Borst, P., Ethidium DNA agarose gel electrophoresis: how it started, *IUBMB Life* 57, 745–747, 2005.

Ethyl Alcohol	Ethanol	46.07	Solvent; used to adjust solvent polarity; use in plasma protein fractionation.

CHEMICALS COMMONLY USED IN BIOCHEMISTRY AND MOLECULAR BIOLOGY AND THEIR PROPERTIES (Continued)

Common Name	Chemical Name	M.W.	Properties and Comment

Dufour, E., Bertrand-Harb, C., and Haertle, T., Reversible effects of medium dielectric constant on structural transformation of beta-lactoglobulin and its retinol binding, *Biopolymers* 33, 589–598, 1993; Escalera, J.B., Bustamante, P., and Martin, A., Predicting the solubility of drugs in solvent mixtures: multiple solubility maxima and the chameleonic effect, *J. Pharm. Pharmcol.* 46, 172–176, 1994; Gratzer, P.F., Pereira, C.A., and Lee, J.M., Solvent environment modulates effects of glutaraldehyde crosslinking on tissue-derived biomaterials, *J. Biomed. Mater. Res.* 31, 533–543, 1996; Sepulveda, M.R. and Mata, A.M., The interaction of ethanol with reconstituted synaptosomal plasma membrane Ca^{2+}, *Biochim. Biophys. Acta* 1665, 75–80, 2004; Ramos, A.S. and Techert, S., Influence of the water structure on the acetylcholinesterase efficiency, *Biophys. J.* 89, 1990–2003, 2005; Wehbi, Z., Perez, M.D., and Dalgalarrondo, M., Study of ethanol-induced conformation changes of holo and apo alpha-lactalbumin by spectroscopy anad limited proteolysis, *Mol. Nutr. Food Res.* 50, 34–43, 2006; Sasahara, K. and Nitta, K., Effect of ethanol on folding of hen egg-white lysozyme under acidic condition, *Proteins* 63, 127–135, 2006; Perham, M., Liao, J., and Wittung-Stafshede, P., Differential effects of alcohol on conformational switchovers in alpha-helical and beta-sheet protein models, *Biochemistry* 45, 7740–7749, 2006; Pena, M.A., Reillo, A., Escalera, B., and Bustamante, P., Solubility parameter of drugs for predicting the solubility profile type within a wide polarity range in solvent mixtures, *Int. J. Pharm.* 321, 155–161, 2006; Jenke, D., Odufu, A., and Poss, M., The effect of solvent polarity on the accumulation of leachables from pharmaceutical product containers, *Eur. J. Pharm. Sci.* 27, 133–142, 2006.

| **Ethylene Glycol** | 1,2-ethanediol | 62.07 | Solvent/cosolvent; increases viscosity (visogenic osmolyte); perturbant; cryopreservative. |

Tanford, C., Buckley, C.E., III, De, P.K., and Lively, E.P., Effect of ethylene glycol on the conformation of gamma-globulin and beta-lactoglobulin, *J. Biol. Chem.* 237, 1168–1171, 1962; Kay, C.M. and Brahms, J., The influence of ethylene glycol on the enzymatic adenosine triphosphatase activity and molecular conformation of fibrous muscle proteins, *J. Biol. Chem.* 238, 2945–2949, 1963; Narayan, K.A., The interaction of ethylene glycol with rat-serum lipoproteins, *Biochim. Biophys. Acta* 137, 22–30, 1968; Bello, J., The state of the tyrosines of bovine pancreatic ribonuclease in ethylene glycol and glycerol, *Biochemistry* 8, 4535–4541, 1969; Lowe, C.R. and Mosbach, K., Biospecific affinity chromatography in aqueous-organic cosolvent mixtures. The effect of ethylene glycol on the binding of lactate dehydrogenase to an immobilized-AMP analogue, *Eur. J. Biochem.* 52, 99–105, 1975; Ghrunyk, B.A. and Matthews, C.R., Role of diffusion in the folding of the alpha subunit of tryptophan synthase from *Escherichia coli*, *Biochemistry* 29, 2149–2154, 1990; Silow, M. and Oliveberg, M., High concentrations of viscogens decrease the protein folding rate constant by prematurely collapsing the coil, *J. Mol. Biol.* 326, 263–271, 2003; Naseem, F. and Khan, R.H., Effect of ethylene glycol and polyethylene glycol on the acid-unfolded state of trypsinogen, *J. Protein Chem.* 22, 677–682, 2003; Hubalek, Z., Protectants used in the cyropreservation of microorganisms, *Cryobiology* 46, 205–229, 2003; Menezo, Y.J., Blastocyst freezing, *Eur. J. Obstet. Gynecol. Reprod. Biol.* 155 (Suppl. 1), S12–S15, 2004; Khodarahmi, R. and Yazdanparast, R., Refolding of chemically denatured alpha-amylase in dilution additive mode, *Biochim. Biophys. Acta.* 1674, 175–181, 2004; Zheng, M., Li, Z., and Huang, X., Ethylene glycol monolayer protected nanoparticles: synthesis, characterization, and interactions with biological molecules, *Langmuir* 20, 4226–4235, 2004; Bonincontro, A., Cinelli, S., Onori, G., and Stravato, A., Dielectric behavior of lysozyme and ferricytochrome-c in water/ethylene-glycol solutions, *Biophys. J.* 86, 1118–1123, 2004; Kozer, N. and Schreiber, G., Effect of crowding on protein–protein association rates: fundamental differences between low and high mass crowding agents, *J. Mol. Biol.* 336, 763–774, 2004; Levin, I., Meiri, G., Peretz, M. et al., The ternary complex of *Pseudomonas aeruginosa* dehydrogenase with NADH and ethylene glycol, *Protein Sci.* 13, 1547–1556, 2004; Stupishina, E.A., Khamidullin, R.N., Vylegzhanina, N.N. et al., Ethylene glycol and the thermostability of trypsin in a reverse micelle system, *Biochemistry* 71, 533–537, 2006; Nordstrom, L.J., Clark, C.A., Andersen, B. et al., Effect of ethylene glycol, urea, and *N*-methylated glycines on DNA thermal stability: the role of DNA base pair composition and hydration, *Biochemistry* 45, 9604–9614, 2006.

| **Ethyleneimine** | Aziridine | 43.07 | Modification of sulfhydryl groups to produce amine functions; alkylating agent; reacts with carboxyl groups at acid pH; monomer unit for polyethylene amine, a versatile polymer. |

CHEMICALS COMMONLY USED IN BIOCHEMISTRY AND MOLECULAR BIOLOGY AND THEIR PROPERTIES (Continued)

Common Name	Chemical Name	M.W.	Properties and Comment

Raftery, M.A. and Cole, R.D., On the aminoethylation of proteins, *J. Biol. Chem.* 241, 3457–3461, 1966; Fishbein, L., Detection and thin-layer chromatography of derivatives of ethyleneimine. I. *N*-carbamoyl and aziridines, *J. Chromatog.* 26, 522–526, 1967; Yamada, H., Imoto, T., and Noshita, S., Modification of catalytic groups in lysozyme with ethyleneimine, *Biochemistry* 21, 2187–2192, 1982; Okazaki, K., Yamada, H., and Imoto, T., A convenient *S*-2-aminoethylation of cysteinyl residues in reduced proteins, *Anal. Biochem.* 149, 516–520, 1985; Hemminki, K., Reactions of ethyleneimine with guanosine and deoxyguanosine, *Chem. Biol. Interact.* 48, 249–260, 1984; Whitney, P.L., Powell, J.T., and Sanford, G.L., Oxidation and chemical modification of lung beta-galactosidase-specific lectin, *Biochem. J.* 238, 683–689, 1986; Simpson, D.M., Elliston, J.F., and Katzenellenbogen, J.A., Desmethylnafoxidine aziridine: an electrophilic affinity label for the estrogen receptor with high efficiency and selectivity, *J. Steroid Biochem.* 28, 233–245, 1987; Musser, S.M., Pan, S.S., Egorin, M.J. et al., Alkylation of DNA with aziridine produced during the hydrolysis of *N,N',N''*-triethylenethiophosphoramide, *Chem. Res. Toxicol.* 5, 95–99, 1992; Thorwirth, S., Muller, H.S., and Winnewisser, G., The millimeter- and submillimeter-wave spectrum and the dipole moment of ethyleneimine, *J. Mol. Spectroso.* 199, 116–123, 2000; Burrage, T., Kramer, E., and Brown, F., Inactivation of viruses by aziridines, *Dev. Biol.* (Basel) 102, 131–139, 2000; Brown, F., Inactivation of viruses by aziridines, *Vaccine* 20, 322–327, 2001; Sasaki, S., Active oligonucleotides incorporating alkylating agent as potential sequence- and base-selective modifier of gene expression, *Eur. J. Pharm. Sci.* 13, 43–51, 2001; Hou, X.L., Fan, R.H., and Dai, L.X., Tributylphosphine: a remarkable promoting reagent for the ring-opening reaction of aziridines, *J. Org. Chem.* 67, 5295–5300, 2002; Thevis, M., Loo, R.R.O., and Loo, J.A., In-gel derivatization of proteins for cysteine-specific cleavages and their analysis by mass spectrometry, *J. Proteome Res.* 2, 163–172, 2003; Sasaki, M., Dalili, S., and Yudin, A.K., *N*-arylation of aziridines, *J. Org. Chem.* 68, 2045–2047, 2003; Gao, G.Y., Harden, J.D., and Zhang, J.P., Cobalt-catalyzed efficient aziridination of alkenes, *Org. Lett.* 7, 3191–3193, 2005; Hopkins, C.E., Hernandez, G., Lee, J.P., and Tolan, D.R., Aminoethylation in model peptides reveals conditions for maximizing thiol specificity, *Arch. Biochem. Biophys.* 443, 1–10, 2005; Li, C. and Gershon, P.D., pK(a) of the mRNA cap-specific 2′-*O*-methyltransferase catalytic lysine by HSQC NMR detection of a two-carbon probe, *Biochemistry* 45, 907–917, 2006; Vicik R., Helten, H., Schirmeister, T., and Engels, B., Rational design of aziridine-containing cysteine protease inhibitors with improved potency: studies on inhibition mechanism, *ChemMedChem*, 1, 1021–1028, 2006.

Ethylene Oxide

Oxirane   44.05   Sterilizing agent; starting material for ethylene glycol and other products such as nonionic surfactants.

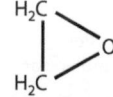

Windmueller, H.G., Ackerman, C.J., and Engel, R.W., Reaction of ethylene oxide with histidine, methionine, and cysteine, *J. Biol. Chem.* 234, 895–899, 1959; Starbuck, W.C. and Busch, H., Hydroxyethylation of amino acids in plasma albumin with ethylene oxide, *Biochim. Biophys. Acta* 78, 594–605, 1963; Guengerich, F.P., Geiger, L.E., Hogy, L.L., and Wright,. P.L., *In vitro* metabolism of acrylonitrile to 2-cyanoethylene oxide, reaction with glutathione, and irreversible binding to proteins and nucleic acids, *Cancer Res.* 41, 4925–4933, 1981; Peter, H., Schwarz, M., Mathiasch, B. et al., A note on synthesis and reactivity towards DNA of glycidonitrile, the epoxide of acrylonitrile, *Carcinogenesis* 4, 235–237, 1983; Grammer, L.C. and Patterson, R., IgE against ethylene oxide-altered human serum albumin (ETO-HAS) as an etiologic agent in allergic reactions of hemodialysis patients, *Artif. Organs* 11, 97–99, 1987; Bolt, H.M., Peter, H., and Fost, U., Analysis of macromolecular ethylene oxide adducts, *Int. Arch. Occup. Environ. Health* 60, 141–144, 1988; Young, T.L., Habraken, Y., Ludlum, D.B., and Santella, R.M., Development of monoclonal antibodies recognizing 7-(2-hydroxyethyl) guanine and imidazole ring-opened 7-(2-hydroxyethyl) guanine, *Carcinogenesis* 11, 1685–1689, 1990; Walker, V.E., Fennell, T.R., Boucheron, J.A. et al., Macromolecular adducts of ethylene oxide: a literature review and a time-course study on the formation of 7-(2-hydroxyethyl)guanine following exposure of rats by inhalation, *Mutat. Res.* 233, 151–164, 1990; Framer, P.B., Bailey, E., Naylor, S. et al., Identification of endogenous electrophiles by means of mass spectrometric determination of protein and DNA adducts, *Environ. Health Perspect.* 99, 19–24, 1993; Tornqvist, M. and Kautianinen, A., Adducted proteins for identification of endogenous electrophiles, *Environ. Health Perspect.* 99, 39–44, 1993; Galaev, I. Yu. and Mattiasson, B., Thermoreactive water-soluble polymers, nonionic surfactants, and hydrogels as reagents in biotechnology, *Enzyme Microb. Technol.* 15, 354–366, 1993; Segerback, D., DNA alkylation by ethylene oxide and mono-substituted expoxides, *IARC Sci. Publ.* 125, 37–47, 1994; Phillips, D.H. and Farmer, P.B., Evidence for DNA and protein binding by styrene and styrene oxide, *Crit. Rev. Toxicol.* 24 (Suppl.), S35–S46, 1994; Marczynski, B., Marek, W., and Baur, X., Ethylene oxide as a major factor in DNA and RNA evolution, *Med. Hypotheses* 44, 97–100, 1995; Mosely, G.A. and Gillis, J.R., Factors affecting tailing in ethylene oxide sterilization part 1: when tailing is an artifact...and scientific deficiencies in ISO 11135 and EN 550, *PDA J. Pharm. Sci. Technol.* 58, 81–95, 2004.

***N*-Ethylmaleimide**

1-ethyl-1*H*-pyrrole-2,5-dione   125.13   Modification of sulfhydryl groups; basic building block for a number of reagents. Mechanism different from alkylating agent in that reaction involves a Michael addition.

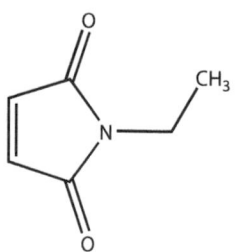

CHEMICALS COMMONLY USED IN BIOCHEMISTRY AND MOLECULAR BIOLOGY AND THEIR PROPERTIES (Continued)

Common Name	Chemical Name	M.W.	Properties and Comment

Lundblad, R.L., *Chemical Reagent for Protein Modification*, 3rd ed., CRC Press, Boca Raton, FL, 2004; Bowes, T.J. and Gupta, R.S., Induction of mitochondrial fusion by cysteine-alkylators ethyacrynic acid and *N*-ethylmaleimide, *J. Cell Physiol.* 202, 796–804, 2005; Engberts, J.B., Fernandez, E., Garcia-Rio, L., and Leis, J.R., Water in oil microemulsions as reaction media for a Diels–Alder reaction between *N*-ethylmaleimide and cyclopentadiene, *J. Org. Chem.* 71, 4111–4117, 2006; Engberts, J.B., Fernandez, E., Garcia-Rio, L., and Leis, J.R, AOT-based microemulsions accelerate the 1,3-cycloaddition of benzonitrile oxide to *N*-ethylmaleimide, *J. Org. Chem.* 71, 6118–6123, 2006; de Jong, K. and Kuypers, F.A., Sulphydryl modifications alter scramblase activity in murine sickle cell disease, *Br. J. Haematol.* 133, 427–432, 2006; Martin, H.G., Henley, J.M., and Meyer, G., Novel putative targets of *N*-ethylmaleimide sensitive fusion proteins (NSF) and alpha/beta soluble NSF attachment proteins (SNAPs) include the Pak-binding nucleotide exchange factor betaPIX, *J. Cell. Biochem.*, 99, 1203–1215, 2006; Carrasco, M.R., Silva, O., Rawls, K.A. et al., Chemoselective alkylation of *N*-alkylaminooxy-containing peptides, *Org. Lett.* 8, 3529–3532, 2006; Pobbati, A.V., Stein, A., and Fasshauer, D., N- to C-terminal SNARE complex assembly promotes rapid membrane fusion, *Science* 313, 673–676, 2006; Mollinedo, F., Calafat, J., Janssen, H. et al., Combinatorial SNARE complexes modulate the secretion of cytoplasmic granules in human neutrophils, *J. Immunol.* 177, 2831–2841, 2006.

Common Name	Chemical Name	M.W.	Properties and Comment
Formaldehyde	Methanal	30.03	Tissue fixation; protein modification; zero-length crosslinking; protein–nucleic acid interactions.

Formaldehyde

$$H_2C=O \quad + \quad H_2O \quad \rightleftharpoons \quad \underset{OH}{\overset{OH}{H-C-H}}$$

gem-diol form

"Paraformaldehyde"

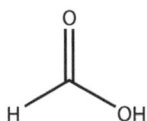

And higher polymers

Feldman, M.Y., Reactions of nucleic acids and nucleoproteins with formaldehyde, *Prog. Nucleic Acid Res. Mol. Biol.* 13, 1–49, 1973; Russell, A.D. and Hopwood, D., The biological uses and importance of glutaraldehyde, *Prog. Med. Chem.* 13, 271–301, 1976; Means, G.E., Reductive alkylation of amino groups, *Methods Enzymol.* 47, 469–478, 1977; Winkelhake, J.L., Effects of chemical modification of antibodies on their clearance for the circulation. Addition of simple aliphatic compounds by reductive alkylation and carbodiimide-promoted amide formation, *J. Biol. Chem.* 252, 1865–1868, 1977; Yamazaki, Y. and Suzuki, H., A new method of chemical modification of N^6-amino group in adenine nucleotides with formaldehyde and a thiol and its application to preparing immobilized ADP and ATP, *Eur. J. Biochem.* 92, 197–207, 1978; Geoghegan, K.F., Cabacungan, J.C., Dixon, H.B., and Feeney, R.E., Alternative reducing agents for reductive methylation of amino groups in proteins, *Int. J. Pept. Protein Res.* 17, 345–352, 1981; Kunkel, G.R., Mehradian, M., and Martinson, H.G., Contact-site crosslinking agents, *Mol. Cell. Biochem.* 34, 3–13, 1981; Fox, C.H., Johnson, F.B., Whiting, J., and Roller, P.P., Formaldehyde fixation, *J. Histochem. Cytochem.* 33, 845–853, 1985; Conaway, C.C., Whysner, J., Verna, L.K., and Williams, G.M., Formaldehyde mechanistic data and risk assessment: endogenous protection from DNA adduct formation, *Pharmacol. Ther.* 71, 29–55, 1996; Masuda, N., Ohnishi, T., Kawamoto, S. et al., Analysis of chemical modifications of RNA from formalin-fixed samples and optimization of molecular biology applications for such samples, *Nucleic Acids Res.* 27, 4436–4443, 1999; Micard, V., Belamri, R., Morel, M., and Guilbert, S., Properties of chemically and physically treated wheat gluten films, *J. Agric. Food Chem.* 48, 2948–2953, 2000; Taylor, I.A. and Webb, M., Chemical modification of lysine by reductive methylation. A probe for residues involved in DNA binding, *Methods Mol. Biol.* 148, 301–314, 2001; Perzyna, A., Marty, C., Facopre, M. et al., Formaldehyde-induced DNA crosslink of indolizino[1,2-b]quinolines derived from the A-D rings of camptothecin, *J. Med. Chem.* 45, 5809–5812, 2002; Yurimoto, H., Hirai, R., Matsuno, N. et al., HxlR, a member of the DUF24 protein family, is a DNA-binding protein that acts as a positive regulator of the formaldehyde-inducible hxlAB operon in *Bacillus subtilis*, *Mol. Microbiol.* 57, 511–519, 2005.

Common Name	Chemical Name	M.W.	Properties and Comment
Formic Acid	Methanoic Acid	46.03	Solvent; buffer component.

CHEMICALS COMMONLY USED IN BIOCHEMISTRY AND MOLECULAR BIOLOGY AND THEIR PROPERTIES (Continued)

Common Name	Chemical Name	M.W.	Properties and Comment

Sarkar, P.B., Decomposition of formic acid by periodate, *Nature* 168, 122–123, 1951; Hass, P., Reactions of formic acid and its salts, *Nature* 167, 325, 1951; Smillie, L.B. and Neurath, H., Reversible inactivation of trypsin by anhydrous formic acid, *J. Biol. Chem* 234, 355–359, 1959; Hynninen, P.H. and Ellfolk, N., Use of the aqueous formic acid-chloroform-dimethylformamide solvent system for the purification of porphyrins and hemins, *Acta Chem. Scand.* 27, 1795–1806, 1973; Heukeshoven, J. and Dernick, R., Reversed-phase high-performance liquid chromatography of virus proteins and other large hydrophobic proteins in formic acid-containing solvents, *J. Chromatog.* 252, 241–254, 1982; Tarr, G.E. and Crabb, J.W., Reverse-phase high-performance liquid chromatography of hydrophobic proteins and fragments thereof, *Anal. Biochem.* 131, 99–107, 1983; Heukeshoven, J. and Dernick, R., Characterization of a solvent system for separation of water-insoluble poliovirus proteins by reversed-phase high-performance liquid chromatography, *J. Chromatog.* 326, 91–101, 1985; De Caballos, M.L., Taylor, M.D., and Jenner, P., Isocratic reverse-phase HPLC separation and RIA used in the analysis of neuropeptides in brain tissue, *Neuropeptides* 20, 201–209, 1991; Poll, D.J. and Harding, D.R., Formic acid as a milder alternative to trifluoroacetic acid and phosphoric acid in two-dimensional peptide mapping, *J. Chromatog.* 469, 231–239, 1989; Klunk W.E. and Pettegrew, J.W., Alzheimer's beta-amyloid protein is covalently modified when dissolved in formic acid, *J. Neurochem.* 54, 2050–2056, 1990; Erdjument-Bromage, H., Lui, M., Lacomis, L. et al., Examination of the micro-tip reversed phase liquid chromatographic extraction of peptide pools for mass spectrometric analysis, *J. Chromatog. A* 826, 167–181, 1998; Duewel, H.S. and Honek, J.F., CNBr/formic acid reactions of methionine- and trifluoromethionine-containing lambda lysozyme: probing chemical and positional reactivity and formylation side reactions of mass spectrometry, *J. Protein Chem.* 17, 337–350, 1998; Kaiser, R. and Metzka, L., Enhancement of cyanogen bromide cleavage yields for methionyl-serine and methionyl-threonine peptide bonds, *Anal. Biochem.* 266, 1–8, 1999; Rodriguez, J.C., Wong, L., and Jennings, P.A., The solvent in CNBr cleavage reactions determines the fragmentation efficiency of ketosteroid isomerase fusion proteins used in the production of recombinant peptides, *Protein Expr. Purif.* 28, 224–231, 2003; Zu, Y., Zhao, C., Li, C., and Zhang, L., A rapid and sensitive LC-MS/MS method for determination of coenzyme Q10 in tobacco (*Nicotiana tabacum* L.) leaves, *J. Sep. Sci.* 29, 1607–1612, 2006; Kalovidouris, M., Michalea, S., Robola, N. et al., Ultra-performance liquid chromatography/tandem mass spectrometry method for the determination of lercaidipine in human plasma, *Rapid Commun. Mass Spectrom.*, 20, 2939–2946, 2006; Wang, P.G., Wei, J.S., Kim, G. et al., Validation and application of a high-performance liquid chromatography-tandem mass spectrometric method for simultaneous quantification of lopinavir and ritonavir in human plasma using semi-automated 96-well liquid–liquid chromatography, *J. Chromatog. A*, 1130, 302–307, 2006.

| **Glutaraldehyde** | Pentanedial | 100.12 | Protein modification; tissue fixation; sterilization agent approved by regulatory agencies; use with albumin as surgical sealant. |

Glutaraldehyde

CHEMICALS COMMONLY USED IN BIOCHEMISTRY AND MOLECULAR BIOLOGY AND THEIR PROPERTIES (Continued)

Common Name	Chemical Name	M.W.	Properties and Comment

Hopwood, D., Theoretical and practical aspects of glutaraldehyde fixation, *Histochem. J.*, 4, 267–303, 1972; Hassell, J. and Hand, A.R., Tissue fixation with diimidoesters as an alternative to aldehydes. I. Comparison of crosslinking and ultrastructure obtained with dimethylsubserimidate and glutaraldehyde, *J. Histochem. Cytochem.* 22, 223–229, 1974; Russell, A.D. and Hopwood, D., The biological uses and importance of glutaraldehyde, *Prog. Med. Chem.* 13, 271–301, 1976; Woodroof, E.A., Use of glutaraldehyde and formaldehyde to process tissue heart valves, *J. Bioeng.* 2, 1–9, 1978; Heumann, H.G., Microwave-stimulated glutaraldehyde and osmium tetroxide fixation of plant tissue: ultrastructural preservation in seconds, *Histochemistry* 97, 341–347, 1992; Abbott, L., The use and effects of glutaraldehyde: a review, *Occup. Health* 47, 238–239, 1995; Jayakrishnan, A. and Jameela, S.R., Glutaraldehyde as a fixative in bioprosthesis and drug delivery matrices, *Biomaterials* 17, 471–484, 1996; Tagliaferro, P., Tandler, C.J., Ramos, A.J. et al., Immunofluorescence and glutaraldehyde fixation. A new procedure base on the Schiff-quenching method, *J. Neurosci. Methods* 77, 191–197, 1997; Cohen, R.J., Beales, M.P., and McNeal, J.E., Prostate secretory granules in normal and neoplastic prostate glands: a diagnostic aid to needle biopsy, *Hum. Pathol.* 31, 1515–1519, 2000; Chae, H.J., Kim, E.Y., and In, M., Improved immobilization yields by addition of protecting agents in glutaraldehyde-induced immobilization of protease, *J. Biosci. Bioeng.* 89, 377–379, 2000; Nimni, M.E., Glutaraldehyde fixation revisited, *J. Long Term Eff. Med. Implants* 11, 151–161, 2001; Fujiwara, K., Tanabe, T., Yabuchi, M. et al., A monoclonal antibody against the glutaraldehyde-conjugated polyamine, putrescine: application to immunocytochemistry, *Histochem. Cell Biol.* 115, 471–477, 2001; Chao, H.H. and Torchiana, D.F., Bioglue: albumin/glutaraldehyde sealant in cardiac surgery, *J. Card. Surg.* 18, 500–503, 2003; Migneault, I., Dartiguenave, C., Bertrand, M.J., and Waldron, K.C., Glutaraldehyde: behavior in aqueous solution, reaction with proteins, and application to enzyme crosslinking, *Biotechniques* 37, 790–796, 2004; Jearanaikoon, S. and Abraham-Peskir, J.V., An x-ray microscopy perspective on the effect of glutaraldehyde fixation on cells, *J. Microsc.* 218, 185–192, 2005; Buehler, P.W., Boykins, R.A., Jia, Y. et al., Structural and functional characterization of glutaraldehyde-polymerized bovine hemoglobin and its isolated fractions, *Anal. Chem.* 77, 3466–3478, 2005; Kim, S.S., Lim, S.H., Cho, S.W. et al., Tissue engineering of heart valves by recellularization of glutaraldehyde-fixed porcine values using bone marrow-derived cells, *Exp. Mol. Med.* 38, 273–283, 2006.

Glutathione	γ-GluCysGly	307.32	Reducing agent; intermediate in phase II detoxification of xenobiotics.

Arias, I.M. and Jakoby, W.B., *Glutathione, Metabolism and Function*, Raven Press, New York, 1976; Meister, A., *Glutamate, Glutamine, Glutathione, and Related Compounds*, Academic Press, Orlando, FL, 1985; Sies, H. and Ketterer, B., *Glutathione Conjugation: Mechanisms and Biological Significance*, Academic Press, London, UK, 1988; Tsumoto, K., Shinoki, K., Kondo, H. et al., Highly efficient recovery of functional single-chain Fv fragments from inclusion bodies overexpressed in *Escherichia coli* by controlled introduction of oxidizing reagent — application to a human single-chain Fv fragment, *J. Immunol. Methods* 219, 119–129, 1998; Jiang, X., Ookubo, Y., Fujii, I. et al., Expression of Fab fragment of catalytic antibody 6D9 in an *Escherichia coli in vitro* coupled transcription/translation system, *FEBS Lett.* 514, 290–294, 2002; Sun, X.X., Vinci, C., Makmura, L. et al., Formation of disulfide bond in p53 correlates with inhibition of DNA binding and tetramerization, *Antioxid. Redox Signal.* 5, 655–665, 2003; Sies, H. and Packer, L., Eds., *Glutathione Transferases and Gamma-Glutamyl Transpeptidases*, Elsevier, Amsterdam, 2005; Smith, A.D. and Dawson, H., Glutathione is required for efficient production of infectious picornativur virions, *Virology*, 353, 258–267, 2006.

Glycine	Aminoacetic Acid	75.07	Buffer component; protein-precipitating agent, excipient for pharmaceutical formulation.

CHEMICALS COMMONLY USED IN BIOCHEMISTRY AND MOLECULAR BIOLOGY AND THEIR PROPERTIES (Continued)

Common Name	Chemical Name	M.W.	Properties and Comment

Sarquis, J.L. and Adams, E.T., Jr., The temperature-dependent self-association of beta-lactoglobulin C in glycine buffers, *Arch. Biochem. Biophys.* 163, 442–452, 1974; Poduslo, J.F., Glycoprotein molecular-weight estimation using sodium dodecyl suflate-pore gradient electrophoresis: comparison of Tris-glycine and Tris-borate-EDTA buffer systems, *Anal. Biochem.* 114, 131–139, 1981; Patton, W.F., Chung-Welch, N., Lopez, M.F. et al., Tris-tricine and Tris-borate buffer systems provide better estimates of human mesothelial cell intermediate filament protein molecular weights than the standard Tris-glycine system, *Anal. Biochem.* 197, 25–33, 1991; Trasltas, G. and Ford, C.H., Cell membrane antigen-antibody complex dissociation by the widely used glycine-HC1 method: an unreliable procedure for studying antibody internalization, *Immunol. Invest.* 22, 1–12, 1993; Nail, S.L., Jiang, S., Chongprasert, S., and Knopp, S.A., Fundamentals of freeze-drying, *Pharm. Biotechnol.* 14, 281–360, 2002; Pyne, A., Chatterjee, K., and Suryanarayanan, R., Solute crystallization in mannitol-glycine systems — implications on protein stabilization in freeze-dried formulations, *J. Pharm. Sci.* 92, 2272–2283, 2003; Hasui, K., Takatsuka, T., Sakamoto, R. et al., Double immunostaining with glycine treatment, *J. Histochem. Cytochem.* 51, 1169–1176, 2003; Hachmann, J.P. and Amshey, J.W., Models of protein modification in Tris-glycine and neutral pH Bis-Tris gels during electrophoresis: effect of gel pH, *Anal. Biochem.* 342, 237–245, 2005.

Glyoxal   Ethanedial   58.04   Modification of proteins and nucleic acids; model for glycation reaction; fluorescent derivates formed with tryptophan.

Nakaya, K., Takenaka, O., Horinishi, H., and Shibata, K., Reactions of glyoxal with nucleic acids. Nucleotides and their component bases, *Biochim. Biophys. Acta* 161, 23–31, 1968; Canella, M. and Sodini, G., The reaction of horse-liver alcohol dehydrogenase with glyoxal, *Eur. J. Biochem.* 59, 119–125, 1975; Kai, M., Kojima, E., Okhura, Y., and Iwaski, M., High-performance liquid chromatography of N-terminal tryptophan-containing peptides with precolumn fluorescence derivatization with glyoxal, *J. Chromatog. A.* 653, 235–250, 1993; Murata-Kamiya, N., Kamiya, H., Kayi, H., and Kasai, H., Glyoxal, a major product of DNA oxidation, induces mutations at G:C sites on a shuttle vector plasmid replicated in mammalian cells, *Nucleic Acids Res.* 25, 1897–1902, 1997; Leng, F., Graves, D., and Chaires, J.B., Chemical crosslinking of ethidium to DNA by glyoxal, *Biochim. Biophys. Acta* 1442, 71–81, 1998; Thrornalley, P.J., Langborg, A., and Minhas, H.S., Formation of glyoxal, methylglyoxal, and 3-deoxyglucosone in the glycation of proteins by glucose, *Biochem. J.* 344, 109–116, 1999; Sady, C., Jiang, C.L., Chellan, P. et al., Maillard reactions by alpha-oxoaldehydes: detection of glyoxal-modified proteins, *Biochim. Biophys. Acta* 1481, 255–264, 2000; Olsen, R., Molander P., Ovrebo, S. et al., Reaction of glyoxal with 2′-deoxyguanosine, 2′-deoxyadenosine, 2′-deoxycytidine, cytidine, thymidine, and calf thymus DNA: identification of the DNA adducts, *Chem. Res. Toxicol.* 18, 730–739, 2005; Manini, P., La Pietra, P., Panzella, L. et al., Glyoxal formation by Fenton-induced degradation of carbohydrates and related compounds, *Carbohydr. Res.* 341, 1828–1833, 2006.

Guanidine   Aminomethanamidine   59.07   Chaotropic agent; guanidine hydrochloride use
Guanidine Hydrochloride (GuCl)   95.53   for study of protein denaturation; GTIC is
Guanidine Thiocyanate (GTIC)   118.16   considered to be more effective than GuCl; GTIC used for nucleic acid extraction.

pKa ~ 12.5

Hill, R.L., Schwartz, H.C., and Smith, E.L., The effect of urea and guanidine hydrochloride on activity and optical rotation of crystalline papain, *J. Biol. Chem.* 234, 572–576, 1959; Appella, E. and Markert, C.L., Dissociation of lactate dehydrogenase into subunits with guanidine hydrochloride, *Biochem. Biophys. Res. Commun.* 6, 171–176, 1961; von Hippel, P.H. and Wong, K.-Y., On the conformational stability of globular proteins. The effects of various electrolytes and nonelectrolytes on the thermal transition ribonuclease transition, *J. Biol. Chem.* 240, 3909–3923, 1965; Katz, S., Partial molar volume and conformational changes produced by the denaturation of albumin by guanidine hydrochloride, *Biochim. Biophys. Acta* 154, 468–477, 1968; Shortle, D., Guanidine hydrochloride denaturation studies of mutant forms of staphylococcal nuclease, *J. Cell Biochem.* 30, 281–289, 1986; Lippke, J.A., Strzempko, M.N., Rai, F.F. et al., Isolation of intact high-molecular-weight DNA by using guanidine isothiocyanate, *Appl. Environ. Microbiol.* 53, 2588–2589, 1987; Alberti, S. and Fornaro, M., Higher transfection efficiency of genomic DNA purified with a guanidinium thiocyanate–based procedure, *Nucleic Acids Res.* 18, 351–353, 1990; Shirley, B.A., Urea and guanidine hydrochloride denaturation curves, *Methods Mol. Biol.* 40, 177–190, 1995; Cota, E. and Clarke, J., Folding of beta-sandwich proteins: three-state transition of a fibronectin type III module, *Protein Sci.* 9, 112–120, 2000; Kok, T., Wati, S., Bayly, B. et al., Comparison of six nucleic

CHEMICALS COMMONLY USED IN BIOCHEMISTRY AND MOLECULAR BIOLOGY AND THEIR PROPERTIES (Continued)

Common Name	Chemical Name	M.W.	Properties and Comment

acid extraction methods for detection of viral DNA or RNA sequences in four different non-serum specimen types, *J. Clin. Virol.* 16, 59–63, 2000; Salamanca, S., Villegas, V., Vendrell, J. et al., The unfolding pathway of leech carboxypeptidase inhibitor, *J. Biol. Chem.* 277, 17538–17543, 2002; Bhuyan, A.K., Protein stabilization by urea and guanidine hydrochloride, *Biochemistry* 41, 13386–13394, 2002; Jankowska, E., Wiczk, W., and Grzonka, Z., Thermal and guanidine hydrochloride-induced denaturation of human cystatin C, *Eur. Biophys. J.* 33, 454–461, 2004; Fuertes, M.A., Perez, J.M., and Alonso, C., Small amounts of urea and guanidine hydrochloride can be detected by a far-UV spectrophotometric method in dialyzed protein solutions, *J. Biochem. Biophys. Methods* 59, 209–216, 2004; Berlinck, R.G., Natural guanidine derivatives, *Nat. Prod. Rep.* 22, 516–550, 2005; Rashid, F., Sharma, S., and Bano, B., Comparison of guanidine hydrochloride (GdnHCl) and urea denaturation on inactivation and unfolding of human placental cystatin (HPC), *Biophys. J.* 91, 686–693, 2006; Nolan, R.L. and Teller, J.K., Diethylamine extraction of proteins and peptides isolated with a mono-phasic solution of phenol and guanidine isothiocyanate, *J. Biochem. Biophys. Methods* 68, 127–131, 2006.

Common Name	Chemical Name	M.W.	Properties and Comment
Hydrazine	N_2H_4	32.05	Reducing agent; modification of aldehydes and carbohydrates; hydrazinolysis used for release of carbohydrates from protein; derivatives such as dinitrophenyl-hydrazine used for analysis of carbonyl groups in oxidized proteins; detection of acetyl and formyl groups in proteins.

Schmer, G. and Kreil, G., Micro method for detection of formyl and acetyl groups in proteins, *Anal. Biochem.* 29, 186–192, 1969; Gershoni, J.M., Bayer, E.A., and Wilchek, M., Blot analyses of glycoconjugates: enzyme-hydrazine — a novel reagent for the detection of aldehydes, *Anal. Biochem.* 146, 59–63, 1985; O'Neill, R.A., Enzymatic release of oligosaccharides from glycoproteins for chromatographic and electrophoretic analysis, *J. Chromatog. A* 720, 201–215, 1996; Routier, F.H., Hounsell, E.F., and Rudd, P.M., Quantitation of the oligosaccharides of human serum IgG from patients with rheumatoid arthritis: a critical evaluation of different methods, *J. Immunol. Methods* 213, 113–130, 1998; Robinson, C.E., Keshavarzian, A., Pasco, D.S. et al., Determination of protein carbonyl groups by immunoblotting, *Anal. Biochem.* 266, 48–57, 1999; Merry, A.H., Neville, D.C., Royle, L. et al., Recovery of intact 2-aminobenzamide-labeled *O*-glycans released from glycoproteins by hydrazinolysis, *Anal. Biochem.* 304, 91–99, 2002; Vinograd, E., Lindner, B., and Seltmann, G., Lipopolysaccharides from *Serratia maracescens* possess one or two 4-amino-4-deoxy-L-arabinopyranose 1-phosphate residues in the lipid A and D-*glycero*-D-*talo*-Oct-ulopyranosonic acid in the inner core region, *Chemistry* 12, 6692–6700, 2006.

Common Name	Chemical Name	M.W.	Properties and Comment
Hydrogen Peroxide	H_2O_2	34.02	Oxidizing agent; bacteriocidal agent.
Hydroxylamine	H_3NO	33.03	
8-Hydroxyquinoline 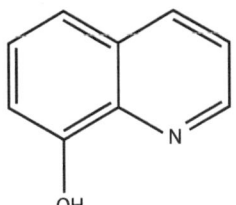	8-quinolinol	145.16	Metal chelator.
Imidazole 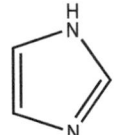	1,3-diazole	69.08	Buffer component.
2-Iminothiolane 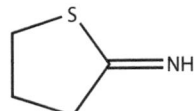	Traut's Reagent (earlier as methyl-4-mercaptobutyrimidate)	137.63	Introduction of sulfhydryl group by modification of amino group; sulfhydryl groups could then be oxidized to form cystine, which served as cleavable protein crosslink.

CHEMICALS COMMONLY USED IN BIOCHEMISTRY AND MOLECULAR BIOLOGY AND THEIR PROPERTIES (Continued)

Common Name	Chemical Name	M.W.	Properties and Comment

Traut, R.R., Bollen, A., Sun, T.-T. et al., Methyl-4-mercaptobutyrimidate as a cleavable crosslinking reagent and its application to the *Escherichia coli* 30S ribosome, *Biochemistry* 12, 3266–3273, 1973; Schram, H.J. and Dulffer, T., The use of 2-iminothiolane as a protein crosslinking reagent, *Hoppe Seylers Z. Physiol.Chem.* 358, 137–139, 1977; Jue, R., Lambert, J.M., Pierce, L.R., and Traut, R.R., Addition of sulfhydryl groups *Escherichia coli* ribosomes by protein modification with 2-iminothiolane (methyl 4-mercaptobutyrimidate), *Biochemistry* 17, 5399–5406, 1978; Lambert, J.M., Jue, R., and Traut, R.R., Disulfide crosslinking of *Escherichia coli* ribosomal proteins with 2-iminothiolane (methyl 4-mercaptobutyrimidate): evidence that the crosslinked protein pairs are formed in the intact ribosomal subunit, *Biochemistry* 17, 5406–5416, 1978; Alagon, A.C. and King, T.P., Activation of polysaccharides with 2-iminothiolane and its use, *Biochemistry* 19, 4341–4345, 1980; Tolan, D.R. and Traut, R.R., Protein topography of the 40 S ribosomal subunit from rabbit reticulocytes shown by crosslinking with 2-iminothiolane, *J. Biol. Chem.* 256, 10129–10136, 1981; Boileau, G., Butler, P., Hershey, J.W., and Traut, R.R., Direct crosslinks between initiation factors 1, 2, and 3 and ribosomal proteins promoted by 2-iminothiolane, *Biochemistry* 22, 3162–3170, 1983; Kyriatsoulis, A., Maly, P., Greuer, B. et al., RNA-protein crosslinking in *Escherichia coli* ribosomal subunits: localization of sites on 16S RNA which are crosslinked to proteins S17 and S21 by treatment with 2-iminothiolane, *Nucleic Acids Res.* 14, 1171–1186, 1986; Uchiumi, T., Kikuchi, M., and Ogata, K., Crosslinking study on protein neighborhoods at the subunit interface of rat liver ribosomes with 2-iminothiolane, *J. Biol. Chem.* 261, 9663–9667, 1986; McCall, M.J., Diril, H., and Meares, C.F., Simplified method for conjugating macrocyclic bifunctional chelating agents to antibodies via 2-iminothiolane, *Bioconjug. Chem.* 1, 222–226, 1990; Tarentino, A.L., Phelan, A.W., and Plummer, T.H., Jr., 2-iminothiolane: a reagent for the introduction of sulphydryl groups into oligosaccharides derived from asaparagine-linked glycans, *Glycobiology* 3, 279–285, 1993; Singh, R., Kats, L., Blattler, W.A., and Lambert, J.M., Formation of *N*-substituted 2-iminothiolanes when amino groups in proteins and peptides are modified by 2-iminothiolanes, *Anal. Biochem.* 236, 114–125, 1996; Hosono, M.N., Hosono, M., Mishra, A.K. et al., Rhenium-188-labeled anti-neural cell adhesion molecule antibodies with 2-iminothiolane modification for targeting small-cell lung cancer, *Ann. Nucl. Med.* 14, 173–179, 2000; Mokotoff, M., Mocarski, Y.M., Gentsch, B.L. et al., Caution in the use of 2-iminothiolane (Traut's reagent) as a crosslinking agent for peptides. The formation of *N*-peptidyl-2-iminothiolanes with bombesin (BN) antagonists (D-trp[6]-leu13-ψ[CH$_2$NH]-Phe[14]BN$_{6-14}$ and D-trp- gln-trp-NH$_2$, *J. Pept. Res.* 57, 383–389, 2001; Kuzuhara, A., Protein structural changes in keratin fibers induced by chemical modification using 2-iminothiolane hydrochloride: a Raman spectroscopic investigation, *Biopolymers* 79, 173–184, 2005.

Indole

	2,3-benzopyrrole	117.15	

Indole-3-acetic Acid

	Indoleacetic Acid; Heteroauxin	175.19	Plant growth regulator.

Kawaguchi, M. and Syono, K., The excessive production of indole-3-acetic and its significance in studies of the biosynthesis of this regulator of plant growth and development, *Plant Cell Physiol.* 37, 1043–1048, 1996; Normanly, J. and Bartel, B., Redundancy as a way of life-IAA metabolism, *Curr. Opin. Plant Biol.* 2, 207–213, 1999; Leyser, O., Auxin signaling: the beginning, the middle, and the end, *Curr. Opin. Plant Biol.* 4, 382–386, 2001; Ljung, K., Hull, A.K., Kowalczyk, M. et al., Biosynthesis, conjugation, catabolism, and homeostasis of indole-3-acetic acid in *Arabidopsis thaliana*, *Plant Mol. Biol.* 49, 249–272, 2002; Kawano, T. Roles of the reactive oxygen species-generating peroxidase reactions in plant defense and growth induction, *Plant Cell Rep.* 21, 829–837, 2003; Aloni, R., Aloni, E., Langhans, M., and Ullrich, C.I., Role of cytokine and auxin in shaping root architecture: regulating vascular differentiation, lateral root initiation, root apical dominance, and root gravitropism, *Ann. Bot.* 97, 882–893, 2006.

Iodoacetamide

	2-iodoacetamide	184.96	Alkylating agents that react with a variety of nucleophiles in proteins and nucleic acids. Reaction is more rapid than the bromo or chloro derivatives.

CHEMICALS COMMONLY USED IN BIOCHEMISTRY AND MOLECULAR BIOLOGY AND THEIR PROPERTIES (Continued)

Common Name	Chemical Name	M.W.	Properties and Comment
Iodoacetic Acid		185.95	

The amide is neutral and is not susceptible to either positive or negative influence from locally charged groups; iodoacetamide is frequently used to modify sulfhydryl groups as part of reduction and carboxymethylation prior to structural analysis. Crestfield, A.M., Moore, S., and Stein, W.H., The preparation and enzymatic hydrolysis of reduced and S-carboxymethylated proteins, *J. Biol. Chem.* 238, 622–627, 1963; Watts, D.C., Rabin, B.R., and Crook, E.M., The reaction of iodoacetate and iodoacetamide with proteins as determined with a silver/silver iodide electrode, *Biochim. Biophys. Acta* 48, 380–388, 1961; Inagami, T., The alkylation of the active site of trypsin with iodoacetamide in the presence of alkylguanidines, *J. Biol. Chem.* 240, PC3453–PC3455, 1965; Fruchter, R.G. and Crestfield, A.M., The specific alkylation by iodoacetamide of histidine-12 in the active site of ribonuclease, *J. Biol. Chem.* 242, 5807–5812, 1967; Takahashi, K., The structure and function of ribonuclease T. X. Reactions of iodoacetate, iodoacetamide, and related alkylating reagents with ribonuclease T, *J. Biochem.* 68, 517–527, 1970; Whitney, P.L., Inhibition and modification of human carbonic anhydrase B with bromoacetate and iodoacetate, *Eur. J. Biochem.* 16, 126–135, 1970; Harada, M. and Irie, M., Alkylation of ribonuclease from *Aspirgillus saitoi* with iodoacetate and iodoacetamide, *J. Biochem.* 73, 705–716, 1973; Halasz, P. and Polgar, L., Effect of the immediate microenvironment on the reactivity of the essential SH group of papain, *Eur. J. Biochem.* 71, 571–575, 1976; Franzen, J.S., Ishman, P., and Feingold, D.S., Half-of-the-sites reactivity of bovine liver uridine diphosphoglucose dehydrogenase toward iodoacetate and iodoacetamide, *Biochemistry* 15, 5665–5671, 1976; David, M., Rasched, I.R., and Sund, H., Studies of glutamate dehydrogenase. Methionione-169: the preferentially carboxymethylated residue, *Eur. J. Biochem.* 74, 379–385, 1977; Ohgi, K., Watanabe, H., Emman, K. et al., Alkylation of a ribonuclease from *Streptomyces erthreus* with iodoacetate and iodoacetamide, *J. Biochem.* 90, 113–123, 1981; Dahl, K.H. and McKinley-McKee, J.S., Enzymatic catalysis in the affinity labeling of liver alcohol dehydrogenase with haloacids, *Eur. J. Biochem.* 118, 507–513, 1981; Syvertsen, C. and McKinley-McKee, J.S., Binding of ligands to the catalytic zinc ion in horse liver alcohol dehydrogenase, *Arch. Biochem. Biophys.* 228, 159–169, 1984; Communi, D. and Erneux, C., Identification of an active site cysteine residue in type Ins(1,4,5)P[3]5-phosphatase by chemical modification and site-directed mutagenesis, *Biochem. J.* 320, 181–186, 1996; Sarkany, Z., Skern, T., and Polgar, L., Characterization of the active site thiol group of rhinovirus 21 proteinase, *FEBS Lett.* 481, 289–292, 2000; Lundblad, R.L., *Chemical Reagents for Protein Modification*, CRC Press, Boca Raton, FL, 2004.

Isatoic Anhydride	3,1-benzoxazine-2,4(1*H*)-dione	163.13	Fluorescent reagents for amines and sulfydryl groups; amine scavenger.

Gelb, M.H. and Abeles, R.H., Substituted isatoic anhydrides: selective inactivators of trypsinlike serine proteases, *J. Med. Chem.* 29, 585–589, 1986; Gravett, P.S., Viljoen, C.C., and Oosthuizen, M.M., Inactivation of arginine esterase E-1 of *Bitis gabonica* venom by irreversible inhibitors including a water-soluble carbodiimide, a chloromethyl ketone, and isatoic anhydride, *Int. J. Biochem.* 23, 1101–1110, 1991; Servillo, L., Balestrieri, C., Quagliuolo, L. et al.,tRNA fluorescent labeling at 3' end including an aminoacyl-tRNA-like behavior, *Eur. J. Biochem.* 213, 583–589, 1993; Churchich, J.E., Fluorescence properties of o-aminobenzoyl-labeled proteins, *Anal. Biochem.* 213, 229–233, 1993; Brown, A.D. and Powers, J.C., Rates of thrombin acylation and deacylation upon reaction with low molecular weight acylating agents, carbamylating agents, and carbonylating agents, *Bioorg. Med. Chem.* 3, 1091–1097, 1995; Matos, M.A., Miranda, M.S., Morais, V.M., and Liebman, J.F., Are isatin and isatoic anhydride antiaromatic and aromatic, respectively? A combined experimental and theoretic investigation, *Org. Biomol. Chem.* 1, 2566–2571, 2003; Matos, M.A., Miranda, M.S., Morais, V.M., and Liebman, J.F., The energetics of isomeric benzoxazine diones: isatoic anhydride revisited, *Org. Biomol. Chem.* 2, 1647–1650, 2004; Raturi, A., Vascratsis, P.O., Seslija, D. et al., A direct, continuous, sensitive assay for protein disulphide-isomerase based on fluorescence self-quenching, *Biochem. J.* 391, 351–357, 2005; Zhang, W., Lu, Y., and Nagashima, T., Plate-to-plate fluorous solid-phase extraction for solution-phase parallel synthesis, *J. Comb. Chem.* 7, 893–897, 2005.

Isoamyl Alcohol	Isopentyl Alcohol; 3-methyl-1-butanol	88.15	Solvent.

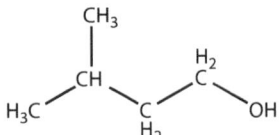

CHEMICALS COMMONLY USED IN BIOCHEMISTRY AND MOLECULAR BIOLOGY AND THEIR PROPERTIES (Continued)

Common Name	Chemical Name	M.W.	Properties and Comment
Isopropanol	2-propanol	60.10	Solvent; precipitation agent for purification of plasmid DNA; reagent in stability test for identification of abnormal hemoglobins.

CH₃ structure (2-propanol)

Brosious, E.M., Morrison, B.Y., and Schmidt, R.M., Effects of hemoglobin F levels, KCN, and storage on the isopropanol precipitation test for unstable hemoglobins, *Am. J. Clin. Pathol.* 66, 878–882, 1976; Bensinger, T.A. and Beutler, E., Instability of the oxy form of sickle hemoglobin and of methemoglobin in isopropanol, *Am. J. Clin. Pathol.* 67, 180–183, 1977; Acree, W.E., Jr. and Bertrand, G.L., A cholesterol-isopropanol gel, *Nature* 269, 450, 1977; Naoum, P.C. Teixeira, U.A., de Abreu Machado, P.E., and Michelin, O.C., The denaturation of human oxyhemoglobin A, A2, and S by isopropanol/buffer method, *Rev. Bras. Pesqui. Med. Biol.* 11, 241–244, 1978; Ali, M.A., Quinlan, A., and Wong, S.C., Identification of hemoglobin E by the isopropanol solubility test, *Clin. Biochem.* 13, 146–148, 1980; Horer, O.L. and Enache, C., 2-propanol dependent RNA absorbances, *Virologie* 34, 257–272, 1983; De Venditis, E., Masullo, M., and Bocchini, V., The elongation factor G carries a catalytic site for GTP hydrolysis, which is revealed by using 2-propanol in the absence of ribosomes, *J. Biol. Chem.* 261, 4445–4450, 1986; Wang, L., Hirayasu, K., Ishizawa, M., and Kobayashi, Y., Purification of genomic DNA from human whole blood by isopropanol-fractionation with concentrated NaI and SDS, *Nucleic Acids Res.* 22, 1774–1775, 1994; Dalhus, B. and Gorbitz, C.H., Glycyl-L-leucyl-L-tyrosine dehydrate 2-propanol solvate, *Acta Crystallogr. C* 52, 2087–2090, 1996; Freitas, S.S., Santos, J.A., and Prazeres, D.M., Optimization of isopropanol and ammonium sulfate precipitation steps in the purification of plasmid DNA, *Biotechnol. Prog.* 22, 1179–1186, 2006; Halano, B., Kubo, D., and Tagaya, H., Study on the reactivity of diarylmethane derivatives in supercritical alcohols media: reduction of diarylmethanols and diaryl ketones to diarylmethanes using supercritical 2-propanol, *Chem. Pharm. Bull.* 54, 1304–1307, 2006.

Isopropyl-β-D-thiogalactoside	IPTG, Isopropyl-β-D-thiogalactopyroa-noside	238.3	"Gratuitous" inducer of the *lac* operon.

(IPTG structure)

Cho, S., Scharpf, S., Franko, M., and Vermeulen, C.W., Effect of isopropyl-β-D-galactoside concentration on the level of *lac*-operon induction in steady state *Escherichia coli, Biochem. Biophys. Res. Commun.* 128, 1268–1273, 1985; Carlsson, U., Ferskgard, P.O., and Svensson, S.C., A simple and efficient synthesis of the induced IPTG made for inexpensive heterologous protein production using the *lac*-promoter, *Protein Eng.* 4, 1019–1020, 1991; Donovan, R.S., Robinson, C.W., and Glick, B.R., Review: optimizing inducer and culture conditions for expression of foreign proteins under control of the *lac* promoter, *J. Ind. Microbiol.* 16, 145–154, 1996; Hansen, L.H., Knudsen, S., and Sorensen, S.J., The effect of the lacy gene on the induction of IPTG-inducible promoters, studied in *Escherichia coli* and *Pseudomonas fluorescens, Curr. Microbiol.* 36, 341–347, 1998; Teich, A., Lin, H.Y., Andersson, L. et al., Amplification of ColE1 related plasmids in recombinant cultures of *Escherichia coli* after IPTG induction, *J. Biotechnol.* 64, 197–210, 1998; Ren, A. and Schaefer, T.S., Isopropyl-β-D-thiogalactoside (IPTG)-inducible tyrosine phosphorylation of proteins in *E. coli, Biotechniques* 31, 1254–1258, 2001; Ko, K.S., Kruse, J., and Pohl, N.L., Synthesis of isobutryl-C-galactoside (IBCG) as an isopropylthiogalactoside (IPTG) substitute for increased induction of protein expression, *Org. Lett.* 5, 1781–1783, 2003; Intasai, N., Arooncharus, P., Kasinrerk, W., and Tayapiwatana, C., Construction of high-density display of CD147 ectodomain on VCSM13 phage via gpVIII: effects of temperature, IPTG, and helper phage infection-period, *Protein Expr. Purif.* 32, 323–331, 2003; Faulkner, E., Barrett, M., Okor, S. et al., Use of fed-batch cultivation for achieving high cell densities for the pilot-scale production of a recombinant protein (phenylalanine dehydrogenase) in *Escherichia coli, Biotechnol. Prog.* 22, 889–897, 2006; Gardete, S., de Laencastre, H., and Tomasz, A., A link in transcription between the native pbpG and the acquired mecA gene in a strain of *Staphylococcus aureus, Microbiology* 152, 2549–2558, 2006; Hewitt, C.J., Onyeaka, H., Lewis, G. et al., A comparison of high cell density fed-batch fermentations involving both induced and noninduced recombinant *Escherichia coli* under well-mixed small-scale and simulated poorly mixed large-scale conditions, *Biotechnol. Bioeng.*, in press, 2006; Picaud, S., Olsson, M.E., and Brodelius, P.E., Improved conditions for production of recombinant plant sesquiterpene synthases in *Escherichia coli, Protein Expr. Purif.*, in press, 2006.

CHEMICALS COMMONLY USED IN BIOCHEMISTRY AND MOLECULAR BIOLOGY AND THEIR PROPERTIES (Continued)

Common Name	Chemical Name	M.W.	Properties and Comment
Maleic Anhydride	2,5-furandione	98.06	Modification of amino groups in proteins. The dimethyl derivative (dimethylmaleic anhydride) is used for ribosome dissociation; monomer for polymer.

Giese, R.W. and Vallee, B.L., Metallocenes. A novel class of reagents for protein modification. I. Maleic anhydride-iron tetracarbonyl, *J. Am. Chem. Soc.* 94, 6199–6200, 1972; Cantrell, M. and Craven, G.R., Chemical inactivation of *Escherichia coli* 30 S ribosomes with maleic anhydride: identification of the proteins involved in polyuridylic acid binding, *J. Mol. Biol.* 115, 389–402, 1977; Jordano, J., Montero, F., and Palacian, E., Relaxation of chromatin structure upon removal of histones H2A and H2B, *FEBS Lett.* 172, 70–74, 1984; Jordano, J., Montero, F., and Palacian, E., Rearrangement of nucleosomal components by modification of histone amino groups. Structural role of lysine residues, *Biochemistry* 23, 4280–4284, 1984; Palacian, E., Gonzalez, P.J., Pineiro, M., and Hernandez, F., Dicarboxylic acid anhydrides as dissociating agents of protein-containing structures, *Mol. Cell. Biochem.* 97, 101–111, 1990; Paetzel, M., Strynadka, N.C., Tschantz, W.R. et al., Use of site-directed chemical modification to study an essential lysine in *Escherichia coli* leader peptidase, *J. Biol. Chem.* 272, 9994–10003, 1997; Wink, M.R., Buffon, A., Bonan, C.D. et al., Effect of protein-modifying reagents on ecto-apyrase from rat brain, *Int. J. Biochem. Cell Biol.* 32, 105–113, 2000.

Common Name	Chemical Name	M.W.	Properties and Comment
2-Mercaptoethanol	β-mercaptoethanol	78.13	Reducing agent; used frequently in the reduction and alkylation of proteins for structural analysis and for preservation of oxidation-sensitive enzymes.

Geren, C.R., Olomon, C.M., Jones, T.T., and Ebner, D.E., 2-mercaptoethanol as a substrate for liver alcohol dehydrogenase, *Arch. Biochem. Biophys.* 179, 415–419, 1977; Opitz, H.G., Lemke, H, and Hewlett, G., Activation of T-cells by a macrophage or 2-mercaptoethanol-activated serum factor is essential for induction of a primary immune response to heterologous red cells *in vitro*, *Immunol. Rev.* 40, 53–77, 1978; Burger, M., An absolute requirement for 2-mercaptoethanol in the *in vitro* primary immune response in the absence of serum, *Immunology* 37, 669–671, 1979; Nealon, D.A., Pettit, S.M., and Henderson, A.R., Diluent pH and the stability of the thiol group in monothioglycerol, *N*-acetyl-L-cysteine, and 2-mercaptoethanol, *Clin. Chem.* 27, 505–506, 1981; Dahl, K.H. and McKinley-McKee, J.S., Enzymatic catalysis in the affinity labeling of liver alcohol dehydrogenase with haloacids, *Eur. J. Biochem.* 118, 507–513, 1981; Righetti, P.G., Tudor, G., and Glanazza, E., Effect of 2-mercaptoethanol on pH gradients in isoelectric focusing, *J. Biochem. Biophys. Methods* 6, 219–227, 1982; Soderberg, L.S. and Yeh, N.H., T-cells and the anti-trinitrophenyl antibody response to fetal calf serum and 2-mercaptoethanol, *Proc. Soc. Exp. Biol. Med.* 174, 107–113, 1983; Ochs, D., Protein contaminants of sodium dodecyl sulfate-polyacrylamide gels, *Anal. Biochem.* 135, 470–474, 1983; Schaefer, W.H., Harris, T.M., and Guengerich, F.P., Reaction of the model thiol 2-mercaptoethanol and glutathione with methylvinylmaleimide, a Michael acceptor with extended conjugation, *Arch. Biochem. Biophys.* 257, 186–193, 1987; Obiri, N. and Pruett, S.B., The role of thiols in lymphocyte responses: effect of 2-mercaptoethanol on interleukin 2 production, *Immunobiology* 176, 440–449, 1988; Gourgerot-Pocidalo, M.A., Fay, M., Roche, Y., and Chollet-Martin, S., Mechanisms by which oxidative injury inhibits the proliferative response of human lymphocytes to PHA. Effect of the thiol compound 2-mercaptoethanol, *Immunology* 64, 281–288, 1988; Fong, T.C. and Makinodan, T., Preferential enhancement by 2-mercaptoethanol of IL-2 responsiveness of T blast cells from old over young mice is associated with potentiated protein kinase C translocation, *Immunol. Lett.* 20, 149–154, 1989; De Graan, P.N., Moritz, A., de Wit, M., and Gispen, W.H., Purification of B-50 by 2-mercaptoethanol extraction from rat brain synaptosomal plasma membranes, *Neurochem. Res.* 18, 875–881, 1993; Carrithers, S.L. and Hoffman, J.L., Sequential methylation of 2-mercaptoenthanol to the dimethyl sulfonium ion, 2-(dimethylthio)ethanol, *in vivo* and *in vitro*, *Biochem. Pharmacol.* 48, 1017–1024, 1994; Paul-Pretzer, K. and Parness, J., Elimination of keratin contaminant from 2-mercaptoethanol, *Anal. Biochem.* 289, 98–99, 2001; Adebiyi, A.P., Jin, D.H, Ogawa, T., and Muramoto, K., Acid hydrolysis of protein in a microcapillary tube for the recovery of tryptophan, *Biosci. Biotechnol. Biochem.* 69, 255–257, 2005; Adams, B., Lowpetch, K., Throndycroft, F. et al., Stereochemistry of reactions of the inhibitor/substrates L- and D-β-chloroalanine with β-mercaptoethanol catalyzed by L-aspartate aminotransferase and D-amino acid amino-transferase, respectively, *Org. Biomol. Chem.* 3, 3357–3364, 2005; Layeyre, M., Leprince, J., Massonneau, M. et al., Aryldithioethyloxycarbonyl (Ardec): a new family of amine-protecting groups removable under mild reducing conditions and their applications to peptide synthesis, *Chemistry* 12, 3655–3671, 2006; Okun, I., Malarchuk, S., Dubrovskaya, E. et al., Screening for caspace-3 inhibitors: effect of a reducing agent on the identified hit chemotypes, *J. Biomol. Screen.* 11, 694–703, 2006; Aminian, M., Sivam, S., Lee, C.W. et al., Expression and purification of a trivalent pertussis toxin-diphtheria toxin-tetanus toxin fusion protein in *Escherichia coli*, *Protein Expr. Purif.* 51, 170–178, 2006.

Common Name	Chemical Name	M.W.	Properties and Comment
(3-Mercaptopropyl)trimethoxysilane	3-(trimethoxysilyl)-1-propanethiol	196.34	Introduction of reactive sulfhydryl onto glass (silane) surface.

CHEMICALS COMMONLY USED IN BIOCHEMISTRY AND MOLECULAR BIOLOGY AND THEIR PROPERTIES (Continued)

Common Name	Chemical Name	M.W.	Properties and Comment

Jung, S.K. and Wilson, G.S., Polymeric mercaptosilane-modified platinum electrodes for elimination of interferants in glucose biosensors, *Anal. Chem.* 68, 591–596, 1996; Mansur, H.S., Lobato, Z.P., Orefice, R.L. et al., Surface functionalization of porous glass networks: effects on bovine serum albumin and porcine insulin immobilization, *Biomacromolecules* 1, 479–497, 2000; Kumar, A., Larsson, O., Parodi, D., and Liang, Z., Silanized nucleic acids: a general platform for DNA immobilization, *Nucleic Acids Res.* 28, E71, 2000; Zhang, F., Kang, E.T., Neoh, K.G. et al., Surface modification of stainless steel by grafting of poly(ethylene glycol) for reduction in protein adsorption, *Biomaterials* 22, 1541–1548, 2001; Jia, J., Wang, B., Wu, A. et al., A method to construct a third-generation horseradish peroxidase biosensor: self-assembling gold nanoparticles to three-dimensional sol-gel network, *Anal. Chem.* 74, 2217–2223, 2002; Abdelghani-Jacquin, C., Abdelghani, A., Chmel, G. et al., Decorated surfaces by biofunctionalized gold beads: application to cell adhesion studies, *Eur. Biophys. J.* 31, 102–110, 2002; Ganesan, V. and Walcarius, A., Surfactant templated sulfonic acid functionalized silica microspheres as new efficient ion exchangers and electrode modifiers, *Langmuir* 20, 3632–3640, 2004; Crudden, C.M., Sateesh, M., and Lewis, R., Mercaptopropyl-modified mesoporous silica: a remarkable support for the preparation of a reusable, heterogeneous palladium catalyst for coupling to reactions, *J. Am. Chem. Soc.* 127, 10045–10050, 2005; Yang, L., Guihen, E., and Glennon, J.D., Alkylthiol gold nanoparticles in sol-gel-based open tabular capillary electrochromatography, *J. Sep. Sci.* 28, 757–766, 2005.

Methanesulfonic Acid		96.11	Protein hydrolysis for amino acid analysis; deprotection during peptide synthesis; hydrolysis of protein substituents such as fatty acids.

Simpson, R.J., Neuberger, M.R., and Liu, T.Y., Complete amino acid analysis of proteins from a single hydrolyzate, *J. Biol. Chem.* 251, 1936–1940, 1976; Kubota, M., Hirayama, T., Nagase, O., and Yajima, H., Synthesis of two peptides corresponding to an alpha-endophin and gamma-endorphin by the methanesulfonic acid deprotecting procedures, *Chem. Pharm. Bull.* 27, 1050–1054, 1979; Yajima, H., Akaji, K., Saito, H. et al., Studies on peptides. LXXXII. Synthesis of [4-Gln]-neurotensin by the methanesulfonic acid deprotecting procedure, *Chem. Pharm. Bull.* 27, 2238–2242, 1979; Sakuri, J. and Nagahama, M. Tryptophan content of *Clostridium perfringens* epsilon toxin, *Infect. Immun.* 47, 260–263, 1985; Malmer, M.F. and Schroeder, L.A., Amino acid analysis by high-performance liquid chromatography with methanesulfonic acid hydrolysis and 9-fluorenylmethyl-chloroformate derivatization, *J. Chromatog.* 514, 227–239, 1990; Weiss, M., Manneberg, M., Juranville, J.F. et al., Effect of the hydrolysis method on the determination of the amino acid composition of proteins, *J. Chromatog. A* 795, 263–275, 1998; Okimura, K., Ohki, K., Nagai, S., and Sakura, N., HPLC analysis of fatty acyl-glycine in the aqueous methanesulfonic acid hydrolysates of N-terminally fatty acylated peptides, *Biol. Pharm. Bull.* 26, 1166–1169, 2003; Wrobel, K., Kannamkumarath, S.S., Wrobel, K., and Caruso, J.A., Hydrolysis of proteins with methanesulfonic acid for improved HPLC-ICP-MS determination of seleno-methionine in yeast and nuts, *Anal. BioAnal. Chem.* 375, 133–138, 2003.

Methanol	Methyl Alcohol	32.04	Solvent.
Methylethyl Ketone (MEK)	2-butanal; 2-butanone	72.11	Solvent; with acid for cleavage of heme moiety of hemeproteins for preparation of apoproteins.

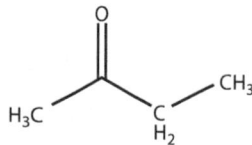

Teale, F.W., Cleavage of haem-protein link by acid methylethylketone, *Biochim. Biophys. Acta* 35, 543, 1959; Tran, C.D. and Darwent, J.R., Characterization of tetrapyridylporphyrinatozinc (II) apomyoglobin complexes as a potential photosynthetic model, *J. Chem. Soc. Faraday Trans. II*, 82, 2315–2322, 1986.

CHEMICALS COMMONLY USED IN BIOCHEMISTRY AND MOLECULAR BIOLOGY AND THEIR PROPERTIES (Continued)

Common Name	Chemical Name	M.W.	Properties and Comment
Methylglyoxal	Pyruvaldehyde; 2-oxopropanal	72.06	Derived from oxidative modification of triose phosphate during glucose metabolism; model for glycation of proteins; reacts with amino groups in proteins and nucleic acids; involved in advanced glycation endproducts.

Szabo, G., Kertesz, J.C., and Laki, K., Interaction of methylglyoxal with poly-L-lysine, *Biomaterials* 1, 27–29, 1980; McLaughlin, J.A., Pethig, R., and Szent-Gyorgyi, A., Spectroscopic studies of the protein-methylglyoxal adduct, *Proc. Natl. Acad. Sci. USA* 77, 949–951, 1980; Cooper, R.A., Metabolism of methylglyoxal in microorganisms, *Annu. Rev. Microbiol.* 38, 49–68, 1984; Richard, J.P., Mechanism for the formation of methylglyoxal from triosephosphates, *Biochem. Soc. Trans.* 21, 549–553, 1993; Riley, M.L. and Harding, J.J., The reaction of methylglyoxal with human and bovine lens proteins, *Biochim. Biophys. Acta* 1270, 36–43, 1995; Thornalley, P.J., Pharmacology of methylglyoxal: formation, modification of proteins and nucleic acids, and enzymatic detoxification — a role in pathogenesis and antiproliferative chemotherapy, *Gen. Pharmacol.* 27, 565–573, 1996; Nagaraj, R.H., Shipanova, I.N., and Faust, F.M., Protein crosslinking by the Maillard reaction. Isolation, characterization, and *in vivo* detection of a lysine–lysine crosslink derived from methylglyoxal, *J. Biol. Chem.* 271, 19338–19345, 1996; Shipanova, I.N., Glomb, M.A., and Nagaraj, R.H., Protein modification by methylglyoxal: chemical nature and synthetic mechanism of a major fluorescent adduct, *Arch. Biochem. Biophys.* 344, 29–34, 1997; Uchida, K., Khor, O.T., Oya, T. et al., Protein modification by a Maillard reaction intermediate methylglyoxal. Immunochemical detection of fluorescent 5-methylimidazolone derivatives *in vivo*, *FEBS Lett.* 410, 313–318, 1997; Degenhardt, T.P., Thorpe, S.R., and Baynes, J.W., Chemical modification of proteins by methylglyoxal, *Cell. Mol. Biol.* 44, 1139–1145, 1998; Izaguirre, G., Kikonyogo, A., and Pietruszko, R., Methylglyoxal as substrate and inhibitor of human aldehyde dehydrogenase: comparison of kinetic properties among the three isozymes, *Comp. Biochem. Physiol. B Biochem. Mol. Biol.* 119, 747–754, 1998; Lederer, M.O. and Klaiber, R.G., Crosslinking of proteins by Maillard processes: characterization and detection of lysine–arginine crosslinks derived from glyoxal and methylglyoxal, *Bioorg. Med. Chem.* 7, 2499–2507, 1999; Kalapos, M.P., Methylglyoxal in living organisms: chemistry, biochemistry, toxicology, and biological implications, *Toxicol. Lett.* 110, 145–175, 1999; Thornalley, P.J., Landborg, A., and Minhas, H.S., Formation of glyoxal, methylglyoxal, and 3-deoxyglucose in the glycation of proteins by glucose, *Biochem. J.* 344, 109–116, 1999; Nagai, R., Araki, T., Hayashi, C.M. et al., Identification of N-epsilon-(carboxyethyl)lysine, one of the methylglyoxal-derived AGE structures, in glucose-modified protein: mechanism for protein modification by reactive aldehydes, *J. Chromatog. B Analyt. Technol. Biomed. Life Sci.*788, 75–84, 2003.

Methyl Methanethiosulfonate (MMTS)	S-methyl Methanethiosulfonate	126.2	Modification of sulfhydryl groups.

Smith, D.J., Maggio, E.T., and Kenyon, G.L., Simple alkanethiol groups for temporary sulfhydryl groups of enzymes, *Biochemistry* 14, 766–771, 1975; Nishimura, J.S., Kenyon, G.L., and Smith, D.J., Reversible modification of the sulfhydryl groups of *Escherichia coli* succinic thiokinase with methanethiolating reagents, 5,5′-dithio-bis(2-nitrobenzoic acid), *p*-hydroxymercuribenzoate, and ethylmercurithiosalicylate, *Arch. Biochem. Biophys.* 170, 407–430, 1977; Bloxham, D.P., The chemical reactivity of the histidine-195 residue in lactate dehydrogenase thiomethylated at the cysteine-165 residue, *Biochem. J.* 193, 93–97, 1981; Gavilanes, F., Peterson, D., and Schirch, L., Methyl methanethiosulfate as an active site probe of serine hydroxymethyltransferase, *J. Biol. Chem.* 257, 11431–11436, 1982; Daly, T.J., Olson, J.S., and Matthews, K.S., Formation of mixed disulfide adducts as cysteine-281 of the lactose repressor protein affects operator- and inducer-binding parameters, *Biochemistry* 25, 5468–5474, 1986; Salam, W.H. and Bloxham, D.P., Identification of subsidiary catalytic groups at the active site of β-ketoacyl-CoA thiolase by covalent modification of the protein, *Biochim. Biophys. Acta* 873, 321–330, 1986; Stancato, L.F., Hutchison, K.A., Chakraborti, P.K. et al., Differential effects of the reversible thiol-reactive agents arsenite and methyl methanethiosulfonate on steroid binding by the glucocorticoid receptor, *Biochemistry* 32, 3739–3736, 1993; Hou, L.X. and Vollmer, S., The activity of *S*-thiolated modified creatine kinase is due to the regeneration of free thiol at the active site, *Biochim. Biophys. Acta* 1205, 83–88, 1994; Jensen, P.E., Shanbhag, V.P., and Stigbrand, T., Methanethiolation of the liberated cysteine residues of human α-2-macroglobulin treated with methylamine generates a derivative with similar functional characteristics as native β-2-macroglobulin, *Eur. J. Biochem.* 227, 612–616, 1995; Trimboli, A.J., Quinn, G.B., Smith, E.T., and Barber, M.J., Thiol modification and site-directed mutagenesis of the flavin domain of spinach NADH: nitrate reductase, *Arch. Biochem. Biophys.* 331, 117–126, 1996; Quinn, K.E. and Ehrlich, B.E., Methanethiosulfonate derivatives inhibits current through the rynodine receptor/channel, *J. Gen. Physiol.* 109, 225–264, 1997;

CHEMICALS COMMONLY USED IN BIOCHEMISTRY AND MOLECULAR BIOLOGY AND THEIR PROPERTIES (Continued)

Common Name	Chemical Name	M.W.	Properties and Comment

Hashimoto, M., Majima, E., Hatanaka, T. et al., Irreversible extrusion of the first loop facing the matrix of the bovine heart mitochondrial ADP/ATP carrier by labeling the Cys(56) residue with the SH-reagent methyl methanethiosulfonate, *J. Biochem.* 127, 443–449, 2000; Spelta, V., Jiang, L.H., Bailey, R.J. et al., Interaction between cysteines introduced into each transmembrane domain of the rat P2X2 receptor, *Br. J. Pharmacol.* 138, 131–136, 2003; Britto, P.J., Knipling, L., McPhie, P., and Wolff, J., Thiol-disulphide interchange in tubulin: kinetics and the effect on polymerization, *Biochem. J.* 389, 549–558, 2005; Miller, C.M., Szegedi, S.S., and Garrow, T.A., Conformation-dependent inactivation of human betaine-homocysteine *S*-methyltransferase by hydrogen peroxide *in vitro*, *Biochem. J.* 392, 443–448, 2005.

Common Name	Chemical Name	M.W.	Properties and Comment
N-Methylpyrrolidone	1-methyl-2-pyrrolidone	99.13	Polar solvent; transdermal transport of drugs.

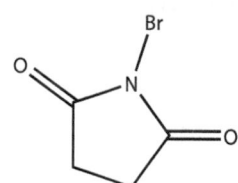

Barry, B.W. and Bennett, S.L., Effect of penetration enhancers on the permeation of mannitol, hydrocortisone, and progesterone through human skin, *J. Pharm. Pharmacol.* 39, 535–546, 1987; Forest, M. and Fournier, A., BOP reagent for the coupling of pGlu and Boc-His(Tos) in solid phase peptide synthesis, *Int. J. Pept. Protein Res.* 35, 89–94, 1990; Sasaki, H., Kojima, M., Nakamura, J., and Shibasaki, J., Enhancing effect of combining two pyrrolidone vehicles on transdermal drug delivery, *J. Pharm. Pharmacol.* 42, 196–199, 1990; Uch, A.S., Hesse, U., and Dressman, J.B., Use of 1-methyl-pyrrolidone as a solubilizing agent for determining the uptake of poorly soluble drugs, *Pharm. Res.* 16, 968–971, 1999; Zhao, F. Bhanage, B.M., Shirai, M., and Arai, M., Heck reactions of iodobenzene and methyl acrylate with conventional supported palladium catalysts in the presence of organic and/or inorganic bases without ligands, *Chemistry* 6, 843–848, 2000; Lee, P.J., Langer, R., and Shastri, V.P., Role of *n*-methyl pyrrolidone in the enhancement of aqueous phase transdermal transport, *J. Pharm. Sci.* 94, 912–917, 2005; Tae, G., Kornfield, J.A., and Hubbell, J.A., Sustained release of human growth hormone from *in situ* forming hydrogels using self-assembly of fluoroalkyl-ended poly(ethylene glycol), *Biomaterials* 26, 5259–5266, 2005; Babu, R.J. and Pandit, J.K., Effect of penetration enhancers on the transdermal delivery of bupranolol through rat skin, *Drug Deliv.* 12, 165–169, 2005; Luan, X. and Bodmeier, R., *In situ* forming microparticle system for controlled delivery of leuprolide acetate: influence of the formulation and processing parameters, *Eur. J. Pharm. Sci.* 27, 143–149, 2006; Lee, P.J., Ahmad, N., Langer, R. et al., Evaluation of chemical enhancers in the transdermal delivery of lidocaine, *Int. J. Pharm.* 308, 33–39, 2006; Ruble, G.R., Giardino, O.X., Fossceco, S.L. et al., *J. Am. Assoc. Lab. Anim. Sci.* 45, 25–29, 2006.

Common Name	Chemical Name	M.W.	Properties and Comment
NBS	*N*-bromosuccinimide; 1-bromo-2,5-pyrrolidinedione	178	Protein modification reagent; bromination of olefins; analysis of a variety of other compounds.

Sinn, H.J., Schrenk, H.H., Friedrich, E.A. et al., Radioiodination of proteins and lipoproteins using *N*-bromosuccinimide as oxidizing agent, *Anal. Biochem.* 170, 186–192, 1988; Tanemura, K., Suzuki, T., Nishida, Y. et al., A mild and efficient procedure for α-bromination of ketones using *N*-bromosuccinimide catalyzed by ammonium acetate, *Chem. Commun.* 3, 470–471, 2004; Lundblad, R.L., *Chemical Reagents for Protein Modification*, 3rd ed., CRC Press, Boca Raton, FL, 2004; Edens, G.J., Redox titration of antioxidant mixtures with *N*-bromosuccinimide as titrant: analysis by nonlinear least-squares with novel weighting function, *Anal. Sci.* 21, 1349–1354, 2005; Abdel-Wadood, H.M., Mohamed, H.A., and Mohamed, F.A., Spectrofluorometric determination of acetaminophen with *N*-bromosuccinimide, *J. AOAC Int.* 88, 1626–1630, 2005; Krebs, A., Starczyewska, B., Purzanowska-Tarasiewicz, H., and Sledz, J., Spectrophotometric determination of olanzapine by its oxidation with *N*-bromosuccinimide and cerium(IV) sulfate, *Anal. Sci.* 22, 829–833, 2006; Braddock, D.C., Cansell, G., Hermitage, S.A., and White, A.J., Bromoiodinanes with a I(III)-Br bond: preparation, X-ray crystallography, and reactivity as electrophilic brominating agents, *Chem. Commun.* 13, 1442–1444, 2006; Chen, G., Sasaki, M., Li, X., and Yudin, A.K., Strained enamines as versatile intermediates for stereocontrolled construction of nitrogen heterocycles, *J. Org. Chem.* 71, 6067–6073, 2006; Braddock D.C., Cansell, G., and Hermitage, S.A., Ortho-substituted iodobenzenes as novel organocatalysts for the transfer of electrophilic bromine from *N*-bromosuccinmide to alkenes, *Chem. Commun.* 23, 2483–2485, 2006.

CHEMICALS COMMONLY USED IN BIOCHEMISTRY AND MOLECULAR BIOLOGY AND THEIR PROPERTIES (Continued)

Common Name	Chemical Name	M.W.	Properties and Comment
NHS	N-hydroxysuccinimide; 1-hydroxy-2,5-pyrrolidinedione	111.1	Use in preparation of active esters for modification of amino groups (with carbodiimide); structural basis for reagents for amino group modification.

Anderson, G.W., Callahan, F.M., and Zimmerman, J.E., Synthesis of N-hydroxysuccinimide esters of acyl peptides by the mixed anhydride method, *J. Am. Chem. Soc.* 89, 178, 1967; Lapidot, Y., Rappoport, S., and Wolman, Y., Use of esters of N-hydroxysuccinimide in the synthesis of N-acylamino acids, *J. Lipid Res.* 8, 142–145, 1967; Holmquist, B., Blumberg, S., and Vallee, B.L., Superactivation of neutral proteases: acylation with N-hydroxysuccinimide esters, *Biochemistry* 15, 4675–4680, 1976; 't Hoen, P.A., de Kort, F., van Ommen, G.J., and den Dunnen, J.T., Fluorescent labeling of cRNA for microarray applications, *Nucleic Acids Res.* 31, e20, 2003; Vogel, C.W., Preparation of immunoconjugates using antibody oligosaccharide moieties, *Methods Mol. Biol.* 283, 87–108, 2004; Cooper, M., Ebner, A., Briggs, M. et al., Cy3B: improving the performance of cyanine dyes, *J. Fluoresc.* 14, 145–150, 2004; Lundblad, R.L., *Chemical Reagents for Protein Modification*, 3rd ed., CRC Press, Boca Raton, FL, 2004; Zhang, R., Tang, M., Bowyer, A. et al., A novel pH- and ionic-strength-sensitive carboxy methyl dextran hydrogel, *Biomaterials* 26, 4677–4683, 2005; Tyan, Y.C., Jong, S.B., Liao, J.D. et al., Proteomic profiling of erythrocyte proteins by proteolytic digestion chip and identification using two-dimensional electrospray ionization tandem mass spectrometry, *J. Proteome Res.* 4, 748–757, 2005; Lovrinovic, M., Spengler, M., Deutsch, C., and Niemeyer, C.M., Synthesis of covalent DNA-protein conjugates by expressed protein ligation, *Mol. Biosyst.* 1, 64–69, 2005; Smith, G.P., Kinetics of amine modification of proteins, *Bioconjug. Chem.* 17, 501–506, 2006; Yang, W.C., Mirzael, H., Liu, X., and Regnier, F.E., Enhancement of amino acid detection and quantitation by electrospray ionization mass spectrometry, *Anal. Chem.* 78, 4702–4708, 2006; Yu, G., Liang, J., He, Z., and Sun, M., Quantum dot-mediated detection of gamma-aminobutyric acid binding sites on the surface of living pollen protoplasts in tobacco, *Chem. Biol.* 13, 723–731, 2006; Adden, N., Gamble, L.J., Castner, D.G. et al., Phosphonic acid monolayers for binding of bioactive molecules to titanium surfaces, *Langmuir* 22, 8197–8204, 2006.

Ninhydrin	1-*H*-indene-1,2,3-trione Monohydrate	178.14	Reagent for amino acid analysis; reagent for modification of arginine residues in proteins; reaction with amino groups and other nucleophiles such as sulfhydryl groups.

Duliere, W.L., The amino-groups of the proteins of human serum. Action of formaldehyde and ninhydrin, *Biochem. J.* 30, 770–772, 1936; Schwartz, T.B. and Engel, F.L., A photometric ninhydrin method for the measurement of proteolysis, *J. Biol. Chem.* 184, 197–202, 1950; Troll, W. and Cannan, R.K., A modified photometric ninhydrin method for the analysis of amino and imino acids, *J. Biol. Chem.* 200, 803–811, 1953; Moore, S. and Stein, W.H., A modified ninhydrin reagent for the photometric determination of amino acids and related compounds, *J. Biol. Chem.* 211, 907–913, 1954; Rosen, H., A modified ninhydrin colorimetric analysis for amino acids, *Arch. Biochem. Biophys.* 67, 10–15, 1957; Meyer, H., The ninhydrin reactions and its analytical applications, *Biochem. J.* 67, 333–340, 1957; Whitaker, J.R., Ninhydrin assay in the presence of thiol compounds, *Nature* 189, 662–663, 1961; Grant, D.R., Reagent stability in Rosen's ninhydrin method for analysis of amino acids, *Anal. Biochem.* 6, 109–110, 1963; Shapiro, R. and Agarwal, S.C., Reaction of ninhydrin with cytosine derivatives, *J. Am. Chem. Soc.* 90, 474–478, 1968; Moore, S., Amino acid analysis: aqueous dimethylsulfoxide as solvent for the ninhydrin reaction, *J. Biol. Chem.* 243, 6281–6283, 1968; McGrath, R., Protein measurement by ninhydrin determination of amino acids released by alkaline hydrolysis, *Anal. Biochem.* 49, 95–102, 1972; Lamothe, P.J. and McCormick, P.G., Role of hydrindantin in the determination of amino acids using ninhydrin, *Anal. Chem.* 45, 1906–1911, 1973; Quinn, J.R., Boisvert, J.G., and Wood, I., Semi-automated ninhydrin assay of Kjeldahl nitrogen, *Anal. Biochem.* 58, 609–614, 1974; Chaplin, M.R., The use of ninhydrin as a reagent for the reversible modification of arginine residues in proteins, *Biochem. J.* 155, 457–459, 1976; Takahashi, K., Specific modification of arginine residues in proteins with ninhydrin, *J. Biochem.* 80, 1173–1176, 1976; Yu, P.H. and Davis, B.A., Deuterium isotope effects in the ninhydrin reaction of primary amines, *Experientia* 38, 299–300, 1982; D'Aniello, A., D'Onofrio, G., Pischetola, M., and Strazzulo, L., Effect of various substances on the

CHEMICALS COMMONLY USED IN BIOCHEMISTRY AND MOLECULAR BIOLOGY AND THEIR PROPERTIES (Continued)

Common Name	Chemical Name	M.W.	Properties and Comment

colorimetric amino acid–ninhydrin reaction, *Anal. Biochem.* 144, 610–611, 1985; Macchi, F.D., Shen, F.J., Keck, R.G., and Harris, R.J., Amino acid analysis, using postcolumn ninhydrin detection, in a biotechnology laboratory, *Methods Mol. Biol.* 159, 9–30, 2000; Moulin, M., Deleu, C., Larher, F.R., and Bouchereau, A., High-performance liquid chromatography determination of pipecolic acid after precolumn derivatization using domestic microwave, *Anal. Biochem.* 308, 320–327, 2002; Pool, C.T., Boyd, J.G., and Tam, J.P., Ninhydrin as a reversible protecting group of amino-terminal cysteine, *J. Pept. Res.* 63, 223–234, 2004; Schulz, M.M., Wehner, H.D., Reichert, W., and Graw, M., Ninhydrin-dyed latent fingerprints as a DNA source in a murder case, *J. Clin. Forensic Med.* 11, 202–204, 2004; Buchberger, W. and Ferdig, M., Improved high-performance liquid chromatographic determination of guanidine compounds by precolumn derivatization with ninhydrin and fluorescence detection, *J. Sep. Sci.* 27, 1309–1312, 2004; Hansen, D.B., and Joullie, M.M., The development of novel ninhydrin analogues, *Chem. Soc. Rev.* 34, 408–417, 2005.

Nitric Acid	HNO_3	63.01	Strong acid.
***p*-Nitroaniline (PNA)**	4-nitroaniline	138.13	Signal from cleavage of chromogenic substrate.

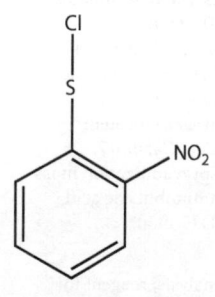

2-Nitrobenzylsulfenyl Chloride	*o*-nitrophenylsulfenyl Chloride	189.6	Modification of tryptophan in proteins.

Fontana, A. and Scofone, E., Sulfenyl halides as modifying reagents for peptides and proteins, *Methods Enzymol.* 25B, 482–494, 1972; Sanda, A. and Irie, M., Chemical modification of tryptophan residues in ribonuclease form a *Rhizopus* sp., *J. Biochem.* 87, 1079–1087, 1980; De Wolf, M.J., Fridkin, M., Epstein, M., and Kohn, L.D., Structure-function studies of cholera toxin and its A and B protomers. Modification of tryptophan residues, *J. Biol. Chem.* 256, 5481–5488, 1981; Mollier, P., Chwetzoff, S., Bouet, F. et al., Tryptophan 110, a residue involved in the toxic activity but in the enzymatic activity of notexin, *Eur. J. Biochem.* 185, 263–270, 1989; Cymes, C.D., Iglesias, M.M., and Wolfenstein-Todel, C., Selective modification of tryptophan-150 in ovine placental lactogen, *Comp. Biochem. Physiol. B* 106, 743–746, 1993; Kuyama, H., Watanabe, M., Toda, C. et al., An approach to quantitate proteome analysis by labeling tryptophan residues, *Rapid Commun. Mass Spectrom.* 17, 1642–1650, 2003; Lundblad, R.L., *Chemical Reagents for Protein Modification*, 3rd ed., CRC Press, Boca Raton, FL, 2004; Matsuo, E., Toda, C., Watanabe, M., et al., Selective detection of 2-nitrobenzensulfenyl-labeled peptides by matrix-assisted laser desorption/ionization-time-of-flight mass spectrometry using a novel matrix, *Proteomics* 6, 2042–2049, 2006; Ou, K., Kesuma, D., Ganesan, K. et al., Quantitative labeling of drug-assisted proteomic alterations by combined 2-nitrobenzenesulfenyl chloride (NBS) isotope labeling and 2DE/MS identification, *J. Proteome Res.* 5, 2194–2206, 2006.

***p*-Nitrophenol**	4-nitrophenol	139.11	Popular signal from indicator enzymes such as alkaline phosphatase.
***n*-Octanol**	1-octanol; Caprylic Alcohol	130.23	Partitioning between octanol and water is used to determine lipophilicity; a factor in QSAR studies.

CHEMICALS COMMONLY USED IN BIOCHEMISTRY AND MOLECULAR BIOLOGY AND THEIR PROPERTIES (Continued)

Common Name	Chemical Name	M.W.	Properties and Comment

Marland, J.S. and Mulley, B.A., A phase-rule study of multiple-phase formation in a model emulsion system containing water, *n*-octanol, *n*-dodecane, and a non-ionic surface-active agent at 10 and 25 degrees, *J. Pharm. Pharmacol.* 23, 561–572, 1971; Dorsey, J.G. and Khaledi, M.G., Hydrophobicity estimations by reversed-phase liquid chromatography. Implications for biological partitioning processes, *J. Chromatog.* 656, 485–499, 1993; Vailaya, A. and Horvath, C., Retention in reversed-phase chromatography: partition or adsorption? *J. Chromatog.* 829, 1–27, 1998; Kellogg, G.E. and Abraham, D.J., Hydrophobicity: is logP(o/w) more than the sum of its parts? *Eur. J. Med. Chem.* 35, 651–661, 2000; van de Waterbeemd,H., Smith, D.A., and Jones, B.C., Lipophilicity in PK design: methyl, ethyl, futile, *J. Comput. Aided Mol. Des.* 15, 273–286, 2001; Bethod, A. and Carda-Broch, S., Determination of liquid–liquid partition coefficients by separation methods, *J. Chromatog. A* 1037, 3–14, 2004.

Common Name	Chemical Name	M.W.	Properties and Comment
Octoxynol	Triton X-100™; Igepal CA-630™		Nonionic detergent; surfactant.

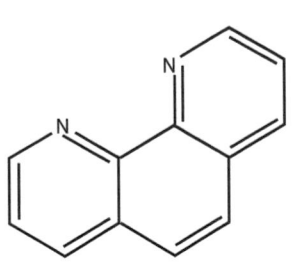

Octoxynol, n = 5–15

Common Name	Chemical Name	M.W.	Properties and Comment
Peroxynitrite			
Petroleum Ether	Mixture of Pentanes and Hexanes	N/A	
Perchloric Acid	$HClO_4$	100.5	Oxidizing agent.
1,10-Phenanthroline Monohydrate	*o*-phenanthroline Hydrate	198.21	Chelating agent; inhibitor for metalloproteinases; use in design of synthetic nucleases and proteases.

CHEMICALS COMMONLY USED IN BIOCHEMISTRY AND MOLECULAR BIOLOGY AND THEIR PROPERTIES (Continued)

Common Name	Chemical Name	M.W.	Properties and Comment

Hoch, F.L., Willams, R.J., and Vallee, B.L., The role of zinc in alcohol dehydrogenases. II. The kinetics of the instantaneous reversible inactivation of yeast alcohol dehydrogenase by 1,10-phenanthroline, *J. Biol. Chem.* 232, 453–464, 1958; Sigman, D.S. and Chen, C.H., Chemical nucleases: new reagents in molecular biology, *Annu. Rev. Biochem.* 59, 207–236, 1990; Pan, C.Q., Landgraf, R., and Sigman, D.S., DNA-binding proteins as site-specific nucleases, *Mol. Microbiol.* 12, 335–342, 1994; Galis, Z.S., Sukhova, G.K., and Libby, P., Microscopic localization of active proteases by *in situ* zymography: detection of matrix metalloproteinase activity in vascular tissue, *FASEB J.* 9, 974–980, 1995; Papavassiliou, A.G., Chemical nucleases as probes for studying DNA–protein interactions, *Biochem. J.* 305, 345–357, 1995; Perrin, D.M., Mazumder, A., and Sigman, D.S., Oxidative chemical nucleases, *Prog. Nucleic Acid Res. Mol. Biol.* 52, 123–151, 1996; Sigman, D.S., Landgraf, R., Perrin, D.M., and Pearson, L., Nucleic acid chemistry of the cuprous complexes of 1,10-phenanthroline and derivatives, *Met. Ions Biol. Syst.* 33, 485–513, 1996; Cha, J., Pedersen, M.V., and Auld, D.S., Metal and pH dependence of heptapeptide catalysis by human matrilysin, *Biochemistry* 35, 15831–15838, 1996; Kidani, Y. and Hirose, J., Coordination chemical studies on metalloenzymes. II. Kinetic behavior of various types of chelating agents towards bovine carbonic anhydrase, *J. Biochem.* 81, 1383–1391, 1997; Marini, I., Bucchioni, L., Borella, P. et al., Sorbitol dehydrogenase from bovine lens: purification and properties, *Arch. Biochem. Biophys.* 340, 383–391, 1997; Dri, P., Gasparini, C., Menegazzi, R. et al., TNF-induced shedding of TNF receptors in human polymorphonuclear leukocytes: role of the 55-kDa TNF receptor and involvement of a membrane-bound and non-matrix metalloproteinase, *J. Immunol.* 165, 2165–2172, 2000; Kito, M. and Urade, R., Protease activity of 1,10-phenanthroline-copper systems, *Met. Ions Biol. Syst.* 38, 187–196, 2001; Winberg, J.O., Berg, E., Kolset, S.O. et al., Calcium-induced activation and truncation of promatrix metalloproteinase-9 linked to the core protein of chondroitin sulfate proteoglycans, *Eur. J. Biochem.* 270, 3996–4007, 2003; Butler, G.S., Tam, E.M., and Overall, C.M., The canonical methionine 392 of matrix metalloproteinase 2 (gelatinase A) is not required for catalytic efficiency or structural integrity: probing the role of the methionine-turn in the metzincin metalloprotease superfamily, *J. Biol. Chem.* 279, 15615– 15620, 2004; Vauquelin, G. and Vanderheyden, P.M., Metal ion modulation of cystinyl aminopeptidase, *Biochem. J.* 390, 351–357, 2005; Schilling, S., Cynis, H., von Bohlen, A. et al., Isolation, catalytic properties, and competitive inhibitors of the zinc-dependent murine glutaminyl cyclase, *Biochemistry* 44, 13415–13424, 2005; Vik, S.B. and Ishmukhametov, R.R., Structure and function of subunit a of the ATP synthase of *Escherichia coli*, *J. Bioenerg. Biomembr.* 37, 445–449, 2005.

Common Name	Chemical Name	M.W.	Properties and Comment
Phenol	Hydroxybenzene; Phenyl Hydroxide	94.11	Solvent; nucleic acid purification.

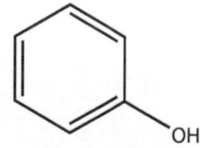

Braun, W., Burrous, J.W., and Phillips, J.H., Jr., A phenol-extracted bacterial deoxyribonucleic acid, *Nature* 180, 1356–1357, 1957; Habermann, V., Evidence for peptides in RNA prepared by phenol extraction, *Biochim. Biophys. Acta* 32, 297–298, 1959; Colter, J.S., Brown, R.A., and Ellem, K.A., Observations on the use of phenol for the isolation of deoxyribonucleic acid, *Biochim. Biophys. Acta* 55, 31–39, 1962; Lust, J. and Richards, V., Influence of buffers on the phenol extraction of liver microsomal ribonucleic acids, *Anal. Biochem.* 20, 65–76, 1967; Yamaguchi, M., Dieffenbach, C.W., Connolly, R. et al., Effect of different laboratory techniques for guanidinium-phenol-chloroform RNA extraction on A260/A280 and on accuracy of mRNA quantitation by reverse transcriptase-PCR, *PCR Methods Appl.* 1, 286–290, 1992; Pitera, R., Pitera, J.E., Mufti, G.J., Salisbury, J.R., and Nickoloff, J.A., Sepharose spin column chromatography. A fast, nontoxic replacement for phenol: chloroform extraction/ethanol precipitation, *Mol. Biotechnol.* 1, 105–108, 1994; Finnegan, M.T., Herbert, K.E., Evans, M.D., and Lunec, J., Phenol isolation of DNA yields higher levels of 8-deoxodeoxyguanosine compared to pronase E isolation, *Biochem. Soc. Trans.* 23, 430S, 1995; Beaulieux, F., See, D.M., Leparc-Goffart, I. et al. Use of magnetic beads versus guanidium thiocyanate-phenol-chloroform RNA extraction followed by polymerase chain reaction for the rapid, sensitive detection of enterovirus RNA, *Res. Virol.* 148, 11–15, 1997; Fanson, B.G., Osmack, P., and Di Bisceglie, A.M., A comparison between the phenol-chloroform method of RNA extraction and the QIAamp viral RNA kit in the extraction of hepatitis C and GB virus-C/hepatitis G viral RNA from serum, *J. Virol. Methods* 89, 23–27, 2000; Kochl, S., Niederstratter, N., and Parson, W., DNA extraction and quantitation of forensic samples using the phenol-chloroform method and real-time PCR, *Methods Mol. Biol.* 297, 13–30, 2005; Izzo, V., Notomista, E., Picardi, A. et al., The thermophilic archaeon *Sulfolobus solfatarius* is able to grow on phenol, *Res. Microbiol.* 156, 677–689, 2005; Robertson, N. and Leek, R., Isolation of RNA from tumor samples: single-step guanidinium acid-phenol method, *Methods Mol. Biol.* 120, 55–59, 2006.

Common Name	Chemical Name	M.W.	Properties and Comment
Phenoxyethanol	2-phenoxyethanol	138.16	Biochemical preservative; preservative in personal care products.

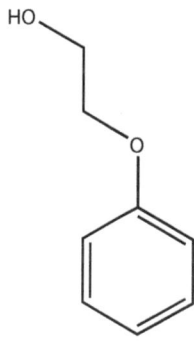

CHEMICALS COMMONLY USED IN BIOCHEMISTRY AND MOLECULAR BIOLOGY AND THEIR PROPERTIES (Continued)

Common Name	Chemical Name	M.W.	Properties and Comment

Nakahishi, M., Wilson, A.C., and Nolan, R.A., Phenoxyethanol: protein preservative for taxonomists, *Science* 163, 681–683, 1969; Frolich, K.W., Anderson, L.M., Knutsen, A., and Flood, P.R., Phenoxyethanol as a nontoxic substitute for formaldehyde in long-term preservation of human anatomical specimens for dissection and demonstration purposes, *Anat. Rec.* 208, 271–278, 1984.

Phenylglyoxal	Phenylglyoxal Hydrate	134.13	Modification of arginine residues.

Takahashi, K., The reaction of phenylglyoxal with arginine residues in proteins, *J. Biol. Chem.* 243, 6171–6179, 1968; Bunzli, H.F. and Bosshard, H.R., Modification of the single arginine residue in insulin with phenylglyoxal, *Hoppe Seylers Z. Physiol. Chem.* 352, 1180–1182, 1971; Cheung, S.T. and Fonda, M.L., Reaction of phenylglyoxal with arginine. The effect of buffers and pH, *Biochem. Biophys. Res. Commun.* 90, 940–947, 1979; Srivastava, A. and Modak, M.J., Phenylglyoxal as a template site-specific reagent for DNA or RNA polymerases. Selective inhibition of initiation, *J. Biol. Chem.* 255, 917–921, 1980; Communi, D., Lecocq, R., Vanweyenberg, V., and Erneux, C., Active site labeling of inositol 1,4,5-triphosphate 3-kinase A by phenylglyoxal, *Biochem. J.* 310, 109–115, 1995; Eriksson, O., Fontaine, E., and Bernardi, P., Chemical modification of arginines by 2,3-butanedione and phenylglyoxal causes closure of the mitochondrial permeability transition pore, *J. Biol. Chem.* 273, 12669–12674, 1998; Redowicz, M.J., Phenylglyoxal reveals phosphorylation-dependent difference in the conformation of *Acanthamoeba* myosin II active site, *Arch. Biochem. Biophys.* 384, 413–417, 2000; Kucera, I., Inhibition by phenylglyoxal of nitrate transport in *Paracoccus denitrificans*; a comparison with the effect of a protonophorous uncoupler, *Arch. Biochem. Biophys.* 409, 327–334, 2003; Johans, M., Milanesi, E., Frank, M. et al., Modification of permeability transition pore arginine(s) by phenylglyoxal derivatives in isolated mitochondria and mammalian cells. Structure-function relationship of arginine ligands, *J. Biol. Chem.* 280, 12130–12136, 2005.

Phosgene	Carbonyl Chloride; Carbon Oxychloride	98.92	Reagent for organic synthesis; preparation of derivatives for analysis.

Wilchek, M., Ariely, S., and Patchornik, A., The reaction of asparagine, glutamine, and derivatives with phosgene, *J. Org. Chem.* 33, 1258–1259, 1968; Hamilton, R.D. and Lyman, D.J., Preparation of *N*-carboxy-α-amino acid anhydrides by the reaction of copper(II)-amino acid complexes with phosgene, *J. Org. Chem.* 34, 243–244, 1969; Pohl, L.R., Bhooshan, B., Whittaker, N.F., and Krishna, G., Phosgene: a metabolite of chloroform, *Biochem. Biophys. Res. Commun.* 79, 684–691, 1977; Gyllenhaal, O., Derivatization of 2-amino alcohols with phosgene in aqueous media: limitations of the reaction selectivity as found in the presence of *O*-glucuronides of alprenolol in urine, *J. Chromatog.* 413, 270–276, 1987; Gyllenhaal, O. and Vessman, J., Phosgene as a derivatizing reagent prior to gas and liquid chromatography, *J. Chromatog.* 435, 259–269, 1988; Noort, D., Hulst, A.G., Fidder, A., et al. *In vitro* adduct formation of phosgene with albumin and hemoglobin in human blood, *Chem. Res. Toxicol.* 13, 719–726, 2000; Lemoucheux, L. Rouden, J., Ibazizene, M. et al., Debenylation of tertiary amies using phosgene or triphosgen: an efficient and rapid procedure for the preparation of carbamoyl chlorides and unsymmetrical ureas. Application in carbon-11 chemistry, *J. Org. Chem.* 68, 7289–7297, 2003.

Picric Acid	2,4,6-trinitrophenol	229.1	Analytical reagent.

CHEMICALS COMMONLY USED IN BIOCHEMISTRY AND MOLECULAR BIOLOGY AND THEIR PROPERTIES (Continued)

Common Name	Chemical Name	M.W.	Properties and Comment

De Wesselow, O.L., The picric acid method for the estimation of sugar in blood and a comparison of this method with that of MacLean, *Biochem. J.* 13, 148–152, 1919; Newcomb, C., The error due to impure picric acid in creatinine estimations, *Biochem. J.* 18, 291–293, 1924; Davidsen, O., Fixation of proteins after agarose gel electrophoresis by means of picric acid, *Clin. Chim. Acta* 21, 205–209, 1968; Gisin, B.F., The monitoring of reactions in solid-phase peptide synthesis with picric acid, *Anal. Chim. Acta* 58, 248–249, 1972; Hancock, W.S., Battersby, J.E., and Harding, D.R., The use of picric acid as a simple monitoring procedure for automated peptide synthesis, *Anal. Biochem.* 69, 497–503, 1975; Vasiliades, J., Reaction of alkaline sodium picrate with creatinine: I. Kinetics and mechanism of formation of the mono-creatinine picric acid complex, *Clin. Chem.* 22, 1664–1671, 1976; Somogyi, P. and Takagi, H., A note on the use of picric acid-formaldehyde-glutaraldehyde fixative for correlated light and electron microscopic immunocytochemistry, *Neuroscience* 7, 1779–1783, 1982; Meyer, M.H., Meyer, R.A., Jr., Gray, R.W., and Irwin, R.L., Picric acid methods greatly overestimate serum creatinine in mice: more accurate results with high-performance liquid chromatography, *Anal. Biochem.* 144, 285–290, 1985; Knisley, K.A. and Rodkey, L.S., Direct detection of carrier ampholytes in immobilized pH gradients using picric acid precipitation, *Electrophoresis* 13, 220–224, 1992; Massoomi, F., Mathews, H.G., III, and Destache, C.J., Effect of seven fluoroquinolines on the determination of serum creatinine by the picric acid and enzymatic methods, *Ann. Pharmacother.* 27, 586–588, 1993.

Common Name	Chemical Name	M.W.	Properties and Comment
Polysorbate	Tween 20		Nonionic detergent; surfactant.

Polysorbates

Common Name	Chemical Name	M.W.	Properties and Comment
Polyvinylpyrrolidone (PVP)	Povidone	N/A	Pharmaceutical; excipient; phosphate analysis.

Morin, L.G. and Prox, J., New and rapid procedure for serum phosphorus using *o*-phenylenediamine as reductant, *Clin. Chim. Acta.* 46, 113–117, 1973; Ohnishi, S.T. and Gall, R.S., Characterization of the catalyzed phosphate assay, *Anal. Biochem.* 88, 347–356, 1978; Steige, H. and Jones, J.D., Determination of serum inorganic phosphorus using a discrete analyzer, *Clin. Chim. Acta.* 103, 123–127, 1980, Plaizier-Vercammen, J.A. and De Neve, R.E., Interaction of povidone with aromatic compounds. II: evaluation of ionic strength, buffer concentration, temperature, and pH by factorial analysis, *J. Pharm. Sci.* 70, 1252–1256, 1981; van Zanten, A.P. and Weber, J.A., Direct kinetic method for the determination of phosphate, *J. Clin. Chem. Clin. Biochem.* 25, 515–517, 1987; Barlow, I.M., Harrison, S.P., and Hogg, G.L., Evaluation of the Technicon Chem-1, *Clin. Chem.* 34, 2340–2344, 1988; Giulliano, K.A., Aqueous two-phase protein partitioning using textile dyes as affinity ligands, *Anal. Biochem.* 197, 333–339, 1991; Goldenheim, P.D., An appraisal of povidone-iodine and wound healing, *Postgrad. Med. J.*, 69 (Suppl. 3), S97–S105, 1993; Vemuri, S., Yu, C.D., and Roosdorp, N., Effect of cryoprotectants on freezing, lyophilization, and storage of lyophilized recombinant alpha 1-antitrypsin formulations, *PDA J. Pharm. Sci. Technol.* 48, 241–246, 1994; Anchordoquy, T.J. and Carpenter, J.F., Polymers protect lactate dehydrogenase during freeze-drying by inhibiting dissociation in the frozen state, *Arch. Biochem. Biophys.* 332, 231–238, 1996; Fleisher, W., and Reimer, K., Povidone-iodine in antisepsis — state of the art, *Dermatology* 195 (Suppl. 2), 3–9, 1997; Fernandes, S., Kim, H.S., and Hatti-Kaul, R., Affinity extraction of dye- and metal ion-binding proteins in polyvinalypyrrolidone-based aqueous two-phase system, *Protein Expr. Purif.* 24, 460–469, 2002; D'Souza, A.J., Schowen, R.L., Borchardt, R.T. et al., Reaction of a peptide with polyvinylpyrrolidone in the solid state, *J. Pharm. Sci.* 92, 585–593, 2003; Kaneda, Y., Tsutsumi, Y., Yoshioka, Y. et al., The use of PVP as a polymeric carrier to improve the plasma half-life of drugs, *Biomaterials* 25, 3259–3266, 2004; Art, G., Combination povidone-iodine and alcohol formulations more effective, more convenient versus formulations containing either iodine or alcohol alone: a review of the literature, *J. Infus. Nurs.* 28, 314–320, 2005; Yoshioka, S., Aso, Y., and Miyazaki, T., Negligible contribution of molecular mobility to the degradation of insulin lyophilized with poly(vinylpyrrolidone), *J. Pharm. Sci.* 95, 939–943, 2006.

CHEMICALS COMMONLY USED IN BIOCHEMISTRY AND MOLECULAR BIOLOGY AND THEIR PROPERTIES (Continued)

Common Name	Chemical Name	M.W.	Properties and Comment
Pyridine	Azine	79.10	Solvent.

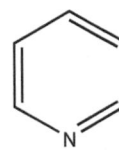

Klingsberg, E. and Newkome, G.R., Eds., *Pyridine and Its Derivatives*, Interscience, New York, 1960; Schoefield, K., *Hetero-aromatic Nitrogen Compounds; Pyrroles and Pyridines*, Butterworths, London, 1967; Hurst, D.T., *An Introduction to the Chemistry and Biochemistry and Pyrimidines, Purines, and Ptreridines*, J. Wiley, Chichester, UK, 1980; Plunkett, A.O., Pyrrole, pyrrolidine, pyridine, piperidine, and azepine alkaloids, *Nat. Prod. Rep.* 11, 581–590, 1994; Kaiser, J.P., Feng, Y., and Bollag, J.M., Microbial metabolism of pyridine, quinoline, acridine, and their derivatives under aerobic and anaerobic conditions, *Microbiol. Rev.* 60, 483–498, 1996.

Pyridoxal-5-phosphate (PLP)	Pyridoxal-5-(dihydrogen phosphate)	247.14	Selective modification of amino groups in proteins; affinity label for certain sites based on phosphate group.

Hughes, R.C., Jenkins, W.T., and Fischer, E.H., The site of binding of pyridoxal-5'-phosphate to heart glutamic-aspartic transaminase, *Proc. Natl. Acad. Sci. USA* 48, 1615–1618, 1962; Finseth, R. and Sizer, I.W., Complexes of pyridoxal phosphate with amino acids, peptides, polylysine, and apotransaminase, *Biochem. Biophys. Res. Commun.* 26, 625–630, 1967; Pages, R.C., Benditt, E.P., and Kirkwood, C.R., Schiff base formation by the lysyl and hydroxylysyl side chains of collagen, *Biochem. Biophys. Res. Commun.* 33, 752–757, 1968; Whitman, W.B., Martin, M.N., and Tabita, F.R., Activation and regulation of ribulose bisphosphate carboxylase-oxygenase in the absence of small subunits, *J. Biol. Chem.* 254, 10184–10189, 1979; Howell, E.E. and Schray, K.J., Comparative inactivation and inhibition of the anomerase and isomerase activities of phosphoglucose isomerase, *Mol. Cell. Biochem.* 37, 101–107, 1981; Colanduoni, J. and Villafranca, J.J., Labeling of specific lysine residues at the active site of glutamine synthetase, *J. Biol. Chem.* 260, 15042–15050, 1985; Peterson, C.B., Noyes, C.M., Pecon, J.M. et al., Identification of a lysyl residue in antithrombin which is essential for heparin binding, *J. Biol. Chem.* 262, 8061–8065, 1987; Diffley, J.F., Affinity labeling the DNA polymerase alpha complex. Identification of subunits containing the DNA polymerase active site and an important regulatory nucleotide-binding site, *J. Biol. Chem.* 263, 19126–19131, 1988; Perez-Ramirez, B. and Martinez-Carrion, M., Pyridoxal phosphate as a probe of the cytoplasmic domains of transmembrane proteins: application to the nicotinic acetylcholine receptor, *Biochemistry* 28, 5034–5040, 1989; Valinger, Z., Engel, P.C., and Metzler, D.E., Is pyridoxal-5'-phosphate an affinity label for phosphate-binding sites in proteins? The case of bovine glutamate dehydrogenase, *Biochem. J.* 294, 835–839, 1993; Illy, C., Thielens, N.M., and Arlaud, G.J., Chemical characterization and location of ionic interactions involved in the assembly of the C1 complex of human complement, *J. Protein Chem.* 12, 771–781, 1993; Hountondji, C., Gillet, S., Schmitter, J.M. et al., Affinity labeling of *Escherichia coli* lysyl-tRNA synthetase with pyridoxal mono- and diphosphate, *J. Biochem.* 116, 502–507, 1994; Brody, S., Andersen, J.S., Kannangara, C.G. et al., Characterization of the different spectral forms of glutamate-1-semialdehyde aminotransferase by mass spectrometry, *Biochemistry* 34, 15918–15924, 1995; Kossekova, G., Miteva, M., and Atanasov, B., Characterization of pyridoxal phosphate as an optical label for measuring electrostatic potentials in proteins, *J. Photochem. Photobiol. B* 32, 71–79, 1996; Kim S.W., Lee, J., Song, M.S. et al., Essential active-site lysine of brain glutamate dehydrogenase isoproteins, *J. Neurochem.* 69, 418–422, 1997; Martin, D.L., Liu, H., Martin, S.B., and Wu, S.J., Structural features and regulatory properties of the brain glutamate decarboxylase, *Neurochem. Int.* 37, 111–119, 2000; Jaffe, M. and Bubis, J., Affinity labeling of the guanine nucleotide binding site of transducin by pyridoxal 5'-phosphate, *J. Protein Chem.* 21, 339–359, 2002.

Sodium Borohydride	NaBH$_4$	37.83	Reducing agent for Schiff bases; reduction of aldehydes; other chemical reductions.

CHEMICALS COMMONLY USED IN BIOCHEMISTRY AND MOLECULAR BIOLOGY AND THEIR PROPERTIES (Continued)

Common Name	Chemical Name	M.W.	Properties and Comment

Chaykin, S., King, L., and Watson, J.G., The reduction of DPN+ and TPN+ with sodium borohydride, *Biochim. Biophys. Acta* 124, 13–25, 1966; Cerutti, P. and Miller, N., Selective reduction of yeast transfer ribonucleic acid with sodium borohydride, *J. Mol. Biol.* 26, 55–66, 1967; Tanzer, M.L., Collagen reduction by sodium borohydride: effects of reconstitution, maturation, and lathyrism, *Biochem. Biophys. Res. Commun.* 32, 885–892, 1968; Phillips, T.M., Kosicki, G.W., and Schmidt, D.E., Jr., Sodium borohydride reduction of pyruvate by sodium borohydride catalyzed by pyruvate kinase, *Biochim. Biophys. Acta* 293, 125–133, 1973; Craig, A.S., Sodium borohydride as an aldehyde-blocking reagent for electron microscope histochemistry, *Histochemistry* 42, 141–144, 1974; Miles, E.W., Houck, D.R., and Floss, H.G., Stereochemistry of sodium borohydride reduction of tryptophan synthase of *Escherichia coli* and its amino acid Schiff's bases, *J. Biol. Chem.* 257, 14203–14210, 1982; Kumar, A., Rao, P., and Pattabiraman, T.N., A colorimetric method for the estimation of serum glycated proteins based on differential reduction of free and bound glucose by sodium borohydride, *Biochem. Med. Metab. Biol.* 39, 296–304, 1988; Lenz, A.G., Costabel, U., Shaltiel, S., and Levine, R.L., Determination of carbonyl groups in oxidatively modified proteins by reduction with tritiated sodium borohydride, *Anal. Biochem.* 177, 419–425, 1989; Yan, L.J. and Sohal, R.S., Gel electrophoresis quantiation of protein carbonyls derivatized with tritiated sodium borohydride, *Anal. Biochem.* 265, 176–182, 1998; Azzam, T., Eliyahu, H., Shapira, L. et al., Polysaccharide-oligoamine-based conjugates for gene delivery, *J. Med. Chem.* 45, 1817–1824, 2002; Purich, D.L., Use of sodium borohydride to detect acyl-phosphate linkages in enzyme reactions, *Methods Enzymol.* 354, 168–177, 2002; Bald, E., Chwatko, S., Glowacki, R., and Kusmierek, K., Analysis of plasma thiols by high-performance liquid chromatography with ultraviolet detection, *J. Chromatog. A* 1032, 109–115, 2004; Eike, J.H. and Palmer, A.F., Effect of NABH$_4$ concentration and reaction time on physical properties of glutaraldehyde-polymerized hemoglobin, *Biotechnol. Prog.* 20, 946–952, 2004; Zhang, Z., Edwards, P.J., Roeske, R.W., and Guo, L., Synthesis and self-alkylation of isotope-coded affinity tag reagents, *Bioconjug. Chem.* 16, 458–464, 2005; Studelski, D.R., Giljum, K., McDowell, L.M., and Zhang, L., Quantitation of glycosaminoglycans by reversed-phase HPLC separation of fluorescent isoindole derivatives, *Glycobiology* 16, 65–72, 2006; Floor, E., Maples, A.M., Rankin, C.A. et al., A one-carbon modification of protein lysine associated with elevated oxidative stress in human substantia nigra, *J. Neurochem.* 97, 504–514, 2006; Kusmierek, K., Glowacki, R., and Bald, E., Analysis of urine for cysteine, cysteinylglycine, and homocysteine by high-performance liquid chromatography, *Anal. BioAnal. Chem.* 385, 855–860, 2006.

Sodium Chloride	Salt; NaCl	58.44	Ionic strength; physiological saline.
Sodium Cholate		430.55	Detergent.

Lindstrom, J., Anholt, R., Einarson, B. et al., Purification of acetylcholine receptors, reconstitution into lipid vesicles, and study of agonist-induced channel regulation, *J. Biol. Chem.* 255, 8340–8350, 1980; Gullick, W.J., Tzartos, S., and Lindstrom, J., Monoclonal antibodies as probes of acetylcholine receptor structure. 1. Peptide mapping, *Biochemistry* 20, 2173–2180, 1981; Henselman, R.A. and Cusanovich, M.A., The characterization of sodium cholate solubilized rhodopsin, *Biochemistry* 13, 5199–5203, 1974; Ninomiya, R., Masuoka, K., and Moroi, Y., Micelle formation of sodium chenodeoxycholate and solublization into the micelles: comparison with other unconjugated bile salts, *Biochim. Biophys. Acta* 1634, 116–125, 2003; Simoes, S.I., Marques, C.M., Cruz, M.E. et al., The effect of cholate on solubilization and permeability of simple and protein-loaded phosphatidylcholine/sodium cholate-mixed aggregates designed to mediate transdermal delivery of macromolecules, *Eur. J. Pharm. Biopharm.* 58, 509–519, 2004; Reis, S., Moutinho, C.G., Matos, C. et al., Noninvasive methods to determine the critical micelle concentration of some bile acid salts, *Anal. Biochem.* 334, 117–126, 2004; Nohara, D., Kajiura, T., and Takeda, K., Determination of micelle mass by electrospray ionization mass spectrometry, *J. Mass Spectrom.* 40, 489–493, 2005; Guo, J., Wu, T., Ping, Q. et al., Solublization and pharmacokinetic behaviors of sodium cholate/lecithin-mixed micelles containing cyclosporine A, *Drug Deliv.* 12, 35–39, 2005; Bottari, E., Buonfigli, A., and Festa, M.R., Composition of sodium cholate micellar solutions, *Ann. Chim.* 95, 479–490, 2005; Schweitzer, B., Felippe, A.C., Dal Bo, A. et al., Sodium dodecyl sulfate promoting a cooperative association process of sodium cholate with bovine serum albumin, *J. Colloid Interface Sci.* 298, 457–466, 2006; Burton, M.I., Herman, M.D., Alcain, F.J., and Villalba, J.M., Stimulation of polyprenyl 4-hydroxybenzoate transferase activity by sodium cholate and 3- [(cholamidopropyl)dimethylammonio]-1-propanesulfonate, *Anal. Biochem.* 353, 15–21, 2006; Ishibashi, A. and Nakashima, N., Individual dissolution of single-walled carbon nanotubes in aqueous solutions of steroid of sugar compounds and their Raman and near-IR spectral properties, *Chemistry*, 12, 7595–7602, 2006.

Sodium Cyanoborohydride	NaBH$_3$(CN)	62.84	Reducing agent; considered more selective than NaBH$_4$.

Rosen, G.M., Use of sodium cyanoborohydride in the preparation of biologically active nitroxides, *J. Med. Chem.* 17, 358–360, 1974; Chauffe, L. and Friedman, M., Factors affecting cyanoborohydride reduction of aromatic Schiff's bases in proteins, *Adv. Exp. Med. Biol.* 86A, 415–424, 1977; Baues, R.J. and Gray, G.R., Lectin purification on affinity columns containing reductively aminated disaccharides, *J. Biol. Chem.* 252, 57–60, 1977; Jentoft, N. and Dearborn, D.G., Labeling of proteins by reductive methylation using sodium cyanoborohydride, *J. Biol. Chem.* 254, 4359–4365, 1979; Jentoft, N., and Dearborn, D.G., Protein labeling by reductive methylation with sodium cyanoborohydride: effect of cyanide and metal ions on the reaction, *Anal. Biochem.* 106, 186–190, 1980; Bunn, H.F. and Higgins, P.T., Reaction of monosaccharides with proteins: possible evolutionary significance, *Science* 213, 222–224, 1981; Geoghegan, K.F., Cabacungan, J.C., Dixon, H.B., and Feeney, R.E., Alternative reducing agents for reductive methylation of amino groups in proteins, *Int. J. Pept. Protein Res.* 17, 345–352, 1981; Habeeb, A.F., Comparative studies on radiolabeling of lysozyme by iodination and reductive methylation, *J. Immunol. Methods* 65, 27–39, 1983; Prakash, C. and Vijay, I.K., A new fluorescent tag for labeling of saccharides, *Anal. Biochem.* 128, 41–46, 1983; Acharya, A.S. and Sussman, L.G., The reversibility of the ketoamine linkages of aldoses with proteins, *J. Biol. Chem.* 259, 4372–4378, 1984; Climent, I., Tsai, L., and Levine, R.L., Derivatization of gamma-glutamyl semialdehyde residues in oxidized proteins by fluorescamine, *Anal. Biochem.* 182, 226–232, 1989; Hartmann, C. and Klinman, J.P., Reductive trapping of substrate to methylamine oxidase from *Arthrobacter* P1, *FEBS Lett.* 261, 441–444, 1990; Meunier, F. and Wilkinson, K.J., Nonperturbing fluorescent labeling of polysaccharides, *Biomacromolecules* 3, 858–864, 2002; Webb, M.E., Stephens, E., Smith, A.G., and Abell, C., Rapid screening by MALDI-TOF mass spectrometry to probe binding specificity at enzyme active sites, *Chem. Commun.* 19, 2416–2417, 2003; Sando, S., Matsui, K., Niinomi, Y. et al., Facile preparation of DNA-tagged carbohydrates, *Bioorg. Med. Chem. Lett.* 13, 2633–2636, 2003; Peelen, D. and Smith, L.M., Immobilization of anine-modified oligonucleotides on aldehyde-terminated alkanethiol monolayers on gold, *Langmuir* 21, 266–271, 2005; Mirzaei, H. and Regnier, F., Enrichment of carbonylated peptides using Girard P reagent and strong cation exchange chromatography, *Anal. Chem.* 78, 770–778, 2006.

CHEMICALS COMMONLY USED IN BIOCHEMISTRY AND MOLECULAR BIOLOGY AND THEIR PROPERTIES (Continued)

Common Name	Chemical Name	M.W.	Properties and Comment
Sodium Deoxycholate	Desoxycholic Acid, Sodium Salt	414.55	Detergent; potential therapeutic use with adipose tissue.

Bril, C., van der Horst, D.J., Poort, S.R., and Thomas, J.B., Fractionation of spinach chloroplasts with sodium deoxycholate, *Biochim. Biophys. Acta* 172, 345–348, 1969; Smart, J.E. and Bonner, J., Selective dissociation of histones from chromatin by sodium deoxycholate, *J. Mol. Biol.* 58, 651–659, 1971; Part, M., Tarone, G., and Comoglio, P.M., Antigenic and immunogenic properties of membrane proteins solubilized by sodium desoxycholate, papain digestion, or high ionic strength, *Immunochemistry* 12, 9–17, 1975; Johansson, K.E. and Wbolewski, H., Crossed immunoelectrophoresis, in the presence of tween 20 or sodium deoxycholate, or purified membrane proteins from *Acholeplasma laidlawii, J. Bacteriol.* 136, 324–330, 1978; Lehnert, T. and Berlet, H.H., Selective inactivation of lactate dehydrogenase of rat tissues by sodium deoxycholate, *Biochem. J.* 177, 813–818, 1979; Suzuki, N., Kawashima, S., Deguchi, K., and Ueta, N., Low-density lipoproteins form human ascites plasma. Characterization and degradation by sodium deoxycholate, *J. Biochem.* 87, 1253–1256, 1980; Robern, H., The application of sodium deoxycholate and Sephacryl S-200 for the delipidation and separation of high-density lipoprotein, *Experientia* 38, 437–439, 1982; Nedivi, E. and Schramm, M., The beta-adrenergic receptor survives solubilization in deoxycholate while forming a stable association with the agonist, *J. Biol. Chem.* 259, 5803–5808, 1984; McKernan, R.M., Castro, S., Poat, J.A., and Wong, E.H., Solubilization of the N-methyl-D-aspartate receptor channel complex from rat and porcine brain, *J. Neurochem.* 52, 777–785, 1989; Carter, H.R. Wallace, M.A., and Fain, J.N., Activation of phospholipase C in rabbit brain membranes by carbachol in the presence of GTP gamma S: effects of biological detergents, *Biochim. Biophys. Acta* 1054, 129–134, 1990; Shivanna, B.D. and Rowe, E.S., Preservation of the native structure and function of Ca2 +-ATPase from sarcoplasmic reticulum: solubilization and reconstitution by new short-chain phospholipid detergent 1,2-diheptanoyl-*sn*-phosphatidylcholine, *Biochem. J.* 325, 533–542, 1997; Arnold, U. and Ulbrich-Hofmann, R., Quantitative protein precipitation from guandine hydrochloride-containing solutions by sodium deoxycholate/trichloroacetic acid, *Anal. Biochem.* 271, 197–199, 1999; Haque, M.E., Das, A.R., and Moulik, S.P., Mixed micelles for sodium deoxycholate and polyoxyethylene sobitan monooleate (Tween 80), *J. Colloid Interface Sci.* 217, 1–7, 1999; Srivastava, O.P. and Srivastava, K., Characterization of a sodium deoxycholate-activable proteinase activity associated with betaA3/A1-crystallin of human lenses, *Biochim. Biophys. Acta* 1434, 331–346, 1999; Rotunda, A.M., Suzuki, H., Moy, R.L., and Kolodney, M.S., Detergent effects of sodium deoxycholate are a major feature of an injectable phosphatidylcholine formulation used for localized fat dissolution, *Dermatol. Surg.* 30, 1001–1008, 2004; Asmann, Y.W., Dong, M., and Miller, L.J., Functional characterization and purification of the secretin receptor expressed in baculovirus- infected insect cells, *Regul. Pept.* 123, 217–223, 2004; Ranganathan, R., Tcacenco, C.M., Rosseto, R., and Hajdu, J., Characterization of the kinetics of phospholipase C activity toward mixed micelles of sodium deoxycholate and dimyristoyl-phophatidylcholine, *Biophys. Chem.* 122, 79–89, 2006.

Sodium Dodecylsulfate	Sodium Lauryl Sulfate, SDS	288.38	Detergent.

Sodium dodecylsulfate, SDS, lauryl sulfate, sodium salt

Shapiro, A.L., Vinuela, E., and Maizel, J.V., Jr., Molecular weight estimation of polypeptide chains by electrophoresis in SDS-polyacrylamide gels, *Biochem. Biophys. Res. Commun.* 28, 815–820, 1967; Shapiro, A.L., and Maizel, J.V., Jr., Molecular weight estimation of polypeptides by SDS-polyacrylamide gel electrophoresis: further data concerning resolving power and general considerations, *Anal. Biochem.* 29, 505–514, 1969; Weber, K. and Osborn, M., The reliability of molecular weight determinations of dodecyl sulfate-polyacrylamide gel electrophoresis, *J. Biol. Chem.* 244, 4406–4412, 1969; Weber, K. and Kuter, D.J., Reversible denaturation of enzymes by sodium dodecyl sulfate, *J. Biol. Chem.* 246, 4504–4509, 1971; de Haen, C., Molecular weight standards for calibration of gel filtration and sodium dodecyl sulfate-polyacrylamide gel electrophoresis: ferritin and apoferritin, *Anal. Biochem.* 166, 235–245, 1987; Smith, B.J., SDS polyacrylamide gel electrophoresis of proteins, *Methods Mol. Biol.* 32, 23–34, 1994; Guttman, A., Capillary sodium dodecyl sulfate-gel electrophoresis of proteins, *Electrophoresis* 17, 1333–1341, 1996; Bischoff, K.M., Shi, L., and Kennelly, P.J., The detection of enzyme activity following sodium dodecyl sulfate-polyacryalamide gel electrophoresis, *Anal. Biochem.* 260, 1–17, 1998; Maizel, J.V., SDS polyacrylamide gel electrophoresis, *Trends Biochem. Sci.* 35, 590–592, 2000; Robinson, J.M. and Vandre, D.D, Antigen retrieval in cells and tissues: enhancement with sodium dodecyl sulfate, *Histochem. Cell Biol.* 116, 119–130, 2001; Todorov, P.D., Kralchevsky, P.A., Denkov, N.D. et al., Kinetics of solublization of *n*-decane and benzene by micellar solutions of sodium dodecyl sulfate, *J. Colloid Interface Sci.* 245, 371–382, 2002; Zhdanov, S.A., Starov, V.M., Sobolev, V.D., and Velarde, M.G., Spreading of aqueous SDS solutions over nitrocellulose membranes, *J. Colloid Interface Sci.* 264, 481–489, 2003; Santos, S.F., Zanette, D., Fischer, H., and Itri, R., A systematic study of bovine serum albumin (BSA) and sodium dodecyl sulfate (SDS) interactions by surface tension and small angle X-ray scattering, *J. Colloid Interface Sci.* 262, 400–408, 2003; Biswas, A. and Das, K.P., SDS-induced structural changes in alpha-crystallin and its effect on refolding, *Protein J.* 23, 529–538, 2004; Jing, P., Kaneta, T., and Imasaka, T., On-line concentration of a protein using denaturation by sodium dodecyl sulfate, *Anal. Sci.* 21, 37–42, 2005; Choi, N.S., Hahm, J.H., Maeng, P.J., and Kim, S.H., Comparative study of enzyme activity and stability of bovine and human plasmins in electrophoretic reagents, β-mercaptoethanol, DTT, SDS, Triton X-100, and urea, *J. Biochem. Mol. Biol.* 38, 177–181, 2005; Miles, A.P. and Saul, A., Quantifying recombinant proteins and their degradation products using SDS-PAGE and scanning laser densitometry, *Methods Mol. Biol.* 308, 349–356, 2005; Thongngam, M. and McClements, D.J., Influence of pH, ionic strength, and temperature on self-association and interactions of sodium dodecyl sulfate in the absence and presence of chitosan, *Langmuir* 21, 79–86, 2005; Romani, A.P., Gehlen, M.H., and Itri, R., Surfactant-polymer aggregates formed by sodium dodecyl sulfate, poly(N-vinyl-2-pyrrolidone), and poly(ethylene glycol), *Langmuir* 21, 1271–1233, 2005; Gudiksen, K.L., Gitlin, I., and Whitesides, G.M., Differentiation of proteins based on characteristic patterns of association and denaturation in solutions of SDS, *Proc. Natl. Acad. Sci. USA* 103, 7968–7972, 2006; Freitas, A.A., Paulo, L., Macanita, A.L, and Quina, F.H., Acid-base equilibria and dynamics in sodium dodecyl sulfate micelles: geminate recombination and effect of charge stabilization, *Langmuir* 22, 7986–7893, 2006.

CHEMICALS COMMONLY USED IN BIOCHEMISTRY AND MOLECULAR BIOLOGY AND
THEIR PROPERTIES (Continued)

Common Name	Chemical Name	M.W.	Properties and Comment
Sodium Metabisulfite	Sodium Bisulfite	190.1	Mild reducing agent; converts unmethylated cytosine residues to uracil residues (DNA methylation).

Miller, R.F., Small, G., and Norris, L.C., Studies on the effect of sodium bisulfite on the stability of vitamin E, *J. Nutr.* 55, 81–95, 1955; Hayatsu, H., Wataya, Y., Kai, K., and Iida, S., Reaction of sodium bisulfite with uracil, cytosine, and their derivatives, *Biochemistry* 9, 2858–2865, 1970; Seno, T., Conversion of *Escherichia coli* tRNATrp to glutamine-accepting tRNA by chemical modification with sodium bisulfite, *FEBS Lett.* 51, 325–329, 1975; Tasheva, B. and Dessev, G., Artifacts in sodium dodecyl sulfate-polyacrylamide gel electrophoresis due to 2-mercaptoethanol, *Anal. Biochem.* 129, 98–102, 1983; Draper, D.E., Attachment of reporter groups to specific, selected cytidine residues in RNA using a bisulfite-catalyzed transamination reaction, *Nucleic Acids Res.* 12, 989–1002, 1984; Oakeley, E.J., DNA methylation analysis: a review of current methodologies, *Pharmacol. Ther.* 84, 389–400, 1999; Geisler, J.P., Manahan, K.J., and Geisler, H.E., Evaluation of DNA methylation in the human genome: why examine it and what method to use, *Eur. J. Gynaecol. Oncol.* 25, 19–24, 2004; Thomassin, H., Kress, C., and Grange, T., MethylQuant: a sensitive method for quantifying methylation of specific cytosines within the genome, *Nucleic Acids Res.* 32, e168, 2004; Derks, S., Lentjes, M.H., Mellebrekers, D.M. et al., Methylation-specific PCR unraveled, *Cell. Oncol.* 26, 291–299, 2004; Galm, O. and Herman, J.G., Methylation-specific polymerase chain reaction, *Methods Mol. Biol.* 113, 279–291, 2005; Ogino, S., Kawasaki, T., Brahmandam, M. et al., Precision and performance characteristics of bisulfite conversion and real-time PCR (MethylLight) for quantitative DNA methylation analysis, *J. Mol. Diagn.* 8, 209–217, 2006; Yang, I., Park, I.Y., Jang, S.M. et al., Rapid quantitation of DNA methylation through dNMP analysis following bisulfite PCR, *Nucleic Acids Res.* 34, e61, 2006; Wischnewski, F., Pantel, K., and Schwazenbach, H., Promoter demethylation and histone acetylation mediate gene expression of MAGE-A1, -A2, -A3, and -A12 in human cancer cells, *Mol. Cancer Res.* 4, 339–349, 2006; Zhou, Y., Lum, J.M., Yeo, G.H. et al., Simplified molecular diagnosis of fragile X syndrome by fluorescent methylation-specific PCR and GeneScan analysis, *Clin. Chem.* 52, 1492–1500, 2006.

| **Succinic Anhydride** | Butanedioic Anhydride; 2,5-diketotetrahydrofuran | 100.1 | Protein modification; dissociation of protein complexes. |

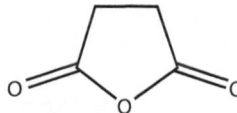

Habeeb, A.F., Cassidy, H.G., and Singer, S.J., Molecular structural effects produced in proteins by reaction with succinic anhydride, *Biochim. Biophys. Acta* 29, 587–593, 1958; Hass, L.F., Aldolase dissociation into subunits by reaction with succinic anhydride, *Biochemistry* 3, 535–541, 1964; Scanu, A., Pollard, H., and Reader, W., Properties of human serum low-density lipoproteins after modification by succinic anhydride, *J. Lipid Res.* 9, 342–349, 1968; Vasilets, I.M., Moshkov, K.A., and Kushner, V.P., Dissociation of human ceruloplasmin into subunits under the action of alkali and succinic anhydride, *Mol. Biol.* 6, 193–199, 1972; Tedeschi, H., Kinnally, K.W., and Mannella, C.A., Properties of channels in mitochondrial outer membrane, *J. Bioenerg. Biomembr.* 21, 451–459, 1989; Palacian, E., Gonzalez, P.J., Pineiro, M., and Hernandez, F., Dicarboxylic acid anhydrides as dissociating agents of protein-containing structures, *Mol. Cell. Biochem.* 97, 101–111, 1990; Pavliakova, D., Chu, C., Bystricky, S. et al., Treatment with succinic anhydride improves the immunogenicity of *Shigella flexneri* type 2a O-specific polysaccharide-protein conjugates in mice, *Infect. Immun.* 67, 5526–5529, 1999; Ferretti, V., Gilli, P., and Gavezzotti, A., X-ray diffraction and molecular simulation study of the crystalline and liquid states of succinic anhydride, *Chemistry* 8, 1710–1718, 2002.

| **Sucrose** | | 342.30 | Osmolyte; density gradient centrifugation. |

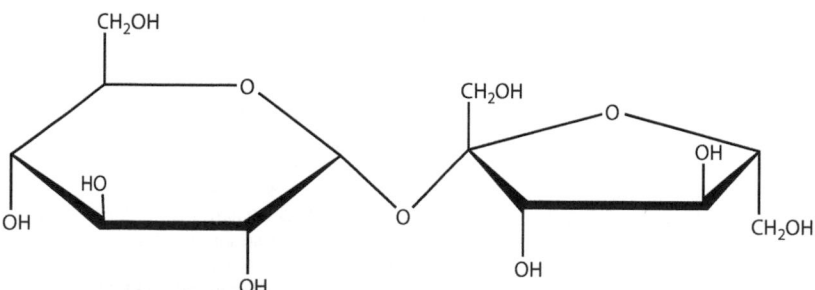

Cann, J.R., Coombs, R.O., Howlett, G.J. et al., Effects of molecular crowding on protein self-association: a potential source of error in sedimentation coefficients obtained by zonal ultracentrifugation in a sucrose gradient, *Biochemistry* 33, 10185–10190, 1994; Camacho-Vanegas, O., Lorein, F., and Amaldi, F., Flat absorbance background for sucrose gradients, *Anal. Biochem.* 228, 172–173, 1995; Ben-Zeev, O. and Doolittle, M.H., Determining lipase subunit structure by sucrose gradient centrifugation, *Methods Mol. Biol.* 109, 257–266, 1999; Lustig, A., Engel, A., Tsiotis, G. et al., Molecular weight determination of membrane proteins by sedimentation equilibrium at the sucrose of nycodenz-adjusted density of the hydrated detergent micelle, *Biochim. Biophys. Acta* 1464, 199–206, 2000; Kim, Y.S., Jones, L.A., Dong, A. et al., Effects of sucrose on conformational equilibria and fluctuations within the native-state ensemble of proteins, *Protein Sci.* 12, 1252–1261, 2003; Srinivas, K.A., Chandresekar, G., Srivastava, R., and Puvanakrishna, R., A novel protocol for the subcellular fractionation of C3A hepatoma cells using sucrose-density gradient centrifugation, *J. Biochem. Biophys. Methods* 60, 23–27, 2004; Richter, W., Determining the subunit structure of phosphodiesterase using gel filtration and sucrose-density gradient centrifugation, *Methods Mol. Biol.* 307, 167–180, 2005; Cioni, P., Bramanti, E., and Strambini, G.B., Effects of sucrose on the internal dynamics of azurin, *Biophys. J.* 88, 4213–4222, 2005; Desplats, P., Folco, E. and Salerno, G.L., Sucrose may play an additional role to that of an osmolyte in *Synechocystis* sp. PCC 6803 salt-shocked cells, *Plant Physiol. Biochem.* 43, 133–138, 2005; Chen, L., Ferreira, J.A., Costa, S.M. et al., Compaction of ribosomal protein S6 by sucrose occurs only under native conditions, *Biochemistry* 21, 2189–2199, 2006.

CHEMICALS COMMONLY USED IN BIOCHEMISTRY AND MOLECULAR BIOLOGY AND THEIR PROPERTIES (Continued)

Common Name	Chemical Name	M.W.	Properties and Comment
Sulfuric Acid	H_2SO_4	98.1	Strong acid; component of piranha solution with hydrogen peroxide.
Tetrabutylammonium Chloride		277.9	Ion-pair reagent for extraction and HPLC.

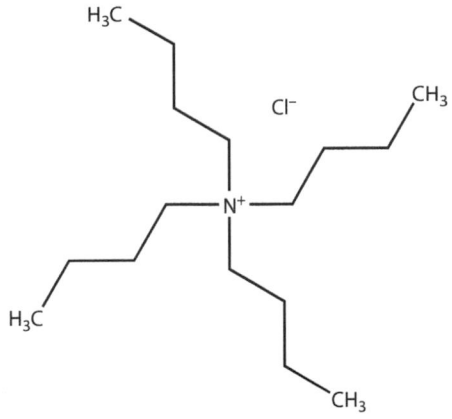

Walseth, T.F., Graff, G., Moos, M.C., Jr., and Goldberg, N.D., Separation of 5′-ribonucleoside monophosphates by ion-pair reverse-phase high-performance liquid chromatography, *Anal. Biochem.* 107, 240–245, 1980; Ozkul, A. and Oztunc, A., Determination of naprotiline hydrochloride in tables by ion-pair extraction using bromthymol blue, *Pharmzie* 55, 321–322, 2000; Cecchi, T., Extended thermodynamic approach to ion interaction chromatography. Influence of the chain length of the solute ion; a chromatographic method for the determination of ion-pairing constants, *J. Sep. Sci* 28, 549–554, 2005; Pistos, C., Tsantili-Kakoulidou, A., and Koupparis, M., Investigation of the retention/pH profile of zwitterionic fluoroquinolones in reversed-phase and ion-interaction high-performance liquid chromatography, *J. Pharm. Biomed. Anal.* 39, 438–443, 2005; Choi, M.M., Douglas, A.D., and Murray, R.W., Ion-pair chromatographic separation of water-soluble gold monolayer-protected clusters, *Anal. Chem.* 78, 2779–2785, 2006; Saradhi, U.V., Prarbhakar, S., Reddy, T.J., and Vairamani, M., Ion-pair solid-phase extraction and gas chromatography mass spectrometric determination of acidic hydrolysis products of chemical warfare agents from aqueous samples, *J. Chromatog. A*, 1129, 9–13, 2006.

Tetrahydrofuran	Trimethylene Oxide	72.1	Solvent; template for combinatorial chemistry.

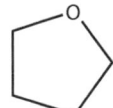

Leuty, S.J., Rapid dehydration of plant tissues for paraffin embedding; tetrahydrofuran vs. t-butanol, *Stain Technol.* 44, 103–104, 1969; Tandler, C.J. and Fiszer de Plazas, S., The use of tetrahydrofuran for delipidation and water solubilization of brain proteolipid proteins, *Life Sci.* 17, 1407–1410, 1975; Dressman, J.B., Himmelstein, K.J., and Higuchi, T., Diffusion of phenol in the presence of a complexing agent, tetrahydrofuran, *J. Pharm. Sci.* 72, 12–17, 1983; Diaz, R.S., Regueiro, P., Monreal, J., and Tandler, C.J., Selective extraction, solubilization, and reversed-phase high-performance liquid chromatography separation of the main proteins from myelin using tetrahydrofuran/water mixtures, *J. Neurosci. Res.* 29, 114–120, 1991; Santa, T., Koga, D., and Imai, K., Reversed-phase high-performance liquid chromatography of fullerenes with tetrahydrofuran-water as a mobile phase and sensitive ultraviolet or electrochemical detection, *Biomed. Chromatogr.* 9, 110–111, 1995; Lee, J., Kang, J.H., Lee, S.Y. et al., Protein kinase C ligands based on tetrahydrofuran templates containing a new set of phorbol ester pharmacophores, *J. Med. Chem.* 42, 4129–4139, 1999; Edwards, A.A., Ichihara, O., Murfin, S. et al., Tetrahydrofuran-based amino acids as library scaffolds, *J. Comb. Chem.* 6, 230–238, 2004; Baron, C.P., Refsgaard, H.H., Skibsted, L.H., and Andersen, M.L., Oxidation of bovine serum albumin initiated by the Fenton reaction — effect of EDTA, tert-butylhydroperoxide, and tetrahydrofuran, *Free Radic. Res.* 40, 409–417, 2006; Bowron, D.T., Finney, J.L., and Soper, A.K., The structure of liquid tetrahydrofuran, *J. Am. Chem. Soc.* 128, 5119–5126, 2006; Hermida, S.A., Possari, E.P., Souza, D.B. et al., 2′-deoxyguanosine, 2′-deoxycytidine, and 2′-deoxyadenosine adducts resulting from the reaction of tetrahydrofuran with DNA bases, *Chem. Res. Toxicol.* 19, 927–936, 2006; Li, A.C., Li, Y., Guirguis, M.S., Advantages of using tetrahydrofuran-water as mobile phases in the quantitation of cyclosporine A in monkey and rat plasma by liquid chromatography-tandem mass spectrometry, *J. Pharm. Biomed. Anal.* 43, 277–284, 2007.

CHEMICALS COMMONLY USED IN BIOCHEMISTRY AND MOLECULAR BIOLOGY AND THEIR PROPERTIES (Continued)

Common Name	Chemical Name	M.W.	Properties and Comment
Tetraphenylphosphonium Bromide		419.3	Membrane-permeable probe; determination of metal ions.

Boxman, A.W., Barts, P.W., and Borst-Pauwels, G.W., Some characteristics of tetraphenylphosphonium uptake into *Saccharomyces cerevisiae, Biochim. Biophys. Acta* 686, 13–18, 1982; Flewelling, R.F. and Hubbell, W.L., Hydrophobic ion interactions with membranes. Thermodynamic analysis of tetraphenylphosphonium binding to vesicles, *Biophys. J.* 49, 531–540, 1986; Prasad, R. and Hofer, M., Tetraphenylphosphonium is an indicator of negative membrane potential in *Candida albicans, Biochim. Biophys. Acta* 861, 377–380, 1986; Aiuchi, T., Matsunada, M., Nakaya, K., and Nakamura, Y., Calculation of membrane potential in synaptosomes with use of a lipophilic cation (tetraphenylphosphonium), *Chem. Pharm. Bull.* 37, 3333–3337, 1989; Nhujak T. and Goodall, D.M., Comparison of binding of tetraphenylborate and tetraphenylphosphonium ion to cyclodextrins studied by capillary electrophoresis, *Electrophoresis* 22, 117–122, 2001; Yasuda, K., Ohmizo, C., and Katsu, T., Potassium and tetraphenylphosphonium ion-selective electrodes for monitoring changes in the permeability of bacterial outer and cytoplasmic membranes, *J. Microbiol. Methods* 54, 111–115, 2003; Min, J.J., Biswal, S., Deroose, C., and Gambhir, S.S., Tetraphenylphosphonium as a novel molecular probe for imaging tumors, *J. Nucl. Med.* 45, 636–643, 2004.

Thionyl Chloride	Sulfurous Oxychloride	118.97	Preparation of acyl chlorides.

Rodin, R.L. and Gershon, H., Photochemical alpha-chlorination of fatty acid chlorides by thionyl chloride, *J. Org. Chem.* 38, 3919–3921, 1973; DuVal, G., Swaisgood, H.E., and Horton, H.R, Preparation and characterization of thionyl chloride-activated succinamidopropyl-glass as a covalent immobilization matrix, *J. Appl. Biochem.* 6, 240–250, 1984; Molnar-Perl, I., Pinter-Szakacs, M., and Fabian-Vonsik, V., Esterification of amino acids with thionyl chloride acidified butanols for their gas chromatographic analysis, *J. Chromatog.* 390, 434–438, 1987; Stabel, T.J., Casele, E.S., Swaisgood, H.E., and Horton, H.R., Anti-IgG immobilized controlled pore glass. Thionyl chloride-activated succinamidopropyl-gas as a covalent immobization matrix, *Appl. Biochem. Biotechnol.* 36, 87–96, 1992; Chamoulaud, G. and Belanger, D., Chemical modification of the surface of a sulfonated membrane by formation of a sulfonamide bond, *Langmuir* 20, 4989–4895, 2004; Porjazoska, A.,Yilmaz, O.K., Baysal, K. et al., Synthesis and characterization of poly(ethylene glycol)-poly(D,L-lactide-co-glycolide) poly(ethylene glycol) tri-block co-polymers modified with collagen: a model surface suitable for cell interaction, *J. Biomater. Sci. Polym. Ed.* 17, 323–340, 2006; Gao, C., Jin, Z.Q., Kong, H. et al., Polyurea-functionalized multiwalled carbon nanotubes: synthesis, morphology, and Ramam spectroscopy, *J. Phys. Chem. B* 109, 11925–11932, 2005; Chen, G.X., Kim, H.S., Park, B.H., and Yoon, J.S., Controlled functionalization of multiwalled carbon nanotubes with various molecular-weight poly(L-lactic acid), *J. Phys. Chem. B* 109, 22237–22243, 2005.

Thiophosgene	$CSCl_2$	115	
Thiourea	Thiocarbamide	76.12	Chaotropic agent; useful for membrane proteins; will react with haloacetyl derivatives such as iodoacetamide; protease inhibitor.

CHEMICALS COMMONLY USED IN BIOCHEMISTRY AND MOLECULAR BIOLOGY AND THEIR PROPERTIES (Continued)

Common Name	Chemical Name	M.W.	Properties and Comment

Maloof, F. and Soodak, M., Cleavage of disulfide bonds in thyroid tissue by thiourea, *J. Biol. Chem.* 236, 1689–1692, 1961; Gerfast, J.A., Automated analysis for thiourea and its derivatives in biological fluids, *Anal. Biochem.* 15, 358–360, 1966; Lippe, C., Urea and thiourea permeabilities of phospholipid and cholesterol bilayer membranes, *J. Mol. Biol.* 39, 588–590, 1966; Carlsson, J., Kierstan, M.P., and Brocklehurst, K., Reactions of L-ergothioneine and some other aminothiones with 2,2'- and 4,4'-dipyridyl disulphides and of L-ergothioneine with iodoacetamide, 2-mercaptoimidazoles, and 4-thiopyridones, thiourea, and thioacetamide as highly reactive neutral sulphur nucleophiles, *Biochem. J.* 139, 221–235, 1974; Filipski, J., Kohn K.W., Prather, R., and Bonner, W.M., Thiourea reverses crosslinks and restores biological activity in DNA treated with dichlorodiaminoplatinum (II), *Science* 204, 181–183, 1979; Wasil, M., Halliwell, B., Grootveld, M. et al., The specificity of thiourea, dimethylthiourea, and dimethyl sulphoxide as scavengers of hydroxyl radicals. Their protection of alpha-1-antiproteinase against inactivation by hypochlorous acid, *Biochem. J.* 243, 867–870, 1987; Doona, C.J. and Stanbury, D.M., Equilibrium and redox kinetics of copper(II)–thiourea complexes, *Inorg. Chem.* 35, 3210–3216, 1996; Rabilloud, T., Use of thiourea to increase the solubility of membrane proteins in two-dimensional electrophoresis, *Electrophoresis* 19, 758–760, 1998; Musante, L., Candiano, G., and Ghiggeri, G.M., Resolution of fibronectin and other uncharacterized proteins by two-dimensional polyacrylamide electrophoresis with thiourea, *J. Chromatog. B* 705, 351–356, 1998; Nagy, E., Mihalik, R., Hrabak, A. et al., Apoptosis inhibitory effect of the isothiourea compound, tri-(2-thioureido-S-ethyl)-amine, *Immunopharmacology* 47, 25–33, 2000; Galvani, M., Rovatti, L., Hamdan, M. et al., Protein alkylation in the presence/absence of thiourea in proteome analysis: a matrix-assisted laser

desorption/ionization-time-of-flight-mass spectrometry investigation, *Electrophoresis* 22, 2066–2074, 2001; Castellanos-Serra, L. and Paz-Lago, D., Inhibition of unwanted proteolysis during sample preparation: evaluation of its efficiency in challenge experiments, *Electrophoresis* 23, 1745–1753, 2002; Tyagarajan, K., Pretzer, E., and Wiktorowicz, J.E., Thiol-reactive dyes for fluorescence labeling of proteomic samples, *Electrophoresis* 24, 2348–2358, 2003; Fuerst, D.E., and Jacosen, E.N., Thiourea-catalyzed enantioselective cyanosilylation of ketones, *J. Am. Chem. Soc.* 127, 8964–8965, 2005; Gomez, D.E., Fabbrizzi, L., Licchelli, M., and Monzani, E., Urea vs. thiourea in anion recognition, *Org. Biomol. Chem.* 3, 1495–1500, 2005; George, M., Tan, G., John, V.T., and Weiss, R.G., Urea and thiourea derivatives as low molecular-mass organochelators, *Chemistry* 11, 3243–3254, 2005; Limbut, W., Kanatharana, P., Mattiasson, B. et al., A comparative study of capacitive immunosensors based on self-assembled monolayers formed from thiourea, thioctic acid, and 3-mercaptopropionic acid, *Biosens. Bioelectron.* 22, 233–240, 2006.

TNBS	Trinitrobenzenesulfonic Acid	293.2	Reagent for the determination of amino groups in proteins; also reacts with sulfydryl groups and hydrazides; used to induce animal model of colitis.

Habeeb, A.F., Determination of free amino groups in proteins by trinitrobenzenesulfonic acid, *Anal. Biochem.* 14, 328–336, 1966; Goldfarb, A.R., A kinetic study of the reactions of amino acids and peptides with trinitrobenzenesulfonic acid, *Biochemistry* 5, 2570–2574, 1966; Scheele, R.B. and Lauffer, M.A., Restricted reactivity of the epsilon-amino groups of tobacco mosaic virus protein toward trinitrobenzenesulfonic acid, *Biochemistry* 8, 3597–3603, 1969; Godin, D.V. and Ng, T.W., Trinitrobenzenesulfonic acid: a possible chemical probe to investigate lipid–protein interactions in biological membranes, *Mol. Pharmacol.* 8, 426–437, 1972; Bubnis, W.A. and Ofner, C.M., III, The determination of epsilon-amino groups in soluble and poorly soluble proteinaceous materials by a spectrophotometric method using trinitrobenzenesulfonic acid, *Anal. Biochem.* 207, 129–133, 1992; Cayot, P. and Tainturier, G., The quantification of protein amino groups by the trinitrobenzenesulfonic acid method: a reexamination, *Anal. Biochem.* 249, 184–200, 1997; Neurath, M., Fuss, I., and Strober, W., TNBS-colitis, *Int. Rev. Immunol.* 19, 51–62, 2000; Lindsay, J., Van Montfrans, C., Brennen, F. et al., IL-10 gene therapy prevents TNBS-induced colitis, *Gene Ther.* 9, 1715–1721, 2002; Whittle, B.J., Cavicchi, M., and Lamarque, D., Assessment of anticolitic drugs in the trinitrobenzenesulfonic acid (TNBS) rat model of inflammatory bowel disease, *Methods Mol. Biol.* 225, 209–222, 2003; Necefli, A., Tulumoglu, B., Giris, M. et al., The effects of melatonin on TNBS-induced colitis, *Dig. Dis. Sci.* 51, 1538–1545, 2006.

TNM	Tetranitromethane	196.03	Modification of tyrosine residues in proteins; crosslinking a side reaction as a reaction with cysteine; antibacterial and antiviral agent.

CHEMICALS COMMONLY USED IN BIOCHEMISTRY AND MOLECULAR BIOLOGY AND THEIR PROPERTIES (Continued)

Common Name	Chemical Name	M.W.	Properties and Comment

Sokolovsky, M., Riordan, J.F., and Vallee, B.L., Tetranitromethane. A reagent for the nitration of tyrosyl residues in proteins, *Biochemistry* 5, 3582–3589, 1966; Nishikimi, M. and Yagi, K., Reaction of reduced flavins with tetranitromethane, *Biochem. Biophys. Res. Commun.* 45, 1042–1048, 1971; Kunkel, G.R., Mehrabian, M., and Martinson, H.G., Contact-site crosslinking agents, *Mol. Cell. Biochem.* 34, 3–13, 1981; Rial, E. and Nicholls, D.G., Chemical modification of the brown-fat-mitochondrial uncoupling protein with tetranitromethane and *N*-ethylmaleimide. A cysteine residue is implicated in the nucleotide regulation of anion permeability, *Eur. J. Biochem.* 161, 689–694, 1986; Prozorovski, V., Krook, M., Atrian, S. et al., Identification of reactive tyrosine residues in cysteine-reactive dehydrogenases. Differences between liver sorbitol, liver alcohol, and *Drosophila* alcohol dehydrogenase, *FEBS Lett.* 304, 46–50, 1992; Gadda, G., Banerjee, A., and Fitzpatrick, P.F., Identification of an essential tyrosine residue in nitroalkane oxidase by modification with tetranitromethane, *Biochemistry* 39, 1162–1168, 2000; Hodges, G.R. and Ingold, K.U., Superoxide, amine buffers, and tetranitro-methane: a novel free radical chain reaction, *Free Radic. Res.* 33, 547–550, 2000; Capeillere-Blandin, C., Gausson, V., Descamps-Latscha, B., and Witko-Sarsat, V., Biochemical and spectrophotometric significance of advanced oxidation protein products, *Biochim. Biophys. Acta* 1689, 91–102, 2004; Lundblad, R.L., *Chemical Reagents for Protein Modification*, CRC Press, Boca Raton, FL, 2004; Negrerie, M., Martin, J.L., and Nghiem, H.O., Functionality of nitrated acetylcholine receptor: the two-step formation of nitrotyrosines reveals their differential role in effectors binding, *FEBS Lett.* 579, 2643–2647, 2005; Carven, G.J. and Stern, L.J., Probing the ligand-induced conformational change in HLA-DR1 by selective chemical modification and mass spectrometry mapping, *Biochemistry* 44, 13625–13637, 2005.

Common Name	Chemical Name	M.W.	Properties and Comment
Trehalose	α-D-glucopyrano-glucopyranosyl-1,1-α-D-glucopyranoside; Mycose	342.3	A nonreducing sugar that is found in a variety of organisms where it is thought to protect against stress such as dehydration; there is considerable interest in the use of trehalose as a stabilizer in biopharmaceutical proteins.

Elbein, A.D., The metabolism of alpha, alpha-trehalose, *Adv. Carbohydr. Chem. Biochem.* 30, 227–256, 1974; Wiemken, A., Trehalose in yeast, stress protectant rather than reserve carbohydrate, *Antonie Van Leeuwenhoek*, 58, 209–217, 1990; Newman, Y.M., Ring, S.G., and Colaco, C., The role of trehalose and other carbohydrates in biopreservation, *Biotechnol. Genet. Eng. Rev.* 11, 263–294, 1993; Panek, A.D., Trehalose metabolism — new horizons in technological applications, *Braz. J. Med. Biol. Res.* 28, 169–181, 1995; Schiraldi, C., Di Lernia, I., and De Rosa, M., Trehalose production: exploiting novel approaches, *Trends Biotechnol.* 20, 420–425, 2002; Elbein, A.D., Pan, Y.T., Pastuszak, I., and Carroll, D., New insights on trehalose: a multifunctional molecule, *Glycobiology* 13, 17R–27R, 2003; Gancedo, C. and Flores, C.L., The importance of a functional trehalose biosynthetic pathway for the life of yeasts and fungi, *FEMS Yeast Res.* 4, 351–359, 2004; Cordone, L., Cottone, G., Giuffrida, S. et al., Internal dynamics and protein-matrix coupling in trehalose-coated proteins, *Biochim. Biophys. Acta* 1749, 252–281, 2005.

Common Name	Chemical Name	M.W.	Properties and Comment
Trichloroacetic Acid		163.4	Protein precipitant.

Common Name	Chemical Name	M.W.	Properties and Comment

Chang, Y.C., Efficient precipitation and accurate quantitation of detergent-solubilized membrane proteins, *Anal. Biochem.* 205, 22–26, 1992; Sivaraman, T., Kumar, T.K., Jayaraman, G., and Yu. C., The mechanism of 2,2,2-trichloroacetic acid-induced protein precipitation, *J. Protein Chem.* 16, 291–297, 1997; Arnold, U. and Ulbrich-Hoffman, R., Quantitative protein precipation form guandine hydrochloride-containing solutions by sodium deoxycholate/ trichloroacetic acid, *Anal. Biochem.* 271, 197–199, 1999; Jacobs, D.I., van Rijssen, M.S., van der Heijden, R., and Verpoorte, R., Sequential solubilization of proteins precipitated with trichloroacetic acid in acetone from cultured *Catharanthus roseus* cells yields 52% more spots after two-dimensional electrophoresis, *Proteomics* 1, 1345–1350, 2001; Garcia-Rodriguez, S., Castilla, S.A., Machado, A., and Ayala, A., Comparison of methods for sample preparation of individual rat cerebrospinal fluid samples prior to two-dimensional polyacrylamide gel electrophoresis, *Biotechnol. Lett.* 25, 1899–1903, 2003; Chen, Y.Y., Lin, S.Y., Yeh, Y.Y. et al., A modified protein precipitation procedure for efficient removal of albumin from serum, *Electrophoresis* 26, 2117–2127, 2005; Zellner, M., Winkler, W., Hayden, H. et al., Quantitative validation of different protein precipitation methods in proteome analysis of blood platelets, *Electrophoresis* 26, 2481–2489, 2005; Carpentier, S.C., Witters, E., Laukens, K. et al., Preparation of protein extracts from recalcitrant plant tissues: an evaluation of different methods for two-dimensional gel electrophoresis analysis, *Proteomics* 5, 2497–2507, 2005; Manadas, B.J., Vougas, K., Fountoulakis, M., and Duarte, C.B., Sample sonication after trichloroacetic acid precipitation increases protein recovery from cultured hippocampal neurons, and improves resolution and reproducibility in two-dimensional gel electrophoresis, *Electrophoresis* 27, 1825–1831, 2006; Wang, A., Wu, C.J., and Chen, S.H., Gold nanoparticle-assisted protein enrichment and electroelution for biological samples containing low protein concentration — a prelude of gel electrophoresis, *J. Proteome Res.* 5, 1488–1492, 2006.

Common Name	Chemical Name	M.W.	Properties and Comment
Triethanolamine	Tris(2-hydroxyethyl)amine	149.2	Buffer; transdermal transfer reagent.

pKa approx. 9.5

Triethanolamine   Triethanolamine hydrochloride

Fitzgerald, J.W., The Tris-catalyzed isomerization of potassium D-glucose 6-*O*-sulfate, *Can. J. Biochem.* 53, 906–910, 1975; Buhl, S.N., Jackson, K.Y., and Graffunder, B., Optimal reaction conditions for assaying human lactate dehydrogenase pyruvate-to-lactate at 25, 30, and 37 degrees C, *Clin. Chem.* 24, 261–266, 1978; Myohanen, T.A., Bouriotas, V., and Dean, P.D., Affinity chromatography of yeast alpha-glucosidase using ligand-mediated chromatography on immobilized phenylboronic acids, *Biochem. J.* 197, 683–688, 1981; Shinomiya, Y., Kato, N., Imazawa, M., and Miyamoto, K., Enzyme immunoassay of the myelin basic protein, *J. Neurochem.* 39, 1291–1296, 1982; Arita, M., Iwamori, M., Higuchi, T., and Nagai, Y., 1,1,3,3-tetramethylurea and triethanolamine as a new useful matrix for fast atom bombardment mass spectrometry of gangliosides and neutral glycosphingolipids, *J. Biochem.* 93, 319–322, 1983; Cao, H. and Preiss, J., Evidence for essential arginine residues at the active site of maize branching enzymes, *J. Protein Chem.* 15, 291–304, 1996; Knaak, J.B., Leung, H.W., Stott, W.T. et al., Toxicology of mono-, di-, and triethanolamine, *Rev. Environ. Contim. Toxicol.* 149, 1–86, 1997; Liu, Q., Li, X., and Sommer, S.S., pK-matched running buffers for gel electrophoresis, *Anal. Biochem.* 270, 112–122, 1999; Sanger-van de Griend, C.E., Enantiomeric separation of glycyl dipeptides by capillary electrophoresis with cyclodextrins as chiral selectors, *Electrophoresis* 20, 3417–3424, 1999; Fang, L., Kobayashi, Y., Numajiri, S. et al., The enhancing effect of a triethanolamine-ethanol-isopropyl myristate mixed system on the skin permeation of acidic drugs, *Biol. Pharm. Bull.* 25, 1339–1344, 2002; Musial, W. and Kubis, A., Effect of some anionic polymers of pH of triethanolamine aqueous solutions, *Polim. Med.* 34, 21–29, 2004.

Common Name	Chemical Name	M.W.	Properties and Comment
Triethylamine	*N,N*-diethylethanamine	101.2	Ion-pair reagent; buffer.

CHEMICALS COMMONLY USED IN BIOCHEMISTRY AND MOLECULAR BIOLOGY AND THEIR PROPERTIES (Continued)

Common Name	Chemical Name	M.W.	Properties and Comment

Brind, J.L., Kuo, S.W., Chervinsky, K., and Orentreich, N., A new reversed-phase, paired-ion thin-layer chromatographic method for steroid sulfate separations, *Steroids* 52, 561–570, 1988; Koves, E.M., Use of high-performance liquid chromatography-diode array detection in forensic toxicology, *J. Chromatog. A* 692, 103–119, 1995; Cole, S.R. and Dorsey, J.G., Cyclohexylamine additives for enhanced peptide separations in reversed-phase liquid chromatography, *Biomed. Chromatog.* 11, 167–171, 1997; Gilar, M. and Bouvier, E.S.P., Purification of crude DNA oligonucleotides by solid-phase extraction and reversed-phase high-performance liquid chromatography, *J. Chromatog. A* 890, 167–177, 2000; Loos, R. and Barcelo, D., Determination of haloacetic acids in aqueous environments by solid-phase extraction followed by ion-pair liquid chromatography-electrospray ionization mass spectrometric detection, *J. Chromatog. A* 938, 45–55, 2001; Gilar, M., Fountain, K.J., Budman, Y. et al., Ion-pair reversed-phase high-performance liquid chromatography analysis of oligonucleotides: retention prediction, *J. Chromatog. A* 958, 167–182, 2002; El-dawy, M.A., Mabrouk, M.M., and El-Barbary, F.A., Liquid chromatographic determination of fluoxetine, *J. Pharm. Biomed. Anal.* 30, 561–571, 2002; Yang, X., Zhang, X., Li, A. et al., Comprehensive two-dimensional separations based on capillary high-performance liquid chromatography and microchip electrophoresis, *Electrophoresis* 24, 1451–1457, 2003; Murphey, A.T., Brown-Augsburger, P., Yu, R.Z. et al., Development of an ion-pair reverse-phase liquid chromatographic/tandem mass spectrometry method for the determination of an 18-mer phosphorothioate oligonucleotide in mouse liver tissue, *Eur. J. Mass Spectrom.* 11, 209–215, 2005; Xie, G., Sueishi, Y., and Yamamoto, S., Analysis of the effects of protic, aprotic, and multi-component solvents on the fluorescence emission of naphthalene and its exciplex with triethylamine, *J. Fluoresc.* 15, 475–483, 2005.

Trifluoroacetic Acid   114.0   Ion-pair reagent; HLPC; peptide synthesis.

Rosbash, D.O. and Leavitt, D., Decalcification of bone with trifluoroacetic acid, *Am. J. Clin. Pathol.* 22, 914–915, 1952; Katz, J.J., Anhydrous trifluoroacetic acid as a solvent for proteins, *Nature* 174, 509, 1954; Uphaus, R.A., Grossweiner, L.I., Katz, J.J., and Kopple, K.D., Fluorescence of tryptophan derivatives in trifluoroacetic acid, *Science* 129, 641–643, 1959; Acharya, A.S., di Donato, A., Manjula, B.N. et al., Influence of trifluoroacetic acid on retention times of histidine-containing tryptic peptides in reverse phase HPLC, *Int. J. Pept. Protein Res.* 22, 78–82, 1983; Tsugita, A., Uchida, T., Mewes, H.W., and Ataka, T., A rapid vapor-phase acid (hydrochloric and trifluoroacetic acid) hydrolysis of peptide and protein, *J. Biochem.* 102, 1593–1597, 1987; Hulmes, J.D. and Pan, Y.C., Selective cleavage of polypeptides with trifluoroacetic acid: applications for microsequencing, *Anal. Biochem.* 197, 368–376, 1991; Eshragi, J. and Chowdhury, S.K., Factors affecting electrospray ionization of effluents containing trifluoroacetic acid for high-performance liquid chromatography/mass spectrometry, *Anal. Chem.* 65, 3528–3533, 1993; Apffel, A., Fischer, S., Goldberg, G. et al., Enhanced sensitivity for peptide mapping with electrospray liquid chromatography-mass spectrometry in the presence of signal suppression due to trifluoroacetic acid- containing mobiles phases, *J. Chromatog. A* 712, 177–190, 1995; Guy, C.A. and Fields, G.B., Trifluoroacetic acid cleavage and deprotection of resin-bound peptides following synthesis by Fmoc chemistry, *Methods Enzymol.* 289, 67–83, 1997; Morrison, I.M. and Stewart, D., Plant cell wall fragments released on solubilization in trifluoroacetic acid, *Phytochemistry* 49, 1555–1563, 1998; Yan, B., Nguyen, N., Liu, L. et al., Kinetic comparison of trifluoroacetic acid cleavage reactions of resin-bound carbamates, ureas, secondary amides, and sulfonamides from benzyl-, benzhyderyl-, and indole-based linkers, *J. Comb. Chem.* 2, 66–74, 2000; Ahmad, A., Madhusudanan, K.P., and Bhakuni, V., Trichloroacetic acid- and trifluoroacetic acid-induced unfolding of cytochrome C: stabilization of a nativelike fold intermediate(1), *Biochim. Biophys. Acta* 1480, 201–210, 2000; Chen, Y., Mehok, A.R., Mant, C.T. et al., Optimum concentration of trifluoroacetic acid for reversed-phase liquid chromatography of peptide revisited, *J. Chromatog. A* 1043, 9–18, 2004.

Tris(2-carboxyethyl) phosphine   TCEP   250.2   Reducing agent.

CHEMICALS COMMONLY USED IN BIOCHEMISTRY AND MOLECULAR BIOLOGY AND THEIR PROPERTIES (Continued)

Common Name	Chemical Name	M.W.	Properties and Comment

Gray, W.R., Disulfide structures of highly bridged peptides: a new strategy for analysis, *Protein Sci.* 2, 1732–1748, 1993; Gray, W.R., Echistatin disulfide bridges: selective reduction and linkage assignment, *Protein Sci.* 2, 1749–1755, 1993; Han, J.C. and Han, G.Y., A procedure for quantitative determination of Tris(2-carboxyethyl)phosphine, an odorless reducing agent more stable and effective than dithiothreitol, *Anal. Biochem.* 220, 5–10, 1994; Wu, J., Gage, D.A., and Watson, J.T., A strategy to locate cysteine residues in proteins by specific chemical cleavage followed by matrix-assisted laser desorption/ionization-time-of-flight mass spectrometry, *Anal. Biochem.* 235, 161–174, 1996; Han, J., Yen. S., Han, G., and Han, F., Quantitation of hydrogen peroxide using Tris(2-carboxyethyl) phosphine, *Anal. Biochem.* 234, 107–109, 1996; Han, J., Clark, C., Han, G. et al., Preparation of 2-nitro-5-thiobenzoic acid using immobilized Tris(2-carboxyethyl) phosphine, *Anal. Biochem.* 268, 404–407, 1999; Anderson, M.T., Trudell, J.R., Voehringer, D.W. et al., An improved monobromobimane assay for glutathione utilizing Tris-(2-carboxyethyl)phosphine as the reductant, *Anal. Biochem.* 272, 107–109, 1999; Shafer, D.E., Inman, J.K. and Lees, A. Reaction of Tris(2-carboxyethyl)phosphine (TCEP) with maleimide and alpha-haloacyl groups: anomalous elution of TCEP by gel filtration, *Anal. Biochem.* 282, 161–164, 2000; Rhee, S.S. and Burke, D.H., Tris(2-carboxyethyl)phosphine stabilization of RNA: comparison with dithiothreitol for use with nucleic acid and thiophosphoryl chemistry, *Anal. Biochem.* 325, 137–143, 2004; Legros, C., Celerier, M.L., and Guette, C., An unusual cleavage reaction of a peptide observed during dithiothreitol and Tris(2-carboxyethyl)phosphine reduction: application to sequencing of HpTx2 spider toxin using nanospray tandem mass spectrometry, *Rapid Commun. Mass Spectrom.* 19, 1317–1323, 2004; Xu, G., Kiselar, J., He, Q., and Chance, M.R., Secondary reactions and strategies to improve quantitative protein footprinting, *Anal. Chem.* 77, 3029–3037, 2005; Valcu, C.M. and Schlink, K., Reduction of proteins during sample preparation and two-dimensional gel electrophoresis of woody plant samples, *Proteomics* 6, 1599–1605, 2006; Scales, C.W., Convertine, A.J., and McCormick, C.L., Fluorescent labeling of RAFT-generated poly(*N*-isopropylacrylamide) via a facile maleimide-thiol coupling reaction, *Biomacromolecules* 7, 1389–1392, 2006.

Urea	Carbamide	60.1	Chaotropic agent.

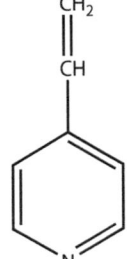

Edelhoch, H., The effect of urea analogues and metals on the rate of pepsin denaturation, *Biochim. Biophys. Acta* 22, 401–402, 1956; Steven, F.S. and Tristram, G.R., The denaturation of ovalbumin. Changes in optical rotation, extinction, and viscosity during serial denaturation in solution of urea, *Biochem. J.* 73, 86–90, 1959; Nelson, C.A. and Hummel, J.P., Reversible denaturation of pancreatic ribonuclease by urea, *J. Biol. Chem.* 237, 1567–1574, 1962; Herskovits, T.T., Nonaqueous solutions of DNA; denaturation by urea and its methyl derivatives, *Biochemistry* 2, 335–340, 1963; Subramanian, S., Sarma, T.S., Balasubramanian, D., and Ahluwalia, J.C., Effects of the urea–guanidinium class of protein denaturation on water structure: heats of solution and proton chemical shift studies, *J. Phys. Chem.* 75, 815–820, 1971; Strachan, A.F., Shephard, E.G., Bellstedt, D.U. et al., Human serum amyloid A protein. Behavior in aqueous and urea-containing solutions and antibody production, *Biochem. J.* 263, 365–370, 1989; Gervais, V., Guy, A., Teoule, R., and Fazakerley, G.V., Solution conformation of an oligonucleotide containing a urea deoxyribose residue in front of a thymine, *Nucleic Acids Res.* 20, 6455–6460, 1992; Smith, B.J., Acetic acid-urea polyacrylamide gel electrophoresis of proteins, *Methods Mol. Biol.* 32, 39–47, 1994; Buck, M., Radford, S.E., and Dobson, C.M., Amide hydrogen exchange in a highly denatured state. Hen egg-white lysozyme in urea, *J. Mol. Biol.* 237, 247–254, 1994; Shirley, B.A., Urea and guanidine hydrochloride denaturation curve, *Methods Mol. Biol.* 40, 177–190, 1995; Bennion, B.J. and Daggett, V., The molecular basis for the chemical denaturation of proteins by urea, *Proc. Natl. Acad. Sci. USA* 100, 5142–5147, 2003; Soper, A.K., Castner, E.W., and Luzar, A., Impact of urea on water structure: a clue to its properties as a denaturant? *Biophys.Chem.*105, 649–666, 2003; Smith, L.J., Jones, R.M., and van Gunsteren, W.F., Characterization of the denaturation of human alpha-1-lactalbumin in urea by molecule dynamics simulation, *Proteins* 58, 439–449, 2005; Idrissi, A., Molecular structure and dynamics of liquids: aqueous urea solutions, *Spectrochim. Acta A Mol. Biomol. Spectrosc.* 61, 1–17, 2005; Chow, C., Kurt, N., Murphey, R.M., and Cavagnero, S., Structural characterization of apomyoglobin self-associated species in aqueous buffer and urea solution, *Biophys. J.* 90, 298–309, 2006.

Vinyl Pyridine	4-vinylpyridine	105.1	Modification of cysteine residues in protein.

CHEMICALS COMMONLY USED IN BIOCHEMISTRY AND MOLECULAR BIOLOGY AND THEIR PROPERTIES (Continued)

Common Name	Chemical Name	M.W.	Properties and Comment
Water	Hydrogen Oxide	18.0	Solvent.

Lumry, R. and Rajender, S., Enthalpy-entropy compensation phenomena in water solutions of proteins and small molecules: a ubiquitous property of water, *Biopolymers* 9, 1125–1227, 1970; Cooke, R. and Kuntz, I.D., The properties of water in biological systems, *Annu. Rev. Biophys. Bioeng.* 3, 95–126, 1974; Fettiplace, R. and Haydon, D.A., Water permeability of lipid membranes, *Physiol. Rev.* 60, 510–550, 1980; Lewis, C.A. and Wolfenden, R., Antiproteolytic aldehydes and ketones: substituent and secondary deuterium isotope effects on equilibrium addition of water and other nucleophiles, *Biochemistry* 16, 4886–4890, 1977; Wolfenden, R.V., Cullis, P.M., and Southgate, C.C., Water, protein folding, and the genetic code, *Science* 206, 575–577, 1979; Wolfenden, R., Andersson, L., Cullis, P.M., and Southgate, C.C., Affinities of amino acid side chains for solvent water, *Biochemistry* 20, 849–855, 1981; Cullis, P.M. and Wolfenden, R., Affinity of nucleic acid bases for solvent water, *Biochemistry* 20, 3024–3028, 1981; Radzicka, A., Pedersen, L., and Wolfenden, R., Influences of solvent water on protein folding: free energies of salvation of *cis* and *trans* peptides are nearly identical, *Biochemistry* 27, 4538–4541, 1988; Dzingeleski, G.D. and Wolfenden, R., Hypersensitivity of an enzyme reaction to solvent water, *Biochemistry* 32, 9143–9147, 1993; Timasheff, S.N., The control of protein stability and association by weak interactions with water: how do solvents affect these processes? *Annu. Rev. Biophys. Biomol. Struct.* 22, 67–97, 1993; Wolfenden, R. and Radzcika, A., On the probability of finding a water molecule in a nonpolar cavity, *Science* 265, 936–937, 1994; Jayaram, B. and Jain, T., The role of water in protein–DNA recognition, *Annu. Rev. Biophys. Biomol. Struct.* 33, 343–361, 2004; Pace, C.N., Trevino, S., Prabhakaran, E., and Scholtz, J.M., Protein structure, stability, and solubility in water and other solvents, *Philos. Trans. R. Soc. Lond. B Biol. Sci.* 359, 1225–1234, 2004; Rand, R.P., Probing the role of water in protein conformation and function, *Philos. Trans. R. Soc. Lond. B Biol. Sci.* 359, 1277–1284, 2004; Bagchi, B., Water dynamics in the hydration layer around proteins and micelles, *Chem. Rev.* 105, 3179–3219, 2005; Raschke, T.M., Water structure and interactions with protein surfaces, *Curr. Opin. Struct. Biol.* 16, 152–159, 2006; Levy, Y. and Onuchic, J.N., Water mediation in protein folding and molecular recognition, *Annu. Rev. Biophys. Biomol. Struct.* 35, 389–415, 2006; Wolfenden, R., Degrees of difficulty of water-consuming reactions in the absence of enzymes, *Chem. Rev.* 106, 3379–3396, 2006.

COMMON DETERGENTS USED IN BIOCHEMICAL RESEARCH

Name	Type	Composition	Form	CMC*	Cloud Point	Solubility	Applications
Brij 35	Nonionic	Polyoxyethylene lauryl ether (E_{23})	Solid white wax; density 1.18–1.22 (6)	0.058 g/1 (4)	100°C (4)	Soluble in H_2O and (6) most organic solvents insoluble in oils	Column chromatography (7)
Tergitol TMN	Nonionic	Polyoxyethylene trimethyl nonanol (E_6)	Pale yellow liquid, 90%; density, 1.024 (6)	—	36°C (4)	Completely soluble in H_2O (6)	Membrane solubilization (2)
Triton X-45	Nonionic	Polyoxyethylene octylphenol (E_5)	Amber liquid, 100% (6)			Soluble in most organic solvents; insoluble in H_2O (6)	Membrane solubilization (2)
Triton X-100	Nonionic	Polyoxyethylene tert-octylphenol (E_{10})	Amber liquid (6)	0.16 g/l (4)	64°C (5)	Soluble in H_2O and (6) alcohols; slightly soluble in aromatic solvents	Membrane solubilization (2) gel electrophoresis (9)
Tween 20 (Polysorbate 20)	Nonionic	Polyoxyethylene sorbitan monolaurate (E_{22})	Yellow oily liquid (6)	0.14 g/l	95°C (4)	Soluble in H_2O and organic solvents (6)	Solubilizer (1, 4)
Tween 80 (Polysorbate 80)	Nonionic	Polyoxyethylene sorbitan monooleate (E_{25})	Amber liquid; density 1.05–1.10 (6)		93°C (4)	Soluble in H_2O and most organic solvents; insoluble in oils (6)	Solubilizer (1, 4)
CTAB	Cationic	Cetyltrimethyl-ammonium bromide	Creamy-white voluminous powder (13)	0.33 g/l (10)		Soluble in H_2O and organic solvents (13)	Membrane solubilization (2)
SDS	Anionic	Sodium dodecyl (lauryl) sulfate	White crystals, flakes, or powder (13)	2.3 g/l (10)		Soluble in H_2O	Protein solubilization (11), gel electrophoresis (12)
Cholate	Anionic	3, 7, 12-Trihydroxy-5 cholanate	White Powder			Partially soluble in H_2O; soluble in most organic solvents (13)	Membrane solubilization (2)
Deoxycholate	Anionic	3, 12-Dihydroxy-5 cholanate	White Powder			Partially soluble in H_2O; soluble in most organic solvents (13)	Membrane solubilization (2)
Lubrol W	Nonionic	A fatty alcohol ethylene oxide condensate	Fawn colored waxy solids (6)		H_2O, 25°C	Soluble in H_2O, vegetable oils and fatty acids (6)	Membrane solubilization (14)
Atlas G	Nonionic	Polyoxyethylene (sorbitol) hexanolate					Membrane solubilization (14)
Span 20	Nonionic	Sorbitan mono-laurate					Membrane solubilization (14)

Compiled by A. Fulmer.

* Critical micelle concentration in H_2O, 25°C.

References

1. Elworthy, Florence, and Macfarlane, *Solubilization by Surface-Active Agents*, Chapman and Hall Ltd., London, 1968.
2. Foxx and Keith, *Membrane Molecular Biology*, Sinauer Associates, Stamford, Conn., 1972.
3. Swanson, Bradford, and McIlwain, *Biochem. J.*, 92, 235 (1964).
4. Schönfeldt, *Surface-Active Ethylene Oxide Adducts*, Pergamon Press, New York, 1969.
5. Shinoda, Nakagawa, Tamamuchi, and Isemura, *Colloidal Surfactants*, Academic Press, New York, 1963.
6. Sisley and Wood, *Encyclopedia of Surface-Active Agents*, Chemical Publishing, New York, 1964.
7. Morris and Morris, *Separation Methods in Biochemistry*, Pitman Publishing, New York, 1963.
8. Roodyn, *Biochem J.*, 85,177 (1962).
9. Alfageme, Zweider, Mahowald, and Cohen, *J. Biol. Chem.*, 249, 3729 (1974).
10. Mukerjee and Mysels, *Critical Micelle Concentrations of Aqueous Surfactants Systems*, Natl. Stand. Ref. Data Ser., Natl. Bureau Stand., 1971.
11. Reynolds and Tanford, *Proc. Natl. Acad. Sci. U.S.A.*, 66, 1002, (1970).
12. Dunder and Reukert, *J. Biol. Chem.*, 244, 5074 (1969).
13. Stecher, Ed., *The Merck Index of Chemicals and Drugs*, 7th ed., Merck & Co., Rahway, N.J., 1960.
14. Umbreit and Strominger, *Proc. Natl. Acad. Sci. U.S.A.*, 70, 2997 (1973).

General References for Surfactants and Detergents

Siskey, J.P.(trans. P.J. Wood), *Encyclopedia of Surface-Active Agents*, Chemical Publishing Company, New York, NY, USA, 1952.

Ferguson, L.N., On the water solubilities of ethers, *J.Amer.Chem.Soc.* 77, 5288–5289, 1955.

Nonionic Surfactants, ed. M.J. Schick, Marcel Dekker, New York, NY, USA, 1966.

Jungermann, E., *Cationic Surfactants*, Marcel Dekker, New York, NY, USA, 1970.

Cabane, B., Structure of some polymer-detergent aggregates in water, *J.Phys.Chem.* 81, 1639–1645, 1977.

Helenius, A., McCaslin, D.R., Fries, E., and Tanford, C., Properties of detergents, *Methods Enzymol.* 56, 734–749, 1979.

Membranes Detergents, and Receptor Solubilization, ed. J.C. Venter and L.C. Harrison, A.R.Liss, New York, NY, USA, 1984.

Industrial Applications of Surfactants II, ed. D.R. Karsa, Royal Society of Chemistry, Cambridge, UK, 1990.

Neugebauer, J.M., Detergents: an overview, *Methods Enzymol.* 182, 239–253, 1990.

Industrial Applications of Surfactants III, ed. D.R. Karsa, Royal Society of Chemistry, Cambridge, UK, 1992.

Surfactants in Lipid Chemistry: Recent Synthetic, Physical and Biodegradation Studies, ed. J.H.P. Tyman, Royal Society of Chemistry, Cambridge, UK, 1992.

Lawrence, M.J., Surfactant systems: Their use in drug delivery, *Chem.Soc. Rev.* 23, 417–223, 1994.

Porter, M.R., *Handbook of Surfactants*, 2nd edn., Blackie Academic & Professional, Glasgow, UK, 1994.

Structure and Flow in Surfactant Solutions, ed. C.A. Herb and R.K. Prud'homme, American Chemical Society, Washington, DC, 1994.
- Chapter 23 (pps 320–336), Li, Y. and Dubin, P.L., Polymer-surfactant complexes.
- Chapter 26 (pps. 370–379), Smith, B.C., Chou, L.–C., Lu, B., and Zakin, J.L., Effect of counterion structure in flow birefringence and dray reduction behavior of quaternary ammonium salt cationic surfactants.
- Chapter 27 (pps. 380–393), Burgess, D.J. and Sahin, N.O., Interfacial rheology of β-casein solutions.

Stevens, L., Solutions used in enzymology, in *Enzymology LabFax*, ed. P.C. Engel, Bios Scientific Publishers, Oxford, UK, Chaper 9, pps. 269–289, 1996.

Cogdell, R.J. and Lindsay, J.G., Integral Membrane Proteins, in *Protein LabFax*, ed. N.C. Price, Bios Scientific Publishers, Oxford, UK, Chapter 10, pps. 101–107, 1996.

Jönsson, B., Lindman, B., Holmberg, K., and Kronberg, B., *Surfactants and Polymers in Aqueous Solution*, John Wiley & Sons, Chichester, UK, 1998.

Tsujii, K., *Surface Activity Principles, Phenomena, and Applications*, Academic Press, San Diego, CA, USA, 1998.

Holmberg, K., *Novel Surfactants Preparations, Applications and Biodegradability*, Marcel Dekker, New York, NY, USA, 1998.

Hill, R.M., *Silicone Surfactants*, Marcel Dekker, New York, NY, 1999.

Industrial Applications of Surfactants IV, ed. D.R. Karsa, Royal Society of Chemistry, Cambridge, UK, 1999.

Specialist Surfactants, ed. I.D. Robb, Blackie Academic & Professional, London, UK, 1997.

Liposomes Rational Design, ed. A.S. Janoff, Marcel Dekker, New York, NY, USA, 1999.

Hummel, D.O., *Handbook of Surfactant Analysis. Chemical, Physico-Chemical and Physical Methods*, John Wiley & Sons, Ltd., Chichester, UK, 2000.

Corrigan, O.I. and Healy, A.M., Surfactants in pharmaceutical products and systems, in *Encyclopedia of Pharmaceutical Technology*, ed. J. Swarbrick and J.C. Boylan, Marcel Dekker, New York, NY, Volume 3, pp. 2639–2653, 2002.

Encyclopedia of Surface and Colloid Science, ed. A.T. Hubbard, Marcel Dekker, Inc, New York, NY, USA, 2002.
- Hirata, H. Surfactant molecular complexes, Volume 4, pps. 5178–5204.
- Imamura, T., Surfactant-protein interactions, Volume 4, pps. 5230–5243.

Rosen, M.J., *Surfactants and Interfacial Phenomena*, Wiley-Interscience, Hoboken, NJ, USA, 2004.

Goodwin, J.W., *Colloids and Interfaces with Surfactants and Polymers: An Introduction*, John Wiley, Hoboken, NJ, USA, 2004.

Tadros, T.F., *Applied Surfactants. Principles and Applications*, Wiley-VCH, Weinheim, Germany, 2005.

Handbook of Functional Lipids, ed. C.C. Akoh, CRC Press/Taylor & Francis Group, Boca Raton, FL, USA, 2006.

SOME PROPERTIES OF DETERGENTS AND SURFACTANTS USED IN BIOCHEMISTRY AND MOLECULAR BIOLOGY

Structures for these compounds may be found on p. 816–818.

Detergent/Surfactant	Molecular Weight	Classification	Key References
Tween 20[a]		nonionic	1–5
Tween 80[b]	1,300	nonionic	6–10
Triton X-100[c]	650	nonionic	11–15
Nonidet P-40[d]	650	nonionic	16–20
Brij Deterents[e] (polyoxyethylene derivatives)		nonionic	21–25
Lubrol[f]	582	nonionic	26–30
Sodium dodecyl dulfate (SDS)[g]	288.4	anionic	31–35
Sodium deoxycholate[h]	432	anionic	36–40
Cetylpyridinium chloride[i]	340.0	cationic	41–45
Cetyltrimethylammonium bromide[j]	364.5	cationic	46–50
Tetradecyltrimethyl-ammonium bromide[k]	336	cationic	51–55
Betainesulfonate,[l] sulfobetaine, alkylsulfobetaine derivatives		zwitterionic	56–60
CHAPS[m]	614.9	zwitterionic	61–65
CHAPSO[n]	630.9	zwitterionic	66–70

Footnotes

[a] Tween 20 is a polysorbate surfactant (polyoxyethylene sorbitan fatty acid ester) useful in immunoassays and pharmaceutical development. Tween 20 reduced protein interaction and protein binding to surfaces. It is related to Tween 80. The Tween surfactants are condensation products of mono-substituted fatty acyl derivatives of sorbitan (SPAN®; a registered trademark of Atlas Chemical) and ethylene oxide. Span® 20 is sorbitan monolaurate and Tween® 20 (polyethoxyethylene (20) sorbitan monolaurate) is derived from Span® 20. Tween®20 has a viscosity of 200–400 cp at 25°C.

[b] Tween® 80 (polysorbate 80) is a polysorbate surfactant (polyoxyethylene sorbitan mono-oleate) is used in pharmaceutical formulation where it stabilizes proteins and in various diagnostics tests. Tween® 80 was added early to bacterial culture media and was also demonstrated to enhance the anti-bacterial activity of certain antibiotics. Tween® 80 has also been used for protein membrane studies and were originally manufactured by Atlas Power Company. Tween 80 has a viscosity of 600–800 cp at 25°C.

[c] Triton X-100 is a nonionic detergent known as octoxynol, octylphenoxy polyethoxyethanol. The Triton family of surfactants which is manufactured by the condensation of ethylene oxide with alkylphenols and contain between 5 and 15 ethylene oxide units; with Triton X-100, there is 9 or 10 ethylene oxide units while Triton X-30 contains three ethyloxide groups. Triton X-100 is also known as Igepal CA or Polydetergent G. These alkylaryl polyether alcohols were first manufacture by I.G. Farbenindustrie as Igepal products and subsequently manufactured and marketed in the United States as Triton. Triton X-100 is used for the lysis of cells and preparation of subcellular fractions and in the study of membrane proteins.

[d] Nonidet® is a registered trademark of the Shell Oil Company; however, it is not clear that Shell Oil Company is still associated with the manufacture and/or distribution of this material. A search of the Shell Oil website did not a result for Nonidet. Nonidet® P-40 [octyl phenolpoly(ethyleneglycolether)] is a popular alkylphenyl ethoxylate nonionic detergent; also referred to as nonylphenylpolyethylene glycol; polyethyleneglycol-p-isooctylphenyl ether; octylphenoxy polyethoxy ethanol; Igepal CO 630. There is question as to the relation of nonidet P-40 to NP-40. Related to the Triton surfactants. It is useful to assure the provenance of a product labeled Nonidet P40 or NP-40.

[e] Brij® detergents are a series of polyoxyethylene ethers such as lauryl polyoxyethylene (dodecyl polyoxyethylate). This class of surfactants is referred to as poloxamers and includes polyoxypropylene. The number of ethylene oxide units determines the solubility of the dodecyl alcohol derivative:

Moles Ethylene Oxide/ Dodecyl Alcohol	Approximate Solubility of Product
0	Insoluble
2	Insoluble
4	Somewhat miscible
6	Slightly soluble
7	Soluble

[f] Lubrol® is a trademark of ICI referring to a series of nonionic surfactants similar to the Brij® surfactants in being a series of polyoxyethylene alkyl ethers. Lubrol® surfactants are used for membrane solubilization and more recently in the study of lipid rafts. While there are similarities between the various nonionic surfactants, there are also distinct differences.

[g] Sodium Dodecyl Sulfate; also known as sodium lauryl sulfate. An anionic detergent used for membrane solubilization and protein denaturation. Used in a popular electrophoretic procedure, SDS-gel electrophoresis where separation is presumed to occur on the basis of molecular weight; there are some exceptions to this assumption (Noel, D., Nikaido, K., and Ames, G.F., A single amino acid substitution in a histidine-transport protein drastically alters its mobility in sodium dodecyl sulfate-polyacrylamide gel electrophoresis, *Biochemistry* 18, 4159–4165, 1979; Briggs, M.M., Klevit, R.E., and Schachat, F.H., Heterogeneity of contractile proteins-purification and characterization of 2 species of troponin-T from rabbit fast skeletal-muscle, *J.Biol.Chem.* 259, 10369–10375, 1984; Sakakura, Y., Hirabayashi, J.,. Oda, Y. *et al.*, Structure of chicken 16-kDa β-galactoside-binding lectin-complete amino-acid-sequence, cloning of cDNA, and production of recombinant lectin, *J.Biol.Chem.* 265, 21573–21579, 1990; Okumura, N., Terasawa, F., Fujita, K. *et al.*, Difference in electrophoretic mobility and plasmic digestion profile between four recombinant fibrinogens, gamma 308K, gamma 3081, gamma 308A, and wild type (gamma 308N), *Electrophoresis* 21, 2309–2315, 2000). The counterion to the lauryl sulfate moiety can also influence the interaction with proteins (Kubo, K. and

Takagi, T., Modulation of the behavior of a protein in polyacrylamide gel electrophoresis in the presence of dodecyl sulfate by varying the cations, *Anal.Biochem.* 224, 572–579, 1995; Kubo, K., Effect of incubation of solutions of proteins containing sodium dodecyl sulfate on the cleavage of peptide bonds by boiling, *Anal. Biochem.* 225, 351–353, 1995).

[h] Deoxycholic acid (3,12-dihydroxycholan-24-oic acid (3α, 5β, 12α), MW 392.6) is relatively insoluble, the sodium salt is more soluble. Deoxychlolate (desoxycholate) is used for membrane solubilization. A natural constituent of bile secretions in man and other mammals.

[i] Cetylpyridinium chloride (1-hexadecylpyridinium chloride) is a cationic detergents which has pharmaceutical use as a preservative and a topical disinfectant. There has been significant use of this material as an active ingredient in mouthwashes. The interaction of cetylpyridinium chloride with glycosaminoglycans such as heparin is useful for characterization. Cetylpyridinium chloride has been used for the isolation of glycosaminoglycans and for the histochemical staining of glycosaminoglycans.

[j] Cetyltrimethylammonium bromide (*N,N,N*-trimethylhexadecaaminium bromide; CTAB; cetrimonium bromide) was developed as a disinfectant and antiseptic. It has been used as detergent in a manner similar to SDS in the determination of protein molecular weight. CTAB is also used for the isolation and assay of nucleic acids.

[k] Tetradecyltrimethyl-ammonium bromide (TTABr). TTABr is one of the components of Cetrimide®, a disinfectant. TTABr has seen occasional use for membrane protein solubilization and in the preparation of mixed micelles.

[l] The "parent" compound for this class of surfactants is betaine sulfonate (sulfobetaine). There are non-detergent sulfobetaines (non detergent sulfobetaines such as 3-(1-pyridino)-1-propanesulfonate; NDSB 201)) which have been useful in preventing unwanted protein-protein aggregation (Vuillard, L., Braun-Breton, C., and Rabilloud, T., Non-detergent sulfobetaines: a new class of mild solubilization agents for protein purification, *Biochem.J.* 305, 337–343, 1995; Collins, T., D'Amico, S., Georlette, D., *et al.*, A nondetergent sulfobetaine prevents protein aggregation in microcalorimetric studies, *Anal.Biochem.* 352, 299–301,2006). Detergent sulfobetaines such Zwittergent® 3–12 (*n*-Dodecyl-N,N-dimethyl-3-ammonio-1-propanesulfonate) contain a long chain alkyl function (Wollstadt, K.H., Karkhanis, Y.D., Gnozzio, M.J. *et al.*, Potential of the sulfobetaine detergent Zwittergent 3-12 as a desorbing agent in biospecific and bioselective affinity chromatography, *J.Chromatog.* 497, 87–100, 1989). The CHAPS class of detergents are derivatives of sulfobetaine which contain a cholamide function.

[m] 3-[(3-cholamidopropyl)dimethylamino]propanesulfonic acid

[n] 3-[(3-cholamidopropyl)dimethylammonio]-2-hydroxy-1-propanesulfonate

References for Table

1. Liljas, L., Lundahl, P., and Hjerten, S., Selective solubilization with Tween 20 of proteins from water-extracted human erythrocyte membranes. Analysis by gel electrophoresis in dodecylsulfate and in Tween 20, *Biochim.Biophys.Acta.* 352, 327–337, 1974.
2. Hoffman, W.L., and Jump, A.A., Tween 20 removes antibodies and other proteins from nitrocellulose, *J.Immunol.Methods* 94, 191–196, 1986.
3. Vandenberg, E.T. and Krull, U.J., The prevention of adsorption of interferents to radiolabeled protein by Tween 20, *J.Biochem. Biophys.Methods* 22, 269–277, 1991.
4. Feng, M., Morales, A.B., Poot, A., et al., Effects of Tween 20 on the desorption of protein from polymer surfaces, *J.Biomater.Sci. Polym.Ed.* 7, 415–424, 1995.
5. Kreilgaard, L., Jones, L.S., Randolph, T.W., et al., Effect of Tween 20 on freeze-thawing- and agitation-induced aggregation of recombinant human factor XIII, *J.Pharm.Sci.* 87, 1597–1603, 1998.
6. Youmans, A.S. and Youmans, G.P., The effect of "tween 80" in vitro on the bacteriostatic activity of twenty compounds for *Mycobacterium tuberculosis, J.Bacteriol.* 56, 245–252, 1948.
7. Young, M., Dinda, M., and Singer, M., Effect of Tween 80 on lipid vesicle permeability, *Biochim. Biophys.Acta.* 735, 429–432, 1983.
8. Kerwin, B.A., Heller, M.C., Levin, S.H., and Randolph, T.W., Effects of Tween 80 and sucrose on acute short-term stability and long-term storage at –20°C of a recombinant hemoglobin, *J.Pharm.Sci.* 87, 1062–1068, 1998.
9. Arakawa, T. and Kita, Y., Protection of bovine serum albumin from aggregation by Tween 80, *J.Pharm.Sci.* 89, 646–651, 2000.
10. Hillgren, A., Lindgren, J., and Alden, M., Protection mechanism of Tween 80 during freeze-thawing of a model protein, LDH, *Int.J.Pharm.* 237, 57–69, 2002.
11. De Duve, C. and Wattiaux, R., Tissue fractionation studies. VII. Release of bound hydrolases by means of triton X-100, *Biochem.J.* 63, 606–608, 1956.
12. Ashani, Y. and Catravas, G.N., Highly reactive impurities in Triton X-100 and Brij 35: partial characterization and removal, *Anal. Biochem.* 109, 55–62, 1980.
13. Labeta, M.O., Fernandez, N., and Festenstein, H., Solubilization effect of Nonidet P-40, Triton X-100 and CHAPS in the detection of MHC-like glycoproteins, *J.Immunol.Methods* 112, 133–138, 1988.
14. Partearroyo, M.A., Urbaneja, M.A., and Goni, F.M., Effective detergent/lipid ratios in the solubilization of phosphatidylcholine vesicles by Triton X-100, *FEBS Lett.* 302, 138–140, 1992.
15. Blonder, J., Yu, L.R., Radeva, G., et al., Combined chemical and enzymatic stable isotope labeling for quantitative profiling of detergent-insoluble membrane proteins isolated membrane proteins isolated using Triton X-100 and Brij-96, *J.Proteome Res.* 5, 349–360, 2006.
16. Schwartz, B.D. and Nathenson, S.G., Isolation of H-2 alloantigens solubilized by the detergent NP-40, *J.Immunol.* 107, 1363–1367, 1971.
17. Hosaka, Y. and Shimizu, Y.K., Artificial assembly of envelope particles of HVJ (Sendai virus). I. Asssembly of hemolytic and fusion factors from envelopes solubilized by Nonidet P40, *Virology* 49, 627–639, 1972.
18. Hart, D.A., Studies on nonidet P40 lysis of murine lymphoid cells. I. Use of cholera toxin and cell surface Ig to determine degree of dissociation of the plasma membrane, *J.Immunol.* 115, 871–875, 1975.
19. Soloski, M.J., Cabrera, C.V., Esteban, M., and Holowczak, J.A., Studies concerning the structure of and organization of the vaccinia virus nucleod. I. Isolation and characterization of subviral particles prepared by treating virions with guanidine-HCl, nonidet-P40, and 2-mercaptoethanol, *Virology* 99, 209–217, 1979.
20. Lanuti, P., Marchisio, M., Cantilena, S., et al., A flow cytometry procedure for simultaneous characterization of cell DNA content and expression of intracellular protein kinase C-zeta, *J.Immunol. Methods* 315, 37–48, 2006.
21. Godson, G.N. and Sinsheimer, R.L., Use of Brij as a general method to prepare polyribosomes from *Escherichia coli., Biochim.Biophys. Acta* 149, 489–495, 1967.
22. Ashani, Y. and Catravas, G.N., Highly reactive impurities in Triton X-100 and Brij 35: partial characterization and removal, *Anal. Biochem.* 109, 55–62, 1980.
23. Krause, M., Rudolph, R., and Schwartz, E., The non-ionic detergent Brij 58P mimics chaperone effects, *FEBS Lett.* 532, 253–255, 2002.
24. Lee, Y.C., Simamora, P., and Yalkowsky, S.H., Effect of Brij-78 on systemic delivery of insulin from an ocular device, *J.Pharm.Sci.* 86, 430–433, 1997.
25. Chakraborty, T., Ghosh, S., and Moulik, S.P., Micellization and related behavior of binary and ternary surfactant mixtures in aqueous medium: cetyl pyridinium chloride (CPC) cetyl trimethyl ammonium bromide (CTAB), and polyoxythelene (10) cetyl ether (Brij-56) derived system,

26. Flawia, M.M. and Torres, H.N., Adenylate cyclase activity in lubrol-treated membranes from *Neurospora crassa*, *Biochim. Biophys.Acta* 289, 428–432, 1972.

27. Young, J.L. and Stansfield, D.A., Solubilization of bovine corpus-luteum adenylate cyclase in Lubrol-PX, triton X-100 or digitonin and the stabilizing effect of sodium fluoride present in the solubilization medium, *Biochem.J.* 173, 919–924, 1978.

28. Hommes, F.A., Eller, A.G., Evans, B.A., and Carter, A.L., Reconstitution of ornithine transport in liposomes with Lubrol extracts of mitochondria, *FEBS Lett.* 170, 131–134, 1984.

29. Chamberlain, L.H., Detergents as tools for the purification and classification of lipid rafts, *FEBS Lett.* 559, 1–5, 2004.

30. Gil, C., Cubi, R., Blasi, J., and Aguilera, J., Synaptic proteins associate with a sub-set of lipid rafts when isolated from nerve endings at physiological temperature, *Biochem.Biophys.Res.Commun.* 348, 1334–1342, 2006.

31. Emerson, M.F. and Holtzer, A., The hydrophobic bond in micellar systems. Effects of various additives on the stability of micelles of sodium dodecyl sulfate and of *n*-dodecyltrimethylammonium bromide, *J.Phys.Chem.* 71, 3320–3330, 1967.

32. Fish, W.W., Reynolds, J.A., and Tanford, C., Gel chromatography of proteins in denaturing solvents. Comparison between sodium dodecyl sulfate and guanidine hydrochloride as denaturants, *J.Biol.Chem.* 245, 5166–5168, 1970.

33. Weber, K. and Kuter, D.J., Reversible denaturation of enzymes by sodium dodecyl sulfate, *J.Biol.Chem.* 246, 4504–4509, 1971.

34. Dai, S. and Tam, K.C., Effects of cosolvents on the binding interaction between poly(ethylene oxide) and sodium dodecyl sulfate, *J.Phys.Chem.B Condens Mater Surf Interfaces Biophys.*, 110, 20794–20800, 2006.

35. Keller, S., Heerklotz, H., Jahnke, N., and Blume, A., Thermodyanamics of lipid membrane solubilization by sodium dodecyl sulfate, *Biophys.J.* 90, 4509–4521, 2006.

36. Benzonana, G., Study of bile salts micelles: properties of mixed oleate-deoxycholate solutions at pH 9.0, *Biochim.Biophys.Acta.* 176, 836–848, 1969.

37. Olsenes, S., Removal of structural proteins from ribosomes by treatment with sodium dexoycholate I the presence of EDTA, *FEBS Lett.* 7, 211–213, 1970.

38. Ehrhart, J.C., and Chaveau, J., Differential solubilization of proteins, phospholipids, free and esterified cholesterol of rat liver cellular membranes by sodium deoxycholate, *Biochim.Biophys.Acta* 375, 434–445, 1975.

39. Robinson, N.C. and Tanford, C., The binding of deoxycholate, Triton X-100, sodium dodecyl sulfate, and phosphatidylcholine vesicles to cytochrome b5, *Biochemistry* 14, 369–378, 1975.

40. Ranganathan, R., Tcacenco, C.M., Rossetto, R., and Hajdu, J., Characterization of the kinetics of Phospholipase C activity toward mixed micelles of sodium deoxycholate and dimyristoylphosphatidylcholine, *Biophys.Chem.* 122, 79–89, 2006.

41. Malchiodi Albedi, F., Cassano, A.M., Ciaralli, F., et al., Influence of cetylpyridinium chloride on the ultrastructural appearance of sulphated glycosaminoglycans in human colonic mucosa, *Histochemistry* 89, 397–401, 1988.

42. Chardin, H., Septier, D., and Goldberg, M., Visualization of glycosaminoglycans in rat incisor predentin and dentin with cetylpyridinium chloride-glutaraldehyde as fixative, *J.Histochem. Cytochem.* 38, 885–894, 1900.

43. Savolainen, H., Isolation and separation of proteoglycans, *J.Chromatogr.B Biomed. Sci.Appl.* 722, 255–262, 1999.

44. Benamor, M., Aguersif, N., and Draa, M.T., Spectrophotometric determination of cetylpyridinium chloride in pharmaceutical products, *J.Pharm.Biomed.Anal.* 26, 151–154, 2001.

45. Arrigler, V., Kogej, K., Majhenc, J., and Svetina, S., Interaction of cetylpyridinium chloride with giant vesicles, *Langmuir* 21, 7653–7661, 2005.

46. Davies, G.E., Quaternary ammonium compounds: a new technique for the study of their bactericidal action and the results obtained with cetavlon (cetyltrimethylammonium bromide), *J.Hyg.*(Lond), 47, 271–277, 1949.

47. Akin, D.T., Shapira, R., and Kinkade, J.M., Jr., The determination of molecular weights of biologically active proteins by cetyltrimethylammonium bromide-polyacrylamide gel electrophoresis, *Anal. Biochem.* 145, 170–176, 1985.

48. Jost, J.P., Jiricny, J. and Saluz, H., Quantitative precipitation of short oligonucleotides with low concentrations of cetyltrimethylammonium bromide, *Nucleic Acid Res.* 17, 2143, 1989.

49. Li, Y.F., Shu, W.Q., Feng, P., et al., Determination of DNA with cetyltrimethylammonium bromide by the measurement of resonance light scattering, *Anal.Sci.* 17, 693–696, 2001.

50. Carra, A., Gambino, G., and Schubert, A., A cetyltrimethylammonium bromide-based method to extract low-molecular-weight RNA from polysaccharide-rich plant tissues, *Anal.Biochem.* 360, 318–320, 2007.

51. Hayakawa, K., Santerre, J.P., and Kwak, J.C, The binding of cationic surfactants by DNA, *Biophys.Chem.* 17, 175–181, 1983.

52. Castedo, A., Castillo, J.L.D., Suarez-Filloys, M.J., and Rodriguez, J.R., Effect of temperature on the mixed micellar tetradecyltrimethylammonium bromide-butanol system, *J.Colloid Interface Sci.* 196, 148–156, 1997.

53. Medrzycka, K. and Zwierzykowski, W., Adsorption of alkyltrimethylammonium bromides at the various interfaces, *J.Colloid Interface Sci.* 230, 67–72, 2000.

54. Stodghill, S.P., Smith, A.E., and O'haver, J.H., Thermodynamics of micellization and adsorption of three alkyltrimethylammonium bromides using isothermal titration calorimetry, *Langmuir* 20, 11387–11392, 2004.

55. Rasmussen, C.D., Nielsen, H.B., and Andersen, J.E., Analysis of the purity of cetrimide by titrations, *PDA J. Pharm.Sci.Technol.* 60, 104–110, 2006.

56. Sims, N.R, Horvath, L.B., and Carnegie, P.R., Detergent solubilization and solubilization of 2':3'-cyclic nucleotide 3'-phosphodiesterase from isolated myelin and c6 cells, *Biochem.J.* 181, 367–375, 1979.

57. Wong, R.K., Nichol, C.P., Sekar, M.C., and Roufogalis, B.D., The efficiency of various detergents for extraction and stabilization of acetylcholinesterase from bovine erythrocytes, *Biochem.Cell Biol.* 65, 8–18, 1987.

58. Wydro, P. and Paluch, M., A study of the interaction of dodecyl sulfobetaine with cationic and anionic surfactant in mixed micelles and monolayers at the air/water interface, *J.Colloid Interface Sci.* 286, 387–391, 2005.

59. Nyuta, K., Yoshimura, T., and Esumi, K., Surface tension and micellization of heterogemini surfactants containing quaternary ammonium salt and sulfobetaine moiety, *J.Colloid Interface Sci.* 301, 267–273, 2006.

60. Zanna, L. and Haeuw, J.F., Separation and quantitative analysis of alkyl sulfobetaine-type detergents by high-performance liquid chromatography and light-scattering detection, *J.Chromatog.B Analyt. Technol.Biomed.Life Sci.*, in press, 2007.

61. Hjelmeland, L.M., A nondenaturing zwitterionic detergent for membrane biochemistry: Design and synthesis, *Proc.Nat.Acad. Sci.USA* 77, 6368–6370, 1980.

62. Ray, J.P., Mernoff, S.T., Sangameswaran, L., and de Blas, A.L., The Stokes Radius of the CHAPS-solubilized benzodiazepine receptor complex, *Neurochem.Res.* 10, 1221–1229, 1985.

63. Labeta, M.O., Fernandez, N., and Festenstein, H., Solubilisation effect of Nonidet P-40, Triton X-100 and CHAPS in the detection of MHC-like glycoprotein, *J.Immunol.Methods* 112, 133–138, 1988.

64. Banerjee, P., Buse, J.T., and Dawson, G., Asymmetric extraction of membrane lipids by CHAPS, *Biochim.Biophys.Acta* 1044, 305–314, 1990.

65. Rouvinski, A., Gahali-Sass, I., Stav, I., et al., Both raft- and non-raft proteins associate with CHAPS-insoluble complexes: some APP in large complexes, *Biochem.Biophys.Res.Commun.* 308, 750–758, 2003.

66. Womack, M.D., Kendall, D.A., and MacDonald, R.C., Detergent effects on enzyme activity and solubilization of lipid bilayer membranes, *Biochim.Biophys.Acta.* 733, 210–215, 1983.

67. Saunders, C.R., 2nd and Prestegard, J.H., Magnetically orientable phospholipid bilayers containing small amounts of a bile salt analogue CHAPSO, *Biophys.J.* 58, 447–460, 1990.

68. Gartner, W., Ullrich, D. and Vogt, K., Quantum yield of CHAPSO-solubilized rhodopsin and 3-hydroxy retinal containing bovine opsin, *Photochem.Photobiol.* 54, 1047–1055, 1991.

69. Banerjee, P., Joo, J.B., Buse, J.T., and Dawson, G., Differential solubilization of lipids along with membrane proteins by different classes of detergents, *Chem.Phys.Lipids* 77, 65–78, 1995.

70. Gehrig-Burger, K., Kohout, L., and Gimpl, G., CHAPSETEROL. A novel cholesterol-based detergent, *FEBS J.* 272, 800–812, 2005.

Tween

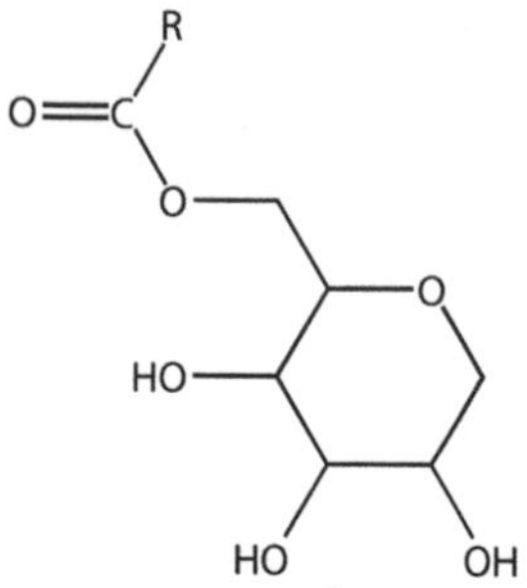

Where R = fatty acid

Sorbitan Fatty Acid Ester, SPAN®

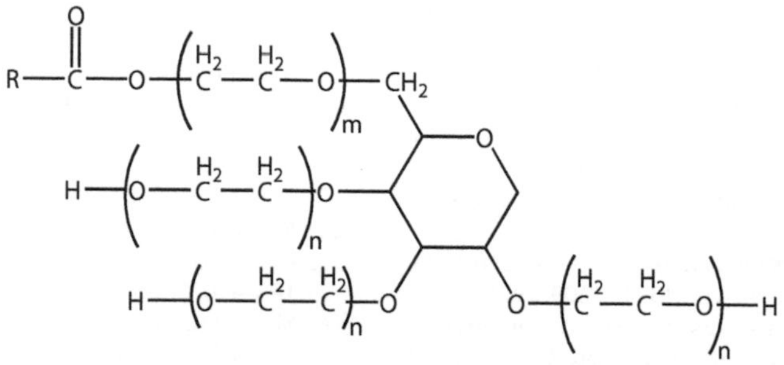

Polysorbate (Tween)

Triton Detergents

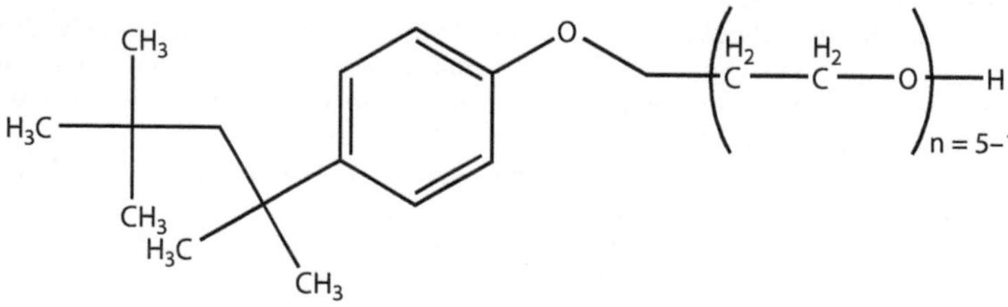

$n = 5\text{--}15$, usually 9

Octoxynol, Triton X®, Igepal® CA

Alkylphenoxy ethoxylate nonionic detergent

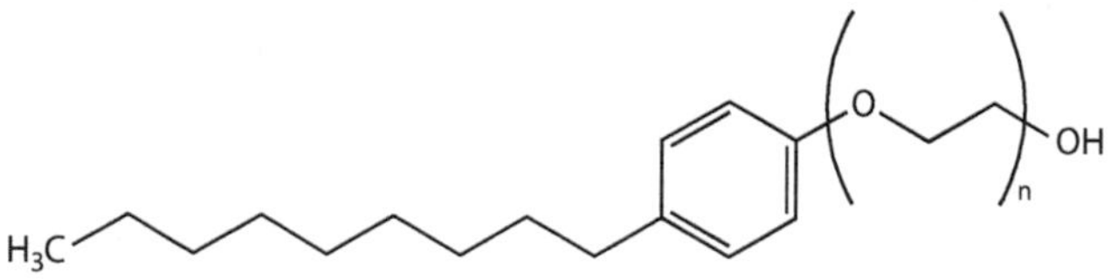

nonoxynol; non-ionic detergent

Polyoxyethyleneglycol Ethers (Polyoxyethylene ethers)

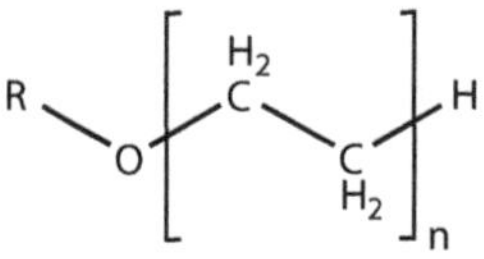

R=alkyl such as cetyl, dodecyl

Sodium dodecylsulfate, SDS, lauryl sulfate, sodium salt

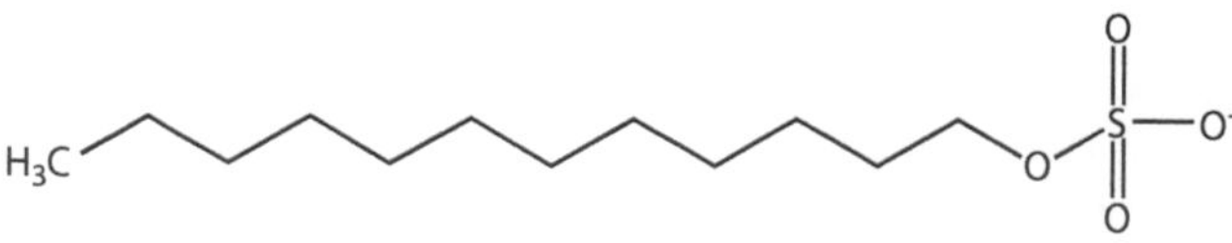

Sodium deoxycholate

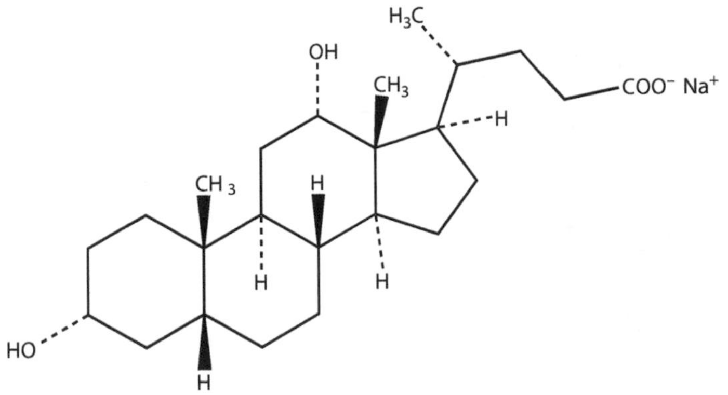

Cetylpyridinium Chloride

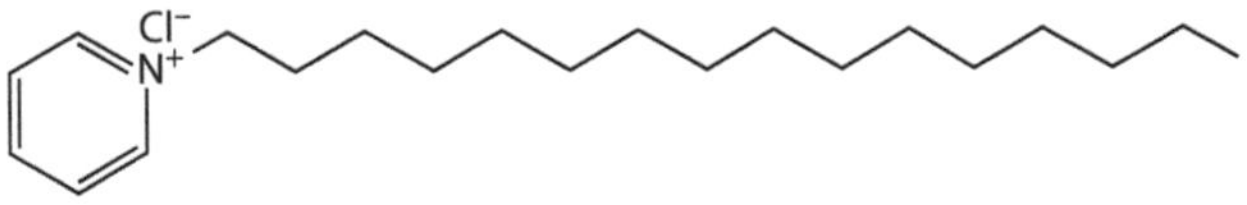

Betaine

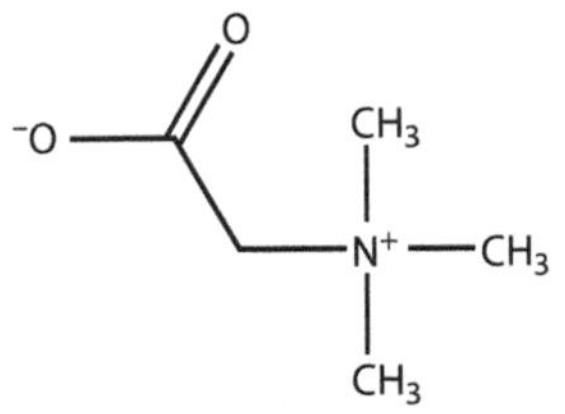

Betaine

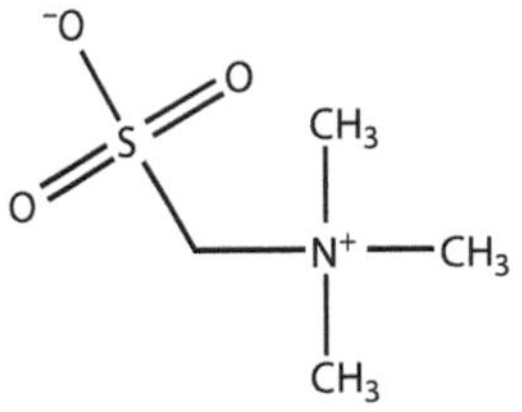

Sulfobetaine

Sulfobetaine Derivatives

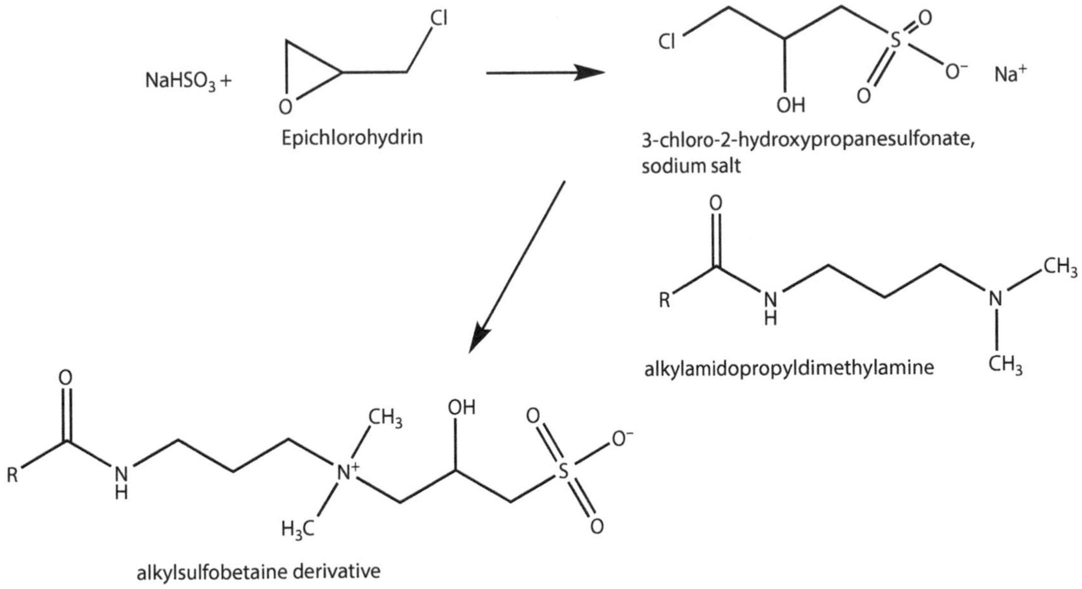

NaHSO$_3$ +

Epichlorohydrin

3-chloro-2-hydroxypropanesulfonate, sodium salt

alkylamidopropyldimethylamine

alkylsulfobetaine derivative

3-[(3-cholamidopropyl)dimethylammonio]-1-propanesulfonate (CHAPS)

BigChap
N,N-bis(3-gluconamidopropyl)cholamide

CHAPSO

3-[(3-cholamidopropyl)dimethylammonio]-2-hydroxy-1-propanesulfonate (CHAPSO)

SOME BIOLOGICAL STAINS AND DYES

Name

Description

Acridine Orange MW 320 as the chloride hydrate

Acridine dyes are strongly yellow fluorescent dyes; stains for nucleic acids and is used for identification of the malaria parasite. Acridine orange is weakly basic, is permeable to membranes and tends to accumulate in intracellular acidic regions. Some use in photodynamic therapy for tumors. The binding of acridine orange to nucleic acids has been extensively studied.

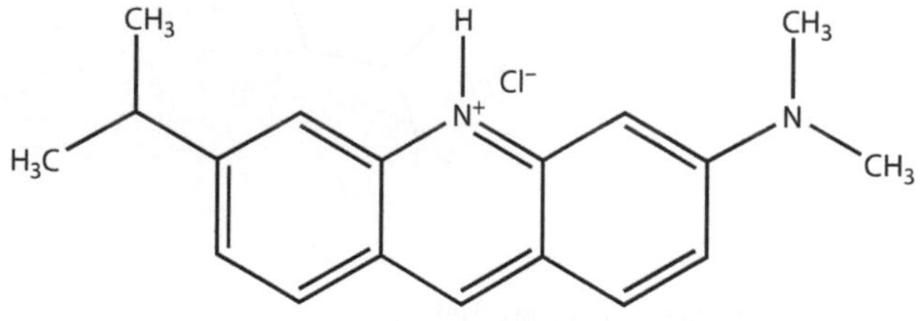

Steiner, R.F. and Beers, R.F., Jr., Spectral changes accompanying binding of acridine orange by polyadenylic acid, *Science* 127, 335–336, 1958; Mayor, H.D. and Hill, N.O., Acridine orange staining of a single-stranded DNA bacteriophage, *Virology* 14, 264–266, 1961; Boyle, R.E., Nelson, S.S., Dollish, F.R., and Olsen, M.J., The interaction of deoxyribonucleic acid and acridine orange, *Arch.Biochem.Biophys.* 96, 47–50, 1962; Leith, J.D., Jr., Acridine orange and acriflavine inhibit deoxyribonuclease action, *Biochim.Biophys.Acta.* 72, 643–644, 1963; Morgan, R.S. and Rhoads, D.G., Binding of acridine orange to yeast ribosomes, *Biochim.Biophys.Acta* 102, 311–313, 1965; Yamabe, S., A spectrophotometric study on binding of acridine orange with DNA, *Mol.Pharmacol.* 3, 556–560, 1967; Stewart, C.R., Broadening by acridine orange of the thermal transition of DNA, *Biopolymers* 6, 1737–1743, 1968; Clerc, S. and Barenholz, Y., A quantitative model for using acridine orange as a transmembrane pH gradient probe, *Anal.Biochem.* 259, 104–111, 1998; Zoccarto, F., Cavallini, L., and Alexandre, A., The pH-sensitive dye acridine orange as a tool to monitor exocytosis/endocytosis, *J.Neurochem.* 72, 625–633, 1999; Lyles, M.B., Cameron, I.L., and Rawls, H.R., Structural basis for the binding efficiency of xanthines with the DNA intercalator acridine orange, *J.Med. Chem.* 44, 4650–4660, 2001; Lyles, M.B. and Cameron, I.L., Interactions of the DNA intercalator acridine orange, with itself, with caffeine, and the double stranded DNA, *Biophys.Chem.* 96, 53–76, 2002; Keiser, J., Utzinger, J., Premji, Z. *et al.*, Acridine orange for malaria diagnosis: its diagnostic performance, its promotion and implementation in Tanzania, and the implications for malaria control, *Ann.Trop.Med.Paristol.* 96, 643–654, 2002; Lauretti, F., Lucas de Mel, F., Benati, F.J., *et al.*, Use of acridine orange staining for the detection of rotavirus RNA in polyacrylamide gels, *J.Virol.Methods* 114, 29–35, 2003; Ueda, H., Murata, H., Takeshita, H., *et al.*, Unfiltered xenon light is useful for photodynamic therapy with acridine orange, *Anticancer Res.* 25, 3979–3983, 2005; Wang, F., Yang, J., Wu, X., *et al.*, Improvement of the acridine orange–protein-surfactant system for protein estimation based on aromatic ring stacking effect of sodium dodecyl benzene sulphonate, *Luminescence* 21, 186–194, 2006; Hiruma, H., Katakura, T., Takenami, T., *et al.*, Vesicle disruption, plasma membrane bleb formation, and acute cell death caused by illumination with blue light in acridine orange-loaded malignant melanoma cells, *J.Photochem.Photobiol.B* 86, 1–8, 2007.

Alizarin Blue MW 292

a carbonyl dye; used as a pH indicator and a stain for copper

Meloan, S.N. and Puchtler, H., Iron alizarin blue S stain for nuclei, *Stain Technol.* 49, 301–304, 1974; Rosenthal, A.R. and Appleton, B., Histochemical localization of intraocular copper foreign bodies, *Am.J.Ophthalmol.* 79, 613–625, 1975; Rao, N.A., Tso, M.O., and Rosenthal, A.R., Chalcosis in the human eye. A clinicopathologic study, *Arch Ophthalmol.* 94, 1379–1384, 1976; Amin, A.S. and Dessouki, H.A., Facile colorimetric methods for the quantitative determination of tetramisole hydrochloride, *Spectrochim.Acta A. Mol.Biomol.Spectros.* 58, 2541–2546, 2002.

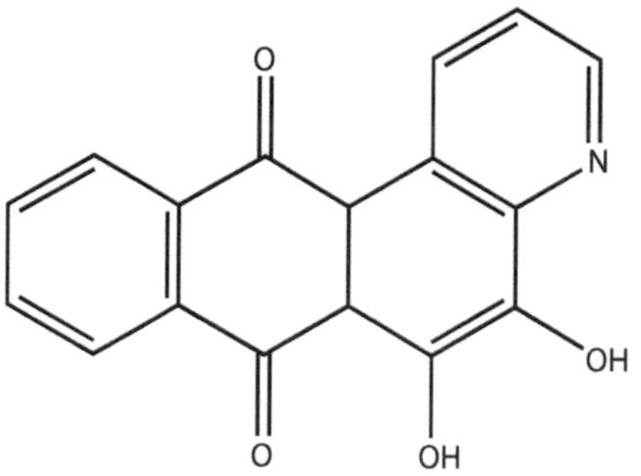

SOME BIOLOGICAL STAINS AND DYES (Continued)

Name

Description

Amido Black 10B(Naphthal Blue Black; Amido Schwarz) MW 617 as sodium salt

Protein staining; originally developed as stain for collagen; protein determination.

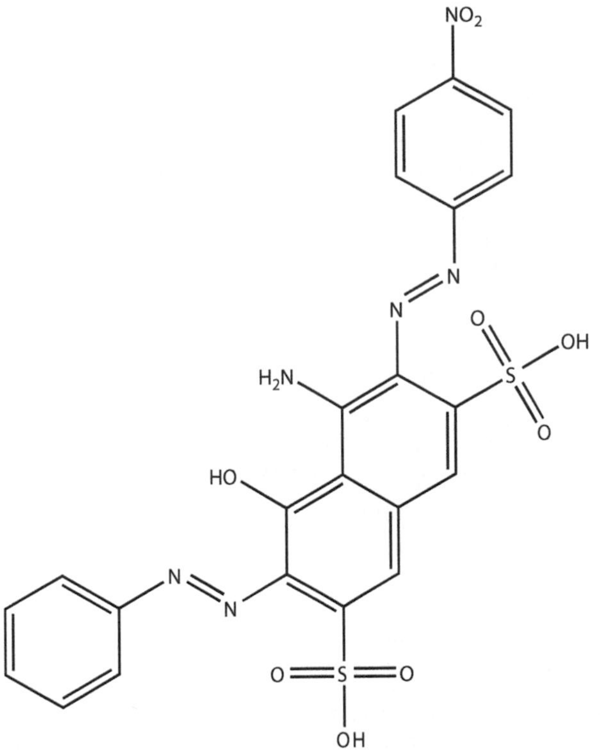

Mundkar, B. and Brauer, B., Selective localization of nucleolar protein with amido black 10B, *J.Histochem.Cytochem.* 14, 94–103, 1966; Mundkar, B. and Greenwood, H., Amido black 10B as a nucleolar stain for lymph nodes in Hodgkin's disease, *Acta Cytol.* 12, 218–226, 1968; Schaffner, W. and Weissmann, C., A rapid, sensitive, and specific method for the determination of protein in dilute solution, *Anal.Biochem.* 56, 502–514, 1973; Kolakowski, E., Determination of peptides in fish and fish products. Part 1. Application of amido black 10B for determination of peptides in trichloroacetic acid extracts of fish meat, *Nahrung* 18, 371–383, 1974; Kruski, A.W. and Narayan, K.A., Some quantitative aspects of the disc electrophoresis of ovalbumin using amido black 10B stain, *Anal.Biochem.* 60, 431–440, 1974; Wilson, C.M., Studies and critique of Amido Black 10B, Coomassie Blue R, and Fast Green FCT as stains for protein after polyacrylamide gel electrophoresis, *Anal.Biochem.* 96, 263–278, 1979; Kaplan, R.S. and Pedersen, P.L., Determination of microgram quantities of protein in the presence of milligram levels of lipid with amido black 10B, *Anal.Biochem.* 150, 97–104, 1985; Nettleton, G.S., Johnson, L.R., and Sehlinger, T.E., Thin layer chromatography of commercial samples of amido black 10B, *Stain Technol.* 61, 329–336, 1986; Tumakov, S.A., Elanskaia, L.N., Esin, M.S., and Drozdova, N.I., Quantitative determination of protein in small volumes of biological substances using amido black 10B(article in Russian), *Lab.Delo.* (5), 54–56, 1988; Schulz, J., Dettlaff, S., Fritzsche, U., *et al.,* The amido black assay: a simple and quantitative multipurpose test of adhesion, proliferation, and cytotoxicity in microplate cultures of keratinocytes (HaCaT) and other cell types growing adherently or in suspension, *J.Immunol.Methods* 167, 1–13, 1994; Gentile, F., Bali, E., and Pignalosa, G., Sensitivity and applications of the nondenaturing staining of proteins on polyvinylidene difluoride membranes with Amido Black 10B in water followed by destaining in water, *Anal.Biochem.* 245, 260–262, 1997; Plekhanov, A.Y., Rapid staining of lipids on thin-layer chromatograms with amido black 10B and other water-soluble stains, *Anal.Biochem.* 271, 186–187, 1999; Butler, P.J.G., Ubarretxene-Belandia, I., Warne, T., and Tate, C.G., The *Escherichia coli* multidrug transporter EmrE is a dimer in the detergent-solubilised state, *J.Mol.Biol.* 340, 797–808,. 2004.

Azure Dyes (Azure A, Azure B or azure blue)

Cationic dyes which are used to stain nucleic acid and sulfated glycosaminoglycans such as heparin. The sensitivity for staining sulfated glycosaminoglycans is increased with the presence of silver.

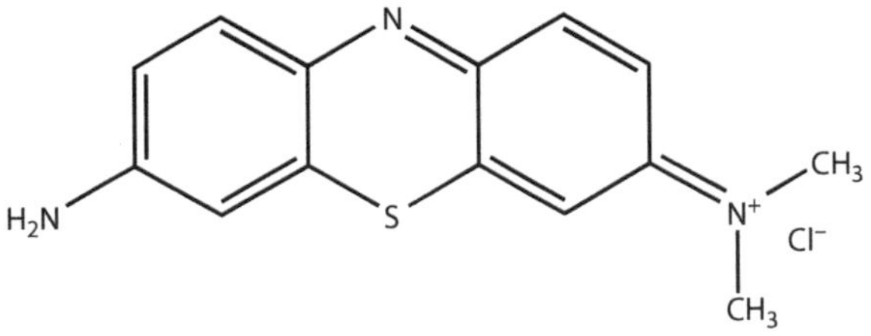

SOME BIOLOGICAL STAINS AND DYES (Continued)

Name

Description

Klein, F. and Szirmai, J.A., Quantitative studies on the interaction of azure A with deoxyribonucleic acid and deoxyribonucleoprotein, *Biochim.Biophys. Acta* 72, 48–61, 1963; Goldstein, D.J., A further note on the measurement of the affinity of a dye (Azure A) for histological substrates, *Q.J.Microsc.Sci.* 106, 299–306, 1965; Wollin, A. and Jaques, L.B., Analysis of heparin—azure A metachromasy in agarose gel, *Can.J.Physiol.Pharmacol.* 50, 65–71, 1972; Lohr, W., Sohmer, I., and Wittekind, D., The azure dyes: their purification and physicochemical properties. I. Purification of azure A, *Stain Technol.* 49, 359–366, 1974; Bennion, P.J., Horobin, R.W., and Murgatroyd, L.B., The use of a basic dye (azure A or toluidine blue) plus a cationic surfactant for selective staining of RNA: a technical and mechanistic study, *Stain Technol.* 50, 307–313, 1975; Dutt, M.K., Staining of DNA-phosphate groups with a mixture of azure A and acridine orange, *Microsc.Acta* 82, 285–289, 1979; Tadano-Aritomi, K., and Ishizuka, I., Determination of peracetylated sulfoglycolipids using the azure A method, *J.Lipid Res.* 24, 1368–1375, 1983; Gundry, S.R., Klein, M.D,. Drongowski, R.A., and Kirsh, M.M., Clinical evaluation of a new rapid heparin assay using the dye azure A, *Am.J.Surg.* 148, 191–194, 1984; Lyon, M. and Gallagher, J.T., A general method for the detection and mapping of submicrogram quantities of glycosaminoglycan oligosaccharides on polyacrylamide gels by sequential staining with azure A and ammoniacal silver, *Anal.Biochem.* 185, 63–70, 1990; van de Lest, C.H., Versteeg, E.M., Veerkamp, J.H. and van Kuppevelt, T.H., Quantification and characterization of glycosaminoglycans at the nanogram level by a combined azure A-silver staining in agarose gels, *Anal.Biochem.* 221, 356–361, 1994; Wang, L., Malsch, P. and Harenberg, J., Heparins, low-molecular weight heparins, and other glycosaminoglycans analyzed by agarose gel electrophoresis and azure A-silver staining, *Semin.Throm.Hemost.* 23, 11–16, 1997.

Biebrich Scarlet (Ponceau B), MW 556 as disodium salt

Anionic diazo dye used as cytoplasmic stain and a stain for basic proteins. Biebrich scarlet also binds specifically to lysozyme and chymotrypsin in a specific manner and inhibits enzyme activity

Douglas, S.D., Spicer, S.S., and Bartels, P.H., Microspectrophotometric analysis of basic protein rich sites stained with Biebrich scarlet, *J.Histochem. Cytochem.* 14, 352–360, 1966; Winkelman, J.W. and Bradley, D.F., Binding of dyes to polycations. I. Biebrich scarlet and histone interaction parameters, *Biochim.Biophys.Acta* 126, 536–539, 1966; Saint-Blancard, J., Allary, M., and Jolles, P., Influence of Biebrich scarlet on the lysis kinetics of *Micrococcus lysodeikticus* by several lysozymes, *Biochemie* 54, 1375–1376, 1972; Holler, E., Rupley, J.A., and Hess, G.P., Productive and unproductive lysozyme-chitosaccharide complexes. Equilibrium measurements, *Biochemistry* 14, 1088–1094, 1975; Giannini, I. and Grasselli, P., Proton transfer to a charged dye bound to the alpha-chymotrypsin active site studied by laser photolysis, *Biochim.Biophys.Acta* 445, 420–425, 1976; Clark, G. and Spicer, S.S., The assessing of acidophilia with Biebrich scarlet, ponceau de zylidine and woodstain scarlet, *Stain Techol.* 54, 13–16, 1979; Smith-Gill, S.J., Wilson, A.C., Potter, M., *et al.*, Mapping the antigenic epitope for a monoclonal antibody against lysozyme, *J.Immunol.* 128, 314–322, 1982; Mlynek, M.L., Comparative investigations on the specificity of Adams' reaction and the Biebrich scarlet stain for the demonstration of eosinophilic granules, *Klin.Wochenschr.* 63, 646–647, 1985; Garvey, W., Fathi, A., Bigelow, F., *et al.*, A combined elastic, fibrin and collagen stain, *Stain Technol.* 62, 365–368, 1987; Allcock, H.R. and Ambrosio, A.M., Synthesis and characterization of pH-sensitive poly(organophosphazene)hydrogels, *Biomaterials* 17, 2295–2302, 1996; Ma, F., Koike, K., Higuchi, T., *et al.*, Establishment of a GM-CSF-dependent megakaryoblastic cell line with the potential to differentiate into an eosinophilic linage in response to retinoic acids, *Br.J.Haematol.* 100, 427–435, 1998; Tan, K., Li, Y., and Huang, C., Flow-injection resonance light scattering detection of proteins at the nanogram level, *Luminescence* 20, 176–180, 2005.

SOME BIOLOGICAL STAINS AND DYES (Continued)

Name	Description
Blue tetrazolium; (Tetrazolium blue, bimethoxyneotetrazolium), MW 728 as the dichloride salt. Also nitro blue tetrazolium and tetranitro blue tetrazolium	A relatively large hydrophobic cation; histochemical stain, used for oxidoreductases. Forms a blue color in the presence of reducing agents which provided the basis for the early use of sulfydryl groups and other reducing compounds. Also used to measure free radicals, superoxide, and Amadori glycation products.

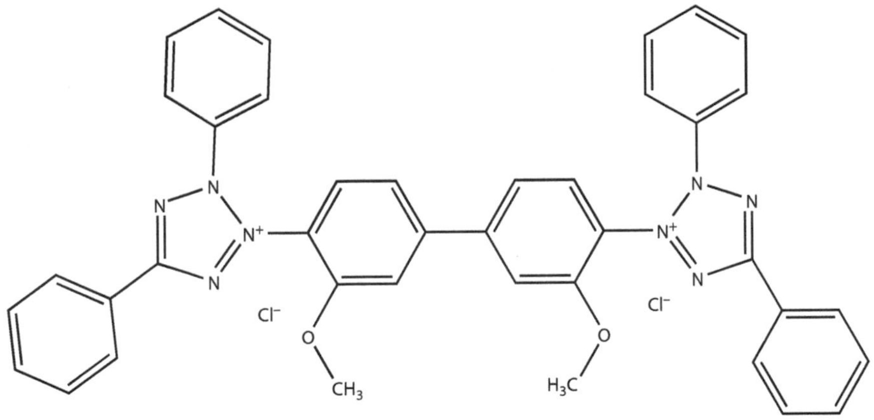

Tetrazolium Blue

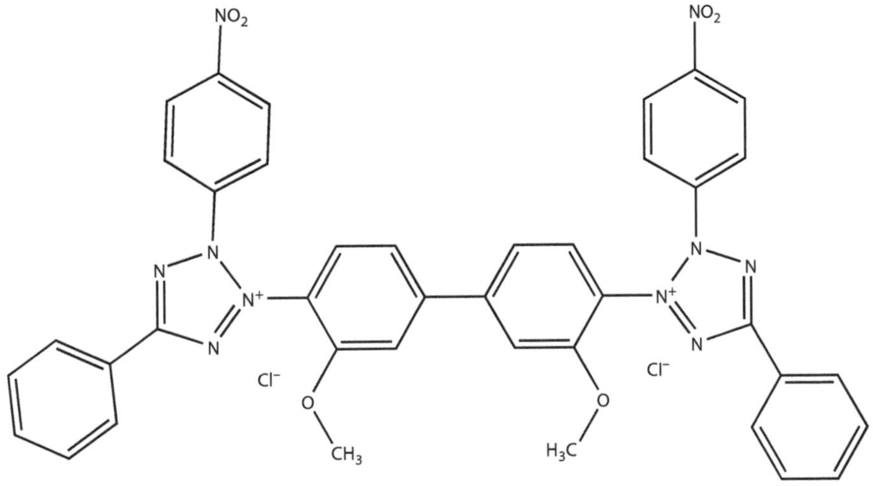

Nitro Blue Tetrazolium

Sulkowitch, H., Rutenburg, A.M., Lesses, M.F., *et al.,* Estimation of urinary reducing corticosteroids with blue tetrazolium, *N.Engl.J.Med.* 252, 1070–1075, 1955; Litteria, M. and Recknagel, R.O., A simplified blue tetrazolium reaction, *J.Lab.Clin.Med.* 48, 463–468, 1956; Leene, W. and van Iterson, W., Tetranitro—blue tetrazolium reduction in *Bacillus subtilis, J.Cell Biol.* 27, 237–241, 1965; Sedar, A.W. and Burde, R.M., The demonstration of the succinic dehydrogenase system in *Bacillus subtilis* using tetranitro—blue tetrazolium combined with techniques of electron microscopy, *J.Cell Biol.* 27, 53–66, 1965; Bhatnagar, R.S. and Liu, T.Z., Evidence for free radical involvement in the hydroxylation of proline: inhibition by nitro blue tetrazolium, *FEBS Lett.* 26, 32–34, 1972; Graham, R.E., Biehl, E.R., Kenner, C.T., *et al.,* Reduction of blue tetrazolium by corticosteroids, *J.Pharm.Sci.* 64, 226–230, 1975; DeChatelet, L.R. and Shirley, P.S., Effect of nitro blue tetrazolium dye on the hexose monophosphate shunt activity of human polymorphonuclear leukocytes, *Biochem.Med.* 14, 391–398, 1975; Oteiza, R.M., Wooten, R.S., Kenner, C.T., *et al.,* Kinetics and mechanism of blue tetrazolium reaction with corticosteroids, *J.Pharm.Sci.* 66, 1385–1388, 1977; DeBari, V.A. and Needle, M.A., Mechanism for transport of nitro-blue tetrazolium into viable and non-viable leukocytes, *Histochemistry* 56, 155–163, 1978; Biehl, E.R., Wooten, R., Kenner, C.T., and Graham, R.E., Kinetic and mechanistic studies of blue tetrazolium reaction with phenylhydrazines, *J.Pharm.Sci.* 67, 927–930, 1978; Schopf, R.E., Mattar, J., Meyenburg, W., *et al.,* Measurement of the respiratory burst in human monocytes and polymorphonuclear leukocytes by nitro blue tetrazolium reduction and chemiluminescence, *J.Immunol. Methods* 67, 109–117, 1984; Jue, C.K. and Lipke, P.N., Determination of reducing sugars in the nanomole range with tetrazolium blue, *J.Biochem. Biophys.Methods* 11, 109–115, 1985; Walker, S.M., Howie, A.F., and Smith, A.F., The measurement of glycosylated albumin

SOME BIOLOGICAL STAINS AND DYES (Continued)

Name	Description

by reduction of alkaline nitro-blue tetrazolium, *Clin.Chim.Acta* 156, 197–206, 1986; Ghiggeri, G.M., Candiano, G., Ginevri, F., *et al.*, Spectrophotometric determination of browning products of glycation of protein amino groups based on their reactivity with nitro blue tetrazolium salts, *Analyst* 113, 1101–1104, 1988; Brenan, M. and Bath, M.L., Indoxyl-tetranitro blue tetrazolium method for detection of alkaline phosphatase in immunohistochemistry, *J.Histochem.Cytochem.* 37, 1299–1301, 1989; Issopoulos, P.B., Sensitive colorimetric assay of cardidopa and methyldopa using tetrazolium blue chloride in pharmaceutical products, *Pharm.Weekbl.Sci.* 11, 213–217, 1989; Fattorossi, A., Nisini, R., Le Moli, S., *et al.*, Flow cytometric evaluation of nitro blue tetrazolium (NBT) reduction in human polymorphonuclear leukocytes, *Cytometry* 11, 907–912, 1990; Albiach, M.R., Guerri, J., and Moreno, P., Multiple use of blotted polyvinylidene difluoride membranes immunostained with nitro blue tetrazolium, *Anal. Biochem.* 221, 25–28, 1994; Chanine, R., Huet, M.P., Oliva, L., and Nadeau, R., Free radicals generated by electrolysis reduces nitro blue tetrazolium in isolated rat heart, *Exp.Toxicol.Pathol.* 49, 91–95, 1997.

Bromophenol Blue (bromphenol blue); tetrabromophenolsulfonphthalein, MW sultone, 670; sodium salt of sulfonic acid, 692	A vital stain; used for determination of protein, pH indicator. There are reports of specific binding to sites on proteins.

Bromophenol Blue (sultone)

Bjerrum, O.J., Interaction of bromophenol blue and bilirubin with bovine and human serum albumin determined by gel filtration, *Scand.J.Clin.Invest.* 22, 41–48, 1968; Ramalingam, K. and Ravidranath, M.H., An evaluation of the metachromasia of bromophenol blue, *Stain Technol.* 47, 179–184, 1972; Harruff, R.C. and Jenkins, W.T., The binding of bromophenol blue to aspartate aminotransferase, *Arch.Biochem.Biophys.* 176, 206–213,1976; Krishnamoorthy, G. and Prabhananda, B.S., Binding site of the dye in bromophenol blue-lysozyme complex. Protein magnetic resonance study in aqueous solutions, *Biochim.Biophys.Acta* 709, 53–57, 1982; Ahmad, H. and Saleemuddin, M., Bromophenol blue protein assay: improvement in buffer tolerance and adaptation for the measurement of proteolytic activity, *J.Biochem.Biophys.Methods* 7, 335–343, 1983; Subrahanian, M., Sheshadri, B.S., and Venkatappa, M.P., Interaction of lysozyme with dyes. II. Binding of bromophenol blue, *J.Biochem.* 96, 245–252, 1984; Ma, C.Q., Li, K.A., and Tong, S.Y., Microdetermination of proteins by resonance light scattering spectroscopy with bromophenol blue, *Anal.Biochem.* 239, 86–91, 1996; Cathey, J.C., Schmidt, C.A., and DeWoody, J.A., Incorporation of bromophenol blue enhances visibility of polyacrylamide gels, *BioTechniques* 22, 222, 1997; Trivedi, V.D., On the role of lysine residues in the bromophenol blue-albumin interaction, *Ital.J.Biochem.* 46, 67–73, 1997; Bertsch, M., Mayburd, A.L., and Kassner, R.J., The identification of hydrophobic sites on the surface of proteins using absorption difference spectroscopy of bromophenol blue, *Anal. Biochem.* 313, 187–195, 2003; Li, J., Chatterjee, K., Medek, A., *et al.*, Acid-base characteristics of bromophenol blue-citrate buffer systems in the amorphous state, *J.Pharm.Sci.* 93, 697–712, 2004; Sarma, S. and Dutta, R.K., Electronic spectral behavior of bromophenol blue in oil in water microemulsions stabilized by sodium dodecyl sulfate and *n*-butanol, *Spectrochim.Acta A Mol.Biomol.Spectrosc.* 64, 623–627, 2006; You, L., Wu, Z., Kim, T., and Lee, K., Kinetics and thermodynamics of bromophenol blue adsorption by a mesoporous hybrid gel derived from tetraethoxysilane and bis(trimethoxysilyl)hexane, *J.Colloid Interface Sci.* 300, 526–535, 2006; Zeroual, Y., Kim, B.S., Kim, C.S., *et al.*, A comparative study on biosorption characteristics of certain fungi for bromophenol blue dye, *Appl.Biochem.Biotechnol.* 134, 51–60, 2006.

SOME BIOLOGICAL STAINS AND DYES (Continued)

Name	Description
Bromothymol Blue or Bromthymol Blue; dibromothymolsulfonphthalein, MW as sultone, 624; as sodium salt, 646	A lipophilic dye; serves as a vital stain to trace fluid movements; used as an ion pair reagent for the measurement of certain drugs; extensive use as pH indicator as there is a change from yellow to blue as pH changes from 6 to 8.0.

Azzone, G.F., Piemonte, G., and Massari, S., Intramembrane pH changes and bromthymol blue translocation in liver mitochondria, *Eur.J.Biochem.* 6, 207–212, 1968; Mitchell, P., Moyle, J., and Smith, L., Bromthymol blue as a pH indicator in mitochondrial suspensions, *Eur.J.Biochem.* 4, 9–19, 1968; Das Gupta, V. and Cadwallader, D.E., Determination of first pKa' value and partition coefficients of bromthymol blue, *J.Pharm.Sci.* 57, 2140–2142, 1968; Jackson, J.B. and Crofts, A.R., Bromothymol blue and bromocresol purple as indicators of pH changes in chromatophores of *Rhodospirillum rubrum*, *Eur.J.Biochem.* 10,226–237, 1969; Gromet-Elhanan, Z. and Briller, S., On the use of bromthymol blue as an indicator of internal pH changes in chromatophores from *Rhodospirillum rubrum*, *Biochem.Biophys.Res.Commun.* 37, 261–265, 1969; Smith, L., Bromthymol blue as a pH indicator in mitochondrial suspensions, *Ann.N.Y.Acad.Sci* 147, 856, 1969; Lowry, J.B., Direct spectrophotometric assay of quaternary ammonium compounds using bromthymol blue, *J.Pharm.Sci.* 68, 110–111, 1979; Mashimo, T., Ueda, I., Shieh, D.D., *et al.*, Hydrophilic region of lecithin membranes studied by bromothymol blue and effects of an inhalation anesthetic, enflurane, *Proc.Natl.Acad.Sci.USA* 76, 5114–5118, 1979; Yamamoto, A., Utsumi, E., Sakane, T. *et al.*, Immunological control of drug absorption from the gastrointestinal tract: the mechanism whereby intestinal anaphylaxis interferes with the intestinal absorption of bromothymol blue in the rat, *J.Pharm.Pharmacol.* 38, 357–362, 1986; Dean, V.S., Dingley, J., and Vaughan, R.S., The use of bromothymol blue and sodium thiopentone to confirm tracheal intubation, *Anaesthesia* 51, 29–32, 1996; Gorbenko, G.P., Bromothymol blue as a probe for structural changes of model membranes induced by hemoglobin, *Biochim.Biophys.Acta* 1370, 107–118, 1998; Ramesh, K.C., Gowda, B.G., Melwanki, M.B., *et al.*, Extractive spectrophotometric determination of antiallergic drugs in pharmaceutical formulations using bromopyrogallol and bromothymol blue, *Anal.Sci.* 17, 1101–1103, 2001; Rahman, N., Ahmed Khan, N. and Hejaz Azmi, S.N., Extractive spectrophotometric methods for the determination of nifedipine in pharmaceutical formulations using bromocresol green, bromophenol blue, bromothymol blue and eriochrome black T, *Farmaco* 59, 47–54, 2004; Erk, N., Spectrophotometric determination of indinavir in bulk and pharmaceutical formulations using bromocresol purple and bromothymol blue, *Pharmazie* 59, 183–186, 2004;

SOME BIOLOGICAL STAINS AND DYES (Continued)

Name	Description
Congo Red (C.I. direct red 28); 696.7 as the disodium salt	Developed as acid-base indicator (Congo Red paper, Riegel's paper); more recent use to detect amyloid peptide aggregates and other fibril structures (crossed β structures); also cellulose surfaces. See also thioflavin T.

Glenner, G.G., The basis of the staining of amyloid fibers: their physico-chemical nature and the mechanism of their dye-substrate interaction, *Prog. Histochem.Cytochem.* 13, 1–37, 1981; Elghetany, M.T. and Saleem, A., Methods for staining amyloid in tissues: a review, *Stain Technol.* 63, 201–212, 1988; Lorenzo, A. and Yankner, B.A., Amyloid fibril toxicity in Alzheimer's disease and diabetes, *Ann.N.Y.Acad.Sci.* 777, 89–95, 1996; Sipe, J.D. and Cohen, A.S., Review: history of the amyloid fibril, *J.Struct.Biol.* 130, 88098, 2000; Piekarska, B., Konieczny, L, Rybarska, J., *et al.*, Intramolecular signaling in immunoglobulins—new evidence emerging from the use of supramolecular protein ligands, *J.Physiol.Pharmacol.* 55, 487–501, 2004; Nilsson, M.R., Techniques to study amyloid fibril formation in vitro, *Methods* 34, 151–160, 2004; Ho, M.R., Lou, Y.C., Lin, W.C., *et al.*, Human pancreatitis-associated protein forms fibrillar aggregates with a native-like conformation, *J.Biol.Chem.* 281, 33566–33576, 2006; Hatters, D.M., Zhong, N., Rutenber, E., and Weisgraber, K.H., Amino-terminal domain stability mediates apolipoprotein E aggregation into neurotoxic fibrils, *J.Mol.Biol.* 361, 932–944, 2006; McLaughlin, R.W., De Stigter, J.K., Sikkink, L.A., *et al.*, The effects of sodium sulfate, glycosaminoglycans, and Congo red on the structure, stability, and amyloid formation of an immunoglobulin light-chain protein, *Protein Sci.* 15, 1710–1722, 2006; Sladewski, T.E., Shafer, A.M., and Hoag, C.M., The effect of ionic strength on the UV-vis spectrum of congo red in aqueous solution, *Spectrochim.Acta A Mol.Biomol.Spectrosc.* 65, 985–987, 2006; Eisert, R., Felau, L., and Brown, L.R., Methods for enhancing the accuracy and reproducibility of Congo Red and thioflavin T assays, *Anal.Biochem.* 353, 144–146, 2006; Sereikaite, J. and Bumelis, V.A., Congo red interaction with α-proteins, *Acta Biochim.Pol.* 53, 87–92, 2006; Frid, P., Anisimov, S.V. and Popovic, N., Congo red and protein aggregation in neurodegenerative diseases, *Brain Res.Brain Res.Rev.* 53, 135–160, 2007; Goodrich, J.D. and Winter, W.T., Alpha-chitin nanocrystals prepared from shrimp shells and their specific surface area measurement, *Biomacromolecules* 8, 252–257, 2007; Lencki, R.W., Evidence for fibril-like structure in bovine casein micelles, *J.Dairy Sci.* 90, 75–89, 2007.

Name	Description
Diaminobenzidine (DAB); 3,3'-dimethyl-aminobenzidine; 3,3',4,4'-tetraaminobiphenyl; MW 214; 360 as the tetrahydrochloride	Histochemical demonstration of peroxidases, oxidases, catalases where DAB serves as electron acceptor forming a polymeric brown product; also used for Western blotting.

Seligman, A.M., Karnovsky, M.J., Wasserkrug, H.L., and Hanker, J.S., Nondroplet ultrastructural demonstration of cytochrome oxidase activity with a polymerizing osmiophilic reagent, diaminobenzidine (DAB), *J.Cell Biol.* 38, 1–14, 1968; Novikoff, A.B., and Goldfischer, S., Visualization of peroxisomes (microbodies) and mitochondria with diaminobenzidine, *J.Histochem.Cytochem.* 17, 675–680, 1969; Ekes, M., The use of diaminobenzidine (DAB) for the histochemical demonstration of cytochrome oxidase activity in unfixed plant tissues, *Histochemie* 27, 103–108, 1971; Herzog, V. and Fahimi, H.D., A new sensitive colorimetric assay for peroxidase using 3,3'-diaminobenzidine as hydrogen donor, *Anal.Biochem.* 55, 554–562, 1973; Nishimura, E.T. and Cooper, C., Peroxidatic reaction of catalase-antibody complex of leukocyte demonstrated by diaminobenzidine, *Cancer Res.* 34, 2386–2392, 1974; Pelliniemi, L.J., Dym, M., and Karnovsky, M.J., Peroxidase histochemistry using diaminobenzidine tetrahydrochloride stored as a frozen solution, *J.Histochem.Cytochem.* 28, 191–192, 1980; van Bogaert, L.J., Quinones, J.A., and van Craynest, M.P., Difficulties involved in diaminobenzidine histochemistry of endogenous peroxidase, *Acta Histochem.* 67, 180–194, 1980; Perotti, M.E., Anderson, W.A., and Swift, H., Quantitative cytochemistry of the diaminobenzidine cytochrome oxidase reaction product in mitochondria of cardiac muscle and pancreas, *J.Histochem.Cytochem.* 31, 351–365, 1983; Bosman, F.T., Some recent developments in immunocytochemistry, *Histochem.J.* 15, 189–200, 1983; Deimann, W., Endogenous peroxidase activity in mononuclear phagocytes, *Prog. Histochem.Cytochem.* 15, 1–58, 1984; Kugler, P., Enzyme histochemical applied in the brain, *Eur.J.Morphol.* 28, 109–120, 1990; Deitch, J.S., Smith, K.L., Swann, J.W., and Turner, J.N., Parameters affecting imaging of the horseradish-peroxidase-diaminobenzidine reaction product in the confocal scanning laser microscope, *J.Microsc.* 160, 265–278, 1990; Ludany, A.,Gallyas, F., Gaszner, B. *et al.*, Skimmed-milk blocking improves silver staining post-intensification of peroxidase-diaminobenzidine staining on nitrocellulose membrane in immunoblotting, *Electrophoresis* 14, 78–80, 1993; Fritz, P., Wu, X., Tuczek, H., *et al.*, Quantitation in immunohistochemistry. A research method or a diagnostic tool in surgical pathology?, *Pathologica* 87, 300–309, 1995; Werner, M., Von Wasielewski, R. and Komminoth, P., Antigen retrieval, signal amplification and intensification in immunohistochemistry, *Histochem.Cell Biol.* 105, 253–260, 1996; Horn, H., Safe diaminobenzidine (DAB) disposal, *Biotech.Histochem.* 77, 229, 2002; Kiernan, J.A., Stability and solubility of 3,3'-diaminobenzidine (DAB), *Biotech. Histochem.* 78, 135, 2003; Rimm, D.L., What brown cannot do for you, *Nat. Biotechnol.* 24, 914–916, 2006.

SOME BIOLOGICAL STAINS AND DYES (Continued)

Name	Description
Dichlorofluorescin diacetate (2,7'-dichlorofluorescin diacetate) MW 487	Histochemical demonstration of peroxidases and esterases; detection of reactive oxygen species (ROS). Not be confused with the fluorescein derivatives

Hassan, N.F., Campbell, D.E., and Douglas, S.D., Phorbol myristate acetate induced oxidation of 2,7'-dichlorofluorescin by neutrophils from patients with chronic granulomatous disease, *J.Leukoc.Biol.* 43, 317–322, 1988; Rosenkranz, A.R., Schmaldienst, S., Stuhlmeier, K.M., *et al.*, A microplate assay for the detection of oxidative products using 2,7'-dichlorofluorescin diacetate, *J.Immunol.Methods* 156, 39–45, 1992; Royall, J.A. and Ischiropoulos, H., Evaluation of 2,7'-dichlorofluorescin and dihydrorhodamine 123 as fluorescent probes for intracellular H_2O_2 in cultured endothelial cells, *Arch.Biochem.Biophys.* 302, 348–355, 1993; Kooy, N.W., Royall, J.A., and Ishiropoulos, H., Oxidation of 2,7'-dichlorofluorescin by peroxynitrite, *Free Radic.Res.* 27, 245–254, 1997; van Reyk, D.M., King, N.J., Dinauer, M.C., and Hunt, N.M., The intracellular oxidation of 2,7'-dichlorofluorescin in murine T lymphocytes, *Free Rad.Biol.Med.* 30, 82–88, 2001; Burkitt, M.J. and Wardman, P., Cytochrome C is a potent catalyst of dichlorofluorescin oxidation: implications for the role of reactive oxygen species in apoptosis, *Biochem.Biophys.Res.Commun.* 282, 329–333, 2001; Chignell, C.F. and Sik, R.H., A photochemical study of cells loaded with 2,7'-dichlorofluorescin: implications for the detection of reactive oxygen species generated during UVA irradiation, *Free Rad.Biol.Med.* 34, 1029–1034, 2003; Afzal, M. Matsugo, S., Sesai, M. *et al.*, Method to overcome photoreaction , a serious drawback to the use of dichlorofluorescin in evaluation of reactive oxygen species, *Biochem.Biophys.Res. Commun.* 304, 619–624, 2003; Lawrence, A., Jones, C.M., Wardman, P., and Burkitt, M.J., Evidence for the role of a peroxidase compound I-type intermediate in the oxidation of glutathione, NADH, ascorbate, and dichlorofluorescein by cytochrome c/H_2O_2. Implications for oxidative stress during apoptosis, *J.Biol.Chem.* 278, 29410–29419, 2003; Myhre, O., Andersen, J.M., Aarnes, H., and Fonnum, F., Evaluation of the probes 2,7'-dichlorofluorescin diacetate, luminol, and lucigenin as indicators of reactive species formation, *Biochem.Pharmacol.* 65, 1575–1582, 2003; Laggner, H., Hermann, M., Gmeincr, B.M., and Kapiotis, S., Cu^{2+} and Cu^+ bathocuproine disulfonate complexes promote he oxidation of the ROS-detecting compound dichlorofluorescin (DCFH), *Anal.Bioanal.Chem.* 385, 959–961, 2006; Matsugo, S., Sasai, M., Shinmori, H. *et al.*, Generation of a novel fluorescent product, monochlorofluorescein from dichlorofluorescin by photo-irradiation, *Free Radic.Res.* 40, 959–965, 2006.

Name	Description
3,3'-Dimethyl-9-methyl-4,5,4',5'-dibenzothiacarbocyanine; DBTC; "Stains all"; MW 560	A cationic dye with a broad specificity for interaction including glycosaminoglycans and nucleic acids. DBTC has been used to stain for calmodulin and other calcium-binding proteins.

SOME BIOLOGICAL STAINS AND DYES (Continued)

Name	Description

Scheres, J.M., Production of C and T bands in human chromosomes after heat treatment at high pH and staining with "stains-all", *Humangenetik*, 23, 311–314, 1974; Green, M.R. and Pastewka, J.V., The cationic carbocyanine dyes Stains-all, DBTC, and Ethyl-stains-all, DBTC-3,3'9-triethyl, *J.Histochem. Cytochem.* 27, 797–799, 1979; Caday, C.G. and Steiner, R.F., The interaction of calmodulin with the carbocyanine dye (Stains all), *J.Biol.Chem.* 260, 5985–5990, 1985; Caday, C.G., Lambooy, P.K., and Steiner, R.F., The interaction of Ca^{2+}-binding proteins with the carbocyanine dye stains-all, *Biopolymers* 25, 1579–1595, 1986; Sharma, Y., Rao, C.M. Rao, S.C., *et al.*, Binding site conformation dictates the color of the dye stains-all. A study of the binding of this dye to the eye lens proteins crystallins, *J.Biol.Chem.* 264, 20923–20927, 1989; Lu, M., Guo, Q., Seeman, N.C. and Kallenbach, N.R., Drug binding by branched DNA: selective interaction of the dye stains-all with an immobile junction, *Biochemistry* 29, 3407–3412, 1990; Nakamura, K., Masuyama, E., Wada, S., and Okuno, M., Applications of stains' all staining to the analysis of axonemal tubulins: identification of beta-tubulin and beta-isotubulins, *J.Biochem.Biophys.Methods* 21, 237–245, 1990; Gruber, H.E. and Mekikian, P., Application of stains-all for demarcation of cement lines in methacrylate embedded bone, *Biotech.Histochem.* 66, 181–184, 1991; Sharma, Y., Gapalakrishna, A., Balasubramanian, D., *et al.*, Studies on the interaction of the dye, stains-all, with individual calcium-binding domains of calmodulin, *FEBS Lett.* 326, 59–64, 1993; Lee, H.G. and Cowman, K., An agarose gel electrophoretic method of analysis of hyaluronan molecular weight distribution, *Anal.Biochem.* 219, 278–287, 1994; Myers, J.M., Veis, A., Sabsay, B., and Wheeler, A.P., A method for enhancing the sensitivity and stability of stains-all for Phosphoproteins separated in sodium dodecyl sulfate-polyacrylamide gels, *Anal. Biochem.* 240, 300–302, 1996; Goldberg, H.A. and Warner, K.J., The staining of acidic proteins on polyacrylamide gels: enhanced sensitivity and stability of "Stains All" staining in combination with silver nitrate, *Anal.Biochem.* 251, 227–233, 1997; Volpi, N., and Maccari, F., Detection of submicrogram quantities of glycosaminoglycans on agarose gels by sequential staining with toluidine blue and Stains All, *Electrophoresis* 23, 4060–4066, 2002; Volpi, N., Macari, F., and Titze, J., Simultaneous detection of submicrogram quantities of hyaluronic acid and dermatan sulfate on agarose-gel by sequential staining with toluidine blue and Stains All, *J.Chromatog.B. Analyt. Technol. Biomed.Life Sci.* 820, 131–135, 2005.

Evans Blue (C.I. Direct Blue 53); MW 961 as tetrasodium salt.

Early use as a method for determining blood volume; histochemical use as a protein stain, extensive use as a vital stain; more recent use to demonstrate vascular leakage and surgical dye.

Gibson, J.G., and Evans, W.A., Clinical studies of the blood volume. I. Clinical application of a method employing the azo dye "Evans Blue" and the spectrophotometer, *J.Clin.Invest.* 16, 301–316, 1937; Morris, C.J., The determination of plasma volume by the Evans blue method: the analysis of haemolyzed plasma, *J.Physiol.* 102, 441–445, 1944; Morris, C.J., Chromatographic determination of Evans blue in plasma and serum, *Biochem.J.* 38, 203–204, 1944; McCord, W.M. and Ezell, H.K., Cell volume determinations with Evans blue, *Proc.Soc.Exptl.Biol.Med.* 76, 727–728, 1951; Caster, W.O., Simon, A.B., and Armstrong, W.D., Evans blue space in tissues of the rat, *Am.J.Physiol.* 183, 317–321, 1955; Clausen, D.F. and Lifson, N., Determination of Evans blue dye in blood in tissues, *Proc.Soc.Exp.Biol.Med.* 91, 11–14, 1956; Larsen, O.A. and Jarnum, S., The Evans Blue test in amyloidosis, *Scand.J.Clin. Lab.Invest.* 17, 287–294, 1965; Rabinovitz, MK. and Schen, R.J., The characteristics of certain alpha globulins in immunoelectrophoresis of human serum, using Evans blue dye, *Clin.Chim.Acta* 17, 499–503, 1967; Crippen, R.W. and Perrier, J.L., The use of neutral red and Evans blue for live-dead determination of marine plankton (with comments on the use of rotenone for inhibition of grazing), *Stain Technol.* 49, 97–104, 1974; Fry, D.L., Mahley, R.W., Weisgraber, K.H. and Oh, S.Y., Simultaneous accumulation of Evans blue dye and albumin in the canine aortic wall, *Am.J.Physiol.* 233, H66–H79, 1977; Shoemaker, K., Rubin, J., Zumbro, G.L., and Tackett, R., Evans blue and gentian violet: alternatives to methylene blue as a surgical marker dye, *J.Thorac. Cardiovasc.Surg.* 112, 542–544, 1996; Skowronek, M., Roterman, Konieczny, L., *et al.*, The conformational characteristics of Congo Red, Evans blue and Trypan blue, *Comput.Chem.* 24, 429–450, 2000; Hamer, P.W., McGeachie, J.M., Davies, M.J., and Grounds, M.D., Evans Blue dye as an *in vivo* marker of myofibre damage: optimizing parameters for detecting initial myofibre membrane permeability, *J.Anat.* 200, 69–79, 2002; Kaptanoglu, E., Okutan, O., Akbiyik, F., *et al.*, Correlation of injury severity and tissue Evans glue content, lipid peroxidation and clinical evaluation in acute spinal cord injury in rats, *J.Clin.Neurosci.* 11, 879–885, 2004; Green, M., Frashid, G., Kollias, J. *et al.*, The tissue distribution of Evans blue dye in a sheep model of sentinel node biopsy, *Nucl.Med.Commun.* 27, 695–700, 2006.

SOME BIOLOGICAL STAINS AND DYES (Continued)

Name   **Description**

Fast Green (Fast Green FCF; C.I. food green 3) M.W.   A histochemical cytoplasmic counterstain; a stain for protein; used to demonstrate histones;
809 as the trisodium salt   marker dye; a food dye FD & C fast green 3).

Bryan, J.H., Differential staining with a mixture of safranin and fast green FCF, *Stain Technol.* 30, 153–157, 1955; Garcia, A.M., Studies on deoxyribonucleoprotein in leukocytes and related cells of mammals. VII. The fast green histone content of rabbit leukocytes after hypertonic treatment, *Stain Technol.* 30, 153–157, 1955; Hunt, D.E. and Caldwell, R.C., Use of fast green in agar-diffusion microbiological assays, *Appl.Microbiol.* 18, 1098–1099, 1969; Gorovsky, M.A., Carlson, K., and Rosenbaum, J.L., Simple method for quantitative densitometry of polyacrylamide gels using fast green, *Anal. Biochem.* 35, 359–370, 1970; Entwhistle, K.W., Congo red-fast green fcf as a supra-vital stain for ram and bull spermatozoa, *Aust.Vet.J.* 48, 515–519, 1972; Noeske, K., Discrepancies between cytophotometric alkaline Fast Green measurements and nuclear histone protein content, *Histochem.J.* 5, 303–311, 1973; McMaster-Kaye, R. and Kaye, J.S., Staining of histones on polyacrylamide gels with amido blank and fast green, *Anal.Biochem.* 61, 120–132, 1974; Medugorac, I., Quantitative determination of cardiac myosin subunits stained with fast green in SDS-electrophoretic gels, *Basic Res. Cardiol.* 74, 406–416, 1979; Glimore, L.B. and Hook, G.E., Quantitation of specific proteins in polyacrylamide gels by the elution of Fast Green FCF, *J.Biochem.Biophys.Methods* 5, 57–66, 1981; Smit, E.F., de Vries, E.G., Meijer, C., *et al.*, Limitations of the fast green assay for chemosensitivity testing in human lung cancer, *Chest* 100, 1358–1363, 1991; Li, Y.F., Huang, C.Z., and Li, M., A resonance light-scattering determination of proteins with fast green FCF, *Anal.Sci.* 18, 177–181, 2002; Tsuji, S., Yoshii, K., and Tonogai, Y. Identification of isomers and subsidiary colors in commercial Fast Green FCF (FD & C Green No. 3, Food Green No. 3) by liquid chromatography-mass spectrometry and comparison between amounts of the subsidiary colors by high-performance liquid chromatography and thin-layer chromatography-spectrometry, *J.Chromatog.A.* 1101, 214–221, 2006; Luo, S., Wehr, N.B., and Levine, R.L., Quantitation of protein on gels and blots by infrared fluorescence of Coomassie glue and Fast Green, *Anal.Biochem.* 350, 233–238, 2006; Ali, M.A. and Bashier, S.A., Effect of fast green dye on some biophysical properties of thymocytes and splenocytes of albino mice, *Food Addit.Contam.* 23, 452–561, 2006.

SOME BIOLOGICAL STAINS AND DYES (Continued)

Name

Description

Fluorescein (C.I. solvent yellow 94) MW as free acid is 332 while the disodium salt is 376.

Fluorescein is an acidic hydroxyxanthene which exists in a variety of forms. Depending on pH, fluorescein is in equilibrium the free acid and a dianion form. When the dianion is present as the sodium salt, the term uranin has been used to describe the molecule. Fluorescein has a broad range of use including use in large quantities to trace environment water flow. Fluorescein has been used to vascular flow with particular interest in ophthalmology. Fluorescein has been modified to include reactive functional groups (isothiocyanate; for covalent insertion of fluorescent probes into protein and other biological macromolecules. Care must be taken to avoid confusion with fluorescin.

Fluorescein

Uranin

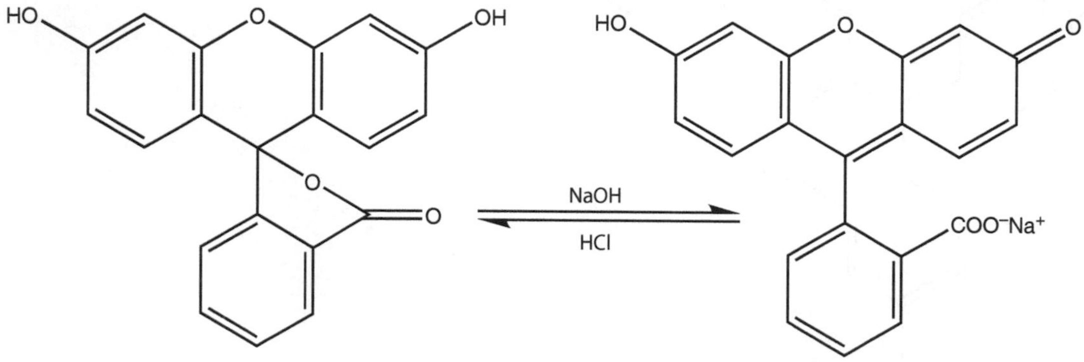

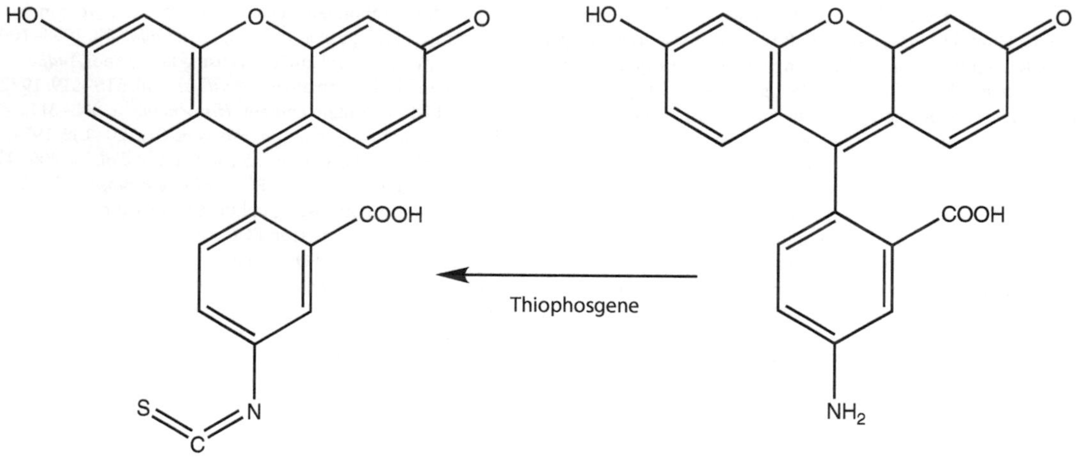

NaOH

HCl

Thiophosgene

Fluorescein Isothiocyanate

SOME BIOLOGICAL STAINS AND DYES (Continued)

Name	Description

Ray, R.R. and Binkhorst, R.D., The diagnosis of papillary block by intravenous injection of fluorescein, *Am.J.Ophthamol.* 61, 480–483, 1966; Hill, D.W., Fluorescein angiography in fundus diagnosis, *Br.Med.Bull.* 26, 161–165, 1970; Gass, J.D., Fluorescein angiography. An aid in the differential diagnosis of intraocular tumors, *Int.Ophthalomol.Clin.* 12, 85–120, 1972; Ohkuma, S., Use of fluorescein isothiocynate-dextran to measure proton pumping in lysosomes and related organelles, *Methods Enzymol.* 174, 131–154, 1989; Klose, A.D. and Gericke, K.R., Fluorescein as a circulation determinant, *Ann. Pharmacother.* 28, 891–893, 1994; Wischke, C. and Borchert, H.H., Fluorescein isothiocyanate labelled bovine serum albumin (FITC-BSA) as a model protein drug: opportunities and drawbacks, *Pharmazie* 61, 770–774, 2006; Berginc, K., Zakelj, S., Levstik, L., *et al.,* Fluorescein transport properties across artificial lipid membranes, Caco-2 cell monolayers and rat jejuna, *Eur.J.Pharm.Biopharm.,* in press, 2006.

Malachite Green (Victoria Green, C.I. basic green 4); MW leukobase, 330; carbinol free base as the hydrochloride, 383)

A cationic diaminotriphenylmethane which is used to stain a variety of cells including bacterial spores, pH indicators, stain for phospholipid; measurement of inorganic phosphate.

Malachite Green
Victoria Green B

Leukomalachite green
Leuko form

Malachite Green Carbinol Chloride

SOME BIOLOGICAL STAINS AND DYES (Continued)

Name	Description

Norris, D., Reconstitution of virus X-saturated potato varieties with malachite green, *Nature* 172, 816, 1953; Kanetsuna, F., A study of malachite green staining of leprosy bacilli, *Int.J.Lepr.* 32, 185–194, 1964; Solari, A.A., Herrero, M.M., and Painceira, M.T., Use of malachite green for staining flagella in bacteria, *Appl.Microbiol.* 16, 792, 1968; Teichman, R.J., Takei, G.H., and Cummins, J.M., Detection of fatty acids, fatty aldehydes, phospholipids, glycolipids and cholesterol on thin-layer chromatograms stained with malachite green, *J.Chromatog.* 88, 425–427, 1974; Singh, E.F., Moawad, A., and Zuspan, F.P., Malachite green—a new staining reagent for prostaglandins, *J.Chromatog* 105, 194–196, 1975; Nefussi, J.R., Septier, D., Sautier, J.M. *et al.,* Localization of malachite green positive lipids in the matrix of bone nodule formed in vitro, *Calif.Tissue Int.* 50, 273–282, 1992; Henderson, A.L., Schmitt, T.C., Heinze, T.M., and Cerniglia, C.E., Reduction of malachite green to leucomalachite green by intestinal bacteria, *Appl.Environ.Microbiol* 63, 4099–4101, 1997; Nguyen, D.H., DeFina, S.C., Fink, W.H., and Dieckmann, T., Binding to an RNA aptamers changes the charge distribution and conformation of malachite green, *J.Am.Chem.Soc.* 124, 15081–15084, 2002; Dutta, K., Bhattacharjee, S., Chauduri, B., and Mukhopadhyay, S., Oxidative degradation of malachite green by Fenton generated hydroxyl radicals in aqueous acidic media, *J.Environ.Sci.Health A. Tox. Hazard Subst. Environ.Eng.* 38, 1311–1326, 2003; Jadhav, J.P. and Govindwar, S.P., Biotransformation of malachite green by *Saccharomyces cerevisiae* MTCC 463, *Yeast* 23, 315–323, 2006.

Methylene Blue, MW 374 as the chloride monohydrate

A weakly hydrophilic cationic diaminothiazine. Methylene blue is used for a variety of purposes including development of the Romanowsky stain, bacterial staining, assay of redox reactions, vital staining, photooxidation of proteins, surgical marker (this use appears to undergoing serious reconsideration), and determination of cell wall permeability. Methylene blue with UV irradiation is used for the inactivation of pathogens in blood plasma.

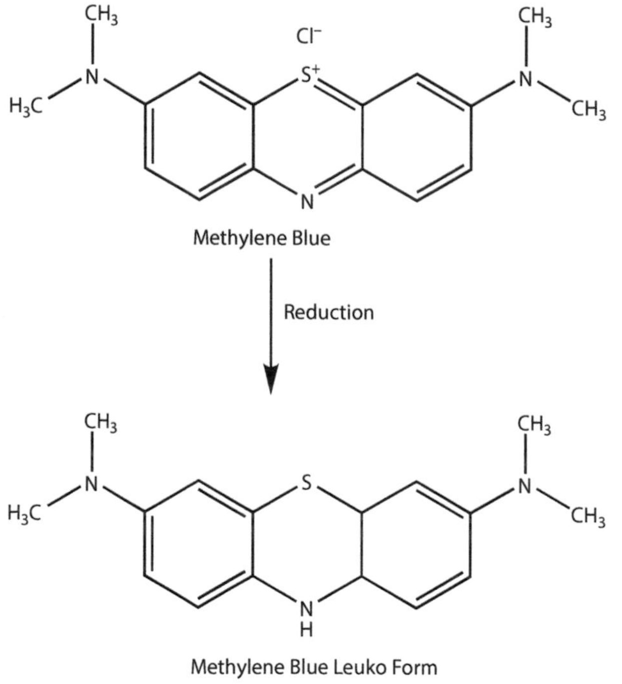

Methylene Blue

Reduction

Methylene Blue Leuko Form

Name	Description

Wishart, G.M., On the reduction of methylene blue by tissue extracts, *Biochem.J.* 17, 103–114, 1923; Whitehead, H.R., The reduction of methylene blue in milk: The influence of light, *Biochem.J.* 24, 579–584, 1930; Worley, L.G., The relation between the Golgi apparatus and "Droplets" in the cell stainable vitally with methylene blue, *Proc.Natl.Acad.Sci.USA* 29, 228–231, 1943; Weil, L., Gordon, W.G., and Buchert, A.R., Photooxidation of amino acids in the presence of methylene blue, *Arch.Biochem.* 33, 90–109, 1951; Moore, T., Sharman, I.M., Ward, R.J., The vitamin E activity of substances related to methylene blue, *Biochem.J.* 54, xvi–xvii, 1953; Yamazaki, I., Fujinaga, K., and Takehara, I., The reduction of methylene blue catalyzed by the turnip peroxidase, *Arch.Biochem.Biophys.* 72, 42–48, 1957; Borzani, W. and Vairo, M.L., Adsorption of methylene blue as a means of determining cell concentration of dead bacteria in suspensions, *Stain Technol.* 35, 77–81, 1960; Tinne, J.E., A methylene blue medium for distinguishing virulent mycobacteria, *Scott.Med.J.* 4, 130–132, 1959; Barbosa, P. and Peters, T.M., The effects of vital dyes on living organisms with special reference to methylene blue and neutral red, *Histochem.J.* 3, 71–93, 1971; Bentley, S.A., Marshall, P.N., and Trobaugh, F.E., Jr., Standardization of the Romanowksy staining procedure: an overview, *Anal.Quant.Cytol.* 2, 15–18, 1980; Wittekind, D.H. and Gehring, T., On the nature of Romanowsky-Giemsa staining and the Romanowsky-Giemsa effect. I. Model experiments on the specificity of azure B-eosin Y stain as compared with other thiazine dye – eosin Y combinations, *Histochem.J.* 17, 263–289, 1985; Schulte, E. and Wittekind, D., The influence of Romanowsky-Giemsa type stains on nuclear and cytoplasmic features of cytological specimens, *Anal.Cell Pathol.* 1, 83–86, 1989; Tuite, E.M. and Kelly, J.M., Photochemical interactions of methylene blue and analogues with DNA and other biological substrates, *J.Photochem.Photobiol.B.* 21, 103–124, 1993; Bradbeer, J.N., Riminucci, M., and Bianco, P., Giemsa as a fluorescent stain for mineralized bone, *J.Histochem.Cytochem.* 42, 677–680, 1994; Wainwright, M. and Crossley, K.B., Methylene blue – a therapeutic dye for all seasons?, *J.Chemother.* 14, 431–443, 2002; Inamura, K., Ikeda, E., Nagayasu, T., *et al.*, Adsorption behavior of methylene blue and its congeners on a stainless steel surface, *J.Colloid Interface Sci.* 245, 50–57, 2002; Floyd, R.A., Schneider, J.E., Jr., and Dittmern, D.P., Methylene blue photoinactivation of RNA viruses, *Antiviral Res.* 61, 141–151, 2004; Rider, K.A. and Flick, L.M., Differentiation of bone and soft tissues in formalin-fixed, paraffin-embedded tissue by using methylene blue/acid fuchsin stain, *Anal.Quant.Cytol.Histol.* 26, 246–248, 2004; Rider, K.A. and Flick, L.M., Differentiating of bone and soft tissues in formalin-fixed, paraffin-embedded tissue by using methylene blue/acid fuchsin stain, *Anal.Quant.Cytol. Histol.* 26, 246–248, 2004; Papin, J.F., Floyd, R.A., and Dittmer, D.P., Methylene blue photoinactivation abolishes West Nile virus infectivity *in vivo*, *Antiviral Res.* 68, 84–87, 2005; Dilgin, Y. and Nisli, G., Fluorometric determination of ascorbic acid in vitamin C tablets using methylene blue, *Chem.Pharm.Bull.* 53, 1251–1254, 2005; Itoh, K., Decolorization and degradation of methylene blue by *Arthrobacter globiformis*, *Bull.Environ.Contam.Toxicol.* 75, 1131–1136, 2005; D'Amico, F., A polychromatic staining method for epoxy embedded tissues: a new combination of methylene blue and basic fuchsine for light microscopy, *Biotech.Histochem.* 80, 207–210, 2005; Cheng, Y., Liu, W.F., Yan, Y.B., and Zhou, H.M., A nonradiometric assay for poly(a)-specific ribonuclease activity by methylene blue colorimetry, *Protein Pept.Lett.* 13, 125–128, 2006; Jurado, E., Fernandez-Serrano, M., Nunez-Olea, J., *et al.*, Simplified spectrophotometric method using methylene blue for determining anionic surfactants: applications to the study of primary biodegradation in aerobic screening tests, *Chemosphere* 65, 278–285, 2006; Dinc, S., Ozaslan, C., Kuru, B., *et al.*, Methylene blue prevents surgery-induced peritoneal adhesions but impairs the early phase of anastomotic wound healing, *Can.J.Surg.* 49, 321–328, 2006; Appadurai, I.R. and Scott-Coombes, D., Methylene blue for parathyroid localization, *Anaesthesia* 62, 94, 2007; Mihai, R., Mitchell, E.W., and Warwick, J., Dose-response and postoperative confusion following methylene blue infusion during parathyroidectomy, *Can.J.Anaesth.* 54, 79–81, 2007; McCullagh, C. and Robertson, P., Effect of polyethyleneimine, a cell permeabiliser, on the photo-sensitised destruction of algae by methylene blue and nuclear fast red, *Photochem.Photobiol.*, in press, 2007.

Methyl Orange, Orange III, Gold Orange, C.I. Orange 52; MW 327 as sodium salt	An azo dye with limited use in histology; use for the assay of redox reactions. Used for the study of protein conformation; early use for assay of albumin; binding to cationic proteins.

Wetlaufer, D.B. and Stahmann, M.A., The interaction of methyl orange anions with lysine polypeptides, *J.Biol.Chem.* 203, 117–126, 1953; Colvein, J.R., The adsorption of methyl orange by lysozyme, *Can.J.Biochem.Physiol.* 32, 109–118, 1954; Lundh, B., Serum albumin as determined by the methyl orange method and by electrophoresis, *Scand.J.Clin.Lab.Invest.* 17, 503–504, 1965; Barrett, J.F., Pitt, P.A., Ryan, A.J., and Wright, S.E., The demethylation of *m*-methyl orange and methyl orange *in vivo* and *in vitro*, *Biochem.Pharmacol.* 15, 675–680, 1966; Shikama, K., Denaturation and renaturation of binding sites of bovine serum albumin for methyl orange, *J.Biochem.* 64, 55–63, 1968; Lang, J., Auborn, J.J., and Eyring, E.M., Kinetic studies of the interaction of methyl orange with beta-lactoglobulin between pH 3.7 and 2.0, *J.Biol.Chem.* 246, 5380–5383, 1971; Browner, C.J. and Lindup, W.E., Decreased plasma protein binding of *o*-methyl red methyl orange and phenytoin (diphenylhydantoin) in rats with acute renal failure,

SOME BIOLOGICAL STAINS AND DYES (Continued)

Name	Description

Br.J.Pharmacol. 63, 367P, 1978; Ford, C.L. and Winzor, D.J., A recycling gel partition technique for the study of protein-ligand interactions: the binding of methyl orange to bovine serum albumin, *Anal.Biochem.* 114, 146–152, 1981; Chung, K.T., Stevens, S.E., Jr., and Cerniglia, C.E., The reduction of azo dyes by the intestinal microflora, *Crit.Rev.Microbiol.* 18, 175–190, 1992; Yang Y. Jung, D.W., Bai, D.G., *et al.*, Counterion-dye staining method for DNA in agarose gels using crystal violet and methyl orange, *Electrophoresis* 22 855–859, 2001; Nam, W., Kim, J., and Han, G., Photocatalytic oxidation of methyl orange in a three-phase fluidized bed reactor, *Chemosphere* 47, 1019–1024, 2002; Marci, G., Augugliaro, V., Bianco Prevot, A., *et al.*, Photocatalytic oxidation of methyl-orange in aqueous suspension: comparison of the performance of different polycrystalline titanium dioxide, *Ann.Chim.* 93, 639–648, 2003; Del Nero, J., de Araujo, R.E., Gomes, A.S., and de Melo, C.P., Theoretical and experimental investigation or the second hyperpolarizabilities of methyl orange, *J.Chem.Phys.* 122, 104506, 2005; de Oliveira, H.P., Oliveira, E.G., and de Melo, C.P., *J.Colloid Interface Sci.* 303, 444–449, 2006; Bejarano-Perez, N.J. and Suarez-Herrera, M.F., Sonophotocatalytic degradation of congo red and methyl orange in the presence of TiO₂ as a catalyst, *Ultrason. Sonochem.* in press, 2006;

Methyl Red (2-[[4-(dimethylamino)-phenyl]azo] benzoic acid; C.I. acid red 2) MW 270; 306 as the hydrochloride

pH indicator; use as signal in redox reactions; rare use in histochemistry; some use for staining protozoa and other bacteria; standard for spectroscopy.

Cowan, S.T., Micromethod for the methyl red test, *J.Gen.Microbiol.* 9, 101–109, 1953; Ljutov, V., Technique of methyl red test, *Acta Pathol.Microbiol. Scand.* 51, 369–380, 1961; Barry, A.L., Berhsohn, K.L., Adams, A.P., and Thrupp, L.D., Improved 18–hour methyl red test, *Appl.Microbiol.* 20, 866–870, 1970; Korzun, W.J. and Miller, W.G., Monitoring the stability of wavelength calibration of spectrophotometers, *Clin.Chem.* 32, 162–165, 1986; Chung, K.T., Stevens, S.E., Jr., and Cerniglia, C.E., The reduction of azo dyes by the intestinal microflora, *Crit.Rev.Microbiol.* 18, 175–190, 1992; Miyajima, M., Sagami, I., Daff, S., *et al.*, Azo reduction of methyl red by neuronal nitric oxide synthase: the important role of FMN in catalysis, *Biochem.Biophys.Res.Commun.* 275, 752–758, 2000; Kashida, H., Tanaka, M., Baba, S., *et al.*, Covalent incorporation of methyl red dyes into double-stranded DNA for their ordered clustering, *Chemistry* 12, 777–784, 2006; Kalyuzhnyi, S., Yemashova, N., and Fedorovich, V., Kinetics of anaerobic biodecolourisation of azo dyes, *Water Sct.Technol.* 54, 73–79, 2006; Katsuda, T. Ooshima, H., Azuma, M., and Kato, J., New detection method for hydrogen gas for screening hydrogen-producing microorganisms using water-soluble Wilkinson's catalyst derivative, *J.Biosci.Bioeng.* 102, 220–226, 2006; Hsueh, C.C. and Chen, B.Y., Comparative study on reaction selectivity of azo dye decolorization by *Pseudomonas luteola,, J.Hazard.Mater.*, in press, 2006.

Methyl Violet (C.I. Basic violet 1); Molecular weight depends on the degree of methylation

Methyl violet is a mixture of *N*-methylated pararoanilines which is used a pH indicator and a biological stain. The term gentian violet is used for this mixture in Europe and for crystal violet (methyl violet 10B, the hexamethyl derivative) in the United States. There is some use of methyl violet for staining DNA. The industrial use is for dyeing fabrics blue and violet. The depth of color is dependent on the degree of methylation.

Methyl Violet

SOME BIOLOGICAL STAINS AND DYES (Continued)

Name	Description

Bancroft, J.D., Methyl green as a differentiator and counterstain in the methyl violet technique for demonstration of amyloid in fresh cryostat sections, *Stain Technol.* 38, 336–337, 1963; Campbell, L.M. and Roth, I.L., Methyl violet: a selective agent for differentiation of *Klebsiella pneumonia* from *Enterobacter aerogenes* and other gram-negative organisms, *Appl.Microbiol.* 30, 258–261, 1975; Dutt, M.K., Staining of depolymerized DNA in mammalian tissues with methyl violet 6B and crystal violet, *Folia Histochem.Cytochem.* 18, 79–83, 1980; Liu, Y., Ma, C.Q., Li, K.A., *et al.*, Rayleigh light scattering study on the reaction of nucleic acids and methyl violet, *Anal.Biochem.* 268, 187–192, 1999; Dogan, M. and Aikan, M., Removal of methyl violet from aqueous solution by perlite, *J.Colloid Interface Sci.* 267, 32–41, 2003; Jin, L.T. and Choi, J.K., Usefulness of visible dyes for the staining of protein of DNA in electrophoresis, *Electrophoresis* 25, 2429–2438, 2004.

Neutral Red (C.I. Basic Red 5; nuclear fast red; 3-amino-7-dimethylamino-2-methylphenazine hydrochloride; toluylene red as the unprotonated form), MW 289 as the hydrochloride

pH indicator, histological stain for Golgi, nuclear. Also a vital stain for intracellular organelles and cytotoxicity testing.

Lepper, E.H. and Martin, C.J., The protein error in estimating pH with neutral red and phenol red, *Biochem.J.* 21, 356–361, 1927; Morse, W.C., Dail, M.C., and Olitzky, I., A study of the neutral red reaction for determining virulence of *Mycobacteria*, *Am.J.Public Health* 43, 36–39, 1953; Vivian, D.L. and Belkin, M., Unexpected anomalies in the behavior of neutral red and related dyes, *Nature* 178, 154, 1956; Darnell, J.E., Jr., Lockart, R.Z., Jr., and Sawyer, T.K., The effect of neutral red on plaque formation in two virus-cell systems, *Virology* 6, 567–568, 1958; Crowther, D. and Melnick, J.L., The incorporation of neutral red and acridine orange into developing poliovirus particles making them photosensitive, *Virology* 14, 11–21, 1961; Boyer, M.G., The role of tannins in neutral red staining of pine needle vacuoles, *Stain Technol.* 38, 117–120, 1967; Sawicki, W., Kieler, J., and Briand, P., Vital staining with neutral red and trypan blue of ^{3}H-thymidine-labeled cells prior to autoradiography, *Stain Technol.* 42, 143–146, 1967; Barbosa, P. and Peters, T.M., The effects of vital dyes on living organisms with special reference to methylene blue and neutral red, *Histochem.J.* 3, 71–93, 1971; Gutter, B., Speck, W.T., and Rosenkranz, H.S., Light-induced mutagenicity of neutral red (3-amino-7-dimethylamino-2-methylphenazine hydrochloride), *Cancer Res.* 37, 1112–1114, 1977; Nemes, Z., Dietz, R., Luth, J.B., *et al.*, The pharmacological relevance of vital staining with neutral red, *Experientia* 35, 1475–1476, 1979; Gray, D.W., Millard, P.R., McShane, P., and Morris, P.J., The use of the dye neutral red as a specific, non-toxic, intra-vital stain of islets of Langerhans, *Br.J.Exp.Pathol.* 64, 553–558, 1983; LaManna, J.C., Intracellular pH determination by absorption spectrophotometry of neutral red, *Metab.Brain Dis* 2, 167–182, 1987; Elliott, W.M. and Auersperg, N., Comparison of the neutral red and methylene blue assays to study cell growth in culture, *Biotech. Histochem.* 68, 29–35, 1993; Fautz, R., Husein, B., and Hechenberger, C., Application of the neutral red assay (NR assay) to monolayer cultures of primary hepatocytes: rapid colorimetric viability determination for the unscheduled DNA synthesis test (UDS), *Mutat.Res.* 253, 173–179, 1991; Kado, R.T., Neutral red: a specific fluorescent dye in the cerebellum, *Jpn.J.Physiol.* 43(Suppl 1), S161–S169, 1993; Ishiyama, M., Tominaga, H. Shiga, M., A combined assay of cell viability and in vitro cytotoxicity with a highly water-soluble tetrazolium salt, neutral red and crystal violet, *Biol.Pharm.Bull.* 19, 1518–1520, 1996; Ciapetti, G., Granchi, D., Verri, E., *et al.*, Application of a combination of neutral red and amido black staining for rapid, reliable cytotoxicity testing of biomaterials, *Biomaterials* 17, 1259–1264, 1996; Sousa, C., Sá e Melo, T., Geze, M., *et al.*, Solvent polarity and pH effects on the spectroscopic properties of neutral red: application to lysosomal microenvironment probing in living cells, *Photochem.Photobiol.* 63, 601–607, 1996; Baker, C.S., Crystallization of neutral red vital stain from minimum essential medium due to pH instability, *In Vitro Cell.Dev.Biol.Anim.* 34, 607–608, 1998; Okada, D., Neutral red as a hydrophobic probe for monitoring neuronal activity, *J.Neurosci.Methods* 101, 85–92, 2000; Zuang, V., The neutral red release assay: a review, *Altern.Lab. Anim.* 29, 575–599, 2001; Svendsen, C., Spurgeon, D.J., Hankard, P.K., and Weeks, J.M., A review of lysosomal membrane stability measured by neutral red retention: is a workable earthworm biomarker?, *Ecotoxicol.Environ.Saf.* 57, 20–29, 2004.

SOME BIOLOGICAL STAINS AND DYES (Continued)

Name

Description

Nile Red (Nile pink); MW 318

A lipophilic benzooxazone used for lipid staining and as a hydrophobic probe for proteins; Nile red has been used as a stain for protein on acrylamide gel. The fluorescence of Nile red is very dependent on solvent. Nile red is poorly soluble in aqueous systems but the recent development of water-soluble derivatives has improved utility.

Greenspan, P., Mayer, E.P., and Fowler, S.D., Nile red; a selective fluorescent stain for intracellular lipid droplets, *J.Cell Biol.* 100, 965–973, 1985; Fowler, S.D. and Greenspan, P., Application of Nile red, a fluorescent hydrophobic probe, for the detection of neutral lipid deposits in tissue sections: comparison with oil red O, *J.Histochem.Cytochem.* 33, 833–836, 1985; Sackett, D.L. and Wolff, J., Nile red as a polarity-sensitive fluorescent probe of hydrophobic protein surfaces, *Anal.Biochem.* 167, 229–234, 1987; Brown, W.J., Warfel, J., and Greenspan, P., Use of Nile red stain in the detection of cholesteryl ester accumulation in acid lipase-deficient fibroblasts, *Arch.Pathol.Lab.Med.* 112, 295–297, 1988; Brown, W.J., Sullivan, T.R., and Greenspan, P, Nile red staining of lysosomal phospholipid inclusions, *Histochemistry* 97, 349–354, 1992; Brown, M.B., Miller, J.N., and Seare, N.J., An investigation of the use of Nile red as a long-wavelength fluorescent probe for the study of alpha 1-acid glycoprotein-drug interactions, *J.Pharm.Biomed. Anal.* 13 1011–1017, 1995; Alba, F.J., Bermudez, A., Bartolome, S. and Daban, J.R,. Detection of five nanograms of protein by two-minute nile red staining of unfixed SDS gels, *BioTechniques* 21, 625–626, 1996; Daban, J.R., Fluorescent labeling of proteins with Nile red and 2-methoxy-2,4-diphenyl-3(2H)-furanone: physicochemical basis and application to the rapid staining of sodium dodecyl sulfate polyacrylamide gels and western blots, *Electrophoresis* 22, 874–880, 2001; Hendriks, J., Gensch, T., Hviid, L., *et al.*, Transient exposure of hydrophobic surface in the photoactive yellow protein monitored with Nile red, *Biophys.J.* 82, 1632–1643, 2002; Prokhorenko, I.A., Dioubankova, N.N., and Korshun, V.A., Oligonucleotide conjugates of Nile Red, *Nucleosides Nucleotides Nucleic Acids* 23, 509–520, 2004; Yablon, D.G. and Schilowitz, A.M., Solvatochromism of Nile Red in nonpolar solvents, *Appl.Spectros.* 58, 843–847, 2004; Genicot, G., Leroy, J.L., Soom, A.V., and Donnay, I., The use of a fluorescent dye, Nile red, to evaluate the lipid content of single mammalian oocytes, *THeriogeneology* 63, 1181–1194, 2005; Sebok-Nagy, K., Miskoczy, Z. and Biczok, L., Interaction of 2-hydroxy-substituted Nile red fluorescent probe with organic nitrogen compounds, *Photochem.Photobiol.* 81, 1212–1218, 2005; Thomas, K.J., Sherman, D.B., Amiss, T.J., *et al.*, A long-wavelength fluorescent glucose biosensor based on bioconjugates on galactose/glucose binding protein and Nile red derivatives, *Diabetes Technol.Ther.* 8, 261–268, 2006; Jose, J. and Burgess, K., Syntheses and properties of water-soluble Nile red derivatives, *J.Org.Chem.* 71, 7835–7839, 2006; Mukherjee, S., Raghuraman, H., and Chattopadhyay, A., Membrane localization and dynamics of Nile red: effect of cholesterol, *Biochim.Biophys.Acta* 1768, 59–66, 2007.

Oil Red O (Sudan Red 5B; C.I. Solvent Red 27)   An extremely lipophilic dye; used for the demonstration of lipid depositions.

Moran, P. and Heyden, G., Enzyme histochemical studies on the formation of hyaline bodies in the epithelium of odontogenic cysts, *J.Oral Pathol.* 4, 120–127, 1975; Merrick, J.M., Schifferle, R., Zadarlik, K., *et al.*, Isolation and partial characterization of the heterophile antigen of infectious mononucleosis from bovine erythrocytes, *J.Supramol.Struct.* 6, 275–290, 1977; Anderson, L.C. and Garrett, J.R., Lipid accumulation in the major salivary glands of streptozotocin-diabetic rats, *Arch.Oral Biol.* 31, 469–475, 1986; Chastre, J,. Fagon, J.Y., Soler, P., *et al.*, Bronchoalveolar lavage for rapid diagnosis of the fat embolism syndrome in trauma patients, *Ann.Intern.Med.* 113, 583–588, 1990; Aleksic, I., Ren, M., Popov, A., *et al.*, In vivo liposome-mediated transfection of HLA-DR alpha-chain gene into pig hearts, *Eur.J.Cardiothorac.Surg.* 12, 792–797, 1997.

SOME BIOLOGICAL STAINS AND DYES (Continued)

Name	Description

Rhodamine B (C.I. Basic Violet 10) MW 479

An aminoxanthene which is a lipophilic cation in acid solution and a lipophilic anion in basic solution. Metal binding reagent, a neutral stain; a fluorescent lipid stain; stain for Phosphoproteins for gel electrophoresis. Isothiocyanate derivative used for labeling proteins.

Martin, G., Colorimetric determination of zinc by thiocyanate derivatives; a new method using rhodamine B, *Bull.Soc.Chim.Biol.* 34, 1174–1177, 1952; Webb, J.M., Hansen, W.H., Desmond, A., and Fitzhugh, O.G., Biochemical and toxicological studies of rhodamine B and 3,6-diaminofluroan, *Toxicol.Appl. Pharmacol.* 3, 696–706, 1961; Miketukova, V., Detection of metals on paper chromatograms with Rhodamine B., *J.Chromatog.* 24, 302–304, 1966; Liisberg, M.F., Rhodamine B as an extremely specific stain for cornification, *Acta Anat.* 69, 52–57, 1968; Shelley, W.B., Fluorescent staining of elastic tissue with Rhodamine B and related xanthene dyes, *Histochemie* 20, 244–249, 1969; Oshima, G.T. and Nagasawa, K., Fluorometric method for determination of mercury(II) with Rhodamine B, *Chem.Pharm.Bull.* 18, 687–692, 1970, Zahradnicek, L., Kratochvila, J., and Garcis, A., Determination of inorganic phosphorus using Rhodamine B by the continuous-flow technique, *Clin.Chim.Acta* 80, 431–433, 1977; Wessely, Z., Shapiro, S.H., Klavins, J.V., and Tinberg, H.M., Identification of Mallory bodies with rhodamine B fluorescence and other strains for keratin, *Stain Technol.* 56, 169–176, 1981; Debruyne, I., Inorganic phosphate determination: colorimetric assay based on the formation of a rhodamine B-phosphomolybdate complex, *Anal.Biochem.* 130, 454–460, 1983; Debruyne, I., Staining of alkali-labile Phosphoproteins and alkaline phosphatases on polyacrylamide gels, *Anal.Biochem.* 133, 110–115, 1983; Balcerzak, M., Sensitive spectrophotometric determination of osmium with tin(II) chloride and rhodamine B after flotation using cyclohexane, *Analyst* 113, 129–132, 1988; Glimcher, M.J. and Lefteriou, B., Soluble glycosylated phosphoproteins of cementum, *Calcif.Tissue Int.* 45, 165–172, 1989; Fernandez-Busquets, X. and Burger, M.M., Use of rhodamine B isothiocyanate to detect proteoglycan core proteins in polyacrylamide gels, *Anal.Biochem.* 227, 394–396, 1995; Jung, D.W., Yoo, G.S. and Choi, J.K., Mixed-dye staining method for protein detection in polyacrylamide gel electrophoresis using calconcarboxylic acid and rhodamine B, *Electrophoresis* 19, 2412–2415, 1998; Pal, J.K., Godbole, D., and Sharma, K., Staining of proteins on SDS polyacrylamide gels and on nitrocellulose membranes by Alta, a colour used as a cosmetic, *J.Biochem.Biophys.Methods* 61, 339–347, 2004; dos Santos Silva, A.L, Joekes, I., Rhodamine B diffusion in hair as a probe for structural integrity, *Colloids Surf.B.Biointerfaces* 40, 19–24, 2005; Moreno-Villoslada, I., Jofre, M., Miranda, V., *et al.*, pH dependence of the interaction between rhodamine B and the water-soluble poly(sodium 4-styrenesulfonate), *J.Phys.Chem.B Condens. Mater. Surf.Interfaces Biophys.* 110, 11809–11812, 2006.

Rose Bengal (Rose Bengal B; rose bengale; C.I. acid red 94; the disodium salt is referred to as rose Bengal extra); MW 1049 as dipotassium salt and 1018 as disodium salt

An acidic hydroxyxanthene soluble in water used as a cellular stain; diagnostic aid in ophthalmology; source of singlet oxygen in photooxidation; use as a probe for surface protein structure; early use of the radioactive derivative as a tracer for liver function.

SOME BIOLOGICAL STAINS AND DYES (Continued)

Name	Description

Conn, H.J., Rose Bengal as a general bacterial stain, *J.Bacteriol.* 6, 253–254, 1921; Forster, H.W., Jr., Rose Bengal test in diagnosis of deficient tear formation, *AMA Arch.Ophthalmol.* 45, 419–424, 1951; Rippa, M. and Picco, C., Rose Bengal as a reporter of the polarity and acidity of the TPN binding site in 6-phosphoglucoonate dehydrogenase, *Ital.J.Biochem.* 19, 178–192, 1970; Lyons, A.B. Ashman, L.K., The Rose Bengal assay for monoclonal antibodies to cell surface antigens: comparisons with common hybridoma screening methods, *J.Immunoassay* 6, 325–345, 1985; Hederstedt, L. and Hatefi, Y., Modification of bovine heart succinate dehydrogenase with ethoxyformic anhydride and rose Bengal: evidence for essential histidyl residues protectable by substrates, *Arch.Biochem.Biophys.* 247, 346–354, 1986; Allen, M.T., Lynch, M., Lagos, A. *et al.*, A wavelength dependent mechanism for rose bengal-sensitized photoinhibition of red cell acetylcholinesterase, *Biochim.Biophys.Acta.* 1075, 42–49, 1991; Feenstra, R.P. and Tseng, S.C., What is actually stained by rose bengal?, *Arch.Ophthalmol.* 110, 984–993, 1992; Shan, M.A. and Ali, R., Modification of pig kidney diamine oxidase with ethoxyformic anhydride and rose bengal: evidence for essential histidine residue at the active site, *Biochem.Mol.Biol.Int.* 33, 9–19, 1994; Tseng, S.C. and Zhang, S.H., Interaction between rose bengal and different protein components, *Cornea* 14, 427–435, 1995; Singh, R.J., Hogg, N. and Kalyanaraman, B., Interaction of nitric oxide with photoexcited rose bengal: evidence for one-electron reduction of nitric oxide to nitroxyl anion, *Arch.Biochem.Biophys.* 324, 367–373, 1995; Bottiroli, G., Croce, A.C., Balzarini, P., *et al.*, Enzyme-assisted cell photosensitization: a proposal for an efficient approach to tumor therapy and diagnosis. The rose bengal fluorogenic substrate, *Photochem.Photobiol.* 66, 374–383, 1997; Perez-Ruiz, T., Martinez-Lozano, C., Tomas, V. and Fenoll, J., Determination of proteins in serum by fluorescence quenching of rose bengal using the stopped-blow mixing technique, *Analyst* 125, 507–510, 2000; Lin, W., Garnett, M.C., Davis, S.S., *et al.*, Preparation and characterization of rose Bengal-loaded surface-modified albumin nanoparticles, *J.Control. Res.* 71, 117–126, 2001; Posadez, A., Biasutti, A., Casale, C., *et al.*, Rose Bengal-sensitized photooxidation of the dipeptides L-tryptophyl-L-phenylalanine, L-trytophyl-L-tyrosine and L-tryptophyl-L-tryptophan: kinetics, mechanism and photoproducts, *Photochem.Photobiol.* 80, 132–138, 2004; Luiz, M., Biasutti, M.A., and Garcia, N.A., Effect of reverse micelles on the Rose Bengal-sensitized photo-oxidation of 1– and 2-hydroxynaphthalene, *Redox Rep.* 9, 199–205, 2004; Khan-Lim, D. and Berry, M., Still confused about rose bengal?, *Curr.Eye Res.* 29, 311–317, 2004; Soldani, C., Bottone, M.G., Croce, A.C., *et al.*, The Golgi apparatus is a primary site of intracellular damage after photosensitization with Rose Bengal acetate, *Eur.J.Histochem.* 48, 443–449, 2004; de Lima Santos, H., Forest Rigos. C., Claudio Tedesco, A., and Ciancaglini, P., Rose Bengal located within liposome do not affect the activity of inside-out oriented Na,K-ATPase, *Biochim.Biophys.Acta* 1715 96–103, 2005; Miller, J.S., Rose bengal-stimulated photooxidation of 2-chlorophenol in water using solar simulated light, *Water Res.* 39, 412–422, 2005; Shimizu, O., Watanabe, J., Naito, S. and Shibata, Y., Quenching mechanism of Rose Bengal triplet state involved in photosensitization of oxygen in ethylene glycol, *J.Phys.Chem.A Mol.Spectrosc.Kinet.Environ.Gen.Theory* 110, 1735–1739, 2006; Seitzman, G.D., Cevallos, V. and Margolis, T.P., Rose bengal and lissamine green inhibit detection of herpes simplex virus by PCR, *Am.J.Ophthalmol.* 141,756–758, 2006; Fini, P., Loseto, R., Catucci, L., *et al.*, Study on the aggregation and electrochemical properties of Rose Bengal in aqueous solution of cyclodextrins, *Bioelectrochemistry* 70, 44–49, 2007.

SITS (stilbene isothiocyanate sulfonic acid; 4-Acetamido-4'-isothiocyanostilbene-,2'-disulfonic acid); MW 498 as disodium salt	Fluorescent stain; use on fixed tissues. Reactive groups permits use as a label for antibodies. Also used as a vital stain and as general cytoplasmic stain; used to characterize membrane anion-transport processes.

Benjaminson, M.A. and Katz, I.J., Properties of SITS (4-acetamido-4'-isothiocyanostilbene-2,2'-disulfonic acid): fluorescence and biological staining, *Stain Technol.* 45, 57–62, 1970; Rothbarth, P.H., Tanke, H.J., Mul, N.A., *et al.*, Immunofluorescence studies with 4–acetamido-4'-isothiocyanato stilbene -2–2'-disulphonic acid (SITS), *J.Immunol.Methods* 19,101–109, 1978; Schmued, L.C. and Swanson, L.W., SITS: a covalently bound fluorescent retrograde tracer that does not appear to taken up by fibers-of-passage, *Brain Res.* 249, 137–141, 1982; Gilbert, P., Kettenmann, H., Orkland, R.K., and Schachner, M., Immunocytochemical cell identification in nervous system culture combined with intracellular injection of a blue fluorescing dye (SITS), *Neurosci.Lett.* 34, 123–128, 1982; Ploem, J.S., van Driel-Kulker, A.M., Goyarts-Veldstra, L., *et al.*, Image analysis combined with quantitative cytochemistry. Results and instrumental developments for cancer diagnosis, *Histochemistry* 84, 549–555, 1986; Pedini, V., Ceccarelli, P., and Gargiulo, A.M., A lectin histochemical study of the zygomatic salivary gland of adult dogs, *Vet.Res.Commun.* 19, 363–375, 1995; Papageorgiou, P. ,Shmukler, B.E., Stuant-Tilley, A.K., *et al.*, AE anion exchangers in atrial tumor cells, *Am.J.Physiol.Heart Circ.Physiol.* 280, H937–H945, 2001; Quilty, J.A., Cordat, E., and Reithmeier, R.A., Impaired trafficking of human kidney anion exchanger (kAE1) caused by hetero-oligomer formation with a truncated mutant associated with distal renal tubular acidosis, *Biochem.J.* 368, 895–903, 2002. For SITS-sensitive anion transport see Villereal, M.L. and Levinson, C., Chloride-stimulated sulfate efflux in Ehrlich ascites tumor cells: evidence for 1:1 coupling, *J.Cell Physiol.* 90, 553–563, 1977; Kimelberg, H.K., Bowman, C.L., and Hirata, H., Anion transport in astrocytes, *Ann.N.Y.Acad.Sci.* 481, 334–353, 1986; Montrose, M., Randles, J., and Kimmich, G.A., SITS-sensitive Cl⁻ conductance pathway in chick intestinal cells, *Am.J.Physiol.* 253, C693–C699, 1987; Bassnett, S., Stewart, S., Duncan, G., and Crogha, P.C., Efflux of chloride from the rat lens: influence of membrane potential and intracellular acidification, *Q.J.Exp.Physiol.* 73, 941–949, 1988; Ishibashi, K., Rector, F.C., Jr., and Berry, C.A., Chloride transport across the basolateral membrane of rabbit proximal convoluted tubules, *Am.J.Physiol.* 258, F1569–F1578, 1990; Wilson, J.M., Laurent, P., Tufts, B.L. *et al.*, NaCl uptake by the branchial epithelium I freshwater teleost fish: an immunological approach to ion-transport protein localization, *J.Exp.Biol.* 203, 2279–2296, 2000; Small, D.L. and Tauskela, J., and Xia, Z., Role for chloride but not potassium channels in apoptosis in primary rat cortical cultures, *Neurosci.Lett.* 334, 95–98, 2002.

SOME BIOLOGICAL STAINS AND DYES (Continued)

Name   **Description**

Texas Red (TR, sulphorhodamine 101 acid chloride; MW 625

The presence of a reactive sulfonyl chloride function allows the labeling of protein amino groups. General probe for proteins and other molecules including DNA and carbohydrate to follow cellular transit.

Titus, J.A., Haugland, R., Sharrow, S.O., and Segal, D.M., Texas Red, a hydrophilic, red-emitting fluorophore for use with fluorescein in dual parameter flow microfluorimetric and fluorescence microscopic studies, *J.Immunol.Methods* 50, 193–204, 1982; Schneider, H., Differential intracellular staining of identified neurones in Locusta with texas red and lucifer yellow, *J.Neurosci.Methods* 30, 107–115, 1989; Leonce, S. and Cudennec, C.A., Modification of membrane permeability measured by Texas-Red during cell cycle progression and differentiation, *Anticancer Res.* 10, 369–374, 1990; Srour, E.F., Lemmhuis, T., Brandt, J.E, *et al.*, Simultaneous use of rhodamine 123, phycoerythrin, Texas red, and allophycocyanin for the isolation of human hematopoietic progenitor cells, *Cytometry* 12, 179–183, 1991; Wessendorf, M.W. and Brelje, T.C., Which fluorophore is brightest? A comparison of the staining obtained using fluorescein, tetramethylrhodamine, lissamine rhodamine, Texas red, and cyanine 3.18, *Histochemistry* 98, 81–85, 1992; Belichenko, P.V. and Dahlstrom, A., Dual channel confocal laser scanning microscopy of Lucifer yellow-microinjected human brain cells combined with Texas red immunofluorescence, *J.Neurosci.Methods* 52, 111–118, 1994; Brismar, H., Trepte, O. and Ulfhake, B., Spectra and fluorescence lifetimes of lissamine rhodamine, tetramethylrhodamine isothiocyanate, texas red, and cyanine 3.18 fluorophores: influences of some environmental factors recorded with a confocal laser scanning microscope, *J.Histochem.Cytochem.* 43, 699–707, 1995; Anees, M., Location of tumour cells in colon tissue by Texas red labelled pentosan polysulphate, an inhibitor of a cell surface protease, *J.Enzyme Inhib.* 10, 203–214, 1996; Simon, S., Reipert, B., Eibl, M.M., Steinkasserer, A., Detection of phosphatidylinositol glycan class A gene transcripts by RT in situ PCR hybridization. A comparative study using fluorescein, Texas Red, and digoxigenin-11 dUTP for color detection, *J.Histochem.Cytochem.* 45, 1659–1664, 1997; Larramendy, M.L., El-Rifai, W., and Knutila, S., Comparison of fluorescein isothiocyanate- and Texas red-conjugated nucleotides for direct labeling in comparative genomic hybridization, *Cytometry* 31,174–179, 1998; Hembry, R.M., Detection of focal proteolysis using Texas-red-gelatin, *Methods Mol.Biol.* 151, 417–424, 2001; Kahn, E., Lizard, G., Frouin, F., *et al.*, Confocal analysis of phosphatidylserine externalization with the use of biotinylated annexin V revealed with streptavidin-FITC, -europium, -physcoerythrin or –Texas Red in oxysterol-treated apoptotic cells, *Anal.Quant.Cytol.Histol.* 23, 47–55, 2001; Alba, F.J. and Daban, J.R., Detection of Texas red-labelled double-stranded DNA by non-enzymatic peroxyoxalate chemiluminescence, *Luminescence* 16, 247–249, 2001; Watanabe, K. and Hattori, S., Real-time dual zymographic analysis of matrix metalloproteinases using fluorescein-isothiocyanate-labeled gelatin and Texas-red-labeled casein, *Anal.Biochem.* 307, 390–392, 2002; Tan, H.H., Thornhill, J.A., Al-Adhami, B.H., *et al.*, A study of the effect of surface damage on the uptake of Texas Red-BSA by schistosomula of *Shistosoma mansoni*, *Paristology* 126, 235–240, 2003; Wippersteg, V., Ribeiro, F., Liedtke, S., *et al.*, The uptake of Texas Red-BSA in excretory system of schistosomes and its colocalisation with ER60 promoter-induced GFP in transiently transformed adult males, *Int.J.Parasitol.* 33, 1139–1143, 2003; Unruh, J.R., Gokulrangan, G., Wilson, G.S., and Johnson, C.K., Fluorescence properties of fluorescein, tetramethylrhodamine and Texas Red linked to a DNA aptamer, *Photochem.Photobiol.* 81, 682–690, 2005.

Thioflavin T (Basic Yellow 1; 318.9)

Fluorescent dye use to detect β-sheet structures such as amyloid protein; also used to detect conformational changes in therapeutic proteins on drying.

SOME BIOLOGICAL STAINS AND DYES (Continued)

Name	Description

Rogers, D.R., Screening for amyloid with the thioflavin-T fluorescent method, *Am.J.Clin.Pathol.* 44, 59–61, 1965; Saeed, S.M. and Fine, G., Thioflavin-T for amyloid detection, *Am.J.Clin.Pathol.* 47, 588–593, 1967; De Ferrari, G.V., Mallender, W.D., Inestrose, N.C. and Rosenberry, T.L., Thioflavin T is a fluorescent probe of the acetylcholinesterase peripheral site that reveals conformational interactions between the peripheral and acylation sites, *J.Biol. Chem.* 276, 23282–23287, 2001; Mathis, C.A. Bacskai, B.J., Kajdasz, S.T., *et al.*, A lipophilic thioflavin-T derivative for positron emission tomography (PET) imaging of amyloid in brain, *Bioorg.Med.Chem.Lett.* 12, 295–298, 2002; Kramenburg, O., Bouma, B., Kroon-Batenberg, M.J., *et al.*, Tissue-type plasminogen activator is a multiligand cross-β structure receptor, *Curr.Biol.*12, 1833–1839, 2002: Bouma, B., Loes, M., Kroon-Batenberg, M.J., *et al.*, Glycation induced formation of amyloid cross-β-structure, *J.Biol.Chem.* 278, 41810–41819, 2003; Krebs, M.R., Bromley, E.H., and Donald, A.M., The binding of thioflavin-T to amyloid fibrils: localization and implications, *J.Struct.Biol.* 149, 30–37, 2005; Khurana, R., Coleman, C., Ionescu-Zanetti, C., *et al.*, Mechanism of thioflavin T binding to amyloid fibrils, *J.Struct.Biol.* 151, 229–238, 2005; Inbar, P., Li, C.Q., Takayama, S.A., *et al.*, Oligo (ethylene glycol) derivatives of Thioflavin T as inhibitors of protein-amyloid interactions, *Chem.Bio.Chem* 7, 1563–1566, 2006; Okuno, A., Kato, M., and Taniguchi, Y., The secondary structure of pressure- and temperature-induced aggregation of equine serum albumin studied by FT-IR spectroscopy, *Biochim.Biophys.Acta* 1764, 1407–1412, 2006; Groenning, M., Olsen, L,. van de Weert, M., *et al.*, Study on the binding of Thioflavin T to β-sheet-rich and non-β-sheet cavities, *J.Struct.Biol.*, in press, 2006; Maskevich, A.A., Stsiapura, V.I., Kuzmitsky, V.A., *et al.*, Spectral properties of Thioflavin-T in solvents with different dielectric properties and in a fibril-incorporated form, *J.Proteome Res.*, in press, 2007; Maas, C., Hermeling, S., Bouma, B., *et al.*, A role for protein misfolding in immunogenicity of biopharmaceuticals, *J.Biol.Chem.* 282, 2229–2236, 2007.

Toluidine Blue (C.I. Basic Blue 17; Methylene Blue T5O, TBO, toluidine blue O, tolonium chloride) MW 306	A diaminothiazine which can exist in a cation form which is hydrophilic. Used for metachromatic staining of biological molecules such as mucins and macromolecular structures. Used for demarcation of tumor tissue for surgery. Very early use for heparin neutralization in blood coagulation.

Haley, T.J. and Rhodes, B., Effect of toluidine blue on the coagulation of fibrinogen by thrombin, *Science* 117, 604–606, 1953; Ball, J. and Jackson, D.S., Histological, chromatographic and spectrophotometric studies of toluidine blue, *Stain Technol.* 28, 33–40, 1953; Gustafsson, B.E. and Cronberg, S., The effect of hyaluronidase and toluidine blue on the mast cells in rats and hamsters, *Acta Rheumatol.Scand.* 5, 179–189, 1959; Schueller, E., Peutsch, M., Bohacek, L.G., and Gupta, R.K., A simplified toluidine blue stain for mast cells, *Can.J.Med.Technol.* 29, 137–138, 1967; Itzhaki, R.F., Binding of polylysine and Toluidine Blue to deoxyribonucleoprotein, *Biochem.J.* 121, 25P-26P, 1971; Sakai, W.S., Simple method for differential staining of paraffin embedded plant material using toluidine blue O, *Stain Technol.* 48, 247–249, 1973; Koski, J.P. and McGarvey, K.E., Toluidine blue as a capricious dye, *Am.J.Clin. Pathol.* 73, 457, 1980; Busing, C.M. and Pfiester, P., Permanent staining of rapid frozen section with toluidine blue, *Pathol.Res.Pract.* 172, 211–215, 1981; Drzymala, R.E., Liebman, P.A. and Romhanyi, G., Acid polysaccharide content of frog rod outer segments determined by metachromatic toluidine blue staining, *Histochemistry* 76, 363–379. 1982; O'Toole, D.K., The toluidine blue-membrane filter method: absorption spectra of toluidine blue stained bacterial cells and the relationship between absorbance and dry mass of bacteria, *Stain Technol.* 58, 357–364, 1983; Waller, J.R., Hodel, S.L., and Nuti, R.N., Improvement of two toluidine blue O-mediated techniques for DNase detection, *J.Clin.Microbiol.* 21, 195–199, 1985; Lior, H. and Patel, A., Improved toluidine blue-DNA agar for detection of DNA hydrolysis by campylobacters, *J.Clin.Microbiol.* 25, 2030–2031, 1987; Paardekooper, M., De Bruijne, A.W., Van Steveninck, J., and Van den Broek, P.J., Inhibition of transport systems in yeast by photodynamic treatment with toluidine blue, *Biochim.Biophys.Acta* 1151, 143–148, 1993; Passmore, L.J., and Killeen, A.A., Toluidine blue dye-binding method for measurement of genomic DNA extracted from peripheral blood leukocytes, *Mol.Diagn.* 1, 329–334, 1996; Korn, K., Greiner-Stoffele, T. and Hahn, U., Ribonuclease assays utilizing toluidine blue indicator plates, methylene blue, or fluorescence correlation spectroscopy, *Methods Enzymol.* 341, 142–153, 2001; Sanchez, A., Guzman, A., Ortiz, A.. *et al.*, Toluidine blue-O of prion protein deposits, *Histochem.Cell Biol.* 116, 519–524, 2001; Prat, E., Camps, J., del Rey, J., *et al.*, Combination of toluidine blue staining and in situ hybridization to evaluate paraffin tissue sections, *Cancer Genet.Cytogenet.* 155, 89–91, 2004; Kaji, Y., Hiraoka, T., and Oshika, T., Vital staining of squamous cell carcinoma of the conjunctive using toluidine blue, *Acta Ophthalmol.Scand.* 84, 825–826, 2006; Missmann, M., Jank, S., Laimer, K., and Gassner, R., A reason for the use of toluidine blue staining in the presurgical management of patients with oral squamous cell carcinomas, *Oral Surg.Oral Med. Oral Pathol. Oral Radiol.Endod.* 102, 741–743, 2006.

SOME BIOLOGICAL STAINS AND DYES (Continued)

Name	Description
Trypan Blue (diamine blue; C.I. Direct Blue 14) MW 961 as tetrasodium salt	A tetrasulfated anionic dye composed of a large planar aromatic system. Moderately soluble in water, more soluble in ethylene glycol but essentially insoluble in ethanol. Used a biological stain with particular interest as vital stain. Used in the early polychrome stains. Current use also as surgical stain for cataract surgery.

Menkin, V., Effects of ACTH on the mechanism of increased capillary permeability to trypan blue in inflammation, *Am.J.Physiol.* 166, 518–523, 1951; Wislocki, G.B. and Leduc, E.H., Vital staining of the hematoencephalic barrier by silver nitrate and trypan blue, and cytological comparisons of the neurohypophysis, pineal body, area postrema, intercolumnar tubercule and supraoptic crest, *J.Comp.Neurol.* 96, 371–413, 1952; Auskaps, A.M. and Shaw, J.H., Vital staining of calcifying bone and dentin with trypan blue, *J.Dent.Res.* 34, 452–459, 1955; Ferm, V.H., Permeability of the rabbit blastocyst to trypan blue, *Anat.Rec.* 125, 745–759, 1956; Kelly, J.W., Staining reactions of some anionic disazo dyes and histochemical properties of the red impurity in trypan blue, *Stain Technol.* 33, 89–94, 1958; Tennant, J.R., Evaluation of the trypan blue technique for determination of cell viability, *Transplantation* 2, 685–694, 1964; Holl, A., Vital staining by trypan blue: its selectivity for olfactory receptor cells of the brown bullhead, *Ictalurus natalis*, *Stain Technol.* 40, 269–273, 1965; Estupinan, J. and Hanson, R.P., Congo red and trypan blue as stains for plaque assay of Newcastle disease virus, *Avian Dis.* 13, 330–339. 1969; Lloyd, J.B. and Field, F.E., The red impurity in trypan blue, *Experientia* 26, 868–869, 1970; Dickinson, J.P. and Apricio, S.G., Trypan blue: reaction with myelin, *Biochem.J.* 122, 65P-66P, 1971; Davies, M., The effect of triton WR-1339 on the subcellular distribution of trypan blue and ^{125}I-labelled albumin in rat liver, *Biochem.J.* 136, 57–65, 1973; Davis, H.W. and Sauter, R.W., Fluorescence of Trypan Blue in frozen-dried embryos of the rat, *Histochemistry* 54, 177–189, 1977; Loike, J.D. and Silverstein, S.C., A fluorescence quenching technique using trypan blue to differentiate between attached and injested glutaraldehyde-fixed red blood cells in phagocytosing murine macrophages, *J.Immunol.Methods.* 57, 373–379, 1983; Boiadjieva, S., Hallberg, C., Hogstrom, M., and Busch, C., Methods in laboratory investigation. Exclusion of trypan blue from microcarriers by endothelial cells: an in vitro barrier function test, *Lab.Invest.* 50, 239–246, 1984; Lee, R.M., Chambers, C., O'Brodovich, H., and Forrest, J.B., Trypan blue method for the identification of damage to airway epithelium due to mechanical trauma, *Scan.Electron Microsc.* (Pt. 3), 1267–1271, 1984; Shen, W.C., Yang, D., and Ryser, H.J., Colorimetric determination of microgram quantities of polylysine by trypan blue precipitation, *Anal.Biochem.* 142, 521–524, 1984; Perry, S.W., Epstein, L.G., and Gelbard, H.A., *In situ* trypan blue staining of monolayer cell cultures for permanent fixation and mounting, *Biotechniques* 22, 1020–1024, 1997; Mascotti, K., McCullough, J., and Burger, S.R., HPC viability measurement: trypan blue versus acridine orange and propidium iodide, *Transfusion* 40, 693–696, 2000; Igarashi, H. Nagura, K., and Sugimura, H., Trypan blue as a slow migrating dye for SSCP detection in polyacrylamide gel electrophoresis, *Biotechniques* 29, 42–44, 2000.

Zincon; 2-[1-(2-hydroxy-5-sulfonatophenyl)-3-phenyl-5-formazano] benzoic acid, sodium salt MW 462	A metal complexing formazan dye which is used in histochemistry to demonstrate the presence of zinc; zincon is also used to stain for zinc proteins on solid support electrophoresis. Zincon is also used to demonstrate the presence of zinc in solution using spectrophotometric estimation of the zinc-dye complex.

SOME BIOLOGICAL STAINS AND DYES (Continued)

Name   **Description**

Corns, C.M., A new colorimetric method for the measurement of serum calcium using a zinc-zincon indicator, *Ann.Clin.Biochem.* 24, 591–597, 1987; Richter, P., Toral, M.I., Tapia, A.E., and Fuenzalida, E., Flow injection photometric determination of zinc and copper with zincon based on the variation of the stability of the complexes with pH, *Analyst.* 122, 1045–1048, 1997; Choi, J.K., Tak, K.H., Jin, L.T., *et al.*, Background-free, fast protein staining in sodium dodecyl sulfate polyacrylamide gel using counterion dyes, zincon and ethyl violet, *Electrophoresis* 23, 4053–4059, 2002; Smejkal, G.B. and Hoff, H.F., Use of the formazan dye zincon for staining proteins in polyacrylamide gels, *Biotechniques* 34, 486–468, 2003; Choi, J.K., Chae, H.Z., Hwang, S.Y., *et al.*, Fast visible dye staining of proteins in one- and two-dimensional sodium dodecyl sulfate-polyacrylamide gels compatible with matrix assisted laser desorption/ionization-mass spectrometry, *Electrophoresis* 25, 1136–1141, 2004; Morais, I.P., Souto, M.P., and Rangel, A.O., A double-line sequential injection system for the spectrophotometric determination of copper, iron, manganese, and zinc in waters, *J.AOAC Int.* 88, 639–644, 2005; Ribiero, M.F., Dias, A.C., Santos, J.L., *et al.*, Fluidized beds in flow analysis: use with ion-exchange separation for spectrophotometric determination of zinc in plant digests, *Anal.Bioanal.Chem.* 384, 1019–1024, 2006.

Biological Stains and Dyes – General References

The Chemistry of Synthetic Dyes and Pigments, ed. H.A. Lubs, American Chemical Society, Reinhold Publishing, New York, NY, USA, 1955.

Kiernan, J.A., Classification and naming of dyes, stains and fluorochromes, *Biotech.Histochem.* 76, 261–278, 2001.

Conn's Biological Stains a Handbook of Dyes, Stains, and Fluorochromes for use in Biology and Medicine, ed. R.W. Horobin and J.A. Kiernan, Bios, Oxford University Press, Oxford, UK, 2002.

MORDANT DYES

Mordant dye is a dye that interacts with a tissue, cell, or subcellular organelle via an interaction with a substance, a mordant, which interacts with the substrate and the dye. The interaction may involve covalent interaction. A mordant can be defined as a substance which interacts with both the substrate (for example tissue, cell, subcellular organelle) and the dye.[1] Most mordants are metal salts such ferric chloride and those of chromium and vanadium. Other compounds such as tannic acid[1] and galloylglucoses[2] can serve as mordants. Hematoxylin used in Hematoxylin and eosin (H and E) staining which contains a mixture of chelates formed between hematein and aluminum ions.[3,4] Mordant blue 3 (Chromoxane cyanine R) uses iron.[5] There has been a significant increase in our understanding of mordant dyes.[4,6]

References

1. Afzelius, B.A., Section staining for electron microscopy using tannic acid as a mordant: a simple method for visualization of glycogen or collagen, *Microsc.Res.Tech.* 21, 65–72, 1992.
2. Simionescu, N. and Simionescu, M., Galloylgluose of low molecular weight as mordant in electron microscopy. I. Procedure, and evidence mordanting effect, *J.Cell Biol.* 70, 608–621, 1976.
3. Bettinger, C. and Zimmermann, H.W., New investigations on hematoloxylin, hematein and hematein-aluminum complexes. 2. Hematein-aluminum complexes and hemalum staining, *Histochemistry* 96, 215–228, 1991.
4. Horobin, R.W., Biological staining: mechanisms and theory, *Biotechnic & Histochemistry* 77, 3–13, 2002.
5. Kiernan, J.A., Chromoxane cyanine R. I. Physical and chemical properties of the dye and of some of its iron complexes, *J.Microsc.* 134, 13–23, 1984.
6. Dapson, R.W., Dye-tissue interactions: mechanisms, quantification and bonding parameters for dyes used in biological staining, *Biotech.Histochem.* 80, 49–72, 2005.

General References for Mordant Dyes

Conn's Biological Stains, 10th edn., ed. R.W. Horobin and J.A. Kiernan, Bios Scientific Publishers, Oxford, UK, 2002.

MORDANT DYES

Dye Name	Metal Ion Specificity[a]	Comments
Mordant Blue 1; chrome azurol A; chromoxane pure blue B	Al, B, Ca	Calcium staining in histochemistry
Mordant Blue 3; eriochrome cyanine R; chromoxane cyanine R	Al, Cr, Fe	Iron staining in histochemistry; also Al
Mordant Blue 10; Gallocyanine;	Cr, Fe, Pb	Chromium complex for staining DNA and RNA
Mordant Blue 14; Celestine blue;	Fe	Complex with iron use as nuclear stain
Mordant Blue 29; chromoxane pure blue BLD	Be	Be staining in histochemistry
Mordant Blue 45; Gallamine blue	Al, Ca	Al complex for staining nuclei
Mordant Blue 80; Chromotrope 2R	Cr	Cytoplasmic counterstain
Mordant Red 3; Alizarin red S	Al, Ca	Calcified tissue stain
Mordant Violet 39; aurin tricarboxylic acid (ATA); aluminon; chrome violet TG	Al, Be, Cr, Fe	Aluminum staining in histochemistry

[a] Metal ion specificity is broad with most mordant stains so other metal ions can be complexed by the respective mordant stain.

Mordant blue 1; Chrome azurol B

Mordant blue 14; Celestine blue

Mordant blue 3; Eriochrome cyanine R

Mordant blue 29; Chromoxane pure blue

Mordant blue 10; Gallocyanine

Mordant blue 45; Gallamine blue

Mordant blue 80; Chromotrope 2R

Mordant Violet 39; Aurin Tricarboxylic Acid

Mordant red 3; Alizarin red S

METAL CHELATING AGENTS[a]

Name	M.W.	Description
BAPTA [1,2-bis(*o*-aminophenoxy)ethane, *N,N,N',N'*-tetraacetic acid]	476.4	Chelating agent with higher affinity for zinc than calcium can be used as with EGTA for chelation of intracellular metal ions. BAPTA-AM, the acetoxymethyl ester, is a useful derivative.

Harrison, S.M. and Bers, D.M., The effect of temperature and ionic strength on the apparent Ca-affinity of EGTA and the analogous Ca-chelators BAPTA and dibromo-BAPTA, *Biochim.Biophys.Acta.* 925, 133–143, 1987; Minta, A., Kao, J.P., and Tsien, R.Y., Fluorescent indicators for cytosolic calcium based on rhodamine and fluorescein chromophores, *J.Biol.Chem.* 264, 8171–8178, 1989; Csermely, P., Sandor, P., Radics, L., and Somogyi, J., Zinc forms complexes with higher kinetic stability than calcium, 5-F-BAPTA as a good example, *Biochem.Biophys.Res.Commun.* 165, 838–844, 1989; Marks, P.W. and Maxfield, F.R., Preparation of solutions with free calcium concentration is the nanomolar range using 1,2-*bis*(*o*-aminophenoxy)ethane-*N,N,N',N'*-tetraacetic acid, *Anal.Biochem.* 193, 61–71, 1991; Brooks, S.P. and Storey, K.B., Bound and determined: a computer program for making buffers of defined ion concentrations, *Anal.Biochem.* 201, 119–126, 1992; Dieter, P., Fitzke, E., and Duyster, J., BAPTA induces a decrease of intracellular free calcium and a translocation and inactivation of protein kinase C in macrophages, *Biol.Chem.Hoppe Seyler* 374, 171–174, 1993; Natarajan, V., Scribner, V.M., and Taher, M.M., 4-Hydroxynonenal, a metabolite of lipid peroxidation, activates phospholipase D in vascular endothelial cells, *Free Radic.Biol.Med.* 15, 365–375, 1993; Bers, D.M., Patton, C.W., and Nuccitelli, R., A practical guide to the preparation of Ca^{2+} buffers, *Methods Cell Biol.* 40, 3–29, 1994; Oiki, S., Yamamoto, T., and Okada, Y., A simultaneous evaluation method of purity and apparent stability constant of Ca-chelating agents and selectivity coefficient of Ca-selective electrodes, *Cell Calcium* 15, 199–208, 1994; Aballay, A., Sarrouf, M.N., Colombo, M.I., *et al.*, Zn^{2+} depletion blocks endosome fusion, *Biochem.J.* 312, 919–923, 1995; Britigan, B.E., Rasmussen, G.T., and Cox, C.D., Binding of iron and inhibition of iron-dependent oxidative cell injury by the "calcium chelator" 1,2-bis(2-aminophenoxy)ethane, *N,N,N',N'*-tetraacetic acid, *Biochem.Pharmacol.* 55, 287–295, 1998; Kim-Park, W.K., Moore, M.A., Hakki, Z.W., and Kowolik, M.J., Activation of the neutrophil respiratory burst requires both intracellular and extracellular calcium, *Ann.N.Y.Acad.Sci.* 832, 394–404, 1997; Barbouti, A., Doulias, P.T., Zhu, B., *et al.*, Intracellular iron, but not copper, plays a critical role in hydrogen peroxide-induced DNA damage, *Free Radic.Biol.Med.* 31, 490–498, 2001; Nielsen, A.D., Fuglsang, C.C., and Westh, P., Isothermal titration calorimetric procedure to determine protein-metal ion binding parameters in the presence of excess metal ion or chelator, *Anal.Biochem.* 314, 227–234, 2003; Gee, K.R., Rukavishnikov, A. and Rothe, A., New Ca^{2+} fluoroionophores based on the BODIPY fluorophore, *Comb.Chem.High Throughput Screen.* 6, 363–366, 2003; Swystum, V., Chen, L., Factor, P., *et al.*, Apical trypsin increases ion transport and resistance by a phospholipase C-dependent rise of Ca^{2+}, *Am.J.Physiol.Lung Cell.Mol.Physiol.* 288, L820–L830, 2005; Lazzaro, M.D., Cardenas, L., Bhatt, A.P., *et al.*, Calcium gradients in conifer pollen tube; dynamic properties differ from those seen in angiosperms, *J.Exp.Bot.* 56, 2619–2628, 2005.

Name	M.W.	Description
α-Benzoin oxime (cupron); 2-hydroxy-1,2-diphenylethanone oxime	227.3	Complexes cupric ions, molybdenum, chromium, lead, or tungsten as well as other metal ions. Used for the analysis of these metal ions. More recently, α-Benzoin oxime has been immobilized and used as a chelating resin for concentration and separation of metal ions. Copper complexes have been used as biocidal agent.

alpha-benzoin oxime

beta-benzoin oxime

benzoin

METAL CHELATING AGENTS (Continued)

Name	M.W.	Description

Borkow, G. and Gabbay, J., Putting copper into action-impregnated products with potent biocidal activities, *FASEB J.* 18, 1728–1730, 2004; Borkow, G. and Gabbay, J., Copper as a biocidal tool, *Curr.Med.Chem.* 12, 2163–2175, 2005; Ghaedi, M., Asadpour, E., and Vafaie, A., Sensitized spectrophotometric determination of Cr(III) ion for speciation of chromium ion in surfactant media using α-benzoin oxime, *Spectrochim.Acta A Mol.Biomol.Spectrosc.* 63, 182–188, 2006; Soylak, M. and Tuzen, M., Dianion SP-850 resin as a new solid phase extractor for preconcentration-separation of trace metal ions in environmental samples, *J.Hazard.Mater.* 137, 1496–1501, 2006.

Chromotropic acid; 4,5-dihydroxy-2,7-naphthalenedisulfonic acid   320.3   Chelation and fluorometric determination of aluminum and other metal ion. Also used for the analysis formaldehyde.

Metal Ions: Durham, A.C. and Walton, J.M., A survey of the available colorimetric indicators for Ca^{2+} and Mg^{2+} ions in biological experiments, *Cell Calcium* 4, 47–55, 1983; Prestel, H., Gahr, A., and Niessner, R., Detection of heavy metals in water by fluorescence spectroscopy: on the way to a suitable sensor system, *Fresenius J.Anal.Chem.* 368, 182–191, 2000; Destandau, E., Alain, V., and Bardez, E., Chromotropic acid, a fluorogenic chelating agent for aluminum(III), *Anal.Bioanal.Chem.* 378, 402–410, 2004; Themelis, D.G. and Kika, F.S., Flow and sequential injection methods for the spectrofluorometric determination of aluminum in pharmaceutical products using chromotropic acid as chromogenic reagent, *J.Pharm.Biomed.Anal.* 41, 1179–1185, 2006; Lemos, V.A., Santos, L.N., Alves, A.P., and David, G.T., Chromotropic acid-functionalized polyurethane foam: A new sorbent for on-line preconcentration and determination of cobalt and nickel in lettuce samples, *J.Sep.Sci.* 29, 1197–1204, 2006; Formaldehyde: Manius, G.J., Wen, L.F., and Palling, D., Three approaches to the analysis of trace formaldehyde in bulk and dosage from pharmaceuticals, *Pharm.Res.*10, 449–453, 1993; Flyvholm, M.A., Tiedmann, E., and Menne, T., Comparison of 2 tests for clinical assessment of formaldehyde exposure, *Contact Dermatitis* 34, 35–38, 1996; Pretto, A., Milani, M.R., and Cardoso, A.A., Colorimetric determination of formaldehyde in air using a hanging drop of chromotropic acid, *J.Environ.Monit.* 2, 566–570, 2000.

Citric acid (2-hydroxy-1,2,3-propanetricarboxylic acid.   192.1   Moderately strong chelating agent. Used frequently for calcium and iron.

Hopkins, E.W. and Herbst, E.J., An explanation for the apparent chelation of calcium by tetrodotoxin, *Biochem.Biophys.Res.Commun.* 30, 528–533, 1968; Steinmetz, W.L., Glick, M.R., and Oei, T.O., Modified aca method for determination of iron chelated by deferoxamine and other chelators, *Clin.Chem.* 26, 1593–1597, 1980; Ford, W.C. and Harrison, A., The role of citrate in determining the activity of calcium ions in human semen, *Int.J.Androl.* 7, 198–202, 1984; Lund, A.J. and Aust, A.E., Iron mobilization from asbestos by chelators and ascorbic acid, *Arch.Biochem.Biophys.* 278, 61–64, 1990; Francis, B., Seebart, C., and Kaiser, I.I., Citrate is an endogenous inhibitor of snake venom enzymes by metal-ion chelation, *Toxicon* 30, 1239–1246, 1992; Morgan, J.M., Navabi, H., Schmid, K.W., and Jasani, B., Possible role of tissue-bound calcium ions in citrate-mediated high temperature antigen retrieval, *J.Pathol.* 174, 301–307, 1994; Rhee, S.H. and Tanaka, J., Effect of citric acid on the nucleation of hydroxyapatite in a simulated body fluid, *Biomaterials* 20, 2155–2160, 1999; Engelmann, M.D., Bobier, R.T., Hiatt, T., and Cheng, I.F., Variability of the Fenton reaction characteristics of the EDTA, DTPA, and citrate complexes of iron, *Biometals* 16, 519–527, 2003; Fernandez, V. and Winkelmann, G., The determination of ferric iron in plants by HPLC using the microbial iron chelator desferrioxamine E, *Biometals* 18, 53–62, 2005; Matinaho, S., Karhumäki, P., and Parkkinen, J., Bicarbonate inhibits the growth of *Staphylococcus epidermidis* in platelet concentrates by lowering the level of non-transferrin-bound iron, *Transfusion* 45, 1768–1773, 2005; Reynolds, A.J., Haines, A.H., and Russell, D.A., Gold glyconanoparticles for mimics and measurement of metal ion-mediated carbohydrate-carbohydrate interactions, *Langmuir* 22, 1156–1163, 2006.

METAL CHELATING AGENTS (Continued)

Name	M.W.	Description
Cupferron; *N*-hydroxy-*N*-nitrosobenzene, ammonium salt	155.2	Chelation of and precipitation of iron, copper, zinc, vanadium.

Kolthoff, I.M. and Liberti, A., Amperometric titration of copper and ferric iron with cupferron, *Analyst* 74, 635–641, 1949; Ahuja, B.S., Kiran, U., and Sudershan, *In vivo* & *in vitro* inhibition of mung bean superoxide dismutase by cupferron, *Indian J. Biochem.Biophys.* 18, 86–87, 1981; Walsh, K.A., Daniel, R.M., and Morgan, H.W., A soluble NADH dehydrogenase (NADH: ferricyanide oxidoreductase) from *Thermus aquaticus* strain T351, *Biochem.J.* 209, 427–433, 1983; Danzaki, Y., Use of cupferron as a precipitant for the determination of impurities in high-purity iron by ICP-AES, *Anal.Bioanal.Chem.* 356, 143–145, 1996; Heinemann, G. and Vogt, W., Quantification of vanadium in serum by electrothermal atomic absorption spectrometry, *Clin.Chem.* 42, 1275–1282, 1996; Oztekin, N. and Erim, F.B., Separation and direct UV detection of lanthanides complexed with cupferron by capillary electrophoresis, *J.Chromatog.A.* 895, 263–268, 2000; Hou, Y., Xie, W., Janczuk, A.J., and Wang, P.G. *O*-Alkylation of cupferron: aiming at the design and synthesis of controlled nitric oxide releasing agents, *J.Org.Chem.* 65, 4333–4337, 2000; Bourque, J.R., Burley, R.K., and Bearne, S.L., Intermediate analogue inhibitors of mandelate racemase: *N*-hydroxyformanilide and cupferron, *Bioorg.Med.Chem.Lett.* 17, 105–108, 2007.

Name	M.W.	Description
Sodium diethyldithiocarbamate; Diethyldithiocarbamate, sodium salt (Dithio carb sodium); diethyl-carbamothioic acid, sodium salt; diethyldithiocarbamic acid sodium salt	171.2	Chelation of zinc, copper, mercury, and nickel.

Rigas, D.A., Eginitis-Rigas, C. and Head, C., Biphasic toxicity of diethyldithiocarbamate, a metal chelation, to T lymphocytes and polymorphonuclear granulocytes: reversal by zinc and copper, *Biochem.Biophys.Res.Commun.* 88, 373–379, 1979; Khandelwal, S., Kachru, D.N., and Tandon, S.K., Chelation in metal intoxication. IX. Influence of amino and thiol chelators on excretion of manganes in poisoned rabbits, *Toxicol.Lett.* 6, 131–135, 1980; Marciani, D.J. Wilkie, S.D., and Schwartz, C.L., Colorimetric determination of agarose-immobilized proteins by formation of copper-protein complexes, *Anal.Biochem.* 128, 130–137, 1983; O'Callaghan, J.P. and Miller, D.B., Diethyldithiocarbamate increases distribution of cadmium to brain but prevents cadmium-induced neurotoxicity, *Brain Res.* 170, 354–358, 1986; Khandelwal, S., Kachru, D.N., and Tandon, S.K., Influence of metal chelators on metalloenzymes, *Toxicol. Lett.* 37, 213–219, 1987; Tandon, S.K., Hashmi, N.S., and Kashru, D.N., The lead-chelating effects of substituted dithiocarbamates, *Biomed.Environ.Sci.* 3, 299–305, 1990; Borrello, S., De Leo, M.E., Landricina, M. *et al.*, Diethyldithiocarbamate treatment up regulates manganese superoxide dismutase gene expression in rat liver, *Biochem.Biophys.Res.Commun.* 220, 546–552, 1996.

Name	M.W.	Description
Dimethylglyoxime; 2,3-butanedionedioxime; diacetyldioxime	116.1	Primary for chelation and detection of nickel; also for separation of lead and chelation of copper.

METAL CHELATING AGENTS (Continued)

Name	M.W.	Description

Lee, D.W. and Halmann, M., Selective separation of nickel (II) by dimethylglyoxime-treated polyurethane foam, *Anal.Chem.* 48, 2214–2218, 1976; Dixon, N.E., Gazzola, C., Asher, C.J. *et al.*, Jack Bean urease (EC 3.5.1.5)-II. The relationship between nickel, enzymatic activity, and the "abnormal" ultraviolet spectrum. The nickel content of jack beans, *Can.J.Biochem.* 58, 474–480, 1980; Huber, K.R., Sridhar, R., Griffith, E.H., *et al.*, Superoxide dismutase-like activities of copper(II) complexes tested in serum, *Biochim.Biophys.Acta* 915, 267–276, 1987; Heo, J., Staples, C.R., Halbleib, C.M., and Ludden, P.W., Evidence for a ligand CO that is required for catalytic activity of CO dehydrogenase from *Rhodospirilum rubrum*, *Biochemistry* 39, 7956–7963, 2000; Celo, V., Murimboh, J., Salam, M.S., and Chakrabarti, C.L., A kinetic study of nickel complexation in model systems by adsorptive catholic stripping voltammetry, *Environ.Sci.Technol.* 35, 1084–1089, 2001; Ponnuswamy, T. and Chyan, O., Detection of Ni^{2+} by a dimethylglyoxime probe using attenuated total-reflection infrared spectrometry, *Anal.Sci.* 18, 449–453, 2002.

Dithizone; diphenylthiocarbazone   256.3   Chelating and measurement of mercury, zinc, cobalt, copper, and lead. Extensive use for the histochemical detection of zinc.

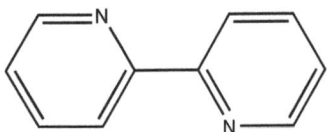

Landry, A.S., Optimum range for maximum accuracy in biological lead analyses by dithizone, *Ind.Health Mon.* 11, 103, 1951; Mager, M., McNary, W.F., Jr., and Lionetti, F., The histochemical detection of zinc, *J.Histochem.Cytochem.* 1, 493–504, 1953; McNary, W.F., Jr., Dithizone staining of myeloid granules, *Blood* 12, 644–648, 1957; Butler, E.J., and Newman, G.E., An absorptiometric method for the determination of traces of copper in biological materials with dithizone, *Clin.Chim.Acta* 11, 452–460, 1965; Shendriker, A.D. and West, P.W., Microdetermination of lead with dithizone and the ring-oven technique, *Anal.Chim.Acta* 61, 43–48, 1972; Nabrzyski, M., Spectrophotometric method for copper and mercury determination in the same food sample using dithizone and lead diethyldithiocarbamate, *Anal.Chem.* 47, 552–553, 1975; Song, M.K., Adham, N.F., and Rinderknecht, R., A simple, highly sensitive colorimetric method for the determination of zinc in serum, *Am.J.Clin.Pathol.* 65, 229–233, 1976; Holmquist, B., Elimination of adventitious metals, *Methods Enzymol.* 158, 6–12, 1988; Goldberg, E.D., Eschenko, V.A., and Bovt, V.D., Diabetogenic activity of chelators in some mammalian species, *Endocrinologie* 28, 51–55, 1990; Kawamura, C., Kizaki, M., Fukuchi, Y., and Ikeda, Y., A metal chelator, diphenylthiocarbazone, induces apoptosis, in acute promyelocytic leukemia (APL): cells mediated by a caspase-dependent pathway with a modulation of retinoic acid signaling pathways, *Leuk.Res.* 26, 661–668, 2002; Shaw, M.J., Jones, P., and Haddad, P.R., Dithizone derivatives as sensitive water soluble chromogenic reagents of the ion chromatographic determination of inorganic and organo-mercury in aqueous matrices, *Analyst* 128, 1209–1212, 2003; Santos, I.G., Hagenbach, A., and Abram, U., Stable gold(III) complexes with thiosemicarbazone derivatives, *Dalton Trans.* (4), 677–682, 2004; Khan, R., Ahmed, M.J., and Bhanger, M.I., A rapid spectrophotometric method for the determination of trace level lead using 1,5-diphenylthiocarbazone in aqueous micellar solutions, *Anal.Sci.* 23, 193–199, 2007.

α,α-Dipyridyl; 2,2'-dipyridyl; bipyridyl; BIPY   156.2   Used for chelation of ferrous iron and other divalent metal cations.

Fredens, K. and Danscher, G., The effect of intravital chelation with dimercaprol, calcium disodium edentate, 1-10-phenanthroline and 2,2'-dipyridyl on the sulfide silver strainability of the rat brain, *Histochemie* 37, 321–331, 1973; Evans, S.A. and Shore, J.D., The role of zinc-bound water in liver alcohol dehydrogenase catalysis, *J.Biol.Chem.* 255, 1509–1514, 1980; Rao, G.H., Cox, A.C., Gerrard, J.M., and White, J.G., Effects of 2,2'-dipyridyl and related compounds on platelet prostaglandin synthesis and platelet function, *Biochim.Biophys.Acta* 628, 468–479, 1980; Ikeda, H., Wu, G.Y., and Wu, C.H., Evidence that an iron chelator regulates collagen synthesis by decreasing the stability of procollagen mRNA, *Hepatology* 15, 282–287, 1992; Hales, N.J. and Beattie, J.F., Novel inhibitors of prolyl 4-hydroxylase. 5. The intriguing structure-activity relationships seen with 2,2'-bipyridine and its 5,5'-dicarboxy acid derivatives, *J.Med.Chem.* 36, 3853–3858, 1993; Henley, R. and Worwood, M., The enhancement of iron-dependent luminal peroxidation by 2,2'-dipyridyl and nitrilotriacetate, *J.Biolumin.Chemilumin.* 9, 245–250, 1994; Nocentini, G. and Barzi, A., The 2,2'-bipyridyl-6-carbothioamide copper (II) complex differs from the iron(II) complex in its biochemical effects in tumor cells, suggesting possible differences in the mechanism leading to cytotoxicity, *Biochem.Pharmacol.* 52, 65–71, 1996; Romeo, A.M., Christen, L, Niles, E.G., and Kosman, D.J., Intracellular chelation of iron by bipyridyl inhibits DNA virus replication: ribonucleotide reductase maturation as a probe of intracellular iron pools, *J.Biol.Chem.* 276, 24301–24308, 2001; Slingsby, R.W., Bordunov, A, and Grimes, M., Removal of metallic impurities from mobile phases in reversed-phase high-performance liquid chromatography by the use of an in-line chelation column, *J.Chromatog. A.* 913, 159–163, 2001; Huang, K., Dai, J., Fournier, J., *et al.*, Ferrous ion autooxidation and its chelation in iron-loaded human liver HepG2 cells, *Free Radic.Biol.Med.* 32, 84–92, 2002; Pfister, A. and Fraser, C.L., Synthesis and unexpected reactivity of iron tris(bipyridine) complexes with poly(ethylene glycol) macroligands, *Biomacromolecules* 7, 459–468, 2006.

METAL CHELATING AGENTS (Continued)

Name	M.W.	Description
EDTA (ethylenediaminetetraacetic acid)	292	General chelation agent[b] Structure serves as the basis for therapeutic agents which deliver radioactive materials to tumor cells. EDTA is used to detach adherent cells from tissue culture surfaces. Frequently included in protease inhibitor "cocktails." The affinity for metal ions decrease as pH decreases and there may be a change in the relative affinity for specific metal ions.[b]

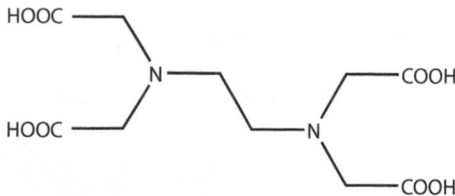

Sakabe, I., Paul, S., Mitsumoto, T., *et al.*, A factor that prevents EDTA-induced cell growth inhibition: purification of transethyretin from chick embryo brain, *Endocr.J.* 44, 375–391, 1999; Rocken, C. and Roessner, A., An evaluation of antigen retrieval procedures for immunoelectron microscopic classification of amyloid deposits, *J.Histochem.Cytochem.* 47, 1385–1394, 1999; Sciaudone, M.P., Chattopadhyay, S., and Freake, H.C., Chelation of zinc amplifies induction of growth hormone mRNA levels in cultured rat pituitary tumor cells, *J.Nutr.* 130, 158–163, 2000; Welch, K.D., Davis, T.Z., and Aust, S.D., Iron autoxidation and free radical generation: effects of buffers, ligands, and chelators, *Arch.Biochem.Biophys.* 397, 360–369, 2002; Breccia, J.D., Andersson, M.M., and Hatti-Kaul, R., The role of poly(ethyleneimine) in stabilization against metal-catalyzed oxidation of proteins: a case study with lactate dehydrogenase, *Biochim.Biophys.Acta* 1570, 165–173, 2002; Cowart, R.E, Reduction of iron by extracellular iron reductases: implications for microbial iron acquisition, *Arch.Biochem.Biophys.* 430, 273–281, 2002; Geebelen, W., Vangronaveld, J., Adriano, D.C., *et al.*, Effects of Pb-EDTA and EDTA on oxidative stress reactions and mineral uptake in *Phaseolus vulgaris*, *Physiol.Plant* 115, 377–382, 2002; Powis, D.A. and Zerbes, M., *In situ* chelation of Ca(2+) in intracellular stores induces capacitative Ca(2+) entry in bovine adrenal chromaffin cells, *Ann.N.Y.Acad.Sci.* 971, 150–152, 2002; Tarasov, K.A., O'Hare, D., and Isupov, V.P., Solid-state chelation of metal ions by ethylenediaminetetraacetate intercalated in a layered double hydroxide, *Inorg.Chem.* 42, 1919–1927, 2003; Nichols, N.M., Benner, J.S., Martin, D.D., and Evans, T.C., Jr., Zinc ion effects on individual Ssp DnaE intein-splicing steps: regulating pathway progression, *Biochemistry* 42, 5301–5311, 2003; Conzone, S.D., Hall, M.M., Day, D.E., and Brown, R.F., Biodegradable radiation delivery system utilizing glass microspheres and ethylenediaminetetraacetate chelation therapy, *J.Biomed.Mater.Res.A.* 70, 256–264, 2004; Reynolds, A.J., Haines, A.H., and Russell, D.A., Gold glyconanoparticles for mimics and measurement of metal ion-mediated carbohydrate-carbohydrate interactions, *Langmuir* 22, 1156–1163, 2006; Fernandes, C.M., Zamuner, S.R., Zuliani, J.P., *et al.*, Inflammatory effects of BaP1: a metalloproteinase isolated from *Bothrops asper* snake venom: leukocyte recruitment and release of cytokines, *Toxicon* 47, 549–559, 2006; Pajak, B. and Orzechowski, A., Ethylenediaminetetraacetic acid affects subcellular expression of clusterin protein in human colon adenocarcinoma COLO 205 cell line, *Anticancer Drugs* 18, 55–63, 2007.

EGTA (ethyleneglycoltetraacetic acid)	380.4	Chelating agent with much greater affinity for calcium ions than for magnesium.

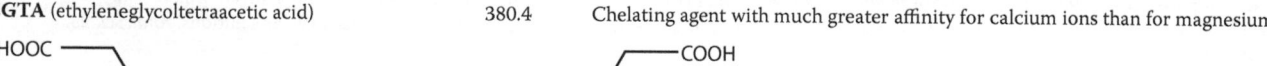

Schor, S.L., The effects of EGTA and trypsin on the serum requirements for cell attachment to collagens, *J.Cell Sci.* 40, 271–279, 1979; Bers, D.M., A simple method for the accurate determination of free [Ca] in Ca-EGTA solutions, *Am.J.Physiol.* 242, C404–408, 1982; Miller, D.J. and Smith, G.L., EGTA purity and the buffering of calcium ions in physiological solutions, *Am.J.Physiol.* 246, C160–C166, 1984; Sulakhe, P.V. and Hoehn, E.K., Interaction of EGTA with a hydrophobic region inhibits particular adenylate cyclase from rat cerebral cortex: a study of an EGTA-inhibitable enzyme by using alamethicin, *Int.J.Biochem.* 16, 1029–1035, 1984; Bryant, D.T. and Andrews, P., High-affinity binding of Ca^{2+} to bovine α-lactalbumin in the absence and presence of EGTA, *Biochem.J.* 220, 617–620, 1984; Smith, G.L. and Miller, D.J., Potentiometric measurements of stoichiometric and apparent affinity constants of EGTA for protons and divalent cations including calcium, *Biochim.Biophys.Acta* 839, 287–299, 1985; Marini, M.A., Evans, W.J., and Berger, R.L., The determination of binding constants with a differential thermal and potentiometric titration apparatus. II. EDTA, EGTA and calcium, *J.Biochem.Biophys. Methods* 12, 135–146, 1986; Harrison, S.M. and Bers, D.M., The effect of temperature and ionic strength on the apparent Ca-affinity of EGTA and the analogous Ca-chelators BAPTA and dibromo-BAPTA, *Biochim.Biophys.Acta* 925, 133–143, 1987; Guan, Y.Y., Kwan, C.Y., and Daniel, E.E., The effects of EGTA on vascular smooth muscle contractility in calcium-free medium, *Can.J.Physiol.Pharmacol.* 66, 1053–1056, 1988Youatt, J., Calcium and microorganisms, *Crit.Rev.Microbiol.* 19, 83–97, 1993; Yingst, D.R., and Barrett, V.E., Binding and elution of EGTA to anion exchange columns: implications for study of (Ca+Mg)-ATPase inhibitors, *Biochim.Biophys.Acta* 1189, 113–118, 1994; Lee, Y.C., Fluorometric determination of EDTA and EGTA using terbium-salicylate complex, *Anal.Biochem.* 293, 120–123, 2001; Rothen-Rutishauser, B., Riesen, F.K., Braun, A., *et al.*, Dynamics of tight and adherens junctions under EGTA treatment, *J.Membr.Biol.* 188, 151–162, 2002; Chen, J.L., Ahluwalia, J.P., and Stamnes, M., Selective effects of calcium chelators on anterograde and retrograde protein transport in the cell, *J.Biol.Chem.* 277, 35682–35687, 2002; Fisher, A.E., Hague, T.A., Clarke, C.L., and Naughton, D.P., Catalytic superoxide scavenging by metal complexes of the calcium chelator EGTA and contrast agent EHPG, *Biochem.Biophys.Res. Commun.* 323, 163–167, 2004; Dweck, D., Reyes-Alfonso, A., Jr., and Potter, J.D., Expanding the range of free calcium regulation in biological solutions, *Anal.Biochem.* 347, 303–315, 2005; Ellis-Davies, G.C. and Barsotti, R.J., Tuning caged calcium: photolabile analogues of EGTA with improved optical and chelation properties, *Cell Calcium* 39, 75–83, 2006; Zhou, J.L., Li, X.C., Garvin, J.L., *et al.*, Intracellular ANG II induces cytosolic Ca^{2+} mobilization by stimulating intracellular AT1 receptors in proximal tubule cells, *Am.J.Physiol.Renal Physiol.* 290, F1382–1390, 2006.

METAL CHELATING AGENTS (Continued)

Name	M.W.	Description
Oxalic Acid	126.1 as hydrate	Modest chelator; history of use in blood and in dentistry.

Lu, H., Mou, S., Yan, Y., *et al.*, On-line pretreatment and determination of Pb, Cu and Cd at the μ l^{-1} level in drinking water by chelation ion chromatography, *J.Chromatog.A.* 800, 247–255, 1998; Bruer, W, Ronson, A., Slotki, I.N., *et al.*, The assessment of serum nontransferrin-bound iron in chelation therapy and iron supplementation, *Blood* 95, 2975–2982, 2000; Salovaara, S., Sandberg, A.S., and Andlid, T., Combined impact of pH and organic acids on iron uptake by Caco-2 cells, *J.Agric.Food Chem.* 51, 7820–7824, 2003; Gerken, B.M., Wattenbach, C., Linke, D., Tweezing-absorptive bubble separation. Analytical method for the selective and high enrichment of metalloenzymes, *Anal.Chem.* 77, 6113–6117, 2005.

o-**Phenanthroline**; 1,10-phenanthroline	198.2 as hydrate	Moderately strong chelating agent. Historical use for zinc. More recent studies have copper and iron complexes as specific nuclease activity and there is some evidence to indicate protease activity. Possible role of metal complexes as oxidizing agents.[d]

o-phenanthroline; 1,10-phenanthroline

Sytkowski, A.J. and Vallee, B.L., Chemical reactivities of catalytic and noncatalytic zinc or cobalt atoms of horse liver alcohol dehydrogenase: differentiation by their thermodynamic and kinetic properties, *Proc.Nat.Acad.Sci.USA.* 73, 344–348, 1976; Kidani, Y. and Hirose, J., Coordination chemical studies on metalloenzyme. II. Kinetic behavior of various types of chelating agents towards bovine carbonic anhydrase, *J.Biochem.* 81, 1383–1391, 1977; Evans, C.W., The spectrophotometric determination of micromolar concentrations of Co^{2+} using *o*-phenanthroline, *Anal.Biochem.* 135, 335–339, 1983; Wu, H.B. and Tsou, C.L., A comparison of Zn(II)_ and Co(II) in the kinetics of inactivation of aminoacylase by 1,10-phenanthroline and reconstitution of the apoenzyme, *Biochem.J.* 296, 435–441, 1993; Auld, D.S., Removal and replacement of metal ions in metallopeptidases, *Methods Enzymol.* 248, 228–242, 1995; Leopold, I. and Fricke, B., Inhibition, reactivation and determination of metal ions in membrane metalloproteases of bacterial origin using high-performance liquid chromatography coupled on-line with inductively coupled plasma mass spectrometry, *Anal.Biochem.* 252, 277–285, 1997; Ciancaglini, P., Pizauro, J.M., and Leone, F.A., Dependence of divalent metal ions on phosphotransferase activity of osseous plate alkaline phosphatase, *J.Inorg.Biochem.* 66, 51–55, 1997.

METAL CHELATING AGENTS (Continued)

Name	M.W.	Description
8-Quinolinol; 8-hydroxyquinoline	145.2	Metal chelating agent with higher affinity for Fe, Cu, and Zn. Lower affinity for Ca and Mg. Therapeutic use as antiseptic/bacteriostatic agent.

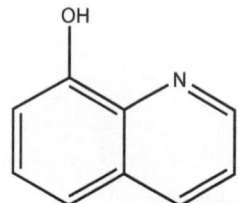

Fayez, M. and El-Tarras, M., Potentiometric titration of 8-hydroxyquinoline with Cu(II) using Cu(II)sulphide-ion selective electrode, *Pharmazie* 30, 799, 1975; Eskeland, T., The effect of various metal ions and chelating agents on the formation of noncovalently and covalently linked IgM polymers, *Scand.J.Immunol.* 6, 87–95, 1977; Albro, P.W., Corbett, J.T. and Schroeder, J.L., Generation of hydrogen peroxide by incidental metal ion-catalyzed autoxidation of glutathione, *J.Inorg.Biochem.* 27, 191–203, 1986; Yasui, T., Yuchi, A., Wade, H., and Nagagawa, S., Reversed-phase high-performance liquid chromatography of several metal-*S*-quinolinethiol complexes, *J.Chromatog.* 596, 73–78, 1992; Vieira, N.E., Yergey, A.L., and Abrams, S.A., Extraction of magnesium from biological fluids using 8-hydroxyquinoline and cation-exchange chromatography for isotopic enrichment using thermal ionization mass spectrometry, *Anal.Biochem.* 218, 92–97, 1994; Zachariouis, M., and Hearn, M.T., Adsorption and selectivity characteristics of several human serum proteins with immobilized hard Lewis metal ion-chelate adsorbents, *J.Chromatog.A.* 890, 95–116, 2000; Anfossi, L., Giraudi, G., Grassi, G., *et al.*, Binding properties of a polyclonal antibody directed against toward lead complexes, *Ann.Chim.* 93, 499–512, 2003; Yamada, H., Hayashi, H., and Yasui, T., Utility of 1-octanol/octane mixed solvents for the solvent extraction of aluminum(III), gallium(III), and indium(III) with 8-quinolinol, *Anal.Sci.* 22, 371–376, 2006; Song, K.C., Kim, J.S., Park, S.M., *et al.*, Fluorogenic Hg^{2+}-selective chemodosimeter derived from 8-hydroxyquinoline, *Org.Lett.* 8, 3413–3416, 2006; Mittal, S.K., Kumar, A., Gupta, N., *et al.*, 8-Hydroxyquinoline based neutral tripodal ionophore as a Cu(II) selective electrode and the effect of remote substituents on electrode properties, *Anal.Chim.Acta* 585, 161–170, 2007.

---

[a] Metal chelating systems can be viewed as metal ion buffer systems.

- MY = metal chelate complex; M is metal and Y is chelating agent. Metal ion are electron acceptors can be viewed as Lewis acids while chelating agents donate electrons and are Lewis bases. Also, chelating agents are polydentate
  - $MY^{n-m} = M^{+n} + M^{-m}$
  - $K_{MY} = [MY^{n+m}]/[M^{+n}][Y^{-m}]$
  - $pM = \log K_{MY} + \log [Y^{-m}]/[MY^{n-m}]$

The values for stability(association constants presented below are dependent of solvent conditions such as pH as well as relative amounts of chelating agent and metal ion.

[b] Stability of some metal ion complexes with EDTA

Metal Ion	Log K (MY)
Ca^{2+}	10.96
V^{+2}	12.70
Mn^{+2}	14.04
Fe^{2+}	14.33
Fe^{3+}	25.1
Co^{2+}	16.31
Ni^{2+}	18.62
Cu^{2+}	18.80
Zn^{2+}	16.50

Adapted from Mingos, D.M.P., *Essential Trends in Inorganic Chemistry*, Oxford University Press, Oxford, United Kingdom, 1998.

[c] Influence of pH on pM for EDTA where pK_1, 2.0; pK_2, 2.67; pK_3, 6.16; pK_4 11.26.

pH	Cu(II)	Zn(II)	Mg(II)	Ca(II)	Mn(II)	Fe(III)
4	8.4	6.7	2.0	2.3	4.5	15.7
6	12.6	10.5	3.8	5.5	7.3	19.5
8	15.0	12.8	5.4	7.3	10.1	21.8
10	16.8	14.6	7.2	9.2	12.0	23.7

Adapted from Chaberek, S. and Martell, A.F., *Organic Sequestering Agents. A Discussion of the Chemical Behavior and Applications of Metal Chelate Compounds in Aqueous Systems*, John Wiley & Sons, London, UK, 1959.

[d] Nuclease activity: Que, B.G., Downey, K.M., and So, A.G., Degradation of deoxyribonucleic acid by a 1,10–phenanthroline-copper complex: the role of hydroxyl radicals, *Biochemistry* 19, 5987–5891, 1980; Goldstein, S. and Czapski, G., The role and mechanism of metal ions and their complexes in enhancing damage in biological systems or in protecting these systems from the toxicity of O^{2-}, *J.Free Radic.Biol.Med.* 2, 3–11, 1986; Sigman, D.S. and Chen, C.H, Chemical nucleases: new reagents in molecular biology, *Annu.Rev.Biochem.* 59, 207–236, 1990; Sigman, D.S., Chemical nucleases, *Biochemistry* 29, 9097–9105, 1990; Montenay-Garestier, T., Helene, C., and Thuong, N.T., Design of sequence-specific bifunctional nucleic acid ligands, *Ciba. Found.Sym.* 158, 147–157, 1991; Pan, C.Q., Landgraf, R., and Sigman, D.S., DNA-binding proteins as site-specific nucleases, *Mol.Microbiol.* 12, 335–342, 1994. Protease activity: Kito, M. and Urade, R., Protease activity of 1,10-phenanthroline-copper systems, *Met.Ions Biol.Syst.* 38, 187–196, 2001. Oxidation: McArdle, J.V., Gray, H.B., Creutz, C., and Sutin, N., Kinetic studies of the oxidation of ferrocytochrome c from horse heart and *Candida krusei* by tris(1,10-phenanthroline) cobalt(3), *J.Amer.Chem.Soc.* 96, 5737–5741, 1974; McArdle, J.V., Coyle, C.L., Gray, H.B., Yoneda, G.S., and Holwerda, R.A., Kinetics studies of the oxidation of blue copper proteins by tris(1-,10-phenanthroline)cobalt(III) ions, *J.Amer.Chem.Soc.* 99, 2483–2389, 1977; Lau, O.W. and Luk, S.F., Spectrophotometric determination of ascorbic acid in canned fruit juices, cordials, and soft drink with iron(III) and 1,10-phenanthroline as reagents, *J.Assoc.Off.Anal.Chem.* 70, 518–520, 1987; Mandal, S., Kazmi, N.H., and Sayre, L.M., Ligand dependence in the copper-catalyzed oxidation of hydroquinones, *Arch.Biochem.Biophys.* 435, 21–31, 2005; Hung, M. and Stanbury, D.W., Oxidation of thioglycolate by [Os(phen)3]$^{3+}$: an unusual example of redox-mediated aromatic substitution, *Inorg.Chem.* 44, 9952–9960, 2005; Ishrat, Q.U. and Iftikhar, A., Kinetics of copper(II) catalyzed oxidation of iodide by iron(III)orthophenanthroline complex in aqueous solution, *Pak.J.Pharm.Sci.* 18, 20–24, 2005; Ozyurek, M., Guglu, K., Bektasoglu, B., and Apak, R., Spectrophotometric determination of ascorbic acid by the modified CUPRAC method with extractive separation of flavonoids-La(III) complexes, *Anal.Chim.Acta* 588, 88–95, 2007.

Some Stability Constants for Divalent Metal Ion Chelate Complexes (log k)

Chelating Agent	Ca	Mg	Zn	Fe	Cu
BAPTA	6.8			6	
EDTA	10.6	8.7	16.4	14.2	18.8
EGTA	11.0	5.2	12.9	11.8	12.9
8-Hydroxyquinoline	3.3	4.7	8.5	8.0	8.5
1,10-Phenanthroline	0.5	1.5	6.4	5.8	6.3
Citrate	3.6	3.6	5.0	4.4	5.9
Oxalate	3.0	2.6	4.9	4.7	4.4

General References for Metal Chelating Agents

Analytical Uses of Ethylene Diamine Tetraacetic Acid, D. Van Nostrand, Princeton, NJ, USA, 1950.

Martell, A.E. and Calvin, M., *Chemistry of the Metal Chelate Compounds*, Prentice-Hall, Englewood Cliffs, NJ, USA, 1952.

Chelating Agents and Metal Chelates, ed. F.P. Dwyer and D.P. Mellon, Academic Press, New York, NY, USA, 1964.

Data for Biochemical Research, ed. R.M.C. Dawson, Clarendon Press, Oxford, UK, 1986.

Handbook on Metals in Clinical and Analytical Chemistry, ed. H.G. Seiler, A. Sigel, and H. Sigel, Marcel Dekker, New York, NY, USA, 1994.

Bertini, I., Gray, H.B., Strefel, E.I., and Valentine, J.S., *Biological Inorganic Chemistry. Structure and Reactivity*, University Science Books, Sausalito, CA, USA, 2007.

METALLOMICS: GUIDELINES FOR TERMINOLOGY AND CRITICAL EVALUATION OF ANALYTICAL CHEMISTRY APPROACHES (IUPAC TECHNICAL REPORT)

Ryszard Lobinski[1,2], J. Sabine Becker[3], Hiroki Haraguchi[4], and Bibundhendra Sarkar[5]

[1]*CNRS/UPPA, UMR5254, Laboratory of Analytical, Bio-Inorganic, and Environmental Chemistry, Hélioparc, 2, av. Pr. Angot, 64053 Pau, France*
[2]*Department of Chemistry, Warsaw University of Technology, ul. Noakowskiego 3, 00-664 Warszawa, Poland*
[3]*Central Division of Analytical Chemistry, Research Centre Jülich, D-52425 Jülich, Germany*
[4]*Graduate School of Engineering, Nagoya University, Nagoya, 464-8603, Japan*
[5]*The Hospital for Sick Children, University of Toronto, 555 University Avenue, Toronto, Ontario M5G 1X8, Canada*

*Sponsoring body: IUPAC Analytical Chemistry Division: see more details on p. 818.

Abstract: Definitions for the terms *metallome* and *metallomics* are proposed. The state of the art of analytical techniques and methods for systematic studies of metal content, speciation, localization, and use in biological systems is briefly summarized and critically evaluated.

Keywords: metals; metabolomics; metallomics; proteomics; speciation.

1. Rationale and History of the Use of the Terms Regarding the Metal-Related -*Omics*

The knowledge of the complete genetic blueprint of an increasing number of organisms has resulted in efforts aimed at the global analysis and functional study of a particular class of components of a living organism and the emergence of different "-omics". The concepts of genomics (the study of genes and their function) and proteomics (the study of the set of proteins produced by an organism, their localization, structure, stability, and interaction) have become part of the everyday language of life sciences [1,2].

Metal ions are a vital component of the chemistry of life [3]. One-third of all proteins is believed to require a metal cofactor, such as copper, iron, zinc, or molybdenum [4], delivered as a simple or complex ion or as a metal-containing compound (e.g., methylcobalamin). The intracellular concentration of several metals, their distribution among the various cell compartments, and their incorporation in metalloproteins are tightly controlled [5]. The understanding of mechanisms by which a metal is sensed, stored, or incorporated as a cofactor requires, in addition to the identification of metalloproteins, the characterization of the pool of non-protein molecules (products of enzymatic or biochemical reactions) interacting with metal ions or of metabolites of exogenous metallocompounds, such as metallodrugs. A systematic approach to the study of metal content, speciation, localization, and use in biological systems is becoming increasingly important [6].

The term *metallome* was coined by Williams who referred to it as an element distribution, equilibrium concentrations of free metal ions, or as a free element content in a cellular compartment, cell, or organism [7]. The latter would therefore be characterized not only by its genome or proteome but also by the metallome, their inorganic complement. The meaning of the term *metallome*

was then proposed to be extended to the entirety of metal and metalloid species present in a cell or tissue type [8,9]. The characterization of the pool of metal-containing species in living organisms and of their interactions with the genome, transcriptome, proteome, and metabolome requires dedicated analytical approaches to in vivo detection, localization, identification, and quantification, in vitro functional analysis and "in silico" prediction using bioinformatics [10]. The term *metallomics* was coined by Haraguchi to denote the ensemble of research activities related to metals of biological interest [11,12] (Figure 1).

Metallomics has been the topic of a number of reviews [13–15], special issues of edited journals [9,16,17] and of a Royal Society of Chemistry journal dedicated to the field, *Metallomics*. The terms *metallome* and *metallomics* have been used in different contexts. In addition, a number of related definitions proliferated, such as ionomics [18], heteroatom-tagged proteomics [19], or elementomics [20]. This report attempts to define the terms *metallome* and *metallomics*, critically evaluates the available relevant

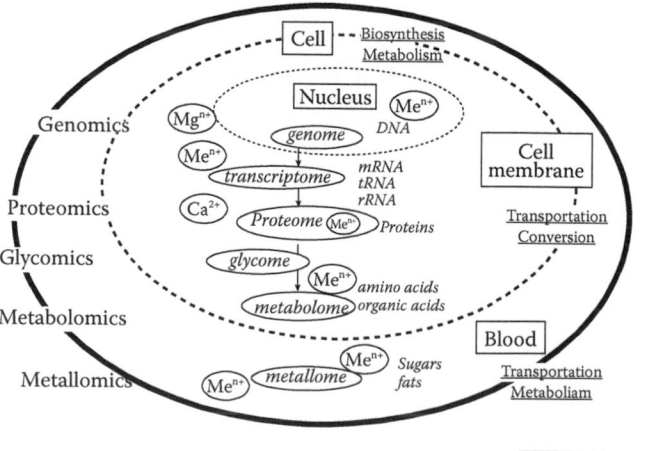

FIGURE 1 Simplified model of biological system and related -omics sciences. The outer area surrounded with the continuous line is showing, for example, an organ or whole body, and the inner area surrounded with the dotted line is showing a biological cell. Biological fluid, for example, blood, is circulating in the intermediate area. The Mg^{2+} and Ca^{2+} ions are given as examples because of their large affinities with DNA and proteins, respectively, in the biological cell. Reproduced from Ref. [12] with some modification.

Reproduced from:
Pure & Appl. Chem., Vol. 82, No. 2, pp. 493–504, 2010. © 2010 IUPAC

analytical methodology, and highlights the concerned disciplines and research areas.

2. Definitions of Terms

Metallome

Entirety of metal and metalloid species* present in a biological system, defined as to their identity and/or quantity.

Note 1: The metallome can be determined in a bulk biological sample representative of the system [or its component(s)] or at specific location(s).

Note 2: The metallome can be characterized with different degrees of approximation, such as

- a set of total element concentrations,
- a set of metal complexes with a given class of ligands, for example, proteins or metabolites, or
- a set of all the species of a given element (e.g., copper metallome).

Note 3: In contrast to the genome of which the analysis has a specific endpoint (the determination of a finite number of DNA sequences), the description of a metallome, like that of a proteome or metabolome [21], can never be complete. In particular, the numerous known and possible metal coordination complexes with biological ligands can be described only in terms of kinetic constants with defined thermodynamic equilibria.

Metallomics

Study of the metallome, interactions, and functional connections of metal ions and other metal species with genes, proteins, metabolites, and other biomolecules in biological systems.

A metallomics study is expected to imply

- a focus on metals (e.g., copper, zinc, iron, manganese, molybdenum, nickel, calcium, ..., cadmium, lead, mercury, uranium) or metalloids (e.g., arsenic, selenium, and antimony) in a biological context;
- a link between the set of element concentrations or element speciation with the genome. This link may be statistical (an enrichment of an element coincides with the presence of a particular gene), structural (sequence of a metalloprotein is traceable to a gene) or functional (the presence of a bioligand is the result of a gene-encoded mechanism); or
- a systematic or comprehensive approach. The identification of a single metal species, however important, without specifying its significance and contribution to the system should not be referred to as metallomics.

3. Methodological Approaches to the Metal-Related -Omics

3.1 Determination of the Elemental Composition of a Biological System

The elemental composition of a biological system has been used in the literature as the basis of the following two types of "-omics" studies:

- *Ionomics* It is based on the building up of a large collection of mutants (differing by deletion of a particular gene) of a model organism, analyzing them for a considerable number of elements and linking the set of element concentrations with DNA sequences in order to detect metal-regulated genes [18,24].
- *Metallogenomics*: It is based on the purification of a large number of open reading frames from a given organism, heterologous expression of proteins and screening for those which contain metals in order to identify the metal-functional genes [25].

The data are acquired by the high-throughput analysis of bulk samples (often microsamples) but multielement analysis with spatial micro- or sub-micrometer resolution (e.g., tissue or cell elemental imaging) is becoming increasingly feasible and is of growing interest.

3.1.1 Bulk Analysis

The most suitable analytical technique is inductively coupled plasma-mass spectrometry (ICP-MS). It is based on the conversion of all forms of an element present in a sample into element ions (usually singly charged) which are separated in a mass analyzer and counted by an ion detector [26]. The technique offers many advantages including femtogram-level detection limits, which are practically independent of the chemical form and the presence of matrix components, multielement and multiisotopic measurement capacity, and a large (10^9) dynamic range [26]. For these reasons, ICP-MS has practically replaced other techniques, such as ICP-atomic emission spectroscopy (AES), X-ray fluorescence (XRF), and instrumental neutron activation analysis (INAA), used in the past for the multielement determination of trace elements. State-of-the-art ICP-MS provides high-throughput analysis of microliter or sub-microliter samples in the continuous or flow-injection mode using dedicated micro- and nanoflow nebulizers [27].

ICP-MS suffers from interferences on a considerable number of isotopes. The understanding and awareness of these interferences by the analyst is a must. The use of a sector-field mass spectrometer at a required mass resolution or an ICP-MS equipped with a collision-cell is strongly recommended. The certitude that the analytically used signal corresponds to the expected isotope only is mandatory even in comparative analyses. The use of a certified reference material with the composition as close as possible to that of the analyzed sample is recommended for method validation and periodic quality assurance. Common sources of error are the selective or nonquantitative transfer of elements to the solution which requires a careful optimization of the sample digestion and minimizing contamination.

3.1.2 Spatially Resolved Analysis

A quantitative imaging (mapping) of the spatial distribution of elements in a solid sample (e.g., a thin section of a biological tissue) is possible by using a microanalytical technique, such as X-ray absorption spectroscopy (XAS), particle-induced X-ray emission spectrometry, or laser ablation (LA) ICP-MS [28]. The analysis is usually not species-specific, although some specificity in terms of the oxidation state or the metal coordination environment can, in some cases (XAS), be obtained.

The high signal-to-noise ratio of ICP-MS makes it possible to acquire quantitative multielement concentration data (images) in thin (ca. 20 μm) section of biological tissues using direct LA with 10–150 μm resolution [29]. The image of the elemental distribution (ion current intensity as a function of tissue x and y

---

* Specific form of an element defined as to isotopic composition, electronic or oxidation state, and/or complex or molecular structure [22].

coordinates and *m/z* ratios) for essential metals (e.g., iron, copper, zinc, manganese, molybdenum, cobalt, and nickel), metalloids (selenium), and non-metals (phosphorous, sulfur, carbon) in the cross-section of analyzed tissue (e.g., brain, liver, kidney) can reveal some unique information for biological and medical research [30,31]. Inhomogeneous (often layered) site-specific metal distribution in tissue sections (as demonstrated in human brain different regions) can be obtained. The resolution can be decreased to the 100-nm level using nano-secondary-ion mass spectrometry (SIMS), nanoprobe synchrotron XRF, or near-field LA-ICP-MS [32], paving the way to metal distribution imaging in single cells and cell organelles.

Technically speaking, a commercial LA system using an Nd:YAG laser is usually coupled to a quadrupole ICP-MS without or with collision cell or double-focusing sector field ICP-MS. Modern commercial LA systems support the imaging of elements in tissues. LA-ICP-MS data are evaluated using dedicated imaging software developed in several laboratories. Detection limits of imaging LA-ICP-MS at the low µg g⁻¹ and upper ng g⁻¹ levels were reported. The measurement time for imaging LA-ICP-MS of biological tissues (up to several hours) depends on the size of the analyzed area and the laser scan speed applied (varied from 20 µm/s up to 100 µm/s). For quantitative analysis, well-defined matrix-matched laboratory standards are required [33].

3.2 Analysis for Metal-Containing or Metal-Binding Biomolecules

The analytical technique should produce a signal specific to a metal-containing biomolecule allowing its detection, identification, and quantification. The metallobiomolecules can be probed directly in a solid sample by XAS or in a sample extract by electrospray MS. The ultimate resolution and sensitivity are offered by hyphenated (coupled) techniques which combine a separation by chromatography or electrophoresis with elemental or molecular MS detection.

3.2.1 X-Ray Absorption Spectroscopy

XAS in the edge region, usually referred to as XANES (X-ray absorption near-edge spectroscopy), provides information about oxidation number, covalence (the number of pairs of electrons which a given atom shares with its neighbors), molecular symmetry of the site, and, hence, coordination number. The analysis beyond the edge region, referred to as EXAFS (extended X-ray absorption fine structure) [34], provides structural information about the atomic neighborhood of a metal (metalloids) being probed, such as the coordination number (number of ligands), the identity of the ligand atoms, and the distance between the metal and each ligand.

XAS is a quantitative technique but it is not particularly sensitive (a minimum analyte concentration at several tens of µg g⁻¹ level is required). In the case of a mixture of different species of the probed element present, the interpretation of the spectra becomes rapidly difficult so the technique is ideal when a single or maximum two dominant species are present. Identification (oxidation state or coordination center) is made by the comparison of the spectrum with that of a reference compound. XAS is invaluable for probing the kinetically labile complexes, which can readily dissociate or exchange ligands during sample handling, and for the differentiation of the oxidation state, which in some cases [e.g., As^III/As^V] is readily modified during any extraction step. A representative example of applications includes the determination of quantitative distribution of zinc among the complexes with phosphate, cysteine, and histidine in plant (XANES) [35] or

the identification of citrate as the major nickel-binding ligand in *Leptoplax* leaves (EXAFS) [36].

XAS, which is becoming popular owing to the increasing access to synchrotrons, gives the comfort of avoiding sample preparation, but its areas of application are limited. It can only confirm the presence of expected species (of a single element at a time) in a sample, but not find new ones.

3.2.2 Chromatography and Capillary Electrophoresis (CE) with Element-Specific Detection

The most favored tool for a rapid semi-quantitative screening for the presence of metal-biomolecule complexes in biological samples has been the coupling of size-exclusion liquid chromatography (LC) and ICP-MS (for reviews of applications, see Refs. [13,37]). The elution is monitored in the multielement (multiisotopic) mode, and as the column can be calibrated in terms of molecular mass, a chromatogram allows the fractionation of the metallobiomolecules as a function of size prior to detection. Fairly concentrated samples (e.g., 3–5 times diluted cytosol) can be analyzed, and conditions for non-denaturing separations can be readily optimized.

The resolution of size-exclusion chromatography (SEC) is low, and the chromatographic purity of peaks is usually poor. The matching of the elution volume with that of a standard cannot be considered as a definitive proof of the species identity. Also, the control of the adsorbed metal ions on the stationary phase is important as they can exchange with the metal ions already complexed or can be scavenged by ligands from the sample leading to ghost peaks.

Among other types of non-denaturing chromatography (preserving the metal–biomolecule bond), anion-exchange high-performance liquid chromatography (HPLC) of metalloproteins [38] and hydrophilic interaction liquid chromatography (HILIC) [39] of metal-containing metabolites have attracted particular attention. They offer much higher resolution than size-exclusion LC, and, especially, HILIC can be readily coupled with electrospray ionization (ESI)-MS for species identification.

Capillary electrophoresis (CE) offers a number of incontestable advantages for metal species analysis such as a small sample size (in the nanoliter range) required, high resolution, and the absence of stationary phase, and hence, the possibility of analysis of labile complexes. The development and commercialization of a dedicated CE-ICP-MS interface eliminated most of the problems of the earlier laboratory-made designs [40].

The rapidly developing application areas of CE-ICP-MS include metal-binding studies with pure compounds of biological origin, for example, recombinant proteins [41,42], the determination of stoichiometry of metal–protein complexes [43–45], and the use of CE for fine (2nd or 3rd dimension) separations of metal-containing fractions isolated by chromatography [46,47].

The potential of some non-chromatographic techniques, such as the coupling of field flow fractionation (FFF) with ICP-MS and high-field asymmetric waveform ion mobility spectrometry (FAIMS) for metallomic-type applications, merits a deeper insight.

3.2.3 Identification of Metal-Containing Species By Molecular Mass Spectrometry

Electrospray ionization allows the production of ions of metal complexes in the gas phase, which can be then analyzed by mass spectrometry. The accurate mass determination should allow the determination of the empiric formula (and thus the metal-ligand stoichiometry), whereas the collision-induced dissociation (CID) mass spectra should deliver information on the structure of the ligand [48]. Paradoxically, the number of reports on the successful use of ESI-MS for the identification of metal complexes has been remarkably scarce [13].

The problem is the vulnerability of ESI-MS to the presence of concomitant ions generated by matrix components which suppress the ionization of the species of interest. This concerns in particular the currently used quadrupole time-of-flight (QTOF) mass spectrometers for which the intrascan dynamic range is small. The ionization efficiency is critically dependent on the analyte chromatographic purity. Even if a single species of a given element is present (as detected by ICP-MS), hundreds of matrix compounds, transparent to the ICP-MS detection, may co-elute. Therefore, a purification step, using an orthogonal separation mechanism, is required prior to electrospray MS [49]. ICP-MS offers the possibility of monitoring the purification of the metalloprotein while accounting for its integrity (monitoring of the metal or, in some cases, the metal-to-sulfur ratio).

Column techniques (chromatography or CE) with the parallel ICP-MS and ESI-MS detection seem to offer the most adequate tool for the in vivo identification of metal–biomolecule complexes at the pico- and nanomolar levels, although the number of successful identifications to date has been limited and concerned relatively small proteins, such as metallothioneins. Further progress in the use of ESI-MS for the identification of metal–bioligand complexes is expected with the wider availability of Fourier transform mass spectrometers, using either ion cyclotron resonance or electrostatic orbital traps, which offer a larger intrascan range and the possibility of the multi-stage fragmentation and mass spectrometry facilitating the species identification.

3.2.4 Gel Electrophoresis with Element-Specific Detection

Polyacrylamide gel electrophoresis (PAGE), employed either in the monodimensional or 2D mode, is considered the most adequate technique for the separation of proteins. The principal difficulty in its use for metalloproteomics is the need for the preservation of the metal–protein bond. Many metal complexes with proteins are labile and can be destroyed by exchange with the metal impurities of the gel during separation and staining. Among the recommended precautions, the most important are (i) the use of non-denaturing separation protocols, (ii) avoiding the presence of metal impurities in gels, and (iii) avoiding staining or the use of ultrapure staining reagents (as, e.g., in BlueNative electrophoresis [50]).

Metal-specific detection in the gels has enjoyed considerable interest for a long time, the principal techniques including autoradiography with its inherent use of radioactive isotopes (e.g., selenium-75), and synchrotron radiation XRF and proton-induced X-ray emission (PIXE) with the need for hardly available facilities. LA-ICP-MS imaging, pioneered by Nielsen et al. [51], offers a competitive alternative for the in situ probing of the protein spots for the presence of metals and metalloids. The ablated analytes are swept into the ICP by a continuous stream of argon, and the ions are analyzed by MS. As a result, an electropherogram is obtained in which the quantity of a given element is a function of its position in the gel. Detection by LA-ICP-MS is a potentially fast and fairly robust technology, because no further reaction or derivatization step is involved, and the signal is, theoretically, directly proportional to the quantity of the analyte element in the gel [52].

LA-ICP-MS detection in 1D gel electrophoresis can be carried out in the lane scan mode [28]. In the spot-to-spot hopping mode [53], protein spots present in a 2D gel must be visualized prior to ablation. An alternative is the imaging mode [54]. The high stability and precision of LA-ICP-MS makes it possible to scan a gel in raster mode and thus to acquire element images. The analysis in the imaging mode is time-consuming. Scanning a gel of 2 cm^2 with a 100-μm resolution takes several hours, but the technique allows the identification of areas with increased metal concentrations regardless of the presence of intense protein spots. As the whole gel is scanned, the metalloproteins do not need to be visualized in either lane or imaging mode by staining, which minimizes the risk of metal loss.

Proteins containing covalently incorporated metals (e.g., selenoproteins) can be recovered from the gel and analyzed using the canonical proteomics protocols. The recovery of an intact metal–protein complex is much more difficult. Unless a mass spectrum of the metal–protein complex is provided, there is always a risk that the protein identified by the spot digestion and peptide mapping is different from that binding the metal in the same spot. Auxiliary data such as the presence of metallated peptides in mass spectra in-gel EXAFS showing the metal–protein bond [55] or the desorption of the metalloprotein from the gel (or the blot) are required.

3.3 Analysis for Biomolecules with Metal-Binding Capacity

There is a class of analytical methods which does not target intact metal complexes but simply biomolecules showing an affinity to bind metals. Such molecules are typically isolated by immobilized metal affinity chromatography (IMAC). The analysis is qualitative and concerns the ligand only. The existence of the metal–ligand bond in vivo is assumed on the basis of the characteristics of the separation step.

IMAC resins use chelating agents (e.g., tridentate iminodiacetic acid) immobilized on a sorbent. Prior to use, metal ions are immobilized on the IMAC resin and are supposed to react with specific protein ligands in the sample. An IMAC protocol includes the saturation of an IMAC support (column/chip/chip array) with the metal of interest, washing off the excess of metal, introduction of a metal-depleted sample (metal depletion results in unoccupied metal-binding sites of proteins which facilitate binding to the IMAC metal), and the removal of the non-bound sample components followed by the elution of the retained proteins (with the metal-binding affinity) with a competing complexing agent. The proteins with the metal-binding affinity are recovered as apo (demetallated forms) and can be analyzed by any of the classic proteomics approach.

Alternatively, the retained proteins can be digested on-column. The metal-coordination center is expected to be preserved by the retention of the metal–peptide complex after the digestion of the protein [56,57], which seems to be a convenient way for the identification of the metal-binding motives.

The IMAC approach enjoys a growing popularity with recent applications referring to the analysis of the zinc [56,57] and copper [56–58] proteomes in human hepatoma cell lines, uranyl proteome in human serum [59], bismuth proteome in *Helicobacter pylori* cell extracts [60], and Ni-proteome in human keratinocytes [61,62] and *Arabidopsis thaliana* roots [63].

IMAC does provide information on the presence of proteins with metal-binding sites but not on the metal–protein complexes present. Also, metalloproteins with a high metal affinity at functional sites, such as superoxide dismutase (SOD), are likely to pass through the IMAC column due to occupation of binding sites by physiological metals [57]. The IMAC approach is not quantitative, and minor proteins are likely to be masked by major ones.

3.4 Bioinformatics and Prediction of the Metal-Binding Patterns

This approach consists of searching metal-binding motives (which are expected to be preserved regardless of the organism studied) in putatively expressed proteins based on genome sequences present in data banks [64,65].

Substantial progress has been recently achieved for the identification of selenoproteins in a number of organisms, including humans. The original computer algorithms were based on the use of the canonical SECIS (selenocysteine insertion sequence) element (AUGA_AA_GA) as a signature for mammalian selenoproteins [66] and then refined to search for SECIS-containing genes with in-frame UGA codons [67]. The vast majority of genes encoding selenocysteine-containing proteins could be identified in this way.

Methods allowing the search for entire sets of metal-binding proteins are less advanced. Bertini et al. proposed an approach taking advantage of known consensus sequences, that is, taking into account the nature and spacing of amino acids present in the metal-binding region; the distribution of iron-, copper-, and zinc-binding proteins in several archaea, bacteria, and eukaryotes was thus described [65]. The bioinformatic analysis of the protein sequence (by correlation with the relevant gene) allows the finding of the conserved metal-binding motifs and provides important clues to function and metal site structure [68]. This approach is critically dependent on the availability of consensus sequences for the binding of different metals.

Bioinformatics is also useful for the prediction of a metal-binding site based on a known 3D structure. It is possible owing to the conserved nature of the metal-binding site and its usual compact size [69]. The number of 3D protein structures is still limited but increases with the progress of structural genomics projects. Metal-binding sites can also be predicted by the combination of low-resolution structural data with sequence information [70].

The bioinformatic methods largely facilitate the identification of seleno- and metalloproteins but do not replace in vivo analysis, which is the sole way to say whether a given protein was actually biosynthesized or not.

4. Interest Areas for Metal-Related -Omics

Metal-related "-omics" are transdisciplinary research areas with an impact on biogeochemistry, clinical physiology and pharmacology, plant and animal physiology, and nutrition. An example of interdisciplinary interest is the detection, quantification, isolation, and characterization of metalloenzymes playing fundamental roles in a number of biological processes, including photosynthesis, respiration, and nitrogen fixation [71].

Biogeochemistry and Environmental Chemistry. Metals represent a link between the chemistry of the atmosphere and oceans from which life has evolved and the genomes and proteomes of living organisms [3]. The role of transition metals in microbial metabolism has been discussed with a particular focus on the deduction of geochemical signatures and phylogenetic relationships of prokaryotes from whole genome sequences and on the

use of this link to infer geochemical aspects of the biosphere through time [72]. Model proteomes were reported to contain putative imprints of ancient shifts in trace metal geochemistry [73]. In environmental chemistry, a systematic view of the transition-metal metabolism requires an understanding of how organisms sense, adapt, and use these metals within the biodiversity characteristic of each specific ecosystem [6]. Environmental pollution with metals leads to the evolution of the protein expression signature and spurs the assignment of some proteins as environmental pollution biomarkers [14]. The correlation of sentinel organism proteomes with the metal contamination is one of the areas of environmental proteomics [14].

Plant Biochemistry and Physiology. The primary concern is the search for mechanisms responsible for the (i) mobilization of low solubility metals from soil, (ii) translocation within the plant, and (iii) sequestering metal ions in cytosol or in cellular compartments. Consequently, the identification and quantification of low-molecular, metal-containing metabolites is of interest in studies of (i) uptake and bioavailability of essential elements, mainly iron and zinc with the aim to combat the micronutrient malnutrition in developing countries [74]; (ii) metal hyperaccumulation with a focus on phytoremediation and/or phytomining [75]; and (iii) plant defense mechanisms against heavy metal stress (including volatilization, appearance of inorganic insoluble forms, or induction of phytochelatins) [76].

Clinical Chemistry and Pharmacology. Despite their vital role as regulatory cofactors, metals can also be highly toxic and involved in pathophysiology of several diseases and human health risk assessment [77]. Most diseases associated with copper, iron, and zinc result from mutations in the genes encoding for metal-transporting proteins which can be identified by proteomics approaches [61,78]. A number of pharmaceuticals contain a metal in their structure and are referred to as metallodrugs [79]. They have anti-neoplastic (e.g., cisplatin or ruthenium compounds), anti-inflammatory (gold), anti-bacterial (bismuth), and other functions. Metallomics studies will focus on the metabolism of these drugs, their transport, and interactions with biologically relevant molecules.

Nutrition and Essential Elements Supplementation. The essential role of many trace elements, their implication in prevention of a number of diseases, and the low levels of some of these elements in the diet in many countries are leading to increasing interest in the supplementation of food and feed with mineral elements, such as selenium [80], zinc, iron, manganese, and chromium. The relevant metallomics studies focus, on one hand, on the characterization of the chemical forms and their bioavailability in the supplements and, on the other hand, on the transport and fate in the target organisms, such as animals (meat, milk, and eggs from selenium-supplemented animals become functional food themselves) and humans [81,82].

5. Membership of Sponsoring Body

Membership of the IUPAC Analytical Chemistry Division Committee for the period 2008–2009 was as follows:

President: A. Fajgelj (Slovenia); ***Titular Members:*** W. Lund (Norway); B. Hibbert (Australia); R. Lobinski (France); P. De Bièvre (Belgium); J. Labuda (Slovakia); M. F. Camões (Portugal); Z. F. Chai (China); Z. Mester (Canada); S. Motomizu (Japan); ***Associate Members:*** P. DeZorzi (Italy); A. Felinger (Hungary); M. Jarosz (Poland); P. Minkkinen (Finland); M. Pingarron (Spain); ***National Representatives:*** S. K. Aggarwal (India);

R. Apak (Turkey); M. S. Iqbal (Pakistan); H. Kim (Korea); T. A. Maryutina (Russia); R. M. Smith (UK); N. Trendafilova (Bulgaria); *Provisional Member:* N. Torto (Botswana).

6. Acknowledgments

The authors acknowledge the valuable comments and suggestions from A. Anbar, M. A. Arruda, J. Bettmer, I. Bertini, J. Caruso, Z. F. Chai, J. L. Gomez-Ariza, R. Grimm, G. Hieftje, M. Jarosz, D. Koppenaal, W. Lund, Z. Mester, E. Roberts, D. Salt, J. Szpunar, and J. Zaleski during the different stages of the preparation of this report.

7. References

1. W. P. Blackstock, M. P. Weir. *Trends Biotechnol.* **17**, 121 (1999).
2. N. L. Anderson, N. G. Anderson. *Electrophoresis* **19**, 1853 (1998).
3. R. J. P. Williams, J. J. R. Frausto Da Silva. *J.Chem. Educ.* **81**, 738 (2004).
4. J. A. Tainer, V. A. Roberts, E. D. Getzoff. *Curr. Opin. Biotechnol.* **2**, 582 (1991).
5. C. E. Outten, T. V. O'Halloran. *Science* **292**, 2488 (2001).
6. D. J. Thiele, J. D. Gitlin. *Nat. Chem. Biol.* **4**, 145 (2008).
7. R. J. P. Williams. *Coord. Chem. Rev.* **216–217**, 583 (2001).
8. J. Szpunar. *Anal. Bioanal. Chem.* **378**, 54 (2004).
9. D. W. Koppenaal, G. M. Hieftje. *J.Anal. At. Spectrom.* **22**, 855 (2007).
10. S. Mounicou, J. Szpunar, R. Lobinski. *Chem. Soc. Rev.* **38**, 1119 (2009).
11. H. Haraguchi, T. Matsuura. In *Bio-Trace Elements 2002 (BITREL 2002)*, E. Enomoto (Ed.), RIKEN (Research Institute of Physics and Chemistry), Wako, 2002.
12. H. Haraguchi. *J. Anal. At. Spectrom.* **19**, 5 (2004).
13. J. Szpunar. *Analyst* **130**, 442 (2005).
14. J. Lopez-Barea, J. L. Gomez-Ariza. *Proteomics* **6**, S51 (2006).
15. W. Shi, M. R. Chance. *Cell. Mol. Life Sci.* **65**, 3040 (2008).
16. N. Jakubowski, R. Lobinski. L. Moens. *J. Anal. At. Spectrom.* **19**, 1 (2004).
17. H. Haraguchi (Ed.). *Pure Appl. Chem.* **80**(12) (2008).
18. B. Lahner, J. Gong, M. Mahmoudian, E. L. Smith, K. B. Abid, E. E. Rogers, M. L. Guerinot, et al. *Nat. Biotechnol.* **21**, 1215 (2003).
19. A. Sanz-Medel. *Anal. Bioanal. Chem.* **381**, 1 (2005).
20. N. Jakubowski, G. M. Hieftje. *J. Anal. At. Spectrom.* **23**, 13 (2007).
21. J. H. Duffus, M. Nordberg, D. M. Templeton. *Pure. Appl. Chem.* **79**, 1153 (2007).
22. D. M. Templeton, F. Ariese, R. Cornelis, L. G. Danielsson, H. Muntau, H. P. Van Leeuwen, R. Lobinski. *Pure Appl. Chem.* **72**, 1453 (2000).
23. D. E. Salt, I. Baxter, B. Lahner. *Annu. Rev. Plant Biol.* **59**, 709 (2008).
24. D. J. Eide, S. Clark, T. M. Nair, M. Gehl, M. Gribskov, M. L. Guerinot, J. F. Harper. *Genome Biol.* **6**, R77 (2005).
25. R. A. Scott, J. E. Shokes, N. J. Cosper, F. E. Jenney, M. W. W. Adams. *J.Synchrotron Rad.* **12**, 19 (2005).
26. A. Montaser. *Inductively Coupled Plasma Mass Spectrometry*, Wiley, New York, 1998.
27. J. S. Becker, *Inorganic Mass Spectrometry. Principles and Applications*, Wiley, Chichester, 2007.
28. R. Lobinski, C. Moulin, R. Ortega. *Biochimie* **88**, 1591 (2006).
29. J. S. Becker, M. Zoriy, B. Wu, A. Matusch, J. Su. Becker. *J. Anal. At. Spectrom.* **23**, 1275 (2008).
30. J. S. Becker, M. V. Zoriy, C. Pickhardt, N. Palomero-Gallagher, K. Zilles. *Anal. Chem.* **77**, 3208 (2005).
31. J. S. Becker, M. Zoriy, J. Su. Becker, J. Dobrowolska, A. Matusch. *J. Anal. At. Spectrom.* **22**, 736 (2007).
32. J. S. Becker, A. Gorbunoff, M. Zoriy, A. Izmer, M. Kayser. *J. Anal. At. Spectrom.* **21**, 19 (2006).
33. J. S. Becker, A. Matusch, C. Depboylu, J. Dobrowolska, M. V. Zoriy. *Anal. Chem.* **79**, 6074 (2007).
34. J. Kawai. In *Encyclopedia of Analytical Chemistry*, R. A. Meyers (Ed.), p. 13288, Wiley, Chichester, 2000.
35. R. Terzano, Z. Al Chami, B. Vekemans, K. Janssens, T. Miano, P. Ruggiero. *J. Agric. Food Chem.* **56**, 3222 (2008).
36. E. Montarges-Pelletier, V. Chardot, G. Echevarria, L. J. Michot, A. Bauer, J. L. Morel. *Phytochemistry* **69**, 1695 (2008).
37. J. Szpunar. *Analyst* **125**, 963 (2000).
38. M. E. Del Castillo Busto, M. Montes-Bayon, A. Sanz-Medel. *Anal. Chem.* **78**, 8218 (2006).
39. L. Ouerdane, S. Mari, P. Czernic, M. Lebrun, R. Lobinski. *J. Anal. At. Spectrom.* **21**, 676 (2006).
40. D. Schaumlöffel, A. Prange. *Fresenius' J. Anal. Chem.* **364**, 452 (1999).
41. K. Polec, J. Szpunar, O. Palacios, P. Gonzalez-Duarte, S. Atrian, R. Lobinski. *J. Anal. At. Spectrom.* **16**, 567 (2001).
42. K. Polec-Pawlak, O. Palacios, M. Capdevilla, P. Gonzalez-Duarte, R. Lobinski. *Talanta* **57**, 1011 (2002).
43. K. Polec-Pawlak, D. Schaumlöffel, J. Szpunar, A. Prange, R. Lobinski. *J. Anal. At. Spectrom.* **17**, 908 (2002).
44. A. Hagege, T. Baldinger, M. Martin-Jouet, F. Zal, M. Leroy, E. Leize, A. V. Dorsselaer. *Rapid Commun. Mass Spectrom.* **18**, 735 (2004).
45. V. Van Lierde, K. Strijckmans, M. Galleni, B. Devreese, J. Van Beeumen, F. Vanhaecke, L. Moens. *LC-GC Europe* **9**, 617 (2003).
46. D. Schaumlöffel, L. Ouerdane, B. Bouyssiere, R. Lobinski. *J. Anal. At. Spectrom.* **18**, 120 (2003).
47. S. Mounicou, S. McSheehy, J. Szpunar, M. Potin-Gautier, R. Lobinski. *J. Anal. At. Spectrom.* **17**, 15 (2002).
48. H. Chassaigne, V. Vacchina, R. Lobinski. *Trends Anal. Chem.* **19**, 300 (2000).
49. J. Szpunar, R. Lobinski. *Anal. Bioanal. Chem.* **373**, 404 (2002).
50. I. Wittig, H.-P. Braun, H. Schaegger. *Nat. Protocols* **1**, 418 (2006).
51. J. L. Neilsen, A. Abildtrup, J. Christensen, P. Watson, A. Cox, C. W. McLeod. *Spectrochim. Acta, Part B* **53**, 339 (1998).
52. R. Ma, C. W. McLeod, K. Tomlinson, R. K. Poole. *Electrophoresis* **25**, 2469 (2004).
53. J. S. Becker, M. Zoriy, J. Su. Becker, C. Pickhardt, M. Przybylski. *J.Anal. At. Spectrom.* **19**, 149 (2004).
54. J. Su. Becker, R. Lobinski, J. S. Becker. *Metallomics* **1**, 312 (2009).
55. S. Chevreux, S. Roudeau, A. Fraysse, A. Carmona, G. Devès, P. L. Solari, T. C. Weng, R. Ortega. *J. Anal. At. Spectrom.* **23**, 1117 (2008).
56. Y. M. She, S. Narindrasorasak, S. Yang, N. Spitale, E. A. Roberts, B. Sarkar. *Mol. Cell. Proteomics* **2**, 1306 (2003).
57. S. D. Smith, Y. M. She, E. A. Roberts, B. Sarkar. *J. Proteome Res.* **3**, 834 (2004).
58. H. Roelofsen, R. Balgobind, R. J. Vonk. *J. Cell. Biochem.* **93**, 732 (2004).
59. C. Basset, A. Dedieu, P. Guérin, E. Quéméneur, D. Meyer, C. Vidaud. *J. Chromatogr., A* **1185**, 233 (2008).
60. R. Ge, X. Sun, Q. Gu, R. M. Watt, J. A. Tanner, B. C. Y. Wong, H. H. Xia, J.-D. Huang, Q.-Y. He, H. Sun. *J. Biol. Inorg. Chem.* **12**, 831 (2007).
61. H. J. Thierse, S. Helm, P. Pankert. *Methods Mol. Biol.* **425**, 139 (2008).
62. K. Heiss, C. Junkes, N. Guerreiro, M. Swamy, M. M. Camacho-Carvajal, W. W. A. Schamel, I. D. Haidl, D. Wild, H. U. Weltzien, H. J. Thierse. *Proteomics* **5**, 3614 (2005).
63. C. C. S. Kung, W. N. Huang, Y. C. Huang, K. C. Yeh. *Proteomics* **6**, 2746 (2006).
64. V. N. Gladyshev, G. V. Kryukov, D. E. Fomenko, D. L. Hatfield. *Annu. Rev. Nutr.* **24**, 579 (2004).
65. I. Bertini, A. Rosato. *Eur. J. Inorg. Chem.* 2546 (2007).
66. G. V. Kryukov, V. M. Kryukov, V. N. Gladyshev. *J. Biol. Chem.* **274**, 33888 (1999).
67. S. Castellano, N. Morozova, M. Morey, M. J. Berry, F. Serras, M. Corominas, R. Guigo. *EMBO Rep.* **2**, 697 (2001).
68. W. Shi, C. Zhan, A. Ignatov, B. A. Manjasetty, N. Marinkovic, M. Sullivan, R. Huang, M. R. Chance. *Structure* **13**, 1473 (2005).

69. J. W. H. Schymkowitz, F. Rousseau, I. C. Martins, J. Ferkinghoff-Borg, F. Stricher, L. Serrano. *Proc. Natl Acad. Sci. U. S. A.* **102**, 10147 (2005).

70. J. S. Sodhi, K. Bryson, L. J. McGuffin, J. J. Ward, L. Wernisch, D. T. Jones. *J. Mol. Biol.* **342**, 307 (2004).

71. C. Andreini, I. Bertini, G. Cavallaro, G. L. Holliday, J. M. Thornton, *J. Biol. Inorg. Chem.* **13**, 1205 (2008).

72. A. L. Zerkle, C. H. House, S. L. Brantley. *Am. J. Sci.* **305**, 467 (2005).

73. C. L. Dupont, S. Yang, B. Palenik, P. E. Bourne. *Proc. Natl Acad. Sci. U. S. A.* **103**, 17822 (2006).

74. J. E. Mayer, W. H. Pfeiffer, P. Beyer. *Curr. Opin. Plant Biol.* **11**, 166 (2008).

75. K. Shah, J. M. Nongkynrih. *Biologia Plantarum* **51**, 618 (2007).

76. S. Clemens. *Planta* **212**, 475 (2001).

77. WHO/IPCS. *Environmental Health Criteria 234.* Elemental Speciation in Human Health Risk Assessment, Geneva, 2006.

78. P. P. Kulkarni, Y. M. She, S. D. Smith, E. A. Roberts, B. Sarkar. *Chem. Eur. J.* **12**, 2410 (2006).

79. Z. Guo, P. J. Sadler. *Angew. Chem. Int. Ed.* **38**, 1513 (1999).

80. G. N. Schrauzer. *J. Nutr.* **130**, 1653 (2000).

81. K. T. Suzuki. *J. Health Sci.* **51**, 107 (2005).

82. K. T. Suzuki, Y. Ogra. *Food Add. Contam.* **19**, 974 (2002).

WATER

Water Purity and Water Purity Classification

Water Type	Resistance[a] Megohm @25°C	Bioburden (cfu)[b]	Dissolved Solids (mg/L)
Deionized	0.05	—	10
Purified	0.2	100	1
Apyrogenic	0.8	0.1	1
High Purity	10	1	0.5
Ultrapure	18	1	0.005

[a] Resistance (R), determined by conductivity(A/V[c]), measured in siemans (S), R is measured in ohms (V/A[d]) (Ω).
[b] Colony-forming units.
[c] SI unit for conductivity – $m^{-2} \cdot kg^{-1} \cdot s^{-3} \cdot A^2$; one S equal to the conductance of one ohm^{-1}.
[d] SI unit for resistance – $m^{-2} \cdot kg^{-1} \cdot s^{-3} \cdot A^{-2}$; one R is equal to one ohm.

Some Definitions of Pharmaceutical Water (FDA/ORA)

- Non-potable
- Potable
- USP purified
- USP water for injection (WFI)
- USP sterile water for injection
- USP bacteriostatic water for injection
- USP sterile water for irrigation

See 2007 USP/NF. *The Official Compendia of Standards*, US Pharmacopeia, Rockville, MD, USA, 2007, http://www.usp.org;

British Pharmacopoeia 2007, TSO Norwich, Norwich, UK, 2007; http://www.pharmacopoeia.org.uk

Process water is defined as that water which is used during the pharmaceutical manufacturing process. A higher purity water may be required for formulation of the final drug product and/or reconstitution of final product prior to use. A high purity water is required for a product which is to be injected as opposed to an oral administered product. http://www.fda.gov/ora/inspect_ref/itg/itg46.html

Meltzer, T.H., *High Purity Water Preparation*, Tall Oaks Publications, Littleton, CO, 1993.

Fischbacher, C., Quality assurance in analytical chemistry, in *Encyclopedia of Analytical Chemistry*, ed. R.A. Meyers, Wiley, New York, NY, USA, pps 13563-13587, 2000.

Environmental water quality issues are a separate issue with different classification issues

- Kannel, P.R., Lee, S., Lee, Y.S., *et al.*, Application of water quality indices and dissolved oxygen as indicators for river water classification and urban impact assessment, *Environ. Monit.Assess.*, in press, 2007.
- Kowalkowski, T., Zhytniewski, R., Szpejna, J., and Buszewski, B., Application of chemometrics in river water classification, *Water Res.* 40, 7544–752, 2006.

WATER PURIFICATION

The Following is a Representation of Estimates of Effectiveness

Technique[a]	Effectiveness of Removal of Contaminant/Impurity			
	Inorganic or Ionized Organic	Organic	Pyrogens	Particulates
Activated Carbon	Partial	Partial	No	No
Ion Exchange	Yes	No	No	No
Distillation	Yes	Yes[b]	Yes	Yes
Reverse Osmosis	Partial	Partial	Yes	Yes
Ultrafiltration	Partial	Partial	Good	Yes

[a] In general, a combination of technologies is required–For example,
  1. Input water (outside line)
  2. Filtration/settling (depends on quality of input water)
  3. Distillation
  4. Reverse osmosis
  5. Terminal filtration (e.g. 0.2 µ filter)Other techniques such as ultraviolet irradiation may be used
[b] Effectiveness of separation depends on vapor pressure (boiling point) differences between water and specific contaminant impurity and lack of formation of a azeotropic mixture.
  http://www.fda.gov/ora/inspect_ref/igs/high.html

PROPERTIES OF WATER

Absorption of Light (adapted from Morton, R.A., *Biochemical Spectroscopy*, Wiley, New York, NY, USA, 1975)

Wavelength (nm)	Absorbance[a]	Wavelength(nm)	Absorbance[a]
220	1.1	500	0.02
250	0.8	600	0.1
280	0.4	700	0.8
300	0.3	800	2.4
320	0.2	1000	40.0
340	0.2	1500	194.0
400	0.1	1800	170.0

Water Quality and Water Analysis References

Water General References

Dorsey, N.E., *Properties of Ordinary Water-Substance*, Reinhold Publishing Company, New York, NY, USA, 1940.

Eisenberg, D. and Kauzmann, W., *The Structure and Properties of Water*, Oxford University Press, New York, NY, USA, 1969.

Water: A Comprehensive Treatise, ed. F. Frank, Plenum Press, London, 1972.

Water and Aqueous Solutions, ed, G.W. Nelson and J.E. Enderby, Adam Hilger, Bristol, UK, 1985.

Robison, G.W., Zhu, S.B., Singh, S., and Evans, M.W., *Water in Biology, Chemistry, and Physics Experimental Overviews and Computational Methodologies*, World Scientific Press, Singapore, 1996.

Frank, F., *Water, 2nd edition, A Matrix of Life*, Royal Society of Chemistry, Cambridge, UK, 2000.

Water Purity

Swaddle, T.W., *Applied Inorganic Chemistry*, University of Calgary Press, Calgary, Alberta, Canada, Chapter 12 (Water conditioning), 1990.

Afshar, A., Zhao, X., Heckert, R.A., and Trotter, H.C., Suitability of autoclaved tap water for preparation of ELISA reagents and washing buffer, *J.Virol.Methods* 46, 275–278, 1994.

Stewart, K.K. and Ebel, R.E., *Chemical Measurements in Biological Systems*, John Wiley & Sons, New York, NY, USA, Chapter 2 (Water, pH, and Buffers), 2000.

Mabic, S. and Kano, I., Impact of purified water quality on molecular biology experiments, *Clin.Chem.Lab.Med.* 41, 486–491, 2003.

Regnault, C., Kano, I., Darbouret, D., and Mabic, D., Ultrapure water for liquid chromatography-mass spectrometry studies, *J.Chromatog.A.* 1030, 289–295, 2004.

Bennett, A., Process Water: Analyzing the lifecycle cost of pure water, *Filtration & Separation*, March, 2006.

Water Analysis

Water analysis, in *Encyclopedia of Analytical Sciences*, ed A. Townshend, Academic Press, London, UK, Volume 9, pps. 5445–5559, 1995.

Fischbacher, C., Quality assurance in analytical chemistry, in *Encyclopedia of Analytical Chemistry*, ed. R.A. Meyers, Wiley, New York, NY, USA, pps 13563–13587, 2000.

Reid, D., Water determination in food, in *Encyclopedia of analytical chemistry*, ed. R.H. Meyers, Wiley, New York, NY, USA, pps. 4318–4332, 2000.

Spectroscopy of Water

Morton, R.A., *Biochemical Spectroscopy*, Wiley, New York, NY, USA, 1975.

Symans, M.C.R., Spectroscopic studies of water and aqueous solutions, in *Water and Aqueous Solutions*, ed G.W. Nelson and J.E. Enderby, Adam Hilger, Bristol, UK, pps. 41–55, 1985.

Googin, P.L. and Carr, C., Far infrared spectroscopy and aqueous solutions, in *Water and Aqueous Solutions*, ed. G.W. Nelson and J.E., Enderby, Adam Hilger, Bristol, UK, pps. 149–161, 1985.

Mehrotra, R., Infrared spectroscopy, gas chromatography/infrared in food analysis, in *Encyclopedia of Analytical Chemistry*, ed. R.H. Meyers, pps. 4007–4024, 2000.

GENERAL INFORMATION ON SPECTROSCOPY

Spectroscopy – the study of the interaction of electromagnetic radiation with matter – excluding chemical effects.

Spectrophotometer – an instrument which measures the relationship between the absorption of light by a substance and the wavelength of the incident light.

Spectrometer – an instrument which measures the distribution of wavelengths in electromagnetic radiation; also an instrument which measures the energies and masses in a distribution of particles as in a mass spectrometer.

Beer's Law (Beer-Lambert Law or Beer-Lambert-Bouguer Law) – states that while the relationship between transmittance and concentration is non-linear, the relationship between absorbance and concentration is linear. The practical consequence is that with high absorbance values, one is measuring small differences in large numbers with attendant inaccuracies.

I/I_0 (Transmittance)	%Transmittance ($I/I_0 \times 100$)	Absorbance (A)
1.0	100	0
0.1	10	1.0
0.01	1	2.0
0.001	0.1	3.0
0.0001	0.01	4.0
0.00001	0.001	5.0
0.000001	0.0001	6.0

$\log_{10} (I/I_0) = \varepsilon c l = A$; where I is the intensity of transmitted light; I_0 is the intensity of incident light; ε is the molar extinction coefficient (L mol^{-1} cm^{-1}), c is concentration (mol L^{-1}), l is pathlength (cm); and A is absorbance.

Electromagnetic Radiation Ranges Frequently Used in Biochemistry and Molecular Biology

Definition	Range (Wavelength)	Range (Wavenumber)	Comments
Ultraviolet (UV)	190–360 nm		Qualitative and Quantitative
Visible (Vis)	360–780 nm		Qualitative and Quantitative
Near Infrared (NIR)	780–2500 nm	12,800 – 4000 cm^{-1}	Qualitative and Quantitative
Infrared (IR)	2500–40,000 nm[a]	4000 – 250 cm^{-1}	Mostly Qualitative
Far Infrared (FIR)	4×10^4–10^6 nm[a]	250 – 10^{-cm}	Mostly Qualitative

[a] Usually used reciprocal centimeters (cm^{-1}) for wavelength description. This quantity is the wave number (reciprocal of the wavelength in cm^{-1}).

Hyperchromic – increase in absorbance
Hypochromic – decrease in absorbance
Hypsochromic – decrease in wavelength; also known as a "blue" shift
Bathochromic – increase in wavelength; also known as a "red" shift

UV-Vis Spectroscopy

Absorbance Data for Common Solvents

Solvent	UV-VIS "Cut-Off" Wavelength[a]
CHCl$_3$	240 nm
Hexanes	200 nm
MeOH/EtOH	205 nm
H$_2$O	190 nm
Dioxane	205 nm
Acetonitrile	190 nm

[a] In this context, "cut-off" is the lowest wavelength at which the solvent can be used; solvent absorbance is sufficiently high below this wavelength to marginalize results.

Water transmits light satisfactorily between 400 nm and 800 nm; from 600 nm to 900 nm, above 900 nm, transmission decreases by a factor 50 and above 1.3 µm, transmission decreases more rapidly; transmission increases from 400 to 220 while a further decrease in wavelength results in markedly decreased transmission.

- Opticalx Properties of Water (Morton, R.A., *Biochemical Spectroscopy*, John Wiley & Sons (A Halsted Press Book), New York, New York, 1975.)

Optical Properties of Plastics Used For Microplate Assays[a,b]

Material	UV "Cut-off"[c]
Quartz	180 nm
Polystyrene[d]	300 nm
Polypropylene[e]	300 nm
Polyvinyl chloride (PVC)	300 nm

[a] These are values for the "common" microplate thickness; with thin-thickness (10 µ), the "cut-off" value of polyethylene is 180 nm (Andrady, A.L., Ultraviolet radiation and polymers, in *Physical Properties of Polymers Handbook*, ed. J.E. Mark, American Institute of Physics, AIP Press, Woodberry, NY, USA, 1996).

[b] There are a number of UV-transparent microplates available on the market. These are made of proprietary plastics; most likely unique blends. The microplates will permit use at 260 nm and 280 nm making them useful for biochemical analyses. However, since the composition of these microplates is proprietary, the microplates must be evaluated for any unique binding properties.

[c] In this context, "cut-off" is the lowest wavelength at which the microplate can be used; the zero absorbance of the microplate is sufficiently high such to marginalize results.

[d] Tends to be hydrophilic so an aqueous sample tends to "film" and stick the sides of well (surface tension effect)

[e] Tends to be hydrophobic so aqueous sample tends to "bead."

Near Infrared Spectroscopy

- The spectra of water
  - Symons, M.C.R., Spectroscopy of aqueous solutions: protein and DNA interactions with water, *Cell.Mol. Life Sci.* 57, 999–1007, 2000.
  - Gregory, R.B., Protein hydration and glass transition behavior, in *Protein-Solvent Interactions*, ed. R.B. Gregory, Marcel Dekker, Inc., New York, New York, USA, Chapter 3, pps 191–264, 1995.

- Application to human tissue
  - Chance, B., Nioka, S., Warren, W., and Yurtsever, G., Mitochondrial NADH as the bellwether of tissue O_2 delivery, *Adv.Exp.Med. Biol.* 566, 231–242, 2005.
  - Cerussi, A.E., Berger, A.J., Bevilacqua, F., Sources of absorption and scattering contrast for near-infrared optical mammography, *Academic Radiology* 8, 211–218, 2001.
  - Eikje, N.S., Ozaki, Y., Aizawa, K., and Arase, S., Fiber optic near-infrared Raman spectroscopy for clinical noninvasive determination of water content in diseased skin and assessment of cutaneous edema, *J.Biomed.Opt.* 10, 14013, 2005.
  - Pickup, J.C., Hussain, F., Evans, N.D., and Sachedina, N., In vivo glucose monitoring: the clinical reality and the promise, *Biosens.Bioelectron.* 20, 1897–1902, 2005.
  - Hielscher, A.H., Bluestone, A.Y., Abdoulaev, G.S., et al., Near-infrared diffuse optical tomography, *Dis. Markers* 18, 313–337, 2002.
  - Christian, N.A., Milone, M.C., Ranka, S.S., et al., Tat-functionalized near-infrared emissive polymerosomes for dendritic cell labeling, *Bioconjug.Chem.* 18, 31–40, 2007.
- Process Monitoring
  - Liu, J., Physical characterization of pharmaceutical formulations in frozen and freeze-dried solid states: techniques and applications in freeze-drying development, *Pharm.Dev.Technol.* 11, 3–28, 2006.
  - Scaftt, M., Arnold, S.A., Harvey, L.M., and McNeil, B., Near infrared spectroscopy for bioprocess monitoring and control: current status and future trends, *Crit.Rev. Biotechnol.* 26, 17–39, 2006.
  - Reich, G., Near-infrared spectroscopy and imaging: basic principles and pharmaceutical applications, *Adv. Drug Deliv.Rev.* 57, 1109–1143, 2005.
  - Suehara, K., and Yano, T., Bioprocess Monitoring using near-infrared spectroscopy, *Adv.Biochem.Eng. Biotechnol.* 90, 173–198, 2004.
- General
  - Ferrari, M., Mottola, L., and Quaresima, V., Principles, techniques, and limitations of near infrared spectroscopy, *Can.J.Appl.Physiol.* 29, 463–487. 2004.
  - McWhorter, S. and Soper, S.A., Near-infrared laser-induced fluorescence detection in capillary electrophoresis, *Electrophoresis* 21, 1267–1280, 2000.
  - Symons, M.C., Spectroscopy of aqueous solutions: proteins and DNA interactions with water, *Cell Mol. Life Sci.* 57, 999–1007, 2000.
  - Nir, S., Nicol, F., and Szoka, F.C., Jr., Surface aggregation and membrane penetration by peptides: relation to pore formation and fusion, *Mol.Membr.Biol.* 16, 95–101, 1999.

Some Spectrometer Window Materials for Infrared Spectroscopy

Material	Wavelength Range (cm⁻¹)	Refractive Index	Characteristics
NaCl	40,000 – 600	1.52	Soluble in H_2O, Etoh
KBr	43,500 – 400	1.54	Soluble in H_2O, EtOH
BaF$_2$	66,666 – 800	1.45	Insoluble in H_2O, soluble in acid
ZnSe	20,000 – 500	2.43	Insoluble in H_2O
Si	8,333 – 33	3.42	Insoluble in H_2O

General References for Spectrometry

Twyman, F. and Allsop, C.B., *The Practice of Absorption Spectrophotometry*, Adam Hilger, London, 1934.

Brode, W.R., *Chemical Spectroscopy*, John Wiley & Sons, New York, New York, 1943.

Analytical Absorption Spectroscopy, ed. M.G. Mellon, John Wiley & Sons, New York, New York, 1950.

Morton, R.A. *Biochemical Spectroscopy*, John Wiley & Sons (A Halsted Press Book), New York, New York, 1975.

Campbell, L.D. and Dwek, R.A., *Biological Spectroscopy*, Benjamin/Cummings, Menlo Park, California, 1984.

Practical Absorption Spectroscopy, ed A. Knowles and C. Burgess (UV Spectrometry Group), Chapman & Hall, London, UK, 1984.

Osborne, B.G., Fearn, T., and Hindle, P.H., *Practical NIR Spectroscopy with Applications in Food and Beverage Analysis*, Longman Scientific and Technical, Harrow, Essex, UK, 1993.

UV Spectroscopy Techniques, Instrumentation, Data Handling, UV Spectrometry Group, ed. B.J. Clark, T. Frost, and M.A. Russell, Chapman & Hall, London, UK, 1993.

Stuart, B., *Biological Applications of Infrared Spectroscopy*, ACOL Series, Wiley, Chichester, UK, 1997.

Standards and Best Practices in Absorption Spectrometry, ed. C. Burgess and T. Frost (UVSG), Blackwell Science, Oxford, UK, 1999.

Stewart, K.K. and Ebel, R.E., *Chemical Measurements in Biological Systems*, John Wiley & Sons, New York, NY, USA, 2000.

Workman, J., Jr., *Handbook of Organic Compounds. NIR, IR, Raman, and UV-Vis Featuring Polymers and Surfactants*, Academic Press, San Diego, California, 2001. Volume 1 Methods and Interpretation, Volume 2 UV-Vis and NIR Spectra, Volume 3 IR and Raman Spectra.

Near-Infrared Spectroscopy, ed. H.W. Siesler, Ozaki, Y., Kawate, S., and Heise, H.M., Wiley-VCH, Weinheim, Germany, 2002.

Stuart, B.H., *Infrared Spectroscopy: Fundamentals and Applications*, John Wiley & Sons, Ltd., Chichester, UK, 2004.

Burns, D.A. and Ciurczak, E.W., *Handbook of Near-Infrared Analysis, Third Edition*, CRC Press, Boca Raton, USA, 2007.

Workman, J. and Weyer, L., *Practical Guide to Interpretive Near-Infrared Spectroscopy*, CRC Press, Boca Raton, USA, 2007.

PLASTICS

Plastics are a group of materials which are used extensively in biochemistry and molecular biology. Plastics can be defined as non-metallic polymeric materials which can be molded or extruded into a shape. A plastic can be a single polymeric component such as polypropylene, a blend of several polymers or a block copolymer consisting of joined segments of two or more individual polymers such as a block copolymer of polybutadiene and poly(ethylene oxide). The physical properties of a plastic are a combination of the polymeric composition and additives such as plasticizers. Plasticizers are high molecular weight liquids or solids melting a low temperature which are blended with thermoplastic resins such as polyvinyl chloride to change physical properties. Plasticizers including phthalate derivatives such as di(2-ethyl)hexylphthalate, derivatives of organic acids such as di-2-ethylhexyladipate, and polyglycols (polyethylene glycol). Other materials included in the manufacture of plastics include antioxidants, lubricants, stabilizers, and colorants. All of these components can influence the property of the final plastic product. It must be emphasized that the biomedical market for plastics is quite small in volume compared to the overall market. Thus, unless a vendor makes their own raw material, most suppliers to biochemistry and molecular biology purchase bulk product from a large chemical company. As a result there can be batch-to-batch and vendor-to-vendor variation in product. Another issue which confounds the use of plastics is the addition of stabilizers. Stabilizers are chemicals such as hydroxybenzophenones and hydroxyphenylbensotriazoles which are added to prevent damage from ultraviolet irradiation. These compounds do absorb ultraviolet light in the 200-400 nm range and do present problems in biochemical analyses. The careful investigator will assure the source of the plastics used in products such as microplates and incubation flasks (Clinchy, B., Youssefi, M.R., and Håkansson, L., Differences in adsorption of serum proteins and production of IL-1ra by human monocytes incubated in different tissue culture microtiter plates, *J.Immunol.Methods* 282, 53–61, 2003).

General References for Plastics

Dubois, J.H., and John, F.W., *Plastics*, 5th Edn, Van Nostrand Reinhold, New York, NY, USA, 1974.

Billmeyer, F.W., *Textbook of Polymer Science*, Wiley, New York, NY, 1984.

Griffin, G.J.L., *Chemistry and Technology of Biodegradable Polymers*, Blackie Academic & Professional, London, UK, 1994.

Physical Properties of Polymers Handbook, ed. J.E. Mark, American Institute of Physics, AIP Press, Woodberry, NY, USA, 1996.

Araki, T. and Qui, T-C., *Structure and Properties of Multiphase Polymeric Materials*, Marcel Dekker, New York, NY, 1998.

Polymer Data Book., ed. J.E. Mark, Oxford University Press, Oxford, UK, 1999.

Plastics Additives Handbook, 5th edn., ed. H. Zweifel, Hanser Publications, Munich, Germany, 2001.

Bart, J.C.J., *Plastics Additives. Advanced Industrial Analysis*, IOS Press, Amsterdam, Netherlands, 2006.

Chiellini, E., *Biomedical Polymers and Polymer Therapeutics*, Kluwer Academic, New York, NY, USA, 2002.

Ramakrishna, S., *An Introduction to Biocomposites*, Imperial College Press, London, UK, 2004.

Carraher, C.A., Jr., *Introduction to Polymer Chemistry*, CRC Press, Boca Raton, FL, USA, 2006.

Polymeric Nanofibers, ed. D.H. Reneker and H. Fong, American Chemical Society, Washington, DC, USA, 2006.

American Chemical Council; http://www.plasticsresource.com.

Plasticizers

Crawford, R.R. and Esmerian, O.K., Effect of plasticizers on some physical properties of cellulose acetate phthalate films, *J.Pharm.Sci.* 60, 312–314, 1971.

Ekwall, B., Nordensten, C., and Albanus, L., Toxicity of 29 plasticizers to HeLa cells in the MIT-24 system, *Toxicology* 24, 199–210, 1982.

Goldstein, D.B., Feistner, G.J., Faull, K.F., and Tomer, K.B., Plasticizers as contaminants in commercial ethanol, *Alcohol Clin.Exp.Res.* 11, 521–524, 1987.

Sager, G. and Little, C., The effect of tris-(2-butoxyethyl)-phosphate (TBEP) and di-(2-ethylhexyl)-phthalate (DEHP) and the β-adrenergic receptor-blockers [3H]-(-)-dihydroalprenolol ([3H]-(-)-DHA) and [3H-(-)-CGP 12177 were tested for their ability to interact with β-adrenergic binding to α 1-acid glycoprotein and mononuclear leukocytes, *Biochem.Pharmacol.* 38, 2551–2557, 1989.

Baker, J.K., Characterization of phthalate plasticizers by HPLC/thermospray mass spectrometry, *J.Pharm.Biomed.Anal.* 15, 145–148, 1996.

Wahl, H.G., Hoffman, A., Haring, H.U., and Liebich, H.M., Identification of plasticizers in medical products by a combined direct thermodesorption—cooled injection system and gas chromatography—mass spectrometry, *J.Chromatog.A* 847, 1–7, 1999.

Cano, J.M., Marin, M.L., Sanchez, A., and Hernandis, V., Determination of adipate plasticizers in poly(vinyl chloride) by microwave-assisted extraction, *J.Chromatog.A* 963, 401–409, 2002.

Siepmann, F., le Brun, V., and Siepmann, J., Drugs acting as plasticizers in polymeric systems: a quantitative treatment, *J.Control.Release* 115, 298–306, 2006.

Some Properties of Plastics Used in Biochemistry and Molecular Biology

Structures for these plastics may be found on p. 866–868

Plastic	Uses	References
Acrylonitrile-Butadiene elastomers (Nitrile rubber)	Soft rubber applications such as gloves and pharmaceutical stoppers	1–4
Nylon (aliphatic polyamides)	Matrix for tissue engineering, suture material, matrix for adsorptive technologies	6–10
Polyacrylamide	Primary use as a matrix for protein electrophoresis (PAGE, polyacrylamide gel electrophoresis). Early use as gel filtration matrix; more recent use as a hydrogel and implant material	11–18
Polyacrylate (PA; polyacrylic acid)[1]	Dental cement, use for manufacture of microparticles and nanoparticles	19–24
Polybutadiene	Chromatographic matrix such as polybutadiene-coated zirconia, microarray plates	25–31
Polycarbonate	Matrix for biological assays; material for tissue culture flasks; implants; filters; use as "solid" component of copolymers; tyrosine-derived polycarbonate used in tissue engineering	32–42
Polyethylene	Implants, tubing	43–45
Polyethylene oxide (PEO)	Component of hydrogels; some use in implant biology; use in copolymers	46–51
Poly(ethylene terephthalate) (PET)	Matrix for tissue engineering; cell culture matrix; used in block copolymers	52–57

Some Properties of Plastics Used in Biochemistry and Molecular Biology (Continued)

Plastic	Uses	References
Poly(methacrylate)[1]	Used in monolithic chromatographic columns	58
Polypropylene	Fiber used in surgery	59–61
Polypropylene oxide	Hydrogels, block copolymers,	62–64
Polystyrene	Microplates, can be modified by irradiation for covalent binding of probes; chromatographic matrices; microbeads for assays; frequently a copolymer with divinylbenzene	65–82
Poly(vinyl chloride)	Use in biosensors; use as flexible tubing when phthalate stabilizers are used; use as copolymer for encapsulation	83–88

[1]. The nomenclature for acrylic acid and derivatives can be confusing. The following definitions are used in this text.
Acrolein (2-propenal)
Acrylamide (2-propenamide)
Acrylic acid (propenoic acid)
Acrylonitrile (2-propenenitrile)
Methacrylic acid (2-methylpropenoic acid)
Methyl methacrylic acid (2-methylpropenoic acid methyl ester)

References

1. Shanker, J., Gibaldi, M., Kanig, J.L. et al., Evaluation of the suitability of butadiene-acrylonitrile rubbers as closures for parenteral solutions, J.Pharm.Sci. 56, 100–108, 1967.

2. Williams, J.R., Permeation of glove materials by physiologically harmful chemicals, Am.Ind.Hyg.Assoc.J. 40, 877–882, 1979.

3. Parker, S. and Braden, M., Soft prosthesis materials based on powdered elastomers, Biomaterials 11, 482–490, 1990.

4. Walsh, D.L., Schwerin, M.R., Kisielewski, R.W., et al., Abrasion resistance of medical glove materials, J.Biomed.Mater.Res.B Appl. Biomater. 68, 81–87, 2004.

5. McConway, M.G. and Chapman, R.S., Application of solid-phase antibodies to radioimmunoassay. Evaluation of two polymeric microparticles, Dynospheres and nylon, activated by carbonyldiimidazole or tresyl chloride, J.Immunol.Methods 95, 259–266, 1986.

6. Absolom, D.R., Zingg, W., and Neumann, A.W., Protein adsorption to polymer particle: role of surface properties, J.Biomed.Mater.Res. 21, 161–171, 1987.

7. Alicata, R., Mantaudo, G., Puglisi, C., and Samperi, F. Influence of chain end groups on the matrix-assisted laser desorption/ionization spectra of polymer blends, Rapid Commun.Mass. Spectrom. 16, 248–260, 2002.

8. Zhu, X., Cai, J., Yang, J., et al., Films coated with molecular imprinted polymers for the selective stir bar sorption extraction of monocrotophos, J.Chromatog.A. 1131, 37–44, 2006.

9. Dennes, T.J., Hunt, G.C., Schwarzbauer, J.E., and Schwartz, J., High-yield activation of scaffold polymer surfaces to attach cell adhesion molecules, J.Am.Chem.Soc. 129, 93–97, 2007.

10. Friedrich, J., Zalar, P., Mororcic, M., et al., Ability of fungi to degrade synthetic polymer nylon-6, Chemosphere, in press, 2007.

11. Hjerten, S. and Mosbach, R., "Molecular-sieve" chromatography of proteins on columns of cross-linked polyacrylamide, Anal. Biochem. 3, 109–118, 1962.

12. Goodfriend, T., Ball, D., and Updike, S., Antibody in polyacrylamide gel, a solid phase reagent for radioimmunoassay, Immunochemistry 6, 481–484, 1969.

13. John, M., Skrabei, H., and Dellweg, H., Use of polyacrylamide gel columns for the separation of nucleotides, FEBS Lett. 5, 185–186, 1969.

14. Bovin, M.V., Polyacrylamide-based glycoconjugates as tools in glycobiology, Glycoconj. J. 15, 431–446, 1998.

15. Patrick, T., Polyacrylamide gel in cosmetic procedures: experience with Aquamid®, Semin.Cutan.Med.Surg. 23, 233–235, 2004.

16. Plieva, F., Bober, B., Dainiak, M., et al., Macroporous polyacrylamide monolithic gels with immobilized metal affinity ligands: the effect of porous structure and ligand coupling chemistry on protein binding, J.Mol.Recognit. 19, 305–312, 2006.

17. Sairam, M., Babu, V.R., Vijaya, B., et al., Encapsulation efficiency and controlled release characteristics of crosslinked polyacrylamide particles, Int.J.Pharm. 320, 131–136, 2006.

18. Sefton, M.V. and Broughton, R.L., Microencapsulation of erythrocytes, Biochim.Biophys.Acta 717, 473–477, 1982.

19. Stevenson, W.T. and Sefton, M.V., Graft copolymer emulsions of sodium alginate with hydroxylalkyl methacrylates for microencapsulation, Biomaterials 8, 449–457, 1987.

20. Laemmli, U.K., Characterization of DNA condensates induced by poly(ethylene oxide) and polylysine, Proc.Nat.Acad.Sci.USA 72, 4288–4292, 1975.

21. Sefton, M.V. and Nishimura, E., Insulin permeability of hydrophilic polyacrylate membranes, J.Pharm.Sci. 69, 208–209, 1980.

22. Svensson, A., Norrman, J., and Piculell, L., Phase behavior of polyion-surfactant ion complex salts: effects of surfactant chain length and polyion length, J.Phys.Chem.B Condens.Matter Mater. Surf. Interface Biophys. 110, 10332–10340, 2006.

23. Turos, E., Shim, J.Y., Wang, Y., et al., Antibiotic-conjugated polyacrylate nanoparticles: new opportunities for development of anti-MRSA agents, Bioorg.Med. Chem Lett. 17, 53–56, 2007.

24. Herdt, A.R., Kim, B.S., and Taton, T.A., Encapsulated magnetic nanoparticles as supports for proteins and recyclable biocatalysts, Bioconjug.Chem. 18, 183–189, 2007.

25. Sun, L. and Carr, P.W., Chromatography of proteins using polybutadiene-coated zirconia, Anal.Chem. 67, 3717–3721, 1995.

26. Alvarez, C., Strumia, M. and Bertorello, H., Synthesis and characterization of a biospecific adsorbent containing bovine serum albumin as a ligand and its use for bilirubin retention, J.Biochem. Biophys.Methods 49, 649–656, 2001.

27. Davoras, E.M. and Coutsolelos, A.G., Efficient biomimetic catalytic epoxidation of polyene polymers by manganese porphyrins, J.Inorg.Biochem. 94, 161–170, 2003.

28. Erhardt, R., Zhang, M., Boker, A., et al., Amphiphilic Janus particles with polystyrene and poly(methacrylic acid) hemispheres, J.Am.Chem.Soc. 125, 3260–3267, 2003.

29. Xu, J. and Zubarev, E.R., Supramolecular assemblies of starlike and V-shaped PB-PEO amphiphiles, Angew.Chem.Int.Ed.Engl. 43, 5491–5496, 2004.

30. Geng, Y., Discher, D.E., Justynska, J., and Schlaad, H., Grafting short peptides onto polybutadiene-block-poly(ethylene oxide): a platform for self-assembling hybrid amphiphiles, Angew.Chem.Int. Ed.Engl. 45, 7578–7581, 2006.

31. Kassu, A., Taguenang, J.M., and Sharma, A., Photopatterning of butadiene substrates by interferometric ultraviolet lithography: fabrication of phospholipid microarrays, Appl.Opt. 46, 489–494, 2007.

32. Chandy, T. and Sharma, C.P., Changes in protein adsorption on polycarbonate due to L–ascorbic acid, Biomaterials 6, 416–420, 1985.

33. Hough, T., Singh, M.B., Smart, I.J., and Knox, R.B., Immunofluorescent screening of monoclonal antibodies to surface antigens of animal and plant cells bound to polycarbonate membranes, J.Immunol.Methods 92, 103–107, 1986.

34. Thelu, J., and Ambroise-Thomas, P., A septate polycarbonate cell culture unit used for Plasmodium falciparum and hybridomas, Trans.R.Soc.Trop.Med.Hyg. 82, 360–362, 1988.

35. Bignold, L.P., Rogers, S.D., and Harkin, D.G., Effects of plasma proteins on the adhesion, spreading, polarization in suspension, random motility and chemotaxis of neutrophil leukocytes on polycarbonate (Nucleopore) filtration membranes, Eur.J.Cell Biol. 53, 27–34, 1990.

36. Lee, J.H., Lee, S.J., Khang, G., and Lee, H.B., Interaction of fibroblasts on polycarbonate membrane surfaces with different micropore sizes and hydrophilicity, J.Biomater.Sci.Poly.Ed. 10, 283–294, 1999.

37. Liu, Y., Ganser, D., Schneider, A., et al., Microfabricated polycarbonate CE devices for DNA analysis, Anal.Chem. 73, 4196–4201, 2001.

38. Liu, J., Zeng, F., and Allen, C., Influence of serum protein on polycarbonate-based copolymer micelles as a delivery system for a hydrophobic anti-cancer agents, *J.Control Release* 103, 481–487, 2005.

39. Meechaisue, C., Dubin, R., Supaphol, P., *et al.*, Electrospun mat of tyrosine-derived polycarbonate fibers for potential use as tissue scaffolding material, *J.Biomater.Sci. Polym.Ed.* 17, 1039–1056, 2006.

40. Li, Y., Wang, Z., Ou, L.M., and Yu, H.Z., DNA detection on plastic: surface activation protocol to convert polycarbonate substrates to biochip platforms, *Anal.Chem.* 79, 426–433, 2007.

41. Carion, O., Souplet, V., Olivier, C., *et al.*, Chemical micropatterning of polycarbonate for site-specific peptide immobilization and biomolecular interactions, *ChemBioChem* 8, 315–322, 2007.

42. Tripathi, A., Wang, J., Luck, J.A., and Suni, L.L., Nanobiosensor design utilizing a periplasmic *E.coli* receptor protein immobilized within Au/polycarbonate nanopores, *Anal.Chem.* 79, 1266–1270, 2007.

43. Raff, R.A.V. and Allison, J.B., *Polyethylene*, Interscience Publishers, New York, NY, USA, 1956.

44. Bhat, S.V., *Biomaterials*, Kluwer Academic Publishers, Boston, MA, USA, 2002.

45. Shanbhag, A. and Rubash, H.E., *Joint Replacement and Bone Resorption: Pathology, Biomaterials, and Clinical Practice*, Taylor & Francis, New York, NY, USA, 2006.

46. Desai, N.P. and Hubbell, J.A., Biological responses to polyethylene oxide modified polyethylene terephthalate surfaces, *J.Biomed. Mater.Res.* 25, 829–843, 1991.

47. Lopina, S.T., Wu, G., Merrill, E.W., and Griffith-Cima, L., Heptocyte culture on carbohydrate-modified star polyethylene oxide hydrogels, *Biomaterials* 17, 559–569, 1996.

48. Vereschagin, E.I., Han, D.H., Troitsky, A.W., *et al.*, Radiation technology in the preparation of polyethylene oxide hydrophilic gels and immobilization of proteases for use in medical practice, *Arch. Pharm.Res.* 24, 229–233, 2001.

49. Liu, L.S. and Berg, R.A., Adhesion barriers of carboxymethylcellulose and polyethylene oxide composite gels, *J.Biomed.Mat.Res.* 63, 326–332, 2002.

50. Wu, N., Wang, L.S., Tan, D.C., *et al.*, Mathematical modeling and in vitro study of controlled drug release via a highly swellable and dissoluble polymer matrix: polyethylene oxide with high molecular weights, *J.Control.Release* 102, 569–581, 2005.

51. Unsworth, L.D., Sheardown, H., and Brash, J.L., Polyethylene oxide surfaces of variable chain density by chemisorption of PEO-thiol on gold: adsorption of proteins from plasma studied by radiolabeling and immunoblotting, *Biomaterials* 26, 5927–5933, 2005.

52. Nair, P.D. and Sreenivasan, K., Effect of steam sterilization on polyethylene terephthalate, *Biomaterials* 5, 305–306, 1984.

53. Dadsetan, M., Mirzadeh, H., Sharifi-Sanjani, N., and Daliri, M., Cell behavior on laser surface-modified polyethylene terephthalate in vitro, *J.Biomed.Mater.Res.* 57, 183–189, 2001.

54. Cenni, E., Granchi, D., Ciapetti, G., *et al.*, Interleukin-6 expression by cultured human endothelial cells in contact with carbon coated polyethylene terephthalate, *J.Mater.Sci.Mater.Med.* 12, 365–369, 2001.

55. Neves, A.A., Medcalf, N., and Brindle, K.M., Influence of stirring-induced mixing on cell proliferation and extracellular matrix deposition in meniscal cartilage constructs based on polyethylene terephthalate scaffolds, *Biomaterials* 26, 4828–4836, 2005.

56. Basu, S. and Yang, S.T., Astrocyte growth and glial cell line-derived neurotrophic factor secretion in three-dimensional polyethylene terephthalate fibrous matrices, *Tissue Eng.* 11, 940–952, 2005.

57. Alisch-Mark, M., Herrmann, A., and Zimmermann, W., Increase of the hydrophilicity of polyethylene terephthalate fibres by hydrolases from *Thermomospora fusca* and *Fusarium solani f.sp.pisi*, *Biotechnol.Lett.* 28, 681–685, 2006.

58. Jungbauer, A. and Hahn, R., Polymethacrylate monoliths for preparative and industrial separation of biomolecular assemblies, *J.Chromatog.A.* 1184, 62–79, 2008.

59. Peter, F.H., *Polypropylene*, Gordon and Breach Science Publishers, New York, NY, USA, 1968.

60. Karger-Kocsis, J., *Polypropylene: Structure, Blends and Composites*, Chapman & Hall, London, UK, 1995.

61. Karger-Kocsis, J., *Polypropylene an A-Z Reference*, Dordrecht, Netherlands, 1998.

62. Topchieva, I.N. and Efremova, N.V., Conjugates of proteins with block co-polymers of ethylene and polypropylene oxides, *Biotechnol.Genet.Eng.Rev.* 12, 357–382, 1994.

63. Newman, M.J., Actor, J.K., Balusubramanian, M., and Jagannath, C., Use of nonionic block copolymers in vaccines and therapeutics, *Crit.Rev.Ther.Drug Carrier Syst.* 15, 89–142, 1998.

64. Gutowska, A., Jeong, B., and Jasionowski, M., Injectable gels for tissue engineering, *Anat.Rec.* 263, 342–349, 2001.

65. Catarero, L.A., Butler, J.E., and Osborne, J.W., The adsorptive characteristics of proteins for polystyrene and their significance in solid-phase immunoassays, *Anal.Biochem.* 105, 375–382, 1980.

66. Zouali, M. and Stollar, B.D., A rapid ELISA for measurement of antibodies to nucleic acid antigens using UV-treated polystyrene microplates, *J.Immunol.Methods* 90, 105–110, 1986.

67. Piskin, E., Tuncel, A., Denizli, A., and Ayhan, H., Monosize microbeads based on polystyrene and their modified forms for some selected medical and biological applications, *J.Biomater.Sci.Polym. Ed.* 5, 451–471, 1994.

68. Kochanowska, I.E., Rapak, A., and Szewczuk, A., Effect of pretreatment of wells in polystyrene plates on adsorption of some human serum proteins, *Arch.Immunol.Ther.Exp.(Warsz.)* 42, 135–139, 1994.

69. Staak, C., Salchow, R., Clausen, P.H., and Luge, E., Polystyrene as an affinity chromatography matrix for the purification of antibodies, *J.Immunol.Methods* 194, 141–146, 1996.

70. Davankov, V., Tsyurupa, M., Ilyin, M., and Pavlova, L., Hypercrosslinked polystyrene and its potential for liquid chromatography: a mini-review, *J.Chromatog.A.* 965, 65–73, 2002.

71. Gessner, A., Lieske, A., Paulke, B.R., and Muller, R.H., Functional groups on polystyrene model nanoparticles: influence on protein adsorption, *J.Biomed.Mater.Res.A.* 65, 319–326, 2003.

72. Saitoh, T., Hattori, N., and Hiraide, M., Protein separation with surfactant-coated polystyrene involving Cibacron Blue 3GA-conjugated Triton X-100, *J.Chromatog.A.* 1028, 149–153, 2004.

73. van Kooten, T.G., Spijker, H.T., and Busscher, H.J., Plasma-treated polystyrene surfaces: model surfaces for studying cell-biomaterial interactions, *Biomaterials* 25, 1735–1747, 2004.

74. Recknor, J.B., Recknor, J.C., Sakaguchi, D.S., and Mallapragada, S.K., Oriented astroglial cell growth on micropatterned polystyrene substrates, *Biomaterials* 25, 2753–2767, 2004.

75. Turner, S.F., Clarke, S.M., Rennie, A.R., *et al.*, Adsorption of gelatin to a polystyrene /water interface as a function of concentration, pH, and ionic strength, *Langmuir* 21, 10082–10088, 2005.

76. Rosado, E., Caroll, H., Sanchez, O., and Peniche, C., Passive adsorption of human antirrabic immunoglobulin onto a polystyrene surface, *J.Biomater.Sci.Polym.Ed.* 16, 435–448, 2005.

77. Carvalho, R.S., Ianzer, D.A., Malavolta, L., *et al.*, Polystyrene-type resin used for peptide synthesis: application for anion-exchange and affinity chromatography, *J.Chromatog.B.Analyt.Technol. Biomed.Life Sci.* 817, 231–238, 2005.

78. Jodar-Reyes, A.B., Ortega-Vinuesa, J.L., and Martin-Rodriguez, A., Adsorption of different amphiphilic molecules onto polystyrene latices, *J.Colloid Interface Sci.* 282, 439–447, 2005.

79. Mitchell, S.A., Davidson, M.R., and Bradley, R.H., Improved cellular adhesion to acetone plasma modified polystyrene surfaces, *J.Colloid Interface Sci.* 281, 122–129, 2005.

80. Cao, Y.C., Hua, X.F., Zhu, X.X., *et al.*, Preparation of Au coated polystyrene beads and their application in an immunoassay, *J.Immunol.Methods* 317, 163–170, 2006.

81. Tirri, M.E., Wahlroos, R., Meltola, N.J., *et al.*, Effect of polystyrene microsphere surface to fluorescence lifetime under two-photon excitation, *J.Fluoresc.* 16, 809–816, 2006.

82. Baker, S.C., Atkin, N., Gunning, P.A., *et al.*, Characterization of electrospun polystyrene scaffolds for three-dimensional *in vitro* biological studies, *Biomaterials* 27, 3136–3146, 2006.

83. Titow, W.V., *PVC Technology*, Elsevier Applied Science, London, UK, 1984.

84. *Encyclopedia of PVC*, ed. L.I. Nass and C.A. Heiberger, Marcel Dekker, New York, NY, USA, 1986.
85. Cha, G.S., Liu, D., Meyerhoff, M.E., *et al.*, Electrochemical performance, biocompatibility, and adhesion of new polymer matrices for solid-state ion sensors, *Anal.Chem.* 63, 1666–1672, 1991.
86. Zielinski, B.A. and Aebischer, P., Chitosan as a matrix for mammalian cell encapsulation, *Biomaterials* 15, 1049–1056, 1994.
87. *Immobilization of Enzymes and Cells,* ed. G.F. Bickerstaff, Humana Press, Totowa, NJ, USA, 1997.
88. Karakus, E., Pekyardimci, S., and Esma, K., Urea biosynthesis based on PVC membrane containing palmitic acid, *Artif.Cells Blood Substit.Immobil.Biotechnol.* 33, 329–341, 2005.

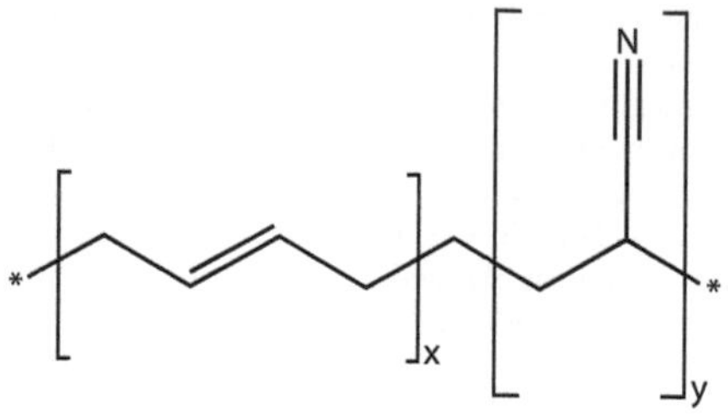

Acrylonitrile-butadiene (Nitrile)

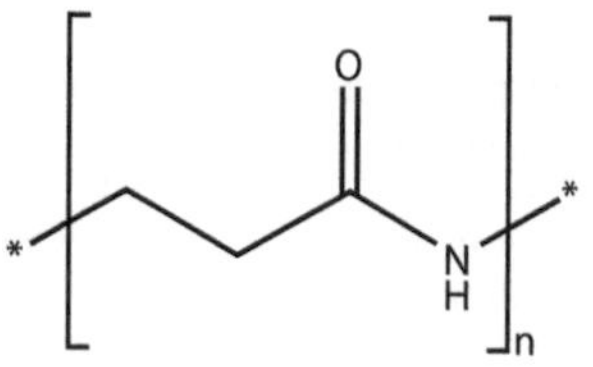

Nylon 3

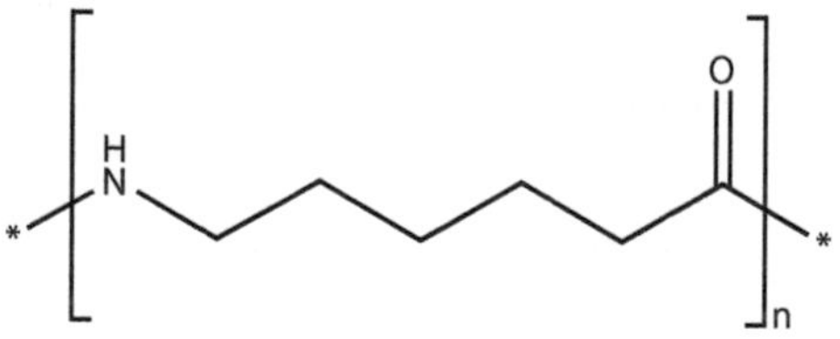

Nylon 6

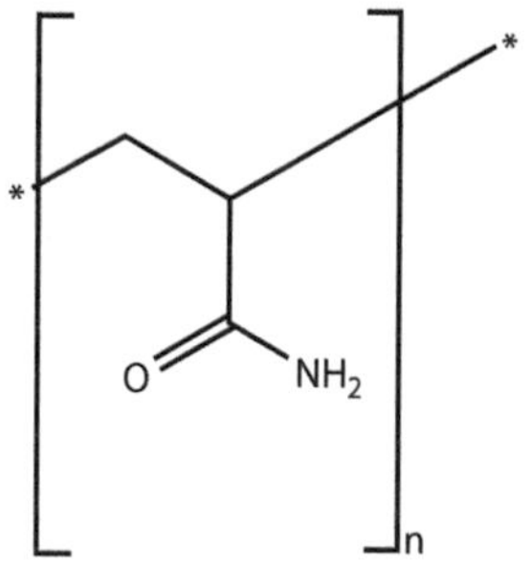

Polyacrylamide

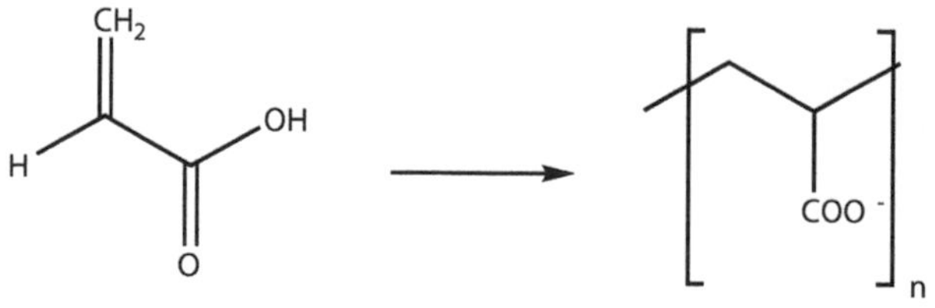

Acrylic Acid

Polyacrylic acid
(usually as sodium salt

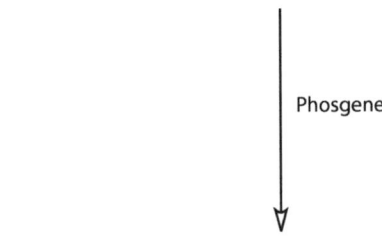

1,3-butadiene

Polybutadiene
(one of several structures shown)

bisphenol A

Phosgene

polycarbonate

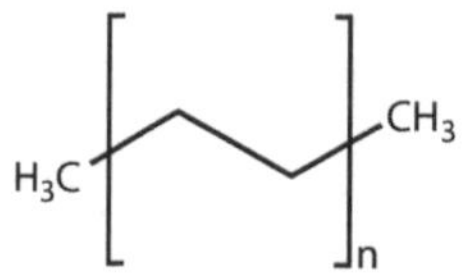

Polyethylene

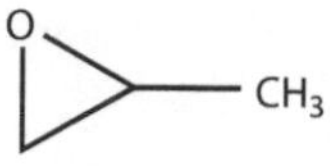

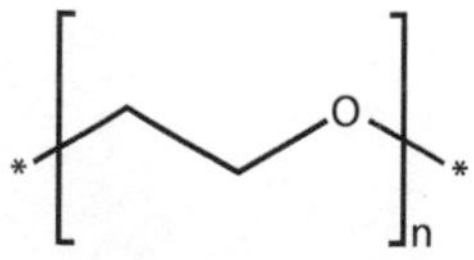

Polyethylene oxide

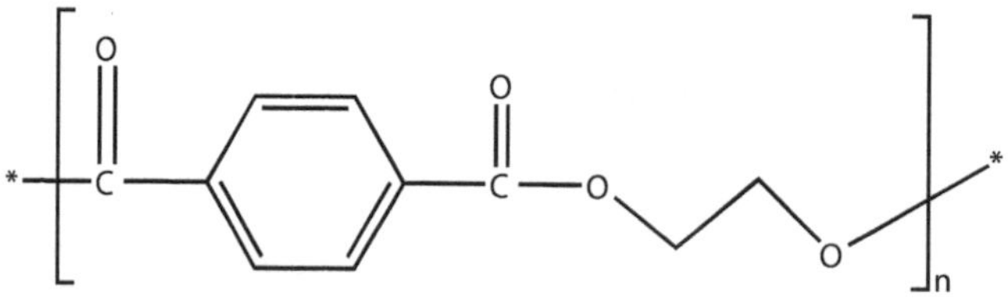

poly(ethylene)terephthalate (PET)

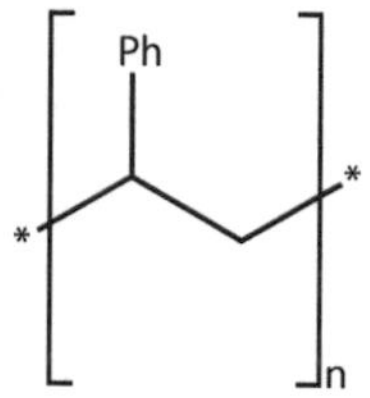

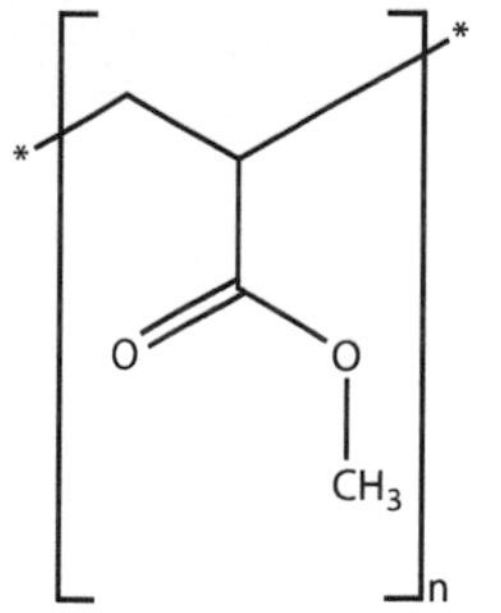

Poly(methyl acrylate)

Polypropylene

Propylene Oxide

KOH

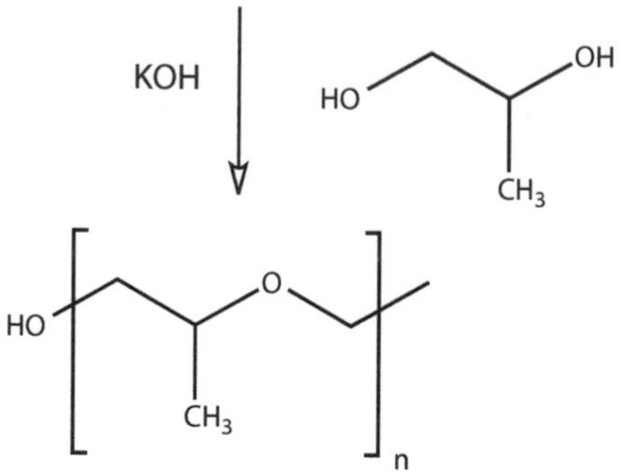

Polypropylene Oxide
(Polypropylene Glycol)

Polystyrene

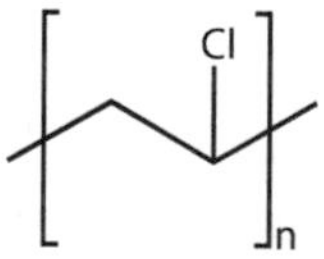

Polyvinyl chloride

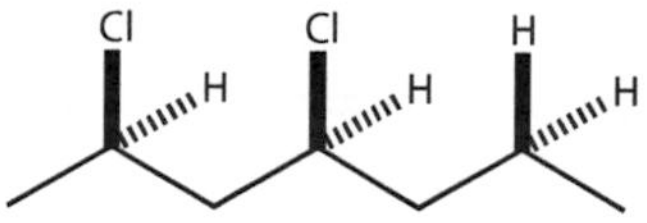

Isotactic

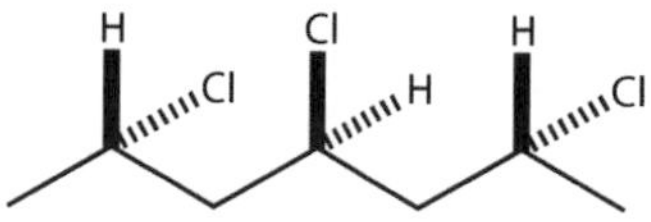

Syndiotactic

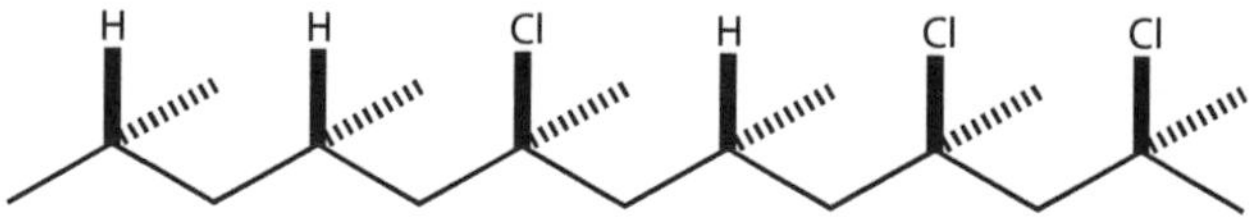

Atactic (an irregular)

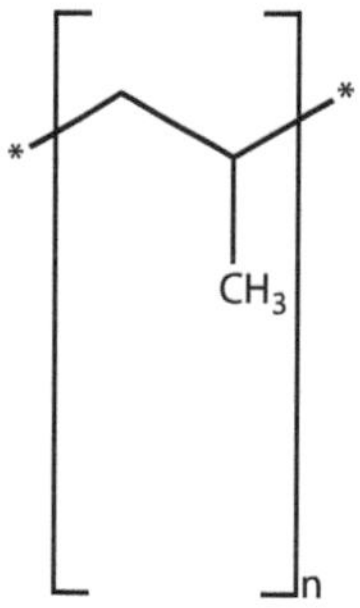

CHEMICAL AND PHYSICAL PROPERTIES OF VARIOUS COMMERCIAL PLASTICS

	Polyethylene Low Density	Polyethylene High Density	Polypropylene Copolymer	Polypropylene	Polymethyl-Pentene	TeflonFEP	Polycarbonate	Polyphenylene Oxide	Polystyrene General Purpose	Styrene-Acrylonitrile	Polyvinyl Chloride
PHYSICAL PROPERTIES											
Temperature Limit, °C	80	120	130	135	175	205	135	135	70	95	70
Specific Gravity	0.92	0.95	0.90	0.90	0.83	2.15	1.20	1.06	1.07	1.07	1.34
Tensile Strength, psi	2,000	4,000	2,900	5,000	4,000	3,000	8,000	9,600	6,000	11,000	6,500
Brittleness Temperature, °C	−100	−100	−40	0	—	−270	−135	—	Brittle[a]	−25	−30
Water Absorption, %	0.01	0.01	0.02	0.02	0.01	0.01	0.35	0.07	0.05	0.23	0.06
Flexibility	Excellent	Rigid	Slight	Rigid	Rigid	Excellent	Rigid	Rigid	Rigid	Rigid	Rigid
Transparency	Translucent	Opaque	Translucent	Translucent	Clear	Translucent	Clear	Opaque	Clear	Clear	Clear
Relative O_2 Permeability	0.40	0.08	0.20	0.11	2.0	0.59	0.15	—	0.11	0.03	0.01
Autoclavable	No	Withcaution	Yes	Yes	Yes	Yes	Yes	Yes	No	No	No
CHEMICAL RESISTANCE[b]											
Acids, inorganic	E	E	E	E	E	E	E	G	N	E	G
Acids, organic	E	E	E	E	E	E	G	E	G	E	G
Alcohols	E	E	E	E	E	E	G	E	G	G	G
Aldehydes	G	G	G	G	G	E	F	G	N	F	F
Amines	G	G	G	G	E	E	N	F	G	G	N
Bases	E	E	E	E	E	E	N	E	G	E	E
Dimethyl sulfoxide (DMSO)	E	E	E	E	E	E	N	E	N	N	N
Esters	E	E	E	G	E	E	N	F	N	N	F
Ethers	G	G	G	G	G	E	F	N	F	N	F
Foods	E	E	E	E	E	E	E	G	E	G	G
Glycols	E	E	E	G	E	E	G	E	G	G	F
Hydrocarbons, aliphatic	G	G	G	G	G	E	F	G	N	E	F
Hydrocarbons, aromatic	G	G	G	G	F	E	N	N	N	N	N
Hydrocarbons, halogenated	G	G	G	G	F	E	N	N	N	N	N
Ketones	G	G	G	E	G	E	N	N	N	G	N
Mineral oil	E	E	E	E	G	E	E	E	G	G	E
Oils, essential	G	G	G	G	G	E	G	F	N	F	N
Oils, lubricating	G	G	E	E	E	E	G	E	G	G	E
Oils, vegetable	E	E	E	E	E	E	E	G	G	E	G
Proteins, unhydrolyzed	E	E	E	E	E	E	E	E	G	E	G
Salts	E	E	E	E	E	E	E	E	E	G	E
Silicones	G	E	E	E	E	E	E	E	G	E	G
Water	E	E	E	E	E	E	E	E	E	E	E

a Normally somewhat brittle at room temperatures.
b E, Excellent. Long exposures (up to one year) at room temperatures have no effect. G, Good. Short exposures (less than 24 hours) at room temperature cause no damage. F, Fair. Short exposures at room temperature cause little or no damage under unstressed conditions. N, Not recommended. Short exposures may cause permanent damage.

By permission of Thermo Fisher Scientific.

CHEMICAL RESISTANCE OF PLASTICS

CHEMICAL RESISTANCE OF PLASTICS USED IN THE MANUFACTURE OF ULTRACENTRIFUGE TUBES

	Cellulose Nitrate	Polyallomers	Polycarbonate	Polyethylene	Polypropylene
Acetaldehyde	N	G	N	G	G
Acetic acid (10%)	E	E	E	E	E
Acetic acid (glacial)	N	E	N	E	E
Acetic anhydride	U		N	N	E
Acetone	N	E	N	G	F
Acetophenone		G	N	G	G
Aluminum salts	E	E	E	G	E
Ammonium salts	E	E	E	E	
Ammonium hydroxide (10%)	N	E	N	E	E
Ammonium hydroxide (conc.)	N	E	N	E	E
Amyl acetate	N	F	N	F	F
Amyl alcohol	N	G	E	G	F
Amyl chloride				F	
Aniline				G	N
Aqua Regia	N		N		N
Asphalt	E		E	E	
Barium salts		E	E	E	E
Benzaldehyde		G	F	F	G
Benzene	E	N	N	N	N
Benzoic acid	E	E	E	E	E
Benzyl alcohol	E	E	N	E	E
Borax	E	E	E	E	
Boric acid	E	E	E	E	E
Butyl acetate	N	E	E	E	G
Butyl alcohol	N	E	E	E	E
Calcium salts	E	E	G	E	E
Carbon disulfide					N
Carbon tetrachloride	E	N	N	F	F
Chlorobenzene	N	N	N	F	F
Chlorine (aqueous solution)			E	F	G
Chloroform	F	N	N	N	F
Chlorosulfonic acid		N	N	N	F
Chromic acid	N	G	E	G	G
Chromic acid (30%)	N	G	G	G	G
Citric acid	E	E	E	E	E
Copper salts		E	E	G	E
Cottonseed oil	E	E	E	E	E
Creosote	E	E		E	E
Cresol			N		
Cyclohexanol		G	N	F	G
Cyclohexanone		G	N	N	F
Decalin				N	
Dibutyl phthalate				F	
Diethyl ester	N	N	N	G	G
Diethyl ketone	N	N	N	G	G
Dioxane		F	N	N	F
Ethyl acetate	N	F	N	E	F
Ethyl alcohol 50%	E	E	E	E	E
Ethyl alcohol 95%	N	E	E	E	E
Ethylene chlorohydrin	N	F	N	F	F
Ethylene dichloride	N	F	N	F	F
Ethylene glycol	E	E	G	E	E
Ferric salts		E	E	E	E
Ferrous salts		E	E	E	E
Formaldehyde (40%)	E	E	E	E	E
Formic acid	E	E	F	E	E
Gasoline	N	N	F	N	N
Glycerin	E	E	E	E	E
Hydrochloric acid (10%)	E	E	E	E	E
Hydrochloric acid (conc.)	N	E	F	E	G
Hydrocyanic acid	E	E	E	E	E
Hydrofluoric acid (10%)	G	E	G	E	E

CHEMICAL RESISTANCE OF PLASTICS USED IN THE MANUFACTURE OF ULTRACENTRIFUGE TUBES (Continued)

	Cellulose Nitrate	Polyallomers	Polycarbonate	Polyethylene	Polypropylene
Hydrofluoric acid (50%)	N	E	N	E	E
Hydrogen peroxide (3%)	E	E	E	G	G
Hydrogen sulfide (aqueous solution)	E	E	E	E	E
Iodine (tincture)		E	F	G	G
Isopropyl alcohol	N	E	E	G	
Kerosene	E	N	E	N	N
Lacquer	N		N	G	
Lactic acid (20%)		E	E	F	E
Linseed oil	E	E	E	G	E
Magnesium salts	E	E	E	E	E
Malic acid		E	E	G	E
Manganese salts		E	E	E	E
Mercury salts	E	E	E	E	E
Methyl alcohol (abs.)	N	E	N	G	G
Methyl ethyl ketone	N	E	N	F	F
Methylene chloride	N	F	N	F	F
Nickel salts	E	E	E	E	E
Nitric acid (10%)	E	E	E	G	E
Nitric acid (conc.)	N	E	N	N	F
Nitrobenzene		F	N	N	F
Oils, vegetable	E	E	E	G	E
Oleic acid	E	E	E	G	
Oxalic acid	E	E	E	E	E
Palmitic acid		E	E	G	G
Perchloric acid		E	N	E	E
Phenol		E	N	G	N
Phosphoric acid (10%)	E	E	E	E	E
Phosphoric acid (conc.)	F	E	G	G	F
Picric acid				G	
Potassium salts	E	E	E	E	E
Potassium hydroxide (5%)	E	E	N	E	E
Potassium hydroxide (conc.)	E	E	N	E	E
Sodium salts	E	E	F	E	E
Sodium hydroxide (1%)	E	E	N	G	E
Sodium hydroxide (10%)	N	E	N	G	G
Sodium hydroxide (conc.)	N	E	N	G	F
Stearic acid		E	F	G	E
Sucrose solutions	E	E	E	E	E
Sulfuric acid (10%)	E	E	N	E	E
Sulfuric acid (conc.)	N	E	E	N	E
Sulfurous acid				G	E
Tannic acid	F	G		G	E
Tartaric acid		E		E	E
Tetra hydrofurane				N	
Thiopen				N	
Toluene	E	N	N	G	N
Trichloroethylene		N	N	N	N
Turpentine		F	N	N	F
Urea	E		E	E	E
Xylene	N	N	N	N	N
Zinc salts	E	E	E	E	E

Source: From Iscotables with permission of the copyright owner, Instrumentation Specialties Company, Inc., Lincoln, Nebraska.
N, not recommended; F, fair; G, good.
The above table is based on information extracted from current literature and is intended to be used solely as a guide in selecting the proper tube material. The user is urged to make preliminary tests under actual conditions of use.

GENERIC SOURCE-BASED NOMENCLATURE FOR POLYMERS

(IUPAC Recommendations 2001)

Prepared by a Working Group consisting of

R. E. Bareiss (Germany), R. B. Fox (USA), K. Hatada (Japan), K. Horie (UK), A. D. Jenkins (UK), J. Kahovec (Czech Republic), R Kubisa (Poland), E. Maréchal (France), I. Meisel (Germany), W. V. Metanomski (USA), I. Mita (Japan), R. F. T. Stepto (UK), and E. S. Wilks (USA)

Prepared for publication by

E. Maréchal[1] and E. S. Wilks[2]

[1] *Université Pierre et Marie Curie (Paris VI), Laboratoire de Synthèse Macromoléculaire, Boîte 184, 4 Place Jussieu F-75252, Paris Cédex 05, France;*
[2] *113 Meriden Drive, Canterbury Hills, Hockessin, DE 19707 USA*

*Membership of the Commission during the preparation of this report (1993–1999) was as follows:

Titular Members: R. E. Bareiss (Germany, 1983–1993); M. Barón (Argentina, from 1996, Secretary from 1998); K. Hatada (Japan, 1989–1997); M. Hess (Germany, from 1998); K. Horie (Japan, from 1997); J. Kahovec (Czech Republic, to 1999); P. Kubisa (Poland, from 1999); E. Maréchal (France, from 1994); I. Meisel (Germany, from 2000); W. V. Metanomski (USA, 1994–1999); C. Noël (France, to 1997); V. P. Shibaev (Russia, to 1995); R. F. T. Stepto (UK, 1989–1999, Chairman to 1999); E. S. Wilks (USA, from 2000); W. J. Work (USA, 1987–1999, Secretary, 1987–1997); ***Associate Members:*** M. Barón (Argentina, 1991–1995); K. Hatada (Japan, 1998–1999); J.-I. Jin (Korea, from 1993); M. Hess (Germany, 1996–1997); O. Kramer (Denmark, from 1996); P. Kubisa (Poland, 1996–1998); E. Maréchal (France, 1991–1993); I. Meisel (Germany, 1997–1999); S. Penczek (Poland, from 1994); L. Shi (China, 1987–1995); V. P. Shibaev (Russia, 1996–1999); E. S. Wilks (USA, 1998–1999).

Abstract: The commission has already published two documents on the source-based names of linear copolymers and nonlinear polymers; however, in some cases this nomenclature leads to ambiguous names. The present document proposes a generic source-based nomenclature that solves these problems and yields clearer source-based names. A generic source-based name comprises two parts:

1. polymer class (generic) name followed by a colon
2. the actual or hypothetical monomer name(s), always parenthesized in the case of a copolymer

The formula, the structure-based name, the source-based name, and the generic source-based name of the polymer are given for each example in the document. In some cases, only generic source-based give unambiguous names, for example, when a polymer has more than one name or when it is obtained through a series of intermediate structures. The rules concern mostly polymers with one or more types of functional group or heterocyclic system in the main chain, but to some extent they are also applicable to polymers with side-groups, carbon-chain polymers such as vinyl or diene polymers, spiro and cyclic polymers, and networks.

Contents

1. Introduction

The IUPAC Commission on Macromolecular Nomenclature has published three documents [1–3] on the structure-based nomenclature for polymers that enable most polymers, except networks, to be named. The Commission has also produced two documents [4,5] on the source-based nomenclature of linear copolymers and nonlinear polymers. In general, source-based names are simpler and less rigorous than structure-based names. However, there are cases in which the simplicity of the source-based nomenclature leads to ambiguous names for polymers. For example, the condensation of a dianhydride (A) with a diamine (B) gives first a polyamide-acid, which can be cyclized to a polyimide; however, both products have the same name poly(A-*alt*-B) according to current source-based nomenclature. If the class name of the polymer "amide-acid" or "imide" is incorporated in the name, differentiation is easily accomplished. Even in cases where only a single product is formed, use of the class name (generic name) may help to clarify the structure of the polymer, especially if it is very complex.

Examples of ambiguous names exist also for homopolymers. The source-based name "polybutadiene" does not indicate whether the structure is 1,2-, 1,4-*cis*-, or 1,4-*trans*-; supplementary information is needed to distinguish between the possibilities.

It is the objective of the present document to introduce a generic nomenclature system to solve these problems, and to yield better source-based names.

Most trivial names, such as polystyrene, are source-based names. Hitherto, the Commission has not systematically recommended source-based names for homopolymers because it considered that the more rigorous structure-based names were more appropriate for scientific communications. However, since the publication of "Nomenclature of Regular Single-Strand Organic Polymers" in 1976, scientists, in both industry and academia, have continued to use trivial names. Even the Commission itself adopted (1985) a source-based nomenclature for copolymers owing to its simplicity and practicality. Based on these facts, the Commission has now decided to recommend source-based nomenclature as an alternative official nomenclature for homopolymers. In this document, the rules for generating source-based names for homopolymers are described. Consequently, source-based and structure-based names are available for most polymers.

Names of the monomers in the source-based names of polymers should preferably be systematic but they may be trivial if well established by usage. Names of the organic groups, as parts of constitutional repeating units (CRU) in structure-based names, are those based on the principles of organic nomenclature and recommended by the 1993 *A Guide to IUPAC Nomenclature of Organic Compounds* [6].

2. Source-Based Nomenclature for Homopolymers

RULE 1

The source-based name of a homopolymer is made by combining the prefix "poly" with the name of the monomer. When the latter consists of more than one word, or any ambiguity is anticipated, the name of the monomer is parenthesized.

Example 1.1

Source-based name: Polystyrene
Structure-based name: poly(1-phenylethylene)

Example 1.2

Source-based name: poly(vinyl chloride)
Structure-based name: poly(1-chloroethylene)

3. Generic Nomenclature

3.1 Fundamental Principles

The basic concept for generic source-based nomenclature is very simple; just add the polymer class name to the source-based name of the polymer. Addition of the polymer class name is frequently OPTIONAL; in some cases, the addition is necessary to avoid ambiguity or to clarify. However, the addition is undesirable if it fails to add clarification.

The system presented here can be applied to almost all homopolymers, copolymers, and others, such as networks. However, generic source-based nomenclature should not be considered as a third nomenclature system to be added to the other two systems of nomenclature; it must be considered as an auxiliary system and a simple extension of current source-based nomenclature. When the generic part of the name is eliminated from the name of a polymer, the well-established source-based name remains.

3.2 General Rules

RULE 2

A generic source-based name of a polymer has two components in the following sequence: (1) a polymer class (generic) name (polyG) followed by a colon and (2) the actual or hypothetical monomer name(s) (A, B, etc.), always parenthesized in the case of a copolymer. In the case of a homopolymer, parentheses are introduced when it is necessary to improve clarity.

polyG: A   polyG: (B)   polyG: (A-*co*-B)   polyG: (A-*alt*-B)

Note 1 The polymer class name (generic name) describes the most appropriate type of functional group or heterocyclic ring system.

Note 2 All the rules given in the two prior documents on source-based nomenclature [4,5] can be applied to the present nomenclature system, with the addition of the generic part of the name.

Note 3 A polymer may have more than one name; this usually occurs when it can be prepared in more than one way.

Note 4 If a monomer or a pair of complementary monomers can give rise to more than one polymer, or if the polymer is obtained through a series of intermediate structures, the use of generic nomenclature is essential (see examples 2.1, 2.3, and 2.4).

Example 2.1

Generic source-based name:
  I. polyalkylene:vinyloxirane
  II. polyether:vinyloxirane

862

Handbook of Biochemistry and Molecular Biology

Source-based names:
I and II have the same source-based name:poly(vinyloxirane).

Structure-based names:
I. poly(1-oxiranylethylene)
II. poly[(oxy(1-vinylethylene)]

Example 2.2

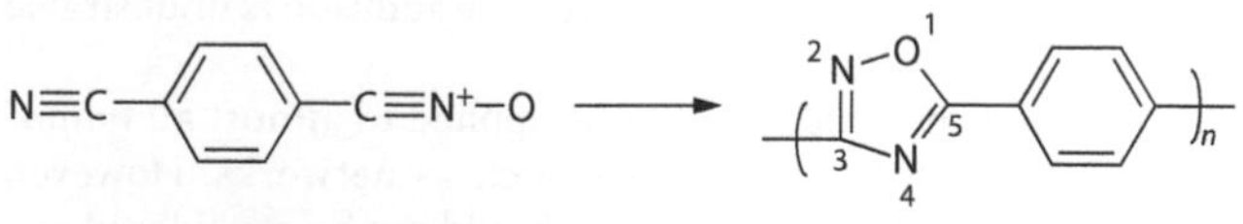

Generic source-based name:
   polyoxadiazole:(4-cyanobenzonitrile *N*-oxide)

Structure-based name:
   poly(1,2,4-oxadiazole-3,5-diyl-1,4-phenylene)

Example 2.3

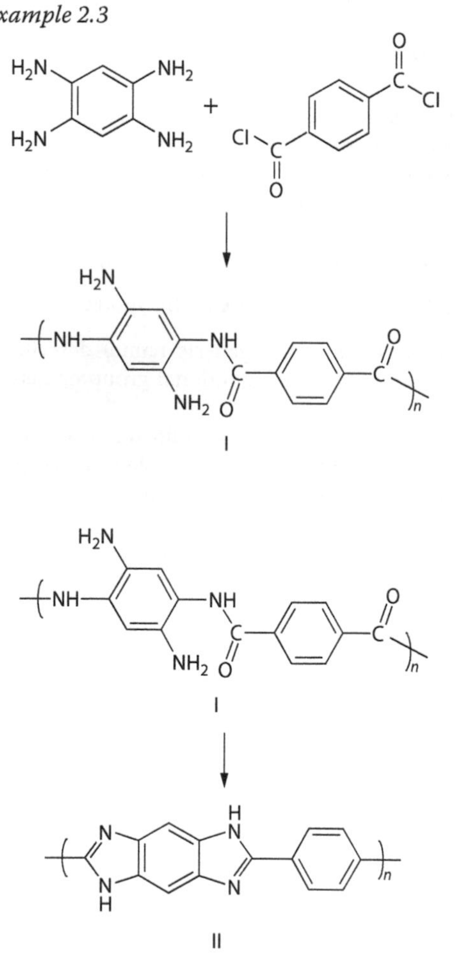

Generic source-based name:
I. polyamide:[(terephthaloyl dichloride)-*alt*-benzene-1,2,4, 5-tetramine]
II. polybenzimidazole:[(terephthaloyl dichloride)-*alt*-benzene-1,2,4,5-tetramine]

Source-based name:
   I and II have the same source-based name:

poly[(terephthaloyl dichloride)-*alt*-benzene-1,2,4,5- tetramine]

Structure-based names:
I. poly[imino(2,5-diamino-1,4-phenylene)iminotereph-thaloyl]
II. poly[(1,5-dihydrobenzo[1,2-*d*:4,5-*d*′]diimidazole-2,6-diyl)-1,4-phenylene]

Example 2.4

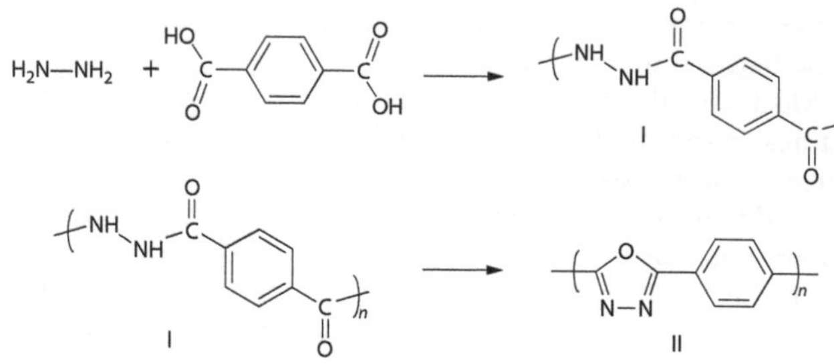

Generic source-based names:
I. polyhydrazide:[hydrazine-*alt*-(terephthalic acid)]
II. polyoxadiazole:[hydrazine-*alt*-(terephthalic acid)]

Source-based name:
   I and II have the same source-based name: poly[hydrazine-*alt*-(terephthalic acid)]

Structure-based names:
I. poly(hydrazine-1,2-diylterephthaloyl)
II. poly(1,3,4-oxadiazole-2,5-diyl-1,4-phenylene)

Example 2.5

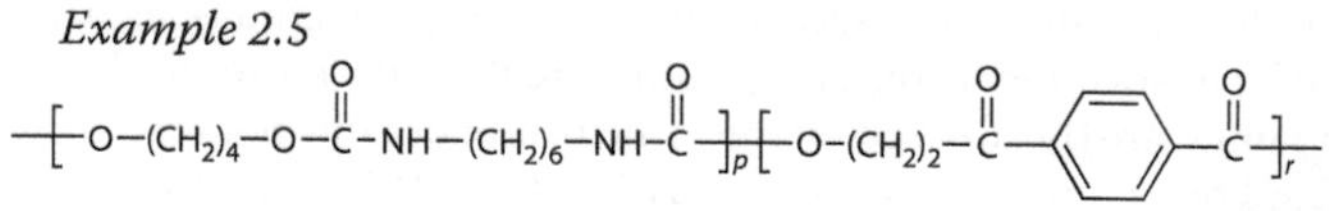

Generic source-based names:
   polyurethane:[butane-1,4-diol-*alt*-(hexane-1,6-diyl diisocyanate)]-*block*-polyester:[(ethylene glycol)-*alt*-(terephthalic acid)]

Structure-based name:
   poly(oxybutane-1,4-diyloxycarbonyliminohexane-1,6-diyliminocarbonyl)-*block*-poly(oxyethyleneoxytere-phthaloyl)

Example 2.6

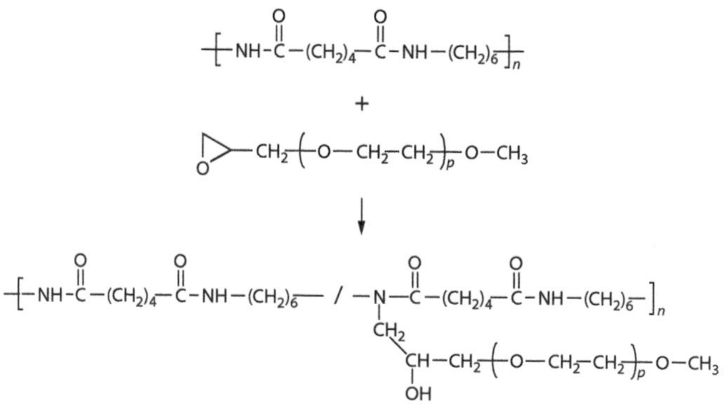

Generic source-based name:
polyamide:[hexane-1,6-diamine-*alt*-(adipicacid)]-*graft*-polyether: (ethylene oxide)

Note 5 It is assumed that this reaction is limited to only one graft for each CRU.

RULE 3

When more than one type of functional group or heterocyclic system is present in the polymer structure, names should be alphabetized; for example, poly(GG′):(A-*alt*-B).

Note 6 It is preferable, but not mandatory, to cite all generic classes.

Example 3.1

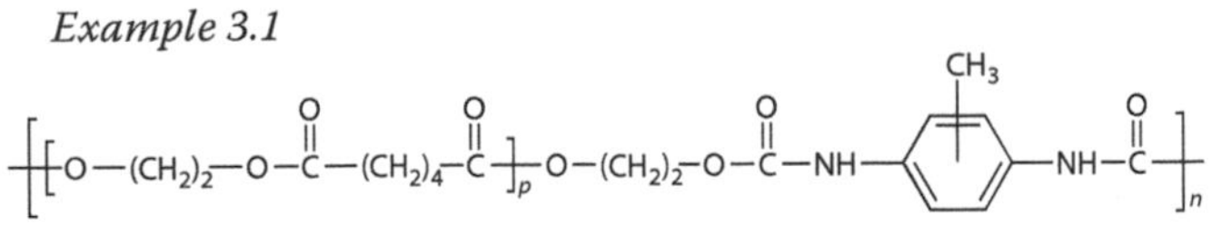

Generic source-based name:
polyesterurethane:(α,ω-dihydroxyoligo[(ethylene glycol)-*alt*-(adipic acid)]-*alt*-(2,5-tolylene diisocyanate)}

Structure-based name:
poly{[oligo(oxyethyleneoxyadipoyl)]oxyethyleneoxycarbonylimino(x-methyl-1,4-phenylene)iminocarbonyl)}

Example 3.2

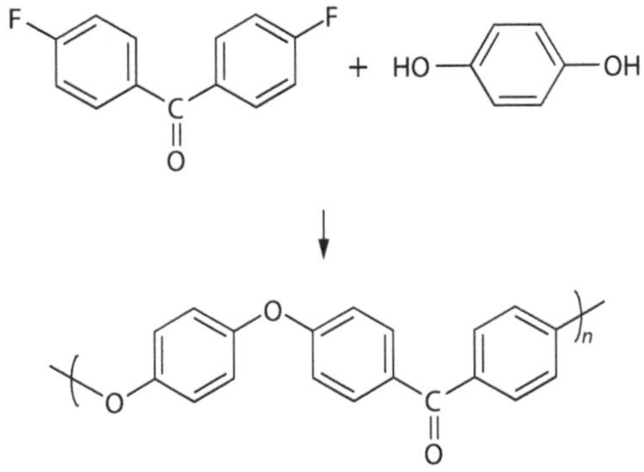

Generic source-based name:
polyetherketone:(4,4′-difluorobenzophenone-*att*-hydroquinone)

Structure-based name:
poly(oxy-1,4-phenyleneoxy-1,4-phenylenecarbonyl-1,4-phenylene)

RULE 4

Polymer class names relevant only to the main chain are specified in the name; names of side-chain functional groups may also be included after a hyphen if they are formed during the polymerization reaction.

Example 4.1

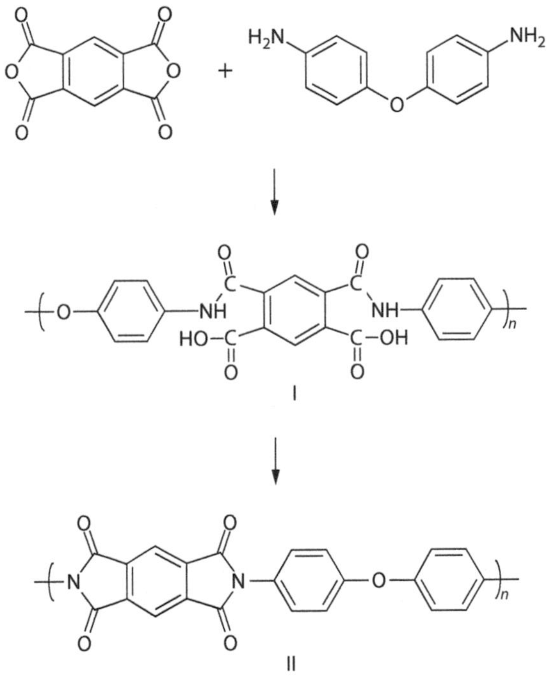

Generic source-based names:
I. poly(amide-acid):[(pyromellitic dianhydride)-*alt*-(4,4′-oxydianiline)] (Both carboxy groups result from the polymerization reaction.)
II. polyimide: [(pyromellitic dianhydride)-*alt*-(4,4′-oxydiani-line)]

Structure-based names:
I. poly[oxy-1,4-phenyleneiminocarbonyl(4,6-dicarboxy-1,3-henylene)carbonylimino-1,4-phenylene]
II. poly[(5,7-dihydro-1,3,5,7-tetraoxobenzo[1,2-*c*:4,5-*c*′]dipyrrole-2,6(1*H*,3*H*)-diyl)-1,4-phenyleneoxy-1,4-phenylene]

Example 4.2

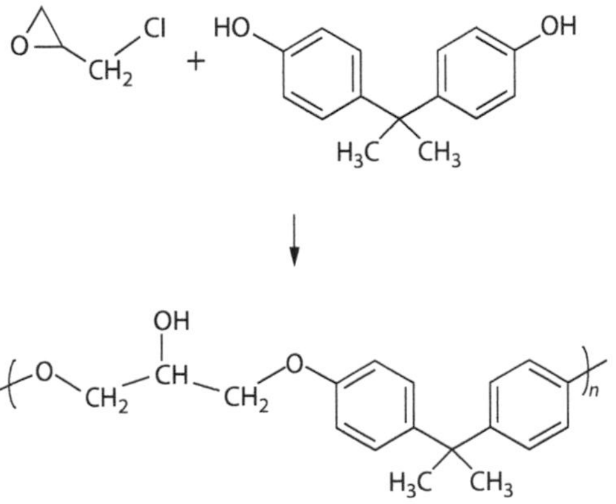

Generic source-based names:
    poly(ether-alcohol):(epichlorohydrin-*alt*-bisphenol A)

Structure-based name:
    poly[oxy(2-hydroxypropane-1,3-diyl)oxy-1,4-phenylene
    (1-methylethane-1,1-diyl)-1,4-phenylene]

RULE 5

In the case of carbon-chain polymers such as vinyl polymers or diene polymers, the generic name is to be used only when different polymer structures may arise from a given monomeric system.

Example 5.1

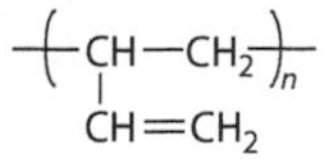

Generic source-based name:
    polyalkylene:(buta-1,3-diene)

Source-based name: poly(buta-1,3-diene)
    Structure-based name: poly(1-vinylethylene)

Example 5.2

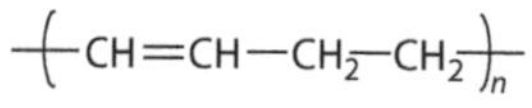

Generic source-based name:
    polyalkenylene:buta-1,3-diene

Source-based name:poly(buta-1,3-diene)
    Structure-based name: poly(but-1-ene-1,4-diyl)

Example 5.3

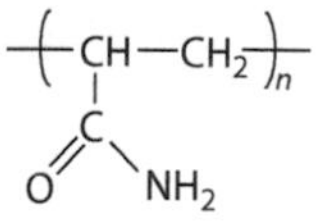

Generic source-based name:
    polyalkylene: acrylamide

Structure-based name: poly[1-(aminocarbonyl)ethylene]

Example 5.4

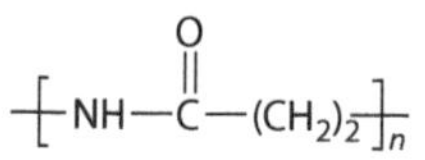

Generic source-based name: polyamide:acrylamide

Structure-based name: poly[imino(1-oxopropane-1,3-diyl)]

Note 7   The terms polyalkylene and polyalkenylene have been defined in ref. 7, p. 149.

4. Further Applications of Generic Names

Generic source-based nomenclature can be extended to more complicated polymers such as spiro and cyclic polymers and networks.

Example 6.1

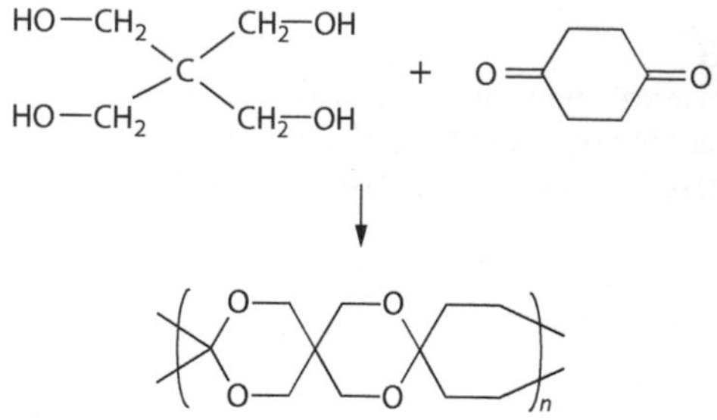

Generic source-based name:
    polyspiroketal:{[2,2-bis(hydroxymethyl)-propane-1,3-diol]-
    alt-cyclohexane-1,4-dione} or polyspiroketal: (pentae-
    rythritol-*alt*-cyclohexane-1,4-dione)

Structure-based name:
    poly[2,4,8,10-tetraoxaspiro[5.5]undecane-3,3,9,9-tetrayl-
    9,9-bis(ethylene)]

Example 6.2

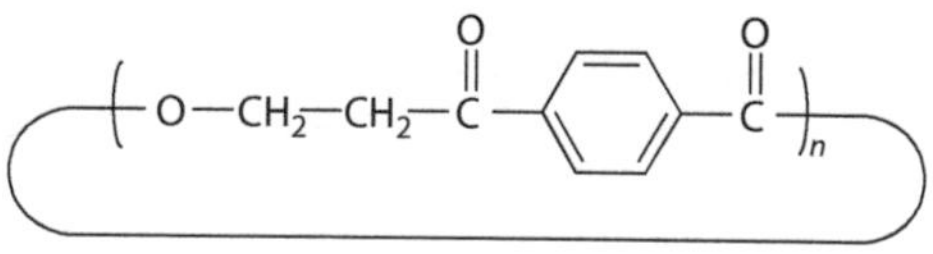

Generic source-based name:
    cyclo-polyester: [(ethylene glycol)-*alt*-(terephthalic acid)]

Note 8   There is no IUPAC nomenclature for cyclic polymers.

Example 6.3

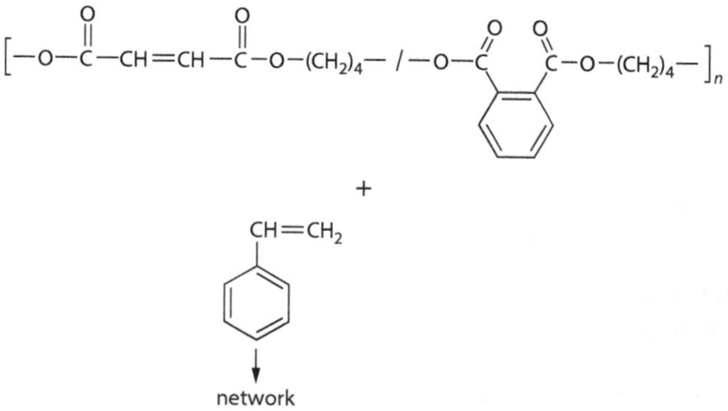

Generic source-based name:
    polyester: {butane-1,4-diol-*alt*-[(maleic anhydride);(phthalic
    anhydride)]}-*net*-polyalkylene: (maleic anhydride)-*co*-
    styrene]

5. References

1. "Nomenclature of regular single-strand organic polymers, 1975", *Pure Appl. Chem.* **48**, 373–385 (1976). Reprinted as chapter 5 in Ref. 7.
2. "Nomenclature of regular double-strand (ladder and spiro) organic polymers 1993", *Pure Appl. Chem.* **65**, 1561–1580 (1993).
3. "Structure-based nomenclature for irregular single-strand organic polymers 1994", *Pure Appl. Chem.* **66**, 873–889 (1994).
4. "Source-Based Nomenclature for Copolymers 1985", *Pure Appl. Chem.* **57**, 1427–1440 (1985). Reprinted as chapter 7 in Ref. 7.
5. "Source-based nomenclature for non-linear macromolecules and macromolecular assemblies", *Pure Appl. Chem.* **69**, 2511–2521 (1997).
6. *A Guide to IUPAC Nomenclature of Organic Compounds*, R. Panico, W. H. Powell, J-C. Richer (Eds.), Blackwell Scientific Publications, Oxford (1993).
7. *Compendium of Macromolecular Nomenclature*, W. V. Metanomski (Ed.), Blackwell Scientific Publications, Oxford (1991).

DEFINITIONS OF TERMS RELATING TO REACTIONS OF POLYMERS AND TO FUNCTIONAL POLYMERIC MATERIALS

(IUPAC Recommendations 2003)

Prepared by a Working Group consisting of

K. Horie[1], M. Barón[2], R. B. Fox[3], J. He[4], M. Hess[5], J. Kahovec[6], T. Kitayama[7], P. Kubisa[8], E. Maréchal[9], W. Mormann[10], R. F. T. Stepto[11], D. Tabak[12], J. Vohlídal[13], E. S. Wilks[14], and W. J. Work[15]

*Members of the Commission on Macromolecular Nomenclature (1997–2001) and the Subcommittee on Macromolecular Nomenclature (2002–2003) contributing to this report were:

G. Allegra (Italy); M. Barón (Argentina, Commission and Subcommittee Secretary); A. Fradet (France); K. Hatada (Japan); J. He (China); M. Hess (Germany, Commission and Subcommittee Chairman); K. Horie (Japan); A. D. Jenkins (UK); J.-I. Jin (Korea); R. G. Jones (UK, Subcommittee Secretary); J. Kahovec (Czech Republic); T. Kitayama (Japan); P. Kratochvíl (Czech Republic); P. Kubisa (Poland); E. Maréchal (France); I. Meisel (Germany); W. V. Metanomski (USA); G. Moad (Australia); W. Mormann (Germany); S. Penczek (Poland); L. P. Rebelo (Portugal); M. Rinaudo (France); I. Schopov (Bulgaria); M. Schubert (USA); V. P. Shibaev (Russia); S. Slomkowski (Poland); R. F. T. Stepto (UK, Commission Chairman); D. Tabak (Brazil); J. Vohlídal (Czech Republic); E. S. Wilks (USA); W. J. Work (USA, Commission Secretary); *Other Contributors:* K. Dorfner (Germany); J. M. J. Fréchet (USA); W. I. Harris (USA); P. Hodge (UK); T. Nishikubo (Japan); C. K. Ober (USA); E. Reichmanis (USA); D. C. Sherrington (UK); M. Tomoi (Japan); D. Wöhrle (Germany).

[1]Department of Organic and Polymer Materials Chemistry, Tokyo University of Agriculture and Technology, 2-24-16 Nakacho, Koganei-shi, Tokyo 184-8588, Japan; [2]Facultad de Ciências Exactas y Naturales, Universidad de Belgrano, Villanueva 1324, Buenos Aires 1426, Argentina; [3]6115 Wiscasset Road, Bethesda, MD 20816, USA; [4]State Key Laboratory of Engineering Plastics, The Chinese Academy of Sciences, Institute of Chemistry, Beijing 100080, China; [5]Fachbereich 6: Physikalische Chemie, Universitat Duisburg-Essen, D-47048 Duisburg, Germany; [6]Ústav Makromolekulární Chemie, Akademie ved Ceské Republiky, Heyrovského námestí 2, CZ-162 06 Praha 6, Czech Republic; [7]Department of Chemistry, Osaka University, Toyonaka, Osaka 560-8531, Japan; [8]Centrum Badan Molek. i Makromolek., Polska Akademia Nauk, Sienkiewicza 112, PL-90 363 Lódz, Poland; [9]Laboratoire de Synthèse Macromoléculaire, Université Pierre et Marie Curie (Paris VI), Boîte 184 - Tour 54, 4e étage, 4 place Jussieu, F-75252 Paris Cédex 05, France; [10]Makromolekulare Chemie, Universität - Gesamthochschule Siegen, Adolf Reichwein Strasse 2, D-57068 Siegen, Germany; [11]Polymer Science and Technology Group (MMSC), University of Manchester and UMIST, Grosvenor Street, Manchester M1 7HS, UK; [12]Praca Pio X, 78 Sala 1213 - Candelaria, Rio de Janerio - RJ 20091-040, Brazil; [13]Katedra Fyzikalni a Makromolekularni Chemie, Universita Karlova, Albertov 2030, CZ-128 40 Praha 2, Czech Republic; [14]113 Meriden Drive, Canterbury Hills, Hockessin, DE 19707, USA; [15]1288 Burnett Road, Huntingdon Valley, PA 19006, USA.

Abstract: The document defines the terms most commonly encountered in the field of polymer reactions and functional polymers. The scope has been limited to terms that are specific to polymer systems. The document is organized into three sections. The first defines the terms relating to reactions of polymers. Names of individual chemical reactions are omitted from the document, even in cases where the reactions are important in the field of polymer reactions. The second section defines the terms relating to polymer reactants and reactive polymeric materials. The third section defines the terms describing functional polymeric materials.

Contents

Introduction

Chemical reactions of polymers have received much attention during the last two decades. Many fundamentally and industrially important reactive polymers and functional polymers are prepared by the reactions of linear or cross-linked polymers and by the introduction of reactive, catalytically active, or other groups onto polymer chains. Characteristics of polymer reactions may be appreciably different from both reactions of low-molar-mass compounds and polymerization reactions. Basic definitions of polymerization reactions have been included in the original [1] and revised [2] documents on basic terms in polymer science published by the IUPAC Commission on Macromolecular Nomenclature. Furthermore, the basic classification and definitions of polymerization reactions [3] and some polymer reactions such as degradation, aging, and related chemical transformations of polymers have been defined [4]. However, in spite of the growing importance of the field, a clear and uniform terminology covering the field of

Reproduced from:
Pure Appl. Chem., Vol. 76, No. 4, pp. 889–906, 2004.
© 2004 IUPAC.

reactions and the functionalization of polymers has not been presented until now. For example, combinatorial chemistry using reactive polymer beads has become a new field in recent years. The development of a uniform terminology for such multidisciplinary areas can greatly aid communication and avoid confusion.

This document presents clear concepts and definitions of general and specific terms relating to reactions of polymers and functional polymers. The document is divided into three sections. In Section 1 terms relating to reactions of polymers are defined. Names of individual chemical reactions (e.g., chloromethylation) are omitted from this document, even in cases where the reactions are important in the field of polymer reactions, because such names are usually already in widespread use and are well defined in organic chemistry and other areas of chemistry [5]. Sections 2 and 3 deal with the terminology of reactive and functional polymers. The term "functional polymer" has two meanings: (a) a polymer bearing functional groups (such as hydroxy, carboxy, or amino groups) that make the polymer reactive and (b) a polymer performing a specific function for which it is produced and used. The function in the latter case may be either a chemical function such as a specific reactivity or a physical function like electric conductivity. Polymers bearing reactive functional groups are usually regarded as polymers capable of undergoing chemical reactions. Thus, Section 2 deals with polymers and polymeric materials that undergo various kinds of chemical reactions (i.e., show chemical functions). Section 3 deals with terms relating to polymers and polymeric materials exhibiting some specific physical functions. For definitions of some physical functions, see also *Compendium of Chemical Terminology* ("Gold Book") [6].

A functional polymer according to Definition 3.6 of the present document is a polymer that exhibits specified chemical reactivity or has specified physical, biological, pharmacological, or other uses that depend on specific chemical groups. Thus, several terms concerned with properties or the structure of polymers are included in Section 3 whenever they are closely related to specific functions.

Terms that are defined implicitly in the notes and related to the main terms are given in bold type.

1. Reactions Involving Polymers

1.1 Chemical Amplification
Process consisting of a chemical reaction that generates a species that catalyzes another reaction and also the succeeding catalyzed reaction.

Note 1: Chemical amplification can lead to a change in structure and by consequence to a change in the physical properties of a polymeric material.

Note 2: The term "chemical amplification" is commonly used in photoresist lithography employing a **photo-acid generator** or **photo-base generator**.

Note 3: An example of chemical amplification is the transformation of [(*tert*-butoxycarbonyl)oxy]phenyl groups in polymer chains to hydroxyphenyl groups catalyzed by a photo-generated acid.

Note 4: The term "amplification reaction" as used in analytical chemistry is defined in [6], p. 21.

1.2 Chemical Modification
Process by which at least one feature of the chemical constitution of a polymer is changed by chemical reaction(s).

Note: A configurational change (e.g., cis–trans isomerization) is not usually referred to as a chemical modification.

1.3 Cross-Linking
Reaction involving sites or groups on existing macromolecules or an interaction between existing macromolecules that results in the formation of a small region in a macromolecule from which at least four chains emanate.

Note 1: See [6], p. 94 and Definition 1.59 in [2] for cross-link.

Note 2: The small region may be an atom, a group of atoms, or a number of branch points connected by bonds, groups of atoms, or oligomeric chains.

Note 3: A reaction of a reactive chain end of a linear macromolecule with an internal reactive site of another linear macromolecule results in the formation of a branch point, but is not regarded as a cross-linking reaction.

1.4 Curing
Chemical process of converting a prepolymer or a polymer into a polymer of higher molar mass and connectivity and finally into a network.

Note 1: Curing is typically accomplished by chemical reactions induced by heating (**thermal curing**), photo-irradiation (**photo-curing**), or electron-beam irradiation (**EB curing**), or by mixing with a chemical curing agent.

Note 2: Physical aging, crystallization, physical cross-linking, and postpolymerization reactions are sometimes referred to as "curing". Use of the term "curing" in these cases is discouraged.

Note 3: See also Definition 1.22.

1.5 Depolymerization
Process of converting a polymer into its monomer or a mixture of monomers (see [6], p. 106 and Definition 3.25 in [2]).

1.6 Grafting
Reaction in which one or more species of block are connected to the main chain of a macromolecule as side chains having constitutional or configurational features that differ from those in the main chain.

Note: See [6], p. 175 and Definition 1.28 in [2] for graft macromolecule.

1.7 Interchange Reaction
Reaction that results in an exchange of atoms or groups between a polymer and low-molar-mass molecules, between polymer molecules, or between sites within the same macromolecule.

Note: An interchange reaction that occurs with polyesters is called **transesterification**.

1.8 Main-Chain Scission
Chemical reaction that results in the breaking of main-chain bonds of a polymer molecule.

Note 1: See [6], p. 64 and Definition 3.24 in [2] for chain scission.

Note 2: Some main-chain scissions are classified according to the mechanism of the scission process: **hydrolytic, mechanochemical, thermal, photochemical**, or **oxidative scission**. Others are classified according to their location in the backbone relative to a specific structural feature, for example, **α-scission** (a scission of the C-C bond alpha to the carbon atom of a photo-excited carbonyl group) and **β-scission** (a scission of the C-C bond beta to the carbon atom bearing a radical), etc.

1.9 Mechanochemical Reaction

Chemical reaction that is induced by the direct absorption of mechanical energy.

Note: Shearing, stretching, and grinding are typical methods for the mechanochemical generation of reactive sites, usually macroradicals, in polymer chains that undergo mechanochemical reactions.

1.10 Photochemical Reaction

Chemical reaction that is caused by the absorption of ultraviolet, visible, or infrared radiation ([6], p. 302).

Note 1: Chemical reactions that are induced by a reactive intermediate (e.g., radical, carbene, nitrene, or ionic species) generated from a photo-excited state are sometimes dealt with as a part of photochemistry.

Note 2: An example of a photochemical reaction concerned with polymers is **photopolymerization.**

Note 3: See also Definitions 1.1, 1.18, 3.14, and 3.25.

1.11 Polymer Complexation Polymer Complex Formation

Process that results in the formation of a polymer–polymer complex or a complex composed of a polymer and a low-molar-mass substance.

1.12 Polymer Cyclization

Chemical reaction that leads to the formation of ring structures in or from polymer chains.

Note 1: Examples of cyclization along polymer chains are: (a) cyclization of polyacrylonitrile, (b) acetalization of poly(vinyl alcohol) with an aldehyde, (c) cyclization of polymers of conjugated dienes such as polyisoprene or polybutadiene leading to macrocycles.

Note 2: Examples of cyclization of polymer molecules are: (a) cyclization of poly(dimethylsiloxane), (b) back-biting reaction during ionic polymerizations of heterocyclic monomers.

1.13 Polymer Degradation

Chemical changes in a polymeric material that usually result in undesirable changes in the in-use properties of the material.

Note 1: In most cases (e.g., in vinyl polymers, polyamides) degradation is accompanied by a decrease in molar mass. In some cases (e.g., in polymers with aromatic rings in the main chain), degradation means changes in chemical structure. It can also be accompanied by cross-linking.

Note 2: Usually, degradation results in the loss of, or deterioration in useful properties of the material. However, in the case of **biodegradation** (degradation by biological activity), polymers may change into environmentally acceptable substances with desirable properties (see Definition 3.1).

Note 3: See Definition 16 in [4] for degradation.

1.14 Polymer Functionalization

Introduction of desired chemical groups into polymer molecules to create specific chemical, physical, biological, pharmacological, or other properties.

1.15 Polymer Reaction

Chemical reaction in which at least one of the reactants is a high-molar-mass substance.

1.16 Polymer-Supported Reaction

Chemical reaction in which at least one reactant or a catalyst is bound through chemical bonds or weaker interactions such as hydrogen bonds or donor-acceptor interactions to a polymer.

Note 1: The easy separation of low-molar-mass reactants or products from the polymer-supported species is a great advantage of polymer-supported reactions.

Note 2: Typical examples of polymer-supported reactions are: (a) reactions performed by use of polymer-supported catalysts, (b) solid-phase peptide synthesis, in which intermediate peptide molecules are chemically bonded to beads of a suitable polymer support.

1.17 Protection of a Reactive Group

Temporary chemical transformation of a reactive group into a group that does not react under conditions where the nonprotected group reacts.

Note: For example, **trimethylsilylation** is a typical transformation used to protect reactive functional groups such as hydroxy or amino groups from their reaction with growing anionic species in anionic polymerization.

1.18 Radiation Reaction

Chemical reaction that is induced by ionizing radiation with γ-ray, X-ray, electron, or other high-energy beams.

Note 1: Radiation reactions involving polymers often lead to chain scission and cross-linking.

Note 2: A **photochemical reaction** (see Definition **1.10**) is sometimes regarded as a type of radiation reaction.

1.19 Reactive Blending

Mixing process that is accompanied by the chemical reaction(s) of components of a polymer mixture.

Note 1: Examples of reactive blending are: (a) blending accompanied by the formation of a polymer-polymer complex, (b) the formation of block or graft copolymers by a combination of radicals formed by the mechanochemical scission of polymers during blending.

Note 2: Reactive blending may also be carried out as reactive extrusion or reaction injection molding (RIM).

1.20 Sol-Gel Process

Formation of a polymer network by the reaction of monomer(s), liquid or in solution, to form a gel, and in most cases finally to form a dry network.

Note: An inorganic polymer (e.g., silica-gel or organic-inorganic hybrid) can be prepared by the sol-gel process.

1.21 Surface Grafting

Process in which a polymer surface is chemically modified by grafting or by the generation of active sites that can lead to the initiation of a graft polymerization.

Note 1: Peroxidation, ozonolysis, high-energy irradiation, and plasma etching are methods of generating active sites on a polymer surface.

Note 2: See also Definition 1.6.

1.22 Vulcanization

Chemical cross-linking of high-molar-mass linear or branched polymer or polymers to give a polymer network.

Note 1: The polymer network formed often displays rubber-like elasticity. However, a high concentration of cross-links can lead to rigid materials.

Note 2: A classic example of vulcanization is the cross-linking of *cis*-polyisoprene through sulfide bridges in the thermal treatment of natural rubber with sulfur or a sulfur-containing compound.

2. Polymer Reactants and Reactive Polymeric Materials

2.1 Chelating Polymer

Polymer containing ligand groups capable of forming bonds (or other attractive interactions) between two or more separate binding sites within the same ligand group and a single atom.

Note 1: Chelating polymers mostly act as ion-exchange polymers specific to ions that form chelates with chelating ligands of the polymer.

Note 2: See [6], p. 68 for chelation.

2.2 Ion-Exchange Polymer

Polymer that is able to exchange ions (cations or anions) with ionic components in solution.

Note 1: See [6], p. 208 for ion exchange.

Note 2: An ion-exchange polymer in ionized form may also be referred to as a **polyanion** or a **polycation.**

Note 3: Synthetic ion-exchange organic polymers are often network polyelectrolytes.

Note 4: A membrane having ion-exchange groups is called an **ion-exchange membrane.**

Note 5: Use of the term "ion-exchange resin" for "ion-exchange polymer" is strongly discouraged.

2.3 Living Polymer

Polymer with stable, polymerization-active sites formed by a chain polymerization in which irreversible chain transfer and chain termination are absent.

Note 1: See [6], p. 236 and Definition 3.21 in [2] for living polymerization.

2.4 Macromonomer

Polymer or oligomer whose molecules each have one end-group that acts as a monomer molecule, so that each polymer or oligomer molecule contributes only a single monomer unit to a chain of the product polymer.

Note 1: The homopolymerization or copolymerization of a macromonomer yields a comb or graft polymer.

Note 2: In the present definition, Definition 2.35 in [2] has been combined with Definition 1.9 in [2]. See also [6], p. 241.

Note 3: Macromonomers are also sometimes referred to as macromers'. The use of the term "macromer" is strongly discouraged.

2.5 Polymer Catalyst

Polymer that exhibits catalytic activity.

Note 1: Certain synthetic polymer catalysts can behave like enzymes.

Note 2: Poly(4-vinylpyridine) in its basic form and sulfonated polystyrene in its acid form are examples of polymers that can act as catalysts in some base- and acid-catalyzed reactions, respectively.

2.6 Polymer-Metal Complex

Complex comprising a metal and one or more polymeric ligands.

2.7 Polymer Phase-Transfer Catalyst

Polymer that acts as a phase-transfer catalyst and thereby causes a significant enhancement of the rate of a reaction between two reactants located in neighboring phases owing to its catalysis of the extraction of one of the reactants across the interface to the other phase where the reaction takes place.

Note 1: Polymer phase-transfer catalysts in the form of beads are often referred to as **triphase catalysts** because such catalysts form the third phase of the reaction system.

Note 2: See [6], p. 299 for phase-transfer catalyst.

2.8 Polymer-Supported Catalyst

Catalyst system comprising a polymer support in which catalytically active species are immobilized through chemical bonds or weaker interactions such as hydrogen bonds or donor-acceptor interactions.

Note 1: Polymer-supported catalysts are often based on network polymers in the form of beads. They are easy to separate from reaction media and can be used repeatedly.

Note 2: Examples of polymer-supported catalysts are: (a) a polymer-metal complex that can coordinate reactants, (b) colloidal palladium dispersed in a swollen network polymer that can act as a hydrogenation catalyst.

Note 3: **Polymer-supported enzymes** are a type of polymer-supported catalysts.

2.9 Polymer Reactant Polymer Reagent Polymer-Supported Reagent

Reactant (reagent) that is or is attached to a high-molar-mass linear polymer or a polymer network.

Note: The attachment may be by chemical bonds, by weaker interactions such as hydrogen bonds, or simply by inclusion.

2.10 Prepolymer

Polymer or oligomer whose molecules are capable of entering, through reactive groups, into further polymerization and thereby contributing more than one structural unit to at least one type of chain of the final polymer.

Note: Definition 2.37 in [2] has been combined with Definition 1.11 in [2]. See also [6], p. 318.

2.11 Reactive Polymer

Polymer having reactive functional groups that can undergo chemical transformation under the conditions required for a given reaction or application.

2.12 Redox Polymer Electron-Exchange Polymer Oxidation-Reduction Polymer

Polymer containing groups that can be reversibly reduced or oxidized.

Note 1: Reversible redox reaction can take place in a polymer main-chain, as in the case of polyaniline and quinone/hydroquinone polymers, or on side-groups, as in the case of a polymer carrying ferrocene side-groups.

Note 2: See [7] p. 346.

Note 3: Use of the term "redox resin" is strongly discouraged.

2.13 Resin

Soft solid or highly viscous substance, usually containing prepolymers with reactive groups.

Note 1: This term was used originally because of its analogy with a natural resin (rosin) and designated, in a broad sense, any polymer that is a basic material for plastics, organic coatings, or lacquers. However, the term is now used in a more narrow sense to refer to prepolymers of thermosets (thermosetting polymers).

Note 2: The term is sometimes used not only for prepolymers of thermosets, but also for cured thermosets (e.g., epoxy resins, phenolic resins). Use of the term for cured thermosets is strongly discouraged.

Note 3: Use of the term "resin" to describe the polymer beads used in solid-phase synthesis and as polymer supports, catalysts, reagents, and scavengers is also discouraged.

2.14 Telechelic Polymer Telechelic Oligomer

Prepolymer capable of entering into further polymerization or other reactions through its reactive end-groups.

Note 1: Reactive end-groups in telechelic polymers come from initiator or termination or chain-transfer agents in chain polymerizations, but not from monomer(s) as in polycondensations and polyadditions.

Note 2: See [6], p. 414 and the Note to Definition 1.11 in [2] for telechelic molecule.

2.15 Thermosetting Polymer

Prepolymer in a soft solid or viscous state that changes irreversibly into an infusible, insoluble polymer network by curing.

Note 1: Curing can be by the action of heat or suitable radiation, or both.

Note 2: A cured thermosetting polymer is called a **thermoset**.

3. Functional Polymeric Materials

3.1 Biodegradable Polymer

Polymer susceptible to degradation by biological activity, with the degradation accompanied by a lowering of its molar mass.

Note 1: See also Note 2 to Definition 1.13.

Note 2: See [6], p. 43 for biodegradation. In the case of a polymer, its biodegradation proceeds not only by catalytic activity of enzymes, but also by a wide variety of biological activities.

3.2 Conducting Polymer

Polymeric material that exhibits bulk electric conductivity.

Note 1: See [6], p. 84 for conductivity.

Note 2: The electric conductivity of a conjugated polymer is markedly increased by doping it with an electron donor or acceptor, as in the case of polyacetylene doped with iodine.

Note 3: A polymer showing a substantial increase in electric conductivity upon irradiation with ultraviolet or visible light is called a **photoconductive polymer**; an example is poly (*N*-vinyl-carbazole) (see [6], p. 302 for photoconductivity).

Note 4: A polymer that shows electric conductivity due to the transport of ionic species is called an **ion-conducting polymer**; an example is sulfonated polyaniline. When the transported ionic species is a proton as, e.g., in the case of fuel cells, it is called a **proton-conducting polymer**.

Note 5: A polymer that shows electric semiconductivity is called a **semiconducting polymer** (See [6], p. 372 for semiconductor).

Note 6: Electric conductance of a nonconducting polymer can be achieved by dispersing conducting particles (e.g., metal, carbon black) in the polymer. The resulting materials are referred to as *conducting* **polymer composites** or **solid polymer-electrolyte composites**.

3.3 Electroluminescent Polymer

Polymeric material that shows luminescence when an electric current passes through it such that charge carriers can combine at luminescent sites to give rise to electronically excited states of luminescent groups or molecules.

Note 1: Electroluminescent polymers are often made by incorporating luminescent groups or dyes into conducting polymers.

Note 2: Electrogenerated chemiluminescence (see [6], p. 130) directly connected with electrode reactions may also be called electroluminescence.

3.4 Ferroelectric Polymer

Polymer in which spontaneous polarization arises when dipoles become arranged parallel to each other by electric fields.

Note 1: See [6], p. 153 for ferroelectric transition.

Note 2: Poly(vinylidene fluoride) after being subjected to a corona discharge is an example of a ferroelectric polymer.

3.5 Ferromagnetic Polymer

Polymer that exhibits magnetic properties because it has unpaired electron spins aligned parallel to each other or electron spins that can easily be so aligned.

3.6 Functional Polymer

(a) Polymer that bears specified chemical groups

or

(b) Polymer that has specified physical, chemical, biological, pharmacological, or other uses which depend on specific chemical groups.

Note: Examples of functions of functional polymers under definition (b) are catalytic activity, selective binding of particular species, capture and transport of electric charge carriers or energy, conversion of light to charge carriers and vice versa, and transport of drugs to a particular organ in which the drug is released.

3.7 Impact-Modified Polymer

Polymeric material whose impact resistance and toughness have been increased by the incorporation of phase microdomains of a rubbery material.

Note: An example is the incorporation of soft polybutadiene domains into glassy polystyrene to produce high-impact polystyrene.

3.8 Liquid-Crystalline Polymer

Polymeric material that, under suitable conditions of temperature, pressure, and concentration, exists as a liquid crystalline mesophase (Definition 6.1 in [7]).

Note 1: See [4], p. 235 for liquid-crystal.

Note 2: A liquid-crystalline polymer can exhibit one or more liquid state(s) with one- or two-dimensional, long-range orientational order over certain ranges of temperatures either in the melt (**thermotropic liquid-crystalline polymer**) or in solution (**lyotropic liquid-crystalline polymer**).

3.9 Macroporous Polymer

Glass or rubbery polymer that includes a large number of macropores (50 nm–1 μm in diameter) that persist when the polymer is immersed in solvents or in the dry state.

Note 1: Macroporous polymers are often network polymers produced in bead form. However, linear polymers can also be prepared in the form of macroporous polymer beads.

Note 2: Macroporous polymers swell only slightly in solvents.

Note 3: Macroporous polymers are used, for example, as precursors for ion-exchange polymers, as adsorbents, as supports for catalysts or reagents, and as stationary phases in size-exclusion-chromatography columns.

Note 4: Porous polymers with pore diameters from ca. 2 to 50 nm are called **mesoporous polymers.**

3.10 Nonlinear Optical Polymer

Polymer that exhibits an optical effect brought about by electromagnetic radiation such that the magnitude of the effect is not proportional to the irradiance.

Note 1: See [6], p. 275 for nonlinear optical effect.

Note 2: An example of nonlinear optical effects is the generation of higher harmonics of the incident light wave.

Note 3: A polymer that exhibits a nonlinear optical effect due to anisotropic electric susceptibilities when subjected to electric field together with light irradiation is called an **electro-optical polymer.** A polymer that exhibits electro-optical behavior combined with photoconductivity is called a **photorefractive polymer.**

3.11 Optically Active Polymer

Polymer capable of rotating the polarization plane of a transmitted beam of linear-polarized light.

Note 1: See [6], p. 282 for optical activity.

Note 2: The optical activity originates from the presence of chiral elements in a polymer such as chiral centers or chiral axes due to long-range conformational order in a polymer (helicity) (see [6], p. 182 for helicity).

3.12 Photoelastic Polymer

Polymer that under stress exhibits birefringence.

3.13 Photoluminescent Polymer

Polymer that exhibits luminescence (i.e., fluorescence or phosphorescence arising from photo-excitation).

Note: See [6], p. 304 for photoluminescence.

3.14 Photosensitive Polymer

Polymer that responds to ultraviolet or visible light by exhibiting a change in its physical properties or its chemical constitution.

Note 1: Examples of the changes in photosensitive polymers are a change in molecular shape (**photoresponsive polymer**), a change in its constitution (**photoreactive polymer**), and a reversible change in color (**photochromic polymer**).

Note 2: Photosensitivity in photosensitive polymers means that the polymers are sensitive to the irradiated light leading to some change in properties or structure. It is different from photo-sensitization defined in [6], p. 307.

Note 3: See [6], p. 307 for photoreaction and [6], p. 302 for photochromism.

3.15 Piezoelectric Polymer

(a) Polymer that exhibits a change in dielectric properties on application of pressure

or

(b) Polymer that shows a change in its dimensions when subjected to an electric field.

3.16 Polyelectrolyte

Polymer composed of molecules in which a portion of the constitutional units has ionizable or ionic groups, or both.

Note 1: A polymer bearing both anionic and cationic groups in the same molecule is called an **amphoteric polyelectrolyte.**

Note 2: A polymer bearing acid or basic groups is called a polymer acid or a polymer base, respectively.

Note 3: A polymer acid or a polymer base can be used as a matrix for ion-conducting polymers.

Note 4: Definition 2.38 in [2] has been combined with Definition 1.65 in [2]. The present definition replaces the one in [6], p. 312.

3.17 Polymer Compatibilizer

Polymeric additive that, when added to a blend of immiscible polymers, modifies their interfaces and stabilizes the blend.

Note: Typical polymer compatibilizers are block or graft copolymers.

3.18 Polymer Drug

Polymer that contains either chemically bound drug molecules or pharmacologically active moieties.

Note: A polymer drug is usually used to provide drug delivery targeted to an organ and controlled release of an active drug at the target organ.

3.19 Polymer Gel

Gel in which the network component is a polymer network.

Note 1: A gel is an elastic colloid or polymer network that is expanded throughout its whole volume by a fluid.

Note 2: The polymer network can be a network formed by covalent bonds or by physical aggregation with region of local order acting as network junctions.

Note 3: An example of covalent polymer gels is *net*-poly(*N*-isopropylacrylamide) swollen in water, which shows volume phase transition during heating.

Note 4: Examples of physically aggregated polymer gels are poly(vinyl alcohol) gel and agarose gel, which show reversible sol-gel transitions.

Note 5: See Definition 1.58 in [2] for network.

Note 6: The definition for gel in [6], p. 170 does not include a polymer gel.

3.20 Polymer Membrane

Thin layer of polymeric material that acts as a barrier permitting mass transport of selected species.

Note: See [6], p. 251 for membrane.

3.21 Polymer Solvent

Polymer that acts like a solvent for compounds of low molar mass.

Note: An example of a polymer solvent is poly(oxyethylene); it can dissolve various inorganic salts by complexation.

3.22 Polymer Sorbent

Polymer that adsorbs or absorbs a certain substance or certain substances from a liquid or a gas.

Note 1: A polymer sorbent may be a **polymer adsorbent** or a **polymer absorbent.** The former acts by surface sorption and the latter by bulk sorption.

Note 2: See [6], p. 383 for sorption, [6], p. 11 for adsorption, and [6], p. 3 for absorption.

3.23 Polymer Support

Polymer to or in which a reagent or catalyst is chemically bound, immobilized, dispersed, or associated.

Note 1: A polymer support is usually a network polymer.

Note 2: A polymer support is usually prepared in bead form by suspension polymerization.

Note 3: The location of active sites introduced into a polymer support depends on the type of polymer support. In a **swollen-gel-bead polymer support** the active sites are distributed uniformly throughout the beads, whereas in a **macroporous-bead polymer support** they are predominantly on the internal surfaces of the macropores.

3.24 Polymer Surfactant

Polymer that lowers the surface tension of the medium in which it is dissolved, or the interfacial tension with another phase, or both.

Note: See [6], p. 409 for surfactant.

3.25 Resist Polymer

Polymeric material that, when irradiated, undergoes a marked change in solubility in a given solvent or is ablated.

Note 1: A resist polymer under irradiation either forms patterns directly or undergoes chemical reactions leading to pattern formation after subsequent processing.

Note 2: A resist material that is optimized for use with ultraviolet or visible light, an electron beam, an ion beam, or X-rays is called a **photoresist** (see [6], p. 307), **electron-beam resist, ion-beam resist,** or **X-ray resist,** respectively.

Note 3: In a **positive-tone resist**, also called a **positive resist**, the material in the irradiated area not covered by a mask is removed, which results in an image with a pattern identical with that on the mask. In a **negative-tone resist**, also called a **negative resist**, the non-irradiated area is subsequently removed, which results in an image with a pattern that is the complement of that on the mask.

3.26 Shape-Memory Polymer

Polymer that, after heating and being subjected to a plastic deformation, resumes its original shape when heated above its glass-transition or melting temperature.

Note: Crystalline *trans*-polyisoprene is an example of a shape-memory polymer.

3.27 Superabsorbent Polymer

Polymer that can absorb and retain extremely large amounts of a liquid relative to its own mass.

Note 1: The liquid absorbed can be water or an organic liquid.

Note 2: The swelling ratio of a superabsorbent polymer can reach the order of 1000:1.

Note 3: Superabsorbent polymers for water are frequently polyelectrolytes.

References

1. IUPAC. *Compendium of Macromolecular Nomenclature*, (the IUPAC "Purple Book"), prepared for publication by W. V. Metanomski, Chap. 1, Blackwell, Oxford (1991); IUPAC. "Basic definitions of terms relating to polymers (1974)", *Pure Appl. Chem.* **40**, 477–491 (1974).
2. A. D. Jenkins, P. Kratochvíl, R. F. T. Stepto, U. W. Suter. "Glossary of basic terms in polymer science (IUPAC Recommendations 1996)", *Pure Appl. Chem.* **68**, 2287–2311 (1996).
3. I. Mita, R. F. T. Stepto, U. W. Suter. "Basic classification and definitions of polymerization reactions (IUPAC Recommendations 1994)", *Pure Appl. Chem.* **66**, 2483–2486 (1994).
4. K. Hatada, R. B. Fox, J. Kahovec, E. Maréchal, I. Mita, V. Shibaev. "Definitions of terms relating to degradation, aging, and related chemical transformations of polymers (IUPAC Recommendations 1996)", *Pure Appl. Chem.* **68**, 2313–2323 (1996).
5. R. A. Y. Jones and J. F. Bunnett. "Nomenclature for organic chemical transformations (IUPAC Recommendations 1989)", *Pure Appl. Chem.* **61**, 725–768 (1989).
6. IUPAC. *Compendium of Chemical Terminology: IUPAC Recommendations*, (the IUPAC "Gold Book"), 2nd ed., compiled by A. D. McNaught and A. Wilkinson, Blackwell, Oxford (1997).
7. C. Noël, V. P. Shibaev, M. Barón, M. Hess, A. D. Jenkins, Jung-Il Jin, A. Sirigu, R. F. T. Stepto, W. J. Work. "Definitions of basic terms relating to low-molar-mass and polymer liquid-crystals (IUPAC Recommendations 2001)", *Pure Appl. Chem.* **73**, 845–895 (2001).

Alphabetical Index of Terms

Term	Definition No.	Term	Definition No.
αα-scission	1.8	polyanion	2.2
β-scission	1.8	polycation	2.2
amphoteric polyelectrolyte	3.16	polyelectrolyte	3.16
biodegradable polymer	3.1	polymer absorbent	3.22
biodegradation	1.13	polymer acid	3.16
chelating polymer	2.1	polymer adsorbent	3.22
chemical amplification	1.1	polymer base	3.16
chemical modification	1.2	polymer catalyst	2.5
conducting polymer	3.2	polymer compatibilizer	3.17
conducting polymer composite	3.2	polymer complex formation	1.11
cross-linking	1.3	polymer complexation	1.11
curing	1.4	polymer cyclization	1.12
depolymerization	1.5	polymer degradation	1.13
EB curing	1.4	polymer drug	3.18
electro-optical polymer	3.10	polymer functionalization	1.14
electroluminescent polymer	3.3	polymer gel	3.19
electron-beam resist	3.25	polymer membrane	3.20
electron-exchange polymer	2.12	polymer phase-transfer catalyst	2.7
ferroelectric polymer	3.4	polymer reactant	2.9
ferromagnetic polymer	3.5	polymer reaction	1.15
functional polymer	3.6	polymer reagent	2.9
grafting	1.6	polymer solvent	3.21
hydrolytic scission	1.8	polymer sorbent	3.22
impact-modified polymer	3.7	polymer support	3.23
interchange reaction	1.7	polymer surfactant	3.24
ion-beam resist	3.25	polymer-metal complex	2.6
ion-conducting polymer	3.2	polymer-supported catalyst	2.8
ion-exchange membrane	2.2	polymer-supported enzyme	2.8
ion-exchange polymer	2.2	polymer-supported reaction	1.16
liquid-crystalline polymer	3.8	polymer-supported reagent	2.9
living polymer	2.3	positive resist	3.25
lyotropic liquid-crystalline polymer	3.8	positive-tone resist	3.25
macromonomer	2.4	prepolymer	2.10
macroporous-bead polymer support	3.23	protection of a reactive group	1.17
macroporous polymer	3.9	proton-conducting polymer	3.2
main-chain scission	1.8	radiation reaction	1.18
mechanochemical reaction	1.9	reactive blending	1.19
mechanochemical scission	1.8	reactive polymer	2.11
mesoporous polymer	3.9	redox polymer	2.12
negative resist	3.25	resin	2.13
negative-tone resist	3.25	resist polymer	3.25
nonlinear-optical polymer	3.10	semiconducting polymer	3.2
optically active polymer	3.11	shape-memory polymer	3.26
oxidation-reduction polymer	2.12	sol-gel process	1.20
oxidative scission	1.8	solid polymer-electrolyte composite	3.2
photo-acid generator	1.1	superabsorbent polymer	3.27
photo-base generator	1.1	surface grafting	1.21
photo-curing	1.4	swollen-gel-bead polymer support	3.23
photochemical reaction	1.10, 1.18	telechelic oligomer	2.14
photochemical scission	1.8	telechelic polymer	2.14
photochromic polymer	3.14	thermal curing	1.4
photoconductive polymer	3.2	thermal scission	1.8
photoelastic polymer	3.12	thermoset	2.15
photoluminescent polymer	3.13	thermosetting polymer	2.15
photopolymerization	1.10	thermotropic liquid-crystalline polymer	3.8
photoreactive polymer	3.14	transesterification	1.7
photorefractive polymer	3.10	trimethylsilylation	1.17
photoresist	3.25	triphase catalyst	2.7
photoresponsive polymer	3.14	vulcanization	1.22
photosensitive polymer	3.14	X-ray resist	3.25
piezoelectric polymer	3.15		

DEFINITIONS OF TERMS RELATED TO POLYMER BLENDS, COMPOSITES, AND MULTIPHASE POLYMERIC MATERIALS

(IUPAC Recommendations 2004)

Prepared by a Working Group consisting of

W. J. Work[1, ‡], K. Horie[2], M. Hess[3], and R. F. T. Stepto[4]

Prepared for publication by

W. J. WORK

[1]*11288 Burnett Road, Huntingdon Valley, PA 19006, USA;* [2]*6-11-21, Kozukayama, Tarumi-ku, Kobe 655-0002, Japan;* [3]*Universitat Duisburg-Essen, Fachbereich 6: Physikalische Chemie, D-47048 Duisburg, Germany;* [4]*University of Manchester and UMIST, Polymer Science and Technology Group (MMSC), Grosvenor Street, Manchester, M1 7HS, UK*

*Membership of the Commission on Macromolecular Nomenclature (extant until 2002) during the preparation of this report (1993–2003) was as follows:

Titular Members: R. E. Bareiss (Germany, to 1993); M. Barón (Argentina, Associate Member to 1995, Titular Member from 1996, *Secretary* from 1998); K. Hatada (Japan, to 1997, Associate Member to 1999); M. Hess (Germany, Associate Member from 1996, Titular Member from 1998, *Chairman* from 2000); K. Horie (Japan, Associate Member from 1996, Titular Member from 1998); R. G. Jones (UK, Pool Titular Member to 1997, Titular Member from 1998); J Kahovec (Czech Republic, to 1999); P. Kubisa (Poland, Associate Member from 1996, Titular Member from 2000); E. Maréchal (France, Associate Member 1992–1993, 2000–2001, Titular Member 1994–1999); I Meisel (Germany, Associate Member from 1998, Titular Member from 2000); W. V. Metanomski (USA, to 1999); C. Noël (France, to 1997); V. P. Shibaev (Russia, to 1995, Associate Member to 1999); R. F. T. Stepto (UK, *Chairman* to 1999); E. S. Wilks (USA, Associate Member from 1998, Titular Member from 2000); W. J. Work (USA, *Secretary* to 1997).

Associate Members contributing to this report: J.-I. Jin (Korea, National Representative to 1993, Associate Member from 1994); T. Kitayama (Japan, from 2000); S. Penczek (Poland, from 1994); J. Vohlídal (Czech Republic, from 2000). ***National Representatives contributing to this report:*** W. Mormann (Germany, from 2000).

**Membership of the Subcommittee on Macromolecular Terminology (extant from 2002) during the preparation of this report (1993–2003) was as follows:

M. Hess (Germany, *Chairman*); M. Barón (Argentina, *Secretary*); G. Allegra (Italy); A. Fradet (France); J. He (China); K. Horie (Japan); A. D. Jenkins (UK); J.-II Jin (Korea); R. G. Jones (UK); J. Kahovec (Czech Republic); T. Kitayama (Japan); P. Kratochvíl (Czech Republic); P. Kubisa (Poland); I. Meisel (Germany); W. V. Metanomski (USA); G. Moad (Australia); W. Mormann (Germany); S. Penczek (Poland); L. P. Rebelo (Portugal); M. Rinaudo (France); I. Schopov (Bulgaria); M. Schubert (USA); V. P. Shibaev (Russia); S. Slomkowski (Poland); R. F. T. Stepto (UK); D. Tabak (Brazil); J. Vohlídal (Czech Republic); E. S. Wilks (USA); W. J. Work (USA).

Other contributors to this report: S. Akiyama (Japan); P. Avakian (USA); K. Binder (Germany); C. Bucknall (UK); R. Gilbert (Australia); J. He (China); J. S. Higgins (UK); T. Inoue (Japan); B.-J. Jungnickel (Germany); R. Koningsveld (Netherlands); J. Lertola (USA); T. Nishi (Japan); T. Nose (Japan); D. Paul (USA); I. Plotzker (USA); L. A. Utracki (Canada); B. Wood (USA).

Abstract: The document defines the terms most commonly encountered in the field of polymer blends and composites. The scope has been limited to mixtures in which the components differ in chemical composition or molar mass and in which the continuous phase is polymeric. Incidental thermodynamic descriptions are mainly limited to binary mixtures although, in principle, they could be generalized to multicomponent mixtures.

The document is organized into three sections. The first defines terms basic to the description of polymer mixtures. The second defines terms commonly encountered in descriptions of phase domain behavior of polymer mixtures. The third defines terms commonly encountered in the descriptions of the morphologies of phase-separated polymer mixtures.

Contents

Reproduced from:
Pure Appl. Chem., Vol. 76, No. 11, pp. 1985–2007, 2004.
© 2004 IUPAC
‡ Corresponding author

Introduction

It is the intent of this document to define the terms most commonly encountered in the field of polymer blends and composites. The scope has been limited to mixtures in which the components differ in chemical composition or molar mass or both and in which the continuous phase is polymeric. Many of the materials described by the term "multiphase" are two-phase systems that may show a multitude of finely dispersed phase domains. Hence, incidental thermodynamic descriptions are mainly limited to binary mixtures, although they can be and, in the scientific literature, have been generalized to multi-component mixtures. Crystalline polymers and liquid-crystal polymers have been considered in other documents [1,2] and are not discussed here.

This document is organized into three sections. The first defines terms basic to the description of polymer mixtures. The second defines terms commonly encountered in descriptions of phase-domain behavior of polymer mixtures. The third defines terms commonly encountered in the descriptions of the morphologies of phase-separated polymer mixtures.

General terms describing the composition of a system as defined in ref. [3] are used without further definition throughout the document. Implicit definitions are identified in boldface type throughout the document.

1. Basic Terms in Polymer Mixtures

1.1 Polymer Blend

Macroscopically homogeneous mixture of two or more different species of polymer [3,4].

Notes:

1. 1. See the Gold Book, p. 312 [3].
2. In most cases, blends are homogeneous on scales larger than several times the wavelengths of visible light.
3. In principle, the constituents of a blend are separable by physical means.
4. No account is taken of the miscibility or immiscibility of the constituent macromolecules, i.e., no assumption is made regarding the number of phase domains present.
5. The use of the term "polymer alloy" for "polymer blend" is discouraged, as the former term includes multiphase copolymers but excludes incompatible polymer blends (see **1.3**).
6. The number of polymeric components which comprises a blend is often designated by an adjective, viz., binary, ternary, quaternary,

1.2 Miscibility

Capability of a mixture to form a single phase over certain ranges of temperature, pressure, and composition.

Notes:

1. Whether or not a single phase exists depends on the chemical structure, molar-mass distribution, and molecular architecture of the components present.
2. The single phase in a mixture may be confirmed by light scattering, X-ray scattering, and neutron scattering.
3. For a two-component mixture, a necessary and sufficient condition for stable or metastable equilibrium of a homogeneous single phase is

$$\left(\frac{\partial^2 \Delta_{mix} G}{\partial \phi^2} \right)_{T,p} > 0$$

where $\Delta_{mix} G$ is the Gibbs energy of mixing and ϕ the composition, where ϕ is usually taken as the volume fraction of one of the components. The system is unstable if the above second derivative is negative. The borderline (spinodal) between (meta)stable and unstable states is defined by the above second derivative equalling zero. If the compositions of two conjugate (coexisting) phases become identical upon a change of temperature or pressure, the third derivative also equals zero (defining a critical state).

4. If a mixture is thermodynamically metastable, it will demix if suitably nucleated (see **2.5**). If a mixture is thermodynamically unstable, it will demix by spinodal decomposition (see **2.8**) or by nucleation and growth if suitably nucleated, provided there is minimal kinetic hindrance.

1.3 Miscible Polymer Blend
Homogeneous Polymer Blend

Polymer blend that exhibits miscibility (see **1.2**).

Notes:

1. For a polymer blend to be miscible, it must satisfy the criteria of miscibility (see **1.2**).
2. Miscibility is sometimes erroneously assigned on the basis that a blend exhibits a single T_g or optical clarity.
3. A miscible system can be thermodynamically stable or metastable (see note 4 in **1.2**).
4. For components of chain structures that would be expected to be miscible, miscibility may not occur if molecular architecture is changed, e.g., by crosslinking.

1.4 Homologous Polymer Blend

Mixture of two or more fractions of the same polymer, each of which has a different molar-mass distribution.

1.5 Isomorphic Polymer Blend

Polymer blend of two or more different semi-crystalline polymers that are miscible in the crystalline state as well as in the molten state.

Notes:

1. Such a blend exhibits a single, composition-dependent glass-transition temperature, T_g, and a single, composition-dependent melting point, T_m.
2. This behavior is extremely rare; very few cases are known.

1.6 Polymer-Polymer Complex

Complex, at least two components of which are different polymers [3].

Notes:

1. See the Gold Book, p. 313 [3].
2. A **complex** is a molecular entity formed from two or more components that can be ionic or uncharged (see the Gold Book, p. 81) [3].
3. Although the intrinsic binding energy between the individual interacting sites giving rise to the complex is weaker than a covalent bond, the total binding energy for any single molecule may exceed the energy of a single covalent bond.
4. The properties of a complex defined here differ from those given in ref. [3] because, owing to the repeating nature of a polymer molecule, many interacting sites may be present, which together will provide stronger bonding than a single covalent bond.

1.7 Metastable Miscibility

Capability of a mixture to exist for an indefinite period of time as a single phase that is separated by a small or zero energy barrier from a thermodynamically more stable multiphase system.

Notes:

1. See the Gold Book, p. 255 [3].
2. Mixtures exhibiting metastable miscibility may remain unchanged or they may undergo phase separation, usually by nucleation or spinodal decomposition.

1.8 Metastable Miscible Polymer Blend

Polymer blend that exhibits metastable miscibility.*Note*: In polymers, because of the low mobility of polymer chains, particularly in a glassy state, metastable mixtures may exist for indefinite periods of time without phase separation. This has frequently led to confusion when metastable miscible polymer blends are erroneously claimed to be miscible.

1.9 Interpenetrating Polymer Network

Recommended acronym: IPN

Polymer comprising two or more polymer networks which are at least partially interlaced on a molecular scale, but not covalently bonded to each other and cannot be separated unless chemical bonds are broken [4].

Notes:

1. See the Gold Book, p. 205 [3].
2. A mixture of two or more preformed polymer networks is not an interpenetrating polymer network.
3. An IPN may be further described by the process by which it is synthesized. When an IPN is prepared by a process in which the second component network is polymerized following the completion of polymerization of the first component network, the IPN may be referred to as a **sequential IPN**. When an IPN is prepared by a process in which both component networks are polymerized concurrently, the IPN may be referred to as a **simultaneous IPN**.

1.10 Semi-Interpenetrating Polymer Network

Recommended acronym: SIPN

Polymer comprising one or more polymer network(s) and one or more linear or branched polymer(s) characterized by the penetration on a molecular scale of at least one of the networks by at least some of the linear or branched chains [4].

Notes:

1. See the Gold Book, p. 372 [3].
2. Semi-interpenetrating polymer networks are different from interpenetrating polymer networks because the constituent linear-chain or branched-chain macromolecule(s) can, in principle, be separated from the constituent polymer network(s) without breaking chemical bonds, and, hence, they are polymer blends.
3. Semi-interpenetrating polymer networks may be further described by the process by which they are synthesized. When an SIPN is prepared by a process in which the second component polymer is polymerized or incorporated following the completion of polymerization of the first component polymer, the SIPN may be referred to as a **sequential SIPN**. When an SIPN is prepared by a process

in which both component polymers are polymerized concurrently, the SIPN may be referred to as a **simultaneous SIPN**. (This note has been changed from that which appears in ref. [4] to allow for the possibility that a linear or branched polymer may be incorporated into a network by means other than polymerization, e.g., by swelling of the network and subsequent diffusion of the linear or branched chain into the network.).

1.11 Immiscibility

Inability of a mixture to form a single phase.

Notes:

1. Immiscibility may be limited to certain ranges of temperature, pressure, and composition.
2. Immiscibility depends on the chemical structures, molar-mass distributions, and molecular architectures of the components.

1.12 Immiscible Polymer Blend
Heterogeneous Polymer Blend

Polymer blend that exhibits immiscibility.

1.13 Composite

Multicomponent material comprising multiple different (non-gaseous) phase domains in which at least one type of phase domain is a continuous phase (see **3.12**).

Note: Foamed substances, which are multiphased materials that consist of a gas dispersed in a liquid or solid, are not normally considered to be composites.

1.14 Polymer Composite

Composite in which at least one component is a polymer.

1.15 Nanocomposite

Composite in which at least one of the phases has at least one dimension of the order of nanometers.

1.16 Laminate

Material consisting of more than one layer, the layers being distinct in composition, composition profile, or anisotropy of properties.

Notes:

1. Laminates may be formed by two or more layers of different polymers.
2. Composite laminates generally consist of one or more layers of a substrate, often fibrous, impregnated with a curable polymer, curable polymers, or liquid reactants.
3. The substrate is usually a sheet-like woven or nonwoven material (e.g., glass fabric, paper, copper foil).
4. A single layer of a laminate is termed a **lamina**.

1.17 Lamination

Process of forming a laminate.

1.18 Delamination

Process that separates the layers of a laminate by breaking their structure in planes parallel to those layers.

1.19 Impregnation

Penetration of monomeric, oligomeric, or polymeric liquids into an assembly of fibers.

Notes:

1. The term as defined here is specific to polymer science. An alternative definition of "impregnation" applies in some other fields of chemistry (see the Gold Book, p. 197) [3].
2. Impregnation is usually carried out on a woven fabric or a yarn.

1.20 Prepreg
Sheets of a substrate that have been impregnated with a curable polymer, curable polymers, or liquid reactants, or a thermoplastic, and are ready for fabrication of laminates.

Notes:

1. See **1.16** notes 2 and 3.
2. During the impregnation the curable polymer, curable polymers, or liquid reactants may be allowed to react to a certain extent (sometimes termed **degree of ripening**).

1.21 Intercalation
Process by which a substance becomes transferred into pre-existing spaces of molecular dimensions in a second substance.

Note: The term as defined here is specific to polymer science. An alternative definition of "intercalation" applies in some other fields of chemistry (see the Gold Book, p. 202 [3]).

1.22 Exfoliation
Process by which thin layers individually separate from a multilayered structure.*Note*: In the context of a nanocomposite material, the individual layers are of the order of at most a few nanometers in thickness.

1.23 Wetting
Process by which an interface between a solid and a gas is replaced by an interface between the same solid and a liquid.

1.24 Adhesion
Holding together of two bodies by interfacial forces or mechanical interlocking on a scale of micrometers or less.

1.25 Chemical Adhesion
Adhesion (see **1.25**) in which two bodies are held together at an interface by ionic or covalent bonding between molecules on either side of the interface.

1.26 Interfacial Adhesion
Adhesion (see **1.25**) in which interfaces between phases or components are maintained by intermolecular forces, chain entanglements, or both, across the interfaces.

Notes:

1. Interfacial adhesion is also referred to as **tack**.
2. **Adhesive strength** (recommended symbol: F_a, unit: N m^{-2}) is the force required to separate one condensed phase domain from another at the interface between the two phase domains divided by the area of the interface.
3. **Interfacial tension** (recommended symbol: γ, unit: N m^{-1}, J m^{-2}) is the change in Gibbs energy per unit change in interfacial area for substances in physical contact.
4. Use of the term **interfacial energy** for interfacial tension is not recommended.

1.27 Interfacial Bonding
Bonding in which the surfaces of two bodies in contact with one another are held together by inter-molecular forces.

Note: Examples of intermolecular forces include covalent, ionic, van der Waals, and hydrogen bonds.

1.28 Interfacial Fracture
Brittle fracture that takes place at an interface.

1.29 Craze
Crack-like cavity formed when a polymer is stressed in tension that contains load-bearing fibrils spanning the gap between the surfaces of the cavity.

Note: Deformation of continua occurs with only minor changes in volume; hence, a craze consists of both fibrils and voids.

1.30 Additive
Substance added to a polymer.

Notes:

1. The term as defined here is specific to polymer science. An alternative definition of "additive" applies in some other fields of chemistry (see the Gold Book, p. 10) [3].
2. An additive is usually a minor component of the mixture formed and usually modifies the properties of the polymer.
3. Examples of additives are antioxidants, plasticizers, flame retardants, processing aids, other polymers, colorants, UV absorbers, and extenders.

1.31 Interfacial Agent
Additive that reduces the interfacial energy between phase domains.

1.32 Compatibility
Capability of the individual component substances in either an immiscible polymer blend (see **1.12**) or a polymer composite (see **1.14**) to exhibit interfacial adhesion (see **1.27**).

Notes:

1. Use of the term "compatibility" to describe miscible systems is discouraged.
2. Compatibility is often established by the observation of mechanical integrity under the intended conditions of use of a composite or an immiscible polymer blend.

1.33 Compatibilization
Process of modification of the interfacial properties in an immiscible polymer blend that results in formation of the interphases (see **3.6**) and stabilization of the morphology, leading to the creation of a polymer alloy.

Note: Compatibilization may be achieved by addition of suitable copolymers or by chemical modification of interfaces through physical treatment (i.e., irradiation or thermal) or reactive processing.

1.34 Degree of Compatibility
Measure of the strength of the interfacial bonding between the component substances of a composite or immiscible polymer blend (see **1.12**).

Notes:

1. Estimates of the degree of compatibility are often based upon the mechanical performance of the composite, the interphase thickness (see "Interfacial region interphase"), or the sizes of the phase domains present in the composite,

relative to the corresponding properties of composites lacking compatibility.

2. The term **degree of incompatibility** is sometimes used instead of degree of compatibility. Such use is discouraged as incompatibility is related to the weakness of interfacial bonding.

1.35 Compatible Polymer Blend

Immiscible polymer blend (see **1.12**) that exhibits macroscopically uniform physical properties throughout its whole volume.

Note: The macroscopically uniform physical properties are usually caused by sufficiently strong interactions between the component polymers.

1.36 Compatibilizer

Polymer or copolymer that, when added to an immiscible polymer blend (see **1.12**), modifies its inter-facial character and stabilizes its morphology.

Note: Compatibilizers usually stabilize morphologies over distances of the order of micrometers or less.

1.37 Coupling Agent Adhesion Promoter

Interfacial agent comprised of molecules possessing two or more functional groups, each of which exhibits preferential interactions with the various types of phase domains in a composite.

Notes:

1. A coupling agent increases adhesion between phase domains.
2. An example of the use of a coupling agent is in a mineral-filled polymer material where one part of the coupling agent molecule can chemically bond to the inorganic mineral while the other part can chemically bond to the polymer.

1.38 Polymer Alloy

Polymeric material, exhibiting macroscopically uniform physical properties throughout its whole volume, that comprises a compatible polymer blend (see **1.35**), a miscible polymer blend (see **1.3**), or a multiphase copolymer (see **3.3**).

Note: See note 5 in **1.1**.

1.39 Dispersion

Material comprising more than one phase where at least one of the phases consists of finely divided phase domains (see **3.2**), often in the colloidal size range, distributed throughout a continuous phase domain.

Notes:

1. The term as defined here is specific to polymer science. An alternative definition of "dispersion" applies in some other fields of chemistry (see the Gold Book, p. 118) [3].
2. Particles in the colloidal size range have linear dimensions [3] between 1 nm and 1 μm.
3. The finely divided domains are called the dispersed or discontinuous phase domains (see **3.13**).
4. For a definition of continuous phase domain, see **3.12**.
5. A dispersion is often further characterized on the basis of the size of the phase domain as a **macrodispersion** or a **microdispersion**. To avoid ambiguity when using these terms, the size of the domain should also be defined.

1.40 Dispersing Agent Dispersing Aid Dispersant

Additive (see **1.30**), exhibiting surface activity, that is added to a suspending medium to promote uniform and maximum separation of extremely fine solid particles, often of colloidal size (see note 2 in **1.39**).

Note: Although dispersing agents achieve results similar to compatibilizers (see **1.36**), they function differently in that they reduce the attractive forces between fine particles, which allows them to be more easily separated and dispersed.

1.41 Agglomeration Aggregation

Process in which dispersed molecules or particles form clusters rather than remain as isolated single molecules or particles.

Note: See the Gold Book, p. 13 [3].

1.42 Agglomerate Aggregate

Clusters of dispersed molecules or particles that results from agglomeration (see **1.41**).

Note: The term as defined here is specific to polymer science. An alternative definition of "aggregate" is used in some other fields of chemistry (see the Gold Book, p. 13) [3].

1.43 Extender

Substance, especially a diluent or modifier, added to a polymer to increase its volume without substantially altering the desirable properties of the polymer.

Note: An extender may be a liquid or a solid.

1.44 Filler

Solid extender.

Notes:

1. The term as defined here is specific to polymer science. An alternative definition of "filler" applies in some other fields of chemistry (see the Gold Book, p. 154) [3].
2. Fillers may be added to modify mechanical, optical, electrical, thermal, flammability properties, or simply to serve as extenders.

1.45 Fill Factor

Recommended symbol: ϕ_{fill}

Maximum volume fraction of a particulate filler that can be added to a polymer while maintaining the polymer as the continuous phase domain.

1.46 Thermoplastic Elastomer

Melt-processable polymer blend or copolymer in which a continuous elastomeric phase domain is reinforced by dispersed hard (glassy or crystalline) phase domains that act as junction points over a limited range of temperature.

Notes:

1. The behavior of the hard phase domains as junction points is thermally reversible.
2. The interfacial interaction between hard and soft phase domains in a thermoplastic elastomer is often the result of covalent bonds between the phases and is sufficient to prevent the flow of the elastomeric phase domain under conditions of use.
3. Examples of thermoplastic elastomers include block copolymers and blends of plastics and rubbers.

2. Phase Domain Behavior

2.1 Miscibility Window

Range of copolymer compositions in a polymer mixture, at least one component substance of which is a copolymer, that gives miscibility (see **1.2**) over a range of temperatures and pressures.

Notes:

1. Outside the miscibility window immiscible mixtures are formed.
2. The compositions of the copolymers within the miscibility window usually exclude the homopolymer compositions of the monomers from which the copolymers are prepared.
3. The miscibility window is affected by the molecular weights of the component substances.
4. The existence of miscibility windows has been attributed to an average force between the monomer units of the copolymer that leads to those units associating preferentially with the monomer units of the other polymers.

2.2 Miscibility Gap

Area within the coexistence curve of an isobaric phase diagram (temperature vs. composition) or an isothermal phase diagram (pressure vs. composition).

Note: A miscibility gap is observed at temperatures below an upper critical solution temperature (UCST) (see **2.15**) or above the lower critical solution temperature (LCST) (see **2.14**). Its location depends on pressure. In the miscibility gap, there are at least two phases coexisting.

2.3 Flory–Huggins Theory Flory–Huggins–Staverman Theory

Statistical thermodynamic mean-field theory of polymer solutions, formulated independently by Flory, Huggins, and Staverman, in which the thermodynamic quantities of the solution are derived from a simple concept of combinatorial entropy of mixing and a reduced Gibbs-energy parameter, the "χ interaction parameter" (see **2.4**).

Notes:

1. See the Gold Book, p. 158 [3].
2. The Flory–Huggins theory has often been found to have utility for polymer blends; however, there are many equation-of-state theories that provide more accurate descriptions of polymer–polymer interactions.
3. The present definition has been modified from that which appears in ref. [5] to acknowledge the contributions of Staverman and to further clarify the statistical basis of the theory.

2.4 χ Interaction Parameter

Recommended symbol: χ

Interaction parameter, employed in the Flory–Huggins theory (see **2.3**), to account for the contribution of the noncombinatorial entropy of mixing and the enthalpy of mixing to the Gibbs energy of mixing.

Notes:

1. The definition and the name of the term have been modified from that which appears in ref. [5] to reflect its broader use in the context of polymer blends. In its simplest form, the χ parameter is defined according to the Flory–Huggins equation for binary mixtures

$$\frac{\Delta_{mix}G}{RT} = n_1 \ln \phi_1 + n_2 \ln \phi_2 + \chi x_1 n_1 \phi_2,$$

for a mixture of amounts of substance n_1 and n_2 of components denoted 1 and 2, giving volume fractions ϕ_1 and ϕ_2, with the molecules of component 1 each conceptually consisting of x_1 segments whose Gibbs energy of interaction with segments of equal volume in the molecules of component 2 is characterized by the interaction parameter χ.

2. The χ interaction parameters characterizing a given system vary with composition, molar mass, and temperature.
3. B is an alternative parameter to χ, where $B = \chi RT/V_m$, in which V_m is the molar volume of one of the components of the mixture.

2.5 Nucleation of Phase Separation

Initiation of phase domain formation through the presence of heterogeneities.

Notes:

1. See the Gold Book, p. 277 [3].
2. In a metastable region of a phase diagram (see **1.2**), phase separation is initiated only by nucleation.

2.6 Binodal Binodal Curve Coexistence Curve

Curve defining the region of composition and temperature in a phase diagram for a binary mixture across which a transition occurs from miscibility of the components to conditions where single-phase mixtures are metastable or unstable (see note 4 in **1.2**).

Note: Binodal compositions are defined by pairs of points on the curve of Gibbs energy of mixing vs. composition that have common tangents, corresponding to compositions of equal chemical potentials of each of the two components in two phases.

2.7 Spinodal Spinodal Curve

Curve defining the region of composition and temperature for a binary mixture across which a transition occurs from conditions where single-phase mixtures are metastable to conditions where single-phase mixtures are unstable and undergo phase separation by spinodal decomposition (see **2.8**).

Notes:

1. The spinodal curve for a binary mixture is defined as the geometrical locus of all states with

$$\left(\frac{\partial^2 \Delta_{mix}G}{\partial \phi^2} \right)_{T,P} = 0 \text{ (see 1.2, note 4)}$$

2. In the unstable region bounded by the spinodal curve, phase domain separation is spontaneous, i.e., no nucleation step is required to initiate the separation process.

2.8 Spinodal Decomposition Spinodal Phase-Demixing

Long-range, diffusion-limited, spontaneous phase domain separation initiated by delocalized concentration fluctuations occurring in an unstable region of a mixture bounded by a spinodal curve.

Note: Spinodal decomposition occurs when the magnitude of Gibbs energy fluctuations with respect to composition are zero.

2.9 Cloud Point

Experimentally measured point in the phase diagram of a mixture at which a loss in transparency is observed due to light scattering caused by a transition from a single- to a two-phase state.

Notes:

1. The phenomenon is characterized by the first appearance of turbidity or cloudiness.
2. A cloud point is heating rate- or cooling rate-dependent.

2.10 Cloud-Point Curve

Curve of temperature vs. composition defined by the cloud points (see **2.9**) over range of compositions of two substances.

Note: Mixtures are observed to undergo a transition from a single- to a two-phase state upon heating or cooling.

2.11 Cloud-Point Temperature

Temperature at a cloud point (see **2.9**).

2.12 Critical Point

Point in the isobaric temperature-composition plane for a binary mixture where the compositions of all coexisting phases become identical.

Notes:

1. An alternative definition of "critical solution point" refers strictly to liquid-vapor equilibria (see the Gold Book, p. 93) [3].
2. Unless specified atmospheric pressure is assumed.
3. In a phase diagram, the slope of the tangent to the spinodal is zero at this point.
4. At a critical point, binodals and spinodals coincide.
5. Although the definition holds strictly for binary mixtures, it is often erroneously applied to multicomponent mixtures.
6. See note 3 in **1.2**.

2.13 Lower Critical Solution Temperature

Recommended acronym: LCST
Critical temperature below which a mixture is miscible.

Notes:

1. See the Gold Book, p. 93 [3].
2. Below the LCST and above the UCST (see **2.14**), if it exists, a single phase exists for all compositions.
3. The LCST depends upon pressure and the molar-mass distributions of the constituent polymer(s).
4. For a mixture containing or consisting of polymeric components, these may be different polymers or species of different molar mass of the same polymer.

2.14 Upper Critical Solution Temperature

Recommended abbreviation: UCST
Critical temperature above which a mixture is miscible.

Notes:

1. See the Gold Book, p. 93 [3].
2. Above the UCST and below the LCST (see **2.13**), if it exists, a single phase exists for all compositions.
3. The UCST depends upon the pressure and molar-mass distributions of the constituent polymer(s).

4. For a mixture containing or consisting of polymeric components, these may be different polymers or species of different molar mass of the same polymer.

2.15 Phase Inversion

Process by which an initially continuous phase domain becomes the dispersed phase domain and the initially dispersed phase domains become the continuous phase domain.

Notes:

1. See the Gold Book, p. 299 [3].
2. Phase inversion may be observed during the polymerization or melt processing of polymer blend systems.
3. The phenomenon is usually observed during polymerization of a monomer containing a dissolved polymer.

2.16 Interdiffusion

Process by which homogeneity in a mixture is approached by means of spontaneous mutual molecular diffusion.

2.17 Blooming

Process in which one component of a polymer mixture, usually not a polymer, undergoes phase separation and migration to an external surface of the mixture.

2.18 Coalescence

Process in which two phase domains of essentially identical composition in contact with one another form a larger phase domain.

Notes:

1. See the Gold Book, p. 75 [3].
2. Coalescence reduces the total interfacial area.
3. The flocculation of a polymer colloid, through the formation of aggregates, may be followed by coalescence.

2.19 Morphology Coarsening Phase Ripening

Process by which phase domains increase in size during the aging of a multiphase material.

Notes:

1. In the coarsening at the late stage of phase separation, volumes and compositions of phase domains are conserved.
2. Representative mechanisms for coarsening at the late stage of phase separation are: (1) material flow in domains driven by interfacial tension (observed in a co-continuous morphology), (2) the growth of domain size by evaporation from smaller droplets and condensation into larger droplets, and (3) coalescence (fusion) of more than two droplets. The mechanisms are usually called (1) Siggia's mechanism, (2) Ostwald ripening (or the Lifshitz-Slyozov mechanism), and (3) coalescence.
3. Morphology coarsening can be substantially stopped by, for example, vitrification, crosslinking, and **pinning**, the slowing down of molecular diffusion across domain interfaces.

3. Domains and Morphologies

Many types of morphologies have been reported in the literature of multiphase polymeric materials. It is the intent of this document to define only the most commonly used terms. In addition, some morphologies have historically been described by very imprecise terms that may not have universal meanings. However, if such terms are widely used they are defined here.

3.1 Morphology
Shape, optical appearance, or form of phase domains in substances, such as high polymers, polymer blends, composites, and crystals.

Note: For a polymer blend or composite, the morphology describes the structures and shapes observed, often by microscopy or scattering techniques, of the different phase domains present within the mixture.

3.2 Phase Domain
Region of a material that is uniform in chemical composition and physical state.

Notes:

1. A phase in a multiphase material can form domains differing in size.
2. The term "domain" may be qualified by the adjective microscopic or nanoscopic or the prefix micro- or nano- according to the size of the linear dimensions of the domain.
3. The prefixes micro-, and nano- are frequently incorrectly used to qualify the term "phase" instead of the term "domain"; hence, "microphase domain", and "nanophase domain" are often used. The correct terminology that should be used is **phase microdomain** and **phase nanodomain**.

3.3 Multiphase Copolymer
Copolymer comprising phase-separated domains.

3.4 Domain Interface Domain Boundary
Surface forming a boundary between two phase domains.

Note: A representation of the domain interface as a two-dimensional surface over-simplifies the actual structure. All interfaces have a third dimension, namely, the interphase or interfacial region (see **3.6**).

3.5 Domain Structure
Morphology of individual phase domains in a multiphase system.

Note: Domain structures may be described for phase domains or domains that are themselves multiphased structures.

3.6 Interfacial Region Interphase
Region between phase domains in an immiscible polymer blend in which a gradient in composition exists.

Note: See the Gold Book, p. 205 [3].

3.7 Phase Interaction
Molecular interaction between the components present in the interphases of a multiphase mixture.

Note: The **interphase elasticity** is the capability of a deformed interphase to return to its original dimensions after the force causing the deformation has been removed.

3.8 Interfacial-Region Thickness Interphase Thickness Interfacial Width
Linear extent of the composition gradient in an interfacial region.

Notes:

1. See the Gold Book, p. 203 [3].

2. The width at half the maximum of the composition profile across the interfacial region (see **3.6**) or the distance between locations where $d\phi/dr$ (with ϕ the composition of a component and r the distance through the interfacial region) has decreased to $1/e$ are used as measures of the interfacial-region thickness.

3.9 Hard-Segment Phase Domain
Phase domain of microscopic or smaller size, usually in a block, graft, or segmented copolymer (see **3.11**), comprising essentially those segments of the polymer that are rigid and capable of forming strong intermolecular interactions.

Note: Hard-segment phase domains are typically of 2–15 nm linear size.

3.10 Soft-Segment Phase Domain
Phase domain of microscopic or smaller size, usually in a block, graft, or segmented copolymer (see **3.11**), comprising essentially those segments of the polymer that have glass transition temperatures lower than the temperature of use.

Note: Soft-segment phase domains are often larger than hard-segment phase domains and are often continuous.

3.11 Segmented Copolymer
Copolymer containing phase domains of microscopic or smaller size, with the domains constituted principally of single types of structural unit.

Note: The types of domain in a segmented copolymer usually comprise hard- and soft-segment phase domains.

3.12 Continuous Phase Domain Matrix Phase Domain
Phase domain (see **3.2**) consisting of a single phase in a heterogeneous mixture through which a continuous path to all phase domain boundaries may be drawn without crossing a phase domain boundary.

Note: In a polymer blend, the continuous phase domain is sometimes referred to as the **host polymer, bulk substance**, or **matrix**.

3.13 Discontinuous Phase Domain Discrete Phase Domain Dispersed Phase Domain
Phase domain in a phase-separated mixture that is surrounded by a continuous phase but isolated from all other similar phase domains within the mixture.

Note: The discontinuous phase domain is sometimes referred to as the **guest polymer**.

3.14 Dual Phase Domain Continuity Co-Continuous Phase Domains
Topological condition, in a phase-separated, two-component mixture, in which a continuous path through either phase domain may be drawn to all phase domain boundaries without crossing any phase domain boundary.

3.15 Core-Shell Morphology
Two-phase domain morphology, of approximately spherical shape, comprising two polymers, each in separate phase domains, in which phase domains of one polymer completely encapsulate the phase domains of the other polymer.

Note: This morphology is most commonly observed in copolymers or blends prepared in emulsion polymerization by the sequential addition and polymerization of two different monomer compositions.

3.16 Cylindrical Morphology

Phase domain morphology, usually comprising two polymers, each in separate phase domains, in which the phase domains of one polymer are of cylindrical shape.

Notes:

1. Phase domains of the constituent polymers may alternate, which results in many cylindrical layers surrounding a central core domain.
2. Cylindrical morphologies can be observed, for example, in triblock copolymers.

3.17 Fibrillar Morphology

Morphology in which phase domains have shapes with one dimension much larger than the other two dimensions.

Note: Fibrillar phase domains have the appearance of fibers.

3.18 Lamellar Domain Morphology

Morphology in which phase domains have shapes with two dimensions much larger than the third dimension.

Note: Plate-like phase domains have the appearance of extended planes that are often oriented essentially parallel to one another.

3.19 Microdomain Morphology

Morphology consisting of phase microdomains.

Notes:

1. See **3.2**.
2. Microdomain morphologies are usually observed in block, graft, and segmented copolymers.
3. The type of morphology observed depends upon the relative abundance of the different types of structural units and the conditions for the generation of the morphology. The most commonly observed morphologies are spheres, cylinders, and lamellae.

3.20 Nanodomain Morphology

Morphology consisting of phase nanodomains.

Note: See **3.2**.

3.21 Onion Morphology

Multiphase morphology of roughly spherical shape that comprises alternating layers of different polymers arranged concentrically, all layers being of similar thickness.

3.22 Ordered Co-Continuous Double Gyroid Morphology

Co-continuous morphology in which a set of two gyroid-based phase domains exhibits a highly regular, three-dimensional lattice-like morphology with Ia3d space group symmetry.

Notes:

1. The domains are composed of tripoidal units as the fundamental building structures.
2. The two domains are interlaced.

3.23 Multicoat Morphology

Morphology observed in a blend of a block copolymer with the homopolymer of one of the blocks and characterized by alternating concentric shells of the copolymer and the homopolymer.

Note: The morphology is identical to onion morphology (see **3.21**) within a matrix of homopolymer [6].

3.24 Rod-Like Morphology

Morphology characterized by cylindrical phase domains.

3.25 Multiple Inclusion Morphology Salami-Like Morphology

Multiphase morphology in which dispersed phase domains of one polymer contain and completely encapsulate many phase domains of a second polymer that may have the same composition as the continuous phase domain (see **3.12**).

References

1. IUPAC. "Definitions of terms relating to crystalline polymers (IUPAC Recommendations 1988)" *Pure Appl. Chem.* **61**, 769–785 (1989).
2. IUPAC. "Definitions of basic terms relating to low-molar-mass and polymer liquid crystals (IUPAC Recommendations 2001)", *Pure Appl. Chem.* **75**, 845–895 (2001).
3. IUPAC. *Compendium of Chemical Terminology* (the "Gold Book"), compiled by A. D. McNaught and A. Wilkinson, 2nd ed., Blackwell Science, Oxford (1997).
4. IUPAC. "Glossary of basic terms in polymer science (IUPAC Recommendations 1996)", *Pure Appl. Chem.* **68**, 2287–2311 (1996).
5. D. K. Carpenter. "Solution properties", in *Encyclopedia of Polymer Science and Engineering*, Vol. 15, 2nd ed., J. I. Kroschwitz (Ed.), pp. 419–481, Wiley Interscience, New York (1989).
6. J. M. G. Cowie. "Miscibility", in *Encyclopedia of Polymer Science and Engineering*, 2nd ed., J. I. Kroschwitz (Ed.), Supplement, pp. 455–480, Wiley Interscience, New York (1989).

Bibliography

1. IUPAC. "Definitions of terms relating to degradation, aging, and related chemical transformations of polymers (IUPAC Recommendations 1996)", *Pure Appl. Chem.* **68**, 2313–2323 (1996).
2. *ASTM Glossary of ASTM Definitions*, 2nd ed., American Society for Testing and Materials, Philadelphia, PA (1973).
3. IUPAC. *Compendium of Macromolecular Nomenclature* (the "Purple Book"), prepared for publication by W. V. Metanomski, Blackwell Scientific, Oxford (1991).
4. A. N. Gent and G. R. Hamed. "Adhesion", in *Encyclopedia of Polymer Science and Engineering*, Vol. 1, 2nd ed., J. I. Kroschwitz (Ed.), pp. 476–517, Wiley Interscience, New York (1985).
5. L. Leibler. "Phase transformations", in *Encyclopedia of Polymer Science and Engineering*, Vol. 11, 2nd ed., J. I. Kroschwitz, (Ed.), pp. 30–45, Wiley Interscience, New York (1988).
6. J. Koberstein. "Interfacial properties", in *Encyclopedia of Polymer Science and Engineering*, Vol. 8, 2nd ed., J. I. Kroschwitz (Ed.), pp. 237–279, Wiley Interscience, New York (1987).
7. D. W. Fox and R. B. Allen. "Compatibility", in *Encyclopedia of Polymer Science and Engineering*, Vol. 3, 2nd ed., J. I. Kroschwitz (Ed.), pp. 758–775, Wiley Interscience, New York (1985).
8. R. A. Orwoll. "Solubility of polymers", *Encyclopedia of Polymer Science and Engineering*, Vol. 15, 2nd ed., J. I. Kroschwitz (Ed.), pp. 380–402, Wiley Interscience, New York (1989).
9. L. H. Sperling. "Microphase structure", in *Encyclopedia of Polymer Science and Engineering*, Vol. 9, 2nd ed., J. I. Kroschwitz (Ed.), pp. 760–788, Wiley Interscience, New York (1987).

10. D. R. Paul, J. W. Barlow, and H. Keskkula. "Polymer blends", in *Encyclopedia of Polymer Science and Engineering*, Vol. 12, 2nd ed., J. I. Kroschwitz (Ed.), pp. 399–461, Wiley Interscience, New York (1988).

11. D. R. Paul and S. Newman. *Polymer Blends*, Academic Press, New York (1978).

12. D. R. Paul and C. B. Bucknall. *Polymer Blends: Formulation and Performance*, John Wiley, New York (1999).

13. L. A. Utracki. *Polymer Alloys and Blends*, Hanser Publishers, New York (1990).

Alphabetical Index of Terms

Alphabetical Index of Terms (Continued)

Term	Definition No.	Term	Definition No.
phase domain	3.2	sequential SIPN	1.10
phase interaction	3.7	semi-interpenetrating polymer network (SIPN)	1.10
phase inversion	2.15	simultaneous IPN	1.9
phase microdomain	3.2	simultaneous SIPN	1.10
phase nanodomain	3.2	soft-segment phase domain	3.10
phase ripening	2.19	spinodal	2.7
pinning	2.19	spinodal curve	2.7
polymer alloy	1.38	spinodal decomposition	2.8
polymer blend	1.1	spinodal phase-demixing	2.8
polymer composite	1.14	tack	1.26
polymer–polymer complex	1.6	thermoplastic elastomer	1.46
prepreg	1.20	upper critical solution temperature	2.14
rod-like morphology	3.24	(UCST)	
salami-like morphology	3.25	wetting	1.23
segmented copolymer	3.11	χ interaction parameter	2.4
sequential IPN	1.9		

TERMINOLOGY FOR BIORELATED POLYMERS AND APPLICATIONS (IUPAC RECOMMENDATIONS 2012)*

Michel Vert[1,‡], Yoshiharu Doi[2], Karl-Heinz Hellwich[3], Michael Hess[4], Philip Hodge[5], Przemyslaw Kubisa[6], Marguerite Rinaudo[7], and François Schué[8]

[1]University Montpellier 1-CNRS, Montpellier, France;
[2]RIKEN, Saitama, Japan;
[3]Postfach 10 07 31, Offenbach, Germany;
[4]Universität Siegen, Siegen, Germany;
[5]University of Manchester, Manchester, UK;
[6]Polish Academy of Sciences, Łódz, Poland;
[7]CERMAV-CNRS, Grenoble, France;
[8]University Montpellier 2, Montpellier, France

Abstract: Like most of the materials used by humans, polymeric materials are proposed in the literature and occasionally exploited clinically, as such, as devices or as part of devices, by surgeons, dentists, and pharmacists to treat traumata and diseases. Applications have in common the fact that polymers function in contact with animal and human cells, tissues, and/or organs. More recently, people have realized that polymers that are used as plastics in packaging, as colloidal suspension in paints, and under many other forms in the environment, are also in contact with living systems and raise problems related to sustainability, delivery of chemicals or pollutants, and elimination of wastes. These problems are basically comparable to those found in therapy. Last but not least, biotechnology and renewable resources are regarded as attractive sources of polymers. In all cases, water, ions, biopolymers, cells, and tissues are involved. Polymer scientists, therapists, biologists, and ecologists should thus use the same terminology to reflect similar properties, phenomena, and mechanisms. Of particular interest is the domain of the so-called "degradable or biodegradable polymers" that are aimed at providing materials with specific time-limited applications in medicine and in the environment where the respect of living systems, the elimination, and/or the bio-recycling are mandatory, at least ideally.

Keywords: biodegradability; biomaterials; biomedicine; bioresorbability; degradability; dentistry; environment; IUPAC Polymer Division; polymers; pharmacology.

Contents

Introduction

For thousands of years, humans have been using available substances for applications as materials, i.e., as substances of practical interest to achieve specific functions. As soon as they became industrially available, man-made polymers (as opposed to natural polymers) have been tested to serve in therapy, several having found clinical and commercial applications, thanks to the development of medical grades. Examples of such compounds are ultra-high-molar-mass polyethylene (UHMWPE), polytetrafluoroethylene (PTFE), poly(methyl methacrylate) (PMMA), and other acrylics and methacrylics, silicones, polyurethanes, etc., that are successfully used for applications such as total hip prosthesis (UHMWPE), vascular grafts (PTFE, silicones), intraocular lenses [PMMA and poly(2-hydroxyethyl methacrylate) (PHEMA) and silicones], dentistry (PMMA and other methacrylics), etc. Among these applications, some require

a therapeutic aid for a limited period of time, namely, the healing period. Ideally, the temporary therapeutic aid must disappear from the body after healing in order to avoid storage of unnecessary foreign material. Indeed, skin, mucosa, and various endothelia are semi-permeable barriers that are closed to macromolecular compounds with molar mass higher than ca. 10^3 g·mol^{-1}. Accordingly, high-molar-mass molecules introduced in the gastrointestinal (GI or enteral compartment) tract cannot be absorbed by the intestinal mucosa, whereas those introduced in parenteral (between skin and mucosa) compartments of animal or human bodies are entrapped. There are only two exits available. The first is the kidneys via complex filtration, but molecules have to be soluble in blood. The second is the lungs, but molecules have to be metabolized and converted to water and carbon dioxide. Exceptionally, cyst formation can lead to expulsion through the skin. Therefore, any high-molar-mass macromolecule or polymer that is to be used parenterally for a limited period of time has to be first degraded, in terms of molar mass decrease, and turned into soluble low-molar-mass compounds to be excretable, unless degradation byproducts can be biochemically

* Sponsoring body: IUPAC Polymer Division: see more details on p. 874.
  Reproduced from: *Pure & Appl. Chem.*, Vol. 84, No. 2, pp. 377–410, 2012.

processed and transformed into carbon dioxide, water, and biomass. The demand of surgical life-respecting polymers was progressively extended to domains like pharmacology (drug delivery systems, bioactive macromolecules) and dentistry (bone augmentation, periodontal membranes). The most recent research is oriented toward tissue engineering and medicated temporary prostheses, i.e., temporary prostheses that are associated with drugs or other bioactive substances, including macromolecules (DNA, genes, proteins, and peptides). Therefore, biology is also implicated.

More recently, humans have started to pay attention to the fact that, in outdoor applications, nonnatural polymers are also in contact with living systems. Initially selected for their resistance to the attack by microorganisms, industrial polymers are now sources of problems related to their biostability in connection with the concept of time-limited applications after which a material becomes waste. In the environment, there are two different problems related to the use of bioresistant polymers and derived objects: (i) littering with its hidden form of water-soluble and water-dispersed macromolecular compounds that are found in detergents, cosmetics, paints, and washings products and (ii) industrial treatment of corresponding collected wastes in water-treatment and in composting plants. Basically, the elimination of environmental wastes and that of biomedical residues left after healing are comparable.

Science and applications of biorelated polymers require people of different disciplines and scien-tific domains. From the terminology viewpoint, polymer-based substances and devices aimed at working in contact with living systems are firstly relevant to terms and definitions recommended to polymer scientists, producers, and users by IUPAC through its various publications. However, scientists and users of other fields of application have often developed incoherent terminologies.

The aim of the following recommendations is to provide a terminology usable without any confusion in the various domains dealing with biorelated polymers, namely, medicine, surgery, pharmacology, agriculture, packaging, biotechnology, polymer waste management, etc. This is necessary because (i) human health and environmental sustainability are more and more interdependent, (ii) research, applications, norms, and regulations are still developed independently in each sector, and (iii) nonspecialists like journalists, politicians, and partners of complementary disciplines are more and more implicated and need a common language.

Within each definition, terms defined elsewhere in the glossary are indicated by italics upon their first use.

Terms Common to All Domains

1. **abiotic abiological**
   Not associated with living systems [1].

2. **absorption (chemistry)**
   Process of penetration and diffusion of a substance (absorbate) into another substance (absorbent) as a result of the action of attractive phenomena.

   Note 1: Modified from [2]. The definition given in [2] does not reflect the dynamic of absorption and creates confusion with *adsorption* (surface phenomenon).

   Note 2: The attractive phenomena can be a gradient of concentration, affinity for the absorbent, etc.
   Note 3: In pharmacology, absorption means transfer of a *drug* from the enteral to the parenteral compartments.

3. **adhesion**
   Process of attachment of a substance to the surface of another substance.

   Note 1: Adhesion requires energy that can come from chemical and/or physical linkages, the latter being reversible when enough energy is applied.

   Note 2: In biology, adhesion reflects the behavior of cells shortly after contact to a surface.

   Note 3: In surgery, adhesion is used when two tissues fuse unexpectedly.

4. **adsorption**
   Increase in the concentration of a substance at the interface of a condensed and a liquid or gaseous layer owing to the operation of surface forces [1].

   Note 1: Adsorption of proteins is of great importance when a *material* is in contact with blood or body fluids. In the case of blood, albumin, which is largely predominant, is generally adsorbed first, and then rearrangements occur in favor of other minor proteins according to surface affinity against mass law selection (Vroman effect).
   Note 2: Adsorbed molecules are those that are resistant to washing with the same solvent medium in the case of adsorption from solutions. The washing conditions can thus modify the measurement results, particularly when the interaction energy is low.

5. **aggregate agglomerate**
   Scrambled auto-assembly of otherwise isolated single molecules or particles.

   Note 1: Adapted from definitions in [2–4] to reflect the absence of order.

   Note 2: Comb-like amphiphilic *macromolecules* form aggregates and not *micelles*, in contrast to diblock amphiphilic copolymers.

6. **artificial**
   Qualifier for something that is made by human activity, rather than occurring naturally [5].

7. **artificial polymer**
   Man-made *polymer* that is not a *biopolymer*.

   Note 1: Artificial polymer should also be used in the case of chemically modified biopolymers.

   Note 2: Biochemists are now capable of synthesizing copies of biopolymers that should be named synthetic biopolymers to make a distinction with true biopolymers.

   Note 3: *Genetic engineering* is now capable of generating non-natural analogues of biopolymers that should be referred to as artificial biopolymers, e.g., artificial protein, artificial polynucleotide, etc.

8. **autocatalytic reaction**
   Chemical reaction in which a product (or a reaction intermediate) also functions as a *catalyst* [2].

   Note: In such a reaction, the observed rate of reaction is often found to increase with time from its initial value.

9. **bioactive**
Qualifier for a substance that provokes any response from a living system.

> *Note*: Modified from [6]. The given definition *"material which has been designed to induce specific biological activity"* is limited to material made bioactive on purpose. However, the concept of *bioactivity* does not imply beneficial action only, although the term is often used positively, i.e., to reflect a beneficial action.

10. **bioactivity biological activity**
Capability of a substance, such as a *drug* or a vaccine, to provoke a response from a living matter.

> *Note 1*: Modified from [5]. The definition is more general.
> *Note 2*: There is no *polymer* (solid or in solution) that is inert in contact with a living system, because of *adsorption* and/or physical-chemical interactions with life elements (*biopolymers*, cells, and tissues).

> *Note 3*: *Stealth* is often used to reflect the absence of recognition by defense proteins of the complement, and more generally opsonins that serve as binding enhancers for the process of phagocytosis.

11. **bioadhesion bioattachment**
Adhesion of cells or tissues to the surface of a *material* [6].

> *Note 1*: Cell adhesion is generally followed by proliferation as a *biofilm* or as a tissue.

> *Note 2*: Assessing of adhesion is made after washing to eliminate unattached cells.

> *Note 3*: The use of the term "bioattachment" is discouraged.

12. **bioalteration (polymer)**
Cell-mediated chemical modification without main *chain scission*. (See *biodegradation*.)

13. **bioassay**
Measurement used to determine the concentration or *bioactivity* of a substance (e.g., vitamin, hormone, plant growth factor, and antibiotic) by measuring its effect on an organism or tissue compared to a standard preparation [2].

14. **bioassimilation**
Conversion of a substance into *biomass* by biochemical processes.

15. **bioavailability**
Property of being accessible to a living system to achieve or undergo a specific biological action.

> *Note 1*: Modified from [1,2] to be general and correspond to a property and not to a quantity.

> *Note 2*: The use of biological availability and physiological availability suggested in [1] as synonymous is not recommended.

> *Note 3*: In general, how much a substance or part of a substance is bioavailable is reflected by the quantification of the achieved or undergone action. (See *biodegradation, degree of biodegradation, degree of biofragmentation*, for instances.)

> *Note 4*: In *pharmacology*, fraction of an administered dose of unchanged drug that reaches the systemic circulation, one of the principal *pharmacokinetic* parameters of drugs [7].

16. **biobased**
Composed or derived in whole or in part of biological products issued from the *biomass* (including plant, animal, and marine or forestry *materials*).

> *Note*: A biobased *polymer* or polymeric device is not necessarily *environmentally friendly* nor *biocompatible* nor *biodegradable*, especially if it is similar to a petro-based (oil-based) polymer.

17. **biocatalyst**
Molecule or molecular complex consisting of, or derived from, an organism or cell culture (in cell-free or whole-cell forms) that catalyses metabolic reactions in living organisms and/or substrate conversions in various chemical reactions.

> *Note*: Modified from [2] to be consistent with the definition of *enzyme*.

18. **biocompatibility**
Ability to be in contact with a living system without producing an adverse effect.

19. **biodegradability**
Capability of being degraded by biological activity.

> *Note*: In vitro activity of isolated *enzymes* cannot be considered as *biological activity*. (See *biodegradation* and *enzymatic degradation*.)

20. **biodegradable**
Qualifier for a substance or device that undergoes *biodegradation*.

21. **biodegradable (biorelated polymer)**
Qualifier for *macromolecules* or polymeric substances susceptible to *degradation* by *biological activity* by lowering of the molar masses of *macromolecules* that form the substances.

> *Note 1*: Adapted from [8] to include the notion of decrease of molar mass in the definition.

> *Note 2*: It is important to note that in the field of *biorelated polymers*, a biodegradable compound is *degradable* whereas a *degradable polymer* is not necessarily biodegradable.

> *Note 3*: Degradation of a polymer in vivo or in the environment resulting from the sole water without any contribution from living elements is not *biodegradation*. The use of *hydrolysis* is recommended. (See also *degradation*.)

22. **biodegradation**
Degradation caused by enzymatic process resulting from the action of cells.

> *Note*: Modified from [8] to exclude *abiotic enzymatic* processes.

23. **biodegradation (biorelated polymer)**
Degradation of a polymeric item due to cell-mediated phenomena [9].

> *Note 1*: The definition given in [2] is misleading because a substance can be degraded by *enzymes* in vitro and never be degraded in vivo or in the environment because of a lack of proper enzyme(s) in situ (or simply a lack of water). This is the reason why *biodegradation* is referred to as limited to degradation resulting from cell activity.

(See *enzymatic degradation*.) The definition in [2] is also confusing because a compounded *polymer* or a copolymer can include bioresistant additives or moieties, respectively. *Theoretical biodegradation* should be used to reflect the sole organic parts that are *biodegradable*. (See *theoretical degree of biodegradation* and *maximum degree of biodegradation*.)

Note 2: In vivo, degradation resulting solely from hydrolysis by the water present in tissues and organs is not biodegradation; it must be referred to as *hydrolysis* or *hydrolytic degradation*.

Note 3: *Ultimate biodegradation* is often used to indicate complete transformation of organic compounds to either fully oxidized or reduced simple molecules (such as carbon dioxide/methane, nitrate/ammonium, and water. It should be noted that, in case of partial biodegradation, residual products can be more harmful than the initial substance.

Note 4: When biodegradation is combined with another degrading phenomenon, a term combining prefixes can be used, such as oxo-biodegradation, provided that both contributions are demonstrated.

Note 5: Biodegradation should only be used when the mechanism is proved, otherwise degradation is pertinent.

Note 6: *Enzymatic degradation* processed abiotically in vitro is not biodegradation.

Note 7: Cell-mediated chemical modification without main *chain scission* is not biodegradation. (See *bioalteration*.)

24. **biodisintegration**
Disintegration resulting from the action of cells.

25. **bioerosion**
Surface *degradation* resulting from the action of cells.

Note 1: *Erosion* is a general characteristic of *biodegradation* by cells that adhere to a surface and the molar mass of the bulk does not change, basically. (See *heterogeneous degradation*.)

Note 2: Chemical degradation can present the characteristics of cell-mediated *erosion* when the rate of chemical *chain scission* is greater than the rate of penetration of the cleaving chemical reagent, like diffusion of water in the case of hydrolytically *degradable polymer*, for instance.

Note 3: Erosion with constancy of the bulk molar mass is also observed in the case of in vitro abiotic enzymatic degradation.

Note 4: In some cases, bioerosion results from a combination of cell-mediated and chemical degradation, actually.

26. **biofilm**
Aggregate of microorganisms in which cells that are frequently embedded within a self-produced matrix of extracellular polymeric substance (EPS) adhere to each other and/or to a surface.

Note 1: A biofilm is a fixed system that can be adapted internally to environmental conditions by its inhabitants.

Note 2: The self-produced matrix of EPS, which is also referred to as slime, is a polymeric conglomeration generally composed of extracellular *biopolymers* in various structural forms.

27. **biofragmentation**
Fragmentation resulting from the action of cells.

28. **biomacromolecule**
Macromolecule (including proteins, nucleic acids, and polysaccharides) formed by living organisms.

Note: Not to be confused with *biopolymer*, although this term is often used as a synonym. In [2] the same definition is assigned to biopolymer. This is not recommended. (See *macromolecule* and *polymer*.)

29. **biomass**
Living systems and collection of organic substances produced by living systems that are exploitable as *materials*, including recent postmortem residues. (See *material*.)

Note 1: Modified from [2] to be more general.

Note 2: In energy, fossil substances like oil and coal that are issued from the long-term transformation of substances of the biomass are sometime considered as parts of the biomass.

Note 3: Living systems also produce minerals that are not integrated in biomass.

30. **biomaterial**
Material exploited in contact with living tissues, organisms, or microorganisms.

Note 1: The notion of exploitation includes utility for applications and for fundamental research to understand reciprocal perturbations as well.

Note 2: The definition "non-viable material used in a medical device, intended to interact with biological systems" recommended in [6] cannot be extended to the environmental field where people mean "material of natural origin".

Note 3: This general term should not be confused with the terms *biopolymer* or *biomacromolecule*. The use of "polymeric biomaterial" is recommended when one deals with *polymer* or polymer device of therapeutic or biological interest.

31. **biomineralization**
Mineralization caused by cell-mediated phenomena [9].

Note: Biomineralization is a process generally concomitant to *biodegradation*.

32. **biopolymer**
Substance composed of one type of *biomacromolecules*.

Note 1: Modified from the definition given in [2] in order to avoid confusion between *polymer* and *macromolecule* in the fields of proteins, polysaccharides, polynucleotides, and bacterial aliphatic polyesters.

Note 2: The use of the term "biomacromolecule" is recommended when molecular characteristics are considered.

33. **bioreactor**
Apparatus used to grow and/or take advantage of cells or microorganisms or of biochemically active compounds derived from these living systems to produce or modify substances by biochemical processes.

Note: Modified from the definition given in [2]. The definition proposed here is more general.

34. **biorelated**
Qualifier for actions or substances that are connected to living systems.

35. **biostability**
Resistance to the deleterious action of living systems that allows preservation of the initial characteristics of a substance.

   Note: If the substance is involved in an application, the term has to be related to a desired duration of performance, because almost any *material* ages in contact with living systems and biochemical processes regardless of the domain.

36. **biotechnology**
Integration of natural sciences and engineering in order to achieve the application of organisms, cells, parts thereof, and their molecular analogues for products and services [2].

37. **biotic**
Pertaining to, or produced by, living cells or organisms.

38. **bulk degradation**
Homogeneous *degradation* affecting the volume of a sample.

   Note 1: Modified from [9]. The definition given therein is not general.

   Note 2: The molar mass of the whole sample decreases progressively as opposed to the constancy observed in the case of *erosion* and *bioerosion*.

   Note 3: This expression is often used when degradation is faster inside than at the surface. This is not appropriate. Nevertheless, it should be adopted specifically in opposition to erosion. In this case, the molar mass distribution becomes rapidly bimodal.

   Note 4: Generally, degradation is faster inside because of autocatalysis by entrapped degradation byproducts or by the presence of a chain-cleaving reagent entrapped within the matrix.

39. **catalyst**
Substance that increases the rate of a reaction without modifying the overall standard Gibbs energy change in the reaction.

40. **chain scission chain cleavage**
Chemical reaction resulting in the breaking of skeletal bonds [2]. (See *degradation*.)

   Note: In the field of *biorelated polymers*, chain scission and degradation are interchangeable although the latter is more commonly used.

41. **chiral**
Having the property of *chirality* [2].

   Note: As applied to a molecule, the term has been used differently by different workers. Some apply it exclusively to the whole molecule, whereas others apply it to parts of a molecule. For example, according to the latter view, a meso compound is considered to be composed of two chiral parts of opposite chirality sense; this usage is to be discouraged.

42. **chirality**
Property of an object (or spatial arrangement of points or atoms) of being non-superposable on its mirror image; such an object has no symmetry elements of the second kind (a mirror plane, $\int = S_1$, a centre of inversion, $i = S_2$, a rotation-reflection axis, S_{2n}).

   Note 1: Modified from [2] to avoid reference to geometry.

   Note 2: If the object is superposable on its mirror image, the object is described as being achiral [2].

   Note 3: In chemistry, the object can be an atom holding a set of ligands, a molecule, or a *macromolecule* with blocked nonplanar conformation, or a self-assembled plurimolecular system like liquid crystals, although the use of the term is not recommended in this case [2].

43. **conjugate**
Molecule obtained by covalent coupling of at least two chemical entities, one of them having a special function.

   Note 1: Modified from [1] to emphasize the notion of function.

   Note 2: The specific function may, for example, be exerted by a drug, a dye, or a chemical reagent.

   Note 3: One of the chemical entities can be a macromolecule or a polymer. (See *prodrug, drug carrier*, and *macromolecular prodrug*.)

44. **controlled delivery**
Supply of a substance according to desired rate and amount over time.

   Note: If only a delayed or prolonged release is obtained without matching a desired release profile, the expression *sustained delivery* is to be used.

45. **controlled release**
Progressive appearance of a substance outgoing from an including system according to desired characteristics.

   Note 1: The control is generally obtained by designing the system adequately.

   Note 2: If the progressive appearance is spontaneous, the expression *sustained release* is to be used.

46. **degradability**
Capability of undergoing *degradation*.

47. **degradable**
Qualifier to a substance that can undergo physical and/or chemical deleterious changes of some properties especially of integrity under stress conditions.

48. **degradable macromolecule**
Macromolecule that is able to undergo *chain scissions* under specific conditions, resulting in a decrease of molar mass.

49. **degradable polymer**
Polymer in which *macromolecules* are able to undergo *chain scissions*, resulting in a decrease of molar mass. (See *degradation* (biorelated polymer).)

50. **degradation**

Progressive loss of the performance or of the characteristics of a substance or a device. (See *degradable*.)

Note: The process of degradation may be specified by a prefix or an adjective preceding the term "degradation". For example, degradation caused by the action of water is termed "hydrodegradation" or *hydrolysis*; by visible or ultraviolet light is termed "photodegradation"; by the action of oxygen or by the combined action of light and oxygen is termed "oxidative degradation" or "photooxidative degradation", respectively; by the action of heat or by the combined effect of chemical agents and heat is termed "thermal degradation" or "thermochemical degradation", respectively; by the combined action of heat and oxygen is termed "thermooxidative degradation".

51. **degradation (biorelated polymer)**

Degradation that results in desired changes in the values of in-use properties of the *material* because of *macromolecule* cleavage and molar mass decrease.

Note 1: Adapted from [8] where the definition is general. For *biorelated polymers*, the definition is purposely and specifically limited to the chemical degradation of macromolecules in order to make a clear distinction with the physical degradation of the material. (See *fragmentation* and *disintegration*.)

Note 2: In any condition, degradation must be used instead of *biodegradation* when the mechanism of *chain scission* is not known or demonstrated as cell-mediated.

Note 3: Degradation can result from the action of *enzymes* (see *enzymatic degradation*), or from the action of cells, organisms, and/or microorganisms. (See *biodegradation*.)

52. **degree of bioassimilation**

Mass fraction of a substance that is bioassimilated [9].

53. **degree of biodegradation**

Mass fraction of a substance that is biodegraded under specified conditions as measured through specified phenomena or techniques sensitive to mineral and *biomass* formations [9].

Note: Expressions like degree of *biodegradability*, extent of biodegradability, etc., are improper because a property reflected by the suffix "ity" cannot be quantified contrary to a deed reflected by "tion".

54. **degree of biodisintegration**

Mass fraction of a biodisintegrated substance [9].

55. **degree of biofragmentation**

Mass fraction of the original *material* that is biofragmented [9].

56. **degree of biomineralization**

Mass fraction of a substance that is biomineralized [9].

57. **degree of degradation (biorelated polymer)**

Mass fraction of a *polymer* that is degraded under specified conditions as measured through a specified phenomenon sensitive to molecular dimensions [9]. (See *degradation (biorelated polymer)*.)

58. **degree of disintegration**

Mass fraction of the particles of defined size issued from a fragmented substance [9].

Note: The size is generally defined by sieving. It is a practical characteristic in composting.

59. **degree of fragmentation**

Mass fraction of a substance that is fragmented [9].

60. **degree of mineralization**

Mass fraction of a substance that is mineralized [9].

61. **denaturation**

Process of partial or total alteration of the native secondary, and/or tertiary, and/or quaternary structures of proteins or nucleic acids resulting in a loss of *bioactivity*.

Note 1: Modified from the definition given in [2].

Note 2: Denaturation can occur when proteins and nucleic acids are subjected to elevated temperature or to extremes of pH, or to nonphysiological concentrations of salt, organic solvents, urea, or other chemical agents.

Note 3: An *enzyme* loses its catalytic activity when it is denaturized.

62. **depolymerase**

Enzyme that is able to catalyse the depolymerization of a *biomacromolecule*.

Note 1: A depolymerase does not necessarily convert all the *macromolecules* to monomer molecules, occasionally, a specific oligomer is the end-product, depending on the mechanism.

Note 2: This term is generally used in the case of macromolecules produced by bacteria, because bacteria have the potential to degrade the *biopolymers* they synthesized.

63. **depolymerization**

Process of converting a *macromolecule* into monomer or a mixture of monomers [2].

Note 1: This term is recommended when the formation of a macromolecule depends on an equilibrium with the monomer.

Note 2: Depolymerization can be caused by an *enzyme*. (See *depolymerase*.)

Note 3: In the absence of recovery of monomers, using *degradation* is recommended.

64. **deterioration**

Deleterious alteration of a *material* in quality, serviceability, or vigor.

Note 1: Deterioration can result from physical and/or chemical phenomena.

Note 2: Deterioration is connected to a loss of performances and thus to the function, whereas *degradation* is connected with a loss of properties.

Note 3: *Polymer* deterioration is more general than *polymer degradation*, which reflects loss of properties resulting from chemical cleavage of *macromolecules* only. (See *degradation*.)

65. **disintegration**
Fragmentation to particles of a defined size [9].

> *Note*: The limiting size is generally defined according to sieving conditions.

66. **dissolution (polymer)**
Process of dispersion of *macromolecules* in a liquid medium where they are solvated.

> *Note 1*: Modified from the definitions in [2,9] to take into account the particular thermodynamic behavior of macromolecules.

> *Note 2*: Nanosized *micelles* and *aggregates* in a visually transparent liquid medium are not solubilized, the use of dispersion is recommended.

> *Note 3*: This definition is not appropriate in the case of simultaneous *degradation*. In this case, the use of degradation is recommended.

67. **durability**
Ability of a *material* to retain the values of its properties under specified conditions [8].

68. **enzymatic degradation enzymatic decomposition**
Degradation caused by the catalytic action of *enzymes* [9].

> *Note 1*: Modified from [2]. The presented definition is more general.

> *Note 2*: Sometimes called enzymic degradation.

> *Note 3*: Degradation caused by *enzymes* can be observed under *biotic* or *abiotic* conditions but only degradation due to cell *bioactivity* can be called *biodegradation*, otherwise enzymatic degradation is to be used, especially in the case of in vitro abiotic conditions.

69. **enzyme**
Macromolecule, mainly protein in nature, which functions as *biocatalyst*.

> *Note 1*: Modified from [2].

> *Note 2*: Often, an enzyme catalyses only one reaction type (reaction specificity) and operates on only one type of substrate (substrate specificity). Substrate molecules are attacked at the same site (regioselectivity) and only one or preferentially one of the enantiomers of chiral substrates or in racemates is attacked (enantioselectivity).

> *Note 3*: Some enzymes like lipases or cutinases are able to function as *biocatalysts* on a range of substances that are not specific substrates.

> *Note 4*: In the case of *polymer enzymatic degradation*, the enzyme can cleave links between constitutional repeating units within the chain more or less at random (endoenzyme) or from chain extremity (exoenzyme).

> *Note 5*: Some *biomacromolecules* that are not protein in nature are now known to behave as catalysts (e.g., RNA in the case of ribozymes).

> *Note 6*: Enzymes or immobilized enzymes can react unusually in an organic solvent, such as in the case of

lactone and hydroxy acid *polymerization* in the presence of some immobilized lipases.

70. **erosion**
Degradation that occurs at the surface and progresses from it into the bulk.

> *Note 1*: Modified from [9] to be more precise.

> *Note 2*: See *enzymatic degradation*. In the case of *polymers*, water-soluble *enzymes* can hardly diffuse into the macromolecular network, except, maybe, in some hydrogels. They adhere to surfaces to cause erosion.

> *Note 3*: Erosion can also result from chemical degradation when the degrading reagent reacts faster than it diffuses inside. There is a risk of confusion that can be eliminated after careful and detailed investigation of the degradation mechanism. (See *bioerosion*.)

> *Note 4*: The wording *bulk erosion* is incorrect and its use therefore discouraged.

71. **fragmentation**
Breakdown of a *material* to particles regardless of the mechanism and the size of fragments.

> *Note*: Modified from [9] in order to remove size limitation. (See *disintegration*.)

72. **genetic engineering**
Process of inserting new genetic information into existing cells in order to modify a specific organism for the purpose of changing its characteristics.

> *Note*: Adapted from [10].

73. **heterogeneous degradation**
Degradation or *biodegradation* occurring at different rates depending on the location within a matrix [9].

74. **homogeneous degradation**
Degradation that occurs at the same rate regardless of the location within a polymeric item [9].

75. **hydrolases**
Enzymes that catalyse the cleavage of C−O, C−N, and other bonds by reactions involving the addition or removal of water.

> *Note*: Modified from [2] to consider the fact that C−C bonds are not directly hydrolysed by hydrolases.

76. **hydrolysis**
Bond cleavage by the action of water. (See also *solvolysis*.)

> *Note 1*: Modified from the definition given in [2]. Hydrolysis can occur in a water-containing solid or solvent.

> *Note 2*: Hydrolysis can be catalysed and autocatalysed. (See *autocatalytic reaction*.)

77. **inhibitor**
Substance that diminishes the rate of a chemical reaction [2].

> *Note 1*: The process is called inhibition [2].

> *Note 2*: Inhibitors are sometimes called negative *catalysts*, but since the action of an inhibitor is fundamentally different from that of a catalyst, this terminology

is discouraged. In contrast to a catalyst, an inhibitor may be consumed during the course of a reaction.

> *Note 3*: In *enzyme*-catalysed reactions, an inhibitor frequently acts by binding to the enzyme, in which case it may be called an enzyme inhibitor.

> *Note 4*: Inhibitors may decrease enzyme (or other) activity simply by competing for the active (recognition) site.

78. **macromolecule polymer molecule**
Molecule of high relative molar mass, the structure of which essentially comprises the multiple repetitions of units derived, actually or conceptually, from molecules of low relative molar mass [2].

> *Note 1*: In many cases, especially for synthetic *polymers*, a macromolecule can be regarded as having a high relative molar mass if the addition or removal of one or a few of the units has a negligible effect on the molecular properties. This statement fails in the case of certain macromolecules for which the properties may be critically dependent on fine details of the molecular structure (e.g., a protein).

> *Note 2*: If a part or the whole of the molecule has a high relative molar mass and essentially comprises the multiple repetition of units derived, actually or conceptually, from molecules of low relative molar mass, it may be described as either macromolecular or polymeric, or by *polymer* used adjectivally.

79. **material**
Substance that is exploited by humans in their practical activities.

> *Note*: Sand on the beach is a substance, sand in concrete is a *material*.

80. **maximum degree of biodegradation**
Greater value of the degree of *biodegradation* that can be reached under selected experimental conditions [9].

> *Note 1*: This expression reflects the fact that some *biodegradable* parts of a *biodegradable material* may not be accessible to biodegradation.

> *Note 2*: Not to be confused with *ultimate degradation*.

81. **micelle (polymers)**
Organized auto-assembly formed in a liquid and composed of amphiphilic *macromolecules*, generally amphiphilic dior triblock copolymers made of solvophilic and solvophobic blocks.

> *Note 1*: An amphiphilic behavior can be observed for water and an organic solvent or between two organic solvents.

> *Note 2*: Polymeric micelles have a much lower critical micellar concentration (CMC) than soap or surfactant micelles, but are nevertheless at equilibrium with isolated macromolecules called unimers. Therefore, micelle formation and stability are concentration-dependent.

82. **microcapsule**
Hollow *microparticle* composed of a solid shell surrounding a core-forming space available to permanently or temporarily entrapped substances.

> *Note*: The substances can be drugs, pesticides, dyes, etc.

83. **microparticle**
Particle with dimensions between 1×10^{-7} and 1×10^{-4} m.

> *Note 1*: The lower limit between microand nano-sizing is still a matter of debate. (See*nanoparticle*.)

> *Note 2*: To be consistent with the prefix "micro" and the range imposed by the definition, dimensions of microparticles should be expressed in μm.

84. **microsphere**
Microparticle of spherical shape without membrane or any distinct outer layer. (See *microcapsule*.)

> *Note*: The absence of outer layer forming a distinct phase is important to distinguish micro-spheres from microcapsules because it leads to first-order diffusion phenomena, whereas diffusion is zero order in the case of microcapsules.

85. **mineralization**
Process through which an organic substance becomes impregnated by or turned into inorganic substances.

> *Note 1*: A particular case is the process by which living organisms produce and structure minerals often to harden or stiffen existing tissues. (See *biomineralization*.)

> *Note 2*: In the case of *polymer biodegradation*, this term is used to reflect conversion to CO_2 and H_2O and other inorganics. CH_4 can be considered as part of the mineralization process because it comes up in parallel to the minerals in *anaerobic composting*, also called methanization [9].

86. **nanocapsule**
Hollow *nanoparticle* composed of a solid shell that surrounds a core-forming space available to entrap substances.

87. **nanoparticle**
Particle of any shape with dimensions in the 1×10^{-9} and 1×10^{-7} m range.

> *Note 1*: Modified from definitions of nanoparticle and nanogel in [2,3].

> *Note 2*: The basis of the 100-nm limit is the fact that novel properties that differentiate particles from the bulk *material* typically develop at a critical length scale of under 100 nm.

> *Note 3*: Because other phenomena (transparency or turbidity, ultrafiltration, stable dispersion, etc.) are occasionally considered that extend the upper limit, the use of the prefix "nano" is accepted for dimensions smaller than 500 nm, provided reference to the definition is indicated.

> *Note 4*: Tubes and fibers with only two dimensions below 100 nm are also nanoparticles.

88. **nanosphere**
Nanoparticle of spherical shape without membrane or any distinct outer layer.

> *Note*: A nanosphere is composed of a matrix where substances can be permanently or temporarily embedded, dissolved, or covalently bound. (See *microsphere*.)

89. **plastic**
Generic term used in the case of polymeric *material* that may contain other substances to improve performance and/or reduce costs.

Note 1: The use of this term instead of *polymer* is a source of confusion and thus is not recommended.

Note 2: This term is used in polymer engineering for materials often compounded that can be processed by flow.

90. **polymer**
Substance composed of *macromolecules* [2].

> *Note*: Applicable to substance macromolecular in nature like cross-linked systems that can be considered as one macromolecule.

91. **polymerase**
Enzyme that is able to catalyse the addition of units in the process of *macromolecule* formation.

92. **polymerisation**
Process in which a monomer, or a mixture of monomers, is converted into *macromolecules*.

> *Note 1*: Modified from [2] to be more precise.

> *Note 2*: Two major types of polymerization are chain growth and step growth. The chain growth mechanism of unsaturated or cyclic monomers must not be confused with the step growth mechanism as in polycondensation and polyaddition reactions [2].

> *Note 3*: It is important to note that a *polymer* made by ring-opening polymerization of a cyclic monomer using an initiator and that made by polycondensation of the corresponding bifunctional open cycle are not necessarily similar compounds. The resulting macromolecules may differ at chain ends because of the presence of initiator residues in the case of the initiated *polymerization*, a difference that can have significant consequences in case chain ends play an important role in a subsequent chemical process. (See *autocatalytic reaction*.)

93. **resorption**
Total elimination of a substance from its initial place caused by physical and/or chemical phenomena.

> *Note*: The resorption of a polymer, like its dissolution in a solvent medium, does not mean that *macromolecules* are degraded. (See *bioresorption*.)

94. **solid dispersion (polymer)**
Solid multiphasic mixture with at least one *polymer* component dominating.

> *Note 1*: The nonpolymeric components can act as fillers [4].

> *Note 2*: The dispersed compounds can be in clusters of particles.

> *Note 3*: Solid dispersion is commonly prepared by three different methods, namely, solventbased, fusion-melt, and hybrid fusion-solvent methods.

> *Note 4*: In pharmaceutical preparations, incompatible polymer-drug mixtures are generally solid dispersions.

95. **solid solution**
Solid in which components are compatible and form a unique phase.

> *Note 1*: The definition "crystal containing a second constituent which fits into and is distributed in the lattice of the host crystal" given in [2,11] is not general and, thus, is not recommended.

> *Note 2*: The expression is to be used to describe a solid phase containing more than one substance when, for convenience, one (or more) of the substances, called the solvent, is treated differently from the other substances, called solutes.

> *Note 3*: One or several of the components can be *macromolecules*. Some of the other components can then act as plasticizers, i.e., as molecularly dispersed substances that decrease the glass-transition temperature at which the amorphous phase of a *polymer* is converted between glassy and rubbery states.

> *Note 4*: In pharmaceutical preparations, the concept of solid solution is often applied to the case of mixtures of *drug* and *polymer*.

> *Note 5*: The number of drug molecules that do behave as solvent (plasticizer) of polymers is small.

96. **solvolysis**
Generally reaction with a solvent, or with a lyonium ion or lyate ion, involving the rupture of one or more bonds in the reaction solute [2]. (See lyonium ion and lyate ion in [2].)

97. **stimulus-responsive polymer smart polymer**
Polymer that responds or that is designed to respond to a stimulus like pH, light, heat, etc. change, and provides a predetermined action.

> *Note 1*: The generated action can be unique or cyclic. It generally results from cooperative phenomena.

> *Note 2*: The stimulus can affect *macromolecules* or macromolecule assemblies forming the polymer.

98. **sustained delivery prolonged delivery**
Supply of a substance from a container where it is temporarily entrapped for the sake of achieving a prolonged action.

> *Note 1*: In some cases, the container is a *polymer* processed as *implant*, film, *microparticle*, or *nanoparticle*, auto-assembly of molecules, or a *macromolecule*.

> *Note 2*: The substance can be temporarily embedded, dissolved, or covalently bound.

> *Note 3*: The term is relevant to the release of substances like pesticides, dyes, *drugs*, etc.

> *Note 4*: In the case of sustained delivery according to required specifications, the use of *controlled delivery* is recommended.

99. **swelling**
Increase in volume of a gel or solid associated with the uptake of a liquid or gas [2].

100. **synthetic biopolymer**
Copy of a *biopolymer* man-made using *abiotic* chemical routes. (See *artificial* and *biopolymer*.)

101. **theoretical degree of biodegradation**
Degree of biodegradation that corresponds to conversion of all the organic matter present in an original *polymer*-based item to minerals and *biomass* [9]. (See *bioavailability*.)

Note: This expression is used as reference to assess *biodegradable* components that are not accessible to biodegradation from those that are bioavailable.

102. **toxicity**
Consequence of adverse effects caused by a substance on a living system.

> *Note 1*: Modified from [1,2] to be general.

> *Note 2*: The adverse effects depend on the quantity of substances, the way in which the substance contacts the living system (single or repeated administrations), the type and severity of the reaction, the time needed to produce the reaction, the nature of the organism(s) affected, and other relevant conditions.

> *Note 3*: The adverse effects are usually quantified according to the physiological response of the living system, and/or to local tissue and cell responses and/or to survival tests.

> *Note 4*: A prefix can be used to specify the living system: "hemo" for blood, "cardio" for heart, "phyto" for plant, "bacterio" for bacteria, etc.

103. **ultimate biodegradation**
Complete breakdown of a compound to either fully oxidized or reduced simple molecules (such as carbon dioxide/methane, nitrate/ammonium, and water) [2].

> *Note 1*: This term reflects the end-products of *biodegradation*. As such, it differs from the *theoretical degree of biodegradation*, which depends on the presence of non-*biodegradable* components.

> *Note 2*: The use of this expression is not recommended.

Polymers of Biological and Biomedical Interest

1. **acute toxicity**
Toxicity occurring within a short time of dosing or exposure.

> *Note 1*: Modified from [1].

> *Note 2*: Usually, adverse effects are monitored up to 14 days after administration of a single exposure to a test substance (amount, dose, or concentration) or after multiple exposures, usually within 24 h of a starting point (which may be exposure to the toxicant, or loss of reserve capacity, or developmental change, etc.).

> *Note 3*: The adverse effect is usually quantified according to the physiological behavior of the living system, to local tissue and cell responses, and/or to survival tests as lethal dose in percentage of dead animals in the test population (LD_{50} for 50 %) or as lethal concentration (e.g., LC_{50}).

2. **artificial organ**
Medical device that replaces, in part or in whole, the function of one of the organs of the body [6].

3. **biocompatibility (biomedical therapy)**
Ability of a *material* to perform with an appropriate host response in a specific application [6].

> *Note*: The more general definition (**18**) could be adopted by the biomedical field.

4. **biomedical**
Qualifier for a domain grouping scientific and practical activities related to therapy.

> *Note*: The term is relevant to therapy in surgery, medicine, pharmacology, dentistry, etc.

5. **bioprosthesis**
Implantable prosthesis that consists totally or substantially of nonviable, treated donor tissue [6].

6. **bioresorbability**
Ability to be eliminated from an animal or human body through natural pathways.

> *Note 1*: Natural pathways are kidneys through glomerular filtration and lungs after metabolization.

> *Note 2*: *Bioassimilation* with formation of novel *biomass* is a particular means of elimination often combined with the other pathways.

7. **bioresorbable**
Qualifier used to indicate that a compound or a device is bioresorbed, i.e., totally eliminated or bioassimilated by an animal or a human body.

> *Note*: To be qualified as bioresorbable, demonstration must be made of the elimination or *bioassimilation*, the best tool being radioactivity labeling.

8. **bioresorption**
Disappearance of a substance from an organism by processes of metabolism, secretion, or excretion.

> *Note 1*: Bioresorption is now considered as pertinent and should be used specifically only when foreign *material* and residues have been shown assimilated or eliminated from the living host, regardless of the followed route, namely, lungs or kidneys or insertion in biochemical processes.

> *Note 2*: In the case of *polymers* or high-molar-mass *macromolecules* that are retained in parenteral compartments, *degradation* or *biodegradation* is necessary prior to bioresorption.

> *Note 3*: This concept does not apply to the environment as everything, including degradation by-products issued from outdoor degradation or biodegradation can only be stored or chemically transformed on Earth, so far.

9. **bone cement**
Synthetic, self-curing organic or inorganic *material* used to fill up a cavity or to create a mechanical fixation.

> *Note 1*: In situ self-curing can be the source of released reagents that can cause local and/or systemic *toxicity* as in the case of the monomer released from methacrylics-based bone cement used in orthopedic surgery.

> *Note 2*: In dentistry, *polymer*-based cements are also used as fillers of cavities. They are generally cured photochemically using UV radiation in contrast to bone cements.

10. **carcinogenicity**
Ability or tendency to produce cancer.

Note: In general, *polymers* are not known as carcinogens or mutagens, however, residual monomers or additives can cause genetic mutations.

11. **chronic toxicity**
Toxicity that persists over a long period of time whether or not adverse effects occur immediately upon exposure or are delayed.

> *Note*: Modified from [1].

12. **complement**
System of multiple proteins part of the nonspecific immune defenses that are activated by foreign microorganisms or *material* surfaces with the aim of lysing essential constituting molecules.

13. **drug medicine**
Any substance that, when absorbed into a living organism, may modify one or more of its functions beneficially.

> Note 1: Modified from [2] to emphasize that the benefit/risk ratio must be positive. (See bioactive.)
>
> Note 2: The term is generally accepted for a substance taken for a therapeutic purpose, but is also commonly used for abused substances.
>
> Note 3: The two terms are also used when the *bioactive* substance is formulated to become a pharmaceutical specialty.
>
> *Note 4*: The use of medicine that is also a discipline is discouraged.

14. **drug carrier (biorelated polymers)**
Macromolecule or *polymer* used to transport a *pharmacologically active* compound to be released later on due to an *abiotic* or *biotic* process. (See *conjugate, sustained release,* and *controlled delivery.*)

> *Note*: A complementary property of a polymeric drug carrier is *targeting*, which can be obtained by specific interactions with a receptor if bearing a specific ligand or by selection depending on other factors such as permeation through membranes or capillaries.

15. **drug delivery**
Process of administration of a *bioactive* substance of *pharmacological* interest. (See *sustained delivery* and *controlled delivery.*)

> *Note 1*: A drug delivery system can be a stationary implant but also an active or passive transport system with or without *targeting* properties.
>
> Note 2: If a drug delivery system fulfills therapeutic and *pharmacokinetic* requirements, one talks of controlled drug delivery. If only a slow release is observed without relation to desired *pharmacokinetic* characteristics, the expression "sustained drug delivery" must be used.

16. **excipient**
Any more or less inert substance added to a drug to give suitable consistency or form to the drug formulation.

> *Note*: Modified from [2]. The presented definition addresses the concept of formulation.

17. **foreign body reaction**
Cellular response of the inflammatory and wound healing processes following introduction of a foreign object in a human or animal body.

> *Note 1*: The foreign object can be a medical device, a *prosthesis*, a particle or any compound introduced accidentally.
>
> *Note 2*: The foreign body reaction results in more or less intense events such as fibrous tissue formation, macrophage activation, giant cells formation, etc.

18. **graft**
Piece of nonviable *material*, viable tissue, or collection of viable cells transferred from a site in a donor to a site in a recipient for the purpose of the reconstruction of the recipient site.

> *Note*: In *polymer* science, *graft* is used to indicate the presence of one or more species of block connected to *macromolecule* main chain as side chains, these side chains having constitutional or configurational features that differ from those in the main chain [2].

19. **host response**
Reaction of a living system to the presence of a substance or a *material*.

> *Note*: Complemented from [6].

20. **hybrid artificial organ**
Artificial organ that is a combination of viable cells and one or more *biomaterials* [6].

21. **immunogenicity**
Ability of a *material* or substance to elicit a cellular immune response and/or antibody production [2].

22. **implant**
Medical device made from one or more *biomaterials* that is intentionally placed within the body, either totally or partially buried beneath an epithelial surface [6].

> *Note*: There are also other devices implanted that are not medical devices, e.g., for cosmetic, cultural, or aesthetic purposes.

23. **macromolecular prodrug**
Prodrug in which the temporary chemical entity is a *macromolecule*.

> *Note*: In this particular case of prodrug, the macromolecule carries several drug molecules generally. These molecules are linked to the carrier through cleavable bonds. (See *conjugate*.)

24. **medical device**
Instrument, apparatus, implement, machine, contrivance, in vitro reagent, or other similar or related article, including any component, part of accessory, which is intended for use in the diagnosis of disease or other conditions, or in the cure, mitigation, treatment, or prevention of disease in man [6].

25. **opsonin**
Antibody in blood serum that attaches to invading microorganisms and other antigens to make them more susceptible to the action of phagocytes [12].

Note: Opsonin molecules include antibodies: IgG and IgA, proteins of the *complement* system: C3b, C4b, and iC3b, mannose-binding lectin (initiates the formation of C3b), etc.

26. **pharmaceutical**
Qualifier for substances or systems, including *polymers*, exploited by the pharmaceutical industry.

> *Note 1*: A pharmaceutical substance can be exploited for its *bioactivity* or as an excipient.

> *Note 2*: The term "pharmaceutical" is also used as short form for a pharmaceutical substance.

27. **pharmacodynamics**
Branch of *pharmacology* concerned with *pharmacological* actions on living systems, including the reactions with and binding to cell constituents, and the biochemical and physiological consequences of these actions.

> *Note*: Modified from [2].

28. **pharmacokinetics**
Branch of *pharmacology* concerned with the uptake of *drugs* by the body, the biotransformation of the drugs and their metabolites in the tissues, and the elimination of the drugs and their metabolites from the body over a period of time.

> *Note 1*: Modified from [2].

> *Note 2*: Pharmacokinetics also includes the distribution of *bioactive* substances within the various compartments present in an animal or human body, especially high-molar-mass *polymers* that cannot cross endothelial or epithelial physiological barriers.

29. **pharmacological   pharmacologic**
Qualifiers for substances, including *macromolecules* or *polymers*, and actions involved in pharmacology.

> Note: A pharmacological polymer can be bioactive by itself or because it is used as a temporary carrier of a bioactive substance of interest in pharmacology. (See macromolecular prodrug.)
> pharmacologically active
> Qualifier for a substance that exhibits *bioactivity* of *pharmacological* interest.

30. **pharmacology**
Science of *drugs* including their origin, composition, *pharmacokinetics*, *pharmacodynamics*, therapeutic use, and toxicology.

31. **polymeric drug   macromolecular drug**
Bioactive macromolecule of *pharmacological* interest.

32. **prodrug**
Compound that undergoes biotransformation before exhibiting *pharmacological* effects.

> *Note 1*: Modified from [13].

> *Note 2*: Prodrugs can thus be viewed as *drugs* containing specialized nontoxic protective groups used in a transient manner to alter or to eliminate undesirable properties in the parent molecule.

33. **prosthesis**
Device that replaces a limb, organ, or tissue of the body [6].

34. **scaffold**
Matrix, generally porous with communicating pores, aimed at culturing cells and forming neotissues to be implanted and integrated in a living organism.

> *Note*: Such a matrix should be *degradable* or *biodegradable* and, ideally, *bioresorbable*.

35. **stealth (biomedical polymer)**
Qualifier for a *macromolecule*, a surface, or a device that is not detected by defense proteins of the *complement* and the Mononuclear Phagocyte System, especially macrophages, after introduction in parental compartments.

> *Note 1*: Detection by natural defenses generally leads to the destruction of the device or of the surrounding tissues.

> *Note 2*: Surfaces are often decorated by chemical entities aimed at suppressing the activation of the natural defense processes.

36. **targeting**
Exploitation of specific or nonspecific interactions to target a particular part of a living system, or a particular type of cells.

37. **therapeutic polymer**
Polymer aimed at helping therapists in treating diseases or trauma.

38. **thrombogenicity**
Property of a *material* (or substance) that induces and/or promotes the formation of a thrombus [6].

39. **tissue engineering**
Use of a combination of cells, engineering and *materials* methods, and suitable biochemical and physico-chemical factors to improve or replace biological functions [7].

> *Note*: While most definitions of tissue engineering cover a broad range of applications, in practice the term is closely associated with applications that repair or replace portions of or whole tissues (i.e., bone, cartilage, blood vessels, bladder, skin, etc.).

40. **transplant**
Complete structure, such as an organ that is transferred from a site in a donor to a site in a recipient for the purpose of the reconstruction of the recipient site [6].

Environmental Polymers and Polymeric Systems

1. **aerobic biodegradation**
Biodegradation in the presence of molecular oxygen.

> *Note 1*: Modified from [2]. The present definition is more general.
> *Note 2*: Oxygen is generally supplied by the atmosphere.

2. **anaerobic biodegradation**
Biodegradation in the absence of oxygen. (See *mineralization*.)

3. **bioplastic**
Biobased polymer derived from the *biomass* or issued from monomers derived from the biomass and which, at

some stage in its processing into finished products, can be shaped by flow.

>   *Note 1*: Bioplastic is generally used as the opposite of polymer derived from fossil resources.
>
>   *Note 2*: Bioplastic is misleading because it suggests that any polymer derived from the biomass is *environmentally friendly*.
>
>   *Note 3*: The use of the term "bioplastic" is discouraged. Use the expression "biobased polymer".
>
>   *Note 4*: A biobased polymer similar to a petrobased one does not imply any superiority with respect to the environment unless the comparison of respective *life cycle assessments* is favourable.

4. **compost**
Solid product resulting from the decomposition of organic wastes by fermentation.

>   *Note*: A compost is generally processed in personal composters or industrially to be used as fertilizer. In the latter case, specifications in structure and quality are to be provided.

5. **composting**
Process of biological decomposition of organic matter performed by microorganisms, mostly bacteria and fungi. (See *biodegradation*.)

>   *Note 1*: Modified from [10] to be more general.
>
>   *Note 2*: Composting can be performed industrially under aerobic or anaerobic conditions or individually (home-composting).
>
>   *Note 3*: If present, earthworms also contribute to composting. They are sometimes cultured purposely in industrial composting facilities. One often talks of lombri-composting.

6. **conditioning film**
Film that is rapidly formed on the surface of a solid in contact with a biological system (in the widest sense) that conditions the surface for subsequent interaction with constituents of the biological system.

>   *Note 1*: Frequently, the conditioning film consists of proteins that prepare almost any surface for subsequent colonization by microorganisms or cells.
>
>   *Note 2*: Not to be confused with conditioning film in packaging.
>
>   *Note 3*: The term can be applied to the surface of any *material* that is in contact with blood or body fluids because the very first event is coverage by more or less denaturated adhering proteins.
>
>   *Note 4*: Not to be confused with *biofilm*, which implies the presence of cells or microorganisms.

7. **ecotoxicity**
Consequence of adverse effects caused by a substance on the environment and on organisms living in it.

>   *Note 1*: Using the term is recommended when adverse effects concern water, air, sediments, etc.
>
>   *Note 2*: If only living organisms (animals, plants, microorganisms) are concerned, the use of *toxicity* is recommended.

8. **environmentally degradable polymer**
Polymer that can be degraded by the action of the environment, through, for example, air, light, heat, or microorganisms [8].

>   *Note*: When it is to be a source of *material*, such a polymer must be designed to degrade into products at a predictable rate compatible with the application. Such products are usually of lower molar mass than the original polymer.

9. **environmentally friendly ecocompatible**
Qualifiers for a substance, device, or process that has minimal deleterious impact on the environment, which is air, water, minerals, living systems, etc.

>   *Note 1*: The assignment of these qualifiers to a *polymer* must be based on a consistent *life cycle assessment*.
>
>   *Note 2*: Ecocompatible is introduced to complement *biocompatible*, whose meaning is limited to living systems.

10. **green chemistry sustainable chemistry**
Design of chemical products and processes that reduce or eliminate the use or generation of substances hazardous to humans, animals, plants, and the environment.

>   *Note 1*: Modified from [14] to be more general.
>
>   *Note 2*: Green chemistry discusses the engineering concept of pollution prevention and zero waste both at laboratory and industrial scales. It encourages the use of economical and *ecocompatible* techniques that not only improve the yield but also bring down the cost of disposal of wastes at the end of a chemical process.

11. **green polymer**
Polymer that conforms to the concept of *green chemistry*.

>   *Note*: Green polymer does not necessarily mean *environmentally friendly* polymer or *biobased polymer* although the confusion is often made in the literature.

12. **life cycle assessment**
Investigation and valuation of the environmental impacts of a given product or service caused or necessitated by its existence [2].

>   *Note 1*: Also known as life cycle analysis, LCA, ecobalance, and cradle-to-grave analysis.
>
>   *Note 2*: Assessing the life cycle of a *polymer* or a *plastic* must take into account all the factors that can be identified from the up-stage raw *material* to the *waste management*.

13. **litter**
Solid *waste* carelessly discarded outside the regular garbage and trash collection [10].

14. **mulching film**
Polymer film aimed at covering seeded area in order to protect the growing plants from weeds and cold and preserve humidity.

>   *Note*: Such film acts as a mobile green house.

15. sustainability

Developments that meet the needs of the present without compromising the ability of future generations to meet their needs [15].

Note: Other definitions are not recommended in the context of *biorelated polymers*.

16. waste

Residue left when a compound or a product reaches the end of its initial usefulness.

Note 1: Modified from [16]. The given definition is not general.

Note 2: Also referred to as rubbish, trash, garbage, or junk depending upon the type of *material* and the regional terminology.

Note 3: In living organisms, waste relates to unwanted substances or toxins that are expelled from them.

17. waste management

Control of the collection, treatment and disposal of *wastes*.

18. weathering

Exposure of a polymeric *material* to a natural or simulated environment [2].

Note 1: Weathering results in changes in appearance or mechanical properties.

Note 2: Weathering in which the rate of change has been artificially increased is termed "accelerated weathering".

Note 3: Weathering in a simulated environment is termed "artificial weathering".

Note 4: The ability of a *polymer* to resist weathering is termed "weatherability".

Membership of Sponsoring Bodies

Membership of the IUPAC Polymer Division Committee for the period 2010–2011 was as follows:

President: C. K. Ober (USA); *Vice President*: M. Buback (Germany); *Secretary*: M. Hess (Germany); *Titular Members*: D. Dijkstra (Germany); R. G. Jones (UK); P. Kubisa (Poland); G. T. Russell (New Zealand); M. Sawamoto (Japan); R. F. T. Stepto (UK), J.-P. Vairon (France); *Associate Members*: D. Berek (Slovakia); J. He (China); R. Hiorns (France); W. Mormann (Germany); D. Smith (USA); J. Stejskal (Czech Republic); *National Representatives*: K.-N. Chen (Taiwan); G. Galli (Italy); J. S. Kim (Korea); G. Moad (Australia); M. Raza Shah (Pakistan); R. P. Singh (India); W. M. Z. B. Wan Yunus (Malaysia); Y. Yagci (Turkey), M. Žigon (Slovenia).

Membership of the Subcommittee on Polymer Terminology (until 2005, the Subcommittee on Macromolecular Terminology) during the preparation of this report (2006–2011) was as follows:

Chair: R. G. Jones (UK); *Secretary*: M. Hess (Germany), 2006–2007; T. Kitayama (Japan) 2008–2009; R. Hiorns (France),

from 2010; *Members*: G. Allegra (Italy); M. Barón (Argentina); T. Chang (Korea); C. dos Santos (Brazil); A. Fradet (France); K. Hatada (Japan); J. He (China); K.-H. Hellwich (Germany); R. C. Hiorns (France); P. Hodge (UK); K. Horie (Japan); A. D. Jenkins (UK); J.-I. Jin (Korea); J. Kahovec (Czech Republic); P. Kratochvíl (Czech Republic); P. Kubisa (Poland); I. Meisel (Germany); W. V. Metanomski (USA); V. Meille (Italy); I. Mita (Japan); G. Moad (Australia); W. Mormann (Germany); C. Ober (USA); S. Penczek (Poland); L. P. Rebelo (Portugal); M. Rinaudo (France); I. Schopov (Bulgaria); M. Schubert (USA); F. Schué (France); V. P. Shibaev (Russia); S Słomkowski (Poland); R. F. T. Stepto (UK); D. Tabak (Brazil); J.-P. Vairon (France); M. Vert (France); J. Vohlídal (Czech Republic); E. S. Wilks (USA); W. J. Work (USA).

References

1. J. H. Duffus, M. Nordberg, D. M. Templeton. *Pure Appl. Chem.* 79, 1153 (2007).
2. IUPAC. *Compendium of Chemical Terminology*, 2nd ed. (the "Gold Book"). Compiled by A. D. McNaught and A. Wilkinson. Blackwell Scientific Publications, Oxford (1997). XML on-line corrected version: http://dx.doi.org/10.1351/goldbook (2006–) created by M. Nic, J. Jirat, B. Kosata; updates compiled by A. Jenkins.
3. J. Alemán, A. V. Chadwick, J. He, M. Hess, K. Horie, R. G. Jones, P. Kratochvíl, I. Meisel, I. Mita, G. Moad, S. Penczek, R. F. T. Stepto. *Pure Appl. Chem.* 79, 1801 (2007).
4. W. J. Work, K. Horie, M. Hess, R. F. T. Stepto. *Pure Appl. Chem.* 76, 1985 (2004).
5. *The American Heritage Dictionary of the English Language*, 4th ed., Houghton Mifflin (2000). Updated in 2009.
6. D. F. Williams (Ed.). *Definitions in Biomaterials, Proceedings of a Consensus Conference of the European Society for Biomaterials*, Elsevier, Amsterdam (2004).
7. J. P. Griffin (Ed.). *The Textbook of Pharmaceutical Medicine*, Wiley-Blackwell (2009).
8. IUPAC. *Compendium of Polymer Terminology and Nomenclature, IUPAC Recommendations 2008 (the "Purple Book")*. Edited by R. G. Jones, J. Kahovec, R. Stepto, E. S. Wilks, M. Hess, T. Kitayama, W. V. Metanomski, RSC Publishing, Cambridge, UK (2008).
9. Europeen Committee for Standarization. *Plastics – Guide for Vocabulary in the Field of Degradable and Biodegradable Polymers and Plastic Items*, CEN/TR 15351:2006 report (2006). <http://esearch.cen.eu/>
10. U.S. EPA online, Terms and Acronyms, <http://www.epa.gov/OCEPAterms/gterms.html>.
11. IUPAC. *Compendium of Analytical Nomenclature*, 3rd ed. (the "Orange Book"). Prepared for publication by J. Inczédy, T. Lengyel, A. M. Ure, Blackwell Science, Oxford (1998).
12. Princeton University. *Wordnet: A Lexical Database for English* <wordnetweb.princeton.edu/ perl/webwn>.
13. C. G. Wermuth, C. R. Ganellin, P. Lindberg, L. A. Mitscher. *Pure Appl. Chem.* 70, 1129 (1998).
14. A. E. Martel, J. A. Davies, W. W. Olson, M. A. Abraham. *Annu. Rev. Environ. Resour.* 28, 401 (2003).
15. Presidio Graduate School. *The Dictionary of Sustainable Development* (<http://www.sustainabil-itydictionary.com/> + entry).
16. European Commission. *Waste Framework Directive* (European Directive 75/442/EC as amended) <http://ec.europa.eu/environment/waste/legislation/a.htm>.

APPENDIX: INDEX IN ALPHABETICAL ORDER

INTRINSIC VISCOSITY OF POLY(ETHYLENE GLYCOL)

Roger L. Lundblad

Intrinsic Viscosity of Poly(Ethylene Glycol) (PEG)[a]

Sample	$[\eta]$ cm^3 g^{-1}	Comment	Reference
PEG1000[b]	6.2	H$_2$O/10°C	1
PEG2000	9.16	H$_2$O/10°C	1
PEG4500	14.4	H$_2$O/10°C	1
PEG7500	19.3	H$_2$O/10°C	1
PEG20000	39	H$_2$O/10°C	1
PEG1000	6.45	8.0 M Urea/10°C	1
PEG2000	9.57	8.0 M Urea/10°C	1
PEG4500	15.7	8.0 M Urea/10°C	1
PEG7500	21	8.0 M Urea/10°C	1
PEG20000	45	8.0 M Urea/10°C	1
PEG300	3.91	H$_2$O/25°C	2
PEG600	5.03	H$_2$O/25°C	2
PEG900	5.84	H$_2$O/25°C	2
PEG1500	7.63	H$_2$O/25°C	2
PEG2000	9.03	H$_2$O/25°C	2
PEG3000	11.50	H$_2$O/25°C	2
PEG6000	17.28	H$_2$O/25°C	2
PEG10000	24.86	H$_2$O/25°C	2
PEG20000	42.02	H$_2$O/25°C	2
PEG35000	55.82	H$_2$O/25°C	2
PEG20000	42.65[c]	H$_2$O:EtOH (95:5, V/V)/9.95°C	3
PEG20000	39.19[c]	H$_2$O:EtOH (95:5, V/V)/19.95°C	3
PEG20000	38.68	H$_2$O:EtOH (95:5, V/V)/29.95°C	3
PEG20000	36.65	H$_2$O:EtOH (95:5, V/V)/39.95°C	3
PEG20000	39.33	H$_2$O:EtOH (95:20, V/V)/39.95°C	3
PEG20000	38.25	H$_2$O:EtOH (95:20, V/V)/39.95°C	3
PEG20000	37.40	H$_2$O:EtOH (95:20, V/V)/39.95°C	3
PEG20000	36.20	H$_2$O:EtOH (95:20, V/V)/39.95°C	3
mPEG[d] (2,800[e])	10.0	H$_2$O/20°C	4
mPEG[d] (4,200[e])	17.3	H$_2$O/20°C	4
mPEG[d] (6,200[e])	20.8	H$_2$O/20°C	4
mPEG[d] (8,350[e])	28.1	H$_2$O/20°C	4
mPEG[d] (15,200[e])	38.7	H$_2$O/20°C	4
mPEG[d] (21,200[e])	49.8	H$_2$O/20°C	4
mPEG[d] (35,600[e])	59.8	H$_2$O/20°C	4
DPMPEG[f] (2,800[e])	9.5	H$_2$O/20°C	4
DPMPEG[f] (6.200[e])	15.5	H$_2$O/20°C	4
DPMPEG[f] (18,600[e])	35.1	H$_2$O/20°C	4
DPMPEG[f] (33,100[e])	58.4	H$_2$O/20°C	4
DPMPEG[f] (48,000[e])	74.2	H$_2$O/20°C	4
IsoFruPEG[g] (1,700[e])	8.3	H$_2$O/20°C	4
IsoFruPEG[g] (3,300[e])	13.6	H$_2$O/20°C	4
IsoFruPEG[g] (4,700[e])	18.1	H$_2$O/20°C	4

[a] Also known as poly(ethylene oxide)(PEO). PEG usually refers to lower molecular polymers and is the terminology used in the life sciences. PEO usually refers to higher molecular polymers and is the terminology used by polymer chemists (Bailey, F.E., Jr., *Poly(ethylene oxide)*, pp. 1–4, Academic Press, New York, 1976).

[b] PEG1000, poly(ethylene glycol), M_w = 1000; the number following PEG is the assigned M_w.

[c] These values obtained through use of the Schulz-Blaschke equation (Schulz, G.V. and Blaschke, F., Molekulargewichsbestimmungen an makromolekularen Stoffen. IX. Eine Gleichung zur Berechnung der Viscositätzahl für sehr kleine Konzentrationen, *J. Prak. Chem.*, 158, 130–135, 1941). These investigators (Reference 3) also reported intrinsic viscosity values obtained by the Huggins equation and Kraemer equation. Intrinsic viscosity values were also obtained at other temperatures and ethanol concentrations.

[d] mPEG, monomethoxy-PEG (prepared by anionic ring opening polymerization) (IVitz, J., Maidanski, T.C., Meier, A., Lutz, P.J., and Schubert, U.S. Polymerization of ethylene oxide under controlled monomer addition *via* a mass controller for tailor made polyethylene oxides, *Polymer Chem.*, 7, 4063–4071, 2016).

[e] M_w obtained from intrinsic sedimentation coefficient and frictional ratio.

[f] DPMPEG, diphenylmethyl PEG (prepared by anionic ring opening polymerization) (IVitz, J., Maidanski, T.C., Meier, A., Lutz, P.J., and Schubert, U.S., Polymerization of ethylene oxide under controlled monomer addition *via* a mass controller for tailor made polyethylene oxides, *Polymer Chem.*, 7, 4063–4071, 2016).

[g] FruPEG, β-ᴅ-Fructopyranosyl PEG (prepared by anionic ring opening polymerization IVitz, J., Maidanski, T.C., Meier, A., Lutz, P.J., and Schubert, U.S., Polymerization of ethylene oxide under controlled monomer addition *via* a mass controller for tailor made polyethylene oxides, *Polymer Chem.* 7, 4063–4071, 2016).

References

1. Hammes, G.G. and Roberts, P.B., Cooperativity of solvent-macromolecule interactions in aqueous solutions of polyethylene glycol and polyethylene glycol-urea, *J. Am. Chem. Soc.* 90, 7119–7122, 1968.
2. Kirinčič, S. and Klofutar, C., Viscosity of aqueous solutions of poly(ethylene glycol)s at 298.15 K, *Fluid Phase Equilibria* 155, 311–325, 1999.
3. Mehrdad, A. and Akbarzadeh, R., Effect of temperature and solvent composition on the intrinsic viscosity of poly (ethylene glycol) in water-ethanol solutions, *J. Chem. Eng. Data* 55, 2537–2541, 2010.
4. Nischang, I., Perevyazko, I., Majdanski, T., et al., Hydrodynamic analysis resolves the pharmaceutically-relevant absolute molar mass and solution properties of synthetic poly (ethylene glycol)s created by varying initiation sites, *Anal. Chem.* 89(2), 1185–1193, 2017.

INTERNATIONAL UNION OF PURE AND APPLIED CHEMISTRY

PHYSICAL CHEMISTRY DIVISION COMMISSION ON
MOLECULAR STRUCTURE AND SPECTROSCOPY*

NMR NOMENCLATURE – NUCLEAR SPIN PROPERTIES
AND CONVENTIONS FOR CHEMICAL SHIFTS

(IUPAC Recommendations 2001)

Prepared for publication by

Robin K. Harris[1], Edwin D. Becker[2], Sonia M. Cabral De Menezes[3], Robin Goodfellow[4], and Pierre Granger[5]

[1]*Department of Chemistry, University of Durham, South Road, Durham, DH1 3LE, UK*

[2]*National Institutes of Health, Bethesda, Maryland 20892-0520, USA*

[3]*PETROBRAS/CENPES/QUÍMICA, Ilha do Fundão, Quadra 7, Cidade Universitária, 21949-900, Rio de Janeiro, R.J., Brazil*

[4]*School of Chemistry, University of Bristol, Cantock's Close, Bristol, BS8 1TS, UK*

[5]*Institut de Chimie, Université Louis Pasteur de Strasbourg, 1 rue Blaise Pascal, 67008 Strasbourg, CEDEX, France*

*Membership of the Commission during the preparation of this report (1994–2001) was as follows:

Chairman: J. E. Bertie (Canada, 1994–2001); *Secretary:* J. F. Sullivan (USA, 1994–1995); P. Klaeboe (Norway, 1996–2001); *Titular Members:* J. E. Boggs (USA, 1998–2001); S. M. Cabral de Menezes (Brazil, 2000–2001); A. M. Heyns (RSA, 1994–2001); N. Hirota (Japan, 1998–2001); R. Janoschek (Austria, 1994–1997, 2000–2001); R. S. McDowell (USA, 1998–2001); P. Klaeboe (Norway, 1994–1995); S. Tsuchiya (Japan, 1994–1997); B. P. Winnewisser (Germany, 1994–1997); *Associate Members:* A. M. Bradshaw (FRG, 1994–1995); S. M. Cabral de Menezes (Brazil, 1994–1999); B. G. Derendjaev (Russia, 1994–1995); E. Hirota (Japan, 1994–1997); J. Kowalewski (Sweden, 1996–2001); A. Oskam (Netherlands, 1994–2001); P. v. R. Schleyer (Germany, 1998–2001); S. Tsuchiya (Japan, 1998–1999); B. J. Van Der Veken (Belgium, 2000–2001); C. Zhang (China, 1994–1997); Q.-S. Zhu (China, 1998–2001); *National Representatives:* B. H. Boo (Korea, 2000–2001); E. Collin (Belgium, 1994–1997); M. Chowdhury (India, 1994–1995); S. Califano (Italy, 1994–1997); D. Escolar (Spain, 1996–1997); T. A. Ford (RSA, 2000–2001); R. K. Harris (UK, 1994–2001); J. P. Hawranek (Poland, 1998–2001); R. Janoschek (Austria, 1998–1999); Y. S. Lee (Republic of Korea, 1994–1999); D. Escolar (Spain, 1991–1997); J. Kowalewski (Sweden, 1994–1995); P. T. Manoharan (India, 1998–2001); S. Suzer (Turkey, 1996–1997); S. Içli (Turkey, 1994–1995); S. L. Spassov (Bulgaria, 2000–2001); J. J. C. Teixeira-Dias (Portugal, 1994–2001); B. J. Van Der Veken (Belgium, 1998–1999).

Reproduced from:
Pure & Appl. Chem., Vol. 73, No. 11, pp. 1795–1818, 2001.

NMR NOMENCLATURE – NUCLEAR SPIN PROPERTIES AND CONVENTIONS FOR CHEMICAL SHIFTS

(IUPAC Recommendations 2001)

Abstract: A unified scale is recommended for reporting the NMR chemical shifts of *all* nuclei relative to the ^{1}H resonance of tetramethylsilane (TMS). The unified scale is designed to provide a precise ratio, Ξ, of the resonance frequency of a given nuclide to that of the primary reference, the ^{1}H resonance of TMS in dilute solution (volume fraction, $\phi < 1\%$) in chloroform. Referencing procedures are discussed, including matters of practical application of the unified scale. Special attention is paid to recommended reference samples, and values of Ξ for secondary references on the unified scale are listed, many of which are the results of new measurements.

Some earlier recommendations relating to the reporting of chemical shifts are endorsed. The chemical shift, δ, is redefined to avoid previous ambiguities but to leave practical usage unchanged. Relations between the unified scale and recently published recommendations for referencing in aqueous solutions (for specific use in biochemical work) are discussed, as well as the special effects of working in the solid state with magic-angle spinning. In all, nine new recommendations relating to chemical shifts are made.

Standardized nuclear spin data are also presented in tabular form for the stable (and some unstable) isotopes of all elements with nonzero quantum numbers. The information given includes quantum numbers, isotopic abundances, magnetic moments, magnetogyric ratios and receptivities, together with quadrupole moments and line-width factors where appropriate.

1. Introduction

A distinguishing feature of nuclear magnetic resonance (NMR) is that signals are isotope-specific. In other words, each signal can be firmly linked to a particular element and nuclide. Two features follow: Firstly, there is a close connection with chemistry and, in particular, with the periodic table, since almost all elements can be studied; secondly, the spin properties of each isotope need to be clearly tabulated and firmly understood. It is a principal purpose of this document to provide such information.

Any scientific discipline relies for its effectiveness upon communication of ideas and results, which can only occur if there is an agreed basis for the meaning of the terminology used. The process of communication is greatly eased if there are universally recognized conventions for measurement and reporting of quantities with their units and symbols. The aim of this document is to set down such a set of meanings and conventions in relation to chemical shifts (and shielding) and to list resonance frequencies for reference signals for each magnetically active nucleus.

Within IUPAC, Commission I.5 has been responsible for molecular structure and spectroscopy. Until now, this Commission has produced only three reports [1–3] specifically relating to NMR. The two earlier reports refer to chemical shifts. The more recent of these two publications is 25 years old, and the NMR world has changed beyond recognition since then. Recently, however, conventions for chemical shifts of five nuclei of wide biochemical interest have been included in "Recommendations for the presentation of NMR structures of proteins and nuclei acids" [4] by Commission I.7, Biophysical Chemistry. The current document addresses the same issue for general chemical usage and extends the conventions to the entire range of active nuclei, providing a more comprehensive guide to the factors important in chemical shift referencing. A unified list of properties of NMR-observable nuclei is also included herein.

2. Nuclear Spin Properties

The phenomenon of NMR is based upon the magnetic properties of various isotopes of elements in the periodic table. It is, therefore, important to have an accessible unified list of these properties. These are contained in Tables 1–3 of this article, which include the following for each stable isotope and each long-lived radioactive isotope with nonzero spin:

(i) The nuclear spin quantum number, I, of the ground state of the nucleus.* This defines the magnitude of the spin angular momentum vector (and hence magnetic dipole moment—see below). The z-component quantum number is then denoted by m_I.

(ii) The standard isotopic natural abundance, x, expressed as a mole fraction in %.

(iii) The magnetic dipole moment, μ, of the nuclide, in terms of the nuclear magneton, μ_N. It should be noted that we have chosen to use the full vector magnitude of μ, given by:

$$|\mu|/\mu_N = |\gamma|\, \hbar[I(I+1)]^{1/2}/\mu_N \qquad (1)$$

where γ is the magnetogyric ratio and $\hbar$ is the Planck constant divided by 2π. Many lists prefer to give only the maximum value of the z-component of μ, namely, $\mu_z = \gamma\, \hbar I$, frequently without explicitly stating this fact. The sign of μ given in Tables 1–3 refers to its direction compared to the related spin angular momentum vector.

(iv) The magnetogyric ratio, γ (sometimes called the gyromagnetic ratio). The SI base units of this quantity are (angular frequency)/(magnetic induction) normally given as rad s^{-1} T^{-1}.

(v) The receptivity, of a nucleus in natural abundance, which influences the NMR signal strength. A common definition [5] involves the proportionality of receptivity to $\gamma^3 x I (I + 1)$. In practice, it is useful to list such receptivities relative to those of the commonly used nuclei ^{1}H (proton) and ^{13}C, giving receptivity ratios D^p and D^C, respectively. Both these quantities are given in Tables 1 and 2.

(vi) The quadrupole moment, Q, for nuclei with spin quantum number $I > 1/2$ (Tables 2 and 3 only). These data fall naturally in the region of 10^{-30} m^2, i.e., fm^2. However, quadrupole moments are often expressed in units of 10^{-28} m^2, called a barn, where 1 barn = 100 fm^2.

---

* NMR is entirely concerned with the nuclear spin in the lowest-energy nuclear state, though Mössbauer spectroscopy involves values of I in higher-energy nuclear states.

TABLE 1: The Spin Properties of Spin- Nuclei[a]

Isotope[b]	Natural abundance,[c] $x/\%$	Magnetic moment,[d] μ/μ_N	Magnetogyric ratio,[d] $\gamma/10^7$ rad s^{-1} T^{-1}	Frequency ratio,[e] $\Xi/\%$	Reference compound	Sample conditions[f]	Literature for Ξ	Relative receptivity[g] D^p	D^c
^{1}H	99.9885	4.837 353 570	26.752 2128	100.000 000[h]	Me$_4$Si	CDCl$_3$, φ = 1%	–	1.000	5.87×10^3
^{3}H[i]	–	5.159 714 367	28.534 9779	106.663 974	Me$_4$Si-t_1	j	10	–	–
^{3}He	1.37×10^{-4}	-3.685 154 336	-20.380 1587	76.179 437	He	gas	11	6.06×10^{-7}	3.56×10^{-3}
^{13}C	1.07	1.216 613	6.728 284	25.145 020	Me$_4$Si	CDCl$_3$, φ = 1%	12,13	1.70×10^{-4}	1.00
^{15}N	0.368	-0.490 497 46	-2.712 618 04	10.136 767	MeNO$_2$	neat/CDCl$_3$[k]	9	3.84×10^{-6}	2.25×10^{-2}
^{19}F	100	4.553 333	25.181 48	94.094 011	CCl$_3$F	j	14	0.834	4.90×10^3
^{29}Si	4.6832	-0.961 79	-5.3190	19.867 187	Me$_4$Si	CDCl$_3$, φ = 1%	15	3.68×10^{-4}	2.16
^{31}P	100	1.959 99	10.8394	40.480 742	H$_3$PO$_4$	j	16	6.65×10^{-2}	3.91×10^2
^{57}Fe	2.119	0.156 9636	0.868 0624	3.237 778	Fe(CO)$_5$	C$_6$D$_6$[l]	9	7.24×10^{-7}	4.25×10^{-3}
^{77}Se	7.63	0.926 775 77	5.125 3857	19.071 513	Me$_2$Se	neat/C$_6$D$_6$[k]	9	5.37×10^{-4}	3.15
^{89}Y	100	-0.238 010 49	-1.316 2791	4.900 198	Y(NO$_3$)$_3$	H$_2$O/D$_2$O[m]	9	1.19×10^{-4}	0.700
^{103}Rh	100	-0.1531	-0.8468	3.186 44$_{n,o}$	Rh(acac)$_3$[p]	CDCl$_3$, sat.	18	3.17×10^{-5}	0.186
(^{107}Ag)	51.839	-0.196 898 93	-1.088 9181	4.047 819	AgNO$_3$	D$_2$O, sat.	9	3.50×10^{-5}	0.205
^{109}Ag	48.161	-0.226 362 79	-1.251 8634	4.653 533	AgNO$_3$	D$_2$O, sat.	9	4.94×10^{-5}	0.290
(^{111}Cd)	12.80	-1.030 3729	-5.698 3131	21.215 480	Me$_2$Cd	neat[l]	19	1.24×10^{-3}	7.27
^{113}Cd[q]	12.22	-1.077 8568	-5.960 9155	22.193 175	Me$_2$Cd	neat[l]	19	1.35×10^{-3}	7.94
(^{115}Sn)	0.34	-1.5915	-8.8013	32.718 749	Me$_4$Sn	neat/C$_6$D$_6$[k]	9	1.21×10^{-4}	0.711
(^{117}Sn)	7.68	-1.733 85	-9.588 79	35.632 259	Me$_4$Sn	neat/C$_6$D$_6$[k]	9	3.54×10^{-3}	20.8
^{119}Sn	8.59	-1.813 94	-10.0317	37.290 632	Me$_4$Sn	neat/C$_6$D$_6$[k]	9	4.53×10^{-3}	26.6
(^{123}Te)	0.89	-1.276 431	-7.059 098	26.169 742	Me$_2$Te	neat/C$_6$D$_6$[k]	9	1.64×10^{-4}	0.961
^{125}Te	7.07	-1.538 9360	-8.510 8404	31.549 769	Me$_2$Te	neat/C$_6$D$_6$[k]	9	2.28×10^{-3}	13.4
^{129}Xe	26.44	-1.347 494	-7.452 103	27.810 186	XeOF$_4$	neat[l]	20,21	5.72×10^{-3}	33.6
^{183}W	14.31	0.204 009 19	1.128 2403	4.166 387	Na$_2$WO$_4$	D$_2$O, 1 M	11	1.07×10^{-5}	6.31×10^{-2}
^{187}Os	1.96	0.111 9804	0.619 2895	2.282 331	OsO$_4$	CCl$_4$, 0.98 M	22	2.43×10^{-7}	1.43×10^{-3}
^{195}Pt	33.832	1.0557	5.8385	21.496 784[n]	Na$_2$WO$_4$	D$_2$O, 1.2 M	9	3.51×10^{-3}	20.7
^{199}Hg	16.87	0.876 219 37	4.845 7916	17.910 822	Me$_2$Hg[r]	neat	11	1.00×10^{-3}	5.89
^{203}Tl	29.524	2.809 833 05	15.539 3338	57.123 200[s]	Tl(NO$_3$)$_3$	j	24	5.79×10^{-2}	3.40×10^2
^{205}Tl	70.476	2.837 470 94	15.692 1808	57.683 838	Tl(NO$_3$)$_3$	j	25	0.142	8.36×10^2
^{207}Pb	22.1	1.009 06	5.580 46	20.920 599	Me$_4$Pb	neat/C$_6$D$_6$[k]	9	2.01×10^{-3}	11.8

a   A complete list for stable nuclei, but excluding the lanthanides, the actinides and most radioactive isotopes.
b   Nuclei in parentheses are considered to be not the most favorable of the element concerned for NMR.
c   Data are "representative isotopic compositions", taken from Rosman et al. [8].
d   Data derived from the compilation in Mills et al. [6], pp. 98–104, which lists values of $|\mu_{max} / \mu_N| = \gamma \hbar I \, \mu_N$. For the error limits, see Mills et al. [6].
e   Ratios of the resonance frequency to that of the protons of TMS at infinite dilution (in practice at φ = 1%) in CDCl$_3$.
f   M ≡ molarity in mol dm^{-3} (solution); m = molality in mol kg^{-1} (solvent). Some results from ref. 9 were initially referenced [7] to a TMS concentration of 4.75 m in CDCl$_3$, but the values are corrected to refer to a dilute (φ = 1 %) solution of TMS in CDCl$_3$.
g D^p is the receptivity [5] relative to that of ^{1}H, whereas D^c is relative to ^{13}C.
h   Value by definition (see the text).
i   Radioactive (half-life 12 y).
j   See literature cited.
k   Small amount of lock substance (φ < 10%) in neat liquid.
l   φ = 20% of C$_6$D$_6$ in Fe(CO)$_5$.
m   H$_2$O/D$_2$O solution, concentration not reported.
n   Alternatively, the precise values 3.160 000 MHz and 21.400 000 have been suggested [17] as the references for ^{103}Rh and ^{195}Pt, respectively.
o   Subject to considerable variation with temperature.
p   acac = acetylacetonato
q   Long-lived radioactive isotope.
r   The high toxicity of this compound means its direct use should be strongly discouraged [23].
s   Deduced from refs. 24 and 25.

TABLE 2: The Spin Properties of Quadrupolar Nuclei[a] (Continued)

Isotope[b]	Spin[c]	Natural abundance,[c] x1%	Magnetic moment,[d] μ/μ_N	Magnetogyric ratio,[d] $\gamma/10^7$ rad s^{-1} T^{-1}	Quadrupole moment[e] Q/fm^2	Frequency ratio,[f] Ξ /%	Reference sample	Sample conditions[g]	Literature for Ξ	Line-width factor,[h] ℓ/fm^4	D^p	D^c
2H/	1	0.0115	1.212 600 77	4.106 627 91	0.2860	15.350 609	(CD$_3$)$_4$Si	neat	15	0.41	1.11×10^{-6}	6.52×10^{-3}
6Li	1	7.59	1.162 5637	3.937 1709	-0.0808	14.716 086	LiCl	D$_2$O, 9.7 m	9	0.033	6.45×10^{-4}	3.79
7Li	3/2	92.41	4.204 075 05	10.397 7013	-4.01	38.863 797	LiCl	D$_2$O, 9.7 m	9	21	0.271	1.59×10^{3}
9Be	3/2	100	-1.520 136	-3.759 666	5.288	14.051 813	BeSO$_4$	D$_2$O, 0.43 m	9	37	1.39×10^{-2}	81.5
10B	3	19.9	2.079 2055	2.874 6786	8.459	10.743 658	BF$_3$.Et$_2$O	CDCl$_3$[k]	29	14	3.95×10^{-3}	23.2
11B	3/2	80.1	3.471 0308	8.584 7044	4.059	32.083 974	BF$_3$.Et$_2$O	CDCl$_3$[k]	29	22	0.132	7.77×10^{2}
14N/	1	99.632	0.571 004 28	1.933 7792	2.044	7.226 317	CH$_3$NO$_2$	neat/CDCl$_3$[ℓ]	9	21	1.00×10^{-3}	5.90
17O	5/2	0.038	-2.240 77	-3.628 08	-2.558	13.556 457	D$_2$O	neat	9	2.1	1.11×10^{-5}	6.50×10^{-2}
21Ne	3/2	0.27	-0.854 376	-2.113 08	10.155	7.894 296[m]	Ne	gas, 1.1 MPa	9	140	6.65×10^{-6}	3.91×10^{-2}
23Na	3/2	100	2.862 9811	7.080 8493	10.4	26.451 900	NaCl	D$_2$O, 0.1 M	9	140	9.27×10^{-2}	5.45×10^{2}
25Mg	5/2	10.00	-1.012 20	-1.638 87	19.94	6.121 635	MgCl$_2$	D$_2$O, 11 M	9	130	2.68×10^{-4}	1.58
27Al	5/2	100	4.308 6865	6.976 2715	14.66	26.056 859	Al(NO$_3$)$_3$	D$_2$O, 1.1 m	9	69	0.207	1.22×10^{3}
33S	3/2	0.76	0.831 1696	2.055 685	-6.78	7.676 000	(NH$_4$)$_2$SO$_4$	D$_2$O, sat.	9	61	1.72×10^{-5}	0.101
35Cl	3/2	75.78	1.061 035	2.624 198	-8.165	9.797 909	NaCl	D$_2$O, 0.1 M	9	89	3.58×10^{-3}	21.0
37Cl	3/2	24.22	0.883 1998	2.184 368	-6.435	8.155 725	NaCl	D$_2$O, 0.1 M	9	55	6.59×10^{-4}	3.87
39K	3/2	93.2581	0.505 433 76	1.250 0608	5.85	4.666 373	KCl	D$_2$O, 0.1 M	9	46	4.76×10^{-4}	2.79
(40K)	4	0.0117	-1.451 3203	-1.554 2854	-7.3	5.802 018	KCl	D$_2$O, 0.1 M	31	5.2	6.12×10^{-7}	3.59×10^{-3}
(41K)	3/2	6.7302	0.277 396 09	0.686 068 08	7.11	2.561 305[n]	KCl	D$_2$O, 0.1 M	31	67	5.68×10^{-6}	3.33×10^{-2}
43Ca	7/2	0.135	-1.494 067	-1.803 069	-4.08	6.730 029[o]	CaCl$_2$	D$_2$O, 0.1 M	32	2.3	8.68×10^{-6}	5.10×10^{-2}
45Sc	7/2	100	5.393 3489	6.508 7973	-22.0	24.291 747	Sc(NO$_3$)$_3$	D$_2$O, 0.06 M	9	66	0.302	1.78×10^{3}
47Ti	5/2	7.44	-0.932 94	-1.5105	30.2	5.637 534	TiCl$_4$	neat[p]	9	290	1.56×10^{-4}	0.918
49Ti	7/2	5.41	-1.252 01	-1.510 95	24.7	5.639 037	TiCl$_4$	neat[p]	9	83	2.05×10^{-4}	1.20
(50V)[q]	6	0.250	3.613 7570	2.670 6490	21.0	9.970 309	voc l$_3$	neat/C$_6$D$_6$[t]	9	17	1.39×10^{-4}	0.818
51V	7/2	99.750	5.838 0835	7.045 5117	-5.2	26.302 948	voc l$_3$	neat/C$_6$D$_6$[t]	9	3.7	0.383	2.25×10^{3}
53Cr	3/2	9.501	-0.612 63	-1.5152	-15.0	5.652 496	K$_2$CrO$_4$	D$_2$O, sat.	9	300	8.63×10^{-5}	0.507
55Mn	5/2	100	4.104 2437	6.645 2546	33.0	24.789 218	KMnO$_4$	D$_2$O, 0.82 m	9	350	0.179	1.05×10^{3}
59Co	7/2	100	5.247	6.332	42.0	23.727 074	K$_3$[Co(CN)$_6$]	D$_2$O, 0.56 m	9	240	0.278	1.64×10^{3}
61Ni	3/2	1.1399	-0.968 27	-2.3948	16.2	8.936 051	Ni(CO)$_4$	neat/C$_6$D$_6$[t]	33	350	4.09×10^{-5}	0.240
63Cu	3/2	69.17	2.875 4908	7.111 7890	-22.0	26.515 473	[Cu(CH$_3$CN)$_4$][ClO$_4$]	CH$_3$CN, sat.[r]	9	650	6.50×10^{-2}	3.82×10^{2}
65Cu	3/2	30.83	3.074 65	7.604 35	-20.4	28.403 693	[Cu(CH$_3$CN)$_4$][ClO$_4$]	CH$_3$CN, sat.[r]	9	550	3.54×10^{-2}	2.08×10^{2}
67Zn	5/2	4.10	1.035 556	1.676 688	15.0	6.256 803	Zn(NO$_3$)$_2$	D$_2$O, sat.	9	72	1.18×10^{-4}	0.692
(69Ga)	3/2	60.108	2.603 405	6.438 855	17.1	24.001 354	Ga(NO$_3$)$_3$	D$_2$O, 1.1 m	34	390	4.19×10^{-2}	2.46×10^{2}
71Ga	3/2	39.892	3.307 871	8.181 171	10.7	30.496 704	Ga(NO$_3$)$_3$	D$_2$O, 1.1 m	34	150	5.71×10^{-2}	3.35×10^{2}
73Ge	9/2	7.73	-0.972 2881	-0.936 0303	-19.6	3.488 315	(CH$_3$)$_4$Ge	neat[s]	35	28	1.09×10^{-4}	0.642
75As	3/2	100	1.858 354	4.596 163	31.4	17.122 614	NaAsF$_6$	CD$_3$CN, 0.5 M	9	1300	2.54×10^{-2}	1.49×10^{2}
(79Br)	3/2	50.69	2.719 351	6.725 616	31.3	25.053 980	NaBr	D$_2$O, 0.01 M	9	1300	4.03×10^{-2}	2.37×10^{2}
81Br	3/2	49.31	2.931 283	7.249 776	26.2	27.006 518	NaBr	D$_2$O, 0.01 M	9	920	4.91×10^{-2}	2.88×10^{2}
83Kr	9/2	11.49	-1.073 11	-1.033 10	25.9	3.847 600[i]	Kr	gas	36	50	2.18×10^{-4}	1.28
(85Rb)	5/2	72.17	1.601 3071	2.592 7050	27.6	9.654 943	RbCl	D$_2$O, 0.01 M	9	240	7.67×10^{-3}	45.0
87Rb[q]	3/2	27.83	3.552 582	8.786 400	13.35	32.720 454	RbCl	D$_2$O, 0.01 M	9	240	4.93×10^{-2}	2.90×10^{2}
87Sr	9/2	7.00	-1.209 0236	-1.163 9376	33.5	4.333 822	SrCl$_2$	D$_2$O, 0.5 M	37	83	1.90×10^{-4}	1.12
91Zr	5/2	11.22	-1.542 46	-2.497 43	-17.6	9.296 298	Zr(C$_5$H$_5$)$_2$Cl$_2$	CH$_2$Cl$_2$, sat.[t]	9	99	1.07×10^{-3}	6.26
93Nb	9/2	100	6.8217	6.5674	-32.0	24.476 170	K[NbCl$_6$]	CH$_3$CN, sat.[u]	22	76	0.488	2.87×10^{3}
95Mo	5/2	15.92	-1.082	-1.751	-2.2	6.516 926	Na$_2$MoO$_4$	D$_2$O, 2 M[v]	34	1.5	5.21×10^{-4}	3.06
(97Mo)	5/2	9.55	-1.105	-1.788	25.5	6.653 695	Na$_2$MoO$_4$	D$_2$O, 2 M[v]	34	210	3.33×10^{-4}	1.95
99Tc[o]	9/2	–	6.281	6.046	-12.9	22.508 326	NH$_4$TcO$_4$	D$_2$O[w]	9	12	–	–
99Ru	5/2	12.76	-0.7588	-1.229	7.9	4.605 151	K$_4$[Ru(CN)$_6$]	D$_2$O, 0.3 M	9	20	1.44×10^{-4}	0.848
101Ru	5/2	17.06	-0.8505	-1.377	45.7	5.161 369	K$_4$[Ru(CN)$_6$]	D$_2$O, 0.3 M	9	670	2.71×10^{-4}	1.59
105pd	5/2	22.33	-0.760	-1.23	66.0	4.576 100	K$_2$PdCl$_6$	D$_2$O, sat.	22	1400	2.53×10^{-4}	1.49
(113In)	9/2	4.29	6.1124	5.8845	79.9	21.865 755	In(NO$_3$)$_3$	D$_2$O, 0.1 M[x]	34	470	1.51×10^{-2}	88.5
115In[q]	9/2	95.71	6.1256	5.8972	81.0	21.912 629	In(NO$_3$)$_3$	D$_2$O, 0.1M[x]	34	490	0.338	1.98×10^{3}
121Sb	5/2	57.21	3.9796	6.4435	-36.0	23.930 577	KSbCl$_6$	CH$_3$CN, sat.[u]	9	410	9.33×10^{-2}	5.48×10^{2}

TABLE 2: The Spin Properties of Quadrupolar Nucleia (Continued)

Isotope[b]	Spin[c]	Natural abundance,[c] x/%	Magnetic moment,[d] μ/μ_N	Magnetogyric ratio,[d] $\gamma/10^7$ rad s^{-1} T^{-1}	Quadrupole moment[e] Q/fm^2	Frequency ratio,[e] Ξ/%	Reference sample	Sample conditions[g]	Literature for Ξ	Line-width factor,[h] ℓ/fm^4	Relative receptivity[i] D^p	D^c
(123Sb)	7/2	42.79	2.8912	3.4892	−49.0	12.959 217	KSbCl$_6$	CH$_3$CN, sat.[u]	9	330	1.99 × 10^{-2}	1.17 × 10^2
127I	5/2	100	3.328 710	5.389 573	−71.0	20.007 486	KI	D$_2$O, 0.01 M	9	1600	9.54 × 10^{-2}	5.60 × 10^2
131Xe	3/2	21.18	0.893 1899	2.209 076	−11.4	8.243 921[v]	XeOF$_4$	neat		170	5.96 × 10^{-4}	3.50
133Cs	7/2	100	2.927 7407	3.533 2539	−0.343	13.116 142	CsNO$_3$	D$_2$O, 0.1 M	9	0.016	4.84 × 10^{-2}	2.84 × 10^2
(135Ba)	3/2	6.592	1.081 78	2.675 50	16.0	9.934 457	BaCl$_2$	D$_2$O, 0.5 M	9,38	340	3.30 × 10^{-4}	1.93
137Ba	3/2	11.232	1.210 13	2.992 95	24.5	11.112 928	BaCl$_2$	D$_2$O, 0.5 M	9,38	800	7.87 × 10^{-4}	4.62
138La	5	0.090	4.068 095	3.557 239	45.0	13.194 300	LaCl$_3$	D$_2$O/H$_2$O[z]	39	120	8.46 × 10^{-5}	0.497
139La	7/2	99.910	3.155 6770	3.808 3318	20.0	14.125 641	LaCl$_3$	D$_2$O, 0.01 M	11	54	6.05 × 10^{-2}	3.56 × 10^2
177Hf	7/2	18.60	0.8997	1.086	336.5	(4.007)[A]	–	–	–	1.5 × 10^4	2.61 × 10^{-4}	1.54
179Hf	9/2	13.62	−0.7085	−0.6821	379.3	(2.517)[A]	–	–	–	1.1 × 10^4	7.45 × 10^{-5}	0.438
181Ta	7/2	99.988	2.6879	3.2438	317.0	11.989 600[B]	KTaCl$_6$	CH$_3$CN, sat.	40	1.4 × 10^4	3.74 × 10^{-2}	2.20 × 10^2
(185Re)	5/2	37.40	3.7710	6.1057	218.0	22.524 600[B]	KReO$_4$	D$_2$O, 0.1 M	40	1.5 × 10^4	5.19 × 10^{-2}	3.05 × 10^2
187Re	5/2	62.60	3.8096	6.1682	207.0	22.751 600[B]	KReO$_4$	D$_2$O, 0.1 M	40	1.4 × 10^4	8.95 × 10^{-2}	5.26 × 10^2
189Os	3/2	16.15	0.851 970	2.107 13	85.6	7.765 400[B]	OsO$_4$	CCl$_4$, 0.98 M	22	9800	3.95 × 10^{-4}	2.32
(191Ir)	3/2	37.3	0.1946	0.4812	81.6	(1.718)[A]	–	–		8900	1.09 × 10^{-5}	6.38 × 10^{-2}
193Ir	3/2	62.7	0.2113	0.5227	75.1	(1.871)[A]	–	–		7500	2.34 × 10^{-5}	0.137
197Au	3/2	100	0.191 271	0.473 060	54.7	(1.729)[A]	–	–		4000	2.77 × 10^{-5}	0.162
201Hg	3/2	13.18	−0.723 2483	−1.788 769	38.6	6.611 583[a]	(CH$_3$)$_2$Hg[D]	neat	41	2000	1.97 × 10^{-4}	1.16
209Bi	9/2	100	4.5444	4.3750	−51.6	16.069 288	Bi(NO$_3$)$_3$	HNO$_3$/D$_2$O/H$_2$O[E]	9	200	0.144	8.48 × 10^2

a Excluding the lanthanides, actinides, and most radioactive isotopes.
b Nuclei in parentheses are considered to be not the most favorable of the element concerned for NMR.
c Data are "representative isotopic compositions", taken from Rosman et al. [8], pp. 98–104. For the error limits on the natural abundances, see Rosman et al. [8].
d Data derived from the compilation in Mills et al.[6] pp. 98–104, which lists values of $\mu_{max} = \mu_N / \gamma \hbar I/\mu_N$. For the error limits, see Mills et al. [6].
e Data from Mills et al. [6], pp. 98–104 (taken mostly from Pyykko [26] and Raghavan [27]) and updated from Pyykko [28]. It should be noted that reported values of Q may be in error by as much as 20–30%. For the error limits, see Pyykko [28].
f Ratio of the resonance frequency to that of the reference to that of the protons of TMS at infinite dilution (in practice at φ = 1%) in CDCl$_3$.
g M = molarity in mol dm^{-3} (solution); m = molality in mol kg^{-1} (solvent). Some results from ref. 9 were initially referenced [7] to a TMS concentration of 4.75 m in CDCl$_3$, but the values are corrected to refer to a dilute (φ = 1%) solution of TMS in CDCl$_3$.
h $\ell = (2I+3)Q^2/I^2(2I-1)$ [5]. The values are quoted, arbitrarily, to 2 significant figures.
i D^p is the receptivity [5] relative to that of ^{1}H whereas D^c is relative to ^{13}C. The values are given to three significant figures only.
j A useful isotope of $I = \frac{1}{2}$ exists.
k 15% by volume of BF$_3$·Et$_2$O in CDCl$_3$.
l Small amount of lock substance (φ < 10%) in neat liquid, except for ^{61}Ni (where φ = ca. 20% of C$_6$D$_6$ is involved).
m Ξ In reasonable agreement with a value deduced from a ratio given in ref. 30.
o Ξ deduced from data in ref. 31.
p Plus C$_6$D$_{12}$ (φ = 10%) for field/frequency lock purposes.
q Radioactive, with a long half-life.
r Containing a little C$_6$D$_6$ (φ < 10%).
s With conversion factors applied by Granger.
t The data in ref. 36 are only accurate to 4 decimal places. The proposal herein is that Ξ (^{83}Kr) is defined to the 6 decimal places given.
u In CH$_3$CN/CD$_3$CN for ^{93}Nb, ^{121}Sb, and ^{123}Sb.
v Plus a small quantity of NaOH.
w Semisaturated in H$_2$O/D$_2$O.
x Plus 0.5 M DNO$_3$.
y Calculated from the value for ^{129}Xe via the ^{129}Xe:^{131}Xe frequency ratio.
z For the solution conditions, see the reference.
A Value calculated from literature data on nuclear magnetic moments.
B The proposal herein is to define to 6 decimal places, but line-widths are generally such that this is unnecessarily accurate.
C Deduced from the ^{201}Hg:^{199}Hg ratio given in ref. 41.
D The high toxicity of this compound means its direct use should be strongly discouraged [23].
E Saturated in conc. HNO$_3$, then diluted with an equal volume of D$_2$O.

TABLE 3: The Spin Properties of Lanthanide and Actinide Nuclei[a]

Isotope	Spin	Natural abundance x/%	Magnetic moment μ /μ_N	Magnetogyric ratio γ /10^7 rad s^{-1} T^{-1}	Quadrupole moment[b] Q/fm^2	NMR frequency c Ξ /%
^{141}Pr	5/2	100	5.0587	8.1907	−5.89	(30.62)
^{143}Nd	7/2	12.2	−1.208	−1.457	−63.0	(5.45)
^{145}Nd	7/2	8.3	−0.744	−0.898	−33.0	(3.36)
^{147}Sm[d]	7/2	14.99	−0.9239	−1.115	−25.9	(4.17)
^{149}Sm	7/2	13.82	−0.7616	−0.9192	7.4	(3.44)
^{151}Eu	5/2	47.81	4.1078	6.6510	90.3	(24.86)
^{153}Eu	5/2	52.19	1.8139	2.9369	241.2	(10.98)
^{155}Gd	3/2	14.80	−0.33208	−0.82132	127.0	(3.07)
^{157}Gd	3/2	15.65	−0.43540	−1.0769	135.0	(4.03)
^{159}Tb	3/2	100	2.600	6.431	143.2	(24.04)
^{161}Dy	5/2	18.91	−0.5683	−0.9201	250.7	(3.44)
^{163}Dy	5/2	24.90	0.7958	1.289	264.8	(4.82)
^{165}Ho	7/2	100	4.732	5.710	358.0	(21.34)
^{167}Er	7/2	22.93	−0.63935	−0.77157	356.5	(2.88)
^{169}Tm	1/2	100	−0.4011	−2.218	–	(8.29)
^{171}Yb	1/2	14.28	0.85506	4.7288	–	17.499306[e]
^{173}Yb	5/2	16.13	−0.80446	−1.3025	280.0	(4.821)
^{175}Lu	7/2	97.41	2.5316	3.0552	349.0	(11.404)
^{176}Lu[d]	7	2.59	3.3880	2.1684	497.0	(8.131)
^{235}U[d]	7/2	0.7200	−0.43	−0.52	493.6	1.841400[f]

[a] These nuclides are sufficiently little used that values for line-width factors and relative receptivities are not listed here. However, for ^{169}Tm, $D^p = 5.70 \times 10^{-4}$ and $D^c = 3.35$, while for ^{171}Yb, $D^p = 7.89 \times 10^{-4}$ and $D^c = 4.63$.

[b] For the limits of accuracy, see ref. 28.

[c] Values in brackets are approximate (calculated from the magnetogyric ratios).

[d] Long-lived radioactive isotope.

[e] Reference: Yb(η-C_5Me_5)$_2$(THF)$_2$, 0.171 M in THF solution (THF ≡ tetrahydrofuran) [42].

[f] Reference: UF$_6$ (with φ = 10% of C_6D_6) [43].

(vii) The line-width factor, l, for quadrupolar nuclei. This is defined [5] by:

$$l = Q^2(2I + 3)/[I^2(2I - 1)] \tag{2}$$

When taken in conjunction with the relative receptivity (e.g., as D^C/l), this quantity gives a guide to the ease with which spectra can be obtained for different quadrupolar nuclei in solution for similar site symmetries and molecular mobilities. However, in practice, both symmetry and mobility may vary widely, thus introducing variations that may amount to several powers of ten.

Table 1 gives the data for the spin $-\frac{1}{2}$ nuclei in the periodic table, whereas Table 2 refers to quadrupolar nuclei. These two tables omit the lanthanide and actinide nuclei, which are separately listed in Table 3. Many of the data in Tables 1–3 have been taken from the IUPAC "Green Book" [6], but additional information is included (particularly on resonance frequencies and quadrupole moments). A version of Tables 1–3 has been published [7]. However, the tables given here contain revised resonance frequencies for consistency with the recommended primary reference, as described in Section 3.5. In addition, some new measurements of resonance frequencies are reported in Tables 1–3, and information about solution conditions and relevant references has been added.

3. Chemical Shifts

3.1 Background

Since the discovery of the chemical shift in 1950, NMR spectroscopy has become of vital importance to chemistry and related disciplines. The term chemical shift refers to a difference in resonance frequency (conventionally expressed as a fraction—see below) between nuclei in different chemical sites (or for samples under different physical conditions). Such effects are caused by variations in shielding by the electronic environment of the nuclei in question, and the concept of chemical shift is described by eq. 3:

$$\nu = \frac{\gamma}{2\pi} B_0 (1 - \sigma) \tag{3}$$

In this equation, the resonance frequency ν (normally in the radio frequency region) is related to the applied magnetic flux density B_0 by the magnetogyric ratio of the nucleus and the shielding constant σ.

In the International System of Units (SI), ν is expressed in hertz, Hz, (and is normally in the range of tens or hundreds of MHz), B_0 is in tesla, T, and σ is a dimensionless fraction (generally reported in parts per million, ppm). Equation 3 is usually applied to the situation in isotropic media (liquids, solutions, and gases), for which σ can be represented as a scalar quantity. However, the value of σ depends on molecular orientation in the applied magnetic field and can be represented by a scalar quantity only because of the averaging caused by rapid isotropic molecular tumbling. Therefore, σ is a second-rank tensor and must be used in that form for many situations in the solid state and in liquid crystals (and their solutions).

Whereas frequencies can be measured very precisely, the same cannot be said of B_0. Thus, although in principle chemists would like to know the absolute value of σ, it has long been recognized that only relative values can normally be obtained with precision. Therefore, from the early days of NMR the concept of a standard reference signal has been developed. This requires a number of choices, among which are:

(i) whether to base chemical shifts on resonance frequencies or on shielding,

(ii) which compound to use as a reference,

(ii) what further conditions to specify for the reference situation, and

(iv) whether to use separate references for different nuclei or to attempt to link them.

These matters will be dealt with in detail below.

In the early days of NMR, resonance was normally achieved by varying the applied field B_0. It therefore seemed natural for positive chemical shifts to refer to situations where the sample resonated at a higher field than that of the reference. Equation 3 shows that this corresponds to greater shielding for the sample than for the reference—a convention that was popular with theoreticians, who are principally concerned with σ. The first clear consensus on an experimental reference compound for proton NMR (by far the most popular nucleus at the time owing to its high sensitivity) was tetramethylsilane (TMS), introduced in 1958 by Tiers [44]. However, both for proton NMR and for other nuclei, various chemical shift scales were used, with some increasing in the direction of increasing magnetic field and others increasing in the direction of decreasing field (which corresponds to increasing frequency).

The convention recommended by IUPAC in the 1972 document [1], which mostly concerned proton NMR, was that given in eq. 4:

$$\delta_{X,sample} = \left(\frac{\nu_{X,sample} - \nu_{X,reference}}{\nu_{X,reference}} \right) \times 10^6 \qquad (4)$$

in which the chemical shift of a resonance for nucleus X is defined. For protons referenced to TMS this convention gives positive values with increasing frequency, and most proton chemical shifts then turn out to be positive. A second IUPAC report [2] in 1976 extended the recommendations to include nuclei other than protons, always with a high-frequency-positive convention.

Of course, since σ is, in principle, a tensor quantity, so is δ. However, the present document deals only with the isotropic average value of δ, which is the usual value of relevance for solution-state NMR. The tensor properties of σ and δ may be the subject of a later document.

3.2 Recommendations Endorsed

At this point, it is appropriate to list those recommendations of the previous two IUPAC reports on NMR which relate to chemical shifts [1,2] (including presentation of spectra) and which we endorse, with one exception noted under item 6. These relate to notational matters and are particularly directed at publications in chemical journals. In several places, we use different wording from the original reports and in some cases extended meanings:

1. The nucleus giving rise to the spectrum concerned should always be explicitly stated in full or in abbreviation (e.g., ^{10}B NMR or boron-10 NMR). The isotopic mass number should be given except in cases without ambiguity. In the case of hydrogen NMR, the *de facto* usage is proton NMR, deuterium NMR, or tritium NMR, in spite of the inconsistency of the wording. Abbreviations such as PMR for proton NMR are strongly discouraged. The term "multinuclear NMR" is clumsy (a repeated word "nuclear") and so is also to be discouraged. Where reference to a variety of nuclei is required, multinuclear magnetic resonance should be written in full.

2. The graphical presentation of spectra should show frequency increasing to the left and positive intensity increasing upwards.

3. The dimensionless scale for chemical shifts should be tied to a reference, which should be clearly stated. The procedures used must be carefully defined.

4. The dimensionless scale factor for chemical shifts should generally be expressed in parts per million, for which ppm is the appropriate abbreviation. The radio frequency of the reference, appropriate to the nucleus in question and to the spectrometer in use, should always be quoted, with sufficient accuracy in relation to the numerical values of shifts listed. Unfortunately, older software supplied by manufacturers to convert from frequency units to ppm in FT NMR sometimes uses the carrier frequency in the denominator instead of the true frequency of the reference, which can lead to significant errors.

5. The chemical shift scale should be defined with respect to resonance frequencies, with the appropriate sign convention (i.e., a positive sign should imply the sample resonates to high frequency from that of the reference). In order to avoid ambiguities of sign, the term "chemical shift" should *not* be used to describe variations in shielding.

6. The symbol δ (lower case Greek delta) should be used for chemical shift scales with the sign convention given above. Such a symbol should *never* be used to refer to shielding. These recommendations cohere with the definition of the δ-scale adopted in refs. 1 and 2. The definition of δ in eq. 4 leads to a value with no units, and the 1972 document recommended that "ppm" be not stated explicitly (e.g., $\delta = 5.00$, *not* $\delta = 5.00$ ppm). However, this convention is widely ignored. Therefore, we do *not* endorse the omission of "ppm" in reporting values of δ (see Section 3.3).

7. The nucleus in question should be indicated as a subscript or in brackets, e.g., δ_C or δ (^{13}C), unless there is no ambiguity.

8. As far as possible, full information should be given in publications regarding any factor that might influence chemical shifts, such as:

(i) The physical state of the sample (solid, liquid, solution, or gas), with additional relevant facts where necessary.

(ii) For solutions, the name of the solvent and the concentration of solute.

(iii) The nature of the reference procedure, e.g., internal, external (coaxial tubes or substitution), absolute frequency. (This aspect is discussed in detail in later sections of this article.)

(iv) The name of the secondary referencing compound local to the nucleus in question and its concentration. Note, however, that no reference compound needs to be added to the sample if the unified scale described in Section 3.5 is used, although a chemical shift value with respect to a recommended secondary reference compound, obtained via the unified scale, may still be quoted. In exceptional cases, where an isotope-specific secondary reference compound must be used in the experimental measurement, a clear description of the referencing procedure should be given.

(v) The temperature and (if different from ambient) the pressure of the sample.

(vi) Whether oxygen and other gases have been removed from the sample.

(vii) Any chemicals present in the sample, in addition to the solvent and the compound under investigation, and details of their concentrations.

3.3 Definition and Reporting of δ Scales

As mentioned above, the IUPAC Recommendation [1] dating from 1972 defined the proton chemical shift scale in such a way that δ has no quoted units but is presumed to be in ppm. However, this recommendation not to use "ppm" has *not* received acceptance in practice. It is a simple matter to rewrite eq. 4 in a general way that can lead validly to the units of ppm. We now *define* the chemical shift (for any nucleus X, using its local reference substance) by eq. 5:

$$\delta_{X,sample} = (\nu_{X,sample} - \nu_{X,reference})/\nu_{X,reference} \tag{5}$$

that is, *without* the factor of 10^6. This leads, in general, to a very small number, $M \times 10^{-n}$. Normal practice has been and will doubtless continue to be to use $n = 6$ and thus to express δ in ppm. With eq. 5 as the *definition* of δ, eq. 6 provides a simple procedure for *calculating* the value of δ in ppm from measured frequencies:

$$\delta_{X,sample}/ppm = \frac{\nu_{X,sample} - \nu_{X,reference}/Hz}{\nu_{X,reference}/MHz} \tag{6}$$

where the *factor* of 10^6 difference in the units of numerator and denominator is appropriately represented by the units ppm.

This redefinition allows values to be quoted also in parts per billion, ppb = 10^{-9}, (as is appropriate for some isotope effects) by expressing the numerator in eq. 6 in millihertz (mHz). Alternatively, the units of eq. 6 could be altered to give % (relevant for some heavy-metal chemical shifts), but ppm will undoubtedly remain as the most common usage. *IUPAC therefore recommends that the chemical shift δ be defined by eq. 5 and that δ normally be expressed in ppm.*

3.4 Referencing Procedures

Accurate and consistent referencing is easy to visualize but hard to implement. For mobile isotropic media (liquids, solutions, and gases) there are several possible methods:

(a) *Internal referencing*, where the reference compound is added directly to the system under study. This method is used almost universally for ^1H and ^{13}C NMR. However, it is clearly limited by the solubility, miscibility, or mutual reactions of the sample components and may be difficult to implement for many samples in which a variety of nuclei are studied.

(b) *External referencing*, involving sample and reference contained separately in coaxial cylindrical tubes. A single spectrum is recorded, which includes signals from both the sample and the reference compound.

(c) *Substitution method*: The use of separate cylindrical tubes for the sample and reference compound, with (in principle) spectra recorded individually for each. It is similar to external referencing in that sample and reference materials are not mixed, but there are significant differences in the two procedures, as described later, which arise because of the common use of precise field/frequency locking (usually via the ^2H signal of a deuterated solvent). If locking is not used, the magnet should not be reshimmed between running the sample and reference solutions, since this changes the applied magnetic field.

(d) Referencing via direct measurement of the absolute frequency of the field/frequency lock signal, usually provided by the ^2H resonance of an internally contained deuterated compound (frequently the solvent). This method is discussed more fully in Section 3.6.

(e) Application of magic-angle spinning, usually with the substitution method, but also conceivably with coaxial tubes—see Section 3.8.

These methods all have various advantages and disadvantages. For (a) the shielding of the reference nucleus depends, to a greater or lesser extent, on the solvent, on the solute under study, and on the concentration of both solute and reference owing to the effects of intermolecular interactions. These effects may be minimized by a judicious choice of solvent and reference compound, but they cannot be eliminated. External reference procedures (b) generally require corrections arising from differences in bulk magnetic susceptibility between sample and reference. These corrections depend on the geometry employed for the sample containers. For the usual coaxial cylindrical arrangement, the correction is [45]

$$\left(\delta_{true}/\delta_{obs}\right) = k\left(\kappa_{sample} - \kappa_{reference}\right) \tag{7}$$

where k refers to the relevant volume magnetic susceptibility (in rationalized units) and ideally $k = +1/6$ for a tube perpendicular to B_0, $k = -1/3$ for a tube parallel to B_0 (as is usual for a superconducting magnet), and $k = 0$ for a tube inclined at the magic angle. These theoretical factors are calculated for infinite cylinders. In practice, they depend on the length of the liquid column and other geometrical factors that are not always under control. No correction is needed for spherical samples, but the production of a truly spherical sample cell is generally not feasible. [Equation 7 is consistent with SI notation. A corresponding expression in cgs form would substitute $k_{cgs} = 4\pi k_{SI}$ along with a $\Delta\chi_V$ term numerically equal to $\Delta\kappa/4\pi$. Many lists of magnetic susceptibility data give χ_V rather than κ.]

The substitution method uses the fact that, with the advent of stable, internally solvent-locked spectrometers, it has become feasible to obtain accurate data by measuring the spectra of sample and reference in two separate experiments. If the sample and the reference compound are each dissolved in the same solvent at low concentration (which, where feasible, we recommend), the substitution method is equivalent to use of an internal reference, except that the reference substance does not contaminate the sample or interact with it, chemically or physically. If the reference compound is a nearly neat liquid with only a small amount of the deuterated "solvent" to serve as a lock, the measured chemical shifts may be slightly different from those obtained with an internal reference because of differing molecular interactions. It might appear that a magnetic susceptibility correction would be needed if the susceptibilities of sample and reference differ, but this is not the case. With the field/frequency lock established via the deuterated solvent, the applied magnetic field simply shifts slightly to maintain the magnetic induction inside the sample tube constant so as to keep the ^2H nuclei on resonance. There is, thus, a distinct difference between the commonly used *internally locked* system, in which the magnetic induction B_0 is maintained constant and an *unlocked* (or *externally locked*) system in which the applied field H_0 is constant.

If the lock signal of the sample differs from that of the reference, a lock correction may need to be applied according to:

$$\left(\delta_{true}/\delta_{measured}\right) + \left(\delta_{sample}^{lock} - \delta_{reference}^{lock}\right) \tag{8}$$

Except for very strongly hydrogen-bonded systems [46–48], no primary isotope effects between proton and deuterium have been firmly established, and none are expected on theoretical grounds. Hence, the difference between deuterium lock frequencies in eq. 8

may be obtained from a table of proton chemical shifts. However, when polyhydrogenated groups are involved, corrections may be needed for secondary isotope effects [46] arising from $^1H \rightarrow {}^2H$ replacement. When high precision is required the measurement of the shift difference between the locks may be obtained via direct observation of the deuterium spectrum of the two solvents, placed in coaxial tubes.

However, for most modern spectrometers, the manufacturers have incorporated compensating procedures for lock changes, largely for the users' convenience of retaining the spectral window in the same position on the screen or chart. Unfortunately, these procedures vary between manufacturers and between spectrometers of different ages from the same manufacturer, so no completely general comments on this question can be made here. NMR spectroscopists must refer to the relevant operating manual for details. In most cases with modern instruments, the effect is to keep the magnetic field inside the samples constant when different lock compounds are used. In such situations, the correction term in brackets in eq. 8 is not necessary. Of course, the accuracy of the result clearly depends on what the manufacturers use for the term in brackets, generally present in a "look-up" table in the spectrometer software. *We recommend that manufacturers give clear, explicit, and accurate guidance on their procedures in this matter and quote their "look-up" tables prominently.*

Another situation where isotope shifts have some effect is when signals of the reference compound are affected, for instance for ^{19}F measurements. In this case, the signal is split into four lines with intensities approximately 27:27:9:1 because the natural-abundance isotopic ratio $^{35}Cl:^{37}Cl$ is ca. 3:1. Since $CFCl_3$ is firmly accepted as the local reference for ^{19}F, it is not reasonable to suggest a new alternative. It is recommended that the reference signal is that of $CF(^{35}Cl)_2(^{37}Cl)$.

Earlier IUPAC documentation [1,2] did not suggest any specific composition for the reference sample, or choice of solvents. Ideally, for most referencing methods, a nonpolar solvent consisting of nearly spherical molecules should be used, and measurements should be extrapolated to zero reference concentration. Clearly, such procedures are not generally feasible, so that caution always needs to be exercised when comparing shift data from different sources.

3.5 Unified Scale

As NMR studies of various nuclei were initiated, each was, of necessity, treated independently, with some substance containing the nuclide being studied selected as a reference compound. The result is a vast collection of data in the literature for multinuclear magnetic resonance based on a large array of reference compounds. The proliferation of reference substances is, however, unnecessary and in some ways unhelpful. In a given magnetic field, all resonance frequencies form a single spectral range, and it is only because different nuclides resonate at markedly different frequencies that use of separate references has arisen. With modern instruments, in which all frequencies are derived from a single source, it is therefore possible to relate the observed frequencies of all nuclides in a particular sample to that of a single primary reference—preferably the proton resonance of TMS.*

There are, however, two reasons for wishing to retain the concept of a separate reference for each nucleus: (*i*) It is convenient

to speak of, say, an aromatic ^{13}C resonance at *x* ppm from the ^{13}C line of TMS, rather than always quoting a frequency to many significant figures, and (*ii*) many data tabulations are available with values only expressed relative to separate heteronuclear references. Thus, for a unified scale to be of practical use, there must be agreed frequency relations between a set of commonly used secondary (heteronuclear) references and the primary reference. Measurements of such relations have been reported sporadically since the time of early double-resonance experiments [49], and it has been proposed to relate the separate reference frequencies to a primary standard originally defined for a magnetic field such that the ^1H TMS signal is at exactly 100 MHz. These frequencies have been given [49] the symbol Ξ (capital Greek xi), and some tabulations have been presented [5,14,50–52]. However, it is clearer and more appropriate for users of modern high-field NMR spectrometers simply *to define Ξ as the ratio of the secondary (isotope-specific) frequency to that of ^1H in TMS in the same magnetic field. Therefore, it is convenient to express Ξ as a percentage by the use of eq. 9:*

$$\Xi\,/\,\% = 100\left(v_X^{obs}\,/\,v_{TMS}^{obs}\right) \qquad (9)$$

where v_{TMS}^{obs} is the measured ^1H frequency of TMS. The use of percentage ensures that values of Ξ with this recommendation are numerically identical to those based on the earlier [49] definition.

Recently, the question of a unified reference has been addressed for multinuclear studies in biomolecular NMR: Wishart *et al.* [53] surveyed the relevant literature, pointed out inconsistencies in existing practices, and proposed the use of a single internal reference—for their purposes, one that is highly soluble in water (sodium 2,2-dimethyl-2-silapentane-5-sulfonate, DSS[†], preferably deuterated at the CH_2 positions). Operationally, as discussed in the following sections, it is often easier to obtain the necessary heteronuclear frequency data directly via the lock signal than to make additional measurements with various reference materials for different nuclei.

IUPAC recommends that a unified chemical shift scale for all nuclides be based on the proton resonance of TMS as the primary reference. This recommendation is in line with the "Recommendations for presentation of NMR structures of proteins and nucleic acids", recently promulgated [4] by IUPAC in conjunction with the International Union of Biochemistry and Molecular Biology and the International Union of Pure and Applied Biophysics, which include recommended Ξ values for several nuclei of importance in such studies for aqueous solutions, but which uses the proton resonance of DSS as the primary standard because of its solubility in water (see Section 3.9).

In conformity with other areas in physical chemistry, it would be desirable to define a precise standard state—for example, pure liquid TMS or TMS at infinite dilution in $CDCl_3$ at 293 K and 1 bar. [Indeed, in principle a better standard might be ^3He or ^{129}Xe in the gaseous state at a very low pressure (see ref. 55 and references therein), but this is not practicable.] However, in this document we concentrate on aspects that are of immediate practical utility. Temperature and pressure effects on chemical shifts for solutions and solid samples are sufficiently small for the lighter elements to be generally ignored for most chemical usage of NMR (largely carried out at ambient probe temperature and pressure), so we make no detailed recommendations regarding these parameters. References 55 and 56 contain some data on

---

* TMS has a low boiling point (28 °C), which can be advantageous in facilitating removal from nonvolatile samples after use, but can in other circumstances be a severe disadvantage. To overcome this problem, a substance such as $[(CH_3)_3Si]_4C$ (m.p. 267 °C), can be used as a reference [54] and the results converted to the TMS standard.

---

† The name sodium 3-(trimethylsilyl)propane-1-sulfonate is strictly the correct one for this compound.

the temperature dependence of ^{1}H and ^{13}C resonances for TMS. Variations of solvent and/or change in sample concentration are known to have important effects on many chemical shifts, but they are relatively small for a symmetrical, nonpolarizable molecule like TMS.

To assess the magnitude of the concentration effect, measurements have been obtained [12] of the proton chemical shift for TMS in solutions of volume fractions, φ = 0.01%, 1%, and 80% in CDCl$_3$ (see the Appendix). The ^{1}H NMR frequency of TMS (φ = 1%) in chloroform is essentially at the infinite dilution level, the value for a φ = 0.01% solution differing by of the order of 10^{-7}% in Ξ, which is normally reported to only 10^{-6}%. However, for a φ = 80% solution Ξ is 9 × 10^{-6}% larger than for a φ = 1% solution. *Therefore, for the primary reference in multinuclear magnetic resonance, we recommend a dilute solution (approximately φ = 1% or less) of TMS in CDCl$_3$. This recommendation does not preclude the use of TMS in other solvents as alternative references for ^{1}H NMR, and it is consistent with the use of DSS in aqueous solutions (see Section 3.7).*

These recommendations should not be taken in any way to preclude the design and implementation of experiments to measure specific properties, such as very high precision relative frequency measurements and special sample arrangements designed to minimize certain molecular interactions. Data will continue to be reported in the most effective way for the purpose at hand, but we believe that adoption of the unified chemical shift scale will facilitate comparison of the vast majority of NMR frequency measurements. The choice of the base reference as the proton signal of TMS is in accord with the virtually universal use of this signal as a reference for proton NMR.*

If the recommendation for use of a unified scale is widely adopted, future measurements should be reported as Ξ values. However, to assure consistency with data already in the literature, it is important to have a set of Ξ values of sufficient accuracy to permit conversion between the primary TMS reference and at least one secondary homonuclear reference for each nuclide (other than ^{1}H). Tables 1–3 list values of Ξ for a number of commonly used secondary references, which are hereby recommended for further use. These values come from a number of sources, as indicated in the tables. However, it should be noted that a number of these compounds are hazardous [for example, Me$_2$Se, Me$_2$Te, Ni(CO)$_4$, and, especially, Me$_2$Hg]. The unified scale has the advantage that its use avoids direct handling of any secondary references (see Section 3.6). For most of the nuclides listed in Table 3, there are few data available, and the values of Ξ are simply approximations based on magnetogyric ratios.

However, for Tables 1 and 2, values of Ξ are stated for almost all nuclides to 10^{-6}%. For 69 of the most commonly studied nuclides, careful measurements of Ξ have been made specifically for the purpose of this tabulation. The frequencies of ^{13}C and ^{29}Si were determined for samples of TMS in dilute solution in CDCl$_3$ [12,13,15]. The remaining 67 measurements were made [9] by the substitution method (as described in the Appendix). Since all observation frequencies and the ^{2}H lock frequency are derived from a single source, the measured frequencies (Ξ) are reproducible to better than 10^{-7}% and are reported to 10^{-6}%. Experimental details are given in the Appendix. Values of Ξ for the remaining

30 nuclides in Tables 1 and 2 are taken from published values, which have been converted to be consistent with the choice of the ^{1}H signal for TMS in very dilute solution as the primary reference. The literature cited should be consulted for details of the experimental procedure and for estimates of experimental precision and accuracy.

For ^{1}H and ^{13}C NMR, internal referencing has been used almost exclusively, primarily to avoid bulk magnetic susceptibility effects, which can be of the same magnitude as some chemical shift differences that are interpretable with regard to chemical structure. The recommended reference for these nuclides is, therefore, TMS in a dilute solution in CDCl$_3$, and for consistency this reference is recommended also for ^{29}Si. For most other nuclides, magnetic susceptibility effects are small relative to chemical shift differences, and many of the published data have been reported relative to an external or replacement reference, often a neat liquid where feasible. To provide maximum utility, most of the entries in Tables 1 and 2 refer to such neat liquids or concentrated solutions, usually with a minimum amount of deuterated substance added to provide a stable lock. Of course, a very large number of such reference materials and lock substances could be used, but as described in Section 3.6, it is relatively simple to convert from one to another if necessary.

Values of Ξ can generally be determined to 10^{-6}%, which represents resonance measurement differences of only 0.01 ppm for nuclides with large values of γ to 0.5 ppm for nuclides with very low γ values (an imprecision that is usually negligible compared with their generally large chemical shift ranges). Under the unified scale, chemical shifts can thus be reported to a precision that is often dependent on line-width or other sample-related factors, rather than instrumental factors. Since literature data for a number of nuclides are usually referred to a secondary reference and hence are often of considerably lower precision, small discrepancies in values of Ξ are of little practical consequence in most instances.

3.6 Practical Application of the Unified Scale

Modern NMR spectrometers invariably include field/frequency locking and frequency synthesizers, so that all frequencies are reliably interrelated by locking to a master clock frequency. There are two ways in which this fact can be used to determine chemical shifts, either directly on the Ξ scale or with respect to a recognized reference for the nucleus in question. These two ways are equivalent to the use of the conventional internal reference and substitution methods, respectively. In the former case, if a nucleus X is to be studied, and the sample can be prepared with a small amount of TMS, then two direct frequency measurements made while maintaining the same ^{2}H locking conditions will provide the chemical shift of X on the unified scale according to eq. 9. If this procedure is applied to a series of samples, the effect is to replace "medium effects" on the shielding of X (given by measurements using a reference compound containing the nuclide X) by medium effects on the shielding of ^{1}H in TMS. In general, this should result in a reduction of medium effects due to the referencing procedure, which is desirable. Clearly, the substitution method can be used similarly and is particularly valuable when it is not convenient to add TMS to the sample. Equation 9 is still pertinent. However, as noted in Section 3.4, medium effects may vary to some extent if different concentrations of sample and reference are used.

In the future, reporting of chemical shift data as Ξ values may become more common and acceptable. Conversion of Ξ values to conventional chemical shifts relative to a reference of an X-containing compound requires only subtraction of the Ξ value

---

* With hindsight, it might have been better to choose the ^{29}Si signal of TMS since that is arguably even less susceptible to outside influence than the ^{1}H resonance (silicon being at the symmetry center of the molecule). However, because of the large amount of literature based on the proton signal, we recommend that the primary reference remain the ^{1}H signal of TMS.

of a suitable homonuclear reference, as given in Tables 1 and 2, followed by division by the Ξ value of the homonuclear reference. Thus:

$$\delta_X \,/\, \text{ppm} = 10^6 \,(\Xi_{X,\text{sample}} - \Xi_{X,\text{reference}}) \,/\, \Xi_{X,\text{reference}} \qquad (10)$$

The widespread use of a ^{2}H lock for NMR measurements on isotropic samples suggests a modification of the substitution approach, since the relevant reference frequency should not vary with time. Thus, the chemical shifts of the X nuclei can, in principle, be determined on the unified (TMS-based) scale merely by measuring the resonance frequency of the sample and using a predetermined reference frequency for the nuclide in question. Thus, only one (sample) tube is required and no reference substance needs to be added. The predetermined reference frequency is obtained by measuring the proton resonance of TMS under similar conditions to the sample (i.e., with the same lock compound) in a single experiment for the spectrometer being used. Then, the frequency of the usual secondary reference for the X nucleus can be calculated using the predetermined value of ν_{TMS}:

$$\nu_{\text{reference}} = \nu_{\text{TMS}} \times \Xi_{\text{reference}} \,/100\% \qquad (11)$$

where $\Xi_{\text{reference}}$ takes the appropriate value given in Tables 1–3. Thence, the chemical shift (or the value of Ξ_X) for the sample can be readily derived. If the lock substance in the sample solution is not the same as that of the reference solution, a lock correction must be applied (eq. 8).

As an example, suppose that a ^{77}Se resonance has been measured on a compound dissolved in acetone-d_6, resulting in a value:

$$\nu_{\text{sample}} = 76\,344\,378 \text{ Hz}$$

On this spectrometer, the ^{1}H resonance of a $\varphi = 1\%$ solution of TMS in CDCl$_3$ has been found at 400 103 342 Hz when the spectrometer was installed. The reference frequency of selenium is then, from Table 1:

$$400\,103\,342 \text{ Hz} \times 19.071\,513 \div 100 = 76\,305\,761 \text{ Hz}$$

The proton chemical shifts of the resonances of the lock compounds are:

$$\delta_H(\text{CHCl}_3) = 7.27 \text{ ppm and } \delta_H(\text{acetone}) = 2.17 \text{ ppm}$$

Then:

$$\begin{aligned}\delta_{\text{Se, sample}} &= (76\,344\,378 - 76\,305\,761)/76.305\,761 + (2.17 - 7.27) \\ &= 501.0 \text{ ppm}\end{aligned}$$

Since this is still basically a substitution method, an error will arise if the ^{2}H frequency of the solvent has been influenced by the particular sample used. For many samples that consist of dilute solutions the error is small, and for many nuclei with large chemical shift ranges the error introduced in this way is probably smaller than would occur if a homonuclear (X) reference were used in the conventional manner.

Reporting of Ξ_X and δ_X measurements in future heteronuclear magnetic resonance studies will ultimately lead to a large set of consistent data, provided that values of $\Xi_{X,\text{ref}}$ are established and used consistently in all future work. Therefore, particularly for comparison with chemical shifts reported relative to a homonuclear (X) reference via conventional internal referencing procedures, it is essential that the values of Ξ in Tables 1 and 2 represent the accepted values for the substances listed (which are the "best" available at the present time). *We therefore recommend that the defined local chemical shift scale zero values are established as those listed in Tables 1 and 2, and that such definitions are not subject to future change arising from remeasurement even where this results in increasing accuracy for the reference compound in question.* However, the values of Ξ for "rare earth" nuclei in Table 3 should be regarded as provisional, pending more accurate measurement.

The Unified Scale offers many advantages over other methods of referencing. However, serious errors can occur in reading and displaying frequencies in some spectrometers unless care is taken. The software in NMR spectrometers is continually evolving, and even some spectrometers of relatively recent vintage are configured to display frequencies that are rounded off or that appear with many digits that do not correctly represent the frequency of a peak indicated by the cursor. The correct information is available in the appropriate parameter tables, but the authors of this document have found that in instruments that are several years old it may be necessary to seek the correct file and not rely on what appears to be an "obvious" display. Although the situation has improved with the latest version of commercial instruments, *we strongly recommend that each user verify that his/her own instrument correctly determines one or more values of Ξ as given in Tables 1–3.*

3.7 Alternative Reference Compounds

Many of the elements have more than one proposed reference compound for the chemical shift scale mentioned in the literature. The majority are secondary reference standards chosen for convenience. Although our recommendation stands for the compounds listed in Tables 1 and 2, there are some situations where an alternative reference has to be used. One of these cases occurs when ^{1}H, ^{13}C, ^{15}N, ^{29}Si, and other nuclei have to be referenced in highly polar solvents such as water, where TMS is only very sparingly soluble. For those situations, DSS or its partially deuterated form, Me$_3$SiCD$_2$CD$_2$CD$_2$SO$_3$Na, is the recommended primary reference [53,57]. {Sodium 3-(trimethylsilyl)propanoate (TSP) is another salt that has been suggested [58].} When DSS is used as a reference, it has been recommended [4] that ^{1}H chemical shifts be denoted by the symbol δ_{DSS} to distinguish them from those referenced to TMS. However, the resonances of DSS and TMS, *both dissolved in the same solvent*, are very close: On the scale with TMS as zero, DSS has a chemical shift of $\delta = 0.0173$ ppm in dilute aqueous solution, while in dilute solution in di[(^{2}H$_3$)methyl] sulfoxide (DMSO-d_6), the chemical shift of DSS is $\delta = -0.0246$ ppm [4]. For most purposes, these differences are negligible (falling well below the anticipated range of solvent effects), and *data from the TMS and DSS scales may be validly compared without correction for the different ^{1}H reference.*

Table 4 repeats the recommended values of Ξ from ref. 4, along with data for additional references proposed in the literature for nitrogen, and compares them with our recommendations in Tables 1 and 2. For ^{13}C studies in aqueous solution, ref. 4 recommends using the ^{13}C methyl resonance of DSS, rather than that of TMS, as the secondary reference. Carbon-13 chemical shifts based on DSS and TMS differ by about 2 ppm, which can cause confusion if not clarified. *We recommend that when ^{13}C chemical shifts are referenced to DSS, that point should be made clear by using a notation such as $\delta_{\text{DSS}}(^{13}\text{C})$.*

Reference 4 recommends use of trimethyl phosphate (internal) as a secondary reference for ^{31}P studies in aqueous solution, whereas Table 1 recommends 85% phosphoric acid (external), which has been used more widely, particularly for chemical

TABLE 4: Alternative Secondary References

Isotope	Alternative secondary references				Recommended secondary references[a]		
	Reference compound	Sample conditions	NMR Frequency Ξ/%	Literature	Reference compound	Sample conditions	NMR Frequency Ξ/%
^{1}H	DSS	Internal	100.000 000	4	TMS	Internal[b]	100.000 000
^{2}H	DSS	Internal	15.350 608	4	TMS	Internal[b]	15.350 609
^{13}C	DSS	Internal	25.144 953	4	TMS	Internal[b]	25.145 020
^{31}P	$(CH_3O)_3PO$	Internal	40.480 864	4	H_3PO_4 (85%)	External	40.480 742
^{15}N	NH_3 (liquid)	External	10.132 912	4	CH_3NO_2	External	10.136 767
^{15}N	$[(CH3)^4N]I$	Internal[c]	10.133 356	59,60			
^{14}N	$[(CH3)^4N]I$	Internal[c]	7.223 885	59	CH_3NO_2	External	7.226 717

[a] See Tables 1 and 2.
[b] Volume fraction $\varphi = 1\%$ in $CDCl_3$.
[c] 0.075 M in DMSO-d_6.

systems where use of an internal reference is not feasible. The two secondary references differ by about 3 ppm, so *it is important to specify which is being used.*

Several reference compounds have been used historically for nitrogen NMR, partly resulting from the very different properties and natural abundances of the two nuclides (^{14}N and ^{15}N). Nitromethane as either an internal or external reference has been the most widely used for ^{14}N and to some extent for ^{15}N, while liquid ammonia has been a popular external reference for ^{15}N. Ammonium and tetramethylammonium salts have been used as internal references for both ^{14}N and ^{15}N. Reference 4 recommends liquid NH_3 as a secondary reference for ^{15}N in aqueous solutions, since most biochemical applications of ^{15}N NMR have used this reference. In Tables 1 and 2 *we recommend nitromethane as a reference,* in line with common usage in many other applications. The values of Ξ for different nitrogen reference compounds are presented in Table 4, along with those for tetramethylammonium iodide, which has been suggested as an internal reference for both ^{14}N and ^{15}N since the tetrahedral geometry results in sharp lines for both isotopomers.

For most of the nuclei listed in Tables 1 and 2, Ξ values are listed for only one homonuclear reference, since conversions to other reference compounds can be readily made from literature values.

3.8 Magic-Angle Spinning

It has been shown [61–63] that, in theory, bulk isotropic magnetic susceptibility effects are eliminated by spinning an infinitely long cylindrical sample with its axis at the magic angle (54.7°) to the static magnetic field of an NMR spectrometer. Therefore, in principle, magic-angle spinning (MAS) can be used in the external referencing method to obtain chemical shifts free from bulk susceptibility problems. Whereas this technique was proposed in the context of solid-state NMR (see below), its utility applies equally well to the solution state [64,65]. In practice, an infinitely long cylinder is not necessary to reduce bulk susceptibility effects on chemical shifts to an acceptable level. Strictly speaking, to correct for *isotropic* bulk magnetic susceptibility effects, it is also not necessary to spin at the magic angle, but merely to orient the cylinder containing the sample at the magic angle (see eq. 7). However, spinning may narrow the lines significantly and so is normally essential for accurate chemical shift measurement.

3.9 Solids

Sample-handling procedures differ substantially for solids from those appropriate for solutions, and there are clear advantages to using suitable solids as secondary references. This is almost always done using sample replacement. However, the spectrometers are generally used without field/frequency locking, so that

the resulting chemical shifts are inevitably less accurate than those for solutions. This is not a significant problem, because linewidths are usually substantially greater than those for solutions and they impose an upper limit to accuracy. High-resolution NMR of solids almost invariably relies on magic-angle spinning, and, as discussed in Section 3.8, this eliminates the effects of differences in bulk isotropic magnetic susceptibilities. Early papers [61,62] addressed this matter, and a recent review by VanderHart [45], which refers to both liquids and solutions, further discusses the influence of MAS for referencing spectra. Unfortunately, the situation is simple only for systems with isotropic magnetic susceptibility. VanderHart [45] discusses the case of anisotropic susceptibility, but there has been to date little experimental work in this area. However, in general it may be taken that, within the accuracy of measurement, referencing by sample replacement under MAS conditions in an unlocked but stable spectrometer is to a good approximation equivalent to the substitution method as described in Section 3.5.

Several papers [66–68] take advantage of the MAS technique to suggest secondary solid standards for practical use in solid-state NMR. For example, the ^{13}C signals of solid adamantane, glycine, hexamethylbenzene, and $[(CH_3)_3Si]_4Si$ have been referenced to those for liquids and solutions using MAS, and data were reported to accuracies in the region of 0.004–0.04 ppm.

Chemical shift referencing for solid-state NMR is not yet at the stage where much further discussion is warranted here, so the only recommendation that we make is for referencing procedures to be always clearly and carefully stated in publications.

4. Summary of Recommendations

In addition to the endorsements of earlier Recommendations stated in Section 3.2 above, IUPAC recommends the following:

(a) Equation 5 should be used to define chemical shift scales, with symbol δ and with ppm (or ppb or %, as appropriate) explicitly stated after the numerical values. Equation 6 provides a simple way to calculate chemical shift values in ppm.

(b) The ^{1}H signal of tetramethylsilane in dilute solution (ca. volume fraction $\varphi = 1\%$ in $CDCl_3$) should be used as the primary *internal* or substitution reference for the resonance frequencies (and hence chemical shifts) for *all* nuclei. However, for aqueous solutions, the recommendations of ref. 4 are supported.

(c) The secondary references listed in Tables 1 and 2 may be used for the nuclei of the various elements, with their Ξ taking the fixed values given (not subject to revision).

(d) Internal referencing may be used for solutions, but its limitations should be recognized.

(e) For solution-state measurements, referencing via an internal ^{2}H lock signal may be used, either to give the value of Ξ directly or to calculate the chemical shift with respect to the relevant secondary reference (via eq. 8, where relevant).

(f) Referencing by the substitution method with field/frequency lock spectrometers may also be used for solutions.

(g) External referencing for either liquids or solids may be carried out with magic-angle spinning.

(h) External referencing by means other than (f) and (g) is to be discouraged unless corrections are applied for bulk magnetic susceptibility effects.

(i) In all circumstances, and especially where strict adherence to these Recommendations is not feasible, details of experimental procedures should be given clearly so that results may be validly intercompared.

Acknowledgments

We thank H. J. C. Yeh (National Institutes of Health), A. M. Kenwright (University of Durham), and B. Ancian (Université de Paris VII) for measurements of Ξ for ^{13}C and ^{29}Si in solutions of TMS in CDCl$_3$. Other special measurements of Ξ have also been made by C. Brevard, R. Hoffman, J. Raya, M. Bourdonneau, T. Meersmann, B. Ancian, and L. Helm. We are also grateful to W. Bremser, who participated in some of the early discussions on the topic of these recommendations, and to J. Kowalewski and G. Martin for comments and encouragement. Specific comments were received from members of IDCNS (W. V. Metanomski, K. Hatada, A. D. Jenkins, J. W. Lorimer, W. H. Powell, S. E. Schwartz, A. J. Thor, H. A. Favre, T. Cvitaš) and a wide range of NMR experts and others (A. D. McNaught, D. L. VanderHart, D. T. Burns, M. Duteil, J. R. Everett, B. E. Mann, W. McFarlane, P. S. Pregosin, B. Mandava, W. von Philipsborn, T. D. W. Claridge, C. Ye, D. Neuhaus, P. Jonsen, Hägele, J. C. Lindon, P. E. Meadows, B. Wrackmeyer, K. Mizuno, T. Richert); we are very grateful for their assistance and guidance. P. Pyykkö very helpfully supplied details of his review of quadrupole moments in advance of publication, and R. Hoffman not only supplied data for Ξ on several nuclei but also made many pertinent and useful suggestions.

Appendix

As noted in the body of this document, a number of new experimental measurements have been made to verify values of Ξ for various nuclides. Experimental details are given here.

Concentration dependence of δ_H (TMS) [12]. Measurements were made with a Varian VXR500S spectrometer, sample at ambient probe temperature (about 23 °C), locked onto the signal for CDCl$_3$. Measured ^{1}H frequencies were as follows:

$\varphi = 0.01\%$:	499.872 5048 MHz
$\varphi = 1\%$:	499.872 5054 MHz
$\varphi = 80\%$:	499.872 5495 MHz

Ξ **for ^{13}C and ^{29}Si.** Three measurements were made of Ξ (^{13}C) for TMS in CDCl$_3$ at $\varphi = 1\%$, all at ambient probe temperature using the following spectrometers: Varian VXR-500S [13], $\Xi = 25.145$ 0188%; Varian Unity-300 [12], $\Xi = 25.145$ 0202%; and Varian Inova-500 [13], $\Xi = 25.145$ 0196%. The reported value [15] (Table 1) of Ξ (^{29}Si) for TMS in CDCl$_3$ at $\varphi = 1\%$ was obtained at ambient probe temperature using a Bruker Avance-400 spectrometer.

Other values of Ξ. Most of the remaining 67 new measurements presented in Tables 1 and 2 were made by the substitution method (as described above) with a Bruker Model MSL spectrometer, operating at a nominal frequency of 300 MHz for ^{1}H, and with corrections applied for the lock signals (see equation 8) [9]. However, Ξ was measured for the following nuclei using a Bruker Avance-400 spectrometer: ^{2}H, ^{17}O, ^{45}Sc, ^{47}Ti, ^{49}Ti, ^{55}Mn, ^{75}As, ^{81}Br, ^{87}Rb, ^{127}I, ^{131}Xe, ^{133}Cs, ^{135}Ba, and ^{137}Ba. The ^{21}Ne value was measured [9] using a Chemagnetics Infinity 600. All 67 measurements were made at ambient probe temperature, approximately 298–300 K. The replacement reference samples used were either a concentrated solution (m = 4.75 mol kg^{-1}, $\varphi = 80\%$) of TMS in CDCl$_3$, or a $\varphi = 1\%$ solution of TMS in CDCl$_3$. In the former case, the values have been converted to refer to TMS ($\varphi = 1\%$) in CDCl$_3$ (see above).

References

1. "Recommendations for the presentation of NMR data for publication in chemical journals", *Pure Appl. Chem.* **29**, 627 (1972).
2. "Presentation of NMR data for publication in chemical journals – B. Conventions relating to spectra from nuclei other than protons", *Pure Appl. Chem.* **45**, 217 (1976).
3. R. K. Harris, J. Kowalewski, S. C. de Menezes. "Parameters and symbols for use in nuclear magnetic resonance", *Pure Appl. Chem.* **69**, 2489 (1997).
4. J. L. Markley, A. Bax, Y. Arata, C. W. Hilbers, R. Kaptein, B. D. Sykes, P. E. Wright, K. Wüthrich. "Recommendations for the presentation of NMR structures of proteins and nucleic acids", *Pure Appl. Chem.* **70**, 117 (1998).
5. *NMR and the Periodic Table*, R. K. Harris and B. E. Mann (Eds.), Academic Press (1978).
6. I. Mills, T. Cvitaš, K. Homann, N. Kallay, K. Kuchitsu. *Quantities, Units and Symbols in Physical Chemistry*, 2nd ed., published for IUPAC by Blackwell Scientific Publications (1993).
7. R. K. Harris. *Encyclopedia of Nuclear Magnetic Resonance*, D. M. Grant and R. K. Harris (Eds.in-Chief), **5**, 3301, Wiley, Chichester (1996).
8. K. J. R. Rosman and P. D. P. Taylor. *Pure Appl. Chem.* **70**, 217 (1998).
9. P. Granger, J. Raya, M. Bourdonneau, L. Helm, T. Meersmann. Measurements previously unpublished in the primary literature. See the Appendix for details.
10. J. P. Bloxsidge, J. A. Elvidge, J. R. Jones, R. B. Mane, M. Saljoughian. *Org. Magn. Reson.* **12**, 574 (1979).
11. R. Hoffman. Private communication.
12. H. J. C. Yeh. Previously unpublished work.
13. A. M. Kenwright. Previously unpublished work.
14. S. Brownstein and J. Bornais. *J. Magn. Reson.* **38**, 131 (1980).
15. H. T. Edzes. *Magn. Reson. Chem.* **30**, 850 (1992).
16. B. Ancian. Previously unpublished work.
17. P. L. Goggin, R. J. Goodfellow, F. J. S. Reed, *J. Chem. Soc., Dalton Trans.* 576 (1974); S. J. Anderson, J. R. Barnes, P. L. Goggin, R. J. Goodfellow. *J. Chem. Res. (M)*, 3601 (1978).
18. R. Benn and A. Rufinska. *Angew. Chem., Int. Ed. Engl.* **25**, 861 (1986).
19. J. D. Kennedy and W. McFarlane. *J. Chem. Soc., Perkin Trans.* **2** 1187 (1977).
20. M. Gerken and G. J. Schrobilgen. *Coord. Chem. Rev.* **197**, 335 (2000).
21. G. A. Schumacker and G. J. Schrobilgen. *Inorg. Chem.* **23**, 2923 (1984).
22. C. Brevard. Previously unpublished work.
23. M. B. Blayney, J. S. Winn, D. W. Nierenberg. *Chem. Eng. News* May 12, 7 (1997); T. Y. Toribara, T. W. Clarkson, D. W. Nierenberg. *Chem. Eng. News* June 16, 6 (1997); D. Love. *Chem. Eng. News* July 14, 7 (1997); R. K. Harris. *Chem. Eng. News* July 14, 7 (1997).
24. J. F. Hinton, G. L. Turner, G. Young, K. R. Metz. *Pure Appl. Chem.* **54**, 2359 (1982).
25. J. F. Hinton and R. W. Briggs. *J. Magn. Reson.* **25**, 555 (1977).
26. P. Pyykkö. *Z. Naturforsch., A* **47**, 189 (1992).
27. P. Raghavan. *At. Data Nucl. Data Tables* **42**, 189 (1989).
28. P. Pyykkö. *Mol. Phys.* **99**, 1617 (2001).

28. J. D. Kennedy. In *Multinuclear NMR*, J. Mason (Ed.), Ch. 8, p. 221, Plenum Press (1987).
29. J. T. LaTourrette, W. E. Quinn, R. F. Ramsey. *Phys. Rev.* **107**, 1202 (1957).
30. W. Sahm and A. Schwenk. *Z. Naturforsch., A* **29**, 1754 (1974).
31. O. Lutz, A. Schwenk, A. Uhl. *Z. Naturforsch., A* **30**, 1122 (1975).
32. N. Hao, M. J. McGlinchey, B. G. Sayer, G. J. Schrobilgen. *J. Magn. Reson.* **46**, 158 (1982).
33. J. Kodweiss, O. Lutz, W. Messner, K. R. Mohn, A. Nolle, B. Stütz, D. Zepf. *J. Magn. Reson.* **43**, 495 (1981).
34. J. Kaufmann, W. Sahm, A. Schwenk. *Z. Naturforsch., A* **26**, 1384 (1971).
35. D. Brinkman. *Helv. Phys. Acta* **41**, 367 (1968).
36. W. Sahm and A. Schwenk. *Z. Naturforsch. A* **29**, 1763 (1974).
37. O. Lutz and H. Oehler. *Z. Physik A* **288**, 11 (1978).
38. O. Lutz and H. Oehler. *J. Magn. Reson.* **37**, 261 (1980).
39. C. Brevard and P. Granger. *Handbook of High Resolution Multinuclear NMR*, Wiley, New York (1981).
40. G. Wu and R. E. Wasylishen. *Magn. Reson. Chem.* **31**, 537 (1993).
41. A. G. Avent, M. A. Edelman, M. F. Lappert, G. A. Lawless. *J. Am. Chem. Soc.* **111**, 3423, (1989).
42. H. LeBail, C. Chachaty, P. Rigny, R. Bougon. *C. R. Acad. Sci.* **297**, 451 (1983).
43. G. V. D. Tiers. *J. Phys. Chem.* **62**, 1151 (1958).
44. D. L. VanderHart. *Encyclopedia of Nuclear Magnetic Resonance*, D. M. Grant and R. K. Harris (Eds.-in-Chief), **5**, 2938, Wiley, Chichester (1996).
45. P. E. Hansen. *Prog. Nucl. Magn. Reson. Spectrosc.* **20**, 207 (1988).
46. D. F. Evans. *J. Chem. Soc., Chem. Comm.* 1226 (1982).
47. L. J. Altman, D. Laungani, G. Gunnarson, H. Wennerström, S. Forsen. *J. Amer. Chem. Soc.* **100**, 8264 (1978).
48. W. McFarlane. *Proc. R. Soc. London, Ser. A* **306**, 185 (1968) and references therein.
49. W. McFarlane. *Annu. Rep. NMR Spectrosc.* **1**, 135 (1968).
50. R. K. Harris and B. J. Kimber. *J. Magn. Reson.* **17**, 174 (1975).
51. D. Canet, C. Goulon-Ginet, J. P. Marchal. *J. Magn. Reson.* **22**, 537 (1976).
52. D. S. Wishart, C. G. Bigam, J. Yao, F. Abildgaard, H. J. Dyson, E. Oldfield, J. L. Markley, B. D. Sykes. *J. Biomol. NMR* **6**, 135 (1995).
53. N. N. Zemlyanskii and O. K. Sokolikova. *Russ. J. Anal. Chem.* **36**, 1421 (1981).
54. C. J. Jameson, A. K. Jameson, S. M. Cohen. *J. Magn. Reson.* **19**, 385 (1975).
55. F. G. Morin, M. S. Solum, J. D. Withers, D. M. Grant. *J. Magn. Reson.* **48**, 138 (1982).
56. G. V. D. Tiers and A. Kowalewsky. Paper presented to the Division of Physical Chemistry, 137th ACS National Meeting, Cleveland, Ohio, 1960; Abstracts, p. 1712; G. V. D. Tiers and R. I. Coon. *J. Org. Chem.* **26**, 2097 (1961).
57. G. V. Tiers and A. Kowalewsky. Division of Physical Chemistry, 137th ACS National Meeting, Cleveland, Ohio, 1960; L. Pohl and M. Ecke. *Angew Chem., Int. Ed. Engl.* **8**, 381 (1969); D. H. Live and S. I. Chan. *Org. Magn. Reson.* **5**, 275 (1973).
58. E. D. Becker. *J. Magn. Reson.* **4**, 142(1971).
59. E. D. Becker, R. B. Bradley, T. Axenrod. *J. Magn. Reson.* **4**, 136 (1971).
60. D. Doskočilová and B. Schneider. *Macromolecules* **5**, 125 (1972).
61. D. Doskočilová, D. D. Tao, B. Schneider. *Czech. J. Phys. B* **25**, 202 (1975).
62. W. L. Earl and D. L. VanderHart. *J. Magn. Reson.* **48**, 35 (1982).
63. A. N. Garroway. *J. Magn. Reson.* **49**, 168 (1982).
64. S. Hayashi, M. Yanagisawa, K. Hayamizu. *Anal. Sci.* **7**, 955 (1991).
65. S. Hayashi and K. Hayamizu. *Bull. Chem. Soc. Jpn.* **62**, 2429 (1989).
66. S. Hayashi and K. Hayamizu. *Bull. Chem. Soc. Jpn.* **64**, 685 (1991).
67. S. Hayashi and K. Hayamizu. *Bull. Chem. Soc. Jpn.* **64**, 688 (1991).

ORGANIC NAME REACTIONS USEFUL IN BIOCHEMISTRY AND MOLECULAR BIOLOGY

Roger L. Lundblad

Akabori Amino Acid Reaction

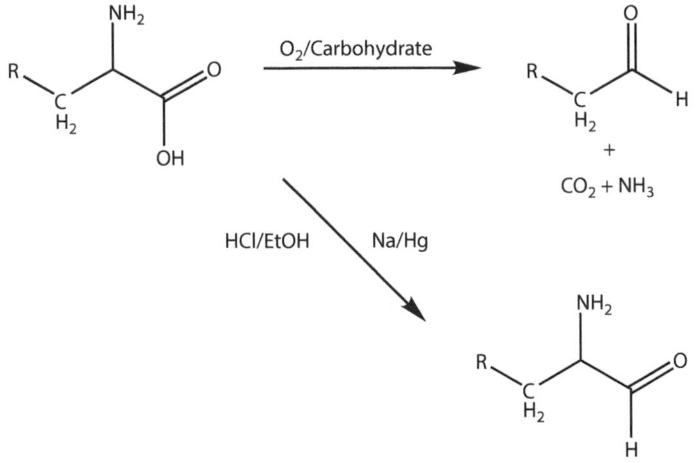

O_2/Carbohydrate

$CO_2 + NH_3$

HCl/EtOH   Na/Hg

Reaction in the presence of hydrazine yields hydrazides which can be coupled to aromatic aldehydes

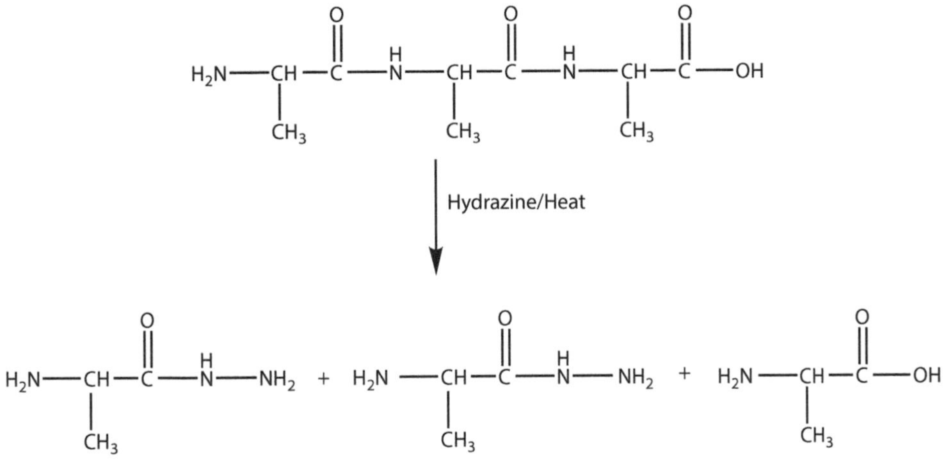

Hydrazine/Heat

Bose, A.K., *et al.*, Microwave enhanced Akabori reaction for peptide analysis, *J.Am.Soc.Mass Spectrom.* **13**, 839–850, 2002

Originally devised as a method for the conversion of amino acids or amino acid esters to aldehydes. The Akabori reaction has been modified for use in the determination of C-terminal amino acids by performing the reaction in the presence of hydrazine and for the production of derivatives useful for mass spectrometric identification. Ambach, E. and Beck, W., Metal-complexes with biologically important ligands. 35. Nickel, cobalt, palladium, and platinum complexes with Schiff-bases of α-amino acids – A contribution to the mechanism of the Akabori reaction, *Chemische Berichte-Recueil* 118, 2722–2737, 1985; Bose, A.K., Ing, Y.H., Pramanik, B.N., *et al.*, Microwave enhanced Akabori reaction for peptide analysis, *J.Am.Soc.Mass Spectrom.* 13, 839–850, 2002; Pramanik, B.N., Ing, Y.H., Bose, A.K., *et al.*, Rapid cyclopeptide analysis by microwave enhanced Akabori reaction, *Tetrahedron Lett.* 44, 2565–2568, 2003; Puar, M.S., Chan, T.M., Delgarno, D., *et al.*, Sch 486058: A novel cyclic peptide of actinomycete origin, *J.Antibiot.* 58, 151–154, 2005.

ORGANIC NAME REACTIONS USEFUL IN BIOCHEMISTRY AND MOLECULAR BIOLOGY (Continued)

Aldol Condensation

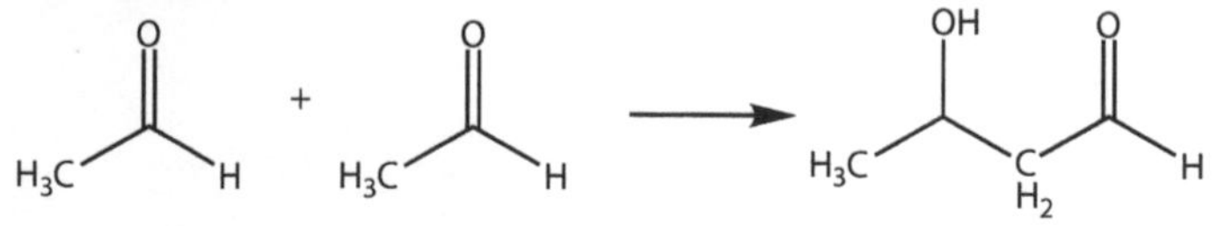

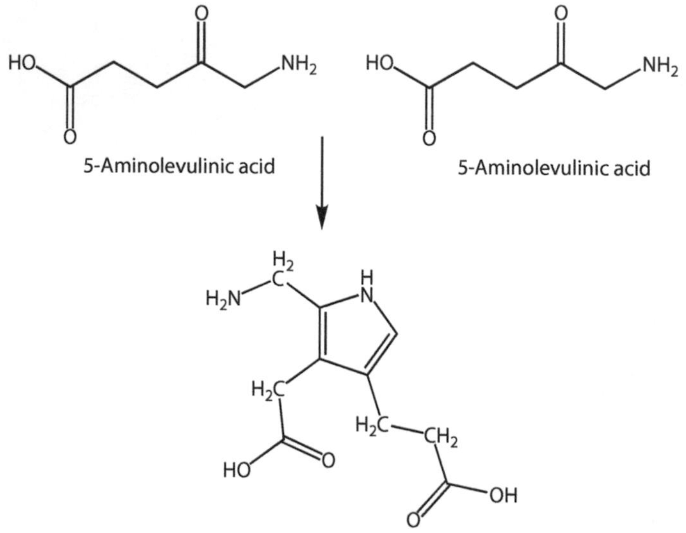

5-Aminolevulinic acid

5-Aminolevulinic acid

Porphobilinogen

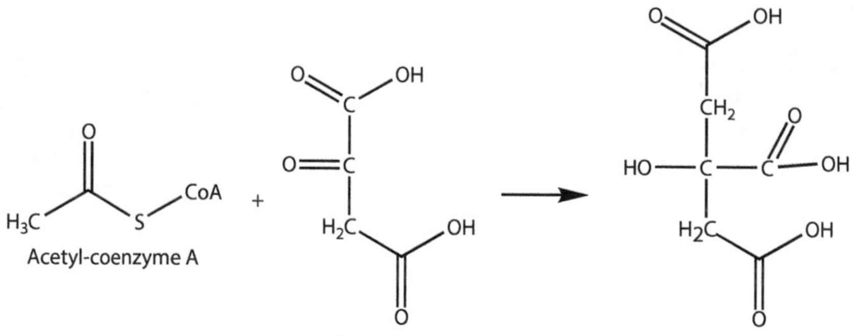

Acetyl-coenzyme A

Oxaloacetic acid

Citrate synthase
an aldol-like condensation

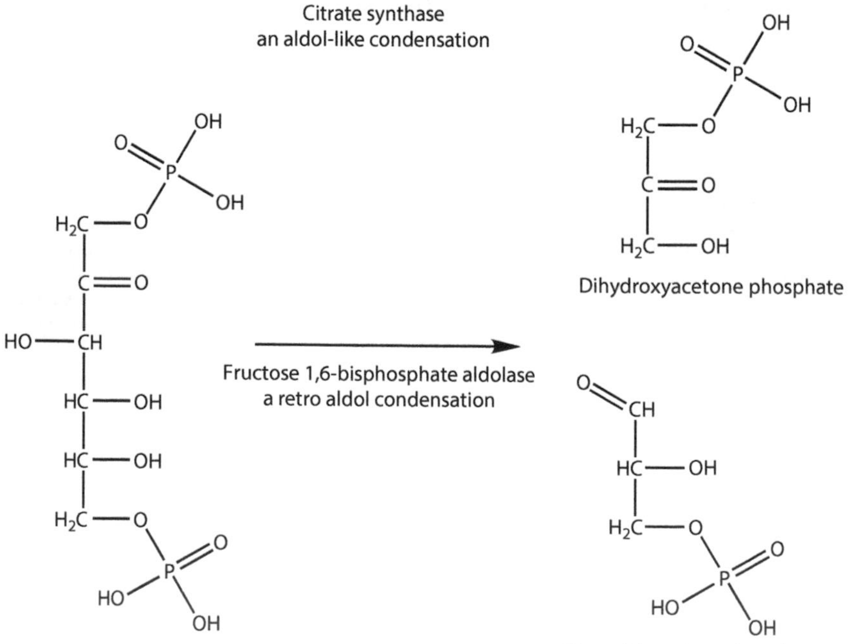

Citrate

Dihydroxyacetone phosphate

Fructose 1,6-bisphosphate aldolase
a retro aldol condensation

Glyceraldehyde-3-phosphate

ORGANIC NAME REACTIONS USEFUL IN BIOCHEMISTRY AND MOLECULAR BIOLOGY (Continued)

Condensation of one carbonyl compound with the enol/enolate form of another to form a β-hydroxyaldehyde; the base-catalyzed reaction proceeds via the enolate form while the acid-catalyzed reaction proceeds via the enol form. The basic chemistry of the aldol condensation is observed in several enzymatic reactions including citrate synthase, fructose-1,6-bisphosphate aldolase, and 2-keto-4-hydroxyglutarate aldolase. See Lane, R.S., Hansen, B.A., and Dekker, E.E., Sulfhydryl groups in relation to the structure and catalytic activity of 2-oxo-4-hydroxyglutarate aldolase from bovine liver, *Biochim.Biophys.Acta* 481, 212–221, 1977; Evans, D.A. and McGee, L.R., Aldol diastereoselection. Zirconium enolates. Product selective, enolate structure independent condensations, *Tetrahedron Lett.* 21, 3975–3978, 1980; Grady, S.R., Wang, J.K., and Dekker, E.E., Steady-state kinetics and inhibition studies of the aldol condensation reaction catalyzed by *Escherichia coli* 2-keto-4-hydroxyglutarate aldolase, *Biochemistry* 20, 2497–2502, 1981; Rokita, S.E., Srere, P.A., and Walsh, C.T., 3-Fluoro-3-deoxycitrate: A probe for mechanistic study of citrate-utilizing enzymes, *Biochemistry* 21, 3765–3774, 1982; Frere, R., Nentwich, M., Gacond, S., *et al.*, Probing the active site of *Pseudomonas aeruginosa* porphobilinogen synthase using newly developed inhibitors, *Biochemistry*, 45, 8243–8253, 2006; Dalsgaard, T.K., Nielsen, J.H., and Larsen, L.B., Characterization of reaction products formed in a model reaction between pentanal and lysine-containing oligopeptides, *J.Agric.Food Chem.* 54, 6367–6373, 2006. A crossed aldol refers to a condensation reaction with two different aldehydes/ketones; the second aldehyde frequently is formaldehyde as it cannot react with itself although this is not a requirement (Kiehlman, E. and Loo, P.W., Orientation in crossed aldol condensation of chloral with unsymmetrical aliphatic ketones, *Canad.J.Chem.* 49, 1588, 1971; Findlay, J.A., Desai, D.N., and McCaulay, J.B., Thermally induced crossed aldol condensations, *Canad.J.Chem.* 59, 3303–3304, 1981; Esmaelli, A.A., Tabas, M.S., Nasseri, M.A., and Kazemi, F., Solvent-free crossed aldol condensation of cyclic ketones with aromatic aldehydes assisted by microwave irradiation, *Monatshefte fur Chemie* 136, 571–576, 2005).

Amadori Rearrangement

Amadori rearrangement

A reaction following the formation of the unstable reaction product between an aldehyde (reducing sugar) and an amino group (formation of a Schiff base, an aldimine) which results in a more stable ketoamine. The Amadori rearrangement is part of the Maillard reaction which is also called the Browning reaction and can result in the formation of advanced glycation end products. See Amadori, M. *Atti.Accad.Nazl.Lincei* 2, 337, 1925; Hodge, J.E., The Amadori rearrangement, *Adv.Carbohydrate Chem.* 10, 169–205, 1955; Acharya, A.S. and Manning, J.M., Amadori rearrangement of glyceraldehyde-hemoglobin Schiff based adducts. A new procedure for the determination of ketoamine adducts in proteins, *J.Biol.Chem.* 255, 7218–7224, 1980; Acharya, A.S. and Manning, J.M., Reaction of glycoaldehyde with proteins: latent crosslinking potential of α-hydroxyaldehydes, *Proc. Natl.Acad.Sci.USA* 80, 3590–3594, 1983; Roper, H., Roper, S., and Meyer, B., Amadori- and N-nitroso-Amadori compounds and their pyrolysis products. Chemical, analytical and biological aspects, *IARC Sci.Publ.* (57), 101–111, 1984; Baynes, J.W., Watkins, N.G., Fisher, C.I. *et al.*, The Amadori product on protein: structure and reactions, *Prog.Clin.Biol.Res.* 304, 43–67, 1989; Nacharaju, P. and Acharya, A.S., Amadori rearrangement potential of hemoglobin at its glycation sites is dependent on the three-dimensional structure of protein, *Biochemistry* 31, 12673–12679, 1992; Zyzak, D.V., Richardson, J.M., Thorpe, S.R., and Baynes, J.W., Formation of reactive intermediates from Amadori compounds under physiological conditions, *Arch. Biochem.Biophys.* 316, 547–554, 1995; Khalifah, R.G., Baynes, J.W., and Hudson, B.G., Amadorins: novel post-Amadori inhibitors of advanced glycation reactions, *Biochem.Biophys.Res.Commun.* 257, 251–158,1999; Davidek, T., Clety, N., Aubin, S., and Blank, I., Degradation of the Amadori compound N-(1-deoxy-D-fructos-1-yl)glycine in aqueous model system, *J.Agric.Food Chem.* 50, 5472–5479, 2002.

Baeyer-Villiger Reaction

Baeyer–Villiger reaction

ORGANIC NAME REACTIONS USEFUL IN BIOCHEMISTRY AND MOLECULAR BIOLOGY (Continued)

The oxidation of a ketone by a peroxy acid to yield an ester. This reaction is catalyzed by bacterial monooxygenases and has proved useful in preparation of optically pure esters and lactones. See Ryerson, C.C., Ballou, D.P. and Walsh, C., Mechanistic studies on cyclohexanone oxygenase, *Biochemistry* 21, 2644–2655, 1982; Bolm, C., Metal-catalyzed asymmetric oxidations, *Med.Res.Rev.* 19, 348–356, 1999; Zambianchi, F., Pasta, P., Carrea, G., *et al.*, Use of isolated cyclohexanone monooxygenase from recombinant *Escherichia coli* as a biocatalyst for Baeyer-Villiger and sulfide oxidations, *Biotechnol.Bioeng.* 78, 489–496, 2002; Alphand, V., Carrea, G., Wohlgemuth, R., *et al.*, Towards large-scale synthetic application of Baeyer-Villiger monooxygenase, *Trends Biotechnol.* 21, 318–323, 2003; Walton, A.Z. and Stewart, J.D., Understanding and improving NADPH-dependent reactions by nongrowing *Escherichia coli* cells, *Biotechnol.Prog.* 20, 403–411, 2004; Malito, E., Alfieri, A., Fraaije, M.W., and Mattevi, A., Crystal structure of a Baeyer-Villiger monooxygenase, *Proc.Nat.Acad.Sci.USA* 101, 13157–13162, 2004; ten Brink, G.J., Arends, I.W., And Sheldon, R.A., The Baeyer-Villiger reaction: new developments toward greener procedures, *Chem.Rev.* 104, 4105–4124, 2004; Boronat, M., Corma. A., Renz, M., *et al.*, A multisite molecular mechanism for Baeyer-Villiger oxidations on solid catalysts using environmentally friendly H_2O_2 as oxidant, *Chemistry* 11, 6905–6915, 2005; Mihovilovic, M.D., Rudroff, E., Winninger, A., *et al.*, Microbial Baeyer-Villiger oxidation: stereopreference and substrate acceptance of cyclohexanone monooxygenase mutants prepared by directed evolution, *Org.Lett.* 8, 1221–1224, 2006; Baldwin, C.V. and Woodley, J.M., On oxygen limitation in a whole cell biocatalytic Baeyer-Villiger oxidation process, *Biotechnol.Bioeng.* 95, 362–369, 2006.

Beckmann Rearrangement

Oxime → Amide (Acid (protic or Lewis))

Beckmann rearrangement

An acid (protic or Lewis)-catalyzed conversion of an oxime to a substituted carboxylic amide. See Darling, C.M. and Chen, C.P., Rearrangement of *N*-benzyl-2-cyano(hydroxyimino)acetamide, *J.Pharm.Sci.* 67, 860–861, 1978; Gayen, A.K., and Knowles, C.O., Penetration and fate of methomyl and its oxime metabolite in insects and two spotted spider mites, *Arch.Environ.Contam.Toxicol.* 10, 55–67, 1981; Mangold, J.B., Mangold, B.L., and Spina, A., Rat liver aryl sulfotransferase-catalyzed sulfation and rearrangement of 9-fluorenone oxime, *Biochim.Biophys.Acta* 874, 37–43, 1986; De Luca, L., Giacomelli, G., and Procheddu, A., Beckmann rearrangement of oximes under very mild conditions, *J.Org.Chem.* 67, 6272–6274, 2002; Torisawa, Y. Nishi, T., and Minamikawa, J., A study on the conversion of indanones into carbostyrils, *Bioorg.Med.Chem.* 11, 2205–2209, 2003; Furuya, Y., Ishihara, K., and Yamamoto, H., Cyanuric chloride as a mild and active Beckmann rearrangement catalyst, *J.Am.Chem.Soc.* 127, 11240–11241, 2005; Yamabe, S., Tsuchida, N., and Yamazaki, S., Is the Beckmann rearrangement a concerted or stepwise reaction? A computational study, *J.Org.Chem.* 70, 10638–10644, 2005; Ichino, T., Arimoto, H., and Uemura, D., Possibility of a non-amino acid pathway in the biosynthesis of marine-derived oxazoles, *Chem.Commun.* (16), 1742–1744, 2006.

Benzoin Condensation

The conversion of benzaldehyde to benzoin (aromatic α-hydroxyketones) via cyanide-mediated condensation; other aromatic aldehydes can participate in this reaction. See Iding, H., Dunnwald, T., Greiner, L., *et al.*, Benzoylformate decarboxylase from *Pseudomonas putida* as stable catalyst for the synthesis of chiral 2-hydroxy ketones, *Chemistry* 6, 1483–1495, 2000; White, M.J. and Leeper, F.J., Kinetics of the thiazolium ion-catalyzed benzoin condensation, *J.Org.Chem.* 66, 5124–5131, 2001; Dunkelmann, P., Kolter-Jung, D., Nitsche, A. *et al.*, Development of a donor-acceptor concept for enzymatic cross-coupling reactions of aldehydes: the first asymmetric cross-benzoin condensation, *J.Am.Chem.Soc.* 124, 12084–12085, 2002; Pohl, M., Lingen, B., and Muller, M., Thiamin-diphosphate-dependent enzymes: new aspects of asymmetric C-C bond formation, *Chemistry* 8, 5288–5295, 2002; Wildemann, H., Dunkelmann, P., Muller, M., and Schmidt, B., A short olefin metathesis-based route to enantiomerically pure arylated dihydropyrans and α, β-unsaturated δ-valero lactones, *J.Org.Chem.* 68, 799–804, 2003; Murry, J.A., Synthetic methodology utilized to prepare substituted imidazole p38 MAP kinase inhibitors, *Curr.Opin.Drug Discov.Devel.* 6, 945–965, 2003; Reich, B.J., Justice, A.K., Beckstead, B.T., *et al.*, Cyanide-catalyzed cyclizations via aldimine coupling, *J.Org.Chem.* 69, 1357–1359, 2004; Sklute, G., Oizerowich, R., Shulman, H., and Keinan, E., Antibody-catalyzed benzoin oxidation as a mechanistic probe for nucleophilic catalysis by an active site lysine, *Chemistry* 10, 2159–2165, 2004; Breslow, R., Determining the geometries of transition states by use of antihydrophobic additives in water, *Acc.Chem.Res.* 37, 471–478, 2004.

ORGANIC NAME REACTIONS USEFUL IN BIOCHEMISTRY AND MOLECULAR BIOLOGY (Continued)

Cannizzaro Reaction

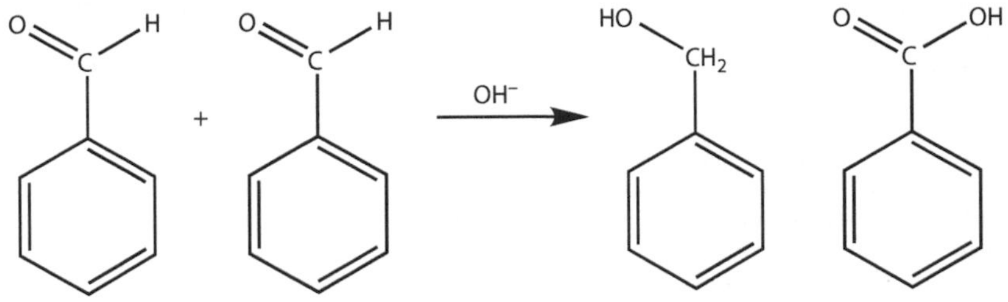

Cannizzaro reaction

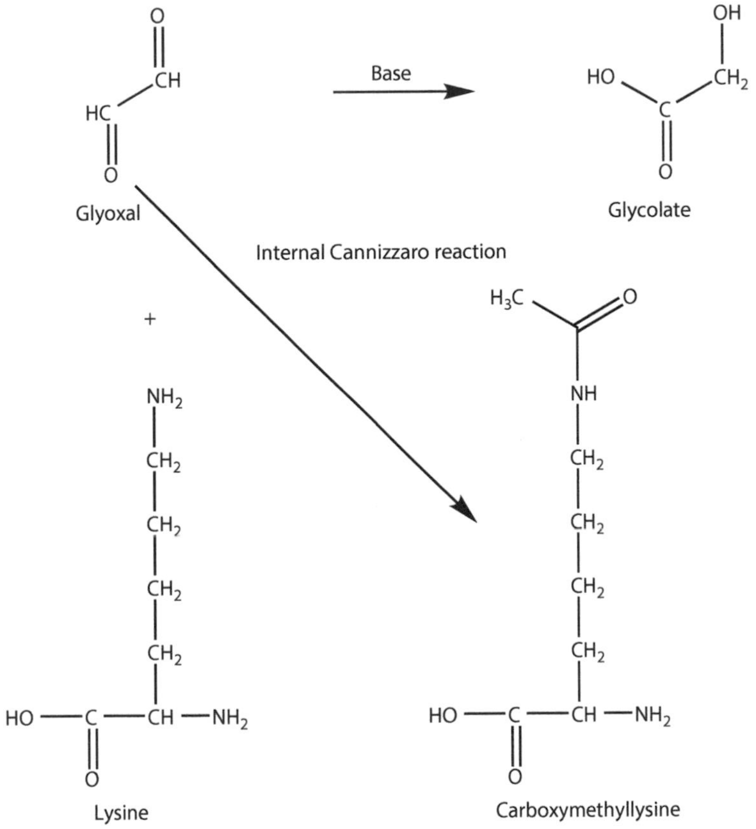

Glyoxal → Glycolate

Internal Cannizzaro reaction

Lysine → Carboxymethyllysine

Base-catalyzed disproportionation of an aldehyde to yield a carboxylic acid and the corresponding alcohol; if an α-hydrogen is present, an aldol condensation is a competing reaction. See Hazlet, S.E. and Stauffer, D.A., Crossed Cannizzaro reactions, *J.Org.Chem.* 27, 2021–2024, 1962; Entezari, M.H. and Shameli, A.A., Phase-transfer catalysis and ultrasonic waves. I. Cannizzaro reaction, *Ultrason.Sonochem.* 7, 169–172, 2000; Matin, M.M., Sharma, T., Sabharwal, S.G., and Dhavale, D.D., Synthesis and evaluation of the glycosidase inhibitory activity of 5-hydroxy substituted isofagomine analogues, *Org. Biomol.Chem.* 3, 1702–1707, 2005; Zhang, L., Wang, S., Zhou, S., *et al.*, Cannizzaro-type disproportionation of aromatic aldehydes to amides and alcohols by using either a stoichiometric amount or a catalytic amount of lanthanide compounds, *J.Org.Chem.* 71, 3149–3153, 2006. Intramolecular Cannizzaro reactions have been described (Glomb, M.A., and Monnier, V.M., Mechanism of protein modification by glyoxal and glycoaldehyde, reactive intermediates of the Maillard reaction, *J.Biol.Chem.* 270, 10017–10026, 1995; Russell, A.E., Miller, S.P., and Morken, J.P., Efficient Lewis acid catalyzed intramolecular Cannizzaro reaction, *J.Org.Chem.* 65, 8381–8383, 2000; Schramm, C. and Rinderer, B., Determination of cotton-bound glyoxal via an internal Cannizzaro reaction by means of high-performance liquid chromatography, *Anal.Chem.* 72, 5829–5833, 2000).

Claisen Condensation

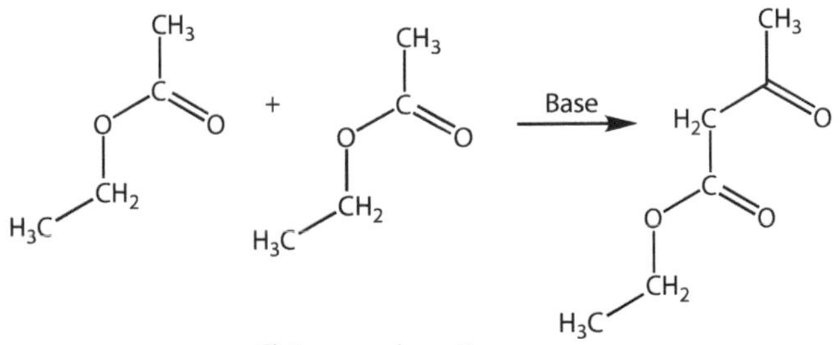

Claisen condensation

ORGANIC NAME REACTIONS USEFUL IN BIOCHEMISTRY AND MOLECULAR BIOLOGY (Continued)

The base-catalyzed condensation of two moles of an ester to give a β-keto ester. Claisen condensations are more favorable with thioesters. This reaction is of great importance in the biosynthesis of fatty acids and polyketides (Haapalainen, A.M., Meriläinen, G., and Wierenga, R.K. The thiolase superfamily: condensing enzymes with diverse reaction specificities, *Trends Biochem.Sci.* 31, 64–71, 2006). For general issues see Dewar, M.J. and Dieter, K.M., Mechanism of the chain extension step in the biosynthesis of fatty acids, *Biochemistry* 27, 3302–3308, 1988; Clark, J.D., O'Keefe, S.J., and Knowles, J.R., Malate synthase: proof of a stepwise Claisen condensation using the double-isotope fractionation test, *Biochemistry* 27, 5961–5971, 1988; Nicholson, J.M., Edafiogho, I.O., Moore, J.A., *et al.*, Cyclization reactions leading to β-hydroxyketo esters, *J.Pharm.Sci.* 83, 76–78, 1994; Lee, R.E., Armour, J.W., Takayama, K., *et al.*, Mycolic acid biosynthesis: definition and targeting of the Claisen condensation step, *Biochim.Biophys.Acta* 1346, 275–284, 1997; Shimakata, T. and Minatogawa, Y., Essential role of trehalose in the synthesis and subsequent metabolism of corynomycolic acid is *Corynebacterium matruchotil, Arch.Biochem.Biophys.* 380, 331–338, 2000; Olsen, J.G., Madziola, A., von Wettstein-Knowles, P., *et al.*, Structures of β-ketoacyl-acyl carrier protein synthase I complexed with fatty acids elucidate its catalytic machinery, *Structure* 9, 233–243, 2001; Klavins, M., Dipane, J., and Babre, K., Humic substances as catalysts in condensation reactions, *Chemosphere* 44, 737–742, 2001; Heath, R.J. and Rock, C.O., The Claisen condensation in biology, *Nat.Prod.Rep.* 19, 581–596, 2002; Takayama, K., Wang, C., and Besra, G.S., Pathway to synthesis and processing of mycolic acids in *Mycobacterium tuberculosis, Clin.Microbiol.Rev.* 18, 81–101, 2005; Ryu, Y., Kim, K.J., Roessner, C.A., and Scott, A.I., Decarboxylative Claisen condensation catalyzed by in vitro selected ribozymes, *Chem.Commun.* (13), 1439–1441, 2006; Kamijo, S. and Dudley, G.B., Claisen-type condensation of vinylogous acyl triflates, *Org.Lett.* 8, 175–177, 2006.

Claisen Rearrangement

Chorismic Acid   Prephenic Acid

Zhang Z. and Bruice T.C., Temperature dependence of the structure of the substrate and active site of the *Thermus thermophilus* chorismate mutase E-S complex, *Biochemistry* **45**, 8562–8567, 2006

The rearrangement of an allyl vinyl ether or the nitrogen or sulfur analogue or allyl aryl ether to yield a γ, δ-unsaturated ketone or an *o*-allyl substituted phenol. See Hilvert, D., Carpenter, S.H., Nared, K.D., and Auditor, M.T., Catalysis of concerted reactions by antibodies: the Claisen rearrangement, *Proc. Nat.Acad.Sci.USA* 85, 4953–4955, 1988; Campbell, A.P., Tarasow, T.M., Massefski, W., *et al.*, *Proc.Nat.Acad.Sci.USA* 90, 8663–8667, 1993; Swiss, K.A. and Firestone, R.A., Catalysis of Claisen rearrangement by low molecular weight polyethylene(1), *J.Org.Chem.* 64, 2158–2159, 1999; Berkowitz, D.B., Choi, S., and Maeng, J.H., Enzyme-assisted asymmetric total synthesis of (-)-podophyllotoxin and (-)-picropodophyllin, *J.Org.Chem.* 65, 847–860, 2000; Itami, K. and Yoshida, J., The use of hydrophilic groups in aqueous organic reactions, *Chem.Rec.* 2 213–224, 2002; Martin Castro, A.M., Claisen rearrangement over the past nine decades, *Chem.Rev.* 104, 2939–3002, 2004; Sparano, B.A., Shahi, S.P., and Koide, K., Effect of binding and conformation on fluorescence quenching in new 2,7'-dichlorofluorescein derivatives, *Org.Lett.* 6, 1947–1949, 2004; Davis, C.J., Hurst, T.E., Jacob, A.M., and Moody, C.J., Microwave-mediated Claisen rearrangement followed by phenol oxidation: a simple route to naturally occurring 1,4-benzoquinones. The first synthesis of verapliquinones A and B and Panicein, A., *J.Org.Chem.* 70, 4414–4422, 2005; Wright, S.K., DeClue, M.S., Mandal, A., *et al.*, Isotope effects on the enzymatic and nonenzymatic reactions of chorismate, *J.Am.Chem.Soc.* 127, 12957–12964, 2005; Declue, M.S., Baldridge, K.K., Kast, P., and Hilvert, D., Experimental and computational investigation of the uncatalyzed rearrangement and elimination reactions of isochorismate, *J.Am.Chem.Soc.* 128, 2043–2051, 2006; Zhang, X. and Bruice, T.C., Temperature dependence of the structure of the substrate and active site of the *Thermus thermophilus* chorismate mutase E-S complex, *Biochemistry* 45, 8562–8567, 2006.

ORGANIC NAME REACTIONS USEFUL IN BIOCHEMISTRY AND MOLECULAR BIOLOGY (Continued)

Criegee Reactions

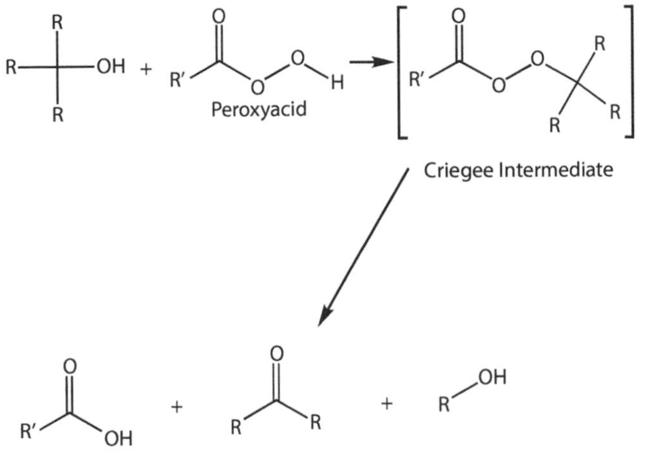

Criegee Intermediate

Mostly the reaction of a peroxyacid with a tertiary alcohol to form a ketone and an alcohol. The intermediate peroxyester is an intermediate (Criegee adduct or Criegee intermediate) in the Baeyer-Villiger reaction. The Criegee intermediate is important in the ozonolysis of alkenes including fatty acids. See Leffler, J.E. and Scrivener, F.E., Jr., The decomposition of cumyl peracetate in nonpolar solvents, *J.Org.Chem.* 37, 1794–1796, 1978; Srisankar, E.V. and Patterson, L.K., Reactions of ozone with fatty acid monolayer: a model system for disruption of lipid molecular assemblies by ozone, *Arch.Environ.Health* 34, 346–349, 1979; Grammer, J.C., Loo, J.A., Edmonds, C.G., *et al.*, Chemistry and mechanism of vanadate-promoted photooxidative cleavage of myosin, *Biochemistry* 35, 15582–15592, 1996; Krasutsky, P.A., Kolomitsyn, I.V., l Kiprof P., *et al.*, Observation of a stable carbocation in a consecutive Criegee rearrangement with trifluoroperacetic acid, *J.Org.Chem.* 65, 3926–3992, 1996; Carlqvist, P., Eklund, P., Hult, K., and Brinck, T., Rational design of a lipase to accommodate catalysis of Baeyer-Villiger oxidation with hydrogen peroxide, *J.Mol.Model.* 9, 164–171, 2003; Deeth, R.J. and Bugg, T.D., A density functional investigation of the extradiol cleavage mechanism in non-heme iron catechol dioxygenease, *J.Biol.Inorg.Chem.* 8, 409–418, 2003; Krasutsky, P.A., Kolomitsyn, I.V., Krasutsky, S.G., and Kiprof, P., Double- and triple-consecutive *O*-insertion into *tert*-butyl and triarylmethyl structures, *Org.Lett.* 6, 2539–2542, 2004.

Curtius Rearrangement

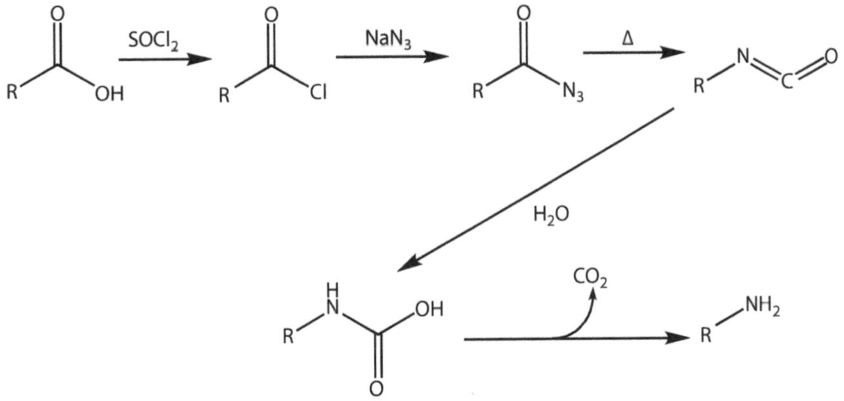

The conversion of a carboxylic acid to an amine via an acid intermediate. See Inouye, K., Watanabe, K., and Shin, M., Formation and degradation of urea derivatives in the azide method of peptide synthesis. Part 1. The Curtius rearrangement and urea formation, *J.Chem.Soc.* (17), 1905–1911, 1977; Chorev, M., and Goodman, M., Partially modified retro-inverso peptides. Comparative Curtius rearrangements to prepare 1, 1-diaminoalkane derivatives, *Int.J.Pept.Protein Res.* 21, 258–268, 1983; Sasmal, S., Geyer, A., and Maier, M.E., Synthesis of cyclic peptidomimetics from aldol building blocks, *J.Org. Chem.* 67, 6260–6263, 2002; Kedrowski, B.L., Synthesis of orthogonally protected (R)- and (S)-2-methylcysteine via an enzymatic desymmeterization and Curtius rearrangement, *J.Org.Chem.* 68, 5403–5406, 2003; Englund, E.A., Gopi, H.N., and Appella, D.H., An efficient synthesis of a probe for protein function: 2,3-diaminopropionic acid with orthogonal protecting groups, *Org.Lett.* 6, 213–215, 2004; Spino, C., Tremblay, M.C., and Gobout, C., A stereodivergent approach to amino acids, amino alcohols, or oxazolidinones of high enantiomeric purity, *Org.Lett.* 6, 2801–2804, 2004; Brase, S., Gil, C., Knepper, K., and Zimmerman, V., Organic azides: an exploding diversity of a unique class of compounds, *Angew.Chem.Int.Ed.Engl.* 44, 5188–5240, 2005; Lebel, H. and Leogane, O., Boc-protected amines via a mild and efficient one-pot Curtius rearrangement, *Org.Lett.* 7, 4107–4110, 2005.

ORGANIC NAME REACTIONS USEFUL IN BIOCHEMISTRY AND MOLECULAR BIOLOGY (Continued)

Dakin Reaction

Conversion of an aromatic ketone or aldehyde to a phenolic derivative with alkaline hydrogen peroxide. The mechanism is thought to be similar to the Baeyer-Villiger reaction possibly proceeding through a peroxyacid intermediate. The presence of an amino group or a hydroxyl group in the position para to the carbonyl function is required. See Corforth, J.W. and Elliott, D.F., Mechanism of the Dakin and West reaction, *Science* 112, 534–535, 1950.

Dakin-West Reaction

Dakin–West reaction

Conversion of amino acids to acetamidoketones via the action of acetic anhydride in base where a carboxyl group is replaced by an acyl group in a reaction proceeding through an oxazolone intermediate. This reaction has been used for the synthesis of enzyme inhibitors and receptor antagonists. See Angliker, H. Wikstrom, P., Rauber, P., *et al.*, Synthesis and properties of peptidyl derivatives of arginylfluoromethanes, *Biochem.J.* 256, 481–486, 1988; Cheng, L., Goodwin, C.A., Schully, M.F., *et al.*, Synthesis and biological activity of ketomethylene pseudopeptide analogues as thrombin inhibitors, *J.Med. Chem.* 35, 3364–3369, 1992; Godfrey, A.B., Brooks, D.A., Hay, L.A., *et al*, Application of the Dakin-West reaction for the synthesis of oxazole-containing dual PPARα/γ agonists, *J.Org.Chem.* 68, 2623–2632, 2003; Loksha, Y.M., el-Barbary, A.A., it-Barbary, M.A., *et al.*, Synthesis of 2-(aminocarbonylmethylthio)-1*H*-imidazoles as novel Capravirine analogues, *Bioorg.Med.Chem.* 13, 4209–4220, 2005.

Diels-Alder Condensation

trans-butadiene   *cis*-butadiene   Maleic anhydride
               diene   dienophile

Diels–Alder condensation

A cycloaddition reaction between a conjugated diene and an alkene resulting in the formation of alkene ring; construction of a six-membered ring with multiple stereogenic centers resulting in a chiral molecule. See Wasserman, A., *Diels-Alder Reactions. Organic Background and Physico-Chemical Aspects*, Elsevier, Amsterdam, Netherlands, 1965; Fringuelli, F., and Taticchi, A., *The Diels-Alder Reaction. Selected Practical Methods*, John Wiley & Sons, Ltd., Chichester, UK, 2002; Stocking, E.M. and Williams, R.M., Chemistry and biology of biosynthetic Diels-Alder reactions, *Angew.Chem.Int.Ed.* 42, 3078–3115, 2003. See also Waller, R.L. and Recknagel, R.O., Determination of lipid conjugated dienes with tetracyanoethylene-[14]C: significance for study of the pathology of lipid peroxidation, *Lipids* 12, 914–921, 1977; Melucci, M., Barbarella, G., and Sotgiu, G., Solvent-free, microwave-assisted synthesis of thiophene oligomers via Suzuki coupling, *J.Org.Chem.* 67, 8877–8884, 2002; Breslow, R., Determining the geometries of transition states by use of antihydrophobic additives in water, *Acc.Chem.Res.* 37, 471–478, 2004; Conley, N.R., Hung, R.J., and Willison, C.G., A new synthetic route to authentic *N*-substituted aminomaleimides, *J.Org.Chem.* 70, 4553–4555, 2005; Boul, P.J., Reutenauer, P., and Lehn, J.M. Reversible Diels-Alder reactions for the generation of dynamic combinatorial libraries, *Org.Lett.* 7, 15–18, 2005. Catalytic antibodies have been used for Diels-Alder reactions (Suckling, C.J., Tedford, C.M., Proctor, G.R., *et al.*, Catalytic antibodies: a new window on protein chemistry, *Ciba Found.Symp.* 159, 201–208, 1991; Meekel, A.A., Resmini, M., and Pandit, U.K., Regioselectivity and enantioselectivity in an antibody catalyzed hetero Diels-Alder reaction, *Bioorg.Med.Chem.* 4, 1051–1057, 1996; Romesberg, F.E., Spiller, B., Schultz, P.G., and Stevens, R.C., Immunological origins of binding and catalysis in a Diels-Alderase antibody, *Science* 279, 1934–1940, 1998; Romesberg, F.E. and Schultz, P.G., A mutational study of a Diels-Alderase catalytic antibody, *Bioorg.Med.Chem.Lett.* 9, 1741–1744, 1999; Chen, J., Deng, Q., Wang, R., *et al.*, Shape complementarity binding-site dynamics, and transition state stabilization: a theoretical study of Diels-Alder catalysis by antibody IE9, *ChemBioChem* 1, 255–261, 2000; Kim, S.P., Leach, A.G., and Houk, K.N., The origins of noncovalent catalysis of intermolecular Diels-Alder reactions by cyclodextrins, self-assembling capsules, antibodies, and RNAses, *J.Org.Chem.* 67, 4250–4260, 2002; Cannizzaro, C.E., Ashley, J.A, Janda, K.D., and Houk, K.N., Experimental determination of the absolute enantioselectivity of an antibody-catalyzed Diels-Alder reaction and theoretical explorations of the origins of stereoselectivity, *J.Am.Chem.Soc.* 125, 2489–2506, 2003.

ORGANIC NAME REACTIONS USEFUL IN BIOCHEMISTRY AND MOLECULAR BIOLOGY (Continued)

Edman Degradation

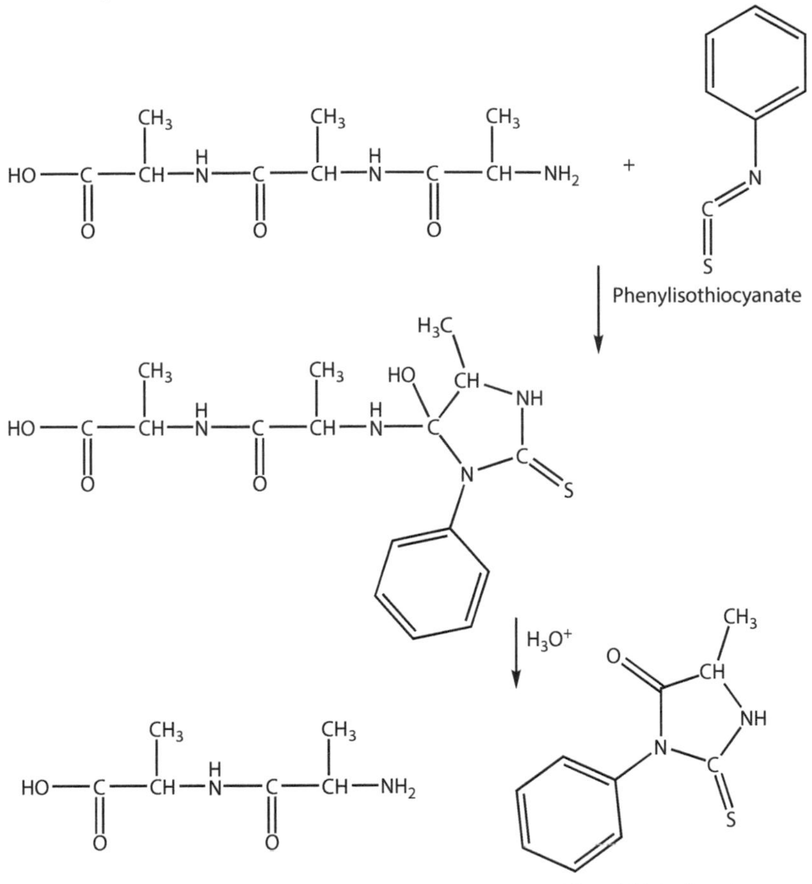

Phenylisothiocyanate

Phenylthiohydantoin

The stepwise degradation of a peptide chain from the amino-terminal via reaction with phenylisothiocyanate. This process is used for the chemical determination of the amino acid sequence of a peptide or protein. See Edman, P., Sequence determination, *Mol.Biol.Biochem.Biophys.* 9, 211–255, 1970; Heinrikson, R.L., Application of automated sequence analysis to the understanding of protein structure and function, *Ann.Clin.Lab.Sci.* 8, 295–301, 1978; Tsugita, A., Developments in protein microsequencing, *Adv.Biophys.* 23, 91–113, 1987; Han, K.K. and Martinage, A., Post-translational chemical modifications of proteins – III. Current developments in analytical procedures of identification and quantitation of post-translational chemically modified amino acid(s) and its derivatives, *Int.J.Biochem.* 25, 957–970, 1993; Masiarz, F.R. and Malcolm, B.A., Rapid determination of endoprotease specificity using peptide mixtures and Edman degradation analysis, *Methods Enzymol.* 241, 302–310, 1994; Gooley, A.A., Ou, K., Russell, J., *et al.*, A role for Edman degradation in proteome studies, *Electrophoresis* 18, 1068–1072, 1997; Wurzel, C., and Wittmann-Liebold, B., A wafer based micro reaction system for the Edman degradation of proteins and peptides, *J.Protein Chem.* 17, 561–564, 1998; Walk, T.B., Sussmuth, R., Kempter, C., *et al.*, Identification of unusual amino acids in peptides using automated sequential Edman degradation coupled to direct detection by electrospray-ionization mass spectrometry, *Biopolymers* 49, 329–340, 1999; Lauer-Fields, J.L., Nagase, H. and Fields, G.B., Use of Edman degradation sequence analysis and matrix-assisted laser desorption/ionization mass spectrometry in designing substrates for matrix metalloproteinases, *J.Chromatog.A.* 890, 117–125, 2000; Hajdu, J., Neutze, R., Sjogren, T., *et al.*, Analyzing protein functions in four dimensions, *Nat.Struct.Biol.* 7, 1006–1012, 2000; Shively, J.E., The chemistry of protein sequence analysis, *EXS* 88, 99–117, 2000; Wang, P., Arabaci, G., and Pei, D., Rapid sequencing of library-derived peptides by partial Edman degradation and mass spectrometry, *J.Comb.Chem.* 3, 251–254, 2001; Brewer, M., Oost, T., Sukonpan, C., *et al.*, Sequencing hydroxylethyleneamine-containing peptides via Edman degradation, *Org.Lett.* 4, 3469–3472, 2002; Sweeney, M.C. and Pei, D., An improved method for rapid sequencing of support-bound peptides by partial Edman degradation and mass spectrometry, *J.Comb.Chem.* 5, 218–222, 2003; Buda, F., Ensing, B., Gribnau, M.C., and Baerends, E.J., O₂ evolution in the Fenton reaction, *Chemistry* 9, 3436–3444, 2003; Liu, Q., Berchner-Pfannschmidt, U., Moller, U., *et al.*, A Fenton reaction at the endoplasmic reticulum is involved in the redox control of hypoxia-inducible gene expression, *Proc.Nat.Acad.Sci.USA* 101, 4302–4307, 2004; Maksimovic, V., Mojovic, M., Neumann, G., and Vucinic, Z., Nonenzymatic reaction of dihydroxyacetone with hydrogen peroxide enhanced via a Fenton reaction, *Ann.N.Y.Acad.Sci.* 1048, 461–465, 2005; Lu, C. and Koppenol, W.H., Inhibition of the Fenton reaction by nitrogen monoxide, *J.Biol.Inorg.Chem.* 10, 732–738, 2005; Baron, C.P., Refsgaard, H.H., Skibsted, H., and Andersen, M.L., Oxidation of bovine serum albumin initiated by the Fenton reaction—effect of EDTA, *tert*-butylhydroperoxide and tetrahydrofuran, *Free Radic.Res.* 40, 409–417, 2006; Thakkar, A., Wavreille, A.S., and Pei, D., Traceless capping agent for peptide sequencing by partial Edman degradation and mass spectrometry, *Anal.Chem.* 78, 5935–5939, 2006.

ORGANIC NAME REACTIONS USEFUL IN BIOCHEMISTRY AND MOLECULAR BIOLOGY (Continued)

Eschweiler-Clarke Reaction

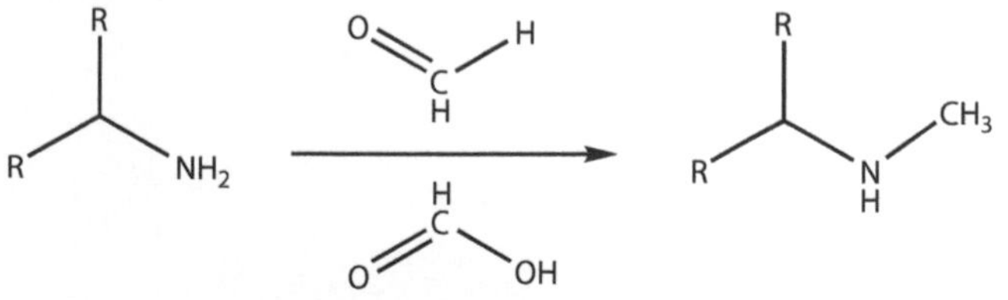

Eschweiler–Clarke reaction

The reductive methylation of amines with formaldehyde in the presence of formic acid. See Lindeke, B., Anderson, B., and Jenden, D.J., Specific deuteromethylation by the Escheweiler-Clarke reaction. Synthesis of differently labelled variants of trimethylamine and their use of the preparation of labelled choline and acetylcholine, *Biomed.Mass Spectrom.* 3, 257–259, 1976; Boldavalli, F., Bruno, O., Mariani, E., *et al.*, Esters of *N*-methyl-*N*-(2-hydroxyethyl or 3-hydroxypropyl)-1,3,3-trimethylbicyclo[2.2.1] heptan-2-endo-amine with hypotensive activity, *Farmaco* 42, 175–183, 1987; Lee, S.S., Wu, W.N., Wilton, J.H., *et al.*, Longiberine and *O*-methyllogiberine, dimeric protoberberine-benzyl tetrahydroisoqunioline alkaloids from *Thalictrum longistrylum*, *J.Nat.Prod.* 62, 1410–1414, 1999; Suma, R and Sai Prakash, P.K., Conversion of sertraline to *N*-methyl sertraline in embalming fluid: a forensic implication, *J.Anal.Toxicol.* 30, 395–399, 2006. The reaction can be accomplished with sodium borohydride or sodium cyanoborohydride and is related to the reductively methylation/ alkylation of lysine residues in proteins (Lundblad, R.L., *Chemical Reagents for the Modification of Proteins*, 3rd edn., CRC Press, Boca Raton, FL, 2004).

Favorskii Rearrangement

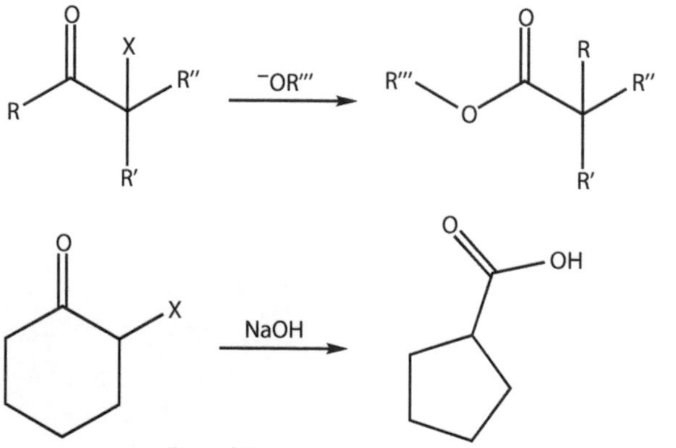

Favorskii rearrangement

The rearrangement of an α-ketone in the presence of an alkoxide to form a carboxylic ester; cyclic α-ketone undergo ring contraction. March, J. *Advanced Organic Chemistry. Reactions, Mechanisms, and Structures*, 3rd edn. John Wiley & Sons, New York, New York, 1985; Gardner, H.W., Simpson, T.D., and Hamberg, M., Mechanism of linoleic acid hydroperoxide reaction with alkali, *Lipids* 31, 1023–1028, 1996; Xiang, L., Kalaitzis, J.A., Nilsen, G. *et al.*, Mutational analysis of the enterocin favorskii biosynthetic rearrangement, *Org.Lett.* 4, 957–960, 2002; Zhang, L. and Koreeda, M., Stereocontrolled synthesis of kelsoene by the homo-favorskii rearrangement, *Org.Lett.* 4, 3755–3788, 2002; Grainger, R.S., Owoare, R.B., Tisselli, P., and Steed, J.W., A synthetic alternative to the type-II intramolecular 4 + 3 cycloaddition, *J.Org.Chem.* 68, 7899–7902, 2003.

Fenton Reagent/Reaction

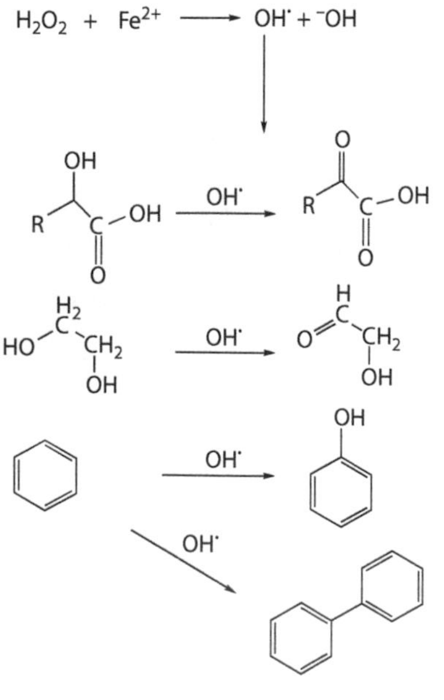

ORGANIC NAME REACTIONS USEFUL IN BIOCHEMISTRY AND MOLECULAR BIOLOGY (Continued)

The reaction of ferrous ions and hydrogen peroxide to yield a hydroxyl radical. See Aust, S.D., Morehouse, L.A., and Thomas, C.E., Role of metals in oxygen radical reactions, *J.Free Radic.Biol.Med.* 1, 3–25, 1985; Goldstein, S., Meyerstein, D. and Czapski, G., The Fenton reagents, *Free Radic.Biol.Med.* 15, 435–445, 1993; Wardman, P. and Candeias, L.P., Fenton chemistry: an introduction, *Radiat.Res.* 145, 523–531, 1996; Held, K.D., Sylvester, F.C., Hopcia, K.L., and Biaglow, J.E., Role of Fenton chemistry in the thiol-induced toxicity and apoptosis, *Radiat.Res.* 145, 542–553, 1996; Merli, C., Petrucci, E., Da Pozzo, A., and Pernetti, M., Fenton-type treatment: state of the art, *Ann.Chim.* 93, 761–770, 2003; Groves, J.T., High-valent iron in chemical and biological oxidations, *J.Inorg.Biochem.* 100, 434–447, 2006.

Fischer Carbene Complexes

$$Cr(CO)_6 \text{ (Chromium carbonyl)} \xrightarrow[R_2X]{R_1Li} Cr(CO)_5=C(OR_2)(R_1) \text{ (Fischer carbene complex)}$$

A Fischer carbene complex consists of a transition metal with a formal carbon-metal bond containing a carbene in the singlet state; stabilization of the carbene is provided by the metal interaction. The Fischer carbene complex is electrophilic as the carbene carbon as opposed to the Schrock complex which is in the triplet state and nucleophilic at the carbene carbon. The Fischer carbene complex is high reactivity and is used in many synthetic procedures. A example is provided by the α,β-unsaturated carbenepentacarbonylchromium complex (de Meijere, A., Schirmer, H., and Duetsch, M., Fischer carbene complexes as chemical multitalents: The incredible range of products from carbenepentacarbonylmetal α,β-unsaturated complexes, *Angew.Chem.Int.Ed.* 39, 3964–4002, 2000). See also Salmain, M., Blais, J.C., Tran-Huy, H., *et al*, Reaction of hen egg white lysozyme with Fischer-type metallocarbene complexes. Chacterization of the conjugates and determination of the metal complex binding sites, *Eur.J.Biochem.* 268, 5479–5487, 2001; Merlic, C.A. and Doroh, B.C., Amine-catalyzed coupling of aldehydes and ketenes derived from Fischer carbene complexes: formation of beta-lactones and enol ethers, *J.Org.Chem.* 68, 6056–6069, 2003; Barluenga, J., Santamaria, J., and Tomas, M., Synthesis of heterocycles via group VI Fischer carbene complexes, *Chem.Rev.* 104, 2259–2283, 2004; Barluenga, J., Fananas-Mastral, M., and Aznar, F., A new synthesis of allyl sulfoxides via nucleophilic addition of sulfinyl carbanions to group 6 Fischer carbene complexes, *Org.Lett.* 7, 1235–1237, 2005; Lian, Y. and Wulff, W.D., Iron in the service of chromium: the o-benzannulation of *trans,trans*-dienyl Fischer carbene complexes, *J.Am.Chem.Soc.* 127, 17162–17163, 2005; Barluenga, J., Mendoza, A., Dieguez, A., *et al.*, Umpolung reactivity of alkenyl Fischer carbene complexes, copper enolates, and electrophiles, *Angew.Chem.Int.Ed.Engl.* 45, 4848–4850, 2006; Samanta, D., Sawoo, S. and Sarkar, A., *In situ* generation of gold nanoparticles on a protein surface: Fischer carbene complex as reducing agent, *Chem.Commun.* (32), 3438–3440, 2006; Rawat, M., Prutyanov, V., and Wulff, W.D., Chromene chromium carbene complexes in the syntheses of naphthoyran and naphthopyrandione units present in photochromic materials and biologically active natural products, *J.Am.Chem.Soc.* 128, 11044–11053, 2006. For general information on carbenes including Fischer carbene complexes and Schrock carbene complexes, see *Carbene Chemistry. From Fleeting Intermediates to Powerful Reagents*, ed. G. Bertrand, Fontis Media/Marcel Dekker, New York, New York, 2002.

ORGANIC NAME REACTIONS USEFUL IN BIOCHEMISTRY AND MOLECULAR BIOLOGY (Continued)

Fischer Indole Synthesis

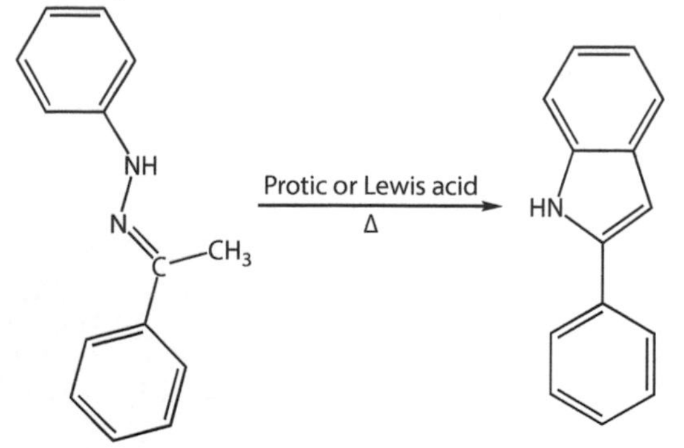

Fischer indole synthesis

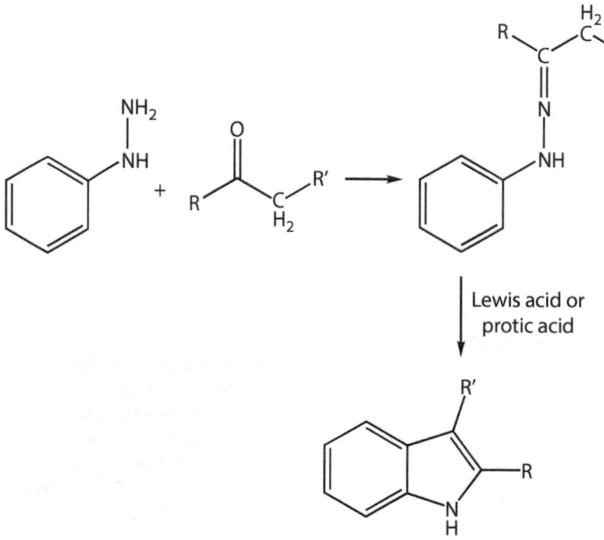

The thermal conversion of arylhydrazones in the presence of a protic acid or a Lewis acid to form an indole ring. See Owellen, R.J., Fitzgerald, J.A., Fitzgerald, B.M., *et al.*, The cyclization phase of the Fischer indole synthesis. The structure and significance of Pleininger's intermediate, *Tetrahedron Lett.* 18, 1741–1746, 1967; Kim, R.M., Manna, M., Hutchins, S.M. *et al.*, Dendrimer-supported combinatorial chemistry, *Proc.Natl.Acad.Sci.USA* 93, 10012–10017, 1996; Brase, S., Gil, C., and Knepper, K., The recent impact of solid-phase synthesis on medicinally relevant benzoannelated nitrogen heterocycles, *Bioorg.Med.Chem.* 10, 2415–2437, 2002; Rosenbaum, C., Katzka, C., Marzinzik, A., and Waldmann, H., Traceless Fischer indole synthesis on the solid phase, *Chem.Commun.* (15), 1822–1823, 2003; Mun, H.S., Ham, W.H., and Jeong, J.H., Synthesis of 2,3-disubstituted indole on solid phase by the Fischer indole synthesis, *J.Comb.Chem.* 7, 130–135, 2005; Narayana, B., Ashalatha, B.V., Vijaya Raj, K.K., *et al.*, Synthesis of some new biologically acivie 1,3,4-oxadiazolyl nitroindole and a modified Fischer indole synthesis of ethyl nitro indole-2-carboxylates, *Bioorg.Med.Chem.* 13, 4638–4644, 2005; Schmidt, A.M. and Eilbracht, P., Tandem hydroformylation-hydrazone formation-Fischer indole synthesis: a novel approach to tryptamides, *Org.Biomol.Chem.* 3, 2333–2343, 2005; Linnepe Nee Kohling, P., Schmidt, A.M., and Eilbracht, P., 2,3-Disubstituted indoles from olefins and hydrazines via tandem hydroformylation-Fischer indole synthesis and skeletal rearrangement, *Org.Biomol.Chem.* 4, 302–313, 2006; Landwehr, J., George, S., Karg, E.M., *et al.*, Design and synthesis of novel 2-amino-5-hydroxyindole derivatives that inhibit human 5-lipooxygenase, *J.Med.Chem.* 49, 4327–4332, 2006.

ORGANIC NAME REACTIONS USEFUL IN BIOCHEMISTRY AND MOLECULAR BIOLOGY (Continued)

Friedel-Crafts Reaction

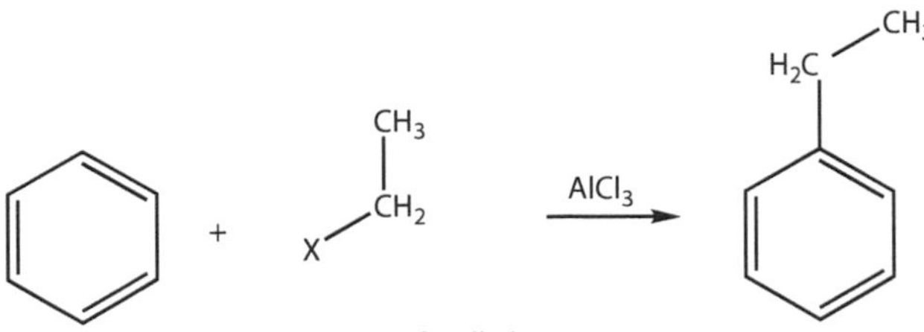

Friedel-Crafts alkylation

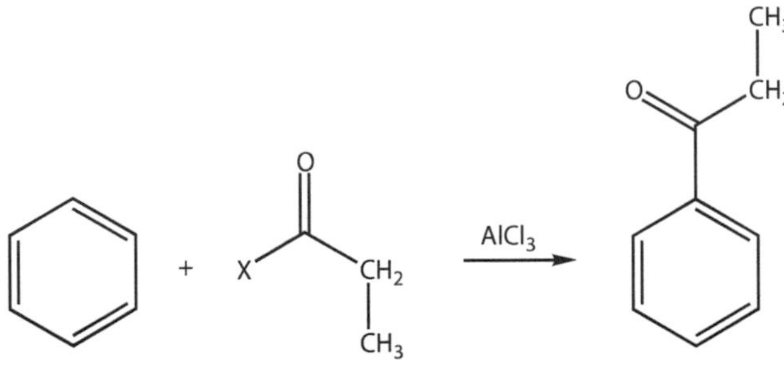

Friedel-Crafts acylation

The alkylation of an aromatic ring by an alkyl halide (order of reactivity F>Cl>Br>I) in the presence of a strong Lewis acid such as aluminum chloride; the acylation of an aromatic ring by an acyl halide (order of reactivity usually is I>Br>Cl>F) in the presence of a strong Lewis acid. Acids and acid anhydrides can replace the acyl halides. A related reaction is the Derzen-Nenitzescu ketone synthesis. See Olah, G.A., *Friedel-Crafts Chemistry*, John Wiley & Sons, New York, New York, 1973; Roberts, R.M. and Khalaf, A.A., *Friedel-Krafts Alkylation Chemistry: A Century of Discovery*, Marcel Dekker, New York, New York, 1989. See also Retey, J., Enzymatic catalysis by Friedel-Crafts-type reactions, *Naturwissenschaften* 83, 439–447, 1996; White, E.H., Darbeau, R.W., Chen, Y. *et al.*, A new look at the Friedel-Crafts alkylation reaction(1), *J.Org.Chem.* 61, 7986–7987, 1996; Studer, J., Purdie, N., and Krouse, J.A., Friedel-Crafts acylation as a quality control assay for steroids, *Appl.Spectrosc.* 57, 791–796, 2003; Retey, J., Discovery and role of methylidene imidazolone, a highly reactive electrophilic prosthetic group, *Biochim.Biophys.Acta* 1647, 179–184, 2003; Bandini, M., Melloni, A., and Umani-Ronchi, A., New catalytic approaches in the stereoselective Friedel-Crafts alkylation reaction, *Angew.Chem.Int.Ed.Engl.* 43, 550–556, 2004; Poppe, L. and Retey, J., Friedel-Crafts-type mechanism for the enzymatic elimination of ammonia from histidine and phenylalanine, *Angew.Chem.Int.Ed.Engl.* 44, 3668–3688, 2005; Keni, M., and Tepe, J.J., One-pot Friedel-Crafts/Robinson-Gabriel synthesis of oxazoles using oxazolone templates, *J.Org.Chem.* 70, 4211–4213, 2005; Movassaghi, M. and Ondrus, A.E., Enantioselective total synthesis of tricyclic myrmicarin alkaloids, *Org.Lett.* 7, 4423–4426, 2005; Paizs, C., Katona, A., and Retey, J., The interaction of heteroaryl-acrylates and alanines with phenylalanine ammonia-lyase form parsley, *Chemistry* 12, 2739–2744, 2006. Cuprous ions have been observed to promote a Friedel-Crafts acylation reaction (Kozikowski, A.P. and Ames, A., Copper(I) promoted acylation reactions. A transition metal mediated version of the Friedel-Crafts reaction, *J.Am.Chem.Soc.* 102, 860–862, 1980).

Friedländer Synthesis

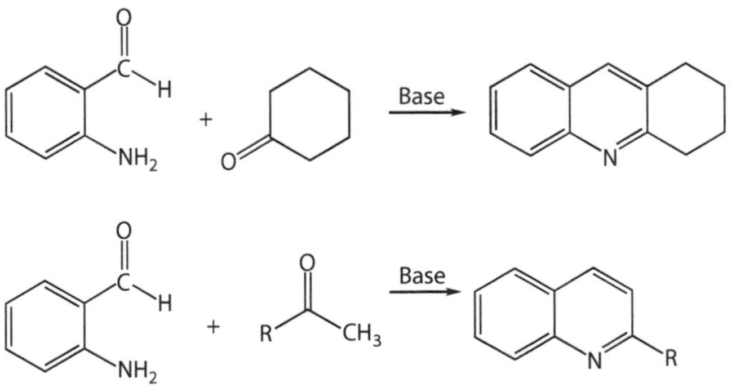

Friedlander synthesis

The base-catalyzed formation of quinoline derivatives by condensation of an o-aminobenzaldehyde with a ketone; also referred to as the Friedländer quinoline synthesis. The general utility of the reaction is somewhat limited by the availability of o-aminobenzaldehyde derivatives. See Maguire, M.P., Sheets, K.R., McVety, K., *et al.*, A new series of PDGF receptor tyrosine kinase inhibitors: 3-substituted quinoline derivatives, *J.Med.Chem.* 37, 2129–2137, 1994; Lindstrom, S., Friedlander synthesis of the food carcinogen 2-amino-1-methyl-6-phenylimidazo[4,5-b]pyridine, *Acta Chem.Scand.* 49, 361–363, 1995; Gladiali, S., Chelucci, G., Mudadu, M.S., *et al.*, Friedlander synthesis of chiral alkyl-substituted 1,10-phenanthrolines, *J.Org.Chem.* 66, 400–405, 2001; Patteux, C., Levacher, V., and Dupas, G., A novel traceless solid-phase Friedlander synthesis, *Org.Lett.* 5, 3061–3063, 2003; McNaughton, B.R. and Miller, B.L., A mild and efficient one-step synthesis of quinolines, *Org.Lett.* 5, 4257–4259, 2003; Yasuda, N., Hsiao, Y., Jensen, M.S., *et al.*, An efficient synthesis of an $\alpha_v\beta_3$ antagonist, *J.Org.Chem.* 69, 1959–1966, 2004.

ORGANIC NAME REACTIONS USEFUL IN BIOCHEMISTRY AND MOLECULAR BIOLOGY (Continued)

Fries Rearrangement

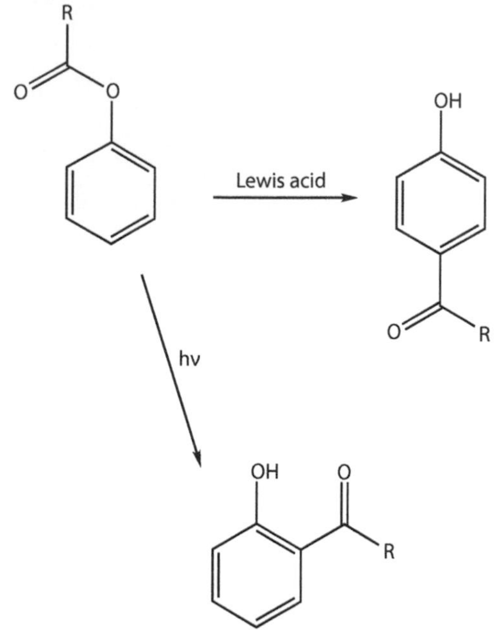

Rearrangement of a phenolic ester to yield *o*- and *p*-acylphenols. The distribution of products between the *ortho* and *para* acyl derivates depends on reaction conditions. The presence of solvent and a Lewis acid, the *para* product is preferred; with the photolytic process or at high temperature in the absence of solvent, the *ortho* derivative is preferred. See Sen, A.B. and Bhattacharji, S., Fries' rearrangement of aliphatic esters of β-naphthol, *Curr.Sci.* 20, 132–133, 1951; Iwasaki, S., Photochemistry of imidazolides. I. The photo-Fries-type rearrangement of *N*-substituted imidazoles, *Helv.Chim.Acta* 59, 2738–2752, 1976; Castell, J.V., Gomez, M.J., MIrabet, V., *et al.*, Photolytic degradation of benorylate: effects of the photoproducts on cultured hepatocytes, *J.Pharm.Sci.* 76, 374–378,1987; Climent, M.J. and Miranda, M.A. Gas chromatographic-mass spectrometric study of photodegradation of carbamate pesticides, *J.Chromatog.A.* 738, 225–231, 1996; Kozhevnikova, E.F., Derouane, E.G., and Kozhevnikov, I.V., Heteropoly acid as a novel efficient catalyst for Fries rearrangement, *Chem.Commun.* (11), 1178–1179, 2002; Dickerson, T.J., Tremblay, M.R., Hoffman, T.Z. *et al.*, Catalysis of the photo-Fries reaction: antibody-mediated stabilization of high energy states, *J.Am.Chem.Soc.* 125, 15395–15401, 2003; Seijas, J.A., Vazquez-Tato, M.P., and Carballido-Reboredo, R., Solvent-free synthesis of functionalized flavones under microwave irradiation, *J.Org.Chem.* 70, 2855–2858, 2005;Canle Lopez, M., Fernandez, M.I., Rodriguez, S., *et al.*, Mechanisms of direct and TiO$_2$-photocatalyzed degradation of phenylurea herbicides, *Chemphyschem* 6, 2064–2074, 2005; Slana, G.B. de Azevedo, M.S., Lopes, R.S., *et al.*, Total syntheses of oxygenated brazanquinones via regioselective homologous anionic Fries rearrangement of benzylic *O*-carbamates, *Beilstein J.Org.Chem.* 2, 1, 2006.

Gabriel Synthesis

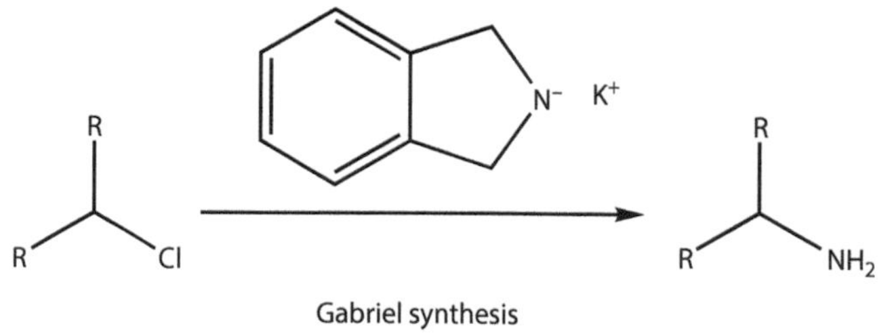

Gabriel synthesis

The conversion of an alkyl halide to alkyl amine mediated by potassium phthalimide. The intermediate product of the reaction of the alkyl halide and phthalimide is hydrolyzed to the product amine by acid or by reflux in ethanolic hydrazine. See Mikola, H. and Hanninen, E., Introduction of aliphatic amino and hydroxy groups to keto steroids using *O*-substituted hydroxylamines, *Bioconjugate Chem.* 3, 182–186, 1992; Groutas, W.C., Chong, L.S., Venkataraman, R., *et al.*, Mechanism-based inhibitors of serine proteinases based on the Gabriel-Colman rearrangement, *Biochem.Biophys.Res.Commun.* 194, 1491–1499, 1993; Konig, S., Ugi, I., and Schramm, H.J., Facile syntheses of C$_2$-symmetrical HIV-1 protease inhibitor, *Arch.Pharm.* 328, 699–704, 1995; Zhang, X.X. and Lippard, S.J., Synthesis of PDK, a novel porphyrin-linked dicarboxyate ligand, *J.Org.Chem.* 65, 5298–5305, 2000; Scozzafava, A. Saramet, I., Banciu, M.D., and Supuran, C.T., Carbonic anhydrase activity modulators: synthesis of inhibitors and activators incorporating 2-substituted-thiazol-4-yl-methyl scaffolds, *J.Enzyme Inhib.* 16, 351–358, 2001; Nicolaou, K.C., Hao, J., Reddy, M.V., *et al.*, Chemistry and biology of diazonamide A: second total synthesis and biological investigations, *J.Am.Chem.Soc.* 126, 12897–12906, 2004; Remond, C., Plantier-Royon, R., Aubry, N., and O'Donohue, M.J., An original chemoenzymatic rotue for the synthesis of β-D-galactofuranosides using an α-L-arabinofuranosidase, *Carbohydr.Res.* 340, 637–644, 2005; Pulici, M., Quartieri, F., and Felder, E.R., Trifluoroacetic acid anhydride-mediated solid-phase version of the Robison-Gabriel synthesis of oxazoles, *J.Comb.Chem.* 7, 463–473, 2005.

ORGANIC NAME REACTIONS USEFUL IN BIOCHEMISTRY AND MOLECULAR BIOLOGY (Continued)

Greiss Reaction

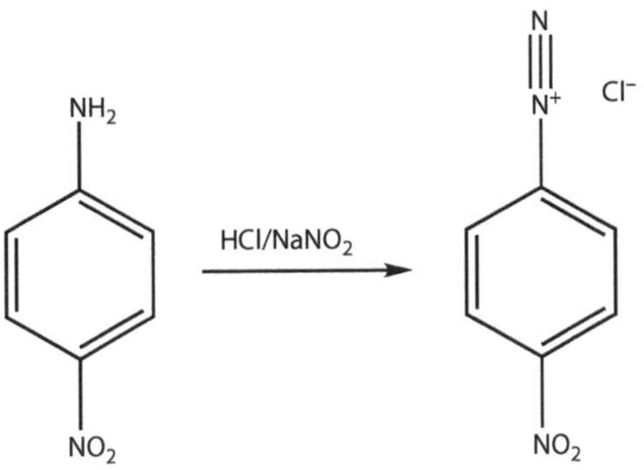

Greiss reaction

Greiss reaction as used for the measurement of nitrite

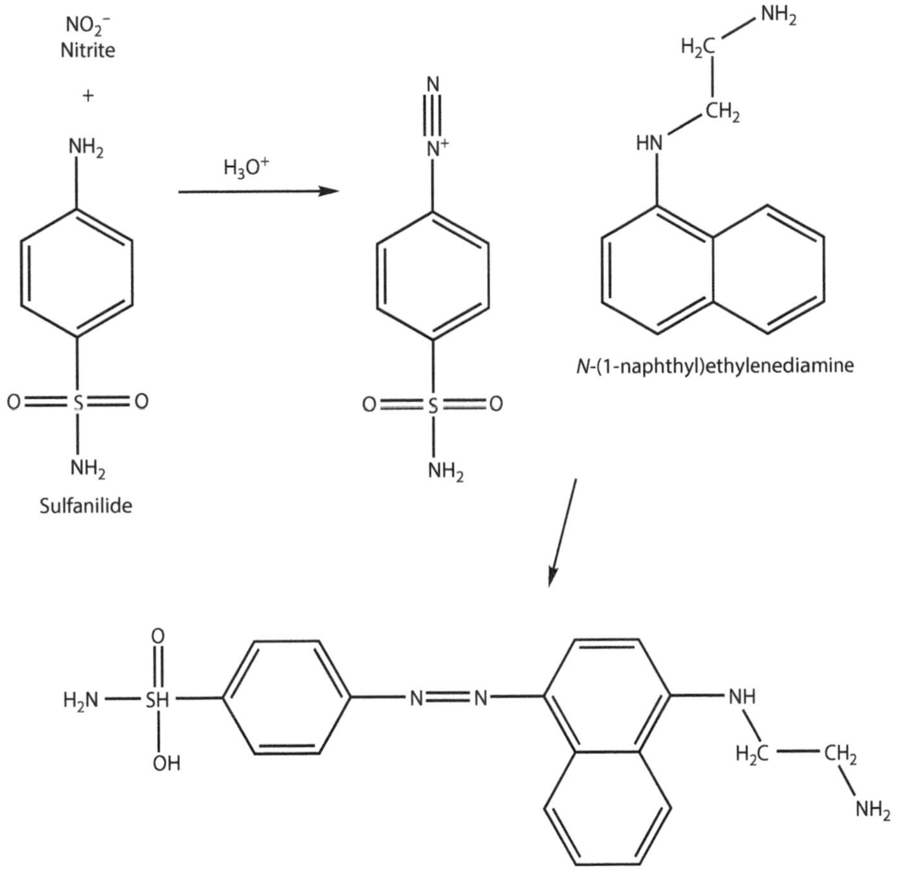

N-(1-naphthyl)ethylenediamine

Sulfanilide

Azo product measured at 520 nm

Diazotization of aromatic amines; used for the assay of nitrites in nitric oxide research. The assay for nitrates uses diazotization of sulfanilamide with subsequent coupling to an aromatic amine (N-1-naphthylethylenediamine) to form an chromophoric azo derivative. See Greenberg, S.S., Xie, J., Spitzer, J.J. *et al.*, Nitro containing L-arginine analogs interfere with assays for nitrate and nitrite, *Life Sci.* 57, 1949–1961, 1995; Pratt, P.F., Nithipatikom, K., and Campbell, W.B., Simultaneous determination of nitrate and nitrite in biological samples by multichannel flow injection analysis, *Anal.Biochem.* 231, 383–386, 1995; Tang, Y., Han, C. and Wang, X., Role of nitric oxide and prostaglandins in the potentiating effects of calcitonin gene-related peptide on Lipopolysaccharide-induced interleukin-6 release from mouse peritoneal macrophages, *Immunology* 96, 171–175, 1999; Baines, P.B., Stanford, S., Bishop-Bailey, D., *et al.*, Nitric oxide production in meningococcal disease is directly related to disease severity, *Crit.Care.Med.* 27, 1163–1165, 1999; Rabbani, G.H., Islam, S., Chowdhury, A.K., *et al.*, Increased nitrite and nitrate concentrations in sera and urine of patients with cholera or shigellosis, *Am.J.Gastroenterol.* 96, 467–472, 2001; Lee, R.H., Efron, D., Tantry, U. and Barbul, A., Nitric oxide in the healing wound: a time-course study, *J.Surg.Res.* 101, 104–108, 2001; Stark, J.M., Khan, A.M., Chiappetta, C.L., *et al*, Immune and functional role of nitric oxide in a mouse model of respiratory syncytial virus infection, *J.Infect.Dis.* 191, 387–395, 2005; Bellows, C.F., Alder, A., Wludyka, P., and Jaffe, B.M., Modulation of macrophage nitric oxide production by prostaglandin D2, *J.Surg.Res.* 132, 92–97, 2006. Diazotization of aromatic amines is also used for the the modification of proteins (Lundblad, R.L., *Chemical Reagents for Protein Modification*, CRC Press, Boca Raton, FL, 2004; Kennedy, J.H., Kricka, L.J., and Wilding, P., Protein-protein coupling reactions and the application of protein conjugates, *Clin.Chim.Acta* 70, 1–31, 1976; Sinnott, M.L., Affinity labeling via deamination reactions, *CRC Crit. Rev.Biochem.* 12, 327–372, 1982; Blair, A.H. and Ghose, T.I., Linkage of cytotoxic agents to

ORGANIC NAME REACTIONS USEFUL IN BIOCHEMISTRY AND MOLECULAR BIOLOGY (Continued)

immunoglobulins, *J.Immunol.Methods* 59, 129–143, 1983). While alkyl azides are unstable, carbonyl azides such as diazoacetyl derivatives have been used in the modification of proteins (Lundblad, R.L. and Stein, W.H., On the reaction of diazoacetyl compounds with pepsin, *J.Biol.Chem.* 244, 154–160, 1969; Keilova, H. and Lapresle, C., Inhibition of cathepsin E by diazoacetyl-norleucine methyl ester, *FEBS Lett.* 9, 348–350, 1970; Giraldi, T. and Nisi, C., Effects of cupric ions on the antitumour activity of diazoacetyl-glycine derivatives, *Chem.Biol.Interact.* 11,59–61, 1975; Kaehn, K., Morr, M., and Kula, M.R., Inhibition of the acid proteinase from *Neurospora crassa* by diazoaetyl-DL-norleucine methyl ester, 1,2-epoxy-3- (4-nitrophenoxy)propane and pepstatin, *Hoppe Seylers Z. Physiol.Chem.* 360, 791–794, 1979; Ouihia, A., René, L., Guilhem, J., *et al.*, A new diazoacylating reagent: Preparation, structure, and use of succinimidyl diazoacetate, *J.Org.Chem.* 58, 1641–1642, 1993.

Grignard Reagent or Grignard Reaction

The reaction of alkyl or aryl halides with magnesium in dry ether to yield derivatives which can be used in a variety of organic synthetic reactions. See Nagano, T. and Hayashi, T., Iron-catalyzed Grignard cross-coupling with alkyl halides possessing beta-hydrogens, *Org.Lett.* 6, 1297–1299, 2004; Querner, C., Reiss, P., Bleuse, J., and Pron, A., Chelating ligands for nanocrystals' functionalization, *J.Am.Chem.Soc.* 126, 11574–11582, 2004; Agarwal, S. anad Knolker, H.J., A novel pyrrole synthesis, *Org.Biomol.Chem.* 2, 3060–3062, 2004; Hatano, M., Matsumara, T., and Ishihara, K., Highly alkyl-selective addition to ketones with magnesiumate complexes derived from Grignard reagents, *Org.Lett.* 7, 573–576, 2005; Itami, K., Higashi, S., Mineno, M., and Yoshida, J., Iron-catalyzed cross-coupling of alkenyl sulfides with Grignard reagents, *Org.Lett.* 7, 1219–1222, 2005; Wang, X.J., Zhang, L., Sun, X., *et al.*, Addition of Grignard reagents to aryl chlorides: an efficient synthesis of aryl ketones, *Org.Lett.* 7, 5593–5595, 2005; Hoffman-Emery, F., Hilpert, H., Scalone, M., and Waldmeier, F., Efficient synthesis of novel NK1 receptor antagonists: selective 1,4-additional of Grignard reagents to 6-chloronicotinic acid derivatives, *J.Org.Chem.* 71, 2000–2008, 2006; Werner, T. and Barrett, A.G., Simple method for the preparation of esters from Grigard reagents and alkyl 1-imidazolecarboxylates, *J.Org.Chem.* 71, 4302–4304, 2006; Demel, P., Keller, M., and Breit, B., o-DPPB-directed copper mediated and –catalyzed allylic substitution with Grignard reagents, *Chemistry* 12, 6669–6683, 2006.

Knoevenagel Reaction or Knoevenagel Condensation

Knoevenagel condensation

EWG = electron-withdrawing group such as CHO, COOH, COOR, CN, NO$_2$

ORGANIC NAME REACTIONS USEFUL IN BIOCHEMISTRY AND MOLECULAR BIOLOGY (Continued)

An amine-catalyzed reaction between active hydrogen compounds of the type Z-CH$_2$-Z where Z can be a CHO, COOH, COOR, NO$_2$SOR, or related electron withdrawing groups and an aldehyde or ketone. For example, the reaction of malonic acid or malonic acid esters and an aldehyde or ketone to yield an α,β-unsaturated derivative. With malonic acid (Z is carboxyl group), decarboxylation occurs *in situ*. See March, J. *Advanced Organic Chemistry. Reactions, Mechanisms, and Structure*, 3rd edn., John Wiley & Sons, New York, New York, 1985; Klavins, M., Dipane, J., and Babre, K., Humic substances as catalysts in condensation reactions, *Chemosphere* 44, 737–742, 2001; Lai. S.M., Martin-Aranda, R., and Yeung, K.L., Knoevenagel condensation reaction in a membrane bioreactor, *Chem.Commun.* (2), 218–219, 2003; Pivonka, D.E. and Empfield, J.R., Real-time *in situ* Ramen analysis of microwave-assisted organic reactions, *Appl.Spectrosc.* 58, 41–46, 2004; Strohmeier, G.A., Haas, W., and Kappe, C.O., Synthesis of functionalized 1,3-thiazine libraries combining solid-phase synthesis and post-cleavage modification reactions, *Chemistry* 10, 2919–2926, 2004; Wirz, R., Ferri, D. and Baiker, A., ATR-IR spectroscopy of pendant NH$_2$ groups on silica involved in the Knoevenagel condensation, *Langmuir* 22, 3698–3706, 2006.

Leuckart Reaction

Leuckart reaction

The reductive amination of carbonyl groups by ammonium formate or amine salts of formic acid; formamides may also be used in the reaction. See Matsueda, G.R. and Stewart, J.M., A *p*-methylbenzhydrylamine resin for improved solid-phase synthesis of peptide amides, *Peptides* 2, 45–50, 1981; Agwada, V.C. and Awachie, P.I., Intermediates in the Leuckart reaction of benzophenone with formamide, *Tetrahedron Lett.* 23, 779–780, 1982; Loupy, A., Monteux, D., Petit, A., *et al.*, Toward the rehabilitation of the Leuckart reductive amination reaction using microwave technology, *Tetrahedron Lett.* 37, 8177–8180, 1996; Adger, B.M., Dyer, U.C., Lennon, I.C., *et al.*, A novel synthesis of *tert*-leucine via a Leuckart type reaction, *Tetrahedron Lett.* 38, 2153–2154, 1997; Lejon, T. and Helland, I., Effect of formamide in the Leuckart reaction, *Acta Chem.Scand.* 53, 76–78, 1999; Kitamura, M.. Lee, D., Hayashi, S., *et al.*, Catalytic Leuckart-Wallach type reductive amination of ketones, *J.Org.Chem.* 67, 8685–8687, 2002; Swist, M., Wilamowski, J., and Parczewski, A., Basic and neutral route specific impurities in MDMA prepared by different synthesis methods. Comparison of impurity profiles, *Forensic Sci. Int.* 155, 100–111, 2005; Tournier, L. and Zard, S.Z., A practical variation on the Leuckart reaction, *Tetrahedron Lett.* 46, 971–973, 2005.

ORGANIC NAME REACTIONS USEFUL IN BIOCHEMISTRY AND MOLECULAR BIOLOGY (Continued)

Lossen Rearrangement

Active Site Serine

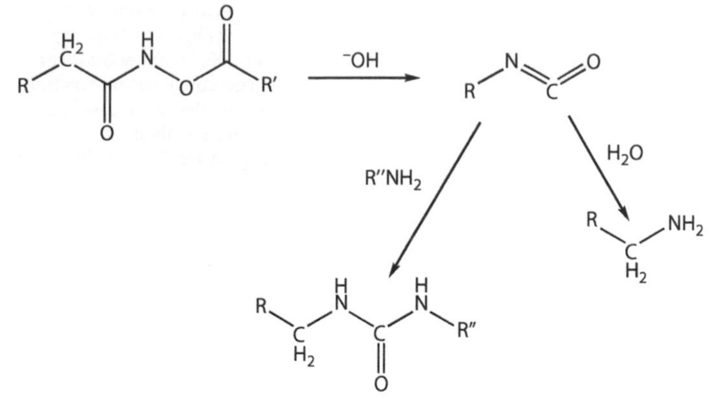

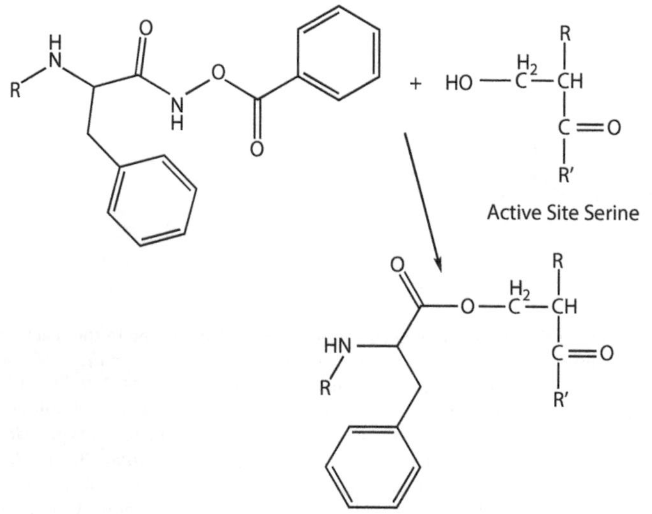

The formation of isocyanates on heating of *O*-acyl derivatives of hydroxamic acids or treatment by base. The isocyanate frequently adds water *in situ* to form an amine one carbon shorter that the parent compound; in the presence of amines, there is the formation of ureas. Andersen, W., The synthesis of phenylcarbamoyl derivatives by Lossen rearrangement of dibenzohydroxamic acid, *C.R.Trav.Lab.Carlsberg.* 30, 79–103, 1956; Gallop, P.M., Seifter, S., Lukin, M., and Meilman, E. Application of the Lossen rearrangement of dintirophenylhydroxamates to analysis of of carboxyl groups in model compounds and gelatin, *J.Biol.Chem.* 235, 2619–2627, 1960; Hoare, D.G., Olson, A., and Koshland, D.E., Jr., The reaction of hydroxamic acids with water-soluble carbodiimides. A Lossen rearrangement, *J.Am.Chem.Soc.* 90, 1638–1643, 1968; Dell, D., Boreham, D.R., and Martin, B.K., Estimation of 4-butoyphenylacetohydroxamic acid utilizing the Lossen rearrangement, *J.Pharm.Sci.* 60, 1368–1370, 1971; Harris, R.B. and Wilson, I.B., Glutamic acid is an active site residue of angiotensin I-converting enzyme. Use of the Lossen rearrangement for identification of dicarboxylic acid residues, *J.Biol.Chem.* 258, 1357–1362, 1983; Libert, R., Draye, J.P., Van Hoof, F., *et al.*, Study of reactions induced by hydroxylamine treatment of esters for organic acids and of 3-ketoacids: application to the study of urines from patients under valproate therapy, *Biol.Mass.Spectrom.* 20, 75–86, 1991; Neumann, U. and Gutschow, M., *N*-(sulfonyloxy)phthalimides and analogues are potent inactivators of serine proteases, *J.Biol.Chem.* 269, 21561–21567, 1994; Steinmetz, A.C., Demuth, H.U., and Ringe, D., Inactivation of subtilisin Carlsberg by *N*-[(*t*-butoxycarbonyl) alanylprolyl-phenylalanyl]-*O*-benzoylhydroxyl-amine: formation of a covalent enzyme-inhibitor linkage in the form of a carbamate derivative, *Biochemistry* 33, 10535–10544, 1994; Needs, P.W., Rigby, N.M., Ring, S.G., and MacDougall, A.J., Specific degradation of pectins via a carbodiimide-mediated Lossen rearrangement of methyl esterified galacturonic acid residues, *Carbohydr.Res.* 333, 47–58, 2001.

ORGANIC NAME REACTIONS USEFUL IN BIOCHEMISTRY AND MOLECULAR BIOLOGY (Continued)

Maillard Reaction

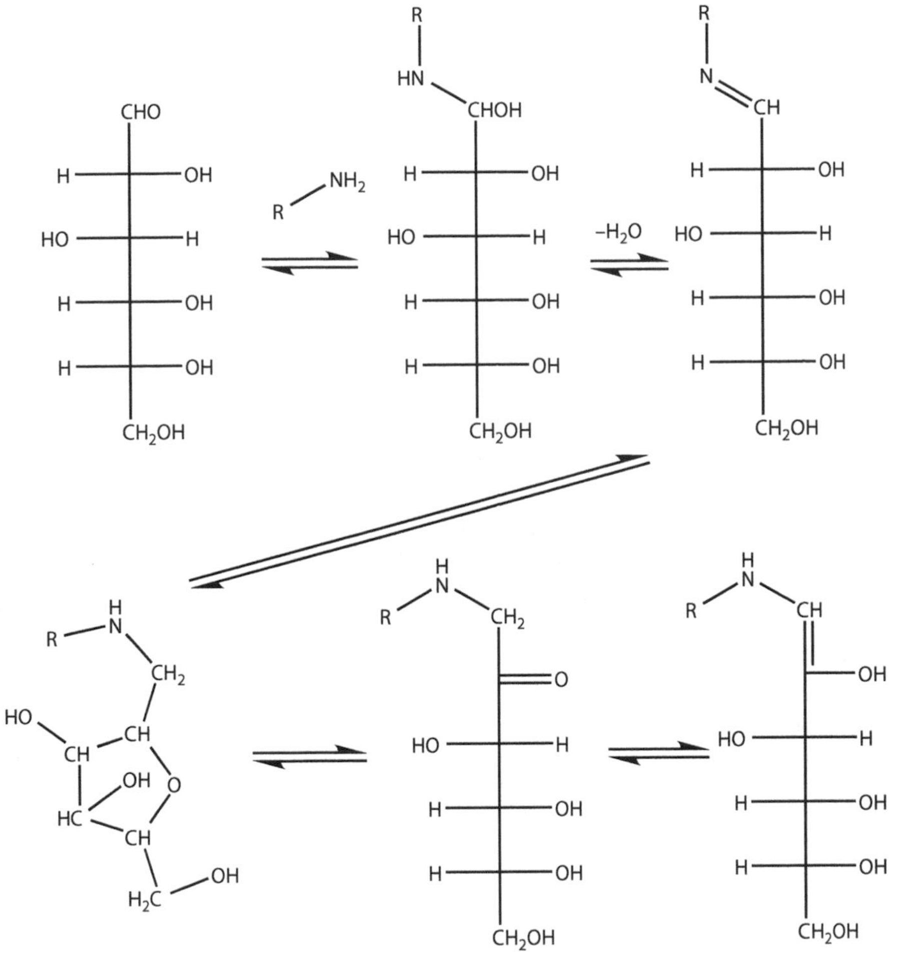

N-substituted glycosamine

Amadori product
N-substituted 1-amino-2-deoxy-2-ketose

The reaction of amino groups with carbonyl groups resulting in the formation of complex products. This process is involved in the tanning of leather and the Browning reaction which is considered unique to the reaction of carbohydrates with proteins and is a critical aspect of food preparation. The Maillard reaction involves the nonenzymatic reaction of sugars with proteins and the formation of advanced glycation end products (AGE products). The Maillard reaction results in the formation of a number of reaction products. See Dills, W.J., Jr., Protein fructosylation: fructose and the Maillard reaction, *Am.J.Clin. Nutr.* 58(Suppl 5), 779S-787S, 1993; Chuyen, N.V., Maillard reaction and food processing. Application aspects, *Adv.Exp.Med.Biol.* 434, 213–235, 1998; van Boekel, M.A., Kinetic aspects of the Maillard reaction: a critical review, *Nahrung* 45, 150–159, 2001; Horvat, S. and Jakas, A., Peptide and amino acid glycation: new insights into the Maillard reaction, *J.Pept.Sci.* 10, 119–137, 2004; Fay, L.B. and Brevard, H., Contribution of mass spectrometry to the study of the Maillard reaction in food, *Mass Spectrom.Rev.* 24, 487–507, 2005; Yaylayan, V.A., Haffenden, L., Chu, F.L., and Wnorowski, A., Oxidative pyrolysis and post pyrolytic derivatization techniques for the total analysis of Maillard model systems: investigations of control parameters of Maillard reaction pathways, *Ann.N.Y.Acad.Sci.* 1043, 41–54, 2005; Monnier, V.M., Mustata, G.T., Biemel, K.L., *et al.*, Cross-linked of the extracellular matrix by the Maillard reaction in aging and diabetes: an update on "a puzzle nearing resolution", *Ann.N.Y.Acad.Sci.* 1043, 533–544, 2005; Matiacevich, S.B., Santagapita, P.R., and Buera, M.P., Fluorescence from the Maillard reaction and its potential applications in food science, *Crit.Rev.Food Sci.Nutr.* 45, 483–495, 2005; van Boekel, M.A., Formation of flavour compounds in the Maillard reaction, *Biotechnol.Adv.* 24, 230–233, 2006.

ORGANIC NAME REACTIONS USEFUL IN BIOCHEMISTRY AND MOLECULAR BIOLOGY (Continued)

Malaprade Reaction

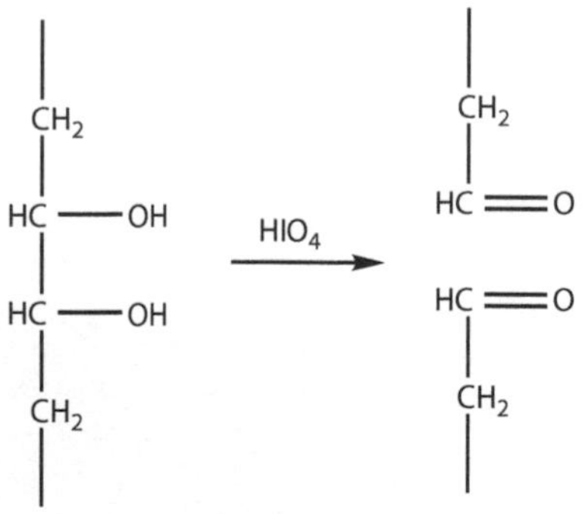

Malaprade reaction

Periodic cleavage of a diol; although this term is seldom used for this extremely common reaction, it would appear to be the correct terminology. Periodic acid is used for the diol cleavage in aqueous solvent while lead tetraacetate can be used in organic solvents. The reaction also occur an amine group vicinal to a hydroxyl function. It would appear that the term Malaprade reaction has been used more in description of analytical techniques for organic diols such as gluconic acid or in the assay of periodate. See Belcher, R., Dryhurst, G., and MacDonal, A.M., Submicro-methods for analysis of organic compounds. 22. Malaprade reaction, *Journal of the Chemical Society*,(July) 3964, 1965; Chen, K,P., Determination of calcium gluconate by selective oxidation with periodate, *J.Pharm.Sci.* 73, 681–683, 1984; Verma, K.K., Gupta, D., Sanghi, S.K., and Jain, A., Spectrophotometric determination of periodate with amodiaquine dihydrochloride and its application to the indirect determination of some organic-compounds via the Malaprade reaction, *Analyst* 112, 1519–1522, 1987; Nevado, J.J.B. and Gonzalez, P.V., Spectrophotometric determination of periodate with salicylaldehyde guanylhydrazone – indirect determination of some organic compounds using the Malaprade reaction, *Analyst* 114, 243–244, 1989; Jie, N,Q., Yang, D.L., Zhang, Q.N., *et al.*, Fluorometric determination of periodate with thiamine and its application to the determination of ethylene glycol and glycerol, *Anal.Chim.Acta* 359, 87–92, 1998; Guillan-Sans, R. and Guzman-Chozas, M., The thiobarbituric acid (TBA) reaction in foods, A review, *Crit.Rev.Food Sci.Nutrition* 38, 315–330, 1998; Pumera, M., Jelinek, I., Jindrich, J., *et al.*, Determination of cyclodextrin content using periodate oxidation by capillary electrophoresis, *J.Chromatog. A* 891, 201–206, 2000; Afkhami, A. and Mosaed, F., Kinetic determination of periodate based on its reaction with ferroin and its application to the indirect determination of ethylene glycol and glycerol, *Microchemical J.* 68, 35–40, 2001; Afkhami, A. and Mosaed, F., Sensitive kinetic-spectrophotometric determination of trace amounts of periodate ion, *J.Anal.Chem.* 58, 588–593, 2003; Mihovilovic, M.D., Spina, M., Muller, B., and Stanetty, P., Synthesis of carbo- and heterocyclic aldehydes bearing an adjacent donor group – Ozonolysis versus OsO$_4$/KIO$_4$-oxidation, *Monatshefte für Chemie* 135, 899–909, 2004.

Malonic Ester Synthesis

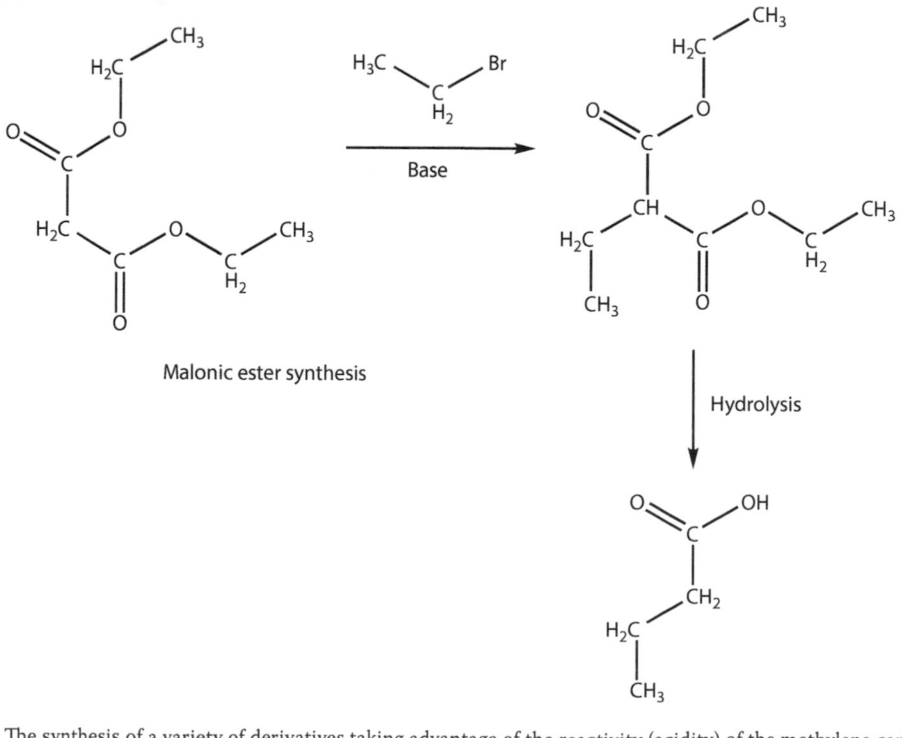

Malonic ester synthesis

The synthesis of a variety of derivatives taking advantage of the reactivity (acidity) of the methylene carbon in malonic esters. The malonic ester synthesis is related to the acetoacetic ester synthesis and the Knoevenagel synthesis. See Mizuno, Y., Adachi, K., and Ikeda, K., Studies on condensed systems of aromatic nitrogenous series. XIII. Extension of malonic ester synthesis to the heterocyclic series, *Pharm.Bull.* 2, 225–234, 1954; Beres, J.A., Varner, M.G., and Bria, C., Synthesis and cyclization of dialkylmalonuric esters, *J.Pharm.Sci.* 69, 451–454, 1980; Kinder, D.H., Frank, S.K., and Ames, M.M. Analogues of carbamyl asparate as inhibitors of dihydroorotase: preparation of boronic acid transition-state analogues and a zinc chelator

ORGANIC NAME REACTIONS USEFUL IN BIOCHEMISTRY AND MOLECULAR BIOLOGY (Continued)

carbamylhomocysteine, *J.Med.Chem.* 33, 819–823, 1990; Groth, T. and Meldal, M., Synthesis of aldehyde building blocks protected as acid labile *N*-boc-*N,O*-acetals: toward combinatorial solid phase synthesis of novel peptide isosteres, *J.Comb.Chem.* 3, 34–44, 2001; Hachiya, I., Ogura, K., and Shimizu, M., Novel 2-pyridine synthesis via nucleophilic addition of malonic esters to alkynyl imines, *Org.Lett.* 4, 2755–2757, 2002; Strohmeier, G.A., Haas, W., and Kappe, C.O., Synthesis of functionalized 1,3-thiazine libraries combining solid-phase synthesis and post-cleavage modification methods, *Chemistry* 10, 2919–2926, 2004.

Mannich Reaction

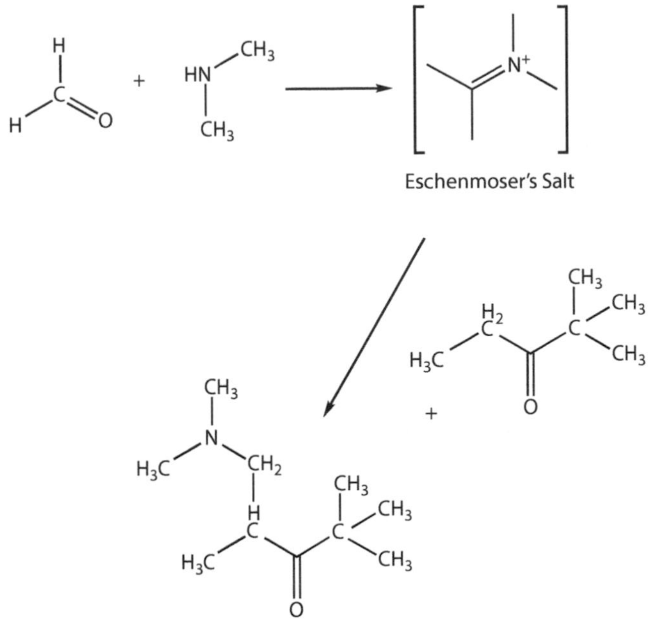

Eschenmoser's Salt

Condensation of an amine with an carbonyl compound which can exist in an enol form, and a carbonyl compound which can not exist as an enol. The reaction frequently use formaldehyde as the carbonyl compound not existing as an enol for condensing with a secondary amine in the first phase of the reaction. See Britton, S.B., Caldwell, H.C., and Nobles, W.L., The use of 2-pipecoline in the Mannich reaction, *J.Am.Pharm.Assoc.Am.Pharm.Assoc.* 43, 641–643, 1954; Nobles, W.L., and Thompson, B.B., Application of the Mannich reaction to sulfones. I. Reactive methylene moiety of sulfones, *J.Pharm.Sci.* 54, 576–580, 1965; Thompson, B.B., The Mannich reaction. Mechanistic and technological considrations, *J.Pharm.Sci.* 57, 715–733, 1968; Nobles, W.L. and Potti, N.D., Studies on the mechanism of the Mannich reaction, *J.Pharm.Sci.* 57, 1097–1103, 1968; Delia, T.J., Scovill, J.P., Munslow, W.D., and Burckhalter, J.H., Synthesis of 5-substituted aminomethyluracils via the Mannich reaction, *J.Med.Chem.* 19, 344–346, 1976; List, B., Pojarliev, P., Biller, W.T., and Martin, H.J., The proline-catalyzed direct asymmetric three-component Mannich reaction: scope, optimization, and application to the highly enantioselective synthesis of 1,2-amino alcohols, *J.Am.Chem.Soc.* 124, 827–833, 2002; Palomo, C., Oiarbide, M., Landa, A., *et al.*, Design and synthesis of a novel class of sugar-peptide hybrids: *C*-linked glyco β-amino acids through a stereoselective "acetate" Mannich reaction as the key strategic element, *J.Am.Chem.Soc.* 124, 8637–8643, 2002; Cordova, A., The direct catalytic asymmetric Mannich reaction, *Acc.Chem.Res.* 37, 102–112, 2004; Azizi, N., Torkiyan, L., and Saidi, M.R., Highly efficient one-pot three-component Mannich reaction in water catalyzed by heteropoly acids, *Org.Lett.* 8, 2079–2082, 2006; Matsuo, J., Tanaki, Y., and Ishibashi, H., Oxidative Mannich reaction of *N*-carbobenzoxy amines 1,3-dicarbonyl compounds, *Org.Lett.* 8, 4371–4374, 2006. Another important example of the Michael addition in biochemistry and molecular biology is the reaction of 4-hydroxynon-2-enal with amines and sulfydryl groups (Winter, C.K., Segall, H.J., and Haddon, W.F., Formation of cyclic adducts of deoxyguanosine with the aldehyde *trans*-4-hydroxy-2-hexenal and *trans*-4-hydroxy-2-nonenal *in vitro*, *Cancer Res.* 46, 5682–5686, 1986; Sayre, L.M., Arora, P.K., Iyer, R.S., and Salomon, R.G., Pyrrole formation from 4-hydroxyonenal and primary amines, *Chem.Res.Toxicol.* 6, 19–22, 1993; Hartley, D.P., Ruth, J.A., and Petersen, D.R., The hepatocellular metabolism of 4-hydroxynonenal by alcohol dehydrogenase, aldehyde dehydrogenase, and glutathione-*S*-transferase, *Arch.Biochem. Biophys.* 316, 197–205, 1995: Engle, M.R., Singh, S.P., Czernik, P.J., *et al.*, Physiological role of mGSTA4–4, a glutathione *S*-transferase metabolizing 4-hydroxynonenal: generation and analysis of mGst4 null mouse, *Toxicol.Appl.Pharmacol.* 194, 296–308, 2004).

Meerwein Reaction

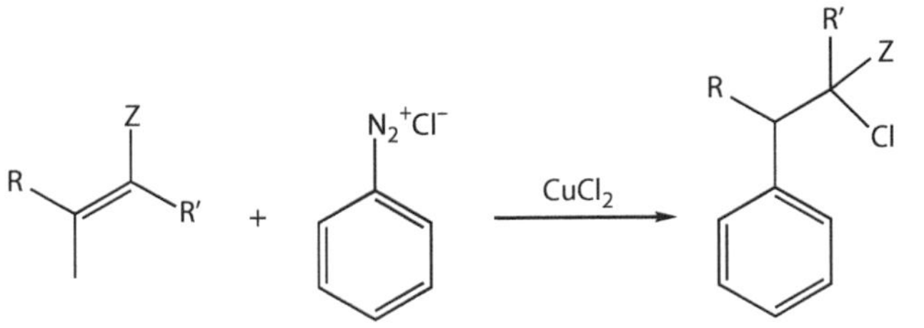

ORGANIC NAME REACTIONS USEFUL IN BIOCHEMISTRY AND MOLECULAR BIOLOGY (Continued)

The reaction of an aryl diazonium halide with an aliphatic unsaturated compound to yield an α-halo-β-phenyl alkene and alkanes. The reaction is performed in the presence of cupric ions. The presence of an electron-withdrawing group is useful in promoting the reactivity of the alkene. See Kochi, J.K., The Meerwein reaction. Catalysis by cuprous chloride, *J.Am.Chem.Soc.* 77, 5090, 1955; Moraes, L.A. and Eberlin, M.N., The gas-phase Meerwein reaction, *Chemistry* 6, 897–905, 2000; Riter, L.S., Meurer, E.C., Handberg, E.S., *et al.*, Ion/molecule reactions peformed in a miniature cylindrical ion trap mass spectrometer, *Analyst* 128, 1112–1118, 2003; Meurer, E.C., Chen, H., Riter, L.S., *et al.*, Meerwein reaction of phosphonium ions with epoxides and thioepoxides in the gas phase, *J.Am.Soc.Mass Spectrom.* 15, 398–405, 2004; Meurer, E.C. and Eberlin, M.N., The atmospheric pressure Meerwein reaction, *J.Mass Spectrom.* 41, 470–476, 2006.

Michael Addition (Michael Condensation)

Michael addition/Michael condensation

Reaction of cysteine with *N*-ethylmaleimide as a Michael addition reaction

4-HNE

Formally a 1, 4 addition/conjugate addition of a resonance-stabilized carbanion (the reaction of an active methylene compound such as a malonate and an α,β-unsaturated carbonyl compound or the reaction of a nucleophile with an "activated unsaturated system; a carbanion defined as an anion with an even number of electrons). The addition of a nucleophile to a conjugated double bond. See Flavin, M. and Slaughter, C., Enzymatic elimination from a substituted four-carbon amino acid coupled to Michael addition of a β-carbon to an electrophilic double bond. Structure of the reaction product, *Biochemistry* 5, 1340–1350, 1966; Fitt, J.J. and Gschwend, H.W., α-Alkylation and Michael addition of amino acid—a practical method, *J.Org.Chem.* 42, 2639–2641, 1977; Powell, G.K., Winter, H.C., and Dekker, E.E., Michael addition of thiols with 4-methyleneglutamic acid: preparation of adducts, their properties and presence in peanuts, *Biochem.Biophys.Res.Commun.* 105, 1361–1367, 1982; Wang, M., Nishikawa, A. and Chung, F.L., Differential effects of thiols on DNA modifications via alkylation and Michael addition by α-acetoxy-*N*-nitrosopyrrolidine, *Chem.Res.Toxicol.* 5, 528–531, 1992; Jang, D.P., Chang, C.W., and Uang, B.J., Highly diastereoselective Michael addition of α-hydroxy acid derivatives and enantioselective synthesis of (+)-crobarbatic acid, *Org.Lett.* 3, 983–985, 2001.

ORGANIC NAME REACTIONS USEFUL IN BIOCHEMISTRY AND MOLECULAR BIOLOGY (Continued)

Naidu, B.N., Sorenson, M.E., Connolly, T.P., and Ueda, Y., Michael addition of amines and thiols to dehydroalanine amides: a remarkable rate acceleration in water, *J.Org.Chem.* 68, 10098–10102, 2003; Ooi, T., Doda, K., and Maruoka, K., Highly enantioselective Michael addition of silyl nitronates to α,β-unsaturated aldehydes catalyzed by designer chiral ammonium bifluorides: efficient access to optically active γ-nitro aldehydes and their enol silyl ethers, *J.Am.Chem.Soc.* 125, 9022–9023, 2003; Weinstein, R., Lerner, R.A., Barbas, C.F., 3rd, and Shabat, D., Antibody-catalyzed asymmetric intramolecular Michael additional of aldehydes and ketones to yield the disfavored *cis*-product, *J.Am.Chem.Soc.* 127, 13104–13105, 2005; Ding, R., Katebzadeh, K., Roman, L., *et al.*, Expanding the scope of Lewis acid catalysis in water: remarkable ligand acceleration of aqueous ytteribium triflate catalyzed Michael addition reactions, *J.Org.Chem.* 71, 352–355, 2006; Pansare, S.V. and Pandya, K., Simple diamine- and triamine-protonic acid catalysts for the enantioselective Michael addition of cyclic ketones to nitroalkenes, *J.Am.Chem.Soc.* 128, 9624–9625, 2006; Dai, H.X., Yao, S.P., and Wang, J., Michael addition of pyrimidine with disaccharide acrylates catalyzed in organic medium with lipase M from *Mucor javanicus, Biotechnol.Lett.* 28, 1503–1507, 2006. One the best examples in biochemistry is the modification of cysteine residues with *N*-alkylmaleimide derivatives (Lundblad, R.L., *Chemical Reagents for Protein Modification*, 3rd edn., CRC Press, Boca Raton, FL, 2004; Heitz, J.R., Anderson, C.D., and Anderson, B.M., Inactivation of yeast alcohol dehydrogenase by *N*-alkylmaleimides, *Arch.Biochem.Biophys.* 127, 627–636, 1968; Smyth, D.B. and Tuppy, H., Acylation reactions with cyclic imides, *Biochim.Biophys.Acta* 168, 173–180, 1968; Lusty, C.J. and Fasold, H., Characterization of sulfhydryl groups of actin, *Biochemistry* 8, 2933–2939, 1969; Bowes, T.J. and Gupta, R.S., Induction of mitochondrial fusion of cysteine-alklyators ethacrynic acid and *N*-ethylmaleimide, *J.Cell Physiol.* 202, 796–804, 2005).

Reformatsky Reaction

Reformatsky reaction

Formation of a complex between zinc and an α-bromoester followed by condensation with an aldehyde yielding a β-hydroxyester; an α,β-unsaturated ester via dehydration following the condensation reaction. See Tanabe, K., Studies on vitamin A and its related compounds. II. Reformatsky reaction of β-cyclocitral with methyl γ-bromosenecioate, *Pharm.Bull.* 3, 25–31, 1955; Ross, N.A. and Bartsch, R.A., High-intensity ultrasound-promoted Reformatsky reactions, *J.Org.Chem.* 68, 360–366, 2003; Jung, J.C., Lee, J.H., Oh., S., Synthesis and antitumor activity of 4-hydroxycoumarin derivatives, *Bioorg.Med. Chem.Lett.* 14, 5527–5531,2004; Kloetzing, R.J., Thaler, T., and Knochel, P., An improved asymmetric Reformatsky reaction mediated by (-)-*N,N*-dimethylaminoisoborneol, *Org.Lett.* 8, 1125–1128, 2006; Moume, R. Laavielle. S., and Karoyan, P., Efficient synthesis of β₂-amino acid by homologation of α-amino acids involving the Reformatsky reaction and Mannich-type imminium electrophile, *J.Org.Chem.* 71, 3332–3334, 2006.

ORGANIC NAME REACTIONS USEFUL IN BIOCHEMISTRY AND MOLECULAR BIOLOGY (Continued)

Rittter Reaction

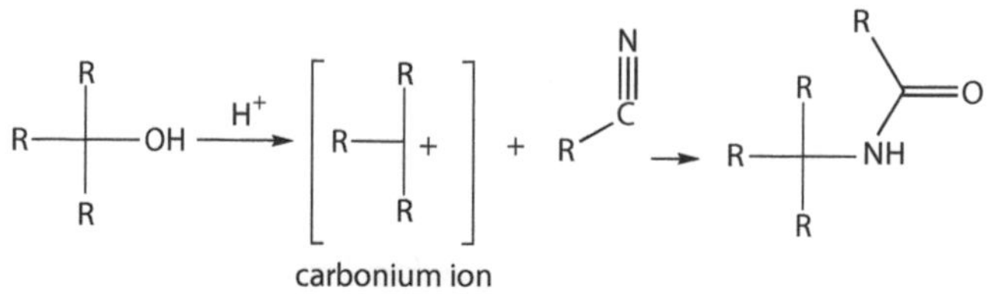

carbonium ion

Acid-catalyzed nucleophilic addition of a nitrile to a carbenium ion generated from alcohol (usually tertiary, primary alcohols other than benzyl alcohol will not react) yielding an amide. Sanguigni, J.A. and Levine, R., Amides from nitriles and alcohols by the Ritter reaction, *J.Med.Chem.* 53, 573–574, 1964; Radzicka, A. and Konieczny, M., Studies on the Ritter reaction. I. Synthesis of 3-/5-bartbituryl/-1propanesulfonic acids with anti-inflammatory activity, *Arch.Immunol.Ther.Exp.* 30, 421–432, 1982; Van Emelen, K., De Wit, T., Hoornaert, G.J., and Compernolle, F., Diastereoselective intramolecular Ritter reaction: generation of a *cis*-fused hexahydro-4a*H*-indeno[1,2-*b*] pyridine ring system with 4a,9b-diangular substituents, *Org.Lett.* 2, 3083–3086, 2000; Concellon, J.M., Reigo, E., Suarez, J.R., *et al.*, Synthesis of enantiopure imidazolines through a Ritter reaction of 2-(1-aminoalkyl)azirdines with nitriles, *Org.Lett.* 6, 4499–4501, 2004; Feske, B.D., Kaluzna, I.A., and Stewart, J.D., Enantiodivergent, biocatalytic routes to both taxol side chain antipodes, *J.Org. Chem.* 70, 9654–9657, 2005; Crich, D. and Patel, M., On the nitrile effect in L-rhamnopyranosylation, *Carbohydr.Res.* 341, 1467–1475, 2006; Fu, Q. and Li, L., Neutral loss of water from the b ions with histidine at the *C*-terminus and formation of the c ions involving lysine side chains, *J.Mass.Spectrom.* 41, 1600–1607, 2006.

Schiff Base

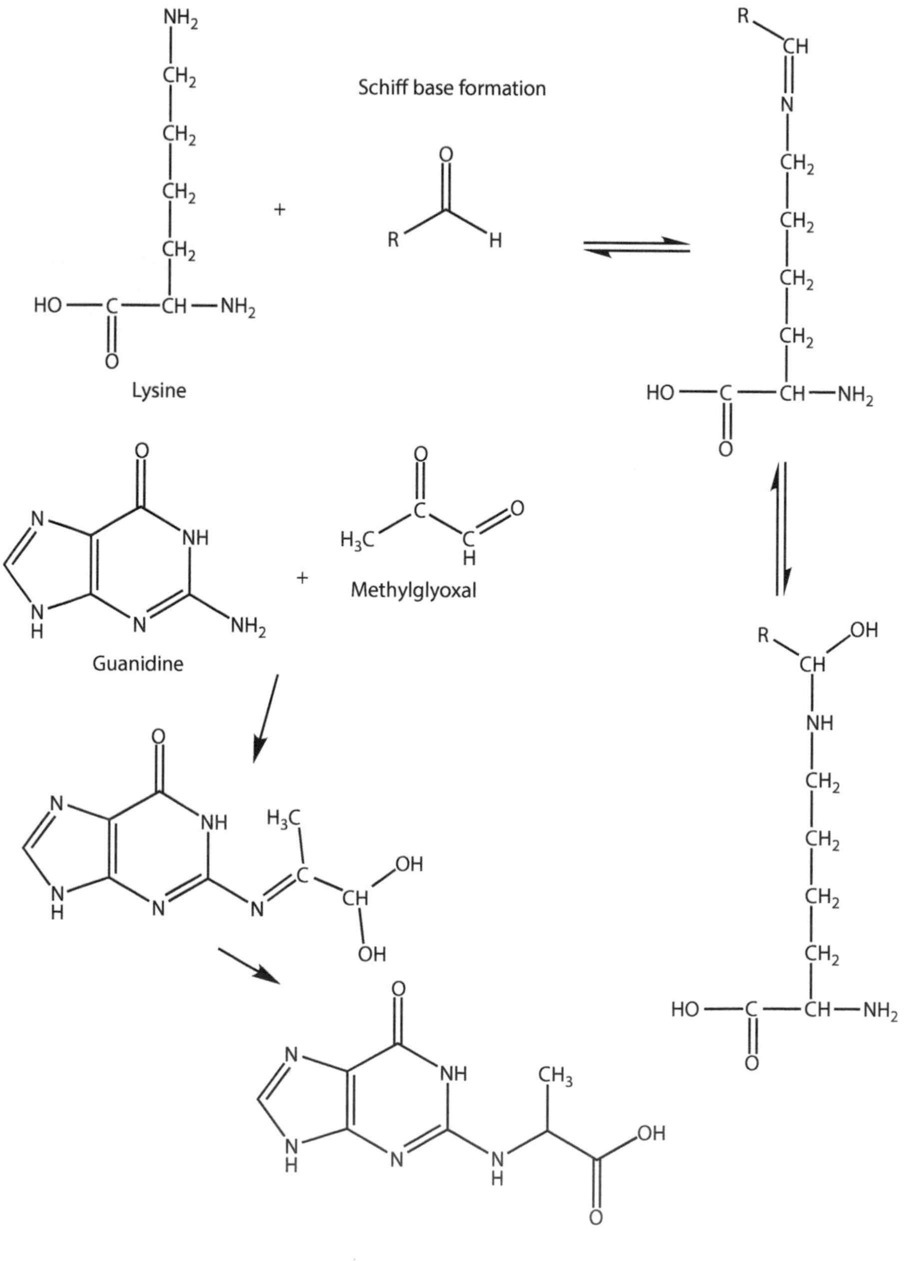

Schiff base formation

Lysine

Guanidine

Methylglyoxal

ORGANIC NAME REACTIONS USEFUL IN BIOCHEMISTRY AND MOLECULAR BIOLOGY (Continued)

The formation of an unstable derivative generally between an carbonyl(usually an aldehyde) and an amino group. The Schiff base can be converted to a stable derivative by reduction with sodium borohydride or sodium cyanoborohydride; Schiff bases appear to be resistant to reduction with sulfhydryl-base reducing agents such as 2-mercaptoethanol or dithiothreitol and phosphines. Schiff bases are involved in a diverse group of biochemical events including the interaction of pyridoxal phosphate with proteins, the interaction of reducing carbohydrates with proteins in reaction leading to AGE products, and reductive alkylation of amino groups in proteins. See Feeney, R.E., Blankenhorn, G., and Dixon, H.B., Carbonyl-amine reactions in protein chemistry, *Adv.Protein.Chem.* 29, 135–203, 1975; Metzler, D.E. Tautomerism in pyridoxal phosphate and in enzymatic catalysis, *Adv.Enzymol. Relat.Areas Mol.Biol.* 50, 1–40, 1979; Puchtler, H. and Meloan, S.N., ON Schiff's bases and aldehyde-fuchsin: a review from H.Schiff to R.D. Lillie, *Histochemistry* 72, 321–332, 1981; O'Donnell, J.P., The reaction of amines with carbonyls: its significance in the nonezymatic metabolism of xenobiotics, *Drug.Metab.Rev.* 13, 123–159, 1982; Stadtman, E.R., Covalent modification reactions are marking steps in protein turnover, *Biochemistry* 29, 6232–6331, 1990; Tuma, D.J., Hoffman, T. and Sorrell, M.F., The chemistry of aldehyde-protein adducts, *Alcohol Alcohol Suppl.* 1, 271–276, 1991; Hargrave, P.A., Hamm, H.E., and Hofmann, K.P., Interaction of rhodopsin with the G-protein, transducin, *Bioessays* 15, 43–50, 1993; Chen, H. and Rhodes, J., Schiff base forming drugs: mechanisms of immune potentiation and therapeutic potential, *J.Mol.Med.* 74, 497–504, 1996; Yim, M.B., Yim, H.S., Lee, C., *et al.*, Protein glycation: creation of catalytic sites for free radication generation, *Ann.N.Y.Acad.Sci.* 928, 48–53, 2001; Gramatikova, S., Mouratou, B., Stetefeld, J. *et al.*, Pyridoxal-5'-phosphate-dependent catatlytic antibodies, *J.Immunol.Methods* 269, 99–110, 2002; Schaur, R.J., Basic aspects of the biochemical reactivity of 4-hydroxynonenal, *Mol.Aspects Med.* 24, 149–159, 2003; Kurtz, A.J. and Lloyd, R.S., 1, N^2-deoxyguanosine adducts of acrolein, crotonaldehyde, and *trans*-4-hydroxynonenal cross-link to peptides via Schiff base linkage, *J.Biol.Chem.* 278, 5970–5975, 2003; Kandori, H., Hydration switch model for the proton transfer in the Schiff base region of bacteriorhodopsin, *Biochim.Biophys.Acta* 1658, 72–79, 2004; Hadjoudis, E. and Mavridis, I.M., Photochomism and thermochromism of Schiff bases in the solid state: structural aspects, *Chem. Soc.Rev.* 33, 579–588, 2004; Stadler, R.H., Acrylamide formation in different foods and potential strategies for reduction, *Adv.Expt.Med.Biol.* 561, 157–169, 2005. There is some interesting chemistry on Schiff bases in inorganic chemistry (Nakoji, M., Kanayama, T., Okino, T., and Takemoto, Y., Chiral phosphine-free Pd-mediated asymmetric allylation of prochiral enolate with a chiral phase-transfer catalyst, *Org.Lett.* 2, 3329–3331, 2001; Walther, D., Fugger, C. Schreer, H., *et al.*, Reversible fixation of carbon dioxide at nickel(0) centers: a route for large organometallic rings, dimers, and tetramers, *Chemistry* 7, 5214–5221, 2001; Benny, P.D., Green, J.L., Engelbrecht, H.P., Reactivity and rhenium(V) oxo Schiff base complexes with phosphine ligands: rearrangement and reduction reactions, *Inorg.Chem.* 44, 2381–2390, 2005).

ORGANIC NAME REACTIONS USEFUL IN BIOCHEMISTRY AND MOLECULAR BIOLOGY (Continued)

Schmidt Reaction/Schmidt Rearrangement

Used to describe the reaction of carboxylic acids, aldehyde and ketones(carbonyl compounds), and alcohols/alkenes with hydrazoic acid. Reaction with carboxylic acids yields amines, carbonyl compounds yield amides in a reaction involving a rearrangement, and alcohols/azides yield alkyl azides. See Rabinowitz, J.L., Chase, G.D., and Kaliner, L.F., Isotope effects of in the decarboxylation of 1–1⁴C-dicarboxylic acids studied by means of the Schmidt reaction, *Anal.Biochem.* 19, 578–583, 1967; Iyengar, R., Schildknegt, K., and Aube, J., Regiocontrol in an intramolecular Schmidt reaction: total synthesis of (+)-aspidospermidine, *Org.Lett.* 2, 1625–1627, 2000; Sahasrabudhe, K., Gracias, V., Furness, K., *et al.*, Asymmetric Schmidt reaction of hydroxyalkyl azides with ketones, *J.Am.Chem.Soc.* 125, 7914–7922, 2003; Wang, W., Mei, Y., Li, H., and Wang, J., A novel pyrrolidine imide catalyzed direct formation of α,β-unsaturated ketones from unmodified ketones and aldehydes, *Org.Lett.* 7, 601–604, 2005; Brase, S., Gil., C., Knepper, K., and Zimmerman, V., Organic azides: an exploding diversity of a unique class of compounds, *Angew.Chem.Int.Ed.Engl.* 44, 5188–5240, 2005; Lang, S. and Murphy, J.A., Azide rearrangements in electron-deficient systems, *Chem.Soc.Rev.* 35, 146–156, 2006; Zarghi, A., Zebardast, T., Hakimion, F., *et al.*, Synthesis and biological evaluation of 1,3-diphenylprop-2-en-1-ones possessing a methanesulfonamido or an azido pharmacophore as cyclooxygenase-1/-2 inhibitors, *Bioorg.Med. Chem.* 14, 7044–7050, 2006.

Ugi Condensation

A four component (aldehyde, amine, isocyanide and a carboxyl group) condensation resulting in an α-aminoacyl amide. See Liu, X.C., Clark, D.S., and Dordick, J.S., Chemoenzymatic construction of a four-component Ugi combinatorial library, *Biotechnol.Bioeng.* 69, 457–460, 2000; Bayer, T., Riemer, C., and Kessler, H., A new strategy for the synthesis of cyclopeptides containing diaminoglutaric acid, *J.Pept.Sci.* 7, 250–261, 2001; Crescenzi, V., Francescangeli, A., Renier, D., and Bellini, D., New cross-linked and sulfated derivatives of partially deacylated hyaluronan: synthesis and preliminary characterization, *Biopolymers* 64, 86–94, 2002; Liu, L., Ping Li, C., Cochran, S., and Ferro, V., Application of the four-component Ugi condensation for the preparation of glycoconjugate libraries, *Bioorg.Med.Chem.Lett.* 14, 2221–2226, 2004; Bu, H., Kjoniksen, A.L., Knudsen, K.D., and Nystrom, B., Rheological and structural properties of aqueous alginate during gelation via the Ugi multicomponent condensation reaction, *Biomacromolecules* 5, 1470–1479, 2004; Tempest, P.A., Recent advances in heterocycle generation using the efficient Ugi multiple-component condensation reaction, *Curr.Opin.Drug Discov.Devel.* 8, 776–788, 2005.

ORGANIC NAME REACTIONS USEFUL IN BIOCHEMISTRY AND MOLECULAR BIOLOGY (Continued)

Wittig Olefination

Wittig reaction/Wittig olefination   Ylide

Synthesis of an alkene from the reaction of an aldehyde or ketone with an ylide (internal salt) generated from a phosphophonium salt. See Jorgensen, M., Iversen, E.H., and Madsen, R., A convenient route to higher sugars by two-carbon chain elongation using Wittig/dihydroxylation reactions, *J.Org.Chem.* 66, 4625–4629, 2001; Magrioti, V., and Constantinou-Kokotou, V., Synthesis of (S)-α-amino oleic acid, *Lipids* 37, 223–228, 2002; van Staden, L.F., Gravestock, D., and Ager, D.J., New developments in the Peterson olefination reaction, *Chem.Soc.Rev.* 31, 195–200, 2002; Han, H., Sinha, M.K., D'Sousa, L.J., *et al.*, Total synthesis of 34-hydroxyasimicin and its photoactive derivative for affinity labeling of the mitochondrial complex I, *Chemistry* 10, 2149–2158, 2004; Rhee, J.U. and Krische, M.J., Alkynes as synthetic equivalents to stabilized Wittig reagents: intra- and intermolecular carbonyl olefinations catalyzed by Ag(1), BF₃, and HBF₄, *Org.Lett.* 7, 2493–2495, 2005; Ermolenko, L. and Sasaki, N.A., Diastereoselective synthesis of all either *l*-hexoses from L-ascorbic acid, *J.Org.Chem.* 71, 693–703, 2006; Halim, R., Brimble, M.A., and Merten, J., Synthesis of the ABC tricyclic fragment of the pectenotoxins via stereocontrolled cyclization of a γ-hydroxyepoxide appended to the AB spiroacetal unit, *Org.Biomol.Chem.* 4, 1387–1399, 2006; Phillips, D.J., Pillinger, K.S., Li, W., *et al.*, Desymmerization of diols by a tandem oxidation/Wittig olefination reaction, *Chem.Commun.* (21), 2280–2282, 2006; Modica, E., Compostella, F. Colombo, D., *et al.*, Stereoselective synthesis and immunogenic activity of the *C*-analogue of sulfatide, *Org.Lett.* 8, 3255–3258, 2006.

BRIEF GUIDE TO THE NOMENCLATURE OF INORGANIC CHEMISTRY

IUPAC Technical Report

Richard M. Hartshorn*, Karl-Heinz Hellwich, Andrey Yerin, Ture Damhus, and Alan T. Hutton

Abstract: This IUPAC Technical Report (PAC-REP-14-07-18) is one of a series that seeks to distil the essentials of IUPAC nomenclature recommendations. The present report provides a succinct summary of the material presented in the publication *Nomenclature of Inorganic Chemistry—IUPAC Recommendations 2005*. The content of this report will be republished and disseminated as a four-sided lift-out document (see supplementary information) which will be available for inclusion in textbooks and similar publications.

Keywords: coordination chemistry; inorganic chemistry; nomenclature; organometallic chemistry.

DOI 10.1515/pac-2014-0718
Received July 24, 2014; accepted February 9, 2015

Article note: Sponsoring body: IUPAC Division of Chemical Nomenclature and Structure Representation.

Karl-Heinz Hellwich: Postfach 10 07 31, 63007 Offenbach, Germany

Andrey Yerin: Advanced Chemistry Development, Ul. Akademika Bakuleva, 6, Str. 1, RF-117513 Moscow, Russia

Ture Damhus: Novozymes A/S, Brudelysvej 32, 6BD1, DK-2880 Bagsvaerd, Denmark

Alan T. Hutton: Department of Chemistry, University of Cape Town, Rondebosch 7701, South Africa

Contents

Preamble

The universal adoption of an agreed chemical nomenclature is a key tool for communication in the chemical sciences, for computer-based searching in databases, and for regulatory purposes, such as those associated with health and safety or commercial activity. The International Union of Pure and Applied Chemistry (IUPAC) provides recommendations on the nature and use of chemical nomenclature [1]. The basics of this nomenclature are shown here, and in companion documents on the nomenclature systems for organic chemistry [2] and polymers [3], with hyperlinks to the original documents. An overall summary of chemical nomenclature can be found in *Principles of Chemical Nomenclature* [4]. Greater detail can be found in the *Nomenclature of Inorganic Chemistry*, colloquially known as the Red Book [5], and in the related publications for organic compounds (the Blue Book) [6] and polymers (the Purple Book) [7]. It should be noted that many compounds may have non-systematic or semi-systematic names (some of which are not accepted by IUPAC for several reasons, for example, because they are ambiguous) and IUPAC rules allow for more than one systematic name in many cases. IUPAC is working towards identification of single names which are to be preferred for regulatory purposes (Preferred IUPAC Names, or PINs).

Note: In this document, the symbol "=" is used to split names that happen to be too long for the column format, unless there is a convenient hyphen already present in the name.

The boundaries between "organic" and "inorganic" compounds are blurred. The nomenclature types described in this document are applicable to compounds, molecules, and ions that do not contain carbon, but also to many structures that do contain carbon (Section 2), notably those containing elements of Groups 1–12. Most boron-containing compounds are treated using a special nomenclature [8].

Reproduced from:
Pure & Appl. Chem., Vol. 87, No. 9–10, pp. 1039–1049, 2015.

1 Stoichiometric or Compositional Names

A **stoichiometric** or **compositional** name provides information only on the composition of an ion, molecule, or compound and may be related to either the empirical or molecular formula for that entity. It does not provide any structural information.

For **homoatomic entities**, where only one element is present, the name is formed (Table 1) by combining the element name with the appropriate **multiplicative prefix** (Table 2). Ions are named by adding charge numbers in parentheses, for example, (1+), (3+), (2−), and for (most) homoatomic anion names, "ide" is added in place of the "en," "ese," "ic," "ine," "ium," "ogen," "on," "orus," "um," "ur," "y," or "ygen" endings of element names [9]. Exceptions include Zn and Group 18 elements ending in "on," where the "ide" ending is added to the element names. For some elements (e.g., Fe, Ag, and Au), a Latin stem is used before the "ide" ending (*cf.* Section 2.3) [9]. Certain ions may have acceptable traditional names (used without charge numbers).

Binary compounds (those containing atoms of two elements) are named stoichiometrically by combining the element names and treating, by convention, the element reached first when following the arrow in the element sequence (Figure 1) as if it were an anion. Thus, the name of this formally "electronegative" element is given an "ide" ending and is placed after the name of the formally "electropositive" element followed by a space (Table 3).

Again, multiplicative prefixes (Table 2) are applied as needed, and certain acceptable alternative names [10] may be used. Stoichiometry may be implied in some cases by the use of oxidation numbers, but is often omitted for common cases, such as in calcium fluoride.

Heteropolyatomic entities in general can be named similarly using compositional nomenclature, but often either substitutive [11] or additive nomenclature (Section 2) is used. In the latter case, information is also provided about the way atoms are connected. For example, $POCl_3$ (or PCl_3O, compositional name phosphorus trichloride oxide) is given an additive name in Table 10.

Certain ions have traditional short names, which are commonly used and are still acceptable (e.g., ammonium, NH_4^+; hydroxide, OH^-; nitrite, NO_2^-; phosphate, PO_4^{3-}; diphosphate, $P_2O_7^{4-}$).

Inorganic compounds in general can be combinations of cations, anions, and neutral entities. By convention, the name of a compound is made up of the names of its component entities: cations before anions and neutral components last (see examples in Table 4).

The number of each entity present has to be specified in order to reflect the composition of the compound. For this purpose, multiplicative prefixes (Table 2) are added to the name of each entity. The prefixes are "di," "tri," "tetra," and so on for use with names for simple entities, or "bis()," "tris()," "tetrakis()," and so on for names of most entities which themselves contain multiplicative prefixes or locants. Care must also be taken in situations when use of a simple multiplicative prefix may be misinterpreted, for example, tris(iodide) must be used for $3I^-$ rather than triiodide (which is used for I_3^-), and bis(phosphate) rather than diphosphate (which is used for $P_2O_7^{4-}$). Examples are shown in Table 4. There is no elision of vowels (e.g., tetraaqua and pentaoxide), except in the special case of monoxide.

Names of neutral components are separated by "em" dashes without spaces. Inorganic compounds may themselves be components in (formal) **addition compounds** (last four examples in Table 4). The ratios of component compounds can be indicated, in general, using a stoichiometric descriptor in parentheses after the name (see the last three examples in Table 4). In the special case of hydrates, multiplicative prefixes can be used with the term "hydrate."

TABLE 1: Examples of Homoatomic Entities

Formula	Name
O_2	dioxygen
S_8	octasulfur
Na^+	sodium(1+)
Fe^{3+}	iron(3+)
Cl^-	chloride(1−) or chloride
I_3^-	triiodide(1−)
O_2^{2-}	dioxide(2−) or peroxide
N_3^-	trinitride(1−) or azide

TABLE 2: Multiplicative Prefixes for Simple and Complicated Entities

No.	Simple	Complicated
2	di	bis
3	tri	tris
4	tetra	tetrakis
5	penta	pentakis
6	hexa	hexakis
7	hepta	heptakis
8	octa	octakis
9	nona	nonakis
10	deca	decakis
11	undeca	undecakis
12	dodeca	dodecakis
20	icosa	icosakis

TABLE 3: Examples of binary compounds

Formula	Name
GaAs	Gallium arsenide
CO_2	Carbon dioxide
CaF_2	Calcium difluoride or calcium fluoride
$FeCl_2$	Iron dichloride or iron(II) chloride
$FeCl_3$	Iron trichloride or iron(III) chloride
H_2O_2	Dihydrogen dioxide or hydrogen peroxide

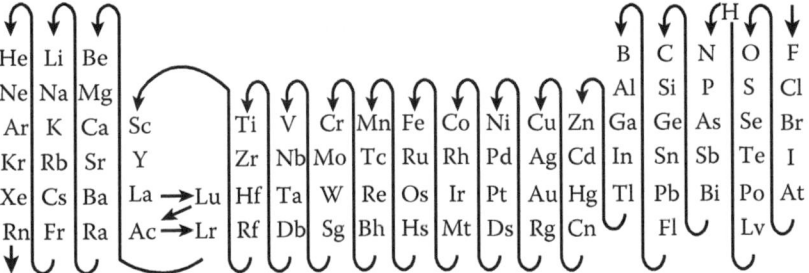

FIGURE 1 Element sequence.

2 Complexes and Additive Nomenclature

2.1 Overall Approach

Additive nomenclature was developed in order to describe the structures of coordination entities, or complexes, but this method is readily extended to other molecular entities as well. Mononuclear complexes are considered to consist of a central atom, often a metal ion, which is bonded to surrounding small molecules or ions, which are referred to as ligands. The names of complexes are constructed (Table 5) by adding the names of the ligands *before* those of the central atoms, using appropriate multiplicative prefixes. Formulae are constructed by adding the symbols or abbreviations of the ligands *after* the symbols of the central atoms (Section 2.7).

2.2 Central Atom(s) and Ligands

The first step is to identify the central atom(s) and thereby also the ligands. By convention, the electrons involved in bonding between the central atom and a ligand are usually treated as belonging to the ligand (and this will determine how it is named).

Each ligand is named as a separate entity using appropriate nomenclature [4]—usually substitutive nomenclature for organic ligands [2,4,6] and additive nomenclature for inorganic ligands. A small number of common molecules and ions are given **special names** when present in complexes. For example, a water ligand is represented in the full name by the term "aqua." An ammonia ligand is represented by "ammine,"

while carbon monoxide bound to the central atom through the carbon atom is represented by the term "carbonyl" and nitrogen monoxide bound through nitrogen is represented by "nitrosyl." Names of **anionic ligands** that end in "ide," "ate," or "ite" are modified within the full additive name for the complex to end in "ido," "ato," or "ito," respectively. Note that the "ido" ending is now used for halide and oxide ligands as well. By convention, a single coordinated hydrogen atom is always considered anionic and it is represented in the name by the term "hydrido," whereas coordinated dihydrogen is usually treated as a neutral two-electron donor entity.

2.3 Assembling Additive Names

Once the ligands have been named, the name can be assembled. This is done by listing the ligand names in alphabetical order before the name of the central atom(s), *without regard* to ligand charge.

If there is more than one ligand of a particular kind bound to a central atom in the same way, the number of such identical ligands is indicated using the appropriate multiplicative prefix for simple or complicated ligands (Table 2), not changing the already established alphabetical order of ligands. The nesting order of enclosing marks, for use in names where more than one set of enclosing marks is required, is (), [()], {[()]}, ({[()]}), and so on.

Any **metal–metal bonds** are indicated by placing the central atom symbols in parentheses, in italics, and connected by an "em" dash, after the name of the complex (without spaces). The **charge number** of the complex or the **oxidation number** of the central atom is appended to the name of the complex. For **anions** that are named additively, the name of the central atom is given the "ate" ending in a similar way to the "ide" endings of homoatomic anions (Section 1). In some cases, by tradition, the Latin stem is used for the "ate" names, such as in ferrate (for iron), cuprate (for copper), argentate (for silver), stannate (for tin), aurate (for gold), and plumbate (for lead) [12]. Finally, the rules of compositional nomenclature (Section 1) are used to combine the additive names of ionic or neutral coordination entities with the names of any other entities that are part of the compound.

2.4 Specifying Connectivity

Some ligands can bind to a central atom through different atoms under different circumstances. Specifying just which ligating (coordinating) atoms are bound in any given complex can be achieved by adding κ-terms to the name of the ligand. The κ-term comprises the Greek letter κ followed by the italicized element symbol of the ligating atom. For more complicated ligands, the κ-term is often placed within the ligand name following the group to which the κ-term refers. Multiple identical links to a central atom can be indicated by the addition of the appropriate numeral as a superscript between the κ and element symbols (see Table 6). These possibilities are discussed in more detail in the Red Book [13]. If the ligating atoms of a ligand are contiguous (i.e., directly bonded to one another), then an η-term is used instead, for example, for many organometallic compounds (Section 2.6) and the peroxido complex in Table 6.

TABLE 4: Use of multiplicative prefixes in compositional names

Formula	Name
$Ca_3(PO_4)_2$	Tricalcium bis(phosphate)
$Ca_2P_2O_7$	Dicalcium diphosphate
BaO_2	Barium(2+) dioxide(2−) or barium peroxide
$MgSO_4 \bullet 7H_2O$	Magnesium sulfate heptahydrate
$CdSO_4 \bullet 6NH_3$	Cadmium sulfate–ammonia (1/6)
$AlK(SO_4)_2 \bullet 12H_2O$	Aluminum potassium bis(sulfate)–water (1/12) or aluminumpotassium bis(sulfate) dodecahydrate
$Al_2(SO_4)_3 \bullet K_2SO_4 \bullet 24H_2O$	Dialuminum tris(sulfate)–dipotassium sulfate–water (1/1/24)

TABLE 5: Producing names for complexes: Simple ligand

Structure to be named		
Central atom(s)	Cobalt(III)	2 × rhenium
Identify and name ligands	Ammonia → ammine	Chloride → chlorido
	Water → aqua	
Assemble name	Pentaammineaquacobalt(III)chloride	Caesium bis(tetrachloridorhenate)(*Re—Re*)(2−)

TABLE 6: Producing names for complexes: Complicated ligands

Structure to be named	Ba²⁺ 2

Central atom	Cobalt(III) → cobaltate(III)	Platinum(II)	
Identify and name ligands	2,2′,2″,2‴-(ethane-1,2-diyldinitrilo)=tetraacetate → 2,2′,2″,2‴-(ethane-1,2-diyldinitrilo)tetraacetato	Chloride → chloridotriphenylphosphane	
Specify ligating atoms	2,2′,2″,2‴-(ethane-1,2-diyldinitrilo-κ²N)=tetraacetato-κ⁴O	*Not required for chloride*triphenylphosphane-κ*P*	
Assemble name	barium [2,2′,2″,2‴-(ethane-1,2-diyldinitrilo-κ²N)tetraacetato-κ⁴O] cobaltate(III)	Dichloridobis(triphenylphosphane-κ*P*) =platinum(II)	

Structure to be named		

Central atom	Cobalt(III)	Molybdenum(III)
Identify and name ligands	Ethane-1,2-diamine	Chloride → chlorido
	Peroxide → peroxido	1,4,8,12-tetrathiacyclopentadecane
Specify ligating atoms	Ethane-1,2-diamine-κ²N	*Not required for chloride*
	η²-peroxido	1,4,8,12-tetrathiacyclopentadecane-κ³S¹, S⁴, S⁸
Assemble name	Bis(ethane-1,2-diamine-κ²N)(η²-peroxido)=cobalt(III)	Trichlorido(1,4,8,12-tetrathiacyclopentadecane-κ³S¹,S⁴,S⁸)molybdenum(III)

A κ-term is required for ligands where more than one coordination mode is possible. Typical cases are thiocyanate, which can be bound through either the sulfur atom (thiocyanato-κ*S*) or the nitrogen atom (thiocyanato-κ*N*), and nitrite, which can be bound through either the nitrogen atom (M–NO₂, nitrito-κ*N*) or an oxygen atom (M–ONO, nitrito-κ*O*). The names pentaammine(nitrito-κ*N*)cobalt(2+) and pentaammine(nitrito-κ*O*)cobalt(2+) are used for each of the isomeric nitrito complex cations. More examples of constructing names using κ-terms to specify the connectivity of ligands are shown in Table 6. A κ-term may also be used to indicate to which central atom a ligand is bound if there is more than one central atom (Section 2.5).

2.5 Bridging Ligands

Bridging ligands are those bound to more than one central atom. They are differentiated in names by the addition of the prefix "μ" (Greek mu), with the prefix and the name of the bridging ligand being separated from each other, and from the rest of the name by hyphens. This is sufficient if the ligand is monoatomic, but if the ligand is more complicated it may be necessary to specify which ligating atom of the ligand is attached to which central atom. This is certainly the case if the ligating atoms are of different kinds, and κ-terms can be used for this purpose.

Di-μ-chlorido-bis[di
chloridoaluminium(III)]
[Cl₂Al(μ-Cl)₂AlCl₂]

μ-peroxido-1κO¹,2κO²-bis(tri
oxidosulfate)(2–)
[O₃S(μ-O₂)SO₃]²⁻

2.6 Organometallic Compounds

Organometallic compounds contain at least one bond between a metal atom and a carbon atom. They are named as coordination compounds, using the additive nomenclature system (see above).

The name for an organic ligand **binding through one carbon atom** may be derived either by treating the ligand as an anion or as a neutral substituent group. The compound [Ti(CH₂CH₂CH₃)Cl₃] is thus named as trichlorido(propan-1-ido)titanium or as trichlorido(propyl)titanium. Similarly, "methanido" or "methyl" may be used for the ligand –CH₃.

When an organic ligand forms **two or three metal–carbon single bonds** (to one or more metal centers), the ligand may be treated as a di- or tri-anion, with the endings "diido" or "triido" being used, with no removal of the terminal "e" of the name of the parent hydrocarbon. Again, names derived by regarding such ligands as substituent groups and using the suffixes "diyl" and "triyl" are still commonly encountered. Thus, the bidentate ligand –CH₂CH₂CH₂– would be named propane-1,3-diido (or propane-1,3-diyl) when chelating a metal center, and μ-propane-1,3-diido (or μ-propane-1,3-diyl) when bridging two metal atoms.

Organometallic compounds containing a **metal–carbon multiple bond** are given substituent prefix names derived from the parent hydrides which end with the suffix "ylidene" for a metal–carbon double bond and with "ylidyne" for a triple bond. These suffixes either replace the ending "ane" of the parent hydride or, more generally, are added to the name of the parent hydride with the insertion of a locant and the elision of the terminal "e," if present. Thus, the entity CH₃CH₂CH= as a ligand is named propylidene and (CH₃)₂C= is called propan-2-ylidene. The "diido"/"triido" approach, outlined above, can also be used in this situation. The terms "carbene" and "carbyne" are not used in systematic nomenclature.

dichlorido(phenylmethylidene)bis(tricyclohexylphosphane-κP)ruthenium,
dichlorido(phenylmethanediido)bis(tricyclohexylphosphane-κP)ruthenium,
or (benzylidene)dichloridobis(tricyclohexylphosphane-κP)ruthenium

The special nature of the bonding to metals of unsaturated hydrocarbons in a "side-on" fashion *via* their π-electrons requires the **eta (η) convention**. In this "hapto" nomenclature, the number of *contiguous* atoms in the ligand coordinated to the metal (the hapticity of the ligand) is indicated by a right superscript on the eta symbol, for example, η^3 ("eta three" or "trihapto"). The η-term is added as a prefix to the ligand name, or to that portion of the ligand name most appropriate to indicate the connectivity, with locants if necessary.

(η^6-benzene)[(1,2,5,6-η)-cycloocta-1,3,5,7-tetraene]cobalt(1+)

tris(η^3-prop-2-en-1-ido)chromium,
tris(η^3-prop-2-en-1-yl)chromium
or tris(η^3-allyl)chromium

A list of many π-**bonding unsaturated ligands**, neutral and anionic, can be found in the Red Book [14].

Note that the ubiquitous ligand η^5-C$_5$H$_5$, strictly η^5-cyclopenta-2,4-dien-1-ido, is also acceptably named η^5-cyclopentadienido or η^5-cyclopentadienyl. When cyclopenta-2,4-dien-1-ido coordinates through one carbon atom *via* a σ bond, a κ-term is added for explicit indication of that bonding. The symbol η^1 should not be used, as the eta convention applies only to the bonding of contiguous atoms in a ligand.

Dicarbonyl(η^5-cyclopentadienido)(cyclopenta-2,4-dien-1-ido-κC^1)iron **or** dicarbonyl(η^5-cyclopentadienyl)(cyclopenta-2,4-dien-1-yl-κC^1)iron

Discrete molecules containing two *parallel* η^5-cyclopentadienido ligands in a "sandwich" structure around a transition metal, as in bis(η^5-cyclopentadienido)iron, [Fe(η^5-C$_5$H$_5$)$_2$], are generically called **metallocenes** and may be given "ocene" names, in this case ferrocene. These "ocene" names may be used in the same way as parent hydride names are used in substitutive nomenclature, with substituent group names taking the forms "ocenyl," "ocenediyl," "ocenetriyl" (with insertion of appropriate locants).

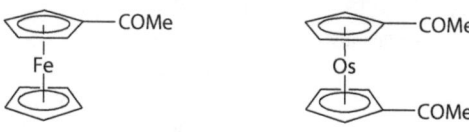

1-ferrocenylethan-1-one   1,1'-(osmocene-1,1'-diyl)di(ethan-1-one)

By convention, "organoelement" compounds of the **main group elements** are named by substitutive nomenclature if derived from the elements of Groups 13–16, but by additive nomenclature if derived from the elements of Groups 1 and 2. In some cases, compositional nomenclature is used if less structural information is to be conveyed. More detail is provided in the Red Book [15].

TABLE 7: Producing line formulae for complexes

Structure		
Central atom(s)	Co	2 × Re
Ligands	NH$_3$, OH$_2$	Cl
Assemble formula	[Co(NH$_3$)$_5$(OH$_2$)]Cl$_3$	Cs$_2$[Cl$_4$ReReCl$_4$]
Structure		
Central atom(s)	Co	Pt
Abbreviate ligands	2,2',2'',2'''-(ethane-1,2-diyl)=dinitrilotetraacetate → edta	Cl triphenylphosphane → PPh3
Assemble formula	Ba[Co(edta)]$_2$	[PtCl$_2$(PPh$_3$)$_2$]

TABLE 8: Examples of inorganic oxoacids and derivatives

Formula	Traditional or organic name	Additive name
H_2SO_4 or $[S(O)_2(OH)_2]$	Sulfuric acid	Dihydroxidodioxidosulfur
$(CH_3)_2SO_4$ or $[S(O)_2(OMe)_2]$	Dimethyl sulfate	Dimethoxidodioxidosulfur or dimethanolatodioxidosulfur
H_2PHO_3 or $[P(H)(O)(OH)_2]$	Phosphonic acid*	Hydridodihydroxidooxidophosphorus
$PhP(O)(OH)_2$	Phenylphosphonic acid	Dihydroxidooxido(phenyl)phosphorus

* The term "phosphorous acid" has been used in the literature for both the species named phosphonic acid in Table 8 and that with the formula $P(OH)_3$, trihydroxidophosphorus. It is used in organic nomenclature in the latter sense.

TABLE 9: Examples of derivatives of inorganic oxoacids and anions formed by functional replacement

Formula	Name indicating functional replacement	Additive name
H_3PS_4 or $[P(S)(SH)_3]$	Tetrathiophosphoric acid or phosphorotetrathioic acid	Tris(sulfanido)sulfidophosphorus
H_2PFO_3 or $[PF(O)(OH)_2]$	Fluorophosphoric acid or Phosphorofluoridic acid	Fluoridodihydroxidooxidophosphorus
$S_2O_3{}^{2-}$ or $[S(O)_3(S)]^{2-}$	Thiosulfate or sulfurothioate	Trioxidosulfidosulfate(2–)
$[O_3S(\mu\text{-}O_2)SO_3]^{2-}$	Peroxydisulfate	See Section 2.5

TABLE 10: Examples of functional class names and corresponding additive names

Formula	Functional class name	Additive name
PCl_3O	Phosphoryl trichloride	Trichloridooxidophosphorus
SCl_2O_2	Sulfuryl dichloride	Dichloridodioxidosulfur
$S(NH_2)_2O_2$	Sulfuric diamide	Diamidodioxidosulfur

2.7 Formulae of Coordination Compounds

Line formulae for coordination entities are constructed within square brackets to specify the composition of the entity. The overall process is shown in Table 7. The symbol for the central atom is placed first and is then followed by the symbols or abbreviations for the ligands (in alphabetical order according to the way they are presented in the formula). Where possible the coordinating (ligating) atom should be placed nearer the central atom in order to provide more information about the structure of the complex. If possible, bridging ligands should be placed between central atom symbols for this same reason (see examples in Section 2.5). Generally, ligand formulae and abbreviations are placed within enclosing marks (unless the ligand contains only one atom), remembering that square brackets are reserved to define the coordination sphere. Multiple ligands are indicated by a right subscript following the enclosing marks or ligand symbol.

2.8 Inorganic Oxoacids and Related Compounds

Inorganic oxoacids, and the anions formed by removing the acidic **hydrons** (H^+) from them, have traditional names, many of which are well-known and can be found in many textbooks: sulfuric acid, sulfate; nitric acid, nitrate; nitrous acid, nitrite; phosphoric acid, phosphate; arsenic acid, arsenate; arsinous acid, arsinite; silicic acid, silicate; and so on. These names are retained in IUPAC nomenclature, firstly because they almost invariably are the names used in practice, and secondly because they play a special role in organic nomenclature when names are needed for organic derivatives. However, all the oxoacids themselves and their derivatives may be viewed as coordination entities and named systematically using additive nomenclature (Table 8) [16].

The traditional oxoacid names may be modified according to established rules for naming derivatives formed by **functional replacement** [16]: thus, "thio" denotes replacement of =O by =S; prefixes "fluoro," "chloro," and so on and infixes "fluorid," "chlorid," and so on denote replacement of –OH by –F, –Cl, and so on; "peroxy"/"peroxo" denote replacement of –O– by –OO–; and so forth (Table 9).

If all hydroxy groups in an oxoacid are replaced, the compound is no longer an acid and is not named as such, but will have a traditional **functional class name** [16] as, for example, an acid halide or amide. Such compounds may again be systematically named using additive nomenclature (Table 10).

A special construction is used in **hydrogen names**, which allows the indication of hydrons bound to an anion without specifying exactly where. In such names, the word "hydrogen" is placed at the front of the name with a multiplicative prefix (if applicable) and with no space between it and the rest of the name, which is placed in parentheses. For example, dihydrogen(diphosphate)(2–) denotes $H_2P_2O_7{}^{2-}$, a diphosphate ion to which two hydrons have been added, with the positions not known or at least not being specified.

One may view the common names for partially dehydronated oxoacids, such as hydrogenphosphate, $HPO_4{}^{2-}$, and dihydrogenphosphate, $H_2PO_4{}^-$, as special cases of such hydrogen names. In these simplified names, the charge number and the parentheses around the main part of the name are left out. Again, these particular anions may be named systematically by additive nomenclature. The word "hydrogen" is placed *separately* in forming analogous names in organic nomenclature, for example, dodecyl hydrogen sulfate, $C_{12}H_{25}OS(O)_2OH$. This difference between the two systems has the consequence that the important carbon-containing ion HCO_3– can be named equally correctly as "hydrogen carbonate" and as "hydrogencarbonate" (but not as bicarbonate).

3 Stereodescriptors

The approximate geometry around the central atom is described using a **polyhedral symbol** placed in front of the name. The symbol is made up of italicized letter codes for the geometry and a number that indicates the coordination number. Frequently used polyhedral symbols are *OC*-6 (octahedral), *SP*-4 (square-planar), *T*-4 (tetrahedral), *SPY*-5 (square-pyramidal), and *TBPY*-5 (trigonal-bipyramidal). More complete lists are available [17].

The relative positions of ligating groups around a central atom can be described using a **configuration index** that is determined in a particular way for each geometry [18], based on the Cahn–Ingold–Prelog priorities of the ligating groups [19,20], and it may change if the ligands change, even if the geometry remains the same. The absolute configuration can also be described. Generally, configuration indices are used only if there is more than one possibility and a particular stereoisomer is to be identified. The full stereodescriptors for the particular square-planar platinum complexes shown below are (*SP*-4-2) and (*SP*-4-1), for the *cis* and *trans* isomers, respectively. Alternatively, a range of traditional stereodescriptors may be used in particular situations. Thus, the isomers that are possible when a square-planar center is coordinated by two ligating groups of one type and two of another are referred to as *cis*- (when the identical ligands are coordinated next to each other) or *trans*- (when they are coordinated opposite to each other).

cis-diamminedichloridoplatinum(II)   trans-diamminedichlorido-
                                                    platinum(II)

Octahedral centers with four ligands of one kind and two of another can also be referred to as *cis*-(when the two identical ligands are coordinated next to each other) or *trans*- (when they are coordinated opposite each other). Octahedral centers with three of each of two kinds of ligand can be described as *fac*-(facial), when the three ligands of a particular kind are located at the corners of a face of the octahedron, or *mer*- (meridional), when they are not.

4 Summary

This document provides an outline of the essential nomenclature rules for producing names and formulae for inorganic compounds, coordination compounds, and organometallic compounds. The complementary document for nomenclature systems of organic chemistry [2] will also be useful to the reader.

Names and formulae have only served half their role when they are created and used to describe or identify compounds, for example, in publications. Achieving their full role requires that the reader of a name or formula is able to interpret it successfully, for example, to produce a structural diagram. The present document is also intended to assist in the interpretation of names and formulae.

Finally, we note that IUPAC has produced recommendations on the graphical representation of chemical structures and their stereochemical configurations [21,22].

5 Membership of Sponsoring Body

Membership of the IUPAC Division of Chemical Nomenclature and Structure Representation (Division VIII) for the period 2014–2015 is as follows:

President: K.-H. Hellwich (Germany); **Secretary:** T. Damhus (Denmark); **Past President:** R. M. Hartshorn (New Zealand); **Titular Members:** M. A. Beckett (UK); P. Hodge (UK); A. T. Hutton (South Africa); R. S. Laitinen (Finland); E. Nordlander (Sweden); A. P. Rauter (Portugal); H. Rey (Germany); **Associate Members:** K. Degtyarenko (Spain); Md. A. Hashem (Bangladesh); M. M. Rogers (USA); J. B. Todd (USA); J. Vohlídal (Czech Republic);

A. Yerin (Russia); **National Representatives:** V. Ahsen (Turkey); D. J. Choo (Republic of Korea); G. A. Eller (Austria); W. Huang (China); T. L. Lowary (Canada); J. Nagy (Hungary); M. Putala (Slovakia); S. Tangpitayakul (Thailand); L. Varga-Defterdarović (Croatia); **Ex Officio:** G. P. Moss (UK).

Note: Republication or reproduction of this report or its storage and/or dissemination by electronic means is permitted without the need for formal IUPAC or De Gruyter permission on condition that an acknowledgment with full reference to the source, along with use of the copyright symbol ©, the name IUPAC, the name De Gruyter, and the year of publication, are prominently visible. Publication of a translation into another language is subject to the additional condition of prior approval from the relevant IUPAC National Adhering Organization and De Gruyter.

Supplemental Material: The online version of this article (DOI: 10.1515/pac-2014-0718) offers as supplementary material a four-sided lift-out document readily available for inclusion in textbooks and similar publications.

References

1. Freely Available at: http://www.iupac.org/publications/pac/; http://www.chem.qmul.ac.uk/iupac/.
2. K.-H. Hellwich, R. M. Hartshorn, A. Yerin, T. Damhus, A. T. Hutton, *Pure Appl. Chem.*, in preparation.
3. R. C. Hiorns, R. J. Boucher, R. Duhlev, K.-H. Hellwich, P. Hodge, A. D. Jenkins, R. G. Jones, et al., *Pure Appl. Chem.* **84**, 2167 (2012).
4. *Principles of Chemical Nomenclature – A Guide to IUPAC Recommendations, 2011 Edition*, G. J. Leigh (Ed.), Royal Society of Chemistry, Cambridge, UK.
5. *Nomenclature of Inorganic Chemistry – IUPAC Recommendations 2005*, N. G. Connelly, T. Damhus, R. M. Hartshorn, A. T. Hutton (Eds.), Royal Society of Chemistry, Cambridge, UK.
6. *Nomenclature of Organic Chemistry – IUPAC Recommendations and Preferred Names 2013*, H. A. Favre, W. H. Powell (Eds.), Royal Society of Chemistry, Cambridge, UK.
7. *Compendium of Polymer Terminology and Nomenclature – IUPAC Recommendations 2008*, R. G. Jones, J. Kahovec, R. Stepto, E. S. Wilks, M. Hess, T. Kitayama, W. V. Metanomski (Eds.), Royal Society of Chemistry, Cambridge, UK.
8. Reference 4, Chapter 10.
9. Reference 5, Table IX.
10. Reference 4, Table P10.
11. Reference 5, Chapter IR-6.
12. Reference 5, Table X.
13. Reference 5, Section IR-9.2.4.
14. Reference 5, Table IR-10.4.
15. Reference 5, Section IR-10.3.
16. Reference 5, Chapter IR-8.
17. Reference 4, Table P5; Reference 5, Tables IR-9.2 and IR-9.3.
18. Reference 5, Section IR-9.3.3.
19. R. S. Cahn, C. Ingold, V. Prelog. *Angew. Chem., Int. Ed. Engl.* **5**, 385, 511 (1966).
20. V. Prelog, G. Helmchen. *Angew. Chem., Int. Ed. Engl.* **21**, 567 (1982).
21. J. Brecher, K. N. Degtyarenko, H. Gottlieb, R. M. Hartshorn, G. P. Moss, P. Murray-Rust, J. Nyitrai, et al., *Pure Appl. Chem.* **78**, 1897 (2006).
22. J. Brecher, K. N. Degtyarenko, H. Gottlieb, R. M. Hartshorn, K.-H. Hellwich, J. Kahovec, G. P. Moss, et al., *Pure Appl. Chem.* **80**, 277 (2008).

PROPERTIES OF FLUORESCENT PROBES COMMONLY USED FOR MEMBRANE STUDIES

Compound	Conditions	λ_{ex}	$\lambda_{f,m}$	Q	P_0	τ	Temp.	Ref.
Octadecylnaphthylamine sulfonate	Ethanol	349	408				22	2
	Phosphatidylcholine vesicles		419			12.7	22	2
Perylene	Cyclohexane	437	467	0.94		6.4	25	1
	Propylene glycol	435	445		0.46		−50	17
12-(9-Anthroyl) stearic acid	Hexane		444			8.5	22	2
	Benzene		448				22	2
	Ethanol	381	458			3.4	22	2
	Phosphatidylcholine vesicles		445			12.4	22	2
	Erythrocyte ghosts pH 7.4	386	442			12.7	37	18
Atebrine	Tris buffer pH 7.5	420	490				25	9
	Ethanol	419	497				25	9
	Phosphate buffer pH 9.0, 50 mM					5.6	25	10, 26
	Phosphate buffer pH 6.0					3.4	25	10
Pyrene	Cyclohexane	336	385	0.32				1
	Dimyristoyl lecithin	334	386 (monomer)					12
	Vesicle (air saturated)		480 (dimer)			135	25	
Pyrene-3-sulphonate	Electron transport	340	380 (monomer)					10, 11
	Particle, pH 7.4		490 (dimer)					
Retinol	Cyclohexane	325	520	0.02		5.0		19
	Ethanol	325	520	0.011		3.5		19
	Dipalmitoyl lecithin vesicles	325	520	0.013		7.0		19
1,4-Sulfonaphthylhydrazone of hellebrigenin (cardiac glycoside)	95% ethanol	330	410					22
1,4-Sulfonaphthyl-hydrazone of dianhydrostrophanthidin (cardiac glycoside)	95% ethanol	330	410					22
A 23187 (ionophore)	50% v/v aq. ethanol sarcoplasmic reticulum	380	440				24	23
		380	440		4.4(Ca²⁺)		24	23
					11(No Ca²⁺)			
Tetracydine								33
Filipin	Dimethylformanide	360	480					27
1-Anilinonaphthalene-8-sulfonate	Cardiolipin–water	366	470	0.20				14
	Phosphatidyl inositol–water	366	468	0.30				14
1-Anilinonaphthalene-7-sulfonate	H_2O	347	516	0.0091				3
	Ethanol	352	443	0.56				3
	Dioxane	352	432	0.68				3
1,N^6-Ethenoadenosine triphosphate	H_2O	275 or 300	410				25	4
2-Methylanthracene	Tetradecane	378	386	0.42				17
9-Vinylanthracene	Ethanol	384	405	0.41				17
Leucensomycin	Red blood cell membranes	330	410				24	25
1,6-Diphenyl-1,3,5-hexatriene					0.362	11.4		35
7-Chloro-4-nitrobenzo-2-oxa-1,3-diazole	Submitochondrial particles	470	520				25	37
2-Toluidinonaphtha-lene-6-sulfonyl chloride	Submitochondrial particles	332–370	445				25	37
1-Dimethylamino-naphthalene-6-sulfonate	Water	366	500	0.0008			25	7
	Methanol	366	443	0.34			25	7
	Ethanol	366	429	0.52			25	7
	Glycerol	366	465	0.24	0.403		25	7
Chlortetracycline calcium complex	90% methanol	380	530					34
Chlortetracycline magnesium complex	90% methanol	370	520					34
1-Dimethylamino-naphthalene-5-sulfonamidoethyltrimethyl ammonium perchlorate	chloroform	340	540					33

Compiled by Jane Vanderkooi.

References

1. Berlman, *Handbook of Fluorescence Spectra of Aromatic Molecules*, Academic Press, New York, 1965.
2. Waggoner and Stryer, *Proc. Natl. Acad. Sci. U. S. A.*, 67, 579 (1970).
3. Turner and Brand, *Biochemistry*, 7, 3381 (1968).
4. Secrist, Barrio, and Leonard, *Science*, 175, 646 (1972).
5. Ygeurabide and Stryer, *Proc. Natl. Acad. Sci. U. S. A.*, 68, 1217 (1971).
6. Czikkaly, Dreizler, Försterling, Kahn, Sondermann, Tillmann, and Wiegand, *Z. Naturforsch.*, 24a, 1821 (1969).
7. McClure and Edelman, *Biochemistry*, 5, 1908 (1966).
8. Brand, Seliskar, and Turner, *Probes of Structure and Function of Macromolecules and Membranes*, Chance, Lee, and Blaisie, Eds., Academic Press, New York, 1971, 17.
9. Lee, *Biochemistry*, 10, 4375 (1971).
10. Döller, *Z. Phys. Chem.*, 34, 151 (1962).
11. Brocklehurst, Freedman, Hancock, and Radda, *Biochem, J.*, 116, 721 (1970).
12. Vanderkooi and Callis, *Biochemistry*, 13, 4000 (1974).
13. Radda and Vanderkooi, *Biochim. Biophys. Acta*, 265, 509 (1972).
14. Gulik-Krzywicki, Schechter, Iwatsubo, Ranck, and Luzzati, *Biochim. Biophys. Acta*, 219, 1 (1970).
15. Oster and Nishijima, *J. Am. Chem. Soc.*, 78, 1581 (1956).
16. Weber and Lawrence, *Biochem. J.*, 56, 31P (1954).
17. Shinitzky, Dianoux, Gitler, and Weber, *Biochemistry*, 10, 2106 (1971).
18. Vanderkooi, Fischkoff, Chance, and Cooper, *Biochemistry*, 13, 1589 (1974).
19. Radda and Smith, *FEBS Lett.*, 287 (1970).
20. Badley, Martin, and Schneider, *Biochemistry*, 12, 268 (1973).
21. Bucher, Wiegand, Snavely, Beck, and Kuhn, *Chem. Phys. Lett.*, 3, 508 (1969).
22. Yoda and Hokin, *Mol. Pharmacol.*, 8, 30 (1972).
23. Case, Vanderkooi, and Scarpa, *Arch. Biochem. Biophys.*, 162, 174 (1974).
24. Chang and Penefsky, *J. Biol. Chem.*, 248, 2746 (1973).
25. Crifo, Strom, Scioscia, and Mondovi, *FEBS Lett.*, 17, 121 (1971).
26. Deamer, Prince, and Crofts, *Biochim. Biophys. Acta*, 274, 323 (1972).
27. Drabikowski, Lagwinska, and Sarzola, *Biochim. Biophys. Acta*, 291, 61 (1973).
28. Gitler, Rubalcava, and Caswell, *Biochim. Biophys. Acta*, 193, 479 (1969).
29. Azzi and Santato, *Biochem. Biophys. Res. Commun.*, 44, 211 (1971).
30. Haynes and Pressman, *J. Membr. Biol.*, 16, 195 (1974).
31. Layton, Azzi, and Graziotti, *FEBS Lett.*, 36, 87 (1973).
32. Cohen and Changeux, *Biochemistry*, 12, 4855 (1973).
33. Weber, Borris, DeRobertis, Barrantes, LeTorre, and deCarlin, *Mol. Pharmacol.*, 7, 530 (1971).
34. Caswell and Hutchison, *Biochem. Biophys. Res. Commun.*, 42, 43 (1971).
35. Schinitzky and Inbar, *J. Mol. Biol.*, 85, 603 (1974).
36. Schinitzky, Dianox, Gitler, and Weber, *Biochemistry*, 10, 2106 (1971). (Perylene or methyl anthracene.)
37. Brocklehurst, Cierkosz, and Lee, *Biochem. Biophys. Acta*, 314, 136 (1973).

CHROMATOGRAPHY

Roger L. Lundblad

Introduction

Chromatography has become an essential tool in biochemistry and molecular biology since the establishment of basic principles by Martin and Synge in 1941.[1] The basic principle is the same for both liquid chromatography and gas chromatography, the specific distribution of a solute between a mobile phase and a stationary phase. This distribution process may be called partitioning or adsorption, and there is an excellent collection of articles that provide basic information on chromatography.[2] The coupling of these separation technologies with mass spectrometry resulting in "hyphenated technologies" (e.g., LC-MS and GC-MS)[3,4] has been critical for progress in proteomics and metabolomics.

TABLE 1: Some Derivatization Reagents for Gas Chromatography[a]

Reagent	Chemistry and uses	References
Alkylating agents		
Pentafluorobenzyl bromide (PFB-Br)	PFB-Br is an alkylating reagent which can be used to modify hydroxyl groups, carboxyl groups, sulfhydryl groups, and amines.[1] PFB-Br can also be used to measure nitrite and peroxynitrite.[2] It is a versatile reagent.[3–5]	1–5
Dimethyl formamide dialkylacetal (DMFDA)	DMFDA is a commonly used reagent.[1,6–8] The dibutylacetal derivative was found to be more useful than the dimethyl derivative for the analysis of heterocyclic amines in meat.[9] The dimethylacetal derivative has been of particular interest in space research.[10]	1,6–10
Trialkylanilinium	Trimethylanilinium hydroxide is the most common reagent in this type of organic ammonium salts.[1,11,12] Other reagents used are tetramethylammonium hydroxide and m-(trifluoromethylphenyl)trimethylammonium hydroxide.[13] The acetate salt[14] and fluoride salt[15] have also been reported.	1,11–15
Boron trihalide-methanol	Boron trifluoride-methanol is the most common reagent in this group[1,16–19] although the boron trichloride has been reported.[20] Boron trifluoride-methanol is used most often for the preparation of fatty acid esters for GC analysis.	1,16–20
Acylating agents		
Acid anhydrides	There are a variety of acid anhydrides that are used to prepare derivatives for gas chromatography under aqueous[21] and non-aqueous conditions.[1] Reagents include acetic anhydride,[22–24] trifluoroacetic anhydride,[25–27] pentafluoropropionic anhydride,[28–30] and heptafluorobutyric anhydride.[31,32] Pentafluropropionic acids, or other acid anhydrides can be used in combination with alcohols (e.g. 2,2,3,3,3-pentafluoro-1-propanol) to modify a greater range of functional groups in a process involving transesterification.[28]	1,21–32
Methylchloroformate (MCF) (Figure 1)	MCF is one of the several chloroformates which has broad use in the preparation of derivatives of alcohols, phenols, amines, carboxyl groups, and sulfhydryl groups.[33–35] MCF has the advantage of use in both aqueous and non-aqueous conditions.[21] MCF has been used in metabolomics.[36]	1,21,33–36
Acyl halides	Acetyl chloride is used for the derivatization of fatty acids by transesterification.[37–41] Other acyl chlorides such as n-butyryl chloride are also used.[42,43]	37–43
Pentafluorobenzoyl chloride	Pentafluorobenzoyl chloride can be used for the derivatization of a variety of analytes including biological amines.[44–46] There is an extensive use for the derivatization of lipids.[47–52]	44–52
Silylation		
Trimethylsilyl chloride (TMCS)	Trialkyl silyl chloride is the most extensively used derivatization reagent for gas chromatography.[53] The reactions are generally performed under anhydrous conditions[53] although reactions can be performed on samples obtained from water-containing samples.[54,55] There are considerable opportunities for artifacts stemming from a variety of reasons including off-target reactions with aldehydes and ketones.[56] The rate of reaction of TMCS with nucleophilic targets is comparatively slow compared to other alkylsilyl chlorides and requires the presence of a base catalyst such as pyridine.[53] TMCS is included as a catalyst with other trialkylsilyl reagent such N,O-bis-(trimethylsilyl)trifluoroacetamide (BSA)[57] or N-methyl-N-(trimethylsilyl)trifluoroacetamide (MSTFA).[58] The order of functional group reactivity is alcohols>phenols>carboxylic acids>amines>amides.[53]	53–58
N-(trimethylsilyl) imidazole (TMSim)	TMSim is quite reactive with hydroxyl groups in a variety of analytes including a variety of lipids.[59–61] As with other derivatization reactions,[62] microwave heating can greatly improve process efficiency.[60]	59–62
N,O-bis(trimethylsilyl)-acetamide (BSA)	BSA is frequently used with TMCS as a catalyst to modify a variety of functional groups[53] including carboxyl groups.[63–65] In one novel application, BSA was used to measure carboxypeptidase activity by forming derivatives which could be determined by gas chromatography.[65] BSA has been used to prepare derivatives of steroids[59,66] and glucocorticoids.	63–67
N,O-bis(trimethylsilyl)-trifluoroacetamide (BSTFA)	BSTFA is similar to BSA in specificity of modification and there are several studies which have used both reagents.[57,68] One study[57] found BSTFA superior to BSA in product stability and yield of derivative. Another study[68] compared several trimethylsilyl donors for end-capping of silica and observed that BSTFA was more reactive than BSA but less reactive than TMCim. Both BSA and BSTFA were used to prepare trimethylsilyl derivatives of pyrimidines and purines.[69] Current work has used BSTFA for metabolomics analysis of urine,[70] for the measurement[71] of khatamines (psychoactive amines of khat (*Catha edulis* Forsk[72]), and for the measurement of acrylamide in cocoa.[73]	57,68–73

[a] Derivatization reagents are used to increase the volatility and in some cases to provide a signal to analytes. The structures of some selected reagents are shown in Figure 1.

Alkylating Agents

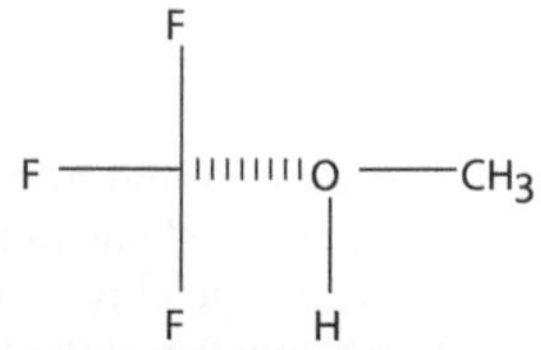

Boron Trifluoride-methanol

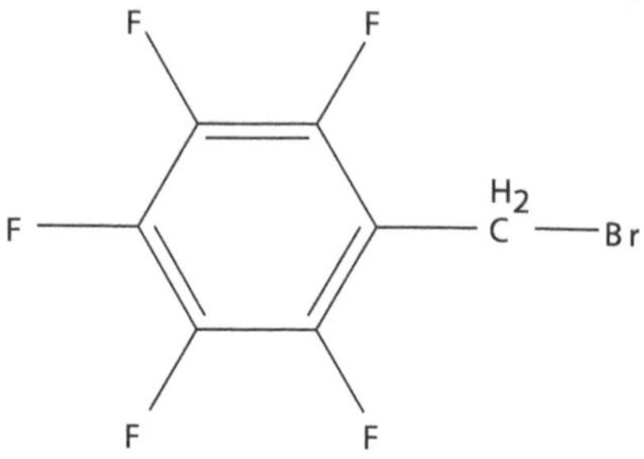

Pentafluorobenzyl bromide

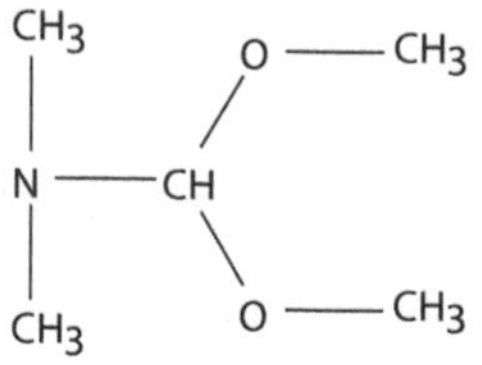

N, N-dimethyformamide dimethylacetal

Acylating Agents

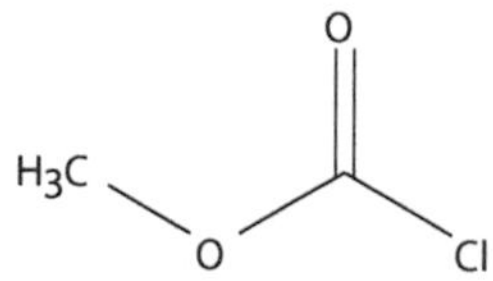

Methyl chloroformate

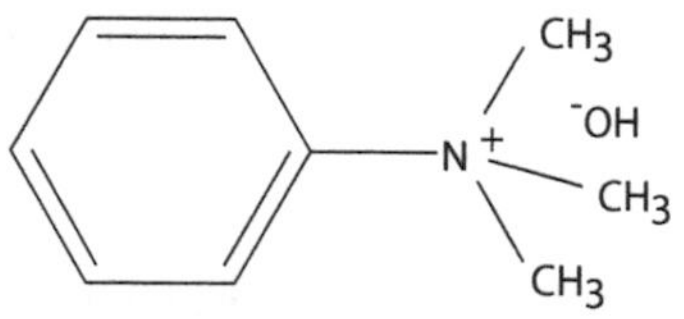

Trimethylanilinium hydroxide
phenyltrimethylammonium hdroxide
trimethylphenylamine hydroxide

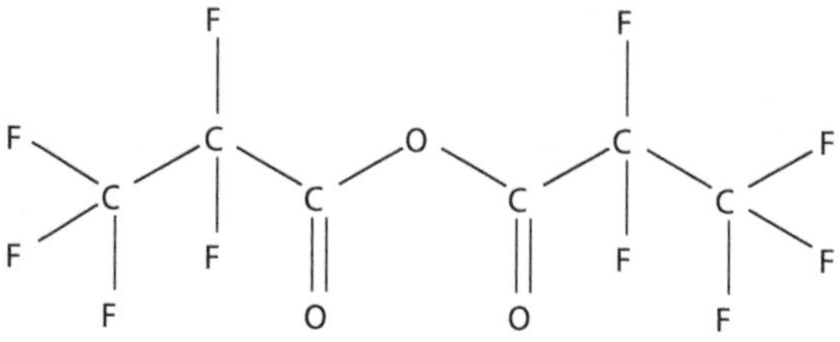

Pentafluoropropionic anhydride

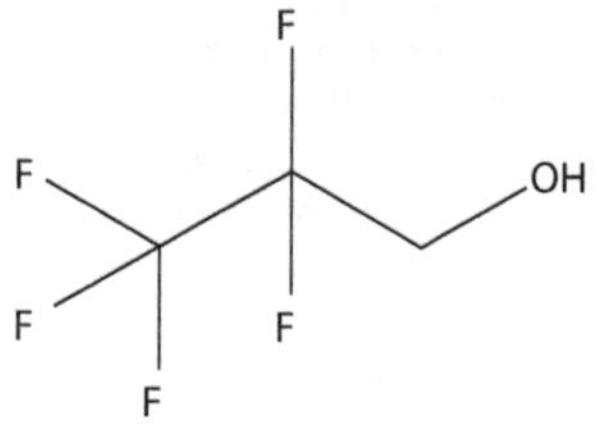

2,2,3,3,3-pentafluoro-1-propanol

Silylation Reagents

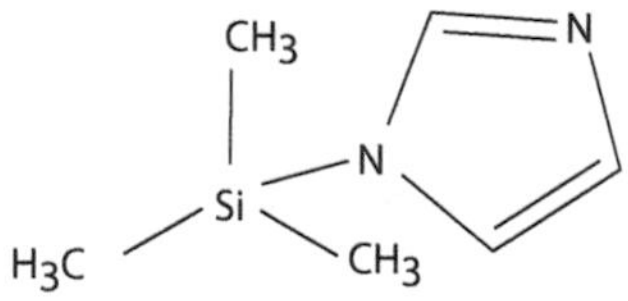

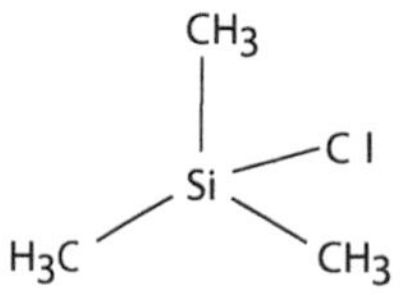

Trimethylsilylchloride

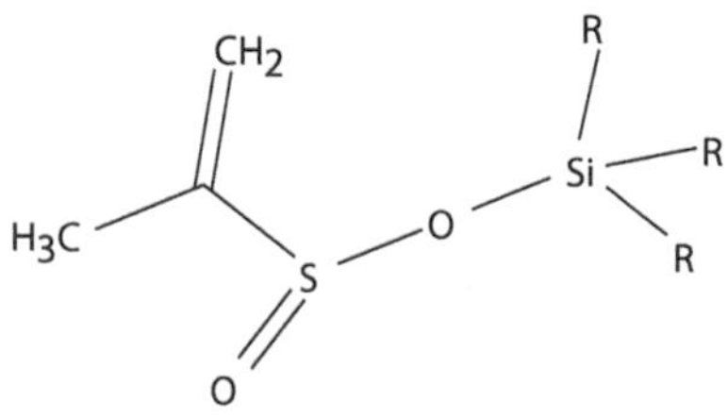

N-trimethylsilylimidazole

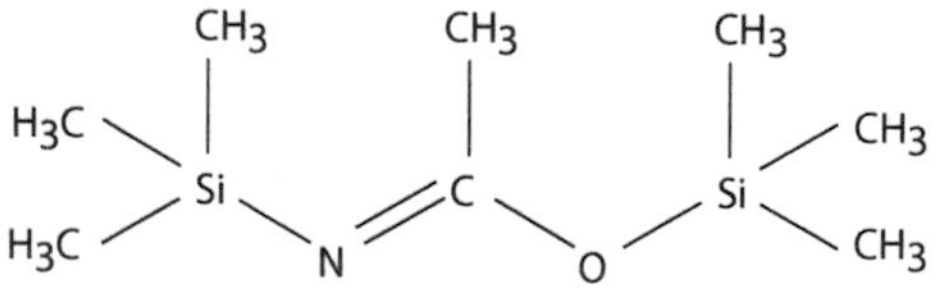

N,O-bis(trimethylsilyl)acetamide

Silyl 2-methylprop-2-ene-1-sulfinate

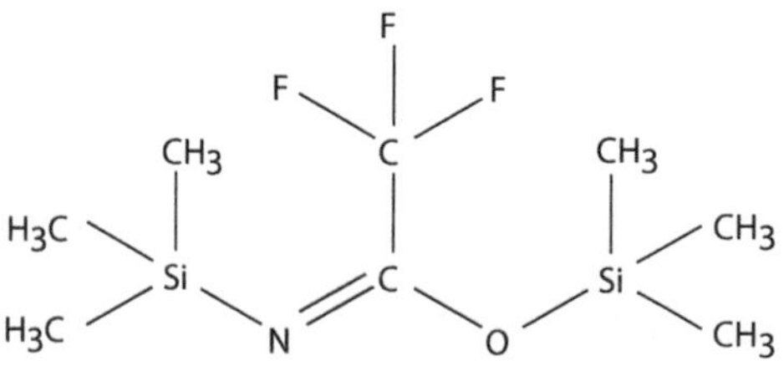

N,O-bis(trimethylsilyl)trifluoroacetamide

FIGURE 1 Reagents for the derivatization of analytes for gas chromatography. The figure shows several examples of reagents used to prepare volatile derivatives of analytes for gas chromatographic analysis. Shown at the top are some examples of alkylating reagents (Wells, R.J., Recent advances in non-silylation derivatization techniques for gas chromatography, *J. Chromatog. A* 841, 1–18, 1999; Fressinet, C., Buch, A., Sternberg, R., et al., Search for evidence of life in space: Analysis of enantiomeric organic molecules by *N,N*-dmethylformamide dimethylacetal derivative dependent gas chromatography-mass spectrometry, *J. Chromatog. A* 1217, 731–740, 2010). Pentafluorobenzyl bromide has been used for the derivatization of peroxynitrite for GC analysis (Tsikas, D., GC-MS and HPLC methods for peroxynitrite (ONOO⁻ and O¹⁵NOO⁻) analysis: A study on stability, decomposition to nitrite and nitrate, laboratory synthesis, and formation of peroxynitrite from *S*-nitrosoglutathione (GSNO) and KO$_2$, *Analyst* 136, 979–987, 2011). Chloroformates are used to prepare ester derivatives (Hušek, P. and Simek, P., Alkylchloroformates in sample derivatization strategies for GC analysis. Review on a decade use of the reagents as esterifying agents, *Curr. Pharm. Anal.* 2, 23–43, 2006). Trimethylanilinium hydroxide is used to prepare methyl ester derivatives of organic acids including fatty acids (Ranz, A. and Lankmayr, E., Screening and optimization of the derivatization of polar herbicides with trimethylanilinium hydroxide for GC-MS analysis, *J. Biochem. Biophys. Methods* 69, 3–14, 2006). Trifluoroacid anhydrides (pentafluoropropionic acid is shown) can be used with homologous alcohols (2,2, 2,3,3-pentafluoro-1-propanol) to prepare derivatives of amino acids and other polar analytes in a "one-pot" reaction (Deyrup, C.L., Chang S.-M., Weintraub, R.A., and Moye, H.A., Simultaneous esterification and acylation of pesticides for analysis by gas chromatography. 1. Derivatization of glyphosate and (aminomethyl)phosphonic acid with fluorinated alcohols-perfluorinated anhydrides, *J. Agric. Food Chem.* 33, 944–947, 1985; Karamani, A.A., Fiamegos, Y.Ch., Vartholomatos, G., and Stalikas, C.D., Fluoroacetylation/fluoroethylesterification as a derivatization approach for gas chromatography-mass spectrometry in metabolomics: Preliminary study of lymphohyperplastic diseases, *J. Chromatog. A* 1302, 125–132, 2013). Silylating reagents are the most common reagents used in GC (Poole, C.F., Alkysilyl derivatives for gas chromatography, *J. Chromatog. A* 1296, 2–14,2013). *N,O*-bis(trimethylsilyl)acetamide (Milkovska-Stamenova, S., Schmidt, R., Frolov, A., and Birkemeyer, C., GC-MS method of the quantitation of carbohydrate intermediates in glycation systems, *J. Agric. Food Chem.* 63, 5911–5911, 2015) and silyl-2-methylprop-2-ene-1-1sulfinate (Marković, D., Tchawou, W.A., Novosjova, I., et al., Applications of silyl-2-methylprop-2-ene-1-sulfinates in preparative sialylation and GC-derivatization reactions of polyols and carbohydrates, *Chemistry* 22, 4196–4205, 2016).

General References for Derivatization Reagents

Ahmed, H., Poole, C.F., and Kozeski, G.E., Determination of descriptors for organosilicon compounds by gas chromatography and non-aqueous liquid-liquid partitioning, *J. Chromatog. A* 1169, 179–192, 2007.

Black, R.M. and Muir, B., Derivatisation reactions in the chromatographic analysis of chemical warfare agents and their degradation products, *J. Chromatog. A* 1000, 253–281, 2003.

Bruheim, P., Kvitvang, H.F.N., and Villas-Boas, S.G., Stable isotope coded derivatizing reagents as internal standards in metabolite profiling, *J. Chromatog. A* 1296, 196–203, 2013.

Damm, M., Rechberger, G., Kollroser, M., and Kappe, C.O., An evaluation of microwave-assisted derivatization procedures using hyphenated mass spectrometric techniques, *J. Chromatog. A* 1216, 5875–5881, 2009.

Handbook of Derivatives for Chromatography, eds. K. Blau and G.S. King, Heyden, London, England, 1978.

Lin, D.-L., Wang, S.-M., Wu, C.-H., et al., Chemical derivatization for the analysis of drugs by GC-MS and LC-MS, *Forensic Sci. Rev.* 28, 18–35, 2016.

Tsikas, D., Identifying and quantifying contaminants contributing to endogenous analytes in gas chromatography/mass spectrometry, *Anal. Chem.* 82, 7835–7841, 2010

Ruiz-Matute, A.J., Hernández-Hernández, O., Rodríguez-Sánchez, S., Sanz, M.L., and Martínez-Castro, I., Derivatization of carbohydrates for GC and GC-MS analyses, *J. Chromatog. B* 879, 1226–1240, 2011.

References to Table 1

1. Davidson, N.D., Gallagher, P.D., and Bao, J.J., Chemical reagents and derivatization reactions in drug analysis, in *Encyclopedia of Analytical Chemistry*, ed. R.A. Meyers, pp. 7042–7046, Wiley, Chichester, England, 2000.
2. Tsikas, D., GC-MS and HPLC methods for peroxynitrite (ONOO⁻) and O^{15}NOO⁻ analysis: A study in on stability, decomposition to nitrite and nitrate, laboratory synthesis and formation of peroxynitrite from *S*-nitrosoglutathione (GSNO) and KO$_2$, *Analyst* 136, 979–987, 2011.
3. Quehenberger, O., Amando, A.M., and Dennis, E.A., High sensitivity quantitative lipidomics analysis of fatty acids in biological samples by gas chromatography-mass spectrometry, *Biochim. Biophys. Acta* 1811, 648–656, 2011.
4. Mabuchi, R., Kunita, A., Miyoshi, N., et al., Analysis of *N*ε-ethyllysine in human plasma proteins by gas chromatography-negative ion chemical ionization/mass spectrometry as a biomarker for exposure to acetaldehyde and alcohol, *Alcohol. Clin. Exp. Res.* 36, 1013–1020, 2012.
5. Musumeci, L.E., Ryona, I., Pan, B.S., et al., Quantification of polyfunctional thiols in wine by HS-SPME-BC-MS following extractive isolation, *Molecules* 20, 12280–12299, 2015.
6. Montrade, M.-P., Maume, D., Le Bizac, B., Pouponneau, K., and Andre, F., Mass spectrometric study of a specific derivatization reaction between *N,N*.-dimethylformamide dimethylacetal and the ethanolamine moiety of β-agonistic drugs, *J. Mass Spectrometry* 32, 626–644, 1997.
7. David, H., Morkeberg Krogh, A., Christophe, A., Akesson, M., and Nielsen, J., CreA influences the metabolic fluxes of *Aspergillus nidulans* during growth on glucose and zylose, *Microbiology* 151, 2209–2221, 2005.
8. Freissinet, C., Buch, A., Sternberg, R., et al., Search for evidence of life in space: Analysis of enantiomeric organic molecules by *N,N*-dimethylformamide dimethylacetal derivative dependent gas chromatography-mass spectrometry, *J. Chromatog. A* 1217, 731–740, 2010.
9. Barcelo-Barrachina, E., Santos, F.J., Puignou, L., and Galceran, M.T., Comparison of dimethylformamide dialkylacetal derivatization reagents for the analysis of heterocyclic amines in meat extracts by gas chromatography-mass spectrometry, *Anal. Chim. Acta* 545, 209–217, 2005.
10. David, M., Musadji, N.-Y., Labanowski, J., Sternberg, R., and Geffroy-Rodier, C., Pilot for validation of online pretreatments for analyses of organics by gas chromatography-mass spectrometry: Application to space research, *Anal. Chem.* 88, 5137–5144, 2016.
11. Menck, R.A., Oliveira, C.D.R., Lima, D.S., et al., Hollow fiber-liquid phase microextraction of barbiturates in liver samples, *Forensic Toxicol.* 31, 31–36, 2013.
12. Levine, B., Phipps, R.J., Naso, C., Fahie, K., and Fowler, D., Tissue distribution of newer anticonvulsant drugs in postmortem cases, *J. Anal. Toxicol.* 34, 506–509, 2010.
13. Drechsel, D., Dettmer, K., and Engewald, W., Studies of thermally assisted hydrolysis and methylation- GC-MS of fatty acids and triglycerides using different reagents and injection systems, *Chromographia* 57(Suppl), S283–S289, 2003.
14. Beiner, K., Plewka, A., Haferkorn, S., et al., Quantification of organic acids in particulate matter by coupling of thermally assisted hydrolysis and methylation with thermodesorption-gas chromatography-mass spectrometry, *J. Chromatog. A* 1216, 6642–6650, 2009.
15. Amijee, M., Cheung, J., and Wells, R.J., Direct on-column derivatization in gas chromatography II. Comparison of various on-column methylation reagents and the development of a new selective methylation reagent, *J. Chromatog. A* 738, 43–55, 1996.
16. Antolin, E.M., Delange, D.M., and Canavaciolo, V.G., Evaluation of five methods for derivatization and GC determination of a mixture of very long chain fatty acids (C24:0-C36:0), *J. Pharm. Biomed. Anal.* 46, 194–199, 2008.

17. Armstrong, J.M., Metherel, A.H., and Stark, K.D., Direct microwave transesterification of fingertip prick blood samples for fatty acid determinations, *Lipids* 43, 187–196, 2008.

18. Chivall, D., Berstan, R., Bull, I.D., and Evershed, R.P., Isotope effects associated with the preparation and methylation of fatty acids by boron trifluoride in methanol for compound-specific stable hydrogen isotope analysis via gas chromatography/thermal conversion/isotope mass spectrometry, *Rapid Commun. Mass Spectrom.* 26, 1232–1240, 2012.

19. Yamazaki, I., Kimura, F., Nakagawa, K., et al., Heterogeneity of the fatty acid composition of Japanese placentae for determining the perinatal fatty acid status: A methodological study, *J. Oleo Sci.* 64, 905–914, 2015.

20. Araujo, P., Nguyen, T.-T., Froyland, L., Wang, J., and Kang, J.X., Evaluation of a rapid method for the quantitative analysis in various matrices, *J. Chromatog. A* 1212, 106–113, 2008.

21. Casas Ferreira, A.M., Fernández Laespada, M.E., Pérez Pavón, J.L., and Moreno Cordero, B., *In situ* aqueous derivatization as sample preparation technique for gas chromatographic determinations, *J. Chromatog. A* 1296, 70–83, 2013.

22. Bringmann, G., Gassen, M., and Schneider, S., Toxic aldehydes formed by lipid peroxidation I. Sensitive, gas chromatography-based stereoanalysis of 4-hydroxyalkenals, toxic products of lipid peroxidation, *J. Chromatog. A* 670, 153–160, 1994.

23. Owen, A.W., McAulay, E.A., Nordon, A., et al., Monitoring of an esterification reaction by on-line direct liquid sampling mass spectrometry and in-line mid infrared spectrophotometry with an attenuated total reflectance probe, *Anal. Chim. Acta* 849, 12–18, 2014.

24. Moerdijk-Poortvliet, T.C.W., Schierbeek, H., Houtekamer, M., et al., Comparison of gas chromatography/isotope ratio mass spectrometry and liquid chromatography/isotope ratio mass spectrometry for carbon stable-isotope analysis of carbohydrates, *Rapid Commun. Mass Spectrom.* 29, 1205–1214, 2015.

25. Garda-Buffon, J. and Badiale-Furlong, E., Kinetics of deoxynivalenol degradation by *Aspergillus oryzae* and *Rhizopus oryzae* in submerged fermentation, *J. Braz. Chem. Soc.* 21, 710–714, 2010.

26. Karamani, A.A., Fiamegos, Y.Ch., Vartholomatos, G., and Stalikas, C.D., Fluoroacetylation/fluoroethylesterification as a derivatization approach for gas chromatography-mass spectrometry in metabolomics: Preliminary study of lymphohyperplastic diseases, *J. Chromatog. A* 1302, 125–132, 2013.

27. Fox, S., Strasdeit, H., Haasmann, S., and Brückner, H., Gas chromatographic separation of stereoisomers of non-protein amino acids on modified γ-cyclodextrin stationary phase, *J. Chromatog. A* 1411, 101–109, 2015.

28. Eckstein, J.A., Ammerman, G.M., Reveles, J.M., and Ackermann, B.L., Simultaneous profiling of multiple neurochemical pathways from a single cerebrospinal fluid sample using GC/MS/MS method with electron capture detection, *J. Mass Spectrom.* 43, 782–790, 2008.

29. Waldhier, M.C., Dettmer, K., Gruber, M.A., and Oefner, P.J., Comparison of derivatization and chromatographic methods for GC-MS analysis of amino acid enantiomers in physiological samples, *J. Chromatog. A* 878, 1103–1112, 2010.

30. Sano, M., Ferchaud-Roucher, V., Nael, C., et al., Simultaneous detection of stable isotope-labeled and unlabeled L-tryptophan and its main metabolites, L-kynurenine, serotonin and quinolinic acid, by chromatography/negative ion chemical ionization mass spectrometry, *J. Mass Spectrom.* 49, 128–135, 2014.

31. Zanetta, J.-P., Timmerman, P., and Leroy, Y., Gas-liquid chromatography of the heptafluorobutyrate derivatives of the O-methyl-glycosides on capillary columns: A method for the quantitative determination of the monosaccharide composition of glycoproteins and glycolipids, *Glycobiology* 9, 255–266, 1999.

32. Pons, A., Richet, C., Robbe, C., et al., Sequential GC/MS analysis of sialic acids, monosaccharides, and amino acids of glycoproteins on a single sample as heptafluorobutyrate derivatives, *Biochemistry* 42, 8342–8353, 2003.

33. Hušek, P., Chloroformates in gas chromatography as general purpose derivatization, *J. Chromatog. B* 717, 57–91, 1998.

34. Hušek, P. and Šimek, P., Alkiyl chloroformates in sample derivatization strategies for GC analysis. Review on a decade of use of the reagents as esterifying agents, *Curr. Pharm. Anal.* 2, 23–43, 2006.

35. Villas-Bôas, S.G., Smart, K.F., Sivakumaran, S., and Lane, G.A., Alkylation or sialylation for analysis of amino and non-amino organic acids by GC-MS?, *Metabolites* 1, 3–20, 2011.

36. Jäpelt, K.B., Chistensen, J.H., and Villas-Bôas, S.G., Metabolic fingerprinting of *Lactobacillus paracasei*: The optimal quenching strategy, *Microb. Cell Fact.* 14, 132, 2015.

37. Masood, A., Stark, K.D., and Salem, N., Jr., A simplified and efficient method for the analysis of fatty acid methyl esters suitable for large clinical studies, *J. Lipid Res.* 46, 2299–2305, 2005.

38. Amusquivar, E., Schiffner, S., and Herrera, E., Evaluation of two methods for plasma fatty acid analysis by GC, *Eur. J. Lipid Sci. Technol.* 113, 711–716, 2011.

39. Lin, Y.H., Hanson, J.A., Strandjord, S.E., et al., Fast transmethylation of total lipids in dried blood by microwave irradiation and its application to a population study, *Lipids* 49, 839–851, 2014.

40. Castro-Gomez, P., Fontecha, J., and Rodriguex-Alcala, L.M., A high-performance direct transmethylation method for total fatty acids assessment in biological and foodstuff samples, *Talanta* 128, 518–523, 2014.

41. Chiu, H.-H., Tasi, S.-J., Tseng, Y.J., et al., An efficient and robust fatty acid profiling method for plasma metabolomic studies by gas chromatography-mass spectrometry, *Clin. Chim. Acta* 451, 183–190, 2015.

42. Angers, P. and Arui, J., A simple method for regiospecific analysis of triacylglycerols by gas chromatography, *J. Am. Oil. Chem. Soc.* 76, 481–484, 1999.

43. Destaillats, F., Arui, J., Simon, J.E., Wolff, R.L., and Angers, P., Dibutyrate derivatization of monoacylglycerols for the resolution of regioisomers of oleic, petroselinic, and *cis*-vaccenic, acids, *Lipids* 37, 111–116, 2002.

44. Clements, R.L.H., Holt, A., Gordon, E.S., Todd, K.G., and Baker, G.B., Determination of rat hepatic polyamines by electron-capture gas chromatography, *J. Pharmacol. Toxicol. Methods* 50, 35–39, 2004.

45. Moawad, M., Khoo, C.S., Lee, S., and Hennell, J.R., Simultaneous determination of eight sympathomimetic amines in urine by gas chromatography/mass spectrometry, *J. AOAC Int.* 93, 116–122, 2010.

46. Singh, D.K., Sanghi, S.K., Gowri, S., Chandra, N., and Sanghi, S.B., Determination of aliphatic amines by gas chromatography-mass spectrometry after in-syringe derivatization with pentafluorobenzoyl chloride, *J. Chromatog. A* 1218, 5683–5687, 2011.

47. Balazy, M. Braquet, P., and Bazan, N.G., Determination of platelet-activating factor and alkyl-ether phospholipids by gas chromatography-mass spectrometry via direct derivatization, *Anal. Biochem.* 196, 1–10, 1991.

48. Shindo, K. and Hashimoto, Y., Quantitative analysis of platelet activating factor treated with pentafluorobenzoyl chloride using gas chromatography/negative ion chemical ionization mass spectrometry, *Drugs Under Exp. Clin. Res.* 17, 343–349, 1991.

49. Falardeau, P., Robillard, M., and Hui, R., Quantification of diacylglycerols by capillary gas chromatography-negative ion chemical ionization-mass spectrometry, *Anal. Biochem.* 208, 311–316, 1993.

50. Wang, Y., Krull, I.S., Liu, C., and Orr, J.D., Derivatization of phospholipids, *J. Chromatog. B* 791, 3–14, 2003.

51. Jenske, R. and Vetler, W., Gas chromatography/electron-capture negative ion mass spectrometry for the quantitative determination of 2- and 3-hydroxy fatty acids in bovine milk fat, *J. Agric. Food Chem.* 56, 5500–5505, 2008.

52. Bowden, J.A, and Ford, D.A., An examination of pentafluorobenzoyl derivatization strategies for the analysis of fatty alcohols using gas chromatography/electron capture negative ion chemical ionization-mass spectrometry, *J. Chromatogr. B. Analyt. Technol. Biomed. Life Sci.* 879, 1375–1383, 2011.

53. Poole, C.F., Alkylsilyl derivatives for gas chromatography, *J. Chromatog. A* 1296, 2–14, 2013.

54. González, A., Avivar, J., and Cerdà, V., Estrogens determination in wastewater samples by automatic in-syringe dispersive liquid-liquid microextraction prior to sialylation and gas chromatography, *J. Chromatog. A* 1413, 1–8, 2015.

55. Saraji, M. and Ghambari, H., Suitability of dispersive liquid-liquid microextraction for the in situ sialylation of chlorophenols in water samples before gas chromatography with mass spectrometry, *J. Sep. Sci.* 38, 3552–3559, 2015.

56. Little, J.L., Artifacts in trimethylsilyl derivatization reactions and ways to avoid them, *J. Chromatog. A* 844, 1–22, 1999.

57. Jurado-Sánchez, B., Ballesteros, E., and Gellego, M., Determination of carboxylic acids in water by gas chromatography-mass spectrometry after continuous extraction and derivatisation, *Talanta* 93. 224–232, 2012.

58. Kwiecien, N.W., Bailey, D.J., Rush, M.J.P., et al., High-resolution filtering for improved small molecule identification via GC/MS, *Anal. Chem.* 87, 8328–8335, 2015.

59. Iida, T., Hirosaka, M., Goto, J., and Nambara, T., Capillary gas chromatographic behavior of *tert.*-hydroxylated steroids by trialkylsilylation, *J. Chromatog. A* 937, 97–105, 2001.

60. Casals, G., Marcos, J., Pozo, O.J., et al., Microwave-assisted derivatization: Application to steroid profiling by gas chromatography/mass spectrometry, *J. Chromatogr. B. Analyt. Technol. Biomed. Life Sci.* 960, 8–13, 2014.

61. Haraguchi, H., Yamada, K., Miyashita, R., et al., Determination of carbon isotopic measurement conditions for ceramide in skin using gas chromatography-combustion-isotope ratio mass spectrometry, *J. Oleo Sci.* 63, 1283–1291, 2014.

62. Cunha, S.C., Pena, A., and Fernandes, J.O., Dispersive liquid-liquid microextraction followed by microwave-assisted sialylation and gas chromatography-mass spectrometry analysis for simultaneous trace quantification of bisphenol A and 13 ultraviolet filters in wastewaters, *J. Chromatog. A* 1414, 10–21, 2015.

63. Haoi, P.M., Tsunoi, S., Ike, M., et al., Dicarboxylic degradation products of nonylphenol polyethoxylates: Synthesis and identification of by gas chromatography-mass spectrometry using electron and chemical ionization modes, *J. Chromatog. A* 1061, 115–121, 2004.

64. Vakhrushev, M.K., Revelsky, A.I., Olenin, A.Y., and Beloborodova, N.V., Development of conditions for the derivatization of phenyl carboxylic acids isolated from blood using gas-chromatography/mass spectrometry, *J. Anal. Chem.* 67, 1050–1056, 2012.

65. Lough, F., Perry, J.D., Stanforth, S.P., and Dean, J.R., Determination of carboxypeptidase activity in clinical pathogens by gas chromatography-mass spectrometry, *Anal. Lett.* 49, 1272–1277, 2016.

66. Bowden, J.A., Colosi, D.M., Stutts. W.L., et al., Enhanced analysis of steroid by gas chromatography/mass spectrometry using microwave-accelerated derivatization, *Anal. Chem.* 81, 6725–6734, 2009.

67. Amendola, L., Garribba, F., and Botre, F., Determination of endogenous and synthetic glucocorticoids in human urine by gas chromatography-mass spectrometry following microwave-assisted derivatization, *Anal. Chim. Acta* 489, 233–243, 2003.

68. McMurtrey, K.D., Reaction of silica gel with trimethylsilyl donors under conditions useful for end-capping HPLC bonded phase packing, *J. Liquid Chromatog.* 113375–113384, 1988.

69. White, E., Krueger, V.P.M., and McCloskey, J.A., Mass spectra of trimethylsilyl derivatives of pyrimidine and purine bases, *J. Org. Chem.* 37, 430–438, 1972.

70. Abbiss, H., Rawlinson, C., Maker, G.L., and Trengove, R., Assessment of automated derivatization protocols for GC-MS-based untargeted metabolomics analysis of urine, *Metabolomics* 11, 1908–1921, 2015.

71. Geisshüsler, S. and Brenneisen, R., The content of psychoactive phenylpropyl and pentapenteyl khatamines in *Cathia edulis* Forsk. Of different origin, *J. Ethnopharmacology* 19, 269–277, 1987.

72. Molnár, B., Fodor, B., Boldizsár, I., and Molnár-Perl, I., Trimethylsilyl speciations of cathine, cathinone and norepinephrine followed by gas chromatography mass spectrometry: Direct sample preparation and analysis of khatamines, *J. Chromatog. A* 1440, 172–178, 2016.

73. Surma, M., Sadowska-Roiek, A., and Cieślik, E., Development of a sample preparation method for acrylamide determination in cocoa via sialylation, *Anal. Methods* 8, 5874–5880, 2016.

Gas Chromatography

Gas chromatography is an analytical system consists of a tube or column passing through a heated chamber. The sample is introduced in a volatile form which frequently requires a process referred to as derivatization to convert the analyte into a volatile form (Table 1). An inert gas such as helium, argon, or nitrogen is the mobile phase[5] and the stationary phase may either be a liquid on the luminal wall of the chromatography column, a liquid adsorbed onto a porous support on the luminal wall of the chromatography column, or a liquid adsorbed onto a material packed into the column.[6–9]

- *Capillary column*: A column (open tubes) with an ID less than 1 mm and not containing packing. The stationary phase is coated on the luminal surface as liquid resulting in thin film or introduced as a porous layer.[10] It is estimated that 90% of gas chromatographic analysis uses capillary columns. The majority of capillary columns are composed of fused silica with a thin film of liquid referred to as a wall-coated open tubular tube (WCOT)[11] Two other types of capillary columns are support-coated open tubular column (SCOT)[12,13] and porous layer open tubular column (PLOT).[14,15]

- *Mobile phase*: This is also referred to as the carrier gas. Nitrogen, hydrogen, and helium are the most common carrier gases.[5]

- *Stationary phase*: A liquid distributed onto the luminal wall of a chromatography column of a solid support packed into the column.[7–9] Ionic liquids[16,17] are used in capillary columns.

- *Packed chromatographic column*: A packed column, defined as a gas chromatographic column, with an ID greater than 1 mm which contain a solid porous support such as graphitized carbon or diatomaceous earth which serves as support for the liquid stationary phase.[18] Most packed columns have an ID between 2 mm and 4 mm. There are some literature on micro-packed columns but the size overlaps with capillary columns.[19,20] The difference is that capillary column do not contain packing.

- *Retention factor (also retention time; retention volume in liquid chromatography)*: The extent to which a solute is retained on the column relative to the column dead volume.

- *Selectivity factor* (α): A measure of how well two solutes are separated in the column. It can be considered as a ratio of the retention factor of two solutes. If $\alpha = 1$, the solutes will not be resolved; if $\alpha \neq 1$, the solutes may be resolved. Selectivity is not unique to gas chromatography but is applicable to liquid chromatography.

- *Resolution factor*: A measure of how well two substances are separated in a column and is dependent on the selectivity factor which is a measure of separation at maximum peak height and the width of peaks. Resolution is not unique to gas chromatography but is applicable to liquid chromatography.

- *Sample preparation*: The sample must either be volatile or have the structural capability to be converted to a volatile derivative by reaction with a suitable reagent.[21] Alkylsilylation is the most common derivatization reaction.[22,23] Other reagents use alkylation, acylation, and condensation to obtain derivatives for gas chromatography.[24–26]

- *Detector systems*: Several detector systems have a long history[27] but current practice is dominated by mass spectrometry.[28]

Liquid Chromatography

Current liquid chromatography is dominated by instrumentation and the physical nature of the solid support. The development of HPLC (high-performance liquid chromatography; high pressure chromatography) was a major technical advance leading to current technologies such as uHPLC.[29,30] These advances in separation technology resulted in increased sensitivity and analysis speed, and together with advances in electrophoresis and mass spectrometry permitted the development of proteomics as a discipline. The early work of Martin and Synge[1] was based on the partition of solute between two liquids, a liquid deposited on a solid phase, defined as the stationary phase, and a liquid mobile phase This is was not the case as there was mixing of the stationary phase and the liquid mobile phase.   This problem was solved by chemically bonding the stationary phase to the solid support provide a product referred to as bonded phase.[31,32] There are a variety of liquid chromatographic methods based on the type of matrix or resin and solvent (Table 2). These variety of solid supports allow multidimensional chromatographic approaches to serve as orthogonal methods of separation (Table 3). The term multidimensional defines the use or two or more chromatographic columns such as size-exclusion followed by reversed-phase chromatography.[33] Multimodal chromatography (Table 4) refers to one matrix demonstrating two or more two mechanisms of separation[34] such as HILIC which can use both ion-exchange and reversed-phase processes. While not referred to as such, gel filtration media can resolve on the basis of hydrophobicity and charge in addition to size and ion-exchanged media can also bind on the basis of hydrophobicity. The development of HPLC and, more recently, uHPLC requires a consideration of sample size and composition.[35] While this has always been a consideration, the scale and sensitivity of new methods makes consideration of sample solvent and size critical. The addition of organic solvents such as methanol and acetonitrile to aqueous buffers does affect solvent pH.

Column efficiency decreases with increasing flow rate, and linear flow velocity (cm min^{-1}) increases proportionally to radius square of the column. Flow must be adjusted to maintain the same resolution over a range of column sizes (Table 5).[33] A plot of height of equivalent theoretic plate (HETP) versus linear flow rate velocity is known as a van Deemter plot which is useful for evaluating column operation efficiency.[36,37]

Table 2: Comparison of liquid chromatographic methods

Method	Matrix	Initial solvent	Comment	Reference
Ion-exchange[a]	Charged functional group on organic matrix such as polystyrene/divinyl-benzene (Figures 2-3) crosslinked dextran,[b] or silica	Usually aqueous dilute salt solution containing buffer to control pH	Binding to the solid phase is based on electrostatic interaction between charged groups on the solid phase with oppositely charged groups on the solute. Elution can be isocratic or with either gradient or stepwise change in pH or increase in ionic strength. While electrostatic interactions predominate, interaction with the matrix can occur.	1–3
Normal-phase	Silica-alumina-bonded phases such as amino, nitro, cyano, and diol	Non-polar organic solvents such as *n*-hexane, non-polar organic solvents containing small of a less polar solvent such as 2-propanol	The term *normal-phase chromatography* refers to a chromatographic process where solutes are bound to a relatively polar stationary phase in the presence of a non-polar solvent (i.e., hexane) and eluted by isocratic elution of by decreasing the increasing the polarity of the mobile phase by addition of a more polar organic solvent.[4–9] Normal phase is sometimes referred to as adsorption chromatography. The use of a bonded silica phase (Figure 4) reduces the number of free silanol groups and reduces the amount of water which could be bound by "dry" solvents thus improving reproducibility; the variable presence of water in solvents can have an influence on separations with a silica solid phase. The free silanol groups (Figure 4) are in three pKa groups, pKa = 3.8, pKa = 5.2, and pKa ~ 9.[9] Unprotonated silanol groups can bind basic solutes.[10] Normal phase chromatography is used mostly for low-molecular organic compounds such as drugs and pesticides.	4–10
Aqueous normal-phase chromatography (ANPC)	Most applications use a silica hydride solid phase; other solid phases have also been used.	Organic solvents such as Acn with water may contain an additive such as formic acid or ammonium formate	In ANPC, the solid phase surface such as silica hydride is hydrophobic relative to the water-containing mobile phase however still capable of adsorbing water from the aqueous/organic mobile phase.[11,12] The amount of water adsorbed to the surface is dependent on the polarity of the surface.[13,14] Aqueous normal phase chromatography has been considered closely related to hydrophilic interaction chromatography (HILIC)[12,15] or separated from HILIC.[16] ANPC is useful for separating polar compounds[17] and can be considered orthogonal to reversed-phase chromatography.[18] ANPC solvent conditions have been used for solid-phase extraction (SPE).[19]	11–19
Reverse-phase chromatography (RPC)	Alkyl or aryl-modified silica. The most common are C_4(butyl) or C_{18}(octadecyl) hydrocarbon chains	Water with dilute weak acid such as 0.1% trifluoroacetic acid or 0.1 % formic acid	RPC is a process where the solute is thought to be partitioned between a hydrophobic matrix and a mobile phase.[20] The matrices are based on a silica gel matrix with alkyl chains attached (Figure 4) and matrices are defined by the chain length of the alkyl chains such as C_4 or C_{18}.[21] Elution is accomplished by increasing the amount of non-polar material (usually acetonitrile) in water with an organic modifier (i.e. 0.1% trifluoroacetic acid); isocratic elution is also used. The matrices used for RPC are similar to those used for HIC but there are differences in solvent conditions and mechanisms of binding .[22] There are studies which have used RPC and HIC in tandem for protein purification.[23,24] Solutes can bind to a reversed-phase matrix by several different mechanisms[25]; one mechanism can be described as solvophobic where solutes would move from the aqueous mobile phase into the bonded hydrophobic solid phase.[26] RPC8 a second would be adsorption to the bonded hydrophobic solid phase,[27] while the third would be partitioning into an adsorbed layer of solvent from the solution phase. It is recognized that these mechanisms are not mutually exclusive.[28] Carboxylic acids are bound the RPC columns through binding to vicinal silanol groups (Figure 4).[29]	20–29
Hydrophobic interaction chromatography (HIC)	Aryl (e.g., Phenyl)- or Alkyl (Butyl)-modified silica	High-salt such as 1-2 M $(NH_4)_2SO_4$	Hydrophobic interaction chromatography (HIC) is the current terminology used to describe "salting-out" chromatography.[30] Salting-out chromatography is a chromatographic technique based on the salt-promoted binding of molecule to an substituted matrix such as agarose[31] or cellulose.[32] Recent use appears to be confined to paper chromatography and thin layer chromatography.[33] HIC used salt-promoted binding of solute to a matrix such as phenyl-agarose. Elution is accomplished by decreasing salt concentration. One major issue with HIC has been the problem with the presence of non-volatile salts precluding subsequent analysis by top-down proteomics. There is recent work using non-volatile salts[34,35] which will make direct analysis by mass spectrometry possible.	30–35

Table 2: Comparison of liquid chromatographic methods (Continued)

Method	Matrix	Initial solvent	Comment	Reference
Hydrophilic interaction chromatography (HILIC)	Polar matrix such unmodified silica or a bonded phase such as cyanopropyl, amino, or diol.	Polar organic solvent such as ACN with H_2O or a buffer such as ammonium formate.	HILIC can be considered to be an extension of normal phase chromatography where there is a polar stationary phase, either unmodified silica or a bonded phase such as an amide, carbamate, or sulfobetaine and mobile phase consisting of water and a miscible organic such as acetonitrile.[36–39] There is a wide variety of potential stationary phases for HILIC.[36] As with RPC, HILIC has the advantage of using volatile solvents permitting a facile interface to mass spectrometry. In an isocratic application, retention can be adjusted by the varying water (buffer) content in the mobile phase or, conversely the amount of an organic solvent such as acetonitrile.[36,40] Retention of solutes on HILIC can result from both partitioning and adsorption.[36,41] HILIC has been useful for the isolation of glycopeptides[43] and for the analysis of polar pharmaceutical products.[43] HILIC is also useful for studies in metabolomics.[44–45]	36–45
Electrostatic repulsion-hydrophilic interaction chromatography (ERLIC)	Polar matrix such unmodified silica, anion- and cation-exchange matrix,	Organic solvent such as used in HILIC with a buffer salt	ERLIC can be described as mixed-mode chromatographic method based on hydrophilic interaction and electrostatic interaction. ERLIC has been useful in the isolation of phosphopeptides and glycopeptides. ERLIC has been suggested as a chromatographic method orthogonal to RPC.	46–48
Gel filtration	Cross-linked dextran, agarose or polyacrylamide matrix	Aqueous solvent with physiological ionic strength	While molecular size[49] is the major factor, electrostatic interaction[50] and/or hydrophobic interaction[51] with the matrix can occur. Gel filtration can be used to obtain a discrete protein fraction for analysis by top-down proteomics[52]	49–52
Gel permeation	Crosslinked polystyrene divinylbenzene (Styragel®) is major matrix.[53,54] Other supports can be used depending on stability in solvent.	Organic solvent such as chloroform, DMSO, or DMac	Also referred to as organic size exclusion chromatography.[54] The major use is the characterization of polymers such as methacrylates and cellulose.[55,56] Size exclusion chromatography has also been used for the characterization of starch and glycogen.[57,58]	53–58
Hydroxyapatite	Hydroxyapatite which can also less frequently be referred to as calcium phosphate or hydroxylapatite	Aqueous solvents most frequently containing sodium phosphate buffer although other solvent systems can be used	Early work with hydroxyapatite was frustrated by slow flow rates.[59] While there were early attempts to mitigate this problem[60,61] it was not until the development of ceramic calcium phosphate that this technique saw extensive use.[62] Most use is for proteins with particular interest in monoclonal antibodies.[63–65] Hydroxyapatite is also used for the purification of nucleic acids[60,66] and lipids.[67]	59–67
Affinity chromatography.	A specific Ligand attached to a matrix (usually dextran or agarose).	Usually aqueous with elution by change in solvent composition.	There are a variety of ligands which can be used in affinity chromatography including immobilized metal ions.[68] High-performance affinity chromatography is used to measure drug-protein interactions.[69,70] There are several recent reviews.[71,72] It should be recognized that affinity chromatography is unique based upon individual properties of the solid phase.	68–72
Supercritical fluid chromatography	Original matrix was silica.[73] Now many difference matrices with ligands such as 2-ethyl pyridine, fluorophenyl as well as ligands such as octadecyl and other matrices used for other forms of liquid chromatography.[74]	Supercritical fluids with CO_2 the most common with the addition of another solvent such as methanol.[75–77]	There is a good collection of reviews on supercritical fluids[73–77] and another work focusing on the use of supercritical fluids in the extraction of food product.[78] The more recent use of supercritical fluids in chromatography has been assisted by the development of systems which are compatible with the conditions (temperature, pressure) required for the use of supercritical fluids. Use of SFC has focused on metabolomics[79,80] and pharmaceutical products.[81,82]	73

[a] Ion-exchange chromatography is occasionally included in discussions of ion chromatography (Haddad, P.R. and Jackson, P.E., *Ion Chromatography Principles and Applications*, Elsevier, Amsterdam, Netherlands, 2000).

[b] Cellulose-based ion-exchange matrices were the earliest matrices to replace the polystyrene -divinylbenezene for the chromatography of proteins (Bates, R.W. and Condliffe, P.G., Chromatography of thyroid stimulating hormone on carboxymethylcellulose, *J. Biol. Chem.* 223, 843–852, 1956).

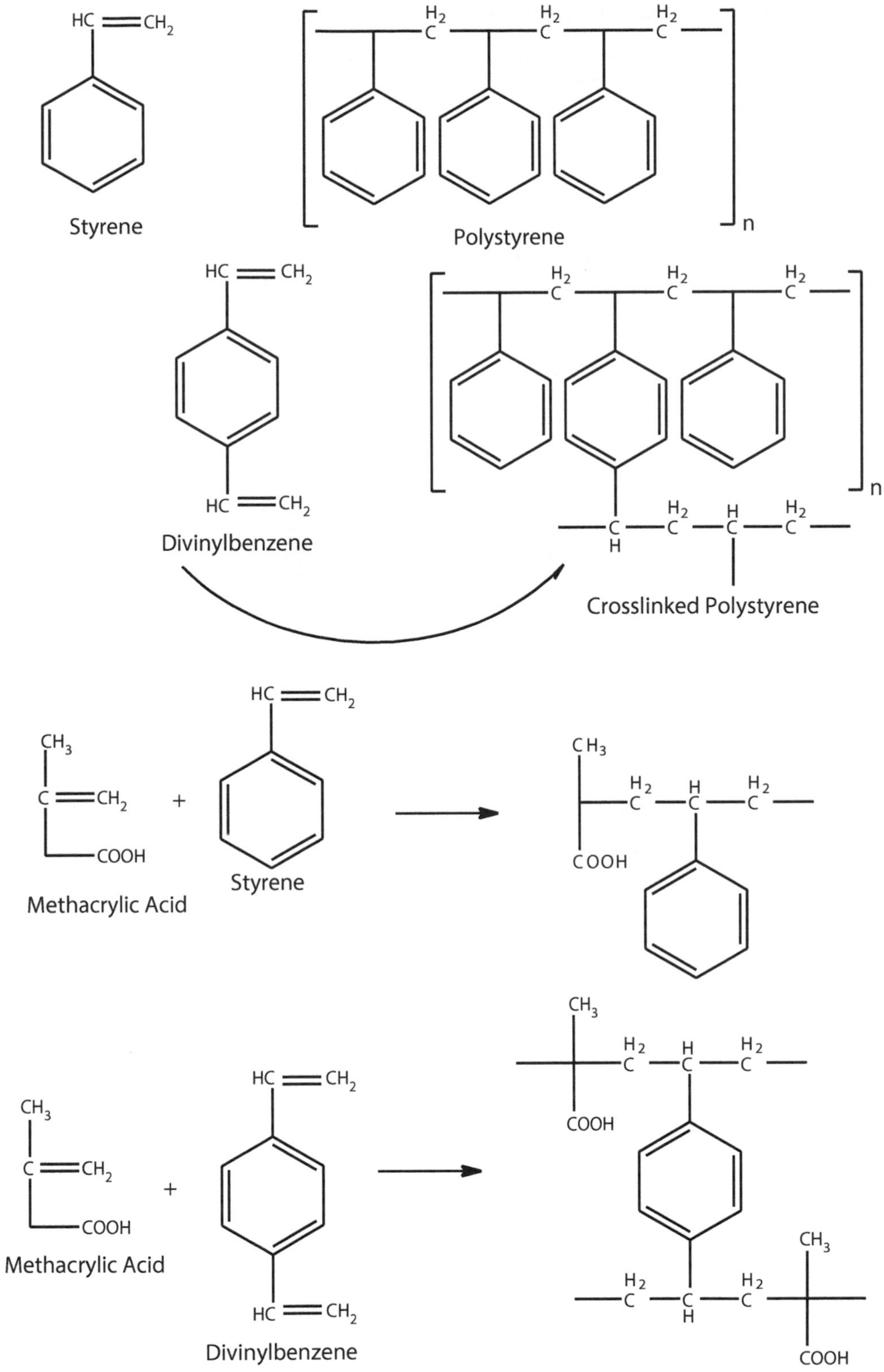

FIGURE 2 Preparation of synthetic ion exchange resins. The figure shows the chemistry for the preparation of resin matrix use for the preparation of strong anion exchange (SAX) (Figure 2), weak anion exchange (WAX), and strong cation exchange (SCX) resins (Figure 3). A weak cation exchange resin (WCX) is shown in this figure. Styrene is the precursor chemical which is polymerized to form polystyrene, a plastic. The use of divinylbenzene permits the formation of a cross-linked polystyrene matrix. The degree of cross-linkage influences resin performance (Kunin, R., *Ion Exchange Resins*, ed. R.E. Krieger, Huntington, New York, 1972). Shown at the bottom is the use methacrylic acid with either styrene or divinylbenzene to prepare a weak cation exchange (WCX) resin based on carboxylic acid functional groups (Paul, C.N., Synthesis of ion-exchange resins, *Ann. N. Y. Acad. Sci.* 57, 67–78, 1953; Stenholm, A., Lindgren, H., and Shaffie, J., Comparison of amine-selective properties of weak and strong cation-exchangers, *J. Chromatog.* 1128, 73–78, 2006).

General References for Chromatography

Chromatography A Laboratory Handbook of Chromatographic and Electrophoretic Methods, ed. E. Heftmann, Van Nostrand Reinhold, New York, 1975.

Encyclopedia of Chromatography, 2nd edn., ed. J. Cazes, Marcel Dekker, New York, 2001.

Encyclopedia of Chromatography, 3nd edn., ed. J. Cazes, CRC Press, Boca Raton, FL, 2010.

Kitchener, J.A., *Ion-Exchange Resins*, London, United Kingdom, 1957.

Liquid Chromatography Fundamentals and Instrumentation, eds. S. Fanai, P.R. Haddad, C.F. Poole, P. Schoenmakers, and D.Lloyd, Elsevier, Netherland, 2013.

Patterson, R., *An Introduction to Ion Exchange*, Heyden/Sadtler, London, United Kingdom, 1970.

Romand, S., Rudaz, S., and Guillarme, D., Separation of substrates and closely related glucuronide metabolites using various chromatographic media, *J. Chromatog. A* 1435, 54–65, 2016.

References for Table 2

1. Jungbauer, A. and Hahn, R., Ion-exchainge chromatography, *Methods Enzymo.* 463, 349–371, 2009.
2. Cook, K. and Thayer, J., Advantages of ion exchange chromatography for oligonucleotide analysis, *Bioanalysis* 3, 1109–1120, 2011.
3. Fekete, S., Beck, A., Veuthy, J.L., and Guillarme, D., Ion-exchange chromatography for the characterization of biopharmaceuticals, *J. Pharm. Biomed. Anal.* 10, 43–55, 2015.
4. Abbott, S.R., Practical aspects of normal-phase chromatography, *J. Chromatog. Sci.* 18, 540–550, 1980.
5. Fallon, A., Booth, R.F.G., and Bell, L.D., High performance normal phase chromatography, in *Applications of HPLC in Biochemistry*, Elsevier, Amsterdam, Netherlands, 1987.
6. Rabel, F.M., Normal-phase chromatography, in *Encylopedia of Chromatography*, ed. J. Cazes, pp 550–553, New York, Marcel Dekker, 2001.
7. Lobrutto, R., Normal-phase stability packings, in *Encyclopedia of Chromatography*, ed. J. Cazes, pp. 553–556, New York, Marcel Dekker, 2001.
8. Borówko, M. and Ościk-Mendyk, B., Adsorption model for retention in normal-phase liquid chromatography with ternary mobile phases, *Adv. Colloid Interface Sci.* 118, 113–124, 2005.
9. Darlington, A.M. and Gibbs-Davis, J.M., Bimodal or trimodal? The influence of Starling pH on site identity and distribution at low salt aqueous/silica interface, *J. Phys. Chem.* 199, 16560–16567.
10. Köhler, J., Chase, D.B., Farlee, R.D., Vega, A.J., and Kirkland, J.J., Comprehensive characterization of some silica-based stationary phase for high-performance liquid chromatography, *J. Chromatog.* 352, 275–305, 1986.
11. Pesek, J.J., Matyska, M.T., Boysen, R.I., Yang, Y., and Hearn, M.T.W., Aqueous normal-phase chromatography using silica-hydrid-based stationary phases, *TRAC* 42, 64–73, 2013.
12. Soukup, J., Janás, P., and Jandera, P., Gradient elution in aqueous normal-phase chromatography on hydrosilated silica-based stationary phases, *J. Chromatog. A* 1286, 111–118, 2013.
13. Soukup, J. and Jandera, P., Adsorption of water from aqueous acetonitrile on silica-based stationary phases in aqueous normal-phase liquid chromatography, *J. Chromatog. A* 1374, 102–111, 2014.
14. Borlan, S., Rychlicki, G., Mayyska, M., Pesek, J., and Buszewski, B., Study of hydration process on silica hydrid surfaces by microcalorimetry and water adsorption, *J. Colloid Interface Sci.* 416, 1551–156, 2014.
15. Soukup, J. and Jandera, P., Comparison of nonaqueous hydrophilic interaction chromatography with aqueous normal-phase chromatography on hydrosilated silica-based stationary phase, *J. Sep. Sci.* 36, 2753–2759, 2013.
16. Pesek, J. and Matyska, M.T., A comparison of two separation modes: HILIC and aqueous normal phase chromatography, *LCGC* 25, 480–490, 2007.

17. Pesek, J.J., Matyska, M.T., Fischer, S.M., and Sana, T.R., Analysis of hydrophilic metabolites by high-performance liquid chromatography-mass spectrometry using siiica hydride-based stationary phase, *J. Chromatog. A* 1204, 49–55, 2008.
18. Deng, Y., Zhang, H., Wu, J.-T., and Olah, T.V., Tandem mass spectrometry with online high-flow reversed phase extraction and normal-phase chromatography on silica columns with aqueous-organic mobile phase for quantitation of polar compounds in biological fluids, *Rapid Commun. Mass Spect.* 19, 2929–2934, 2005.
19. Naidong, W., Shou, W.Z., Addison, T., Maleki, S., and Jiang, X., Liquid chromatography/tandem mass spectrometric bioanalysis using normal-phase columns with aqueous/organic mobile phases – A novel approach of eliminating evaporation and reconstitution steps in 96-well SPE, *Rapid Commun. Mass Spect.* 16, 1965–1973, 2002.
20. Pesek, J.J. and Matyska, M.T., Reversed-phase chromatography: Description and applications, in *Encyclopedia of Chromatography*, ed. J. Cazes, pp. 719–722, Marcel Dekker, New York, 2001.
21. Pesek, J.J. and Matyska, M.T., Reversed-phase stationary phases, in *Encyclopedia of Chromatography*, ed. J. Cazes, pp. 723–725, Marcel Dekker, New York, 2001.
22. Chang, J., Guo, L., Feng, W., and Geng, X., Studies on the correlation of chromatographic behavior of biopolymers between reversed-phase and hydrophobic interaction chromatography. Testing the stoichiometric displacement between biopolymer and displacing agent, *Chromatographia* 32, 589–596, 1992.
23. Ribeiro, J.M.C., Schneider, M., and Guimaraes, J.A., Purification and characterization of prolixin S(nitrophorin 2), the salivary anticoagulant of the blood-sucking bug *Rhodnius prolixus*, *Biochem. J.* 308, 243–249, 1995.
24. Valeja, S.G., Xiu, L., Gregorich, Z.R., et al., Three-dimensional liquid chromatography coupling ion exchange chromatography/hydrophobic interaction chromatography/reverse phase chromatography for effective protein separation in top-down proteomics, *Anal. Chem.* 87, 5363–5371, 2015.
25. Tuzimski, T. and Soczewiński, E., Method development of chromatography, relation-eluent composition relationships and application to the analysis of pesticides, in *High Performance Liquid Chromatography in Pesticide Residue Analysis*, eds. T. Tuzimski and J. Sherma, pp. 77–98, CRC Press/Taylor & Francis, Boca Raton, FL, 2015.
26. Horváth, C., Melander, W., and Molnár, I., Solvophobic interactions in liquid chromatography with nonpolar stationary phases, *J. Chromatog.* 125, 129–156, 1976.
27. Andrzjewska, A., Gritti, F., and Guiochon, G., Investigation of the adsorption mechanism of a peptide in reversed phase liquid chromatography, from pH controlled and uncontrolled solutions, *J. Chromatog. A* 1216, 3992–4004, 2009.
28. Rafferty, J.L., Zhang, L., Siepmann, J.I., and Schure, M.R., Retention mechanism in reversed-phase liquid chromatography: A molecular perspective, *Anal. Chem.* 79, 6551–6558, 2007.
29. Carr, P.W., Dolan, J.W., Dorsey, J.G., Snyder, L.R., and Kirkland, J.J., Contributions to reversed-phase column selectivity III. Column hydrogen-bond basicity, *J. Chromatog. A* 1395, 57–64, 2015.
30. Lascu, I., Abrudan, I., Muresan, L., et al., Salting-out chromatography on unsubstituted Sepharose CL-6B as a convenient method for purifying proteins from dilute crude extracts. Application to horseradish peroxidase, *J. Chromatog.* 357, 436–439, 1986.
31. Kuhn, A.O. and Lederer, M., Adsorption chromatography on cellulose. I. Salting-out chromatography of organic compounds, *J. Chromatog.* 406, 389–404, 1987.
32. Komsta, L., Skibinski, R., Bojarczuk, A., and Radon, M., Salting-out chromatography – A practical review, *Acta Chromatographica* 23, 191–203, 2011.
33. McCue, J.T., Theory and use of hydrophobic interaction chromatography in protein purification applications, *Methods Enzymol.* 463, 405–414, 2009.
34. Xiu, L., Valeja, S.G., Alpert, A.J., Jin, S., and Ge, Y., Effective protein separation by coupling hydrophobic interaction and reverse phase chromatography for top-down proteomics, *Anal. Chem.* 86, 7899–7906, 2014.

35. Chen, B., Peng, Y., Valeja, S.G., et al., Online hydrophobic interaction chromatography-mass spectrometry for top-down proteomics, *Anal. Chem.* 88, 1885–1891, 2016.

36. Jandera, P., Stationary phases for hydrophilic interaction chromatography, their characterization and implementation into multidimensional chromatography concepts, *J. Sep. Sci.* 31, 1421–1437, 2008.

37. Cavazzini, A. and Felinger, A., Hydrophilic interaction liquid chromatography, in *Liquid Chromatography Fundamentals and Instrumentation*, eds. S. Fanai, P.R. Haddad, C.F. Poole, P. Schoenmakers, and D. Lloyd, pp. 105–119, Elsevier, Amsterdam, Netherland, 2013.

38. Gama, M.R., de Costa Silva, R.G., Collins, C.H., and Bottoli, C.B.G., Hydrophilic interaction chromatography, *TRAC Trends Anal. Chem.* 37, 48–60, 2012.

39. Heaton, J.C. and McCalley, D.V., Some factors that can lead to poor peak shape in hydrophilic interaction chromatography, and possibilities for their remediation, *J. Chromatog. A* 1427, 37–44, 2016.

40. Wijekoon, A., Gangoda, M.E., and Gregory, R.B., Characterization and multi-mode liquid chromatographic application of 4-propylaminomethyl benzoic acid bonded silica-A zwitterionic stationary phase, *J. Chromatog. A* 1270, 212–218, 1270.

41. Kumar, A., Heaton, J.C., and McCalley, D.V., Practical investigation of the factors the affect the selectivity of in hydrophilic interaction chromatography, *J. Chromatog. A* 1270, 33–40, 2013.

42. Zauner, G., Deelder, A.M., and Wuhrer, M., Recent advances in hydrophilic interaction liquid chromatography (HILIC) for structural glycomics, *Electrophoresis* 32, 3456–3466, 2011.

43. Isokawa, M., Kanamori, T., Funatsu, T., and Tsundoa, M., Recent advances in hydrophilic interaction chromatography for quantitative analysis of endogenous and pharmaceutical compounds in plasma samples, *Bioanalysis* 6, 2421–2439, 2014.

44. Spagou, K., Tsoukali, H., Raikos, N., et al., Hydrophilic interaction chromatography coupled to MS for metabolomic/metabolomic studies, *J. Sep. Sci.* 33, 716–727, 2010.

45. García-Cañaveras, J.C., López, S., Castell, J.V., et al., Extending metabolome coverage for untargeted metabolite profiling of adherent cultured hepatic cells, *Anal. Bioanal. Chem.* 408, 1217–1230, 2016.

46. Alpert, A.J., Electrostatic repulsion hydrophilic interaction chromatography for isocratic separation of charged solutes and selective isolation of phosphopeptides, *Anal. Chem.* 80, 62–70, 2008.

47. Zhang, H., Guo, T., Li, X., et al., Simultaneous characterization of glyco- and phosphoproteomes of mouse brain membrane proteome with electrostatic repulsion hydrophilic interaction chromatography, *Mol. Cell. Proteomics* 9, 635–647, 2010.

48. Tze-Yang, N., Piliang, H., and Sie Kwan, S., The use of electrostatic repulsion-hydrophilic interaction chromatography (ERLIC)for proteomics research, *Mass Spect. Lett.* 5, 95–103, 2014.

49. Kyte, J., Counting polypeptides, in *Structure of Protein Chemistry*, 2nd edn., pp. 407–449, Garland Science/Taylor and Francis, New York, 2007.

50. Dublin, P., Electrostatic effects, in *Aqueous Size Exclusion Chromatography*, ed. P. Dublin, pp. 55–75, Elsevier, Amsterdam, Netherlands, 1988.

51. Janado, M., Partitioning: Hydrophobic interactions, in *Aqueous Size Exclusion Chromatography*, ed. P. Dublin, pp. 23–54, Elsevier, Amsterdam, Netherlands, 1988.

52. Chen, X. and Ge, Y., Ultrahigh pressure fast size exclusion chromatography for top-down proteomics, *Proteomics* 13, 2563–2566, 2013.

53. Pacco, J.M. and Mukherji, A.K., Determination of polychlorinated biphenyls in a polymer matrix by gel permeation chromatography using micro-Styragel® columns, *J. Chromatog.* 144, 113–117, 1977.

54. Meehan, E., Semirigid polymer gels for size-exclusion chromatography, in *Handbook of Size Exclusion Chromatography*, 2nd edn., ed. C.-S. Wu, pp. 25–44, Marcel Dekker, New York, 2004

55. Prokai, L., Stevens, S.M., Jr., and Simonsick, W.J., Jr., Size-exclusion chromatography coupled to mass spectrometry and tandem mass spectrometry for oligomer analysis, *ACS Symp. Ser.* 895, 196–207, 2005.

56. Mari, S. and Barth, H.G., Synthetic Polymers, in *Size Exclusion Chromatography*, pp. 131–153, Springer-Verlag, Berlin, Germany, 1999.

57. Gilberg, R.G., Size-separation characterization of starch and glycogen for biosynthesis-structure-property relationships, *Anal. Bioanal. Chem.* 399, 1425–1438, 2011.

58. Tan, X., Sullivan, M.A., Gao, F., et al., A new non-degradative method to purify glycogen, *Carbohydrate Polymers* 147, 165–170, 2016.

59. Levin, Ö., Column chromatography of proteins: Calcium phosphate, *Methods Enzymol.* 5, 27–32, 1962.

60. Main, R.K., Wilkins, M.J., and Cole, L.J., A modified calcium phosphate for column chromatography of polynucleotides and proteins, *J. Am. Chem. Soc.* 81, 6490–6495, 1959.

61. Siegelman, H.W., Wieczorek, G.A., and Turner, B.C., Preparation of calcium phosphate for protein chromatography, *Anal. Biochem.* 13, 402–404, 1965.

62. Cummings, L.J., Snyder, M.A., and Brisack, K., Protein chromatography on hydroxyapatite columns, *Methods Enzymol.* 463, 387–404, 2009.

63. Gagnon, P., Improved antibody aggregate removal by hydroxyapatite chromatography in the presence of polyethylene glycol, *J. Immunol. Methods* 336, 222–228, 2008.

64. Cummings, L.J., Hydroxyapatite chromatography: Purification strategies for recombinant proteins, *Methods Enzymol.* 541, 67–83, 2014.

65. Saito, M., Yoshitake, T., and Okuyama, T., Separation and analysis of charged isomers of monoclonal immunoglobulin G by ceramic hydroxyapatite chromatography, *Prep. Biochem. Biotechnol.* 46, 215–221, 2016.

66. Freitag, R. and Hilbrig, F., Isolation and purification of recombinant proteins, antibodies and plasmid DNA with hydroxyapatite chromatography, *Biotechnol. J.* 7, 90–102, 2012.

67. Pinto, G., Caira, S., Mamone, G., et al., Fractionation of complex lipid mixtures by hydroxyapatite chromatography for lipidomics purposes, *J. Chromatog.* 1360, 82–92, 2014.

68. Block, H., Maertens, B., Spriestersbach, A., et al., Immobilized-metal affinity chromatography (IMAC): A review, *Methods Enzymol.* 463, 439–473, 2009.

69. Bi, C., Beeram, S., LI, Z., Zheng, X., and Hage, D.S., Kinetic analysis of drug-protein interactions by affinity chromatography, *Drug Discov. Today Technol.* 17, 16–21, 2015.

70. Li, Z., Beeram, S.R., Bi, C., et al., High-performance affinity chromatography: Applications in drug-protein binding studies and personalized medicine, *Adv. Protein Chem. Struct. Biol.* 102, 1–39, 2015.

71. *Handbook of Affinity Chromatography*, ed. D.S. Hage, CRC Press/Taylor & Francis Group, Boca Raton, FL, 2006.

72. *Affinity Chromatography Methods and Protocols*, ed. S. Reichelt, Springer/Humana, New York, 2015.

73. Berger, T.A. and Wilson, W.H., Packed column supercritical fluid chromatography with 220 000 plates, *Anal. Chem.* 65, 1451–1455, 1992.

74. Khater, S., West , C., and Lesellier, E., Characterization of five chemistries and three particle sizes of stationary phases used in supercritical fluid chromatography, *J. Chromatog. A* 1319, 148–159, 2013.

75. Aasberg, D., Enmark, M., Samuelsson, J., and Fornstedt, T., Evaluation of co-solvent fraction, pressure and temperature effects in analytical and preparative supercritical fluid chromatography, *J. Chromatog. A* 1374, 254–260, 2014.

76. de Mas, N., Natalie, K., Quiroz, F., et al., A partial classical resolution/preparative chiral supercritical fluid chromatography method for the rapid preparation of the pivotal intermediate in the synthesis of two nonsteroidal glucocorticoid receptor modulators, *Org. Process Res. Dev.* 20, 934–939, 2016.

77. *Supercritical Fluids. Fundamentals and Applications*, eds. E. Kiran, P.G. Debenedetti, and C.J. Peters, Kluwer Academic, Dordrecht, Netherlands, 2000.

78. *Modern Extraction Techniques. Food and Agricultural Samples*, ed. C. Turner, Oxford University Press/American Chemical Society, Washington, DC, 2006.

79. Jones, M.D., Rainville, P.D., Isaac, G., et al., Ultra high resolution SFC-MS as a high throughput platform for metabolic phenotyping: Application to metabolic profiling of rat and dog bile, *J. Chromotag. B. Analyt. Technol. Biomed. Life Sci.* 966, 200–207, 2014.

80. Taguchi, K., Fukusaki, E., and Bamba, T., Supercritical fluid chromatography/mass spectrometry in metabolite analysis, *Bioanalysis* 6, 1679–1689, 2014.

81. Desfontaine, V., Guiillarme, D., Francotte, E., and Nováková, L., Supercritical fluid chromatography in pharmaceutical analysis, *J. Pharmaceut. Biomed. Analysis* 113, 56–71, 2015.

82. Lemasson, E., Bertin, S., and West, C., Use and practice of achiral and chiral supercritical fluid chromatography in pharmaceutical analysis and purification, *J. Sep. Sci.* 39, 212–233, 2016.

Table 3: Multidimensional chromatographic systems[a]

Chromatographic system	Use	References
RP-RP[b] Two C_{18} columns with the first run under basic conditions (ammonium formate with acetonitrile step gradient) and second under acid conditions (trifluoroacetic acid with acetonitrile gradient). Analysis was performed on tryptic peptides (bottom-up proteomics).	Detection of host cell protein impurities in monoclonal antibodies	1
RP-SCX-RP C_{18} (basic conditions) followed by strong cation-exchange (SCX)[c] followed by C_{18} column (acid conditions). These investigators also used high pH RP followed by low pH RP	Peptide analysis is shotgun proteomics	2
Silica column with n-hexane/isopropanol followed by a cellulose-based chiral column[d] in the same solvent	Determinations of chiral coumarins and furocoumarins in *Citrus* essential oils	3
A biphasic column consisting of a SCX column packed above a C_{18} matrix (RP) is used to separate peptides. Stepwise elution is used to elute a discrete group of peptides which are then fractionated on the C_{18} column for subsequent analysis by mass spectrometry	This is an "online" process where there is no separate transfer of sample with direct application to the mass spectrometry. This concept was named multidimensional protein identification technology (MudPIT). After the salt fraction is eluted from the SCX column on the RP column, the initial solvent for the RP step (0% B) is used to remove the salt prior to use of the RP gradient. A second salt elution step then elutes more peptides onto the RP column. The single column reduces sample loss.	4
A triphasic column consisting of an RP, an SCX, and a RP segment	Direct loading of sample on triphasic column reduces sample loss when compared to a biphasic column and a separate RP column	5
SCX column coupled with RP (C_{18}) for protein identification	Rat liver homogenate subjected to chromatography on SCX column (first phase) with discrete fractions collected and chromatographed on a RP column. High abundance proteins ($A_{215} > 0.1$) were digested with trypsin and analysis by MS/MS. Fractions with $A_{215} < 0,1$ were subjected to further RP fractionation and MS/MS.	6
RP(C_{18}) followed by carboxymethylated β-cyclodextran bonded to silica	Separation of flavanone-7-*O*glycoside diastereomers in citrus juice	7
Comparison of SCX with isoelectric focusing (IEF) for first step followed by RP with analysis by MS (LC-MS)[e]	Shotgun proteomics[f] analysis of adenocarcinoma tissue found IEF superior for peptide prefractionation prior to LC-MS.	8
Albumin affinity column followed by Protein G column followed by target affinity column with RP (styrene-divinyl benzene) column for a trap.	Clusterin was purified from plasma. Albumin and IgG were removed by tandem affinity columns. Clusterin was captured from depleted plasma samples by an affinity column and collected in the effluent with a reversed phase column. Final characterization of the clusterin was performed by electrophoresis.	9
First phase with a bonded silica matrix (cyano and C_8) and a second phase of a C_{18} matrix.	The first phase is a bonded silica phase in an SDS containing solvent; the first phase serves as capture step for drug substances with a second phase in a C_{18} matrix in as SDS buffer serving as the analytical step. SDS is described a micellar modifier for the two systems._	10
C_{18} capture followed by derivatization with a second column phenylhexyl silica column	Determination of ursodeoxycholic acid and the glycine-conjugate of ursodeoxycholic acid in serum by initial capture with a C_{18} matrix followed by derivatization with phenacyl bromide. A phenylhexyl silica column (RP) is used for analysis of the derivatives.	11
Anion-exchange chromatography followed by anion exchange for solutes not retained by anion exchange chromatography or anion exchange chromatography for solutes retained by the initial anion exchange column	Identification of water-soluble arsenic compounds. An anion exchange column (DEAE-A25 Sephadex®) was used as the initial capture step. Solutes not retained on this column were chromatographed on an SCX column Solutes retained on the initial anion exchange column were chromatographed on a trimethylamine silica column.	12

[a] Multidimensional chromatography refers to the use of two or more separate steps or columns in the chromatographic fractionation of a sample. In some studies, an electrophoretic step may provide a separate fractionation step. The important point is that there are two or more physically separate orthogonal fractionation steps.

[b] RP, reversed phase; SCX, strong cation-exchange.

[c] SCX is polysulfoethyl A™, a silica-based matrix with a bonded polymer, poly(2-sulfoethylaspartamide).

[d] Astec cellulose dimethylphenylcarbamate (Ikeda, K., Hamasaki, T., Kohno, H., et al., Direct separation of enantiomers by reversed-phase high performance liquid chromatography on cellulose tris (3,5-dimethylphenylcarbamate), *Chem. Lett.*, 6, 1089–1090, 1989).

[e] LC-MS is C_{18} liquid chromatography followed by mass spectrometry.

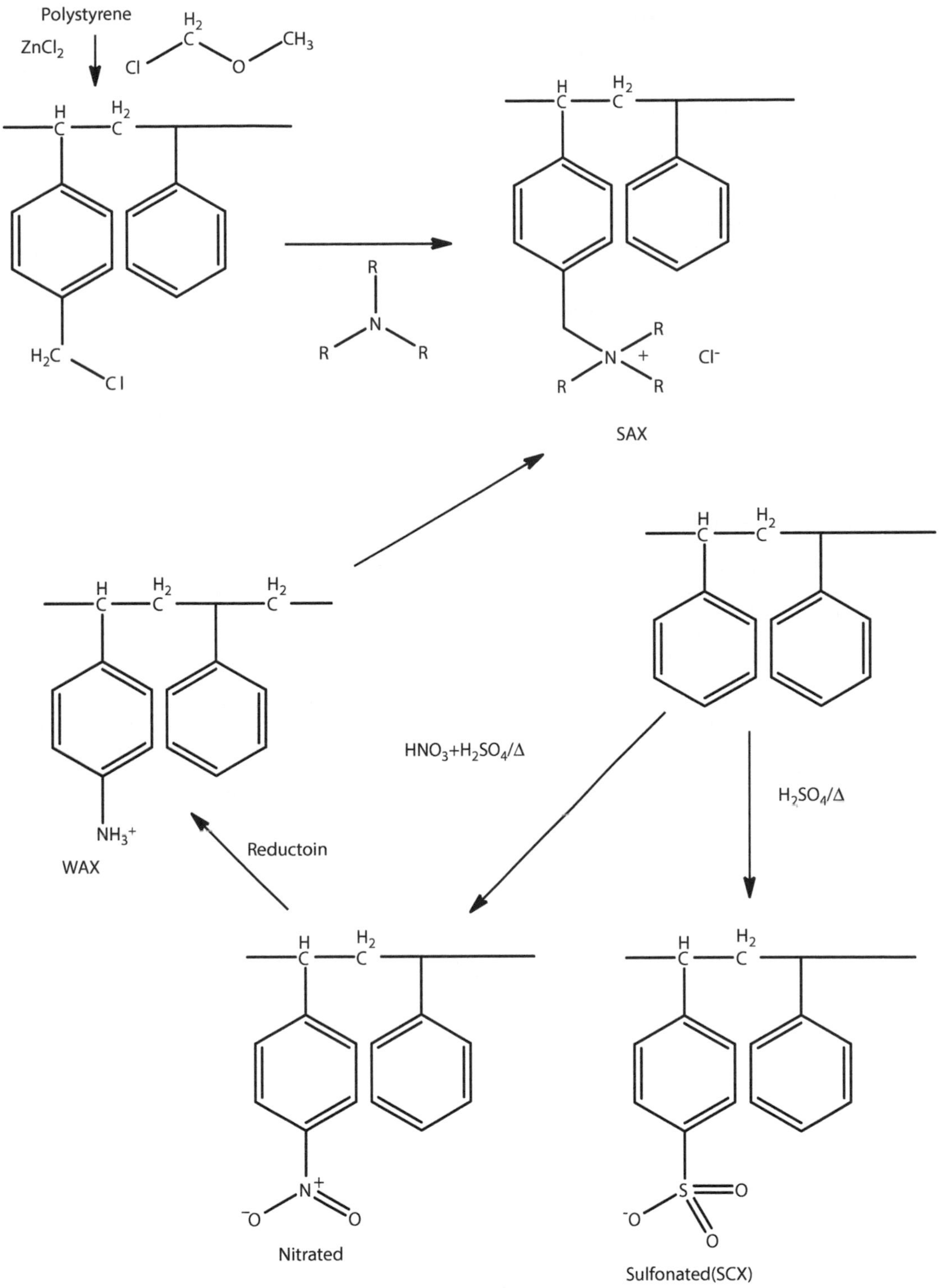

FIGURE 3 Functional groups present on ion exchange resins. With the exception of the carboxylic acid resins (Figure 2), the functional groups have to be added to the ion exchange resin prepared as described in Figure 2. The reaction shown depicts the sulfonation of polystyrene which is crosslinked (Figure 2) to yield a strong cation exchange (SCX) resin such as BioRad AG50 (Strehlow, F.W.E., Victor, A.H., van Zyl, C.R., and Eloff, C., Distribution coefficients and cation exchange behavior of elements in hydrochloric acid-acetone, *Anal. Chem.* 43, 870–876, 1971; Khym, J.X., *Analytical Ion-Exchange Procedures in Chemistry and Biology Theory, Equipment, Techniques,* Prentice-Hall, Englewood Cliffs, NJ, 1974). Concentrated sulfuric acid is used for the sulfonation reaction. Also shown is the nitration of polystyrene with nitric acid (Phillippides, A., Budd, P.M., Price, C., and Cucliffe, A.V., The nitration of polystyrene, *Polymer* 34, 3509–3513, 1993) can use nitric acid, a nitrating mixture (38% nitric acid and 61% sulfuric acid + water). There is an alternative procedure using a mixture of nitric oxide (NO) and nitrogen peroxide (NO_2) (Sinha, S. and Kumar, A., Preparation of high capacity chloroethylated strong base anion exchange resin using NO_x, *Separation Sci. Technol.* 37, 895–918, 2002). The nitro group can be reduced to produce an amine derivative (WAX) which can be alkylated to yield a SAX.

General References for Multidimensional Chromatography

Dugo, P., Cacciola, F., Kumm, T, Dugo, G., and Mondello, L., Comprehensive multidimensional liquid chromatography: Theory and applications, *J. Chromatogr.* 1183, 353–368, 2008.

Franco, M.S., Padovan, R.N., Fumes, B.H., and Lancas, F.M., An overview of multidimensional liquid phase separations in food analysis, *Electrophoresis* 37, 1768–1783, 2016.

Horvatovich, P., Hoekman, B, Govorukhina, N., and Bischoff, R., Multidimensional chromatography coupled to mass spectrometry in analyzing complex proteomic samples, *J. Sep. Sci.* 33, 1421–1437, 2010.

Kitz, P. and Radke, W., Application of two-dimensional chromatography to the characterization of macromolecules and biomacromolecules, *Anal. Bioanal. Chem.* 407, 193–215, 2015.

Stoll, D.R., O'Neill, K., and Harmes, D.C., Effects of pH mismatch between the two dimensions of reversed phase x reversed phase two-dimensional separations on second dimension separation quality for ionogenic compounds – I. Carboxylic acids, *J. Chromatog. A* 1383, 25–34, 2015.

References to Table 3

1. Doneanu, C.E., Anderson, M., Williams, B.J., et al., Enhanced detection of low-abudance host cell protein impurities in high-purity monoclonal antibodies down to 1 ppm using ion mobility mass spectrometry coupled with multidimensional liquid chromatography, *Anal. Chem.* 87, 10283–10291, 2015.
2. Law, H.C.H., Kong, R.P.W., Szeto, S.S.W., et al., A versatile reversed phase-strong cation exchange -reversed phase (RP-SCX-RP) multidimensional liquid chromatography platform for qualitative and quantitative shotgun proteomics, *Analyst* 140, 1237–1252, 2015.
3. Dugo, P., Russo, M., Sarò, M., et al., Multidimensional liquid chromatography for the determination of chiral coumarins and furo-coumarins in *Citrus* essential oils, *J. Sep. Sci.* 35, 1828–1836, 2012.
4. Link, A.J., Eng, J., Schieltz, D.M., et al., Direct analysis of protein complexes using mass spectrometry, *Nat. Biotechnol.* 17, 676–682, 1999.
5. Magdeldin, S., Moresco, J.J., Yamamoto, T., and Yates, J.R., III, Off-line liquid chromatography and auto sampling result in sample loss in LC/LC-MS/MS, *J. Proteome Res.* 13, 3826–3836, 2014.
6. Gao, M., Zhang, J., Deng, C., et al., Novel strategy of high-abundance protein depletion using multidimensional liquid chromatography, *J. Proteome Res.* 5, 2653–2860, 2006.
7. Aturki, Z., Brandi, V., and Sinibaldi, M., Separation of flava-none-7-O-glycoside diastereomers and analysis in citrus juices by multidimensional liquid chromatography coupled with mass spectrometry, *J. Agr. Food Chem.* 52, 5303–5308, 2004.
8. Slebos, R.J., Brock, J.W.C., Winters, N.F., et al., Evaluation of strong cation exchange versus isoelectric focusing of peptides for multidimensional liquid chromatography-tandem mass spectrometry, *J. Proteome Res.* 7, 5286–5294, 2008.
9. Tous, F., Bones, J., Iliopoulos, O., Hancock, W.S., and Hincapie, M., Multidimensional liquid chromatography platform for profiling alterations of clusterin N-glycosylation in the plasma of patients with renal cell carcinoma, *J. Chromatog. A* 1256, 121–128, 2012.
10. Posluszny, J.V. and Weinberger, R., Determination of drug substance in biological fluids by direct injection multidimensional liquid chromatography with a micellar cleanup and reversed-phase chromatography, *Anal. Chem.* 60, 1953–1958, 1988.
11. Choi, S.J., Jeong, C.K., Lee, H.M., et al., Simultaneous determination of ursodeoxycholic acid and its glycine-conjugate in serum as phenacyl esters using multidimensional liquid chromatography, *Chromatographia* 50, 96–100, 1999.
12. McSheehy, S. and Mester, Z., Arsenic speciation in marine certified reference materials Part 1. Identification of water-soluble arsenic species using multidimensional liquid chromatography combined with inductively coupled plasma, electrospray and electrospray high-field asymmetric waveform ion mobility spectrometry with mass spectrometry detection, *J. Anal. Atom. Spectrom.* 19, 373–380, 2004.

TABLE 4: Multimodal Chromatography[a]

Chromatographic systems	Use	References
A C_8 substituent and either phenylsulfonyl or phenyltrimethylamine were bonded to a silica matrix followed by end capping (Figure 4)[1]	Separation of oligonucleotides, DNA fragments[2] and various drugs[3]	1–3
HILIC with a β-cyclodextrin structure bonded to a silica matrix or a covalently bonded macrocyclic antibiotic	Chiral separation of drug substances and amino acids by HILIC.	4
Arginine as an effective eluotropic agent in multimodal chromatography	It is suggested that arginine is an eluotropic agent from a multiple mode column with 4-mercaptoethylpyridine (Figure 5) as the ligand[5] as well as for columns with Capto™ MMC (Figure 5) as the ligand.[6]	5,6
Capto™ MMC resin[b] (Figure 5) with pH gradient	A pH gradient is shown to be more effective than a salt gradient in improving resolution of proteins on a Capto™ MMC resin	7
Capto™ adhere resin[c] (Figure 5) with a salt gradient	Single stranded DNA could be separated from double stranded DNA. The order of elution was poly(dA), poly(dC),poly(dG),poly (dT)	8
Capto™ adhere resin with stepwise salt elution	Separation of plasmid DNA topoisomers (supercoiled and open circular)	9
Capto™ MMC resin	Capture of VEGF from conditioned media from a bacterial fermentation with stepwise elution with arginine	10
Capto™S and Capto™MMC resin	Comparison of Capto™ S and Capto™MMC for antibody purification from condition media (CHO cells). Both resins were effective in capturing product from the conditioned media; the Capto™MMC resin appeared to be more selective	11
Capto™ MMC and Nuvia™ cPrime	Comparison of protein (lysozyme and a MAB) adsorption by Capto™MMC and Nuvia™cPrime. Hydrophobic interaction dominates at low pH and electrostatic binding at pH above 6. It is suggested that Nuvia™cPrime has a higher dynamic binding capacity	12

[a] Multimodal chromatography refers to the use of two different mechanisms in the separation of analytes on a single chromatography column. Reversed-phase chromatography and ion-exchange are the two most common mechanisms.
[b] *N*-benzoyl-2-amino-4-mercaptobutyric acid.
[c] *N*-benzoyl-*N*-methylethanolamine.

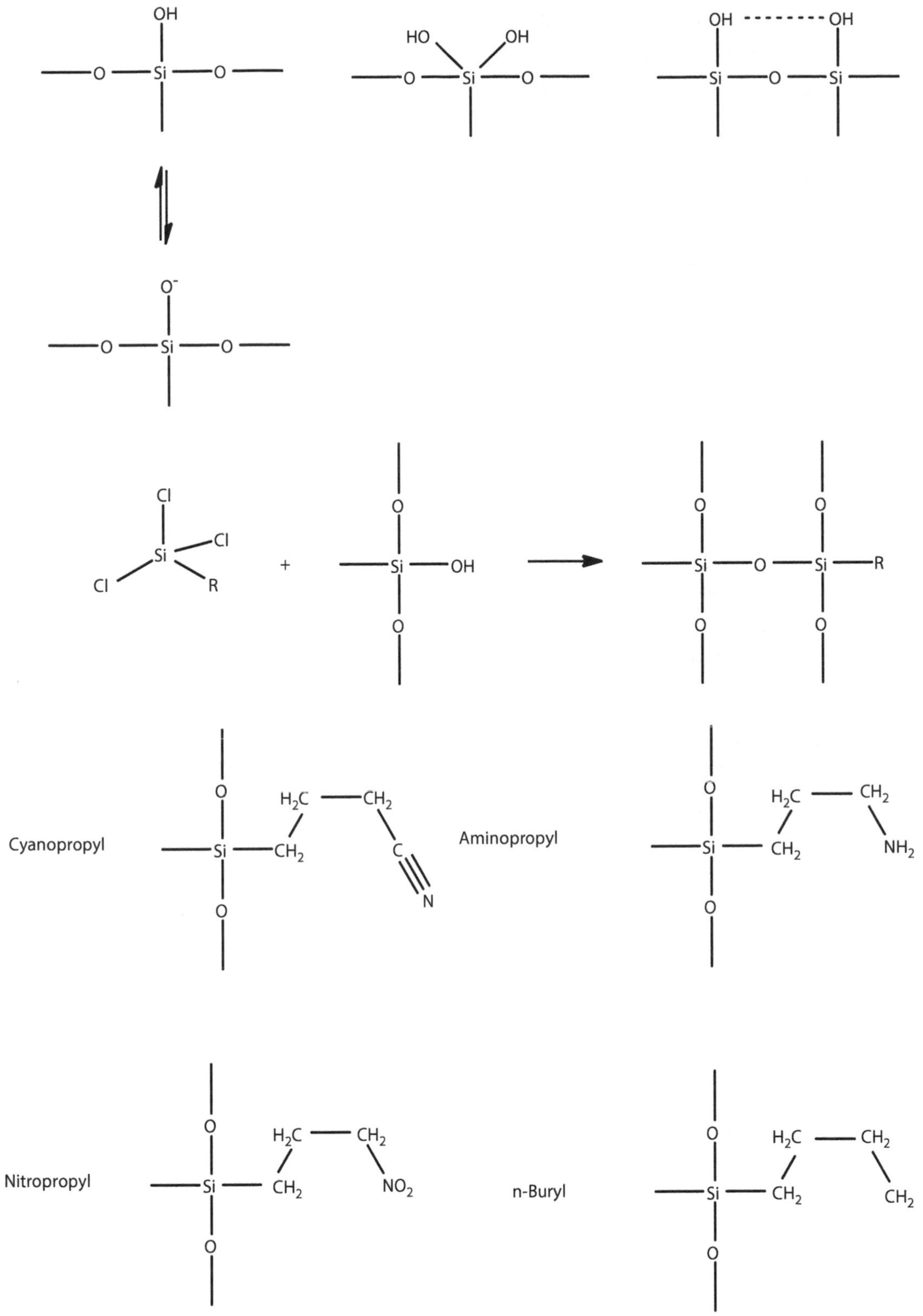

FIGURE 4 Silica-based chromatography matrices. Shown at the top is the structure of various silanol groups. The unmodified silanol hydroxyl is acidic and dissociates to provide a negative charge (Davies, N.H., Euerby, M.R., and McCalley, D.V., Study of overload for basic compounds in reversed-phase high performance liquid chromatography as a function of mobile phase pH, *J. Chromatog. A.* 1119, 11–19, 2006; Dalington, A.M. and Gibbs-Davies, J.M., Bimodal or trimodal? The influence of starting pH on site identify and distribution at the low salt aqueous/silica interface, *J. Phys. Chem.* 119, 16560–16567, 2015). Shown below is the reaction of n-alkyltrichlorosilane with silica gel to prepare an n-alkyl-bonded phase (Pesek, J.J. and Matyska, M.T., Reversed-phase stationary phases, in *Encyclopedia of Chromatography*, ed. J. Cazes, pp. 723–725, Marcel Dekker, New York, 2001). Various silica derivatives are shown which provide stationary phases which can also be used for reverse-phase chromatography. Much of the specificity is derived from the solvent.

General References for Multimodal Chromatography

Chhatre, S., Konstantinidis, S., Ji,Y., et al., The simplex algorithm for the rapid identification of operating conditions during early bioprocess development: Case studies in Fab' precipitation and multimodal chromatography, *Biotechnol. Bioengineer.* 108, 2162–170, 2011.

Heinitz, M.L., Kennedy, L., Kopaciewicz, W., and Regnier, F.E., Chromatography of proteins on hydrophobic interaction and ion-exchange chromatographic matrices: Mobile phase contributions to selectivity, *J. Chromatog. A* 443, 173–182, 1988.

Hou, Y. and Cramer, S.M., Evaluation of selectivity in multimodal anion exchange systems: *A priori* prediction of protein retention and examination of mobile phase modifier effects, *J. Chromatog. A* 1218, 7813–7820, 2011.

Karkov, H.S., Krogh, B.O., Woo, J., et al., Investigation of protein selectivity in multimodal chromatography using *in silico* designed Fab fragment variants, *Biotechnol. Bioengineer.* 112, 2305–2315, 2015.

Kennedy, L.A., Kopaciewicz, W., and Regnier, F.E., Multimodal chromatography columns for the separation of proteins in either the anion exchange or hydrophobic-interaction mode, *J. Chromatog.* 359, 73–84, 1986.

Lee, S.-C. and Whitaker, J.R., Are molecular weights of proteins determined by Superose 12 column chromatography correct?, *J. Agrc. Food Chem.* 52, 4948–4962, 2004.

Melander, W.R., El Rassi, Z., and Horvath, C., Interplay of hydrophobic and electrostatic interactions in biopolymer chromatography effect of salts on the retention of proteins, *J. Chromatog.* 469, 3–27, 1989.

Pujar, N.S. and Zydney, A.L., Electrostatic effects of protein partitioning in size-exclusion chromatography and membrane ultrafiltration, *J. Chromatog. A* 796, 229–238, 1998.

Srinivasan, K., Parimal, S., Lopez, M.M., McCallum, S.A., and Cramer, S.M., Investigation into the molecular and thermodynamic basis of protein interactions in multimodal chromatography using functionalized nanoparticles, *Langmuir* 30, 13205–13215, 2014.

Wolfe, L.S., Barringer, C.P., Mostafa, S.S., and Shukla, A.A., Multimodal chromatography: Characterization of protein binding and selectivity enhancement through mobile phase modulators, *J. Chromatog. A* 1340, 151–156, 2014.

References for Table 4

1. Crowther, J.B. and Hartwick, R.A., Chemically bonded multifunctional stationary phases for high-performance liquid chromatography, *Chromatographia* 16, 349–354, 1982.
2. Floyd, T.R., Cicero, S.E., Fazio, S.D., et al., Mixed-mode hydrophobic ion exchange for the separation of oligonucleotides and DNA fragments using HPLC, *Anal. Biochem.* 154, 570–577, 1986.
3. Lloyd, J.R., Cotter, M.L., Ohori, D., and Oyler, A.R., Mixed-mode column thermospray liquid chromatography/mass spectrometry, *Anal. Chem.* 59, 2533–2534, 1987.

4. Risley, D.S. and Strege, M.A., Chiral separations of polar compounds by hydrophobic interaction chromatography with evaporative light scattering detection, *Anal. Chem.* 72, 1736–1739, 2000.
5. Hirano, A., Maruyama, T., Shiraki, K., Arakawa, T., and Kameda, T., Mechanism of protein desorption from 4-mercaptoethylpyridine resins by arginine solutions, *J. Chromatog. A* 1373, 141–145, 2014.
6. Hirano, A., Arakawa, T., and Kameda, T., Interaction of arginine with Capto MMC in multimodal chromatography, *J. Chromatog. A* 1338, 58–66, 2014.
7. Holsten, M.A., Nikfetrat, A.A.M., Gaga, M., Hirsh, A.G., and Cramer, S.M., Improving selectivity in multimodal chromatography using controlled pH gradient elution, *J. Chromatog. A* 1233, 152–155, 2012.
8. Matos, T., Queiroz, J.A., and Bülow, L., Binding and elution behavior of small deoxyribonucleic acid fragments on a strong anion-exchanger multimodal chromatography resin, *J. Chromatog. A* 1302, 40–44, 2013.
9. Silva-Santo, A.R., Alves, C.P.A., Prazeres, D.M.F., and Azevdo, A.M., Separation of plasmid DNA topoisomers by multimodal chromatography, *Anal. Biochem.* 503, 68–70, 2016.
10. Kaleas, K.A., Schmelzer, C.H., and Pizarro, S.A., Industrial case study: Evaluation of a mixed mode resind for selective capture of a human growth factor recombinantly expressed in *E. coli*, *J. Chromatog. A* 1217, 235–242, 2010.
11. Le Sénéchal, G.J.C., Bégorre, M., Garbay, B., Santarelli, X., and Cabanne, C., Cation exchange versus multimodal cation exchange resins for antibody capture from CHO supernatants: Identification of contaminating host cell proteins by mass spectrometry, *J. Chromatog. B* 942–943, 126–133, 2013.
12. Zhu, M. and Carta, G., Protein adsorption equilibrium and kinetics in multimodal cation exchange resins, *Adsorption* 22, 165–179, 2016.

TABLE 5: Equivalent flows rates for different sized columns[a]

Column ID (mm)	Flow rate (mL/min)
100	480
50	120
25	30
10	4.8
5	1.2
3	0.43
2.0	0.19
1.0	0.05

[a] This was adapted from Buszewski, B. and Bocian, S., Selection of the mode of stationary phases and columns for analysis of pesticides, in *High Performance Liquid Chromatography in Pesticide Analysis*, eds. T. Tuzinski and J. Sharma, pp. 139–166, CRC Press/Taylor & Francis, Boca Raton, FL, 2015.

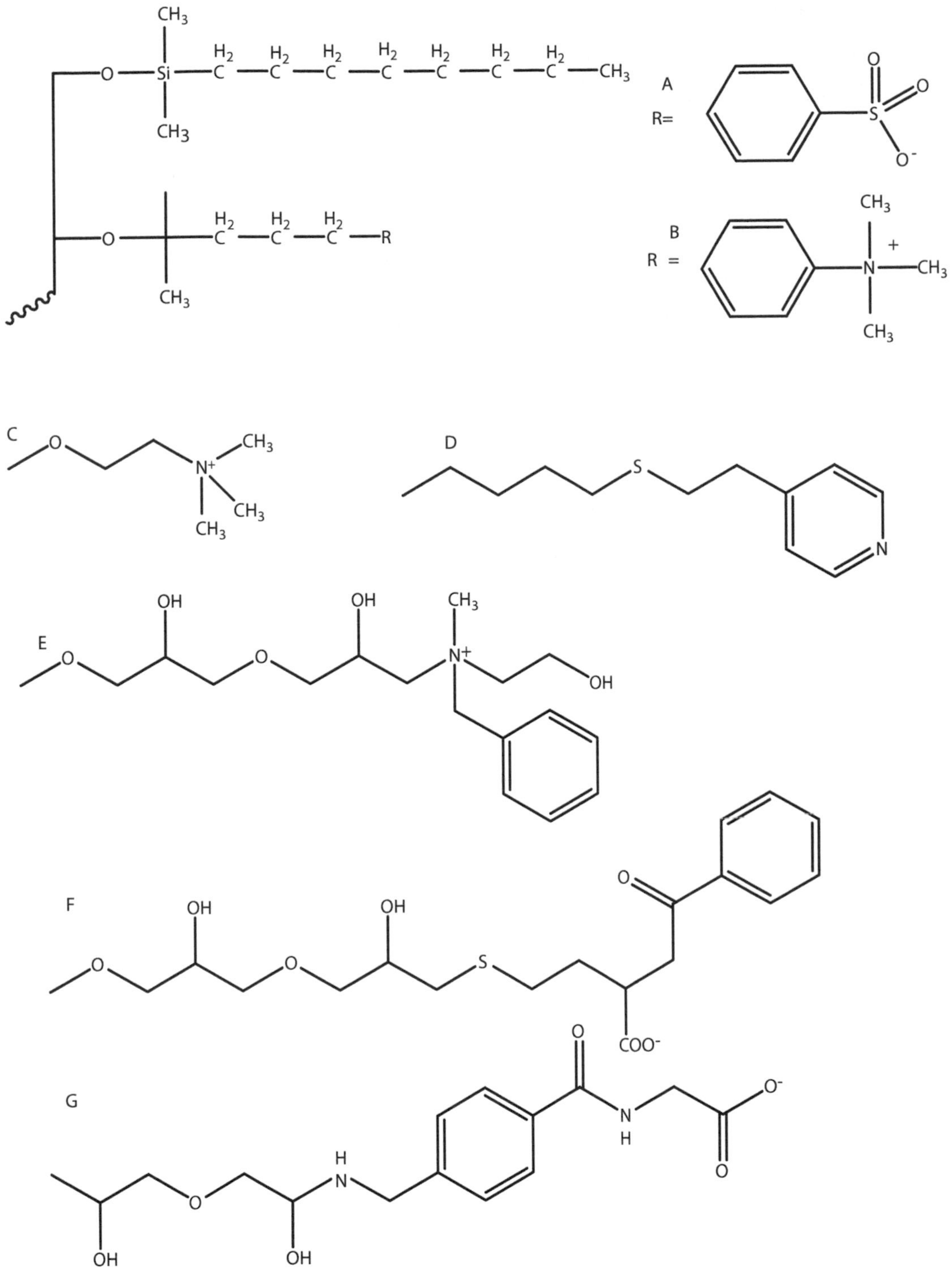

FIGURE 5 Ligands used for multimodal chromatography. Shown are some ligands used for multimodal chromatography. A and B are bound to a silica matrix. D is bound to high porosity cross-linked cellulose; C, E, and F are bound to a crosslinked dextran. A and B represent cation-exchange and anion-exchange multimodal resins including a hydrophobic C_8(octyl function) (Crowther, J.B. and Hartwick, R.A., Chemically bonded multifunctional stationary phases for high-performance liquid chromatography, *Chromatographia* 16, 349–353, 1982); C is Q-Sepharose and E is Capto-adhere(*N*-benzoyl-*N*-methylethanolamine) (Hou, Y. and Cramer, S.M., Evaluation of selectivity in multimodal anion exchange systems: *A priori* prediction of protein retention and examination of mobile phase modifier effects, *J. Chromatog. A* 1218, 7813–7820, 2011); D is 4-mercaptoethylpyrdine (Hirano, A., Maruyama, T., Shiraki, K., Arakawa, T., and Kameda, T., Mechanism of protein desorption from 4-mercaptoethylpyridine resins by arginine solutions, *J. Chromatog. A* 1373, 141–145, 2014) and F is Capto MMC resin (*N*-benzoyl-2-aminobutyric acid) (Holsten, M.A., Nikferrat, A.A.M., Gage, M., Hirsh, A.G., and Cramer, S.M., Improving selectivity in multimodal chromatography using controlled pH gradient elution, *J. Chromatog. A* 1233, 152–155, 2012). G is Nuvia™cPrime where the functional ligand is hippuric acid coupled to the resin. (Yan, J., Zhang, Q.L., Lin, D.Q., and Yao, S.J., Protein adsorption behavior and immunoglobulin separation with a mixed-mode resin based on *p*=hippuric acid, *J. Sep. Sci.* 37, 2474–2480, 2014).

References

1. Martin, A.J. and Synge, R.L., A new form of chromatogram employing two liquid phases 1. A theory of chromatography. 2. Application to the microdetermination of the higher mono-amino-acids in proteins, *Biochem. J.* 35, 1358–1368, 1941.
2. *Encyclopedia of Chromatography*, ed. J. Cazes, Marcel Dekker, New York, 2001.
3. Sarker, S.U. and Nahar, L., Hyphenated techniques, in *Natural Products Isolation*, eds. S.U. Sarkar and L. Nahar, pp. 223–267, Sprinter/Humana, Totowa, NJ, 2005.
4. Theodoridis, G. and Wilson, I.D., Hyphenated techniques for global metabolite profiling, *J. Chromatog. B* 871, 141–142, 2008.
5. Berezkin, V.G., Carrier gas in capillary gas-liquid chromatography, *Adv. Chromatog.* 41, 337–377, 2001.
6. *Practical Gas Chromatography*, eds. K. Dettmer-Wilde and W. Engewald, Springer, Heidelberg, Germany, 2014.
7. Poole, C.F., The column in gas chromatography, in *The Essence of Chromatography*, pp. 79–170, Elsevier, Amsterdam, 2003.
8. Miller, J.M., Gas Chromatography, in *Chromatography Concepts and Contrasts*, 2nd edn., pp. 141–182, Wiley-Interscience, Hoboken, NJ, 2005.
9. Barry, E.F. and Grob, R.L., *Columns for Gas Chromatography Performance and Selection*, Wiley, Hoboken, NJ, 2007.
10. McNair, H.M., Miller, J.M., and Settle, F.A., Capillary columns and inlets, in *Basic Gas Chromatography*, ed. H.M. Mcnair pp. 84–103, Wiley Interscience, Hoboken, NJ, 2009.
11. Arrendale, R.F., Severson, R.F., and Chorytk, O.T., Preparation of fused-silica polar stationary phase wall coated open tubular columns, *J. Chromatog.* 254, 63–68, 1983.
12. Pullarkat, R.K. and Reha, H., Fatty-acid composition of rat brain lipids. Determined by support-coated open-tubular gas chromatography, *J. Chromatog. Sci.* 14, 25–28, 1976.
13. Willis, D.E., Multidimensional gas chromatographic analysis of hexane hydroformylation products using support-coated open tubular columns with column sequence reversal("foreflushing"), *J. Chromatog. Sci.* 24, 417–422, 1986.
14. Hao, Y., Lee, M.L., and Markides, K.E., Charcoal porous layer open tubular column gas chromatography for permanent gas analysis, *J. Microcolumn Sep.* 7, 207–212, 1995.
15. Nesterenko, R.P., Burke, M., de Bosset, C, et al., Monolithic porous layer open tubular (monoPLOT) capillary columns for gas chromatography, *RCS Adv.* 5, 7890–7896, 2015.
16. Poole, C.F. and Lenca, N., Gas chromatography on wall-coated open-tubular columns with ionic liquid stationary phases, *J. Chromatog. A* 1357, 87–109, 2014.
17. Johnson, K.E., What's an ionic liquid?, *Electrochemical Society Interface* 16, 38–41, 2007.
18. McNair, H.M., Miller, J.M., and Settle, E.A., *Basic Gas Chromatography*, Wiley-Interscience, Hoboken, NJ, 2007.
19. Haudebourg, R., Matouk, Z., Zoghlami, E., et al., Sputtered alumina as a novel stationary phase for micro machined gas chromatography columns, *Anal. Bioanal. Chem.* 406, 1245–1247, 2014.
20. Sun, J.H., Guan, F.Y., Zhu, X.F., et al., Micro-fabricated packed gas chromatography column based on laser etching technology, *J. Chromatog. A* 1429, 311–316, 2016.
21. David, M., Nusadji, N.-Y., Labanowski, J., Sternberg, R., and Geffroy-Rodier, C., Pilot for validation of online pretreatments for analyses of organics by gas chromatography-mass spectrometry: Application to space research, *Anal. Chem.* 88, 5137–5144, 2016.
22. Poole, C.F., Alkylsilyl derivatives for gas chromatography, *J. Chromatog. A* 1296, 2–14, 2011.
23. Little, J.L., Artifacts in trimethylsilyl derivatization reactions and ways to avoid them, *J. Chromatog. A* 844, 1–22, 1999.
24. Wells, R.J., Recent advances in non-silylation derivatization techniques for gas chromatography, *J. Chromatog. A* 843, 1–18, 1999.
25. Danielson, N.D., Gallagher, P.A., and Bao, J.J., Chemical reagents and derivatization reactions in drug analysis, in *Encyclopedia of Analytical Chemistry*, ed. R.A. Meyers, Wiley, Chichester, United Kingdom, 2000, 7042–7076.
26. Ferreira, A.M., Laespada, M.E., Pavón, J.L., and Cordero, B.M., *In situ* aqueous derivatization as sample preparation technique for gas chromatographic determinations, *J. Chromatog. A* 1296, 70–83, 2013.
27. Andersson, J.T., Detectors, in *Practical Gas Chromatography*, eds. K. Dettmer-Wilde and W. Engewald, pp. 206–249, Springer, Heidelberg, Germany, 2014.
28. Moeder, M., Gas chromatography-mass spectrometry, in *Practical Gas Chromatography*, eds. K. Dettmer-Wilde and W. Engewald, pp. 303–250, Springer, Heidelberg, Germany, 2014.
29. Lippert, J.A., Xin, B., Wu, N., and Lee, M.L., Fast ultrahigh-pressure liquid chromatography: On-column UV and time-of-flight mass spectrophotometric detection, *J. Microcolumn Sep.* 11, 631–643, 1999.
30. Wu, N., Collins, D.C., Lippert, J.A., Ziang, Y., and Lee, M.L., Ultrahigh pressure liquid chromatography/time-of-flight mass spectrometry for fast applications, *J. Microcolumn Sep.* 12, 462–469, 2000.
31. Majors, R.E. and Hopper, M.S., Studies of siloxane phases bonded to silica gel for use in high-performance liquid chromatography, *J. Chromatog. Sci.* 12, 767–778, 1974.
32. Cox, G.B., Practical aspects of bonded phase chromatography, *J. Chromatog. Sci.* 15, 385–397, 1977.
33. Horvatovich, P., Hoekman, B., Govorukhina, N., and Bischoff, R., Multidimensional chromatography coupled to mass spectrometry in analysing complex proteomics samples, *J. Sep. Sci.* 33, 1421–1437, 2010.
34. Wolfe, L.S., Barringer, C.P., Mostafa, S.S., and Shukla, A.A., Multimodal chromatography: Characterization of protein binding and selectivity enhancement through mobile phase modulators, *J. Chromatog. A* 1340, 151–156, 2014.
35. Heaton, J.C. and McCalley, D.V., Some factors that can lead to poor peak shape in hydrophilic interaction chromatography, and possibilities for their remediation, *J. Chromatog. A* 1427, 37–44, 2016.
36. McCoy, R.W. and Pauls, R.E., Comparison of commercial column types in liquid chromatography, *J. Liquid Chromatog.* 5, 1869–1897, 1982.
37. Matthias, R., Gillet, F., Heege, S., et al., Combined Yamamoto approach for simultaneous estimation of adsorption isotherm and kinetic parameters in ion-exchange chromatography, *J. Chromatog. A* 1413, 68–76, 2015.

BLOTTING TECHNOLOGIES

BLOTTING TECHNOLOGIES IN THE CHARACTERIZATION OF BIOLOGICAL POLYMERS

Technology	Description	References
Southern blotting	The Southern blot is an analytical process by which regions of DNA immobilized on a membrane are identified with a specific probe.[1] Early work used radioactive probes,[1,2] whereas more recent work uses non-radioactive probes such as biotin.[3,4]	1–4
Northern blotting	Northern blotting is an analytical process where RNA is immobilized on a membrane, and specific probes, frequently a labeled DNA, are used to detect specific regions on the RNA.[5–7] The use of northern blots peaks in the middle 1990s and has steadily decreased in use. RT-PCR is more sensitive than a northern blot.[8]	5–8
Western blotting	Western blotting is a technique where protein immobilized on nitrocellulose after transfer from polyacrylamide gel electrophoresis (PAGE) is detected with antibody.[9,10] Current work uses polyvinylidene fluoride (PDVF) membrane in addition to nitrocellulose.[11,12]	9–12
Far-Western blotting	Far-western blotting is a technique related to western blotting where the protein(prey)[a] is immobilized on nitrocellulose[13–15] or polyvinylidene fluoride[15] after separation on PAGE. The prey is then incubated with the bait protein to form a prey–bait complex which is then detected with an anti-bait antibody (e.g., rat monoclonal anti-bait) which is detected with the secondary probe (e.g., peroxidase-labeled goat anti-rat antibody).[13] GST fusion proteins are detected with anti-GST immunoblotting.[14]	13–15
Southwestern blotting	Southwestern blotting is a technique similar to western blotting where the proteins are immobilized on a nitrocellulose or polyvinylidene membrane after separation on PAGE. Specific interactions are identified with labeled DNA oligonucleotide probes.[16–18] Since most DNA probes are based on radioactive phosphate (^{32}P DNA), the use of alkaline phosphatase permits repeated probing of an electrophoretogram.[18]	16–18
Eastern blot	The term *eastern blotting* describes an analytical process where an antibody, usually monoclonal in nature, is used to identify low molecular compounds transferred from thin-layer chromatography plates to nitrocellulose. The antibody is usually detected with a secondary antibody. A far-eastern blot[22] has been described which appears similar to the eastern blot using high-performance thin layer chromatography.[23] Double eastern blotting refers to the use of two antibodies on the same blot.[24]	19–21

[a] A general article on blotting technology (Nicholas, M.W. and Nelson, K., North, south, or east? Blotting techniques, *J. Invest. Dermatol.*, 133, e10, 2013).

[b] The concept of a prey protein and a bait protein is derived from the yeast two-hybrid system where a bait protein is used to identify interactions with a number of potential binding partners referred to as prey proteins expressed in a yeast system (McAliste-Henn, L., Gibson, N., and Panisko, E., Applications of the yeast two-hybrid system, *Methods*, 19, 330–337, 1999; Fashena, S.J., Serebriski, I., and Golemis, E.A., The continued evolution of two-hybrid screening approaches in yeast: how to outwit different preys with different baits *Gene*, 250, 1–14, 2000).

References

1. Southern, E.M., Detection of specific sequences among DNA fragments separated by gel electrophoresis, *J. Mol. Biol.* 98, 503–517, 1975.
2. Cariani, E. and Bréchet, C., Detection of DNA sequences by Southern blot, *Ric. Clin. Lab.* 18, 161–170, 1988.
3. Zavala, A.G., Kulkarni, A.S., and Fortunato, E.A., A dual color Southern blot visualize two genomics or genic regions simultaneously, *J. Virol. Methods* 198, 64–68, 2014.
4. Aravalli, R.N., Park, C.W., and Steer, C.J., Detection of Sleeping Beauty transposition in the genome of host cells by non-radioactive Southern blot analysis, *Biochem. Biophys. Res. Comnun.* 477, 317–328, 2016.
5. Alwine, J.C., Kemp, D.J., and Stark, G.R., Method for detection of specific RNAs in agarose gels by transfer to diazobenzylmethyl-paper and hybridization with DNA probes, *Proc. Natl. Acad. Sci. U. S. A.* 74, 5350–5354, 1977.
6. Rohde, W. and Sänger, H.L., Detection of complementary RNA intermediates of viroid replication by Northern blot hybridization, *Biosci. Rep.* 1, 327–336, 1981.
7. Ferrer, M., Henriet, S., Chamotin, C., Lainé, S., and Mougel, M., From cells to virus particles: Quantitative methods to monitor RNA packaging, *Viruses* 8(8), E239, 2016.
8. Chwetzoff, S. and d'Andrea, S., Ubiquitin is physiologically induced by interferons in luminal epithelium of porcine uterine endometrium in early pregnancy: Global RT-PCR cDNA in place of RNA for differential display screening, *FEBS Lett.* 405, 148–152, 1997.
9. Towbin, H., Staehelin, T., and Gordon, J., Electrophoretic transfer of protein from polyacrylamide gels to nitrocellulose sheets: Procedure and some applications, *Proc. Natl. Acad. Sci. U. S. A.* 76, 4350–4554, 1979.
10. Sixma, J.J., Schiphorst, M.E., Verhoeckx, C., and Jockusch, B.M., Peripheral and integral proteins of human blood platelet membranes α-Actinin is not identical to glycoprotein III, *Biochim. Biophys. Acta* 704, 333–344, 1982.
11. MacPhee, D.J., Methodological considerations for improving western blot analysis *J. Pharmacol. Toxicol. Methods* 61, 171–177, 2010.
12. Taylor, S.C. and Posch, A., The design of a quantitative western blot experiment, *Biomed. Res. Int.* 2014, 362590, 2014.
13. Grässer, F.A., Sauder, C., Haiss, P., et al., Immunological detection of proteins associated with Epstein-Barr virus nuclear antigen 2A, *Virology* 195, 550–560, 1993.
14. Duprez, V., Blank, U., Chrétien, S., Gisselbrecht, S. and Mayeux, P., Physical and functional interaction between p72^{syk} and erythropoietin receptor, *J. Biol. Chem.* 267, 10670–10675, 1998.
15. Wu, Y., Li, Q., and Chen, X.-Z., Detecting protein-protein interactions by far western blotting, *Nat. Protoc.* 2(12), 3278–3284, 2007.
16. Bowen, B., Steinberg, J, Laemmli, U.K., and Weintraub, H., The detection of DNA-binding proteins by protein blotting, *Nucleic Acids Res.* 8, 1–20, 1980.
17. Siu, F.K.Y., Lee, L.T.O., and Chow, B.K.C., Southwestern blotting in investigating transcriptional regulation, *Nat. Protoc.* 3, 51–58, 2008.
18. Jia, Y., Daifeng, J., and Jarrett, H.W., Repeated probing of southwestern blots using alkaline phosphatase stripping, *J. Chromatog. A* 1217, 7177–7181, 2010.
19. Bogdanov, M., Sun, J., Kaback, H.R., and Dowhan, W., A phospholipid acts as a chaperone in assembly of a membrane transport protein, *J. Biol. Chem.* 271, 11615–11618, 1996.

20. Shan, S., Tanaka, H., and Shoyama, Y., Enzyme-linked immuno-sorbent assay for glycyrrhizin using anti-glycyrrhizin monoclonal antibody and an eastern blotting technique for glucuronides of glycyrrhetic acid, *Anal. Chem.* 73, 5784–5790, 2001.

21. Li, X.W., Morinaga, O., Tian, M., et al., Development of an eastern blotting technique for the visual detection of aristolochic acids in *Aristolochia* and *Asarum* species by using a monoclonal antibody against aristolochic acids I and II, *Phytochem. Anal.* 24, 645–653, 2013.

22. Taki, T., Gonzalez, T.V., Goto-Inoue, N., Hayasaka, T., and Setou, M., TLC-blot (Far-Eastern Blot) and its applications, *Methods Mol. Biol.* 536, 545–556, 2009.

23. Rabel, F. and Sherma, J., New TLC/HPTLC commercially prepared and laboratory prepared plates: A review, *J. Liq. Chromatogr. Relat. Technol.* 39, 385–393, 2016.

24. Fujii, S., Morinaga, O., Uto, T., Nomura, S., and Yukihiro, S., Development of double eastern blotting for major licorice components, glycyrrhizin and liquiritin for chemical quality control of licorice using anti-glycyrrhizin and anti-liquiritin monoclonal antibodies, *J. Agric. Food Chem.* 64, 1087–1093, 2016.

OXIDATION OF THIOLS

Roger L. Lundblad

REDOX POTENTIALS OF THIOLS AND RELATED COMPOUNDS[a]

Compound/system	$E^{o\prime}(V)$[b]	Reference	Compound/system	$E^{o\prime}(V)$[b]	Reference
Dithiothreitol	−0.33	1	2,3-Dimercaptopropan-1-ol[g]	−0.298	3
Dithiothreitol	−0.323	2	1.3-Dimercaptopropan-2-ol	−0.279	3
Dithiothreitol	−0.323	3	1,3-Dimercaptopropane	−0.296	3
Dithioerythreitol	−0.319	3	1,4-Dimercaptobutane	−0.328	3
2-Mercaptoethanol	−0.231	2	2,2′-Oxydiethanethiol	−0.314	3
2-Mercaptoethanol	−0.207	3	Glycol dimercaptoacetate	−0.227	3
Cysteine[c]	0.223	2	1,5-Dimercapto-2,4-pentandiol	−0.283	3
Cysteine	−0.21	1	1,6-Dimercapto-2,5-hexanediol	−0.279	3
Cysteine	−0.241	2	Selenocysteine[h]	−0.388	6
Cysteine	−0.22	4	Selenocysteine[h]	−0.488	10
Cysteine	−0.233	5	Selenocysteine[h]	−0.488	5
Selenocysteine[d]	−0.388	6	Selenocystamine[h]	−0.368[i]	11
Tellurocysteine	−0.850[e]	7	Selenocystamine[h]	−0.368[i]	11
Dihydrolipoic acid	−0.288	2	NADPH	−0.327	10
Dihydrolipoic acid	−0.32	4	NADPH	−0.324	12
Dihydrolipoamide (Lipo[red])	−0.288	3	NADH	−0.320	12
Reduced glutathione	−0.244	2	FADH$_2$	−0.283	10
Reduced glutathione	−0.24	4	Thioredoxin	−0.270	11
Reduced glutathione	−0.205	3	Glutaredoxin	−0.233	11
Reduced glutathione	−0.240	5	Tryparedoxin	−0.249	11
Reduced glutathione	−0.407	5	Protein disulfide isomerase	−0.127	11
Thiophenol	−0.31	8	Dsba	−0.125	11
Ergothionine	−0.06	8	Hydrated electron	−2.9	13
Thioredoxin	−0.20	8	Benzenethiol	−0.31	12
NADH$_2$	−0.32	8	Phenylmethylthiol	−0.272	13
Reduced insulin	−0.38[f]	9			

[a] IUPAC definitions and nomenclature (De Bolster, M.W.G., Glossary of terms used in bioinorganic chemistry, *Pure Appl. Chem.*, 69, 1251–1303, 1997).

[b] Shown is the potential as reducing agent. Results obtained at pH(pD) 7.0 unless otherwise indicated versus hydrogen electrode unless otherwise indicated.

[c] Also known as 2-sulfanylethan-1-ol (IUPAC definitions).

[d] Sulfur and selenium are chalcogens. Chalcogen is a term used to describe members of the Group VIa of the periodic table. Tellurium and polonium are other members of this group.

[e] Versus Ag/AgCl electrode; -0.640 for selenocysteine in the same system.

[f] Weitzman suggested that data obtained from polarographic studies (Cecil, R. and Weitzman, P.D.J., The electroreduction of the disulphide bonds of insulin and other proteins, *Biochem. J.*, 93, 1–11, 1964) supports a value of -0.24 to 0.26 volts for reduction potential for various reduced proteins such as RNAse, chymotrypsin, and bovine serum albumin.

[g] Also known as British anti-Lewisite (BAL) which was developed as defense against chemical warfare agents during WWII. It is still used for treatment of heavy metal poisoning and arsenic poisoning (Vilensky, J.A. and Redman, K., British anti-Lewisite (dimercaprol): An amazing history, *Ann. Emerg. Med.*, 41, 378–383, 2003).

[h] There is difficulty in the accurate determination of oxidation/reduction potentials for selenium (Wessjohann, L.A., Schneider, A., Abbas, M., and Brandt, W., Selenium in chemistry and biochemistry in comparison to sulfur, *Biol. Chem.*, 386, 997–1006, 2007).

[i] (SeCya$_{ox}$/2SeCya) (SeCya, selenocystamine).

[j] (Hemiselenocysteine$_{ox}$/cysteine, selenocysteine).

References

1. Cleland, W.W., Dithiothreitol, a new protective reagent for SH groups, *Biochemistry* 3, 482–484, 1964.

2. Rabenstein, D.L., Redox potentials of cysteine residues in peptides and proteins: Methods for their determination, in *Oxidative Folding of Peptides and Proteins*, eds. J. Buchner and L. Moroder, RSC Publishing, Cambridge, United Kingdom, 2009.

3. Szakewski, R.P. and Whitesides, G.M., Rate constants and equilibrium constants for thiol-disulfide interchange reactions involving oxidized glutathione, *J. Am. Chem. Soc.* 102, 2011–2026, 1980.

4. Jocelyn, P.C., The standard redox potential of cysteine-cystine from the thiol-disulphide exchange reaction with glutathione and lipoic acid, *Eur. J. Biochem.* 2, 327–331, 1967.

5. Muttenthaler, M. and Alewood, P.F., Selenocysteine peptides-synthesis, folding and application, in *Oxidative Folding of Peptides and Proteins*, eds. J. Buchner and L. Moroder, pp. 396–418, RSC Publishing, Cambridge, United Kingdom, 2009.

6. Nauser, T., Dockheer, S., Kissner, R., and Koppenol, W.H., Catalysis of electron transfer by selenocysteine, *Biochemistry* 45, 6038–6043, 2006.

7. Liu, X., Silks, L.A., Liu, C., et al., Incorporation of tellurocysteine into glutathione transferase generates high glutathione peroxidase efficiency, *Angew.Chem. Int. Ed.* 48, 2020–2023, 2009.

8. Jocelyn P.C., *Biochemistry of the SH group*, Academic Press, London, United Kingdom, 1972.

9. Weitzman, P.D.J., The standard reduction potential and free energy change of disulfide bonds in proteins, *Biochim. Biophys. Acta* 107, 146–148, 1965.

10. Jacob, C., Giles, G.I., Giles, N.M., and Sies, H., Sulfur and selenium. The role of oxidation state in protein structure and function, *Angew. Chem. Int. Ed.* 42, 4742–4758, 2003.

11. Steinmann, D., Nauser, T., and Koppenol, W.H., Selenium and sulfur in exchange reactions: A comparative study, *J. Org. Chem.* 75, 6696–6699, 2010.

12. Lees, W.J. and Whitesides, G.M., Equilibrium constants for thiol-disulfide interchange reactions: A coherent, corrected set, *J. Org. Chem.* 53, 642–647, 1993.

13. Sibanda, S., Parsons, B.J., Houee-Levin, C., et al., One-electron oxidation and reduction of glycosaminoglycan chloramides: A kinetic study, *Free Rad. Biol. Med.* 63, 126–134, 2013.

Redox Potential

Any oxidation–reduction (redox) reaction can be divided into two half reactions: one in which a chemical species undergoes oxidation and one in which another chemical species undergoes reduction. If a half-reaction is written as reduction, the driving force is the reduction potential. If the half-reaction is written as oxidation, the driving force is the oxidation potential related to the reduction potential by a sign change. So, the redox potential is the reduction/oxidation potential of a compound measured under standard conditions against a standard reference half-cell.

In biological systems, the standard redox potential is defined at pH = 7.0 versus the hydrogen electrode and partial pressure of hydrogen = 1 bar. See also *electrode potential*.

Electrode Potential

The so-called electrode potential of an electrode is defined as the electromotive force (emf) of a cell in which the electrode on the left is a standard hydrogen electrode and the electrode on the right is the electrode in question. See also *redox potential*.

Rate of oxidation of thiols and dithiols

Thiol or Dithiol	Conditions	Rate	Reference
10 μM 2,3-dimercaptopropan-1-ol[a]	50 mM phosphate, pH 7.1, 38°C	9.8×10^{-3} min$^{-1,b}$	1
10 μM 2,3-dimercaptopropan-1-ol[a]	50 mM phosphate, pH 7.1, 38°C; HCN, 5×10^{-4} M	5.6×10^{-3} min$^{-1,b}$	1
10 μM 2,3-dimercaptopropan-1-ol[a]	50 mM phosphate, pH 7.1, 38°C; CuCl$_2$, 2×10^{-4} M	7.8×10^{-2} min$^{-1,b}$	1
10 μM 2,3-dimercaptopropan-1-ol[a]	50 mM phosphate, pH 7.1, 38°C; FeCl$_3$, 2×10^{-4} M	1.6×10^{-2} min$^{-1,b}$	1
10 μM 2,3-dimercaptopropan-1-ol[a]	50 mM phosphate, pH 7.1, 38°C; MnSO$_4$, 2×10^{-4} M	9.8×10^{-3} min$^{-1,b}$	1
10 μM 2,3-dimercaptopropan-1-ol[a]	50 mM phosphate, pH 7.1, 38°C; CoSO$_4$, 2×10^{-4} M	9.8×10^{-3} min$^{-1,b}$	1
10 μM 2,3-dimercaptopropan-1-ol[a]	50 mM phosphate, pH 7.1, 38°C; NiSO$_4$, 2×10^{-4} M	9.8×10^{-3} min$^{-1,b}$	1
10 μM 2,3-dimercaptopropan-1-ol[a]	50 mM phosphate, pH 7.1, 38°C; iron protoporphyrin	1.4×10^{1} min^{-1}	1
20 μM 2,3-dimercaptopropan-1-ol[a]	30 mM phosphate, pH 7.0, 22.4°C; CuCl$_2$, 2×10^{-4} M	6.6×10^{-2} min^{-1}	1
20 μM 1.3-dimercaptopropan-2-ol	30 mM phosphate, pH 7.0, 22.4°C; CuCl$_2$, 2×10^{-4} M	2.7×10^{-2} min^{-1}	1
20 μM 1,3-dimercaptopropane	30 mM phosphate, pH 7.0, 22.4°C; CuCl$_2$, 2×10^{-4} M	2×10^{-3} min^{-1}	1
20 μM 1,5-dimercaptohexane	30 mM phosphate, pH 7.0, 22.4°C; CuCl$_2$, 2×10^{-4} M	1.4×10^{-3} min^{-1}	1
20 μM 1,2,3-dimercaptopropane	30 mM phosphate, pH 7.0, 22.4°C; CuCl$_2$, 2×10^{-4} M	5.6×10^{-3} min^{-1}	1
20 μM 2,3-dimercaptopropylacetate	30 mM phosphate, pH 7.0, 22.4°C; CuCl$_2$, 2×10^{-4} M	5.1×10^{-1} min^{-1}	1
20 μM 2,3-dimercaptopropyl ethyl ether	30 mM phosphate, pH 7.0, 22.4°C; CuCl$_2$, 2×10^{-4} M	4.1×10^{-3} min^{-1}	1
20 μM 3,4-dimercaptobutan-1-ol	30 mM phosphate, pH 7.0, 22.4°C; CuCl$_2$, 2×10^{-4} M	2.3×10^{-3} min^{-1}	1
200 μM Cystamine	50 mM Tris, pH 7.5, 25°C; CuSO$_4$, 40 mM	›1.4 min^{-1}	2
200 μM L-cysteine	50 mM Tris, pH 7.5, 25°C; CuSO$_4$, 40 mM	›1.4 min^{-1}	2
200 μM 2-mercaptoproteomic acid	50 mM Tris, pH 7.5, 25°C; CuSO$_4$, 40 mM	›1.4 min^{-1}	2
200 μM D-penicillamine	50 mM Tris, pH 7.5, 25°C; CuSO$_4$, 40 mM	›1.4 min^{-1}	2
200 μM N-acetylcysteine	50 mM Tris, pH 7.5, 25°C; CuSO$_4$, 40 mM	2.1×10^{-2} min^{-1}	2
200 μM Dithiothreitol	50 mM Tris, pH 7.5, 25°C; CuSO$_4$, 40 mM	6.2×10^{-3} min^{-1}	2
200 μM Reduced glutathione	50 mM Tris, pH 7.5, 25°C; CuSO$_4$, 40 mM	1.5×10^{-2} min^{-1}	2
200 μM Homocysteine	50 mM Tris, pH 7.5, 25°C; CuSO$_4$, 40 mM	1.5×10^{-2} min^{-1}	2
200 μM 2-mercaptoethanol	50 mM Tris, pH 7.5, 25°C; CuSO$_4$, 40 mM	1.1×10^{-2} min^{-1}	2
200 μM 3-mercaptopropionic acid	50 mM Tris, pH 7.5, 25°C; CuSO$_4$, 40 mM	0.14 min^{-1}	2
2-Methcaptoethanol	Methylcob(III)alamine, sodium potassium phosphate, pH 7.0[d]	3×10^{-3} s$^{-1,e}$	3
2-Methcaptoethanol	Adenosylcob(III)alamine, broad pH dependence[d]	3×10^{-3} s^{-1}	3
2-Methcaptoethanol	Cyanocob(III)alamine(Vitamin B$_{12}$), Tris hydrochloride, pH 8.0[d]	8×10^{-2} s^{-1}	3
2-Methcaptoethanol	Aquacob(III)alamine(Vitamin B$_{12a}$), Tris hydrochloride, pH 8.4[d]	1.8×10^{-1} s^{-1}	3
2-Methcaptoethanol	Methylaquacob(III)inamide, sodium carbonate, pH 9–11[d]	5.6×10^{-1} s^{-1}	3
2-Methcaptoethanol	Adenosylaquacob(III)inamide, sodium carbonate, pH 8.9[d]	2.3×10^{-1} s^{-1}	3
2-Methcaptoethanol	Cyanoaquacob(III)inamide, Tris/carbonate, pH 8.5–9.5[d]	191	3
2-Methcaptoethanol	Diaquacob(III)inamide, Tris/carbonate, pH 8.8[d]	211	3
Dithioerythritol	Adenosylcob(III)alamine, broad pH dependence[d]	1×10^{-3} s^{-1}	3
Dithioerythritol	Aquacob(III)alamine (Vitamin B$_{12a}$), sodium potassium phosphate, pH 7.5[d]	6.4×10^{-1} s^{-1}	3
Dithioerythritol	Adenosylaquacob(III)inamide, pH 7.5–9.5[d]	4.6×10^{-1} s^{-1}	3
Dithioerythritol	Diaquacob(III)inamide, sodium potassium phosphate, pH 7.5[d]	725	3
Cysteine	HOSCN[f]	7.8×10^{4} M^{-1} s^{-1}	4
Cysteine	HNOOH	3.8×10^{3} M^{-1} s^{-1}	4
Cysteine	HO$^-$	~4×10^{10} M^{-1} s^{-1}	4
Selenocysteine	HOSCN[f]	1.24×10^{6} M^{-1} s^{-1}	4
Selenocysteine	HNOOH	1.8–4.5×10^{4} M^{-1} s^{-1}	4
Reduced glutathione	HOSCN[f]	2.5×10^{4} M^{-1} s^{-1}	4
Reduced selenoglutathione	HOSCN[f]	5.8×10^{6} M^{-1} s^{-1}	4
Cystamine	HOSCN[f]	7.1×10^{4} M^{-1} s^{-1}	4
Selenocystamine	HOSCN[f]	5.8×10^{6} M^{-1} s^{-1}	

[a] Also known as British anti-Lewisite (BAL) which was developed as defense against chemical warfare agents during WWII. It is still used for the treatment of heavy metal poisoning and arsenic poisoning (Oehme, F.W., British anti-Lewisite (BAL), the classic heavy metal antidote, *Clin. Toxicol.*, 5, 215–222, 1972).

[b] Rate of oxidation determined by oxygen uptake (manometric).

[c] 10 μM.

[d] Ionic strength, 0.2; all buffers contained 0.001 M EDTA. When buffer species is missing, only pH range is given.

[e] Rate of oxidation determined by oxygen uptake (polarographic).

[f] A highly reactive oxidant produced by the action of peroxidase on thiocyanate (Tenovuo, J., Pruitt, K.M., Mansson-Rahemtulla, B., Harrington, P., and Haldone, D.C., Products of thiocyanate peroxidation: Properties and reaction mechanisms, *Biochim. Biophys. Acta* 870, 377–384, 1986.

References

1. Barron, E.S.G., Miller, Z.B., and Kalnitsky, G., The oxidation of dithiols, *Biochem. J.* 41, 62–68, 1947.
2. Smith, R.C., and Reed, V.D., Inhibition by thiols of copper(II)-induced oxidation of oxyhemoglobin, *Chem. Biol. Interact.* 82, 209–217, 1992.
3. Jacobsen, D.W., Troxell, L.S., and Brown, K.L., Catalysis of thiol oxidation by cobalamins and cobinamides: Reaction products and kinetics, *Biochemistry* 23, 2017–2025, 1984.
4. Rahmanto, A.S. and Davies, M.J., Selenium-containing amino acids as direct and indirect antioxidants, *IUBMB Life* 64, 863–871, 2012.

pKa values for thiol groups

Thiol group	pKa	Reference	Thiol group	pKa	Reference
Cysteine	8.5	1	Penicillamine	8.60[a]	2
Cysteine	8.91[a]	2	2-Amino-2-methyl-1-propanethiol	8.78[a]	2
Cysteine	8.50	3	Coenzyme A	9.83[a]	2
Selenocysteine	5.2	1	Captopril	10.31[a]	2
Cystamine	8.67[a]	2	2-Mercaptoethylamine	8.35	3
Homocysteine	9.65[a]	2	Thioglycolic acid	10.55	3
2-Mercaptoethanol	10.14[a]	2	3-Mercaptopropylamin	9.35	3
Reduced glutathione	9.33[a]	2	4-Mercaptobutrylamine	9.60	3
3-Mercaptopropionic acid	10.83[a]	2			

References

1. Jacob, C., Giles, G.I., Giles, N.M., and Sies, H., Sulfur and selenium. The role of oxidation state in protein structure and function, *Angedw. Chem. Int. Ed.* 42, 4742–4758, 2003.
2. Keire, D.A., Strauss, E., Guo, W., Noszál, B., and Rabenstein, D.L., Kinetics and equilibria of thiol/disulfide interchange reactions of selected biological thiols and related molecules with oxidized glutathione, *J. Org. Chem.* 57, 123–127, 1992.
3. Bagiyan, G.A., Koroleva, I.K., Soroka, N.V., and Ufimtsev, A.V., Oxidation of thiol compounds by molecular oxygen in aqueous solution, *Russ. Chem. Bull. Int. Ed.* 52, 1135–1141, 2003.

PARTIAL VOLUMES FOR SOME SELECTED COMPOUNDS

PARTIAL MOLAR VOLUMES OF SOME NUCLEIC ACID BASES, NUCLEOSIDES AND RELATED BIOCHEMICALS[a]

Substance	Reference							
	1	2	2[e]	2[f]	3	3[g]	3[h]	4[i]
Acetyl-CoA	545.3[c]							
Acetyl-CoA	500.9[d]							
FMN(Na)								281.5
NAD(Free Acid)[b]								409.4
NAD(Na)[b]								394.3
Cytosine		73.6	74.14	72.61		74.3	75.8	
Cytidine		154.19	155.37	155.7		156.7	157.4	
Uracil		72.29	71.74	71.58		72.9	73.3	
Uridine		152.32	153.39	153.25		153.6	154	
Thymine		88.75	86.37	87.07		88.6	87.4	
Thymidine		168.03	168.74	169.19		168.3	168.6	
Adenine		90.49	86.41					
Adenosine		171.43	171.08	171.49		170.6	172.3	
AMP(Na)					189.1	203		
ATP(2Na)					238.9	257.7	271.3	

[a] Values at 298.15 K (25°C) unless otherwise indicated.
[b] 20°C.
[c] Free acid.
[d] Sodium salt.
[e] 1 molal glucose.
[f] 1 molal sucrose.
[g] 1 molal NaCl.
[h] 1 molal CaCl$_2$.
[i] This study contains calculated and experimental partial molal volume data for a large number of chemicals.

References

1. Durchschlag, H. and Zipper, P., Calculation of partial specific volumes and other volumetric properties of small molecules and polymers. *J. Appl. Cryst.* 30, 803–807, 1997.
2. Kishore, N., Bhat, R., and Ahluwalia, J.C., Thermodynamics of some nucleic acid bases and nucleosides in water, and their transfer to aqueous glucose solutions at 298.15 K. *Biophys. Chem.* 33, 227–236, 1989.
3. Kishore, N. and Ahluwalia, J.C., Partial molar heat capacities and volumes of transfer of nucleic acid bases, nucleosides and nucleotides from water to aqueous solutions of sodium and calcium chloride at 25°C. *J. Solution Chem.* 19, 51–64, 1990.
4. Durchschlag, H. and Zipper, P., Calculation of the partial volume of organic compounds and polymers. *Prog. Colloid Polymer Sci.* 94, 20–39, 1994.

PARTIAL VOLUMES FOR SOME BIOCHEMICALS[a]

Substance	Reference					
	1[b]	2[c]	3[c]	4[c]	5[c]	6[b,d]
	cm³ m⁻¹					
α-Aminobutyric acid	75.5		75.5	76.5		
ε-Aminocaproic acid				104.9		
Urea		44.23		44.3	44.23	
Thioacetamide		66.42			66.42	44.2
Thiourea					54.79	
Dextrose		112.04			112.04	
D-Fructose						110.2
D-Glucose						110.3
D-Ribose		95.21			95.21	95.8
Sucrose		211.32			211.32	
Succinic acid		82.67			82.67	
Norleucine			107.93			
Norvaline			91.7			
Formic acid				34.7		
Foramide				38		
Acetic acid				50.7		
Acetamide		55.6		55	55.6	
Propionic acid				67.9		
Butyric acid				84.3		
Glycine				43.5		
Glycinamide				60.3		
Leucinamide				123.8		
Pyridine				76.7		
1,4-Dioxane					80.94	

a Values at 298.15 K (25°C).
b Partial molar volume.
c Partial molal volume.
d This study contains partial molal volume data for a large number of chemicals including detergents.

References

1. Singh, S.K. and Kishore, N., Volumetric properties of amino acids and hen-egg white lysozyme in aqueous Triton X-100 at 298.15 K, *J. Solution Chem.* 33, 1411–1427, 2004.
2. Milero, F.J. and Huang, F., The partial molal volumes and compressibilities of nonelectrolytes and amino acids in 0.725 M NaCl, *Aquat. Geochem.* 22, 1–16, 2016.
3. Mishra, A.K. and Abluwalla, J.C., Apparent molal volumes of amino acids, N-acetylamino acids, and peptides in aqueous solution. *J. Phys. Chem* 88, 86–92, 1984.
4. Edsall, J.T., Apparent molal volume, heat capacity, compressibility and surface tension of dipolar ions in solutions, in *Proteins, Amino Acids and Peptides as Ions and Dipolar Ions*, eds. J.T. Edsall and E.J. Cohn, pp. 155–176, Reinhold Publishing, New York, 1943.
5. Lo Surdo, A., Chin, C., and Millero, F.J., The apparent molal volumes and adiabatic compressibility of some organic solutes in water at 25°C, *J. Chem. Eng. Data* 23, 197–201, 1978.
6. Durchschlag, H. and Zipper, P., Calculation of the partial volume of organic compounds and polymers, *Prog. Colloid Polymer Sci.* 94, 20–39, 1994.

APPENDIX A: ABBREVIATIONS AND ACRONYMS

2D-DIGE: two-dimensional difference gel electrophoresis

2DE: two-dimensional electrophoresis

A: absorbance

A1AT: α-antitrypsin

A1GP: α-1-glycoprotein

A23187: a calcium ionophore, Calcimycin

AAAA: Association Against Acronym Abuse

AAG box: an upstream *cis*-element

AAS: aminoalkylsilane; atomic absorption spectroscopy

AAT: amino acid transporter; alpha-1-antitrypsin

AAV: adenoassociated virus

ABA: Abscisic acid, a plant hormone

ABC: ATP-Binding Cassette; antigen-binding cell

ABC-A1: ABC transporter A1

ABC-Transporter Proteins: ATP-binding cassette transporter proteins

ABE: acetone butanol ethanol

Abl: retroviral oncogene derived from Abelson murine leukemia

ABRC: ABA response complex

ABRE: ABA response element

7-ACA: 7-aminocephalosporanic acid

ACES: 2-[(2-amino-2-oxyethyl)amino]-ethanesulfonic acid

ACSF: Artificial cerebrospinal fluid

ACS: active sequence collection; acute coronary syndrome

Ach (AcCho): acetylcholine

AChR (AcChoR): acetylcholine receptor

ACME: arginine catabolic mobile element

ACTH: adrenocorticotropin

ACN: acetonitrile

Acrylodan: 6-acryloyl-2-(dimethylamino)-napthalene

AD: adverse event

ADA: adenosine deaminase; antidrug antibody

ADAM: a disintegrin and metalloproteinase

ADAMTS: a subfamily of disintegrin and metalloproteinase with thrombospondin motifs.

ADCC: antibody-dependent cell-mediated cytotoxicity as in NK cells attacking antibody-coated cells

ADH: alcohol dehydrogenase; antidiuretic hormone

ADME: adsorption, distribution, metabolism, excretion

ADME/T: adsorption, distribution, metabolism, excretion/ toxicology

AdoMet: *S*-adenosyl-l-methionine

ADR: adverse drug reaction

AE: adverse event

AEC: alveolar epithelial cell

AFLP: amplified fragment length polymorphism

AFM: atomic force microscopy

AGE: advanced glycation endproducts

AGO: argonaute protein family

AGP: acid glycoprotein

AID: activation-induced cytodine deaminase

AKAP: A-kinase anchoring proteins

Akt: a protein kinase

Akt: a retroviral oncogene derived from AKT8 murine T cell lymphoma

Alk: anaplastic lymphoma kinase; receptor member of insulin superfamily

ALL: acute lymphocytic leukemia

ALP: alkaline phosphatase

ALS: anti-lymphocyte serum

ALT: alanine aminotransferase

altORF: alternative open reading frame

ALV: avian leukosis virus

AML: acute myeloid leukemia

AMPK: AMP-activated protein kinase

AMS: accelerator mass spectrometry

AMT: accurate mass tag

AAA: abdominal aortic aneurysm; AAA+. ATPases associated with various cellular activities:

ANDA: Abbreviated New Drug Application

ANOVA: analysis of variables (factorial analysis of variables)

ANS: 1-anilino-8-napthlenesulfonate; autonomic nervous system

ANTH: AP180 N-terminal homology as in ANTH-domain

2-AP: 2-aminopyridine

6-APA: 6-aminopenicillanic acid

APAF1: apoptotic protease activating factor 1

Apg1: a serine/threonine protein kinase required for vesicle formation which is essential for autophagy

API: Active pharmaceutical ingredient

APL: acute promyelocytic leukemia

ApoB: apolipoprotein B

APPs: acute phase proteins

AQP: adenosine tetraphosphate

ARAP3 : a dual Arf and Rho GTPase activating protein

ARD: acute respiratory disease; acireductone dioxygenase; automatic relevance determination; acid rock drainage

ARE: AU-rich elements

ARF: ADP-ribosylation factor

ARL: Arf-like

ARM: arginine-rich motif

ARS: automatic replicating sequence or autonomously replicating sequence

ART: mono-ADP-ribosyltransferase; family of proteins, large group of A-B toxins

AS: antisense

ASD: alternative splicing database; http://www.ebi.ac.uk/asd

ASPP: ankyrin-repeat, SH3-domain and proline-rich-region-containing proteins

AST: aspartate aminotransferase

ATC: aspartate transcarbamylase domain

ATCase: aspartate transcarbamylase

ATP: adenosine-5'-triphosphate

ATD: Arrival time distribution

ATPg S: adenosine-5'-3-*O*-(thiotriphosphate)

ATR-FTIR: attenuated total reflectance-Fourier transform infrared

ATR-IR: attenuated total reflection infrared

AVT: arginine vasotocin

Axl: anexceleko; used in reference to a receptor kinase related to the Tyro 3 family

BA: betaine aldehyde

BAC: bacterial artificial chromosome; also blood alcohol concentration

BAD: a member of the Bcl02 protein family considered to be a proapoptotic factor

BADH: betaine aldehyde dehydrogenase

BAEC: bovine aortic endothelial cells

BAEE: Benzoyl-arginine ethyl ester[a]

BALT: bronchial associated lymph tissue

BBB: blood brain barrier

B-CAM: basal cell adhesion molecule

BCG: bacille-Calmette-Guérin

BCR: breakpoint cluster region; B-cell receptor

BCR-ABL: BCR-ABL is the fused gene that results from the *Philadelphia chromosome*, The BCR-ABL gene produces the *Bcr-ABl tyrosine kinase*

Bcl-2: protein family regulating apoptosis

BCIP: 5-bromo, 4-chloro, 3-indoyl phosphate

BCS: biopharmaceutical classification system for describing the gastrointestinal absorption of drugs; also Budd-Chiari syndrome

BDH: d-*b*-butyrate dehydrogenase

BDNF: brain-derived growth factor

BEBO: an unsymmetrical cyanine dye for binding to the minor grove of DNA; 4-[(3-methyl-6-(6-methyl-benzothiazol-2-yl)-2,3,-dihydro(benzo-1,3-thiazole)-2-methylidene)]-1-methyl-pyridinium iodide.

BET: refers to an isotherm for adsorption phenomena in chromatography; acronym derived from Stepen Brunauer, Paul Emmet, and Edward Teller

BEVS: bacillus expression vector system

B/F: bound/free

bFGF: basic fibroblast growth factor

BFP: blue fluorescent protein

BFS: blow-finish-seal

BGE: background electrolyte

Bicine: *N,N*-bis(2-hydroxyethyl)glycine

BiFC: bimolecular fluorescence complementation

BIND: biomolecular interaction network database

BiP: immunoglobulin heavy chain-binding protein

Bis-TRIS: 2,2-bis-(hydroxymethyl)-2,2',2" nitriloethanol

BHK: baby hamster kidney

BLA: Biologic License Application

BLAST: basic local alignment search tool

BME: 2-mercaptoethanol; *b*-mercaptoethanol

BMP: bone morphogenic protein

BopA: a secreted protein required for biofilm formation

BPTI: bovine pancreatic trypsin inhibitor

BCRA-1: breast cancer 1; a tumor suppressor gene associated with breast cancer

BRE-luc: a mouse embryonic stem cell line used to study bone morphogenetic protein.

BRET: bioluminescence resonance energy transfer

BrdU: bromodeoxyuridine

Brig: polyoxyethylene lauryl ether

BSA: bovine serum albumin

BsAB: bispecific antibody

BTEX: benzene, toluene, ethylbenzene, and *o-/p*-xylene

BUN: blood urea nitrogen

bZIP: basic leucine zipper transcription factor

C1INH: C1 inhibitor; inhibitor of activated complement component 1, missing in hereditary angioneurotic edema.

CA125: cancer antigen 125; a glycoprotein marker used for prognosis in ovarian cancer; also referred to as MUC16

CAD: multifuntional protein which is responsible for the *de novo* pyrimidine biosynthesis; caspases-activated DNAse; charged aerosol detection

CAK: Cdk-activating kinase

CALM: clathrin assembly lymphoid myeloid leukemia as in CALM gene

CAM (CaM): calmodulin; cell adhesion molecule

CAMK: calmodulin kinase, isoforms I, II, III

CaMK: Ca^{2+}/calmodulin-dependent protein kinase

CAPA: corrective and protective action

CAPS: cleavable amplified polymorphic sequences; also cationic antimicrobial peptide

CAR: chimeric antigen receptor

CAR-T: chimeric antigen receptor T cell

CArG: a promoter element [CC(A/T)$_6$G] gene for smooth muscle *a*-actin

CASP: critical assessment of structural prediction

CASPASE: cysteine-dependent aspartate-specific protease

CAT: catalase; chloramphenicol acetyl transferase

CATH: class, architecture, topology, homologous superfamily; hierarchical classification of protein domain structure; informal for catheter

CATP: chloramphenicol acetyltransferase

CBE: changes being effected

CBER: Center for Biologics Evaluation and Research

Cbl: a signal transducing protein downstream of a number of receptor-couple tyrosine kinases; a product of the *c-cbl* proto-oncogene

Cbs: chromosomal breakage sequence

CBz: carbobenzoxy

CCC: concordance correlation coefficient

CCD: charge-coupled device

CCK: choleocystokinin

CCS: Rotationally average collision cross section

CCV: clathrin-coated vesicles

CD: clusters of differentiation; circular dichroism; cyclodextrin

CDC: complement-dependent cytotoxicity; complement-mediated cell death

CDK (cDK): cyclin-dependent kinase

cDNA: complementary DNA

CDR: complementary determining region

CDTA: 1,2-cyclohexylenedinitriloacetic acid

CE: capillary electrophoresis

CDS: coding sequence

CEC: capillary electrochromatography

CE-SDS: capillary electrophoresis in the presence of sodium dodecyl sulfate

CELISA: cellular enzyme-linked immunosorbent assay; enzyme-linked immunosorbent assay on live cells

CERT: ceramide transport protein

CEPH: Centre d'Etude du Polymorphisme Humain

CEX: cation exchange

CFA: complete Freund's adjuvant

CFP: Cyan Fluorescent Protein

CFR: Code of Federal Regulations

CFTR: cystic fibrosis transmembrane conductance region

Cfuc: colony forming unit

CGE: capillary gel electrophoresis

CGH: comparative genome hybridization

CGN: *cis*-Golgi network

CH: calponin homology

CHAPS: 3-[(3-cholamidopropyl)dimethylammonio]-1-propane-sulfonic acid

CHCA: *a*-cyano-4-hydroxycinnamic acid

CHEF: chelation-enhanced fluorescence

CHES: 2-(*N*-cyclohexylamino)ethanesulfonic acid

ChiP: chromatin immunoprecipitation

CHMP: Committee for medicinal products for human use

CHO: chinese hamster overy; carbohydrate

CIC: circulating immune complex

CIC: Capicua transcriptional repressor gene

CID: collision-induced dissociation; collision-induced dimerization

CIDEP: chemically induced dynamic electron polarization

CIDNP: chemically induced dynamic nuclear polarization

CIEEL: chemically initiated electron exchange luminescence

CIP: Clean in place

CLIP: class-II-associated invariant chain (Ii) peptide

CLT: clotvinazole [1-(a2-chlorotrityl)imidazole]

CLU: clusterin

CLUSTALW: A general purpose program for structural alignment of proteins and nucleic acids http://www.ebi.ac.uk/clustalw/

cM: centimorgan

CM: carboxymethyl

CMC: Chemistry, manufacturing and controls; critical micelle concentration

CMCA: competitive metal capture analysis

CML: chronic myelogenous leukemia

CML: carboxymethyl lysine

CMO: Contract manufacturing organization

CNA: bacterial cell wall collagen-binding protein

Cn: calcineurin

CNC: Cap'n'Collar family of basic leucine zipper proteins

CNE: conserved non-coding elements

dCNE: duplicated CNE

COACH: comparison of alignments by constructing hidden Markow models

CoA: coenzyme A

COA(CofA): Certificate of Analysis

COFFEE: consistency based objective function for alignment evaluation

COFRADIC: combined fractional diagonal chromatography

COG: conserved oligomeric Golgi; cluster of orthologous groups

COPD: chronic obstructive pulmonary disease

COS: cell line derived from African green monkeys

Cot ½ DNA: a method for measuring genome complexity by determining the time required for one-half of DNA in a sample to renature compared a standard sample (not currently in use as determined by literature search)

COX: cytochrome C oxidase

Cp: ceruloplasmin

Cp and Cpk: Measures of process capability

CPA: carboxypeptidase A

CPB: carboxypeptidase B

CPD: cyclobutane pyrimidine dimer

CPDK: calcium-dependent protein kinase

CpG: cytosine-phosphate-guanine

CpG-C: cytosine-phosphate-guanine class C

COG: cluster of orthologous genes

CPP: cell penetrating peptide; combinatorial protein pattern; critical process parameter

CPSase: carbamoyl-phosphate synthetase

CPY: carboxypeptidase Y

CQA: critical process attribute

CRAC: calcium-release activated calcium (channels)

CRE: cyclicAMP response element

Cre1: cytokine response 1; a membrane kinase

CREA: creatinine

CREB: cAMP-response element binding protein

CRISPR: clustered regularly interspaced single palindromic repeats

CRM: certified reference material

CRO: contract research organzation

CRP: C-reactive protein; cAMP receptor protein

CRY: chaperone

CS: chondroitin sulfate

CSF: colony stimulating factor; cerebral spinal fluid

CSP: cold-shock protein

CSR: cluster-situated regulator; class-switch recombination

CSSL: chromosome segment substitution lines

Ct: chloroplast

CT: charge transfer

CTB: cholera toxin B subunit

CTD: C-terminal domain

CTL: cytotoxic T lymphocytes

CTL: cytotoxic T lymphocyte

CTLA: cytotoxic T lymphocyte-associated antigen

CTLL: cytotoxic T-cell lines

CTPSase: CTP synthetase

CtrA: a master regulator of cell cycle progression

CV: coefficient of variation

CV-1: cell line derived from African green monkey.

Cvt: cytosome to vacuole targeting

CW: continuous wave(non-pulsed source of electromagnetic radiation)

CYP: cytochrome P450 enzyme

Cst3: cystatin 3

CZE: capillary zone electrophoresis

D: diffusion

D_{ax}: axial dispersion coefficient

DAB(p-dab): p-dimethyl amino azo benzene

dABs: domain antibodies

DABSYL: N,N-dimethylaminoazobenzene-4'-sulfonyl-usually as the chloride, DABSYL chloride

DAD: diaphanous-autoregulatory domain

DAF: decay accelerating factor

DAG: diacyl glycerol

DALI: distance matrix alignment; http://www2.ebi.ac.uk/dali/

DANSYL: 5-dimethylaminonapthalene-1-sulfonyl; usually as the chloride (DANSYL chloride)

DAP: DNAX-activation protein; also diaminopimelic acid;

DAP12: DNAX activating protein of 12kDa mass

DAS: distributed annotated system; downstream activation site

DAVID: database for annotation, visualization and integrated discovery

DBMB: Dulbecco's modified Eagles Medium

DBD-PyNCS: 4-(3-isocyanatopyrrolidin-1-yl)-7-(N,N-dimethylaminosulfonyl)-2-benzoxadiazole

DBS: dried blood spot

DBTC: "Stains All"; 4,5,4',5'-dibenzo-3,3'-diethyl-9-methylthiacarbocyanine bromide

DC: dendritic cell

DCC: dicyclohexylcarbodiimide

DCCD: N,N'-dicyclohexylcarbodimide

DD: Differential Display

DDA: data directed analysis

DDBJ: DNA Databank of Japan; http://www.ddbj.nig.ac.jp

DDRs: discoidin domain receptors (DDR1, DDR2)

DDR1: discoidin domain receptor1, CAK, CD167a, PTK3, Mck10

DDR2: discoidin domain receptor2, NTRK3, TKT, Tyro10

DEAE: diethylaminoethyl

DEG: differentially expressed gene(s)

DEP: diethylpyrocarbonate (ethoxyformic anhydride)

DEX: dendritic-cell-derived exosomes

DFF: DNA fragmentation factor

DFP: diisopropylphosphorylfluoridate (diisopropylfluorophosphate, isofluorophate)

DHFR: dihydrofolate reductase

DHO: dihydroorotase domain

DHOase: dihydroorotase

DHPLC(dHPLC): denaturing HPLC

DHS: Dnase I hypersensitivity site

DI: deionized as in DI water (**DIW**)

DIP: database of interacting proteins – http://dip.doe-mbi.ucla. edu; also dictionary of interfaces in proteins – http://drug-redesign.de/superposition.html; also used to designate an enzyme inactivated by diisopropylphosphoryl floridate(DFP) such as DIP-trypsin

Dipso: 3-[*N,N*.-bis(2-hydroxyethyl)amino]-2-hydroxypropane-sulfonic acid

DLS: dynamic light scattering

DM: an accessory protein located in the lysosome associated with MHC-class-II antigen presentation. It is located in the endosomal/lysosomal system of APC

DMBA: 7,12-dimethylbenzo[*a*]anthracene

DMD: Duchenne muscular dystrophy; also Doctor of Dental Medicine

DMF: dimethylformamide; decayed, missing, filled(dentistry); drug master file

DMS: dimethyl sulfate; dried media spot

DMSO: dimethyl sulfoxide

DMT1: divalent metal transporter 1

ssDNA: single-stranded DNA

DNAa: a bacterial replication initiation factor

DNAX: DNAase III, tau and gamma subunits

dNPT: deoxynucleoside triphosphate

DNase I: Deoxyribonuclease I

DO: an accessory protein located in the lysosome associated with MHC-class-II antigen presentation. DO has an accessory role to DM

DOAC: direct oral anticoagulants; also known as NOAC (new/novel oral anticoagulants)

DOE: design of experiments

DOTA: tetraazacyclodedecanetetraacetic acid

DPE: downstream promoter element

DPI: dual polarization interferometry

DPM: disintegrations per minute

DPN: diphosphopyridine dinucleotide (currently NAD);

DPPC: dipalmitoylphosphatidylcholine

DPPE: 1,2-dipalmitoyl-*sn*-glycerol-3-phosphoethanolamine

DPTA: diethylenetriaminepentaacetic acid

DQ: design qualification

dsDNA: double-stranded DNA

dsRNA: double-stranded RNA

dsRBD: double-stranded RNA binding domain

DRE: dehydration response element; dioxin response element

DRT: dimensionless retention time (a value for chromatography)

DSA: donor-specific anti-HLA antibodies

DSB: DNA double-strand break

DSC: differential scanning calorimetry

DSP: downstream processing

DTAF: dichlorotriazinyl aminofluorescein

DTE: dithioerythritol

DTNB: 5,5'-dithio-bis(2-nitrobenzoic acid) Ellman's Reagent

DTT: dithiothreitol

DUP: a duplicated yeast gene family

DVDF: polyvinyl difluoride

E1: ubiquitin-activating enzyme

E2: ubiquitin carrier protein

E3: ubiquitin-protein isopeptide ligase

E-64: *trans*-epoxysuccinyl-l-leucylamino-(4-guanidino)-butane, proteolytic enzyme inhibitor

EAA: excitatory amino acid

EBA: expanded bead adsorption

EBV: Epstein-Barr virus

EBPR: enhanced biological phosphate removal

EDC(EADC): 1-ethyl-3-(3-dimethylaminopropyl) carbodiimide; *N*-ethyl-*N*'-(3-dimethyl-aminopropyl) carbodiimide

ECD: electron-capture detection

ECF: extracytoplasmic factor; extracellular fluid

ECM: extracellular matrix

EDC: 1-ethyl-(3-dimethylaminopropyl)-carbodiimide

EDI: electrodeionization

EDTA: ethylenediaminetetraacetic acid, Versene, (ethylenedinitrilo) tetraacetic acid;

EEO: electroendoosmosis

EEOF: electroendoosmotic flow

EF: electrofiltration

EGF: epidermal growth factor

EGFR: epidermal growth factor receptor; Erb*b*-1; HER1

EGTA: ethyleneglycol-bis(*b*-aminoethylether)-*N,N,N',N'*-tetraacetic acid;

eIF: eukaryotic initiation factor

EK: electrokinetic

EKLF: erythroid Krüppel-like factor

ELSD: evaporative light scattering detection

ELISA: enzyme-linked immunosorbant assay (enzyme-linked immunoassay)

EM: electron microscopy

EMA: European Medicines Agency (formerly EMEA)

EMBL: European Molecular Biology Laboratory

EMCV: encephalomyocarditis virus

EMF: electromotive force

EMMA: enhanced mismatch mutation analysis

EMSA: electrophoretic mobility shift assay

ENaC: epithelial Na channel

EndoG: endonuclease G

ENTH: epsin *N*-terminal homology as ENTH-domain

ENU: *N*-ethyl-*N*-nitrosourea

EO: ethylene oxide

EOF: electroosmotic flow

EPC: endothelial progenitor cell

Eph: a family of receptor tyrosine kinases; function as receptors/ ligands for ephrins

EPL: expressed protein ligation

EPO: erythropoietin

Epps: 4-(2-hydroxyethyl)-1-piperazinepropanesulfonic acid

EPR: electron paramagnetic resonance

ER: endoplasmic reticulum

ERAD: endoplasmic reticulum-associated protein degradation

ErbB2: epidermal Growth Factor Receptor, HER2

ErbB3: epidermal Growth Factor Receptor, HER3

ErbB4: epidermal Growth Factor Receptor, HER4

ERK: Extracellular-regulated kinase

Erk ½: P 42/44 extracellular signal-regulated kinase

Ero1p: a thiol oxidase which generates disulfide bonds inside in the endoplasmic reticulum

ERSE: endoplasmic reticulum(ER) stress response element

ES: embryonic stem as in embryonic stem cell

ESC: embryonic stem cell
ESI: electrospray ionization
ESR: electron spin resonance; erthyrocyte sedimentation rate
ESS: exonic splicing silencer
EST: expressed sequence tag
ETAAS: electrothermal atomic absorption
5,6-ETE: 5,6-epoxyeicosatrienoic acid
ETD: electron transfer dissociation
ETS: family of transcription factors
EUROFAN: European functional analysis network – http://mips.gsf.de/proj/eurofan/; also European Programme for the Study and Prevention of Violence in Sport
Exo1: exonuclease 1
EXP1: expansion gene
FAAH: fatty acid amide hydrolase
Fab: an antigen binding fragment from immunoglobulin; consists of a light chain and segment of the heavy chain amino-terminal to the hinge region linked by a disulfide bond; obtained from the papain digestion of IgG.
Fab': an antigen binding fragment from immunoglobulin; consists of a light chain and segment of the heavy chain containing the hinge region; linked by a disulfide bond and obtained by reduction of an F(ab')$_2$ obtained from the pepsin digestion of IgG. A dimeric derivative as compared to Fab or Fab'. contains two antigen binding sites
FAB: fast atom bombardment
FAB-MS/MS: fast atom bombardment-mass spectrometry/mass spectrometry
FACE: fluorophore-assisted carbohydrate electrophoresis
FACS: fluorescence-activated cell sorting
FADD: Fas association death domain
FAD: flavin adeninine dinucleotide
FAK: focal adhesion kinase
FAME: fatty acid methyl ester
FAR: failure analysis report
FBS: fetal bovine serum
Fc: region of an immunoglobulin representing the C-terminal and contains various effector functions such as activation of cells.
FcR: cell surface receptor for the Fc domain of IgG; separate types are FcαR and FcγR.
FcRn: neonatal Fc receptor
FDA: fluorescein diacetate; Food and Drug Administration
FDA483: A form prepared at the end of an FDA inspection which contains a list of observations which may be violations of law. Since this information is accessible under the FOA act, it may also be used to obtain competitive intelligence.
FDC: follicular dendritic cells
FDP: fibrin/fibrinogen degradation products
FCCP: carbonyl cyanide *p*-trifluoromethoxyphenyl-hydrazine
FD&C: Food Drug and Cosmetic Act
FEAU: 2'-fluoro-2'-deoxy-*b*-D-arabinofuranosyl-5-ethyluracil
FEN: flap endonuclease
FERM: as in FERM-domain (four-point-one; ezrin, radixin, moesin).
FFAT: two phenylalanyl residues in an acidic tract
FIAU: 2'-fluoro-2'-deoxy-*b*-D-arabinofuranosyl-5-iodouracil
FecA: ferric citrate transporter
FEN: flap endonuclease
Fes: retroviral oncogene derived from ST and GA feline sarcoma
FFAP: free fatty acid phase

FFPE: formalin-fixed, paraffin-embedded
FGF: fibroblast growth factor
FGFR: fibroblast growth factor receptor
Fgr: retroviral oncogene derived from GR feline sarcoma
FIBC: flexible intermediate bulk container
FIGE: field-inversion gel electrophoresis
FITC: fluoroscein isothiocyanate
FTIR: Fourier-transformed infrared reflection
FTIR-ATR: Fourier-transformed infrared reflection-attenuated total reflection
FLAG™: an epitope "tag" which can be used as a fusion partner for recombinant protein expression and purification.
FlhB: a component of the flagellum-specific export apparatus in bacteria.
FLIP: fluorescence loss in photobleaching
FLK-1: receptor for vascular endothelial growth factor(VEGF)
FLT-1: receptor for vascular endothelial growth factor receptor
FMEA: Failure mode evaluation and analysis
fMLP(FMLP): *N*-formyl methionine leucine phenylalanine
fMOC: 9-Fluorenzylmethyloxycarbonyl
Fms: retroviral oncogene derived from SM feline sarcoma
FB: fibronectin
Fok1: a type IIS restriction endonuclease derived from *Flavobacterium okeanokoites*
Fos: retroviral oncogene derived from FBJ murine osteosarcoma
FOX: forkhead box
FpA: fibrinopeptide A
FPC: fingerprinted contigs
FPLC: fast protein liquid chromatography
Fps: retroviral oncogene from Fujiami avian sarcoma
FRAP: fluorescence recovery after photobleaching
FRET: fluorescence resonance energy transfer; Förster resonance energy transfer
FSSP: fold classification based on structure alignment of proteins; http://www2.ebi.ac.uk/dali/fssp/fssp.html
FT: Fourier Transform
FTE: full-time equivalent
FT-IR: Fourier Transform-InfraRed
FU: aluorescence unit
5-Fu: 5-fluorouracil
Fur: ferric uptake receptor
Fur: gene for Fur
FYVE: a zinc-binding motif; acronym derived from four proteins containing this domain
G: guanine
Ga: heterotrimeric G protein, *a*-subunit
Gb: heterotrimeric G protein, *b*-subunit
Gg: heterotrimeric G protein, *g*-subunit
G-6-PD: glucose-6-phosphate dehydrogenase
GABA: gamma (*g*)-aminobutyric acid
GAG: glycosaminoglycan
Gal-3: galactan-3 as in galactin-3 protein
GalNac: *N*-acetylgalactosamine
GALT: gut-associated lymphoid tissues
GALV: gibbon ape leukemia virus
GAMP: good automated manufacturing product
GAPDH: glyceraldehyde 3-phosphate dehydrogenase
GAPS: GTPase activating proteins
GAS6: a protein, member of the vitamin K-dependent protein family
GASP: Genome Annotation Assessment Project; http://www.fruitfly.org/GASP1/; also growth advantage in stationary phase

GBD: GTPase binding domain

GC: gas chromatography; granular compartment

GC-MS: gas chromatography-mass spectroscopy

GC-MSD: gas chromatography-mass selective detector

GcrA: A master regulator of cell cycle progression

G-CSF: granulocyte colony stimulating factor

GCP: Good Clinical Practice

GDH: glutamate Dehydrogenase

GDNF: glial-derived neurotrophic factor

GdnHCl: guanidine hydrochloride

GDUFE: generic drug user fee amendments

GEFs: guanine nucleotide exchange factors

GF-AAS: graphite furnace atomic absorption spectroscopy

GFC: gel filtration chromatography

GFP: green fluorescent protein

GGDEF: a protein family

GGT: gamma-glutamyl transferase

GGTC: German Gene Trap Consortium; a reference library of gene trap sequence tags (GTST) http://www.genetrap.de/

GHG: greenhouse gas

GI: gastrointestinal; genomic islands

cGK: cyclic GMP (cGMP)-dependent protein kinase

GLC: gas-liquid chromatography

GlcNac: N-acetylglucosamine

GLD: gelsolin-like domain

GLP: Good Laboratory Practice(s)

GLPC: gas-liquid phase chromatography

GlpD: glyceraldehyde-3-phosphate dehydrogenase

GLUT: a protein family involves in the transport of hexoses into mammalian tissues

Glut4: facilitative glucose transporter which is insulin-sensitive

Glut5: a fructose transporter, catalyzes the uptake of fructose

GM: genetically modified

GM-CSF: granulocyte-macrophage colony stimulating factor

GMP: current good manufacturing practice; cGMP, current good manufacturing practice

GMP-PDE(cyclic GMP-PDE): cyclic GMP-phosphodiesterase

GNSO: 5-nitrosoglutathione

GPC: gel permeation chromatography

GPCR: G-protein coupled receptor

GPI: glycosyl phosphatidylinositol

GPx: glutathione peroxidase

GRAS: generally regarded as safe

GRIP: a Golgi-targeting protein domain

GRP: glucose-regulated protein

Grp78: a glucose regulated protein; identical with BiP

GSC: gas-solid chromatography; glioma stem cell; glioblastoma stem-like cell

GSH: glutathione

GST: glutathione-S-transferase; gene trap sequencing tag

GTF: general Transcription factor

GTST(GST): gene trap sequence tags

GTP (cGTP): good tissue practice (current good tissue practice)

GUS: beta-glucuronidase

GVDH: graft-versus-host disease

GXP(s): A generic acronym for good .... practices including but not limited to good clinical practice, good laboratory practice, good manufacturing processes.

HA: hemaglutin-A; hyaluronic acid; hydroxyapaptite, $Ca_{10}(PO_4)_6(OH)_2$

HABA: [2-(4'-hydroxyazobenzene)] benzoic acid;

HACCP: hazard analysis, critical control point

HAPT: haptoglobin

HAS: hyaluronan synthase

HAT: histone acetyltransferase; hypoxanthine, aminopterin and thymidine

HBSS: Hanks Balanced Salt Solution

H/D: hydrogen/deuterium exchange

HAD: heteroduplex analysis

HCP: host cell protein, refers to protein derived from the cell line used to expressed recombinant proteins

HCIC: hydrophobic charge induction chromatography

HDAC: histone deacetylase

HDL: high-density lipoprotein

HDLA: human leukocyte differentiation antigen

HD-ZIP: homeodomain-leucine zipper proteins

HEPT: height equivalent to plate number

HeLa cells: a immortal cell line derived from human cervical cancer cells, acronym is from the patient's name, Henrietta Lacks

HEPA: high-efficiency particulate air as in HEPA-filtration

ERV: human endogenous retrovirus

20-HETE: 20-hydroxyeicosatetranenoic acid

HETP: plate height (chromatography);

HexNac: N-acetylhexosamine

HP-LPME: hollow-fiber liquid-phase microextraction

HGH: human growth hormone

HGP: human genome project

HH: hereditary hemochromatosis

HHM: hidden Markov models

HIC: hydrophobic interaction chromatography

HILIC: hydrophilic interaction liquid chromatography

His-Tag(His$_6$; H$_6$): histidine tag – a hexahistidine sequence

HLA: human leukocyte associated antigen

HLA-DM: enzyme responsible for loading peptides onto MHC class II molecules

HLA-DO: protein factor which modulates the action of HLA-DM

HMGR: 3-hydroxy-3-methylglutamyl-coenzyme A reductase

HMP: herbal medicinal product(s)

HMT: histone

hnRNA: heterologous nuclear RNA

HOG: high-osmolarity glycerol

HOPE: Hepes-glutaminic acid-buffer mediated organic solvent protein effect

HOX(_HOX_, _hox_): describing a family of transcription factors

HPAED-PAD: high performance anion-exchange chromatography-pulsed amperometric detection

5-HPETE: 5-hydroperoxyeicosatetranenoic acid

HPRD: human protein reference database

HPRT: hypoxanthine phosphoribosyl transferase

HRP: horse radish peroxidase

HRR: homologous recombination repair

HPLC: high performance liquid chromatography (high pressure liquid chromatography)

uHPLC: ultra high performance liquid chromatography

HS: heparan sulfate

HSA: human serum albumin

HSB: homologous synteny blocks

HSC: hematopoietic stem cell

HSCQ: heteronuclear single quantum correlation

HSCT: hematopoietic stem cell transplantation

HSE: heat shock element

Hsp: heat-shock protein

Hsp70: heat shock protein 70

HS-SDME: head space-single-drop microextraction

HS-SPME: head space solid-phase microextraction

5-HT: 5-hydroxytryptamine

HTF: *Hpa*II tiny fragments; distinct fragments from the *Hpa*II digestion of DNA; *Hpa*II is a restriction endonuclease

HTH: helix-turn-helix

HTS: high-throughput screening

htSNP: haplotype single nucleotide polymorphism

HUGO: human genome organization

HUVEC: human umbilical vein endothelial cells

IAA: iodoacetic acid

IAEDANS: *N*-iodoacetyl-*N'*-(5-sulfo-1-napthyl) ethylenediamine

IBD: identical-by-descent; also inflammatory bowel disease

IC: ion chromatography

ICAM: intercellular adhesion molecule

ICAT: isotope-coded affinity tag

ICH: intracerebral hemorrhage; a gene related to *Ice* involved in programmed cell death; historically, international chick unit; International Conference for Harmonisation

ICPMS: inductively coupled plasma mass spectrometry

ID: internal diameter

IDA: interaction defective allele

IdeS: a protease from *Streptococcus .pyogenes* which specifically cleaves IgG on the carboxyl side of the hinge region in a manner similar to pepsin.

IDMS: isotope dilution mass spectrometry

IEC: ion-exchange chromatography

IEF: isoelectric focusing

IES: internal eliminated sequences

IFE: immunofixation electrophoresis

IFN: interferon

IFN: interferon

IEX: ion-exchange chromatography

Ig: immunoglobulin

IGF: insulin-like growth factor

IGFR: insulin-like growth factor receptor

Ihh: indian hedgehog

I*k***B:** NF-*k*B inhibitor

I*k***K:** I*k*B kinase

IL: Interleukin, e.g., **IL-2**, interleukin-2; **IL-6**, interleukin-6

iLAP: integrated lysis and purification

ILGF: insulin-like growth factor

ILGFR: insulin-like growth factor receptor

ILK: integrin-linked kinase

IMAC: immobilized metal-affinity chromatography

IMINO: Na^+-dependent alanine-insensitive proline uptake system (SLC6A20)

IMMS: ion mobility mass spectrometry

IMP: integrin-mobilferrin pathway membrane protein system involves in the transport of ferric iron; also inosine-5'-monophosphate

IMS: ion mobility separation

IND: investigation new drug application

IP$_3$: inositol 1,4,5-triphosphate

IPG: immobilized pH gradient

IPTG: isopropylthio-*b*-d-galactopyranoside

IQ: installation qualification

IR: inverted repeat; insulin receptor

IRB: institutional review board

IRES: internal ribosome entry site

IRS: insulin receptor substrate

ISE: ion-specific electrode

ISO: International Standards Organization

ISS: immunostimulatory sequence; also intronic splicing silencer

ISS-ODN: immunostimulatory sequence-oligodeoxynucleotide

ISSR: inter-simple sequence repeats

IT: isotocin

ITAF: IRES trans-acting factor

ITAM: immunoreceptor tyrosine-based activation motif

ITC: isothermal titration calorimetry

iTRAQ: isobaric tags for relative and absolute quantitation of proteins in proteomic research

JAK: Janus Kinase

JNK: *c*-Jun *N*-terminal kinase

KARAP: killer cell activating receptor-associated protein

Kb, kb: kilobase

KDR: kinase insert domain-containing receptor; KDR is the human homolog of the mouse FLK-1 receptor. The KDR and FLK-1 receptors are also known as VEGFR2. See VEGFR

KEGG: kyoto encyclopedia of genes and genomes

Kit: mast/stem cell growth factor receptor, CD 117

***Kit*:** retroviral oncogene derived from HZ4 feline sarcoma

KLF5: Kruppel-like factor 5, a transcription factor

KRED: aldo/keto reductases

LAK: lymphokine-activated killer cells

LAL: limulus amebocyte lysate (assay)

LATE-PCR: linear-after-the-expotential-PCR

LB: Luria-Bertani

Lck: member of the Src family of protein kinases

LC$_{50}$: median lethan concentration in air

LC/MS: liquid chromatography/mass spectrometry

LC/MS/MS: liquid chromatography/mass spectrometry/mass spectrometry

LCR: low-copy repeat; locus control region; low complexity region

LCST: lower critical solution temperature

LD: as in LD motif, a leucine/aspartic acid-rich protein-binding domain; also used to refers to peptidases without sterospecificity; also longin domain; linkage disequilibrium; lactate dehydrogenase

LD$_{50}$: median lethal dose

LDL: low-density lipoprotein

LEAC: linear elution adsorption chromatography

LECE: ligand exchange capillary electrophoresis

LED: light emitting diode

Lek: lymphocyte-specific protein tyrosine kinase

LFA: lymphocyte function-associated antigen

LGIC: ligand-gated ion channel

LH: luteinizing hormone

LIF: laser-induced fluorescence

LIM : a domain involved in protein-protein interaction, originally described in transcription factors LIN1, ISL1, and MED3.

LIMS: laboratory information management systems

LINE: long interspersed nuclear element

LLC: liquid-liquid chromatography

LLE: liqud-liquid extraction

LLOD: lower limit of detection

LLOQ: lower limit of quantification

Lnr: initiator element

lncRNA: long, noncoding RNA

lnRNP: large nuclear ribonucleoprotein

LOD: limit of detection; log_{10} of odds

LOLA: list of lists - annotated

LOT: the entire content of a production batch of a therapeutic product (drug or biologic)

LOQ: limit of quantitation

LP: lysophospholipid

LPA: lysophosphatidic acid

LPH: lipotropic hormone

LPME: liquid-phase microextraction

LPS: lipopolysaccharide

LR: linear range

LTB$_4$: leukotriene B$_4$

LTH: luteotropic hormone

Ltk: leukocyte tyrosine kinase

LRP: low-density lipoprotein receptor-related protein

LSC: liquid-solid chromatography

LSPR: localized surface plasmon resonance

LTR: long terminal repeat

LUCA: last universal cellular ancestor

Lys-C: a protease with specificity for cleavage at lysine carboxyl group

LZ: leucine/isoleucine zipper

M13: a bacteriophage used in phage display

MΦ: macrophage

Mab: monoclonal antibody

MAC: membrane attack complex

MAD: multiwavelength anomalous diffraction

Maf: retroviral oncogene derived from AS42 avian sarcoma

MAGE: microarray and gene expression

MALDI-TOF: matrix-assisted laser desorption ionization time of flight mass spectrometry

MALLS: multiangle laser light scattering

MAP: mitogen-activated protein; usually referring to a protein kinase such MAP-kinase

MAPK: MAP-kinase

MAPKK: MAP-kinase kinase

MAPKKK: MAP-kinase kinase kinase

MAR: matrix attachment region

MASE: matrix-solid phase extraction

Mb, mb: megabase (10^6)

MB: molecular beacon

MBL: mannose-binding lectin;

MBP: myelin basic protein; maltose-binding protein

MCA: 4-methylcoumaryl-7-acetyl

MCAT: mass coded abundance tag

MCD: magnetic circular dichroism

MCM: mini-chromosome maintenance

MCS: multiple cloning site

M-CSF: M-colony stimulating factor (Macrophage-colony stimulating factor)

MDA: malondialdehyde

MDMA: 3,4-methylenedioxymethamphetamine

MDCK: Madin-Darby canine kidney

MEF: mouse embryonic fibroblasts

MEF-2: myocyte enhancer factor 2

MEGA-8: octanoyl-N-methylglucamide

MEGA-10: decanoyl-N-methylglucamide

MEK: mitogen-activated protein kinase/extracellular signal-regulated kinase kinase; also methylethyl ketone

MELC: microemulsion liquid chromatography

MELK: multi-epitope-ligand-kartographie

MEM: minimal essential medium

Mer: a receptor protein kinase; also Mertk, Mer tyrosine kinase

MES: 2-(N-morpholinoethanesulfonic acid)

Met: receptor for hepatocyte growth factor

MFB: membrane fusion protein

MGO: methylglyoxal

MGUS: monoclonal gammopathy of undetermined significance

MHC: major histocompatibility complex

MIAME: minimum information about a microarray experiment

Mil: retroviral oncogene derived from Mill Hill-2 chicken carcinoma

MIP: molecularly imprinted polymer; macrophage inflammatory protein; methylation induced premeiotically

MIPS: Munich Information Center for Protein Sequences

MIS: Mullerian Inhibiting Substance

MLCK: myosin light chain kinase

MLCP: myosin light chain phosphatase

MMP: matrix metalloproteinase

MMR: mismatch repair

MMTV: mouse mammary tumor virus

MOPS: 3-(N-morpholino)propanesulfonic acid; 4-morpholinopropanesulfonic acid

MOPSo: 3-(N-morpholino)-2-hydroxypropanesulfonic acid

Mos: retroviral oncogene derived from Moloney murine sarcoma

MPD: 2-methyl-2,4-pentanediol

MPSS: massively parallel signature sequencing

MR: magnetic resonance

MRI: magnetic resonance imaging

MRM: multiple reaction monitoring

mRNA: messenger RNA

miRNA: microRNA

MRP: migratory inhibitory factor-related protein

MRTF: myocardin-related transcription factor

MS: mass spectrometry, also mechanosensitive (receptors), multiple sclerosis

MS/MS: mass spectrometry/mass spectrometry

MS^3: tandem mass spectrometry/mass spectrometry/mass spectrometry

MSDS: Material safety data sheet(s)

MSP: macrophage stimulating protein

Mt: mitochondrial

mt-DNA: mitochondrial DNA

MTBE: methyl-t-butyl ether

MTOC: microtubule organizing center

mTOR: a eukaryotic regulatory of cell growth and proliferation; mechanistic target of rapamycin

MTSP: membrane type serine proteases

mTRAQ: MRM tags for relative and absolute quantitation

MTT: methylthiazoletetrazolium

MTX: methotrexate

MU: Miller Units

Mu: Mutator

MUSK: muscle skeletal receptor tyrosine kinase

MuDPiT: multidimensional protein identification technology

MuLV: Muloney leukemia virus

MWCO: molecular weight cut-off

My: million years

Myb: retroviral oncogene derived from avian myeloblastosis

Myc: retroviral oncogene derived from MC29 avian myelocytomatosis

MYPT: myosin phosphatase-targeting

Mys: myristoylation site

NAA: neutron activation analysis

Nabs: neutralizing antibodies

nAChR (nAcChoR): nicotinic acetylcholine receptor

NAD: nicotinamide adenine dinucleotide (DPN)

NADP: nicotinamide adeninine dinucleotide phosphate (TPN)

NAO: non-animal origin

NASH: non-alcoholic steatohepatitis

NAT: nucleic acid amplification testing; nucleic acid testing.

Nbs$_2$: Ellman's Reagent; 5,5'-dithiobis(2-nitrobenzene acid)

NBD: nucleotide-binding domain

NBD-PyNCS: 4-(3-isothiocyanato pyrrolidin-1-yl)-7-nitro-2,1,3-benzoxadiazole

NBE: new biological entity

NBS: *N*-bromosuccinimide

NBT: nitroblue tetrazolium

NCBI: National Center for Biotechnology Information

NCE: new chemical entity

NCED: 9-*cis*-epoxycarotenoid dioxygenase

ncRNA: noncoding RNA

NDA: New Drug Application

n-DAMO: nitrite-dependent anaerobic methane oxidation

NDB: nucleic acid databank

NDMA: *N*-methyl-d-aspartate

NDSB: 3-(1-pyridinio)-1-propanesulfonate (non-detergent sulfobetaine)

NEM: *N*-ethylmaleimide

NEO: Neopterin

NEP: nucleous-encoded polymerase (RNA polymerase)

NeuAc: *N*-acetylneuraminic acid

NeuGc: *N*-glycolylneuraminic acid

NF: National Formulary

NFAT: nuclear factor of activated T cells, a transcription factor

NF-*k*B: nuclear factor kappa B, a nuclear transcription factor

NGF: nerve growth factor

NGFR: nerve growth factor receptor

NGS: next generation sequencing

NHEJ: non-homologous end-joining

NHS: *N*-hydroxysuccinimide

Ni-NTA: nickel-nitrilotriacetic acid

NIR: near infrared

NIRF: near infrared fluorescence

NIST: National Institute of Standards and Technology

NK: natural killer (as in cytotoxic T cell)

NKCF: natural killer cytotoxic factor

NKF: *N*-formylkynurenine

NMDA: *N*-methyl-d-aspartate

NME: new molecular entity

NMM: nicotinamide mononucleotide

NMR: nuclear magnetic resonance

NO: nitric oxide

NOE: nuclear Overhauser effect

NOESY: nuclear Overhauser effect spectroscopy

NOHA: N^w-hydroxy-l-arginine

NORs: specific chromosomal sites of nuclear reformulation

NOS: nitric oxide synthetase

iNOS: inducible oxide synthetase

NPC: nuclear pore complex

***p*NPP:** *p*-Nitrophenyl phosphate

NSAID: non-steroid anti-inflammatory drug(s)

NSF: *N*-ethylmaleimide sensitive factor; National Science Foundation; *N*-ethylmaleimide-sensitive fusion

Nt,nt: nucleotide

NTA: nitriloacetic acid

NTPDases: nucleoside triphosphate diphosphohydrolases; also known as apyrases, E-ATPases

NuSAP: nucleolar spindle-associated protein

OCED: Organization for Economic Cooperation and Development

OCT: optical coherence tomography

ODMR: optically detected magnetic resonance

ODN: oligodeoxynucleotide

OFAGE: orthogonal-field-alternation gel electrophoresis

OHQ: 8-hydroxyquinoline

OLED: organic light emitting diode

OMG: Object Management Group

OMIM: online Mendelian Inheritance in Man (database) OMIM220100 located at http://www.ncbi.nlm.nih.gov

OMP: outer membrane protein; A protein family associated with membranes

OMT: outer membrane transport

OOS: out of specification

OOT: out-of-tolerance; out-of-trend

OPG: Osteoprotegerin

OPV: organic photovoltaic as in organic photovoltaic cells

ORC: origin recognition complex

ORD: optical rotatory dispersion

ORF: open reading frame

ORFan: orphan open-reading frame

ORFeome: the protein-coding ORFs of an organism

uORF: upstream open reading frame

OSBP: oxysterol-binding proteins

OTCE: optically transparent carbon electrodes

OTFT: organic thin-film transistor

OTU: operation taxonomic unit

OVA: Ovalbumin

OQ: operational qualification

OXPHOS: oxidative phosphorylation

OYE: Old Yellow Enzyme

p53: A nuclear phosphoprotein which functions as a tumor suppressor.

PA: peptide amphiphile

PAC: P1-derived artificial chromosome

PACAP: pituitary adenyl cyclase-activating polypeptide

PAD: peptidylarginine deiminase; protein argininine deiminase (EC 3.5.5.15)

PADGEM: platelet activator-dependent granule external membrane protein; GMP-140

PAGE: polyacrylamide gel electrophoresis

PAH: polycyclic aromatic hydrocarbon

PAK: P21-activated kinase

PAO: A redundant gene family (seripaoparin)

PAR: protease-activated receptor; proven acceptable range

PARP: poly(ADP-ribose) polymerase

PAS: preautophagosomal structure; periodic acid Schiff; preapproval supplement (prior approval supplement)

PAT: process analytical technology /process analytical technologies

PAT1: H$^+$-coupled amino acid transporter (slc36a1)

PAZ: a protein interaction domain; PIWI-argonaute-zwille

PBP: periplasmic binding protein

PBM: PDZ-binding protein

PBS: phosphate-buffered saline

PBST: phosphate-buffered saline with Tween-20

PC: polycystin; phosphatidyl choline

PCA: principal component analysis

PCAF: p300/CBP-associated factor, a histone acetyltransferase

PCB: polychlorinated biphenyl

PCNA: proliferating Cell Nuclear Antigen; processing factor

PCOOH: phosphatidyl choline hydroperoxide

PCR: polymerase chain reaction
PDB: Protein Data Bank
PDE: phosphodiesterase
PDGF: platelet-derived growth factor
PDGFR: platelet-derived growth factor receptor
pDNA : plasmid DNA
PDI: protein disulfide isomerase
PDMA: polydimethylacrylamide
PDMS: polydimethylsiloxane
PDZ: as in PDZ domains; acronym derived from the first three proteins: **p**ostsynaptic density protein 95 (PSD-95), **d**isks large (Dlg), and **z**ona occludens 1 (ZO-1) proteins
PE: phycoerythrin; polyethylene
PEC: photoelectrochemistry
PECAM-1: platelet/endothelial cell adhesion molecule-1
PEEK: polyether ether ketone
PEF: polyethylene furanoate
PEG: poly(ethylene) glycol
PEI: polyethyleneimine
PEL: permissible exposure limit
PEND protein: a DNA-binding protein in the inner envelope membrane of the developing chloroplast
PEP: phosphoenol pyruvate
PEPCK-C: phosphoenolpyruvate carboxykinase, cytosolic form
PERK: double-stranded RNA-activated protein kinase-like ER kinase
PES: photoelectron spectroscopy
PET: positron emission tomography; polyethylene terephthalate
PEP: plastid-encoded polymerase (RNA polymerase)
Pfam: a protein family database; protein families database of alignments
PFE: pressure-fluid extraction
PFGE: pulsed-field gel electrophoresis;
PFK: phosphofructokinase
PFU: plaque forming unit
PG: phosphatidyl glycerol; prostaglandin,
3-PGA: 3-phospho-d-glycerate
PGO: phenylglyoxal
PGP-Me: archaetidylglycerol methyl phosphate
PGT box: an upstream *cis*-element
PGx(PGX): pharmacogenetics (PGx) is the use of genetic information to guide drug choice; prostaglandins(PGX) include thromboxanes and prostacyclins.
PH: pleckstrin homology
PHA: polyhydroxyalkanoates
PHD: plant homeodomain
pHB(*p*-HB): 4-hydoxybenzoic acid (*p*-hydroxybenzoate)
PI: propidium iodide
Pi: isoelectric point
PIC: pre-initiation complex – complex of GTFs
PINCH: PINCH-protein; particularly interesting cis-his-rich protein
PIP$_3$: phosphatidylinositol-3,4,5-triphosphate
PIP$_n$: polyinositol polyphosphate
PIP$_n$S: polyinositol polyphosphates
Pipes: 1,4-piperzainediethanesulfonic acid
PIRL*b*: paired immunoglobulin-like type 2 receptor *b*
PKA: protein kinase A; cAMP-dependent kinase; pKa, acid dissociation constant
PKC: protein kinase C
PKG: cGMP-dependent protein kinase
Pkl: paxillin kinase linker
PLA: polylactide

PLL: poly-l-Lysine
PLOT: porous-layer open-tubular
PLP: pyridoxal-5-phosphate
PMA: phenyl mercuric acetate; phorbol-12-myristate-13 acetate;
PMCA: plasma membrane Ca^{2+} as PMCA-ATPase, a PMCA pump
PMSF: phenylmethylsulfonyl fluoride
PNA: peptide nucleic acid; *p*-nitroanilide
PNGase: endoglycosidase
PNGase-F: peptide N-glcyanase-F
PNP: *p*-nitrophenol (4-nitrophenol)
POD: peroxidase
POET: pooled ORF expression technology
POINT: prediction of interactome database
Pol II: RNA polymerase II
POTRA: polypeptide translocation associated
PP: polypropylene
PPAR: peroxisome proliferator activated receptor
PPase: phosphoprotein phosphatase
PQ: performance qualification
PQL: protein quantity loci
PS: position shift polymorphism
PS-DVB polystyrene-divinylbenzene
PSG: pregnancy-specific glycoprotein(s)
PS-1: presenilin-1
PSI: photosystem I
psi: pounds per square inch
PSI-BLAST: position specific interative BLAST; position-shife iterated BLAST (software program)
PSII: photosystem II
PTB: polypyrimidine-tract-binding protein; a repressive regulator of protein splicing; also pulmonary tuberculosis
PTC: point to consider, plasma thromboplastin component (alternative name for blood coagulation factor IX, Christmas factor)
PTD: protein transduction domain
PTEN: phosphatase and tensin homolog deleted on chromosome 10
PTFE: polytetrafluoroethylene
PTH: phenylthiohydantoin
PTGS: post-transcriptional gene silencing
PTK: protein-tyrosine kinase
PTM: post-translational modification
PTPase: protein tyrosine phosphatase
PUFAs: polyunsaturated fatty acids
PVA: polyvinyl alcohol
PVDF: polyvinylidine difluoride
QA: quality assurance
QC: quality control
QMA: quaternary methyl amine
QP: qualified person (also responsible protein)
QSAR: Quantitive Strucure-Activity Relationship(s)
Q-TOF: quadrupole time-of-flight
QTL: quantitative trait loci
R$_f$: retardation factor
RA: rheumatoid Arthritis
RAB-GAP: Rab-GTPase-activing protein
RACE: rapid amplification of cDNA ends
***raf*:** retroviral oncogene derived from 3611 murine sarcoma
RAGE: receptors for Advanced Glycation Endproducts; receptors for AGE; recombinase-activated gene expression
RAMP: receptor activity modified protein

RANK: receptor activator of NF-kB

RANK-L: receptor activator of NF-kB ligand

Rap: a family of GTPase-coupled signal transduction factors which are part of the RAS superfamily

Rap1: a small GTPase involved in integrin activation and cell adhesion

RAPD : randomly amplified polymorphic DNA

RARE: RecA-assisted restriction endonuclease

RAS: GTP-binding signal transducers

H-ras: retroviral oncogene derived from Harvey murine sarcoma

K-ras: retroviral oncogene derived from Kirsten murine sarcoma

RC: recombinant cogenic

RCA: rolling circle amplification

RCCX: RP-C4-CYP21-TNX module

RCFP: reef coral fluorescent protein

RCR: rolling circle replication

RDP: receptor component protein

rDNA: ribosomal DNA

REA: restriction enzyme analysis

Rel: avian reticuloendotheliosis

REMI: restriction enzyme-mediated integration

REMS: risk evaluation and mitigation strategy

RET: receptor for the GDNF family

RF: a transcription factor, RFX family

Rfactor: final crystallographic residual

RFID: radio frequency identification device

RFLP: restriction fragment length polymorphism

RFP: request for proposal(s)

RGD: a signature peptide sequence-arginine-glycine-aspartic acid found in protein which bind integrins

RGS: regulator of G-protein signaling

RHD: Rel homology domain

Rheb: Ras homologue enriched in brain

RhoA: Ras homologous; signaling pathway

RLD: reference listed drug

RI: random integration

RIP: repeat-induced point mutation

RIS: radioimmunoscintigraphy

RISC: RNA-induced silencing complex

RIT: radioimmunotherapy

RM: reference material

RNA: ribonucleic acid

RNA-Seq: RNA sequencing by NGS technology for analysis of transcriptome

RNAi: RNA interference

dsRNA: double-stranded RNA

hpRNAi: hairpin RNA interference

ncRNA: non-coding RNA

rRNA: ribosomal RNA

shRNA: small hairpin RNA

siRNA: small interfering RNA

snRNA: small nuclear RNA

snoRNA: small nuceolar RNA

stRNA: small temporal RNA

RNAse/RNAase: ribonuclease

RNAse III: a family of ribonucleases (RNAses)

RNC: ribosome-nascent chain complex

snRNP: small nuclear ribonucleoprotein particle

RNS: reactive nitrogen species

RO: reverse osmosis

ROCK (ROK): Rho kinase

ROESY: rotating frame Overhauser effect spectroscopy

RON: receptor for macrophage stimulating protein

ROS: reactive oxygen species

RP: reverse-phase; a nuclear serine/threonine protein kinase; responsible person (RP)

RP-CEC: reverse-phase capillary electrochromatography

RP-HPLC: reverse-phase high performance liquid chromatography

RPA: replication protein A

RPEL: a protein motif involved in the cytoskeleton

RPC: reverse-phase chromatography

RPMC: reverse phase microcapillary liquid chromatography

RPMI 1640: growth media for eukaryotic cells

RPTP: receptor protein-tyrosine kinase

RRM: RNA-recognition motif

RRS: Ras recruitment system; resonance Raleigh scattering

R,S: designating optical activity of chiral compounds where R is rectus (right) and S is sinester (left)

RSD: root square deviation; relative standard deviation

RT: reverse transcriptase; also room temperature

RTD: residence time distribution

RTK: receptor tyrosine kinase

RT-PCR: reverse transcriptase-polymerase chain reaction

RTX: repeat in toxins; pore-forming toxin of *E.coli* type (RTX toxin); also rituximab, resiniteratoxin, renal transplantation

Rub1: a ubiquitin-like protein, Nedd8

S1P: sphingosine-1-phosphate

S100 : S100 protein family

SA: salicylic acid

SAGE: serial analysis of gene expression

SALIP: saposin-like proteins

SAM: self-assembling monolayers

SAMK: A plant MAP kinase

SAMPL: selective amplification of microsatellite polymorphic loci

Sap: Saposin

SAP: sphingolipid activator protein; also serum amyloid P, shrimp alkaline phosphatase

SAR: scaffold associated region; structure-activity relationship

SATP: heterobifunctional crosslinker; *N*-succinimidyl-*S*-acetylthiopropionate

SAXS: small angle x-ray scattering

scFv: single chain Fv fragment of an antibody

SCF: supercritical fluid

SCID: severe combined immunodeficiency

SCOP: structural classification of proteins; http://scop.mrc-lmb.cam.ac.uk/scop

SCOPE: structure-based combinatorial protein engineering

SDS: sodium dodecyl sulfate

SDS-PAGE: Sodium dodecyl sulfate-polyacrylamide gel electrophoresis

SEC: secondary emission chamber for pulse radiolysis; size exclusion chromatography

Sec-: secretory – usually related to protein translocation

SELDI: surface-enhanced laser desorption/ionization

SELEX: systematic evolution of ligands by exponential enrichment

SEM: scanning electron microscopy

SERCA: sarco/endoplasmic reticulum Ca^{2+}as in SERCA-ATPase, a calcium pump

SERS: surface-enhanced Ramen Spectroscopy

SFC: supercritical fluid chromatography

SHAP: serum-derived hyaluron-associated protein

SH2: *Src* homology domain 2

SH3: *Src* homology domain 3

Shh: sonic hedgehog

shRNA: small hairpin RNA

SHO: yeast osmosensor

SILAC: stable-isotope labeling with amino acids in cell culture

(p)SILAC: pulsed stable isotope labeling with amino acid in cell culture

SIMK: a plant MAP kinase

SINE: short interspersed nuclear element

SINS: sequenced insertion sites

SIP: steam-in-place

SIPK: salicylic-acid induced protein kinase

SIRS: systemic inflammatory response syndrome

Sis: retroviral oncogene derived from simian sarcoma

SISDC: Sequence-independent site-directed chimeragenesis

Ski: retroviral oncogene derived from avian SK77

Skp: a chaperone protein

S+/L−: indicator cell line contain murine sarcoma virus (S+) but does not contain murine leukemia virus (L-)

SLAC: serial Lectin Affinity Chromatography

SLE: systemic lupus erythematosus; supported liquid extraction

SLICE: seamless ligation cloning extract

SLN1: yeast osmosensor

S/MAR: scaffold and matrix attachment region

Smad: small mothers against decapentaplegic(proteins)

SMC: smooth muscle cell

SNAP-tag: a modified form of the DNA repair enzyme, O^6-alkylguanine-DNA-alkyltransferase which can execute a self-labeling reaction with O^6-benzylguanine derivatives.

SNAREs: soluble *N*-ethylmaleimide-sensitive factor (NSF; *N*-ethylmaleimide-sensitive factor) protein attach ment protein receptors; can be either R-SNAREs or Q-SNARES depending on sequence homologies

SNDA: supplemental new drug application

SNM: SNARE motif

SNP: Single nucleotide polymorphism

snRNA: small nuclear RNA

snoRNA: small nucleolar RNA

snRNP: small nuclear ribonucleoprotein particle

SNV: single nucleotide variant

SOC: soil organic carbon; store-operated channel

SOCS: suppressors of cytokine signalling

SOD: superoxide dismutase

SOD1s: CuZn-SOD enzyme (Intracellular)

SOP: standard operating procedure

sORF: short open reading frame

SOS: responseofacellto DNAdamage; saltoverlysensitive(usually plants); son of Sevenless (signaling cascade protein)

SPA: scintillation proximity assay

SPC: statistical process control

SPE: solid-phase extraction

SPECT: sporozite mineneme protein essential for transversal; also single-photon emission computed tomography

SPIN: surface properties of protein-protein interfaces (database)

SPP: signal peptide peptidase; superficial porous particles

SPR: surface plasmon resonance

SQL: structured query language

SR: as in the SR protein family (serine- and arginine-rich proteins); also sarcoplasmic reticulum; also scavenger receptor

SRCD: synchrotron radiation circular dichroism

SRP: signal recognition particle

SRF: serum response factor, a ubiquitous transcription factor

SRM: selected reaction monitoring

SRPK: SR protein kinase

SPR: structure-property relationship

SRS: sequence retrieval system; SOS recruitment system

SRWC: short rotation woody crop

SSA: serum amyloid protein

SSC: saline sodium citrate

ssDNA: single-stranded DNA

SSLP: simple sequence length polymorphism

SSR: simple sequence repeats

STAT: signal transducers and activators of transcription

STC: sequence-tagged connector

STL: stereolithography

STM: sequence-tagged mutagenesis

STORM: systematic tailored ORF-data retrieval and management; stochastic optical reconstruction microscopy

STR: short tandem repeats

STREX: stress-axix related exon

STRING: search tool for the retrieval of interacting genes/ proteins

stRNA: small temporal RNA

SUB: single use bioreactor

SUMO: small ubiquitin-like (UBL) modifier; small ubiquitin-related modifier; sentrin

SUPAC: scale-up and post-approval changes

SurA: A chaperone protein

SUS: single use system

SV40: simian virus 40

SVS: seminal vesicle secretion

$S_{w,20}$: sedimentation coefficient corrected to water at 20°C

SWI/SNF: Switch/sucrose-non fermenting

TAC: transcription-competent artificial chromosome

TACE: tumor necrosis factor −*a*-converting enzyme; also transcatheter arterial chemoembolization

TAFs: TBP-associated factors

TAFE: transversely alternating-field electrophoresis

TAFI: thrombin-activatable fibrinolysis inhibitor

TAG: triacyl glycerol

TAME: tosyl-arginine methyl ester

TAP: tandem affinity purification; also transporter associated with antigen processing

TAR: transformation-associated recombination; *trans*-activation response region

TAT: *trans*-activator of transcription

TATA: as in the TATA box which is a TATA-rich region located upstream from the initiation RNA-synthesis initiation site in eukaryotes and within the promoter region for the gene in question. Analogous to the Pribnow box in prokaryotes.

TBA-Cl: tetrabutylammonium chloride

TBP: TATA-binding protein; telomere-binding protein

TCA: trichloroacetic acid; tricarboxylic acid

TCEP: tris (2-carboxyethyl)phosphine hydrochloride

TCR: T-cell receptor

TE: therapeutic equivalence; transposable elements

TEA: triethylamine

TEAA: triethylammonium acetate

TEF: toxic equivalency factor

TEM: transmission electron microscopy

TEMED (TMPD): *N,N,N′,N′*-tetramethylethylenediamine

TEV: tobacco etch protease

TF: tissue factor; transcription factor
TFA: trifluoroacetic acid
TFIIIA: transcription factor IIIA
TGN: *trans*-Golgi network
TGS: transcriptional gene silencing
TH: thyroid hormone
THF: tetrahydrofuran
TIGR: The Institute for Genomic Research
TIM: translocase of inner mitochondrial membrane
TIP: tonoplast intrinsic protein(s)
TIR: toll/IL-1 receptor
TI-VAMP: tetanus neurotoxin-insensitive VAMP
TLCK: tosyl-lysyl chloromethyl ketone
TLR: toll-like receptor
T_m: tubular membrane
TM: transmembrane
TMAO: trimethylamine oxide
TMD: *trans*-membrane domain
TMS: trimethylsilyl; thimersol
TMV: tobacco mosaic virus
TNA: treose nucleic acid
TNB: 5-thio-2-nitrobenzoate
TNBS: trinitrobenzenesulfonic acid
TnC: troponin C
TNF: tumor necrosis factor
TnI: troponin l
TnT: troponin T
TNF-*a* (TNF*a*): tumor necrosis factor-*a*
TNR: transferrin receptor
TNX: tenascin-X
TPD: temperature programmed desorption
TOC: total organic carbon
TOCSY: total correlated spectroscopy
TOF: time-of-flight (in mass spectrometry)
TOP: 5′ tandem oligopyrimidine (terminal oligopyrimidine) tract
TOPRIN: Topoisomerase and Primase in reference to a domain
OR: target of rapamycin; mTOR, mammalian target of rapamycin; dTOR, *Drosophila* target of rapamycin
TORCOID: TORC1 organized in inhibited domains
TOX: toxicology
TPCK: tosylphenylalanylchloromethyl ketone
TPEN: *N′,N′*-tetrakis-(2-pyridyl-methyl)ethylenediamine
TPN: triphosphopyridine dinucleotide (now NADP)
TRADD: a scaffold protein
TRAP: tagging and recovery of associated proteins as in RNA-TRAP; also thrombin receptor activation peptide
TRE: thyroid hormone response elements
TRH: thyrotropin-releasing hormone
TRI: as in TRI reagents such as TRIZOL™ reagents used for RNA purification from cells and tissues
TRIC: trimeric intracellular cation (channel)
Tricine: *N*-(2-hydroxy-1,1-bis(hydroxymethyl)ethyl) glycine
TRIF: TIR domain-containing adaptor-inducing interferon-*b*
Tris: tris-(hydroxymethyl)aminomethyl methane; 2-amino-2-hydroxymethyl-1,3-propanediol
bis-Tris: 2-[bis(2-hydroxyethyl)amino]-2-(hydroxymethyl) propane-1,3-diol
Trk: neurotrophic tyrosine kinase receptor
TRL: time-resolved luminescence
TRP: transient receptor potential as in TRP-protein
TRs: thyroid receptors
Trx: thioredoxin

TSE: transmissible spongiform encephalopathy
TSP: thrombospondin; traveling salesman problem
TTSP: transmembrane type serine proteases
TUSC: Trait Utility System for Corn
Tween: polyoxyethylsorbitan monolaurate
TWIG: traveling wave ion guide
TX: thromboxane, also treatment
TyroBP: tyro protein tyrosine kinase binding protein, DNAX-activation protein 12, DAP12, KARAP
UAS: upstream activation site
UBL: ubiquitin-like modifiers
UCDS: universal conditions direct sequencing
UDP: ubiquitin-domain proteins; uridine diphosphate
UDP-GlcNAc: uidine-5′-diphospho-*N*-acetylglucosamine
UNG: uracil DNA glycosylase
UPA: universal protein array; urokinse-like plasminogen activator
UPR: unfolded protein response
URL: uniform resource locator
URS: upstream repression site
USP: United States Pharmacopeia
USP-NF: United States Pharmacopeia-national formulary
USPS: ubiquitin-based split protein sensor
UTR: untranslated region
VAMP: vesicle-associated membrane protein
VAP: VAMP-associated protein
VASP: vasodilator-stimulate phosphoprotein
VDAC: voltage-dependent anion-selective channel
VCAM: vascular cellular adhesion molecule
VDJ: variable diversity joining; regions of DNA joined in recombination during lymphocyte development; see VDJ recombination.
VDR: vitamin D receptor
VEGF: vascular endothelial growth factor
VEGFR: vascular endothelial growth factor receptor
VGH: non-acronymial use; a neuronal peptide
V_H: variable heavy chain domain
VICKZ: A family of RNA-binding proteins recognizing specific *cis*-acting elements
VIGS: virus-induced gene silencing
VIP: vasoactive intestinal peptide
VLP: virus-like particle
VLDL: very low density lipoprotein
VNC (VNBC): viable, but not-cultivatable (bacteria)
VNTR: variable number tandem repeat; variable number of tandem repeats
VOC: volatile organic carbon
VPAC: VIP PACAP receptors
VSG: variable surface glycoproteins
VSP: vesicular sorting pathway
Vsp10: a type I transmembrane receptor responsible for delivery of protein to lysozyme/vacuole
vsp10: gene for Vsp10
WBOT: wide-bore open-tubular
WGA: whole-genome amplification
WFI: water for injection
WT, Wt: wild type
XBP: x-box binding protein
XO: xanthine oxidase
XPS: x-ray photoelectron spectroscopy
Y2H: yeast two-hybrid
YAC: yeast artificial chromosome
YCp: yeast centromere plasmid

YEp: yeast episomal plasmid
YFP: yellow fluorescent protein
Z: benzyloxycarbonyl
ZDF: Zucker diabetic factor
Zif: zinc finger domain peptides (i.e. Zif-1, Zif-3)
ZIP: leucine zipper
b-ZIP: basic leucine zipper
ZZ Domain: a tandem repeat dimer of the immunoglobulin-
      binding protein A from *Staphylococcus aureus*

It is recognized that there are likely some omissions in this list.
Many journals (e.g. *Journal of Biological Chemistry*) have a list
of abbreviations/acronyms show which can be used in a title and
which may restricted to use in text). The works cited below discuss some of the issues with the use of acronyms.

Bettuzzi, S., Introduction: Clusterin, *Adv.Cancer Res.* 104, 1–8, 2009.

Anon., NUAP (No unnecessary acronyms please), *Nature Methods* 8, 521, 2011.

Stohner, J. and Quack, M., Conventions, symbols, quantities, units and constants for high-resolution molecular spectroscopy, in *Handbook of High-Resolution Spectroscopy*, ed. M. Quack and Merkl, F., Vol. 1, pps. 263–324, John Wiley and Sons, Hoboken, New Jersey, USA, 2011.

Charde, M., Shukla, A., Bukhariya, V., Mehta, J., and Chakole, R., A review on the significance of microwave-assisted techniques in green chemistry, *Int.J.Phytopharm.* 2, 39–50, 2012.

Ali, H. and Ali-Mulla, F., Defining umbilical cord blood stem cells, *Stem Cell Discovery* 2, 15–23, 2012.

Murray, K.K., Boyd, R.K., Eberlin, M.N., *et al.*, Definition of terms relating to mass spectrometry (IUPAC recommendations 2013), *Pure Appd.Chem.* 85, 1515–1609, 2013.

Seah, M.P., Summary of ISO/TC 201 standard – ISO 18115-1:2013-surface chemical analysis -vocabulary-general terms and terms used in spectroscopy, *Surface Interface Analysis* 46, 357–360, 2013.

Seah, M.P., Summary of ISO/TC 201 standard: ISO 18115-2:2013-surface chemical analysis – vocabulary – terms used in scanning probe microscopy, *Surface Interface Analysis* 46, 361–364, 2013.

O'Conner, P.B., Dreiseward, K., Strupat, K., and Hillenkamp, F., MALDI mass spectrometry interpreted, in *MALDI MS*, ed. F. Hillenkamp and P. Katalinic, Wiley/Blackwell, Weinheim, Germany, 2014.

Dobson, G.P., Letson, H.L., Sharma, R., Sheppard, F.R., and Cap, A.P., Mechanisms of early trauma-induced coagulopathy: The clot thickens or not?, *J.Trauma Acute Care Surg.* 79, 301–309, 2015.

Jones, D.S.J., Pujado, P.R., and Treese, S.A., Dictionary of abbreviations, acronyms, expressions, and terms used in petroleum processing and refining, in *Handbook of Petroleum Processing*, ed. S.A. Tresse, P.R., Pujado, and D.S.J. Jones, Springer AG, Switzerland, 2015.

Linecker, M., Kron, P., Lang, H., de Santibañes, E., and Clavien, P.A. Too many languages in the ALPPS: preventing another tower of Babel?, *Ann.Surg.* 263, 837–838, 2016.

Pinh, N., and Kunej, T., Toward a taxonomy for multi-Omics science? Terminology development for whole genome study approaches by Omics technology and hierarchy, *OMICS* 21, 1–16, 2017.

Freire, C., Fernandes, D.M., Nunes, M., and Araujo, M., Polyoxometalate-based modified electrodes for electrocatalysis: From molecular sensing to renewable energy-related applications, in *Advanced Electrode Materials*, ed. A. Tiwani, F. Kuralay, and Uzun, L., pps. 147–212, John Wiley and Sons, Hoboken, New Jersey, 2017.

INDEX

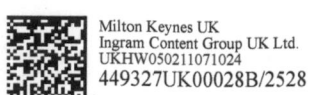